Tietz Fundamentals of
CLINICAL CHEMISTRY AND MOLECULAR DIAGNOSTICS

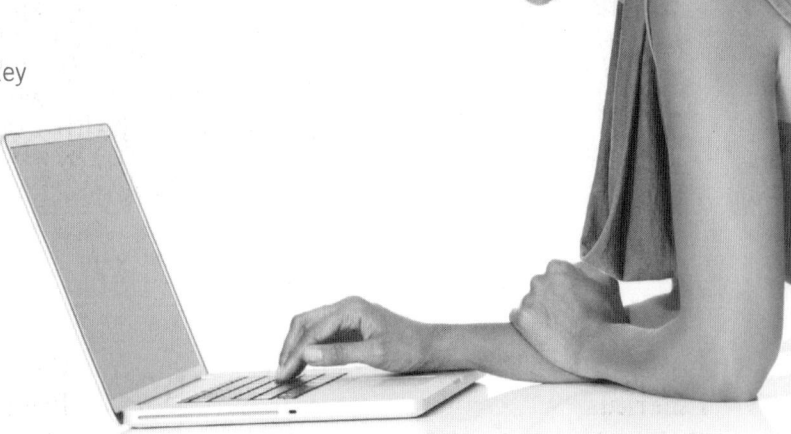

Tietz Fundamentals of
CLINICAL CHEMISTRY AND MOLECULAR DIAGNOSTICS

Seventh Edition

Carl A. Burtis, Ph.D.
Emeritus
Oak Ridge National Laboratory
Oak Ridge, Tennessee
Clinical Professor of Pathology
University of Utah School of Medicine
Salt Lake City, Utah

David E. Bruns, M.D.
Professor of Pathology
University of Virginia School of Medicine
Director of Clinical Chemistry and
    Associate Director of Molecular
    Diagnostics
University of Virginia Health System
Charlottesville, Virginia

Consulting Editor
**Barbara G. Sawyer, Ph.D., M.L.S.
(A.S.C.P.)CM, MB (A.S.C.P.)CM**
Professor, Clinical Laboratory Science/
    Molecular Pathology
Texas Tech University Health Sciences
    Center
Lubbock, Texas

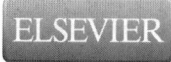

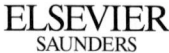

3251 Riverport Lane
St. Louis, Missouri 63043

Content Development Manager: Ellen Wurm-Cutter
Content Development Specialist: Andrea Hunolt
Publishing Services Manager: Julie Eddy
Senior Project Managers: Andrea Campbell, Celeste Clingan
Design Direction: Paula Catalano

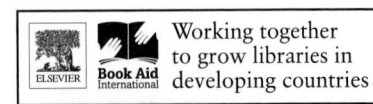

Printed in the United States of America

Last digit is the print number: 9 8 7 6 5 4 3 2 1

Dedication to Seventh Edition

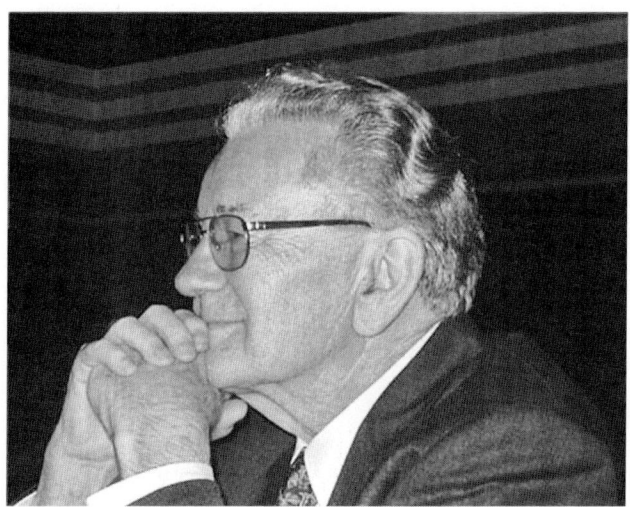

Mentor, Colleague, Friend

On behalf of the worldwide community of clinical laboratorians, we are pleased to dedicate this edition of the **Tietz Fundamentals of Clinical Chemistry and Molecular Diagnostics** to Professor Norbert W. Tietz, Ph.D. Through his many scientific, educational, and editorial efforts, Professor Tietz has had a significant and worldwide impact on the profession, practice, and teaching of clinical laboratory medicine.

Professor Tietz is internationally known for creating and subsequent editing of one of the first books produced for clinical laboratorians, the internationally acclaimed **Fundamentals of Clinical Chemistry.** It was the first modern textbook that integrated clinical chemistry with the basic medical sciences and pathophysiology. Dr. Tietz also edited the first edition of the **Textbook of Clinical Chemistry**, a reference text that bridges the gap between the clinical laboratory and medical management by relating pathophysiology to analytical results in health and disease. He has also edited the **Clinical Guide to Laboratory Tests** and the **Applied Laboratory Medicine**.

In summary, Professor Tietz has been and continues to be a strong advocate of clinical chemistry, and through his energetic scientific, educational, and editorial efforts he has encouraged countless clinical chemists, clinical pathologists, and medical technologists to advance their profession by linking progress in laboratory medicine with the practice of medicine. The name of Tietz is synonymous with the profession and practice of quality laboratory medicine. It is our distinct pleasure to dedicate this edition of the **Fundamentals of Clinical Chemistry and Molecular Diagnostics** to an individual who has had such a significant impact on our profession and our careers.

Contributors

Thomas M. Annesley, Ph.D.
Emeritus Professor
University of Michigan Medical School
Ann Arbor, Michigan;
Deputy Editor, *Clinical Chemistry*
Washington, D.C.
Mass Spectrometry

Fred S. Apple, Ph.D.
Medical Director of Clinical Laboratories
Hennepin County Medical Center,
Professor of Laboratory Medicine and Pathology
University of Minnesota School of Medicine
Minneapolis, Minnesota
Cardiovascular Disease

Edward R. Ashwood, M.D.
Professor of Pathology
University of Utah School of Medicine;
President and Chief Executive Officer
ARUP Laboratories
Salt Lake City, Utah
Clinical Evaluation of Methods

Michael N. Badminton, M.B., Ch.B., Ph.D., F.R.C.Path.
Honorary Consultant and Clinical Lead,
National Acute Porphyria Service (Cardiff)
Medical Biochemistry & Immunology
University Hospital of Wales;
Senior Lecturer
Institute of Molecular and Experimental Medicine
School of Medicine, Cardiff University
Heath Park, Cardiff
Porphyrins and Porphyrias

Renze Bais, Ph.D., F.F.Sc. (R.C.P.A.)
rbaisconsulting.com
Sydney, NSW Australia
Enzyme and Rate Analyses; Serum Enzymes

James C. Barton, M.D.
Director, Southern Iron Disorders Center;
Clinical Professor of Medicine
Department of Medicine
University of Alabama at Birmingham
Birmingham, Alabama
Hemoglobin, Iron, and Bilirubin

Lindsay A.L. Bazydlo, Ph.D.
Co-Director Clinical Chemistry, University of Florida Health
    Shands Hospital
Director Clinical Toxicology, University of Florida Health PathLabs
Assistant Professor
Department of Pathology, Immunology, and Laboratory Medicine
University of Florida College of Medicine
Gainesville, Florida
Electrophoresis

Laura K. Bechtel, Ph.D., D.A.B.C.C.
Laboratory Director
Forensic Laboratories, Inc.
Denver, Colorado
Clinical Toxicology

Roger L. Bertholf, Ph.D.
Professor of Pathology
Director of Clinical Chemistry, Toxicology, and Point of Care
    Testing
University of Florida Health Science Center
Jacksonville, Florida
*Disorders of the Pituitary; Disorders of the Adrenal Cortex; Thyroid
    Disorders*

Patrick M.M. Bossuyt, Ph.D.
Professor of Clinical Epidemiology
Academic Medical Center
University of Amsterdam
Amsterdam, The Netherlands
Evidence-Based Laboratory Medicine

James C. Boyd, M.D.
Associate Professor of Pathology
Chief, Division of Clinical Pathology
University of Virginia Medical School
Director of Systems Engineering and Core Lab Automation
Associate Director of Clinical Chemistry and Toxicology
University of Virginia Health System
Charlottesville, Virginia;
Deputy Editor, Clinical Chemistry
Washington, D.C.
*Selection and Analytical Evaluation of Methods—With Statistical
    Techniques; Automation*

David E. Bruns, M.D.
Professor of Pathology
University of Virginia School of Medicine
Director of Clinical Chemistry and Associate Director of Molecular
   Diagnostics
University of Virginia Health System
Charlottesville, Virginia
Clinical Chemistry, Molecular Diagnostics, and Laboratory Medicine;
*   Clinical Evaluation of Methods; Evidence-Based Laboratory Medi-*
*   cine; Reference Information*

Carl A. Burtis, Ph.D.
Emeritus
Oak Ridge National Laboratory
Oak Ridge Tennessee
Clinical Professor of Pathology
University of Utah School of Medicine
Salt Lake City, Utah
Clinical Chemistry, Molecular Diagnostics, and Laboratory Medicine;
*   Chromatography; Reference Information*

Daniel W. Chan, Ph.D., D.A.B.C.C., F.A.C.B.
Professor of Pathology, Oncology, Radiology, and Urology
Director of Clinical Chemistry Division
Department of Pathology,
Director, Center for Biomarker Discovery
Johns Hopkins Medical Institutions
Baltimore, Maryland
Tumor Markers and Cancer Genes

Rossa W.K. Chiu, M.B.B.S, Ph.D., F.R.C.P.A., F.H.K.A.M.
(Pathology)
Professor
Department of Chemical Pathology
The Chinese University of Hong Kong
Honorary Consultant
Department of Chemical Pathology
Prince of Wales Hospital
Hong Kong, SAR, China
Principles of Molecular Biology

Allan C. Deacon, Ph.D., F.R.C.Path.
Consultant Clinical Scientist
Clinical Biochemistry Department
Bedford Hospital
Bedfordshire, United Kingdom
Porphyrins and Porphyrias

Michael P. Delaney, B.Sc., M.D., F.R.C.P.
Consultant Nephrologist
East Kent Hospitals
NHS Foundation Trust
Canterbury, Kent, United Kingdom
Kidney Disease

Mari L. DeMarco, Ph.D.
Clinical Assistant Professor
University of British Columbia,
Clinical Chemist
St. Paul's Hospital
Department of Pathology and Laboratory Medicine
Vancouver, British Columbia, Canada
Reproduction-Related Disorders

Paul D'Orazio, Ph.D.
Director
Critical Care Analytical Instrumentation Laboratory Co.
Bedford, Massachusetts
Electrochemistry and Chemical Sensors

Basil T. Doumas, Ph.D.
Professor Emeritus
Department of Pathology
Medical College of Wisconsin
Milwaukee, Wisconsin
Hemoglobin, Iron, and Bilirubin

D. Robert Dufour, M.D.
Consultant, Pathology and Hepatology
Veterans Affairs Medical Center,
Emeritus Professor of Pathology
George Washington University Medical Center
Washington, D.C.
Liver Disease

John H. Eckfeldt, M.D.
Vice Chair for Clinical Affairs
Department of Laboratory Medicine and Pathology
University of Minnesota Medical School
Minneapolis, Minnesota
Hemoglobin, Iron, and Bilirubin

Graeme Eisenhofer, Ph.D.
Professor
Department of Medicine III
Institute of Clinical Chemistry and Laboratory Medicine
Chief, Division of Clinical Neurochemistry
University Hospital Carl Gustav Carus Dresden at the Dresden
   University of Technology
Dresden, Germany
Catecholamines and Serotonin

George H. Elder, M.D., F.R.C.P., F.R.C.Path.
Emeritus Professor
Department of Medical Biochemistry and Immunology
School of Medicine, Cardiff University
Cardiff, United Kingdom
Porphyrins and Porphyrias

Jens Peter Goetze, M.D., D.M.Sc.
Professor, Chief Physician
Department of Clinical Biochemistry
Rigshospitalet
University of Copenhagen and Aarhus
Copenhagen, Denmark
Cardiovascular Disease

David G. Grenache, Ph.D., M.T. (A.S.C.P.), D.A.B.C.C., F.A.C.B.
Associate Professor of Pathology
University of Utah School of Medicine
Medical Director, Special Chemistry
ARUP Laboratories
Salt Lake City, Utah
Pregnancy and Prenatal Testing

Ann M. Gronowski, Ph.D.
Professor, Department of Pathology and Immunology
Professor, Department of Obstetrics and Gynecology
Washington University School of Medicine
St. Louis, Missouri
Reproduction-Related Disorders

Amy R. Groszbach, M.E.D., M.L.T., M.B. (A.S.C.P.)CM
Education Program Coordinator
Molecular Genetics Laboratory, Mayo Clinic
Program Director, Molecular Genetics Technology Internship
    Program
Mayo School of Health Science
Mayo Clinic
Rochester, Minnesota
Specimen Collection, Processing, and Other Preanalytical Variables

Doris M. Haverstick, Ph.D., D.A.B.C.C.
Associate Professor of Pathology
University of Virginia
Charlottesville, Virginia
Specimen Collection, Processing, and Other Preanalytical Variables

Charles D. Hawker, Ph.D., M.B.A., F.A.C.B.
Adjunct Professor of Pathology
University of Utah School of Medicine
ARUP Laboratories
Salt Lake City, Utah
Automation

Trefor Higgins, M.Sc., F.C.A.C.B.
Director of Clinical Chemistry
GynaLIFE$_{DX}$
Clinical Professor
Department of Laboratory Medicine and Pathology
Faculty of Medicine
University of Alberta
Edmonton, Alberta
Hemoglobin, Iron, and Bilirubin

Peter G. Hill, Ph.D., F.R.C.Path.
Emeritus Consultant Clinical Biochemistry
Royal Derby Hospital
Derby, United Kingdom
Gastrointestinal and Pancreatic Diseases

Christopher P. Holstege, M.D.
Chief, Division of Medical Toxicology
Associate Professor, Department of Emergency Medicine and
    Pediatrics
University of Virginia School of Medicine
Medical Director, Blue Ridge Poison Center
University of Virginia Health System
Charlottesville, Virginia
Clinical Toxicology

Gary L. Horowitz, M.D.
Associate Professor of Pathology
Harvard Medical School
Director of Clinical Chemistry
Beth Israel Deaconess Medical Center
Boston, Massachusetts
Establishment and Use of Reference Values

Glen L. Hortin, M.D., Ph.D.
Clinical Pathology Medical Director, Southeast Region
Quest Diagnostics
Tampa, Florida
Chromatography; Amino Acids, Peptides, and Proteins

Allan S. Jaffe, M.D.
Consultant in Cardiology and Laboratory Medicine
Professor of Medicine
Professor of Laboratory Medicine and Pathology
Chair, CCLS Division of Laboratory Medicine and Pathology
Mayo Clinic and Medical School
Rochester, Minnesota
Cardiovascular Disease

Ishwarlal Jialal, M.D., Ph.D., F.R.C.Path. (London), D.A.B.C.C.
Robert E. Stowell Endowed Chair in Experimental Pathology
Director of the Laboratory for Atherosclerosis and Metabolic Research
Distinguished Professor of Pathology and Internal Medicine
    (Endocrinology, Diabetes, and Metabolism)
University of California Davis Medical Center
Sacramento, California
Disorders of the Pituitary; Disorders of the Adrenal Cortex

George G. Klee, M.D., Ph.D.
Emeritus Professor of Laboratory Medicine and Pathology
College of Medicine
Department of Laboratory Medicine and Pathology
Mayo Clinic
Rochester, Minnesota
Quality Management

Michael Kleerekoper, M.D., F.A.C.B., F.A.C.P., M.A.C.E.
Clinical Professor of Internal Medicine/Endocrinology
College of Medicine and Life Sciences
University of Toledo
Toledo, Ohio
Hormones; Disorders of Bone and Mineral Metabolism

Larry J. Kricka, D.Phil, F.A.C.B., C.Chem., F.R.S.C., F.R.C.Path.
Professor
University of Pennsylvania
Department of Pathology and Laboratory Medicine
Director of General Chemistry and the Critical Care Laboratory
Hospital of the University of Pennsylvania
Philadelphia, Pennsylvania
Optical Techniques; Immunochemical Techniques

Noriko Kusukawa, Ph.D.
Director, New Technology Assessment and Licensing
ARUP Laboratories
Adjunct Associate Professor of Pathology
University of Utah School of Medicine
Salt Lake City, Utah
*Nucleic Acid Techniques and Applications; Genomes and Nucleic Acid
    Variations*

Edmund J. Lamb, Ph.D., F.R.C.Path.
Head, Department of Clinical Biochemistry
East Kent Hospitals
NHS Foundation Trust
Canterbury, Kent, United Kingdom
Kidney Function Tests—Creatinine, Urea, and Uric Acid; Kidney Disease

Geralyn Lambert-Messerlian, Ph.D., F.A.C.B.
Professor
Department of Pathology and Laboratory Medicine
Alpert Medical School of Brown University
Director
Division of Medical Screening and Special Testing
Women and Infants Hospital
Providence, Rhode Island
Pregnancy and Prenatal Testing

James P. Landers, Ph.D.
Professor of Chemistry
Professor of Mechanical Engineering
University of Virginia
Associate Professor of Pathology
University of Virginia Health System
Charlottesville, Virginia
Electrophoresis

Loralie Langman, Ph.D., F.C.A.C.B., D.A.B.C.C.
(C.C., M.B., T.C.), D.A.B.F.T.
Director, Toxicology and Drug Monitoring Laboratory
Department of Laboratory Medicine and Pathology
Mayo Clinic
Associate Professor of Laboratory Medicine and Pathology
Mayo Clinic College of Medicine
Rochester, Minnesota
Clinical Toxicology

Vicky A. LeGrys, Ph.D., Dr.A., M.T. (A.S.C.P.) C.L.S. (N.C.A.)
Professor
Division of Clinical Laboratory Science
School of Medicine
University of North Carolina at Chapel Hill
Chapel Hill, North Carolina
Electrolytes and Blood Gases

Kristian Linnet, M.D., Ph.D.
Professor, Chief, Section of Forensic Chemistry
Department of Forensic Medicine
Faculty of Health Sciences
University of Copenhagen
Copenhagen, Denmark
Selection and Analytical Evaluation of Methods—With Statistical Techniques

Stanley F. Lo, Ph.D., D.A.B.C.C., F.A.C.B.
Associate Professor of Pathology
Medical College of Wisconsin
Associate Director, Clinical Laboratories
Children's Hospital of Wisconsin
Milwaukee, Wisconsin
Principles of Basic Techniques and Laboratory Safety

Y.M. Dennis Lo, M.A., D.M., D.Phil., F.R.C.P., F.R.C.Path., F.R.S.
Li Ks Shing Professor of Medicine
Professor of Chemical Pathology
Department of Chemical Pathology
The Chinese University of Hong Kong
Prince of Wales Hospital
Hong Kong S.A.R., China
Principles of Molecular Biology

Nicola Longo, M.D., Ph.D., F.A.C.M.G.
Professor of Pediatrics and Pathology
Chief, Division of Medical Genetics
Department of Pediatrics, Medical Co-Director, ARUP Biochemical Genetics Laboratory, University of Utah
Salt Lake City, Utah
Newborn Screening and Inborn Errors of Metabolism

Gwendolyn A. McMillin, Ph.D., D.A.B.C.C. (C.C., T.C.)
Assistant Professor (Clinical) of Pathology
University of Utah School of Medicine
Medical Director, Toxicology, Trace Elements, Pharmacogenomics
ARUP Laboratories
Salt Lake City, Utah
Therapeutic Drugs and Their Management; Pharmacogenetics; Reference Information

Mark E. Meyerhoff, Ph.D.
Philip J. Elving Professor of Chemistry
Department of Chemistry
The University of Michigan
Ann Arbor, Michigan
Electrochemistry and Chemical Sensors

Thomas P. Moyer, Ph.D.
Professor of Laboratory Medicine
Department of Laboratory Medicine & Pathology
Mayo College of Medicine
Mayo Clinic
Rochester, Minnesota
Toxic Metals

Mauro Panteghini, M.D.
Professor of Clinical Biochemistry and Clinical Molecular Biology
Department of Biomedical and Clinical Sciences "Luigi Sacco"
University of Milan
Director, Clinical Pathology Laboratory
Ospedale "Luigi Sacco"
Milan, Italy
Enzyme and Rate Analyses; Serum Enzymes

Jason Y. Park, M.D., Ph.D., F.C.A.P.
Assistant Professor
Department of Pathology
University of Texas Southwestern Medical Center
Director
Advanced Diagnostics Laboratory
Children's Medical Center
Dallas, Texas
Optical Techniques; Immunochemical Techniques

Marzia Pasquali, Ph.D., F.A.C.M.G.
Professor of Pathology
University of Utah School of Medicine
Medical Director, Biochemical Genetics and Supplemental Newborn Screening
ARUP Laboratories
Salt Lake City, Utah
Newborn Screening and Inborn Errors of Metabolism

Christopher P. Price, Ph.D., F.R.S.C., F.R.C.Path.
Visiting Professor in Clinical Biochemistry
Department of Primary Care Health Sciences
University of Oxford
Oxford, United Kingdom
*Evidence-Based Laboratory Medicine; Point-of-Care Instrumentation;
   Kidney Function Tests—Creatinine, Urea, and Uric Acid; Kidney
   Disease*

Alex J. Rai, Ph.D., D.A.B.C.C., F.A.C.B.
Director, Special Chemistry Laboratory New York Presbyterian
   Hospital
Associate Professor of Pathology and Cell Biology
Chief Scientific Officer, Center for Advanced Laboratory Medicine
Department of Pathology and Cell Biology
Columbia University Medical Center
New York, New York
Tumor Markers and Cancer Genes

Alan T. Remaley, M.D., Ph.D.
Department of Laboratory Medicine
National Institutes of Health
Bethesda, Maryland
Lipids, Lipoproteins, Apolipoproteins, and Other Cardiac Risk Factors

Nader Rifai, Ph.D.
The Louis Joseph Gay-Lussac Chair in Laboratory Medicine
Director of Clinical Chemistry
Boston Children's Hospital
Professor of Pathology
Harvard Medical School
Boston, Massachusetts
Lipids, Lipoproteins, Apolipoproteins, and Other Cardiac Risk Factors

Juha Risteli, M.D, Ph.D., F.E.B.M.B.
Professor of Clinical Chemistry
Department of Clinical Chemistry
Institute of Diagnostics
University of Oulu
Oulu, Finland
Disorders of Bone and Mineral Metabolism

Leila Risteli, M.D., Ph.D., M.A., F.E.B.M.B.
Chief Physician
Northern Finland Laboratory Centre (NordLab)
Adjunct Professor of Medical Biochemistry
University of Oulu
Oulu, Finland
Adjunct Professor of Clinical Chemistry
University of Tampere
Tampere, Finland
Disorders of Bone and Mineral Metabolism

Norman B. Roberts, M.Sc., Ph.D., C.Chem.
Consultant Clinical Scientist
Department of Clinical Biochemistry
The Royal Liverpool and Broadgreen University Hospitals
Honorary Reader, *Clinical Chemistry*
The University of Liverpool
Liverpool, United Kingdom
Vitamins, Trace Elements, and Nutritional Assessment

Alan L. Rockwood, Ph.D., D.A.B.C.C.
Scientific Director for Mass Spectrometry
ARUP Laboratories
Professor (Clinical) of Pathology
University of Utah School of Medicine
Salt Lake City, Utah
Mass Spectrometry

Thomas G. Rosano, Ph.D., D.A.B.F.T., D.A.B.C.C.
Head of Clinical Laboratory Services
Director of Clinical Chemistry and Forensic Toxicology
Albany Medical Center Hospital and College
Albany, New York
Catecholamines and Serotonin

Francois A. Rousseau, M.D., M.S., F.R.C.P.C.
Head, Department of Medical Biology
Faculty of Medicine
University of Laval
Quebec, Canada
Clinical Chemistry, Molecular Diagnostics, and Laboratory Medicine

David B. Sacks, M.D., Ch.B., F.R.C.Path.
Adjunct Professor
Department of Medicine
Division of Endocrinology and Metabolism
Georgetown University
Washington, D.C.
Carbohydrates; Diabetes

Desmond Schatz, M.D.
Professor and Associate Chairman
Department of Pediatrics
Division of Endocrinology
Medical Director, Diabetes Center
University of Florida
Gainesville, Florida
Thyroid Disorders

Emily I. Schindler, M.D., Ph.D.
Resident Physician
Department of Pathology and Immunology
Barnes Jewish Hospital
St. Louis, Missouri
*Electrolytes and Blood Gases; Physiology and Disorders of Water,
   Electrolyte, and Acid-Base Metabolism*

Mitchell G. Scott, Ph.D.
Professor of Pathology and Immunology
Co-Medical Director, Clinical Chemistry
Division of Laboratory and Genomic Medicine
Washington University School of Medicine
St. Louis, Missouri
*Electrolytes and Blood Gases; Physiology and Disorders of Water,
   Electrolyte, and Acid-Base Metabolism*

Alan Shenkin, Ph.D., F.R.C.P., F.R.C.Path.
Emeritus Professor
Unit of Clinical Chemistry
School of Clinical Sciences
University of Liverpool
Liverpool, United Kingdom
Vitamins, Trace Elements, and Nutritional Assessment

Nicholas E. Sherman, Ph.D.
Research Associate Professor
Director of Mass Spectrometry
University of Virginia
Charlottesville, Virginia
Mass Spectrometry

Christine L.H. Snozek, Ph.D., D.A.B.C.C.
Assistant Professor
Mayo Clinic College of Medicine
Director of Chemistry, Collections/Processing, and Point-of-Care
    Testing
Department of Laboratory Medicine and Pathology
Mayo Clinic in Arizona
Scottsdale, Arizona
Therapeutic Drugs and Their Management

Lori J. Sokoll, Ph.D., F.A.C.B.
Associate Professor of Pathology, Oncology, and Urology
Associate Director, Clinical Chemistry Division
Department of Pathology
Johns Hopkins Medical Institutions
Baltimore, Maryland
Tumor Markers and Cancer Genes

Andrew St. John, Ph.D.
ARC Consulting
Mt. Lawley Western Australia, Australia
Point-of-Care Instrumentation

G. Russell Warnick, M.S., M.B.A.
Executive Director
Foundation for Health Information and Technology
Chief Science Officer
Health Diagnostic Laboratory
Richmond, Virginia
Lipids, Lipoproteins, Apolipoproteins, and Other Cardiac Risk Factors

James O. Westgard, Ph.D.
Professor
Department of Pathology and Laboratory Medicine
University of Wisconsin Medical School
Madison, Wisconsin
Quality Management

Sharon D. Whatley, Ph.D.
Clinical Biochemist
Medical Biochemistry Department
University Hospital of Wales,
Cardiff, United Kingdom
Porphyrins and Porphyrias

Ronald J. Whitley, Ph.D., F.A.C.B., D.A.B.C.C.
Professor
Department of Pathology and Laboratory Medicine
University of Kentucky
Director of Clinical Chemistry, Toxicology, and Core Laboratories
University of Kentucky Medical Center College of Medicine
Lexington, Kentucky
Catecholamines and Serotonin

William E. Winter, M.D., D.A.B.C.C., F.A.C.B., F.C.A.P.
Professor
Departments of Pathology, Immunology & Laboratory Medicine,
    Pediatrics, and Molecular Genetics & Microbiology
Principle Investigator, Type 1 Diabetes TrialNet ICA Core
    Laboratory
Director, UF Pathology Laboratories, Endocrine Autoantibody
    Laboratory
University of Florida
Gainesville, Florida
*Disorders of Bone and Mineral Metabolism; Disorders of the Pituitary;
    Disorders of the Adrenal Cortex; Thyroid Disorders*

Carl T. Wittwer, M.D., Ph.D.
Professor of Pathology
University of Utah School of Medicine
Salt Lake City, Utah
*Nucleic Acid Techniques and Applications; Genomes and Nucleic Acid
    Variations*

Foreword

As a practitioner and instructor of clinical chemistry for over 20 years, I have observed many innovative changes in the clinical laboratory, from implementation of new analytical techniques to dependence on laboratory informatics to the inclusion of molecular testing and its unique practice standards. I have worked with the editors and publishers of *Tietz Fundamentals of Clinical Chemistry and Molecular Diagnostics* as consulting editor for three editions and have followed each edition as they reflect the numerous advances in laboratory science. In the area of education, such updates are crucial for informing students of what they should expect in their careers as professional laboratorians or as other practitioners in health care. As with previous editions, the seventh edition of *Tietz Fundamentals of Clinical Chemistry and Molecular Diagnostics* presents information that today's clinical chemistry students and practicing laboratorians must know to succeed in this discipline and in the contemporary world of pathology.

The true purpose of education must go beyond providing the knowledge necessary to be successful in a particular field. It must also stimulate and encourage students to investigate knowledge beyond that presented in the formal classroom setting. The highly regarded authors of the seventh edition of *Tietz Fundamentals of Clinical Chemistry and Molecular Diagnostics* excel at presenting essential knowledge. Their updates and revisions of traditional topics and the addition of new chapters, such as "Pharmacogenetics" and "Genomes and Nucleic Acid Alterations," provide interesting and indispensable material for the active learner. To inspire students to seek information beyond that provided in the various chapters, the seventh edition provides end-of-chapter multiple-choice questions that encourage continued review and study. Updated websites within each chapter offer further sources of data to increase understanding of the subject matter. Thought-provoking figures that illustrate chapter concepts and innovative algorithms that provide a unique way of examining diagnostic issues have been added to this edition.

For both the educator and the student, improved and testable objectives have been designed and related Test Bank questions have been added, revised, or modified. For the laboratory science student, the professional laboratorian, and the practicing pathologist, this textbook serves as an outstanding resource for (1) the study of basic laboratory operations, (2) understanding clinical chemistry analytes, and (3) comprehending fundamental pathophysiology. The last chapter "Reference Information for the Clinical Laboratory" provides an excellent source of reference intervals for analytes of clinical relevance. As with previous editions of *Tietz Fundamentals of Clinical Chemistry and Molecular Diagnostics*, this textbook provides something of interest for anyone who is involved in the field of medical laboratory science.

It is a privilege and an honor to have been invited to take part in the continuation of such a quality endeavor as this exceptional textbook. To observe and comment on its continued growth and maturation is both rewarding and stimulating. I find it truly fulfilling to know that students, educators, managers, and pathologists use this text as a primary resource in the classroom, laboratory, and clinic for information regarding the field of clinical chemistry. Maintaining the highest standards of quality while providing crucial contemporary information that is both concise and readable, this volume continues in the tradition of excellence set by previous editions of *Tietz Fundamentals of Clinical Chemistry and Molecular Diagnostics*.

Barbara G. Sawyer, Ph.D., M.L.S.(A.S.C.P.)[CM]**,**
M.B.(A.S.C.P.)[CM]
Professor, Clinical Laboratory Science/Molecular Pathology

Preface

As the discipline of clinical laboratory science and medicine has evolved and expanded, each new edition of *Tietz Fundamentals of Clinical Chemistry* has been revised to reflect these changes. The seventh edition of this series is no exception, as we have made significant revisions in its format and content. First, reflecting the effect that molecular diagnostics has had and continues to have on the practice of clinical chemistry and laboratory medicine, we have retitled the seventh edition as *Tietz Fundamentals of Clinical Chemistry and Molecular Diagnostics*. Consequently, chapters have been added on the topic of molecular diagnostics and many of the other updated chapters now include discussions of genetic testing and descriptions of the genetic basis of diseases.

Second, 47 new authors along with 53 veterans from the sixth edition have joined our company of subject-matter experts to revise and produce chapters that reflect the state-of-the-art in their respective fields. Consequently, this new edition covers many new topics and updates information on older ones. With these changes, the seventh edition now contains 50 chapters that are grouped into sections entitled (I) Principles of Laboratory Medicine, (II) Analytical Techniques and Instrumentation, (III) Analytes, (IV) Pathophysiology, (V) Molecular Diagnostics, and (VI) Reference Information.

Third, learning tools have been added or expanded. For example, a set of objectives and a list of key terms and definitions were included at the beginning of each chapter. (Note: in each chapter key terms are listed in alphabetical order in a bold red font and again when each appears for the first time in their respective chapter.) At the end of each chapter, a list of review questions has been added to assist students in the review of the salient points covered in each chapter. At the end of the book, we have combined the keywords and definitions into a Glossary. Of note, many of these key words and definitions were obtained, in whole or in part, from the 32nd edition of *Dorland's Illustrated Medical Dictionary*, with permission kindly granted by Elsevier.

As with the sixth edition, we have relied on information technology to prepare and produce the seventh edition. For example, each chapter was submitted and edited via Elsevier's "Electronic Manuscript Submission System." In addition, many of the figures, especially those that included chemical structures, were drawn or revised by Ed Ashwood using ChemWindows software. This resulted in a uniform representation of chemical structures and facilitated the integration of figures within the text while reducing errors. Readers will note that references to web-based sources of information are found throughout the text.

To assist us in preparing the seventh edition, we again invited Barbara G. Sawyer, Ph.D., to join our editorial team as an educational consultant. Because of her experience with using *Fundamentals* as a teaching text and her perspective as an educator, Professor Sawyer's advice and assistance were again very useful to us as we produced the seventh edition.

We appreciate the opportunity provided us by Elsevier to prepare the seventh edition of *Tietz Fundamentals of Clinical Chemistry*. It has been an exciting, challenging, and educational experience. We trust that this edition will live up to the reputation and success of its distinguished predecessors. We have enjoyed working with the team of dedicated authors that have spent many hours preparing comprehensive chapters that are authoritative and timely. We thank them sincerely and believe that they have enabled us to produce a textbook that is reflective of the diverse, technical, and practical nature of the current practice of clinical laboratory science and medicine.

We have also benefited from and enjoyed working with the Elsevier staff, especially Sonya Seigafuse, Executive Content Strategist; Ellen Wurm-Cutter, Content Development Manager; and Rachel E. McMullen and Andrea Campbell, Senior Project Managers. Their patience, cooperation, advice, and professional dedication are gratefully acknowledged.

Finally, we thank our valued colleague Ed Ashwood for his years of work as an editor of this book's predecessors. The current product continues to benefit from his many contributions.

Carl A. Burtis
David E. Bruns

Contents

PART VI   REFERENCE INFORMATION

Clinical Chemistry, Molecular Diagnostics, and Laboratory Medicine

David E. Bruns, M.D., Francois A. Rousseau, M.D., and Carl A. Burtis, Ph.D.

Objectives

1. Define the following terms:

   Core laboratory   Molecular diagnostics

   Ethics   Pharmacogenetics

   Laboratory medicine
2. List and explain six reasons for performing a laboratory test.
3. Describe the field of laboratory medicine, including subdisciplines, information handling, and ethical issues.
4. State the contribution of epidemiology to the field of clinical chemistry.
5. State the applications of molecular diagnostics in laboratory medicine.
6. List and explain five ethical issues that confront laboratorians; state the critical importance of maintaining confidentiality in the laboratory.
7. Evaluate a possible confidentiality or conflict of interest issue and determine whether it is an ethics violation.

Key Words and Definitions

Core laboratory A laboratory that provides all of the high-volume and emergency testing in many hospitals.

Ethics Rules or standards governing the conduct of an individual or the members of a profession.

Laboratory medicine A component of laboratory science that is involved in the selection, provision, and interpretation of diagnostic testing of individual specimens.

Laboratory testing A process conducted in a clinical laboratory to rule in or rule out a diagnosis, to select and monitor disease treatment, to provide a prognosis, to screen for a disease, or to determine the severity of and monitor a physiological disturbance.

Molecular diagnostics Use of molecular biology techniques for the purposes of prevention, diagnosis, and follow-up or prognosis of disease; and selection, optimization, and monitoring of therapies.

In this chapter, we begin with a general discussion to introduce the field of laboratory medicine and the disciplines of clinical chemistry (or clinical biochemistry) and molecular diagnostics. This will include a discussion of the meaning of the term *laboratory medicine* and the relationships among (1) clinical chemistry, (2) molecular diagnostics, (3) laboratory medicine, and (4) evidence-based laboratory medicine. The concepts introduced in this chapter are developed in the remaining chapters of this book.

The chapter concludes with a discussion on the ethical issues that clinical chemists/biochemists face in the practice of their profession and issues that they will face in the future.

Laboratory Medicine

The term laboratory medicine refers to the discipline involved in the (1) selection, (2) provision, and (3) interpretation of diagnostic testing that uses primarily samples from patients. This discipline includes (1) research, (2) administration, (3) teaching activities, and (4) clinical service. Testing in laboratory medicine may be directed at (1) confirming a clinical suspicion, which may include making, or ruling in, a diagnosis, (2) excluding, or ruling out, a diagnosis, (3) assisting in selection, optimization, and monitoring of treatment, (4) providing a prognosis, (5) screening for disease in the absence of clinical signs or symptoms, and (6) establishing and monitoring the severity of a physiological disturbance (Box 1-1).

The field of laboratory medicine includes clinical chemistry and its traditional subdisciplines (including toxicology and drug monitoring, endocrine and organ function testing, and "biochemical" and "molecular" genetics) and areas such as microbiology, hematology, hemostasis and thrombosis, blood banking (transfusion medicine), immunology, and identity testing (Box 1-2). In some parts of the world, laboratory medicine also encompasses cytology and anatomic pathology (histopathology). In recent years, molecular diagnostics has become an increasingly important part of all of the specialties of laboratory medicine. Information management and interpretation (including laboratory informatics) are key aspects of the laboratory medicine service, as are activities concerned with maintaining quality, such as (1) quality control, (2) proficiency testing, (3) audit, (4) benchmarking, and (5) clinical governance. Closer links with patients are increasingly attained through the use of telemedicine and tele-healthcare, which includes facets of laboratory medicine such as

---

BOX 1-1   Uses of Testing in the Clinical Laboratory

- Confirming a clinical suspicion (which could include making a diagnosis)
- Excluding a diagnosis
- Assisting in selection, optimization, and monitoring of treatment
- Providing a prognosis
- Screening for disease in the absence of clinical signs or symptoms
- Establishing and monitoring the severity of a physiological disturbance

---

BOX 1-2   Disciplines of the Modern-Day Clinical Laboratory

- Biochemical Genetics
- Cancer Diagnostics
- Clinical Chemistry/Biochemistry
- Clinical Hematology
- Clinical Immunology
- Cytogenetics
- Drug Monitoring
- Endocrinology Testing
- Hemostasis/Thrombosis (Coagulation) Testing
- Identity Testing
- Infectious Disease Testing
- Information Technology
- Laboratory Management
- Microbiology
- Molecular Cytogenetics
- Molecular Diagnostics
- Nutrition
- Organ Transplantation
- Organ Function Testing
- Pharmacogenetics
- Proteomics
- Quality Management
- Toxicology
- Trace Elements
- Transfusion Medicine (Blood Banking)

---

(1) analytical testing, (2) the use of clinical decision support systems, and (3) informatics.

Clinical Chemistry and Laboratory Medicine

The ties between clinical chemistry and other areas of laboratory medicine have deep roots. Individuals working primarily in the area of clinical chemistry/biochemistry have developed tools and methods that have become part of the fabric of laboratory medicine beyond the clinical chemistry laboratory. Examples include (1) the theory and practice of reference intervals (see Chapter 5), (2) the use of both (internal) quality control and proficiency testing (see Chapter 7), (3) the introduction of automation into the clinical laboratory (see Chapter 16), and (4) concepts of diagnostic testing (see Chapters 3 and 4). From physician and patient perspectives, no distinction is evident among these specialties, and invariably the repertoire of more than one specialty will be called upon when a clinical decision is made. Examples of clinical scenarios that require tests from multiple laboratory areas include the diagnosis and management of many diseases and the management of patients in intensive care (see Chapters 33 through 45).

Boundaries between and among the parts of the clinical laboratory have become more blurred with increasing emphasis on the use of chemical and "molecular" (nucleic acid) testing. Molecular diagnostic testing has evolved beyond human genetic testing—an area in which clinical chemists have long been active. Now, clinical chemists in "molecular" laboratories contribute their expertise in laboratory medicine to infectious disease testing, cancer diagnostics, and identity testing—activities that formerly were associated primarily or solely with, respectively, clinical microbiology, hematology, and blood bank laboratories. Successful contributions by clinical chemists to these areas require an understanding of the principles of laboratory medicine and close collaboration with clinical microbiologists, hematologists, and others who have specialized expertise in those areas of laboratory medicine.

The relationship between the clinical chemist and laboratory medicine has evolved further with the advent of **"core" laboratories**. These laboratories provide all of the high-volume and emergency testing in many hospitals. Their efficient and reliable operation depends on automation (see Chapter 16), computers, and high levels of quality control and quality management (see Chapter 7). Clinical chemists, who have long been active in these areas, have assumed increasing responsibility in core laboratories and thus have become more involved in areas such as hematology, coagulation, urinalysis, and even microbiology. Thus a new type of "clinical chemist" has emerged, and again the functions require a broader knowledge of laboratory medicine and greater collaboration with other specialists.

A virtual merger of clinical chemistry and laboratory medicine has been suggested in many ways. For example, journals in the field of clinical chemistry publish articles in all of the areas of laboratory medicine. The current logo of the American Association for Clinical Chemistry reads, "AACC—Improving Healthcare through Laboratory Medicine." Moreover, the

International Federation of Clinical Chemistry Societies is now called the International Federation of Clinical Chemistry and Laboratory Medicine (IFCC). Being active in the field of laboratory medicine today requires, more often than not, familiarity with core concepts in several if not all of the sub-disciplines of the field.

During the past two decades, the field of clinical chemistry has been profoundly influenced by new activities in the fields of clinical epidemiology and evidence-based medicine (see Chapter 4). Clinical epidemiologists have developed study designs to quantify the diagnostic accuracy (as opposed to analytical accuracy) of tests developed in laboratory medicine (see Chapter 3). Moreover, they have introduced methods that are used to evaluate the effects and value of **laboratory testing** in healthcare (see Chapter 2). These developments are expected to play an increasing role in the selection and interpretation of tests. Thus Chapter 4 of this book is devoted to evidence-based laboratory medicine.

Molecular Diagnostics

Molecular diagnostics is defined as the use of the techniques of molecular biology for the purpose of prevention, diagnosis, follow-up, or prognosis of disease. Molecular diagnostics has impacted all fields of laboratory medicine and has delivered several new diagnostic tools of proven clinical utility. After the discovery of DNA as the repository of genetic information in the 1950s, the development of molecular biology methods to study DNA and RNA in the 1970s and 1980s, and the invention of the polymerase chain reaction (PCR) in 1985, analysis of nucleic acids and molecular biology methods have been used to decipher many biological processes of the living cell (see Chapters 46 to 49) in normal and disease states. These discoveries naturally led to the development of the discipline of molecular diagnostics, which entered the realm of laboratory medicine in multiple forms and in multiple fields. Molecular diagnostics has been applied to the study of the constitutive genome (e.g., inherited diseases, histocompatibility, identity assessment, pharmacogenetics; see Chapter 46) and to the study of acquired states (e.g., infectious diseases, grafting, and pregnancy). Molecular diagnostic methods can be qualitative or quantitative in nature, depending on the clinical need.

The field of molecular diagnostics is characterized by very rapidly evolving technology (as the result of massive investments in the human genome project and endeavors that followed), as well as by a rapidly increasing variety of potential clinical applications. Of note, the advent of massively parallel nucleic acid sequencing is opening a wide spectrum of potential new diagnostic applications, where tens to hundreds of millions of different molecules are characterized and quantified in a single experiment and supported by high throughput clinical bioinformatic data analyses. Chapters 47, 48, and 49 provide an overview, respectively, of the Principles of Molecular Biology, Nucleic Acid Techniques and Applications, and Genome and Nucleic Acid Alterations.

One field in which molecular diagnostics has made a significant impact is the study of hematopoietic malignancies such as malignant lymphomas and leukemias. Easy access to malignant cells through a blood or bone marrow sample allowed the development of molecular biomarkers to refine the diagnosis of such tumors. These include genetic rearrangements that are specific to certain types of malignancies and are associated with the aggressiveness and prognosis of the malignancy and, hence, are useful tools for orienting treatment. Further, once the molecular signature of the patient's tumor has been identified, quantitative assays allow monitoring of response to therapy and aid in detection of residual disease in the event of a relapse and confirmation of durable remissions.

Pharmacogenetics (see Chapter 46), or the study of variation in drug metabolism between individuals, has been a field of intensive work and increasing interest because studying the genomic DNA from a patient is simpler than measuring the activity of enzymes in tissues that are not easily accessible but are involved in drug activation and metabolism.

Apart from the study of tissues and nucleated cells, molecular diagnostics has been applied to the study of plasma nucleic acids (or circulating nucleic acids; see Chapter 47). Plasma nucleic acid analysis has been made possible by the discovery that cells in the body release DNA and RNA into the extracellular compartment and ultimately into the bloodstream, where they can be detected and analyzed. Because of their short half-life in the circulation (less than 24 hours), plasma nucleic acids provide a measure of processes that are ongoing at the time of blood sampling. Such processes include the presence of nucleic acids from abnormal tissue (tumor nucleic acids) or the existence of nonhost nucleic acids (microorganisms, graft–donor, and the fetus during pregnancy). It is expected that molecular diagnostic analysis of plasma nucleic acids will enter routine clinical practice for various indications with the appearance of a high-quality evidence base for their clinical utility.

Ethical Issues in Laboratory Medicine

As in other branches of medicine, practitioners in laboratory medicine are faced with ethical issues, often on a daily basis; examples are listed in Box 1-3. The definition of **ethics** varies, but in this chapter, the following definition is relevant: "The rules or standards governing the conduct of an individual or the members of a profession (e.g., laboratory medicine)." Specific ethical issues that pertain to the practice of laboratory medicine include but are not limited to (1) confidentiality of genetic information and patient medical information, (2) allocation

---

BOX 1-3 **Ethical Issues in Clinical Chemistry and Molecular Diagnostics**

- Confidentiality of genetic information
- Confidentiality of patient medical information
- Allocation of resources
- Codes of conduct
- Publishing issues
- Conflict of interest

of healthcare resources, (3) codes of conduct, (4) publishing issues, and (5) conflict of interest.

Confidentiality of Genetic Information

Prominent in the news in the first and second decades of this millennium has been the issue of confidentiality of genetic information. Legislation was considered necessary to prevent denial of health insurance or employment to people found by DNA testing to be at risk of disease. Less appreciated is the fact that the issue of confidentiality of clinical laboratory data predated DNA testing. In fact, many non-DNA tests, old and new, also carry information about risks of illness and death. Clinical laboratorians have long been responsible for maintaining the confidentiality of all laboratory results—a situation made even more critical with the advent of increasingly powerful genetic testing.

Confidentiality of Patient Medical Information

Because new medical tests are constantly needed, laboratory physicians and scientists spend a great deal of time and effort developing new diagnostic tests or evaluating them for use in a specific setting. This process requires use of patient samples and may involve use of patient medical information.[3] Ethical judgments are required regarding the type of informed consent that is needed from patients for use of their samples and clinical information. Clinical laboratory physicians and scientists often serve on institutional review boards that examine proposed research on human subjects. In these discussions, ethical concepts such as equipoise and confidentiality are central to decision making.

Allocation of Healthcare Resources

Because resources are finite, clinical laboratorians must make ethically responsible decisions about allocation of resources in the clinical laboratory and beyond. When a trade-off exists between cost and quality (of testing reagents or analyzers, for example), ethical issues may need to be considered: What is best for patients generally? How can the most good be done with the available resources?

Business Ethics

For laboratorians in business, the newly appreciated area of business ethics comes into play. One example, recently epitomized by scandals associated with names such as Madoff and Enron, involves the area of accounting—a human endeavor that in the public mind had not been much associated with concerns about ethics.

Codes of Conduct

Most professional organizations publish a Code of Conduct that requires adherence by their members. For example, the American Association for Clinical Chemistry (AACC) has published Ethical Guidelines (http://www.aacc.org/about/ethics/Pages/default.aspx#; accessed June 26, 2013) that require AACC members to endorse principles of ethical conduct in their professional activities, including (1) selection and performance of clinical procedures, (2) research and development,

(3) teaching, (4) management, (5) administration, and (6) other forms of professional service.

Publishing Issues

Publication of documents having high scientific integrity depends on authors, editors, and reviewers all working in concert in an environment governed by high ethical standards.[2]

Authors are responsible for honest and complete reporting of original data produced in ethically conducted research studies. Practices such as fraud, plagiarism, and falsification or fabrication of data are unacceptable! The International Committee of Medical Journal Editors (ICMJE)[7] and the Committee on Publication Ethics (COPE)[5] have published policies that address such behavior. Other practices to be avoided include redundant publication, and inappropriate credit for authorship; in addition, ethical policies require that factors that might influence the interpretation of a study must be revealed. Most journals now have conflict of interest policies for both authors and journal editors. For example, *Clinical Chemistry* requires that authors complete a full disclosure form upon manuscript submission. Annually, the Editor and Associate Editors are also required to complete such a form (http://www.clinchem.org/; accessed June 26, 2013).

Conflict of Interest

Concern has been raised over the interrelationships between practitioners in the medical field and commercial suppliers of drugs, devices, equipment, etc., to the medical profession.[8] These concerns led the National Institutes of Health (NIH) in 1995 to require official institutional review of financial disclosure by researchers and management of situations in which disclosure indicates potential conflict of interest and/or conflict of effort in research. In 2009, the Institute of Medicine (IOM) issued a report[6] that questioned inappropriate relationships between pharmaceutical and device companies and physicians and other healthcare professionals.[8] Similarly, the relationships between clinical laboratorians and manufacturers and providers of diagnostic equipment and supplies have been scrutinized.

As a consequence of these concerns and as a result of the enactment of various laws designed to prevent fraud, abuse, and waste in Medicare, Medicaid, and other federal programs, professional organizations that represent manufacturers of in vitro diagnostics (IVD) and other device and healthcare companies have published Codes of Ethics. For example, the Advanced Medical Technology Association (AdvaMed) has revised and published its Code of Ethics that became effective July 1, 2009.[1] Topics discussed in this revised Code include (1) gifts and entertainment, (2) consulting arrangements and royalties, (3) reimbursement for testing, and (4) education. Similarly, the European Diagnostic Manufacturers Association (EDMA) has published its Code of Ethics.[4] In Part A of this document, topics discussed include (1) member-sponsored product training and education, (2) supporting third-party educational conferences, (3) sales and promotional meetings, (4) financial arrangements for consultants (5) gifts, (6) provision of reimbursements and other economic information, and (7) donations for charitable and philanthropic purposes.

Both documents address demands from regulators while nurturing the unique role that laboratorians and other healthcare professionals play in developing and refining new technology.[8]

In closing, it is our opinion that practitioners of clinical chemistry, molecular diagnostics, and laboratory medicine have before them a future full of promises and challenges. New insight into disease and its treatment is exploding, and these insights are based in sciences that are at the heart of the clinical laboratory. The clinical laboratory is the place of translation of these insights into effective healthcare. We honor the important role of ethical laboratory professionals in these efforts and have endeavored to provide in this book chapters prepared by expert authors that help to define the evidence base and the knowledge base of the profession.

Review Questions

1. The clinical laboratory discipline that is used most often to assess inherited disease through study of the constitutive genome is:
   a. transfusion services.
   b. clinical chemistry.
   c. molecular diagnostics.
   d. hematology.
2. The study of the genetic variation between individuals in their ability to metabolize drugs is referred to as:
   a. pharmacogenetics.
   b. molecular diagnostics.
   c. clinical chemistry.
   d. epidemiology.
3. When a practitioner in clinical chemistry has an inappropriate personal relationship with a commercial supplier of medical supplies and chemistry analyzers, there may be a potential issue with:
   a. publication development.
   b. confidentiality.
   c. selection of treatment.
   d. conflict of interest.
4. "Molecular testing" involves the clinical analysis of:
   a. atoms and molecules.
   b. nucleic acids.
   c. cellular components of blood.
   d. the physical structure of compounds.
5. Which one of the following is not considered an ethical issue facing a clinical laboratorian?
   a. Allocation of resources
   b. Conflicts of interest
   c. Discussion of one's salary
   d. Maintenance of confidentiality

References

1. Advanced Medical Technology Association (AdvaMed). Code of Ethics on interactions with health care professionals. Effective July 1, 2009. http://www.advamed.org/ (accessed on June 26, 2013).
2. Annesley TM, Boyd JC, Rifai N. Publication ethics: *Clinical Chemistry* editorial standards. Clin Chem 2009;55:1–4.
3. Council of Europe. Additional protocol to the convention for the protection of human rights and dignity of the human being with regard to the application of biology and medicine on biomedical research. Law Hum Genome Rev 2004;21:201–214.
4. European Diagnostic Manufacturers Association (EDMA). Part A: interaction with health care professionals. http://www.edma-ivd.be/ (accessed June 26, 2013).
5. Graf C, Wager E, Bowman A, Fiack S, Scott-Lichter D, Robinson A. Best practice guidelines on publication ethics: a publisher's perspective. Int J Clin Pract Suppl 2007;61:1–26.
6. Institute of Medicine. Conflict of interest in medical research, education, and practice. http://www.iom.edu (accessed June 26, 2013).
7. International Committee of Medical Journal Editors. Uniform requirements for manuscripts submitted to biomedical journals: writing and editing for biomedical publication. http://www.icmje.org/ (accessed June 26, 2013).
8. Malone B. Ethics code changes for diagnostics manufacturers. Clin Lab News 2009;35(6).

Selection and Analytical Evaluation of Methods—With Statistical Techniques*

Kristian Linnet, M.D., D.M.Sc., and James C. Boyd, M.D.

Objectives

1. Define the following:

Analytical measurement range	Median
Bias	Population
Clinical sensitivity	Precision
Clinical specificity	Random error
Coefficient of variation	Random sample
Correlation coefficient	Regression analysis
Difference plot	Sample
Error model	Standard deviation
Frequency distribution	Systematic error
Gaussian probability distribution	Student *t* distribution
Limit of detection	Trueness
Linearity	Uncertainty
Mean	

2. List and describe three criteria that must be considerations in laboratory method selection, including the specific parameters involved in each criterion.

3. Compare population and sample mean, population parameter and sample statistic, and population standard deviation and sample standard deviation, including a description of each, symbols used to express these, how they are calculated, and the information they provide.

4. State the connection of the following concepts to analytical methods:

Accuracy	Linearity
Analytical sensitivity	Precision
Analytical specificity	Repeatability
Calibration	Reproducibility
Limit of detection	

5. List two common approaches used to objectively analyze data in a methods comparison study.

6. Describe the components of a difference plot, including the plot's use in method comparison and how the plot is interpreted.

7. Discuss assessment of error in an objective analysis of data in method comparison, including how error occurrence relates to an assay's performance characteristics, the difference between random and systematic error, what causes error, and how error is evaluated in a difference plot.

8. For the following types of analyses, list the components of the analysis, its application in method comparison, how it is computed, how outliers affect it, and how the results are interpreted:

Deming regression	Ordinary least-squares regression
Nonparametric regression	Regression

9. Describe the calibration hierarchy, including the tracing of values of routine clinical chemistry measurements to a primary reference, how the values are obtained, and the methods involved; draw a calibration hierarchy given a specific analyte.

10. Discuss the concept of uncertainty in relation to clinical laboratory results, including the components of the standard uncertainty formula and two ways in which uncertainty is assessed.

11. Given appropriate values, state the formula and calculate the following:

Coefficient of variation	Population mean
Coefficient of variation percent	Precision analyses
Deming regression	Standard deviation
Linear regression	Standard uncertainty

Key Words and Definitions

Analyte The substance being analyzed in an analytical procedure.

Analytical sensitivity The ability of an analytical method to assess small variations in the concentration of analyte.

Analytical specificity The ability of an assay procedure to determine specifically the concentration of the target analyte in the presence of potentially interfering substances or factors in the sample matrix.

Bias In an analytical method, the difference between the average value and the true value that is expressed numerically and is inversely related to the trueness.

*The authors gratefully acknowledge the original contributions by Theodore Peters, Robert O. Kringle, and David D. Koch on which portions of this chapter are based.

Key Words and Definitions—cont'd

Calibration In relation to analytical methods, a function that describes the relationship between instrument signal and concentration of analyte.

Commutability The equivalence of the mathematical relationships between the results of different measurement procedures for a reference material and for representative samples from healthy and diseased individuals.

Difference plot A bias plot that shows the dispersion of observed differences between the measurements of two methods as a function of the average concentration of the measurements; also referred to as a "Bland-Altman plot."

Limit of detection An assay characteristic defined as the lowest value that significantly exceeds the measurements of a blank sample.

Matrix In relation to analytical methods, human serum that contains analytes.

Measuring interval The analyte concentration range over which measurements are within the declared tolerances for imprecision and bias; also referred to as "reportable range."

Method comparison Comparison of measurements by two methods that is carried out objectively using statistical procedures and graphics displays.

Ordinary least-squares regression (OLR) analysis A method used to estimate the unknown parameters in a linear regression assessment performed to minimize the sum of squared vertical distances between observed responses and responses predicted by linear approximation.

Population In relation to analytical methods, the complete set of all observations that might occur as the result of performing a particular procedure according to specified conditions.

Random error Error that arises from imprecision of measurement of the type that is described by a Gaussian distribution (e.g., caused by pipetting variability, signal variability).

Reference measurement procedure A procedure of highest analytical quality that has been shown to yield values having an uncertainty of measurement commensurate with its intended use, especially in assessing the trueness of other measurement procedures for the same quantity and in characterizing reference materials.

Regression analysis A statistical analysis that compares measurement relations between two analytical methods.

Systematic error Error in measurement that arises from calibration bias or nonspecificity of an assay and, in the course of a number of analyses of the same analyte, remains constant (y-intercept deviation from zero) or varies in a proportional way (slope deviation from unity) based on the analyte concentration.

Traceability In relation to analytical methods, a concept based on a chain of comparisons of measurements that lead to a known reference value done to ensure reasonable agreement between measurements of routine methods.

Trueness A qualitative term that describes the closeness of agreement between the average value obtained from a large series of results of measurements and a true value.

Uncertainty A parameter associated with the result of a measurement that characterizes the dispersion of the values that could reasonably be attributed to the measure and, or, more briefly, uncertainty is a parameter characterizing the range of values within which the value of the quantity being measured is expected to lie.

The introduction of new or revised methods is a common task for laboratorians working in the clinical laboratory (Figure 2-1). In practice, a new or revised method must be selected carefully and its performance evaluated thoroughly in the laboratory before it is adopted for routine use. The establishment of a new method may also involve an evaluation of the features of the automated analyzer on which the method will be implemented.

Method evaluation in the clinical laboratory is influenced strongly by guidelines (e.g., see the Clinical and Laboratory Standard Institute [CLSI; www.clsi.org/; accessed July 6, 2013] and the International Organization for Standardization [ISO; www.iso.org/; accessed July 6, 2013]). In addition, meeting laboratory accreditation requirements has become an important aspect of the method selection and evaluation process. This chapter presents an overview of considerations in the method selection process, followed by sections on basic statistics, method evaluation, and method comparison. A list of abbreviations used in this chapter is provided in Box 2-1.

Method Selection

Optimal method selection involves consideration of (1) medical usefulness, (2) analytical performance, and (3) practical criteria.

Medical Usefulness Criteria

The selection of appropriate methods for clinical laboratory assays is a vital part of rendering optimal patient care, and advances in patient care are frequently based on the use of new or improved laboratory tests.

Ascertaining what is necessary clinically from a laboratory test is the first step in selecting a candidate method (see Figure 2-1). Key parameters, such as desired turnaround time and necessary clinical utility for an assay, often are derived from discussions between laboratorians and clinicians. When new diagnostic assays are introduced, reliable estimates of clinical **sensitivity** and **specificity** must be obtained by reviewing the literature or by conducting a clinical outcome study. With established analytes (the substances analyzed in an analytical procedure), a common scenario is the replacement of an older, labor-intensive method with a newer, automated assay that is more economical for daily use.

Analytical Performance Criteria

In evaluating the performance characteristics of a candidate method, (1) precision, (2) accuracy (trueness), (3) analytical range, (4) detection limit, and (5) analytical specificity are of prime importance. The sections in this chapter on method evaluation and comparison contain outlines of these concepts and of their assessment. The estimated performance parameters for a method are related to quality goals that ensure acceptable medical use of the test results (see section, "Analytical Goals"). From a practical point of view, the "ruggedness" of the method in routine use is of importance.

When a new clinical analyzer is included in the overall evaluation process, various instrumental parameters also require evaluation, including (1) pipetting precision, (2) specimen-to-specimen carryover, (3) reagent-to-reagent carryover, (4) detector imprecision, (5) time to first reportable result, (6) on-board reagent stability, (7) overall throughput, (8) mean time between instrument failures, and (9) mean time to repair. Information on most of these parameters should be available from the instrument manufacturer.

Other (Practical) Criteria

Various categories of candidate methods may be considered. New methods described in the scientific literature may require "in-house" development. Commercial kit methods, on the other hand, are ready for implementation in the laboratory, often in a "closed" analytical system on a dedicated instrument. When prospective methods are reviewed, attention should be given to the following:

1. The principle of the assay, with original references
2. The detailed protocol for performing the test
3. The composition of reagents and reference materials, the quantities provided, and their storage requirements (e.g., space, temperature, light, and humidity restrictions) applicable both before and after the original containers are opened
4. The stability of reagents and reference materials (e.g., their shelf life)
5. Technologist time and required skills
6. Possible hazards and appropriate safety precautions according to relevant guidelines and legislation
7. The type, quantity, and disposal of waste generated
8. Specimen requirements such as conditions for collection, specimen volume requirements, the necessity for anticoagulants and preservatives, and necessary storage condition
9. The reference interval of the method, including information on how it was derived, typical values obtained in health and disease, and the necessity of determining a reference interval for one's own institution (see Chapter 5 for details on how to generate a reference interval)
10. Instrumental requirements and limitations
11. Cost-effectiveness
12. Computer platforms and interfacing to the laboratory information system
13. The availability of technical support, supplies, and service

Other considerations should be taken into account. For example, is there sufficient space, electrical power, cooling, and plumbing for a new instrument? Does the projected workload match with the capacity of a new instrument? Is the test repertoire of a new instrument sufficient? What is the method of calibration, and what is its frequency? Is staffing of the laboratory sufficient or is training required? What are the appropriate choices of quality control procedures and proficiency testing? What is the estimated cost of performing an assay using the proposed method, including the costs of calibrators, quality control specimens, and technologists' time?

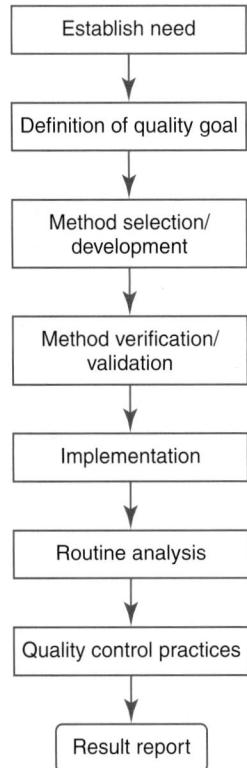

Figure 2-1 Flow diagram that illustrates the process of introducing a new method into routine use. The diagram highlights the key steps of method selection, method evaluation, and quality control.

BOX 2-1	Abbreviations
CI	Confidence interval
CV	Coefficient of variation (=SD/x, where x is the concentration)
CV%	= CV 100%
CV_A	Analytical coefficient of variation
CV_{RB}	Random bias coefficient of variation
ISO	International Organization for Standardization
OLR	Ordinary least-squares regression analysis
SD	Standard deviation
SEM	Standard error of the mean = SD/$\sqrt{N}$)
SD_A	Analytical standard deviation
SD_{RB}	Random bias standard deviation
x_m	Mean

Basic Statistics

In this section, fundamental statistical concepts and techniques are introduced in the context of typical analytical investigations. The basic concepts of populations, samples, parameters, statistics, and probability distributions are defined and illustrated. Two important probability distributions, Gaussian and Student *t*, are introduced and discussed.

Frequency Distribution

A graphical device for displaying a large set of data is the *frequency distribution,* also called a *histogram.* Figure 2-2 shows a frequency distribution displaying the results of serum γ-glutamyltransferase (GGT) measurements of 100 apparently healthy 20- to 29-year-old men. The frequency distribution is constructed by dividing the measurement scale into cells of equal width, counting the number, n_i, of values that fall within each cell, and drawing a rectangle above each cell whose area (and height, because all cell widths are equal) is proportional to n_i. In this example, the selected cells were 5 to 9, 10 to 14, 15 to 19, 20 to 24, 25 to 29, and so on, with 60 to 64 being the last cell. The ordinate axis of the frequency distribution gives the number of values falling within each cell. When this number is divided by the total number of values in the data set, the relative frequency in each cell is obtained.

Often, the position of a subject's value within a distribution of values is useful medically. The *nonparametric* approach is used to determine directly the *percentile* of a given subject. When *N* subjects have been ranked according to their values, the *n*-percentile, $Perc_n$, may be estimated as the value of the $(N[n/100] + 0.5)$ ordered observation. In cases of a noninteger value, interpolation is carried out between neighboring values.

Population and Sample

The purpose of analytical work is to obtain information and draw conclusions about characteristics of one or more populations of values. In the GGT example, the interest involves the location and spread of the population of GGT values for 20- to 29-year-old healthy men. Thus a working definition of a **population** is the complete set of all observations that might occur as a result of performing a particular procedure according to specified conditions.

Most populations of interest in clinical chemistry are infinite in size and so are impossible to study in their entirety. Usually a subgroup of observations is taken from the population as a basis on which conclusions can be formed about the population characteristics. The group of observations that has actually been selected from the population is called a *sample.*

For example, the 100 GGT values represent a sample from a respective population. However, a sample is used to study the characteristics of a population only if it has been properly selected. For instance, if the analyst is interested in the population of GGT values over various lots of materials and some time period, the sample must be selected to be representative of these factors as well as of the age, sex, and health factors. Consequently, exact specification of the population(s) of interest is necessary before a plan can be designed for obtaining the sample(s).

Probability and Probability Distributions

Consider again the frequency distribution in Figure 2-2. In addition to the general location and spread of the GGT determinations, other useful information is easily extracted from this frequency distribution. For instance, 96% (96 of 100) of the determinations are less than 55 U/L, and 91% (91 of 100) are greater than or equal to 10 but less than 50 U/L. Because the cell interval is 5 U/L in this example, statements like these can be made only to the nearest 5 U/L. A larger sample would allow a smaller cell interval and more refined statements. For a sufficiently large sample, the cell interval is made so small that the frequency distribution is approximated by a continuous, smooth curve like that shown in Figure 2-3. In fact, if the sample is large enough, we can consider this a close representation of the true *population frequency distribution.* In general, the functional form of the population frequency distribution curve of a variable *x* is denoted by f(*x*).

The population frequency distribution allows us to make probability statements about the GGT of a randomly selected member of the population of healthy 20- to 29-year-old men. For example, the probability $Pr(x > x_a)$ that the GGT value *x* of a randomly selected 20- to 29-year-old healthy man is greater than some particular value x_a is equal to the area under the population frequency distribution to the right of x_a. If $x_a = 58$, then from Figure 2-3, $Pr(x > 58) = 0.05$. Similarly, the probability $Pr(x_a < x < x_b)$ that *x* is greater than x_a but less than x_b is equal to the area under the population frequency distribution between x_a and x_b. For example, if $x_a = 9$ and $x_b = 58$, then from Figure 2-3, $Pr(9 < x < 58) = 0.90$. Because the population frequency distribution provides all information about the probabilities of a randomly selected member of the population, it is called the *probability distribution of the population.* Although the true probability distribution is never exactly

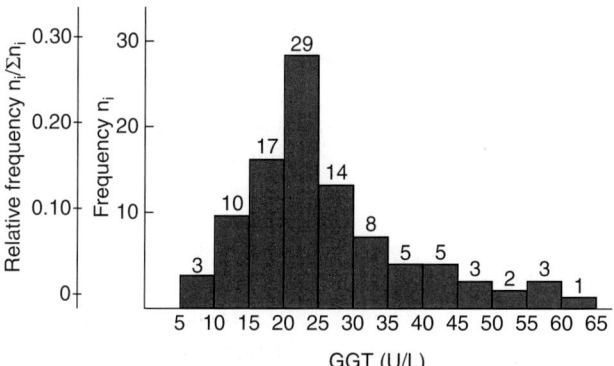

Figure 2-2 Frequency distribution of 100 γ-GGT values.

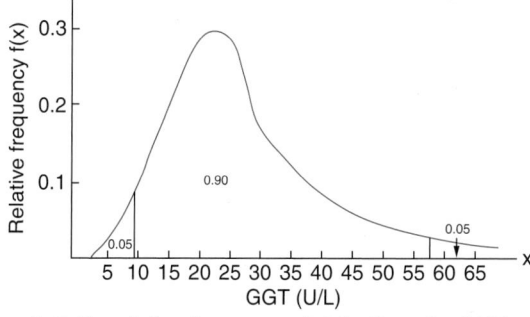

Figure 2-3 Population frequency distribution of γ-GGT values.

known in practice, it is approximated with a large sample of observations.

Parameters: Descriptive Measures of a Population

Any population of values can be described by measures of its characteristics. A *parameter* is a constant that describes some particular characteristic of a population. Although most populations of interest in analytical work are infinite in size, for the following definitions we shall consider the population to be of finite size N, where N is very large.

One important characteristic of a population is its *central location.* The parameter most commonly used to describe the central location of a population of N values is the *population mean* (μ):

$$\mu = \frac{\sum x_i}{N}$$

An alternative parameter that indicates the central tendency of a population is the *median,* which is defined as the 50th percentile, Perc_{50}.

Another important characteristic of a population is the *dispersion* of values about the population mean. A parameter very useful in describing this dispersion of a population of N values is the *population variance* σ^2 (sigma squared):

$$\sigma^2 = \frac{\sum (x_i - \mu)^2}{N}$$

The *population standard deviation* σ, the positive square root of the population variance, is a parameter frequently used to describe the population dispersion in the same units (e.g., mg/dL) as the population values.

Statistics: Descriptive Measures of the Sample

As was noted earlier, the clinical laboratorian usually has available only a few observations from the population of interest. A *statistic* is a value calculated from the observations in a sample to describe a particular characteristic of that sample. The sample mean x_m is the arithmetic average of a sample, which is an estimate of μ. Likewise, the sample standard deviation (SD) is an estimate of σ, and the coefficient of variation (CV) is the ratio of the SD to the mean multiplied by 100%. The equations used to calculate x_m, SD, and CV, respectively, are as follows:

$$x_m = \frac{\sum x_i}{N}$$

$$SD = \sqrt{\frac{\sum (x_i - x_m)^2}{N - 1}} = \sqrt{\frac{\sum x_i^2 - \frac{(\sum x_i)^2}{N}}{N - 1}}$$

$$CV = \frac{SD}{x_m} \times 100\%$$

where x_i is an individual measurement, and N is the number of sample measurements.

Random Sampling

A random selection from a population is one in which each member of the population has an equal chance of being selected. A *random sample* is one in which each member of the sample is considered to be a random selection from the population of interest. Although much of statistical analysis and interpretation depends on the assumption of a random sample from some fixed population, actual data collection often does not satisfy this assumption. In particular, for sequentially generated data, it is often true that observations adjacent to each other tend to be more alike than observations separated in time. A sample of such observations cannot be considered a sample of random selections from a fixed population. Fortunately, precautions can usually be taken in the design of an investigation to validate approximately the random sampling assumption.

The Gaussian Probability Distribution

The *Gaussian* probability distribution, which is illustrated in Figure 2-4, is of fundamental importance in statistics for several reasons. As was mentioned earlier, a particular analytical value x will not usually be equal to the true value μ of the specimen being measured. Rather, associated with this particular value x will be a particular measurement error, $\varepsilon = x - \mu$, which is the result of many contributing sources of error. These measurement errors tend to follow a probability distribution like that shown in Figure 2-4, where the errors are symmetrically distributed, with smaller errors occurring more frequently than larger ones, and with an expected value of 0. This important fact is known as the *central limit effect for distribution of errors*: If a measurement error ε is the sum of many independent sources of error ($\varepsilon_1, \varepsilon_2, \ldots, \varepsilon_k$), several of which are major contributors, the probability distribution of the measurement error ε will tend to be Gaussian as the number of sources of error becomes large.

Another reason for the importance of the Gaussian probability distribution is that many statistical procedures are based on the assumption of a Gaussian distribution of values; this approach is commonly referred to as *parametric*. Furthermore, these procedures usually are not seriously invalidated by departures from this assumption. Finally, the magnitude

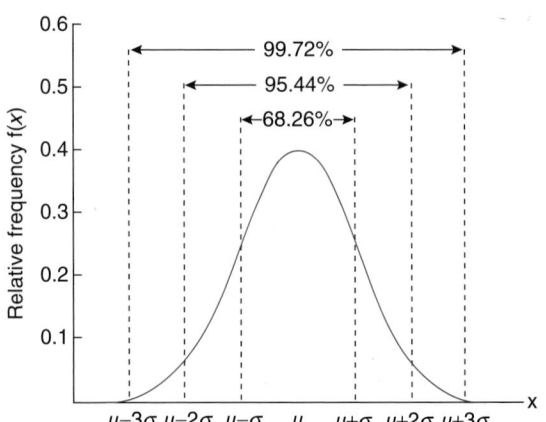

Figure 2-4 The Gaussian probability distribution.

of the uncertainty associated with sample statistics can be ascertained on the basis of the fact that many sample statistics computed from large samples have a Gaussian probability distribution.

The Gaussian probability distribution is completely characterized by its mean μ and variance σ^2. The notation $N(\mu,\sigma^2)$ is often used for the distribution of a variable that is Gaussian with mean μ and variance σ^2. Probability statements about a variable x that follows an $N(\mu,\sigma^2)$ distribution are usually made by considering the variable z:

$$z = \frac{x - \mu}{\sigma}$$

which is called the *standard Gaussian variable*. The variable z has a Gaussian probability distribution with $\mu = 0$ and $\sigma^2 = 1$, that is, z is $N(0,1)$. The probability that x is within 2σ of μ [i.e., $\Pr(x - \mu| < 2\sigma) =$] is 0.9544. Most computer spreadsheet programs can be used to calculate probabilities for all values of z.

Student *t* Probability Distribution

To determine probabilities associated with a Gaussian distribution, it is necessary to know the population standard deviation σ. In actual practice, σ is often unknown, so we cannot calculate z. However, if a random sample is taken from the Gaussian population, it is possible to calculate the sample SD, substitute SD for σ, and compute the value t:

$$t = \frac{x - \mu}{SD}$$

Under these conditions, the variable t has a probability distribution called the *Student* t *distribution*. The t distribution is really a family of distributions depending on the degrees of freedom (v_n) for the sample standard deviation. Several t distributions from this family are shown in Figure 2-5. When the size of the sample and the degrees of freedom for SD are infinite, there is no uncertainty in SD, and so the t distribution is identical to the standard Gaussian distribution. However, when the sample size is small, the uncertainty in SD causes the t distribution to have greater dispersion and heavier tails than the standard Gaussian distribution, as illustrated in Figure 2-5. Most computer spreadsheet programs can calculate probabilities for all values of t, given the degrees of freedom for SD.

Suppose that the distribution of fasting serum glucose values in healthy men is known to be Gaussian and to have a mean of 90 mg/dL. Suppose also that σ (SD) is unknown and that a random sample of size 20 from the healthy men yielded a sample SD = 10.0 mg/dL. Then, to find the probability $\Pr(x > 105)$, we proceed as follows:

1. $t_a = (x_a - \mu)/SD = (105 - 90)/10 = 1.5$
2. $\Pr(t > t_a) = \Pr(t > 1.5) = 0.08$, approximately, from a t distribution with 19 degrees of freedom
3. $\Pr(x > 105) = 0.08$

The Student t distribution is commonly used in significance tests, such as the comparison of sample means or testing of whether a regression slope differs significantly from 1. Descriptions of these tests are found in statistics textbooks and in the *Tietz Textbook of Clinical Chemistry,* 3rd edition, pages 274 to 287.

Basic Concepts in Relation to Analytical Methods

This section defines the basic concepts used in this chapter: (1) *calibration, (2) trueness (accuracy), (3) precision, (4) linearity, (5) limit of detection,* and (6) others.

Calibration

The **calibration** function is the relation between instrument signal *(y)* and concentration of analyte *(x)*, i.e.,

$$y = f(x)$$

The inverse of this function, also called the *measuring function,* yields the concentration from response:

$$x = f^1(y)$$

This relationship is established by measurement of samples with known amounts (the quantity) of analyte (calibrators). One may distinguish between solutions of pure chemical standards and samples with known amounts of analyte present in the typical **matrix** that is to be measured (e.g., human serum). The first situation applies typically to a **reference measurement procedure,** which is not influenced by matrix effects, and the second case corresponds typically to a field method that often is influenced by matrix components and so preferably is calibrated using the relevant matrix. Calibration functions may be linear or curved and in the case of immunoassays often of a special form (e.g., modeled by the four-parameter logistic curve; see Chapter 15). In the case of curved calibration functions, nonlinear regression analysis is applied to estimate the relationship, or a logit transformation is performed to produce a linear form. An alternative, model-free approach is to estimate a smoothed spline curve, which often is performed for immunoassays. The only requirement is that there should be a monotonic relationship between signal and analyte concentration over the analytical measurement range. Otherwise the possibility of error occurs (e.g., the hook effect in noncompetitive immunoassays), caused by a decreasing signal response at very high concentrations.

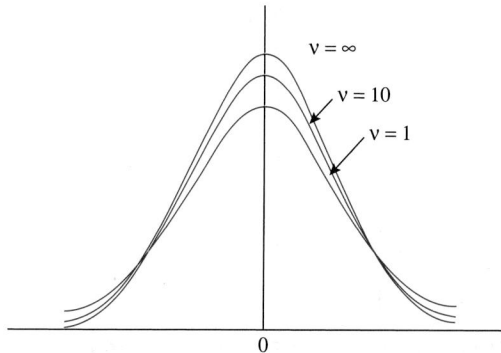

Figure 2-5 The *t* probability distribution for $v = 1$, 10, and ∞.

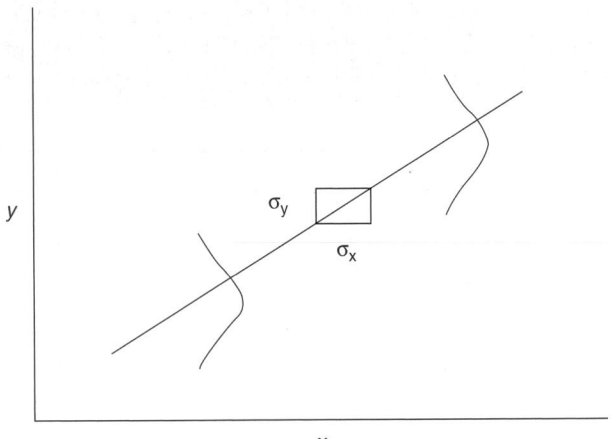

Figure 2-6 Relation between concentration *(x)* and signal response *(y)* for a linear calibration curve. The dispersion in signal response (σ_y) is projected onto the *x*-axis, giving rise to assay imprecision (σ_x).

TABLE 2-1	An Overview of Qualitative Terms and Quantitative Measures Related to Method Performance

Qualitative Concept	Quantitative Measure
Trueness	*Bias*
Closeness of agreement of mean value with "true value"	A measure of the systematic error
Precision	*Imprecision (SD)*
Repeatability (within run)	A measure of the dispersion of random errors
Intermediate precision (long term) Reproducibility (interlaboratory)	
Accuracy	*Error of Measurement*
Closeness of agreement of a single measurement with "true value"	Comprises both random and systematic influences

The precision of the analytical method depends on the stability of the instrument response for a given amount of analyte. In principle, a random dispersion of instrument signal at a given concentration transforms into dispersion on the measurement scale as schematically shown (Figure 2-6). The detailed statistical aspects of calibration are rather complex, but some approximate relations are reviewed here. If the calibration function is linear, and the imprecision of the signal response is the same over the analytical measurement range, the analytical standard deviation (SD_A) of the method tends to be constant over the analytical measurement range (see Figure 2-6). If the imprecision increases proportionally to the signal response level, the analytical SD of the method tends to increase proportionally to the concentration level *(x)*, which means that the *relative* imprecision, CV, is constant over the analytical measurement range—supposing that the intercept of the calibration line is zero.

In modern, automated clinical chemistry instruments/systems, the relation between analyte concentration and signal is often very stable, so that calibration is necessary infrequently (e.g., at intervals of several months). However, in traditional chromatographic analysis (e.g., high-performance liquid chromatography [HPLC]), it is customary to calibrate each analytical series (run), which means that calibration is carried out daily.

Trueness and Accuracy

Trueness of measurement is defined as closeness of agreement between the average value obtained from a large series of results of measurements and a true value.[5] The difference between the average value (strictly, the mathematical expectation) and the true value is the **bias,** which is expressed numerically and so is inversely related to trueness. Trueness in itself is a qualitative term that is expressed as, for example, low, medium, or high. From a theoretical point of view, the exact true value is not available, and instead an "accepted reference value" is considered, which is the "true" value that is determined in practice.[5] Trueness also is evaluated by comparison of measurements by a given (field) method and a reference method. Such an evaluation may be carried out by parallel measurements of a set of patient samples or by measurements of reference materials (see traceability and uncertainty). The ISO has introduced the trueness expression as a replacement for the term "accuracy," which now has gained a slightly different meaning. *Accuracy* is the closeness of the agreement between the result of a measurement and a true concentration of the analyte. Accuracy is thus influenced by both bias and imprecision and in this way reflects the total error. Accuracy, which in itself is a qualitative term, is inversely related to the "uncertainty" of measurement, which is quantified as described later (Table 2-1).

In relation to trueness, the concepts (1) *recovery,* (2) *drift,* and (3) *carryover* may also be considered. Recovery is the fraction or percentage increase of concentration that is measured in relation to the amount added. Recovery experiments are typically carried out in the field of drug analysis. One may distinguish between *extraction recovery,* which often is interpreted as the fraction of compound that is carried through an extraction process, and the recovery measured by the entire analytical procedure, in which the addition of an internal standard compensates for losses in the extraction procedure. A recovery close to 100% is a prerequisite for a high degree of trueness, but it does not ensure unbiased results because possible nonspecificity against matrix components is not detected in a recovery experiment. *Drift* is caused by instrument or reagent instability over time, so that calibration becomes biased. Assay *carryover* also must be close to zero to ensure unbiased results.

Precision

Precision has been defined as the closeness of agreement between independent results of measurements obtained under stipulated conditions.[5] The degree of precision is usually expressed on the basis of statistical measures of imprecision, such as SD or CV, which thus are inversely related to precision. Imprecision of measurements is solely related to the **random error** of measurements and has no relation to the trueness of measurements.

Precision is specified as follows[5]:

Repeatability: closeness of agreement between results of successive measurements carried out under the same conditions (i.e., corresponding to within-run precision).

Reproducibility: closeness of agreement between results of measurements performed under changed conditions of measurements (e.g., time, operators, calibrators, reagent lots). Two specifications of reproducibility are often used: total or between-run precision in the laboratory, often termed *intermediate precision,* and interlaboratory precision (e.g., as observed in external quality assessment schemes [EQAS]) (see Table 2-1).

The total standard deviation (σ_T) may be split into within-run and between-run components by using the principle of analysis of variance components (variance is the squared SD):

$$\sigma_T^2 = \sigma_{Within-run}^2 + \sigma_{Between-run}^2$$

In laboratory studies of analytical variation, it is *estimates* of imprecision that are obtained. The more observations, the more certain are the estimates. Commonly the number 20 is given as a reasonable number of observations. To estimate both within-run imprecision and total imprecision, a common approach is to measure duplicate control samples in a series of runs. For example, one may measure a control in duplicate for more than 20 runs, in which case 20 observations are present with respect to both components. Here one may notice that the dispersion of the means (x_m) of the duplicates is given as

$$\sigma_{x_m}^2 = \sigma_{Within-run}^2/2 + \sigma_{Between-run}^2$$

From the 20 sets of duplicates, we may derive the within-run SD using the shortcut formula:

$$SD_{Within-run}^2 = \sum d_i^2/(2 \times 20)$$

where d_i refers to the difference between the ith set of duplicates. When estimating SDs, the concept degrees of freedom (df) is used. In a simple situation, the number of degrees of freedom equals $N - 1$. For N duplicates, the number of degrees of freedom is $N(2 - 1) = N$. Thus both variance components are derived in this way. The advantage of this approach is that the within-run estimate is based on several runs, so that an average estimate is obtained rather than only an estimate for one particular run, if all 20 observations had been obtained in the same run. The described approach is a simple example of a *variance component analysis.*

There is nothing definitive about the selected number of 20. Generally, the estimate of the imprecision improves as more observations become available. In Table 2-2, factors corresponding to the 95% confidence intervals (CIs) are given as a function of sample size for simple SD estimation according to the X^2 distribution. These factors provide guidance on the validity of estimated SDs for precision. Suppose we have estimated the imprecision to an SD of 5.0 on the basis of $N = 20$ observations. From Table 2-2, we get the 2.5 and 97.5 percentiles:

$$5.0 \times 0.76 < \sigma < 5.0 \times 1.46$$

TABLE 2-2	Factors Corresponding to 95% CI Limits for an SD (the number of degrees of freedom is N − 1)	
	95% CI	
N	**Lower**	**Upper**
20	0.760	1.460
30	0.797	1.346
40	0.819	1.283
50	0.835	1.243
60	0.848	1.217
70	0.857	1.198
80	0.865	1.183
90	0.872	1.171
100	0.878	1.161
150	0.898	1.128
200	0.911	1.109
250	0.919	1.096
300	0.926	1.087

Precision Profile

Precision often depends on the concentration of analyte being considered. A presentation of precision as a function of analyte concentration is the precision profile, which usually is plotted in terms of SD or CV as a function of analyte concentration (Figure 2-7, *A-C*). Some typical examples may be considered. First, the SD may be constant and independent of the concentration, as it often is for analytes with a limited range of values (e.g., electrolytes). When the SD is constant, the CV varies inversely with the concentration and is high in the lower part of the range and low in the high part of the range. For analytes with extended ranges (e.g., hormones), the SD frequently increases as the analyte concentration increases. If a proportional relationship exists, the CV is constant. This may often apply approximately over a large part of the analytical measurement range. Actually, this relationship is anticipated for measurement error arising because of imprecise volume dispensing. Often a more complex relationship exists. Not infrequently, the SD is relatively constant in the low range, so that the CV increases in the area approaching the detection limit. At intermediate concentrations, the CV may be relatively constant and perhaps may decline somewhat at increasing concentrations.

Linearity

Linearity refers to the relationship between measured and expected values over the range of analytical measurements. Linearity may be considered in relation to actual or relative analyte concentrations. In the latter case, a dilution series of a sample may be studied. This is often carried out for immunoassays, in which case it is investigated to find out whether the measured concentration declines as expected according to the dilution factor. Dilution is usually carried out with the appropriate sample matrix (e.g., human serum [individual or pooled serum]).

Evaluation of linearity may be carried out in various ways. A simple, but subjective, approach is to visually assess whether

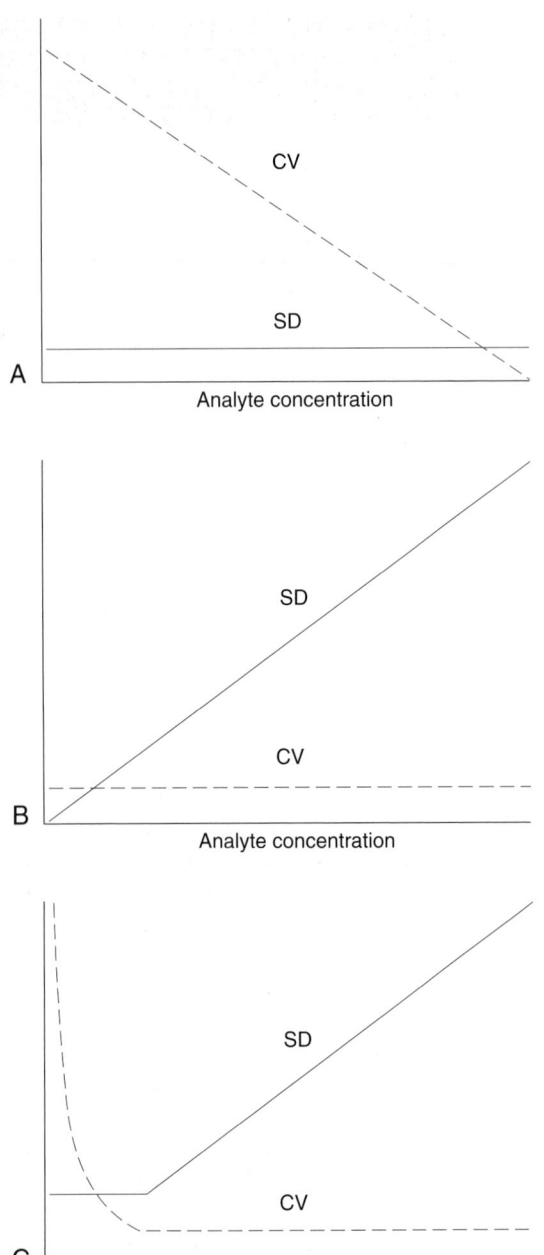

Figure 2-7 Relations between analyte concentration and SD/CV. **A,** The SD is constant so that the CV varies inversely with the analyte concentration. **B,** The CV is constant because of a proportional relationship between concentration and SD. **C,** Illustration of a mixed situation with constant SD in the low range and a proportional relationship in the rest of the analytical measurement range.

the relationship between measured and expected concentrations is linear or not. A more formal evaluation may be carried out on the basis of statistical tests. Various principles may be applied here. When repeated measurements are available at each concentration, the random variation between measurements and the variation around an estimated regression line may be evaluated statistically (by an *F*-test). This approach has been criticized because it only relates the magnitude of random and **systematic error** without taking the absolute deviations

from linearity into account. When significant nonlinearity is found, it may be useful to explore nonlinear alternatives to the linear regression line (i.e., polynomials of higher degrees).[2]

Another commonly applied approach for detecting nonlinearity is to assess the residuals of an estimated regression line and test for whether positive and negative deviations are randomly distributed. This is carried out by a runs test (see "Regression Analysis" section). An additional consideration for evaluating dilution curves is whether or not an estimated regression line passes through zero. Furthermore, testing for linearity is related to assessment of trueness over the analytical measurement range. The presence of linearity is a prerequisite for a high degree of trueness. A CLSI guideline suggests procedure(s) for assessment of linearity.[2]

Analytical Measurement Range and Limits of Quantification

The analytical measurement range (**measuring interval,** reportable range) is the analyte concentration range over which measurements are within declared tolerances for imprecision and bias of the method. Taking drug assays as an example, requirements for a CV% of less than 15% and a bias of less than 15% are common. The measurement range then extends from the lowest concentration (lower limit of quantification [LloQ]) to the highest concentration (upper limit of quantification [UloQ]) for which these performance specifications are fulfilled.

The LloQ is medically important for many analytes. Thyroid-stimulating hormone (TSH) is a good example. As assay methods improved, lowering the LloQ, low TSH results could be distinguished from the lower limit of the reference interval, making the test useful for the diagnosis of hyperthyroidism.

The **limit of detection** (LoD) is another characteristic of an assay. The LoD may be defined as the lowest value that significantly exceeds the measurements of a blank sample. Thus the limit has been estimated on the basis of repeated measurements of a blank sample and has been *reported* as the mean plus 2 or 3 SDs of the blank measurements. In the interval from LoD up to LloQ, one should report a result as "detected" but not provide a quantitative result. More complicated approaches for estimation of the LoD have been suggested.[12]

Analytical Sensitivity

The detection limit of a method should not be confused with its so-called analytical sensitivity. **Analytical sensitivity** is the ability of an analytical method to assess small variations in the concentration of analyte. This is often expressed as the slope of the calibration curve. However, in addition to the slope of the calibration function, the random variation of the calibration function should be taken into account. In fact, analytical sensitivity depends on the ratio between the SD of the calibration function and the slope. As was mentioned previously, the smaller the random variation of the instrument response and the steeper the slope, the greater is the ability to distinguish small differences in analyte concentration. Thus, analytical sensitivity depends on the precision of the method.

Analytical Specificity and Interference

Analytical specificity is the ability of an assay procedure to determine specifically the concentration of the target analyte in the presence of potentially interfering substances or factors in the sample matrix (e.g., hyperlipemia, hemolysis, bilirubin, anticoagulants, antibodies, degradation products). Also, in the context of a drug assay, specificity is of relevance in relation to drug metabolites. Interference from hyperlipemia, hemolysis, and bilirubin is generally concentration dependent and is often quantified as a function of the concentration of the interfering compound. In relation to immunoassays, interference from proteins (usually heterophilic antibodies) should be recognized.

Analytical Goals

Setting goals for analytical quality is based on various principles, and a hierarchy has been suggested on the basis of a consensus conference on the subject[14] (Table 2-3). The top level of the hierarchy specifies goals on the basis of clinical outcome in specific clinical settings, which is a logical principle.

However, analytical goals related to biological variation have attracted considerable interest.[7] Originally, focus was on imprecision, and it was suggested that the analytical SD (σ_A) should be less than half the intraindividual biological variation, $\sigma_{Within-B}$. The rationale for this relation is the principle of adding variances. If a subject is undergoing monitoring of an analyte, random variation from measurement to measurement consists of both analytical and biological components of variation. The total SD for the random variation during monitoring then is determined by the relation

$$\sigma_T^2 = \sigma_{Within-B}^2 + \sigma_A^2$$

where the biological component includes the preanalytical variation. If σ_A is equal to or less than half the $\sigma_{Within-B}$ value, σ_T exceeds $\sigma_{Within-B}$ by less than 12%. Thus, analytical imprecision only adds limited random noise in a monitoring situation.

In addition to imprecision, goals for bias should be considered. The allowable bias is related to the width of the reference interval, which is determined by combined within- and between-subject biological variations, in addition to the analytical variation. On the basis of considerations concerning the included percentage in an interval in the presence of analytical bias, it has been suggested that

$$Bias < 0.25 \left(\sigma_{Within-B}^2 + \sigma_{Between-B}^2 \right)^{0.5}$$

where $\sigma_{Between-B}$ is the between-subject biological SD component.

Another principle that has been used is relating assay goals to the limits set by professional bodies (e.g., the bias goal of 3% for serum cholesterol [originally 5%] set by the National Cholesterol Education Program). Ricos and colleagues have published a comprehensive listing of data on biological variation along with a database that is available at www.westgard.com/guest17.htm (accessed July 6, 2013).

TABLE 2-3	Hierarchy of Procedures for Setting Analytical Quality Specifications for Laboratory Methods
I	Evaluation of the effect of analytical performance on clinical outcomes in specific clinical settings
II	Evaluation of the effect of analytical performance on clinical decisions in general: A. Data based on components of biological variation B. Data based on analysis of clinicians' opinions
III	Published professional recommendations: A. From national and international expert bodies B. From expert local groups or individuals
IV	Performance goals set by: A. Regulatory bodies (e.g., Clinical Laboratory Improvement Amendments) B. Organizers of external quality assessment (EQA) schemes
V	Goals based on the current state of the art: A. Data from EQA/proficiency testing scheme B. Data from current publications on methodology

Qualitative Methods

Qualitative methods, which currently are gaining in use in the form of point-of-care testing (POCT), are designed to distinguish between results below and above a predefined cutoff value (see Chapter 17). Notice that the cutoff point should not be confused with the detection limit. These tests are assessed primarily on the basis of their ability to correctly classify results in relation to the cutoff value.

The probability of classifying a result as positive (exceeding the cutoff) is called *clinical sensitivity* (see Chapter 3). Classifying a result as negative (below the cutoff) is termed *clinical specificity*. Determination of clinical sensitivity and specificity is based on comparison of test results with a "gold" standard. The gold standard may be an independent test that measures the same analyte, but it may also be a clinical diagnosis determined by definitive clinical methods (e.g., radiographic testing, follow-up, outcomes analysis). Clinical sensitivity and specificity may be given as a fraction or as a percentage after multiplication by 100. Standard errors of estimates are derived from the binomial distribution.

One approach for determining the recorded performance of a test in terms of clinical sensitivity and specificity is to determine the true concentration of analyte using an independent reference method. The closer the concentration is to the cutoff point, the larger are the expected error frequencies. Actually the cutoff point is defined in such a way that for samples having a true concentration exactly equal to the cutoff point, 50% of the results will be positive and 50% will be negative. Concentrations above and below the cutoff point at which repeated results are 95% positive or 95% negative, respectively, have been called the "95% interval" for the cutoff point for that method (notice that this is not a CI; Figure 2-8).[4] Thus in an evaluation of a qualitative test, it is important to specify in detail the composition of the samples. A CLSI guideline on the topic[4] recommends that samples should be prepared with

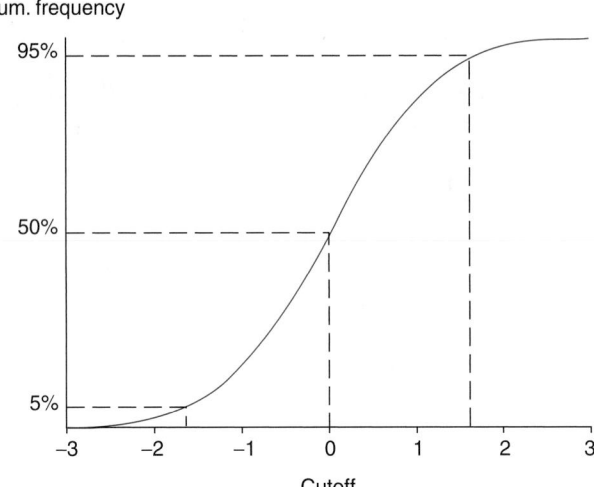

Figure 2-8 Cumulative frequency distribution of positive results. The *x*-axis indicates concentrations standardized to zero at the cutoff point (50% positive results) with unit SD.

a concentration equal to the cutoff point and with concentrations 20% below and above the cutoff point. Twenty replicate measurements are then carried out at each concentration, and the percentages of positive and negative results are recorded. On the basis of these measurements, it is possible to judge whether the 95% interval for the cutoff point is within or outside this interval. In relation to the suggested procedure, one should be aware of the limitations associated with repeated measurements of pools. Measurements of individual patient samples with the specified concentrations are preferable to get a true impression of possible matrix effects.

Method Comparison

Comparison of measurements by two methods is a frequent task in the laboratory. Preferably, parallel measurements of a set of patient samples should be undertaken. To prevent artificial matrix-induced differences, fresh patient samples are the optimal material. A nearly even distribution of values over the analytical measurement range is also preferable. In an ordinary laboratory, comparison of two field methods will be the most frequently occurring situation. Less commonly, comparison of a field method with a reference method is undertaken. When two field methods are compared, the focus is on observed differences. In this situation, it is not possible to establish that one set of measurements is the correct one and then consider deviation of the other set of measurements from the presumed correct concentrations. Rather, the question is whether the new method can replace the existing one without a general change in measurement concentration. To carry out a formal, objective analysis of the data, a statistical procedure with graphics display should be applied. Commonly used approaches include (1) a difference (bias) plot, which shows differences as a function of the average concentration of the measurements (Bland-Altman plot); and (2) a regression analysis. In the following, a general error model is presented, and statistical approaches are demonstrated.

Basic Error Model

The occurrence of measurement error is related to the performance characteristics of the assay. It is important to distinguish between (1) pure, random measurement errors, which are present in all measurement procedures, and (2) errors related to incorrect calibration and nonspecificity of the assay. A reference measurement procedure is associated only with pure, random error, whereas a routine method typically has some additional bias related to errors in calibration and limitations with regard to specificity. An erroneous calibration function gives rise to a systematic error, whereas nonspecificity yields an error that typically varies from sample to sample. The error related to nonspecificity thus has a random character, but in contrast to the pure measurement error, it is not reduced by repeated measurements of a sample. Although errors related to nonspecificity for a group of samples look like random errors, for the individual sample this type of error is a bias. Because this bias varies from sample to sample, it has been called a *sample-related random bias*. In the following section, various error components are incorporated into a formal error model.

Measured Value, Target Value, Modified Target Value, and True Value

Upon taking into account that an analytical method measures analyte concentrations with some random measurement error, one has to distinguish between the actual, measured value and the average result we would obtain if the given sample was measured an infinite number of times. If the method is a reference method without bias and nonspecificity, we have the following, simple relationship:

$$x_i = X_{\text{True}i} + \varepsilon_i$$

where x_i represents the measured value, $X_{\text{True}i}$ is the average value for an infinite number of measurements, and ε_i is the deviation of the measured value from the average value. If we were to undertake repeated measurements, the average of ε_i would be zero and the SD would equal the analytical SD (σ_A) of the reference measurement procedure. Pure, random measurement error will usually be Gaussian distributed.

In the case of a routine method, the relationship between the measured value for a sample and the true value becomes more complicated:

$$x_i = X_{\text{True}i} + \text{Cal-Bias} + \text{Random-Bias}_i + \varepsilon_i$$

The *Cal-Bias* term (calibration bias) is a systematic error related to the calibration of the method. This systematic error may be a constant for all measurements corresponding to an offset error, or it may be a function of the analyte concentration (e.g., corresponding to a slope deviation in the case of a linear calibration function). The *Random-Bias$_i$* term is a bias that is specific for a given sample in relation to nonspecificity of the method. It may arise because of codetermination of substances that vary in concentration from sample to sample. For example, a chromogenic creatinine method codetermines some other components with creatinine in serum. Finally, we have the random measurement error term ε_i.

If we performed an infinite number of measurements of a specific sample by the routine method, the random measurement error term ε_i would be zero. The cal-bias and the random-bias$_i$, however, would be unchanged. Thus, the average value of an infinite number of measurements would equal the sum of the true value and these bias terms. This average value may be regarded as the target value $(X_{Targeti})$ of the given sample for the routine method. We have

$$X_{Targeti} = X_{Truei} + \text{Cal-Bias} + \text{Random-Bias}_i$$

As has been mentioned, calibration bias represents a systematic error component in relation to the true values measured by a reference measurement procedure. In the context of regression analysis, this systematic error corresponds to the intercept and the slope deviation from unity when a routine method is compared with a reference measurement procedure (outlined in detail later). It is convenient to introduce a modified target value expression $(X'_{Targeti})$ for the routine method to delineate this systematic calibration bias, so that

$$X'_{Targeti} = X_{Truei} + \text{Cal-Bias}$$

Thus, for a set of samples measured by a routine method, the $X_{Targeti}$ values are distributed around the respective $X'_{Targeti}$ values with an SD, which is called σ_{RB}.

If the method is a reference method without bias and nonspecificity, the target value and the modified target value equal the true value, that is,

$$X_{Targeti} = X'_{Targeti} = X_{Truei}$$

The error model is outlined in Figure 2-9.

Calibration Bias and Random Bias

For an individual measurement, the total error is the deviation of x_i from the true value, that is,

$$\text{Total error of } x_i = \text{Cal-Bias} + \text{Random-Bias}_i + \varepsilon_i$$

Estimation of the bias terms requires parallel measurements between the method in question and a reference method as outlined in detail later. With regard to calibration bias, one should be aware of the possibility of lot-to-lot variation in analytical kit sets. The manufacturer should provide documentation on this lot-to-lot variation because often it will not be possible for the individual laboratory to investigate a sufficient number of lots to assess this variation. Lot-to-lot variation will show up as a calibration bias that changes from lot to lot.

The previous exposition defines the total error in somewhat broader terms than is often seen. A traditional total error expression is

$$\text{Total error} = \text{Bias} + 2\,SD_A,$$

which often is interpreted as the calibration bias plus 2 SD_A. If a one-sided statistical perspective is taken, the expression is modified to Bias + 1.65 SD_A, indicating that 5% of results are located outside the limit. If a lower percentage is desired, the multiplication factor is increased accordingly, supposing a normal distribution. Interpreting the bias as identical with the calibration bias may lead to an underestimation of the total error.

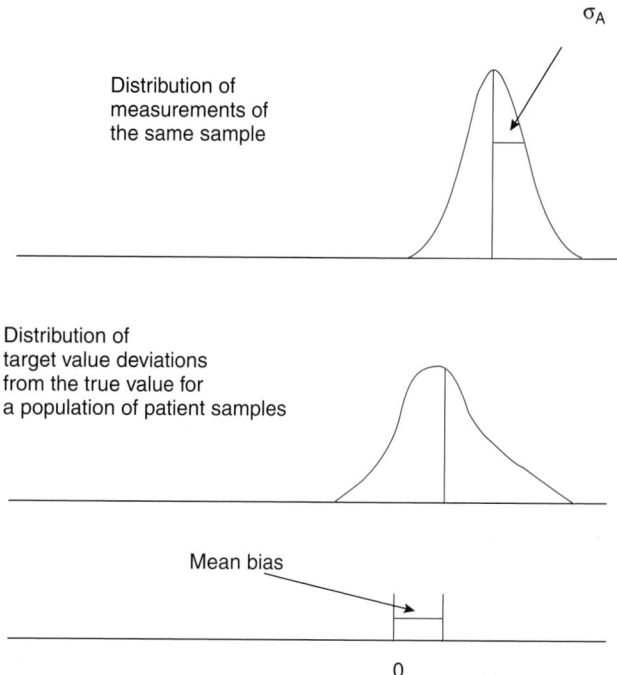

Figure 2-9 Outline of basic error model for measurements by a field method. *Upper part:* The distribution of repeated measurements of the *same* sample, representing a Gaussian distribution around the target value *(vertical line)* of the sample with a dispersion corresponding to the analytical standard deviation, σ_A. *Middle part:* Schematic outline of the dispersion of target value deviations from the respective true values for a population of patient samples. A distribution of an arbitrary form is displayed. The vertical line indicates the mean of the distribution. *Lower part:* The distance from zero to the mean of the target value deviations from the true values represents the calibration bias (Mean bias = Cal-Bias) of the method.

Random bias related to sample-specific interferences may take several forms. It may be a regularly occurring additional random error component, perhaps of the same order of magnitude as the analytical error. In this context, it is natural to quantify the error in the form of an SD or coefficient of variation. The most straightforward procedure is to carry out a **method comparison** study based on a set of patient samples in which one of the methods is a reference method, as outlined later. For example, it has been found that for the Jaffe creatinine method, the random bias constituted 80% of the total random error. This relatively high amount should be interpreted in light of the limited specificity of the Jaffe creatinine measurement principle.

Another form of sample-related random interference is more rarely occurring gross errors, which typically are seen in the context of immunoassays and are related to unexpected antibody interactions (see "Interference" section). Such an error usually will show up as an outlier in method comparison studies. A well-known source is the occurrence of heterophilic antibodies. Outliers should not just be discarded from the data analysis procedure. Outliers must be investigated to identify their cause, which may be an important limitation in using a given method. Supplementary studies may help to clarify such random sample-related interferences and may provide specifications for the assay that limit its application in certain contexts (e.g., with regard to samples from certain patient categories).

Mistakes or Clerical Errors

Another reason for outliers in method comparison studies and in daily practice is *mistakes* (sometimes termed *blunders*) or *clerical errors.* In the past, this type of error usually arose in relation to manual transfer of results. Today, this kind of error typically is related to computer errors originating at interfaces between computer systems. Errors on test order forms or errors related to handling of order forms appear to occur relatively frequently (1% to 5% of recorded cases have been revealed in systematic studies). In the postanalytical phase, inappropriate interpretation may take place (e.g., in relation to erroneous reference intervals).

Method Comparison Data Model

We here consider our error model in relation to the method comparison situation. For a given sample measured by two analytical methods, 1 and 2, we have

$$x1_i = X1_{Target i} + \varepsilon 1_i = X_{True i} + \text{Cal-Bias1} + \text{Random-Bias1}_i + \varepsilon 1_i$$

$$x2_i = X2_{Target i} + \varepsilon 2_i = X_{True i} + \text{Cal-Bias2} + \text{Random-Bias2}_i + \varepsilon 2_i$$

From this general model, we may study some typical situations. First, comparison of a routine method with a reference method will be treated. Second, the more frequently occurring situation—the comparison of two routine methods—is considered.

Comparison of a Routine Method With a Reference Method

The process of comparing the performance of a routine method with that of a reference method begins with considering that method 1 is a reference method. In this case, the bias components per definition disappear, and we have the following situation:

$$x1_i = X1_{Target i} + \varepsilon 1_i = X_{True i} + \varepsilon 1_i$$

$$x2_i = X2_{Target i} + \varepsilon 2_i = X_{True i} + \text{Cal-Bias2} + \text{Random-Bias2}_i + \varepsilon 2_i$$

The paired differences become

$$(x2_i - x1_i) = \text{Cal-Bias2} + \text{Random-Bias2}_i + (\varepsilon 2_i - \varepsilon 1_i)$$

We thus have an expression consisting of a constant term (the calibration bias of method 2) and two random terms. The random bias term is distributed around the calibration bias according to an undefined distribution. The second random term is a difference between two random measurement errors that are independent and, commonly, Gaussian distributed. Under these assumptions, the differences between random measurement errors are also random and Gaussian. However, we remind the reader that the SD for analytical methods often depends on the concentration level, as mentioned earlier. For analytes with a wide analytical measurement range (e.g., some hormones), both random matrix-related interferences and analytical SDs are likely to depend on the measurement concentration, often in a roughly proportional manner. It may then be more useful to evaluate the *relative* differences—$(x2_i - x1_i)/[(x2_i + x1_i)/2]$—and accordingly express calibration and random bias and analytical error as proportions. An alternative is to partition the total analytical measurement range into segments (e.g., three parts), and consider calibration bias, random bias, and analytical error separately for these segments. The segments may preferably be divided in relation to important decision concentrations (e.g., in relation to reference interval limits or treatment decision concentrations or both).

Comparison of Two Routine Methods

In the comparison of two routine methods, the paired differences become

$$\begin{aligned}(x2_i - x1_i) = &\,(\text{Cal-Bias2} - \text{Cal-Bias1}) \\ &+ (\text{Random-Bias2}_i - \text{Random-Bias1}_i) \\ &+ (\varepsilon 2_i - \varepsilon 1_i)\end{aligned}$$

The expression again consists of a constant term, the difference between the two calibration biases, and two random terms. The first random term is a difference between two random bias components that may or may not be independent. If the two routine methods are based on the same measurement principle, the random bias terms are likely to be correlated. For example, two chromogenic methods for creatinine are likely to be subject to interference from the same chromogenic compounds present in a given serum sample. Alternatively, chromogenic and enzymatic creatinine methods are subject to different types of interfering compounds, and the random bias terms may be relatively independent. In the $\varepsilon 2_i - \varepsilon 1_i$ term, the same relationships as described above are likely to apply. One may notice that the general form of the expressed differences is the same in the two situations. Thus the same general statistical principles apply. In the following sections, we will consider the distribution of differences under various circumstances as well as the measurement relations between methods 1 and 2 on the basis of regression analysis.

Planning a Method Comparison Study

In the planning phase of a method comparison study, several points require attention, including (1) the number of samples necessary, (2) the distribution of analyte concentrations (preferably uniform over the analytical measurement range), and (3) the representativeness of the samples. To address point (3), samples from relevant patient categories should be included, so that possible interference phenomena will be discovered. Practical aspects related to storage and treatment of samples (e.g., container) and possible artifacts induced by storage (e.g., freezing of samples) and addition of anticoagulants should be considered. Comparison of measurements preferably should be undertaken over several days (e.g., at least 5 days), so that the comparison of methods does not become dependent on the performance of methods in one particular analytical run. Finally, ethical aspects (e.g., informed consent from patients whose samples will be used) should be considered in relation to existing legislation.

When the comparison protocol is considered, various guidelines may be consulted. The CLSI Evaluation Protocol (EP) guidelines give advice on various aspects. For example, the CLSI guideline EP9-A2-IR, "Method Comparison and Bias Estimation Using Patient Samples,"[3] suggests measurement of 40 samples in duplicate by each method when a new method is introduced in the laboratory as a substitute for an established one.[10] Additionally, it is proposed that the vendor of an analytical test system should have made a comparison study based on at least 100 samples measured in duplicate by each method. The principle of a more demanding requirement for vendors appears reasonable. This initial validation should be comprehensive to disclose the performance of the assay system in detail. Then the requirement for the ordinary user may be more modest. The CLSI EP15-A2 guideline, "User Verification of Performance for Precision and Trueness," suggests a more condensed approach based on a bias or **difference plot,** which does not involve regression analysis and can be carried out using 20 samples. Although these general guidelines on sample size are useful, additional aspects are important. The probability of detecting rarely occurring interferences showing up as outliers should be taken into account when the necessary sample size is considered. Finally, in relation to evaluation of automated methods, special consideration should be given to the sample sequence to evaluate drift, carryover, and nonlinearity (e.g., by a multifactorial design).

Difference (Bland-Altman) Plot

This procedure was originally introduced by Bland and Altman for comparison of measurements in clinical medicine, but the procedure has been adopted also in clinical chemistry.[1] The Bland-Altman plot is usually understood as a plot of the differences against average results of the methods. Thus the difference plot in this version provides information on the relation between differences and concentration, which is useful in evaluating whether problems exist at certain ranges (e.g., in the high range) as the result of nonlinearity of one of the methods. It may also be of interest to observe whether differences tend to increase proportionally with the concentration, or whether they are independent of concentration. The underlying error model outlined previously applies also to the difference plot.

The basic version of the difference plot consists of plotting the differences against the average of the measurements. If one set of measurements is without random measurement error, one may plot the differences against this value. Figure 2-10 shows the plot for an example consisting of $N = 65$ samples measured by two drug assay methods. The interval ± 2 SD of the differences is often delineated around the mean difference that corresponds to the mean and the 2.5 and 97.5 percentiles.

A constant mean bias over the analytical measurement range changes the average concentration away from zero. The presence of random matrix-related interferences increases the width of the distribution. If the mean bias depends on the concentration or if the dispersion varies with the concentration, or both, the relations become more complex, and the interval mean ± 2 SD of the differences may not fit very well as a 95% interval throughout the analytical measurement range.

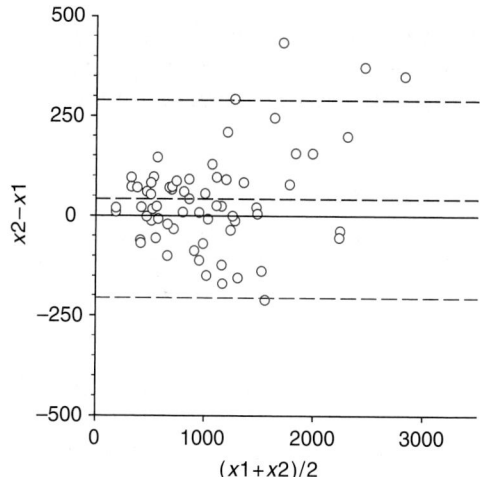

Figure 2-10 Bland-Altman plot of differences for the drug comparison example. The differences are plotted against the average concentration. The mean difference (42 nmol/L) with ± 2 SD of differences is shown *(dashed lines).*

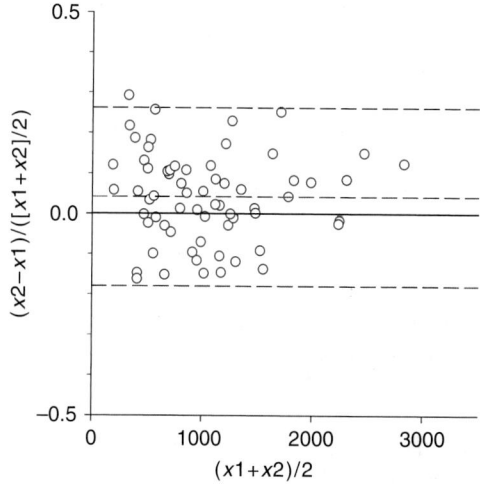

Figure 2-11 Bland-Altman plot of *relative* differences for the drug comparison example. The differences are plotted against the average concentration. The mean relative difference (0.042) with ± 2 SD of relative differences is shown *(dashed lines).*

In the displayed Bland-Altman plot for drug assay comparison data, there is a tendency toward increasing scatter with increasing concentration, which is a reflection of increasing random error with the concentration level. Thus a plot of the *relative* differences against the average concentration is of relevance (Figure 2-11). Now there is a more homogeneous dispersion of values agreeing with the estimated limits for the dispersion (i.e., the relative mean difference $\pm t_{0.025(N-1)} \, \mathrm{SD}_{\mathrm{RelDif}}$).

Difference (Bland-Altman) Plot With Specified Limits

In many situations where a routine method is being considered for implementation, it may be desired primarily to *verify* whether differences in relation to the existing method are located within given specified limits rather than *estimating* the distribution of differences. For example, one may set limits corresponding to $\pm 15\%$ as clinically acceptable and desire that most (e.g., 95% of differences) are located within this interval.

TABLE 2-4	Lower Bounds (One-Sided 95% CI) of Observed Proportions (%) of Results Located Within Specified Limits for Paired Differences That Are in Accordance With the Hypothesis of at Least 95% of Differences Being Within the Limits
N	**Observed Proportions**
20	85
30	87
40	90
50	90
60	90
70	90
80	91
90	91
100	91
150	92
200	93
250	93
300	93
400	93
500	93
1000	94

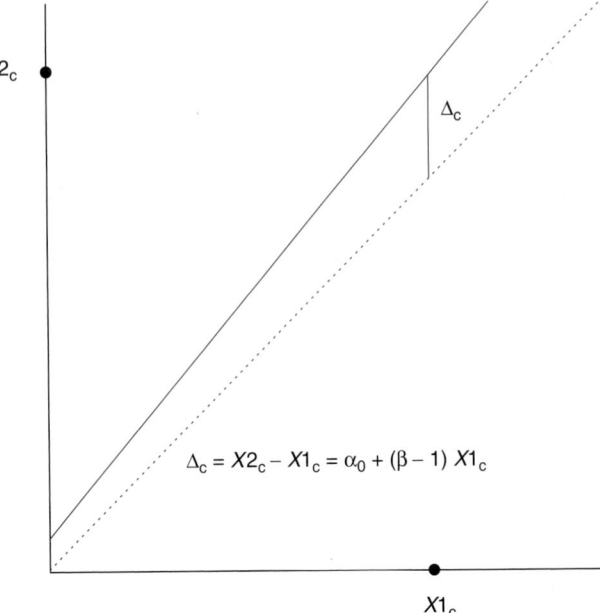

$$\Delta_c = X2_c - X1_c = \alpha_0 + (\beta - 1)\, X1_c$$

Figure 2-12 Illustration of the systematic difference $_c$ between two methods at a given level $X1_c$ according to the regression line. The difference is a result of a constant systematic difference (intercept deviation from zero) and a proportional systematic difference (slope deviation from unity). The dotted line represents the diagonal $X2 = X1$.

By counting, it may be determined whether the expected proportion of results is within the limits (i.e., 95%). One may accept percentages that do not deviate significantly from the supposed percentage at the given sample size derived from the binomial distribution (Table 2-4). For example, if 50 paired measurements have been performed in a method comparison study, and if it is observed that 46 of the results (92%) are within the specified limits (e.g., ±15%), the study supports that the achieved goal has been reached because the lower boundary for acceptance is 90%. It is clear that a reasonable number of observations should be obtained for the assessment to have an acceptable power.

When appropriate limits are considered for a comparison study, one should be aware of the error components of the comparison method. Suppose an imprecision corresponding to an analytical coefficient of variation (CV_A) of 5% is allowed for the new method, and a bias of up to ±3% in relation to the comparison method is reasonable. If the CV_A of the comparison method is 4%, the limits for the differences become ±[3% + 2(5^2 + 4^2)$^{0.5}$] (i.e., ±15.8% [supposing a 95% interval]). Note that here we have ignored the possibility of random matrix-related interferences.

Regression Analysis

Regression analysis is commonly applied in comparing the results of analytical method comparisons. Typically an experiment is carried out in which a series of paired values is collected when a new method is compared with an established method. This series of paired observations ($x1_i$, $x2_i$) is then used to establish the nature and strength of the relationship between the tests. Regression analysis has the advantage that it allows the relation between target values for the two compared

methods to be studied over the full analytical measurement range. If the systematic difference between target values (i.e., the calibration bias difference between the two methods or the systematic error) is related to the analyte concentration, such a relationship may not be clearly shown when the previously mentioned types of difference plots are used. In linear regression analysis, it is assumed that the systematic difference between target values is modeled as a constant systematic difference (intercept deviation from zero) combined with a proportional systematic difference (slope deviation from unity), usually related to a discrepancy with regard to calibration of the methods (Figure 2-12). In situations with constant SDs of random errors, unweighted regression procedures are used (i.e., **ordinary least-squares [OLR]** and Deming regression analyses). For cases with SDs that are proportional to the measurement level, the corresponding weighted regression procedures are optimal.

Error Models in Regression Analysis

As was outlined previously, we distinguish between the measured value (x_i) and the target value ($X_{Target i}$) of a sample subjected to analysis by a given method. In linear regression analysis, we assume a linear relationship between values devoid of random error of any kind. In statistical terminology, a so-called structural relationship is assumed. Thus, to operate with a linear relationship between values without random measurement error and sample-related random bias, we assume a linear relationship between the modified target values:

$$X2'_{Target i} = \alpha_0 + \beta X1'_{Target i}$$

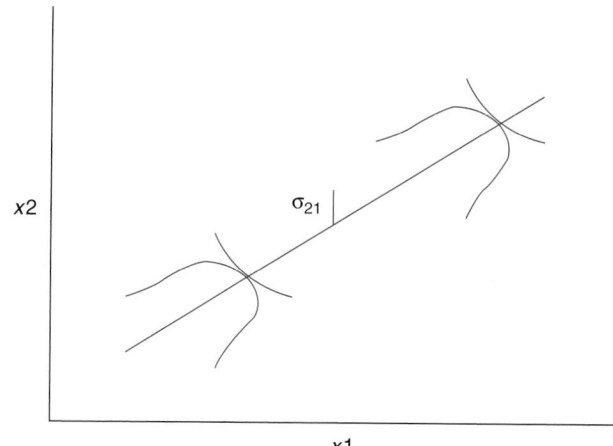

Figure 2-13 Outline of the relation between $x1$ and $x2$ values measured by two methods subject to random error with constant SDs over the analytical measurement range. A linear relationship between the target values ($X1'_{Targeti}$, $X2'_{Targeti}$) is presumed. The $x1_i$ and $x2_i$ values are Gaussian distributed around $X1'_{Targeti}$ and $X2'_{Targeti}$, respectively, as schematically shown. σ_{21} (σ_{yx}) is demarcated.

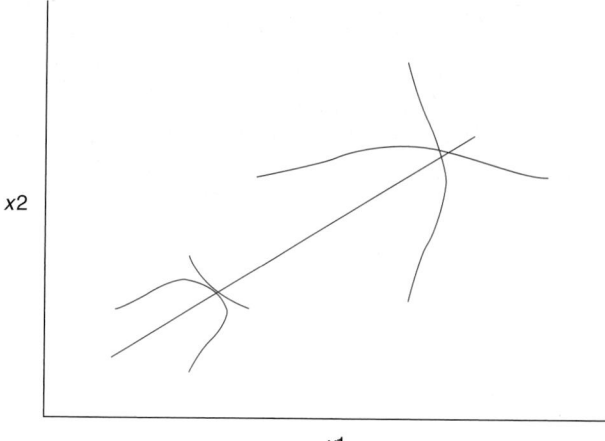

Figure 2-14 Outline of the relation between $x1$ and $x2$ values measured by two methods subject to proportional random errors. A linear relationship between the target values is assumed. The $x1_i$ and $x2_i$ values are Gaussian distributed around $X1'_{Targeti}$ and $X2'_{Targeti}$, respectively, with increasing scatter at higher concentrations as schematically shown.

In this model, α_0 corresponds to a constant difference with regard to calibration, and $(\beta - 1)$ is a proportional deviation. Thus, the systematic error or calibration difference between the measurements corresponds to

$$X2'_{Targeti} - X1'_{Targeti} = \alpha_0 + (\beta - 1)X1'_{Targeti}$$

Because of sample-related random interferences and measurement imprecision (of the type described by a Gaussian distribution, e.g., caused by pipetting variability, signal variability), individually measured pairs of values ($x1_i$, $x2_i$) will be scattered around the line expressing the relationship between $X1'_{Targeti}$ and $X2'_{Targeti}$. Figure 2-13 outlines schematically how the random distribution of $x1$ and $x2$ values occurs around the regression line. We have

$$x1_i = X1_{Targeti} + \varepsilon1_i = X1'_{Targeti} + \text{Random-Bias1}_i + \varepsilon1_i$$

$$x2_i = X2_{Targeti} + \varepsilon2_i = X2'_{Targeti} + \text{Random-Bias2}_i + \varepsilon2_i$$

The random error components may be expressed as SDs, and generally we assume that sample-related random bias (SD σ_{RB}) and analytical imprecision (SD σ_A) are independent for each analyte, yielding the relations

$$\sigma_{x1}^2 = \sigma_{RB1}^2 + \sigma_{A1}^2$$

$$\sigma_{x2}^2 = \sigma_{RB2}^2 + \sigma_{A2}^2$$

where σ_{x1}^2 and σ_{x2}^2 are the total SDs of the distributions of $x1i$ and $x2i$ around their respective modified target values, $X1'_{Targeti}$ and $X2'_{Targeti}$. The sample-related random bias components for methods 1 and 2 may not necessarily be independent. They also may not be Gaussian distributed, contrary to the analytical components. Thus when a regression procedure

is applied, the explicit assumptions to take into account should be considered. In situations without random bias components of any significance, the relationships simplify to

$$\sigma_{x1}^2 = \sigma_{A1}^2$$

$$\sigma_{x2}^2 = \sigma_{A2}^2$$

In this situation, it usually is assumed that the error distributions are Gaussian, and estimates of the analytical SDs may be available from quality control data.

Another methodological problem concerns the question of whether the dispersion of sample-related random bias and the analytical imprecision are constant or change with the analyte concentration, as considered previously in the difference plot sections. In cases with a considerable range (e.g., a decade or longer), this phenomenon should be taken into account when a regression analysis is applied. Figure 2-14 schematically shows how dispersions may increase proportionally with concentration.

Deming Regression Analysis and Ordinary Least-Squares Regression Analysis (Constant SDs)

To reliably estimate the relationship between modified target values (i.e., a_0 for α_0 and b for β), a regression procedure taking into account errors in both $x1$ and $x2$ is preferable (a situation termed *the Deming approach*; see Figure 2-13). Although the OLR procedure is commonly used in method comparison studies, it does not take errors in $x1$ into account but is based on the assumption that only the $x2$ measurements are subject to random error (Figure 2-15). In the Deming procedure, the sum of squared distances from measured sets of values ($x1_i$, $x2_i$) to the regression line is minimized at an angle determined by the ratio between SDs for the random variations of $x1$ and $x2$. It is possible to prove theoretically that, given Gaussian *error* distributions, this estimation procedure is optimal. It should here be

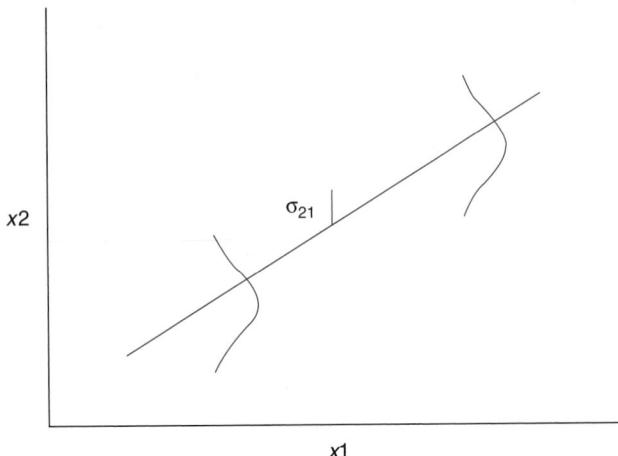

Figure 2-15 The model assumed in ordinary OLR. The $x2$ values are Gaussian distributed around the line with constant SD over the analytical measurement range. The $x1$ values are assumed to be without random error. σ_{21} (σ_{yx}) is shown.

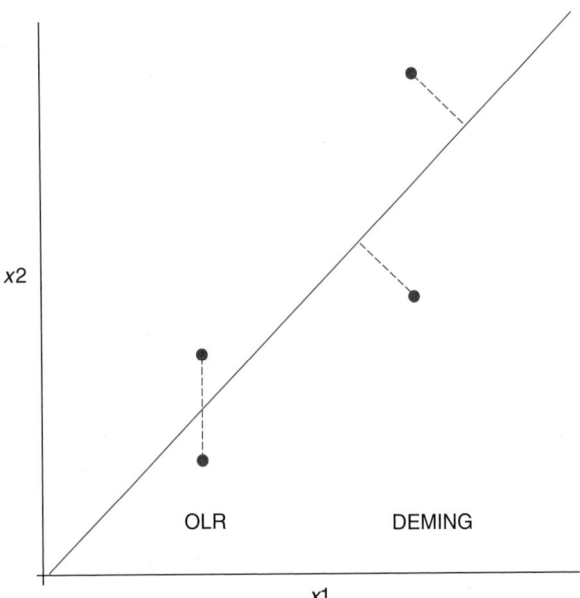

Figure 2-16 In OLR, the sum of squared deviations from the line is minimized in the vertical direction. In Deming regression analysis, the sum of squared deviations is minimized at an angle to the line depending on the random error ratio. Here the symmetric case is displayed with orthogonal deviations. *(Reproduced with permission from Linnet K. The performance of Deming regression analysis in case of a misspecified analytical error ratio,* Clin Chem *1998;44:1024–1031 [Figure 1].)*

noted that it is the *error* distributions that should be Gaussian, not the dispersion of values over the measurement range. This is often misunderstood. In Figure 2-16, the symmetrical case is illustrated with a regression slope of 1 and equal SDs for the random variations of $x1$ and $x2$, in which case the sum of squared distances is minimized orthogonally in relation to the line.

OLR is not recommended except in special situations. In OLR, the sum of squared distances is minimized in the vertical direction to the line (see Figure 2-16). It is possible to prove theoretically that neglect of the random error in $x1$ induces a downward biased slope estimate

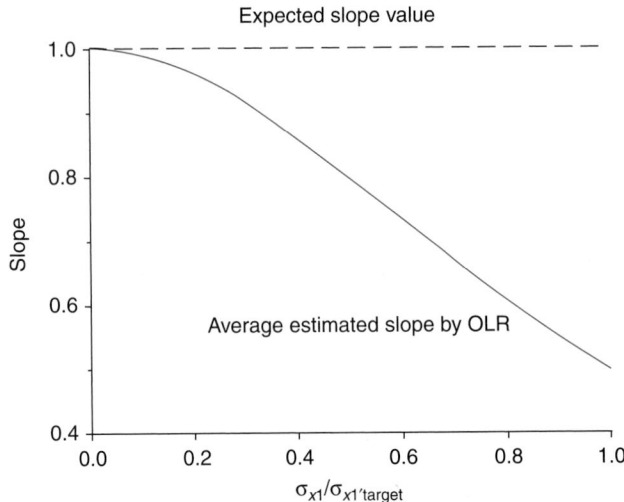

Figure 2-17 Relations between the true (expected) slope value and the average estimated slope by OLR. The bias of the OLR slope estimate increases negatively for increasing ratios of the SD random error in $x1$ to the SD of the $X1$ target value distribution.

$$\beta' = \beta\left[\sigma^2_{x1'target}\Big/\left(\sigma^2_{x1'target} + \sigma^2_{x1}\right)\right]$$

$$= \beta\Big/\left[1 + \left(\sigma_{x1}/\sigma_{X1'target}\right)^2\right]$$

where $\sigma_{X1'target}$ is the SD of $X1'$ target values. The magnitude of the bias depends on the ratio between the SD for the random error in $x1$ and the SD of the $X1'$ target values. Figure 2-17 shows the bias as a function of the ratio of the random error SD to the SD of the $X1'$ target value dispersion. For a ratio up to 0.1, the bias is less than 1%. At a ratio of 0.33, the bias amounts to 10%; it increases further for increasing ratios. In a given case, one takes the analytical SD (e.g., from quality control data) and divides by the SD of the measured $x1$ values, which approximately equals the SD of $X1'$ target values. As an example, a typical comparison study for two serum sodium methods may be associated with a downward directed slope bias of about 10% (Figure 2-18).

In the example presented previously, the ratio of the analytical SD to the SD of the target value distribution is large because of the tight physiological regulation of electrolyte concentrations, which means that the biological variation is limited. Most other types of analytes exhibit wider distributions, and the ratio of error to target value distribution is smaller. For example, for analytes with a distribution of longer than 1 decade and an analytical error corresponding to a CV of 5% at the middle of the analytical measurement range, the OLR slope bias amounts to about −1%.

Computation Procedures for OLR and Deming Regression

Assuming no errors in $x1$ and a Gaussian error distribution of $x2$ with constant SD throughout the analytical measurement range, OLR is the optimal estimation procedure as developed by Carl Friedrich Gauss in the eighteenth century. Given

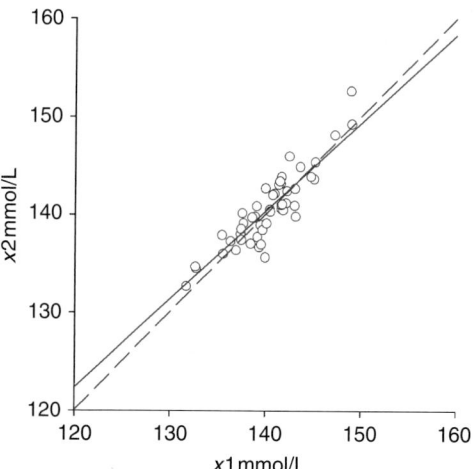

Figure 2-18 Simulated comparison of two sodium methods. The solid line indicates the average estimated OLR line, and the dotted line is the identity line. Even though there is no systematic difference between the two methods, the average OLR line deviates from the identity line corresponding to a downward slope bias of about 10%.

errors in both $x1$ and $x2$, the Deming approach is the method of choice.[10] It should be noted for these parametric procedures that only the error distributions must be Gaussian or normal. The least-squares principle does not presume normality to be applied, but it is optimal under normality conditions, and the nominal Type I errors for the associated statistical tests for slope and intercept hold true under this assumption. The procedures are generally robust toward deviations from normality, but they are sensitive toward outliers because of the squaring principle. Finally, the distributions of the target values of $x1$ and $x2$ do not have to be Gaussian. A uniform distribution over the analytical measurement range is generally of advantage, but the distribution may in principle take any form. For both procedures, we may evaluate the SD of the dispersion in the vertical direction around the line (commonly denoted $SD_{y \cdot x}$ and here given as SD_{21}). We have

$$SD_{21} = \left[\sum \left(x2_i - X2'_{\text{Targetest}i} \right)^2 / (N-2) \right]^{0.5}$$

Further discussion regarding the interpretation of SD_{21} will be given later.

To compute the slope in Deming regression analysis, the ratio between the SDs of the random errors of $x1$ and $x2$ is necessary, that is,

$$\lambda = \left(\sigma_{RB1}^2 + \sigma_{A1}^2 \right) / \left(\sigma_{RB2}^2 + \sigma_{A2}^2 \right)$$

SD_As are estimated from duplicate sets of measurements as

$$SD_{A1}^2 = (1/2N) \sum \left(x1_{2i} - x1_{1i} \right)^2$$

$$SD_{A2}^2 = (1/2N) \sum \left(x2_{2i} - x2_{1i} \right)^2$$

or they may be available from quality control data.

If a specific value for λ is not available and the two field methods that are compared are likely to be associated with random error levels of the same order of magnitude, λ is set to 1. The Deming procedure is generally relatively insensitive to a misspecification of the λ value.

Formulas for computing slope (β), intercept (α_0), and their standard errors are available from other sources[10,11] and will not be repeated here. Commonly available software packages for performing regression analysis by both methods will be reviewed later.

Evaluation of the Random Error Around an Estimated Regression Line

The estimated slope and intercept provide an estimate of the systematic difference or error between two methods over the analytical measurement range. Additionally, an estimate of the random error is important. As has been mentioned, it is commonplace to consider the dispersion around the line in the vertical direction, which is quantified as $SD_{y \cdot x}$ (here denoted SD_{21}). SD_{21} has originally been introduced in the context of OLR, but it may as well be considered in relation to Deming regression analysis.

Interpreting $SD_{y \cdot x}$ (SD_{21}) With Random Errors in Both $x1$ and $x2$

With regard to σ_{21}, we have here without sample-related random interferences

$$\sigma_{21}^2 = \beta^2 \sigma_{A1}^2 + \sigma_{A2}^2$$

Thus σ_{21} reflects the random error in both $x1$ (with a rescaling) and $x2$. Often β is close to unity, and in this case σ_{21}^2 becomes approximately the sum of the individual squared SDs. This relation holds true for both Deming and OLR analyses. Frequently, OLR is applied in situations associated with random measurement error in both $x1$ and $x2$, and in these situations σ_{21} reflects the errors of both.

The presence of sample-related random interferences in both $x1$ and $x2$ gives the following expression:

$$\sigma_{21}^2 = \left[\beta^2 \sigma_{A1}^2 + \sigma_{A2}^2 \right] + \left[\beta^2 \sigma_{RB1}^2 + \sigma_{RB2}^2 \right]$$

Thus the σ_{21} value is influenced by the slope value, the analytical error components σ_{A1} and σ_{A2} (grouped in the first bracket) and σ_{RB1} and σ_{RB2} (grouped in the second bracket). In many cases, the slope is close to unity, in which case we have simple addition of the components. As has been mentioned, the matrix-related random interferences may not be independent. In this case, simple addition of the components is not correct because a covariance term should be included. However, in a real case, we estimate the combined effect corresponding to the bracket term. Information on the analytical components is usually available, either from duplicate sets of measurements or from quality control data. On this basis, the combined random bias term in the second bracket is derived by subtracting the analytical components from σ_{21}. Overall, it is possible to judge whether the total random error is acceptable or not. The systematic difference is adjusted for relatively easily by rescaling of one of the sets of measurements. However, if the random error term is very large, such rescaling does not ensure equivalency of measurements with regard to individual samples. Thus it is important to assess both the systematic difference and the random error when deciding whether a new field method can replace an existing one. In a roughly symmetrical situation with a slope close to unity and two field methods of presumed equal specificity and precision, the total random error expressed as SD_{21} may be subdivided into component errors associated with each test by dividing with the square root of two. One may then assess the random error levels in relation to stated goals.

Assessment of Outliers

The principle of minimizing the sum of squared distances from the line makes the described regression procedures sensitive toward outliers, and an assessment of the occurrence of outliers should be carried out routinely. The distance from a suspected outlier to the line is recorded in SD units, and rejection of the outlier is performed if the distance exceeds a predetermined limit (e.g., 3 or 4 SD units). In the case of OLR, the SD unit equals SD_{21}, and the vertical distance is considered. For Deming regression analysis, the unit is the SD of the deviation of the points from the line at an angle determined by the error variance ratio, λ. A plot of these deviations, a so-called residuals plot, conveniently illustrates the occurrence of outliers.[10,11] Figure 2-19, *A*, illustrates a Deming regression analysis example with occurrence of an outlier and the associated residuals plot *(B)*, which clearly shows the outlier pattern. In this example, the residuals plot was standardized to unit SD. In this example with an outlier limit of 4 SD units, the outlier was rejected and a reanalysis was undertaken. In this example, rejection of the outlier changed the slope from 1.14 to 1.03. With regard to outliers, these measurements should not just be rejected automatically; the reason for their presence should be investigated as a method limitation (e.g., possibly a nonspecificity for the analyte).

The Correlation Coefficient

In addition to outlining the random error components related to regression analysis, some comments on the correlation coefficient may be appropriate. The ordinary correlation coefficient ρ, also called *the Pearson product moment correlation coefficient,* is estimated as *r* from sums of squared deviations for *x1* and *x2* values as follows:

$$r = p/[uq]^{0.5}$$

where

$$p = \sum (x1_i - x1_m)(x2_i - x2_m)$$

$$u = \sum (x1_i - x1_m)^2 \quad q = \sum (x2_i - x2_m)^2$$

and

$$x1_m = \sum x1_i/N \quad x2_m = \sum x2_i/N$$

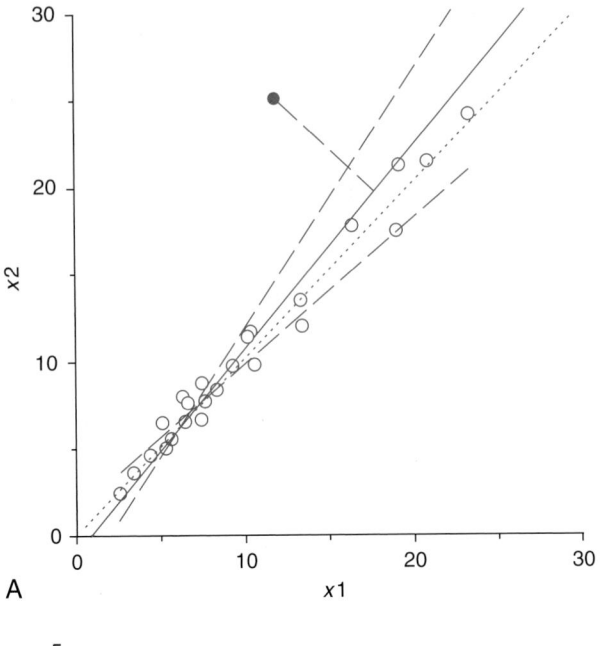

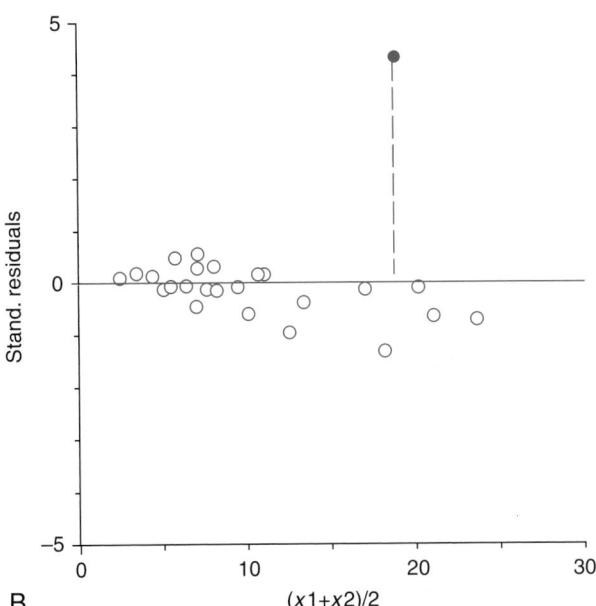

Figure 2-19 A, A scatter plot with the Deming regression line *(solid line)* with an outlier *(filled point)*. The *dotted straight line* is the diagonal, and the *curved dashed lines* demarcate the 95% confidence region. **B,** Standardized residuals plot with indication of the outlier.

Theoretically, ρ is related to the ratio between the SDs of the distributions of target values ($\sigma_{X1'\text{target}}$ and $\sigma_{X2'\text{target}}$) and the associated independent total random error components (σ_{x1} and σ_{x2})

$$\rho = \sigma_{X1'\text{target}}\sigma_{X2'\text{target}} / \left[\left(\sigma^2_{X1'\text{target}} + \sigma^2_{x1} \right) \left(\sigma^2_{X2'1\text{target}} + \sigma^2_{x2} \right) \right]^{0.5}$$

The total random error components comprise both imprecision error and sample-related random interferences (i.e., $\sigma^2_{x1} = \sigma^2_{A1} + \sigma^2_{RB1}$ and $\sigma^2_{x2} = \sigma^2_{A2} + \sigma^2_{RB2}$). Thus ρ is a *relative* indicator of the amount of dispersion around the regression line. If the range of values is narrow, ρ tends to be low and vice versa for a wide range of values. For example, consider simulated examples, where the random errors of $x1$ and $x2$ are the same, but the width of the distributions of target values differs (Figure 2-20, A and B). In (A), the target values are uniformly distributed over the range 1 to 3, and in (B), the range is 1 to 6. The random error SD is presumed constant, and it is in both cases set to 0.15 for both $x1$ and $x2$, corresponding to a CV of 5% at level 3. Given sets of 50 paired measurements, the correlation coefficient is 0.93 in case (A) and 0.99 in case (B). Further, a single point located outside the range of the rest of the observations exerts a strong influence (Figure 2-20, C). In (C), 49 of the observations are distributed within the range 1 to 3 with a single point located apart from the others around the value 6, other factors being equal. The correlation coefficient here takes an intermediate value, 0.97. Thus a single point located away from the rest has a strong influence (a so-called influential point). Notice that it is not an outlying point, just an aberrant point with regard to the range.

Although σ_{21} is the relevant measure for random error in method comparison studies, ρ is still incorrectly used as a supposed measure of agreement between two methods. It should be noted that a systematic difference due to a difference with regard to calibration is expressed not through ρ but solely in the form of an intercept (α_0) deviation from zero and/or a slope (β) deviation from unity. Thus even though the correlation coefficient is very high, a considerable calibration bias may be noted between the measurements of two methods.

Regression Analysis in Case of Proportional Random Errors

As has been discussed in relation to the precision profile, for analytes with wide ranges (e.g., 1 or several decades), the SD_A is seldom constant. Rather, a proportional relationship may apply. This may also be true for the random bias components. In this situation, the regression procedures described previously still may be used, but they are not optimal because the standard errors of slope and intercept become larger than is the case when a weighted form of regression analysis is applied. The optimal approaches are weighted forms of regression analysis that take into account the relationship between random error and analyte concentration.[10,11] Given a proportional relationship, a weighted procedure assigns larger weights to observations in the low range; low-range observations are more precise than measurements at higher concentrations that are subject to larger random errors. More specifically, weights are applied in the computations that are inversely proportional to the squared SDs (variances) that express the random error. In the weighted modification of the Deming procedure, distances from ($x1i$, $x2i$) to the line are inversely weighted according to the squared SDs at a given concentration (Figure 2-21). The regression procedures are most conveniently performed using dedicated software.

Testing for Linearity

Dividing systematic error into a constant and a proportional component depends on the assumption of linearity,

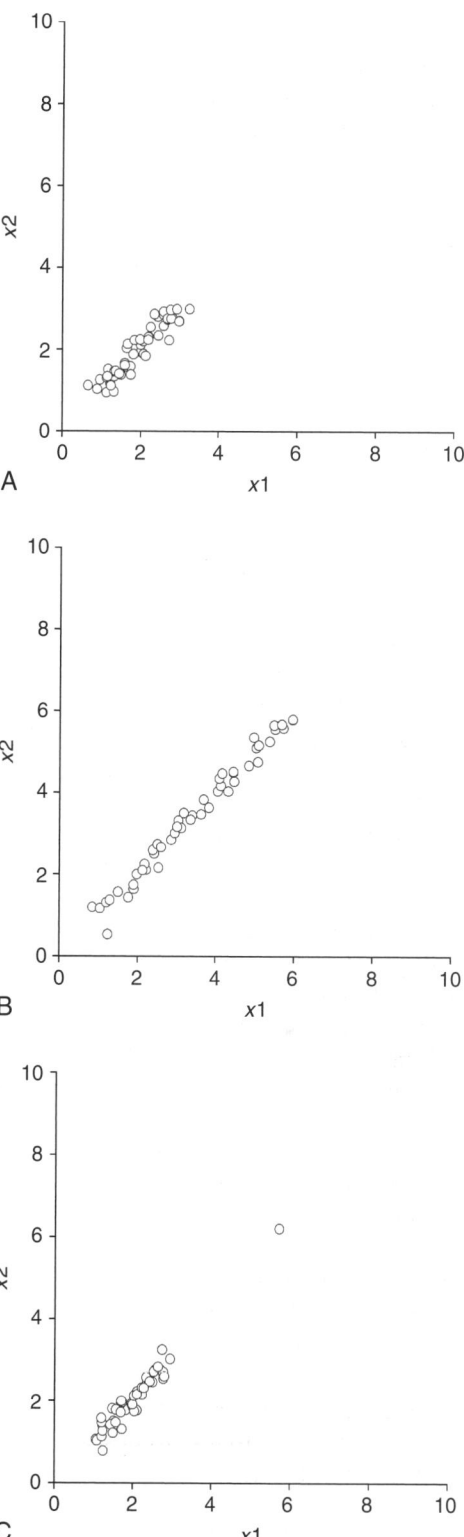

Figure 2-20 Scatter plots illustrating the effect of the range on the value of the correlation coefficient ρ. **A,** The target values are uniformly distributed over the range 1 to 3 with random errors of both $x1$ and $x2$ corresponding to an SD of 5% of the target value at 3 (constant error SDs). **B,** The range is extended to 1 to 6 with the same random error levels. The correlation coefficient equals 0.93 in **A** and 0.99 in **B**. In **C,** the effect of a single aberrant point is shown. Forty-nine of the target values are distributed over the range 1 to 3 with a single point at 6. The correlation coefficient is 0.97.

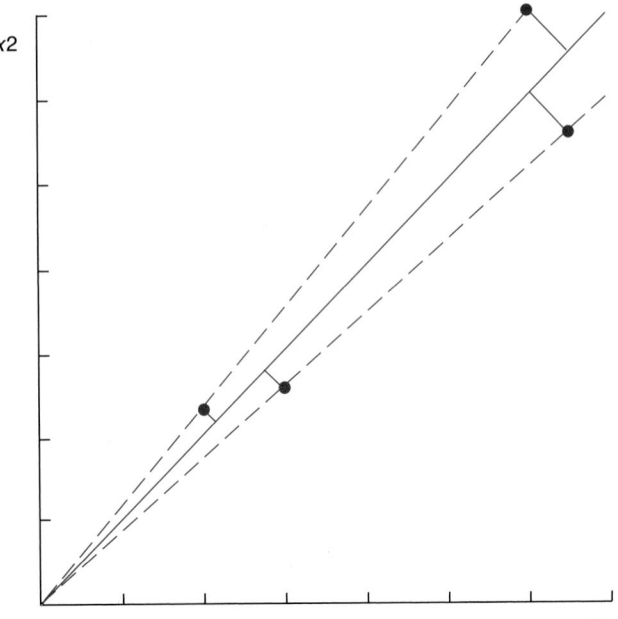

Figure 2-21 Distances from data points to the line in weighted Deming regression, assuming proportional random errors in *x*1 and *x*2. The symmetrical case is illustrated with equal random errors and a slope of unity, yielding orthogonal projections onto the line. *(From Linnet K. Necessary sample size for method comparison studies based on regression analysis,* Clin Chem *1999;45:882-94.)*

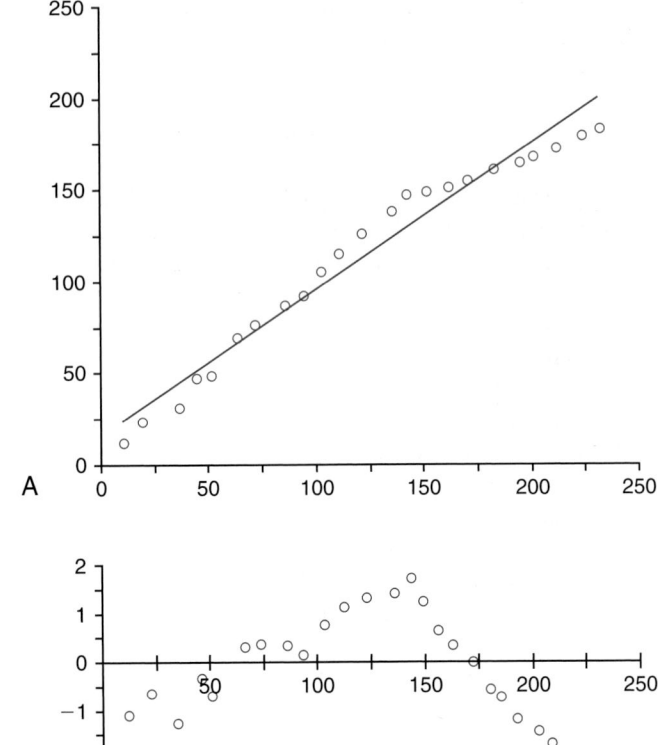

Figure 2-22 *Top,* Scatter plot showing an example of nonlinearity in the form of downward deviating *x*2 values at the upper part of the range. *Bottom,* Plot of residuals showing the effect of nonlinearity. At the upper end of the analytical measurement range, a sequence (run) of negative residuals is present from *x* = 150 to 200.

which should be tested. A convenient test is a runs test, which in principle assesses whether negative and positive deviations from the points to the line are randomly distributed over the analytical measurement range. The term *run* here relates to a sequence of deviations with the same sign. Consider for example the situation with a downward trend of *x*2 values at the upper end of the analytical measurement range (Figure 2-22, *A*). The standardized deviations from the line (i.e., the residuals) will tend to be negative in this area instead of being randomly distributed above and below the line[10] (Figure 2-22, *B*). Given a sufficient number of points, such a sequence will turn out to be statistically significant in a runs test.

Nonparametric Regression Analysis (Passing-Bablok)

The slope and the intercept may be estimated by a nonparametric procedure, which is robust to outliers and requires no assumptions of Gaussian error distributions.[13] Note, however, that parametric regression procedures do not presume Gaussian distributions of *x*1 and *x*2 values over the measurement range, but only of the *error* distributions. Thus the main advantage of the nonparametric procedure is its robust performance in the presence of outliers. The method takes measurement errors for both *x*1 and *x*2 into account, but it presumes that the ratio between random errors is related to the slope in a fixed manner:

$$\lambda = \left(SD_{RB1}^2 + SD_{A1}^2\right)\Big/\left(SD_{RB2}^2 + SD_{A2}^2\right) = 1/\beta^2$$

Otherwise, a biased slope estimate is obtained.[10] The procedure may be applied both in situations with random errors with constant SDs and in cases with proportional SDs. The method is not as efficient as the corresponding parametric procedures (i.e., Deming and weighted Deming procedures).[10,11] Slope and intercept with CIs are provided, together with Spearman's rank correlation coefficient. A software program is required for the procedure.

Interpretation of Systematic Differences Between Methods Obtained on the Basis of Regression Analysis

A systematic difference between two methods is identified if the estimated intercept differs significantly from zero, or if the slope deviates significantly from 1. This is decided on the basis of *t*-tests:

$$t = (a_0 - 0)/SE(a_0)$$

$$t = (b - 1)/SE(b)$$

SE(a_0) and SE(*b*) are the standard errors of the estimated intercept α_0 and the slope *b*, respectively. In practice, standard errors are derived by a computerized resampling principle called *the jackknife procedure,* which is carried out using appropriate software[10] (see section Software Packages).

Having estimated a_0 and b, we have the estimate of the systematic difference between the methods, D_c, at a selected concentration, $X1'_{Targetc}$:

$$D_c = X2'_{Targetestc} - X1'_{Targetc} = a_0 + (b-1)X1'_{Targetc}$$

$X2'_{Targetestc}$ is the estimated $X2'$ target value at $X1'_c$. Note that D_c refers to the *systematic* difference (i.e., the difference between modified target values corresponding to a calibration difference). The standard error of D_c is derived by the jackknife procedure using a software program. By evaluating the standard error throughout the analytical measurement range, a confidence region for the estimated line is displayed. If method comparison is performed to assess the calibration to a reference measurement procedure, correction of a significant systematic difference $Delta_c$ will often be performed by recalibration [$x2_{rec} = (x1 - a_0)/b$]. The associated standard uncertainty is the standard error of $Delta_c$. Even though the intercept and the slope are not significantly different from zero and 1, respectively, the combined expression $Delta_c$ may be significantly different from zero.

Example of Application of Regression Analysis (Weighted Deming Analysis)

Application of weighted Deming regression analysis may be illustrated by the comparison of drug assays example ($N = 65$ [$x1$, $x2$] measurements). As was outlined previously, in this example, the random error of the differences increases with the concentration, suggesting that the weighted form of Deming regression analysis is appropriate. Figure 2-23 shows (A) the estimated regression line with 95% confidence bands and (B) a plot of residuals. The nearly homogeneous scatter in the residuals plot supports the assumed proportional random error model and the assumption of linearity. The slope estimate (1.014) is not significantly different from 1 (95% CI, 0.97 to 1.06), and the intercept is not significantly different from zero (95% CI, −6.7 to 47.4) (Table 2-5). A runs test for linearity does not contradict the assumption of linearity. The amount of random error is quantified in the form of the SD_{21} proportionality factor equal to 0.11 or 11%. In the present example with a slope close to unity and two routine methods with assumed random errors of about the same magnitude, we divide the random error by the square root of two and get $CV_{x1} = CV_{x2} = 7.8\%$. Quality control data in the laboratory have provided CV_As of 6.1% and 7.2% for methods 1 and 2, respectively. Thus in this example, the random error may be attributed largely to analytical error. The assay principle is HPLC for both methods, which generally is a rather specific measurement principle, and considerable random bias effects are not expected in this case. If one or both of the assays had been immunoassays, the situation might have been different.

In the table, the estimated systematic differences at the limits of the therapeutic interval (300 and 2000 nmol/L) are displayed (24.6 and 48.9 nmol/L, respectively). This corresponds to percentage values of 8.2% and 2.4%, respectively. The estimated standard errors by the jackknife procedure yield the 95% CIs as shown in the table. At the low concentration, the difference is significant (95% CI: 5.7 to 44 nmol/L does not include

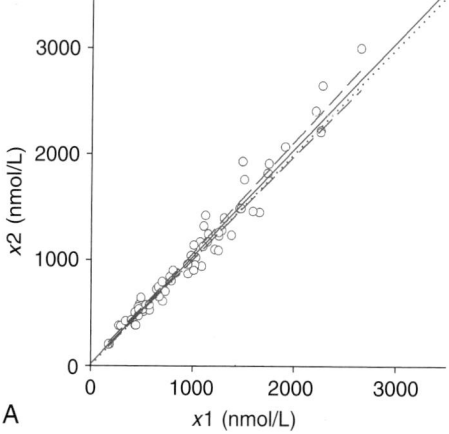

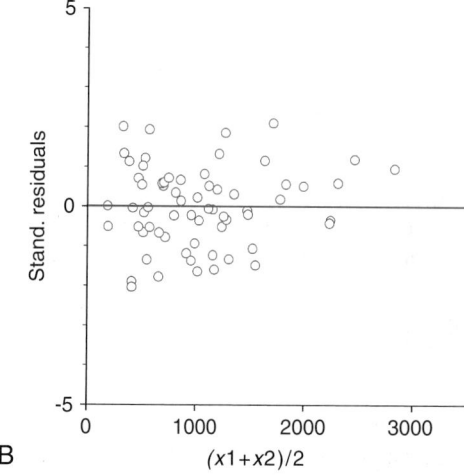

Figure 2-23 An example of weighted Deming regression analysis for the comparison of drug assays. **A,** The *solid line* is the estimated weighted Deming regression line, the *dashed curves* indicate the 95% confidence region, and the *dotted line* is the line of identity. **B** is a plot of residuals standardized to unit SD. The homogeneous scatter supports the assumed proportional error model and the assumption of linearity.

TABLE 2-5	Results of Weighted Deming Regression Analysis for the Comparison of Drug Assays Example, N = 65 (x1, x2) Measurements		
	Estimate	**Standard Error (SE)**	**95% CI**
Slope (b)	1.014	0.022	0.97 to 1.06
Intercept (a_0)	20.3	13.5	−6.7 to 47.4
Weighted correlation coefficient	0.98		
SD_{21} proportionality factor	0.11		
Runs test for linearity	NS		
$Delta_c = X_2 - X_1$ at $X_c = 300$	24.6	9.5	5.72 to 43.6
$Delta_c = X_2 - X_1$ at $X_c = 2000$	48.9	34.2	−19.3 to 117

zero), which is not the case at the high level (95% CI, −19 to 117 nmol/L). Even though the intercept and slope estimates separately are not significantly different from the null hypothesis values of zero and 1, respectively, the combined difference $Delta_c$ is significant at low concentrations in this example. If the difference is considered of medical importance and both methods are to be used simultaneously in the laboratory, recalibration of one of the methods might be considered.

Discussion of Application of Regression Analysis

Generally, it is recommended that Deming or weighted Deming regression analysis should be used with a type of regression analysis that is based on a correct error model. Most published method evaluations are based on unweighted regression analysis; here the use of unweighted analysis is considered in the setting of proportional random errors.

Basically, the Deming procedure provides unbiased estimates of slope and intercept when SDs vary, provided that their ratio is constant throughout the analytical measurement range. This aspect is important and indicates that generally the estimates of slope and intercept are reliable in this frequently encountered situation. However, applying the unweighted Deming analysis in cases of proportional SD_As is less efficient than applying the weighted approach. For uniform distributions of values with range ratios from 2 to 100, 1.2 to 3.7 times as many samples are necessary to obtain the same uncertainty of the slope estimated by the unweighted compared with the weighted approach.[11] Thus the larger the range ratio, the more inefficient is the unweighted method.

Monitoring Serial Results

An important aspect in clinical chemistry is monitoring of disease or treatment (e.g., tumor markers in case of cancer, drug concentrations in case of therapeutic drug monitoring). To assess changes in a rational way, the various imprecision components have to be taken into account.[7,8] Biological within-subject variations ($SD_{Within-B}$) and preanalytical (SD_{PA}) and analytical variations (SD_A) all have to be recognized. Assuming that preanalytical variation is already included in the estimated within-subject variation SD, a total SD (SD_T) is estimated by:

$$SD_T^2 = SD_{Within-B}^2 + SD_A^2$$

The limit for statistically significant changes then is $k\sqrt{2}$ SD_T, where k depends on the desired probability level. When a two-sided 5% level is given, k is 1.96. The corresponding one-sided factor is 1.65. If a higher probability level is desired, k should be increased.

Traceability and Measurement Uncertainty

As was outlined previously in the error model sections, laboratory results are influenced by systematic and random errors of various kinds. Obtaining agreement of measurements between laboratories or agreement over time in a given laboratory often is problematic.

Traceability

To ensure reasonable agreement between measurements of routine methods, the concept of traceability comes into focus. Traceability is based on an unbroken chain of comparisons of measurements leading to a known reference value

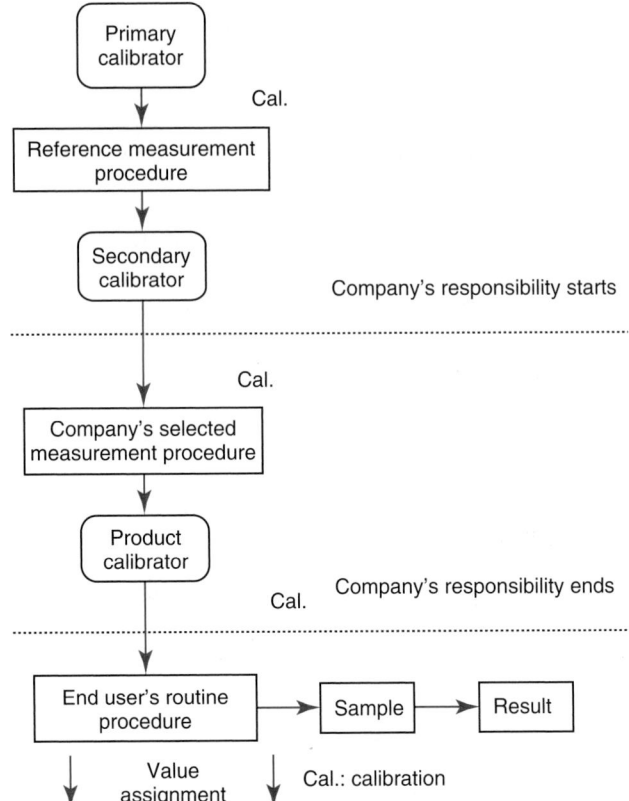

Figure 2-24 The calibration hierarchy from a reference measurement procedure to a routine method. The uncertainty increases from top to bottom.

(Figure 2-24).[15] A hierarchical approach for tracing the values of routine clinical chemistry measurements to reference measurement procedures was proposed by Tietz and has been adapted by the ISO.[9] For well-established analytes, a hierarchy of methods exists with *a reference measurement procedure* at the top, *selected measurement procedures* at an intermediate level, and finally *routine measurement procedures* at the bottom. A reference measurement procedure is a fully understood procedure of highest analytical quality containing a complete uncertainty budget given in SI units. Reference procedures are used to measure the analyte concentration in *secondary reference materials,* which typically have the same matrix as samples that are to be measured by routine procedures (e.g., human serum). Secondary reference materials are usually of high analytical quality, and certified secondary reference materials must be validated for commutability[1] with clinical samples if they are intended for use as trueness controls for routine methods. Otherwise, their use is restricted to those selected measurement procedures for which they are intended. The certificate of analysis should state the methods for which the secondary reference materials have been validated to be commutable with clinical samples. When no information is given

---

[1]Several definitions have been developed for **commutability.** In this chapter, the following definition is used: "The equivalence of the mathematical relationships between the results of different measurement procedures for a reference material and for representative samples from healthy and diseased individuals."

for commutability, it must be assumed that the reference material is not commutable with clinical samples, and the user has the responsibility to validate commutability for the methods of interest. Uncertainty of the measurement procedure results in increases from the top level to the bottom. ISO guidelines (15193 and 15194) address requirements for reference methods and reference materials.[9]

When cortisol is used as an example, the primary reference material is crystalline cortisol with a chemical analysis for impurities (NIST SRM 921, cortisol [hydrocortisone]). A primary calibrator is then a cortisol preparation with a stated mass fraction (purity) (e.g., 0.998 and a 95% CI of ±0.001). The reference measurement procedure is an isotope dilution gas chromatography–mass spectrometry (IDMS) method that is calibrated with the primary calibrator. A panel of individual frozen serum samples that have values assigned by the primary reference measurement procedure is available from the Institute for Reference Materials and Measurements (IRMM) as secondary reference materials (ERM-DA451/IFCC). A manufacturer's *selected measurement* procedure is calibrated with the secondary reference materials and is used for measurement of the quantity in the manufacturer's *product calibrator,* which is the calibrator used for the routine method in clinical laboratories.

Only 25 to 30 of clinical chemistry analytes currently are traceable to SI units, such as electrolytes, some metabolites (glucose, creatinine, and uric acid), steroids, and some thyroid hormones). For plasma proteins, a human reference serum material is available from IRMM with certified mass concentrations of 12 serum proteins (ERM-DA470k/IFCC). With protein hormones, the existence of heterogeneity or microheterogeneity complicates the problem of traceability.[15]

The Uncertainty Concept

To assess in a systematic way errors associated with laboratory results, the *uncertainty* concept has been introduced into laboratory medicine.[6] According to the ISO "Guide to the Expression of Uncertainty in Measurement" (GUM), **uncertainty** is formally defined as "a parameter associated with the result of a measurement that characterizes the dispersion of the values that could reasonably be attributed to the measurand."[5] In practice, this means that the uncertainty is given as an interval around a reported laboratory result that specifies the location of the true value with a given probability (e.g., 95%). In general, the uncertainty of a result, which is traceable to a particular reference, is the uncertainty of that reference together with the overall uncertainty of the traceability chain.[6] Updated information on traceability aspects is available on the website of the Joint Committee on Traceability in Laboratory Medicine (www.bipm.org/en/committees/jc/jctlm/; accessed September 1, 2012).

The Standard Uncertainty (u_{st})

The uncertainty concept is directed toward the end user (clinician) of the result, who is concerned about the total error possible and is not particularly interested in the question of whether the errors are systematic or random. In the outline of the uncertainty concept, it is assumed that any known systematic error components of a measurement method have been corrected, and the specified uncertainty includes uncertainty associated with correction of the systematic error(s).[6] Although this appears logical, one problem may be that some routine methods have systematic errors dependent on the patient category from which the sample originates. For example, kinetic Jaffe methods for creatinine are subject to positive interference by 2-Oxo compounds and to negative interference by bilirubin and its metabolites, which means that the direction of systematic error will be patient dependent and is not generally predictable.

In the theory on uncertainty, a distinction between type A and type B uncertainties is made. Type A uncertainties are frequency-based estimates of SDs (e.g., an SD of the imprecision). Type B uncertainties are uncertainty components for which frequency-based SDs are not available. Instead, uncertainty is estimated by other approaches or by the opinion of experts. Finally, the total uncertainty is derived from a combination of all sources of uncertainty. In this context, it is practical to operate with *standard uncertainties* (u_{st}), which are equivalent to SDs. By multiplication of a standard uncertainty with a *coverage factor (k),* the uncertainty corresponding to a specified probability level is derived. For example, multiplication with a coverage factor of 2 yields a probability level of ≈95%, given a Gaussian distribution. When the total uncertainty of an analytical result obtained by a routine method is considered, (1) preanalytical variation, (2) method imprecision, (3) sample-related random interferences, (4) uncertainty related to calibration and (5) bias corrections (traceability) should be taken into account. In expressing the uncertainty components as standard uncertainties, we have the following general relation:

$$u_{st} = \left[u_{P\ Ast}^2 + u_{Ast}^2 + u_{R\ B\ st}^2 + u_{Trac\ st}^2 \right]^{0.5}$$

where the individual components refer to preanalytical, analytical, and sample-related random bias and traceability uncertainty.

Uncertainty is assessed in various ways; often a combination of procedures is necessary. In principle, uncertainty is judged *directly* from measurement comparisons or *indirectly* from an analysis of individual error sources according to the law of error propagation ("error budget"). Measurement comparison may consist of a method comparison study with a reference method based on patient samples according to the principles outlined previously or by measurement of commutable certified matrix reference materials (CRMs).

Example of Direct Assessment of Uncertainty on the Basis of Measurements of a Commutable Certified Reference Material

Suppose a CRM is available that was validated to be *commutable* with patient samples for a given routine method with a specified value 10.0 mmol/L and a standard uncertainty of

0.2 mmol/L. Ten repeated measurements in independent runs give a mean value of 10.3 mmol/L with SD 0.5 mmol/L. The standard error of the mean is then $0.5/\sqrt{10} = 0.16$ mmol/L. The mean is not significantly different from the assigned value $[t = (10.3 - 10.0)/(0.2^2 + 0.16^2)^{0.5} = 1.17]$. The total standard uncertainty with regard to traceability is then $u_{\text{Trac st}} = (0.16^2 + 0.2^2)^{0.5} = 0.26$ mmol/L. If the bias had been significant, one might have considered making a correction to the method, and the standard uncertainty would then be the same at the given concentration. Thus measurements of the CRM provide an estimate of the uncertainty related to traceability, *given the assumption of commutability with patient samples.* The other components have to be estimated separately. Regarding method imprecision, long-term imprecision (e.g., observed from quality control measurements) should be used rather than the short-term SD observed for CRM material. Here we suppose that the long-term SD_A is 0.8 mmol/L. Data on preanalytical variation is obtained by sampling in duplicates from a series of patients or can be a matter of judgment (type B uncertainty) based on literature data or data on similar analytes. We here suppose that SD_{PA} equals half the analytical SD (i.e., 0.4 mmol/L). Finally, we lack data on a possible sample-related random bias component, which we may choose to ignore in the present example. The standard uncertainty of the results then becomes

$$u_{st} = \left[u_{P\ Ast}^2 + u_{Ast}^2 + u_{R\ B\ st}^2 + u_{Trac\ st}^2 \right]^{0.5}$$

$$= \left[0.4^2 + 0.8^2 + 0.26^2 \right]^{0.5}$$

$$= 0.93\ (\text{mmol/L})$$

In this case, the major uncertainty component is the long-term imprecision in the laboratory.

Indirect Evaluation of Uncertainty by Quantification of Individual Error Source Components

On the basis of a detailed quantitative model of the analytical procedure, the standard approach is to assess the standard uncertainties associated with the individual input parameters and combine them according to the law of propagation of uncertainties.[6] The relationship between the combined standard uncertainty $u_c(y)$ of a value y and the uncertainty of the *independent* parameters $x_1, x_2, \ldots x_n$, on which it depends, is

$$u_c\ [y(x1, x2, \ldots)] = \left[\sum c_i^2 u(x_i)^2 \right]^{0.5}$$

where c_i is a sensitivity coefficient (the partial differential of y with respect to x_i). These sensitivity coefficients indicate how the value of y varies with changes in the input parameters x_i. If the variables are not independent, the relationship becomes

$$u_c\ [y(x_i, x_k, \ldots)] = \sum c_i^2 u(x_i)^2 + \left[\sum c_i c_k u(x_i, x_k)^2 \right]^{0.5}$$

where $u(x_i, x_k)$ is the covariance between x_i and x_k, and c_i and c_k are the sensitivity coefficients. The covariance is related to the correlation coefficient ρ_{ik} by

$$u(x_i, x_k) = u(x_i)u(x_k)\ \rho_{ik}$$

| TABLE 2-6 | Relations Between Standard Deviation and Range for Various Types of Distributions |

Gaussian Distribution	Rectangular Distribution	Triangular Distribution
SD = Half-width of 95% interval/$t_{0.975}(v)$ ≈ Half-width of 95% interval/2	SD = Half-width/$\sqrt{3}$	SD = Half-width/$\sqrt{6}$

This is a complex relationship that usually will be difficult to evaluate in practice. In many situations, however, the contributing factors are independent, thus simplifying the picture. Below, some simple examples of combined expressions are shown. The rules are presented in the form of combining SDs or coefficients of variation (CVs) given *independent* input components.[6A]

$$q = x + y \quad SD(q) = \left[SD(x)^2 + SD(y)^2 \right]^{0.5}$$

$$q = x - y \quad SD(q) = \left[SD(x)^2 + SD(y)^2 \right]^{0.5}$$

$$q = ax \quad SD(q) = aSD(x)\ \text{and}\ CV(q) = CV(x)$$

$$q = x^p \quad CV(q) = p\ CV(x)$$

$$q = xy \quad CV(q) = \left[CV(x)^2 + CV(y)^2 \right]^{0.5}$$

$$q = x/y \quad CV(q) = \left[CV(x)^2 + CV(y)^2 \right]^{0.5}$$

For example, the shown formulas may be used to calculate the combined uncertainty of a calibrator solution from the uncertainties of the reference compound, the weighting, and dilution steps.

Some relations between the SD and non-Gaussian distributions may also be of relevance for uncertainty calculations (Table 2-6). For example, if the uncertainty of a CRM value is given with some percentage, it may be understood as referring to a rectangular probability distribution. In relation to calibration of flasks, the triangular distribution is often assumed.

Software Packages

Statistical analyses today are usually carried out in spreadsheets or by statistical programs. Concerning the latter, large, general program packages or smaller programs more or less specialized toward the field of clinical chemistry may be applied. Various large, general packages are now on the market (e.g., SPSS, SAS, Stata, Systat). Among programs of an intermediate size, GraphPad (www.graphpad.com; accessed July 6, 2013) and SigmaStat should be mentioned. Excel (Microsoft) also contains various statistical routines. The general programs may lack procedures of interest to clinical chemists (e.g., the Deming and Passing-Bablok procedures). Among more or less specialized programs for clinical chemistry, Analyze-it (www.analyze-it.com; accessed July 6, 2013), MedCalc (www.medcalc.be; accessed July 6, 2013), StatisPro (CLSI), and a program distributed by one of the authors (KL), CBstat (www.cbstat.com; accessed July 6, 2013), are available. The latter program includes automated routines for method validation (e.g., the Deming and Passing-Bablok procedures), reference interval estimation, and diagnostic test evaluation.

Review Questions

1. The type of error that occurs when an analytical method is nonspecific for an analyte and is actually considered to be a type of bias is:
   a. systematic error.
   b. nonsystematic error.
   c. random error.
   d. true error.

2. The statistical analysis commonly applied when the results of analytical method comparison that involves a plot of paired observations (one from the established method and the other from the new method) are assessed is:
   a. uncertainty analysis.
   b. traceability analysis.
   c. regression analysis.
   d. difference analysis.

3. In the selection of a new method, the first step in selecting a candidate method is the determination of:
   a. reliability.
   b. total allowable error.
   c. specifics of the assay including reagent stability.
   d. what is necessary clinically from a laboratory test.

4. To categorize whether a systematic error is either constant or proportional, one must assume and test for:
   a. randomness.
   b. linearity.
   c. precision.
   d. accuracy.

5. Which one of the following, when stated as an interval around a reported laboratory result, will specify the location of the true value with a given probability?
   a. Traceability
   b. Coefficient of variation
   c. Trueness
   d. Uncertainty

6. The closeness of agreement between independent results of measurements obtained under specific conditions is:
   a. linearity.
   b. precision.
   c. accuracy.
   d. specificity.

7. Analytical specificity is:
   a. the ability of an assay procedure to determine the concentration of a target analyte in the presence of interfering substances in the sample matrix.
   b. the detection limit of a method.
   c. the ability of an analytical method to assess small variations in the concentration of analyte.
   d. the analyte concentration range over which measurements are within the declared tolerances for imprecision and bias of the method.

8. In a regression analysis that compares results of two methods, the y-intercept is calculated to be 2.0 and the slope is 3. This indicates a(n):
   a. calibration error.
   b. uncertainty.
   c. systematic difference.
   d. interference in one method.

9. A type of regression analysis that is used to estimate slope and intercept and that is acceptant to outlier values in the methods and does not require assumption of a Gaussian distribution is:
   a. weighted Deming regression analysis.
   b. ordinary least-squares regression analysis.
   c. linear regression analysis.
   d. nonparametric regression analysis.

10. In a method comparison analysis, the lowest value of an analyte that significantly exceeds the measurement of a blank sample is referred to as the
   a. limit of detection of a method.
   b. analytical sensitivity.
   c. analytical specificity.
   d. basic error of a method.

References

1. Bland JM, Altman DG. Statistical methods for assessing agreement between two methods of clinical measurement. Lancet 1986; 1:307–310.
2. Clinical Laboratory Standards Institute. Evaluation of the linearity of quantitative measurement procedures: a statistical approach; approved guideline. CLSI Document EP06-A, Wayne, Pa: Clinical and Laboratory Standards Institute, 2003.
3. Clinical Laboratory Standards Institute. Method comparison and bias estimation using patient samples; approved guideline, 2nd edition (interim revision). CLSI Document EP9-A2-IR, Wayne, Pa: Clinical and Laboratory Standards Institute, 2010.
4. Clinical Laboratory Standards Institute. User protocol for evaluation of qualitative test performance; approved guideline, 2nd edition. CLSI Document EP12-A2, Wayne, Pa: Clinical and Laboratory Standards Institute, 2008.
5. Dybkær R. Vocabulary for use in measurement procedures and description of reference materials in laboratory medicine. Eur J Clin Chem Clin Biochem 1997;35:141–173.
6. Ellison SLR, Rosslein M, Williams A, eds. Eurachem/Citac guide, CG 4: quantifying uncertainty in analytical measurement, 2nd edition. EURACHEM/CITAC, 2000: 4, 5, 9, 17. www.measurementuncertainty.org (accessed on March 27, 2013).
6A. Farrance I, Frenkel R. Uncertainty of measurement: a review of the rules for calculating uncertainty components through functional relationships. Clin Biochem Rev 2012;33:49–75.
7. Fraser CG. Biological variation: from principles to practice. Washington, DC: AACC Press, 2001:50–54, 133–141.
8. Harris EK, Boyd JC. Statistical bases of reference values in laboratory medicine. New York: Marcel Dekker, 1995:238–250.
9. International Organization for Standardization (ISO). Medical laboratories—particular requirements for quality and competence (15189). Geneva: ISO, 2007.
10. Linnet K. Evaluation of regression procedures for methods comparison studies. Clin Chem 1993;39:424–432.

11. Linnet K. Necessary sample size for method comparison studies based on regression analysis. Clin Chem 1999;45:882–894.

12. Linnet K, Kondratovich M. Partly nonparametric approach for determining the limit of detection. Clin Chem 2004;50:732–740.

13. Passing H, Bablok W. A new biometrical procedure for testing the equality of measurements from two different analytical methods. J Clin Chem Clin Biochem 1983;21:709–720.

14. Petersen PH, Fraser CG, Kallner A, Kenny D, eds. Strategies to set global analytical quality specifications in laboratory medicine. Scand J Clin Lab Invest, 1999;59: 475–585.

15. Vesper HW, Thienpont LM. Traceability in laboratory medicine. Clin Chem 2009;55:1067–1075.

Clinical Evaluation of Methods

Edward R. Ashwood, M.D., and David E. Bruns, M.D.

Objectives

1. Define the following terms:

Likelihood ratio	Sensitivity
Odds ratio	Specificity
Predictive value	True/false positive
Prevalence	True/false negative
Receiver operating characteristic plot	

2. State the formulas for and calculate, given appropriate information, the following: sensitivity, specificity, predictive value for positive/negative tests, odds ratio, and positive/negative likelihood ratio.

3. State the relationship between high sensitivity and false negatives; state the relationship between high specificity and false positives.

4. Compare dichotomous and continuous tests; include definition, sensitivity/specificity, and a clinical example of each type of test.

5. State how the predictive value of a laboratory test is affected by prevalence.

6. Construct and interpret a receiver operating characteristic plot using data from a diagnostic test study.

7. Describe Bayes' theorem, its usefulness in the clinical laboratory, and its main limitation.

8. Write the formula for and calculate with Bayes' theorem the probability of disease given a positive test result.

9. Describe "combination testing" as it is used in the clinical laboratory; include examples, diagnostic usefulness, and associated problems.

Key Words and Definitions

Likelihood ratio The probability of occurrence of a specific test value given that the disease is present divided by the probability of the same test value if the disease was absent.

Odds ratio The probability of the presence of a specific disease divided by the probability of its absence.

Predictive value of a positive test The proportion of subjects with a positive test who have the disease.

Predictive value of a negative test The proportion of subjects with a negative test who do not have the disease.

Prevalence The frequency of disease in the population examined.

Receiver operating characteristic plot A graph of sensitivity versus 1 − specificity for all possible cutoff values of a diagnostic test; used to estimate sensitivity and specificity for various decision cutoffs.

Sensitivity The proportion of subjects with disease who have a positive laboratory test result.

Specificity The proportion of subjects without disease who have a negative laboratory test result.

Whenever a clinician or a healthcare professional uses a laboratory test, he or she needs to have a clear understanding of the clinical performance characteristics of that test. The extent of agreement of test results with accurate patient diagnosis is represented in several ways, including (1) sensitivity and specificity, (2) predictive values, (3) receiver operating characteristic (ROC) curves, and (4) likelihood ratios.

Sensitivity and Specificity

The **sensitivity** of a test reflects the fraction of those with a specified disease that the test correctly predicts. The specificity is the fraction of those without the disease that the test correctly predicts. Table 3-1 shows the classification of unaffected and diseased individuals by test result. *True positives (TPs)* are those diseased individuals who are correctly classified by the test. *False positives (FPs)* are nondiseased individuals misclassified by the test. *False negatives (FNs)* are those diseased patients misclassified by the test. *True negatives (TNs)* are nondiseased patients correctly classified by the test.

$$Sensitivity = \frac{TP}{TP + FN}$$

TABLE 3-1	Classifications of a Test Result Applied to Unaffected and Diseased Populations	
	Number of Patients with Positive Test Result	Number of Patients with Negative Test Result
Number of patients with disease	TP	FN
Number of patients without disease	FP	TN

FN, False negative (number of diseased patients misclassified by the test); *FP,* false positive (number of nondiseased patients misclassified by the test); *TN,* true negative (number of nondiseased patients correctly classified by the test); *TP,* true positive (number of diseased patients correctly classified by the test).

$$Specificity = \frac{TN}{TN + FP}$$

Both high sensitivity (few FNs) and high specificity (few FPs) are desirable characteristics for a test, but one is typically preferred over the other, depending on the clinical situation.

By design, some tests have only positive or negative results and provide qualitative results. These tests, which are termed *dichotomous,* have a single sensitivity and specificity pair for a designated assay cutoff. If a cutoff value is selected to produce high sensitivity, the specificity often will be compromised. Likewise, cutoffs that maximize specificity lower sensitivity.

An example of a dichotomous test is the human immunodeficiency virus (HIV) screening test. This test detects HIV antibodies, producing results that may be nonreactive (negative) or reactive (positive). False positives occur owing to technical errors such as mislabeling or contamination and the presence of cross-reacting antibodies found in individuals such as multiparous women and multiply transfused patients.[10] False negatives occur because of technical problems such as pipetting errors and sampling determinants such as testing in early infection (3 to 4 weeks) before antibody production. Reported sensitivities and specificities for the HIV screening test vary widely,[9] but reasonable estimates are 96% and 99.8%, respectively. Thus, 4 of 100 HIV-infected subjects will test negative. Only 2 of 1000 noninfected subjects will test positive. The clinical usefulness of an HIV test result from an unknown subject will be explained later in the "Probabilistic Reasoning" section.

As opposed to dichotomous tests, *continuous* tests are those that produce quantitative results. Continuous tests have an infinite number of sensitivity and specificity pairs, as the cutoff varies from lowest to highest decision value.

Figure 3-1 is a dot plot of the performance of a continuous assay for prostatic-specific antigen (PSA) in patients with benign prostatic hyperplasia (BPH) and in those with established carcinoma of the prostate (stages A through D).[5] Often continuous tests are used in a dichotomous fashion by choosing one or more decision cutoffs. Note the two dashed lines crossing the graphs that represent two diagnostic cutoffs. Both tests A and B are PSA tests, but they have different decision cutoffs, namely, 4 µg/L and 10 µg/L. When test A is compared

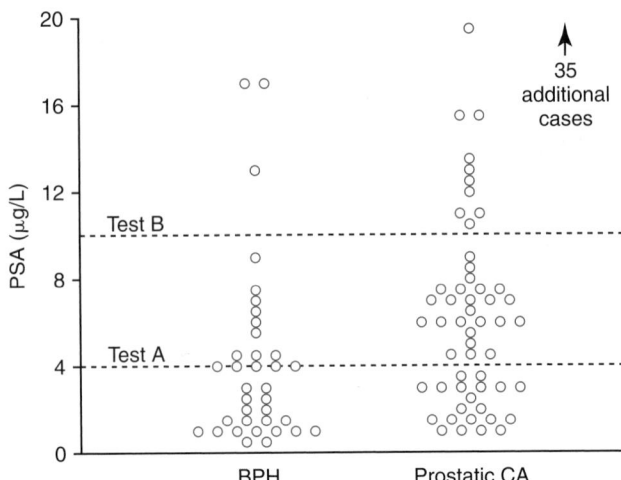

Figure 3-1 Prostate-specific antigen (PSA) concentrations for patients with benign prostatic hyperplasia (BPH) and known prostatic carcinoma (CA) are shown with two decision-level cutoffs.

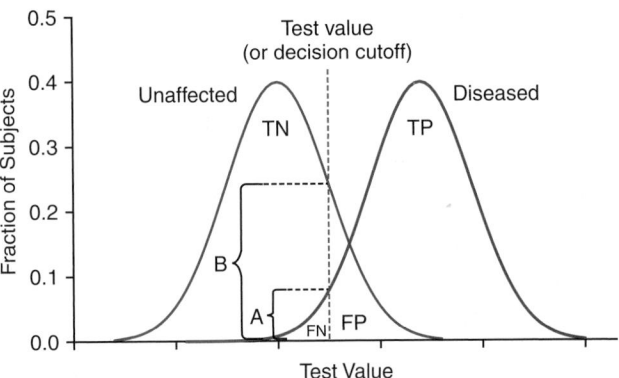

Figure 3-2 Simulated distributions of unaffected and diseased populations. Note that the ratio of diseased patients to healthy patients, A to B, is less than 1 and is very different at the point of decision (the likelihood ratio) from the ratio of TP to FP, which is much greater than 1. *FN,* False negative; *FP,* false positive; *TN,* true negative; *TP,* true positive.

with test B, the decision cutoff of 4 µg/L for test A produces increased sensitivity but at the cost of a decrease in specificity. Thus increased true-positive detection has been traded for an increase in the number of false-positive results. This tradeoff occurs in every test performed in medicine.

Figure 3-2 illustrates a hypothetical test that shows higher results in patients who have a disease compared with those who are unaffected. As the decision cutoff is increased, FPs decrease and FNs increase. At extremely low and extremely high cutoffs, sensitivity and specificity are 100%.

Receiver Operating Characteristic Plots[7]

The dot plot (see Figure 3-1) displays quantitative performance in a limited fashion. For example, one cannot easily estimate sensitivity and specificity for various decision cutoffs using the dot plot. A graphical technique for displaying the same information is called a **receiver operating characteristic (ROC)**

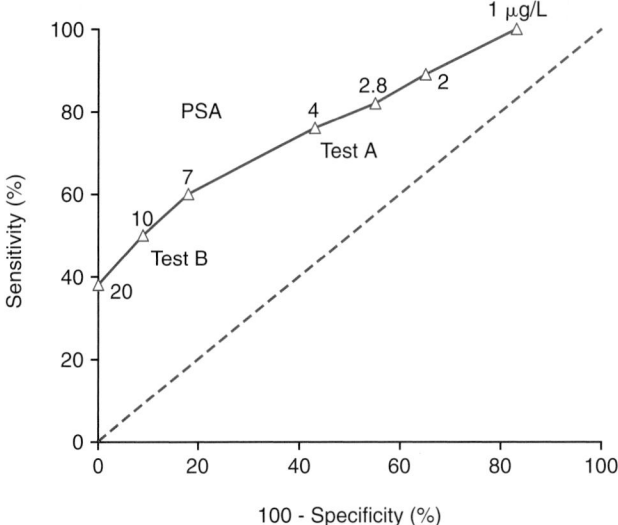

Figure 3-3 Receiver operating characteristic curve of prostate-specific antigen (PSA). Each point on the curve represents a different decision level. The sensitivity and 1 − specificity can be read for tests *A* and *B*, with 4 and 10 μg/L as decision thresholds, respectively.

plot. An ROC curve is generated by plotting sensitivity (*y*-axis) versus 1 − specificity (*x*-axis).[7]

Figure 3-3 shows the ROC curve for the data in Figure 3-1. The *x*-axis plots the fraction of nondiseased patients who were erroneously categorized as positive for a specific decision threshold. This "false-positive rate" is mathematically the same as 1 − specificity. The *y*-axis plots the "true-positive rate" (the sensitivity). A "hidden" third axis is contained within the curve itself: The curve is drawn through points that represent different decision cutoff values. Those decision cutoffs are listed as labels on the curve. The entire curve is a graphical display of the performance of the test.

Tests A and B from Figure 3-3 are displayed as two decision points on the ROC curve. The dotted line extending from the lower left to the upper right represents a test with no discrimination and is designated the random guess line. A curve that is "above" the diagonal line describes performance that is better than random guessing. A curve that extends from the lower left to the upper left and then to the upper right is a perfect test. The area under the curve describes the test's overall performance. The strength of the ROC plot lies in its provision of a meaningful comparison of the diagnostic performance of different tests. In the medical literature, the use of 2 × 2 tables to present the sensitivity and specificity of a test has led to the common logical misconception that a quantitative test has a single sensitivity and specificity. When the initial publication of an assay recommends a cutoff for analysis purposes, the assay is often categorized as sensitive or specific on the basis of this cutoff. Yet, as seen in the ROC curve, every assay will be as sensitive as desired at some cutoff and as specific as desired at another. When two procedures are compared, confusion is avoided by using ROC curves instead of accepting statements such as, "Test A is more sensitive, but test B is more specific."

The area under the ROC curve is a relative measure of a test's performance. A Wilcoxon statistic statistically determines which ROC curve has more area. Area comparisons are particularly helpful when the curves do not intersect. When the ROC curves of two laboratory tests assessing for the same disease intersect, the tests may exhibit different diagnostic performances, even though the areas under the curve are identical. Test performance depends on the region of the curve (e.g., high sensitivity vs. high specificity) chosen.

Probabilistic Reasoning

Although the ROC curve improves our ability to judge a test's performance, a result should not be interpreted in isolation. The clinician must take into account the clinical setting before rendering an interpretation. For example, a positive HIV screening test has a different meaning for an adult as compared with a newborn. In the newborn, antibodies detected by an HIV test are maternal antibodies; thus the result is an indication of the HIV status of the newborn's mother.

Interpretation of almost all laboratory test results is affected by the probability of the disorder before testing. For example, an elevated PSA concentration in a 35-year-old is not interpreted in the same way as in a 70-year-old because the rate of occurrence of prostatic cancer in 35-year-olds is much lower than that in older men.[11] Interpretation must be tempered by knowledge of the prevalence of the disease.

Prevalence

Prevalence is defined as the frequency of disease in the population examined. Several useful techniques have been applied to combine the prevalence with information previously obtained in the results of testing.

Predictive Values

The results of dichotomous tests (and continuous tests used in a dichotomous manner) are interpreted using predictive values. The **predictive value of a positive test** (PV+) is the fraction of subjects with a positive test who have the disease. The **predictive value of a negative test** (PV−) is the fraction of subjects with a negative test who do not have the disease. The predictive value equations are as follows:

$$PV^- = \frac{TN}{TN + FN} \quad PV^+ = \frac{TP}{TP + FP}$$

Predictive values are a function of sensitivity, specificity, and prevalence. It is regrettable that clinicians often confuse sensitivity with PV+. For example, consider a situation where 1,000,000 U.S. residents were randomly chosen and tested for HIV infection using the HIV screening test. The Centers for Disease Control and Prevention estimates that the prevalence of HIV infection in the United States is 330.4 per 100,000 population.[4] On the basis of this prevalence, about 3304 infected individuals would be expected in a population of

1 million. Because the sensitivity of the HIV test is 96%, about 3172 infected individuals would have a positive test result (i.e., TP = 3172). Similarly, because the specificity of the HIV test is 99.8%, about 2 FPs per 1000 subjects would be expected. Thus about 1993 individuals would have false-positive results (i.e., FP = 1993). Therefore, the PV+ is 3172/(3172 + 1993), or 61%. Thus a random individual with a positive test result has a moderate chance of having a false-positive result. Additional testing is necessary to separate TP individuals from FP individuals. Most laboratories automatically test all specimens that have a positive HIV screening result with a confirmatory test such as the HIV Western blot.

In this example, the PV− is much higher than the PV+. Calculations reveal 132 false-negative results (3304 − 3172) and about 994,703 true negatives (99.8% × [1,000,000 − 3304]). Thus, the PV− is 99.987%. Note that many of the FNs could reflect these infected individuals with early HIV infection before antibody development. The limitation of FNs can be overcome by frequent testing of high-risk individuals.

Odds Ratio

The **odds ratio** (OR) is defined as the probability of the presence of a specific disease divided by the probability of its absence. The odds ratio reflects the prevalence of the disease in a population.

$$Odds\ Ratio = \frac{Probability\ of\ event}{1 - Probability\ of\ event}$$

Likelihood Ratio

The **likelihood ratio** (LR) is the probability of occurrence of a specific test value given that the disease is present divided by the probability of the same test value if the disease was absent. Choi[6] describes three different slopes of the ROC curve, which represent LR in different settings (as illustrated in Figure 3-4):

1. The tangent slope, which is equal to the LR of a *continuous* test at a given test value
2. The slope from the origin to a test value equal to a decision cutoff, the LR+ for a positive result of a *dichotomous* test; this slope has a companion slope (which is the slope from the cutoff value to the upper right corner of the ROC plot), which represents the LR− for a negative result of a *dichotomous* test.
3. A slope between any two test values (not illustrated in Figure 3-4), which is termed the *interval* LR and represents the LR of a result that lies between the values; the interval LR is useful for continuous tests that have results grouped into intervals.

For qualitative tests, the *positive likelihood ratio* (LR+) is equal to the sensitivity/(1 − specificity). Conversely, the *negative likelihood ratio* (LR−) is the probability of occurrence of a specific test value given that the disease is absent divided by the probability of the same test value if the disease were present. Thus for qualitative tests, the LR− is specificity/(1 − sensitivity).

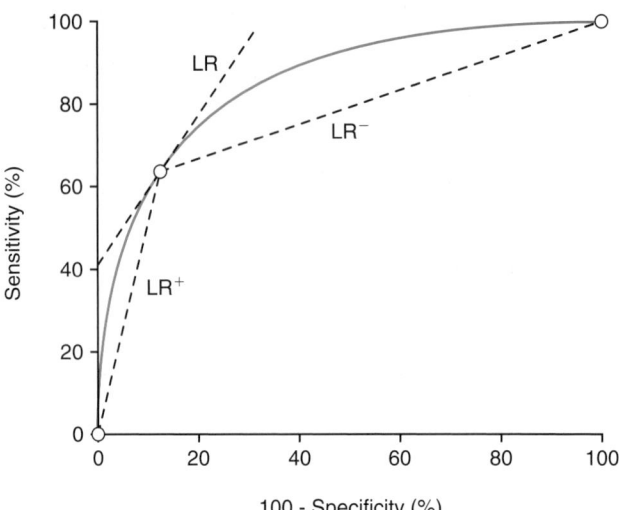

Figure 3-4 Receiver operating characteristic curve illustrating the slopes that define the likelihood ratio (LR) for a continuous test at a specific test result (the gray point) and the positive likelihood ratio (LR+) and the negative likelihood ratio (LR−) of a dichotomous test.[6]

For quantitative tests, the LR is the tangent slope of the ROC curve, which equals the ratio of the heights A and B of the two curves at the test value in Figure 3-2. Note that the areas under each curve in Figure 3-2 are the same. The likelihood ratio does not take disease prevalence or any other prior information into account. To arrive at a final probability, one must adjust for the best estimate of the probability of disease before obtaining the test result.

Bayes' Theorem

Bayes' theorem provides a method of calculating the probability of a disease after new information is added to previously obtained information. The basic theorem is usually written as follows:

$$P(D \mid R) = \frac{P(R \mid D) \times P(D)}{P(R)}$$

where D is disease and R is a positive result. Thus the above equation is "the probability of disease given a particular result is equal to the probability of that result given the disease (i.e., sensitivity) times the probability of disease (i.e., prevalence) divided by the overall probability of having that result." For a dichotomous test, the probability of a positive result is equal to the numerator of the equation plus P(R|not D) × P(not D), or (1 − specificity) × (1 − prevalence). Thus, Bayes' theorem can be rewritten to express the probability of disease given a positive test result as follows:

$$P(D \mid R) = \frac{Sensitivity \times Prevalence}{Sensitivity \times Prevalence + (1 - Specificity) \times (1 - Prevalence)}$$

Bayes' theorem is also applied with the use of the likelihood ratio. The odds ratio of the occurrence of a disease is calculated before the test result is known; this information is then combined with the LR. The final result is again in the form of an odds ratio, which can be converted into a probability, if desired.

$$\text{Odds ratio after testing} = \text{Odds ratio before testing} \\ \times \text{Likelihood ratio of a given test result}$$

The calculation of the post-test probability has also been solved using a convenient nomogram.[3]

Limitations of Bayes' Theorem

Although Bayes' theorem is widely recommended as an aid to refine the probabilistic estimates of disease, it rests on the assumption of *test independence,* which often is not present. As an extreme example of the possible errors that occur when nonindependent tests are used, consider testing the PSA concentration of a BPH patient on three consecutive days. Each day, the PSA value is approximately 10 μg/L. The LR for this result is then estimated from the tangent of the slope at 10 μg/L in Figure 3-2. This slope is approximately 1.2. Using the likelihood form of Bayes' theorem, next multiply the prior odds ratio (assume 10 to 90) by the LR to obtain the odds ratio after 0.13, or a probability of 12% after the first test. The odds ratio is 1.2 × 0.13 = 0.16 after the second test, and finally 0.19 after the third test. This gives a 16% probability of disease. Very little new information has been provided by the second and third tests, yet the probability of disease has apparently increased from 10% to 16%.

Judging independence is difficult without collecting a large set of clinical data and examining them mathematically. A useful approach is to think about the incorrect results given by each test. If both tests tend to yield incorrect results for the same patients, then the tests are not independent, and thus Bayes' theorem cannot be applied to the combination of their results to correctly estimate the probability of disease. If the tests seem intuitively to be independent, then the errors made by assuming independence are likely to be small.

Combination Testing

Panels of tests are commonly used to increase sensitivity and specificity or are used sequentially to decrease costs. For the practicing laboratorian, the value of panels is limited by sparse literature on the performance of combinations of tests. The same issue of test independence addressed in the previous section makes it difficult to calculate the performance of panels of tests. In addition, the use of multiple tests can increase the probability of the occurrence of false-positive or false-negative results, depending on how the tests are combined. The often used maternal serum screening panel described in Chapter 44 uses four tests but combines the results using a log normal covariate distribution model, which adjusts for lack of independence among the tests.[13]

Because most reference intervals exclude a fraction of those patients without disease, there is an expected false-positive rate. As multiple tests are added to panels, the probability

TABLE 3-2	**Combination Test Performance Maximizing Specificity***		
	Sensitivity, %	Specificity, %	Cost
Test A	80	99	$100
Test B	99	80	$100
A followed by B	79.2	99.8	
Prevalence = 0.2			$117
Prevalence = 0.8			$164
B followed by A	79.2	99.8	
Prevalence = 0.2			$136
Prevalence = 0.8			$183

*Results of test A *and* test B must be positive for a positive diagnosis to be made.

of false-positive results increases. Efforts have been made to establish multivariate reference intervals that correct for multiple tests and their interrelationships, but the concept has not found widespread acceptance. Although this concept is mathematically reasonable, those who have investigated the utility of multivariate reference intervals believe that more work is needed before they will prove useful.

The gain in test performance to be achieved by combining test results may be illusory. As demonstrated by the dot plot in Figure 3-1, and by the ROC curve in Figure 3-3, it is possible to increase sensitivity at the expense of decreased specificity. This does not guarantee that the individual test, if the decision threshold were modified to improve sensitivity, would not have comparable performance.

A widely held belief[14] is that one should first test with a sensitive test and then follow up the occurrence of positive results with a specific test for best performance. The logic for this is that if the first test determines which patients are to undergo a second test, the first test should be the more sensitive of the two, to ensure that the disease has not been missed. It is surprising that even when the first test determines which patients will undergo a second test, the order in which the tests are performed does not affect the combination of sensitivity and specificity. However, it does affect the overall cost. In the following examples, two hypothetical tests that are independent are used sequentially. It is assumed that fixed decision limits are used for the two tests and that the two tests cost the same. Although these tests are hypothetical, the principles are generally applicable to other sequential testing situations.

Example 1. Often care is optimized if it is confirmed that a disease is not present. In this case, if screening test A yields a positive result, it will be followed by test B; otherwise, testing stops. If test B yields a positive result, then the overall interpretation is a positive result. Because tests A and B are necessary for the diagnosis, specificity is improved; however, sensitivity decreases compared with the use of test A alone. As shown in Table 3-2, the average cost of the combination varies with disease prevalence; however, note that performance of the more *specific* test first results in lower expected costs. This lower cost would be accentuated if the second test were to cost more than the first.

The net effect of the use of the test combination compared with the use of test A alone has been a fivefold decrease in the

TABLE 3-3	Combination Test Performance Maximizing Sensitivity*		
	Sensitivity, %	Specificity, %	Cost
Test A	80	99	$100
Test B	99	80	$100
A followed by B	99.8	79.2	
Prevalence = 0.2			$183
Prevalence = 0.8			$136
B followed by A	99.8	79.2	
Prevalence = 0.2			$164
Prevalence = 0.8			$117

*Results of test A *or* test B must be positive for a positive diagnosis to be made.

false-positive rate with a decrease of 0.8% in the true-positive rate. Whether this tradeoff is desirable depends on the implications of missing a diagnosis versus generating false-positive results.

Example 2. Diagnosing a curable disease that has a low-cost therapy often increases the relative value of sensitivity over specificity. If the first test result is negative, the second test might still be performed to maximize sensitivity. When either of two tests yields a positive result, this would be interpreted as a positive finding overall. This is more typically seen when tests are done simultaneously, but it also occurs in sequential testing. In Table 3-3, a negative result on the first test is followed by performance of the second test; otherwise, testing ceases. If the result of the second test is negative, the overall interpretation is negative. The cost of performing tests sequentially with this rule varies with prevalence, as can be seen in Table 3-3. When this rule is used, the combination sensitivity increases as the specificity decreases. Note that the strategy of first using the test with *lower* specificity results in lower average cost.

According to the strategy outlined in Table 3-2, the first test's specificity determines the cost of sequential testing. When the strategy is to confirm all negative results of the first test (see Table 3-3), the first test should be the more sensitive, so as to minimize costs. As demonstrated in the two examples presented earlier, the decision rule used preferentially trades off sensitivity at the expense of specificity, or vice versa. Although independent tests have been used in these examples, the conclusions are the same for dependent tests. It should be remembered that it is the interpretive rule and the two tests that determine the overall panel performance and costs; the order of testing does not affect performance but can dramatically affect costs.

Methods of Assessing Diagnostic Accuracy

Most studies of diagnostic accuracy are cross-sectional as opposed to longitudinal, attempting to determine the utility of a test at a single point in time. The results of a new test (often referred to as the *index test,* the test of interest) are compared with those from a "gold standard test" using the same subjects, which is more formally called a *reference standard* (the best current practice for establishing the presence of a disorder). The reference standard often includes many methods of establishing a subject's health status, such as (1) additional laboratory tests, (2) imaging tests, (3) medical history, (4) physical examination, and (5) clinical changes over time.

Around 1980, some investigators realized that most diagnostic accuracy studies contained serious flaws, introducing biases into reported performance characteristics. The work of advocates for improved study design and reporting led to the development of many important assessment tools.[8] Of note are QUADAS (Quality Assessment of Diagnostic Accuracy Studies)[15] and STARD (Standards for Reporting of Diagnostic Accuracy).[1,2] Both QUADAS and STARD are described in greater detail in Chapter 4.

Well-designed studies minimize several sources of bias and variation, including those that affect the selection of study subjects (both patients and controls), verification using the reference standard, observer/technician bias, missing or incomplete patient data, and analysis techniques that affect estimates of diagnostic accuracy. A 2006 meta-analysis concluded that most reported studies have shortcomings that variably affect estimates of diagnostic accuracy.[12] Often, an incomplete study description prevents full assessment of potential sources of bias and variation. Chapter 3 of *Tietz Textbook of Clinical Chemistry and Molecular Diagnostics,* 5th edition, describes how to design a study to assess diagnostic accuracy.

Review Questions

1. A dichotomous laboratory test is one that produces _____ results.
   a. semi-quantitative
   b. quantitative
   c. qualitative
   d. semi-qualitative
2. When a receiver operating characteristic plot is plotted, the *x*-axis plots the:
   a. false-positive rate.
   b. true-positive rate.
   c. false-negative rate.
   d. true-negative rate.
3. The frequency of a disease in a particular population is referred to as its:
   a. predictive value.
   b. likelihood.
   c. probability.
   d. prevalence.
4. The probability of the presence of a specific disease divided by the probability of its absence is the:
   a. likelihood ratio.
   b. odds ratio.
   c. prevalence.
   d. predictive value.
5. True positives /(true positives + false positives) is the formula used to determine the:
   a. predictive value of a positive test.
   b. predictive value of a negative test.
   c. prevalence.
   d. odds ratio.

6. A graphical plot for quantitative analyses that is generated using sensitivity and 1 − specificity and is used to estimate sensitivity and specificity at various decision cutoff values is a:
   a. Bayes' theorem plot.
   b. Levey-Jennings chart.
   c. receiver operating characteristic plot.
   d. dot plot.

7. An important limitation of using Bayes' theorem for determining probabilities of having a particular disease given a specific result is that the theorem assumes:
   a. test dependence.
   b. result independence.
   c. an odds ratio of 50%.
   d. test independence

References

1. Bossuyt PM, Reitsma JB, Bruns DE, Gatsonis CA, Glasziou PP, Irwig LM, et al. Towards complete and accurate reporting of studies of diagnostic accuracy: the STARD initiative. Standards for Reporting of Diagnostic Accuracy. Clin Chem 2003;49:1–6.
2. Bossuyt PM, Reitsma JB, Bruns DE, Gatsonis CA, Glasziou PP, Irwig LM, et al. The STARD statement for reporting studies of diagnostic accuracy: explanation and elaboration. Clin Chem 2003;49:7–18.
3. Boyd JC. Statistical analysis and presentation of data. In: Price CP, Christenson RH, eds. Evidence-based laboratory medicine principles, practice and outcomes, 2nd edtion. Washington DC: AACC Press, 2007:113–140.
4. Centers for Disease Control and Prevention. Cases of HIV infection and AIDS in the United States and dependent areas, by race/ethnicity, 2003-2007. HIV/AIDS Surveillance Supplemental Report 2009;14:1–43.
5. Chan DW. PSA as a marker for prostatic cancer. Lab Mgmt 1988;26:35–39.
6. Choi BC. Slopes of a receiver operating characteristic curve and likelihood ratios for a diagnostic test. Am J Epidemiol 1998;148:1127–1132.
7. Clinical Laboratory Standards Institute. Assessment of the clinical accuracy of laboratory tests using receiver operating characteristic (ROC) plots; approved guideline, 2nd edition. CLSI document GP10-A2. Wayne, Pa: CLSI, 2011.
8. Furukawa TA, Guyatt GH. Sources of bias in diagnostic accuracy studies and the diagnostic process. CMAJ 2006;174:481–482.
9. Guy R, Gold J, Calleja JM, Kim AA, Parekh B, Busch M, et al. Accuracy of serological assays for detection of recent infection with HIV and estimation of population incidence: a systematic review. Lancet Infect Dis 2009;9:747–759.
10. Nuwayhid NF. Laboratory tests for detection of human immunodeficiency virus type 1 infection. Clin Diagn Lab Immunol 1995;2:637–645.
11. Parker SL, Tong T, Bolden S, Wingo PA. Cancer statistics, 1996 CA Cancer J Clin 1996;46:5–27.
12. Rutjes AW, Reitsma JB, Di Nisio M, Smidt N, van Rijn JC, Bossuyt PM. Evidence of bias and variation in diagnostic accuracy studies. CMAJ 2006;174:469–476.
13. Wald NJ, Densem JW, George L, Muttukrishna S, Knight PG. Prenatal screening for Down's syndrome using inhibin-A as a serum marker. Prenat Diagn 1996;16:143–153.
14. Watts NB. Medical relevance of laboratory tests: a clinical perspective. Arch Pathol Lab Med 1988;112:379–382.
15. Whiting P, Rutjes AW, Reitsma JB, Bossuyt PM, Kleijnen J. The development of QUADAS: a tool for the quality assessment of studies of diagnostic accuracy included in systematic reviews. BMC Med Res Methodol 2003;3:25.

Evidence-Based Laboratory Medicine

Christopher P. Price, Ph.D., Patrick M.M. Bossuyt, Ph.D., and David E. Bruns, M.D.

Objectives

1. Define the following terms or acronyms:

Bias	Internal validity
Evidence-based medicine	Meta-analysis
Evidence-based	QALY
laboratory medicine	Quality
External validity	Randomized controlled trial
Index test	STARD

2. State the justification for practicing an evidence-based approach to medicine and evidence-based laboratory medicine; list and describe the five major needs in evidence-based laboratory medicine studies.
3. State the four diagnostic questions addressed by the decision-making process in laboratory medicine.
4. Compare and contrast internal and external validity in relation to a diagnostic accuracy study.
5. Discuss the STARD initiative, including its uses, its components, and its application in the clinical laboratory.
6. Explain the need for and describe the different types of outcome studies in medical practice; compare outcome studies with prognostic value studies.
7. Design a mock randomized controlled trial, including subjects, treatments or interventions, and measurable outcomes.
8. List and describe the key steps of a systematic review of a diagnostic test.
9. List and describe five methods of evaluating the economic impact of a diagnostic test; state how economic evaluations are perceived by patients, laboratory practitioners, clinicians, insurance companies, and society.
10. State the need for clinical practice guidelines and clinical audits; list the steps involved in preparing clinical practice guidelines and problems that might be involved in these steps; list and describe the four components of a clinical audit.

Key Words and Definitions

Bias Systematic error that occurs when there is constant overestimation or underestimation of a measured value as opposed to random error, which is unpredictable.

Clinical audit A review of case histories of patients against the benchmark of current best practice; used as a tool to improve clinical practice.

Clinical practice guidelines Systematically developed statements to assist practitioner and patient decisions about appropriate healthcare for specific clinical circumstances; in the laboratory, goals for accuracy, precision, and turnaround times of tests are included.

Clinical reference standard The best available method for establishing the presence or absence of the target condition; also, the suspected condition or disease for which the target is to be applied.

Diagnostic accuracy The closeness of agreement between values obtained from a diagnostic test (index test) and those of reference standard (gold standard) for a specific disease or condition; these results are expressed in a number of ways, including sensitivity and specificity, predictive values, likelihood ratios, diagnostic odds ratios, and areas under receiver operating characteristic (ROC) curves.

Evidence-based medicine The conscientious, judicious, and explicit use of best evidence in making decisions about the care of individual patients.

Evidence-based laboratory medicine The application of principles and techniques of evidence-based medicine to laboratory medicine; the conscientious, judicious, and explicit use of best evidence in laboratory medicine investigations to assist decision making about the care of individual patients.

Index test In diagnostic accuracy studies, the "new" test or the test of interest.

Outcomes Results related to the quality or quantity of life of patients; examples include mortality, functional status, quality of life, and well-being.

Outcomes studies Studies performed to determine whether a medical intervention (such as a specific laboratory test) will improve patient outcomes.

Key Words and Definitions—cont'd

Randomized controlled trial An experimental study in which study participants are randomly allocated to an intervention (treatment) group or an alternative treatment (control) group.

STARD Standards for Reporting of Diagnostic Accuracy; a project designed to improve the quality of reporting of the results of diagnostic accuracy studies.

Systematic review A methodical and comprehensive review of all published and unpublished information about a specific topic to answer a precisely defined clinical question.

In this chapter, we review the new influences on clinical chemistry and laboratory medicine from the fields of clinical epidemiology and evidence-based medicine (EBM). Key chapter topics include the following:

- How to assess the diagnostic accuracy of tests
- How to use clinical outcomes studies.
- Ways to evaluate the economic value of medical tests.
- How to conduct systematic reviews of diagnostic tests.
- How to use clinical practice guidelines.
- When and how to conduct a clinical audit.

These principles provide a foundation for the rational and appropriate use of diagnostic tests.

Clinical chemists/laboratorians must know (1) how to select tests based on their analytical performance, (2) how well tests perform as diagnostic or prognostic tests, and (3) how use of tests affects the care of patients. Clinical epidemiologists have developed study designs to quantify the diagnostic (and prognostic) accuracy of the tests employed in laboratory medicine. They have also developed study methods that can be used to evaluate the value of laboratory testing and its effect on patient outcomes and, more broadly, on healthcare. Practitioners of Evidence Based Medicine (EBM) focus on using the best available evidence from such well-designed studies in the care of individual patients. In practice, EBM does the following:

- Rephrases problems as structured clinical questions in the clinical care of patients.
- Looks for (or develops) available evidence.
- Evaluates the quality of that evidence (clinical studies).
- Evaluates the clinical implications of the results (including the impact of changes in practice).
- Provides tools to help clinicians use those results, both effectively and efficiently, in the care of individual patients.

Today, these principles are applied in decisions about whether or not to introduce new tests, as well as in the audit of utilization of tests (see later in chapter).

Evidence-Based Medicine—What Is It?

Since the term **evidence-based medicine** was introduced in 1991, EBM has had an important influence on medicine.

Definition and Goals of Evidence-Based Medicine

In this chapter, EBM is defined as "the conscientious, judicious, and explicit use of the best evidence in making decisions about the care of individual patients."[11] The word *judicious* implies the use of skills of experienced clinicians to put evidence in context and to recognize patient individuality and preferences. A goal of EBM is "to incorporate the best evidence from clinical research into clinical decisions."[5] The word *best* implies the necessity for critical appraisal. The words *making decisions* indicate why the principles of EBM must be applied in laboratory medicine, as laboratory medicine is one of the fundamental tools used in making decisions in the practice of medicine.

Justifications for an evidence-based approach to medicine are founded in the following: (1) constant requirement for information; (2) constant addition of new information; (3) recognition of poor quality of access to good information; (4) decline in up-to-date knowledge and/or expertise with advancing years of an individual clinician's practice; (5) limited time available to read the literature; and (6) variability in the values and preferences of individual patients. To this one might add, specifically in relation to laboratory medicine, (1) limited number and poor quality of studies linking test results to patient benefits, (2) poor appreciation of the value of diagnostic tests, (3) relatively limited integration of laboratory medicine services into the care pathway, as witnessed by poor adherence to clinical practice guidelines, (4) ever-increasing demand for tests, and (5) disconnected approach to resource allocation (reimbursement) in laboratory medicine—"silo budgeting," which addresses only laboratory costs without consideration of benefit outside the laboratory. Silo budgeting forces healthcare staff to make decisions that save expense in the laboratory but provide insufficient attention to the needs of patients, caregivers, and payers. Silo budgeting also stifles innovation and inhibits change. EBM is a rational counterforce.

The Practice of Evidence-Based Medicine

Guyatt and colleagues[5] summarized the practice of EBM as follows: "An evidence-based practitioner must (1) understand the patient's circumstances or predicament; (2) identify knowledge gaps and frame questions to fill those gaps; (3) conduct an efficient literature search; (4) critically appraise the research evidence; and (5) apply that evidence to patient care." Glasziou and colleagues described a key objective of EBM as "…trying to improve the quality of the information on which decisions are based," and pointed out that EBM was "…not about mechanisms, but about outcomes…"[4]

Efficient practice of EBM requires the following:

- Knowledge of the *clinical process* and conversion of a clinical need into an answerable question.

- A facility that can generate and critically appraise information to generate knowledge.
- A critically appraised knowledge resource.
- Ability to use that knowledge resource.
- Means of accessing and delivering the knowledge resource.
- Means of assessing application of the knowledge.
- A framework of clinical and economic accountability.
- A framework of quality management.

Evidence-Based Medicine and Laboratory Medicine

The services of laboratory medicine are important tools at the disposal of clinicians for answering diagnostic questions and making decisions.

The tools provided by laboratory medicine are called *diagnostic tests,* but these tests are used for much more than making a diagnosis. As mentioned previously and discussed later, diagnostic tests are also used in (1) making a prognosis, (2) excluding a diagnosis, (3) selecting, (4) guiding, and (5) monitoring a treatment or disease process, and (6) screening for disease. Thus the word *diagnostic* is used in a much broader sense. An alternative phrase would be a *medical test.*

What Is Evidence-Based Laboratory Medicine?

Evidence-based laboratory medicine is the application to laboratory medicine of the principles and techniques of EBM and clinical epidemiology. A clinician or healthcare provider who requests an investigation has a question and must make a decision. These providers hope that the test result will help them answer the question and will assist them in making decisions. Thus a definition of evidence-based laboratory medicine could be "the conscientious, judicious, and explicit use of best evidence from laboratory medicine investigations in decision making about the care of individual patients." It might also be expressed more directly in terms of health outcomes as "ensuring that the best evidence obtained on testing is made available and the clinician is assisted in using the best evidence to ensure that the best decisions are made about the care of individual patients, leading to an increased probability of improved health outcomes." Clearly, this discussion makes the assumption that appropriate action is taken once the decision is made. As is discussed later, outcomes may be (1) clinical, (2) operational, and/or (3) economic.

Types of Diagnostic Questions Addressed in Laboratory Medicine

The decision-making process involves one of four scenarios (Figure 4-1), typified by questions such as these:
- What is the diagnosis?
- Can another diagnosis be ruled out?
- What is this patient's prognosis and disease severity?
- What is the most appropriate treatment intervention?
- How is the patient doing?

In the first scenario, a diagnosis is being sought. Diagnostic conclusions lead to a decision and to some form of action,

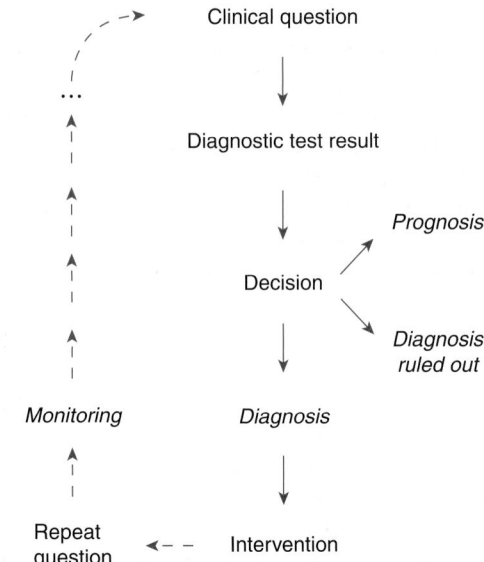

Figure 4-1 Schematic representation of four common decision-making steps in which the result of an investigation is involved.

which often involves an intervention designed to improve outcomes. Thus, when a test for acetaminophen reveals a dangerously high concentration of the drug, administration of *N*-acetyl cysteine will reduce the risk of a fatal outcome. The measurement of acetaminophen in this scenario is referred to as a "rule-in test."

In the second scenario, the test result excludes a diagnosis; this is referred to as a "rule-out test." For example, when a patient is admitted with chest pain and acute myocardial infarction is suspected, a finding that cardiac troponin is undetectable in plasma may be used to rule out acute myocardial necrosis.

The third use of an investigation is for prognosis, which may be considered as the assessment of risk and complements the diagnostic application. For example, measurement of the concentration of human immunodeficiency virus (HIV) RNA in plasma after the initial diagnosis of HIV infection has been used to predict the time interval before immune collapse if the condition is not treated. The test result is used in a similar way to stratify the patient according to disease severity, which may influence the treatment strategy. For example, a patient with diabetes and a hemoglobin A_{1c} (HbA_{1c}) result of 69 mmol/mol (8.5%) may be treated differently than a patient with HbA_{1c} of 55 mmol/mol (7.2%). The fourth and fifth uses of a test result are concerned with patient management, which consists of treatment selection and optimization, and then treatment monitoring. For example, in a patient with breast cancer, a tissue test for Her-2/neu is required to determine candidacy for use of the drug Herceptin. In the case of a patient with a chronic disease, the test result may be used to assist in optimizing and assessing the effectiveness of an intervention, which will also include assessing patient compliance. For example, in a person with diabetes, HbA_{1c} measurements are used to assess glycemic control and thus the effectiveness of therapy. If HbA_{1c} is high, changing treatment should be considered. If HbA_{1c} is not elevated, the current treatment should be maintained. Tests employed in this way are often referred to as "companion diagnostics"; they help to provide "personalized medicine".

In each of these examples, three components are present: (1) a *question,* (2) a *decision,* and (3) an *action.* Identifying these three components proves to be critical in designing studies of outcomes of testing (see later in this chapter). These components are also important in auditing (see later) the use of investigations from the viewpoints of both clinical and financial governance. Recognition of this triad has led to the definition of an *appropriate test request* as one in which there is a clear clinical *question* for which the result will provide an answer, enabling the clinician to make a *decision* and to initiate some form of *action,* leading to a health benefit for the patient. This benefit is extended to the healthcare provider and to society as a whole to encompass more completely the potential for operational and economic benefit.

Examples of questions that specify the amount of detail required to accurately qualify the use of a test result are given in Table 4-1. Criteria for introducing a screening test have been identified for many years but with some degree of variation; one of the key criteria is that valid treatment must be available; furthermore, the combination of test and treatment should do more good than harm.

Using the Test Result

The key criterion for a useful *diagnostic* test is that the result leads to a change in the probability of the presence of the target condition. The change in probability does not, in itself, make the decision. The clinician must use this information along with other findings and clinical judgment to make decisions or recommendations about care.

Test Results Alone Do Not Produce Clinical Outcomes

In most cases, testing must be followed by an appropriate intervention to produce a desired outcome. A test result alone may provide reassurance or an understanding of the origin of one's complaint, but even this may require explanation and further reassurance from a physician or healthcare provider. The value of a test is assessed only by looking at its impact on the patient's health.[3] Because of the difficulty involved in documenting that testing improves patient outcomes, most research in laboratory medicine addresses only the analytical characteristics and diagnostic performance of tests, not the effects of tests on patients' lives. This restricted research leads to a poor understanding and appreciation of the contribution that the test result makes to improved outcomes. For example, a randomized study of a rapid chest pain evaluation protocol that shows that normal results for cardiac markers ruled out myocardial infarction does not address the question of whether testing leads to fewer admissions to the coronary care unit with decreased morbidity and mortality. The consequence of this argument is that the impact of a test on an outcome should be evaluated as a "test-and-act," or "test-and-treat," intervention.

Information Needs in Evidence-Based Laboratory Medicine

Studies in the field of evidence-based laboratory medicine are of five major types:
1. Characterization of the *diagnostic accuracy* of tests by studying groups of patients.
2. Determination of the value of testing for people who are tested *(outcomes).*
3. *Systematic review* of studies of diagnostic accuracy or outcomes of tests to answer a specific clinical question.
4. *Economic evaluation* of tests to assess the economic value of using the test.
5. *Audit* of performance of tests during use to answer questions about their use.

Increasingly, researchers in laboratory medicine are beginning to use computer-based modeling techniques to assess

TABLE 4-1	**Examples of Clinical Questions for Which a Laboratory Assessment May Be of Value, and the Associated Action and Potential Outcome (Benefit)**			
Test	**Question**	**Result**	**Possible Action**	**Potential Outcome**
Rule In TSH	Does this child have hypothyroidism?	12.2 mU/L	Treat with thyroxine	Decreased morbidity and mortality
Rule Out BNP	Is this breathless patient suffering from heart failure?	56 ng/L	Seek alternative diagnosis	Avoid incorrect diagnosis and treatment with their potential for harm
Monitoring HbA$_{1c}$	Is patient complying with treatment protocol?	92 mmol/mol (10.6%) (no change in a year)	Consider changing treatment, closer monitoring of compliance, clinic visits and consultations with diabetes nurse	Persistently high HbA$_{1c}$ carries increased risk of complications; intervention necessary to decrease risk
Prognosis cTnI	What is this patient's risk of a further cardiac event?	0.9 μg/L	Consider intervention	Increased risk without intervention

BNP, B-type natriuretic peptide; *cTnI,* cardiac troponin I; *HbA$_{1c}$,* hemoglobin A$_{1c}$; *TSH,* thyroid-stimulating hormone.

the cost-effectiveness of tests, as well as to assess the impact of process changes on resource utilization. The following sections of this chapter provide brief introductions to the principles of how to gain these critical types of information, which are needed for patient care.

Characterization of Diagnostic Accuracy of Tests

When a new test is developed or an old test is applied to a new clinical question, users need information about the extent of agreement of the test's results with the correct diagnoses of patients. We refer to such studies as **diagnostic accuracy** studies.

Study Design

In studies of diagnostic accuracy, the results of one test (often referred to as the **index test,** the test of interest) are compared with those from the clinical reference standard—the best current practice to arrive at a diagnosis. A reference standard is any method that is used to obtain additional information on a patient's health status. Methods include (1) laboratory tests, (2) imaging tests, (3) function tests, (4) data from the history and physical examination, and (5) genetic data.

The **clinical reference standard** is the best available method of establishing the presence or absence of the target condition—the suspected condition or disease for which the test is to be applied. The reference standard can be a single test or can consist of a combination of methods and techniques, including clinical follow-up of tested patients. In some cases, it is the independent opinion of two experts in the field, as in the case of the diagnosis of heart failure.

There are several potential threats to the internal and external validity of a study of diagnostic accuracy, of which only the major ones will be addressed in this section. Poor *internal validity* (problems in the design of the study) will produce **bias,** or systematic error, because the estimates of diagnostic accuracy differ from those one would have obtained using an optimal design for the study. Poor *external validity* limits the "extent" to which clinical research studies apply to broader populations. A research study has external validity if its results can be generalized to the larger population (Agency for Health Research and Quality Effective Health Care Program; http://effectivehealthcare.ahrq.gov/index.cfm/glossary-of-terms/?pageaction=showterm&termid=26; accessed July 5, 2013).

The ideal diagnostic accuracy study examines a consecutive series of patients by enrolling all consenting patients suspected of the target condition within a specific period. All patients undergo the index test and are evaluated by the reference standard. The term *consecutive* refers to the total absence of any form of selection beyond the definition (determined at the start of the study) of the criteria for inclusion in the study (and exclusion); explicit efforts are required to identify and enroll all patients who qualify for inclusion.

Alternative designs are possible. Some studies first select patients known to have the target condition and then contrast the study results of these patients with those of patients from

a control group. This approach has been used to characterize the performance of tests in settings in which the condition of interest is uncommon, as in maternal serum screening tests for detection of Down syndrome in the fetus. It is also used in preliminary studies to assess the potential of a test before prospective studies of a series of patients are begun. With this design, the selection of the control group is critical. If the control group consists of healthy individuals only, the diagnostic accuracy of the test will tend to be overestimated. The control group should include patients in whom the disease is suspected but has been ruled out.

In the ideal study, the results of all patients in whom the test under evaluation has been performed are contrasted with the results of a single reference standard. If the reference standard is not applied to all patients, partial verification is the result. In a typical case, some patients with negative test results (test-negatives) are not verified by an expensive or invasive reference standard, and those patients are excluded from the analysis. This may result in an underestimation of the number of false-negative results.

A different form of verification bias happens if more than one reference standard is used, and the two reference standards correspond to different manifestations of disease. This study design can produce *differential verification bias.* Suppose the diagnoses in test-positive patients are verified through further testing, but the diagnoses in test-negative patients are verified by clinical follow-up. An example is the verification of suspected appendicitis, with histopathology of the appendix versus follow-up as the two forms of the reference standard. A patient is classified as having a false-positive test result if the additional test does not confirm the presence of disease after a positive index test result. Alternatively, a patient is classified as false-negative if an event compatible with appendicitis is observed during follow-up after a negative test result. Yet these are different definitions of disease because not all patients who have positive test results by the reference standard would have experienced an event during follow-up if they had been left untreated. The use of two reference standards, one pathological and the other based on follow-up, can affect the assessment of diagnostic accuracy and usually leads to inflated estimates of accuracy.[6] This approach also leads to variability among studies when studies differ in the proportions of patients verified by each of the two standards.

Should clinical information be provided to those performing or reading the index test for the study of its diagnostic accuracy? For example, should the radiologist reading the new type of x-ray image know the results of prior tests on the patient? Withholding this information is known as *blinding* or *masking.* Some clinical information is often routinely known by the reader of the test, as when a pathologist is told the site from which a biopsy is obtained. To try to withhold such information in the context of a study of diagnostic accuracy may create an artificial scenario that has no counterpart in routine patient care. For most study questions, however, masking is preferable because knowledge of the results will tend to increase agreement of the results of the studied (index) test with those of the reference standard (test).

Severity of disease in studied patients with the target condition and the range of other conditions in other patients (controls) can affect the apparent diagnostic accuracy of a test. For example, if a test that is designed to detect early cancer is evaluated in patients with clinically apparent cancer, the test is likely to perform better than when used for persons who do not yet show signs of the condition. This problem has been called *spectrum bias*. Similarly, if a test is developed to distinguish patients with the target condition from patients with a similar condition, it may be misleading to use healthy subjects as controls, rather than patients with similar symptoms, when the diagnostic accuracy of the test is evaluated.

Reporting of Studies of Diagnostic Accuracy and the Role of the STARD Initiative

Complete and accurate reporting of studies of diagnostic accuracy should allow the reader to detect the potential for bias in the study and to assess the ability to generalize the results and their applicability to an individual patient or group. In fact, most studies of diagnostic accuracy published in leading general medical journals either showed poor adherence to standards of clinical epidemiologic research or failed to provide information about adherence to those standards. This deficiency led to efforts at the journal *Clinical Chemistry* in 1997 to produce a checklist for reporting of studies of diagnostic accuracy. After this checklist was introduced, the quality of reporting improved in that journal but not in another journal that did not use the checklist.

In 1999, Lijmer et al[6] showed that poor study design and poor reporting are associated with overestimates of the diagnostic accuracy of evaluated tests. This report reinforced the necessity to improve the reporting of studies of diagnostic accuracy for all types of tests, not only those in clinical chemistry. This led to the STARD initiative on Standards for Reporting of Diagnostic Accuracy.

Key components of the STARD document[1] include a checklist of items to be included in reports of studies of diagnostic accuracy and a diagram to document the flow of participants in the study. The checklist contains 25 items that are worth reading and understanding (Figure 4-2). The flow diagram (Figure 4-3) communicates vital information about the *design* of a study—including the method of recruitment and the order of test execution—and about the *flow* of participants.

The STARD document has been endorsed by numerous journals, including all the major journals of clinical chemistry and general medicine. A separate document, referenced in STARD, explains the meaning and rationale of each item and briefly summarizes the available evidence. Most if not all of the content of STARD also applies to studies of tests used for prognosis, monitoring, or screening.

Outcomes Studies

Medical and public health interventions are intended to improve the health of (1) patients, (2) the population at large, or (3) population segments. In terms of therapeutic interventions, patients are interested not only in whether a drug decreases serum cholesterol or blood pressure (risk factors) but, more important, whether it decreases the risk of (1) heart attack, (2) stroke, and (3) cardiovascular death. On the diagnostic side of medicine, most patients have little interest in knowing their serum cholesterol concentration unless that knowledge will lead to actions that improve their quality and/or quantity of life. People want improved outcomes, and healthcare providers and policymakers are increasingly demanding evidence of improved outcomes.

What Are Outcomes Studies?

Outcomes may be defined as results of medical interventions in terms of health or cost; they are often described in terms of (1) clinical, (2) operational, and (3) economic outcomes. "Patient outcomes" are outcomes that are associated with the patient's condition and experience. Examples of outcomes include (1) mortality, (2) morbidity, (3) complication rates, (4) length of stay in the hospital, (5) waiting times at a clinic, (6) cost of care, and (7) patient satisfaction with care. An improved test will improve outcomes when the outcomes depend on making the correct diagnosis. Improved outcomes may be difficult to establish, however, if no effective treatment is available for the diagnosed condition, or if the condition and the conditions with which it is confused are treated in the same way.

Some tests are used as surrogate outcome markers in intervention studies when a strong relationship has been documented between the test result and morbidity or mortality. Examples include the use of HbA_{1c} and the urine albumin-to-creatinine ratio in studies on the management of diabetes mellitus.

Operational and economic outcomes are results of interest to patient care providers, purchasers, and policy makers. A correct diagnosis often saves money. Much recent interest has been focused on rates of re-admission to the hospital for patients with heart failure. Some patients diagnosed with heart failure are suffering from lung disease and vice versa; failure to diagnose and treat the condition that the patient actually has leads to costly re-admissions. Proper use of diagnostically accurate tests reduces these costs. Proper testing also reduces the length of hospital stay, and thus cost, by facilitating early diagnosis and treatment. Point-of-care testing (POCT) in doctors' offices may save patients money by avoiding the need to travel to a laboratory facility.

Outcomes studies must be distinguished from studies of prognosis. Studies of the prognostic value of a test ask the question, "Can the test be used to predict an outcome?" By contrast, outcomes studies ask questions such as, "Does use of the test improve outcomes?" For example, a study of the prognostic ability of a test might ask the question, "Does the concentration of a cardiac troponin I in serum correlate with the mortality rate after myocardial infarction?" An outcomes study might ask, "Is the mortality rate of patients with suspected myocardial infarction decreased when physicians use troponin testing to guide decisions?"

Many test attributes are amenable to studies of outcomes. Such studies address not only the effect of making a test

Section and Topic	Item #		On page #
TITLE/ABSTRACT/ KEYWORDS	1	Identify the article as a study of diagnostic accuracy (recommend MeSH heading sensitivity and specificity).	
INTRODUCTION	2	State the research questions or study aims, such as estimating diagnostic accuracy or comparing accuracy between tests or across participant groups.	
METHODS		Describe	
Participants	3	The study population: The inclusion and exclusion criteria, setting, and locations where the data were collected.	
	4	Participant recruitment: Was recruitment based on presenting symptoms, results from previous tests, or the fact that the participants had received the index tests or the reference standard?	
	5	Participant sampling: Was the study population a consecutive series of participants defined by the selection criteria in items 3 and 4? If not, specify how participants were further selected.	
	6	Data collection: Was data collection planned before the index test and reference standard were performed (prospective study) or after (retrospective study)?	
Test methods	7	The reference standard and its rationale.	
	8	Technical specifications of material and methods involved, including how and when measurements were taken, and/or cite references for index tests and reference standard.	
	9	Definition of and rationale for the units, cutoffs, and/or categories of the results of the index tests and the reference standard.	
	10	The number, training, and expertise of the persons executing and reading the index tests and the reference standard.	
	11	Whether or not the readers of the index tests and reference standard were blind (masked) to the results of the other test and describe any other clinical information available to the readers.	
Statistical methods	12	Methods for calculating or comparing measures of diagnostic accuracy, and the statistical methods used to quantify uncertainty (e.g., 95% confidence intervals).	
	13	Methods for calculating test reproducibility, if done.	
RESULTS		Report	
Participants	14	When study was done, including beginning and ending dates of recruitment.	
	15	Clinical and demographic characteristics of the study population (e.g., age, sex, spectrum of presenting symptoms, comorbidity, current treatments, recruitment centers).	
	16	The number of participants satisfying the criteria for inclusion that did or did not undergo the index tests and/or the reference standard; describe why participants failed to receive either test (a flow diagram is strongly recommended).	
Test results	17	Time interval from the index tests to the reference standard, and any treatment administered between.	
	18	Distribution of severity of disease (define criteria) in those with the target condition; other diagnoses in participants without the target condition.	
	19	A cross tabulation of the results of the index tests (including indeterminate and missing results) by the results of the reference standard; for continuous results, the distribution of the test results by the results of the reference standard.	
	20	Any adverse events from performing the index tests or the reference standard.	
Estimates	21	Estimates of diagnostic accuracy and measures of statistical uncertainty (e.g., 95% confidence intervals).	
	22	How indeterminate results, missing responses, and outliers of the index tests were handled.	
	23	Estimates of variability of diagnostic accuracy between subgroups of participants, readers, or centers, if done.	
	24	Estimates of test reproducibility, if done.	
DISCUSSION	25	Discuss the clinical applicability of the study findings.	

Figure 4-2 STARD checklist.

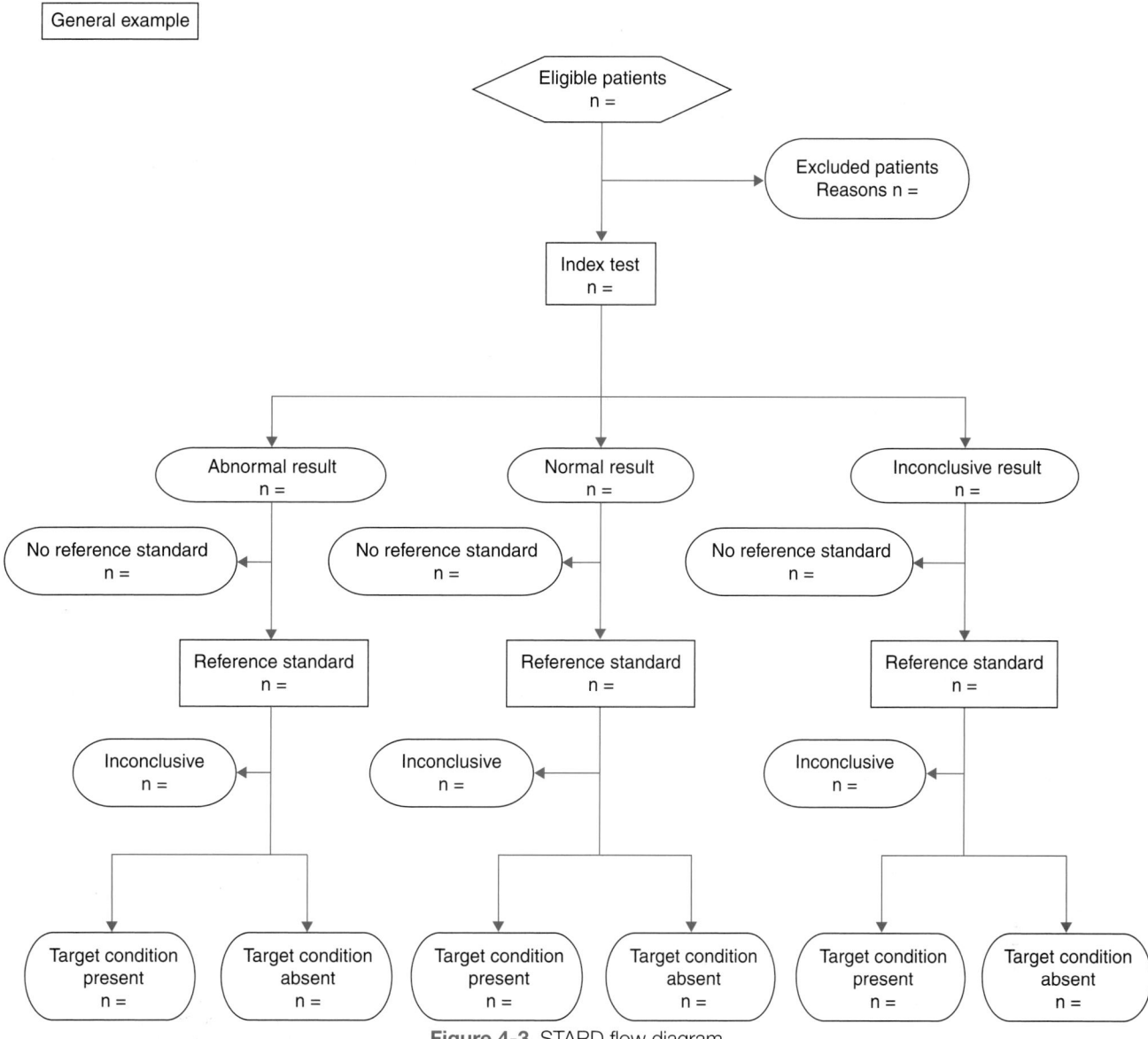

Figure 4-3 STARD flow diagram.

available but also such attributes of tests as (1) the method used to obtain a measurement, (2) the analytical quality of the test performance, (3) turnaround time (as for POCT in the emergency department), (4) the method of reporting test results (e.g., rapid reporting of life-threatening results), and (5) reporting of results with or without extensive interpretation.

Why Outcomes Studies?

Outcomes studies have taken on considerable importance in medicine. On the therapeutic side of medicine, few drugs are approved by modern government agencies (or paid for by healthcare organizations or health insurers) without strong evidence of their safety and effectiveness. Increasingly, diagnostic testing is entering a similar environment, in which individuals or institutions such as (1) physicians, (2) health-care providers, (3) governments, (4) commercial health insurers, and (5) patients demand evidence of effectiveness of diagnostic procedures. To appreciate this, one need

only recall the enormous interest in controversies about the value of mammography and the effectiveness of measuring serum prostate-specific antigen (PSA) in population programs. These issues (and many others) hinge on studies of outcomes.

In the United States, the Joint Commission has defined *quality* as increased probability of desired *outcomes* and decreased probability of undesired *outcomes*. If a healthcare organization, or a unit of it, such as the clinical laboratory, wishes to propose that its quality is high, or that it contributes to the quality of the institution, the message is clear: Demonstrate improved outcomes.

Design of Studies of Medical Outcomes

The **randomized controlled trial (RCT)** is the de facto standard for studies of the health effects of medical interventions. In these studies, patients are randomly assigned to receive either the intervention to be tested (such as a new drug or a new test) or an alternative (typically either a placebo or a conventional drug or test), and an outcome is measured. RCTs have been used to evaluate (1) therapeutic interventions, including drugs, (2) radiation therapy, (3) surgical interventions, and (4) others. Measured outcomes vary from (1) hard measures, such as mortality and morbidity, to (2) softer measures, such as patient-reported satisfaction, or (3) surrogate measures, typified by markers of disease activity (e.g., HbA_{1c}, serum creatinine, urine albumin-to-creatinine ratio).

The high impact of RCTs of therapeutic interventions has led to scrutiny of how they are conducted and reported. An interdisciplinary group (largely editors of medical journals and clinical epidemiologists) developed a guideline known as CONSORT (Consolidated Standards for Reporting Trials)[13] for the conduct of these studies. Although initially designed for trials of therapies, CONSORT provides useful reminders for those designing or appraising outcomes studies of tests in clinical chemistry. As for STARD, the key features of the CONSORT guidelines include a checklist of items to include in the report and a flow diagram of patients in the study.

The optimal design for an RCT of a diagnostic test is not always obvious. A classic design is to randomly assign patients to receive a test or not receive it, and then to take clinical action (from conventional therapy to a different therapy) based on the test result in the tested patients. However, this approach leads to problems in interpretation.[7] For example, if the new therapy is always effective, the tested group will always fare better, even if the test is a coin-toss, because only the tested group had access to the new therapy. The conclusion that the testing was valuable would thus be wrong. By contrast, if the new therapy is always worse than the conventional treatment, patients in the tested group will do worse, and the test will be judged worse than useless, no matter how diagnostically accurate it is. Similarly, if the two treatments are equally effective, the outcomes will be the same with or without testing; this scenario, too, will lead to the conclusion that the test is not good, no matter how diagnostically accurate it is. When a truly better therapy becomes available, the test may prove to be valuable, so it is important to not discount the test's potential based on a study with a new therapy that offers no advantage over the old therapy.

If the treatment choice remains the same in the two arms of a study, these problems do not arise, for example, when a test done in a clinic is compared with a similar (or identical) test done in a laboratory, the treatment choices would not be expected to change. In all cases, however, it is crucial to evaluate the combination of test and treatment as a single intervention.

Alternative designs have been described to address the question of test use in an RCT.[7] In one design, all patients undergo the new test, but the results are hidden during the trial. Patients are randomly assigned to receive or not receive the new therapy. In this design, the new test should be adopted only if a benefit is associated with switching to the new therapy in a subgroup of test results. The test should not be adopted if all patients tested benefit sufficiently, or if none of those tested in the trial benefits sufficiently.

Unfortunately an RCT is not always feasible, and an alternative is used. These studies include those that use historical or contemporaneous control patients in whom the intervention was not undertaken. Uncertainty about the comparability of controls and patients with such designs is a threat to the validity of these studies. Another approach is to use the "before-and-after" approach, that is, to compare clearly identified outcome measures using the existing diagnostic approach with outcome measures after introduction of the new diagnostic (test) approach. Again, problems have been associated with this approach, one of which involves ensuring that the spectrum of patients is similar in both phases of the study. Handling confounders is a challenge, and statistical techniques to improve comparability, such as the use of propensity scores, are considered.

In making decision about whether the results of an **outcome study** are relevant to one's own situation or hospital, it is essential to evaluate if one's situation is comparable with that of the setting where the study was done. Results of outcomes studies performed at a referral hospital may not apply in a community hospital (different spectrum of disease); results of outcomes studies that were done exclusively in men may not apply in women; etc.

Systematic Reviews of Diagnostic Tests

Systematic reviews, in contrast to traditional narrative reviews, aim to answer an exactly defined clinical question and to do so in a way that is transparent and designed to minimize bias. Some of the defining features of systematic reviews are (1) a clear definition of the clinical question to be addressed; (2) an extensive and explicit strategy to find all studies (published or unpublished) that may be eligible for inclusion in the review; (3) explicit criteria by which studies are included and excluded; (4) a mechanism to assess the risk of bias in each study; and, in some cases, (5) synthesis of results with the use of statistical techniques of meta-analysis. By contrast, traditional reviews (1) are subjective, (2) are rarely well focused on a clinical question, (3) lack explicit criteria for selection of studies to be reviewed, (4) do not indicate criteria to assess the quality of included studies, and (5) rarely are amenable to meta-analysis.

The explicit method required for systematic reviews suggests that persons skilled in the art of systematic reviewing should be able to reproduce the data of a systematic review, just as researchers in chemistry or biochemistry expect to be able to reproduce published primary studies in their fields. This concept strengthens the credibility of systematic reviews, and workers in the field of EBM generally consider well-conducted systematic reviews of high-quality primary studies to constitute the highest level of evidence on a medical question.

Why Systematic Reviews?

The medical literature is so vast that no one is able to read, much less digest, all relevant work. This serves as an impetus for systematic reviews. Other motivations include (1) the massive amount of new technology, (2) the poor quality of narrative reviews—especially in relation to guiding practice, and (3) the need to provide an accurate digest for practicing clinicians. Systematic reviews are at the core of health technology assessment (HTA).

In practice, systematic reviews are designed to achieve multiple objectives. For example, they are able to (1) identify the number, scope, and quality of primary studies and (2) provide a summary of available evidence on the diagnostic accuracy of a test. They are also capable of exploring sources of heterogeneity in test results by comparing the diagnostic accuracy of tests across settings or subgroups, or by examining associations between study results and study design features. In this way, they also are able to identify areas that require further research and to recognize questions that are well answered and for which additional studies may not be necessary. In addition, some systematic reviews, by analyzing data on many patients from multiple similar studies, include a sufficient number of patients to achieve the statistical "power" requirements for a reliable assessment of statistical significance of results and for sufficiently precise estimates of diagnostic accuracy; this often is not possible in the individual studies.

Conducting a Systematic Review

Systematic reviewing is time-consuming and requires multiple skills. Usually a team is required, including at least one person experienced in the science and art of systematic reviewing. The team must agree on the clinical problem to be tackled and on the scope of the review.

An early step in preparation for performing a systematic review is to identify whether a similar review has been undertaken recently. Among other things, such a search helps to focus the review. The Cochrane Collaboration provides an excellent resource of reviews, with an increasing number covering diagnostic tests. The Database of Abstracts of Reviews of Effectiveness (DARE), which is run by the Centre for Reviews and Dissemination at the University of York, in the United Kingdom, contains reviews of some diagnostic tests. Other resources include electronic databases, such as PubMed and EMBASE, and recent clinical practice guidelines, which are likely to cite systematic reviews that were available at the time of the guideline's development (see section on guidelines later in this chapter).

The review team must develop a protocol for the project. A protocol should include:

- A title
- Background information
- Composition of the review group
- A timetable
- The clinical question(s) to be addressed in the review
- Search strategy
- Inclusion and exclusion criteria for selection of studies
- Methodology of data extraction and data extraction forms
- Methodology of and checklists for critical appraisal of studies
- Methodology of study synthesis and summary measures to be used.

Description of all of the details is beyond the scope of this chapter, and only some highlights will be discussed. Review of the references cited here, and of references therein,[10,15] is recommended before one embarks on a systematic review.

The Clinical Question and Criteria for Selection of Studies

The most important of the steps (Box 4-1) in conducting a systematic review is the formulation of the clinical question for which the test results are expected to give an answer. This question forms the basis of the review. Two types of questions are addressed in a systematic review in diagnostic medicine: One type is related to the diagnostic accuracy of a test, and the other is related to the value (to patients or to others) of using the test. The questions that arise are similar in structure but require different approaches.

Examples:

Type 1 question regarding diagnostic accuracy of a test: In patients coming to the emergency department with shortness of breath, how well does B-type natriuretic peptide (BNP) or N-terminal pro-BNP (NT-proBNP) predict (identify the presence of) heart failure, as assessed by the independent opinions of two experienced cardiologists?

Type 2 question regarding the value of a test in improving patient outcomes:

In patients admitted to the hospital for treatment of heart failure, how well does use of BNP or NT-proBNP as a guide to therapy reduce the need for subsequent readmission?

Note that each question identifies (1) the patient's problem (shortness of breath or heart failure in a clinical setting [emergency department or hospital]), (2) the test being used (BNP or NT-proBNP), (3) the reference standard for the diagnosis (the independent opinions of two experienced cardiologists) or for the clinical outcome (rate of subsequent re-admission), and (4) the studied attribute of the test (diagnostic accuracy, the ability to detect the presence of heart failure vs. process outcome).

More complex questions often arise. For example, a type 1 question may involve comparing the diagnostic accuracy of two or more tests, or it may address the improvement in diagnostic accuracy that results from adding the results of a new test to those of an existing test or tests. In all cases, however, it

---

BOX 4-1   Selected Key Steps in a Systematic Review of a Diagnostic Test

Identify the clinical question.
Define inclusion and exclusion criteria.
Search the literature.
Identify relevant studies.
Select studies against explicit quality criteria.
Extract data and assess quality.
Analyze and interpret data.
Present and summarize findings.

is recommended that the clinical question be specific, and that it focuses on defined clinical scenarios and clinical settings. This could be considered part of the application of EBM in comparative effectiveness, where the performance of the new test is compared with current practice.

The clinical question leads to inclusion and exclusion criteria for studies to be included in the review. These criteria include the setting in which the test is to be used, as well as the measures to be considered. The setting and the nature of the question affect the diagnostic performance of a test, because they identify a unique population of patients.

Until recently, individuals interested in systematic reviews have focused on studies of the effects of interventions, especially drugs, on patient outcomes. Their work is generally applicable to systematic reviews of diagnostic tests that start with a question of the second type above. Although this discussion is focused on systematic reviews of the diagnostic accuracy of tests, it is important to recognize the increasing literature on reviews of the use of diagnostic tests as part of a "test-and-treat" intervention and their impact on health outcomes.

When the questions to be addressed are defined, the review group must agree on the scope of the review. The review group may do the following:

- Restrict the review to studies of high quality directly applicable to the problem of immediate interest, or
- Explore the effects of variability in study quality and other characteristics (setting, type of population, disease spectrum, etc.) on estimates of accuracy, using subgroup analysis or meta-regression.

The second approach is more complex but allows estimates of such things as the applicability of estimates of diagnostic accuracy to different settings and the effects of study design and inherent patient characteristics (such as age, sex, and symptoms) on estimates of a test's diagnostic accuracy.

Search Strategy
Searching of the primary literature is usually carried out in three ways: (1) an electronic search of literature databases, (2) hand searching of key journals, and (3) review of the references of key review articles. It is usual to search both MEDLINE and EMBASE because the overlap between the two has been as low as 35%. Searching of databases is a detailed exercise, and the help of a librarian or information scientist is recommended. Guidance that is tailored to searching for studies of diagnostic accuracy in the published literature is available in the *Cochrane Handbook for Diagnostic Test Accuracy Reviews* (http://srdta.cochrane.org/handbook-dta-reviews; accessed July 5, 2013). The Agency for Health Research and Quality has also published a comprehensive guide to searching the literature on medical tests for systematic reviews (http://effectivehealthcare.ahrq.gov/index.cfm/search-for-guides-reviews-and-reports/?pageaction=displayproduct&productid=1091; accessed July 5, 2013).

Additional studies may be found in the "grey" literature, such as (1) theses, (2) conference proceedings, (3) technical reports, and (4) monographs. Consultation with individuals active in the field may uncover studies in these sources and studies that are being prepared for publication.

Data Extraction and Critical Appraisal of Studies
Identified papers should be read independently by two persons and data extracted according to a template. A checklist of items to extract from primary studies in preparing a systematic review on test accuracy is available in the *Cochrane Handbook for Diagnostic Test Accuracy Reviews*. The STARD checklist[1] has been used as an additional guide in designing the template.

The quality of studies must be assessed as part of the systematic review. The study design is an important consideration. For many questions related to outcomes, an RCT will be the design of highest quality. For studies of diagnostic accuracy, studies of consecutive series of patients will rank above studies using historical controls. In practice, a study may use a good design but suffer from serious drawbacks in other dimensions, for example, many patients may have been lost to follow-up, or the studied test may have performed poorly during the study, as indicated by high day-to-day imprecision. Thus, adequate grading of the quality of studies must go beyond the categorization of study design. Tools for assessment of studies of diagnostic accuracy include QUADAS (Quality Assessment of Diagnostic Accuracy).[15]

Summarizing the Data
Characteristics and data from critically appraised studies should be presented in tables. Data from studies of diagnostic accuracy should include (1) sensitivities, (2) specificities, and (3) likelihood ratios wherever possible. These are summarized in plots that provide an indication of the variation among studies. The summary should also include an assessment of the quality of each study, using an explicit scoring system such as QUADAS. A review should also present critical analysis of the data highlighted in the review.

Meta-Analysis
A meta-analysis is a statistical way of analyzing data from multiple studies. It may be possible to undertake a meta-analysis if data are available from sufficiently similar studies. Meta-analyses (1) explore sources of variability in the results of clinical studies, (2) increase confidence in the data and conclusions, and (3) signal when no further studies are necessary. The conduct of meta-analyses, however, is beyond the scope of this chapter. Meta-analysis of test accuracy studies is more challenging than for RCTs because tests of accuracy usually produce two statistics (such as sensitivity and specificity)—not one, and these two statistics are correlated over studies. For guidelines on the conduct of meta-analyses of RCTs, see the *Cochrane Handbook for Diagnostic Test Accuracy Reviews* (http://srdta.cochrane.org/handbook-dta-reviews; accessed July 5, 2013) or the overview paper by Reitsma et al.[10]

Economic Evaluations of Diagnostic Testing

Healthcare costs worldwide have surged in recent decades. For example, the United States spent $2.3 trillion, or 17.3% of its gross domestic product, on healthcare in 2010. Although direct laboratory costs are small in comparison, these tests have a profound influence on medical decisions and therefore on total costs.

A Hierarchy of Evidence

A hierarchy of evidence regarding medical tests begins with assessment of the test's technical performance and proceeds through study of the test's clinical performance to clinical effectiveness (an identification of the benefits) and an economic evaluation. This hierarchy of evidence also is seen in the context of the data required to make decisions about the implementation of a test. It therefore lies at the heart of the processes of policy making and service management. Economic evaluation provides a means of evaluating the comparative costs and comparative health effects of alternative care strategies. The use of economic modeling to assess cost-effectiveness after meta-analysis of clinical effectiveness data is increasing.[12]

Methodologies for Economic Evaluations

Health economics is concerned with the *costs* and *consequences* of decisions made in the care of patients. It therefore involves (1) identifying, (2) measuring, and (3) appraising the value of both costs and consequences. The process is complex and is an "inexact science." Approaches to economic evaluation include (1) cost minimization, (2) cost benefit, (3) cost-effectiveness, and (4) cost utility analysis (Table 4-2).

Cost-minimization analysis compares the costs of alternative approaches that produce the same outcome. It is considered the simplest type of economic evaluation. In the area of diagnostic testing, it is applicable to the costs of alternative suppliers of the same (1) test, (2) device, or (3) instrument. It is therefore a technique that is limited to the procurement process, whereby the specifications of the service are already established and the outcomes clearly defined. It might be considered as providing the "cost per test," an often quoted indicator that is not, however, a true economic evaluation because it does not identify an outcome except the provision of a test result.

Cost-benefit analysis determines whether the value of the benefit exceeds the cost of the intervention and therefore whether the intervention is worthwhile. The benefit is assessed in monetary terms, and so is the cost; this is often challenging because it may require the analyst to equate a year of life to a monetary amount. Several methods may be used, including the "human capital approach," which assesses the individual's

productivity (in terms of earnings), and the "willingness to pay approach," which assesses how much money individuals are prepared to pay for a specific benefit.

A variant of cost-benefit analysis is cost-consequences analysis, which measures benefit in different ways and not necessarily in monetary or natural units (see next paragraph). This enables different types of decision makers to make assessments in the context of their own areas of responsibility.

Cost-effectiveness analysis looks at the most efficient way of spending a fixed budget to achieve a certain goal. This goal is expressed in natural units, such as years of life or number of strokes prevented. Surrogate measures with clear relationships to morbidity and mortality have also been used (e.g., change in blood pressure). When an intervention is assessed, the number of cases of disease prevented may be used as a measure of benefit. The analysis evaluates differences in effectiveness between alternative approaches relative to corresponding differences in costs.

Cost-utility analysis focuses on the quality and the quantity of the health outcome. The cost of the intervention is assessed in monetary terms, but the outcomes are expressed in utilities, that is, quantitative expressions of their relative value. An often used metric is *quality-adjusted life-years* (QALYs). The analysis evaluates differences in expected utility between alternative approaches relative to corresponding differences in costs. Cost-utility analysis has been used to evaluate and compare screening programs.

New technology often increases both cost and benefit. When tests increase both the cost and the benefit, decisions about their use will depend on factors such as willingness to pay and other political and individual pressures. A figure of $50,000 per QALY has been used in the United States as a reference point. This reflects a decision by the U.S. Congress to approve dialysis treatment for end-stage renal failure—a treatment with approximately this cost per QALY.

Four possible findings may result from cost-effectiveness or cost-utility analyses and corresponding possible decisions; they are often summarized in an incremental cost-effectiveness plane (Figure 4-4):

- Test is more costly but provides greater benefit—possibly introduce test, depending on overall gain (A).
- Test is more costly but provides less benefit—do not introduce test (B).
- Test is less costly but provides greater benefit—introduce test (C).

TABLE 4-2	Approaches to Economic Evaluation		
Type of Evaluation	**Test Evaluated**	**Effect or Outcome**	**Decision Criteria**
Cost minimization	Alternative tests or delivery options	Identical outcomes	Least expensive alternative
Cost benefit	Alternative tests or delivery options	Improved effect or outcome	Effect evaluated purely in monetary terms
Cost effectiveness	Alternative tests or delivery options	Common unit of effect but differential effect	Cost per unit of effect (e.g., dollars per life-year gained)
Cost utility	Alternative tests or delivery options	Improved effect or outcome	Outcome expressed in terms of survival and quality of life

• Test is less costly but provides less benefit—possibly introduce test, depending on the size of the loss in benefit and the magnitude of savings (D).

Note: This cost may be able to produce a demonstrably greater benefit if spent on a different intervention or test.

Perspectives of Economic Evaluations

The perspective from which an economic evaluation is performed affects the (1) design, (2) conduct, and (3) results of the evaluation, which may prompt the use of cost-consequences analysis. The perspective may, for example, be that of (1) a patient, (2) a provider, (3) a payer (government health agency or health insurance company), or (4) society. The perspective for evaluating cost and benefit may be long term or short term. The questions below illustrate the importance of perspective:

• What is the cost of the test result produced on analyzer A compared with analyzer B?

• What is the cost of the test result produced by laboratory A compared with laboratory B?

• What is the cost of the test result produced by POCT compared with the laboratory?

• Will provision of rapid blood testing for the emergency department reduce the length of patient stays in the department, thus decreasing costs for the hospital?

• Will rapid HbA_{1c} testing in a clinic (rather than in a distant laboratory) save time for patients by providing results at the time of the clinic visit?

• Will it save money for patients' employers by reducing employees' time away from work to go to repeated physician appointments?

• Will it save time for the physician and thus money for the clinic? Will it improve care of diabetes for the patient as indicated by independent measures of glycemic control (perhaps by facilitating counseling at the time of the clinic visit)?

• Will it save money for the healthcare system by improving glycemic control and thus decreasing hospitalizations related to poor glycemic control?

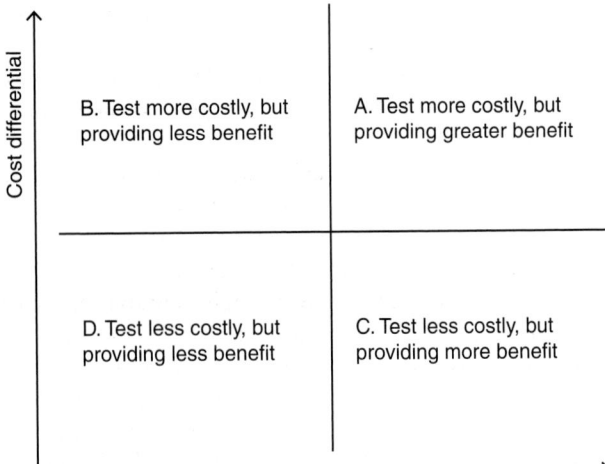

Figure 4-4 A summary of the incremental cost-effectiveness plane.

• Will it provide benefit for society by decreasing society's healthcare costs (for hospitalizations) and increasing patients' functioning and contributions to society?

The first scenario describes the type of evaluation made for equipment-purchasing decisions and is a simple procurement exercise. The outcome is the same—the provision of a given test result to a given standard of accuracy and precision within a given time (the specification). The second question might appear to be the same, but it is not, and it will undoubtedly have to take into account other issues such as the logistical issues associated with sample transport or the level of communication support provided by the laboratories. To make a relevant evaluation in the third scenario concerning the value of POCT, it is important to take into account the implications outside of the laboratory that may result from a delay in sending the sample to the laboratory. The implications of the remaining questions are similar. Note that the clinical complications of poor glycemic control are largely long term and may extend beyond the time frame of the financial interests of those performing an economic analysis. Indeed, rigorous long-term economic evaluations of the use of tests are rare, except in the particular scenario of national screening programs, such as for neonatal hypothyroidism and breast cancer, where they form part of a "test-and-treat" intervention.

Quality of Economic Evaluations

Criteria for evaluating an economic study of a diagnostic test include the following:

• Clear definition of the economic question, including perspective of the evaluation (e.g., perspective of [1] a patient, [2] society, [3] an employer, [4] a health insurance company, or [5] a hospital administrator; long-term versus short-term perspective).

• Description of competing alternatives.

• Evidence of effectiveness of intervention.

• Clear identification and quantification of costs and consequences, including incremental analysis.

• Appropriate consideration of effects of differential timing of costs and benefits.

• Performance of sensitivity analysis (How sensitive are results and conclusions to plausible changes in assumptions or in input [e.g., changes in cost of drugs or benefit in life-years]?).

• Inclusion of summary measure of efficiency, ensuring that all issues are addressed.

Use of Economic Evaluations in Decision Making

The stream of new tests in laboratory medicine requires frequent decisions about whether or not to implement them. Economic evaluations help in making these decisions. The finite resources for healthcare require use of an objective means of determining how resources are allocated and how the efficiency and effectiveness of service delivery are improved.

Economic evaluations are important for laboratories. First, the laboratory budget is usually "controlled" independently of the other costs of healthcare. This is often referred to as "silo budgeting." The budget for testing is established independently of the budgets for services that might achieve benefit if a new diagnostic test is introduced. Second, achievement of a favorable outcome (e.g., a reduction in length of stay, a decrease in admissions to the coronary care unit) is of use from a management standpoint only if that outcome is turned into real money. Third, the introduction of a new test or testing modality (e.g., POCT) will produce benefits only if a corresponding change in practice is implemented. For example, the D-dimer test has been used to exclude diagnoses of thromboembolic disease and thus avoid the need for expensive radiologic procedures. This approach works only if clinicians actually consider the D-dimer results and stop ordering the expensive imaging tests when the D-dimer result and the clinical findings indicate that they are not needed. Finally, even if the desired cost savings are achieved, silo budgeting ensures that the savings are seen in a budget different from that of the laboratory, and the laboratory budget shows only an increased expenditure. Fortunately, the drawbacks of silo budgeting are being recognized, and a broader view of health economics seems to be developing in some healthcare settings. Thus the Office of Health Economics in the UK is asking whether a value-based pricing approach should be taken to molecular diagnostics, the arguments for which could equally be applied to all types of diagnostic tests (http://www.ohe.org/publications/article-/value-based-pricing-and-molecular-diagnostics-117.cfm; accessed July 5, 2013).

Clinical Practice Guidelines

The patient-centered goals of evidenced-based laboratory medicine are not reached by primary studies and systematic reviews alone. The results of these investigations must be turned into action. Increasingly, health systems and professional groups in medicine have turned to the use of clinical practice guidelines. Guidelines are a tool that are used to facilitate implementation of lessons from primary studies and systematic reviews. Important motivations for development of guidelines have been to decrease variability in practice (and improve the use of best practices) and to shorten the (often prolonged) time required for new information to be used for the benefit of patients or for prevention of disease.

The development of practice guidelines for the clinical laboratory is a challenging new area. A limited amount of advice is available on preparing such guidelines,[8] but the applicability of the AGREE (Appraisal of Guidelines for Research and Evaluation) tool has recently been described in preparation of the National Clinical Biochemistry Practice Guidelines.[2]

What Is a Clinical Practice Guideline?

According to the Institute of Medicine, "**Clinical practice guidelines** are systematically developed statements to assist practitioner and patient decisions about appropriate healthcare for specific clinical circumstances". Guidelines of various sorts have long addressed issues of concern to laboratorians, such as requirements or goals for (1) accuracy, (2) precision, and (3) turnaround time of tests and considerations about the

frequency of repeat tests in the monitoring of patients. The focus of modern clinical practice guidelines, such as recent ones on laboratory testing in diabetes and liver disease, is the patient in the "specific clinical circumstances" referred to in the definition of clinical practice guidelines. The tools of EBM and clinical epidemiology allow guidelines to be developed in a more transparent way from thoroughly conducted studies and systematic reviews.

Use of Transparency in the Development of Guidelines

In the absence of a transparent process for the development of a guideline, the credibility of the product is compromised and should be questioned. When guidelines are developed by a professional group (such as specialist physicians or laboratory-based practitioners), the recommendations (e.g., to perform a diagnostic procedure in a given setting) may be suspected of promoting the welfare of that professional group. In contrast, when guidelines are prepared under the auspices of healthcare payers (governments and insurance companies), the recommendations may be suspected of being influenced by cost-control measures, which sometimes may harm patients. In the latter setting, a key danger is that the absence of evidence of benefit from a medical intervention may be interpreted as proof of absence of benefit.

Steps in the Development of Guidelines

The development of guidelines is best undertaken according to a step-by-step plan. One such scheme is shown in Figure 4-5; only selected issues of this will be discussed here. For a more detailed discussion, see Oosterhuis et al[8] or Watine et al.[14]

Selection and Refinement of a Topic

The critical importance of this first step is analogous to the importance of the corresponding step in the development of a systematic review. For example, (1) the scope must not exceed the capabilities in time, funding, and expertise of the group, (2) the topic must not be without evidence (or the guideline will lack credibility), and (3) the area must be one that requires attention (or the guideline will have little value).

Typically such guidelines will address (1) clinical conditions—such as diabetes and liver disease, (2) symptoms—chest pain, (3) signs—abnormal bleeding, or (4) interventions—whether therapeutic (coronary angioplasty and aspirin) or diagnostic (cardiac markers). To decide whether developing a guideline should be considered, the following questions are of help:

- Is there variation in practice that suggests uncertainty?
- Is the issue a matter of public health importance, such as the increasing problems of diabetes and obesity? and
- Is there a perceived necessity for cost reduction?

Refinement of the topic ideally involves a multidisciplinary group that includes (1) clinicians, (2) healthcare providers, (3) laboratory experts, (4) patients, and (5) likely users of the guidelines. The scope will be affected by the support staff (if any) and the financial support available to the guideline group.

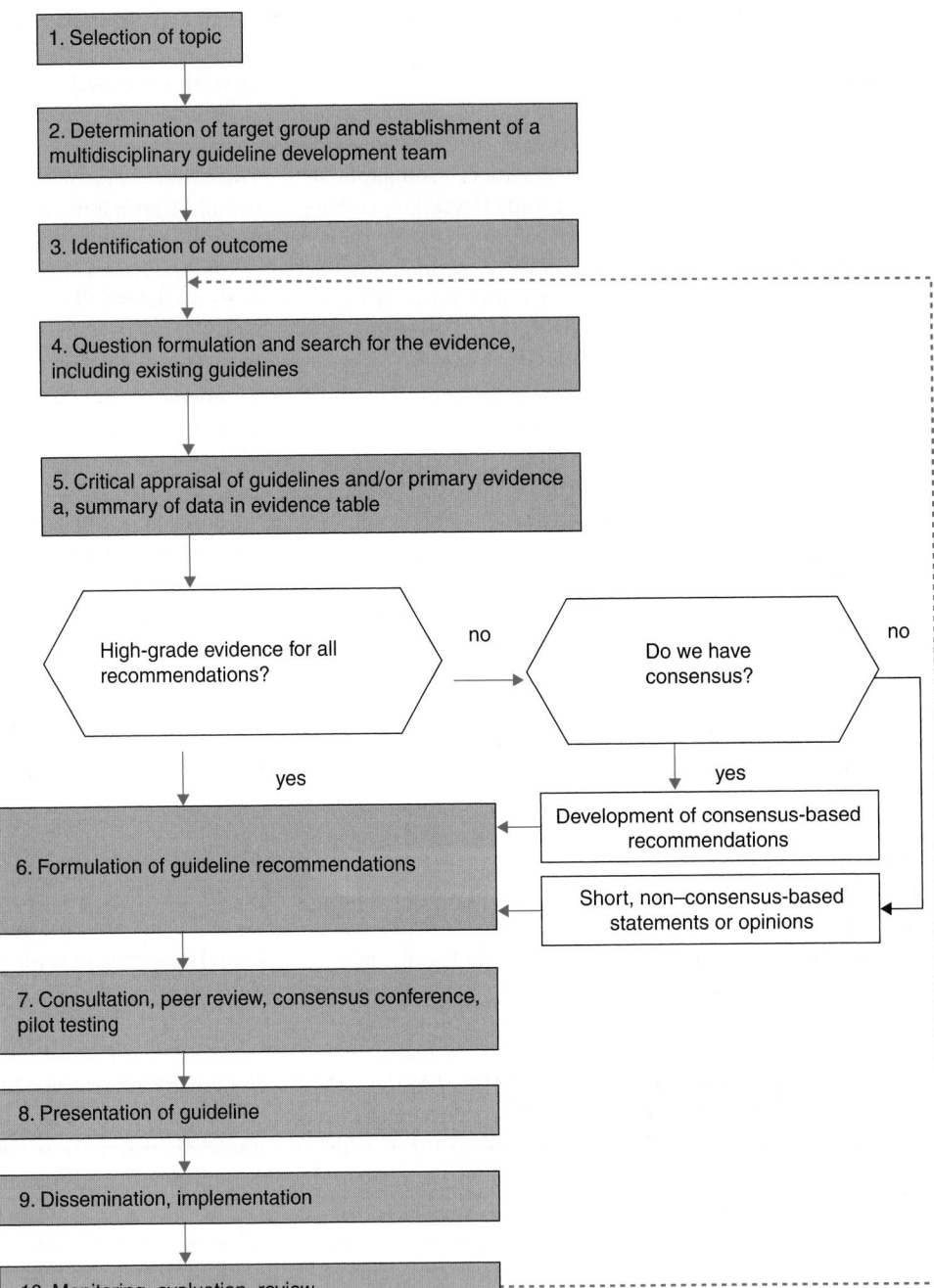

Figure 4-5 Steps in the development of a clinical practice guideline. *(Modified from Oosterhuis WP, Bruns DE, Watine J, Sandberg S, Horvath AR. Evidence-based guidelines in laboratory medicine: principles and methods,* Clin Chem 2004;50:806-818.)

Determination of Target Group and Establishment of a Multidisciplinary Guideline Development Team

The intended audience must be identified. For example, is it (1) nurses, (2) general practice physicians, (3) clinical specialty physicians, (4) healthcare providers, (5) laboratory specialists, or (6) patients?

The guideline development team should include representatives from all key groups involved in management of the target condition. For the development of guidelines in laboratory medicine, teams ideally include (1) relevant medical specialists, (2) laboratory experts, (3) methodologists (for expertise in statistics, literature search, critical appraisal, and guideline development), and (4) those who deliver services (e.g., nurse

practitioners and patients, for guidelines on home monitoring of glucose; laboratory technologists and managers, for a guideline that addresses turnaround times for cardiac markers).

Potential conflicts of interest of all members must be noted. The role, if any, of sponsors (commercial or nonprofit) in the guideline development process must be agreed upon and reported. Ideally, staff support members are available to (1) help arrange meetings and conference calls, (2) retrieve published work, and (3) assist with publication and other forms of dissemination (e.g., audio conferences).

A minimum group size of six has been recommended. Groups consisting of more than 12 to 15 persons will inhibit the airing of each person's views. A recommended tool is the use of subgroups to focus on specific questions, with a steering committee responsible for coordination and production of the final guideline.

Identifying and Assessing the Evidence

When available, well-performed systematic reviews form the most important part of the evidence base for guidelines. Systematic reviews are necessary when variation between studies is expected. When no systematic reviews exist, the group effectively must undertake to produce one. The level of evidence supporting each conclusion in the review will affect the recommendations made in the guidelines.

Translating Evidence Into a Guideline and Grading the Strength of Recommendations

The processes required for preparing recommendations within an expert group are poorly understood; this challenge has been addressed by the Grading of Recommendations Assessment, Development, and Evaluation (GRADE) Working Group (http://www.gradeworkinggroup.org; accessed July 5, 2013). The GRADE process begins when an explicit question is asked, including specification of all important outcomes. After evidence has been collected and summarized, GRADE provides explicit criteria for rating the quality of evidence, including (1) study design, (2) risk of bias, (3) imprecision, (4) inconsistency, (5) indirectness, and (6) magnitude of effect. Recommendations are then characterized as strong or weak according to the quality of the supporting evidence and the balance between desirable and undesirable consequences of the alternative management options.

Developing recommendations for clinical practice guidelines may involve balancing of costs and benefits after values

are assigned and the quality of evidence has been determined. Conclusive evidence for recommendations is not always available. However, authors of guidelines have an ethical responsibility to make very clear the level of evidence that supports each recommendation.

Several schemes are available for rating the evidence. For example, the National Academy of Clinical Biochemistry (NACB) is working with the Professional Practice Committee of the American Diabetes Association to revise the NACB diabetes guidelines. Their goal is to develope a new system that offers a means of both rating the overall quality of evidence and grading the strength of recommendations. This approach is summarized in Table 4-3. The level or rating of evidence does not always predict the strength of a recommendation because recommendations involve assessing changes in outcome and may require extrapolation from study results. For example, multiple studies supporting use of a drug may have been done well and a competent systematic review may be available, so the evidence may be graded as high. However, if the studies were done in adults and the guideline is for children, the strength of the recommendation may be low.

The highest level of evidence is rare in guidelines on the use of diagnostic tests. With many such guidelines, most of the recommendations are based on expert opinion. As more studies are published on the diagnostic accuracy of tests and on the relationships of tests to outcomes, the dependence of guidelines on "opinion" should decrease.

For analytical goal setting or "quality specifications" for analytical methods in guidelines, randomized controlled clinical trials (outcomes studies) are not appropriate. In such situations, a different hierarchy of evidence (Table 4-4) may be useful for grading of such laboratory-related recommendations. The

TABLE 4-3	A Scheme for Rating the Quality of Evidence in Grading the Strength of Recommendations in Clinical Guidelines
Level	**Characteristics**
	Rating scale for quality of evidence
High	Further research is unlikely to change the confidence in the results. Body of evidence from individual studies sufficiently powered provides precise, consistent, and directly applicable results in a relevant population.
Moderate	Further research is likely to have an important impact on confidence in the estimate of effect and may change the estimate and the recommendation. Body of evidence comes from high/moderate-level individual studies sufficient to determine effects, but strength of evidence may be limited by number, quality or consistency of included studies, generalizability to routine practice, or the indirect nature of the evidence.
Low	Further research is very likely to have an important impact on confidence in the estimate of effect and may change the estimate and the recommendation. Body of evidence is of low level with serious design flaws, or evidence is indirect.
Very low	Any estimate of effect is very uncertain. Evidence is insufficient for assessment of effects on health outcomes because of the limited number or power of studies, important flaws in their design or conduct, gaps in the chain of evidence, or lack of information.
	Grading strength of recommendation
	Grading based on rating of evidence and expert agreement on impact on health outcomes and substantial benefit over harm
A	Strongly recommend *for* or *against* adoption
B	Recommend *for* or *against* adoption
C	Insufficient evidence to make a recommendation because of poor quality or lack of evidence
GPP	Good practice point based on expert consensus and mainly applicable to technical matters

For full information, consult Sacks DB, Arnold M, Bakris GL, Bruns DE, Horvath AR, Kirkman MS, et al. Executive summary: guidelines and recommendations for laboratory analysis in the diagnosis and management of diabetes mellitus, Clin Chem 2011;57:793-798.

highest level of evidence is evidence related to medical needs. It is conceivable that even statistical modeling of specific clinical decisions could be considered as a subtype of evidence related to medical needs. For example, simulation modeling of the diagnostic process has been employed to study the impact of rapid turnaround of results for troponin measurements on triage times in the emergency room for patients presenting with chest pain. Monte Carlo simulation has been used to quantify the effects of errors in glucose measurements (imprecision and bias) on the ability of insulin-dosing protocols to control glucose concentrations in patients.

Level 1B in Table 4-4 refers primarily to the concepts of within-individual and among-individual biological variation. Levels of (1) optimum, (2) desirable, and (3) minimum performance for both imprecision and bias have been defined on the basis of these concepts. Meeting these performance goals ensures that the analytical imprecision is small compared with the normal day-to-day variations that occur within an individual. Similarly, the goal for bias is to minimize variation within an individual compared with variation among individuals. Thus, reference intervals for a test in a given reference group will be unaffected by the small amount of analytical error or bias. Use of this type of quality specification for imprecision and bias appears appropriate in guidelines. In practice, failure to use this approach is difficult to justify because data on within-individual and among-individual biological variation are available for virtually all commonly used tests.

Obtaining External Review and Updating the Guidelines

Three types of outside examiners have been used to evaluate guidelines:
- Experts in the clinical content area—to assess completeness of the literature review and the reasonableness of recommendations.
- Experts on systematic reviewing and guideline development—to review the process of guideline development.
- Potential users of the guidelines.

In addition, (1) journals, (2) sponsoring organizations, and (3) other potential endorsers of the guidelines may undertake formal reviews. Each of these reviews adds value.

As part of the guideline development process, a plan for updating should be developed. The importance of this step is underscored by the finding that one of the most common reasons for nonadherence to guidelines is that the guidelines are outdated. About half of published guidelines are outdated in 5 to 7 years, and no more than 90% of conclusions are still valid after 3 to 5 years. These findings suggest that the time interval between completion and review of a guideline should be short.

Clinical Audit

In healthcare, the term *audit* refers to the review of case histories of patients against the benchmark of current best practice. In practice, the **clinical audit** improves clinical practice. However, the effects are typically modest. A more general role for audit, however, is that it is used as part of the wider management exercise of benchmarking of performance with the use of relevant performance indicators against the performance of peers. This is sometimes referred to as *performance management*.

Audits also are used to (1) solve problems, (2) monitor workload in the context of controlling demand, (3) monitor the introduction of a new test and/or change in practice, and (4) monitor the variation between providers and adherence with best practices (e.g., with guidelines).

The components of the audit cycle are depicted in Figure 4-6. All of the audit activities are found in the practice of evidence-based laboratory medicine. There is a clinical question for which the test result should provide an answer, and the answer will lead to a decision being made and an action taken, resulting in an improved health outcome.

Audit to Help Solve Problems

All audits involve the collection of observational data and comparison against a standard or specification. Thus, an audit

TABLE 4-4	Hierarchy of Criteria for Quality Specifications
Level	**Basis**
1A	Medical decision making: use of test in specific clinical situations
1B	Medical decision making: use of test in medicine generally
2	Guidelines—"experts"
3	Regulators or organizers of external quality assurance schemes
4	Published data on state of the art

From Fraser CG, Petersen PH. Analytical performance characteristics should be judged against objective quality specifications, Clin Chem 1999;45:321-323.

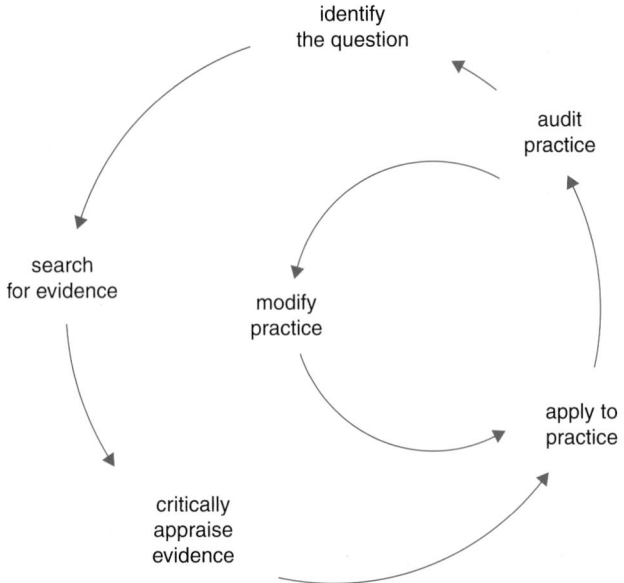

Figure 4-6 The audit cycle. (*From Price CP. Evidence-based laboratory medicine: supporting decision-making,* Clin Chem 2000;46:1041-1050.)

may determine the proportion of test results that are returned within a specified time or standard (such as 45 minutes from receipt). In many cases a standard does not exist, and maybe not even a specification. In such cases, the first step of an auditing process is to establish a specification.

Solving a problem related to a process may first involve collecting data on aspects of the process that are considered to have an influence on the outcome. For example, a study of test result turnaround times might collect data on (1) phlebotomy waiting time, (2) quality of patient identification, (3) transport time, (4) sample registration time, (5) quality of sample identification, (6) sample preparation time, (7) analysis time, (8) test result validation time, and (9) result delivery time.

Audit to Monitor Workload and Demand

The true demand for a test will depend on the number of patients and the spectrum of disease in the group for which the test is appropriate. When an audit of workload for a test is conducted, it is possible to ask a number of questions that address the appropriateness of the test requests. These questions, which typically are asked by questionnaire, include the following:

- What clinical question is being asked?
- What decision will be aided by the results of the test?
- What action will be taken after the decision is made?
- What risks are associated with not receiving the result?
- What are the expected outcomes?
- Is there evidence to support the use of the test in this setting?
- And, for tests ordered urgently, why was this test result required urgently?

This approach is likely to identify (1) unnecessary use of tests, (2) misunderstandings about the use of tests, and (3) instances of use of the wrong test. With the advent of electronic requesting and the electronic patient record, it is possible to build this approach into routine practice.

Actions that may follow from the answers to these questions include (1) feedback of results to users, (2) re-education of users, (3) identification of unmet needs and research to satisfy, for example, a need for advice on an alternative test, (4) creation of an algorithm or guideline on use of the test, and (5) re-audit in 6 months to review for changes in practice. An algorithm may be embedded in the electronic requesting package to provide an automatic bar to inappropriate requesting (e.g., liver function tests being requested every day on a patient).

Audit to Monitor the Introduction of a New Test

An audit is used to ensure (1) that the change in practice that should accompany the introduction of a new test has occurred, and (2) that the outcomes originally predicted are being delivered. The development of any new test should lead to evidence that identifies the way in which the test is going to be used, including:

- Identification of the clinical question(s), the patient cohort, and the clinical setting.

- Identification of preanalytical and analytical requirements for the test.
- Identification of any algorithm into which the test might have to be inserted (e.g., use in conjunction with other tests, signs, or symptoms).
- Identification of the decision(s) likely to be made on receipt of the result.
- Identification of the action(s) likely to be taken on receipt of the result.
- Identification of the likely outcome(s).
- Identification of any risks associated with introduction of a new test.
- The evidence (and the quality of that evidence) that supports the use of the test and the outcomes to be expected.
- Identification of any changes in practice (e.g., deletion of another test from the repertoire, move to POCT, reduction in laboratory workload).

This summary of use and portfolio of evidence forms the basis of the standard operating procedure for (1) the clinical use of the test, (2) the core of the educational material for users of the service, and (3) the basis for conducting the audit.

Before the introduction of a new test is audited, it is obviously important to have ensured that a full program of education of users has been completed, and that any other changes in practice have been accommodated in the clinic and/or ward routines.

Audit to Monitor Variation Between Providers and Adherence to Best Practice

This is the scenario that probably best reflects the way in which the clinical audit was first conceived and practiced. Typically the clinical audit takes two forms: (1) auditing the log of requests for a specific test from users of a service (e.g., HbA_{1c} testing ordered by primary care physicians' practices or hospital clinical departments); (2) auditing randomly selected cases from a clinical team, with the review undertaken by an independent clinician. Both approaches are likely to identify when a test has not been performed and to identify unnecessary testing; the former is possibly of greater interest to the payer. The audit is best performed against some form of benchmark, which may be a local, regional, or national guideline; a guideline will have used the best evidence and thus removed differences of opinion that may exist between clinical teams.

Applying the Principles of Evidence-Based Laboratory Medicine in Routine Practice

The principles of evidence-based laboratory medicine support the manner in which laboratory medicine is practiced, from the discovery of a new diagnostic test through to its application in routine patient care. These principles provide the logic on which all of the elements of practice are founded. The tools of evidence-based laboratory medicine provide the means of delivering the highest quality of service in meeting the needs of patients and the healthcare professionals who serve them, extending from purchase of the service to performance management of the practice.[9] In practice, the application of evidence-based practice is far more complex for laboratory medicine than for therapeutic interventions, but it is critical for success.

Review Questions

1. Meta-analysis:
   a. is a statistical technique that compares results from various studies.
   b. is an extensive and explicit strategy that is used to find all studies (published or unpublished) pertaining to a single assay.
   c. includes the quality and the quantity of the health outcome.
   d. is a tool used to facilitate implementation of lessons from primary studies and systematic reviews.

2. Systematic error produces bias and typically results from a flawed design of a study of diagnostic accuracy. This is caused by poor:
   a. reliability.
   b. external validity.
   c. internal validity.
   d. standardization.

3. In an economic evaluation of a medical test, the determination of whether or not the value of the benefit of performing the test exceeds the cost of the intervention is referred to as:
   a. minimal cost analysis.
   b. cost-effectiveness analysis.
   c. cost-utility analysis.
   d. cost-benefit analysis.

4. The first step in designing clinical practice guidelines that focus on a patient is:
   a. establishing a multidisciplinary guideline development team.
   b. selecting and refining a topic for which to develop guidelines.
   c. translating evidence into a guideline.
   d. obtaining external reviewers to evaluate guidelines.

5. The overall aim of a systematic review is to:
   a. review all literature on a particular subject.
   b. reach a recommendation by an expert group.
   c. answer an exactly defined clinical question with transparency and minimal bias.
   d. develop a recommendation that involves a balance of cost and benefit.

6. Which one of the following IS NOT a component of a clinical audit?
   a. Solving problems associated with a process or outcome
   b. Monitoring workload in the context of controlling demand
   c. Evaluating the costs of alternative approaches that produce the same outcome
   d. Monitoring the introduction of a new test and/or changes in practice

7. A systematically developed statement to assist practitioner and patient decisions about appropriate healthcare for specific clinical circumstances defines:
   a. clinical practice guidelines.
   b. systematic review.
   c. STARD.
   d. evidence-based laboratory medicine.

8. The acronym QALY stands for:
   a. quality of all life-years.
   b. quality assessment of living youth.
   c. quantifiable analysis of life's yields.
   d. quality-adjusted life-year.

9. The de facto standard for research studies of the health effects and outcomes of medical interventions is the:
   a. epidemiologic study.
   b. randomized controlled trial.
   c. open-ended survey.
   d. before-and-after design study.

10. In relation to healthcare, the word *quality* is defined as:
    a. the most expensive care that can be provided to a patient.
    b. the use of the best analyzers and equipment available for diagnostics to improve outcomes.
    c. the increased probability of desired outcomes and the decreased probability of undesired outcomes.
    d. an improved outcome.

References

1. Bossuyt PM, Reitsma JB, Bruns DE, Gatsonis CA, Glasziou PP, Irwig LM, et al. Towards complete and accurate reporting of studies of diagnostic accuracy: the STARD initiative. Standards for Reporting of Diagnostic Accuracy. Clin Chem 2003;49:1–6.
2. Don-Wauchope AC, Sievenpiper JL, Hill SA, Iorio A. Applicability of the AGREE II instrument in evaluating the development process and quality of current National Academy of Clinical Biochemistry guidelines. Clin Chem 2012;58:1426–1437.
3. Ferrante di Ruffano L, Hyde CJ, McCaffery KJ, Bossuyt PM, Deeks JJ. Assessing the value of diagnostic tests: a framework for designing and evaluating trials. BMJ 2012;344:e686.
4. Glasziou P, Del Mar C, Salisbury J. Evidence-based practice workbook, 2nd edition. Oxford, UK: Blackwell Publishing, BMJ Books, 2007.
5. Guyatt GH, Rennie D, eds. Users' guides to the medical literature: a manual for evidence-based clinical practice. Chicago, AMA Press, 2002.
6. Lijmer JG, Mol BW, Heisterkamp S, Bonsel GJ, Prins MH, van der Meulen JH, et al. Empirical evidence of design-related bias in studies of diagnostic tests. JAMA 1999;282:1061–1066.
7. Lord SJ, Irwig L, Bossuyt PM. Using the principles of randomized controlled trial design to guide test evaluation. Med Decis Making 2009;29:E1–12.
8. Oosterhuis WP, Bruns DE, Watine J, Sandberg S, Horvath AR. Evidence-based guidelines in laboratory medicine: principles and methods. Clin Chem 2004;50:806–818.
9. Price CP. Evidence-based laboratory medicine: is it working in practice? Clin Biochem Rev 2012;33:13–19.
10. Reitsma JB, Moons KG, Bossuyt PM, Linnet K. Systematic reviews of studies quantifying the accuracy of diagnostic tests and markers. Clin Chem 2012;58:1534–1545.
11. Sackett DL, Rosenberg WMC, Muir Gray JA, Haynes RB, Richardson WS. Evidence-based medicine: what it is and what it isn't. BMJ 1996;312:71–72.
12. Sutton AJ, Cooper NJ, Goodacre S, Stevenson M. Integration of meta-analysis and economic decision modeling for evaluating diagnostic tests. Med Decis Making 2008;28:650–667.

13. Turner L, Shamseer L, Altman DG, Weeks L, Peters J, Kober T, et al. Consolidated standards of reporting trials (CONSORT) and the completeness of reporting of randomised controlled trials (RCTs) published in medical journals. Cochrane Database Syst Rev 2012, 11. MR000030.

14. Watine J, Oosterhuis WP, Nagy E, Bunting PS, Horvath AR. Formulating and using evidence-based guidelines. In: Price CP, Christenson RH, eds. Evidence-based laboratory medicine: principles, practice and outcomes, 2nd edition. Washington, DC: AACC Press, 2007:275–294.

15. Whiting PF, Rutjes AW, Westwood ME, Mallett S, Deeks JJ, Reitsma JB, et al. QUADAS-2 Group. QUADAS-2: a revised tool for the quality assessment of diagnostic accuracy studies. Ann Intern Med 2011;155:529–536.

Establishment and Use of Reference Values*

Gary L. Horowitz, M.D.

Objectives

1. Define the following terms:

   Clinical sensitivity
   Clinical specificity
   Exclusion criteria
   Interpercentile interval
   Outlier
   Partitioning; partitioning
     criteria
   Population-based
     reference value
   Predictive value
   Prevalence

   Random sample
   Range
   Reference individual
   Reference interval
   Reference limits
   Reference population
   Reference value
   Selection criteria
   Subject-based reference value
   Transferability or transference

2. List three conditions that are essential when a valid comparison of individual laboratory results with reference values is performed; state the need for establishing reference intervals.
3. Give three examples of exclusion criteria used in the production of health-associated reference values; give three examples of partitioning criteria used to subgroup a reference group.
4. State why standardization of specimen collection is important when reference values are established.
5. Compare the terms *reference value* and *reference interval;* list three categories of reference intervals.
6. Briefly state the parametric and nonparametric statistical methods of determining an interpercentile interval; state the important assumption that must be made when parametric statistics are used.
7. State the limitation of using population-based reference intervals instead of subject-based reference intervals, and state a solution to this limitation.
8. Discuss the issue of transferability of reference values with regard to prerequisites and solutions to the issue.
9. State the formulas used in calculating clinical sensitivity, clinical specificity, and predictive value of a laboratory test; given appropriate values, calculate clinical sensitivity, clinical specificity, and predictive value for a laboratory test.
10. State how the predictive value of a laboratory test is affected by prevalence.

Key Words and Definitions

Clinical sensitivity The proportion of subjects with disease who have positive test results.

Clinical specificity The proportion of subjects without disease who have negative test results.

Nonparametric analysis A statistical approach to reference value analysis that requires no assumptions about the nature of the distribution; thus, it can be applied to distributions that are Gaussian or non-Gaussian.

Parametric analysis A statistical approach to reference value analysis that requires specific distributional assumptions. For example, it usually requires that the distribution of values be Gaussian (or that the values be mathematically manipulated so that they become Gaussian).

Partitioning The use of specific criteria in the subclassification of reference groups to reduce the biological variation in each group; the most commonly used criteria are age and sex.

Predictive value The predictive value of a positive laboratory test is the number of true positive results divided by the total number of positive results (true positives plus false positives); the negative predictive value is the number of true negative results divided by the total number of negative results (true negatives plus false negatives).

Prevalence The proportion of subjects in a specified population who have a specified disease or condition.

Reference individual An individual selected as the basis for comparison with individuals under clinical investigation through the use of defined criteria.

Reference interval (population-based) A set of values usually defined by an upper reference limit and a lower reference limit, representing a specified proportion of the reference population; this is frequently the central 95% of values from the reference population.

*The author gratefully acknowledges the original contribution by Helge Eric Solberg on which major portions of this chapter are based.

Key Words and Definitions—cont'd

Reference interval (subject-based) A set of values usually defined by an upper reference limit and a lower reference limit, representing a specified proportion of the values from a reference individual; this is frequently the central 95% of values from the reference individual.

Reference population An undefined number of individuals that represent the demographic for which the reference intervals will be used. Reference individuals are chosen, preferably at random, from this larger population to provide reference samples for the establishment of a reference interval.

Reference value A value obtained by observation or measurement of a particular type of quantity on a reference individual; results

of a certain type of quantity obtained from a single individual or group of individuals corresponding to a stated description.

Selection criteria A set of criteria that define the desired characteristics of a reference individual. The specific criteria chosen will depend of the purpose of the reference interval and the specific population the RI is intended to represent.

Transferibility or Transference The adoption by a laboratory of previously established reference intervals established elsewhere. Procedures for validation of reference intervals must be completed by the adopting laboratory prior to the use of the transferred RI to ensure that they are appropriate to the laboratory's patient population and laboratory methods.

In practice, data collected during (1) medical interviews, (2) clinical examinations, and (3) supplementary investigations are interpreted by comparison with reference data. If the condition of the patient resembles that typical of a particular disease, the clinician or healthcare provider may base the diagnosis on the observation (positive diagnosis). This diagnosis is made more likely if observed symptoms and signs do not fit the patterns that characterize a set of alternative diseases (diagnosis by exclusion).

Interpretation of medical laboratory data is an example of decision making by comparison. We therefore need *reference values* for all tests performed in the clinical laboratory, not only from healthy individuals but from patients with relevant diseases.[8,9,14] Ideally, observed values should be related to several collections of reference values, such as values from (1) healthy people, (2) undifferentiated hospital population, (3) people with typical diseases, or (4) ambulatory individuals, and to previous values from the same subjects.[9] A patient's laboratory result is simply not medically useful if appropriate data for comparison are lacking. Establishment and use of such reference values are the topics of this chapter.

Establishment of Reference Values

Certain conditions are mandatory for ensuring that the comparison of a patient's laboratory results with reference values is valid:

1. All groups of reference individuals should be clearly defined.
2. The patient examined should resemble sufficiently the reference individuals (in all groups selected for comparison) in all respects other than those under investigation.
3. The conditions under which the samples were obtained and processed for analysis should be known.
4. All quantities compared should be of the same type.
5. All laboratory results should be produced with the use of adequately standardized methods under sufficient analytical quality control (see Chapter 7).
6. The clinical sensitivity, clinical specificity, and prevalence in the populations tested should be known so that laboratory tests can be interpreted intelligently (see Chapter 3).

Background

The term *normal values* has been used frequently in the past. Confusion arose because the word *normal* has several very different connotations. Consequently, this term is now considered obsolete and **should not be used!** Instead, the International Federation of Clinical Chemistry and Laboratory Medicine (IFCC)[9] recommends use of the term *reference values* and related terms, such as *reference individual, reference limit, reference interval,* and *observed values.* **Reference values** are results of a certain type of quantity obtained from a single individual or group of individuals corresponding to a stated description, which must be spelled out and made available for use by others.

A short description of qualifiers associated with the term *reference values,* such as *health-associated reference values* (close to what was understood by the obsolete term *normal values*), is convenient. Other examples of such qualifying words are (1) *diabetic patient,* (2) *hospitalized diabetic patient,* and (3) *ambulatory diabetic patient.* These short descriptions prevent the common misunderstanding that reference values are associated only with health.

A further distinction is made between subject-based and population-based reference values. *Subject-based reference values* are previous values from the same individual, obtained when the individual was in a defined state of health. *Population-based reference values* are those obtained from a group of systematically defined reference individuals and are usually the values referred to when the term *reference values* is used with no qualifying words.

Selection of Reference Individuals

A set of explicit criteria should be used to determine which individuals should be included in the group of **reference individuals.** Such criteria include (1) statements describing the source population, (2) specifications of criteria for health, and (3) the disease of interest.[9,14] The selection of reference individuals is based essentially on the application of these defined criteria to the entire group of examined candidates. The required characteristics of the reference values determine which criteria should be used in the selection process.

BOX 5-1	Examples of Exclusion Criteria for Health-Associated Reference Values*

Diseases
Risk Factors
Obesity
Hypertension
Risks from occupation or environment
Genetically determined risks

Intake of Pharmacologically Active Agents
Drug treatment for disease or suffering
Oral contraceptives
Drug abuse
Alcohol
Tobacco

Specific Physiological States
Pregnancy
Stress
Excessive exercise

*This box lists only some major classes of criteria. It should be supplemented with other relevant criteria based on known sources of biological variation.

BOX 5-2	Examples of Partitioning Criteria for Possible Subgrouping of the Reference Group

Age (not necessarily categorized by equal intervals)
Gender
Genetic Factors
Ethnic origin
Blood groups (ABO)
Histocompatibility antigens (HLA)
Genes

Physiological Factors
Stage in menstrual cycle
Stage in pregnancy
Physical condition

Other Factors
Socioeconomic
Environmental
Chronobiological

HLA, Human leukocyte antigen.

As examples, Box 5-1 provides some criteria that should be considered when excluding individuals in the production of health-associated reference values.

Ideally the group of reference individuals should be a *random sample* of all individuals in the parent population who meet the selection criteria. However, a strictly random sampling scheme is impossible to obtain in most situations for a variety of practical reasons. For example, it would imply the examination and application of selection criteria to the entire population (thousands or millions of individuals) and the random selection of a subset of individuals among those accepted. Therefore, using the best reference sample obtained after all practical considerations have been taken into account is necessary. Data then should be used and interpreted with due caution because of the possible bias introduced by the nonrandomness of the sample selection process.

Often, separate reference values for sex, age group, and other criteria are necessary. Thus, it is important to define the *partitioning* criteria for the subclassification of the set of selected reference individuals. Some examples are provided in Box 5-2.[2,3] In practice, each partition could require as many as 120 samples; therefore the number of partitions should usually be kept as small as possible to obtain sufficient sample sizes for the derivation of valid statistical estimates.

Age and sex are the most frequently used criteria for partitioning because several analytes vary significantly among different age and gender groups. Age may be categorized by equal intervals (e.g., by decades) or by intervals that are narrower in the periods of life where greater variation is observed. In addition, the use of qualitative age groups (e.g., [1] postnatal, [2] infancy, [3] childhood, [4] prepubertal, [5] pubertal, [6] adult, [7] premenopausal, [8] menopausal, and [9] geriatric]) often may be appropriate. Height and weight also have been used as criteria for the categorization of children.

Specimen Collection

Preanalytical standardization of (1) preparation of individuals before sample collection, (2) the sample collection itself, and (3) handling of the sample before analysis may eliminate or minimize bias or variation from these factors. These steps may reduce biological "noise" that otherwise may conceal important biological "signals" of (1) disease, (2) risk, or (3) treatment effect.

The magnitudes of preanalytical sources of variation clearly are not equal for different analytes. Therefore one may argue that one should consider only those factors that cause unwanted variation in the biological quantity for which reference value production is intended. Body posture during sample collection is, for instance, highly relevant for the establishment of reference values for nondiffusible analytes, such as albumin in serum, but is irrelevant for diffusible ones, such as serum sodium.

However, performing separate studies to allow for different preanalytical conditions for each constituent is impractical. In addition, several constituents are typically analyzed in the same clinical specimens. For these reasons, standardized procedures are recommended for sample collection, taking into account the requirements that will enable all the constituents under study to be measured accurately.

A special problem is caused by drug ingestion before sample collection. A distinction may be made between indispensable and dispensable medications. The latter category of drugs always should be avoided for at least 2 days before specimen collection. The use of indispensable drugs, such as contraceptive pills or essential medication, may be a criterion for exclusion or partition.

Analytical Procedures and Quality Control

Essential components of the required definition of a set of reference values are specifications concerning (1) analysis method, including information on (a) equipment, (b) reagents, (c) calibrators, (d) types of raw data, and (e) calculation method; (2) quality control (see Chapter 7); and (3) reliability criteria (see Chapter 2). Specifications should be carefully described so that another investigator will be able to reproduce the study and evaluate comparability of the reference values with values obtained by the methods used for production of the patient's values in a routine laboratory. To ensure comparability between reference and observed values, the same analytical method should be used. Alternatively (or in addition), one establishes comparability of methods and populations by analyzing 20 samples from reference individuals and ensuring that no more than two values fall outside the proposed limits.[1]

Statistical Treatment of Reference Values

After the analysis of the reference specimens is performed, the reference values are subjected to a statistical treatment, which includes (1) partitioning of the reference values into appropriate groups, (2) inspection of the distribution of each group, (3) identification of outliers, and (4) determination of reference limits.

Partitioning of Reference Values

The subset of reference individuals and the corresponding reference values may be partitioned according to sex, age, and other characteristics (see Box 5-2). **Partitioning** is also known as (1) *stratification,* (2) *categorization,* or (3) *subgrouping,* and its results are called (1) *partitions,* (2) *strata,* (3) *categories,* (4) *classes,* or (5) *subgroups.* Such partitioning gives rise to narrower and potentially more appropriate reference intervals. For example, testosterone reference intervals for adult males and adult females do not overlap; combining them into a single interval would obscure those differences. Various statistical criteria for partitioning have been suggested,[6] and all feature the need to collect sufficient data to allow evaluation of the partitions separately and then, if appropriate, to combine them. One may, for example, test for differences in means or in standard deviations of the separate distributions. Note, though, that differences in means or differences in variability may be *statistically* significant and still too small *clinically* to justify replacing a single overall reference interval with several class-specific intervals. Harris and Boyd[6] and Lahti and coworkers[11] have developed other criteria for partitioning and statistical methods for this purpose.

In the following sections, a homogeneous reference distribution is assumed to exist—either the complete sample distribution (if partitioning is unnecessary) or a subclass distribution after partitioning.

Inspection of Distribution

It is advisable to display the reference distribution graphically and subsequently to inspect it. A histogram, as shown in Figure 5-1, is prepared manually or by a computer program. Examination of the histogram serves as a safeguard against the misapplication or misinterpretation of statistical methods, and it may provide valuable information about the data. The following characteristics should be sought in an examination of the distribution:

1. Highly deviating values (outliers) may represent erroneous values.
2. Bimodal or polymodal distributions have more than one peak and may indicate that the distribution is

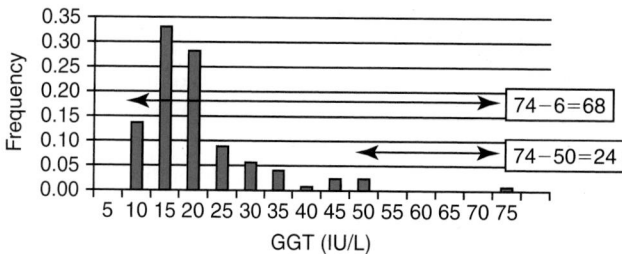

Figure 5-1 Observed distribution of 124 γ-glutamyltransferase (GGT) values in serum (IU/L). This distribution is clearly not Gaussian; it appears skewed to the right. The *upper arrow* indicates the range of observed values (highest − lowest, or 74 − 6 = 68); the *lower arrow* indicates the difference between the highest value and the next highest value (74 − 50 = 24). Because the quotient (24/68 = 0.35) exceeds 0.33, Dixon's range test indicates that the highest value is an outlier and therefore is omitted from all further analyses.

nonhomogeneous because of the mixing of two or more distributions. If nonhomogeneity is the case, the criteria used to select reference individuals should be reevaluated or partitioning of the values according to age, sex, or other relevant factors attempted.
3. The shape of the distribution may be asymmetrical (skewed) or more or less peaked than the symmetrical and bell-shaped Gaussian distribution (non-Gaussian kurtosis).[8,14]
4. Visual inspection may provide initial estimates of the location of reference limits that are useful as checks on the validity of computations.

Identification and Handling of Outliers

An outlier is an erroneous value that deviates significantly from the proper reference values.[15] Visual inspection of a histogram is a reliable method for identification of possible outliers. However, the inspector must keep in mind that values near the farthest point on the long tail of a skewed distribution may easily be misinterpreted as outliers. If the distribution is positively skewed, inspection of a histogram displaying the logarithms of the values may aid in the identification of outliers. Some outliers may be identified by statistical tests[7,9,14] but no single method will detect outliers in every situation that may occur. Two main problems are often encountered:

1. Many tests assume that the type of the true distribution is known before the tests are used. Some tests specifically require that the distribution be Gaussian. However, biological distributions are very often non-Gaussian, and their types seldom are known in advance. The Dixon-Reed range test, described in IFCC's recommendation,[9] is relatively robust and involves identification of the extreme value as an outlier if the difference between the two highest (or lowest) values in the distribution exceeds one-third of the range of all values (see Figure 5-1).
2. Several tests for outliers assume that the data contain only a single outlier. Thus the range test may fail in the presence of several outliers.

A method published in 2005[12] may provide a solution to both of these problems. The algorithm involves mathematically transforming the data so as to approximate a Gaussian distribution, calculating the range of the central 50% of the resulting distribution, and then subtracting 150% of this value from the 25th percentile and adding 150% of this value to the 75th percentile. Any values beyond these limits are considered outliers.

Deviating values identified as possible outliers should not be discarded automatically. Values should be included or excluded on a rational basis. The records of the suspect values should be checked and any errors corrected. In some cases, deviating values should be rejected because uncorrectable causes have been found, such as previously unrecognized conditions that qualify individuals for exclusion from the group of reference individuals.

Determination of Reference Limits

In clinical practice, an observed patient's value usually is compared with the corresponding **reference interval**, which is bounded by a pair of reference limits. This interval, which may be defined in different ways, is a useful condensation of the information carried by the total set of reference values.

The terms *reference limits* and *clinical decision limits* should not be confused. Reference limits describe the reference distribution and provide information about the observed variation of values in the selected set of reference individuals. Thus comparison of new values with these limits only conveys information about similarity to the given set of reference values. In contrast, clinical decision limits provide optimal separation among clinical categories. Such limits usually are based on analysis of reference values from several groups of individuals (e.g., healthy individuals, patients with relevant diseases) and thus are used for the purpose of differential diagnosis. Alternatively, such values are established scientifically on the basis of outcome studies and are used as clinical guidelines for treatment. The National Cholesterol Education Program guidelines for cholesterol is an example of decision limits currently in widespread use.[2]

As discussed earlier, the term *reference range* has been used for the term *reference interval,* but this use should be discouraged because the statistical term *range* denotes the difference (a single value!) between maximum and minimum values in a distribution.

Categories of reference intervals include (1) tolerance interval, (2) prediction interval, and (3) interpercentile interval.[9] The choice from among these three may be important for certain systematically defined statistical problems, but, in practice, their numerical differences are negligible when based on at least 100 reference values.

The interpercentile interval is (1) simple to estimate, (2) more commonly used, and (3) recommended by the IFCC.[9] It is defined as an interval bounded by two percentiles of the reference distribution. A percentile denotes a value that divides the reference distribution such that a specified percentage of its values has magnitudes less than or equal to the limiting value. For example, if 47 IU/L is the 97.5 percentile of serum γ-glutamyltransferase (GGT) values, then 97.5% of the values are equal to or below this value.

The definition of the reference interval as the central 95% interval bounded by the 2.5 and 97.5 percentiles is an arbitrary but common convention as 2.5% of the values are cut off in both tails of the reference distribution.[9] Another size or an asymmetrical location of the reference interval may be more appropriate in particular cases.

Of importance is the degree of uncertainty associated with a given percentile as an estimate of a population value; the magnitude of this uncertainty depends on the size of the number of samples, which increases when the number of observations is low. If the assumption of random sampling is fulfilled, determination of the confidence interval of the percentile (i.e., the limits within which the true percentile is located with a specified degree of confidence) is possible. The 0.90 confidence interval of the 97.5 percentile (upper reference limit) for serum GGT may, for example, be 39 to 50 IU/L. The true percentile would be expected in this interval with a confidence limit of 0.90 if all serum GGT concentrations in the total reference population were measured. The theoretical minimum sample size required for estimation of the 2.5 and 97.5 percentiles is 40 values, but usually at least 120 reference values are required to obtain reliable estimates.

The interpercentile interval has been determined by both parametric and nonparametric statistical techniques. The **parametric** method for the determination of percentiles and their confidence intervals assumes a certain type of distribution, and it is based on estimates of population parameters, such as the mean and standard deviation (SD). For example, a parametric method is used if the true distribution is believed to be Gaussian and reference limits (percentiles) are determined as the values located 2 SDs below and above the mean. Most parametric methods in fact are based on the Gaussian distribution. If the reference distribution has another shape, mathematical functions that transform data to approximately Gaussian shape may be used. In contrast, the **nonparametric** method makes no assumptions concerning the type of distribution and does not use estimates of distribution parameters. The percentiles are determined simply by cutting off the required percentage of values in each tail of the subset reference distribution.

When the results obtained by these two methods are compared, the estimates of the percentiles usually are very similar. In general, the simple and reliable nonparametric method is preferable to the parametric method.

Nonparametric Method

Several nonparametric methods are available,[14] but those based on ranked data are simple and reliable and allow nonparametric estimation of the confidence intervals of the percentiles.[6,9,13,14]

The steps in a nonparametric procedure are as follows:

1. Sort the n reference values in ascending order of magnitude, and rank the values. The minimum value has rank number 1, the next value number 2, and so on, until the maximum value, rank n, is reached. Consecutive rank numbers should be given to two or more values that are equal ("ties"). Spreadsheet software such as EXCEL is often used to sort and rank this type of data.

2. Compute the rank numbers of the 2.5 and 97.5 percentiles as $0.025(n + 1)$ and $0.975(n + 1)$, respectively.

3. Determine the percentiles by finding the original reference values that correspond to the computed rank numbers, provided that the rank numbers are integers. Otherwise, interpolation between the two limiting values is necessary.
4. Finally, determine the confidence interval of each percentile by using the binomial distribution. Table 5-1 facilitates this step for the 0.90 confidence interval of 2.5 and 97.5 percentiles. The bounding rank numbers for each percentile may be located in the table.

Table 5-2, *A* and *B* shows an example of the nonparametric determination of percentiles using the serum GGT values shown in Figure 5-1.

Parametric Method
The parametric method[6,8,9,14] is more complicated than the nonparametric method and usually requires the use of a computer statistics program when large data sets are processed.[13] The parametric method assumes that the true distribution is Gaussian. It is absolutely critical, therefore, to test the goodness-of-fit level of the reference distribution to a hypothetical Gaussian distribution. A simple test is examination of the cumulative frequency plotted on Gaussian probability paper (Figure 5-2, *B*); the plot should be close to a straight line if the distribution is Gaussian. In addition, many statistical computer programs have goodness-of-fit tests (e.g., tests based on coefficients of skewness and kurtosis, the Kolmogorov-Smirnov test, the Anderson-Darling test).[9,13,14]

If the reference distribution does not differ significantly from the Gaussian distribution, the 2.5 and 97.5 percentiles are estimated by values approximately 2 SDs on each side of the mean, or, more precisely:

$$2.5 \text{ percentile} = \bar{x} - 1.96 \times SD$$

$$97.5 \text{ percentile} = \bar{x} + 1.96 \times SD$$

The 0.90 confidence interval of each percentile is estimated by the following two limits:

$$\text{Lower confidence limit} = \text{percentile limit} - 2.81 \times \frac{SD}{\sqrt{n}}$$

$$\text{Upper confidence limit} = \text{percentile limit} + 2.81 \times \frac{SD}{\sqrt{n}}$$

If the reference distribution is non-Gaussian, mathematical transformation of data may adjust the shape to approximate

TABLE 5-1	Nonparametric Confidence Intervals of Reference Limits*	
	Rank Numbers	
Sample Size	**Lower**	**Upper**
119-132	1	7
133-160	1	8
161-187	1	9
188-189	2	9
190-218	2	10
219-248	2	11
249-249	2	12
250-279	3	12
280-307	3	13
308-309	4	13
310-340	4	14
341-363	4	15
364-372	5	15
373-403	5	16
404-417	5	17
418-435	6	17
436-468	6	18
469-470	6	19
471-500	7	19

*The table shows the rank numbers of the 0.90 confidence interval of the 2.5 percentile for samples with 119 to 500 values. To obtain the corresponding rank numbers of the 97.5 percentile, subtract the rank numbers in the table from ($n = 1$), where n is the sample size.
From IFCC.[9]

TABLE 5-2, A	γ-Glutamyltransferase (GGT) Values Used in the Nonparametric Determination of Reference Intervals	
GGT Value (IU/L)	**Frequency**	**Rank Order**
6	1	1
7	2	2, 3
8	6	4-9
9	4	10-13
10	4	14-17
11	9	18-26
12	7	27-33
13	7	34-40
14	9	41-49
15	9	50-58
16	8	59-66
17	11	67-77
18	8	78-85
19	5	86-90
20	3	91-93
21	2	94, 95
22	2	96, 97
23	2	98, 99
24	2	100, 101
25	3	102-104
26	2	105, 106
27	1	107
28	1	108
29	2	109, 110
30	1	111
32	2	112, 113
34	2	114, 115
35	1	116
39	1	117
42	2	118, 119
45	1	120
47	1	121
48	1	122
50	1	123

TABLE 5-2, B	Nonparametric Determination of Reference Interval*

Calculation of Rank Numbers of Percentiles

Lower	0.025 (123 + 1) = 3.1 (i.e., Rank #3)
Upper	0.975 (123 + 1) = 120.9 (i.e., Rank #121)

Original Values Corresponding to These Rank Numbers

Lower limit (2.5 percentile)	7 IU/L
Upper limit (97.5 percentile)	47 IU/L

Rank Numbers and Values of the 0.90 Confidence Limits

Lower Reference Limits

Rank numbers (see Table 5-1)	#1 and #7
Values	#6 and #8 IU/L

Upper Reference Limits

Rank numbers (see Table 5-1)	(123 + 1) − 7 = 117 and (123 + 1) − 1 = 123
Values	39 and 50 IU/L

Summary

Lower reference limit	7 (6 to 8) IU/L
Upper reference limit	47 (39 to 50) IU/L

*The table shows an example using the γ-glutamyltransferase (GGT) results listed in Table 5-2, A.

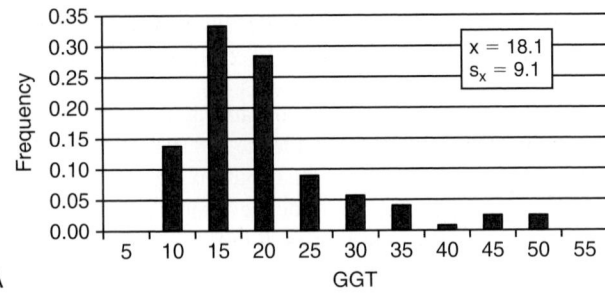

A

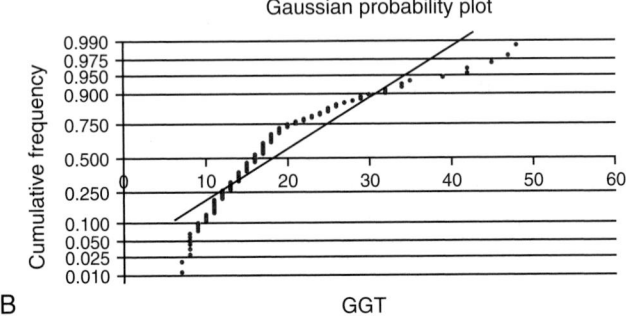

B

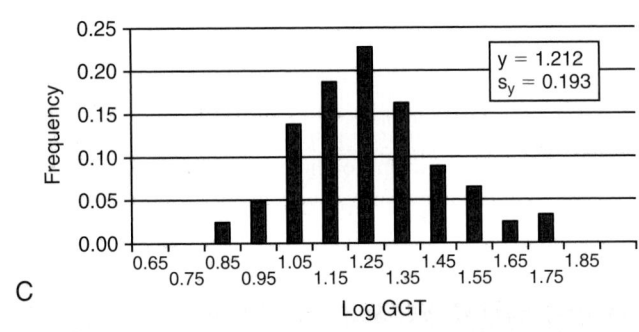

C

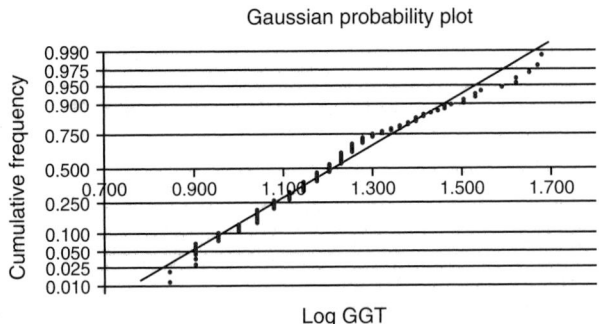

D

Figure 5-2 Distribution of 123 remaining γ-glutamyltransferase (GGT) values from reference subjects. **A,** A histogram of the original, untransformed data. **B,** The cumulative frequency of the data from **A,** plotted on Gaussian probability paper. **C,** A histogram of the logarithmic transformed data. **D,** The cumulative frequency of the data from **C,** plotted on Gaussian probability paper.

the Gaussian distribution. One frequent observation of interest is that logarithmically transformed values of a distribution with a long right tail (positively skewed) fit the Gaussian distribution rather closely (Figure 5-2, *D*). In other cases, square roots of the values better approximate the Gaussian distribution. This information provides the basis for the common use of logarithmic and square root transformations when reference limits are estimated, as described in the following section. If these two functions fail to transform data to fit a Gaussian distribution, more general transformations can be used. Such functions are described in other relevant literature.[6,8,9,14]

To apply the parametric procedure to transformed data, the process is very similar, as shown in the following steps:

1. Transform data with the logarithmic function $y = \log_{10}(x)$ (or $y = \ln[x]$) or by using square roots: $y = \sqrt{x}$. Then test the fit to the Gaussian distribution by using the methods described previously. If both transformations fail, then more general functions, which usually are more complicated, or the simple nonparametric method previously described should be used.

2. Then compute the *mean* ($\bar{y}$) and the standard deviation (SD_y) of the transformed data.

3. Next, estimate the percentiles and their confidence intervals in the transformed scale by using the formulas presented above, substituting $\bar{y}$ for $\bar{x}$ and SD_y for SD.

4. Finally, reconvert the percentiles and their confidence intervals to the original data scale by using inverse functions—antilogarithms or squares, respectively.

As shown in Figure 5-2, *D*, the mean and the SD of the serum GGT values in Figure 5-1 after logarithmic ($\log_{10}$) transformation are $\bar{y} = 1.212$ and $SD_y = 0.193$. The 2.5 percentile is:

$$1.212 - 1.96 \times 0.193 = 0.835$$

$$2.5 \text{ percentile} = 10^{0.835} = 6.84$$

The lower reference limit of serum GGT thus is 7 IU/L. The 0.90 confidence interval of this percentile is:

$$1.212 - 2.81 \times (0.193/\sqrt{123}) = 0.786$$

$$\text{Lower confidence limit} = 10^{0.786} = 6.1$$

$$1.212 + 2.81 \times (0.193/\sqrt{123}) = 0.884$$

$$\text{Upper confidence limit} = 10^{0.884} = 7.7$$

TABLE 5-3   Summary of GGT Reference Interval Determination by Three Methods

Method	Lower Limit (Confidence Interval)	Upper Limit (Confidence Interval)	Values Below Lower Limit	Values Above Upper Limit
Nonparametric	7 (6 to 8)	47 (39 to 50)	1	2
Parametric—untransformed data	0 (−2 to 2)	36 (34 to 38)	0	7
Parametric—transformed data	7 (6 to 8)	40 (35 to 44)	1	6

The table summarizes the 95% reference intervals and associated 90% confidence limits generated by each of three methods for the same data set. The numbers of observed values deemed lower and higher than the corresponding interval for each method are given in the last two columns. Because the original data are positively skewed, note that the parametric techniques generate intervals that are biased low. Note too that the parametric technique on untransformed data has a lower confidence interval, which is actually less than 0.

that is, 6 to 8 IU/L. The 97.5 percentile (and its 0.90 confidence interval) is by the same method found to be 40 IU/L (35 to 44 IU/L).

Table 5-3 demonstrates that the nonparametric method and the parametric method (using the transformed data) result in very similar estimates of reference limits (percentiles).

Other Methods for Calculating Reference Limits

Other methods have been recommended for calculating reference limits, including the so-called bootstrap and robust methods. Neither of these methods makes assumptions about the underlying distribution; it need not be Gaussian. Both require the use of computer software because they involve numerous iterations and somewhat complicated calculations. A brief discussion of these two methods is available elsewhere.[8]

Use of Reference Values

In practice, interpreting medical laboratory data requires comparison of the patient's values with reference values.

Presentation of an Observed Value in Relation to Reference Values

An observed value (patient's value) may be compared with reference values. This comparison is often similar to hypothesis testing, but it is seldom statistical testing in the strict sense. Thus it is advisable to consider the reference values as the yardstick for a less formal assessment than hypothesis testing.

The clinician or healthcare provider should be supplied with as much information about the reference values as necessary for the interpretation.[9] Reference intervals for all laboratory tests may be presented to clinicians or healthcare providers in a booklet, together with information about the analysis methods and their imprecision, along with descriptions of the reference values. A convenient presentation of the observed value and the reference interval on the same report sheet may be helpful for the busy clinician or healthcare provider. For example, the reference intervals may be preprinted on report forms, or the computer system may select the appropriate age- and sex-specific reference interval from the database and print it next to the test result or in graphical form.

An observed value may be classified as low, usual, or high, depending on its location in relation to the reference interval.

On reports, a convenient practice is to flag unusual results (e.g., through use of the letters L and H for low and high, respectively).

Another popular method of classification is expressing the observed value by a mathematical distance measure. For example, the well-known SD unit, or normal equivalent deviation, is such a measure. It is calculated as the difference between the observed value and the mean of the reference values divided by their SD.[2] This measure, however, is unreliable if the distribution of values is skewed. Values beyond ≈2 SD imply that the value is beyond the central 95% of the reference interval. Indeed, by using the SD unit deviation value, one determines the percentile of the observed value (e.g., values greater than 3.0 SD occur in only less than 0.15% of people in the reference distribution).

Subject-Based Reference Values

Figure 5-3 illustrates the inherent problem associated with population-based reference values. The figure shows two hypothetical reference distributions. One represents the common reference distribution based on single samples obtained from a group of several different reference individuals. It has a true (hypothetical) mean μ and an SD of σ. The other distribution is based on several samples collected over time in a single individual, the *i*th individual. Its hypothetical mean is μ_i and the SD, σ_i.

If an observed value is located outside the subject's 2.5 and 97.5 percentiles, the personal or **subject-based reference interval**, the cause may be a change in biochemical status, suggesting the presence of disease. Figure 5-3 demonstrates that such an observed value still may be within the population-based reference interval.[5] The sensitivity of the latter interval to changes in a subject's biochemical status depends accordingly on the location of the individual's mean μ_i relative to the common mean μ and to the relative magnitudes of the corresponding SDs, σ_i and σ. A mean μ_i close to μ and a small σ_i relative to σ may conceal the individual's changes entirely within the population-based reference interval.

Two specific examples may help to clarify this concept. Figure 5-4 depicts immunoglobulin M (IgM) values from several healthy individuals over the course of several days.[16] As illustrated, intraindividual differences are small as compared with interindividual differences. Even though the population-based reference interval might extend from 200 to 1600 mg/dL, in practice it would be unusual (abnormal) for any patient's IgM value to change by more than 200 mg/dL, even if the value remained within the population-based reference interval. Similarly, it is well known that any given patient's serum creatinine value is reasonably constant,[4] and this is related both to glomerular filtration rate (GFR) and to lean muscle mass. If the latter is constant, then changes in GFR are inversely proportional to the serum creatinine (see Chapters 21 and 35), that is, even though a typical (population-based) reference interval for serum creatinine might extend from 62 to 106 μmol/L (0.7 to 1.2 mg/dL), a change from 65 to 105 μmol/L in

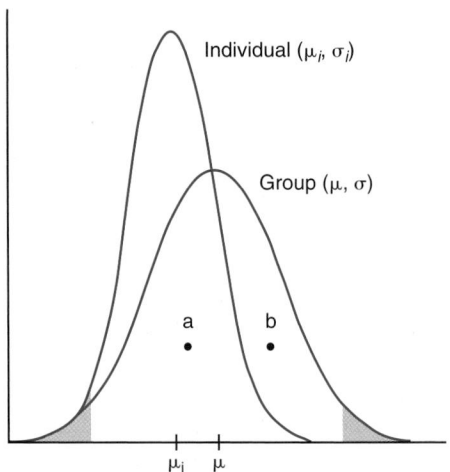

Figure 5-3 The relationship between population-based and subject-based reference distributions and reference intervals. The example is hypothetical, and the two distributions are, for simplicity, Gaussian. Hypothetical means and standard deviations are μ and σ (for the population) and μ_i and σ_i (individual i); x, analysis result. *(Modified from Harris EK. Effects of intra- and interindividual variation on the appropriate use of normal ranges,* Clin Chem *1974;20:1536.)*

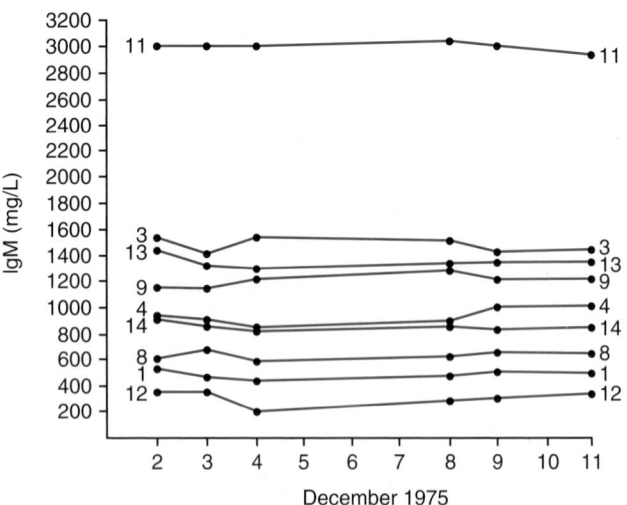

Figure 5-4 Serial immunoglobulin M (IgM) values over several days from reference individuals. Note that intraindividual variability is very small compared with interindividual variability. *(From Statland BE, Winkel P, Killingsworth LM. Factors contributing to intra-individual variation of serum constituents: 6. Physiological day-to-day variation in concentrations of 10 specific proteins in sera,* Clin Chem *1976;22:1635-6.)*

a given patient would be distinctly abnormal, representing loss of almost half of the GFR.

At least one solution is known for the problem of the limitations of population-based reference intervals for certain tests. With this solution, the subject's previous values, obtained in a well-defined state of health, are used as the reference for any future value.[6,14] Application of subject-based reference values becomes more feasible as "health-screening" by laboratory tests and computer storage of results become available to large sections of the general population.

Transferability (Transference) of Reference Values

Determining reliable reference values for each test in the laboratory's repertoire is a major task that is often far beyond the capabilities of the individual laboratory. Therefore, it would be convenient if reference values generated in another laboratory could be used. This is especially important when ethical considerations limit the number of available individuals (e.g., when pediatric reference values are produced). Then, cooperative establishment of reference values may be necessary.

A major prerequisite for transfer of reference values is that the populations must be comparable, and no major ethnic, social, or environmental differences must be noted between them. If they are not comparable, a separate reference interval study must be done.

Other factors that should not be overlooked include adherence to explicit, standardized protocols for (1) qualifying reference individuals, (2) preparing those individuals for specimen collection, and (3) performing specimen collection.

Analytical Issues

In practice, even if the populations are comparable and preanalytical standards are met, the problem of analytical transferability remains. The optimal, but usually very unrealistic, situation assumes that analytical methods, including their calibration and quality assurance, are identical in the laboratories. A more pragmatic approach involves (1) standardization of analytical protocols, (2) common calibration, (3) design of a sufficiently efficient external quality control scheme, and (4) the use of mathematical transfer functions if results still are not directly comparable.

Multicenter Trials

Another way to assist individual laboratories in generating reference values is to pool data from multiple sites to obtain the requisite minimum 120 samples (per partition). *Multicenter production of reference values* is gaining acceptance, both as a theoretical concept and as a practical approach. A Spanish study[3] introduced a cooperative model by simulating a virtual laboratory for 15 biochemical quantities. A project in the Nordic countries (NORIP) has produced common reference intervals for 25 analytes.[12]

Verification of Transfer

Whether a laboratory adopts reference values from (1) a package insert, (2) another laboratory, or (3) a multicenter trial, it is important that the laboratory verify the appropriateness of those values for its own use.[6] This verification serves as the final check that the laboratory has implemented the analytical method correctly and that the laboratory's own population is comparable with that used for the original reference value study.

Comparison of a locally produced, small subset of values with the large set produced elsewhere using traditional statistical tests often is not appropriate because the underlying statistical assumptions are not fulfilled and the sample sizes are unbalanced. A reasonably practical alternative has been

Formulas

	Patients with positive test result	Patients with negative test result	
Patients with disease	True Positives (TP)	False Negatives (FN)	*Clinical sensitivity=* $\frac{TP}{TP+FN}$
Patients without disease	False Positives (FP)	True Negatives (TN)	*Clinical specificity=* $\frac{TN}{FP+TN}$
	Total Positives= TP+FP	*Total Negatives= FN+TN*	
	PV (positive test)= $\frac{TP}{TP+FP}$	*PV (negative test)=* $\frac{TN}{(FN+TN)}$	

A

Test X: Disease prevalence = 50%

	Patients with positive test result	Patients with negative test result	
100	95	5	*Sensitivity= 95/(95+5)=95%*
100	10	90	*Specificity= 90/(90+10)=90%*
	Positives= 95+10=105	*Negatives= 5+90=95*	
	PV (positive)= 95/(95+10)=90%	*PV (negative)= 90/(90+5)=95%*	

B

Test X: Disease prevalence = 5%

	Patients with positive test result	Patients with negative test result	
500	475	25	*Sensitivity= 95%*
9500	950	8550	*Specificity= 90%*
	Positives= 475+950=1425	*Negatives= 25+8550=8575*	
	PV (positive)= 475/1425=5%	*PV (negative)= 8550/8575=100%*	

C

Figure 5-5 A, A basic 2 × 2 table *(bold lines)* facilitates understanding of the concepts of sensitivity, specificity, and predictive value. In the left-hand column, all patients with positive test results are tabulated; in the right-hand column, all patients with negative test results are tabulated. In the top row, patients with the disease under study are divided by their test results; likewise, the bottom row *(show shading symbol)* divides people without the disease by their test results. The top left-hand corner, then, represents patients with disease who have positive results, TRUE POSITIVES. The other three boxes are as labeled. As shown, the clinical sensitivity is calculated using the top row; the clinical specificity is calculated using the bottom row. The predictive value of a positive test is calculated using the data in the left-hand column; the predictive value of a negative test, using the right-hand column. **B,** The calculations described in **A** are done on test X, whose sensitivity and specificity are 95% and 90%, respectively. For this example, the prevalence of the population tested is 50%, reflected in the fact that 100 people with disease and 100 people without disease are tested. Of note, this is frequently the prevalence used when tests are first described in the literature. As shown, the predictive value of a positive test is 90%. **C,** The same calculations are done on the same test X, but the prevalence used is a more realistic, but still quite high, 5%, reflected in the fact that 500 people have the disease and 9500 do not. Although the sensitivity and specificity remain unchanged (95% and 90%, respectively), the predictive value of a positive test is now just 5%, that is, the likelihood that a patient with a positive test result in this population actually has the disease is 5%, or, in other words, 67% of the positive results are FALSE POSITIVES.

recommended by the Clinical Laboratory and Standards Institute (CLSI)[1]: With a sample size of 20 reference values, one verifies the appropriateness of a proposed reference interval so long as no more than two values are outside the proposed limits.

Clinical Sensitivity and Specificity and Predictive Value

When a clinician or a healthcare provider uses a laboratory test to help establish a diagnosis (as opposed to following a trend or evaluating the effectiveness of treatment), knowing the test's sensitivity and specificity can assist with proper interpretation (see Chapter 3). The **clinical sensitivity** of an assay is the fraction of those subjects with a specific disease that the assay correctly predicts. The **clinical specificity** is the fraction of those individuals without the disease that the assay correctly predicts. Figure 5-5, *A*, illustrates pertinent definitions and formulas.

Changing the decision limit of an assay affects both clinical sensitivity and specificity. Consider the case when the disease group has higher assay values than the nondisease group (Figure 5-6). Values above the decision limit are classified as positive; those at or below are negative. Moving the upper decision limit to a lower value increases the clinical sensitivity—but at the cost of a decrease in the clinical specificity. Thus increased true positive detection is traded for an increase in the number of false positive results. This trade-off occurs in most tests performed in medicine.

A separate, perhaps more important and more practical, issue that faces clinicians is this: Given a positive result, what is the likelihood that a patient actually has the disease? The **predictive value** of a positive test answers this question. The predictive value of a test combines disease prevalence with the test's sensitivity and specificity. **Prevalence** is the proportion of the population (or of those being tested) with the disease. The predictive value of a positive test is the number of true positive results divided by the total number of positive results (true positive and false positive results combined). As reflected in Figure 5-5, *B-C*, the proportion of true-positive and false-positive results is a function of the prevalence in the population and of the sensitivity and specificity of the test in question.

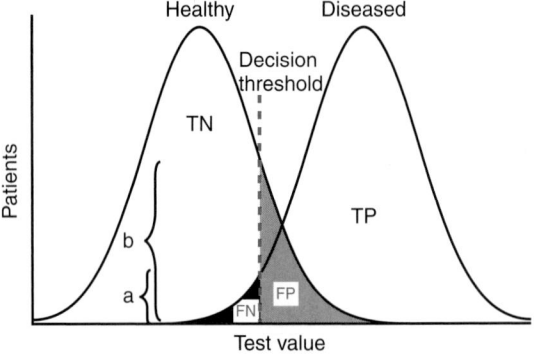

Figure 5-6 Simulated distributions of healthy and diseased populations. Note that at the shown decision threshold, the probability of a subject with disease *(a)* is much less than the probability of a healthy subject *(b)*. *TN,* true negatives; *TP,* true positives; *FN,* false negatives; *FP,* false positives.

As shown in Figure 5-5, *A*, the predictive value of a negative test follows in a similar way. It answers the question, "Given a negative result, how likely is it that a patient does not actually have the disease?" It has been used very effectively in many situations, for example, to reliably exclude, in the appropriate clinical context, deep venous thrombosis and/or pulmonary embolism.[10]

Review Questions

1. A "subject-based" reference value is:
   a. obtained from a group of systematically defined reference individuals.
   b. the type of value referred to when the term *reference value* is used with no qualifying words.
   c. based on several samples collected over time in a single individual.
   d. a random sample of all individuals in the parent population who fulfill the selection criteria.

2. True negatives ÷ (false positives + true negatives) × 100 is the formula for determining:
   a. clinical sensitivity.
   b. clinical specificity.
   c. predictive value.
   d. reference value.

3. The proportion of a population that has the particular disease being studied for establishment of reference values is referred to as the:
   a. prevalence.
   b. predictive value.
   c. positive value.
   d. clinical sensitivity.

4. When reference values are established, the criteria used to determine which individuals should be included in the group of reference individuals are referred to as:
   a. exclusion criteria.
   b. inclusion criteria.
   c. partition criteria.
   d. selection criteria.

5. Calculate the predictive value of a test in which 220 tested individuals with positive test results actually have the disease and 45 tested individuals with positive test results do not have the disease.
   a. 16.9%
   b. 66%
   c. 83%
   d. 120%

6. An example of an exclusion criterion would be a(n):
   a. individual's age.
   b. risk factor such as obesity.
   c. individual's ethnic origin.
   d. individual's sex.

7. In the selection of reference individuals, subclassifying a set of these individuals into homogeneous groups is referred to as:
   a. partitioning.
   b. excluding.
   c. transferring.
   d. including.

8. The number of true positive results divided by the sum of true positive results plus false positive results is referred to as:
   a. clinical sensitivity of a positive result.
   b. clinical specificity of a positive result.
   c. prevalence of the disease.
   d. predictive value of a positive result.

9. When reference limits are determined, the statistical method that assumes that the true distribution of reference values is a Gaussian (normal) distribution is the:
   a. nonparametric method.
   b. parametric method.
   c. interpercentile interval method.
   d. predictive value.

References

1. Clinical and Laboratory Standards Institute. Defining, establishing, and verifying reference intervals in the clinical laboratory. CLSI Document C28-A3c (renumbered as EP28-A3c). Wayne, Pa: Clinical and Laboratory Standards Institute, 2010.
2. Expert Panel on Detection, Evaluation, and Treatment of High Blood Cholesterol in Adults. Executive summary of the Third Report of the National Cholesterol Education Program (NCEP) Expert Panel on Detection, Evaluation, and Treatment of High Blood Cholesterol in Adults (Adult Treatment Panel III). JAMA 2001;285:2486–97.
3. Ferré-Masferrer M, Fuentes-Arderiu X, Alvarez-Funes V, Güell-Miró R, Castiñeiras-Lacambra MJ. Multicentric reference values: shared reference limits. Eur J Clin Chem Clin Biochem 1997;35:715–8.
4. Fraser CG. Biological variation: from principles to practice. Washington, DC: AACC Press, 2001:15–7.
5. Harris EK. Effects of intra- and interindividual variation on the appropriate use of normal ranges. Clin Chem 1974;20:1535–42.
6. Harris EK, Boyd JC. Statistical bases of reference values in laboratory medicine. New York: Marcel Dekker, 1995.
7. Horn PS, Feng L, Li Y, Pesce AJ. Effect of outliers and nonhealthy individuals on reference interval estimation. Clin Chem 2001;47:2137–45.
8. Horowitz GL. Establishment and use of reference values. In: Burtis CA, Ashwood ER, Bruns DE, eds. Tietz textbook of clinical chemistry and molecular diagnostics, 5th edition. St Louis: Saunders, 2012:95–118.
9. International Federation of Clinical Chemistry and Laboratory Medicine (IFCC), Expert Panel on Theory of Reference Values. Approved recommendation on the theory of reference values. Part 1. The concept of reference values. J Clin Chem Clin Biochem 1987;25:337-42. Part 2. Selection of individuals for the production of reference values. J Clin Chem Clin Biochem 1987;25:639-44. Part 3. Preparation of individuals and collection of specimens for the production of reference values. J Clin Chem Clin Biochem 1988;26:593-8. Part 4. Control of analytical variation in the production, transfer, and application of reference values. Eur J Clin Chem Clin Biochem 1991;29:531-5. Part 5. Statistical treatment of collected reference values: determination of reference limits. J Clin Chem Clin Biochem 1987;25:645-56. Part 6. Presentation of observed values related to reference values. J Clin Chem Clin Biochem 1987;25:657–62.
10. Kearon C, Ginsberg JS, Douketis J, Turpie AG, Bates SM, Lee AY, et al. An evaluation of D-dimer in the diagnosis of pulmonary embolism: a randomized trial. Ann Intern Med 2006;144:812–21.
11. Lahti A, Petersen PH, Boyd JC, Rustad P, Laake P, Solberg HE. Partitioning of nongaussian-distributed biochemical reference data into subgroups. Clin Chem 2004;50:891–900.
12. Rustad P, Felding P, eds. Transnational biological reference intervals: procedures and examples from the Nordic Reference Interval Project 2000. Scand J Clin Lab Invest 2004;64:265–441.
13. Solberg HE. The IFCC recommendation on estimation of reference intervals. The RefVal Program. Clin Chem Lab Med 2004;42:710–4.
14. Solberg HE, Gräsbeck R. Reference values. Adv Clin Chem 1989;27:1–79.
15. Solberg HE, Lahti A. Detection of outliers in reference distributions: performance of Horn's algorithm. Clin Chem 2005;51:2326–32.
16. Statland BE, Winkel P, Killingsworth LM. Factors contributing to intraindividual variation of serum constituents: 6. Physiological day-to-day variation in concentrations of 10 specific proteins in sera. Clin Chem 1976;22:1635–8.

CHAPTER
6

Specimen Collection, Processing, and Other Preanalytical Variables*

Doris M. Haverstick, Ph.D., D.A.B.C.C., and Amy R. Groszbach, M.E.D., M.L.T., M.B.(A.S.C.P.)C.M

Objectives

1. Define the following terms:
   - Anticoagulant
   - Controllable preanalytical variable
   - Hemolysis
   - Order of draw
   - Phlebotomy
   - Plasma
   - Preanalytical variable
   - Preanalytical error
   - Serum
   - Uncontrollable preanalytical variable
   - Venipuncture

2. Give two examples of a preanalytical error and two examples of an uncontrollable preanalytical variable.

3. List the types of biological specimens that are analyzed in a clinical laboratory.

4. Summarize the steps that are performed by a phlebotomist in obtaining a blood sample by venipuncture; state the preferred site of venous blood collection, including the practice used when an intravenous line is present.

5. List the general effects on analytes caused by the following:
   - Pumping a fist before venipuncture
   - Stress
   - Collection order (first tube, second tube, etc.)
   - Time of collection related to diurnal variation
   - Prolonged venous occlusion with a tourniquet
   - Not filling collection tube completely

6. Discuss order of draw for multiple blood specimens, including the order required for collecting multiple tubes of blood, color of stopper and associated additive, need for tube filling and inversion, and reason for filling tubes in a specific order.

7. Describe the skin puncture collection technique, including methods of stimulating blood flow; state the reasons for collecting a specimen using skin puncture; and describe the collection procedure for obtaining a blood spot for molecular genetic testing.

8. Explain the difference between serum and plasma.

9. Compare the difference in composition, if any, between serum and plasma specimens of the following analytes:
   - Calcium
   - Cholesterol
   - Albumin
   - Creatinine
   - Total protein
   - Glucose
   - Potassium

10. State how the following anticoagulants prevent blood from coagulating:
    - Heparin
    - EDTA
    - Citrate
    - Oxalate
    - Iodoacetate

11. State the appropriate analytical situations for using evacuated tubes containing various additives; state reasons why blood collected in the same anticoagulants cannot be used for certain analyses.

12. Describe the hemoglobin concentration at which hemolysis is observable in plasma; describe how hemolysis affects measurement of certain analytes and use of certain analytical procedures.

13. List three types of urine specimens and their use in clinical analysis; list two methods of urine preservation and discuss the use of each.

14. Outline the procedure for collecting a timed urine specimen.

15. List the clinical chemistry analyses performed on the following specimen types and the collection procedure name, if any:
    - Feces
    - Cerebrospinal fluid (CSF)
    - Synovial fluid
    - Amniotic fluid
    - Chorionic villus
    - Pleural, pericardial, and ascitic fluids
    - Saliva
    - Buccal cells
    - Hair and nails

16. Summarize each of the four aspects of specimen handling; discuss these in relation to specimen identification on various containers, centrifugation of blood samples, sample storage on ice/at −20 °C/at 4 °C, protection from light, and transport guidelines.

---

*The authors gratefully acknowledge the original contributions by Drs. Donald S. Young and Edward W. Bermes, on which portions of this chapter are based.

Key Words and Definitions

Additives Compounds added to biological specimens to prevent them from clotting or to preserve the constituents of a specimen.

Anticoagulant Any substance that prevents blood from clotting.

Chorionic villus sampling A prenatal test to detect birth defects that is performed at an early stage of pregnancy and involves retrieval and examination of tissue from the chorionic villi. Also called *chorionic villus biopsy.*

Coagulation (clotting) The sequential process by which the multiple coagulation factors of blood interact in the coagulation cascade, resulting in formation of an insoluble fibrin clot.

Diurnal variation Variation that occurs in the amount of a substance during a 24-hour period.

Hemolysis Disruption of the red cell membrane causing release of hemoglobin and other components of red blood cells.

Phlebotomist One who practices phlebotomy; the individual drawing a specimen of blood.

Phlebotomy The puncture of a blood vessel to collect blood; literally, "the letting of blood in the treatment of disease."

Preanalytical errors Factors that affect specimens before tests are performed and that can lead to error if not controlled; they are classified as controllable or uncontrollable.

Preservative A substance or preparation added to a specimen to prevent changes in the constituents of a specimen.

Plasma The noncellular component of anticoagulated whole blood; plasma contains clotting factors.

Serum The watery portion of blood that remains after coagulation has occurred; it is obtained after centrifugation.

Sharps Any object which could readily puncture or cut the skin of an individual when encountered.

Sharps container a container designed for the disposal of sharps; required and regulated by the Occupational Safety and Health Administration (OSHA).

Skin puncture Collection of capillary blood usually from a pediatric patient by making a thin cut in the skin, usually at the heel of the foot.

Specimen A sample or portion of body fluid or tissue collected for examination, study, or analysis.

Venipuncture All of the steps involved in obtaining an appropriate and identified blood specimen from an individual's vein.

Venous occlusion Obstruction of the return of venous blood to the heart and distention of the veins; in phlebotomy, this is a temporary blockage caused by application of pressure, usually from a tourniquet.

Critical factors involved in collecting a valid specimen for analysis in the clinical laboratory include appropriate policies, procedures, and techniques for (1) collection, (2) identification, (3) processing, (4) storage, and (5) transport. Many errors have been known to occur when a specimen is collected; such errors are considered **preanalytical errors**. Other types of errors in laboratory testing are analytical errors (errors made during the testing process, such as [1] running the wrong test, [2] reagent or instrument failure, or [3] technologist error) and postanalytical errors (errors made in interpretation of analytical results, such as a wrong calculation or data entry errors when results are manually entered into the laboratory information system).

Minimizing specifically preanalytical errors through careful adherence to the concepts discussed here and to individual institutional policies will result in more reliable information for use by healthcare professionals in providing quality patient care.

Errors are considered controllable variables; however, uncontrollable variables are also present in the preanalytical phase of testing.[12,22] Such uncontrollable variables may be those associated with the physiology of the particular patient (age, sex, underlying disease, etc.) or variables associated with different specimen types from the same patient. Laboratorians need to understand these issues as well.

Types of Specimens

Types of biological **specimens** that are analyzed in clinical laboratories include (1) whole blood; (2) serum; (3) plasma; (4) urine; (5) feces; (6) saliva; (7) spinal, synovial, amniotic, pleural, pericardial, and ascitic fluids; and (8) various types of solid tissue. The Clinical and Laboratory Standards Institute (CLSI) has published several procedures for collecting many of these specimens under standardized conditions.[3-11] These procedures are updated as required, and the most current versions are listed on the CLSI website (www.CLSI.org; accessed July 5, 2013).

Blood

Blood for analysis may be obtained from (1) veins, (2) arteries, or (3) capillaries. Venous blood is usually the specimen of choice, and venipuncture is the method for obtaining this specimen. Arterial puncture is used mainly for blood gas analyses. In young children and for many point-of-care tests, skin puncture is frequently used to obtain what is mostly capillary blood. The process of collecting blood is known as **phlebotomy** (the letting of blood in the treatment of disease) and should always be performed by a trained **phlebotomist**.

Venipuncture

In the clinical laboratory, **venipuncture** is defined as all of the steps involved in obtaining an appropriate and identified blood specimen from a patient's vein. Patient and phlebotomist safety should be equally balanced during this process. Before any specimen is collected, the phlebotomist must confirm the identity of the patient using at least two methods of identification. In specialized situations, such as paternity testing or other tests of medico-legal importance, establishment of a chain of custody for the specimen may require additional patient identification, such as a photograph, provided as part of the identification process or taken to confirm the identity of the patient. Identification must be an active process, and many hospitals now provide translation services for non–English-speaking patients. In the case of pediatric patients, the parent or guardian should be present and should provide active identification of the child. Finally, for some tests for genetic diseases, the performing laboratory may request a signed consent form from the patient; this should be completed at the time of collection if it was not provided by the requesting physician.

Before collecting a specimen, a phlebotomist should dress in personal protective equipment (PPE),[8] with additional precautions and equipment for patients in isolation as required by institutional policies. If appropriate, the phlebotomist should verify that the patient is fasting, what medications are being taken or have been discontinued as required, and so forth. The patient (1) should be comfortable, (2) should be seated or supine (if sitting is not feasible), and (3) should have been in this position for as long as possible before the specimen is drawn. At no time should venipuncture be performed on a standing patient. Either of the patient's arms should be extended in a straight line from the shoulder to the wrist. An arm with an inserted intravenous line should be avoided, as should an arm with extensive scarring or with a hematoma at the intended collection site. If a woman has had a mastectomy, arm veins on that side of the body should not be used because the surgery may have caused lymphostasis (blockade of normal lymph node drainage), affecting the blood composition. If a woman has had double mastectomies, blood should be drawn from the arm of the side on which the first procedure was performed.

The phlebotomist should estimate the volume of blood to be drawn and should select and collect the appropriate number and types of tubes for the blood, plasma, or serum tests requested. Sections that follow discuss in greater detail the recommended order of draw for multiple specimens and types of tubes. In addition to tubes, an appropriate needle must be selected. All needles must be (1) sterile, (2) sharp, and (3) without barbs. If blood is drawn for trace element measurements, the needle should be stainless steel and should be known to be free from contamination.

The preferred site for collecting venous blood in adults is the median cubital vein in the antecubital fossa, or the crook of the elbow because the vein is large and is close to the surface of the skin.[3,15] If fluid is being infused intravenously into a limb, the fluid should be shut off for 3 minutes before a specimen is obtained and a suitable note made in the patient's chart and on the result report form. Specimens obtained from the opposite arm are preferred. The area around the intended puncture site should be cleaned with whatever cleanser is approved for use by the institution. Cleaning of the puncture site should be done with a circular motion and from the site outward. The skin should be allowed to dry in the air. No alcohol or cleanser should remain on the skin because traces may cause hemolysis and may invalidate test results. Once the skin has been cleaned, it should not be touched until after the venipuncture has been completed.

The time at which a specimen is obtained is important for those blood constituents that undergo marked **diurnal variation** (e.g., corticosteroids, iron) and for those used to monitor drug therapy. For most current molecular diagnostic tests, the time of day is unlikely to contribute to altered or invalid test results.

After the skin is cleaned, a blood pressure cuff or a tourniquet is applied 4 to 6 inches (10 to 15 cm) above the intended puncture site (distance for adults). This obstructs the return of venous blood to the heart and distends the veins (**venous occlusion**). It is rarely necessary to leave a tourniquet in place for longer than 1 minute, but even within this short time, the composition of blood changes. Although the changes that occur in 1 minute are slight, marked changes have been observed after 3 minutes for many chemistry analytes (Table 6-1). No known changes affect molecular diagnostics.

The composition of blood drawn first—that is, the blood closest to the tourniquet—is most representative of the composition of circulating blood. The first-drawn specimen should therefore be used for those analytes such as calcium that are pertinent to critical medical decisions.[20] Blood drawn later shows a greater effect from venous stasis. Thus the first tube may show a 5% increase in protein, whereas the third tube may show a 10% change.[17] The concentration of protein-bound constituents is also influenced by stasis. Prolonged stasis may increase the concentration of protein or protein-bound constituents by as much as 15%.

Pumping of the fist before venipuncture should be avoided because it causes an increase in plasma potassium, phosphate, and lactate concentrations. Lowering of blood pH by accumulation of lactate causes the plasma ionized calcium concentration to increase.[20] The ionized calcium concentration reverts to normal 10 minutes after the tourniquet is released.

Stress associated with blood collection has been known to have effects on patients at any age. As a consequence, plasma concentrations of cortisol and growth hormone may increase. Stress occurs particularly in young children who are (1) frightened, (2) struggling, and (3) held in physical restraint. Collection under these conditions may cause adrenal stimulation, leading to an increased plasma glucose concentration, or may

TABLE 6-1	Changes in Composition of Serum When Venous Occlusion Is Prolonged from 1 Minute to 3 Minutes* †		
Increase	**%**	**Decrease**	**%**
Total protein	4.9	Potassium	6.2
Iron	6.7		
Total lipids	4.7		
Cholesterol	5.1		
Aspartate aminotransferase	9.3		
Bilirubin	8.4		

*To estimate the probable effect of a factor on results, relate percent increase or decrease shown in table to analytical variation (±% CV) routinely found for analytes.
†Mean values obtained from 11 healthy individuals.
From Statland BE, Bokelund H, Winkel P. Factors contributing to intraindividual variation of serum constituents: effects of posture and tourniquet application on variation of serum constituents in healthy subjects. Clin Chem 1974;20:1513-9.

cause increases in the serum activities of enzymes that originate in skeletal muscle.

Order of Draw for Multiple Blood Specimens

Several types of evacuated tubes are used for venipuncture collection. They vary by the presence or absence and type of **additive**, as well as by the volume of the tube. The different types of additives are identified by the color of the stopper used (Table 6-2) and are covered in greater detail later in this section. For a variety of reasons, the most important of which is the possibility of cross-contamination between tube additives, blood should be collected into tubes in the order outlined in Table 6-2. This table also provides the recommended number of inversions for each tube type because it is critical that complete mixing of any additive with the blood collected be accomplished as quickly as possible.

A typical system for collecting blood directly into evacuated tubes includes a single-use device that incorporates a cover designed to be placed over the needle when collection of the blood is complete, thereby reducing the risk of puncture of the phlebotomist by the now contaminated needle.[8] A needle or a winged (butterfly) set is screwed into the collection tube holder, and the tube is then gently inserted into this holder. After the skin has been cleaned, the needle is guided gently into the patient's vein (Figure 6-1); once the needle is in place, the tube is pressed forward into the holder to puncture the stopper and release the vacuum. As soon as blood begins to flow into the tube, the tourniquet should be released without moving the needle (see earlier discussion on venous occlusion). The tube is filled until the vacuum is exhausted. It is critically important that the evacuated tube be filled completely. Many additives are provided in the tube based on a "full" collection; deviation or short draws can be a source of preanalytical error because they can significantly affect test results. Once the tube is filled completely, it should be withdrawn from the holder, mixed gently by inversion, and replaced by another tube, if this is necessary. Collection directly into a syringe follows the same process, except that the needle is attached directly to the syringe, and a single collection is performed.

When blood collection is complete and the needle withdrawn, the patient should be instructed to hold a dry gauze pad over the puncture site, with the arm raised to lessen the likelihood of leakage of blood. With a collection device, such as that described previously, the needle is covered, and the needle and the tube holder are immediately discarded into a **sharps container**. In the event that a winged (butterfly) set is used, the wings are pushed forward to cover the needle, or with newer available equipment, a button is pressed, releasing a spring that retracts the needle. If a syringe was used, the needle and syringe (still attached) should be discarded in a hazardous waste receptacle.

All tubes should be labeled per institutional policy. Most institutions have a written procedure prohibiting the advance labeling of tubes because this is seen as providing the potential for mislabeling, one of the most common sources of preanalytical error. Some institutions recommend showing the labeled tube to the patient to further confirm correct identification. Finally PPE should be discarded and institutional policies for cleaning between patients should be followed if there are additional patients to be drawn.

TABLE 6-2	Recommended Order of Draw for Multiple Specimen Collection With Tube Color Identification	
Stopper Color	**Contents**	**Inversions**
Yellow	Sterile media for blood culture	8
Royal blue	No additive (for trace elements)	0
Clear/red	Non-additive; discard tube if no royal blue used	0
Light blue	Sodium citrate	3-4
Gold/red	Serum separator tube	5
Red/red, orange/yellow, royal blue	Serum tube, with or without clot activator, with or without gel	5
Green	Heparin tube with or without gel	8
Royal blue	Sodium EDTA	8
Lavender, pearl white, pink/pink, tan (plastic)	EDTA tubes, with or without gel	8
Gray	Glycolytic inhibitor	8
Yellow (glass)	ACD for molecular studies and cell culture	8

Modified from information in CLSI. Tubes and additives for venous blood specimen collection; CLSI-approved standard H1-A6, 6th edition. Wayne, Pa: Clinical and Laboratory Standards Institute, 2010 (current document code GP39-A6); Kiechle FL, ed. So you're going to collect a blood specimen: an introduction to phlebotomy, 14th edition. Northfield, Ill: College of American Pathologists, 2013; Becton Dickinson Web page. http:/www.bd.com/ (accessed July 7, 2013).

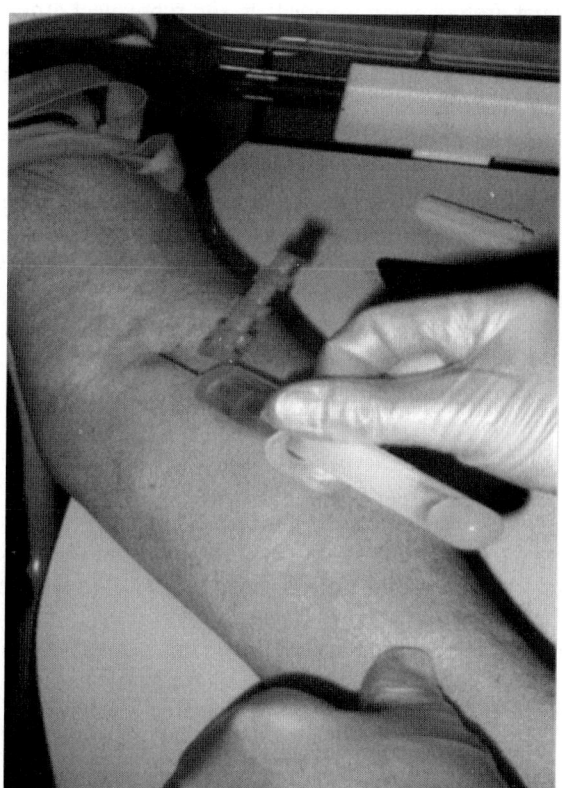

Figure 6-1 Venipuncture. *(Courtesy Ruth M. Jacobsen, Mayo Clinic, Rochester, Minn.)*

Blood Collection Through Skin Puncture

The techniques for venipuncture in children and adults are similar. However, in the pediatric population, alternative collection through skin puncture is often used. **Skin puncture** is an open collection technique in which the skin is punctured by a lancet, and a small volume of blood is collected into a micro-device or directly onto filter paper. Skin puncture blood is more like arterial blood than venous blood. In practice, it is used in situations in which (1) sample volume is limited (e.g., pediatric applications), (2) repeated venipunctures have resulted in severe vein damage, or (3) patients have been burned or bandaged and veins therefore are unavailable for venipuncture. This technique is also commonly used when the sample is to be applied directly to a testing device in a point-of-care testing situation or to filter paper. It is most often performed on (1) the tip of a finger, (2) an earlobe, and (3) the heel or big toe of infants (Figure 6-2).

The same steps of patient identification, appropriate PPE, and cleansing of the area to be pierced are followed as with venipuncture.[4] The skin is quickly punctured by a sharp stab with a lancet. If the finger is the site of puncture, it should be held in such a way that gravity assists collection of blood at the fingertip, and the lancet held to make the incision as close to perpendicular to the fingernail as possible.[15] Massage of the finger, or of any other site used, to stimulate blood flow should be avoided because this causes the outflow of debris and tissue fluid, which does not have the same composition as plasma. To improve circulation of the blood, the area to be pierced may be warmed by application of a warm, wet washcloth or a specialized device, such as a heel warmer, for 3 minutes before the lancet is applied. The first drop of blood is wiped off, and subsequent drops are transferred to the appropriate collection tube by gentle contact. Filling should be done rapidly to prevent clotting, and introduction of air bubbles should be prevented. A variety of collection tubes are commercially available, and available additives generally mirror those of full-sized collection devices. If multiple tubes are to be filled, the correct order of filling is the same as for evacuated blood tubes (see Table 6-2).

For collection of blood specimens on filter paper for molecular genetic testing and neonatal screening, the skin is cleaned and punctured as described previously. The first drop of blood

should be wiped away. Then the filter paper is gently touched against a large drop of blood that is allowed to soak into the paper to fill the marked circle. Only a single application per circle should be made to prevent nonuniform analyte concentration. The filter paper should be air-dried (generally for 2 to 3 hours to prevent mold or bacterial overgrowth) before storage in a properly labeled paper envelope.

Arterial Puncture

Arterial puncture, reserved primarily for arterial blood gas analysis in acid-base measurements during critical illness, requires considerable skill and is usually performed only by physicians or specially trained technicians or nurses.[5] Preferred sites of arterial puncture are, in order, (1) the radial artery at the wrist, (2) the brachial artery in the elbow, and (3) the femoral artery in the groin. Because leakage of blood from the femoral artery tends to be greater, especially in the elderly, sites in the arm are used most often.

Serum and Anticoagulants Used for Plasma Collection

Serum is defined as the liquid portion of blood that remains after **coagulation** has occurred; it is the specimen of choice for many analyses, including viral screening and protein electrophoresis. Samples are collected into tubes with no additive or with a clot activator and must be allowed to complete the coagulation process before further processing. **Plasma** is defined as the noncellular component of anticoagulated whole blood; it is being used increasingly for routine chemistry testing because the ability to immediately centrifuge the sample without waiting for clotting decreases turnaround time. Sometimes considerable differences may be observed between the concentrations of analytes in serum and in plasma, as shown in Table 6-3. Additives used to collect anticoagulated blood are discussed in the following section.

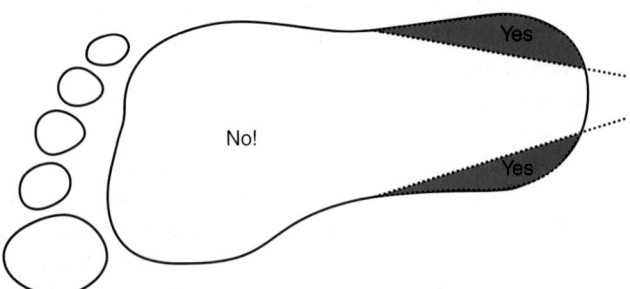

Figure 6-2 Acceptable sites for skin puncture to collect blood from an infant's foot. *(Modified from Blumenfeld TA, Turi GK, Blanc WA. Recommended site and depth of newborn heel punctures based on anatomical measurements and histopathology,* Lancet *1979;1:230-3. Reprinted with permission from Elsevier.)*

TABLE 6-3	Differences in Composition Between Plasma and Serum*			
Plasma Value > Serum Value, %		**No Difference Between Serum and Plasma Values**	**Plasma Value < Serum Value, %**	
Calcium	0.9	Bilirubin	Albumin	1.3
Chloride	0.2	Cholesterol	Alkaline phosphatase	1.6
Lactate dehydrogenase	2.7	Creatinine	Aspartate aminotransferase	0.9
Total protein	4.0		Bicarbonate	1.8
			Creatine kinase	2.1
			Glucose	5.1
			Phosphorus	7.0
			Potassium	8.4
			Sodium	0.1
			Urea	0.6
			Uric acid	0.2

From Ladenson JH, Tsai L-MB, Michael JM, Kessler G, Joist JH. Serum versus heparinized plasma for eighteen common chemistry tests. *Am J Clin Pathol* 1974;62:545-52. Copyright © 1974 by the American Society of Clinical Pathologists.

Heparin

Heparin is the most widely used **anticoagulant** for chemistry and hematology testing. It is a mucoitin polysulfuric acid that is available as (1) sodium (most often used for cytogenetic studies), (2) potassium, (3) lithium, and (4) ammonium salts, all of which adequately prevent coagulation. This anticoagulant accelerates the action of antithrombin III, which neutralizes thrombin and thus prevents the formation of fibrin from fibrinogen.

It should be noted that heparin is unacceptable for most tests performed using the polymerase chain reaction (PCR) because of inhibition of the polymerase enzyme by this large molecule. DNA can be extracted from heparinized samples, but amplification may be reduced.

Ethylenediaminetetraacetic Acid (EDTA)

EDTA is a chelating agent of divalent cations such as Ca^{2+} and Mg^{2+}. Because it preserves the cellular components of blood, it is particularly useful for (1) hematologic examinations, (2) isolation of genomic DNA, and (3) qualitative and quantitative virus determinations by molecular techniques. It is used as the disodium, dipotassium, or tripotassium salt. EDTA prevents coagulation by binding calcium, which is essential for the clotting mechanism. Newer advances using EDTA include the inclusion of a gel barrier to separate plasma from cells (white tubes). In blue/black tubes, incorporation of a density gradient allows recovery of nucleated cells after centrifugation, thus increasing the yield of DNA.

EDTA, probably by chelation of metallic cofactors, inhibits the activity of enzymes that require a metallic cofactor such as (1) alkaline phosphatase, (2) CK, and (3) leucine aminopeptidase. Because it chelates calcium and iron, EDTA is unsuitable for specimens for calcium and iron analyses using photometric or titrimetric techniques.

Sodium Fluoride

Sodium fluoride is a weak anticoagulant that is often added as a preservative for blood glucose. As a preservative, together with another anticoagulant such as potassium oxalate, it is effective at a concentration of approximately 2 g/L of blood. It exerts its **preservative** action by inhibiting the enzyme systems involved in glycolysis, although such inhibition is not immediate[18] and a certain amount of degradation occurs during the first hour after collection. Without an antiglycolytic agent, the blood glucose concentration decreases approximately 10 mg/dL (0.56 mmol/L) per hour at 25 °C. The rate of decrease is faster in newborns because of the increased metabolic activity of their erythrocytes and in leukemic patients because of the high metabolic activity of the white cells. Sodium fluoride is poorly soluble, and blood must be mixed well before effective antiglycolysis occurs. Fluoride is a potent inhibitor of many serum enzymes and in high concentrations also affects urease, which is used to measure urea nitrogen in many analytical systems.

Citrate

Sodium citrate solution, at a concentration of 34 to 38 g/L in a ratio of 1 part to 9 parts of blood, is widely used for coagulation studies, as the anticoagulation effect (chelation of Ca^{2+}) is easily reversible through the addition of Ca^{2+} to the plasma. However, the correct ratio of blood to anticoagulant is critical because modern analyzers add a standard amount of Ca^{2+} that is based on a proper collection volume. This forms the basis of the first step for most modern coagulation assays. A citrate tube is rarely acceptable for chemistry testing but may be acceptable, if not centrifuged, for genomic DNA isolation.

Acid Citrate Dextrose (ACD)

As indicated previously, the collection of specimens into EDTA is often used for isolation of genomic DNA from the patient. However, additional and complementary diagnostic tests, such as cytogenetic testing, may be requested at the same time. For this reason, samples for molecular diagnostics are often collected into ACD anticoagulant, so as to preserve both the form and the function of the cellular components. There are two ACD tube designations: ACD A and ACD B. These differ only by the concentrations of the additives. Both enhance the viability and recovery of white blood cells for several days after collection of the specimen, thus they are suitable for both molecular diagnostic testing and cytogenetic testing.

Oxalates

Sodium, potassium, ammonium, and lithium oxalates inhibit blood coagulation by forming rather insoluble complexes with calcium ions. Potassium oxalate ($K_2C_2O_4 \cdot H_2O$), at a concentration of approximately 1 to 2 g/L of blood, is the most widely used oxalate. At concentrations of greater than 3 g oxalate per liter, hemolysis is likely to occur, so this is another example in which the volume of blood added to the tube is critical.

Iodoacetate

Sodium iodoacetate at a concentration of 2 g/L is an effective antiglycolytic agent (with the caveats mentioned earlier) and a substitute for sodium fluoride. Because it has no effect on urease, it is often used when glucose and urea tests are performed on a single specimen. It inhibits CK but appears to have no notable effects on other clinical tests.

Influence of Site of Collection on Blood Composition

Blood obtained from different sites differs in composition. Skin puncture blood is more like arterial blood than venous blood, although blood obtained by skin puncture is prone to contamination with interstitial and intracellular fluids. Thus there are no clinically significant differences between freely flowing capillary blood and arterial blood in pH, PCO_2, PO_2, and oxygen saturation. The PCO_2 of venous blood is up to 6 to 7 mm Hg (0.8 to 0.9 kPa) higher. Venous blood glucose is as much as 7 mg/L (0.39 mmol/L) less than capillary blood glucose. The major differences between venous serum and capillary serum have been covered elsewhere.[14]

Hemolysis

Hemolysis is defined as disruption of the red cell membrane, resulting in the release of hemoglobin; it may be the consequence of intravascular events (in vivo hemolysis) or may occur subsequent to or during blood collection (in vitro hemolysis). In vitro hemolysis can be caused by (1) alcohol left on the skin, (2) use of small bore needles, (3) underlying red cell disorders, (4) temperature extremes during transport, and (5) other causes. Serum and plasma show visual evidence of hemolysis when the hemoglobin concentration exceeds 50 mg/dL, and once the level exceeds 150 to 200 mg/dL, the plasma will appear bright red to most observers. Slight hemolysis has little effect on most test values. However, a notable effect may be observed on those constituents that are present at a higher concentration in erythrocytes than in plasma. Thus plasma activities or concentrations of (1) lactate dehydrogenase, (2) potassium, (3) magnesium, and (4) phosphate are particularly increased by hemolysis. The inorganic phosphate in serum increases rapidly as the organic esters in the cells are hydrolyzed. An additional band caused by hemoglobin may be observed on serum protein electrophoresis. Because the effect of free hemoglobin following hemolysis may be spectral (i.e., direct interference by the absorbance of hemoglobin at the wavelength at which an assay is measured), most manufacturers now provide data on the effects of hemolysis on the analytical performance of individual tests; this should be evaluated in the selection of individual methods.

In molecular diagnostic testing, hemoglobin may interfere with the amplification reaction, particularly when reverse transcriptase (RT)-PCR is the first step in the analysis of RNA. In some situations, the isolation of nucleic acid is sufficiently selective that free hemoglobin from the ruptured cells is removed and will not cause a problem. However, with hemolyzed blood, alternative or additional extraction methods are usually needed to ensure that RNA is fully and accurately transcribed, and that the greatest amplification of DNA is achieved.

Urine

The type of urine specimen and required preservation during collection are dictated by the tests to be performed. Untimed or random specimens are suitable for only a few chemical tests; usually, urine specimens must be collected over a predetermined interval of time, such as 4, 12, or 24 hours. A clean, early morning, fasting specimen is usually the most concentrated specimen and thus is preferred for microscopic examinations and for the detection of abnormal quantities of constituents, such as proteins, or of unusual compounds, such as chorionic gonadotropin. The clean timed specimen is one obtained at specific times of the day or during certain phases of the act of micturition. Bacterial examination of the first 10 mL of urine voided is most appropriate to detect urethritis, whereas the midstream specimen is best used for investigating bladder disorders. The double-voided specimen is the urine excreted during a timed period after complete emptying of the bladder; it is used, for example, to assess glucose excretion during a glucose tolerance test. Its collection must be timed in relation to the ingestion of glucose. Similarly, in some metabolic disorders, urine must be collected during or immediately after symptoms of the disease appear.

When they are to be tested for their alcohol and drugs of abuse content, urine specimens are often collected under rigorous conditions requiring chain of custody documentation, particularly if the results will be used for forensic purposes.

Catheter specimens are used for microbiological examination in critically ill patients or in those with urinary tract obstruction, but they should not normally be obtained just for examination of chemical constituents. The suprapubic tap specimen is a useful alternative.

Even though tests in the clinical laboratory are not usually affected by lack of sterile collection procedures, the patient's genitalia should be cleaned before each voiding to minimize the transfer of surface bacteria to the urine. Cleansing is essential if the true concentration of white cells is to be obtained.

Currently, urine is not a common specimen type in the molecular diagnostic laboratory for genomic testing, although some tests use urine samples for bladder cancer screening and monitoring of therapy for bladder cancer. Urine is frequently used for molecular testing for infectious agents, such as *Chlamydia*, a common sexually transmitted organism, or BK virus, associated with potential rejection and/or failure of transplanted kidneys. Because most requests involve a specific organism, an untimed or random urine specimen collected into a sterile container with no preservative is usually acceptable.

Timed Urine Specimens

The collection period for timed specimens should be long enough to minimize the influence of short-term biological variations. When specimens are to be collected over a specified period of time, the patient's close adherence to instructions is important. The bladder must be emptied at the time the collection is to begin, and this urine discarded. Thereafter, all urine must be collected until the end of the scheduled time, at which time the bladder should be emptied again as the final collection. If a patient has a bowel movement during the collection period, precautions should be taken to prevent fecal contamination of the urine. If a collection has to be made over several hours, urine should be passed into a separate container at each voiding and then emptied into a larger container for the complete specimen. This two-step procedure prevents the danger of patients splashing themselves with a preservative, such as acid. The large container should be stored at 4 °C during the entire collection period.

Before beginning a timed collection, a patient should be given written instructions with regard to diet or drug ingestion, if appropriate, to avoid interference of ingested compounds with analytical procedures. Urine should not be collected at the same time for two or more tests requiring different preservatives. Aliquots for an analysis such as a microscopic examination should not be removed while a 24-hour collection is in process. Removal of aliquots is not permissible even when the volume removed is measured and corrected, because excretion of most compounds varies throughout the day, and test results will be affected. Appropriate information regarding collection, including warnings with respect to handling of the specimen, should appear on the container label.

Before a specimen is transferred into small containers for each of the ordered tests, it must be thoroughly mixed to ensure homogeneity because the specific gravity, volume, and composition of the urine may vary throughout the collection period.

To obtain a sterile urine specimen for culture from an infant, a suprapubic tap is performed. The collection of specimens from older children is done as in adults, with assistance from a parent when this is necessary.

Urine Preservatives

Urine preservatives have different roles but usually are added to (1) reduce bacterial action, (2) reduce chemical decomposition, or (3) solubilize constituents that otherwise might precipitate out of solution. Some specimens should not have *any* preservatives added because of the possibility of interference with analytical methods.

One of the most acceptable forms of preservation of urine specimens is refrigeration immediately after collection; it is even more successful when combined with chemical preservation. Acidification to below pH 3 through the addition of (1) hydrochloric, (2) acetic, or (3) nitric acid to the specimen container before collection is widely used to preserve 24-hour specimens. Such acidification is particularly useful for specimens requiring determination of (1) calcium, (2) steroids, and (3) vanillylmandelic acid (VMA). However, precipitation of urates will occur, thereby rendering a specimen unsuitable for measurement of uric acid.

Sulfamic acid (10 g/L of urine) has also been used to reduce pH. Boric acid (5 mg/30 mL) has been used, but it too causes precipitation of urates. A mild base, such as sodium bicarbonate or a small amount of sodium hydroxide, is used to preserve (1) porphyrins, (2) urobilinogen, and (3) uric acid. A sufficient quantity should be added to adjust the pH to between 8 and 9.

Feces

A fecal sample is commonly used in the clinical laboratory for the identification of disease-causing organisms. Fecal material is also frequently analyzed to detect the presence of "hidden" blood—also known as "occult" blood. Detecting this blood is considered an effective means of discovering the presence of a bleeding ulcer or malignant disease in the gastrointestinal tract. Tests for occult blood should be done on aliquots of excreted stools rather than on material obtained on the glove of a physician doing a rectal examination, because this procedure may cause enough bleeding to produce a positive result.

In the newborn, the first specimen from the bowel (meconium) may be used for detection of maternal drug use during the gestational period; this requires specific attention to the details of collection and identification. Feces from infants and children may be screened for tryptic activity to detect cystic fibrosis.

In adults, measurement of fecal nitrogen and fat in 72-hour specimens is used to assess the severity of malabsorption; measurement of fecal porphyrins is occasionally required to characterize the type of porphyria. Usually no preservative is added to the feces, but the container should be kept refrigerated throughout the collection period, and care should be taken to prevent contamination from urine.

Testing of patient DNA in stool is uncommon, but DNA isolated from fecal samples is representative of the genetic composition of the colonic mucosa at the time of stool collection. The differential and quantitative analysis of stool DNA integrity has been proposed as a sensitive and specific biomarker that is useful for the detection of colorectal cancer.[1]

Cerebrospinal Fluid

Cerebrospinal fluid (CSF) is normally obtained from the lumbar region, although a physician may occasionally request analysis of fluid obtained during surgery from the cervical region or from a cistern or ventricle of the brain. CSF is examined when there is a question as to the presence of (1) a cerebrovascular accident, (2) meningitis, (3) demyelinating disease, or (4) meningeal involvement in malignant disease. Lumbar punctures should always be performed by a physician. The tubes used for collection do not contain any preservative but must be sterile, especially if microbiological tests are required. Because the initial specimen may be contaminated by tissue debris or skin bacteria, the first tube should be used for chemical or serologic tests, the second for microbiological tests, and the third for microscopic and cytologic examination.

The most common chemical test on CSF is glucose. Antiglycolytic agents are not added to the tube for glucose measurement, as CSF specimens are rapidly processed, thereby ensuring that little metabolism of glucose occurs even in the presence of many bacteria. To allow proper interpretation of spinal fluid glucose values, a simultaneous blood specimen should be obtained. The most common use of spinal fluid in molecular diagnostics is for the rapid identification of an infectious agent and for T- and B-cell gene rearrangements associated with hematologic malignancies.

Synovial Fluid

Synovial fluid is a clear thixotropic fluid that serves as a lubricant in a (1) joint, (2) tendon sheath, or (3) bursa. The technique used to obtain it for examination is called *arthrocentesis*. Synovial fluid is withdrawn from joints to aid characterization of the type of arthritis and to differentiate noninflammatory effusions from inflammatory fluids. Normally, only a very small amount of fluid is present in any joint, but this volume is usually very much increased in the presence of inflammatory conditions. Arthrocentesis should be performed by a physician using sterile procedures, and the technique is modified from joint to joint, depending on the anatomic location and the size of the joint. Sterile plain tubes should be used for culture and for glucose and protein measurements; an EDTA tube is necessary for (1) total leukocyte, (2) differential, and (3) erythrocyte counts.

The most common use of synovial (joint) fluid in molecular diagnostics is to assess the presence of infectious microorganisms that lead to complications of great severity. Examples of organisms that the laboratory may test for include (1) *Borrelia burgdorferi*, the causative agent in Lyme disease; (2) *Staphylococcus aureus* for the presence of a staph infection; and (3) aerobic gram-negative bacilli for the presence of *Salmonella*, *Pasteurella*, or *Pseudomonas*.

Amniotic Fluid

Amniotic fluid is the liquid contained by the amniotic sac of a pregnant woman. It is collected using a technique termed *amniocentesis*—a technique performed by a physician. Amniotic fluid is analyzed (1) for prenatal diagnosis of congenital disorders, (2) to assess fetal maturity, or (3) to look for Rh isoimmunization or intrauterine infection. In addition to chemical analyses, virtually any molecular diagnostic assay has been applied to the DNA from an amniotic fluid specimen. Some of the more common molecular diagnostic assays include tests for (1) cystic fibrosis, (2) sickle cell anemia, (3) Tay-Sachs disease, and (4) thalassemia.

For prenatal determination of genetic disorders, the cellular content of the amniocentesis sample may not provide sufficient nucleic acid for analysis. In this situation, the fluid may be cultured under highly specialized conditions to expand the number of cells. Nine to 12 days of culturing are needed to obtain a sufficient number of cells for DNA extraction.

Chorionic Villus Sampling and Testing

Chorionic villus sampling (CVS) is the technique of inserting a catheter or needle into the placenta and removing some of the chorionic villi, or vascular projections, from the chorion of the womb during early pregnancy. This tissue has the same chromosomal and genetic makeup as the fetus and is used to test for disorders that may be present in the fetus.

In practice, the specimen is examined under a microscope by a physician at the time of collection to determine the (1) quality, (2) quantity, and (3) integrity of the chorionic villi. Once it is received by the laboratory, the quality of the specimen is further assessed by examination for (1) branching, (2) budding, and (3) veining, and for evaluation of maternal cell contamination. The specimen is then placed in culture medium and is allowed to grow for up to 3 weeks before DNA isolation.

CVS and subsequent testing allow for earlier diagnosis of inherited genetic disorders than is possible with amniotic fluid analysis. For example, with CVS, testing is performed at a gestation period of 10 to 12 weeks, whereas with amniotic fluid, testing generally is not performed until weeks 15 to 20 of gestation.

Pleural, Pericardial, and Ascitic Fluids

The (1) pleural, (2) pericardial, and (3) peritoneal cavities normally contain a small amount of serous fluid, which lubricates the opposing parietal and visceral membrane surfaces. Inflammation or infection affecting the cavities causes fluid to accumulate. The fluid may be removed to determine whether it is an effusion or an exudate—a distinction made possible by protein or enzyme analysis with, for example, a protein concentration higher in the fluid, indicating an exudate. The fluid may also be examined for cellular elements. The primary uses of these fluids in the molecular diagnostic laboratory are for infectious agent identification and possibly for the detection of cancer cells.[19]

The collection procedure is called *paracentesis*. When specifically applied to the pleural cavity, the procedure is a *thoracentesis*; if applied to the pericardial cavity, a *pericardiocentesis*. Paracentesis should be performed only by skilled and experienced physicians. Pericardiocentesis has now been largely supplanted by echocardiography.

Saliva

Although measurement of the concentrations of certain analytes in saliva (known formally as oral fluid) has been advocated,[2] clinical application of methods that use saliva has been limited. Exceptions include measurement of blood group substances to determine secretor status and genotype. Measurement of a drug in saliva has been suggested to estimate the free, pharmacologically active concentration of the drug in serum. However, a considerable difference in pH has been noted between saliva and serum, and ratios of bound to free drug may not be the same in the two sample types.

Buccal Cells

Collection of buccal cells (cells of the oral cavity of epithelial origin) has been identified as providing an excellent source of genomic DNA. Collection of buccal cells is often viewed as less invasive than collection of blood. It is particularly useful for collecting cells with the patient's genomic DNA when the patient has had blood transfusions and thus has blood with another person's (or persons') DNA. Similarly, it is useful after bone marrow transplantation when the circulating blood cells are derived wholly or partially from the donor of the bone marrow. Two methods are used commonly to collect buccal cells: rinsing with mouthwash and using swabs or cytobrushes.

Solid Tissue

Traditionally, the solid tissue most often analyzed in the clinical laboratory was malignant tissue from the breast for estrogen and progesterone receptors. During surgery, at least 0.5 to 1 g of tissue is removed and trimmed of fat and nontumor material. This tissue is quickly frozen within 20 minutes, preferably in liquid nitrogen or in a mixture of dry ice and alcohol. A histologic section should always be examined at the time of analysis of the specimen to confirm that the specimen indeed consists of malignant tissue.

The same procedure may be used to obtain and prepare solid tissue for toxicologic analysis; however, when trace element determinations are to be made, all materials used in the collection or handling of the tissue should be made of plastic or materials known to be free of contaminating trace elements.

Somatic gene analyses, such as T-cell receptor rearrangement and clonal expansion, are now providing important information to clinicians. Additionally, mutations in malignant tissues may be used to direct therapy. For these studies, the molecular diagnostic laboratory often receives tissue that has been formalin-fixed and paraffin-embedded (FFPE). In general, neutral buffered formalin, which contains no heavy metals, will not interfere with amplification reactions. DNA can still be extracted from tissue embedded in paraffin, but the DNA will be degraded to low molecular weight fragments, suitable for most PCR reactions but not for Southern blot methods.

Also, it is possible to retain tissue structure without permanent fixation by freezing specimens in an optimal cutting temperature (OCT) compound. This mixture of polyvinyl alcohol and polyethylene glycol surrounds but does not infiltrate the tissue. The sample is then frozen at ≈-80 °C, and sections are prepared for review by a pathologist. OCT is fully water soluble and should be completely removed from a tissue specimen before it is used as a source of DNA. In general, DNA of higher molecular weight can be extracted from OCT-fixed tissues compared with that extracted from FFPE samples.

Hair and Nails

Currently, the use of hair or nail in molecular diagnostics is limited to forensic analysis (genomic DNA identification). Hair and fingernails or toenails have been used for trace metal and drug analyses. However, collection procedures have been poorly standardized, and quantitative measurements are better obtained from blood or urine.

Handling of Specimens for Analysis

Steps that are important for obtaining a valid specimen for analysis include (1) identification, (2) preservation, (3) separation and storage, and (4) transport.

Maintenance of Specimen Identification

Proper identification of the specimen must be maintained at each step of the testing process. All labels should conform to the laboratory's stated requirements to facilitate proper processing of specimens. No specific labeling should be attached to specimens from patients with infectious disease to suggest that these specimens should be handled with special care. All specimens should be treated as if they are potentially infectious.

In practice, every specimen container must be adequately labeled even if the specimen must be placed in ice, or if the container is so small that a label cannot be placed along the tube, as might happen with a capillary blood tube, where the label should be applied as a "flag" on the tube. For small volumes of urine submitted in a screw-cap urine cup and any specimen submitted in a screw-cap test tube or cup, the label should be placed on the cup or tube directly, not on the cap.

Preservation of Specimens

The practitioner must ensure that specimens are collected into the correct container and are properly labeled; in addition, specimens must be properly treated both during transport to the laboratory and from the time the serum, plasma, or cells have been separated until analysis. For some tests, specimens must be kept at 4 °C from the time the blood is drawn until the specimens are analyzed; or until the serum or plasma is separated from the cells. Examples are specimens for (1) ammonia, (2) lactate, (3) certain hormone tests (e.g., gastrin and renin activity) and (4) blood gas determinations, such as PCO_2, PO_2, and blood pH. Transfer of these specimens to the laboratory must be done by placing the specimen container in ice water but in such a way as to maintain label integrity.

For all test constituents that are thermally labile, serum and plasma should be separated from cells in a refrigerated centrifuge. Specimens for bilirubin or carotene and for some drugs, such as methotrexate, must be protected from both daylight and fluorescent light to prevent photodegradation.

Hemolysis may also occur during specimen transport, particularly in pneumatic tube systems unless the tubes are completely filled and movement of the blood tubes inside the specimen carrier is prevented.[21] With many systems, the plasma hemoglobin concentration may be increased, and the serum activity of red cell enzymes, such as lactate dehydrogenase, may also be increased. Nonetheless, the amount of hemolysis is usually so small that it is often ignored. In special cases, such as when the cells of a patient who is undergoing chemotherapy are fragile, samples should be centrifuged before they are placed in the pneumatic tube system or identified as "messenger delivery only."

For the molecular diagnostic laboratory, it is challenging to recover RNA from transported specimens. Depending on the tissue source, RNA yields will vary, primarily because of the amount of RNA present at the time of collection. Specimens from liver, spleen, or heart have large amounts of RNA, but specimens from skin, muscle, and bone have lower RNA content. Increasingly, creative solutions to this issue continue to be produced with collection kits that contain stabilizers and even the first reagents required for extraction, all of which have the effect of maximizing the recoverable nucleic acid. Tissue samples should be frozen immediately. Alternatively, a blood specimen should never be frozen before separation of the cellular elements because of hemolysis and released heme that may interfere with subsequent amplification processes.

For specimens that are collected in a remote facility with infrequent transportation by courier to a central laboratory, proper specimen processing must be done in the remote facility so that appropriately separated and preserved plasma or serum is delivered to the laboratory. This necessitates that the remote facility has ready access to all commonly used preservatives and to wet ice.

Separation and Storage of Specimens

Plasma or serum should be separated from cells, either by removal of the liquid to an aliquot tube or by migration of a gel barrier during centrifugation, as soon as possible and certainly within 2 hours.[16] Premature separation of serum, however, may permit continued formation of fibrin, which will clog sampling devices in testing equipment. If it is impossible to centrifuge a blood specimen within 2 hours, the specimen should be held at room temperature rather than at 4 °C to decrease hemolysis.

For most plasma samples used for molecular diagnostics, the plasma should be removed from the primary tube promptly after centrifugation and held at −20 °C in a freezer capable of maintaining this temperature. Frost-free freezers should be avoided for all specimens because they have a wide temperature swing during the freeze-thaw cycle. Note, however, that 4 °C or −20 °C is not the optimum storage temperature for all tests; some lactate dehydrogenase isoenzymes, for instance, are more stable at room temperature than at 4 °C.

Specimen tubes should be centrifuged with stoppers in place. Closure reduces evaporation, which occurs rapidly in a warm centrifuge with the air currents set up by centrifugation. Stoppers also prevent aerosolization of infectious particles. Specimen tubes containing volatiles, such as ethanol, *must* be stoppered while they are spun. Centrifuging specimens with the stopper in place maintains anaerobic conditions, which are important in the measurement of carbon dioxide and ionized calcium. Removal of the stopper before centrifugation allows loss of carbon dioxide and an increase in blood pH. Control of pH is especially important for the enzymatic measurement of acid phosphatase, which is labile under alkaline conditions engendered by CO_2 loss.

Cryopreservation of white blood cells and DNA is one method of storing and maintaining samples for extended periods. Whole blood specimens can be centrifuged, and white cells removed and cryopreserved at −20 °C until these cells are required for DNA extraction. For even longer periods of storage, isolated DNA can be stored at −70 °C. The extracted DNA should not be exposed to repetitive cycles of freezing and thawing because this can lead to shearing of DNA. After these extracted DNA samples have completely thawed, it is important to fully mix the sample to ensure a homogeneous specimen.

Transport of Specimens

Although the remaining discussion uses the specific example of referral laboratory testing by another laboratory, many of the issues discussed, such as regulations related to shipping, are also relevant to a laboratory that receives specimens from outlying clinics via a (laboratory-owned and/or operated) courier service. This may involve validating specific transport/storage conditions that are in conflict with existing CLSI recommendations.[13]

Before a referral laboratory is used for any tests, the quality of its work should be verified by the referring laboratory. For laboratories accredited by the College of American Pathologists (CAP), it is a requirement that the referring laboratory validate that the referral laboratory is Clinical Laboratory Improvement Amendments (CLIA) certified by obtaining a copy of the CLIA certificate before specimens are shipped. For molecular diagnostic testing, this is of particular importance because often the latest genetic test being requested by a physician has not yet been moved from research interest status to patient care status, and it may not be available in a CLIA-certified laboratory.

Specimen type and quantity and specimen handling requirements of the referral laboratory must be observed, and in laboratories operating under CLIA '88 regulations, test results reported by a referral laboratory must be identified as such when they are filed in a patient's chart.

In situations in which sample delivery for molecular analysis will be delayed, extracted nucleic acid, usually DNA only, is transported in a buffer solution or water, or it is dried down and shipped as a loose powder. With either method, DNA should be transported at ambient temperatures but should not be exposed to extremely high temperatures for an extended period because it will begin to degrade, and testing may be compromised.

Various laws and regulations apply to the shipment of biological specimens. Although these rules theoretically apply only to etiologic agents (known infectious agents), all specimens should be transported as if the same regulations applied. Airlines have rigid regulations covering the transport of specimens. Airlines deem dry ice a hazardous material; therefore the transport of most clinical laboratory specimens is affected by the regulations, and those who package the specimens should be trained in the appropriate regulations, such as those put forth by the U.S. Air International Transport Association (IATA).

The various modes of transport of specimens influence the shipping time and cost, and each laboratory will need to make its own assessment as to adequate service. The objective is to ensure that the properly (1) collected, (2) processed, and (3) identified specimen arrives at the testing facility in time and under the correct storage conditions, so that the analytical phase can then proceed.

Other Preanalytical Variables

Preanalytical variables are classified as either controllable or uncontrollable.[22] Some of the more common ones are discussed here. For additional information on this subject, interested readers are referred to Chapters 6 and 7 in the 5th edition of *Tietz Textbook of Clinical Chemistry and Molecular Diagnostics* and to texts by Young[22] and Guder and colleagues[12] on the subject.

Controllable Variables

Many of the preanalytical variables related to specimen collection discussed previously are examples of controllable variables. Others include physiological variables[12] and those associated with (1) diet, (1) lifestyle, (3) stimulants, (4) drugs, (5) herbal preparations, and (6) recreational drug ingestion.

Physiological Variables

Controllable personal variables that affect analytical results include (1) posture, (2) prolonged bed rest, (3) exercise, (4) physical training, (5) circadian variation, and (6) menstrual cycle.

Posture. In general, concentrations of freely diffusible constituents with molecular weights of less than 5000 Da are unaffected by postural changes. However, a significant increase in potassium (≈0.2 to 0.3 mmol/L) occurs after an individual stands for 30 minutes. Changes in the concentrations of some major serum constituents with change in posture are listed in Table 6-4.

TABLE 6-4	Change in Concentration of Serum Constituents With Change from Lying to Standing

Constituent	Average Increase (%)
Alanine aminotransferase	7
Albumin	9
Alkaline phosphatase	7
Amylase	6
Aspartate aminotransferase	5
Calcium	3
Cholesterol	7
IgA	7
IgG	7
IgM	5
Thyroxine	11
Triglycerides	6

From Felding P, Tryding N, Hyltoft Petersen P, Hørder M. Effects of posture on concentrations of blood constituents in healthy adults: practical application of blood specimen collection procedures recommended by the Scandinavian Committee on Reference Values. Scand J Clin Lab Invest 1980;40:615-21.

TABLE 6-5	Total and Analytical Variation for Serum Tests on Specimens Obtained at 0800 and 1400*

Constituent	Mean	Total Variation, %	Analytical Variation, %
Sodium, mmol/L	141	1.9	1.8
Potassium, mmol/L	4.4	7.1	2.8
Calcium, mg/dL	10.8	3.2	2.7
Chloride, mmol/L	102	3.8	3.4
Phosphate, mg/dL	3.8	10.7	2.4
Urea nitrogen, mg/dL	14	22.5	2.5
Creatinine, mg/dL	1.0	14.5	6.3
Uric acid, mg/dL	5.6	11.5	2.6
Iron, µg/dL	116	36.6	3.4
Cholesterol, mg/dL	193	14.8	5.7
Albumin, g/dL	4.5	5.5	3.9
Total protein, g/dL	7.3	4.8	1.7
Total lipids, g/L	5.3	25.0	3.6
Aspartate aminotransferase, U/L	9	25	6
Alanine aminotransferase, U/L	6	56	17
Acid phosphatase, U/L	3	15	8
Alkaline phosphatase, U/L	63	20	3
Lactate dehydrogenase, U/L	195	16	12

*11 male subjects, age 21-27 years, studied at 0800, 1100, 1400.
From Winkel P, Statland BE, Bokelund H. The effects of time of venipuncture on variation of serum constituents. Am J Clin Pathol 1975;64:433-47. Copyright © 1975 by the American Society of Clinical Pathologists. Reprinted with permission.

Exercise and Physical Training. In considering the effects of exercise, the nature and extent of the exercise should be taken into account. Static or isometric exercise, usually of short duration but of high intensity, uses previously stored ATP and creatine phosphate, whereas more prolonged exercise must use ATP generated by normal metabolic pathways. Changes in concentrations of analytes as a result of exercise are largely due to (1) shifts of fluid between intravascular and interstitial compartments, (2) changes in hormone concentrations stimulated by the change in activity, and (3) loss of fluid due to sweating. The physical fitness of an individual may also affect the extent of change in the concentration of a constituent. Whether any amount of exercise significantly affects laboratory results also depends on how long after an exercise activity a specimen was collected.

Circadian Variation. *Circadian variation* refers to the pattern of (1) production, (2) excretion, and (3) concentrations of analytes each 24 hours. Many constituents of body fluids exhibit cyclical variations throughout the day. Factors contributing to such variations include (1) posture, (2) activity, (3) food ingestion, (4) stress, (5) daylight or darkness, and (6) sleep or wakefulness. These cyclical variations may be quite large; therefore the drawing of the specimen must be strictly controlled. For example, the concentration of serum iron may change by as much as 50% from 0800 to 1400, and that of cortisol by a similar amount from 0800 to 1600. Serum potassium has been reported to decline from 5.4 mmol/L at 0800 to 4.3 mmol/L at 1400. The typical total variation of several commonly measured serum constituents over 6 hours is illustrated in Table 6-5; total variation is listed together with analytical error.

Hormones are secreted in bursts, and this, together with the cyclical variation to which most hormones are subject, may make it very difficult to interpret their serum concentration properly. Additionally, the effects of hormones on other analytes make the time of sample collection extremely important.

For example, basal plasma insulin is higher in the morning than later in the day, and its response to glucose is greatest in the morning and least about midnight. When a glucose tolerance test is given in the afternoon, higher glucose values occur than when the test is given early in the day. Higher plasma glucose occurs in spite of a greater insulin response, which nevertheless is delayed and less effective.

Menstrual Cycle. The plasma concentrations of many female sex hormones and other hormones are affected by the menstrual cycle. On the preovulatory day, the aldosterone concentration may actually be twice that of the early part of the follicular phase. The change in renin activity is almost as great. These changes are usually more pronounced in women who retain fluid before menstruation. Urinary catecholamine excretion increases at midcycle and remains high throughout the luteal phase. These changes within the menstrual cycle make it essential to do repetitive measurements on women at the same time during the cycle.

Travel

Travel across several time zones affects the normal circadian rhythm. Five days is required to establish a new stable diurnal rhythm after travel across 10 time zones. Changes in laboratory test results are generally attributable to altered pituitary and adrenal function. Urinary excretion of catecholamines is usually increased for 2 days; serum cortisol is reduced. During a flight, serum glucose and triglyceride concentrations increase, while glucocorticoid secretion is stimulated. During a prolonged flight, fluid and sodium retention occurs, but urinary excretion returns to normal after 2 days.

Diet

Diet has considerable influence on the composition of plasma. Studies with synthetic diets have shown that day-to-day changes in the amount of protein are reflected within a few days in the composition of the plasma and in the excretion of end products of protein metabolism.

When dietary carbohydrates consist mainly of starch or sucrose rather than other sugars, the serum activities of ALP and LD are increased. Conversely, the plasma triglyceride concentration is reduced when sucrose intake is decreased. Flatter glucose tolerance curves are observed with a bread diet than when a high-sucrose diet is ingested. A high-carbohydrate diet decreases the serum concentrations of very low-density lipoprotein (VLDL) cholesterol, triglycerides, and protein. Individuals who eat many small meals throughout the day tend to have concentrations of total LDL and HDL cholesterol that are lower than when the same type and amount of food is eaten in three meals.

Food Ingestion

The concentration of certain plasma constituents is affected by the ingestion of a meal, with the time between ingestion of a meal and collection of blood affecting the plasma concentrations of many analytes. For example, fasting overnight for 10 to 14 hours noticeably decreases the variability in the concentrations of many analytes; this is seen as the optimal time for fasting around which to standardize blood collections, particularly lipids. The biggest increases in serum concentrations after a meal are seen in glucose, iron, total lipids, and ALP.

Vegetarianism

Concentrations of LDL cholesterol, total lipids, and phospholipids are reduced in individuals who have been vegetarians for a long time; their concentrations of cholesterol and triglycerides may be only two-thirds of those in people on a mixed diet. Both HDL and LDL cholesterol concentrations are affected. In strict vegetarians, the LDL concentration may be 37% less and the HDL cholesterol concentration 12% less than in nonvegetarians.

Malnutrition

In malnutrition, (1) total serum protein, (2) albumin, and (3) β-globulin concentrations are reduced. The increased concentration of γ-globulin does not fully compensate for the decrease in other proteins. Concentrations of (1) complement C3, (2) retinol-binding globulin, (3) transferrin, and (4) prealbumin decrease rapidly with the onset of malnutrition and are measured to define the severity of the condition.

Fasting and Starvation

As a consequence of fasting for longer than 24 hours or in response to starvation, the body attempts to conserve protein at the expense of other sources of energy, such as fat. The blood glucose concentration decreases by as much as 18 mg/dL (1 mmol/L) within the first 3 days of the start of a fast in spite of the body's attempts to maintain glucose production. Insulin secretion is greatly reduced, whereas glucagon secretion may double in an attempt to maintain normal glucose concentration. Lipolysis and hepatic ketogenesis are stimulated. Ketoacids and fatty acids become the principal sources of energy for muscle. This results in an accumulation of organic acids that leads to a metabolic acidosis with reduction of blood pH, PCO_2, and plasma bicarbonate concentrations.

Lifestyle

Smoking and alcohol ingestion are life-style factors that affect the concentrations of commonly measured analytes.

Smoking. Smoking, through the action of nicotine, may affect several laboratory tests. The extent of the effect is related to the number of cigarettes smoked and to the amount of smoke inhaled.

Through stimulation of the adrenal medulla, nicotine increases the concentration of epinephrine in the plasma and the urinary excretion of catecholamines and their metabolites. Glucose concentration may be increased by 10 mg/dL (0.56 mmol/L) within 10 minutes of smoking a cigarette. Typically the plasma glucose concentration is higher in smokers than in nonsmokers, and glucose tolerance is mildly impaired in smokers. The plasma growth hormone concentration is particularly sensitive to smoking. It may increase tenfold within 30 minutes after an individual has smoked a cigarette.

Smoking affects the body's immune response. For example, serum IgA, IgG, and IgM levels are generally lower in smokers than in nonsmokers, whereas the IgE concentration is higher. Smokers, more often than nonsmokers, may show the presence of antinuclear antibodies and may test weakly positive for carcinoembryonic antigen. The sperm count of male smokers is often reduced compared with that of nonsmokers: The number of abnormal forms is greater and sperm motility is less.

Alcohol Ingestion. A single moderate dose of alcohol has few effects on laboratory tests. Ingestion of enough alcohol to produce mild inebriation may increase the blood glucose concentration by 20% to 50%. The increase may be even greater in individuals with diabetes. Over time after ingestion, inhibition of gluconeogenesis occurs and becomes apparent as hypoglycemia and ketonemia as ethanol is metabolized to acetaldehyde and to acetate.

Intoxicating amounts of alcohol stimulate the release of cortisol, although the effect is more related to intoxication than to the alcohol per se. Sympatheticomedullary activity is increased by acute alcohol ingestion but without detectable effect on the plasma epinephrine concentration and with only a mild effect on norepinephrine. With intoxication, plasma concentrations of catecholamines are substantially increased. Acute ingestion of alcohol leads to a sharp reduction in plasma testosterone in men and an increase in the plasma luteinizing hormone concentration.

Chronic alcohol ingestion affects the activity of many serum enzymes. For example, increased activity of γ-glutamyltransferase (GGT) is often used as a marker of persistent drinking. Chronic alcoholism is associated with many characteristic biochemical abnormalities, including (1) abnormal pituitary, (2) adrenocortical, and (3) medullary function. Measurement of carbohydrate-deficient transferrin is used to identify habitual alcohol ingestion. Increased mean cell volume (MCV) has also been used as a marker of habitual alcohol use and may be related to folic acid deficiency or may be a direct toxic effect of alcohol on red blood cell precursors.

Drug Administration

The effects of drugs on laboratory tests are complicated by known and unknown ingestion of (1) prescribed medications, (2) recreational drug use, and (3) herbal preparations.

Prescribed Medications. Typically, hospitalized patients receive medication. For certain medical conditions, more than 10 drugs may be administered at one time. Even many healthy individuals take several drugs regularly, such as (1) vitamins, (2) oral contraceptives, or (3) sleeping tablets. Individuals with chronic diseases often ingest drugs on a continuing basis. It is important to understand the differences between (1) the act of receiving a medication, (2) the physiological effects of the medication, and (3) analytical interference with the specific test method used.

Many drugs, when administered intramuscularly, cause sufficient muscle irritation to increase amounts of enzyme released, such as CK and LD, into the serum. These increased activities may persist for several days after a single injection, and consistently high values may be observed during a course of treatment. This contrasts with the reduction in plasma potassium concentration and the possible hyponatremia that follow prolonged diuretic drug administration because of increased urinary output (physiological response). Analytical interferences vary significantly among test methods.

Recreational Drug Ingestion. Recreational drug ingestion refers to the ingestion of compounds for mood-altering purposes. Many commonly prescribed pain medications have migrated from pharmaceutical use to "drug of abuse" status. Among the more classical drugs of abuse, amphetamines increase the concentration of free fatty acids. Morphine increases the activity of (1) amylase, (2) lipase, (3) ALT, (4) AST, and (5) ALP, as well as the serum bilirubin concentration. Concentrations of gastrin, TSH, and prolactin are also increased. In contrast, concentrations of insulin, norepinephrine, pancreatic polypeptide, and neurotensin are decreased. Heroin increases the plasma concentrations of (1) cholesterol, (2) T_4, and (3) potassium. PCO_2 is increased, but PO_2 is decreased. The plasma albumin concentration is also decreased. Cannabis increases plasma concentrations of (1) sodium, (2) potassium, (3) urea, (4) chloride, and (5) insulin but decreases those of (1) creatinine, (2) glucose, and (3) uric acid.

Herbal Preparations

Herbal preparations are not regulated by standardized manufacturing practices, resulting in great variability in their composition and thus in their reported effects. Long-term use of (1) aloe vera, (2) sandalwood, and (3) cascara sagrada may cause hematuria and albuminuria. Through their laxative effects, prolonged use of (1) aloe vera, (2) Chinese rhubarb, (3) frangula bark, (4) senna, and (5) buckthorn may lead to hypokalemia, provoking hyperaldosteronism. Trailing arbutus may cause hemolytic anemia and liver damage. Green tea has been reported to cause microcytic anemia. Quinine and quinidine have been observed to cause thrombocytopenia. Cayenne (Capsicum annuum) increases fibrinolytic activity and induces hypocoagulability. Hyperthyroidism has been caused by the seaweed bladderwrack.

Many herbal preparations affect liver function. For example, germander has been reported to cause liver cell necrosis, and bishop's weed infrequently causes cholestatic jaundice. Tonka beans have been known to cause reversible liver damage. Comfrey has been associated with one death from liver failure. Bugleweed reduces the plasma concentration of prolactin and reduces the deiodination of T_4. Many of the reported effects of herbal preparation on liver function may be associated with contaminants from the unregulated manufacturing process, rather than the herbs themselves.

Uncontrollable Variables

Examples of uncontrollable preanalytical variables include those related to (1) biological, (2) environmental, and (3) long-term cyclical influences, and (4) those related to underlying medical conditions.

Biological Influences

Age, sex, and race of the patient influence the results of individual laboratory tests, which are discussed individually in various chapters of this book. Reference intervals for various analytes as a function of these biological influences are listed in Chapter 5.

Age. Age has a notable effect on reference intervals (particularly hormones), although the degree of change differs in various reports and may be dependent upon the analytical method used. In general, individuals are considered in four groups—the newborn, the older child to puberty, the sexually mature adult, and the elderly adult. Reference intervals for these age categories for affected analytes are found in Chapter 50 and in earlier editions of this book.

Sex. Until puberty, few differences in laboratory data are noted between young female and male humans. After puberty characteristic changes in the concentrations of sex hormones, including prolactin, become apparent. Also after puberty, higher activity of enzymes originating from skeletal muscle in men is related to their greater muscle mass. After menopause, the activity of ALP increases in women until it is higher than in men. Although total LD activity is similar in men and women, the activities of the LD-1 and LD-3 isoenzymes are higher, and LD-2 is less, in young women than in men. These differences disappear after menopause.

Race. Differentiation of the effects of race from those of socioeconomic conditions is often difficult, as may be the determination of the race of the patient. However, the total serum protein concentration is known to be higher in blacks than in whites. This is largely attributable to a much higher γ-globulin, although usually the concentrations of α_1- and β-globulins are also increased. The serum albumin is typically less in blacks than in whites. In black men, serum IgG is often 40% higher, and serum IgA may be as much as 20% higher, than in white men.

Carbohydrate and lipid metabolism differs in blacks and whites. Glucose tolerance is less in blacks, Polynesians, Native Americans, and Inuits than in comparable age- and sex-matched whites.

Environmental Factors

Environmental factors that affect laboratory results include (1) altitude, (2) ambient temperature, (3) geographical location of residence, and (4) seasonal influences.

Altitude. In individuals living at a high altitude, blood hemoglobin and hematocrit are greatly increased because of reduced atmospheric PO_2. Erythrocyte 2,3-diphosphoglycerate is also increased, and the oxygen dissociation curve is shifted to the right. The increased erythrocyte concentration leads to an increased turnover of nucleoproteins and excretion of uric acid. The fasting basal concentration of growth hormone concentration is high in individuals living at a high altitude, but concentrations of renin and aldosterone are decreased in healthy individuals. Plasma sodium and potassium concentrations are typically unaffected by high altitude, although the osmolality is reduced. Serum concentrations of C-reactive protein, transferrin, and β_2-globulin are notably increased with transition to a high altitude. Complete adaptation to a high altitude takes many weeks, whereas adjustment to lower altitudes takes less time.

Ambient Temperature. Ambient temperature affects the composition of body fluids. Acute exposure to heat causes the plasma volume to expand by an influx of interstitial fluid into the intravascular space and by reduction of glomerular filtration. The plasma protein concentration may decrease by up to 10%. Sweating may cause salt and water loss, but usually no changes in plasma sodium and chloride concentrations are noted. Plasma potassium concentration may decrease by as much as 10% as potassium is taken up by the cells. If sweating is extensive, hemoconcentration rather than hemodilution may occur.

Geographical Location of Residence. The geographical location where individuals live may affect the composition of their body fluids. For example, a statistically significant increase in serum concentrations of (1) cholesterol, (2) triglycerides, and (3) magnesium has been observed in people living in areas with hard water. Trace element concentrations are also affected by geographical location, for example, in areas where there is much ore smelting, serum concentrations of the trace elements involved may be increased. Carboxyhemoglobin concentrations are higher in areas where there is much heavier automobile traffic than in rural areas (as was true for blood lead in the 1970s in the United States). Individuals who primarily work indoors typically have lower concentrations of 25-hydroxy vitamin D than those who work outdoors, leading to higher serum calcium concentrations and greater urinary excretion of calcium.

Seasonal Influences. Seasonal influences on the composition of body fluids are small compared with those related to changes in posture or misuse of a tourniquet. Probable factors are dietary changes as different foods come into season and altered physical activity as more or different forms of exercise become feasible.

Underlying Medical Conditions

Some general medical conditions have an effect on the composition of body fluids and affect laboratory results. These include (1) obesity, (2) blindness, (3) pregnancy), (4) stress, (5) fever, (6) shock and trauma, and (7) transfusions and infusions.

Obesity. Serum concentrations of (1) cholesterol, (2) triglycerides, and (3) β-lipoproteins are positively correlated with obesity. The increase in the concentration of cholesterol is attributable to LDL cholesterol because HDL cholesterol is typically reduced. The serum uric acid concentration is also correlated with body weight, especially in individuals weighing more than 80 kg. Serum LD activity and glucose concentration increase in both sexes with increasing body weight. In men, serum (1) AST, (2) creatinine, (3) total protein, and (4) blood hemoglobin concentration increase with increasing body weight. In women, serum calcium increases with increasing body weight. In both sexes, serum phosphate decreases with increased body mass.

Fasting concentrations of (1) pyruvate, (2) lactate, (3) citrate, and (4) unesterified fatty acids are higher in obese individuals than in those of normal body weight. Serum iron and transferrin concentrations are low.

Blindness. Normal stimulation of the hypothalamic-pituitary axis is reduced with blindness. Consequently, certain features of hypopituitarism and hypoadrenalism may be observed. In some blind individuals, the normal diurnal variation of cortisol may or may not persist. Urinary excretion of 17-ketosteroids and 17-hydroxycorticosteroids is reduced. Plasma sodium and chloride are often low in blind individuals, probably as a result of reduced aldosterone secretion. Plasma glucose may be reduced in blind people, and insulin tolerance is often less. The excretion of uric acid is reduced. Renal function may be slightly impaired, as evidenced by slight increases in serum creatinine and urea nitrogen.

Pregnancy. Many changes in the concentrations of analytes occur during pregnancy, and proper interpretation of test results is dependent on knowledge of the duration of pregnancy.

Substantial hormonal changes occur during pregnancy, including several not normally associated with reproduction. Many of these changes are related to the great increase in blood volume that occurs during pregnancy, from about 2600 mL early in pregnancy to 3500 mL at about 35 weeks. This hemodilution reduces the concentration of plasma proteins. However, the concentration of some transport proteins, including ceruloplasmin and thyroxine-binding globulin, is increased, resulting in increased concentrations of copper and T_4. The concentrations of cholesterol and triglycerides are notably increased. In contrast, pregnancy creates a relative deficiency of iron and ferritin.

Urine volume increases during pregnancy, so that it is typically 25% greater in the third trimester than in the nonpregnant woman. The glomerular filtration rate increases by 50% during the third trimester. This results in increased urinary excretion of hydroxyproline and increased creatinine clearance. Pregnancy triggers many physiological stress reactions and is associated with increased concentrations of acute-phase reactant proteins. The erythrocyte sedimentation rate increases fivefold during pregnancy.

Stress. Physical and mental stress influences the concentrations of many plasma constituents. Anxiety stimulates increased secretion of (1) aldosterone, (2) angiotensin, (3) catecholamines, (4) cortisol, (5) prolactin, (6) renin, (7) somatotropin, (8) TSH, and (9) vasopressin. Plasma concentrations of (1) albumin, (2) cholesterol, (3) fibrinogen, (4) glucose, (5) insulin, and (6) lactate also increase.

Fever. Fever provokes many hormonal responses. For example, hyperglycemia occurs early and stimulates the secretion of insulin. This improves glucose tolerance, but insulin secretion does not necessarily reduce the blood glucose concentration because increased secretion of growth hormone and glucagon occurs. Fever appears to reduce the secretion of T_4, as do acute illnesses even without fever. In response to increased corticotropin secretion, the plasma cortisol concentration is increased and its normal diurnal variation may be abolished. The urinary excretion of (1) free cortisol, (2) 17-hydroxycorticosteroids, and (3) 17-ketosteroids is increased. As acute fever subsides, or if it lessens but still persists for a prolonged period, hormone responses diminish.

Shock and Trauma. Regardless of the cause of shock or trauma, certain characteristic biochemical changes result. For example, corticotropin secretion is stimulated to produce a threefold to fivefold increase in the serum cortisol concentration. 17-Hydroxycorticosteroid excretion is greatly increased, although excretion of 17-ketosteroids and metabolites of adrenal androgens may be unaffected. Aldosterone secretion is stimulated. Plasma renin activity is increased, as are secretions of (1) growth hormone, (2) glucagon, and (3) insulin. Anxiety and stress increase the excretion of catecholamines. The stress of surgery has been shown to reduce the serum T_3 by 50% in patients without thyroid disease. Changes in the concentrations of blood components reflect the physiological response to these hormonal changes. The general metabolic response to shock includes the normal response to stress.

Immediately after an injury, loss of fluid to extravascular tissue results in decreased plasma volume. If the decrease is enough to impair circulation, glomerular filtration is diminished. Diminished renal function leads to the accumulation of urea and other end products of protein metabolism in the circulation. In burned patients, serum total protein concentration falls by as much as 0.8 g/dL because of both loss to extravascular spaces and catabolism of protein. Serum α_1-, α_2-, and β-globulin concentrations are increased but not enough to compensate for the reduced albumin concentration. The plasma fibrinogen concentration responds dramatically to trauma and may double 2 to 8 days after surgery. The concentration of C-reactive protein rises at the same time.

Transfusion and Infusions. The protein-rich fluid lost from the intravascular space after trauma is replaced with protein-poor fluid from the interstitial spaces. Subsequently, this is replaced by a fluid similar in composition to plasma. Transfusion of whole blood or plasma raises the plasma protein concentration; the extent of increase depends on the amount of blood administered. Serum LD activity, primarily LD-1 and LD-2 isoenzymes, and bilirubin are increased by the breakdown of transfused erythrocytes. Transfusions to replace blood lost because of injury reduce sodium, chloride, and water retention precipitated by the injury. Serum iron and transferrin concentrations are reduced immediately after an injury, but extensive blood transfusions have been known to lead to siderosis and an increased serum iron concentration. Serum potassium may increase with transfusion of stored blood.

Normal Biological Variability

Data from studies of biological variation may be used to (1) assess the importance of changes in test values within an individual from one occasion to another, (2) determine the appropriateness of reference intervals, and, in conjunction with data from analytical variation, (3) establish laboratory analytical goals. Application by clinicians of information on biological variability enhances their ability to precisely identify important changes in test results in their patients. Categories of biological variation include (1) within an individual and (2) between individuals. The change in laboratory data around a hemostatic set point from one occasion to another within one person is called *within-subject* or *intraindividual variation*. The difference between the set points of different individuals is called *interindividual variation*. Intraindividual variability is great for different analytes, even within the same biochemical class of compounds.

Mechanisms used to assess variability include the delta check and reference change values.

Delta Check

When a patient's clinical condition is generally stable and differences between repeated test results are small, the difference between successive results may be used as a form of quality assurance. Most clinicians and healthcare providers arbitrarily decide when there is a clinically significant difference between repeated measurements of the same analyte. However, it is possible to address this issue more systematically and logically. The delta check concept is applied to two successive values regardless of the time interval between them. Delta check values are typically generated in one of two ways: The first is derived from differences between collected consecutive values for an analyte in many individuals, which are then plotted in a histogram with the central 95% or 99% of all values used to identify a clinically significant change in values. Delta checks may involve the absolute difference or the percent change between consecutive numbers. The second approach to establishing delta check values relies on a laboratorian's or a clinician's best estimate of an appropriate delta to yield a manageable number of flagged results for follow-up. Rate checks that involve dividing a delta check value by the time interval between successive measurements also are used. Several different delta check methods have been proposed, including (1) delta difference: current result minus previous result; (2) delta percent change: (current result − previous result) × 100%/previous result; (3) rate difference: delta difference/delta time; and (4) rate percent change: delta percent change/delta time (where delta time is the interval between current and previous specimen collection times). Some laboratory information systems include delta checks in the reporting of test results but usually in the simplest way, as in delta difference or delta percent change.

In healthy individuals and in stable patients, the delta value between any two results should be small. Acceptable delta values may be calculated within a population of healthy individuals and then averaged, with the average used as a guide to determine whether a difference of possible clinical significance had occurred between serial measurements in patients.

Reference Change Values

To determine whether the difference between consecutive results for a single analyte in a patient might have clinical significance, Harris and Yasaka developed the concept of reference change values (RCVs). An RCV, also known as *critical difference,* is the value that must be exceeded before a change in consecutive test results is statistically significant at a predetermined probability. This concept introduces a scientific approach to an area where clinicians have largely relied on their intuition and experience. Historically, clinicians' impressions of clinically significant differences have varied significantly. Fraser and colleagues have shown that systematically calculated critical differences for many analytes tend to be less than physicians' assumptions of clinically significant differences.

An RCV takes into account both analytical and within-individual variations. To enhance the utility of the RCV, intraindividual variability should also be minimized with standardization of patient preparation and specimen collection and processing practices. Standardization is more readily achieved in hospital practice, where uniform timing of collections by trained phlebotomists is often possible, than in outpatient practices.

The change in values between successive measurements in a hospitalized patient is generally greater than the change in values reported in the literature derived from studies of healthy individuals because of the change in the patient's medical condition and his or her response to treatment. RCVs are not constant, and a significant change is likely to be smaller over the short term than over a longer time span. Thus application of RCVs from healthy individuals derived over a short time will identify an inappropriately large number of apparently significant changes in hospitalized patients.

Review Questions

1. Which blood specimen, in a multi-draw situation, most closely represents the composition of circulating blood?
   a. The blood drawn first
   b. The final tube drawn
   c. Only the serum tubes
   d. Only the plasma tubes

2. A blood collection tube containing sodium fluoride and an oxalate inhibits *coagulation* by:
   a. binding calcium, which is essential for the clotting mechanism.
   b. accelerating the action of antithrombin III.
   c. forming insoluble complexes with calcium ions.
   d. inhibiting the enzyme systems involved in glycolysis.

3. Why is pumping the fist before venipuncture inappropriate for blood collection?
   a. It causes venous stasis.
   b. It causes increased potassium, lower blood pH, and increased ionized calcium.
   c. It causes increased plasma concentrations of cortisol and growth hormone.
   d. It leads to premature separation of serum and fibrin clot formation.

4. One of the best and most acceptable methods of preserving a urine specimen is:
   a. thymol.
   b. refrigeration.
   c. incubation at 37 °C.
   d. phenol.

5. To allow for early diagnosis of an inherited genetic disorder at a gestational period of 10 to 12 weeks, the best specimen is:
   a. saliva.
   b. synovial fluid.
   c. amniotic fluid.
   d. chorionic villus sampling.

6. After centrifugation, plasma or serum is best separated from cells:
   a. within two hours.
   b. within six hours.
   c. within twelve hours.
   d. when it is convenient for the laboratorian.

7. The difference between serum and plasma is that:
   a. plasma contains all of the cellular elements of blood (WBCs, RBCs, etc.), but serum does not.
   b. plasma contains none of the clotting factors.
   c. serum is obtained by mixing anticoagulants with whole blood.
   d. serum is obtained when whole blood is allowed to clot and then is centrifuged.

8. Hemolysis is defined as:
   a. increased lipids in the blood that give the serum a milky appearance.
   b. excess bilirubin in serum that give it a greenish-yellow appearance.
   c. plasma that has been allowed to clot over time.
   d. damage to red blood cell membranes leading to release of the contents of red cells into the plasma.

9. An evacuated blood collection tube with a light blue stopper contains which of the following additives?
   a. Heparin
   b. EDTA
   c. Sodium citrate
   d. Sterile media for blood culture

10. An example of a *controllable* preanalytical variable for laboratory testing would be:
    a. diet.
    b. sex.
    c. age.
    d. underlying disease.

References

1. Boynton KA, Summerhayes IC, Ahlquist DA, Shuber AP. DNA integrity as a potential marker for stool-based detection of colorectal cancer. Clin Chem 2003;49:2112–3

2. Carroll T, Raff H, Findling JW. Late-night salivary cortisol for the diagnosis of Cushing's syndrome: a meta-analysis. Endocr Pract 2009; 6:1–17

3. Clinical and Laboratory Standards Institute. Procedures for the collection of diagnostic blood specimens by venipuncture; CLSI approved standard H3-A6, ed 6, Wayne, Pa: Clinical and Laboratory Standards Institute, 2007. (Current document code GP41-A6)

4. Clinical and Laboratory Standards Institute. Procedures and devices for the collection of capillary blood specimens; CLSI approved standard H4-A6, 6th edition. Wayne, Pa: Clinical and Laboratory Standards Institute, 2008. (Current document code GP42-A6)

5. Clinical and Laboratory Standards Institute. Procedures for the collection of arterial specimen; CLSI approved standard H11-A4, 4th edition. Wayne, Pa: Clinical and Laboratory Standards Institute, 2004. (Current document code GP43-A4)

6. Clinical and Laboratory Standards Institute. Urinalysis; CLSI approved guideline GP16-A3, 3rd edition. Wayne, Pa: Clinical and Laboratory Standards Institute, 2009.

7. Clinical and Laboratory Standards Institute. Collection, transport, preparation, and storage of specimens for molecular methods; CLSI approved guideline MM13-A, 1st edition. Wayne, Pa: Clinical and Laboratory Standards Institute, 2006.

8. Clinical and Laboratory Standards Institute. Protection of laboratory workers from occupationally acquired infections; CLSI approved guideline M29-A3. Wayne, Pa: National Clinical and Laboratory Standards Institute, 2005.

9. Clinical and Laboratory Standards Institute. Tubes and additives for venous and capillary blood specimen collection; CLSI approved standard H1-A6, 6th edition. Wayne, Pa: National Clinical and Laboratory Standards Institute, 2010. (Current document code GP39-A6)

10. Clinical and Laboratory Standards Institute. Sweat testing: sample collection and quantitative chloride analysis; CLSI approved standard C34-A3, 3rd edition. Wayne, Pa: National Clinical and Laboratory Standards Institute, 2009.

11. Clinical and Laboratory Standards Institute. Procedures for the handling and processing of blood specimens for common laboratory tests; CLSI approved guideline H18-A4, 4th edition. Wayne, Pa: National Clinical and Laboratory Standards Institute, 2010. (Current document code GP44-A4)

12. Guder WG, Narayanan S, Wisser H, Zawta B. Diagnostic samples: from the patient to the laboratory: the impact of preanalytical variables on the quality of laboratory results, 4th ed. London: Wiley Blackwell, 2009.

13. Haverstick DM, Brill LB, Scott MG, Bruns DE. Preanalytical variables in measurement of free (ionized) calcium in lithium heparin-containing blood collection tubes. Clin Chim Acta 2009;403:102–4

14. Haverstick DM, Groszbach A. Specimen collection and processing. In: Burtis CA, Ashwood ER, Bruns DE, eds. Tietz textbook of clinical chemistry and molecular diagnostics. St Louis, Mo: Elsevier, 2012.

15. Kiechle FL, ed. So you're going to collect a blood specimen: an introduction to phlebotomy, 14th edition. Northfield, Ill: College of American Pathologists, 2013.

16. Laessig RH, Indriksons AA, Hassemer DJ, Passkey TA, Schwartz TH. Changes in serum chemical values as a result of prolonged contact with the clot. Am J Clin Pathol 1976;66:598–604

17. McNair P, Nielsen SL, Christiansen C, Axelsson C. Gross errors made by routine blood sampling from two sites using a tourniquet applied at different positions. Clin Chim Acta 1979;98:113–8

18. Mikesh LM, Bruns DE. Stabilization of glucose in blood specimens: mechanism of delay in fluoride inhibition of glycolysis. Clin Chem 2008;54:930–2

19. Natsugoe S, Tokuda K, Matsumoto M. Molecular detection of free cancer cells in pleural lavage fluid from esophageal cancer patients. Int J Mol Med 2003;12:771–5

20. Renoe BW, McDonald JM, Ladenson JH. The effects of stasis with and without exercise on free calcium, various cations, and related parameters. Clin Chim Acta 1980;103:91–100

21. Steige H, Jone JD. Evaluation of pneumatic tube system for delivery of blood specimens. Clin Chem 1971;17:1160–4

22. Young DS. Effects of preanalytical variables on clinical laboratory tests, 3rd edition. Washington, DC: AACC Press, 2007.

Quality Management*

George G. Klee, M.D., Ph.D., and James O. Westgard, Ph.D.

Objectives

1. Define the following terms:

CLIA	Quality assessment
Control materials	Quality control
False rejections	Quality laboratory process
Five-Q framework	Six Sigma process
ISO 9000	Standard deviation interval
JCTLM	Total quality management
Lean production	Waived test
Proficiency testing	Westgard multirules
Quality	

2. List and describe three costs of conformance and three costs of nonconformance.

3. Discuss in-service training programs for laboratory personnel, including the need for such programs, components of a program, methods of program delivery, and implementation of a program.

4. Describe the five laboratory testing processes and potential errors that might occur during each process; relate these processes to preanalytical, analytical, and postanalytical variables that affect laboratory test results.

5. List and describe examples of preanalytical, analytical, and postanalytical variables that affect laboratory test results; state how each of these variables is controlled.

6. Explain the need for and use of control materials in the clinical laboratory; compare random and systematic error with regard to causes; state the usefulness of patient specimen measurements combined with liquid controls in monitoring analytical bias.

7. In considering the use of control charts in the clinical laboratory:
    Explain the need for these charts.
    Describe how control limits are calculated and how data are entered on a control chart.
    Assess a Levey-Jennings control chart for error and out-of-limit control data.
    Evaluate appropriate actions required to resolve errors.

8. List and explain the Westgard multirules used for interpretation of laboratory control data, and discuss how each multirule describes specific types of error; list the steps involved in the multirule procedure.

9. Compare internal quality control with external quality assessment programs, including needs, requirements, and features of each program; state the role of proficiency testing in laboratory accreditation, and calculate and interpret a standard deviation interval.

10. Assess and resolve case studies related to quality management in the laboratory.

Key Words and Definitions

Control procedure Statistical and/or nonstatistical check protocols implemented in a clinical laboratory to assess the performance of an analytical method.

Control rules Decision criteria that define when an analytical run is judged acceptable ("in control") or unacceptable ("out of control").

External quality assessment Procedures and programs that provide information about systematic errors and maintenance of long-term accuracy of analytical methods.

ISO 9000 A set of four standards used to ensure quality management and quality assessment developed by the International Organization for Standardization.

Lean Production A quality process that is focused on creating greater value by eliminating activities that are considered waste.

Levey-Jennings control chart A graphical display with observed control values plotted against an acceptable range of values, indicated on the chart by lines for upper and lower control limits, commonly indicated as the mean control value plus or minus three standard deviations.

Proficiency testing (PT) A process in which simulated patient specimens made from a common pool are analyzed by laboratories to determine the "quality" of laboratories' performance; considered to be part of external quality assessment.

*The authors gratefully acknowledge the original contribution of Susan M. Lehman, Director, Clinical Laboratory Science Program, Mayo Clinic, Rochester, Minnesota, who provided information on personnel competency and training.

Key Words and Definitions—cont'd

Quality Conformance to the requirements of users or customers and the satisfaction of their needs and expectations.

Quality assessment A quality laboratory process that is concerned primarily with broader measures and monitors of laboratory performance such as turnaround times and test utility.

Quality control A quality laboratory process that involves statistical analysis of internal control procedures through use of control materials for method performance assessment and nonstatistical check procedures such as linearity studies and reagent checks.

Six Sigma process control A quantitative framework for evaluating process performance and providing more objective evidence for process improvement, with a goal of having Six Sigmas or six standard deviations of process variation fitting within the tolerance limits of the process.

Total quality management (TQM) A management philosophy and approach that focuses on processes and their improvement as the means to satisfy customer needs and requirements; a quality system that is implemented to ensure quality.

Total testing process A broad definition of the laboratory testing and reporting process that includes preanalytical, analytical, and postanalytical phases.

Turnaround time (TAT) The time between when a test is ordered or a specimen is submitted for analysis and when the test results are reported.

Westgard multirules A series of control rules used to interpret control data.

The principles of quality management, assurance, and control have become the foundation by which clinical laboratories are managed and operated. This chapter begins with a discussion of the fundamentals of total quality management and follows with descriptions of (1) total quality management of the clinical laboratory, (2) control of preanalytical variables, (3) control of analytical variables (with emphasis on statistical quality control and identification of sources of analytical errors), (4) **external quality assessment** and **proficiency testing programs**, and (5) the combined use of liquid controls plus moving averages of patient values for quality control monitoring. The chapter concludes with discussions of new quality initiatives, including **Six Sigma** principles and metrics, **Lean Production**, and the **ISO 9000** certification process.

Fundamentals of Total Quality Management

Quality systems in healthcare organizations continue to evolve, with numerous sources of information available on the Internet.[15] Public and private pressures to contain costs now are accompanied by pressures for quality improvement (QI). The seemingly contradictory pressures for both cost reduction and QI require that healthcare organizations adopt new systems to manage quality. When faced with these same pressures, other industries have implemented a process termed **total quality management** (TQM). This process is also referred to as *total quality control* (QC), *total quality leadership, continuous quality improvement, quality management science,* or, more generally, *industrial quality management.* It provides both a management philosophy for organizational development and a management process for improvement of quality in all aspects of work. Many healthcare organizations have adopted the concepts and principles of TQM.

Concepts

In this chapter, **quality** is defined as conformance to the requirements of users or customers and the satisfaction of their needs and expectations. The universal principles of total quality management include (1) customer focus, (2) management commitment, (3) training, (4) process capability and control, and (5) measurement through quality improvement tools.[28] The focus on users and customers is important, particularly in service industries such as healthcare. Users of healthcare laboratories are often the nurses and the doctors; their customers are the patients and other parties responsible for payment.

Costs must be understood in the context of quality. If quality means conformance to requirements, then "quality costs" must be understood in terms of "costs of conformance" and "costs of nonconformance," as illustrated in Figure 7-1. In industrial terms, costs of conformance are divided into prevention costs and appraisal costs. Costs of nonconformance consist of internal and external failure costs. For a laboratory testing process, calibration is a good example of a cost incurred to prevent problems. Likewise, quality control involves a cost for performance appraisal, a repeat run is an internal failure

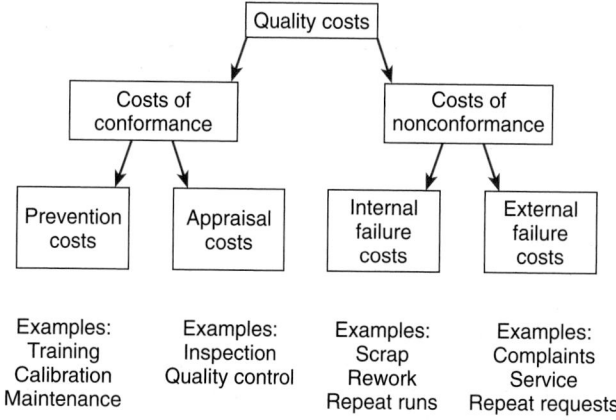

Figure 7-1 The cost of quality in terms of the costs of conformance and the costs of nonconformance to customer requirements. *(From Westgard JO, Barry PL. Cost-effective quality control: managing the quality and productivity of analytical processes. Washington, DC: AACC Press, 1997.)*

cost for poor analytical performance, and repeat requests for tests—because of poor analytical quality—constitute an external failure cost.

This understanding of quality and cost leads to a new perspective on the relationship between these two concepts. Improvements in quality lead to reductions in cost. For example, with better analytical quality, a laboratory eliminates repeat runs and repeat requests for tests. This repeat work is waste. If quality improves, waste is reduced, which, in turn, reduces cost. The father of this fundamental concept was the late W. Edwards Deming, who developed and internationally promulgated the idea that quality improvement reduces waste and leads to improved productivity, which, in turn, reduces costs and provides a competitive advantage.[11]

Methodology

Quality improvement occurs when problems are eliminated permanently. Problems arise primarily from imperfect processes, not from imperfect individuals. Industrial experience has shown that 85% of all problems are process problems, whereas the remaining 15% are problems requiring the action and performance improvement of individual employees. Thus, quality problems are primarily management problems because only management has the power to change work processes.

This emphasis on work processes leads to a new view of the organization as a system of processes (Figure 7-2).[7] For example, various disciplines will have different views of the work processes of a healthcare organization (Box 7-1). The total system for a healthcare organization involves the interaction of all of these processes and others.[15]

Given the primary importance of these processes for the organization, TQM views the organization as a support structure rather than a command structure. The most immediate processes required for delivery of services are those of frontline employees. The role of senior management is to support frontline employees and empower them to identify and solve problems in their own work processes.

The importance of empowerment is understood easily when a problem involves processes from two different departments. For example, if a problem involves the link between process A and process B (see Figure 7-2), the traditional management structure requires that a problem be passed up from the line workers to a section manager or supervisor, a department director, and an organization administrator. The administrator then works back through an equal number of intermediaries in the other department. Direct involvement of line workers and their managers should provide more immediate resolution of the problem.

However, solving such problem requires a carefully structured process to ensure that root causes are identified and proposed solutions are verified. Juran's "project-by-project" quality improvement process provides detailed guidelines that have been adopted widely and integrated into current team problem-solving methodology.[16] As listed in Box 7-2, this

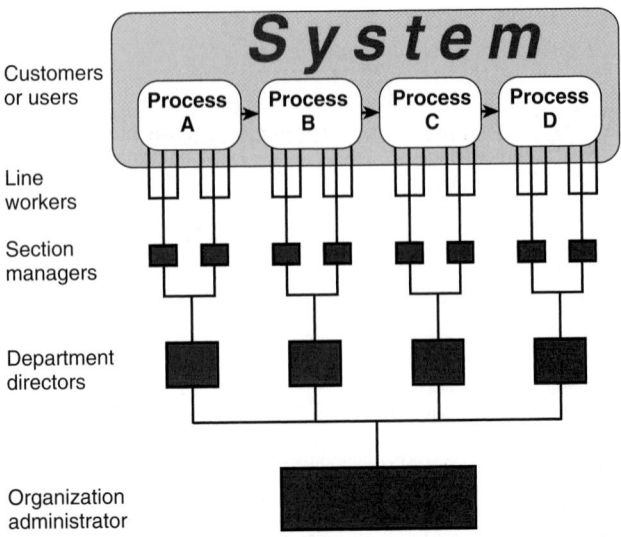

Figure 7-2 The total quality management view of an organization as a system of processes.

BOX 7-1   Different Views of the Work Processes of a Healthcare Organization as a Function of One's Position in the Organization

Physician/Healthcare Provider
- Patient examination
- Patient testing
- Patient diagnosis
- Patient treatment

Healthcare Administrator
- Processes for admission of patients
- Tracking of patient services
- Discharge of patients
- Billing for costs of services

Laboratory Director
- Processes for acquiring specimens
- Processing of specimens
- Analyzing of samples
- Reporting of test results

Laboratorian
- Acquisition of samples
- Analysis of samples
- Quality control measures
- Release of patient test results

BOX 7-2   Elements of a "Project-by-Project" Approach to Quality Improvement

Careful definition of the problem
Establishment of baseline measures of process performance
Identification of root causes of the problem
Identification of a remedy for the problem
Verification that the remedy actually works
"Standardization" or generalization of the solution for routine implementation of an improved process
Establishment of ongoing measures for monitoring and control of the process

methodology outlines distinct steps to be followed in such a quality improvement process.

Implementing TQM

The principles and concepts of TQM have been formalized into a quality management process (Figure 7-3). The traditional framework for quality management in a healthcare laboratory emphasizes establishment of (1) quality laboratory processes (QLPs), (2) quality control (QC), (3) **quality assessment (QA)**, and (4) quality systems (QSs).[7] QLPs include analytical processes, as well as the general policies, practices, and procedures that define how all aspects of the work are done. QC emphasizes statistical **control procedures** but also includes nonstatistical check procedures, such as (1) linearity checks, (2) reagent and standard checks, and (3) temperature monitors. QA, as currently applied, is concerned primarily with broader measures and monitors of laboratory performance, such as (1) **turnaround time**, (2) specimen identification, (3) patient identification, and (4) test utility. Note that *quality assessment* is the proper term for these activities, as opposed to **quality assurance**, which has been used incorrectly to describe these activities. Measuring performance does not by itself improve performance and often does not detect problems in time to prevent harmful effects. Quality assessment requires that causes of problems be identified through QI and eliminated through quality planning (QP), or that QC detect the problems early enough to prevent their consequences.

To provide a fully developed framework for quality management, QI and QP components must be established. QI provides a structured problem-solving process to help identify the root cause of a problem and a remedy for that problem. QP is necessary to (1) standardize the remedy, (2) establish measures for performance monitoring, (3) ensure that the performance achieved satisfies quality requirements, and (4) document the new QLP. The new process then is (1) implemented through QLP, (2) measured and monitored through QC and QA, (3) improved through QI, and (4) replanned through QP. These components, which work together in a feedback loop, illustrate how continuous QI is accomplished and quality assurance is built into laboratory processes.

The *five-Q framework* (see Figure 7-3) also defines how quality is managed objectively with the "scientific method," or the *PDCA cycle* (**p**lan, **d**o, **c**heck, **a**ct). QP provides the planning step, QLP establishes standard processes for the way things are done, QC and QA provide measures for checks on how well things are done, and QI provides a mechanism through which one can act on those measures. The methodology naturally applied in scientific experiments should serve as the basis for objective management decisions.

Objectivity, however, depends on the existence of quantitative quality requirements for evaluating the performance of existing processes and planning the performance of new processes. Laboratories must define their service goals and objectives and establish clinical and analytical quality requirements for process testing. Without such quality goals, no objective way exists to (1) determine whether acceptable quality is being achieved, (2) identify processes that need improvement, or (3) plan or design new processes that ensure the attainment of a specified level of quality.

TQM is considered a quality system that is implemented to ensure quality. For example, a Clinical Laboratory and Standards Institute (CLSI) document describes a quality management system (QMS) as a "set of key quality elements that must be in place for an organization's work operations to function in a manner to meet the organization's stated quality objectives."[7] Essentials of a QS (QSE) are listed in Box 7-3. These depict the infrastructure required by a laboratory to provide quality laboratory services. Details on how to implement QSs are given in the CLSI document.[7]

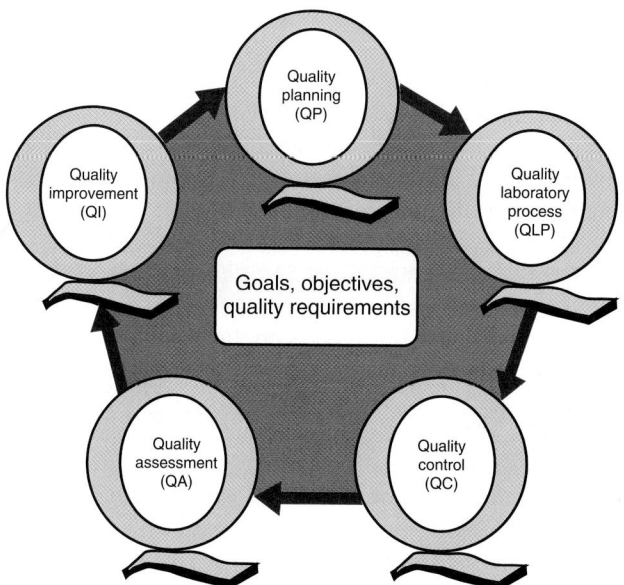

Figure 7-3 Total quality management framework for management of quality in a healthcare laboratory. *(From Westgard JO, Burnett RW, Bowers GN. Quality management science in clinical chemistry: a dynamic framework for continuous improvement of quality, Clin Chem 1990;36:1712-6.)*

BOX 7-3 Essentials of a Quality System

Documents and records
Organization
Personnel
Equipment
Purchasing and inventory
Process control
Information management
Occurrence management
Assessment: external and internal
Process improvement
Customer service

Adapted from Clinical and Laboratory Standards Institute. A quality system model for health care, 2nd edition. CLSI5 Document HS01-A2. Wayne, Pa: Clinical and Laboratory Standards Institute, 2004.

Personnel Competency and Training

People are critical components of a total quality system, and training and education are vital to the performance of personnel. A key factor for successful training and assessment of laboratory staff is the planning and implementation of targeted education programs. CLIA[24] identifies the following six areas as required components of a laboratory competency assessment program: (1) direct observation of routine patient test performance; (2) monitoring of the recording and reporting of test results; (3) review of intermediate test results, QC records, proficiency testing results, and preventive maintenance records; (4) direct observation and performance of instrument maintenance and function checks; (5) assessment of test performance through testing of previously analyzed specimens, internal blind testing of samples, or external proficiency testing of samples; and (6) assessment of problem-solving skills.[4]

Assessment of competence in job tasks as required by CLIA must be conducted semiannually the first year of employment and annually thereafter, and upon implementation of new test methodology before reporting of patient test results. Guidelines to assist in the development and documentation of competency assessment are available from the Clinical and Laboratory Standards Institute (CLSI). The CLSI Guideline, *Training and Competence Assessment,* gives detailed directions on how to develop and implement a training and competency assessment program that meets regulatory requirements, and provides examples of forms for documentation and record keeping.[5]

Design of an in-service training program based on instructional systems design includes the following elements: (1) analysis, (2) design, (3) implementation, and (4) evaluation. The program begins with a needs assessment or gap analysis to (1) determine employee performance requirements, (2) identify deficiencies, and (3) evaluate existing education and training resources. It requires the development of measurable instructional objectives that are based on the specific skills and competencies required of the employee to perform the job or task, and selection of an appropriate teaching strategy. The in-service training program also considers how an instructional program will be delivered and includes a range of organizational factors that may impact successful delivery of the instruction. These include (1) employee participation, (2) scheduling, (3) availability of subject matter experts to teach, (4) budget constraints, and (5) assessment of learning outcomes. It provides ways to evaluate the effectiveness of the instructional program.[10]

In the face of increased pressure to reduce operating costs, including expenses associated with attendance and travel to conferences, Internet education programs provide an effective, cost-efficient way to implement in-service training. Web-based training programs in quality control concepts are available through both professional organizations and private companies. As an example, the Mayo Clinic identified that a gap in academic education on basic quality control concepts existed based on the diversity of their workforce and the varying academic backgrounds required for their highly specialized laboratories. To provide the desired level of academic education to its employees in a way that could be readily accomplished, the Mayo Clinic enrolled employees in the course *Basic QC Practices,* available on the Web through Westgard QC, Inc. The e-learning content of the curriculum included the following modules: (1) statistical quality control; (2) construction and interpretation of **Levey-Jennings control charts**; (3) electronic checks and sources of error; (4) CLIA '88 regulations for QC; (5) control materials and limitations of QC; (6) multirule and multilevel interpretation of QC data; (7) false rejection and error detection; (8) troubleshooting; (9) regulatory guidelines; (10) QC documentation and record keeping; and (11) external quality assessment programs. In addition, the online curriculum was customized to employees' specific needs through the addition of staff lectures, six 2-hour laboratory sessions, assignments tailored to clinical laboratory practice, and pretesting and post-testing to assess competency.

Implementation of this in-house training program in basic quality control by the Mayo Clinic followed the education model designed for the Clinical Laboratory Science program. The didactic component is provided in an e-learning platform that consists of three modalities of learner interaction with content, instructor, and fellow learners. Each lesson plan includes a supplemental laboratory module taught by traditional methods of interaction between instructor and learner, which is closely anchored in the context of the work they perform. And finally, the curricular model implements the "reverse lecture-homework paradigm," whereby learners complete the Web-supported didactic modules asynchronously as "homework" assignments (Figure 7-4, *A*) and complete the laboratory lessons in the classroom (work setting) under the guidance and direction of the instructor/supervisor (Figure 7-4, *B*).

Implementing an e-learning platform allows the curricular model to expand the number of students over time toward an improved economy of scale. For academic programs, this approach allows for a potential increase in class size with minimal additional expenses. For in-service training, an electronic curriculum provides the opportunity to share training across different physical sites within a healthcare delivery system. This sharing (1) eliminates the costs associated with duplication of effort, (2) reduces operating costs to cover additional employees, and (3) decreases startup costs for new academic and in-service programs at additional sites.

The Total Testing Process

Accurate and timely test reports are the responsibility of the laboratory. However, many problems arise before and after submitted specimens are analyzed (see Chapter 6). Therefore the **total testing process** must be managed properly in the (1) preanalytical, (2) analytical, and (3) postanalytical phases. *Note:* These are also known as (1) pre-examination, (2) examination, and (3) post-examination processes.

The many steps or subprocesses that take place from the time of the initial request for a test to the time of final interpretation of the test result are determined through performance of a "systems analysis." Table 7-1 lists the steps or subprocesses of a typical clinical laboratory testing process and the potential errors associated with them. Although such an analysis

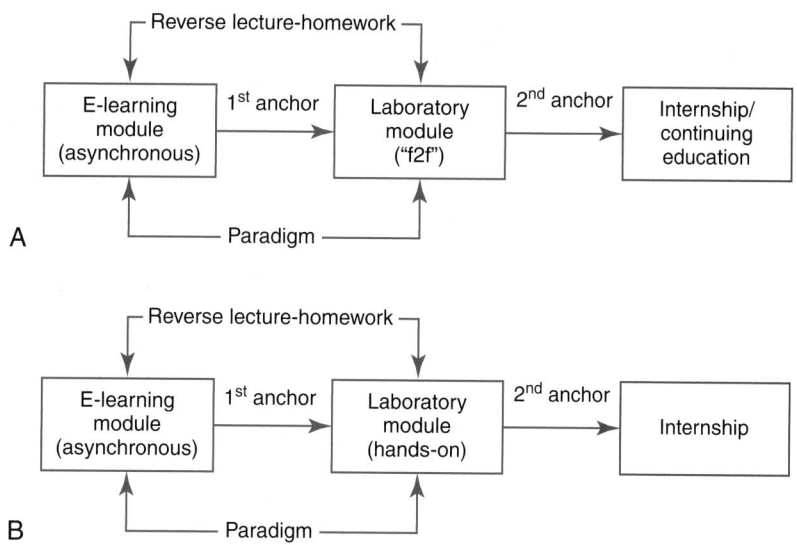

Figure 7-4 Examples of reverse lecture homework paradigms.

TABLE 7-1	Laboratory Testing Processes and Their Potential Errors
Process	**Potential Errors**
Test ordering	Inappropriate test
	Handwriting not legible
	Wrong patient identification
	Special requirements not specified
	Cost or delayed order
Specimen acquisition	Incorrect tube or container
	Incorrect patient identification
	Inadequate volume
	Invalid specimen (e.g., hemolyzed, too dilute)
	Collected at wrong time
	Improper transport conditions
Analytical measurement	Instrument not calibrated correctly
	Specimen mix-up
	Incorrect volume of specimen
	Interfering substance present
	Instrument precision problem
	Poorly written laboratory procedure
Test reporting	Wrong patient identification
	Report not posted in chart
	Report not legible
	Report delayed
	Transcription error
Test interpretation	Interfering substances not recognized
	Specificity of test not understood
	Precision limitations not recognized
	Analytical sensitivity not appropriate
	Previous values not available for comparison

identifies the critical processes for a typical laboratory, each laboratory situation is different, and additional processes and sources of error may be present. Thus, each laboratory should perform a systems analysis of its own laboratory testing system to identify those areas in which errors are likely to occur.

Once the processes have been documented, those processes most susceptible to error should be identified and should receive rigorous attention. Many times the processes that lead to the greatest number of complaints, such as lost specimens or delayed results, are judged most important. However, other factors, such as the appropriateness of test selection and the acceptability of a specimen, may be more important for achieving optimal medical care. Guidelines describing procedures for specimen handling are available from organizations such as the Clinical and Laboratory Standards Institute (CLSI). Documents put forth by accrediting agencies, such as the College of American Pathologists (CAP), the Centers for Disease Control and Prevention (CDC), and state regulatory agencies, are also helpful.[2,7,15]

Control of Preanalytical Variables

Establishing effective methods for monitoring and control of preanalytical variables is difficult because many such variables are outside the traditional laboratory areas (see Chapter 6). Monitoring of preanalytical variables requires the coordinated effort of many individuals and hospital departments, each of which must recognize the importance of these efforts in the maintenance of high-quality service. Accomplishing such monitoring may require support from outside the laboratory, particularly from the institution's clinical practice committee or some similar authority. Important variables for consideration are listed in Box 7-4 and are discussed in the following section of this chapter.

Test Utilization and Practice Guidelines

Traditionally, laboratory test utilization always has been monitored or controlled. However, current emphasis on the cost of medical care and government regulation of medical care have increased the importance of this factor.

Patient Identification

Correct identification of patients and specimens is a major concern for laboratories. The highest frequency of errors occurs with the use of handwritten labels and request forms.

BOX 7-4   Variables in the Preanalytical Process

Test utilization and practice guidelines
Patient identification
Turnaround time
Laboratory logs
Transcription errors
Patient preparation
Specimen collection
Specimen transport
Specimen separation and distribution of aliquots

The use of bar-coding technology for patient identification has minimized this potential source of error (see Chapter 16).

Turnaround Time (TAT)

The turnaround time (TAT) is defined as the time between when a test is ordered or a specimen is submitted for analysis and when the test results are reported. Delayed and lost test requisitions, specimens, and reports are major problems for laboratories. An essential feature of monitoring for the cause of delays is recording of actual times of (1) specimen collection, (2) receipt in the laboratory, and (3) reporting of test results and then calculating the TAT.

Laboratory Logs

When the serum aliquot tubes arrive in the laboratory, a request/report form generally accompanies the specimens. The patient name and identification number and the tests requested on the form should be checked against the information on the label of the specimen tube to ensure that they are the same. In addition, the specimen should be inspected to confirm adequacy of volume and freedom from problems that may interfere with the assay, such as lipemia or hemolysis. The specimens then should be stored appropriately, and the identifying information and arrival time recorded in a master log. In practice, this is now done electronically.

Transcription Errors

In laboratories where electronic identification and tracking have not been implemented, a substantial risk of transcription error is associated with manual entry of data, even when results are double-checked. Computerization reduces this type of transcription error because computerized systems have error detection routines programmed into the terminal entry functions. These routines may include (1) check digits, (2) limit checks, (3) test-correlation checks, and (4) verification checks with master hospital files.

Patient Preparation

Laboratory tests are affected by many patient factors, such as (1) recent intake of food, alcohol, or drugs, (2) smoking, (3) exercise, (4) stress, (5) sleep, (6) posture during specimen collection, and (7) other variables (see Chapter 6). Proper patient preparation is essential for obtaining meaningful test results. The laboratory must define the instructions and procedures for patient preparation and specimen acquisition.

Specimen Collection

The techniques used to acquire a specimen have affected many laboratory tests (see Chapter 6). Improper containers and incorrect preservatives also affect test results and make them inappropriate. One way to monitor and control this aspect of laboratory processing is to assign a specially trained laboratory team to handle specimen collection.

Specimen Transport

The stability of specimens during transport from the patient to the laboratory is critical for some tests performed locally and for most tests sent to regional centers and commercial laboratories. For control of specimen transport, the essential feature is the authority to reject specimens that arrive in the laboratory in an obviously unsatisfactory condition (such as a thawed specimen that should have remained frozen).

Specimen Separation and Distribution of Aliquots

Separation of blood specimens and distribution of aliquots are functions usually performed under the direct control of the laboratory. The main variables are (1) the centrifuges, (2) the containers, and (3) personnel. Centrifuges should be monitored through checks on speed, time, and temperature (see Chapter 8). Sources of calcium and trace metal contamination include (1) collection tubes, (2) pipettes, (3) stoppers, and (4) aliquot tubes; each lot number of materials used should be tested for contamination by calcium and possibly other elements.

Control of Analytical Variables

In practice, analytical variables are carefully controlled to ensure accurate measurements by analytical methods. Reliable analytical methods are identified through a careful process of (1) selection, (2) evaluation, (3) implementation, (4) maintenance, and (5) control (see Chapter 2). Smooth and uninterrupted laboratory service requires many procedures performed to prevent the occurrence of problems. Different laboratories have experienced different problems with the same analytical methods because different amounts of effort were allocated to the care, maintenance, and support of those methods.

Certain variables such as (1) water quality, (2) calibration of analytical balances, (3) calibration of volumetric glassware and pipettes, (4) stability of electrical power, and (5) the temperature of heating baths, refrigerators, freezers, and centrifuges should be monitored on a laboratory-wide basis because they affect many laboratory methods (see Chapter 8). In addition, certain variables specifically affect individual analytical methods, and these require the development of procedures to deal specifically with characteristics of the methods.

Documentation of Analytical Protocols

The CLSI[6] defines a process as a set of interrelated or interacting activities that transform inputs into outputs (ISO 9000; http://www.iso.org/iso/iso_9000/; accessed July 24. 2013). In practice, a process may be documented as a flowchart or a table that describes operations within the laboratory. A procedure document provides step-by-step instructions that a single individual needs to follow to successfully complete one activity in the process. Such a procedure is critical if a method is to achieve the same results when used by different laboratorians over a long time. Box 7-5 outlines the information contained in a procedure document. More detailed guidelines are provided in the CLSI document.[6] Contents required in a laboratory manual are listed in Box 7-6. Such a manual should be reviewed annually and revised whenever changes occur, and this should be documented. In addition, retaining outdated procedures in an archival file (hard copy or electronic) is a good practice.

Monitoring of Technical Competency

Proper training of laboratory personnel to establish uniformity in technique is important, as is scheduling of sufficient routine service to maintain proper techniques. A written list of objectives that outline critical tasks and knowledge is a helpful tool in training of personnel on new analytical methods. These objectives ensure systematic instruction that covers the critical points. Before analyses for clinical use are performed, the technical competence of personnel should be checked and practice runs performed. Periodic monitoring of competency may be difficult, but incident reports and results from internal

and external QC checks will identify specific problems; these problems should be discussed directly with the personnel involved. In-service and continuing education programs help to maintain and improve competence. Employee conferences help to uncover nontechnical problems that may affect work quality.

Statistical Control of Analytical Methods

Performance of analytical methods typically is monitored through analysis of specimens with known concentrations and subsequent comparison of observed values with known values. The known values usually are represented by an interval of acceptable values, or by upper and lower limits for control (control limits). When observed values fall within control limits, the laboratorian is assured that the analytical method is performing properly. When observed values fall outside control limits, the laboratorian is alerted to the possibility of problems in the analytical determination. A variety of available sources of information describe the application of statistical QC in the clinical laboratory.[13,26]

Control Materials

Specimens that are analyzed for QC purposes are known as *control materials.* They need to be available (1) in a stable form, (2) in aliquots or vials, and (3) for analysis over an extended time. In addition, only minimal vial-to-vial variation should exist, so that differences between repeated measurements are attributed to the analytical method alone. The control material preferably should have the same matrix as the test specimens of interest, for example, a protein matrix should be present when serum is the test material to be analyzed by the analytical method. Materials from human sources generally are preferred, but because of limited availability and biohazard considerations, animal materials offer a certain advantage in terms of safety and are often more readily available. The concentration of analyte should be within healthy and abnormal reference intervals, corresponding to concentrations that are critical in the medical interpretation of test results.

In practice, laboratories purchase control materials from one of several companies that manufacture control sera or "control products." These products generally are supplied in lyophilized or freeze-dried forms that are reconstituted by the addition of water or a specific diluent solution. Also available are materials with matrices representing (1) urine, (2) spinal fluid, and (3) whole blood. Liquid control materials also are available and offer the advantage of eliminating errors caused by reconstitution. However, the matrices of these liquid materials contain other materials that constitute a potential source of error with some analytical methods and instruments.

In addition to the product's matrix, several other factors must be considered in the selection of commercial control materials. Stability is critical because the laboratory often purchases a year's supply of one manufacturing lot or batch. Different batches (or lot numbers) of the same material have different concentrations, which require new estimates of the mean and the standard deviation (SD). The size of the aliquots or vials should be convenient for the analytical methods to be monitored. Larger vials generally are less expensive (on a per-milliliter basis), but unused materials may eliminate potential savings. Two or three different materials should be selected to obtain concentrations that monitor performance at different medical decision levels.

Control products are purchased as assayed or unassayed materials. Assayed materials come with a list of values for the concentrations or activities expected for that material. This list often includes both the mean and the SD for several common analytical methods and preferably for a reference method used to measure a particular analyte. Because of the work required to determine these values, the assayed materials are more expensive. Although stated assay values are useful in selection of desired materials, determination of the mean and the SD in the user's laboratory is advisable because this process improves the performance characteristics of statistical control procedures.

General Principles of Control Charts

One method commonly used to compare values observed for control materials with their known values is the use of control charts.[*] Control charts are simple graphical displays in which the observed values are plotted versus the time when the observations are made. Known values are represented by an acceptable range of values, as indicated on the chart by lines for upper and lower control limits. When plotted points fall within control limits, this occurrence generally is interpreted to mean that the method is performing properly; points falling outside control limits are problematic.

Control limits usually are calculated from the mean (x) and the SD (s) obtained from repeated measurements on known specimens by the particular analytical method that is to be controlled (see Chapter 2). When the method is performing properly, initial estimates should be based on measurements obtained over a period of at least 1 month. In practice, this initial estimate may not be entirely reliable because of the low number of data points and possible outliers in the data. Estimates are revised when additional data have been accumulated by recording of n and summations of x_i and (x_i^2), and when cumulative totals in the previous equations are subsequently used to determine cumulative means and SDs. The effects of outliers are minimized by elimination of values exceeding the mean by more than ± 3.1 to 3.8 s's (where the exact factor depends on the total number of data points: 3.14 for $n = 30$; 3.22, $n = 40$; 3.33, $n = 60$; 3.41, $n = 80$; 3.47, $n = 100$; 3.66, $n = 200$; and 3.83, $n = 400$).

Error distribution of the analytical method is assumed to be Gaussian (i.e., symmetrical and bell-shaped; see Chapter 2). The control limits are set to include most of the control values, usually 95% to 99.7%, which correspond to the mean ± 2 or 3 SDs (s). Because observance of a value in the tails of the

distribution should be a relatively rare occurrence (only 1 out of 20 times for 2 s limits, 3 out of 1000 for 3 s limits), such an observation is suspect and suggests that something may have happened to the analytical method. Such an occurrence could have caused a shift in the mean (an accuracy problem), which would result in a higher probability of exceeding the limits, or it could have caused an increase in the SD (a precision problem), which would widen the distribution and result in a higher probability of exceeding the control limits of acceptability.

Figure 7-5, A, illustrates how the distributions of control values appear for three different situations: (1) stable performance in which only an occasional observation exceeds control limits, (2) occurrence of a systematic error that shifts the mean of the distribution and causes a much higher expectation or probability that control values may be observed outside one of the control limits, and (3) occurrence of an increase in random error or imprecision, which widens the distribution and causes a much higher probability that a control value may be observed outside either of the control limits.

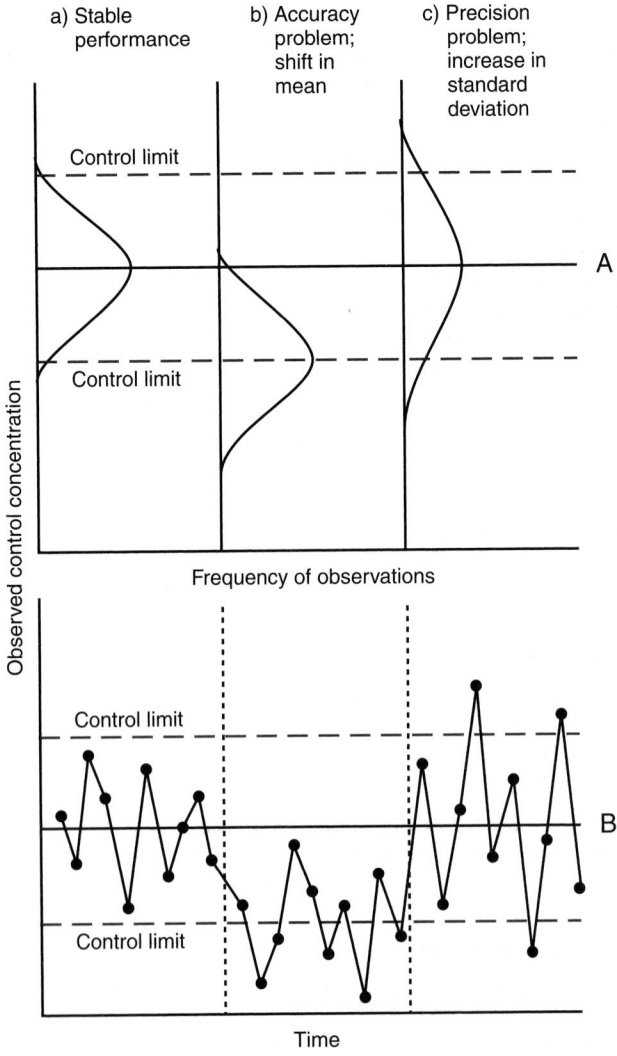

Figure 7-5 Conceptual basis of control charts. **A,** Frequency distributions of control observations for different error conditions. **B,** Display of control values representing those distributions for which concentration is plotted versus time on a control chart.

---

[*]Control charts were introduced into the clinical chemistry laboratory by Levey and Jennings in 1950. They demonstrated how industrial control procedures could be used with the mean and the range of duplicate measurements derived from clinical chemical methods.

In practice, control charts are used to compare observed control values with control limits and to provide a visual display that is inspected and reviewed quickly. On these charts, the concentration or observed value is plotted on the y-axis versus time of observation on the x-axis. Commonly, one month's data are plotted on a chart, usually only one or two points a day, but the time axis should be appropriate for the method being monitored. An example of a Levey-Jennings control chart is shown in Figure 7-5, B, where control values represent the three situations in Figure 7-5, A, with 10 values per situation (for a total of 30 values). If the analytical method is operating properly, control values fall predominantly within control limits. When an accuracy problem exists, control values are shifted to one side and several values in a row may fall outside one of the limits. When a precision problem exists, control values fluctuate much more widely and may exceed both upper and lower control limits.

Interpretation of control data is guided by certain decision criteria or **control rules**, which define when an analytical run is judged "in control" (acceptable) or "out of control" (unacceptable). The term *analytical run* is used in this discussion to refer to that segment of data for which a decision on acceptability is to be made. This is the group of patient results to be reported, based on control results available for inspection at that time. The total number of control observations available for inspection when a decision is to be made on the acceptability of an analytical run is designated as N. For example, when one control observation precedes and one follows a group of 10 patient samples whose results are to be reported, two control observations exist in that analytical run. The control rules are given symbols such as A_L, or n_L, where A is the abbreviation for a statistic, n is the number of control observations, and L refers to the control limits. For example, 1_{3s} refers to a control rule in which 1 observation exceeding the mean ± 3 s control limits is the criterion for rejection of the analytical run. Similarly, 1_{2s} refers to a control rule in which 1 observation exceeds the mean ± 2 s.

Performance Characteristics of a Control Procedure

The different control procedures discussed previously have different performance capabilities, depending on the control rules and the number of control observations chosen. For example, a Levey-Jennings control chart with control limits set as the mean ± 2 s has a high rate of "false alarms" (i.e., rejections when the method is actually performing satisfactorily). Use of 3 s control limits, such as a 1_{3s} control rule, reduces the false alarms to 1% or less; however, the true alarms or error detection also experiences a reduction.

Selection of control rules and the numbers of control measurements are related to the quality goals set by the laboratory.[8] For example, practical knowledge of the performance characteristics of control procedures is necessary to select control rules that detect relevant laboratory problems without causing too many false alarms. Experienced laboratorians often use a series of informal rules or judgments to reduce the number of false alarms without knowing their effects on the detection of real problems or true alarms. Some quantitative assessment of these two characteristics—false alarms and true alarms—should take place whenever capabilities of new control procedures are assessed, or when established control procedures are reviewed.

Recognizing the seriousness of the false-rejection problem and its relationship to the control limits chosen for the Levey-Jennings chart is important. These false rejections are in effect an inherent property of the control procedure. They occur because of the control limits that have been selected, not because of any problems with the analytical method. Therefore the use of 2 s control limits generally is not recommended. With the use of 3 s control limits, the false-rejection problem is eliminated, but error detection unfortunately is reduced.

Westgard Multirule Chart

The "multirule" procedure developed by Westgard and associates[25] uses a series of control rules to interpret control data. The probability for false rejections is kept low through selection of only those rules with low individual probabilities for false rejection (≤0.01). The probability of error detection is improved through selection of those rules that are particularly sensitive to random and systematic errors. The **Westgard multirule procedure** requires a chart with lines for control limits drawn at the mean ± 1 s, 2 s, and 3 s (i.e., adapted to existing Levey-Jennings charts by the addition of one or two sets of control limits).

The following control rules are used:
- 1_{2s}: one control observation exceeding the mean ± 2 s; used only as a "warning" rule that initiates testing of control data by other control rules
- 1_{3s}: one control observation exceeding the mean ± 3 s; primarily sensitive to random error
- 2_{2s}: two consecutive control observations exceeding the same mean plus 2 s or mean minus 2 s limit; sensitive to systematic error
- R_{4s}: one observation exceeding the mean plus 2 s and another exceeding the mean minus 2 s; sensitive to random error
- 4_{1s}: Four consecutive observations exceeding the mean plus 1 s or the mean minus 1 s; sensitive to systematic error
- 10_x: 10 consecutive control observations falling on one side of the mean (above or below, with no other requirement on the size of deviations); sensitive to systematic error

Use of the multirule procedure is similar to use of a Levey-Jennings chart, but data interpretation is more structured and rigorous. In performing the multirule procedure, the following steps are followed:
1. Samples of the control material are analyzed by the analytical method to be controlled on at least 20 different days. Two different materials with appropriate concentrations are recommended. The mean and the SD are calculated for the results for each control material being used.
2. A control chart is constructed for each of the control materials being used. The observed concentration or control value is plotted on the y-axis, setting the range of concentrations to include the mean ± 4 s. Horizontal lines are drawn for the mean, the mean ± 1 s, the mean ± 2 s, and the mean ± 3 s. In practice, the use of different colors for these lines, perhaps green, yellow, and red for the 1 s, 2 s, and 3 s

limits, respectively, is helpful. The *x*-axis is scaled for time, day, or run number and is labeled accordingly.

3. Two control specimens are introduced into each analytical run—one for each of the two concentrations (when two different materials have been selected). Control values are recorded and plotted for each on its respective control chart.

4. When both control observations fall within the 2 *s* limits, the analytical run is accepted and the patient results reported. When one of the control observations exceeds a 2 *s* limit, the patient results are held and additional rules applied. For example, the control data are inspected using the 1_{3s}, 2_{2s}, R_{4s}, 4_{1s}, and 10_x rules. When any of these rules indicates that the run is out of control, the analytical run is rejected, and the patient results are not reported. When all rules indicate that the run is in control, the analytical run is accepted, and the patient results are reported.

5. When a run is out of control, the type of error is determined on the basis of the control rule that has been violated. This involves looking for sources of that type of error. The problem is then corrected, and the analysis of the entire run is repeated, including both control and patient samples.

An example of the application of the multirule procedure is shown in Figure 7-6, where the top chart illustrates a high-concentration control material and the bottom chart

a low-concentration material. Of note is that the R_{4s} rule is applied only within a run, so that between-run systematic errors are not wrongly interpreted as random errors. However, the rule may be applied "across" materials, meaning that one of the observations is on the low material and the other on the high material, as long as they are within the same run. Alternatively, note that the 2_{2s}, 4_{1s}, and 10_x rules are applied across runs and materials. This application effectively increases *n* and improves the error detection capabilities of the procedure.

Identifying Sources of Analytical Errors

Statistical control procedures provide a way to alert the laboratorian to analytical problems that cause the quality of analytical performance to be less than the goals set for the laboratory. However, these control procedures do not identify the sources of the analytical errors and do not solve the control problems. The laboratorian must respond to the out-of-control signal to correct the problem and prevent future occurrences.

QC guidelines from a CLSI document[8] emphasize the importance of problem correction, as opposed to routine repeat of controls, which, in effect, consists of just repeating tests until the controls are within an acceptable range. When control procedures are selected properly on the basis of the quality required for the test and the imprecision and inaccuracy observed with the method, false rejections should be minimized; therefore routine repetition wastes time and effort. Practical tools for selection of appropriate QC procedures have been described in the literature.[26] A laboratorian, when alerted to a control problem, should conduct an inspection of the analytical method, equipment, reagents, and specimens to ensure that the test is performing correctly. An inspection may appear to be a qualitative and sensory technique, but it is a very powerful tool when combined with checklists developed for specific analytical methods. This inspection should include a review of records documenting changes that occur with the instrument and the reagents. Brief instrument function checks often are performed to verify proper system performance and to separate chemical and instrumental sources of error. Experienced laboratorians often spot the problem by performing this kind of inspection, whereas inexperienced laboratorians are aided by formal checklists.

The type of error itself provides a clue to the source of the error. For example, systematic errors often related to calibration problems are listed in Box 7-7. Random errors more likely

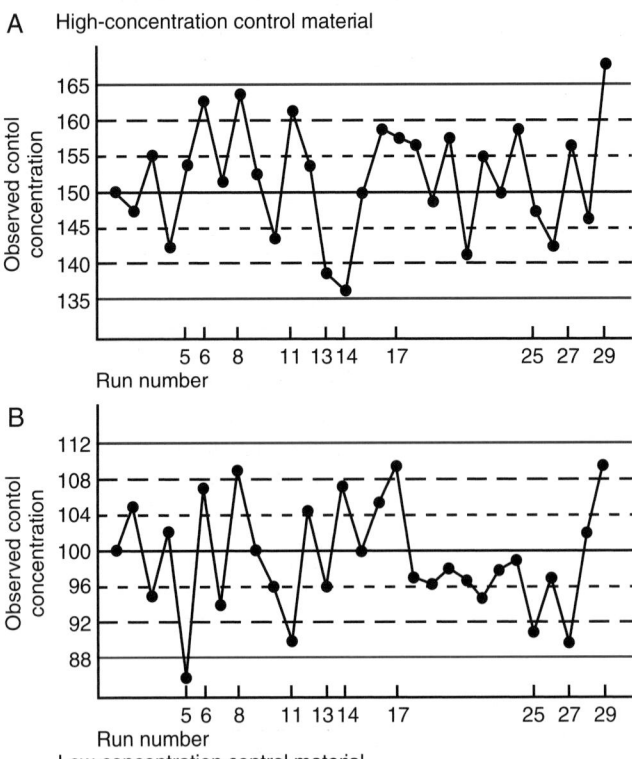

Figure 7-6 Westgard multirule control chart with control limits drawn at the mean ± 1 *s*, 2 *s*, and 3 *s*. Concentration is plotted on the *y*-axis versus time (run number) on the *x*-axis. **A,** Chart for high-concentration control material. **B,** Chart for low-concentration control material. *s,* Standard deviation. *(From Westgard JO, Barry PL, Hunt MR, et al: A multi-rule Shewhart chart for quality control in clinical chemistry,* Clin Chem *1981;27:493-501.)*

BOX 7-7	**Systematic Errors Often Related to Calibration Problems**

Impure calibration materials
Improper preparation of calibrating solutions
Erroneous set point and assigned values
Unstable calibrating solutions
Contaminated solutions
Inadequate calibration techniques
Nonlinear or unstable calibration functions
Inadequate sample blanks
Unstable reagent blanks

are due to (1) lack of reproducibility in the pipetting of samples and reagents, (2) dissolving of reagent tablets and mixing of sample and reagents, and (3) lack of stability of temperature baths, timing regulation, and photometric and other sensors. Individual analytical methods may not be subject to all of these possible sources of error; rather only a few plausible sources may exist for a particular type of error. Experienced laboratorians often know what these common sources are for their particular analytical methods and quickly identify the source once the type of error is known.

A clue to type of error is the control rule that is violated. Different control rules have different sensitivities to detect random and systematic errors. For example, 1_{3s} and R_{4s} rules tend to respond to random error; 2_{2s}, 4_{1s}, and 10_x rules to systematic error. Control procedures that use patient samples rather than stable control materials help identify preanalytical sources of error, such as sample handling and processing. External quality assessment procedures may provide more extensive information about systematic errors than can be obtained from internal procedures. Information derived from all these procedures is complementary and, when used in combination, provides a complete assessment of the types of errors and their possible sources.

Combined Use of Liquid Controls and Moving Averages of Patient Values for Quality Control Monitoring

Distributions of measured test values for patients have been used to supplement traditional liquid controls for monitoring analytical bias. These patient specimen measurements generally have much larger variances than liquid controls because they contain (1) biological, (2) pathophysiological, and (3) preanalytical sources of variation, in addition to analytical variation. However, if some of these sources of variation are controlled, averaging techniques often are used to generate tracking parameters that have variations of the same order of magnitude as liquid controls. Demographic information about specific patients such as (1) age, (2) sex, and (3) medical provider service area has been used to normalize test values, resulting in smaller variances of group means for the monitoring parameters. The larger the window size used for averaging patient values, the smaller the variance. The coefficient of variation (CV) of the group mean decreases approximately proportionately to the square root of the number of samples. Various statistical techniques have been used to average patient values, such as the exponentially adjusted moving mean. In general, a balance is present between decreased variance and increased time for error detection when larger numbers of patient values are used in these moving averages. For most chemistry tests, window sizes that use 50 to 100 sample values often are necessary.[18] An advantage of test value distributions over liquid controls is the inclusion of preanalytical variation caused by specimen collection, transport, and storage. This allows patient value–derived parameters to detect changes in these variables, in addition to changes in analytical testing.

Figure 7-7 illustrates an algorithm for combining liquid controls with a patient value–derived parameter. The same multirule evaluation systems used for liquid controls have been used for tracking the patient value–derived QC statistic. Set points and

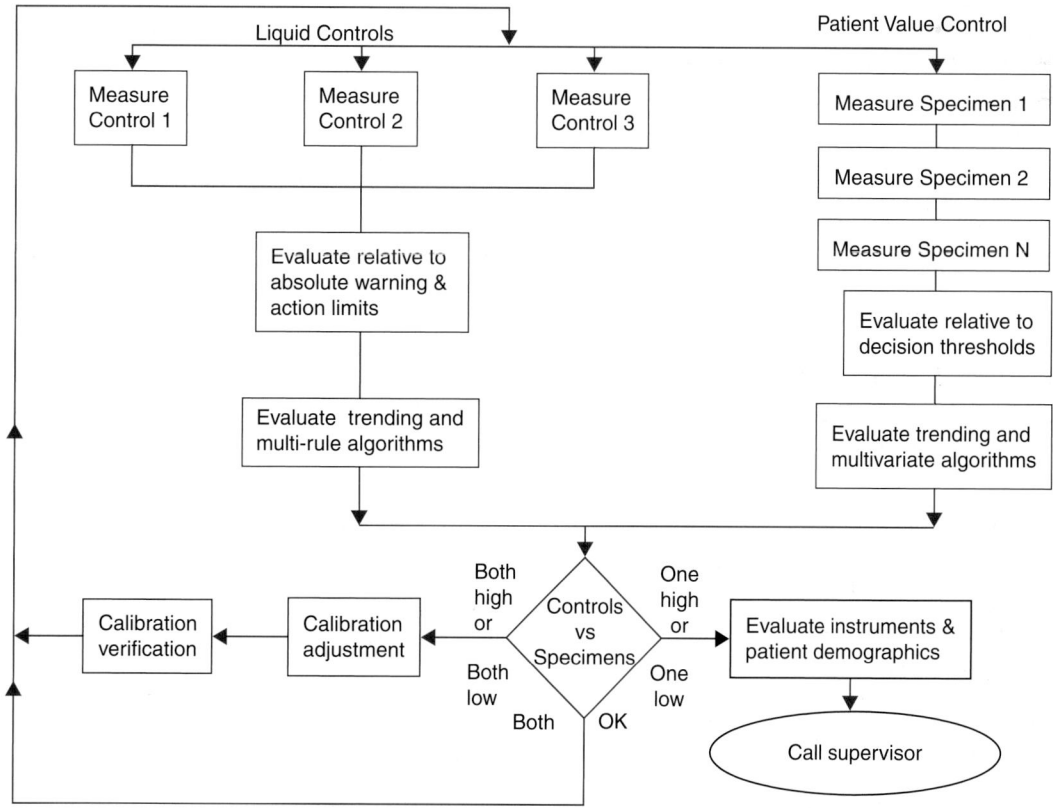

Figure 7-7 Protocol for combining liquid controls and a patient value–derived control.

threshold values are assigned to this derived parameter to optimize the power for error detection for systematic error. Note that the averaging algorithms used to generate these derived parameters average out random errors, so these derived parameters are not useful for detecting random errors. As illustrated in the figure, this combined control protocol is most accurate when both the liquid control and the patient-derived control move in the same direction (both high or both low). When the controls move discordantly, further investigation is necessary to determine whether the problem is related to instability of liquid controls, changes in patient characteristics (such as many sick patients seen at one time), preanalytical test changes, or other causes.

External Quality Assessment and Proficiency Testing Programs

All control procedures described previously have focused on monitoring by a single laboratory. These procedures constitute what is often called *internal QC,* to distinguish them from procedures used to compare the performances of different laboratories, the latter known as *external QA.* The two procedures are complementary: Internal QC is necessary for daily monitoring of the precision and accuracy of the analytical method, and external QA is important for the maintenance of long-term accuracy of analytical methods.

Participation in an external proficiency testing program is required for all U.S. laboratories that perform tests classified by CLIA as *moderate-* and *high-complexity tests.*[24] Many point-of-care testing sites perform some of these tests and must enroll in proficiency testing programs. Current approved providers of proficiency testing programs deliver sets of up to five specimens for analysis by the laboratory 3 times per year. The laboratory reports its results to the provider, who then makes them available to the regulatory agencies.

Features of External Quality Assessment Programs

Several external QA programs available to the clinical laboratory are sponsored by professional societies and manufacturers of control materials. The basic operation of these programs involves all participating laboratories analyzing the same lot of control material, usually daily as part of internal QC activities. The results are tabulated monthly and are sent to the sponsoring group for data analysis. Summary reports are prepared by the program sponsor and are distributed to all participating laboratories.

The reports generated from external QA programs often include extensive data analysis, statistical summaries, and plots. The overall mean of all laboratories in the program or the mean of values of all laboratories is taken as the "true" or correct value and is used for comparison with the individual laboratory's mean. Different programs do this in different ways. For example, the *t*-test is used to test the statistical significance of any differences between an individual laboratory's observed mean and the group mean. When the difference is significant, the laboratory is alerted that its results are biased in comparison with the results of most other laboratories. Another approach is to divide the difference by the overall SD of the group and then express the difference in terms of the number of SDs.

$$SDI = \frac{Lab\ Result - Group\ Mean}{Group\ s}$$

where *SDI* is the standard deviation interval or index, and *group s* is the SD for the group or for a selected subset of the group. Differences greater than 2 indicate that a laboratory is not in agreement with the rest of the laboratories in the program. These calculations reduce all test results to the same values, which makes possible interpretation of the data from different analytes without reference to the exact mean and *s* for each analytical method. For example, a value of ±2.0 has the same meaning for any test, indicating that the value is 2 *s* above or below its established mean.

Additional information about the nature of the systematic error is obtained when two different control materials are analyzed by each laboratory. The laboratory's observed mean for material A is plotted on the *y*-axis versus its observed mean for material B on the *x*-axis. These graphs are called *Youden plots.* Ideally, the point for a laboratory should fall at the center of the plot. Data points falling from the center but on the 45° line suggest a proportional analytical error. Data points falling from the center but not onto the 45° line suggest an error that is constant for both materials or one that occurs with just one material.

The report also may include Levey-Jennings plots of the data, but because this information is not available in real time, it does not effectively serve the purposes of internal QC. Blank control charts set up for each analyte and each control material save the laboratory the time required to prepare these charts manually.

Role of Proficiency Testing in Accreditation

Proficiency testing (PT) is the process by which simulated patient specimens made from a common pool are analyzed by laboratories; the results of this procedure are evaluated to determine the "quality" of the laboratories' performance. In 1988, the U.S. Congress to passed revisions to the Clinical Laboratory Improvement Act of 1967 (CLIA '67) and the Clinical Laboratory Improvement Amendments of 1988 (CLIA '88). One of the revisions mandate PT as a major part of the laboratory accreditation process. The final legislative rule for this legislation was published on January 24, 2003.[21] Additional interpretative guidelines, however, were published by the Centers for Medicare & Medicaid Services (CMS) in January 2004 in the form of the *State Operations Manual.*[24] Appendix C of that document refers specifically to guidelines for laboratories and laboratory testing services.

CLIA requires that all U.S. laboratories register with the government and identify the tests that they perform. Tests may be classified as "waived" or "nonwaived." Waived tests are those that any laboratory is able to perform as long as it follows the manufacturer's directions. No other requirements have been put forth for quality management of those tests. Laboratories that perform "nonwaived" tests are subject to complete CLIA regulations and must be inspected periodically by the government or by certain professional organizations deemed to have standards at least as stringent as CLIA requirements.

Two such organizations are the College of American Pathologists (CAP) and The Joint Commission (TJC). Note that this latter organization was formerly known as the Joint Commission on Accreditation of Healthcare Organizations (JCAHO), and previous to that the Joint Commission on Accreditation of Hospitals (JCAH). The CLIA implementation rules and interpretative guidelines outline the criteria for acceptable performance in laboratory inspection and accreditation.

The CLIA requirements cover several broad classes: (1) Subpart J, Facility Administration; (2) Subpart K, Quality Systems; (3) Subpart M, Personnel; and (4) Subpart Q, Inspection. The final rule dealt mainly with changes to the subpart on Quality Systems,[21] with particular attention to preanalytical, analytical, and postanalytical systems. It places increased emphasis on having quality systems in place to monitor preanalytical and postanalytical processes, yet the biggest impact of the final rule is on analytical quality assessment and analytical quality systems.

The CLIA '88 proposed criteria that group laboratory tests into "specialty" and "subspecialty" categories and specify representative tests to be monitored in each category. To succeed in a given category, a laboratory must produce correct results on four of five specimens for each of the analytes in that category and must score overall at least 80% for three consecutive challenges. If more than two incorrect results are produced for any analyte, the laboratory is considered "on probation." If a laboratory has two or more incorrect results for any analyte or an overall score less than 80% on two of three consecutive surveys, it is classified as "suspended" and must cease testing of all analytes in that specialty category until it is reinstated.

An additional requirement of the final CLIA regulations is that laboratories must perform method validation studies on all new tests introduced after April 24, 2003. Before this time, laboratories that implemented new methods and analytical systems that had been cleared by the U.S. Food and Drug Administration (FDA) could simply follow manufacturers' directions for operation and assume that the manufacturers' performance claims were valid. With the issuance of the final rule, the performance of all new tests must be validated in each laboratory to document (1) reportable range, (2) precision, (3) accuracy, and (4) reference intervals. For some methods, it may also be necessary to (5) determine the detection limit and (6) test for possible interferences.

Another major change in the final rule was the elimination of an earlier provision that would have required the FDA to review a manufacturer's QC instructions. This was a key provision for allowing laboratories to simply follow a manufacturer's directions. However, with elimination of this provision, laboratories now have greater responsibility for establishing effective QC systems that will (1) monitor the complete analytical process, (2) take into account the performance specifications of the method, (3) detect immediate errors, and (4) monitor long-term precision and accuracy.

A controversial change in the final rule was the introduction of "equivalent QC procedures" (EQCs) that allowed laboratories to reduce daily QC to weekly or even monthly QC for analytical systems that have built-in procedural controls. The provision was targeted for point-of-care testing (POCT) or near patient testing (NPT), in cases where personnel lack the skills to perform QC and instead rely on instrument checks, most notably electronic checks or electronic QC. Although at least one example is known of an analytical system with improved QC technology that requires little or no external QC,[27] most analytical systems have yet to demonstrate the performance that would justify reduction of daily QC to only weekly or monthly QC. Because of the controversy involving EQC, CMS announced in 2012 that EQCs would be phased out and recommended that alternative QC procedures be developed on the basis of risk management.[9] The CMS refers to this new approach as an individualized QC plan (IQCP).

However, one should recognize that PT programs are far from ideal monitors of laboratory performance. For example, in a study of PT survey problems at the Mayo Clinic, more than one-half of the errors on surveys were related directly to deficiencies in the surveys (e.g., invalid specimens, inappropriate evaluation criteria), and only 28% could be linked to specific analytical problems.[17]

New Quality Initiatives

Several additional quality initiatives have been developed and implemented to ensure that laboratories incorporate the principles of quality management and QA in their daily operations. These include implementation of the (1) Six Sigma Process, (2) Lean Production, and (3) ISO 9000 standards. In addition, the Joint Committee for Traceability in Laboratory Medicine (JCTLM) has been organized to give guidance on internationally recognized and accepted equivalence of measurements in laboratory medicine and traceability to appropriate measurement standards

The Six Sigma Process

Six Sigma is an evolution in quality management that is being widely implemented in business and industry in the new millennium.[14] Six Sigma metrics are being adopted as the universal measure of quality to be applied to industry processes and the processes of suppliers. The principles of Six Sigma are traceable to Motorola's approach to TQM in the early 1990s and the performance goal that "*6 sigmas or 6 standard deviations of process variation should fit within the tolerance limits for the process*"; hence, the name *Six Sigma* (http://mu.motorola.com/; accessed July 25, 2013).

In practice, the Six Sigma process provides a more quantitative framework for evaluating process performance and more objective evidence for process improvement. The goal for process performance is illustrated in Figure 7-8, which shows an error distribution of a measurement procedure that fits acceptably within tolerance specifications or quality requirements for that measurement. In practice, a process is evaluated in terms of a sigma metric that describes how many sigmas fit within the tolerance limits. For processes in which poor outcomes are counted as errors or defects, the defects are expressed as defects per million (DPM), then are converted to

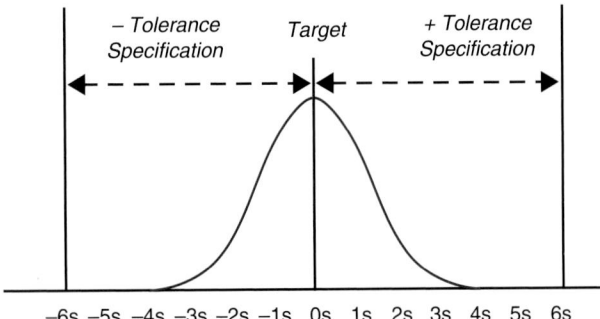

Figure 7-8 Six Sigma goal for process performance "tolerance specification" represents the quality requirement.

a sigma metric using a standard table available in Six Sigma textbooks.[14] As optimizing healthcare outcomes and reducing medical errors are of great interest, Six Sigma provides a general method that can be used to describe process outcomes on the sigma scale. The Six Sigma process is used in many industries[1,20] and institutions, and a primer for healthcare facilities is now available.[3]

Lean Production

Lean Production is a quality process that is focused on creating greater value by eliminating activities that are considered waste. For example, any inefficient activity or process that consumes resources or adds cost or time without creating value is revised or eliminated. In practice, it focuses on "system-level" improvements (as opposed to "point improvements").

Because of its success in increasing efficiency environments, the Lean approach has proven useful wherever a defined set of activities is working to produce a product or service. For example, a "Lean team" at Saint Mary's Hospital, a Mayo Clinic hospital in Rochester, Minnesota, used Lean Production to improve the efficiency of its paper ordering system for lab work in its intensive care unit.[19] Because the goal of Lean Production is to increase efficiency and the Six Sigma process to improve quality, these approaches have been combined and integrated into the management of several organizations, including healthcare facilities and clinical laboratories.[12]

ISO 9000

The International Organization for Standardization (ISO), in Geneva, Switzerland (http://www.iso.ch/; accessed July 25, 2013), has developed and promulgated the ISO 9000 standards. ISO is a worldwide federation of national standards bodies from some 100 countries. The mission of ISO is to promote the development of standardization and related activities in the world with a view toward facilitating the international exchange of goods and services and developing cooperation in the spheres of (1) intellectual, (2) scientific, (3) technological, and (4) economic activities. The work of ISO results in international agreements, which are published as International Standards. The ISO 9000 standards are examples of such standards, and they have been applied worldwide. ISO also has organized several technical advisory groups that address quality issues of interest to clinical laboratorians.

ISO 9000 is a set of four standards enacted to ensure quality management and QA in manufacturing and service industries.[23] They were first published in 1987 and are used worldwide; more than 80 countries have adopted them.

The ISO 9000 standards represent an international consensus on the essential features of a quality system designed to ensure the effective operation of any business, whether a manufacturer or a service provider or any other type of organization, in the public or private sector. ISO certification is provided by accredited organizations known as *registrars*. Registrars review the organization's quality manual and audit the process to ensure that the system documented in the manual is in place and effective.

Preparing for ISO Accreditation

In 2002 Burnett compared ISO standards and synthesized an "ideal standard," which became a practical guide for laboratories preparing for ISO accreditation.[22] In his comparison, Burnett supplements the original ISO standards, illustrates their application, and provides many examples of specific forms and policies that would be appropriate for a laboratory. He provides additional technical information about the quality required for the "intended use" of laboratory tests, which is important if the goal of uniform quality is to be achieved for a patient who moves from place to place and from country to country.

Joint Committee for Traceability in Laboratory Medicine (JCTLM)

Many organizations have been involved in developing a traceable accuracy base for analytes of clinical interest (Figure 7-9). A driver for current efforts to develop such a base is the European Directive 98/79/EC on in vitro diagnostic medical devices (www.ce-mark.com/ivd.pdf/; accessed July 25, 2013), which requires that "the traceability of values assigned to calibrators and/or control materials must be assured through available reference measurement procedures and/or available reference materials of a higher order."

In 2002 the JCTLM was created to meet the requirement for a worldwide platform to promote and give guidance on internationally recognized and accepted equivalence of measurements in laboratory medicine and traceability to appropriate measurement standards (www.bipm.org/en/committees/jc/jctlm/; accessed July 25, 2013). The three principal participants in JCTLM are the International Bureau of Weights and Measures (BIPM), the International Federation for Clinical Chemistry and Laboratory Medicine (IFCC), and the International Laboratory Accreditation Cooperation.

The JCTLM has created two working groups: (1) JCTLM WG-I, Reference Materials and Reference Procedures, and (2) JCTLM WG-II, Reference Laboratory Networks. These groups are responsible for providing practical support to the worldwide in vitro diagnostics (IVD) industry in establishing metrological traceability for values assigned to calibrators and/or control materials as required by the forthcoming European Directive on IVD and by comparable regulations in other countries.

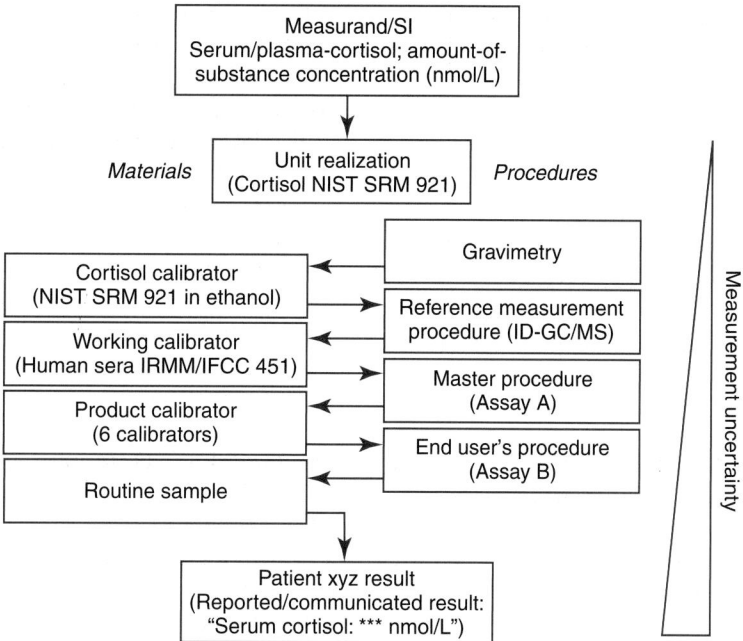

Figure 7-9 Example of a traceability chain developed for serum cortisol measurements. Arrows pointing to the left indicate value assignment activity using the procedure; arrows pointing to the right indicate calibration activity using the material. *(Reproduced from Vesper HW, Thienpont LM. Traceability in laboratory medicine, Clin Chem 2009;55:1067-75. With permission from The American Association for Clinical Chemistry. Publishing for* Clinical Chemistry *Journal.)*

Review Questions

1. The process by which simulated patient specimens made from a common pool are analyzed by laboratories to determine the "quality" of the laboratories' performance is referred to as:
   a. quality control.
   b. proficiency testing.
   c. total quality management
   d. Six Sigma process control.

2. The Westgard multirules for quality control were designed to interpret control data and to aid in troubleshooting analytical processes. The multirule stated as 1_{2s} indicates that:
   a. one control value has exceeded $\pm 2\ s$ from the mean.
   b. two consecutive control values have exceeded $\pm 2\ s$ from the mean.
   c. two consecutive control values have exceeded $\pm 1\ s$ from the mean.
   d. the numerical difference between two control values exceeds $1\ s$.

3. Choosing an incorrect colored-stopper blood collection tube to obtain a blood specimen is referred to as a(n) _____ variable.
   a. statistical
   b. analytical
   c. preanalytical
   d. controlled

4. With regard to statistical quality assessment in the laboratory, a _____ is a graphical plot of data that uses statistically derived means and standard deviations to determine analytical precision and accuracy.
   a. Levey-Jennings chart
   b. Gaussian distribution
   c. normal curve
   d. Youden plot

5. Conformance to the requirements of a laboratory's users (physicians, patients, etc.) is the definition of:
   a. multirules.
   b. cost.
   c. the total quality method.
   d. quality.

6. What is the role of quality improvement in the five-Q framework of quality?
   a. To monitor the laboratory as a whole for result quality
   b. To monitor the statistical analysis of results
   c. To ensure that the laboratory's policies, procedures, and practices are followed
   d. To identify the cause of a problem and find a remedy for that problem

7. Quality assessment, as part of the five-Q framework of total quality management, involves and monitors which of the following?
   a. Statistical control procedures such as Westgard multirules and Levey-Jennings charts
   b. Laboratory performance such as turnaround times, specimen and patient ID procedures, and test usage
   c. General policies and procedures such as manuals and employee handbooks
   d. Identification of the causes of problems in the laboratory and the solutions to those problems

8. Two types of error may be encountered during analysis of a control material. The type of error that reflects imprecision is:
    a. systematic error.
    b. imprecision error.
    c. random error.
    d. analytical error.

9. With regard to costs in the context of quality, which of the following would be considered a cost of conformance?
    a. Cost of analyzer calibration
    b. Cost of repeating analytical runs
    c. Cost of service calls
    d. Cost of repeated test requests

10. Westgard multirule R_{4s} indicates that one control value has exceeded the mean $+2\,s$ and another has exceeded the mean $-2\,s$. This control rule is sensitive to which type of analytical error?
    a. Systematic error
    b. Analytical error
    c. Imprecision error
    d. Random error

References

1. Blumenthal D. The errors of our ways. Clin Chem 1997;43:1305.
2. CAP. Standards for accreditation of medical laboratories. Skokie, Ill: College of American Pathologists, 2013.
3. Carlson RO, Amirahmadi F, Hernandez JS. A primer on the cost of quality for improvement of laboratory and pathology specimen processes. Am J Clin Pathol 2012;138:347–54
4. Centers for Disease Control and Prevention. Prevention CfDCa. Code of Federal Regulations: 42CFR493.1451. Standard: Technical Supervisor Responsibilities. Atlanta, Ga: CDC, 2012.
5. Clinical and Laboratory Standards Institute. Training and competence assessment: CLSI approved guideline, 3rd edition. CLSI Document GP21-A3 (new code QMS03-A3). Wayne, Pa: Clinical and Laboratory Standards Institute, 2009.
6. Clinical and Laboratory Standards Institute. Laboratory documents: development and control, 5th edition. CLSI Document GP-02-A6 (new code QMS02-A6). Wayne, Pa: Clinical and Laboratory Standards Institute, 2006.
7. Clinical and Laboratory Standards Institute. Quality managements System: A model for Laboratory Services , 4th edition. CLSI Document QMS01-A4. Wayne, Pa: Clinical and Laboratory Standards Institute, 2011.
8. Clinical and Laboratory Standards Institute. Statistical quality control for quantitative measurements: principles and definitions, 3rd edition. CLSI Document C24-A3. Wayne, Pa: Clinical and Laboratory Standards Institute, 2006.
9. Clinical and Laboratory Standards Institute. Laboratory quality control based on risk management, 1st edition. CLSI Document EP23-A. Wayne, Pa: Clinical and Laboratory Standards Institute, 2011.
10. Coldeway DO. Instructional systems design. Madison, Wis: University of Wisconsin, Madison, 2005.
11. Deming WE. Out of the crisis. Cambridge, Mass: Center of Massachusetts Institute of Technology, 1987.
12. George ML. Lean Six SIGMA: combining Six SIGMA quality with Lean Production speed, 1st edition. New York: The McGraw-Hill Companies, 2002.
13. Harris EK, Boyd JC. Statistical bases of reference values in laboratory medicine (Statistics: a series of textbooks and monographs). New York: CRC Press, 1995.
14. Harry M, Schroeder R. Six Sigma: the breakthrough manangement strategy revolutionizing the world's top corporations. New York: Doubleday, 2000.
15. Chicago Rush University Medical Center. Internet resources for health care quality, 2012: quality internet resources. http://www.ruch.edu/rumc/page-1277738429568.html (accessed on November 8, 2012).
16. Juran JM, Endres A. Quality improvement for services. Wilton, Conn: Juran Institute, 1986.
17. Klee GG, Forsman RW. A user's classification of problems identified by proficiency testing surveys. Arch Pathol Lab Med 1988;1124:371–3
18. Klee GG, Schryver PG, Bauer GL. Use of patient test values to enhance the quality control of PSA assays. Clin Chem 2003;49(Suppl 6):A94–5
19. Lusky K. Trimming the fat from lab processes. *CAP Today,* 2006.
20. Maisel WH, Moynahan M, Zuckerman BD, et al. Pacemaker and ICD generator malfunctions: analysis of Food and Drug Administration annual reports. JAMA 2006;295:1901–6
21. Medicare, Medicaid, and CLIA programs: laboratory requirements relating to quality systems and certain personnel qualifications. Final rule issued January 24, 2003, with an effective date of April 24, 2003. Washington, DC: US Centers for Medicare & Medicaid Services (CMS), 2003:3640–714
22. Poyser KH, Sherwood RA, eds. A practical guide to accreditation in laboratory medicine. London, UK: ACB Venture Publications, 2002.
23. Rabbitt JT, Bergh AP. Miniguide to ISO 9000, 1st edition. New York: Productivity Press, 1995.
24. US Centers for Medicare & Medicaid Services. Regulations and interpretive guidelines for laboratories and laboratory services, Revision 1. Appendix C of state operations manual. Washington, DC: CMS, May 21, 2004.
25. Westgard JO, Barry PL, Hunt MR, et al. A multi-rule Shewhart chart for quality control in clinical chemistry. Clin Chem 1981;27:493–501
26. Westgard JO, Barry PL. Cost-effective quality control: managing the quality and productivity of analytical processes, 1st edition. Washington, DC: AACC Press, 1997.
27. Westgard JO, Ehrmeyer SS, Darcy TP. CLIA final rules for quality systems: quality assessment issues and answers. Madison, Wis: Westgard QC, 2004.
28. Westgard JO, Fallon KD, Mansouri S. Validation of iQM active process control technology. Point of Care 2003;2:1–7

Principles of Basic Techniques and Laboratory Safety*

CHAPTER

8

Stanley F. Lo, Ph.D., D.A.B.C.C., F.A.C.B.

Objectives

1. Define the following:

Analyte	LOINC system
Buffer	Lyophilization
Centrifugation	Primary/Secondary reference
Dilution	material
Evaporation	Relative centrifugal force/field
Filtration	Solution
Gravimetry	Universal Precautions

2. Describe the expressions of concentrations of solutions, including molarity, % concentration, normality, and molality; convert mg/L to mmol/L; calculate solution concentration, given appropriate data.
3. State the units of measure used in the clinical laboratory; describe metric units and the International System of Units, and relate the differences between units.
4. List and compare the three types of water used in the laboratory, and state the uses of each type; describe three methods of preparing reagent grade water.
5. List and compare the different grades of reagents available, and state which are appropriate for use in a clinical laboratory.
6. Compare the two types of reference materials used in the clinical laboratory, and state the specific uses of each type.
7. List and describe three types of pipettes used in the clinical laboratory; state the proper use and the specific uses of each type.

8. For the process of centrifugation:
   State the principle.
   List six uses of centrifugation in the clinical laboratory.
   Calculate RCF and rpm when given the appropriate information.
   Determine the time required for centrifugation using an alternate rotor.
   Outline proper operation and operation practice of a centrifuge.
9. Describe three types of balances used in the clinical laboratory and how they are calibrated.
10. Compare serial dilutions with simple dilutions; state and calculate the formula used to prepare a solution of lesser concentration from one of greater concentration.
11. List and describe the elements of an OSHA-approved chemical hygiene plan, a hazard exposure plan, and a tuberculosis control plan; describe the Universal Precautions document, including source and specific mandates; state the CAP requirements for a laboratory ergonomics program.
12. For the following hazard types, interpret laboratory hazard signage, and state the appropriate work practice used to control these hazards:
    Biological
    Chemical
    Electrical
    Fire

Key Words and Definitions

Analyte A solute dispersed in a solution that is measured in laboratory practice; also referred to as a *measurand*.

Buffer solution A solution containing either a weak acid and its salt or a weak base and its salt, which is resistant to changes in pH.

Chemical hygiene plan (CHP) An Occupational Safety and Health Administration (OSHA)-required listing of responsibilities for laboratory employers, employees, and a chemical hygiene officer, and including a complete chemical inventory that is updated annually, along with a copy of the Material Safety Data Sheet (MSDS) that defines each chemical as toxic, carcinogenic, or

dangerous, and that must be on file and available to all employees 24 hours a day, 7 days a week.

Centrifugation The process of using centrifugal force to separate the lighter portions of a solution from the heavier portions; a centrifuge is a device by which centrifugation is effected.

CLSI The Clinical and Laboratory Standards Institute (formerly the National Committee for Clinical Laboratory Standards, or NCCLS) that guides the development and implementation of standards and guidelines that help all laboratories fulfill their goals.

*The author gratefully acknowledges the original contributions of Drs. Edward W. Bermes, Jr., Stephen E. Kahn, and Donald S. Young.

107

Key Words and Definitions—cont'd

Ergonomics The study of capabilities in relationship to work demands completed by defining postures that minimize unnecessary static work and reduce the forces working on the body.

Exposure control plan An Occupational Safety and Health Administration (OSHA)-required plan that ensures the protection of laboratory workers against potential exposure to bloodborne pathogens, while ensuring that medical wastes produced by the clinical laboratory are managed and handled in a safe and effective manner.

International System of Units (SI) A system of units for analytical results that is based on the cubic meter as the reference volume and is an internationally (except in the United States) adopted system of measurement. The units of the system are called SI units.

Material Safety Data Sheet (MSDS) A technical bulletin that contains information about a hazardous chemical, such as chemical composition, chemical and physical hazard, and precautions for safe handling and use.

Measurand See *Analyte*.

Metric system A system of weights and measures based on the meter as a standard unit of length, the liter as a standard unit of volume, and the gram as a standard unit of mass.

OSHA Occupational Safety and Health Administration, formed by the federal government of the United States to formally regulate the oversight of employee safety.

pH A measure of acidity and alkalinity of a solution.

Pipette Device used for the transfer of a volume of liquid from one container to another.

Reagent Chemical used in many high-purity applications.

Reference material A material or substance, one or more physical or chemical properties of which are sufficiently well established to be used for the calibration of an apparatus, the verification of a measurement method, or the assigning of values to materials. Certified, primary, and secondary are types of reference materials.

Relative centrifugal force or field (RCF) Force required to separate two phases (liquid and solid) in a centrifuge.

Universal Precautions Approach to infection control that treats all human blood and certain human body fluids as if they were known to be infectious for bloodborne pathogens.

To reliably perform qualitative and quantitative analyses on body fluids and tissue, the clinical laboratorian must understand the basic *principles and procedures* that affect the analytical process and operation of the clinical laboratory. These include knowledge of (1) the concept of solute and solvent; (2) units of measurement; (3) chemicals and **reference materials**; (4) basic techniques, such as (a) volumetric sampling and dispensing, (b) **centrifugation**, (c) gravimetry, (d) thermometry, (e) **buffer solution**, and (f) processing of solutions; and (5) safety.[†]

Concept of Solute and Solvent

Many analyses in the clinical laboratory are concerned with determination of the presence or measurement of concentrations of substances in solutions, the solutions most often being (1) blood, (2) serum, (3) urine, (4) spinal fluid, or (5) other body fluids (see Chapter 6).

Definitions

A *solution* is a homogeneous mixture of one or more *solutes* dispersed molecularly in a sufficient quantity of a dissolving *solvent*. In laboratory practice, solutes are typically measured and are frequently referred to as **analytes** or **measurands**. A solution may be (1) gaseous, (2) liquid, or (3) solid. A clinical laboratorian is concerned primarily with the measurement of gases or solids in liquids, where the amount of solvent is relatively large when compared with the amount of solute.

[†]*Note:* Additional discussions on topics of interest to the clinical laboratorian are found in Lo SF. Principles of basic techniques and laboratory safety. In: Burtis CA, Ashwood ER, eds. Tietz textbook of clinical chemistry, 5th edition. Philadelphia: WB Saunders, 2012:207-31.

Expressing Concentrations of Solutions

In the United States, analytical results typically are reported in terms of mass of solute per unit volume of solution, usually the deciliter. However, the **Système Internationale d'Unités (SI)** recommends the use of moles of solute per volume of solution for analyte concentrations (substance concentrations) whenever possible, and the use of liter as the reference volume.[9] In addition, mass concentration is reported in terms of grams percent or percent. This is typically how concentrations of ethanol in blood are expressed. This terminology indicates an amount of solute per mass of solution (e.g., grams per 100 g) and would be appropriate only if reference materials against which the unknowns were compared were measured in the same terms. An exception to the general expression of analyte concentrations in terms of volume of solution is the measurement of osmolality, in which concentrations are expressed in terms of mass of solvent (mOsmol/kg or mmol/kg).

When both the solution and the solvent are liquids, as in alcohol solutions, the concentration of such a solution is frequently expressed in terms of volume per volume (vol/vol). By adding 70 mL of alcohol to a flask and mixing it to 100 mL with water, a solution whose concentration is 700 mL/L would be achieved. The expression "700 mL/L" is preferred to the alternatives of 70 volumes percent and 70% (vol/vol).

The following equations define the expression of concentrations:

$$\text{Mole} = \frac{\text{mass (g)}}{\text{gram molecular weight (g)}}$$

$$\text{Molarity of a solution} = \frac{\text{number of moles of solute}}{\text{number of liters of solution}}$$

$$\text{Molarity of a solution} = \frac{\text{number of moles of solute}}{\text{number of kilograms of solvent}}$$

$$\text{Normality of a solution} = \frac{\text{number of gram equivalents of solute}}{\text{number of liters of solution}}$$

Gram equivalent weight
$$\text{(as oxidant or reductant)} = \frac{\text{formula weight (g)}}{\text{difference in oxidation state}}$$

For example, using these equations, a 1 *molar* solution of H_2SO_4 contains 98.08 g H_2SO_4 per liter of solution. (*Note:* The symbol M, to denote molarity, is no longer acceptable and has been replaced by mol/L.) A *molal* solution contains 1 mol of solute in 1 kg of solvent. Molality is properly expressed as mol/kg.

In the past, milliequivalent (mEq) was used to express the concentration of electrolytes in plasma. Now, the *recommended* unit for expressing the concentration of an electrolyte in plasma is millimoles per liter (mmol/L). For example, if a sample contains 322 mg of Na per liter, the molar concentration of Na is:

$$\text{mmol/L} = \frac{\text{mg/L}}{\text{mg molecular mass}} = \frac{322 \times 10 \times 1}{23} = 140 \text{ mmol/L}$$

In clinical laboratory practice, a *titer* is thought of as the lowest dilution at which a particular reaction takes place. Titer is customarily expressed as a ratio, for example, 1:10, or 1 to 10.

Regarding gases in solution, Henry's law states that the solubility of a gas in a liquid is directly proportional to the pressure of the gas above the liquid at equilibrium. Thus as the pressure of a gas is doubled, its solubility is also doubled. The relationship between pressure and solubility varies with the nature of the gas. When several gases are dissolved at the same time in a single solvent, the solubility of each gas is proportional to its partial pressure in the mixture. The solubility of most gases in liquids decreases with an increase in temperature, and boiling a liquid frequently drives out all dissolved gases. Traditionally the unit used to describe the concentration of gases in liquids has been percent by volume (vol/vol). Using the SI, gas concentrations are expressed in moles per cubic meter (mol/m^3).

Units of Measurement

A meaningful measurement is expressed with both a number and a unit. The unit identifies the dimension—mass, volume, or concentration—of a measured property. The number indicates how many units are contained in the property.

Traditionally, measurements in the clinical laboratory have been made in metric units. In the early development of the **metric system**, units were referenced to length, mass, and time. The first absolute systems were based on the centimeter, gram, and second (CGS), and then on the meter, kilogram, and second (MKS). The SI is a different system that was accepted internationally in 1960. The *units of the system* are called SI units.

International System of Units

Base, derived, and supplemental units are the three classes of SI units.[13] The eight fundamental base units are listed in Table 8-1. A *derived unit* is derived mathematically from two or more base units (Table 8-2). A *supplemental unit* is a unit

TABLE 8-1	Système Internationale d'Unités (SI) Base Units	
Quantity	**Name**	**Symbol**
Length	meter	m
Mass	kilogram	kg
Time	second	s
Electrical current	ampere	A
Thermodynamic temperature	kelvin	K
Amount of substance	mole	mol
Luminous intensity	candela	cd
Catalytic amount	katal	Kat

TABLE 8-2	Examples of SI-Derived Units Important in Clinical Medicine, Expressed in Terms of Base Units			
Quantity	**Name**	**SI Symbol**	**Expression in Terms of Other SI Units**	**Expression in Terms of SI Base Units**
Volume	cubic meter	m^3		m^3
Mass density	kilogram per cubic meter	kg/m^3		kg/m^3
Concentration of amount of substance	mole per cubic meter	mol/m^3		mol/m^3
Frequency	hertz	Hz		s^{-1}
Force	newton	N		$m \cdot kg \cdot s^{-2}$
Pressure	pascal	Pa	N/m^2	$m^{-1} \cdot kg \cdot s^{-2}$
Energy, work, quantity of heat	joule	J	$N \cdot m$	$m^2 \cdot kg \cdot s^{-2}$
Power	watt	W	J/s	$m^2 \cdot kg \cdot s^{-3}$
Electrical potential, potential difference, electromotive force	volt	V	$W \cdot A^{-1}$	$m^2 \cdot kg \cdot s^{-3} \cdot A^{-1}$

SI, Système Internationale d'Unités.

that conforms to the SI but has not been classified as base or derived. At present only the radian (for plane angles) and the steradian (for solid angles) are classified this way.

The Conférence Générales des Poids et Mésures (CGPM) recognizes that some units outside the SI continue to be important and useful in particular applications. An example is the liter as the reference volume in clinical analyses. Liter is the name of the submultiple (cubic decimeter) of the SI unit of volume, the cubic meter. Considering that 1 cubic meter represents some 200 times the blood volume of an adult human, the SI unit of volume is neither a convenient nor a reasonable reference volume in a clinical context. The minute, hour, and day have had such long-standing use in everyday life that it is

unlikely that SI units derived from the second will supplant them. Some other non-SI units are still accepted; although they are rarely used by most individuals in their daily lives, they have been very important in some specialized fields. Details of the SI system are found in an expanded version of this chapter.[9]

Decimal Multiples and Submultiples

In practical application of units, certain values are too large or too small to be expressed conveniently. Numerical values are brought to convenient size when the unit is appropriately modified by official prefixes (Table 8-3).

Applications of SI in Laboratory Medicine

Many international clinical laboratory organizations and national professional societies have accepted the SI unit in its broad application. The United States is one of the few countries that have yet to accept SI units. A comparison of results of some of the commonly measured serum constituents, at a concentration found in healthy individuals, is shown in Table 8-4.

Standardized Reporting of Test Results

To describe test results properly, it is important that all necessary information be included in the test description. Systems developed for expressing the results produced by the clinical laboratory include the Logical Observation Identifier Names and Codes (LOINC) system and the International Federation of Clinical Chemistry/International Union of Pure and Applied Chemistry (IFCC/IUPAC) system.[10]

LOINC System

The LOINC system is a universal coding system for reporting laboratory and other clinical observations to facilitate electronic transmission of laboratory data within and between institutions (http://loinc.org/; accessed on July 22, 2013).[10]

TABLE 8-3   Metric Prefixes of SI Units*

Factor	Prefix	Symbol	Factor	Prefix	Symbol
10^{24}	yotta	Y	10^{-1}	deci	d
10^{21}	zetta	Z	10^{-2}	centi	c
10^{18}	exa	E	10^{-3}	milli	m
10^{15}	peta	P	10^{-6}	micro	μ
10^{12}	tera	T	10^{-9}	nano	n
10^{9}	giga	G	10^{-12}	pico	p
10^{6}	mega	M	10^{-15}	femto	f
10^{3}	kilo	k	10^{-18}	atto	a
10^{2}	hecto	h	10^{-21}	zepto	z
10^{1}	deka†	da	10^{-24}	yocto	y

SI, Système Internationale d'Unités.

*The Eleventh Conférence Générale des Poids et Mésures (CGPM) (1960, Resolution 12) adopted a first series of prefixes and symbols of prefixes to form the names and symbols of the decimal multiples and submultiples of SI units. Prefixes for 10^{-15} and 10^{-18} were added by the Twelfth CGPM (1964, Resolution 8) and those for 10^{15} and 10^{18} by the Fifteenth CGPM (1975, Resolution 10); those for 10^{21}, 10^{24}, and 10^{-24} were proposed by the Comité International des Poids et Mesures CIPM (1990) for approval by the Nineteenth CGPM (1991).

†Outside the United States, the spelling "deca" is used extensively.

From The International System of Units (SI). Washington, DC: National Institute of Standards and Technology, 1991.

TABLE 8-4   Typical Values for Analytes and Reporting Increments

	Conventional Units	Recommended Units	Rounded Recommended Units	Smallest Recommended Reporting Increment
Albumin	3.8 g/dL	550.6 µmol/L	550.0 µmol/L	10.0 µmol/L
Bilirubin	0.2 mg/dL	3.42 µmol/L	3 µmol/L	2 µmol/L
Calcium	9.8 mg/dL	2.45 mmol/L	2.45 mmol/L	0.02 mmol/L
Cholesterol	200 mg/dL	5.17 mmol/L	5.2 mmol/L	0.05 mmol/L
Creatinine	0.8 mg/dL	90.48 µmol/L	90 mmol/L	10 µmol/L
Glucose	90 mg/dL	5.00 mmol/L	5.0 mmol/L	0.1 mmol/L
Phosphorus	3.0 mg/dL	0.97 mmol/L	1.0 mmol/L	0.05 mmol/L
Thyroxine	7.0 µg/dL	90.09 nmol/L	90 nmol/L	10 nmol/L
Triglycerides	100 mg/dL	1.14 mmol/L	1.15 mmol/L	0.05 mmol/L
Urea nitrogen*	10 mg/dL	3.57 mmol/L	3.5 mmol/L	0.05 mmol/L
Uric acid	5.0 mg/dL	297 µmol/L	300 µmol/L	10 µmol/L

*Urea nitrogen is reported as urea (mmol/L) when SI units are used.

SI, Système Internationale d'Unités.

These codes are intended to be used in context with existing standards, such as ASTM E1238 (American Society for Testing and Materials), HL7 version 2.2 (Health Level Seven; http://www.hl7.org/; accessed July 22, 2013), and the Systematized Nomenclature of Medicine, Reference Technology (SNOMED-RT). A similar standard, known as CEN ENV 1613, is being developed by the European Committee for Standardization of the Comité Européen de Normalisation (CEN) Technical Committee 251 (http://www.cen.eu; accessed July 22, 2013).

The LOINC database currently carries records for more than 30,000 observations.[10] For each observation, (1) a code, (2) a long formal name, (3) a short 30-character name, and (4) synonyms are listed. A mapping program termed "Regenstrief LOINC Mapping Assistant" (RELMA) is available to map local test codes to LOINC codes and to facilitate searching of the LOINC database. Both LOINC and RELMA are available at no cost from http://loinc.org/ (accessed July 22, 2013).

IFCC/IUPAC System

The IFCC/IUPAC system known as the NPU (Nomenclature, Properties, and Units) recommends that the following items be included with each test result:

1. The name of the system or its abbreviation
2. A dash (two hyphens)
3. The name of the analyte (never abbreviated) with an initial capital letter
4. A comma
5. The quantity name or its abbreviation
6. An equals sign
7. The numerical value and the unit or its abbreviation

Application

On April 1, 2009, the owners of LOINC, NPU, and SNOMED CT began an operational trial of prospective divisions of labor in the generation of laboratory test terminology content. It is expected this trial will provide practical experience and important information on opportunities to decrease duplication of effort in the development of laboratory test terminology and to ensure that SNOMED CT works effectively in combination with either LOINC or NPU.

Chemicals

The quality of the analytical results produced by the laboratory is a direct indication of the purity of the chemicals used as analytical **reagents**. The availability and quality of the reference materials used to calibrate assays and to monitor their analytical performance also are important.

Laboratory chemicals are available in a variety of grades. The solutes and solvents used in analytical work are *reagent grade chemicals*, among which water is a solvent of primary importance.

Reagent Grade Water

The preparation of many reagents and solutions used in the clinical laboratory requires "pure" water. Single-distilled water fails to meet the specifications for Clinical Laboratory Reagent Water (CLRW) established by the **Clinical Laboratory and Standards Institute (CLSI)**.[7] Because the term "deionized water" and the term "distilled water" describe preparation techniques, they should be replaced by "reagent grade water," followed by the designation of CLRW, which better defines the specifications of the water and is independent of the method of preparation (Table 8-5).

Preparation of Reagent Grade Water

The following sections describe processes used to prepare reagent grade water. In practice, water is filtered before any of these processes are used.

Distillation

Distillation is the process of vaporizing and condensing a liquid to purify or concentrate a substance or to separate a volatile substance from less volatile substances. However, water

TABLE 8-5	CLSI Specifications for Reagent Water	
	CLRW
Microbiological content,* colony-forming units per mL, cfu/mL (maximum)	<10
pH	NA
Resistivity,† MΩ · centimeter (MΩ·cm), 25 °C	≥10 (in line)
Particulate matter‡‡	Water passed through 0.22-μm filter
Organics ‡	Total Organic Content (TOC) <500 ng/g

*The microbiological content of viable organisms, as determined by total colony count after incubation at 36 ± 1 °C for 14 hours, followed by 48 hours at 25 ± 1 °C, and reported as colony-forming units per mL (cfu/mL).
†Specific resistance or resistivity. The electrical resistance in ohms measured between opposite faces of a 1-cm cube of an aqueous solution at a specified temperature. For these specifications, the resistivity will be corrected for 25 °C and reported in MΩ-cm. The greater the quantity of ionizable materials, the lower the resistivity, and the higher the conductivity.
‡When water is passed through a membrane filter with a mean pore size of 0.22 μm, it is considered to be free of particulate matter. When water is passed through a bed of activated carbon, it is considered to contain minimum organic material.
CLRW, Clinical Laboratory Reagent Water; *CLSI,* Clinical Laboratory Standards Institute; *NA,* not applicable.
From Clinical Laboratory Standards Institute (CLSI): Preparation and testing of reagent water in the clinical laboratory, 4th edition. CLSI Document C3-A4-AMD (new document code GP40-A4-AMD). Wayne, Pa: CLSI, 2006.

treated by distillation alone does not meet the specific conductivity requirement of type I water.

Ion Exchange

Ion exchange is a process that removes ions to produce mineral-free *deionized water*. Such water is most conveniently prepared using commercial equipment. In practice, a single-bed deionizer generally is capable of producing water that has a specific resistance in excess of 1 MΩ·cm. When connected in series, mixed-bed deionizers usually produce water with a specific resistance that exceeds 10 MΩ·cm.

Reverse Osmosis

Reverse osmosis is the process by which water is forced through a semipermeable membrane that acts as a molecular filter. The membrane removes 95% to 99% of organic compounds, bacteria, and other particulate matter and 90% to 97% of all ionized and dissolved minerals but fewer of the gaseous impurities. Although the process is inadequate for producing reagent grade water for the laboratory, it may be used as a preliminary purification method.

Ultraviolet Oxidation

Ultraviolet oxidation is another method that is used as part of a total system. The use of ultraviolet radiation at the biocidal wavelength of 254 nanometers eliminates many bacteria and cleaves many ionizing organics that are then removed by deionization.

Types of Purified Water

Other types of purified water used in the clinical laboratory are defined by the purpose.[7] These types are:
- Special reagent water
- Instrument feed water
- Water supplied by a method manufacturer for use as a diluent or reagent
- Commercially bottled, purified water
- Autoclave and wash water applications

Testing for Water Purity

At a minimum, water should be tested for (1) microbiological content, (2) organic impurities, (3) resistivity, and (4) particulate and colloid content.[7] Once the type of water is validated as fit for its purpose, the frequency of the maintenance of the system should occur no less than manufacturer's recommendations.

Reagent Grade or Analytical Reagent Grade (AR) Chemicals

Chemicals that meet the specifications of the American Chemical Society (ACS) are described as reagent or analytical reagent grade. These specifications have also become the de facto standards for chemicals used in many high-purity applications. They are available in two forms: (1) lot-analyzed reagents, in which each individual lot is analyzed and the actual amount of impurity reported, and (2) maximum impurities reagents, for which maximum impurities are listed. The Committee on Analytical Reagents of the ACS periodically publishes "Reagent Chemicals" listing specifications (http://pubs.acs.org/reagents/index.html; accessed July 22, 2013). These reagent grade chemicals are of very high purity and are recommended for quantitative or qualitative analyses.

Ultrapure Reagents

Many analytical techniques require reagents whose purity exceeds the specifications of those described previously. No uniform designation is used for these chemicals and organic solvents. Terms such as "spectrograde," "nanograde," and "HPLC pure" have been used. Data of interest to the user (e.g., absorbance at a specific ultraviolet [UV] wavelength) are supplied with the reagent.

Reference Materials

A reference material is a material or substance, one or more physical or chemical properties of which are sufficiently well established for it to be used for (1) calibration of instruments, (2) validation of methods, (3) assignment of values to materials, and (4) evaluation of the comparability of results. Reference materials also are of prime importance in establishing *metrological transferability* (http://www.bipm.org/; accessed July 22, 2013), a term defined as "the property of a measurement result whereby the result is related to a reference through a documented unbroken chain of calibrations, each contributing to the measurement uncertainty."

Primary, secondary, standard, and certified are types of reference materials.

Primary Reference Materials

Primary reference materials are highly purified chemicals that are directly weighed or measured to produce a solution whose concentration is exactly known. The IUPAC has proposed a degree of 99.98% purity for primary reference materials. These highly purified chemicals may be weighed out directly for the preparation of solutions of selected concentration or for the calibration of solutions of unknown strength. They are supplied with a certificate of analysis for each lot.

Secondary Reference Materials

Secondary reference materials are solutions whose concentrations cannot be prepared by weighing the solute and dissolving a known amount into a volume of solution. The concentration of secondary reference materials is typically determined by analysis of an aliquot of the solution by an acceptable reference method, using a primary reference material to calibrate the method.

Standard Reference Materials (SRMs)

Standard Reference Materials (SRMs) for clinical and molecular laboratories are available from the National Institute of Standards and Technology (NIST; http://ts.nist.gov/; accessed July 22, 2013). Cholesterol, the first SRM developed by the NIST, was issued in 1967. It should be noted that not all standard reference materials have the properties and the degree of

TABLE 8-6	Standard Reference Materials (SRMs)—Pure Crystalline Standards
SRM Number	**Analyte**
998	Angiotensin 1 (human)
916a	Bilirubin
915b	Calcium carbonate
911c	Cholesterol
921	Cortisol (hydroxycortisone)
914a	Creatinine
917b	D-Glucose (dextrose)
920	D-Mannitol
937	Iron metal (clinical)
928	Lead nitrate
924a	Lithium carbonate
929a	Magnesium gluconate dihydrate
918b	Potassium chloride
919b	Sodium chloride
1595	Tripalmitin
912a	Urea
913a	Uric acid
925	VMA (4-hydroxy-3-methoxy-DL-mandelic acid)
8327	Peptide reference materials (for molecular mass and purity measurements)

From Montgomery RR. NIST standard reference materials catalog, 2012. Washington, DC: National Institute for Standards and Technology, July 23, 2013; and Lo SF. Principles of basic techniques and laboratory safety. In: Burtis CA, Ashwood ER, eds. Tietz textbook of clinical chemistry, 5th edition. Philadelphia: WB Saunders, 2012:207-31.

purity specified for a primary standard, but each has been well characterized for certain chemical or physical properties and is issued with a certificate that gives the results of the characterization. These details may then be used to characterize other materials.

Examples of SRMs available from the NIST for use in clinical and molecular diagnostics laboratories include (1) pure crystalline standards, (2) human-based standards, (3) animal blood standards, (4) standards containing drugs of abuse in urine and human hair, and (5) SRMs used for DNA profiling/crime scene investigations. For example, compounds available as pure crystalline standards are listed in Table 8-6. Other compounds are found in the SRM catalog (Montgomery RR. NIST standard reference materials catalog, 2013. Washington, DC, National Institute for Science and Technology, November 6, 2012).[9]

Certified Reference Materials (CRMs)

Certified reference materials (CRMs) are available for clinical and molecular laboratories from the Institute for Reference Materials and Measurements (IRMM) in Geel, Belgium (http://www.irmm.jrc.be/; accessed July 22, 2013). The IRMM is one of seven institutes of the Joint Research Centre (JRC), a Directorate-General of the European Commission (EC). Other acronyms used to label IRMM reference materials include ERM (European Reference Materials), BCR (Community Bureau of Reference of the Commission of the European Communities), and IFCC (International Federation of Clinical Chemistry). Examples of available IRMM standards are

TABLE 8-7	Reference Materials Available from the Institute for Reference Materials and Measurements
Number	**Description**
BCR-304	Lyophilized Human Serum
BCR-573; 574; & 575	Creatinine in Human Serum
IRMM-468 & 469	Thyroxine (T_4) and Triiodothyronine (T_3), two concentrations each
ERM-DA451/IFCC	Cortisol Reference Panel of Fresh Frozen Human Serum
ERM-DA192 & 193	Cortisol in Human Serum
BCR-348R & BCR-DA347	Progesterone in Human Serum
BCR-576; 577; & 578	17-β-Estradiol in Human Serum
ERM-CE-194; 195; & 196	Pb and Cd in Lyophilized Bovine Blood
BCR-634; 635; & 636	Pb and Cd in Lyophilized Human Blood
BCR-637; 638; & 639	Al, Se, and Zn in Human Serum
BCR-393	Lyophilized APO A1 from Human Serum
BCR-457	Human Thyroglobin (Tg)
BCR-486	Purified Alpha Fetoprotein (AFP)
BCR-613	Prostate-Specific Antigen (PSA) in the Reconstituted Material
BCR-405	Glycated Hemoglobin (HbA_{1c}) in Human Hemolysate
ERM-DA470k	Human Serum Proteins
ERM-DA472/IFCC	C-Reactive Protein (CRP)
BCR-522	Hemiglobincyanide (HCN) in Bovine Blood Lysate
IRMM/IFCC-466 & 467	Hemoglobin Isolated from Whole Blood
BCR-410	Prostatic Acid Phosphatase from Human Prostate
BCR-647	Human Adenosine Deaminase (ADA1) from Human Erythrocytes
BCR-693	Human Pancreatic Lipase from Pancreatic Juice
BCR-6974	Human Pancreatic Lipase (Recombinant)
ERM-AD452/IFCC	γ-Glutamyltransferase from Pig Kidney
ERM-AD453/IFCC	Human Lactate Dehydrogenase Isoenzyme 1
ERM-AD454/IFCC	Alanine Aminotransferase from Pig Heart
ERM-AD455/IFCC	Creatine Kinase (CK-MB) from Human Heart
IRMM/IFCC-456	Human Pancreatic α-Amylase
ERM-AD457/IFCC	Aspartate Transaminase (AST)

From www.irmm.jrc.be/; accessed July 23, 2013.

listed in Table 8-7 and are described in Reference 1. Reference materials also are available from the World Health Organization (WHO; http://www.who.int/biologicals Accessed July 22, 2013. http://ts.nist.gov/; accessed October 17).

Basic Techniques and Procedures

Basic practices used in the clinical and molecular diagnostic laboratories include (1) optical, (2) chromatographic, (3) electrochemical, (4) electrophoretic, (5) mass spectrometric, (6) enzymatic, and (7) immunoassay techniques. These techniques are discussed in detail in Chapters 9 through 15. Here we discuss the basic techniques of (1) volumetric sampling and dispensing, (2) centrifugation, (3) gravimetry, (4) thermometry, (5) control of hydrogen ion concentration, and (6) use of procedures for processing solutions.

Volumetric Sampling and Dispensing

Analytical procedures require accurate volumetric measurements to ensure accurate results. For accurate work, only Class A glassware should be used. Class A glassware is certified to conform to the specifications outlined in NIST Circular C-602.

Pipettes

Pipettes are used for the transfer of a volume of liquid from one container to another. They are designed (1) to contain (TC) a specific volume of liquid or (2) to deliver (TD) a specified volume. Pipettes used in clinical, molecular diagnostic, and analytical laboratories include (1) manual transfer and measuring pipettes, (2) micropipettes, and (3) electronic and mechanical pipetting devices. Developments in improved design of pipetting systems include robotic automation, the capability to provide electronic and personal computer (PC) control of pipetting devices, and careful attention to advanced **ergonomic** design features. Automatic photometric pipette calibration systems are also available that reduce the time required to periodically check pipettes and potentially provide more efficient use of personnel.

Transfer and Measuring Pipettes

A transfer pipette is designed to transfer a known volume of liquid. Measuring and serological pipettes are scored in units such that any volume up to a maximum capacity can be delivered.

Transfer Pipettes. *Transfer pipettes* include both volumetric and Ostwald-Folin pipettes (Figure 8-1). They consist of a cylindrical bulb joined at both ends to narrower glass tubing. A calibration mark is etched around the upper suction tube, and the lower delivery tube is drawn out to a gradual taper.

A volumetric transfer pipette (Figure 8-1, *A*) is calibrated to deliver accurately a fixed volume of a dilute aqueous solution.

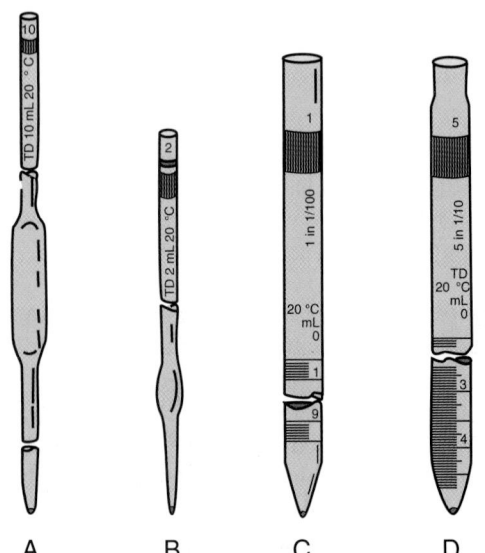

Figure 8-1 Pipettes. **A,** Volumetric (transfer). **B,** Ostwald-Folin (transfer). **C,** Mohr (measuring). **D,** Serological (graduated to the tip).

Ostwald-Folin pipettes (Figure 8-1, *B*) are similar to volumetric pipettes but have their bulb closer to the delivery tip and are used for the accurate measurement of viscous fluids, such as blood or serum. In contrast to a volumetric pipette, an Ostwald-Folin pipette has an etched ring near the mouthpiece, indicating that it is a blow-out pipette. With the use of a pipetting bulb, the liquid is blown out of the pipette only after the blood or serum has drained to the last drop in the delivery tip. When filled with opaque fluids, such as blood, the top of the meniscus is read. Controlled slow drainage is required with all viscous solutions so that no residual film is left on the walls of the pipette.

Measuring Pipettes. The second principal type of pipette is the *graduated* or *measuring pipette* (Figure 8-1, *C*). This is a piece of glass tubing that is drawn out to a tip and is graduated uniformly along its length. Two kinds are available. The Mohr pipette is calibrated between two marks on the stem, whereas the serological pipette has graduated marks down to the tip. The serological pipette (Figure 8-1, *D*) must be blown out to deliver the entire volume of the pipette and has an etched ring (or pair of rings) near the bulb end of the pipette signifying that it is a blow-out pipette. Mohr pipettes require controlled delivery of the solution between the calibration marks. Serological pipettes have a larger orifice than do Mohr pipettes and thus drain faster. In practice, measuring pipettes are principally used for the measurement of reagents and generally are not considered sufficiently accurate for measuring samples and calibrators.

Pipetting Technique

General pipetting techniques apply to the pipettes described previously. For example, pipetting bulbs should always be used, and pipettes must be held in a vertical position when the liquid level is adjusted to the calibration line and during delivery. When it is sighted at eye level, the lowest part of the meniscus should be level with the calibration line on the pipette. The flow of the liquid should be unrestricted when volumetric pipettes are used, and the tips should be touched to the inclined surface of the receiving container for 2 s after the liquid has ceased to flow.

With graduated pipettes, the flow of liquid may have to be slowed during delivery. Serological pipettes are calibrated to the tip, and the etched glass ring on top of the pipette signifies that it is to be blown out. First, the pipette is allowed to drain, and then the remaining liquid is blown out with a pipetting bulb.

Micropipettes

Micropipettes are pipettes that are used for the measurement of microliter volumes. With such devices, the remaining volume that coats the inner wall of a pipette causes notable error. For this reason, most micropipettes are calibrated TC the stated volume rather than TD it. Proper use requires rinsing of the pipette with the final solution after the contents have been delivered into the diluent. Volumes are expressed in microliters (μL); the older term *lambda* is no longer recommended. (One lambda [λ] = 1 μL = 0.001 mL.)

Micropipettes are generally available in small sizes, ranging from 0.2 to 500 µL.

Semiautomatic and Automatic Pipettes and Dispensers
Figure 8-2, *A* and *B,* illustrates two types of adjustable micropipetting devices that demonstrate unique ergonomic design features. These devices are programmable and are used to simultaneously dispense aliquots of liquid into multiple wells. In practice, with the use of disposable plastic tips, they allow simultaneous aspiration and delivery of solutions to multiple sample micro wells. Each channel is piston driven to allow the user to pipette with as few or as many tips as necessary. Aliquots of liquid as small as 0.2 µL are dispensed at three different aspiration or dispense rates.

Semiautomatic manual and electronic versions of pipettes and dispensers are available in sizes from 0.5 µL to 10 mL. Figure 8-2, *C,* illustrates an electronically operated, positive-displacement multichannel pipettor. This device aspirates and dispenses its predefined volumes (from 0.5 to 200 µL) when its plunger is moved through a complete cycle. Its disposable fluid containment tips are made of a plastic material that tends to retain less inner surface film than does glass. Such pipettes (1) avoid the risk of cross contamination among samples, (2) eliminate the necessity for washing between samples, and (3) improve the precision of measurements. Models that allow for digital adjustment of the volumes aspirated and dispensed are available.

Figure 8-3, *A,* shows an automatic dispensing apparatus that aspirates and dispenses preset volumes of two different liquids by means of two motor-driven syringes—one for metering a volume of the sample and one for metering a volume of the diluent. It is possible to adjust this device to aspirate as little as 1 µL of one liquid and to deliver it with as much as 999 µL of the other. This type of device, available as a dilutor or a dispenser, is obtainable as a (1) manual, (2) electronic, or (3) computer-controlled device. The latter is microprocessor controlled and is easily programmed. Twenty-one dispensing programs are stored in memory and retrieved.

A more versatile piece of equipment is the robotic liquid handling workstation shown in Figure 8-3, *B.* This automated pipetting station is used with individual reaction tubes and with 96- and 384-well microtiter plates. Depending on the

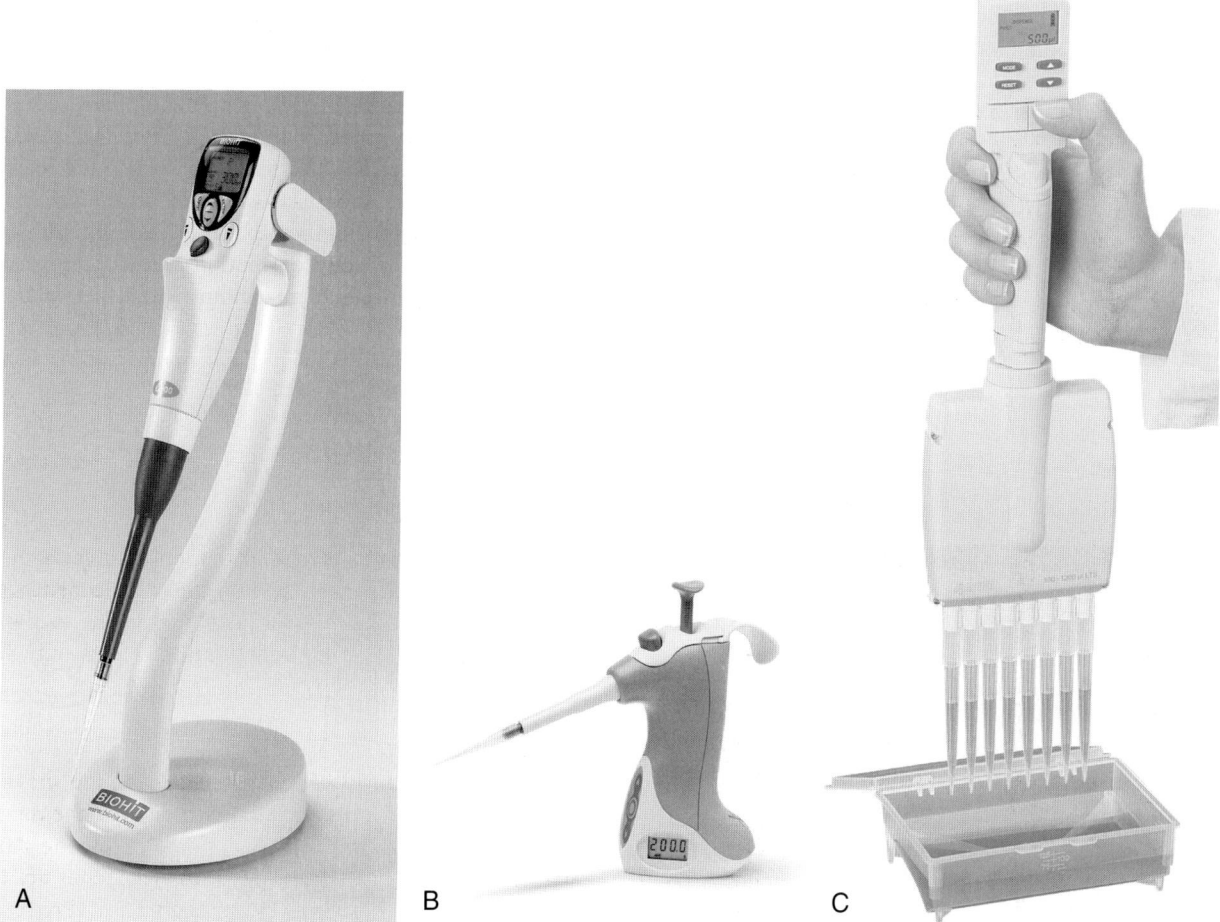

Figure 8-2 A, Adjustable volume micropipetting device with ergonomic design. **B,** Adjustable volume electronic micropipetting device with ergonomic design. **C,** Electronic programmable multichannel pipette. (**A,** *Courtesy Biohit Plc.* **B,** *Courtesy VistaLab Technologies, Inc.* **C,** *Courtesy Rainin Instrument LLC.*)

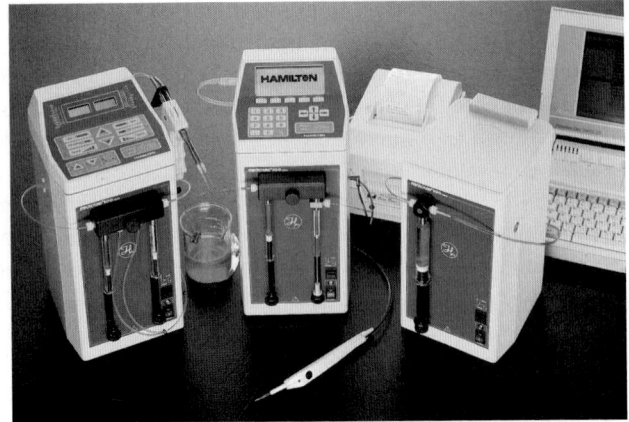

A

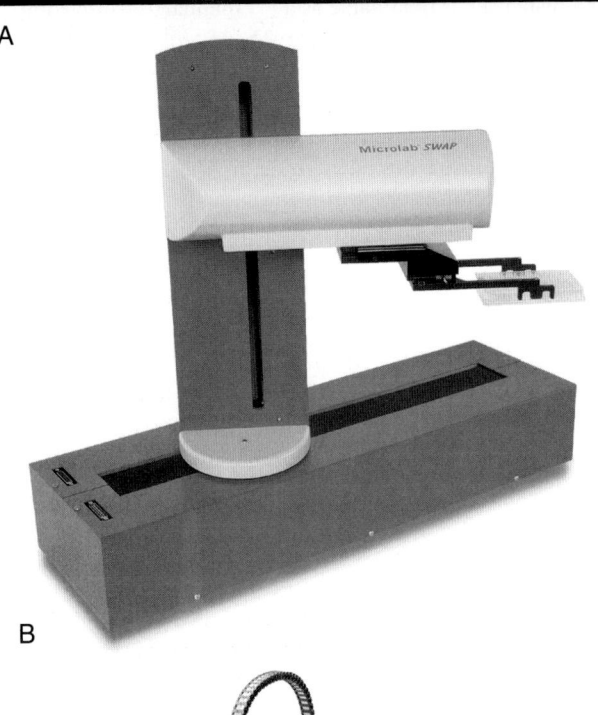

B

design of the system, a single probe or multiple probes may be used rapidly to transfer programmed volumes of solution from one container to a multiple of chambers in one microtiter plate. For example, with a 96-well plate, up to 96 aliquots are transferred to all 96 wells in 1 minute. With some systems, liquid sensing is incorporated into the sample probes to minimize contact with sample and reagents, even though automatic washing of the probes is performed between specimens. Two-dimensional (X-Y) movement of probes and tubes or microtiter plates is built into the pipetting stations to minimize the necessity for operator intervention. This device dispenses programmed volumes from 0.5 μL to 1000 μL in serial dilutions from 4 to 16 channels employing an autoloaded system with bar codes for positive identification.

Volumetric Flasks

Volumetric flasks (Figure 8-4) are used to measure exact volumes; they are commonly found in sizes ranging from 1 to 4000 mL. In practice, they are used primarily to prepare solutions of known concentration, and they are available in various grades. The most accurate are certified to meet standards set forth by the NIST.

An important factor in the use of a volumetric apparatus is the requirement for an accurate adjustment of the meniscus. A small card that is half black and half white is most useful. The card is placed 1 cm behind the apparatus with the white half uppermost and the top of the black area about 1 mm below the meniscus. The meniscus then appears as a clearly defined, thin black line. This device is also useful in reading the meniscus of a burette.

Volumetric equipment should be used with solutions equilibrated to room temperature. Solutions diluted in volumetric flasks should be repeatedly mixed during dilution so that the

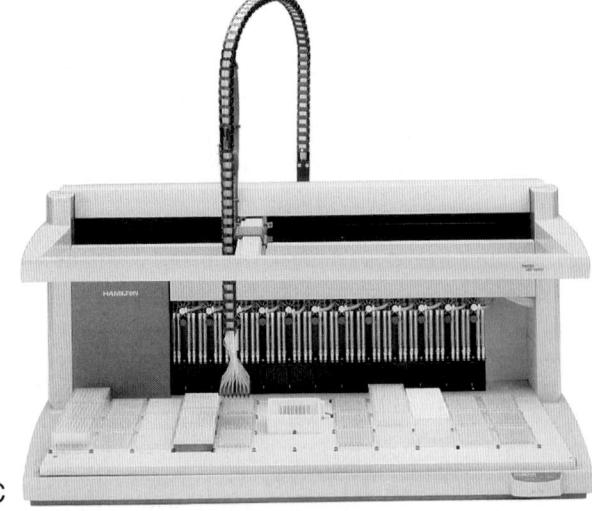

C

Figure 8-3 A, Personal computer (PC)-controlled diluting and/ or dispensing apparatus that aspirates and dispenses preset volumes of one or two different liquids, such as a diluent and a sample, by means of motor-driven syringes. **B** and **C,** Robotic liquid handling workstations. *(Courtesy Hamilton Co.)*

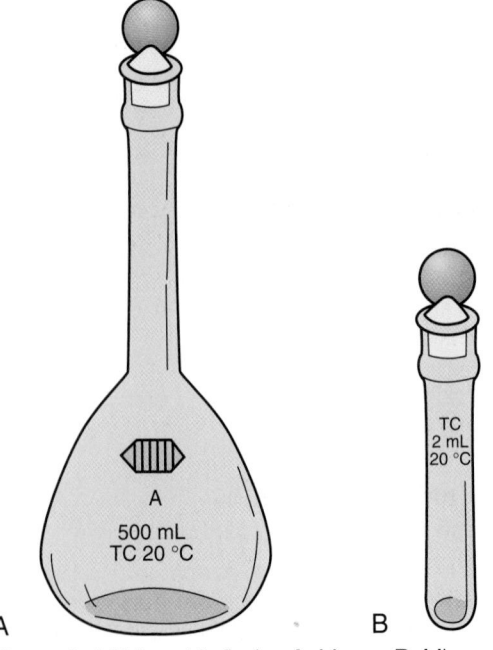

A   B

Figure 8-4 Volumetric flasks. **A,** Macro. **B,** Micro.

contents are homogeneous before the solution is made up to final volume. Errors caused by expansion or contraction of liquids on mixing are thereby minimized.

Volumetric flasks should be thoroughly cleaned and dried before calibration. The flask is then weighed and filled with carbon dioxide–free deionized water until just above the graduation mark. The neck of the flask just above the water level should be kept free of water. The meniscus mark is set at the graduation line by removing excess water, and the flask is reweighed. The final weight is corrected for the equilibrated water and the air temperature to obtain the volume of the flask.

Centrifugation

Centrifugation is the process of using centrifugal force to separate the lighter portions of a solution, mixture, or suspension from the heavier portions. A *centrifuge* is a device by which centrifugation is effected.

In the clinical laboratory, centrifugation is used to:

1. Remove cellular elements from blood to obtain cell-free plasma or serum for analysis (see Chapter 6)
2. Concentrate cellular elements and other components of biological fluids for microscopic examination or chemical analysis
3. Remove chemically precipitated protein from an analytical specimen
4. Separate protein-bound or antibody-bound ligand from free ligand in immunochemical and other assays (see Chapter 15).
5. Extract solutes in biological fluids from aqueous to organic solvents
6. Separate lipid components such as chylomicrons from other components of plasma or serum, and lipoproteins from one another (see Chapter 23).

Types of Centrifuges

Types of centrifuges used in the clinical laboratory include (1) horizontal-head or swinging-bucket, (2) fixed-angle or angle-head, (3) ultracentrifuge, and (4) axial. Automatic balancing centrifuges are also available.

Principles of Centrifugation

The correct term to describe the force required to separate two phases in a centrifuge is *relative centrifugal force* (**RCF**), also called *relative centrifugal field*. Units are expressed as number of times greater than gravity (e.g., $500 \times g$).

RCF is calculated as follows:

$$RCF = 1.118 \times 10^{-5} \times r \times rpm^2$$

where

1.118×10^{-5} = an empirical factor;

r = radius in centimeters from the center of rotation to the bottom of the tube in the rotor cavity or bucket during centrifugation; and

rpm = the speed of rotation of the rotor in revolutions per minute.

The RCF of a centrifuge may also be determined from a nomogram distributed by manufacturers of centrifuges. RCF is derived from the distance from the rotor center to the bottom of the tube, whether the tube is horizontal to, or at an angle to, the rotor center.

The time required to sediment particles depends on (1) rotor speed, (2) radius of the rotor, and (3) effective path length travelled by sedimented particles. Following is a useful formula for calculating the speed required of a rotor whose radius differs from the radius with which a prescribed RCF was originally defined:

$$rpm \text{ (alternate rotor)} = 1000 \times \sqrt{\frac{RCF, \text{ original rotor}}{11.18 \times r \text{ (cm), alternate rotor}}}$$

The length of time for centrifugation is calculated so that running with an alternate rotor of a different size is equivalent to running with the original rotor:

$$time \text{ (alternate rotor)} = \frac{time \times RCF \text{ (original rotor)}}{RCF \text{ (alternate rotor)}}$$

Operation of the Centrifuge

For proper operation of a centrifuge, only those tubes recommended by the manufacturer should be used. The material used for the tube must withstand the RCF to which the tube is expected to be subjected. Polypropylene tubes are generally capable of withstanding RCFs of up to $5000 \times g$. The tubes should have a tapered bottom, particularly if a supernatant is to be removed, and should be of an appropriate size to fit securely into the rack to be centrifuged. The top of the tube should not protrude so far above the bucket that the swing into a horizontal position is impeded by the rotor.

For smooth operation of the centrifuge, the rotor must be properly balanced. The weight of racks, tubes, and their contents on opposite sides of a rotor should not differ by more than 1% or by an acceptable limit established by the manufacturer. Tubes of collected blood should be centrifuged before they are unstoppered to reduce the probability that an aerosol will be produced when the tube is opened. The practice of using a wooden applicator to release a clot stuck to the top of the tube or to its stopper should be avoided; it is a potential cause of hemolysis. Centrifugation at an appropriate RCF usually ensures that the clot is released from the tube wall and is drawn to the bottom of the tube.

Despite years of experience with centrifuges, just a few specific recommendations have been put forth for RCF or time for centrifugation of blood specimens. For example, one tube manufacturer recommends for their non-gel tubes an RCF $\leq 1300 \times g$ for 10 minutes, and for their gel tubes an RCF of 1000 to 1300 $\times g$ for 10 minutes in a swinging bucket or 15 minutes in a fixed-angle centrifuge (http://www.bd.com/vacutainer/faqs/#tubes. Accessed July 22, 2013). CLSI standard H18-A3[2] proposes an RCF of 1000 to 1200 $\times g$ for 10 ± 5 minutes. Standards have not been established for centrifugation of other specimens, such as serum to which a protein precipitant has been added.

Operating Practice

Cleanliness of a centrifuge is important in minimizing the possible spread of infectious agents, such as hepatitis viruses. With proper operation of a centrifuge, few tubes break. In case of breakage, the racks and chamber of the centrifuge must be carefully cleaned. Any spillage should be considered a possible bloodborne pathogen hazard. Gray dust arising from the sandblasting of the chamber by fragments of glass indicates tube breakage and possible contamination, necessitating cleaning of the chamber. Broken glass embedded in cushions of tube holders may be a continuing cause of breakage if cushions are not inspected and replaced in the cleanup procedure.

The speed of a centrifuge should be checked at least once every 6 months. The measured speed should not differ by more than 5% from the rated speed under specified conditions. All speeds at which the centrifuge is commonly operated should be checked. The centrifuge timer should be checked at least once every 6 months against a reference timer (such as a stopwatch) and should not be more than 10% in error. Commutators and brushes should be checked at least every 6 months. Brushes (where used) should be replaced when they show considerable wear. However, in many modern induction-drive motors, brushes have been eliminated, thus removing a source of dust that causes motor failure.

Because centrifuges generate heat, the temperature in the chamber in many centrifuge models may increase by as much as 5 °C after a single run. When the material to be centrifuged has a labile temperature, a refrigerated centrifuge should be used. In the simplest form, a refrigerator unit is mounted beside the centrifuge, and cold air is blown into the rotor chamber. This approach is usually inadequate to stabilize the low temperature. With more sophisticated centrifuges, refrigeration coils around the chamber make it possible to maintain a preset temperature within ± 1 °C. The temperature of a refrigerated centrifuge should be measured at least once every 6 months under reproducible conditions and should be within 2 °C of the expected temperature.

Gravimetry

Gravimetry is the process used to measure the mass of a substance. Weight is a function of mass under the influence of gravity, a relationship expressed by

$$Weight = mass \times gravity$$

Two substances of equal weight and subject to the same gravitational force have equal masses. The determination of mass is made using a balance to compare the mass of an unknown with that of a known mass. This comparison is called *weighing*, and the absolute standards with which masses are compared are called *weights*. In practice, the terms *mass* and *weight* are used synonymously.

The classic form of a balance is a beam poised on an agate knife-edge fulcrum, with a pan hanging from each end of the beam and a rigid pointer hanging from the beam at the poised point.

Principles of Weighing

In practice, two modes of weighing are used: (1) Analytical weights are added to equal the weight of the object being weighed, or (2) the material to be weighed is added to a balance pan to achieve equilibrium with a preset weight. This second mode is used more commonly in clinical laboratories, where the major necessity is to weigh a fixed quantity of chemical so that a calibrator or reagent solution of known concentration may be prepared. Before a sample of the chemical is weighed, the weight of the container must be determined to subsequently allow for deducting the weight of the container from the gross weight of the container plus sample to obtain the net weight of the sample. This is called *taring*. When taring is impractical, the weight of the empty container must be subtracted from the combined weight of the container and the material to obtain the weight of the material alone.

Types of Balances

Double- and single-pan and electronic balances are frequently used in the clinical laboratory.

Double-Pan Balance

A double-pan balance conforms to the classic design, consisting of a single beam with arms of equal length. Standard weights are usually added by hand to the right-side pan to counterbalance the weight of the object on the other, but in some models, a dial or a vernier with chain is used to make fine adjustments to the mass associated with the right-side pan. In *single-pan* balances, the arms are of unequal length. The object to be weighed is placed on the pan attached to the shorter arm. A restoring force is applied mechanically or electronically to the other arm to return the beam to its null position. Double- and triple-beam balances are forms of the unequal-arm balance.

Single-Pan Balance

The single-pan balance is a commonly used balance in the clinical laboratory. It is most often electronically operated and self-balancing. Such a balance may be coupled directly to a computer or recording device. In the electronic single-pan balance, a load on the pan causes the beam to tilt downward. A null detector senses the position of the beam and indicates when the beam has deviated from the equilibrium point.

Electronic Balance

In an electronic balance, an electromagnetic force is applied to return the balance beam to its null position. This force is proportionate to the weight on the pan. Most electronic balances have a built-in provision for taring, so that the mass of the container is subtracted easily from the total mass measured. In addition, in many modern balances, a built-in computer compensates for changes in temperature and provides both automatic zero tracking and calibration.

Analytical Weights. Analytical weights are used to counterbalance the weight of objects weighed on two-pan balances and to verify the performance of both single- and two-pan balances. The NIST recognizes five classes of analytical weights. Class S weights are used for calibrating balances. In the clinical laboratory, balances should be calibrated at least monthly and before very accurate analytical work is conducted. These weights are typically made from brass or stainless steel and are lacquered or plated for protection. The fractional weights of a set of class S standards are usually made of platinum or aluminum. Tolerances of the different weights have been defined by the NIST. For class S weights from 1 to 5 g, the tolerance is ±0.054 mg, from 100 to 500 mg it is ±0.025 mg, and from 1 to 50 mg it is ±0.014 mg.

Thermometry

In the clinical chemistry laboratory, measurements of temperature are made primarily to verify that devices measure within their prescribed temperature limits. Water baths and heated cells where reactions take place are examples of such devices, as are refrigerators, whose temperatures must be measured and recorded daily to meet laboratory regulatory requirements.

The two most popular types of thermometers in the chemistry laboratory are liquid-in-glass thermometers and thermistor probes.

All thermometers must be verified against a certified thermometer before they are placed into use. For example, the NIST SRM 934 is a mercury-in-glass thermometer with calibration points at 0 °C, 25 °C, 30 °C, and 37 °C. Some manufacturers supply liquid-in-glass thermometers that have ranges greater than the SRM thermometer and are verified to have been calibrated against the NIST thermometers. Details of verification of the calibration of a thermometer have been described.[6] The NIST also supplies several materials that melt at a known temperature, including gallium (SRM 1968), which melts at 29.7723 °C, and rubidium (SRM 1969), which melts at 39.3 °C.

Control of Hydrogen Ion Concentration

In the laboratory, hydrogen ion concentration is controlled with buffers. Buffers are defined as a s solution containing either a weak acid and its salt or a weak base and its salt, which is resistant to changes in the **pH** of a system. All weak acids or bases, in the presence of their salts, form buffer systems. The action of buffers and their role in maintaining the pH of a solution are explained with the aid of the Henderson-Hasselbalch equation, which is derived as follows.

Chemically, the ionization of a weak acid, HA, and of a salt of that acid, BA, is represented as:

$$HA \underset{\rightarrow}{\leftarrow} H^+ + A^-$$

$$BA \overset{\leftarrow}{\rightarrow} B^+ + A^-$$

The dissociation constant for a weak acid (K_a) may be calculated from the following equation:

$$K_a = \frac{[H^+] \, [A^-]}{[HA]}$$

Thus

$$[H^+] = K_a \times \frac{[HA]}{[A^-]}$$

or

$$\log[H^+] = \log K_a + \log \frac{[HA]}{[A^-]}$$

where brackets indicate the concentration of the compound contained within. Now multiplying throughout by −1:

$$-\log[H^+] = -\log K_a - \log \frac{[HA]}{[A^-]}$$

By definition, pH= −log [H⁺], and pK_a = −log K_a, therefore

$$pH = pK_a + \log \frac{[A^-]}{[HA]}$$

This equation is known as the Henderson-Hasselbalch equation. Because A⁻ is derived principally from the salt, the equation also is written as:

$$pH = pK_a + \log \frac{[salt]}{[undissociated \ acid]}$$

or simply as:

$$pH = pK_a + \log \frac{[salt]}{[acid]}$$

where [salt] = [A⁻] = concentration of dissociated salt and [acid] = [HA] = concentration of undissociated acid.

This derivation demonstrates that the pH of the system is determined by the pK_a of the acid and the ratio of [A⁻] to [HA]. The buffer has its greatest buffer capacity at its pK_a, that is, that pH at which [A⁻] = [HA].

The capacity of the buffer decreases as the ratio deviates from 1. In general, buffers should not be used at a pH greater than 1 unit from their pK_a. If the ratio is beyond 50:1 or 1:50, the system is considered to have lost its buffering capacity. This point is approximately 1.7 pH units to either side of the pK_a of the acid because

$$pH = pK_a \pm 1.7$$

Use of Procedures for Processing Solutions

Several procedures are routinely used to process solutions in the clinical laboratory, including those for (1) diluting, (2) evaporating (3) lyophilizing, and (4) filtering solutions.

Dilution

Dilution is the process by which the concentration or activity of a given solution is decreased by the addition of solvent. In laboratory practice, most dilutions are made by transferring an exact volume of a concentrated solution into an appropriate flask and then adding water or another diluent to the required volume, with appropriate mixing to ensure homogeneity. A *serial dilution* is a sequential set of dilutions done in mathematical sequence. A given dilution is expressed as the amount, either volume or weight, of a solute (analyte) in a specified volume. For example, a 1:5 volume-to-volume (vol/vol) dilution contains one volume in a total of five volumes (one volume plus four volumes).

To prevent errors that arise when two liquids of very different composition are mixed, the technique of diluting to volume is used. Instead of adding 90 mL of water to 10 mL of concentrated solution, the 10 mL of concentrated solution should be pipetted into a 100-mL volumetric flask. Water is added to bring the volume to the 100-mL mark on the neck of the flask with its contents mixed.

When a dilution is performed, the following equation is used to determine the volume (V_2) necessary to dilute a given volume (V_1) of solution of a known concentration (C_1) to the desired lesser concentration (C_2):

$$C_1 \times V_1 = C_2 \times V_2$$

or

$$V_2 = \frac{C_1 \times V_1}{C_2}$$

Likewise, the equation is used to calculate the concentration of the diluted solution when a given volume is added to the starting solution.

Evaporation

Evaporation is a process used to convert a liquid or a volatile solid into vapor. It is used in the clinical laboratory to remove liquid from a sample, thereby increasing the concentrations of analyte(s) left behind.

Note: Evaporation is also an analytical problem when a sample remains in its cup for too long a time. When this occurs, the concentration of a nonvolatile analyte increases and subsequent measurement yields an inaccurate result.

Lyophilization

Lyophilization (also known as "freeze drying") is used in laboratory medicine for the preparation of (1) calibrators, (2) control materials, (3) reagents, and (4) individual specimens for analysis. Lyophilization first entails freezing a material at −40 °C or less and then subjecting it to a high vacuum. Very low temperatures cause the ice to sublimate to a vapor state. The solid nonsublimable material remains behind in a dried state.

Filtration

Filtration is defined as the passage of liquid through a filter and is accomplished by (1) gravity, (2) pressure, or (3) vacuum. *Filtrate* is the liquid that has passed through the filter. The purpose of filtration is to remove particulate matter from the liquid. Many filtrations in the clinical laboratory are carried out with *filter paper* and with plastic *membranes* of controlled pore size.

Membrane filters have been incorporated into certain disposable tips for use with semiautomatic pipettes. These filters minimize the exchange of aerosol droplets between the tips and the pipette. This is of particular importance for DNA amplification and microbiological procedures. Other membrane filters are designed for ultrafiltration and are available in a variety of pore sizes for selective filtration. *Ultrafiltration* is a technique by which dissolved particles are removed with the use of an extremely fine filter. It is used to concentrate macromolecules, such as proteins, because smaller dissolved molecules pass through the filter.

Safety

In the United States, the Federal Occupational Safety and Health Act of 1970 marked the beginning of formal regulatory oversight of employee safety. Since 1970 the Occupational Safety and Health Administration (**OSHA**) and the Centers for Disease Control and Prevention (CDC) have published numerous safety standards that apply to clinical laboratories. Each year, as The Joint Commission (TJC), formerly known as the Joint Commission on Accreditation of Healthcare Organizations (JCAHO), and the College of American Pathologists (CAP) revise their guidelines, more attention is devoted to safety. Consideration for the health and responsibility for the safety of employees are now accepted as obligations of all employers and laboratory directors. In May of 1988, OSHA expanded the Hazard Communication Standard to apply to hospital workers. Part of this standard is frequently referred to as the "Lab Right to Know Standard."

The safe operation of a clinical laboratory comprises many aspects. Key elements to ensure safety in the clinical laboratory include the following:
1. A formal safety program
2. Documented policies and effective use of mandated plans and/or programs in the areas of (a) chemical hygiene, (b) control of exposure to bloodborne pathogens, (c) tuberculosis control, and (d) ergonomics
3. Identification of significant occupational hazards, such as (a) biological, (b) chemical, (c) fire, and (d) electrical hazards, and clear identification and documentation of policies for employees to deal with each type of hazard (e.g., packaging and shipping of diagnostic specimens and infectious substances)
4. Recognition that additional important and relevant safety areas of concern must be addressed. These areas include effective (a) waste management, (b) bioterrorism, and (c) chemical terrorism response plans in the event of potential threats or casualties involving these types of agents.

Safety Program

Every clinical laboratory must have a comprehensive and effective formal safety program. Regardless of the size of the clinical laboratory, a specific individual should be designated as "Safety Officer" or "Chair of the Safety Committee" and given the responsibility to implement and maintain a safety program. Safety is each employee's responsibility, but responsibility for the entire program begins with the laboratory leadership (directors, administrative directors, supervisors, managers, etc.) and is delegated through the leadership to the safety officer or the safety committee. This individual or committee then has the duties of providing guidance to laboratory leadership on matters related to the provision of a safe workplace for all employees. Although a small institution may have one individual who deals with all safety-related matters for all departments, including the laboratory, OSHA mandates that the laboratory specifically have a chemical hygiene officer who is designated on the basis of training or experience to provide technical guidance in the development of the chemical hygiene plan (CHP) discussed later.

An integral part of the laboratory safety program is the education and motivation of all laboratory employees in all matters related to safety. All new employees should be given a copy of the general laboratory safety manual as part of their orientation. The continuing education program of the laboratory should include periodic talks on safety. Several audiovisual resources are available from a variety of sources to support the continuing education part of the safety program.[3,5]

Another important part of the laboratory safety program relates to ensuring that the laboratory environment meets accepted safety standards. This effort would include, but not be limited to, attention to such items as (1) proper labeling of chemicals, (2) types and locations of fire extinguishers, (3) hoods that are in good working order, (4) proper grounding of electrical equipment, (5) ergonomic issues (which include attention to equipment, such as pipetting devices and laboratory furniture, and prevention of musculoskeletal disorders),[12] and (6) means for the proper handling and disposal of biohazardous materials, including all patient specimens.[4]

Safety Equipment

OSHA requires that institutions provide employees with all necessary personal protective equipment (PPE). Key important safety items include (1) clothing (such as laboratory coats, gowns, and/or scrubs), (2) gloves, and (3) eye protection. These safety items should be used in areas where they are appropriate. Eye washers or face washers should be available in every chemistry laboratory. Many types are available, and some simply connect to existing plumbing. A handheld eye and/or face safety spray is a requisite safety device and is typically placed in a position next to each sink using only a few inches of space. Safety showers, strategically located in the laboratory, must be available and should be tested on a regular basis.

Heat-resistant (nonasbestos) gloves should be available for handling hot glassware and dry ice. Eye safety devices such as (1) safety goggles, (2) glasses, and (4) visors, including some that will fit conveniently over regular eyeglasses, are available in many sizes and shapes. Personnel wearing contact lenses should be aware of the danger of irritants getting under a lens, making it difficult to irrigate the eye properly. Shatterproof safety shields should be used in front of systems posing a potential danger because of implosion (vacuum collapse) or pressure explosions. *Desiccator* guards should be used with vacuum desiccators. Hot beakers should be handled with tongs. Inexpensive polyethylene pumps are available to pump acids from large bottles. Spill kits for acids, caustic materials, or flammable solvents are available in various sizes. Such kits and other appropriate safety materials should be located at convenient and appropriate sites in the laboratory.

A chemical fume hood is a necessity for every clinical chemistry laboratory. The fume hood is used to (1) open any container of a material that gives off harmful vapors, (2) prepare reagents that produce fumes, and (3) heat flammable solvents. In the event of an explosion or a fire in the hood, closing its window contains the fire.

Safety Inspections

It is good laboratory practice to organize a safety inspection team from the laboratory staff. This team is responsible for conducting periodic and scheduled safety inspections of the laboratory.[5]

In the United States, several (1) regulatory, (2) private accreditation, (3) state, and (4) federal organizations may conduct a safety inspection of the laboratory. Some of these safety inspections may occur unannounced. From an external perspective, OSHA inspectors have the authority to enter a clinical laboratory unannounced and, on presentation of credentials, inspect it. The inspection may be regular or may occur as the result of a complaint. In addition, the Commission on Inspection and Accreditation of the CAP inspects clinical laboratories and uses various safety checklists (available to the laboratory before inspection) when evaluating a laboratory for accreditation. Although the TJC will accept CAP accreditation of a laboratory, it still may conduct a safety inspection of the laboratory when it inspects the hospital. The TJC and the CAP conduct their accreditation inspections, which may include a full laboratory or laboratory safety component, unannounced.

Depending on the group designated as responsible for accrediting a particular laboratory, selected laboratories may be subject to inspection for the purposes of accreditation and/or safety only by state agencies or local Center for Medicare & Medicaid Services (CMS) groups. Inspections may be made on a regular basis by state or local health departments or by local fire departments to determine conformance to their particular safety requirements. Currently a laboratory that meets federal or state OSHA requirements is likely to satisfy the standards of any other inspecting agency.

Mandated Plans

In 1991 OSHA mandated that all clinical laboratories in the United States must have a **CHP** and an **exposure control plan**. OSHA has since updated its requirements for the exposure control plan to provide new examples of engineering controls and to place significantly greater responsibility on employers to minimize and manage employee occupational exposure to bloodborne pathogens.[14] Also, the CAP and other groups require that an accredited laboratory have a documented tuberculosis exposure control plan that conforms with biosafety guidelines published by the CDC.[1] In addition, it is now recognized that the workplace setting of a clinical laboratory exposes employees to the occupational risk of developing various musculoskeletal disorders. As a result, the focus of OSHA on laboratories having an effective ergonomics program has caused federal, state, and private accreditation groups to address this area of occupational safety. However, considerable controversy has surrounded this issue, and a final ergonomics rule was published and then withdrawn in 2001.[8]

Chemical Hygiene Plan

Major elements of a CHP include listing of responsibilities for (1) employers, (2) employees, and (3) a chemical hygiene officer. Also, every laboratory must have a complete chemical inventory that is updated annually. A copy of the **Material Safety Data Sheet (MSDS)**, which defines each chemical as (1) toxic, (2) carcinogenic, or (3) dangerous, must be on file and readily accessible and available to all employees 24 hours a day, 7 days a week. The MSDS contains important information for the benefit of laboratory employees. The chemical manufacturer's information as supplied on the MSDS is used to ascertain whether a certain chemical is hazardous. Each MSDS must give the product's identity as it appears on the container label and the chemical and common names of its hazardous components. The MSDS also provides physical data on the product, such as (1) boiling point, (2) vapor pressure, and (3) specific gravity. Easily recognized characteristics of the chemical are listed on the line for "appearance and odor." Information about hazardous properties is given in detail on the MSDS; this includes fire and explosion hazard data and health-related data, including the threshold limit value (TLV), exposure limits, and toxicity values. The TLV is the exposure allowable for an employee during one 8-hour day. It also notes effects of overexposure and provides first aid procedures. Each MSDS also provides information on spill and disposal procedures and on protective personal gear and equipment requirements.

Exposure Control Plan

OSHA regulations require that each laboratory develop, implement, and adhere to a plan that ensures the protection of laboratory workers against potential exposure to bloodborne pathogens[3,5,11,14] and ensures that the medical wastes produced by the laboratory are managed and handled in a safe and effective manner.[3,5,11,14] OSHA regulations also place responsibility on employers (1) to implement new developments in exposure control technology; (2) to solicit the input of employees directly involved in patient care in the identification, evaluation, and selection of these work practice controls; and, in certain instances, (3) to maintain a log for employee percutaneous injuries from sharp devices, such as syringe needles.[14] Organizationally, the plan should include sections on (1) purpose, (2) scope, (3) applicable references, (4) applicable definitions, (5) definitions of responsibilities, and (6) detailed procedural steps.

When implementing the plan, each laboratory employee must be placed into one of three groups. The three classifications are as follows:

Group I: A job classification in which all employees have occupational exposure to blood or other potentially infectious materials

Group II: A job classification in which some employees have occupational exposure to blood or other potentially infectious materials

Group III: A job classification in which employees do not have any occupational exposure to blood or other potentially infectious materials

Tuberculosis Control Plan

The purpose of the tuberculosis control plan is to prevent the transmission of tuberculosis (TB), which occurs when an individual inhales a droplet that contains *Mycobacterium tuberculosis*. *M. tuberculosis* is aerosolized when an infected individual sneezes, speaks, or coughs. Transmission of TB and exposure to TB are greatly diminished by (1) early identification and isolation of patients at risk, (2) environmental controls, (3) appropriate use of respiratory protection equipment, (4) education of laboratory employees, and (5) early initiation of therapy.

An effective tuberculosis control plan will include determination of exposure at regular intervals for all employees who are at occupational risk. Engineering and work practice controls are particularly important in laboratory areas, such as surgical pathology and microbiology. But a risk of exposure from specimens of patients with suspected or confirmed tuberculosis is clearly present in every section of the laboratory, including chemistry.

Ergonomics Program

Several areas of occupational risk for development of musculoskeletal disorders are present in the clinical laboratory. These include (1) routine laboratory activity, (2) functionality of the workspace (including laboratory floor matting, bright lighting, and noise generation), and (3) equipment design (computer keyboards and displays, workstations, and chairs). One particular laboratory function, pipetting and related pipette design, has received considerable attention. As depicted in Figure 8-2, pipettes are being designed with the goal of reducing an employee's risk of developing cumulative stress disorders caused by awkward posture, repetitive motion, and the repeated use of force.

The CAP requires accredited laboratories to have a comprehensive and defined ergonomics program that is designed to prevent work-related musculoskeletal disorders through prevention and engineering controls. The documented ergonomics plan should include (1) elements of employee training regarding areas of risk, (2) engineering controls designed to minimize or eliminate risks, and (3) an assessment process for use in identifying problematic issues for documentation and remediation.

Hazards in the Laboratory

Various types of hazards are encountered in the operation of a clinical laboratory. These hazards must be identified and labeled, and work practices developed for dealing with them. The major categories of hazards encountered include (1) biological, (2) chemical, (3) electrical, and (4) fire hazards.

Identification of Hazards

Clinical laboratories deal with each of the nine classes of hazardous materials. These are classified by the United Nations (UN) as (1) explosives, (2) compressed gases, (3) flammable liquids, (4) flammable solids, (5) oxidizer materials, (6) toxic materials, (7) radioactive materials, (8) corrosive materials, and (9) miscellaneous materials not elsewhere classified.

Shipping and handling of class 6 toxic materials, specifically, biological and potentially infectious materials, has received considerable attention. In 2002 the U.S. Department of Transportation (DOT) released a revised rule with standards for infectious substance hazardous material handling. The impact and requirements of these regulations are described in the section on biological hazards.

Warning labels aid in the identification of chemical hazards during shipment. Under regulations of the DOT, chemicals that are transported in the United States must carry labels based on the UN classification. DOT placards or labels are diamond shaped with a digit imprinted on the bottom corner that identifies the UN hazard class (1 to 9). The hazard is identified more specifically in printed words placed along the horizontal axis of the diamond. Color coding and a pictorial art description of the hazard supplement the identification of hazardous material on the label; the artwork appears in the top corner of the diamond (Figure 8-5, *A*).

This system is used by the DOT for shipping hazardous materials; however, when the hazardous material reaches its destination and is removed from the shipping container, this identification is lost. The laboratory must then label each individual container. Usually the information necessary to classify the contents of the container appropriately is contained on the shipping label and should be noted. Important first aid information is usually provided on this label as well.

In practice, OSHA prescribes the use of labels or other appropriate warnings for hazardous chemicals used in clinical laboratories. Appropriate hazard warnings include any (1) words, (2) pictures, (3) symbols, or (4) combinations that convey the health or physical hazards of the container's contents and must be specific as to the effect of the chemical and the specific target organs involved. The National Fire Protection Association (NFPA) has developed the 704-M Identification System, which classifies hazardous material from 0 to 4 (most hazardous) according to flammability and reactivity (instability). This system uses diamond-shaped labels (Figure 8-5, *B*), which are available from most companies that sell laboratory safety equipment. The labels are color-coded and are divided into quadrants. Three of the quadrants have a characteristic color and represent a particular type of hazard. A number in the quadrant indicates the degree of the hazard. The fourth (lower) quadrant contains information of special interest to firemen.

Biological Hazards

It is essential to minimize the exposure of laboratory workers to infectious agents, such as the hepatitis viruses and human immunodeficiency virus (HIV). Exposure to infectious agents results from (1) accidental puncture with needles, (2) spraying of infectious materials by a syringe or spilling and splattering of these materials on bench tops or floors, (3) centrifuge accidents, and (4) cuts or scratches from contaminated vessels. Any unfixed tissue, including blood slides, must also be treated as potentially infectious material.

OSHA has mandated that all U.S. laboratories have an exposure control plan. In addition, the National Institute for Occupational Safety and Health (NIOSH), a functional unit

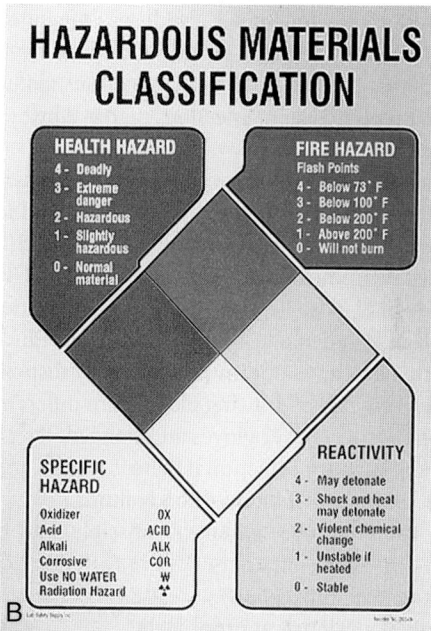

Figure 8-5 A, Department of Transportation label for corrosives. **B,** Labeling identification system of the National Fire Protection Association. *(Courtesy Lab Safety Supply Inc., Janesville, Wis.)*

of the CDC, has prepared and widely distributed a document entitled **Universal Precautions** that specifies how U.S. clinical laboratories should handle infectious agents.[11] In general it mandates that clinical laboratories treat all human blood and other potentially infectious materials as if they were known to contain infectious agents, such as (1) hepatitis B virus (HBV), (2) HIV, and (3) other bloodborne pathogens. These requirements apply to all specimens of (1) blood, (2) serum, (3) plasma, (4) blood products, (5) vaginal secretions, (6) semen, (7) cerebrospinal fluid, (8) synovial fluid, and (9) concentrated HBV or HIV viruses. In addition, any specimen of any type that contains visible traces of blood should be handled using these Universal Precautions.

Universal Precautions also specify that barrier protection must be used by laboratory workers to prevent skin and mucous membrane contamination from specimens. These barriers, also known as personal protective equipment (PPE), include (1) gloves, (2) gowns, (3) laboratory coats, (4) face shields or mask and eye protection, (5) mouthpieces, (6) resuscitation bags, (7) pocket masks, and (8) other ventilator devices. With some individuals, latex allergy is a problem when latex gloves are used for barrier protection. For such individuals, medical grade nonlatex gloves made of materials such as vinyl, nitrile, neoprene, or thermoplastic elastomer are available. If latex gloves are to be used, they should be made of powder-free, low-allergen latex.

New products for improving employee protection against needle sticks include an array of novel containers for sharps (e.g., needles, scalpels, glass) and biological safety disposal bags and needle sheaths that may be closed after venipuncture without physically touching the needle or the sheath.

The CLSI has published a similar set of recommendations,[4,5] several of which are specified as requirements in the OSHA exposure control plan. They include the following:

1. Never perform mouth pipetting and never blow out pipettes that contain potentially infectious material.
2. Do not mix potentially infectious material by bubbling air through the liquid.
3. Use barrier protection, such as gloves, masks, and protective eyewear and gowns, when drawing blood from a patient and when handling all patient specimens. This includes the removal of stoppers from tubes. Gloves must be made of disposable, nonsterile latex or another material that provides adequate barrier protection. Phlebotomists must change gloves and must adequately dispose of them between sessions of drawing blood from different patients.
4. Wash hands whenever gloves are changed.
5. Use facial barrier protection if there is significant potential for the spattering of blood or body fluids.
6. Avoid using syringes whenever possible, and dispose of needles in rigid containers (Figure 8-6, A) without handling them (Figure 8-6, B).
7. Dispose of all sharps appropriately.
8. Wear protective clothing, which serves as an effective barrier against potentially infective materials. When leaving the laboratory, remove protective clothing.
9. Strive to prevent accidental injuries.
10. Encourage frequent hand washing in the laboratory; employees must wash their hands whenever they leave the laboratory.
11. Make a habit of keeping your hands away from your mouth, nose, eyes, and any other mucous membranes. This reduces the possibility of self-inoculation.
12. Minimize spills and spatters.
13. Decontaminate all surfaces and reusable devices after use with appropriate U.S. Environmental Protection Agency (EPA)-registered hospital disinfectants. Sterilization, disinfection, and decontamination are discussed in detail in CLSI publication M29-A3.[3] Do not use warning labels on patient specimens because all should be treated as potentially hazardous.
15. Use biosafety level 2 procedures whenever appropriate.
16. Before centrifuging tubes, inspect them for cracks. Inspect the inside of the trunnion cup for signs of erosion or adhering matter. Be sure that rubber cushions are free from all bits of glass.
17. Use biohazard disposal techniques (e.g., "Red Bag").

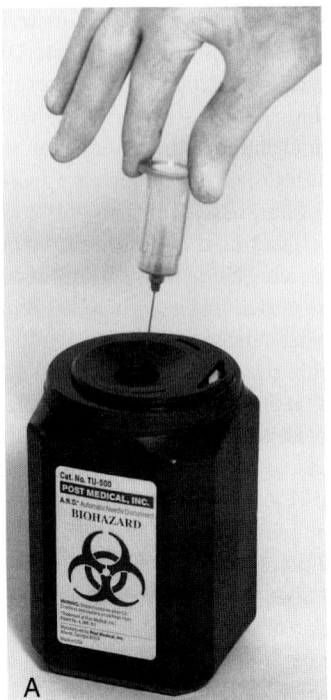

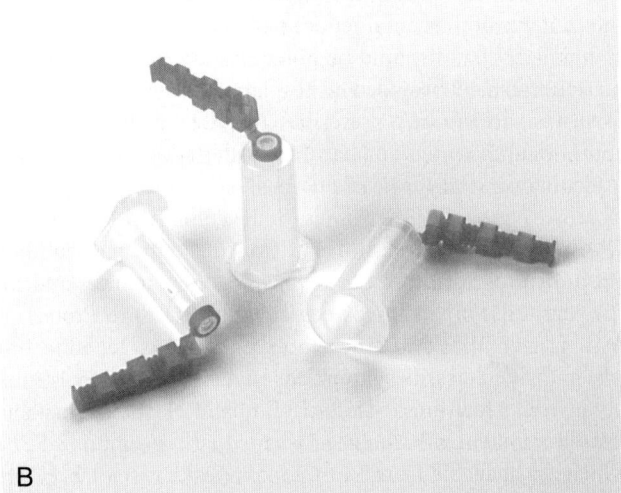

Figure 8-6 A, Convenient needle disposal system for sharps. **B,** Needle sheathing devices for prevention of body contact with needle. *(B, Courtesy MarketLab Inc.)*

18. Never leave a discarded tube or an infected material unattended or unlabeled.
19. Periodically, clean out the freezer and dry-ice chests to remove broken ampules and tubes of biological specimens. Use rubber gloves and respiratory protection during this cleaning.
20. OSHA requires that hepatitis B vaccine be offered to all employees at risk of potential exposure as a regular or occasional part of their duties. CDC's Advisory Committee on Immunization Practices (ACIP) recommends that (1) medical technologists, (2) phlebotomists, and (3) pathologists be vaccinated with hepatitis B vaccine. It is a regulatory mandate that all of the above laboratory employees at a minimum be given the option to receive free hepatitis B vaccine.

Investigation of tragic air accidents in the late 1990s by the U.S. National Transportation Safety Board (NTSB) led to the development of revised and strict requirements for the shipping and handling of hazardous materials by DOT, in cooperation with the International Air Transport Association (IATA) and the International Civil Aviation Organization (ICAO).[4] With continued awareness of the necessity for Universal Precautions, the risk of bloodborne pathogens, and the potentially adverse consequences of serious infection, the shipping and handling of class 6 toxic materials—biological materials—is a critical safety issue.

Federal shipping and packaging guidelines divide potentially infectious specimens or substances into four risk groups that range from low to high risk.

These regulations place particular emphasis on the hazardous material (HAZMAT) training that must be given to laboratory employees for shipping and handling infectious substances. Elements include (1) general awareness and familiarization, (2) function-specific training, and (3) safety training. Proper training, particularly in the areas of package labeling and documentation (including a shipper's declaration of contents for dangerous goods), is mandatory, and documented certification is required from employers that the relevant employees have completed appropriate training programs. Although the adverse impact of improper training can be reflected most by potential human morbidity and mortality, identified violations of these regulations also carry large financial fines and penalties for both the infringing individual and the employer or institution.

Chemical Hazards

Proper storage and use of chemicals is necessary to prevent dangers, such as (1) burns, (2) explosions, (3) fires, and (4) toxic fumes. Thus knowledge of the properties of the chemicals in use and of proper handling procedures greatly reduces dangerous situations. Bottles of chemicals and solutions should also be handled carefully, and a cart should be used to transport heavy or multiple numbers of containers from one area to another. Glass containers with chemicals should be transported in rubber or plastic containers that protect them from breakage and, in the event of breakage, contain the spill. Appropriate spill kits should be available in strategic locations. A general spill kit, such as the Sasco Solidifier Spill Response Kit (http://www.sascochemical.com; accessed July 22, 2013), should contain specific materials to be used with spills of acid or of caustic or organic materials. Directions for use of these materials are contained in the kit.

Spattering from acids, caustic materials, and strong oxidizing agents is a hazard to clothing and eyes and is a potential source of chemical burns. A bottle should never be held by its neck but instead should be held firmly around its body with one or both hands, depending on the size of the bottle. Acids must be diluted by slowly adding them to water while mixing; water should never be added to concentrated acid. When one is working with acid or alkali solutions, safety glasses should be worn. Acids, caustic materials, and strong oxidizing agents should be mixed in the sink. This provides water for cooling

and for confinement of the reagent in the event that the flask or the bottle breaks.

All bottles that contain reagents must be properly labeled. It is good practice to label the container before adding the reagent, thus preventing the possibility of an unlabeled reagent. The label should bear (1) the name and concentration of the reagent, (2) the initials of the person who made up the reagent, and (3) the date on which the reagent was prepared. When appropriate, the expiration date should also be included. Labels should be color-coded or another label added to designate specific storage instructions, such as the requirement for refrigeration or special storage related to a potential hazard. All reagents found in unlabeled bottles should be disposed of in accordance with appropriate procedures and precautions.

Hazardous chemicals such as (1) strong acids, (2) caustic materials, and (3) strong oxidizing agents should be dispensed by a commercially available automatic dispensing device. Under no circumstances is mouth pipetting permitted.

In some instances, all waste materials are not collected in the same container. With certain pieces of equipment, strong acids or other hazardous materials are pumped directly into the drain. This should always be accompanied by a steady flow of water from the faucet. Safety glasses should be used by instrument operators when acids are pumped under pressure.

Perchloric acid, because it is potentially explosive in contact with organic materials, requires careful handling. Perchloric acid should not be used on wooden bench tops, and bottles of this acid should be stored on a glass tray. Disposal may be accomplished by adding the acid dropwise (using a splatter shield) to at least 100 volumes of cold water and pouring the diluted acid down the drain with large amounts of additional cold water. Special perchloric acid hoods, with special washdown facilities, should be installed if large amounts of this acid are used.

Special care is necessary when one is dealing with mercury. Even small drops of mercury on bench tops and floors may poison the atmosphere in a poorly ventilated room. The element's ability to amalgamate with a number of metals is well known. After an accidental spillage of mercury, the spill area should be cleaned carefully until no droplets remain. All containers of mercury should be kept well stoppered. Because it is highly hazardous, most recommend that **no** mercury be used in the laboratory.

The EPA controls the disposal of nonradioactive hazardous wastes. The Resource Conservation and Recovery Act of 1976 (RCRA) states that disposal of materials classifiable within any of the nine UN hazardous materials classes is enforced in such a way that health and safety professionals involved in the disposal of such materials are personally liable for each individual violation.

A CLSI publication[4] covers hazardous waste disposal; however, many municipalities and states have their own regulations. These agencies should be contacted by the laboratory for specifics.

Volatile chemicals and compressed gases pose specific hazards.

Hazards from Volatiles

Use of organic solvents in a clinical laboratory represents a potential fire hazard and hazards to health from inhalation of toxic vapors or skin contact. These solvents should be used in a fume hood. Storage of organic solvents is regulated by rules set down by OSHA. However, some local fire department rules are more stringent. Solvents should be stored in an OSHA-approved metal storage cabinet that is properly vented. The maximum working volume of flammable solvents allowed outside storage cabinets is 5 gallons per room. No more than 60 gallons of type I and II solvents may be stored in a single cabinet. No more than three cabinets may be located in each 5000 square feet of laboratory space.

Vaporization is a major problem in the ignition and spread of fires. Vapors from flammable and combustible liquids and solids form a flammable mixture with air. They are characterized by their flash point, where the flash point is defined as the lowest temperature at which a solvent gives off flammable vapors in the close vicinity of its surface. The mixture at its flash point ignites when exposed to a source of ignition. At temperatures below the flash point, the vapor given off is considered too lean for ignition.

Disposal of flammable solvents in storm sewers or sanitary sewers generally is not allowed. Exceptions include small amounts of those materials that are miscible with water, but even disposal of these should be followed by large amounts of cold water. Other solvents should be collected in safety cans. Separate cans should be used for ether and for chlorinated solvents; all other solvents may be combined in a third can. The cans should be stored, in keeping with storage quantity rules, in a safety cabinet until pickup by a waste disposal firm. A more economical approach is to transfer the solvents to larger cans or drums in an outside storage facility so that pickup is less frequent. Some large institutions have their own in-house disposal facilities.

Hazards from Compressed Gases

DOT regulations cover the labeling of cylinders of compressed gases that are transported by interstate carriers. The diamond-shaped labels described previously are used on all large cylinders and on any boxes containing small cylinders. Some general rules for handling large cylinders of compressed gas follow here:

1. Always transport cylinders using a hand truck to which the cylinder is secured.
2. Leave the valve cap on a cylinder until the cylinder is ready for use, at which time the cylinder should have been secured by a support around the upper one-third of its body. Disconnect the hose or regulator, shut off the valve, and replace the cap before the cylinder is completely empty to prevent the possibility of the development of negative pressure. Place an "empty" sign or label on the cylinder.
3. Chain or secure cylinders at all times even when empty.
4. Always check cylinders for the composition of their contents before connection.
5. Never force threads; if a regulator does not thread readily, something is wrong.

The precautions cited for large refillable gas cylinders also apply to small cylinders that are not refillable. Propane cylinders and cylinders of calibrating gases for blood gas equipment are examples of disposable cylinders. Cylinders in floor-standing base supports require the additional security of a chain or a strap attached to a wall or a fixed piece of furniture. Local fire department regulations (which vary considerably from place to place) govern the disposal of exhausted cylinders.

Electrical Hazards

Electrical wires or connections are potential shock or fire hazards. Worn wires on all electrical equipment should be replaced immediately, and all equipment should be grounded with the use of three-prong plugs. OSHA regulations stipulate that the requirements for grounding of electrical equipment of the National Electrical Code (published by NFPA) must be met. If grounded receptacles are not available, a licensed electrician should be consulted for proper alternative grounding techniques. Some local codes are more stringent than OSHA requirements and do not allow for two-pole mating receptacles with adapters for a three-pole plug.

Use of extension cords is prohibited. This standard is more stringent than any other existing regulation. In some instances, an extension cord may have to be used temporarily. In such cases, the cord should (1) be less than 12 feet long, (2) consist of at least 16 American Wire Gauge (AWG) wire, (3) be approved by the Underwriters Laboratory (UL), and (4) have only one outlet at the end. If several outlets are necessary in an area, a power strip with its own fuse or circuit breaker may be installed at least 3 inches above bench top level. Several manufacturers now sell devices to check for high resistance in neutral or ground wiring or excess voltage in neutral wiring.

Electrical equipment and connections should not be handled with wet hands, nor should electrical equipment be used after liquid has been spilled on it. The equipment must be turned off immediately and dried thoroughly. In the case of a wet or malfunctioning electrical instrument that is used by several people, the plug should be pulled, and a note cautioning coworkers against use should be left on the instrument.

Fire Hazards

NFPA and OSHA publish standards covering subjects from emergency exits (including means of egress) to safety and firefighting equipment. NFPA also publishes the National Fire Codes. Many state and local agencies have adopted these codes (some of which are more stringent than OSHA requirements) and thus make them legally enforceable.

Every laboratory should have the necessary equipment to extinguish or confine a fire in the laboratory and to extinguish a fire on the clothing of an individual. Easy access to safety showers is essential. A safety shower should have a pull chain attached to the wall at a convenient height or hanging down from the shower head; the chain should have a large ring attached, so that the shower may be easily activated, even with eyes closed. Fire blankets for smothering fire on clothing should be available in an easily accessible wall-mounted case. The blanket is unrolled from the case and rolled around the body by taking hold of the rope that is attached to the blanket

TABLE 8-8	Classification of Fires and Fire Extinguisher Requirements	
Type of Hazard	**Class of Fire**	**Recommended Extinguisher Agents**
Ordinary combustibles: wood, cloth, paper	A	Water, dry chemical foam, loaded steam
Flammable liquids and gases: solvents and greases, natural or manufactured gases	B	Dry chemical, carbon dioxide, loaded steam, Halon 1211 or 1301 foam
Electrical equipment: any energized electrical equipment. If electricity is turned off at source, this reverts to a Class A or B	C	Dry chemical, carbon dioxide, Halon 1211 or 1301 foam
Combinations of ordinary combustibles and flammable liquids and gases	A & B	Dry chemical, loaded steam, foam
Combinations of ordinary combustibles and electrical equipment	A & C	Dry chemical
Combinations of flammable liquids and gases and electrical equipment	B & C	Dry chemical, carbon dioxide, Halon 1211 or 1301 foam
Combinations of ordinary combustibles, flammable liquids and gases, and electrical equipment	A, B, & C	Triplex dry chemical

and turning the body around. The location of this equipment and the locations of fire alarms and maps of evacuation routes are dictated by the local fire marshal.

Various types of fire extinguishers are available. The type that should be used depends on the type of fire. Because it is impractical to have several types of fire extinguishers present in every area, dry-chemical fire extinguishers are among the preferred all-purpose extinguishers for laboratory areas. An extinguisher should be provided near every laboratory door and, in a large laboratory, at the end of the room opposite to the door. Everyone in the laboratory should be instructed in the use of these extinguishers and any other firefighting equipment. All fire extinguishers should be tested by qualified personnel at intervals specified by the manufacturer. The three classes of fires and the type of fire extinguisher to be used for each are listed in Table 8-8. Every fire extinguisher is labeled as to the type of fire it should be used to extinguish.

Two additional types of fires, designated "D" and "E," should be handled only by trained personnel. Type "D" fires include those involving powdered metal materials (e.g., magnesium). A special powder is used to fight this hazard. A type "E" fire is one that cannot be put out or is liable to result in a detonation (such as an arsenal fire). A type "E" fire is usually allowed to burn out while nearby materials are appropriately protected.

Many clinical laboratories now have a computer that is housed in a temperature- and humidity-controlled room. The most popular automatic fire control system used in these rooms is Halon 1301 (bromotrifluoromethane). Although this is the least toxic of the halons, NFPA regulations require a warning sign at the entrance to the room and availability of self-contained breathing equipment.

Review Questions

1. One aspect of universal precautions and an OSHA requirement involves the provision of personal protective equipment (PPE) to laboratory employees. PPE includes (but is not limited to) which of the following?
   a. Gloves only
   b. Gloves and a lab coat only
   c. Gloves, eye protection, and a lab coat
   d. Gloves, eye protection, a lab coat, and special footwear

2. The formula for determining how much of a concentrated solution is required to make a specific volume of a less concentrated solution is:
   a. $C_1V_1 = C_2V_2$.
   b. number of moles of solute/number of kilograms of solvent.
   c. mg/L divided by mg molecular mass.
   d. mass in grams/gram molecular weight in grams.

3. The organization that develops and implements standards and guidelines for laboratories in addition to setting certain safety guidelines is:
   a. CAP.
   b. CLSI.
   c. EPA.
   d. DOT.

4. The process by which the concentration or activity of a given solution is decreased by the addition of solvent is referred to as:
   a. solution.
   b. evaporation.
   c. lyophilization.
   d. dilution.

5. The formula used to determine the molarity of a solution is which of the following?
   a. $C_1V_1 = C_2V_2$.
   b. number of moles of solute/number of liters of solution.
   c. mg/L divided by mg molecular mass.
   d. mass in grams/gram molecular weight in grams.

6. The universal coding system for reporting laboratory and other clinical observations to facilitate electronic transmission of laboratory data within and between institutions is referred to as the system.
   a. OSHA
   b. CLIA
   c. LOINC
   d. CLSI

7. Which of the following statements regarding water type is *incorrect*?
   a. Type I water is acceptable for analytical purposes.
   b. Testing that requires minimal interference (such as iron or enzyme analysis) requires the use of type I water.

c. Type I water is distilled water that is acceptable for glassware-washing purposes.

d. Type I water results from ion exchange purification.

8. The two chemical grades that are suitable for use in a clinical chemistry laboratory are:
   a. technical and analytical reagent grades.
   b. ultrapure and technical grades.
   c. technical and National Formulary grades.
   d. ultrapure and analytical reagent grades.

9. RCF is measured in which of the following units?
   a. Gravities (*g*)
   b. Centimeters (cm)
   c. RPMs
   d. Forces (f)

10. Protection of laboratory workers against potential exposure to bloodborne pathogens and assurance that medical waste is handled safely are OSHA requirements that are part of which of the following plans?
    a. Chemical hygiene plan
    b. Exposure control plan
    c. Tuberculosis control plan
    d. Fire safety plan

References

1. Centers for Disease Control and Prevention, and the National Institutes of Health. Biosafety in microbiological and biomedical laboratories, 4th edition. Washington, DC: Department of Health and Human Services, U.S. Government Printing Office, May 1999.

2. Clinical and Laboratory Standards Institute. Procedures for the handling and processing of blood specimens: approved guideline, 3rd edition. CLSI Document H18-A4 (new document code GP44-A4). Wayne, PA: Clinical and Laboratory Standards Institute, 2010.

3. Clinical and Laboratory Standards Institute. Protection of laboratory workers from occupationally acquired infections: approved guideline, 3rd edition. CLSI Document M29-A3. Wayne, PA: Clinical and Laboratory Standards Institute, 2005.

4. Clinical and Laboratory Standards Institute. Clinical laboratory waste Management: approved Guideline, 2nd edition. CLSI Document GP5-A3. Wayne, PA: Clinical and Laboratory Standards Institute, 2011.

5. Clinical and Laboratory Standards Institute. Clinical laboratory safety, 3rd edition. CLSI Document GP17-A3. Wayne, PA: Clinical and Laboratory Standards Institute, 2012.

6. Clinical and Laboratory Standards Institute. Temperature calibration of water baths, instruments, and temperature sensors: approved guideline, 2nd edition. CLSI Document I09-A2. Wayne, PA: Clinical and Laboratory Standards Institute, 1990.

7. Clinical and Laboratory Standards Institute. Preparation and testing of reagent water in the clinical laboratory: approved guideline, 4th edition. CLSI Document C03-A4-AMD (New code GP 40-A4-AMD). Wayne, PA: Clinical and Laboratory Standards Institute, 2006.

8. Ergonomics program. Final rule: removal. Occupational Safety and Health Administration (OSHA). Fed Reg 2001;666:20403.

9. Lo SF. Principles of basic techniques and laboratory safety. In: Burtis CA, Ashwood ER, Bruns D E eds, Tietz textbook of clinical chemistry 5th ed. Philadelphia: WB Saunders, 2012:207–31.

10. McDonald CJ, Huff SM, Suico JG, Hill G, Leavelle D, et al. LOINC, a universal standard for identifying laboratory observations: a 5-year update. Clin Chem 2003;49:624–33.

11. National Institute for Occupational Safety and Health. Guidelines for Prevention of Transmission of Human Immunodeficiency Virus and Hepatitis B Virus of Health-Care and Public Safety Workers. DHSS (NIOSH) Publication No. 89-107. Washington DC: Department of Health and Social Services, February, 1989.

12. National Institute for Occupational Safety and Health (NIOSH). Musculoskeletal disorders and workplace factors: a critical review of epidemiologic evidence for work-related musculoskeletal disorders of the neck, upper extremities, and low back. Centers for Disease Control (NIOSH) Publication No. 97-141. Atlanta, GA: Centers for Disease Control, July, 1997.

13. National Institute of Standards and Technology. The International System of Units (SI). NIST Special Publication 811. Gaithersburg, MD: National Institute of Standards and Technology (http://www.nist.gov/index.html), 1994.

14. Occupational exposure to bloodborne pathogens: needlesticks and other sharps injuries: final rule. Occupational Safety and Health Administration (OSHA). Fed Reg 2001;66:5318–25.

Optical Techniques*

L.J. Kricka, D.Phil., F.A.C.B., C.Chem., F.R.S.C., F.R.C.Path., and Jason Y. Park, M.D., Ph.D.

Objectives

1. Define the following terms:

Absorbance	Phosphorimetry
Atomic absorption	Photometry
Beer's law	Spectral/Natural
Electromagnetic radiation	bandwidth
Flame emission	Spectrophotometry
spectrophotometry	Stokes shift
Fluorescence	Transmittance
Fluorescence polarization	Turbidimetry
Light	Visible/Ultraviolet/Infrared
Nephelometry	spectrum
Percent transmittance	Wavelength

2. Describe the relationship between the light transmitted and the light absorbed by a solution of a compound; state this relationship as a mathematical formula.

3. Express Beer's law mathematically, and define each of the components of the formula; calculate the concentration of a substance in solution using Beer's law.

4. Explain how Beer's law is used to create a calibration curve, and list five conditions that must be met before Beer's law can be applied to a measurement.

5. List the basic components of generic single-beam and double-beam spectrophotometers and state the purpose of each of the components; provide and describe two examples, if appropriate, of each component.

6. State the principle of reflectance photometry and the clinical laboratory applications of this technique.

7. State the principle of atomic absorption spectrophotometry; list the clinical laboratory applications of this technique.

8. List the components of an atomic absorption spectrophotometer and the role each component plays in measurement.

9. Describe and give examples of spectral and nonspectral interferences that might limit measurements made using atomic absorption.

10. State the principle of fluorescence; list the clinical laboratory applications of this technique.

11. Express as an equation the derivation of the Beer-Lambert law in relation to fluorescence intensity and concentration, and define each of the components of this equation.

12. Compare the sensitivity of fluorescence intensity measurements with that of absorbance measurements, and list three reasons why fluorescence measurements are more sensitive.

13. Describe fluorescence polarization and its use in the clinical laboratory.

14. List the components of a generic fluorometer; list and describe four types of fluorometers, including their use in the clinical laboratory.

15. List and describe six possible interferences that influence fluorescence measurements.

16. Explain the basic concepts of chemiluminescence, bioluminescence, and electrochemiluminescence; list the clinical laboratory applications of these techniques.

17. Explain the basic concepts of light scattering, including six factors that affect light scattering.

18. Compare nephelometry and turbidimetry, and list the clinical laboratory applications of these techniques; describe a turbidimeter and a nephelometer.

19. List and describe two possible interferences that might limit light-scattering measurements.

*The authors gratefully acknowledge the original contributions by Dr. Merle A. Evenson and Dr. Thomas O. Tiffany, upon which portions of this chapter are based.

Key Words and Definitions

Absorbance (A) The amount of light absorbed as incident light passes through a sample, which is equivalent to log (1/T) or −log (T), where T is transmittance.

Absorptivity (a) A proportionality constant for a compound that is the measure of the absorption of radiant energy at a given wavelength as it passes through a solution of that compound at a concentration of 1 g/L; expressed mathematically as absorbance divided by the product of the concentration of a substance in g/L and the sample path length in centimeters ($a = A/bc$).

Atomic absorption (AA) spectrophotometry An emission technique in which an element in a sample is dissociated from its chemical bonds (atomized) and placed in an unexcited or ground state (neutral atom); the atom at low energy is able to absorb radiation and the radiant energy given off as the element returns to its ground state is measured.

Bandpass The range of wavelengths passed by a filter or a monochromator at one-half the peak transmittance of that filter.

Beer's law A mathematical equation that states that the concentration of a substance is directly proportional to the amount of light absorbed or is inversely proportional to the logarithm of the transmitted light; mathematically expressed as $A = abc$.

Bioluminescence The emission of light when an electron returns from an excited or higher energy level to a lower energy level in which the excitation event is caused by a biochemical reaction and not by photo illumination; a special form of chemiluminescence in which an enzyme or a photoprotein increases the efficiency of the light emission.

Blank A solution used in photometry/spectrophotometry that is identical to calibrating or unknown solutions except for the substance to be measured.

Chemiluminescence The emission of light when an electron returns from an excited or higher energy level to a lower energy level, in which the excitation event is caused by a chemical reaction and not by photo illumination; the excitation event is caused by the oxidation of an organic compound.

Electrochemiluminescence The emission of light when an electron returns from an excited or higher energy level to a lower energy level, in which the excitation event is a reaction generated electrochemically on the surface of an electrode.

Flow cytometry The measurement of a physical or chemical characteristic of cells or particles made while the cells or particles pass singly through a measuring apparatus in a flowing fluid stream.

Fluorescence The emission of electromagnetic radiation that occurs when a molecule absorbs light at one wavelength and reemits light at a longer wavelength, when it returns to ground state with the excitation event being caused by photo illumination.

Fluorometry The measurement of emitted fluorescence light that occurs when a molecule absorbs light at one wavelength and reemits light at a longer wavelength.

Light Energy transmitted via electromagnetic waves that are characterized by frequency and wavelength; light is composed of photons whose energy is inversely proportional to the wavelength.

Light scattering A physical phenomenon that results from the interaction of light with particles in solution.

Molar absorptivity (ε) A proportionality constant for a compound that is the measure of the absorption of radiant energy at a given wavelength as it passes through a solution of that compound at a concentration of 1 mol/L; expressed mathematically as absorbance divided by the product of the concentration of a substance in mol/L and the sample path length in centimeters ($\varepsilon = A/bc$).

Nephelometry The detection and measurement of light energy scattered or reflected toward a detector that is not in the direct path of the transmitted light; common nephelometers measure scattered light at right angles to the incident light, and some are designed to measure scattered light at an angle other than 90°.

Photometry/Spectrophotometry The measurement of the luminous intensity of light or the amount of luminous light falling on a surface from such a source; spectrophotometry is the measurement of the intensity of light at selected wavelengths.

Reflectance photometry A spectrophotometric technique in which diffused light illuminates a reaction mixture in a carrier containing a substance of interest, and the intensity of the reflected light is measured and compared with a reference; the reflected light is nonlinear in relation to the concentration of the substance and must be converted to a linear format.

Spectral bandwith The width in nanometers of the spectral transmittance curve at a point equal to one-half of the peak transmittance; used to describe the spectral purity of a filter or other monochromator.

Transmittance The intensity of a transmitted light beam divided by the intensity of an incident (incoming) light beam passed through a square cell containing a solution of a compound that absorbs light at a specific wavelength stated as $T = I/I_0$; when compared with a reference cell, the transmitted light is divided by the incident light $(T = I/I_R)$. A reference cell is used to set an arbitrary value of 100 which corresponds to 100% transmittance.

Turbidimetry The detection and measurement of a decrease in intensity of an incident beam of light as it passes through a solution of particles.

Wavelength A characteristic of electromagnetic radiation; the distance between two wave crests that is measured in nanometers.

Many determinations made in the clinical laboratory are based on measurements of radiant energy (1) emitted, (2) transmitted, (3) absorbed, (4) scattered, or (5) reflected under controlled conditions (Table 9-1). The principles involved in such measurements are considered in this chapter.

Photometry and Spectrophotometry

Photometry[5] is the measurement of the luminous intensity of **light** or the amount of luminous light falling on a surface from such a source. **Spectrophotometry** is the measurement of the intensity of light at selected wavelengths. The term *photometric measurement* was defined originally as the process used to measure light intensity independent of wavelength. Modern instruments, however, isolate a narrow wavelength range of the spectrum for measurements. Those that use filters for this purpose are referred to as *filter* photometers, whereas those that use prisms or gratings are called spectrophotometers. The primary analytical utility of filter photometry or spectrophotometry is the isolation and use of discrete portions of the spectrum for purposes of measurement.

Basic Concepts

Energy is transmitted via electromagnetic waves that are characterized by their frequency and **wavelength.** Analytically, the term *wavelength* describes a position within a spectrum. Electromagnetic radiation includes radiant energy that extends from cosmic rays with wavelengths as short as 10^{-9} nm up to radio waves longer than 1000 km. However, in this chapter, the term *light* is used to describe radiant energy from the ultraviolet to the visible light portions of the spectrum (290 to 750 nm).

In addition to possessing wavelength characteristics, light behaves as if it is composed of discrete energy packets called *photons,* whose energy is inversely proportional to the wavelength. For example, *ultraviolet (UV) radiation* at 200 nm possesses greater energy than *infrared (IR) radiation* at 750 nm.

Table 9-2 shows the approximate relationships between wavelengths and color characteristics for the UV, visible, and short IR portions of the spectrum.

Relationship Between Transmittance and Absorbance

When an incident light beam with intensity I_0 passes through a square cell containing a solution of a compound that absorbs light of a specific wavelength, λ (Figure 9-1), given that the intensity of the transmitted light beam is I, the **transmittance** of light is defined as

$$T = \frac{I}{I_0} \qquad (1)$$

Some of the incident light, however, may be reflected by the surface of the cell or absorbed by the cell wall or solvent. These factors are eliminated by using a reference cell identical to the sample cell, except that the compound of interest is

Table 9-1	Scope of Optical Methods
Type	**Example**
Absorption	Atomic absorption, densitometry, Fourier transform infrared spectroscopy, photometry, spectrophotometry, reflectance photometry, x-ray spectroscopy
Emission	Fluorescence correlation spectroscopy (FCS), fluorescence energy transfer spectroscopy (FRET), fluorometry, luminometry (light emission from a bioluminescent, chemiluminescent, or electrochemiluminescent reaction), phosphorimetry, time-resolved fluorimetry
Polarization	Fluorescence polarization spectroscopy, polarimetry
Scattering	Nephelometry, turbidimetry

Table 9-2	Ultraviolet, Visible, and Short Infrared Spectrum Characteristics Colors	
Wavelength, nm	**Region Name**	**Observed***
<380	Ultraviolet[†]	Invisible
380-440	Visible	Violet
440-500	Visible	Blue
500-580	Visible	Green
580-600	Visible	Yellow
600-620	Visible	Orange
620-750	Visible	Red
750-2500	Near-infrared	Not visible
2500-15,000	Mid-infrared	Not visible
15,000-1,000,000	Far-infrared	Not visible

*Owing to the subjective nature of color, the wavelength intervals shown are only approximations.

[†]The ultraviolet (UV) portion of the spectrum is sometimes further divided into "near" UV (220 to 380 nm) and "far" UV (<220 nm). This arbitrary distinction has a practical basis because cuvets made from silica transmit light effectively at wavelengths ≥220 nm.

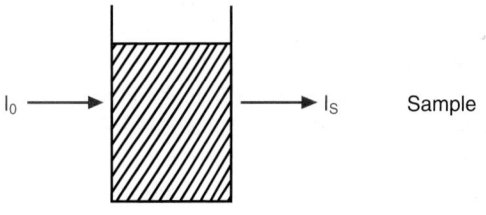

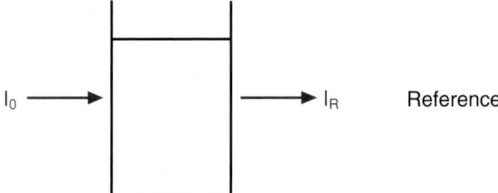

Figure 9-1 Transmittance of light through sample and reference cells. Transmittance of sample versus reference = I/I_R. I_0 = intensity of incident light; I = intensity of transmitted light for compound in solution; I_R = intensity of transmitted light through the reference cell.

omitted from the solvent in the reference cell. The transmittance (T) through this reference cell is I_R divided by I_0; the transmittance for the compound in solution then is defined as I divided by I_R. In practice the reference cell is inserted and the instrument adjusted to an arbitrary scale reading of 100 (corresponding to 100% transmittance), after which the percent transmittance reading is made on the sample. The amount of light absorbed *(A)* as the incident light passes through the sample is equivalent to

$$A = -\log\frac{I}{I_R} = -\log T \qquad (2)$$

Beer's Law

Beer's law states that the concentration of a substance is directly proportional to the amount of light absorbed or is inversely proportional to the logarithm of the transmitted light (Figure 9-2). Mathematically, Beer's law is expressed as

$$A = abc \qquad (3)$$

where

A = absorbance;
a = proportionality constant defined as **absorptivity**;
b = light path in centimeters; and
c = concentration of the absorbing compound, usually expressed in grams per liter.

This equation forms the basis of quantitative analysis by absorption photometry. **Absorbance (A)** values have no units; hence, the units for a are the reciprocal of those for b and c. When b is 1 cm and c is expressed in moles per liter, the symbol ε (epsilon) is substituted for the constant a. The value for ε is a constant for a given compound at a given wavelength under prescribed conditions of solvent, temperature, pH, etc., and is called the **molar absorptivity** (ε). The nomenclature of spectrophotometry is summarized in Table 9-3.

Application of Beer's Law

In practice, the direct proportionality between absorbance and concentration must be established experimentally for a given instrument under specified conditions. Frequently, a linear relationship exists up to a certain concentration or

absorbance. When this relationship occurs, the solution is said to obey Beer's law up to this point. Within this limitation, a calibration constant (K) may be derived and used to calculate the concentration of an unknown solution by comparison with a calibrating solution. From Equation (3),

$$a = \frac{A}{bc} \qquad (4)$$

Therefore,

$$\frac{A_1}{b_1 c_1} = \frac{A_2}{b_2 c_2} \qquad (5)$$

where subscripts 1 and 2 indicate the absorbance *(A)*, path length *(b)*, and concentration *(c)* of calibrating and unknown solutions, respectively.

Because the light path *(b)* remains constant in a given method of analysis with a fixed cuvet size, $b_1 = b_2$, Equation (5) then becomes

$$\frac{A_1}{c_1} = \frac{A_2}{c_2} \text{ or } \frac{A_c}{c_c} = \frac{A_u}{c_u} \qquad (6)$$

where c and u represent calibrator and unknown, respectively.

Solving for the concentration of unknown,

$$c_u = \frac{A_u}{A_c} \times c_c \qquad (7)$$

or the equivalent expression,

$$c_u = A_u \times \frac{c_c}{A_c} = A_u \times K \qquad (8)$$

where $K = c_C/A_C$. The value of the constant K is obtained through measurement of the absorbance (A_C) of a calibrator of known concentration (c_C).

Certain precautions must be observed with the use of such calibration constants. Under no circumstances should the constant be used when the calibrator or unknown readings exceed the linear portion of the calibration curve (i.e., when the curve no longer obeys Beer's law). At least two or preferably more

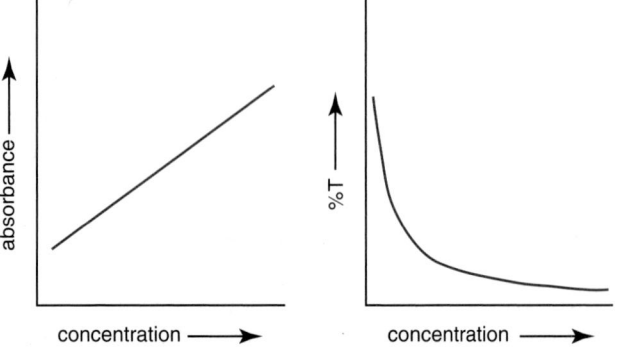

Figure 9-2 Absorbance and %T relationship.

Table 9-3	Spectrophotometry Nomenclature	
Name	**Symbol**	**Definition**
Absorbance	A	$\log T$ or $\log I_0/I$
Absorptivity	a	A/bc (c in g/L)
Molar absorptivity	ε	A/bc (c in mol/L)
Path length	b	Internal cell or sample length, in cm
Transmittance	T	I/I_0*
Wavelength unit	nm	10^{-9} m
Absorption maximum	λmax	Wavelength at which maximum absorption occurs

*I/I_0 is the ratio of the intensity of transmitted light to incident light.

calibrators should be included in the generation of a calibration curve. A nonlinear calibration curve may be used if a sufficient number of calibrators of varying concentrations are included to cover the entire range encountered for readings on unknowns.

In some cases, a pure reference material may not be readily available, and constants may be provided that were obtained on pure materials and reported in the literature. In general, published constants should be used only if the method is followed in detail and measurements are made on a spectrophotometer capable of providing light of high spectral purity at a verified wavelength. Use of broader-band light sources usually leads to some decrease in absorbance. The absorbance of reduced nicotinamide adenine dinucleotide (NADH) at 340 nm, for example, frequently is used as a reference for the determination of enzyme activity, based on a molar absorptivity of 6.22×10^3 (see Chapter 19). This value is acceptable only under the carefully controlled conditions previously described and should not be used unless these conditions are met. Published values for molar absorptivities and absorption coefficients should be used only as guidelines until they are verified by readings on pure reference materials for a given instrument. In addition, Beer's law is followed only if the following conditions are met:

- Incident radiation on the substance of interest is monochromatic.
- The solvent absorption is insignificant, compared with the solute absorbance.
- The solute concentration is within given limits.
- An optical interferant is not present.
- A chemical reaction does not occur between the molecule of interest and another solute or solvent molecule.

Measurement Errors

With most photometers, the response of the detector to a signal of transmitted light is such that any uncertainty in %T is constant over the entire %T scale. The uncertainty derives from electrical and mechanical imperfections in the instrument and individual variations in the use of the instrument.

A fixed distance on the linear scale (e.g., 1% T) represents a greater change in absorbance for low values of %T than for high values of %T. For this reason, the absolute concentration error or uncertainty is greater when readings are taken at high absorbance. However, the relative concentration error is greater for readings at both low and high absorbances. Studies have shown that the relative error is minimal at an absorbance of 0.434 (36.8% T). Consequently, methods should be designed within an absorbance interval of approximately 0.1 and 0.7 (20% and 80% T).

Instrumentation

Modern instruments isolate a narrow wavelength range of the spectrum for measurements. Those that use filters for this purpose are referred to as *filter photometers;* those that use prisms or gratings are called *spectrophotometers.* Spectrophotometers are classified as single- or double-beam.

The major components of a *single-beam spectrophotometer* are shown schematically in Figure 9-3. With such an instrument, a beam of light is passed through a monochromator that isolates the desired region of the spectrum to be used for measurements. Slits are used to isolate a narrow beam of the light and improve its chromatic purity. The light next passes through an absorption cell (cuvet), where a portion of the radiant energy is absorbed, depending on the nature and concentration of the substance in the solution. Any light not absorbed is transmitted to a detector (photocell or phototube), which converts light energy to electrical energy that is registered on a meter or recorder or digitally displayed.

In manual operation, an opaque block is substituted for the cuvet, so that no light reaches the photocell, and the meter is adjusted to read 0% T. Next, a cuvet containing a reagent **blank** is inserted, and the meter is adjusted to read 100% T (zero absorbance). The composition of the reagent blank should be identical to that of calibrating or unknown solutions except for the absorbing substance to be measured. Calibrating solutions containing various known concentrations of the substance are inserted, and readings are recorded. Finally, a reading is made of the unknown solution, and its concentration is determined by comparison with readings obtained on the calibrators. With most spectrophotometers, digital hardware and software are integral components and perform these functions automatically.

Figure 9-4 illustrates schematically a typical double-beam-in-space system in which all components are duplicated except the light source. Another approach is a double-beam-in-time instrument that uses a light-beam chopper (a rotating wheel with alternate silvered sections and cutout sections) inserted after the exit slit (Figure 9-5). A system of mirrors passes the portions of light reflected off the chopper alternately through the sample and a reference cuvet onto a common detector. The chopped-beam approach, using one detector, compensates for light source variation and for sensitivity changes of the detector.

Components

The basic components of a spectrophotometer include (1) a light source, (2) a means to isolate light of a desired wavelength, (3) fiber optics, (4) cuvets, (5) a photodetector, (6) a readout device, (7) a computer, and (8) a recorder.

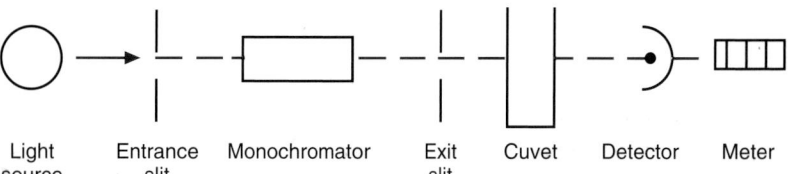

Figure 9-3 Major components of a single-beam spectrophotometer.

Light source | Entrance slit | Monochromator | Exit slit | Cuvet | Detector | Meter

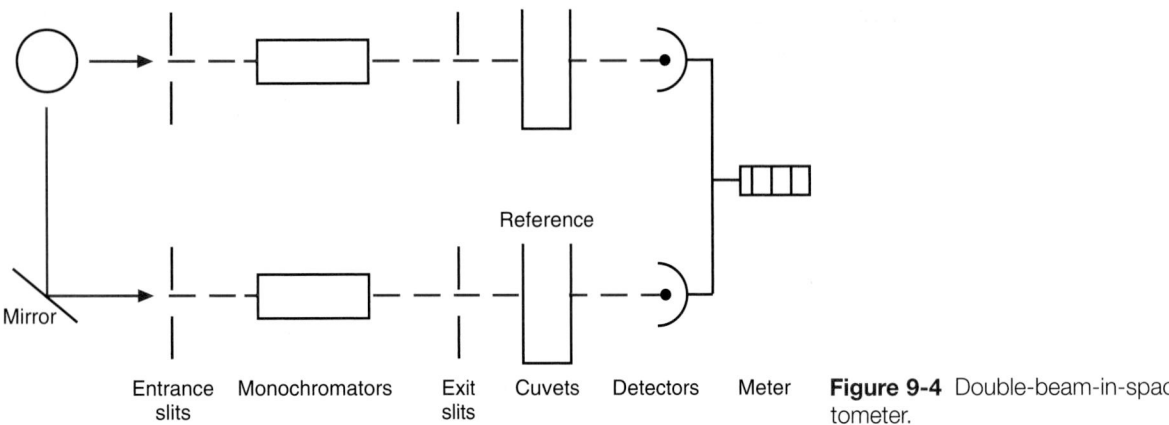

Figure 9-4 Double-beam-in-space spectrophotometer.

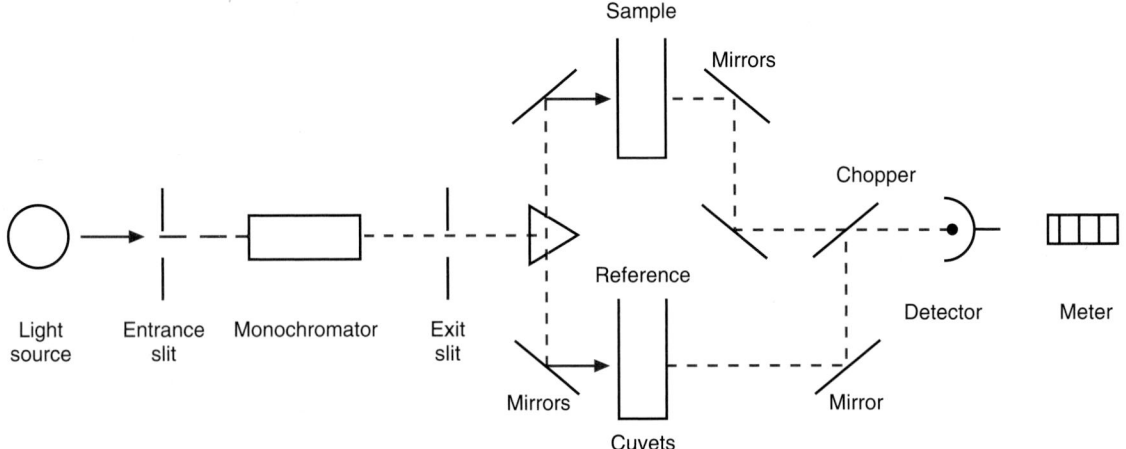

Figure 9-5 Double-beam-in-time spectrophotometer.

Light Sources
Types of light sources used in spectrophotometers include incandescent lamps and lasers.

Incandescent Lamps
The light source for measurements in the visible portion of the spectrum is usually a tungsten light bulb. The lifetime of a tungsten filament is greatly increased by the presence of a low pressure of iodine or bromine vapor within the lamp. An example is the *quartz-halogen* lamp, which has a fused-silica envelope, and which provides high-intensity light over a wide spectrum and for extended operating periods.

A tungsten light source does not supply sufficient radiant energy for measurements below 320 nm. In the UV region of the spectrum, a low-pressure mercury vapor lamp that emits a discontinuous or line spectrum is useful for calibration purposes but is not practical for absorbance measurements because it is used only at certain wavelengths. Hydrogen and deuterium lamps provide sources of continuous spectra in the UV region with some sharp emission lines, as do high-pressure mercury and xenon arc lamps. These sources are more commonly used in UV absorption measurements. A deuterium lamp is more stable and has a longer life than a hydrogen lamp.

A widely used photometer employed as a high-pressure liquid chromatographic (HPLC) detector uses the intense 254-nm resonance line produced by a mercury arc lamp (see Chapter 12). Others employ a miniature hollow cathode lamp as a very-narrow-wavelength intense source. For example, a zinc hollow cathode lamp gives a line at 214 nm that is adequately close to the maximum wavelength of peptide bond absorption (206 nm) and has been used to measure peptides and proteins. Details on the hollow cathode lamp are found in the section on Atomic Absorption Spectrophotometry.

Laser Sources
A laser (*light amplification by stimulated emission of radiation*) is a device that also is used as a light source in spectrophotometers. These devices transform light of various frequencies into an extremely intense, focused, and nearly nondivergent beam of monochromatic light. Through selection of different materials, different wavelengths of light emitted by the laser are obtained (Table 9-4).

Spectral Isolation
A system for isolating radiant energy of a desired wavelength and excluding that of other wavelengths is called a *monochromator*. Devices used for spectral isolation include (1) filters,

Table 9-4	Various Types of Lasers and the Wavelengths at Which They Operate
Laser	**Wavelength, nm**
Argon fluoride	193
Argon fluoride	248
Helium-cadmium	325 or 442
Nitrogen	337
Argon (blue)	488
Argon (green)	514
Helium-neon (green)	543
Light-emitting diode—GaP	550 or 700
Rhodamine 6G dye (tunable)	570-650
Laser diode (AlGaInP, GaAlAs)	634-1660
Helium-neon (red)	633
Ruby (CrAlO$_3$) (red)	694
Light-emitting diode—GaAs	880
Light-emitting diode—Si	1100
Neodymium-YAG (yttrium aluminum garnet)	1064
Carbon dioxide	9300, 9600, 10,300, or 10,600

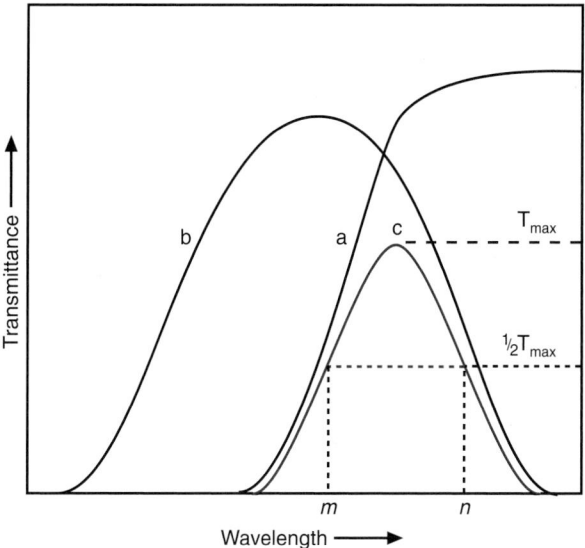

Figure 9-6 Spectral characteristics of a sharp-cutoff filter *(a)* and a wide-bandpass filter *(b)*. The narrow-bandpass filter *(c)* is obtained by combining filters *a* and *b*. The spectral bandwidth of filter *c* (distance n-m) is defined as the width in nanometers of the spectral transmittance curve at a point equal to one-half of maximum transmittance.

(2) prisms, and (3) diffraction gratings. In addition, combinations of lenses and slits are often inserted before or after the monochromatic device to render light rays parallel or to isolate narrow portions of the light beam. Variable slits also are used to permit adjustments in total radiant energy reaching the photocell.

Filters

The simplest type of filter is a thin layer of colored glass. Strictly speaking, a glass filter is not a true monochromator because it transmits light over a relatively wide range of wavelengths. The spectral purity of a filter or other monochromator is usually described in terms of its **spectral bandwidth**. This is defined as the width, in nanometers, of the spectral transmittance curve at a point equal to one-half the peak transmittance (Figure 9-6). Commonly used glass filters have spectral bandwidths of approximately 50 nm and are referred to as *wide-bandpass filters*.

Other glass filters include the narrow-bandpass and sharp-cutoff types (see Figure 9-6). As shown, a cutoff filter typically shows a sharp rise in transmittance over a narrow portion of the spectrum and is used to eliminate light below a given wavelength. Narrow-bandpass filters are constructed by combining two or more sharp-cutoff filters or regular filters.

Interference filters are also used as monochromators. These filters have narrow spectral bandwidths, usually from 5 to 15 nm. Because they also transmit harmonics, or multiples, of the desired wavelength, accessory glass filters are required to eliminate these undesired wavelengths. Thus an interference filter designed for 620 nm will also transmit some radiation at 310 and 1240 nm unless accessory cutoff filters are provided to absorb this undesired stray light.

Prisms and Gratings

Prisms and diffraction gratings are also widely used as monochromators. A *prism* separates white light into a continuous spectrum by refraction with shorter wavelengths that are being bent, or refracted, to a greater extent than longer wavelengths as they pass through the prism. A *diffraction grating* is prepared by depositing a thin layer of aluminum-copper alloy on the surface of a flat glass plate; then, many small parallel grooves are made in the metal coating. Diffraction gratings (1) are extremely accurate, (2) have low light scatter, and (3) are widely used in the spectrophotometers used in analytical instruments. For example, most UV-visible spectrophotometers and virtually all IR spectrophotometers use reflective gratings. In addition, HPLC detectors frequently use a concave holographic reflective grating in their optical system.

Each groove of the grating, when illuminated, gives rise to a tiny spectrum. Wave fronts are formed that reinforce those wavelengths in phase and cancel those not in phase. The net result is a uniform linear spectrum. Some instruments contain diffraction gratings that produce spectral bandwidths of 20 nm or more; higher-priced instruments may have a resolution of 0.5 nm or less.

A grating may also be ruled at a specified angle, so that a maximum fraction of the radiant energy is directed into wavelengths diffracted at a selected angle. This type of grating is called an *echelette* and is said to have been given a *blaze* at a particular angle or to have been blazed at a certain wavelength (e.g., 250 nm).

Selection of a Monochromator

The type of monochromator chosen depends on the analytical purpose for which it is to be used. For example, narrow spectral bandwidths are required in spectrophotometers for resolving and identifying sharp absorption peaks that are closely adjacent. Lack of agreement with Beer's law will occur when a part of the spectral energy transmitted by the monochromator is not absorbed by the substance being measured. This is more commonly observed with wide-bandpass instruments.

Some increase in absorbance and improved linearity with concentration are usually observed with instruments that operate at narrower bandwidths of light. This is especially true for substances that exhibit a sharp peak of absorption. Spectral absorbance curves for a solution of coproporphyrin I (Figure 9-7) demonstrate a notable decrease in maximum absorbance as the spectral bandwidth is increased from 1 to 20 nm. The *natural bandwidth* of an absorbing substance is defined as "the bandwidth of the spectral absorbance curve at a point equal to one-half of the maximum absorbance." *Curve a* in Figure 9-7, scanned at a *spectral* bandwidth of 1 nm, shows a *natural* bandwidth of approximately 10 nm. As a general rule, for peak absorbance readings to be within 99.5% of true values, the spectral bandwidth should not exceed 10% of the natural bandwidth. For example, many chemistry procedures used in the clinical laboratory produce an absorbing species for which the natural bandwidth ranges from 40 to greater than 200 nm. The natural bandwidth of NADH is 58 nm (λmax = 339 nm). Therefore, for accurate measurements of this compound, an instrument should be used that has a spectral bandwidth of 6 nm or less.

In practice, the wavelength selected is usually at the peak of maximum absorbance to achieve maximum sensitivity; however, it may be desirable to choose another wavelength to minimize interfering substances. For example, **turbidity** readings on a spectrophotometer are greater in the blue region than in the red region of the spectrum, but the latter region is chosen for turbidity measurements to avoid absorption of light by bilirubin (460 nm) or hemoglobin (417 and 575 nm). In addition, measurements should not be taken on the steep slope of an absorption curve because a slight error in wavelength adjustment will introduce a significant error in absorbance readings.

Fiber Optics

In the single- and double-beam spectrophotometers shown diagrammatically in Figures 9-4 and 9-5, the positioning of the individual components dictates the path that the light beam must follow as it travels from the source to the detector. This approach places certain restrictions on the (1) design, (2) size, and (3) cost of such instruments. To overcome these restrictions, fiber optics are now integrated into the optical design of spectrophotometers. Fiber optics, also known as *light pipes,* are bundles of thin, transparent fibers of glass, quartz, or plastic that are enclosed in material of a lower index of refraction and that transmit light throughout their lengths by internal reflections. The use of fiber optics in spectrophotometers offers the advantage of better directional control of the beam of light within the geometrical confines of an instrument. This allows for the design and manufacture of miniature and inexpensive optical subsystems for use in automated instruments. For example, a single light source is multiplexed with multiple detectors by fiber optics for optimal positioning of the source and detectors in an automated system. Disadvantages of fiber optics include (1) greater amounts of stray light; (2) refractive index changes in the glass, quartz, or plastic rods; and (3) loss of transmitted energy after continued use in the UV region of the spectrum. This loss of energy is known as *solarization* and results in a decrease in the optical performance of an instrument.

Cuvets

A cuvet (also often termed a cuvette) is a small vessel used to hold a liquid sample to be analyzed in the light path of a spectrometer. Cuvets may be (1) round, (2) square, or 3) rectangular and are constructed from (1) glass, (2) silica (quartz), or (3) plastic. Square or rectangular cuvets have plane-parallel optical surfaces and a constant light path. Most have a 1.0-cm light path, held to close tolerances. Ordinary borosilicate glass cuvets are suitable for measurements in the visible portion of the spectrum. For readings below 340 nm, however, quartz cells are usually required. Some plastic cells have good clarity in both visible and UV ranges but often present problems related to (1) tolerance, (2) cleaning, (4) etching by solvents, and (4) temperature deformation. Many plastic cuvets are designed for disposable, single-use applications.

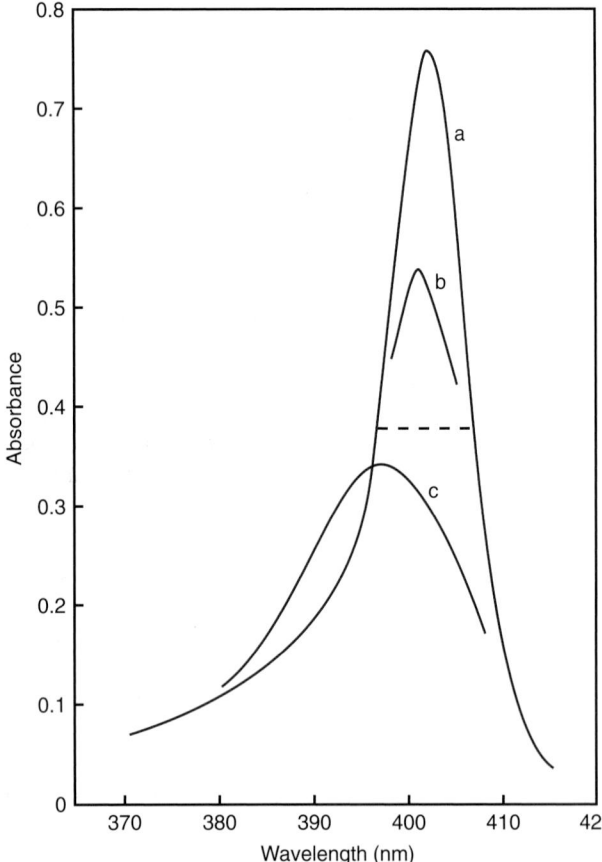

Figure 9-7 Effect of spectral bandwidth (SBW) on the absorption spectrum of coproporphyrin I. Nominal concentration, 1 μg/mL in HCl, 0.1 mol/L. SBW: *curve a,* 1 nm; *curve b,* 10 nm; and *curve c,* 20 nm. The *dotted horizontal line* shows a natural bandwidth of 10 nm for coproporphyrin I when scanned at a spectral bandwidth of 1 nm. The shift of A_{max} to lower wavelengths as SBW is increased is related to skewness of the absorption spectrum to the left.

Cuvets must be clean and optically clear because etching or deposits on the surface affect absorbance values. Cuvets used in the visible range are cleaned by copious rinsing with tap water and distilled water. Alkaline solutions should not be left standing in cuvets for prolonged periods because alkali slowly dissolves glass and produces etching. Cuvets may be cleaned in mild detergent or soaked in a mixture of concentrated HCl/water/ethanol (1:3:4). Cuvets should never be soaked in dichromate cleaning solution because the solution is hazardous and tends to adsorb onto and discolor the glass.

Cuvets used for measurements in the UV region should be handled with special care. Invisible scratches, fingerprints, or residual traces of previously measured substances may be present and may absorb significantly. A good practice is to fill all such cuvets with distilled water and measure the absorbance for each against a reference blank over the wavelengths to be used. This value should be essentially zero.

Photodetectors

Photodetectors are devices that convert light into an electrical signal that is proportional to the number of photons striking its photosensitive surface. The photomultiplier tube (PMT) is a photodetector that is commonly to measure light intensity in UV and visible regions of the spectrum. PMTs (1) have extremely rapid response times, (2) are very sensitive, and (3) are slow to fatigue.

Photodiodes also are used as photodetectors. They are solid-state devices that are fabricated from photosensitive semiconductor materials, such as (1) silicon, (2) gallium arsenide, (3) indium antimonide, (4) indium arsenide, (5) lead selenide, and (6) lead sulfide. These materials absorb light over a characteristic wavelength range (e.g., 250 nm to 1100 nm for silicon). Their development and use as detectors in spectrophotometers have resulted in instruments capable of measuring light at a multitude of wavelengths. When a photodetector consists of two-dimensional arrays of diodes, each of which responds to a specific wavelength, it is known as a *photodiode array*. For example, photodiode arrays have been designed to have a 2-nm resolution per diode from 200 to 340 nm, and a 1-nm resolution per diode from 340 to 800 nm.

Readout Devices

Electrical energy from a detector is displayed on some type of meter or readout system. Historically, analog devices were widely used as readout devices in spectrophotometers. However, they have been replaced by digital readout devices that provide a visual numerical display of absorbance or converted values of concentrations. These operate on the principle of selective illumination of portions of a bank of light-emitting diodes (LEDs), controlled by the voltage signal generated. Visible LEDs incorporate gallium as the major component, and at present, $GaAs_XP_X$ diodes that emit red light are most widely used. Compared with meters, digital readout devices have faster response and are easier to read.

Digital Hardware and Software Computers

Various types of digital hardware, with resident software and processors, are incorporated and integrated into both photometers and spectrophotometers. For example, with a resident computer and software, (1) output from a calibrator is digitally stored, (2) digital signals from blanks are subtracted from calibrators and unknowns, and (3) the concentration of unknowns is automatically calculated. Data from multiple calibrators often are used to (1) store a complete calibration curve, (2) display or print out the curve for visible inspection, and (3) calculate results of unknowns based on the curve or some mathematical transformation of the data. Computers and their resident software also are used to convert kinetic data into concentration or enzyme activity.

Recorders

Historically, spectrophotometers were equipped with recorders in addition to or instead of a digital display. These were synchronized to provide line traces of transmittance or absorbance as a function of time or wavelength. When a continuous tracing of absorbance versus wavelength is recorded, the resultant figure is called an *absorption spectrum*. If a substance absorbs light, distinct peaks of absorbance will be observed. Measuring the absorption spectra of an unknown sample and comparing them with spectra from known compounds is very useful for qualitative purposes. For example, this type of procedure is especially useful for identification of drugs that absorb in the UV region. Several criteria are used, including (1) determination of those wavelengths showing maximum and minimum absorbance in both dilute acid and alkaline solutions; (2) absorptivity at the wavelength of maximum absorbance; and (3) ratios of absorbance at two wavelengths. Finally, the entire spectrum is compared with that of a known sample of the suspected drug.

Performance Parameters

In most spectrophotometric analytical procedures, the absorbance of an unknown is compared directly with that of a calibrator or a series of calibrators. Under these circumstances, (1) minor errors in wavelength calibration, (2) variations in spectral bandwidths, and (3) the presence of stray light are compensated for and do not usually contribute to serious errors. Use of a series of calibrators covering a wide range of concentrations also provides a measure of linearity and validation of agreement with Beer's law for a given procedure and instrument. However, when calculations are based on published or previously determined values for molar absorptivities or absorption coefficients, the spectrophotometer must be checked more rigorously.

The National Institute of Standards and Technology (NIST) provides several standard reference materials (SRMs) for spectrophotometry that are useful in the calibration or verification of the performance of photometers or spectrophotometers (e.g., SRM 930e is used for the verification and calibration of the transmittance and absorbance scales of visible absorption spectrometers) (http://www.nist.gov; accessed July 21, 2013). The Institute for Reference Materials and Measurements

(IRMM), a metrology institute that belongs to the European Commission, also provides reference materials for verification of the performance of photometers or spectrophotometers (http://www.irmm.jrc.be; accessed July 21, 2013).

Reflectance Photometry

In **reflectance photometry,** diffused light illuminates a reaction mixture in a carrier, and the reflected light is measured.[4] Alternatively, the carrier is illuminated and the reaction mixture generates a diffuse reflected light, which is measured. The intensity of the reflected light from the reagent carrier is compared with the intensity of light reflected from a reference surface. Because the intensity of reflected light is nonlinear in relation to the concentration of the analyte, the Kubelka-Munk equation or the Clapper-Williams transformation is commonly used to convert the data into a linear format. The electro-optical components used in reflectance photometry are essentially the same as those required for absorbance photometry. Reflectance photometry is used as the measurement method with dry-film chemistry systems.

Atomic Absorption Spectrophotometry

Atomic absorption (AA) spectrophotometry is used widely in clinical laboratories to measure elements including (1) aluminum, (2) calcium, (3) copper, (4) lead, (5) lithium, (6) magnesium, and (7) zinc.

Basic Concepts

AA is an optical technique in which an element in the sample is excited and the radiant energy produced is measured as the element returns to its lower energy level. However, the element is not appreciably excited in the flame but is merely dissociated from its chemical bonds (atomized) and placed in an unexcited or ground state (neutral atom). Thus, the atom is at a low energy level, at which it is capable of absorbing radiation at a very narrow bandwidth corresponding to its own line spectrum. A hollow-cathode lamp with the cathode made of the material to be analyzed is used to produce a wavelength of light specific for the material. Thus, if the cathode was made of calcium, calcium light at predominantly 423 nm would be emitted by the lamp. When the light from the hollow-cathode lamp enters the flame, some of it is absorbed by the ground-state atoms in the flame, resulting in a net decrease in the intensity of the beam from the lamp. This process is referred to as *atomic absorption.* Owing to the unique specificity of the wavelength from the hollow-cathode lamp, these methods are highly specific for the element being measured.

Instrumentation

The components of an AA spectrophotometer are shown in Figure 9-8. A hollow-cathode lamp serves as the light source for an AA spectrophotometer. Such lamps are made of the metal of the substance to be analyzed; this is different for each metal analysis. When an alloy is used to make the cathode, the result is a multielement lamp.

With *flameless AA* techniques (carbon rod or "graphite furnace"), the sample is placed in a depression on a carbon rod in an enclosed chamber. Strips of tantalum or platinum metal are used as sample cups. In successive steps, the temperature of the rod is raised to dry, char, and finally atomize the sample in the chamber. The atomized element then absorbs energy from the corresponding hollow-cathode lamp. This approach is very sensitive and permits determination of trace metals in small samples of blood or tissue.

With flameless AA, a novel approach called *the Zeeman correction* has been used to correct for background absorption.[10] With Zeeman background correction, the analyte is placed in a strong magnetic field. The intense magnetic field splits the degenerate (i.e., of equal energy) atomic energy levels of equal energy into two components that are polarized parallel and perpendicular to the magnetic field, respectively. The parallel component is at the resonance line of the source, whereas the two perpendicular components are shifted to different wavelengths. The two components interact differently with polarized light. A polarizer is placed between the source and the atomizer, and two absorption measurements are taken at different polarizer settings. One measures both analyte and background absorptions (A_t), the other only background absorption (A_{bc}). The difference between the two absorption readings is the corrected absorbance.

The major advantage of the Zeeman correction method is that the same light source at the same wavelength is used to measure total and background absorption. Implementation is complex and expensive, and the strength of the magnetic field needs to be optimized for every element, but the method gives more accurate results at higher background levels than are associated with other correction techniques.

Limitations of Atomic Absorption Spectrophotometry

Spectral and nonspectral interferences are limitations of AA spectroscopy.

Spectral Interferences
Spectral interferences include (1) absorption by other closely absorbing atomic species, (2) absorption by molecular species, (3) scattering by nonvolatile salt particles or oxides, and

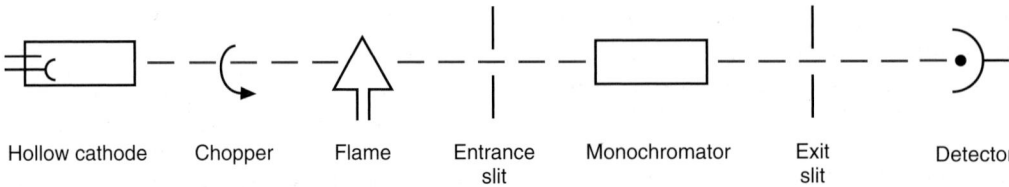

Hollow cathode   Chopper   Flame   Entrance slit   Monochromator   Exit slit   Detector

Figure 9-8 Basic components of an atomic absorption spectrophotometer.

(4) background emission (which is corrected for by electronic filtering). Absorption by other atomic species usually is not a problem because of the extremely narrow bandwidth (0.01 nm) used in absorption measurements. Absorption and scattering by molecular species are particularly problematic in lower atomizing temperatures.

Nonspectral Interferences

Nonspectral interferences may be nonspecific or specific. *Nonspecific interferences* affect nebulization by altering the (1) viscosity, (2) surface tension, or (3) density of the analyte solution, and consequently the sample flow rate. *Specific interferences* (chemical interferences) are analyte dependent. *Solute volatilization interference* refers to the situation in which the contaminant forms nonvolatile species with the analyte. An example is seen in phosphate interference in the determination of calcium that is caused by the formation of calcium-phosphate complexes. The phosphate interference is eliminated by adding a cation, usually lanthanum or strontium that competes with calcium for the phosphate. Enhancement effects are also observed, in which the addition of contaminants increases the volatilization efficiency. Such is the case with aluminum, which normally forms nonvolatile oxides but in the presence of hydrofluoric acid forms more volatile aluminum fluoride. *Dissociation interferences* affect the degree of dissociation of the analyte. Analytes that form oxides or hydroxides are especially susceptible to dissociation interferences. *Ionization interference* occurs when the presence of an easily ionized element, such as K, affects the degree of ionization of the analyte, which leads to changes in the analyte signal. In cases of *excitation interference*, the analyte atoms are excited in the atomizer, with subsequent emission at the absorption wavelength. This type of interference is more pronounced at higher temperatures.

Fluorometry

Fluorescence occurs when a molecule absorbs light at one wavelength and reemits light at a longer wavelength. An atom or molecule that fluoresces is termed a *fluorophore*. **Fluorometry** is defined as the measurement of emitted fluorescence light. Fluorometric analysis is a very sensitive and widely used method of quantitative analysis in the chemical and biological sciences.[5]

Basic Concepts

The relationship between (1) absorption, (2) fluorescence, and (3) phosphorescence is shown in Figure 9-9. As indicated, each molecule contains a series of closely spaced energy levels. Absorption of a quantum of light energy by a molecule causes the transition of an electron from the singlet ground state to one of a number of possible vibrational levels of its first singlet state. The actual number of molecules in the excited state under typical reaction conditions and excited with a typical 150-W light source is very small and is estimated to be about 10^{-13} mole per mole of fluorophore. Once the molecule is in an excited state, it returns to its original energy state by different mechanisms. These include (1) radiation-less vibrational

equilibration, (2) the fluorescence process, (3) quenching of the excited singlet state, (4) radiation-less crossover to a triplet state, (5) quenching of the first triplet state, and (6) the phosphorescence process.

As shown in Figure 9-9, vibrational equilibration before fluorescence results in some loss of excitation energy. The emitted fluorescence light is therefore of less energy or has a longer wavelength than the excitation light. The difference between the maximum wavelength of the excitation light and the maximum wavelength of the emitted fluorescence light is a constant referred to as the *Stokes shift*. This constant is a measure of energy lost during the lifetime of the excited state (radiation-less vibrational deactivation) before return to the ground singlet level (fluorescence emission).

Time Relationships of Fluorescence Emission

The time required for a molecule to absorb radiant energy and to be promoted to an excited state is approximately 10^{-15} s. The length of time needed for vibrational equilibration to occur to the lowest excited state is of the order of 10^{-14} to 10^{-12} s. The length of time required for fluorescence emission to occur is of the order of 10^{-8} to 10^{-7} s. Relatively speaking, there is a considerable time delay between (1) absorption of light energy, (2) return to the lowest excited state, and (3) emission of fluorescence light. This time relationship is shown in Figure 9-10. Phase I represents the time period between absorbance of light energy and radiation-less loss of energy during vibrational rearrangement to the lowest excited energy state. This time period is represented by the up and down arrows in the diagram. Phase II shows the emission and decay of a short-lived (b) and a longer-lived (a) fluorophore. If the fluorescence emission is measured over time following a pulse of light from an excitation source, such as a xenon lamp or laser, the intensity of the emitted light decays as a first-order process similar to radioactive decay. The time required for the emitted light to

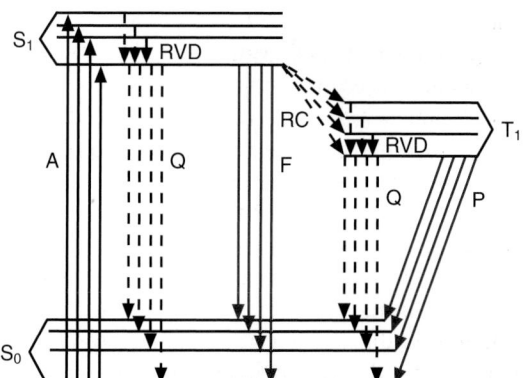

Figure 9-9 Luminescence energy-level diagram of typical organic molecule. S_0 is the ground level singlet state; S_1 is the first excited singlet state; *A* is the absorption process; T_1 is the first excited triplet state; and *RVD* is the radiation-less vibrational deactivation. *Q* is quenching of the excited singlet or triplet state. *F* is the fluorescence process from the first excited singlet state. *P* is the phosphorescence process from the first excited triplet state. *RC* is the radiation-less crossover from the first excited singlet state to the first excited triplet state.

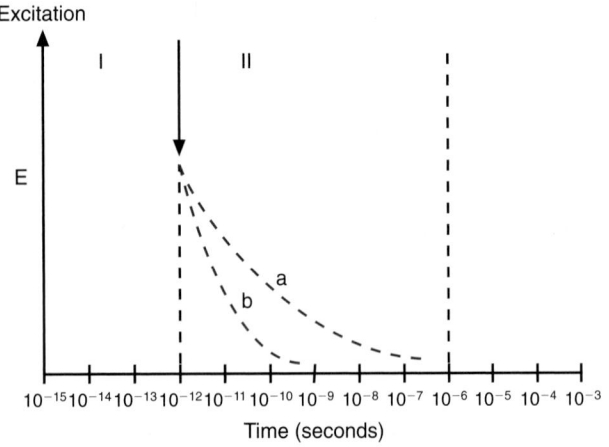

Figure 9-10 Fluorescence decay process: E is the absorption of energy; I is the vibrational deactivation time phase; II is the fluorescence emission time phase; a is long fluorescence decay time; and b is short fluorescence decay time.

reach $1/e$ of its initial intensity, where e is the Naperian base 2.718, is called the *average lifetime of the excited state of the molecule*, or the *fluorescence decay time*.

The time delay between absorption of quanta of energy and fluorescence used in fluorescence instrumentation is called a *time-resolved fluorometer*. Advantages of a time-resolved fluorometer include the elimination of background light scattering and background from short-lived fluorescence. This results in a consequent dramatic increase in the signal-to-noise ratio and detection sensitivity.

Depending on how the fluorescence emission response is measured, time-resolved fluorometry[3] is categorized as pulse or phase fluorometry. In pulse fluorometry, the sample is illuminated with an intense brief pulse of light, and the intensity of the resulting fluorescence emission is measured as a function of time with a fast detector system. In phase fluorometry, a continuous-wave laser illuminates the sample, and the fluorescence emission response is monitored for impulse and frequency response.[6]

Relationship of Concentration and Fluorescence Intensity

The relationship of concentration to the intensity of fluorescence emission is derived from Beer's law and is expressed as:

$$F = \Phi I_0 abc \qquad (9)$$

where

F = relative intensity;
Φ = fluorescence efficiency (i.e., the ratio between quanta of light emitted and quanta of light absorbed);
I_0 = initial excitation intensity;
a = molar absorptivity;
b = volume element defined by geometry of the excitation and emission slits; and
c = the concentration in mol/L.

Equation (9) indicates that fluorescence intensity is directly proportionate to the concentration of the fluorophore and the intensity of the excitation. This relationship holds only for dilute solutions in which absorbance is less than 2% of the exciting radiation. Above 2%, the fluorescence intensity becomes nonlinear. This phenomenon is called the *inner filter effect*, and it is discussed in greater detail in a later section. Other factors influencing the measurement of fluorescence intensity are the sensitivity of the detector and the degree of background light scatter seen by the detector.

Fluorescence intensity measurements are more sensitive than absorbance measurements. The magnitude of absorbance of a chromophore in solution is determined by its concentration and the path length of the cuvet. The magnitude of the fluorescence intensity of a fluorophore is determined by (1) its concentration, (2) the path length, and (3) the intensity of the light source. Comparatively, fluorescence measurements are 100 to 1000 times more sensitive than absorbance measurements. This is due to the use of (1) more intense light sources, (2) digital signal filtering techniques, and (3) sensitive emission photometers.

Frequently, fluorescence measurements are expressed in relative intensity units. The word *relative* is used because the intensity measured is not an absolute quantity. It is a small part of the total fluorescence emission, and its magnitude is defined by (1) instrument slit width, (2) detector sensitivity, (3) monochromator efficiency, and (4) excitation intensity. Because these are instrument-related variables, establishing an absolute intensity unit for a given concentration of a fluorophore that is valid from instrument to instrument is difficult, if not impossible.

Fluorescence Polarization

Light is composed of electrical and magnetic waves at right angles to each other. Light waves produced by standard excitation sources have their electrical vectors oriented randomly. Light waves passed through certain crystalline materials (polarizers) have their electrical vectors oriented in a single plane and are said to be plane-polarized. Fluorophores absorb light most efficiently in the plane of their electronic energy levels. If their rotational relaxation (Brownian movement) is slower than their fluorescence decay time, as is the case for large fluorescent-labeled molecules, the emitted fluorescence light will be polarized. Because small molecules have rotational relaxation times that are much shorter than their fluorescence decay time, their emitted fluorescence light is depolarized. However, if the small fluorescent molecule is attached to a macromolecule, or if it is placed in a viscous solution, the small molecule will emit polarized light. Fluorescence polarization, P, is defined by the following equation:

$$P = \frac{I_v - I_h}{I_v + I_h} \qquad (10)$$

where

I_v = intensity of emitted fluorescence light in the vertical plane; and

I_h = intensity of emitted fluorescence light in the horizontal plane.

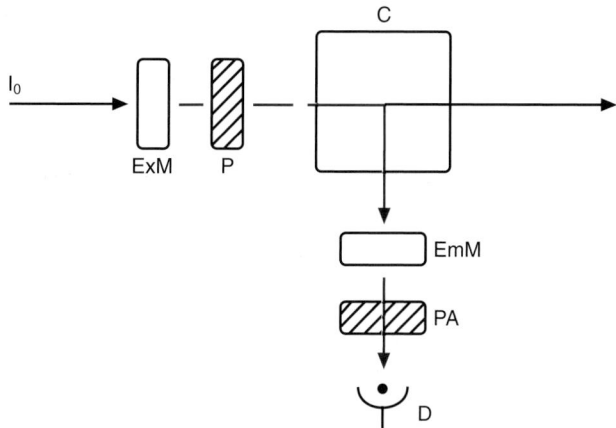

Figure 9-11 Schematic diagram of a fluorescence polarization analyzer. I_0 is the intensity of excitation light. P is the polarizer to provide polarized excitation light. PA is the polarizer analyzer, which is rotated to provide the measurement of parallel and perpendicular polarized fluorescence-emission intensity. ExM is the excitation monochromator, EmM is the emission monochromator, D is the detector, and C is the reaction cell or cuvet.

As indicated, P is the difference between the two observed intensities divided by their sum. Fluorescence polarization is measured by placing a mechanically or electrically driven polarizer between the sample cuvet and the detector. A diagram of a fluorescence polarization measurement system is shown in Figure 9-11. In the normal instrumentation mode, the sample is excited with polarized light to obtain maximum sensitivity. First, the polarization analyzer is positioned to measure the intensity of emitted fluorescence light in the vertical plane (I_v), and then the polarization analyzer is rotated 90° to measure emitted fluorescence light intensity in the horizontal plane (I_h). P is then calculated manually or automatically by using Equation (10).

Fluorescence polarization is used to quantitate analytes by using the change in fluorescence depolarization following immunologic reactions (see Chapter 15). Quantitation is accomplished by adding a known quantity of fluorescent-labeled analyte molecules to a reaction solution containing an antibody specific to the analyte. The labeled analyte binds to the antibody, resulting in a change in its rotational relaxation time and fluorescence polarization. The addition of a nonlabeled analyte, such as an unknown quantity of a therapeutic drug in a serum specimen, will result in competition for binding to the antibody with the fluorescent-labeled analyte. This change in binding of the fluorophore-labeled analyte causes a change in fluorescence polarization that is inversely proportional to the amount of analyte contained in a given sample. Because the change in fluorescence polarization is a direct response to the reaction mixture, the bound fluorophore need not be separated from free fluorophore. Thus fluorescence polarization is applicable to homogeneous assays of low-molecular-weight analytes, such as therapeutic drugs.[7]

Instrumentation

Fluorometers and spectrofluorometers are used to measure fluorescence. Operationally, a fluorometer uses interference

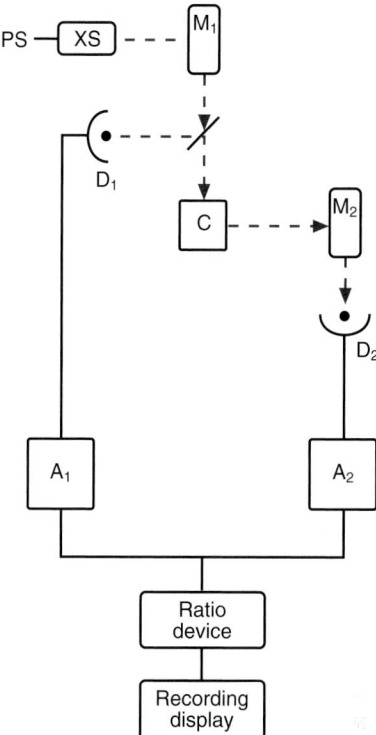

Figure 9-12 Block diagram of a typical spectrofluorometer: XS is the xenon source; PS is the power supply; M_1 is the excitation monochromator; C is the sample cell; M_2 is the emission monochromator. D_1 and D_2 are detectors; D_1 monitors the variation in excitation intensity, and D_2 measures fluorescence emission intensity. A_1 and A_2 are excitation signal and emission signal amplifiers, respectively.

filters or glass filters to produce monochromatic light for sample excitation and for isolation of fluorescence emission, whereas a spectrofluorometer uses a grating or prism monochromator.

Components

Basic components of fluorometers and spectrofluorometers include (1) an excitation source, (2) an excitation monochromator, (3) a cuvet, (4) an emission monochromator, and (5) a detector. In Figure 9-12, these components are shown as they would be configured in a 90° optical system.

With fluorometers and spectrofluorometers, placement of the cuvet and the excitation beam relative to the photodetector is critical in establishing the optical geometry for fluorescence measurements. As fluorescence light is emitted in all directions from a molecule, several excitation/emission geometries are used to measure fluorescence (Figure 9-13). Most commercial spectrofluorometers and fluorometers use the right angle detector approach because it minimizes the background signal that limits analytical detection. The end-on approach allows the adaptation of a fluorescence detector to existing 180° absorption instruments. Its limit of detection is restricted by (1) the quality of the excitation and/or emission interference filter pair, (2) the excitation and/or emission spectral band overlap, and (3) the inner filter effect that is discussed later. The front surface approach provides the greatest linearity over a broad range of concentration because it minimizes the

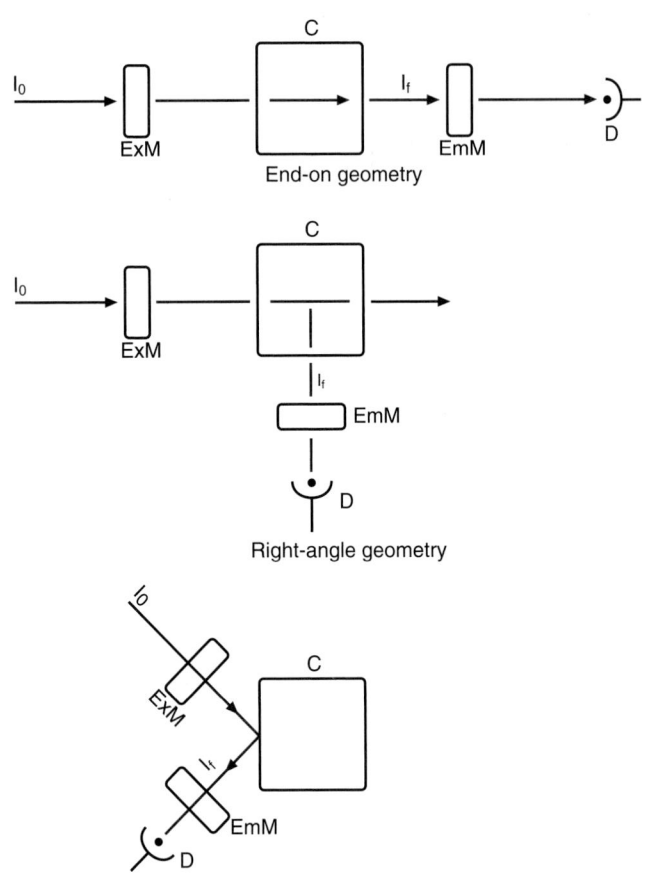

Figure 9-13 Fluorescence excitation/emission geometries: I_0 is the initial excitation energy; *ExM* is the excitation monochromator; *C* is the sample cuvet; I_f is the fluorescence intensity; *EmM* is the emission monochromator; and *D* is the detector.

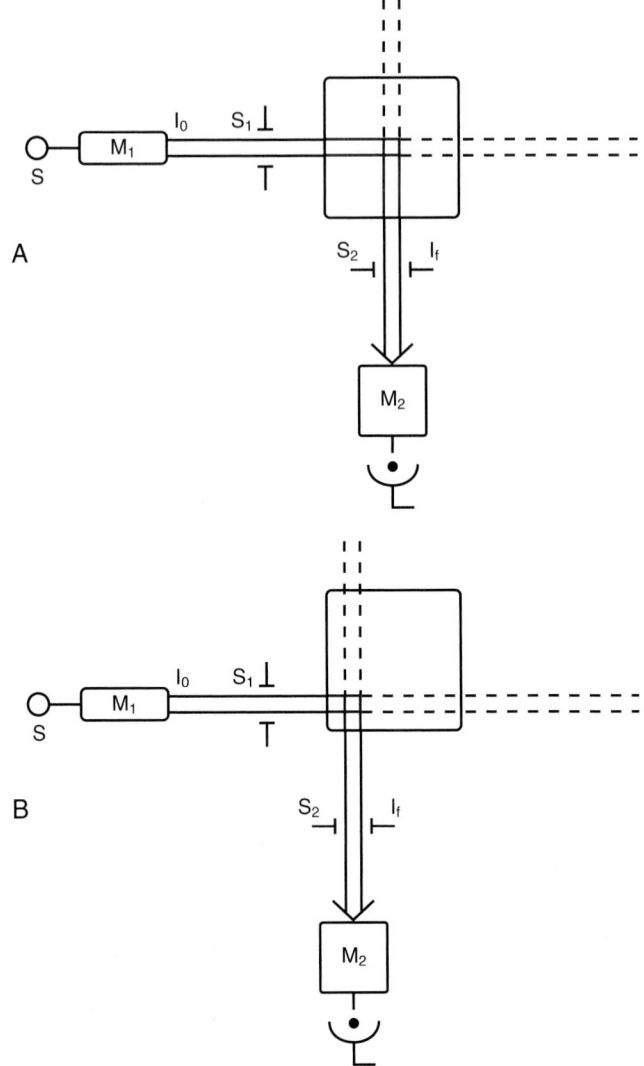

Figure 9-14 Two right-angle fluorescence sample cuvet positions. A shows the standard 90° configuration. B shows the offset positioning of the cuvet to minimize the inner filter effect.

inner filter effect. The front surface approach has a comparable limit of detection to right angle detectors but is more susceptible to background light scatter. Front surface fluorometry has been widely applied to heterogeneous solid phase fluorescence immunoassay systems.

To accommodate these different geometries, the sample cell is oriented at different angles in relation to the excitation source and the detector. Major concerns related to the geometry of the sample cell are (1) light scattering, (2) the inner filter effect, and (3) the sample volume element seen by the detector. Figure 9-14 shows the sample cell and slit arrangement for a conventional fluorescence spectrophotometer with excitation and emission slits oriented at a right angle. S_1 and S_2 designate the excitation and emission slits, respectively. The position of the emission slit and the width of the slit are important. If the emission slit is located near the front edge of the sample cell, as shown in Figure 9-14, *B*, the inner filter effect is minimized. If the emission slit width is increased, the detector will be more sensitive, but specificity may decrease.

Performance Verification

As with spectrophotometers, NIST provides a number of SRMs for use in calibration or verification of the performance of fluorometers or fluorospectrophotometers. These include SRM

936a (quinine sulfate dihydrate) for calibrating such instruments and SRM 1932 (fluorescein) for establishing a reference scale for fluorescence measurements (see http://www.nist.gov; accessed July 21, 2013).

Types of Fluorometers and Spectrofluorometers

Fluorometers and fluorescence spectrophotometers are available that offer a variety of features. These features include (1) ratio referencing, (2) computer-controlled excitation and emission monochromators, (3) pulsed xenon light sources, (4) photon counting, (5) a rhodamine cell for corrected spectra, (6) polarizers, (7) flow cells, (8) front surface viewing adapters, (9) multiple cell holders, and (10) computer-based data reduction systems.

In addition to the basic spectrofluorometer discussed earlier (see Figure 9-12), other types of fluorometric instruments include (1) a ratio-referencing spectrofluorometer, (2) a time-resolved fluorometer, (3) a flow cytometer, and (4) a hematofluorometer.

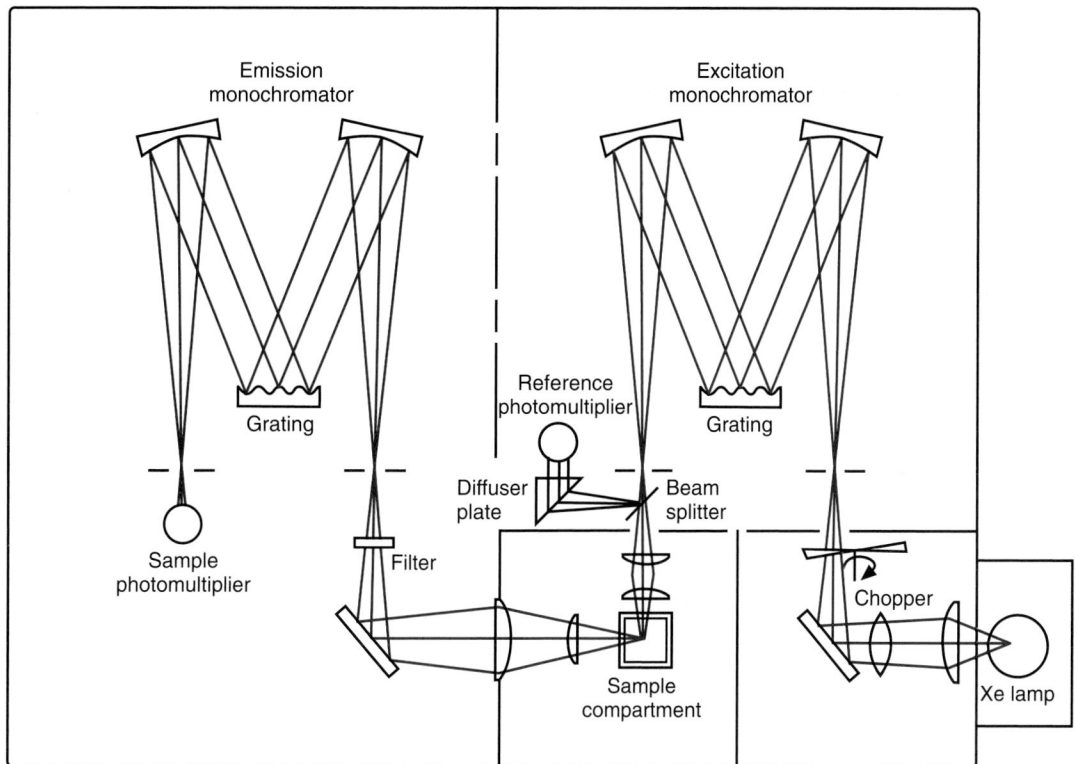

Figure 9-15 Diagram of a typical ratio-referencing spectrofluorometer.

Ratio-Referencing Spectrofluorometer

A typical ratio-referencing spectrofluorometer is illustrated in Figure 9-15. Basically, this is a simple right-angle instrument that uses two monochromators (M1 and M2), two PMT detectors (D1 and D2, the reference and sample PMTs), and a xenon lamp source. The light from the exciter monochromator (M1) is split, and a small portion (10%) is directed to the reference PMT (D1) for ratio-referencing purposes. The remaining excitation light is focused into the sample cuvet (C). Emission optics are positioned at a right angle to the excitation optics. An emission monochromator (M2) is used to select or scan the desired portion of the emission spectra, which is directed to the sample PMT (D2) for measurement of emission intensity. The output signals from the reference and from the sample PMTs are amplified (A1 and A2), and a ratio of the sample to the reference signal is provided by a digital display or a chart recorder. The operational mode of a ratio fluorometer is similar to that of a spectrofluorometer; however, only discrete excitation and emission wavelengths are available, and the use of this type of instrument is precluded from scanning fluorophores to obtain emission and excitation spectra. The ratio filter fluorometer is most useful for obtaining concentration measurements at defined excitation and emission wavelengths.

The ratio-referencing spectrofluorometer is operated at fixed excitation and emission wavelength settings for concentration measurements, or it is used to measure the excitation or emission spectrum of a given compound. Measurement of the concentration of unknowns is accomplished in a similar manner as with a single-beam fluorometer. A blank solution

and a calibrating solution are first measured, and then the unknown samples are measured. The ratio-referencing spectrofluorometer in Figure 9-15 provides two advantages over single-beam spectrofluorometers. First, it eliminates short- and long-term xenon lamp energy fluctuations (i.e., arc flicker and lamp decay), thus minimizing the need for frequent calibration of the instrument during analysis. Second, it provides "essentially" corrected excitation spectra by compensating for wavelength-dependent energy fluctuations.

Time-Resolved Fluorometers

The time-resolved fluorometer was introduced in the mid-1970s, when Weider developed a pulsed nitrogen laser fluorometer in conjunction with a lanthanide-based immunoassay system. This instrument measured fluorescence decay of lanthanide chelates as a means of eliminating background interferences from light scatter and short decay time fluorescence compounds. The time-resolved fluorometer[3] is similar to the ratio-referencing fluorometer, with the exception that the light source is pulsed[9] and the detector monitors, in a fast photon-counting mode, the exponential decay of the fluorescence signal after excitation. Time-resolved fluorometry requires the use of long-lived fluorophores, such as the lanthanide (rare earth) metal ions europium (Eu^{3+}) and samarium (Sm^{3+}). Whereas most fluorescence compounds have decay times of 5 to 100 ns, europium chelates decay in 0.6 to 100 s. Thus time-resolved fluorescence assays take advantage of the difference in the lifetimes of fluorophore and background fluorescence by measuring the decaying fluorescence signal. This eliminates background interferences and at the same time averages the signal to improve the precision of measurement. Detection limits of approximately 10^{-13} mol/L have been achieved with time-resolved fluorometry, for an improvement of about four orders of magnitude compared with conventional fluorometric measurements. For example, Eu^{3+}-labeled nanoparticles in combination with time-resolved fluorometry have been used to develop a highly sensitive immunoassay for free and total prostate-specific antigen with a functional sensitivity of 0.5 ng/L.[11]

Flow Cytometer

Cytometry refers to the measurement of physical and/or chemical characteristics of cells or particles. **Flow cytometry** is a process in which such measurements are made while cells or particles pass, preferably in single file, through the measuring apparatus in a fluid stream. Flow sorting extends flow cytometry by using electrical or mechanical means to divert and collect cells with one or more measured characteristics falling within a range or a ranges of values set by the user.[8,9]

Operationally, flow cytometry combines laser-induced fluorometry and particle light-scattering analysis that allow different populations of (1) molecules, (2) cells, or (3) particles to be differentiated by size and shape using low-light and right-angle light scattering. The use of a laser is ideally suited for low-angle light scattering. These cells, molecules, or particles are labeled with different specific fluorescent labels, such as (1) β-phycoerythrin, (2) fluorescein isothiocyanate, (3) rhodamine-6G, and (4) dye-labeled antibodies. As these elements flow through the flow cell, simultaneous fluorescence and light-scattering measurements are automatically performed by the flow cytometer. Most flow cytometers incorporate two or more fluorescence emission detection systems so that multiple fluorescent labels are able to be used. In this manner, molecules, cells, and particles are classified by (1) size, (2) shape, and (3) type according to their light-scattering and fluorescent properties. A schematic diagram of a flow cytometer is shown in Figure 9-16.

Flow cytometers are able to measure multiple parameters, including (1) cell size (forward scatter), (2) granularity (90° scatter), (3) DNA and RNA content, (4) DNA (AT)/(GC) nucleotide ratios, (5) chromatin structure, (6) antigens, (7) total protein content, (8) cell receptors, (9) membrane potential, and (10) calcium ion concentration as a function of pH. Of particular note have been the development and use of particle-based flow cytometric assays. With this technology, a flow cytometer is combined with microspheres that are used as the solid support for conventional immunoassay, affinity assay, or DNA hybridization assay.[14] The resultant system is very flexible and has led to the development of multiplexed assays that simultaneously measure many different analytes in a small sample volume.

Hematofluorometer

The *hematofluorometer* is a single-channel front surface photofluorometer dedicated to the analysis of zinc protoporphyrin in whole blood (see Chapter 29). A typical hematofluorometer uses a quartz-tungsten lamp, a narrow-bandpass excitation filter (420 nm), front surface optics, a narrow-bandpass filter (594 nm), and a PMT. A drop of whole blood is placed on a small rectangular glass slide that serves as a cuvet.

Limitations of Fluorescence Measurements

Factors that influence fluorescence measurements include (1) concentration effects (e.g., inner filter effect, concentration quenching), (2) background effects (due to Rayleigh and Raman scattering), (3) solvent effects (e.g., interfering nonspecific fluorescence, quenching from the solvent), (4) sample effects (e.g., light scattering, interfering fluorescence, sample adsorption), (5) temperature effects, and (6) photodecomposition (bleaching) of the sample.

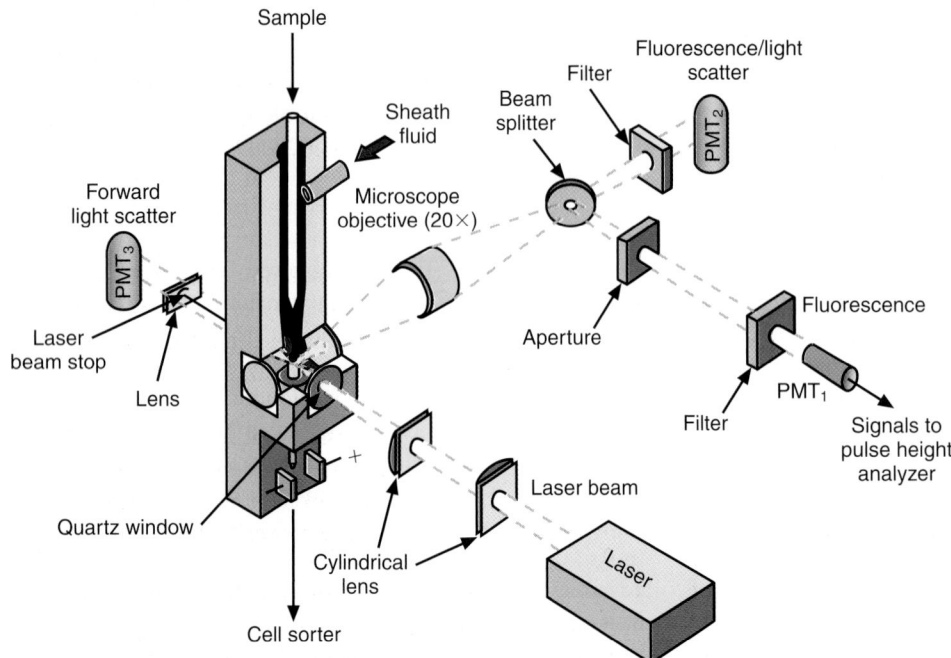

Figure 9-16 Schematic diagram of a flow cytometer.

Inner Filter Effect

The linear relationship between concentration and fluorescence emission (Equation 9) is valid when solutions absorb less than 2% of the exciting light. As the absorbance of the solution increases above this amount, the relationship becomes nonlinear—a phenomenon known as the *inner filter effect*. It is caused by loss of excitation intensity across the cuvet path length as excitation light is absorbed by the fluorophore. Thus, as the fluorophore becomes more concentrated, absorbance of excitation intensity increases, and loss of excitation light as it travels through the cuvet increases. This effect is most often encountered with a right-angle fluorescence instrument, in which the emission slits are set to monitor the center of the sample cell, where absorbance of excitation light is greater than at the front surface of the cuvet. Therefore it is less problematic if a front surface fluorescence instrument is used. However, most fluorescence measurements are made on very dilute solutions, and the inner filter effect therefore is not a problem.

Concentration Quenching

Another related phenomenon that results in a lower quantum yield than expected is called *concentration quenching*. This occurs when a macromolecule, such as an antibody, is heavily labeled with a fluorophore, such as fluorescein isothiocyanate. When this compound is excited, the fluorescence labels are in such close proximity that a radiation-less energy transfer occurs. Thus the resulting fluorescence is much lower than expected for the concentration of the label. This is a common problem in flow cytometry and in laser-induced fluorescence when attempts are made to enhance detection sensitivity by increasing the density of the fluorescing label.

Light Scattering

Light scattering—Rayleigh and Raman—limits the use of fluorescence measurements. Rayleigh scattering occurs with no change in wavelength. For fluorophores with small Stokes shifts, the excitation and emission spectra overlap and are particularly susceptible to loss of detection caused by background light scatter. Rayleigh scatter is controlled by the use of well-defined emission and excitation interference filters or by appropriate monochromator settings and the use of polarizers.

Raman scattering occurs with lengthening of wavelength. This type of light scattering is independent of excitation wavelength and is a property of the solvent. Because Raman light scattering appears at longer wavelengths than the exciting radiation, it is a difficult interference to eliminate when working at very low fluorophore concentrations.

Cuvet Material and Solvent Effects

Certain quartz glass and plastic materials that contain ultraviolet absorbers will fluoresce. Some solvents, such as ethanol, are also known to cause appreciable fluorescence. It is therefore important when developing a fluorescence assay to assess the background fluorescence of all components of the reaction mixture. Fluorescence grade solvents and cuvets with minimum fluorescence emission, which minimize these types of fluorescence background problems, are commercially available.

Sample Matrix Effects

A serum or urine sample contains many compounds that fluoresce. Thus the sample matrix is a potential source of unwanted background fluorescence and must be examined when new methods are developed. The most serious contributors to unwanted fluorescence are proteins and bilirubin. However, because protein excitation maxima are in the spectral region of 260 to 290 nm, their contribution to overall background fluorescence is minor when excitation occurs above 300 nm.

Light scattering of proteins and other macromolecules in the sample matrix has been known to cause unwanted background fluorescence. Lipemic samples, for example, are noted for their intense light scattering, and the relative contribution of lipids to the background signal of a fluorescence measurement should be investigated when a new method is developed.

In addition to background interferences, dilute solutions of some fluorophores in the concentration range of 10^{-9} mol/L and below will absorb to the walls of glass cuvets and other reaction vessels. Also, dilute solutions of fluorophores, when excited over long periods, are susceptible to photodecomposition by intense excitation light. Operationally, these problems are prevented by (1) selecting proper reaction vessels, (2) adding wetting agents, and (3) minimizing the length of time a sample is exposed to the excitation light.

Temperature Effects

The fluorescence quantum efficiency of many compounds is sensitive to temperature fluctuations. Therefore the temperature of the reaction must be regulated to within ±0.1 °C. In general, fluorescence intensity decreases with increasing temperature by approximately 1% to 5% per degree Celsius. Furthermore, collisional quenching decreases with increasing viscosity, thereby reducing the quenching of fluorescence. Operationally, fluorescence intensity is enhanced by increasing reaction viscosity or lowering solvent temperature. Temperature effects are minimized by controlling reaction temperature and warming samples or reagents, or both, if they have been refrigerated.

Photodecomposition

In conventional **fluorometry**, excitation of weakly fluorescing or dilute solutions with intense light sources will cause photochemical decomposition of the analyte (photobleaching).

The following steps help to minimize photodecomposition effects:

1. Always use the longest feasible wavelength for excitation that does not introduce light-scattering effects.
2. Decrease the duration of excitation of the sample by measuring the fluorescence intensity immediately after excitation.
3. Protect unstable solutions from ambient light by storing them in dark bottles.
4. Remove dissolved oxygen from the solution.

In addition, highly intense laser light sources with energy output greater than 5 to 10 mW will rapidly photodecompose some fluorescence analytes. This decomposition introduces nonlinear response curves and loss of most of the sample fluorescence. Fluorescence-based assays for analytes at ultralow concentrations require optimization of laser intensity and use of a sensitive detector. Assays with high energy, photodecomposing light sources include (1) flow cytometry, (2) fluorescence microscopy, and (3) laser-induced fluorescence measurements. This decomposition introduces nonlinear response curves and loss of sample fluorescence. Fluorescence-based assays for analytes at ultralow concentrations require optimization of laser intensity and use of a sensitive detector.

Phosphorimetry

Phosphorimetry is the measurement of phosphorescence, a type of luminescence produced by certain substances after radiant energy or other types of energy are absorbed. Phosphorescence is distinguished from fluorescence in that it continues even after the radiation causing it has ceased. The decay time of emission of phosphorescence light is longer (10^{-4} to 10^{-2} s) than the decay time of fluorescence emission. Decay times are expressed in a time range of several orders of magnitude and vary with the molecule and its solution environment. Phosphorescence shows a larger shift in emitted light wavelength than does fluorescence.

Luminometry

Chemiluminescence, bioluminescence, and **electrochemiluminescence** are types of luminescence in which the excitation event is caused by a chemical, biochemical, or electrochemical reaction, and not by photo illumination. Instruments for measuring this type of light emission are known generically as luminometers.

Basic Concepts

The physical event of light emission in (1) chemiluminescence, (2) bioluminescence, and (3) electrochemiluminescence is similar to fluorescence in that it occurs from an excited singlet state, and the light is emitted when the electron returns to the ground state.

Chemiluminescence and Bioluminescence

Chemiluminescence is the emission of light when an electron returns from an excited or higher energy level to a lower energy level. The excitation event is caused by a chemical reaction with compound such as (1) luminol, (2) isoluminol, (3) acridinium esters, (4) luciferin, (5) hydrogen peroxide, (6) hypochlorite, and (7) oxygen. Light is emitted from the excited product formed in the oxidation reaction. These reactions occur in the presence of catalysts such as (1) enzymes (e.g., alkaline phosphatase, horseradish peroxidase, microperoxidase), (2) metal ions or metal complexes (e.g., Cu^{2+} and Fe^{3+} phthalocyanine complex), and (3) hemin.[2,15]

Bioluminescence is a special form of chemiluminescence found in biological systems. In bioluminescence, an enzyme or a photoprotein increases the efficiency of the luminescence reaction. Luciferase and aequorin are two examples of these biological catalysts. The quantum yield (e.g., total photons emitted per total molecules reacting) is approximately 0.1% to 10% for chemiluminescence and 10% to 30% for bioluminescence.

Chemiluminescence assays are ultrasensitive (attomole-to-zeptomole detection limits) and have wide dynamic ranges. They are now widely used in automated immunoassay and DNA probe assay systems such as (1) acridinium ester and acridinium sulfonamide labels, (2) 1,2-dioxetane substrates for alkaline phosphatase labels, and (3) the enhanced luminol reaction for horseradish peroxidase labels.

Electrochemiluminescence

Electrochemiluminescence differs from chemiluminescence in that the reactive species that produce the chemiluminescent reaction are electrochemically generated from stable precursors at the surface of an electrode.[1] A ruthenium (Ru^{2+}), tris(bipyridyl) chelate is the most commonly used electrochemiluminescence label, and electrochemiluminescence is generated at an electrode via an oxidation reduction type of reaction with tripropylamine. This chelate is very stable and relatively small and has been used to label haptens or large molecules (e.g., proteins, oligonucleotides). The electrochemiluminescence process has been used in both immunoassays and nucleic acid assays. Advantages of this process include (1) improved reagent stability, (2) simple reagent preparation, and (3) enhanced sensitivity. With its use, detection limits of 200 fmol/L and a dynamic range extending over six orders of magnitude have been obtained.

Instrumentation

The basic components of a luminometer include (1) the sample cell housed in a light-tight chamber, (2) the injection system for adding reagents to the sample cell, and (3) the detector.[2,15] The detector is usually a PMT. However, (1) a charged coupled detector (CCD—multichannel device), (2) x-ray film, or (3) photographic film has been used to image bioluminescence or chemiluminescence reactions on a membrane or in the wells of a microplate. For electrochemiluminescence, the reaction vessel incorporates an electrode at which the electrochemiluminescence is generated.

Limitations of Chemiluminescence, Bioluminescence, and Electrochemiluminescence Measurements

Factors that commonly degrade the analytical performance of luminescence measurements include (1) light leaks, (2) light piping, (3) and high background luminescence from assay reagents and reaction vessels (e.g., plastic tubes exposed to light). The ultrasensitive nature of chemiluminescence assays requires stringent controls on the purity of reagents and the solvents (e.g., water) used to prepare reagent solutions. Efficient capture of the light emission from reactions that produce a flash of light requires an efficient injector that provides adequate mixing when the triggering reagent is added to the reaction vessel. Bioluminescence, chemiluminescence, and electrochemiluminescence assays have a wide linear range, usually including several orders of magnitude, but very high-intensity light emission has led to pulse pileup in PMT tubes, and this may lead to a serious underestimation of the true light emission intensity.

Nephelometry and Turbidimetry

Light scattering is a physical phenomenon that results from the interaction of light with particles in solution. **Nephelometry** and **turbidimetry** are analytical techniques that are used to measure scattered light. Light-scattering measurements have been applied to immunoassays of specific proteins and haptens.

Basic Concepts

Light scattering occurs when radiant energy passing through a solution encounters a molecule in an elastic collision, which results in scattering of light in all directions. Unlike fluorescence emission, the wavelength of the scattered light is the same as that of the incident light.

Factors that influence light scattering include (1) effect of particle size, (2) wavelength dependence, (3) distance of observation, (4) effect of polarization of incident light, (5) concentration of the particles, and (6) molecular weight of the particles.

Particle Size

The Rayleigh scattering Equation (11) presented below applies to the scattering of light from small particles with much smaller dimensions than the wavelength of incident light (e.g., particle size $< \lambda/10$). When the dimensions of the particles are much smaller than the wavelength of the incident light, each particle is subjected to the same electrical field strength at the same time. The reradiated or scattered light waves from the small particle are in phase and reinforce each other. As the particles become larger than the incident light wave, the radiated light waves are no longer all in phase. Reinforcement of radiation occurs in some directions, and destructive interference occurs in others. The scattering patterns from these large particles are characteristic of the size and shape of the particle.

Wavelength Dependence of Light Scattering

In 1871 Lord Rayleigh derived the following equation, which demonstrates the relationship of the intensity (I_S) of scattered light to the intensity (I_0) of incident light:

$$\frac{I_S}{I_0} = \frac{16\pi^2 a \sin^2\theta}{\lambda^4 r^2} \tag{11}$$

where

I_S = intensity of scattered light;
I_0 = intensity of excitation light;
a = polarizability of the small particle;
θ = angle of observation;

λ = wavelength of incident light; and
r = distance from light scattering to the detector.

As indicated, the intensity of light scattering increases by the fourth power of the wavelength as the wavelength of the incident light is decreased. Another useful observation from Equation (11) is the fact that light intensity decreases by the square of the distance r from the light-scattering particles to the detector. Thus the detector should be located close to the analytical cell by combining the cell and the detector or by using good collection optics.

Concentration and Molecular Weight Factors in Light Scattering

The direct relationship of light scattering to the concentration of the particles and to the molecular weight of the particles is derived from Equation (11), showing that:

$$\frac{I}{I_0} = \frac{4\pi^2 (dn/dc)^2 Mc \sin^2\theta}{N_a \lambda^4 r^2} \tag{12}$$

where

I = intensity of scattered light from small particles excited by polarized light;
I_0 = incident intensity;
dn/dc = change in refractive index of the solvent with respect to change in solute concentration;
M = molecular weight (g/mol);
c = concentration (g/mL) of the particles;
θ = angle of observation;
N_a = Avogadro's number;
λ = wavelength of the incident light; and
r = distance from light scattering to the detector.

As indicated in Equation (12), there is a direct relationship of light scattering to the concentrations of particles and to their molecular weight.[13]

The Effect of Polarized Light on Light Scattering

Equations (11) and (12) are different forms of the Rayleigh expression for light scattering from small particles if excited by polarized light. Figure 9-17, *A*, shows the effects of polarized and nonpolarized light on light-scattering intensity from small particles as a function of the scattering angle. Curve 2 shows a spherically symmetrical intensity diagram as predicted by Equation (11). Curve 3 is the resultant intensity diagram when Curves 1 and 2 are summed and is the scattering angular intensity diagram obtained when light scatters from small particles excited with nonpolarized light. Curves 1 and 2 represent intensity diagrams from vertically and horizontally polarized light components that are considered to comprise nonpolarized light. The Rayleigh light-scattering expression for small particles excited by nonpolarized light is given by Equation (13):

$$\frac{I}{I_0} = \frac{2\pi^2 (dn/dc)^2 Mc (1 + \cos\theta)}{N_a \lambda^4 r^2} \tag{13}$$

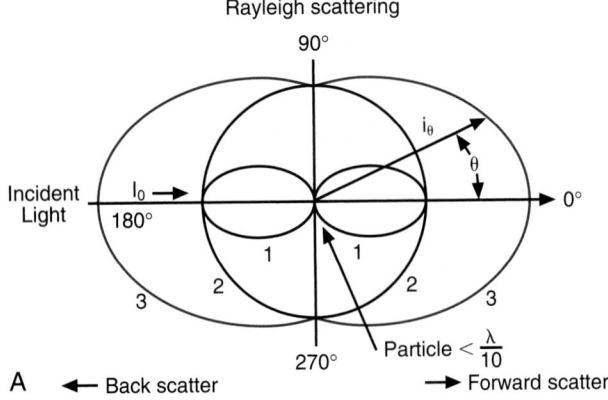

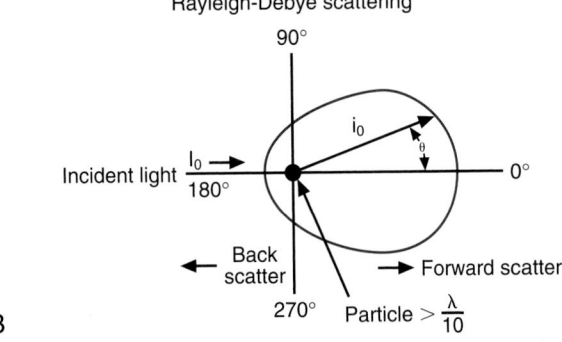

Figure 9-17 The angular dependence of light-scattering intensity with nonpolarized and polarized incident light for small particles **(A)** and the angular dependence of light scattering with nonpolarized light for larger particles **(B)**.

The Angular Dependence of Light Scattering

The angular dependence of light scattering from small particles (less than $\lambda/10$) is represented by Figure 9-17, *A*. As shown in Curve 3, the light scatter intensity for forward scatter and back scatter (I_0 at 0° and 180°) from small particles excited by nonpolarized light is equal. However, light scatter intensity at 90° is much less. As particles become larger (e.g., greater than $\lambda/10$), the angular dependence of light scatter takes on the dissymmetrical relationship shown in Figure 9-17, *B*. In this situation, the light-scattering intensities at forward and back angles are not equal, and the forward-scatter intensity is much greater. Also, the light-scattering intensity at 90° is much less than the intensity at the forward (0°) angle. As particles become even larger, this dissymmetry increases even further. This dissymmetry and the change in angular dependence of light scattering with change in the size of particles are very useful for characterization and differentiation of various classes of macromolecules and cells.

Measurement of Scattered Light

Turbidimetry and nephelometry are methods used to measure scattered light. These techniques have proved useful for the quantitation of serum proteins.

Turbidimetry

Turbidity decreases the intensity of the incident beam of light as it passes through a solution of particles. The measurement of this decrease in intensity is called *turbidimetry*. Analogous to absorption spectroscopy, turbidity is defined as:

$$I = I_0 e^{-bt} \tag{14}$$

or

$$t = \frac{1}{b} \ln \frac{I_0}{I} \tag{15}$$

where

t = turbidity;
b = path length of incident light through the solution of light-scattering particles;
I = intensity of transmitted light; and
I_0 = intensity of incident light.

A turbidimeter is used to measure the intensity of light scattering. Photometers or spectrophotometers are often used as turbidimeters, as turbidimetric measurements are easily performed on them and require little optimization. The principal concern of turbidimetric measurements is signal-to-noise ratio. Photometric systems with electro-optical noise in the range of ±0.0002 absorbance unit or less are useful for turbidity measurements.

Nephelometry

Nephelometry is defined as the detection of light energy scattered or reflected toward a detector that is not in the direct path of the transmitted light. Common nephelometers measure scattered light at right angles to the incident light. Some nephelometers are designed to measure scattered light at an angle other than 90° to take advantage of the increased forward-scatter intensity caused by light scattering from larger particles (e.g., immune complexes).

Fluorometers are often used to perform nephelometric measurements. However, the angular dependence of light-scattering intensity has resulted in the design of special nephelometers. These devices place the PMT detector at appropriate angles to the excitation light beam. The design principle of a nephelometer is similar to the design principle applied in fluorescence measurements. The major operational difference between the fluorometer and the nephelometer is that the excitation and detection wavelengths of a nephelometer will be set to the same value. The principal parameters of light scatter instrumentation are (1) excitation intensity, (2) wavelength, (3) distance of the detector from the sample cuvet, and (4) minimization of external stray light. As shown in Figure 9-18, the basic components of a nephelometer include (1) a light source, (2) collimating optics, (3) a sample cell, and (4) collection optics, which include light-scattering optics, a detector optical filter, and a detector. The schematic diagram also shows the different angles from the incident light beam where the detector, filter, and optics are placed to measure light scattering. Figure 9-18, *a*, shows the straight-through arrangement for turbidimetry, whereas Figure 9-18, *b* and *c*, shows arrangements frequently found in nephelometers. The detector arrangement shown in Figure 9-18, *b*, is used for measurement of

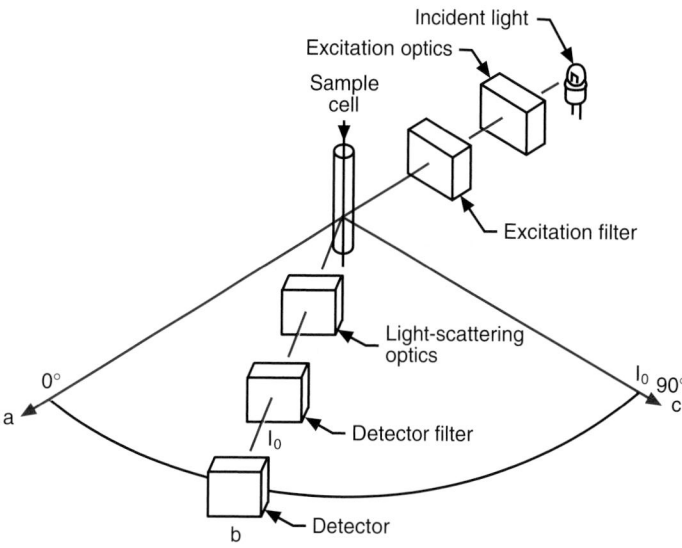

Figure 9-18 Schematic diagram of light-scattering instrumentation shows **(a)** the optics position for a turbidimeter; **(b)** the optics position for a forward-scattering nephelometer; and **(c)** the optics position for a right-angle nephelometer.

(a) = 0° Turbidimeter

(b) = 30° Forward-scattering nephelometer

(c) = 90° Nephelometer

forward scatter at 30°—the optical arrangement used in some commercial nephelometers.

Operationally, the optical components used in turbidimeters and nephelometers are similar to those used in fluorometers or photometers. For example, the light sources commonly used are (1) quartz-halogen lamps, (2) xenon lamps, and (3) lasers. Helium-neon (He-Ne) lasers, which operate at 633 nm, have typically been used for light-scattering applications, such as (1) nephelometric (2) immunoassays, (3) particle size determination, and (4) particle shape determination. The laser beam is used specifically in some nephelometers because of its high intensity; in addition, the coherent nature of laser light makes it ideally suited for nephelometric applications. Ratio-referencing fluorometers are also well suited for nephelometric measurements.

Limitations of Light-Scattering Measurements

Antigen excess and matrix effects are limitations encountered in the use of turbidimeters and nephelometers for measurement of analytes of clinical interest.

Antigen Excess

Antigen-antibody reactions are complex and appear to result in a mixture of aggregate sizes. As turbidity increases during addition of antigen to antibodies, the signal increases to a maximum value and then decreases. The point at which the decrease begins marks the beginning of the phase of antigen excess; this phenomenon is explained in Chapter 15. Consequently, light-scattering methods for quantification of antigen-antibody reactions must provide a method for detecting antigen excess. The kinetics of immune complex formation measured by nephelometry or turbidimetry is sufficiently different in each of the three phases— (1) antibody excess, (2) equivalence, and (3) antigen excess—that computer algorithms have been developed to automatically flag antigen excess.[12]

Matrix Effects

Particles, solvent, and all serum macromolecules scatter light. Lipoproteins and chylomicrons in lipemic serum provide the highest background turbidity or nephelometric intensity. With appropriate dilutions, the relative intensity of light scattering from a lipemic sample is less than that from the antiserum blank. However, as the concentration of the antigen in serum decreases and correspondingly less dilute samples are used, the background interference from lipemic samples becomes greater. An effective method for minimizing this background interference is the use of rate measurements, for which the initial sample blank is eliminated.

Large particles, such as suspended dust, also cause significant background interference. This background interference is controlled by filtering all buffers and diluted antisera before analysis is attempted.

Review Questions

1. What units of measurement are traditionally applied when wavelengths in the electromagnetic spectrum are measured?
   a. Millimeters (mm)
   b. Centimeters (cm)
   c. Nanometers (nm)
   d. Micrometers (μm)
2. Oxidation of an organic compound with resultant light emission is known as:
   a. nephelometry.
   b. turbidimetry.
   c. chemiluminescence.
   d. fluorescence.
3. The expression of the relationship between the concentration of a substance in solution and absorbance of light by

that substance is referred to as Beer's law. This relationship is expressed in a formula as:

a. $\log (1/T)$.

b. $C = abc$.

c. $I_0/I_s \times 100$.

d. $A = abc$.

4. With regard to atomic absorption spectrophotometry (AAS):

a. the light source used emits a wide range of wavelengths.

b. the technique measures concentration through the detection of absorbance of electromagnetic radiation by the atoms of elements instead of compounds.

c. oxidation of an organic compound such as luminol induces an excited state and light is emitted when the electron returns to the ground state

d. the amount of light scattered at right angles to the incident light is directly proportional to the concentration of the analyte of interest.

5. Which component of a single-beam spectrophotometer isolates radiant energy of a specific wavelength and excludes that of other wavelengths?

a. Monochromator

b. Entrance slit

c. Cuvet

d. Light source

6. Measurement of the concentration of a substance that is performed by measuring the decreased intensity of light blocked by particles in solution at 180° from the source is called:

a. fluorometry.

b. atomic absorption.

c. turbidimetry.

d. nephelometry.

7. A solution that is identical to that of calibrating or unknown solutions except that the substance to be measured and that is used to set 100% T (zero absorbance) at the beginning of a photometric analysis is referred to as a:

a. standard solution.

b. calibrating solution.

c. reference blank.

d. reagent blank.

8. In a fluorescence measurement, if an excited macromolecule is heavily labeled by a fluorophore, the label could be in such close proximity to other fluorophores that the resulting fluorescence is much lower than expected. This limitation of fluorescence is referred to as:

a. light scattering.

b. concentration quenching.

c. solvent quenching.

d. the sample matrix effect.

9. In a flameless atomic absorption technique, the sample holder is typically a:

a. carbon rod in an enclosed chamber.

b. flame.

c. borosilicate glass cuvet.

d. reflective surface.

10. The bandwidth of the spectral absorbance curve of an absorbing substance at a point equal to one-half of the maximum absorbance is referred to as the:

a. standard curve.

b. bandpass filter.

c. natural bandwidth.

d. monochromatic bandwidth.

References

1. Blackburn GF, Shah HP, Kenten JH, et al. Electrochemiluminescence: development of immunoassays and DNA probe assays for clinical diagnostics. Clin Chem 1991;37:1534–9.

2. DeLuca M, McElroy WD. Bioluminescence and chemiluminescence, Part B. Methods in enzymology, volume 133. San Diego: Academic Press, 1986:1–649.

3. Diamandis E, Christopoulos TK. Europium chelate labels in time-resolved fluorescence immunoassays and DNA hybridization assays. Anal Chem 1990;62:1149A-57A.

4. Evenson ME. Spectrophotometric techniques. In: Burtis CA, Ashwood ER, eds. Tietz textbook of clinical chemistry, 3rd ed. Philadelphia: WB Saunders Co, 1999:75–93.

5. Gore MG, ed. Spectrophotometry and spectrofluorimetry: a practical approach, 2nd edition. London: Oxford University Press, 2000:1–368.

6. Heiftje GM, Vogelstein EE. A linear response theory approach to time-resolved fluorometry. In: Wehry EL, ed. Modern fluorescence spectroscopy, vol 4. New York: Plenum Press, 1981:25–50.

7. Jolley ME, Stroupe SD, Schwenzer KS, et al. Fluorescence polarization immunoassay. III. An automated system for therapeutic drug determination. Clin Chem 1981;27:1575–9.

8. Patrick CW. Clinical flow cytometry. MLO 2002;34:10–16.

9. Shapiro HM. Practical flow cytometry, 4th edition. Hoboken, NJ: John Wiley & Sons, 2003.

10. Slavin W. Atomic absorption spectroscopy: the present and future. Anal Chem 1982;54:685A-94A.

11. Soukka T, Antonen K, Harma H, et al. Highly sensitive immunoassay of free prostate-specific antigen in serum using Europium(III) nanoparticle label technology. Clin Chim Acta 2003;328:45–58.

12. Sternberg J. A rate nephelometer for measuring specific proteins by immunoprecipitin reactions. Clin Chem 1977;25:1456–64.

13. Tiffany TO. Fluorometry, nephelometry, and turbidimetry. In: Burtis CA, Ashwood ER, eds. Tietz textbook of clinical chemistry, 3rd edition. Philadelphia: WB Saunders Co, 1999:94–112.

14. Vignali DA. Multiplexed particle-based flow cytometric assays. J Immunol Methods 2000;243:244–55.

15. Ziegler MM, Baldwin TO, eds. Bioluminescence and chemiluminescence, Part C. Methods in enzymology, volume 305. San Diego: Academic Press, 2000:1–732.

Electrochemistry and Chemical Sensors*

Paul D'Orazio, Ph.D., and Mark E. Meyerhoff, Ph.D.

Objectives

1. Define the following:

Amperometry	Indicator electrode
Biosensor	Optode
Conductometry	Potentiometry
Coulometry	Reference electrode
Electrochemistry	Voltage potential
Electromotive force	Voltammetry

2. Describe the functions of the components of a basic electrochemical cell, including electrodes, filling solutions, and voltmeter.

3. State the principles and clinical applications of the following measurement techniques:

Voltammetry/Amperometry	Coulometry
Conductometry	Potentiometry

4. List three basic classifications of potentiometric electrodes; for each classification, state the principles, components, and clinical uses of two electrode types; list two types of reference electrodes and two types of indicator electrodes used in each type of measurement.

5. Describe a PCO_2 electrode, including components and internal reactions.

6. List four examples of biosensors and state their uses in the clinical laboratory; state the principle of affinity biosensors and their uses in the clinical laboratory.

7. List three examples of optodes and state their uses in the clinical laboratory.

8. Describe enzyme-based biosensors, including their combination with electrochemical measurements and uses in the clinical laboratory.

9. State the application of the Nernst equation to electrochemical measurements.

10. Compare galvanic and electrolytic electrochemical cells, including components, electrochemistry of each, and reactions involved.

Key Words and Definitions

Activity (of an ion) The concentration of free, unbound ion in solution.

Amperometry An electrolytic electrochemical process in which current is monitored at a fixed (controlled) voltage between working and reference electrodes in an electrochemical cell.

Biosensor A type of chemical sensor consisting of a biological recognition element and a physicochemical transducer, often an electrochemical or an optical device.

Conductometry An electrochemical technique used to determine the quantity of an analyte present in a mixture by measuring its effect on the electrical conductivity of the mixture.

Coulometry An electrochemical technique that measures the electrical charge passing between two electrodes in an electrochemical cell, with the amount of charge passing between the electrodes being directly proportional to oxidation or reduction of an electroactive substance at one of the electrodes.

Electrochemical cell An electrochemical device that consists of two electrodes (electron or metallic conductors) that are connected by an electrolyte solution that conducts ions (galvanic cell), or an electrochemical device in which an external voltage is applied to a polarizable working electrode with the resulting cathodic or anodic current of the cell being monitored (electrolytic cell).

Electrode A half-cell that consists of a single metallic conductor in contact with an electrolyte solution; the indicator (measuring) electrode is one half-cell and the reference electrode is the second half-cell.

Electrode potential The reduction potential for a redox couple that is measured with respect to a standard hydrogen electrode set at zero; the electromotive force of an electrochemical cell.

Ion-selective electrode An electrode that selectively interacts with a single ionic species; the potential produced at the membrane/sample solution interface is proportional to the logarithm of the ionic activity or the concentration of the ion in question.

*The authors gratefully acknowledge the original contributions of Drs. Richard A. Durst and Ole Siggard-Andersen, on which portions of this chapter are based.

Key Words and Definitions—cont'd

Nernst equation The equation used to determine the reduction potential for a given redox couple and used to correlate chemical energy with the electrical potential of an electrochemical cell.

Optode An optical sensor that measures specific substances such as pH, blood gases, and electrolytes using dye immobilization, fluorescence quenching, or phosphorescence.

Potential difference The work required to move an electrical charge and measured in volts.

Potentiometry An electrochemical technique that measures an electrical potential difference between two electrodes (half-cells) in an electrochemical cell.

Redox couple A conjugate pair of substances that consists of any substance that accepts electrons (the oxidant) and any substance that donates electrons (the reductant); redox processes take place only between two redox couples, with electrons transferred from a reductant (Red_1) to an oxidant (Ox_2).

Voltammetry An electrolytic electrochemical process in which a specific oxidation or reduction reaction occurs at the surface of the working electrode; it is the charge transfer at this interface (current flow) that provides analytical information.

Several analytical methods used in the clinical laboratory are based on electrochemical measurements. In this chapter, the fundamental electrochemical principles of (1) potentiometry, (2) voltammetry/amperometry, (3) conductometry, and (4) coulometry will be summarized and clinical applications presented. Optodes and biosensors also are discussed.

Potentiometry

Potentiometric sensors are widely used clinically for the measurement of pH, PCO_2, and electrolytes (Na^+, K^+, Cl^-, Ca^{2+}, Mg^{2+}, Li^+) in whole blood, serum, plasma, and urine, and as transducers for developing biosensors for metabolites of clinical interest.

Basic Concepts

Potentiometry is the measurement of an electrical potential difference between two electrodes (half-cells) in an **electrochemical cell** (Figure 10-1). Such a **galvanic electrochemical cell** consists of two electrodes (electron or metallic conductors) that are connected by an electrolyte solution that conducts ions. An **electrode**, or *half-cell*, consists of a single metallic conductor that is in contact with an electrolyte solution. The ion conductors consist of one or more phases that may be in direct contact with each other or separated by membranes permeable only to specific cations or anions (see Figure 10-1). One of the electrolyte solutions is the sample containing the analyte(s) to be measured. This solution may be replaced by an appropriate reference solution of analyte for calibration purposes. By convention, the cell notation is shown so that the left electrode (M_L) is the reference electrode, and the right electrode (M_R) is the *indicator (measuring) electrode* (see later, Equation 3).[3]

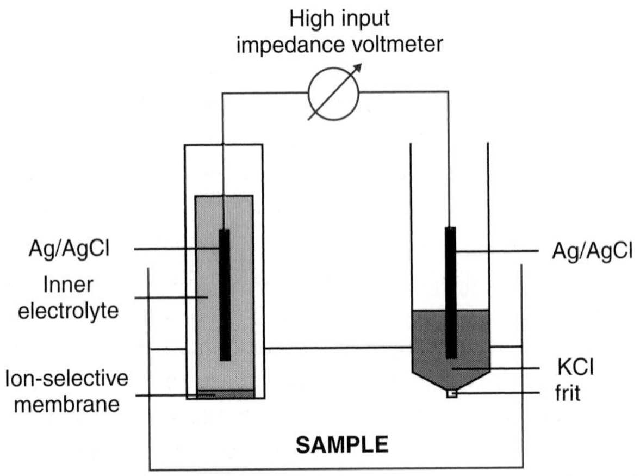

The *electromotive force* (E or EMF) is defined as the maximum difference in potential between the two electrodes (right minus left) obtained when the cell current is zero. The cell potential is measured using a *potentiometer,* of which the common pH meter is a special type. The *direct-reading potentiometer* is a voltmeter that measures the potential across the cell (between the two electrodes); however, to obtain an accurate potential measurement, it is necessary that the current through the cell is essentially zero. This is accomplished by incorporating high resistance within the voltmeter (input impedance $> 10^{12}\ \Omega$). Modern direct-reading potentiometers are accurate and have been modified to provide direct digital display or printouts.

Within any one conductive phase, the potential is constant as long as the current is zero. However, a potential difference arises between two different phases in contact with each other. The overall potential of an electrochemical cell is the sum of all potential differences that exist between adjacent phases of the cell. However, the potential of a single electrode with respect to the surrounding electrolyte and the absolute magnitude of the individual potential gradients between the phases are unknown and cannot be measured. Only the **potential difference** between two electrodes (half-cells) are measured. The potential gradients have been classified as (1) redox potentials, (2) membrane potentials, or (3) diffusion potentials. Generally, it is possible to devise a cell in such a manner that all potential gradients except one are constant. This potential is then related to the activity of a specific ion of interest (e.g., H^+, Na^+).

Types of Electrodes

Different types of potentiometric electrodes are used for clinical applications. They include (1) redox, (2) ion-selective membrane (glass and polymer), and (3) PCO_2 gas-sensing electrodes.

Figure 10-1 Schematic of ion-selective membrane electrode-based potentiometric cell.

Redox Electrodes

Redox potentials are the result of chemical equilibria involving electron transfer reactions:

$$\text{Oxidized form (Ox)} + ne^- \leftrightarrow \text{Reduced form (Red)} \quad (1)$$

where n represents the number of electrons (e^-) involved in the reaction. Any substance that accepts electrons is an *oxidant* (Ox), and any substance that donates electrons is a *reductant* (Red). The two forms, Ox and Red, represent a **redox couple** (conjugate redox pair). Usually, homogeneous redox processes take place only between two redox couples. In such cases, the electrons are transferred from a reductant (Red_1) to an oxidant (Ox_2). In this process, Red_1 is oxidized to its conjugate Ox_1, whereas Ox_2 is reduced to Red_2:

$$Red_1 + Ox_2 \leftrightarrow Ox_1 + Red_2 \quad (2)$$

In an electrochemical cell, electrons may be accepted from or donated to an inert metallic conductor (e.g., platinum). A reduction process tends to charge the electrode positively (remove electrons), and an oxidation process tends to charge the electrode negatively (add electrons). By convention, a heterogeneous redox equilibrium (Equation 2) is represented by the cell

$$M_L \,|\, Red_1 - Ox_1 \,::\, Ox_2 - Red_2 \,|\, M_R \quad (3)$$

A positive potential ($E > 0$) for this cell signifies that the cell reaction proceeds spontaneously from left to right; $E < 0$ signifies that the reaction proceeds from right to left; and $E = 0$ indicates that the two redox couples are at mutual equilibrium.

The **electrode potential** (reduction potential) for a redox couple is defined as the couple's potential measured with respect to the standard hydrogen electrode, which is set equal to zero (see hydrogen electrode later). This potential, by convention, is the electromotive force of a cell, where the standard hydrogen electrode is the reference electrode (left electrode) and the given half-cell is the indicator electrode (right electrode). The reduction potential for a given redox couple is given by the **Nernst equation:**

$$E = E° - \frac{N}{n} \times \log \frac{a_{Red}}{a_{Ox}} = E° - \frac{0.0592V}{n} \times \log \frac{a_{Red}}{a_{Ox}} \quad (4)$$

where

E = electrode potential of the half-cell;
$E°$ = standard electrode potential when $a_{Red}/a_{Ox} = 1$;
n = number of electrons involved in the reduction reaction;
$N = (R \times T \times \ln 10)/F$ (the Nernst factor if $n = 1$);
$N = 0.0592V$ if $T = 298.15$ K (25 °C);
$N = 0.0615V$ if $T = 310.15$ K (37 °C);
R = gas constant (= 8.31431 Joules $\times$ K^{-1} $\times$ mol^{-1}) ;
T = absolute temperature (unit: K, kelvin);
F = Faraday constant (= 96,487 Coulombs $\times$ mol^{-1});
$\ln 10$ = natural logarithm of 10 = 2.303;
a = activity; and
a_{Red}/a_{Ox} = ratio of activities of reduced and oxidized species (also called the reaction quotient)…

Redox electrodes currently in use may be (1) inert metal electrodes immersed in solutions containing redox couples or (2) metal electrodes whose metal functions as a member of the redox couple.

Inert Metal Electrodes

Platinum and *gold* are examples of inert metals used to record the potential of a redox couple dissolved in an electrolyte solution. The *hydrogen electrode* is a special redox electrode for pH measurement. It consists of a platinum or gold electrode that is electrolytically coated (platinized) with highly porous platinum (platinum black) to catalyze the electrode reaction.

$$H^+ + e^- \leftrightarrow \frac{1}{2}H_2 \quad (5)$$

The electrode potential is given by

$$E = E° - N \times \log \frac{(f_{H_2})^{1/2}}{a_{H^+}} \quad (6)$$

Or

$$E = E° - N \times [\log(f_{H_2})^{1/2} - \log a_{H^+}] \quad (7)$$

where

$E° = 0$ at all temperatures (by convention);
f_{H_2} = fugacity of hydrogen gas;
a_{H^+} = activity of hydrogen ions; and
$-\log a_{H^+}$ = negative log of the H$^+$ activity (pa_{H^+} or pH).

When the partial pressure of hydrogen (PH_2) in the solution (and hence f_{H_2}) is maintained constant by bubbling hydrogen through the solution, the potential is a linear function of $\log a_{H^+}$. Because the pH of the solution is $-\log a_{H^+}$, the cell potential is linearly related to the pH. In the *standard hydrogen electrode* (SHE), the electrolyte consists of an aqueous solution of hydrogen chloride with a_{HCl} equal to 1.000 (or c_{HCl} = 1.2 mol/L) in equilibrium with a gas phase, and with f_{H_2} equal to 1.000 (or PH_2 = 101.3 kPa = 1 atm). The SHE is also used as a reference electrode.

Metal Electrodes Participating in Redox Reactions

The silver-silver chloride electrode is an example of a metal electrode that participates as a member of a redox couple. The silver-silver chloride electrode consists of a silver wire or rod coated with $AgCl_{(solid)}$ that is immersed in a chloride solution of constant activity; this sets the half-cell potential. It should be noted that rather than being deposited on the silver electrode, the $AgCl_{(solid)}$ can be dispersed into the solution with fixed chloride activity. The Ag/AgCl electrode itself is considered a potentiometric electrode because its phase boundary potential is governed by an oxidation-reduction electron transfer equilibrium reaction that occurs at the surface of the silver:

$$AgCl_{(solid)} + e^- \leftrightarrow Ag°_{(solid)} + Cl^- \quad (8)$$

The Nernst equation for the reference half-cell potential of an Ag/AgCl reference electrode also is written as:

$$E_{Ag/AgCl} = E_{Ag/AgCl}^\circ + \frac{RT}{nF} \times \ln\frac{a_{AgCl}}{a_{Ag}a_{Cl^-}} \quad (9)$$

Because AgCl and Ag are both solids, their activities are equal to unity ($a_{AgCl} = a^0_{Ag} = 1$). Therefore, from Equation 9, the half-cell potential is controlled by the activity of chloride ion in solution (a_{Cl^-}) contacting the electrode.

The Ag/AgCl electrode is used both as an internal reference element in potentiometric **ion-selective electrodes** (ISEs) and as an external reference electrode half-cell of constant potential, required to complete a potentiometric cell (see Figure 10-1). In both cases, the Ag/AgCl electrode must be in equilibrium with a solution of constant chloride ion activity.

The Ag/AgCl element of the external reference electrode half-cell is in contact with a high-concentration solution of a soluble chloride salt. Saturated potassium chloride is commonly used. A porous membrane or frit is frequently employed to separate the concentrated KCl from the sample solution. The frit serves both as a mechanical barrier to hold the concentrated electrolyte within the electrode and as a diffusional barrier to prevent proteins and other species in the sample from coming into contact with the internal Ag/AgCl element, which could poison and alter its potential. The interface between two dissimilar electrolytes (concentrated KCl/calibrator or sample) occurs within the frit and develops the liquid-liquid junction potential (E_j), which represents a source of error in potentiometric measurements. The difference in liquid-liquid junction potential between calibrator and sample (residual liquid junction potential) is responsible for this error but is minimized and usually is neglected in practice if the compositions of the calibrating solutions are matched as closely as possible to the sample with respect to ionic content and ionic strength. An equitransferent* electrolyte at high concentration as the reference electrolyte further helps to minimize the residual liquid junction potential. Potassium chloride at a concentration ≥2 mol/L is preferred.

The presence of erythrocytes in the sample may affect the magnitude of the residual liquid junction potential in a less predictable manner. For example, erythrocytes in blood of normal hematocrit are estimated to produce approximately 1.8 mmol/L positive error in the measurement of sodium by ISEs when an open, unrestricted liquid-liquid junction is used.[5] This bias may be minimized if a restrictive membrane or frit is used to modify the liquid-liquid junction.

The *saturated calomel electrode* is another example of a metal electrode that participates as a member of a redox couple. The calomel electrode consists of mercury covered by a layer of relatively insoluble calomel (Hg_2Cl_2) (or present as insoluble salt dispersed in the electrolyte), which is in contact with an electrolyte solution containing Cl^-. The oxidation-reduction equilibrium reaction is as shown:

$$Hg_2Cl_2 + 2e^- \leftrightarrow 2Hg^\circ + 2Cl^- \quad (10)$$

As with the Ag/AgCl electrode, the half-cell potential is controlled by the activity of chloride ion contacting the electrode. Calomel electrodes are frequently used as reference electrodes for pH measurements using glass pH electrodes.

Ion-Selective Electrodes

Membrane potentials are caused by the permeability of certain types of membranes to selected anions or cations. Such membranes are used to fabricate ISEs that selectively interact with a single ionic species. The potential produced at the membrane/sample solution interface is proportional to the logarithm of ionic activity or of the concentration of the ion in question. Measurements with ISEs are (1) simple, (2) often rapid, (3) nondestructive, and (4) applicable to a wide range of concentrations.

The ion-selective membrane is the "heart" of an ISE, as it controls the selectivity of the electrode. Ion-selective membranes typically consist of (1) glass, (2) crystalline, or (3) polymeric materials. The chemical composition of the membrane is designed to achieve an optimal permselectivity toward the ion of interest. In practice, other ions exhibit finite interaction with membrane sites and will display some degree of interference for determination of an analyte ion. In clinical practice, if the interference exceeds an acceptable value, a correction is required.

The Nicolsky-Eisenman equation describes the selectivity of an ISE for the ion of interest over interfering ions:

$$E = E^\circ + \left(\frac{2.303RT}{z_iF}\right) \log\left(a_i + \sum_j K_{i/j}a_j^{zi/zj}\right) \quad (11)$$

where

a_i = activity of the ion of interest;

a_j = activity of the interfering ion;

$K_{i/j}$ = selectivity coefficient for the primary ion over the interfering ion. Low values indicate good selectivity for the analyte "i" over the interfering ion "j";

z_i = charge of the primary ion; and

z_j = charge of the interfering ion.

All other terms are identical to those in the Nernst equation (Equation 4).

Glass membrane and polymer membrane electrodes are two types of ISEs that are commonly used in clinical chemistry applications.

The Glass Electrode

Glass membrane electrodes are used to measure pH and Na^+ and as an internal transducer for PCO_2 sensors. The H^+ response of thin glass membranes was first demonstrated in 1906 by Cremer. In the 1930s, practical application of this

---

*An electrolyte is equitransferent if the ions have the same mobility in solution, measured as the ionic equivalent conductivity.

phenomenon for measurement of acidity in lemon juice was made possible by the invention of the pH meter by Arnold Beckman.[3] Glass electrode membranes are formulated from melts of silicon and/or aluminum oxide mixed with oxides of alkaline earth or alkali metal cations. By varying the glass composition, electrodes with selectivity for H^+, Na^+, K^+, Li^+, Rb^+, Cs^+, Ag^+, Tl^+, and NH_4^+ have been produced. However, glass electrodes for H^+ and Na^+ are today the only types with sufficient selectivity over interfering ions to allow practical application in clinical chemistry. A typical formulation for H^+ selective glass is 72% SiO_2; 22% Na_2O; 6% CaO. This formulation has a selectivity order of $H^+ >>> Na^+ > K^+$, and has sufficient selectivity for H^+ over Na^+ to allow error-free measurements of pH in the range of 7.0 to 8.0 ($[H^+] = 10^{-7}$ to 10^{-8} mol/L) in the presence of >0.1 mol/L Na^+. By altering slightly the formulation of the glass membrane to 71% SiO_2; 11% Na_2O; 18% Al_2O_3, its selectivity order becomes $H^+ > Na^+ > K^+$, and the preference of the glass membrane for H^+ over Na^+ is greatly reduced, resulting in a practical sensor for Na^+ at pH values typically found in blood.

Polymer Membrane Electrodes

Polymer membrane ISEs are employed for monitoring pH and for measuring electrolytes, including K^+, Na^+, Cl^-, Ca^{2+}, Li^+, Mg^{2+}, and CO_3^{2-} (for total CO_2 measurements). They are the predominant class of potentiometric electrodes used in modern clinical analysis instruments.

The mechanisms of response of these ISEs fall into three categories: (1) charged, dissociated ion exchanger, (2) charged associated carrier, and (3) neutral ion carrier (ionophore). An early charged associated ion exchanger–type ISE for Ca^{2+} was developed and commercialized for clinical application in the 1960s. This electrode was based on the Ca^{2+}-selective ion exchange/complexation properties of 2-ethylhexyl phosphoric acid dissolved in dioctyl phenyl phosphonate (charged associated carrier). A porous membrane was impregnated with this solution and mounted at the end of an electrode body. This type of sensor was referred to as the *liquid membrane* ISE. Later, a method was devised whereby these ingredients were cast into a plasticized poly(vinyl chloride) (PVC) membrane that was more rugged and convenient to use than its wet liquid predecessor. This same approach is still used today to formulate PVC-based ISEs for clinical use.

A major breakthrough in the development and routine application of PVC-type ISEs was the discovery that the neutral antibiotic valinomycin could be incorporated into organic liquid membranes (and later plasticized PVC membranes), resulting in a sensor with high selectivity for K^+ over Na^+ ($K_{K/Na}$ = 2.5×10^{-4}).[16] The K^+ ISE based on valinomycin is extensively used today for routine measurement of K^+ in blood. A wide linear range of over three orders of magnitude makes this ISE suitable for the measurement of K^+ in blood and urine. The K^+ range in blood is only a small portion of the electrode linear range and is spanned by a total EMF of about 9 mV. Interference from other cations, seen as deviation from linearity, is not apparent at K^+ activities >10^{-4} mol/L. Other, less selective polymer-based ISEs (e.g., for the measurement of Mg^{2+}

and Li^+) are subject to interference from Ca^{2+}/Na^+, and Na^+, respectively, requiring simultaneous determination and correction for the presence of significant concentrations of interfering ions.

Studies regarding the relationship between molecular structure and ionic selectivity have resulted in the development of polymer-based ISEs using a number of naturally occurring and synthetic ionophores, with sufficient selectivity for application in clinical analysis. The chemical structures of several of these neutral ionophores are illustrated in Figure 10-2.

Dissociated anion exchanger–based electrodes employing lipophilic quaternary ammonium salts as active membrane components also are still used commercially for the determination of Cl^- in whole blood, serum, and plasma despite some limitations. Selectivity for this type of ISE is controlled by extraction of the ion into the organic membrane phase and is a function of the lipophilic character of the ion (because, unlike the carriers described previously, no direct binding interaction occurs between the exchanger site and the anion in the membrane phase). Thus the selectivity order for a Cl^- ISE based on an anion exchanger is fixed as $R^- > ClO_4^- > I^- > NO_3^- > Br^- > Cl^- > F^-$, where R^- represents anions that are more lipophilic than ClO_4^-. The application of the Cl^- ion-exchange electrode is therefore limited to samples without significant concentrations of anions more lipophilic than Cl^-. Blood samples containing salicylate or thiocyanate, for example, will produce positive interference for the measurement of Cl^-. Repeated exposure of the electrode to the anticoagulant heparin will lead to loss of electrode sensitivity toward Cl^- caused by extraction of the negatively charged heparin into the membrane. Indeed, this extraction process has been used successfully to devise a method to detect heparin concentrations in blood by potentiometry.[12]

High selectivity for carbonate anion has been achieved using a neutral carrier ionophore possessing trifluoroacetophenone groups doped within a polymeric membrane.[10] Such ionophores form negatively charged adducts with carbonate anions, and the resulting electrodes have proved useful in commercial instruments for determination of total carbon dioxide in serum/plasma after dilution of the blood to a pH value in the range of 8.5 to 9.0, where a significant fraction of total carbon dioxide will exist as carbonate anions.

In practice, the ultimate detection limits of polymer membrane–type ISEs are partially controlled by the leakage of analyte ions from the internal solution to the outer surface of the membrane and into the sample phase in close contact with the membrane.[13] Hence, much lower limits of detection are achieved by decreasing the concentration of the primary analyte ion within the internal solution of the electrode. Further, this leakage of analyte ions, coupled with an ion-exchange process at the membrane/sample interface when the selectivity of the membrane over other ions is assessed, often yields a measured potentiometric selectivity coefficient that underestimates the true selectivity of the membrane. In determining "unbiased" selectivity coefficients by the separate solution method, the membrane should not be exposed to the analyte

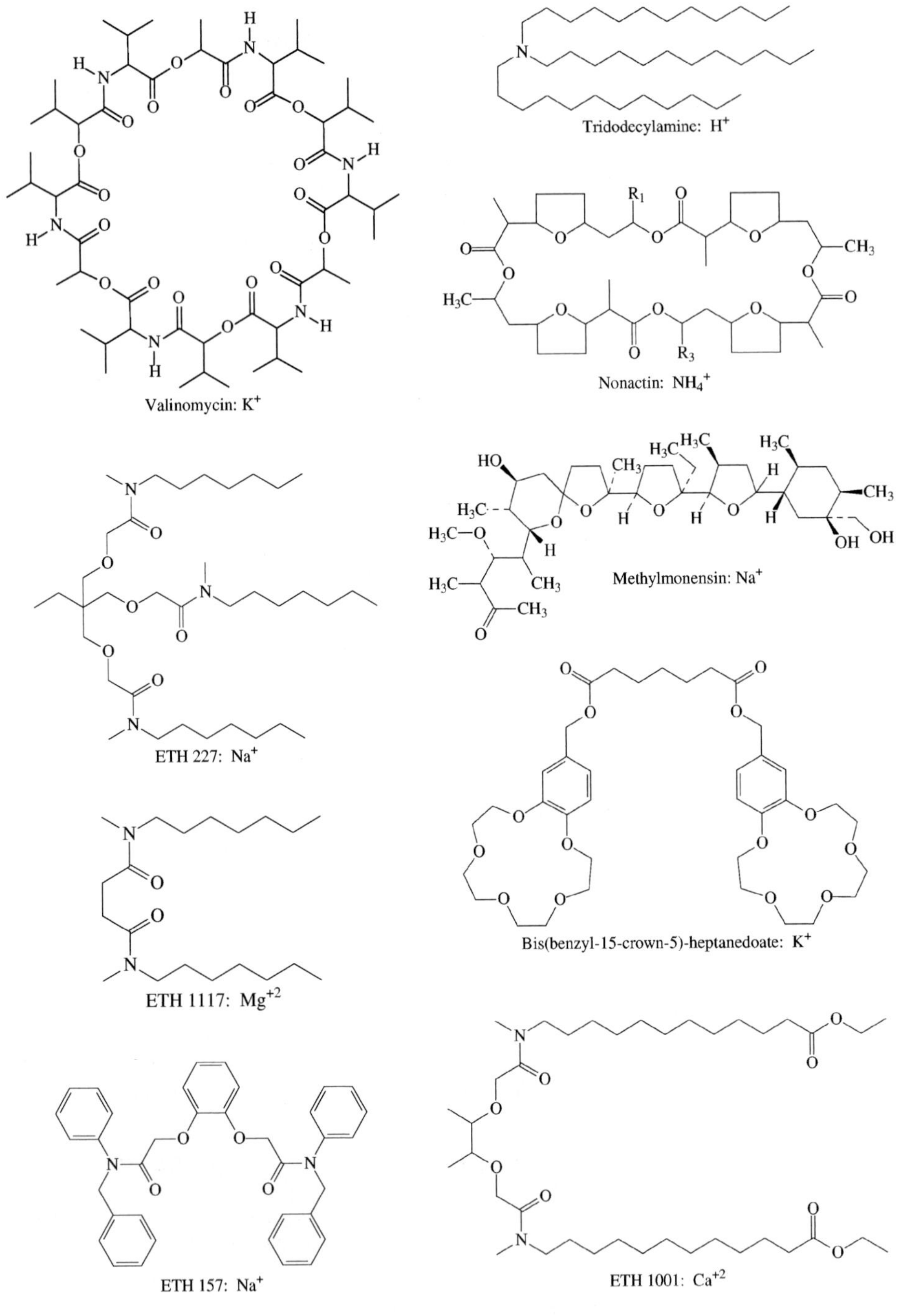

Figure 10-2 Structures of common ionophores used to fabricate polymer membrane types of ion-selective electrodes (ISEs) for clinical analysis.

ion for extended periods, and the concentration of analyte ion in the internal solution should be low.

Electrodes for PCO_2

Electrodes are available that measure PCO_2 in body fluids. The first PCO_2 electrode, developed in the 1950s by Stow and Severinghaus, used a glass pH electrode as the internal element in a potentiometric cell for measurement of the partial pressure of carbon dioxide.[2] This important development led to the commercial availability of the three-channel blood analyzer (pH, PCO_2, PO_2) that clinically provides the complete picture of the oxygenation and acid-base status of blood.

Figure 10-3 shows a diagram of a typical Stow-Severinghaus–style electrode for PCO_2. A thin membrane that is approximately 20 μm thick and is permeable only to gases and water vapor is in contact with the sample. Membranes of silicone rubber, Teflon, and other polymeric materials are suitable for this purpose. On the opposite side of the membrane is a thin electrolyte layer consisting of a weak bicarbonate salt (about 5 mmol/L) and a chloride salt. A pH electrode and an Ag/AgCl reference electrode are in contact with this solution. The PCO_2 electrode is a self-contained potentiometric cell. Carbon dioxide gas from the sample or calibration matrix diffuses through the membrane and dissolves in the internal

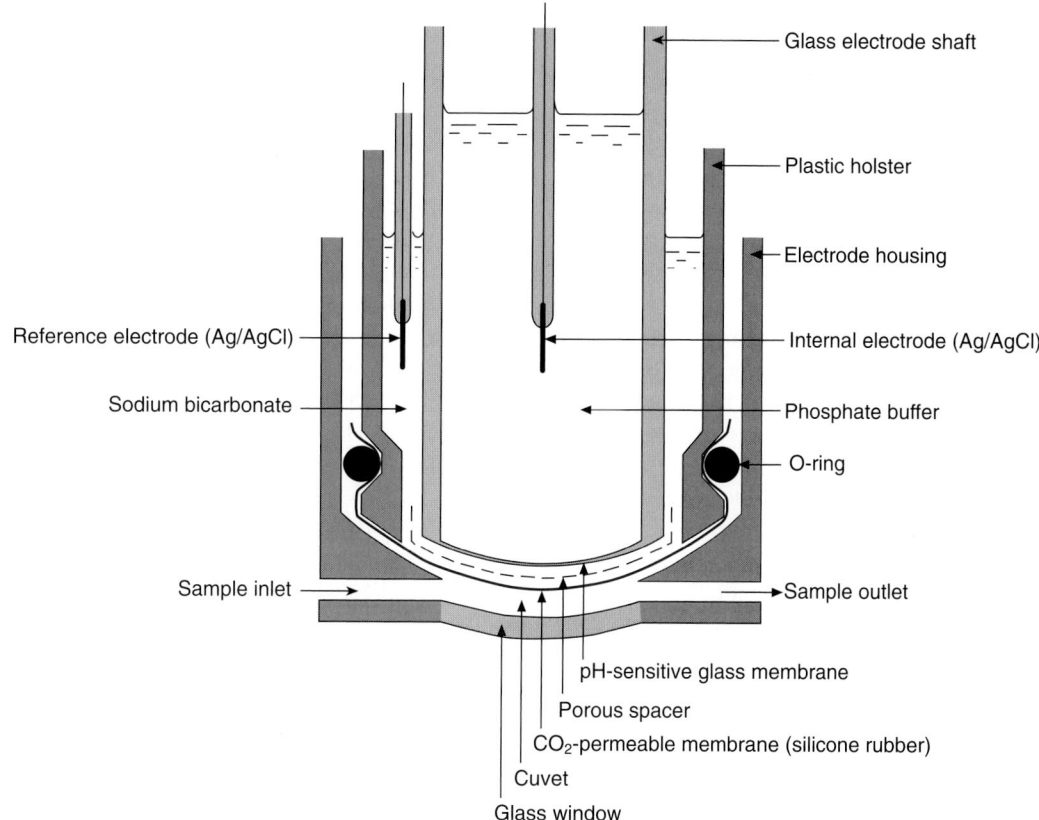

Figure 10-3 Schematic of Stow-Severinghaus–style PCO_2 sensor used to monitor CO_2 concentrations in blood samples. *(From Siggard-Andersen O. The acid-base status of the blood, 4th ed. Baltimore: Williams & Wilkins, 1974:172.)*

electrolyte layer. Carbonic acid is formed and dissociates, shifting the pH of the bicarbonate solution within the internal layer:

$$CO_2 + H_2O \leftrightarrow H_2CO_3 \leftrightarrow H^+ + HCO_3^- \tag{12}$$

and

$$\Delta \log PCO_{2(sample)} \approx \Delta pH_{(internal\ layer)} \tag{13}$$

The relationship between the sample PCO_2 and the signal generated by the internal pH electrode is logarithmic and is governed by the Nernst equation (Equation 4). The electrode may be calibrated using exact gas mixtures or solutions with stable PCO_2 concentrations. Although Stow-Severinghaus–style electrodes for PCO_2 have gained widespread use in modern blood gas analyzers, the format in which such sensors may be constructed is limited by their (1) size, (2) shape, and (3) ability to fabricate the internal pH-sensitive element.

A slightly different potentiometric cell for PCO_2 is shown in Figure 10-4. This cell arrangement uses two PVC-type pH-selective electrodes in a differential mode. The electrode membranes contain a lipophilic amine–type neutral ionophore that exhibits very high selectivity for H^+ (see Figure 10-2). One electrode has an internal layer, which is buffered, and the other is unbuffered, consisting of a low concentration of bicarbonate salt. Carbon dioxide gas from the sample or calibration matrix diffuses across the outer H^+-selective PVC membranes of both sensors. On the unbuffered side, CO_2 diffusion produces a

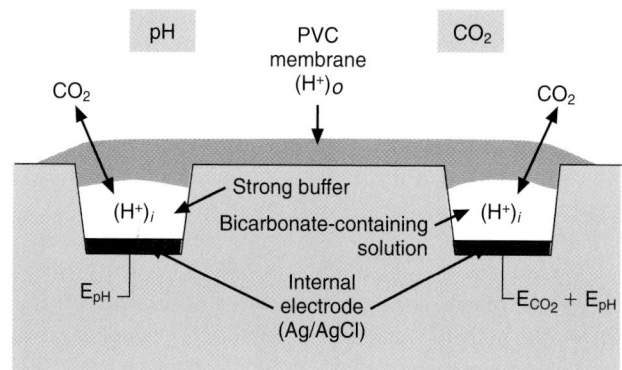

Figure 10-4 Differential planar PCO_2 potentiometric sensor design based on two identical polymeric membrane pH electrodes but with different internal reference electrolyte solutions. Both pH-sensing membranes are prepared with H^+-selective ionophore.

potential shift at the internal interface of the pH-responsive membrane proportional to the sample PCO_2 concentration. The signal at the electrode with the buffered internal layer is unaffected by CO_2 that diffuses across the membrane. Consequently, one-half of the sensor responds to pH alone, and the other half responds to both pH and PCO_2. The signal difference between the two electrodes cancels any contribution of sample pH to the overall measured cell potential. The differential signal is proportional only to PCO_2.

Direct Potentiometry by ISE—Units of Measure and Reporting for Clinical Applications

Most analytical methods measure the total *concentration (c)* of a given ion in the sample, usually expressed in units of millimoles of ion per liter of sample (mmol/L). *Molality (m)* is a measure of the moles of ion per mass of water (mmol/kg) in the sample. With the sodium ion used as an example, the relationship between concentration and molality is given by:

$$c_{Na+} = m_{Na+} \times \rho H_2O \qquad (14)$$

where ρH_2O is the mass concentration of water in kg/L. For blood plasma from healthy individuals, the mass concentration of water is approximately 0.93 kg/L, but in specimens with elevated lipids or protein, the value may be as low as 0.8 kg/L. In these specimens, the difference between concentration and molality may be as great as 20%. A significant advantage of direct potentiometry by ISE for the measurement of electrolytes is that the technique is sensitive to molality and therefore is not affected by variations in the concentration of protein or lipids in the sample. Techniques such as flame photometry and other photometric methods requiring sample dilution are affected by the presence of protein and lipids. With these methods, only the water phase of the sample is diluted, producing results lower than molality as a function of the concentration of protein and lipids in the sample. Thus, there is a risk for error, such as a falsely low Na^+ concentration (pseudohyponatremia), in cases of extremely elevated protein and lipid concentrations.[1]

In addition to the difference between molality and concentration, measurement of ions by direct potentiometry provides yet another unit of measurement known as *activity (a)*, the concentration of free, unbound ion in solution. Unlike methods sensitive to total ion concentration, ISEs do not sense the presence of complexed or electrostatically "hindered" ions in the sample. The relationship between activity and concentration, using, again, sodium ion as an example, is expressed as:

$$a_{Na+} = \gamma_{Na+} \times c_{Na+} \qquad (15)$$

where γ is a dimensionless quantity known as the *activity coefficient*. The activity coefficient is primarily dependent on the ionic strength of the sample as described by the Debye-Hückel equation:

$$\log\gamma = -\frac{\left(A \times z^2 \times I^{1/2}\right)}{1 + \left(B \times a \times I^{1/2}\right)} \qquad (16)$$

where *A* and *B* are temperature-dependent constants (A = 0.5213 and B = 3.305 in water at 37 °C), *a* is the ion size parameter for a specific ion, and *I* is the ionic strength ($I = 0.5\Sigma m \times z^2$, where *z* is the charge number of the ions). Equation 16 shows that a decrease in the activity coefficient occurs with an increase in ionic strength. This effect is more pronounced when the charge *(z)* of the ion is high. Activity coefficients for ions in biological fluids, such as blood and serum, are difficult to calculate with accuracy because of the uncertain contribution of macromolecular ions, such as proteins, to the overall ionic strength. However, if it is assumed that the normal ionic strength of blood plasma is 0.160 mol/kg, then estimates of activity coefficients at 37 °C are as follows: Na^+ = 0.75, K^+ = 0.74, and Ca^{2+} = 0.31. In reference to Equation 15, activity and concentration will differ greatly in samples of physiological ionic strength, especially for divalent ions.

Physiologically, ionic activity is assumed to be more relevant than concentration when chemical equilibria or biological processes are considered. Practically, however, *ionic concentration* is the more familiar term in clinical practice, forming the basis of reference intervals and medical decision concentrations for electrolytes. Early in the evolution of ISEs as practical tools in clinical chemistry, it was decided that changing clinical reference intervals to a system based on activity instead of concentration was impractical and carried the risk for clinical misinterpretation. A pragmatic approach for using ISEs in modern analyzers without changing established concentration-based reference intervals is to formulate calibration solutions with ionic strengths and ionic compositions as close as possible to those of blood plasma from healthy individuals. Thus the activity coefficient of each ion in the calibrating solutions approximates that in the sample matrix, allowing calibration and measurement of electrolytes in units of concentration instead of activity.

Voltammetry/Amperometry

Voltammetric and amperometric techniques are among the most sensitive and widely applicable of all electroanalytical methods.

Basic Concepts

In contrast to potentiometry, voltammetric and amperometric methods are based on electrolytic electrochemical cells, in which an external voltage is applied to a polarizable working electrode (measured vs. a suitable reference electrode: $E_{appl} = E_{work} - E_{ref}$), and the resulting cathodic (for analytical reductions) or anodic (for analytical oxidations) current of the cell is monitored and is proportional to the concentration of analyte present in the test sample. Current flows only if E_{appl} is greater than a certain voltage (decomposition voltage), as determined by the thermodynamics for a given redox reaction of interest (Ox + ne$^-$ ↔ Red; defined by the E° value for that reaction [standard reduction potential]) and the kinetics for heterogeneous electron transfer at the interface of the working electrode. Often, slow kinetics of electron transfer for the redox reaction on a given inert working electrode (Pt, carbon, gold, etc.) requires use of a much more negative (for reductions) or positive (for oxidations) E_{appl} than predicted based merely on the E° for a given redox reaction. This is called an *overpotential* (η). Regardless of whether an overpotential for electron transfer exists, in **voltammetry/amperometry**, a specific oxidation or reduction reaction occurs at the surface of the working electrode, and it is the charge transfer at this interface (current) that provides the analytical information.

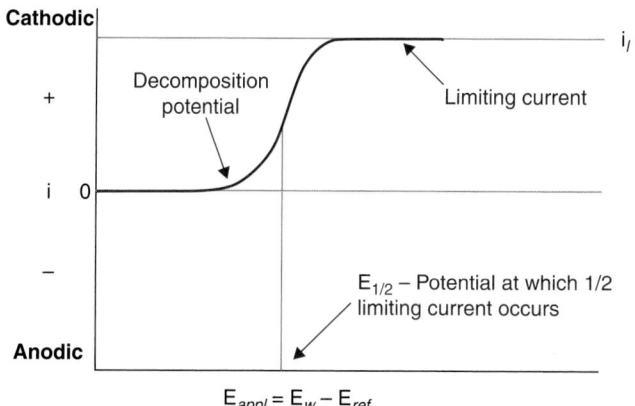

Figure 10-5 Illustration of the current versus voltage curve (voltammogram) obtained for oxidized species (Ox) reduced to Red at the surface of the working electrode, as the E_{appl} is scanned more negative and the solution is stirred to yield a steady state response.

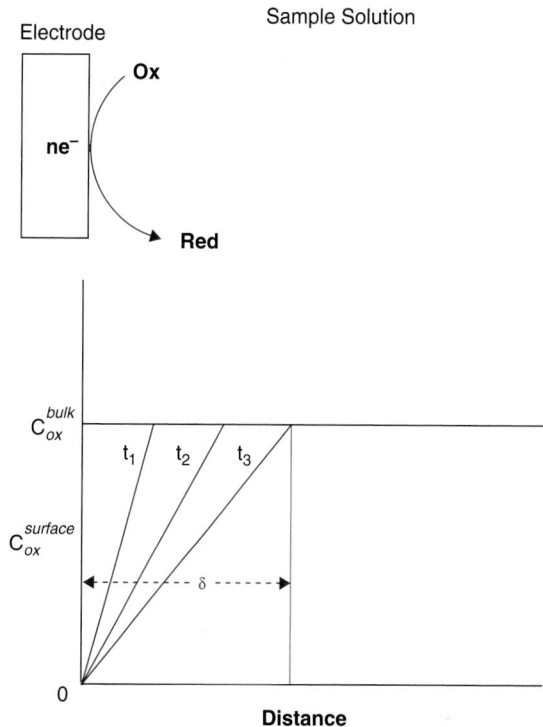

Figure 10-6 Concept of electrochemical reaction increasing diffusion layer thickness (concentration polarization) of the analyte via reduction (or oxidation) at the surface of the working electrode. As time (t) increases, the diffusion layer thickness grows quickly to a value that is determined by degree of convection in the sample solution.

For electrolytic cells that form the basis of voltammetric and amperometric methods:

$$E_{appl} = E_{cell} + \eta - iR_{cell} \tag{17}$$

where E_{cell} is the thermodynamic potential between working and reference electrodes in the absence of an applied external voltage. When the external voltage is greater or less than this equilibrium potential, plus or minus any overpotential (η), then current will flow because of an oxidation or reduction reaction at the working electrode. A voltammogram is simply the plot of observed current, i, versus E_{appl} (Figure 10-5). In amperometry (see later), a fixed voltage is applied, and the resulting current is monitored. The amount of current is inversely related to the resistance of the electrolyte solution and to any "apparent" resistance that develops because of the mass transfer of the analyte species to the surface of the working electrode. Because the electrochemical reactions are heterogeneous and occur only at the surface of the working electrode, the amount of current observed is highly dependent on the surface area (A) of the working electrode.

When a potential is applied to a working electrode that will oxidize or reduce a species in the solution phase contacting the electrode, the electrochemical reaction causes the concentration of electroactive species to decrease at the surface of the electrode (Figure 10-6) through a process termed *concentration polarization*. This in turn causes a concentration gradient of the analyte species between the bulk sample solution and the surface of the electrode. When the bulk solution is stirred, the diffusion layer of analyte grows out from the surface of the electrode very quickly to a fixed distance controlled by how vigorously the solution is stirred. This diffusion layer, which is termed the *Nernst layer,* has a finite thickness (δ) after a relatively short time (see Figure 10-6) when the solution is moving (convection). Voltammetry carried out in the presence of convection (by stirring the solution, rotating the electrode, flowing solution by electrode, etc.) is called *steady state voltammetry*. When the solution is motionless, the diffusion layer is not constant and grows with time, creating larger and

larger δ values. This is termed *non–steady state voltammetry* and often results in peak currents in i versus E_{appl} plots for electrolytic cells.

In steady state voltammetry, when the potential of the working electrode is scanned past a value that will cause an electrochemical reaction, the current will rise rapidly and then eventually will reach a near-constant value, even as E_{appl} changes further. Figure 10-5 illustrates such a wave for a hypothetical reduction of an oxidized species (Ox) via an n electron transfer from a reduced species (Red). When the applied potential is much more negative than required, the current reaches a limiting value (termed the *limiting current, i_l*). This limiting current is proportional to the concentration of the electroactive species (Ox in this case) as expressed by the following equation:

$$i_l = nFA \left(\frac{D}{\delta} \right) C_{ox} \tag{18}$$

where *i* is the measured current in amperes, *n* equals the number of electrons in the electrochemical reaction (reduction in this case), *F* is Faraday's constant (96,487 coulombs/mol), *A* is the electrochemical surface area of the working electrode (in cm^2) (if a planar electrode geometry is assumed), *D* is the diffusion coefficient (in cm^2/s) of the electroactive species (Ox in this case), δ is the diffusion layer thickness (in centimeters), and *C* is the concentration of the analyte species in mol/cm^3. The D/δ term is often denoted as m_o, the mass transfer coefficient of the Ox species to the surface of the working electrode. Note that Equation 18 indicates a linear relationship for limiting current and concentration. The same equation applies for detecting reduced species by an oxidation reaction at the working electrode. In this case, by convention, the resulting anodic current is considered a negative current. As shown in Figure 10-5, the potential of the working electrode that corresponds to a current that is exactly one-half the limiting current is termed the $E_{1/2}$ value. This value is not dependent on analyte concentration but is determined by the thermodynamics ($E°$) of the given redox reaction, the solution conditions (e.g., if protons are involved in reaction, the pH will influence the $E_{1/2}$ value), and any overpotential caused by slow electron transfer, and so forth, at a particular working electrode surface. The $E_{1/2}$ values are indicative of a given species undergoing an electrochemical reaction under specified conditions; hence, the $E_{1/2}$ values enable one to distinguish one electroactive species from another in the same sample. If the $E_{1/2}$ values for various species differ significantly (e.g., >120 mV), then measurement of several limiting currents in a given voltammogram is capable of yielding quantitative results for several different species simultaneously.

Electrochemical cells employed to carry out voltammetric or amperometric measurements typically involve a two- or three-electrode configuration. In the two-electrode mode, the external voltage is applied between the working electrode and a reference electrode, and the current is monitored. Because the current must also pass through the reference electrode, such current flow will alter the surface concentration of electroactive species that poises the actual half-cell potential of the reference electrode, changing its value through a concentration polarization process. For example, if an Ag/AgCl reference electrode were used in a cell in which a reduction reaction for the analyte occurs at the working electrode, an oxidation reaction would take place at the surface of the reference electrode:

$$Ag° + Cl^- \rightarrow AgCl_{(s)} + 1e^- \tag{19}$$

Consequently, the activity/concentration of chloride ions near the surface of the electrode would decrease, which would make the potential of the reference electrode more positive than its true equilibrium value based on the actual activity of chloride ion in the reference half-cell, because the Nernst equation for this half-cell is:

$$E_{Ag/AgCl} = E°_{Ag/AgCl} - 0.059\log\left(a_{Cl^-}^{surface}\right) \tag{20}$$

Such concentration polarization of the reference electrode is prevented by maintaining the current density (J; amperes/cm^2) very low at the reference electrode. This is achieved in practice by making sure that the area of the working electrode in the electrochemical cell is much smaller than the surface area of the reference electrode; consequently, the total current will be limited by this much smaller area, and J values for the reference will be very small, as desired, to prevent concentration polarization.

To completely eliminate changes in reference electrode half-cell potentials, a three-electrode potentiostat is often employed. In simple terms, the potentiostat applies a voltage to the working electrode that is measured versus a reference electrode via a zero current potentiometric-type measurement, but the current flow is between the working electrode and a third electrode, called the *counter electrode*. Thus if reduction takes place at the working electrode, oxidation would occur at the counter electrode, but no net reaction would take place at the surface of the reference electrode, because no current flows through this electrode.

In voltammetric methods, the E_{appl} is varied via some waveform to alter the working electrode potential as a function of time, and the resulting current is measured. The current change occurs at the decomposition potential range, which is expected to be specific for a given analyte. However, the location of the current response as a function of E_{appl} provides information on the nature of the species present (e.g., $E_{1/2}$), along with a concentration-dependent signal. This scan of E_{appl} is linear (linear sweep voltammetry), or it can have more complex shapes that enable greatly enhanced sensitivity to be achieved for monitoring the concentration of a given electroactive species (e.g., normal pulsed voltammetry, differential pulse voltammetry, square wave voltammetry). When a dropping mercury electrode (DME) is used, such voltammetric methods are considered polarographic methods of analysis.

Amperometric methods differ from voltammetry methods in that E_{appl} is fixed, generally at a potential value that occurs in the limiting current plateau region of the voltammogram. The resulting current is proportional to concentration. Amperometry usually is more sensitive than common voltammetric methods because background charging currents that arise from changing the E_{appl} as a function of time in voltammetry do not exist. Hence, when selectivity is ensured at a given E_{appl} value, amperometry may be preferred to voltammetric methods for more sensitive quantitative measurements.

Applications

Molecular oxygen is capable of undergoing several reduction reactions, all with significant overpotentials at solid electrodes, such as Pt, Au, or Ag. For example, the following reaction:

$$O_2 + 2H_2O + 4e^- \rightarrow 4OH^-$$
$$(E° = +0.179 \text{ vs Ag/AgCl};1\text{mol/L Cl}^-) \tag{21}$$

exhibits an $E_{1/2}$ of approximately -0.500 V on a Pt electrode (vs. Ag/AgCl), with a limiting current plateau beginning at approximately -0.600 V. This reaction has been used to monitor the partial pressure of oxygen (PO_2) in blood and is the basis of the widely used Clark style amperometric oxygen sensor (Figure 10-7). This device employs a small area planar platinum electrode as a working electrode (encased in insulating glass or other material) and an Ag/AgCl reference electrode, typically with a cylindrical design (see Figure 10-7). This two-electrode electrolytic cell is placed within a sensor housing on which a gas-permeable membrane (e.g., polypropylene, silicone rubber, Teflon) is held at the distal end. The inner working platinum electrode is pressed tightly against the gas-permeable membrane to

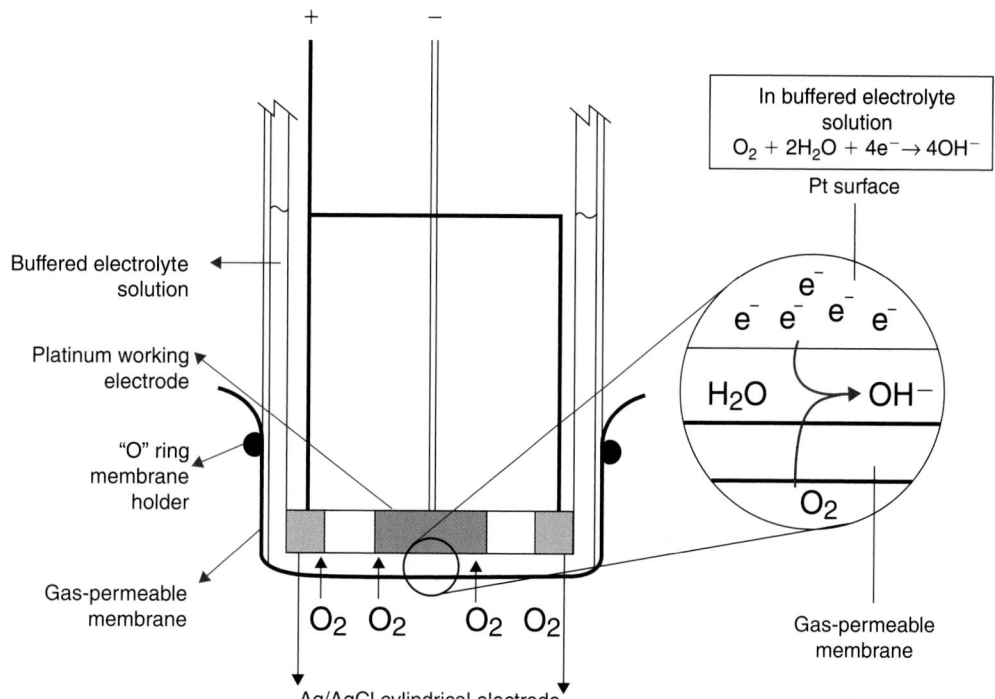

In buffered electrolyte solution
$O_2 + 2H_2O + 4e^- \rightarrow 4OH^-$

Pt surface

Figure 10-7 Design of Clark-style amperometric oxygen sensor used to monitor PO_2 concentrations in blood.

create a thin film of internal electrolyte solution (usually buffer with KCl added). Oxygen in the sample permeates across the membrane and is reduced in accordance with the above electrochemical reaction. An E_{appl} of −0.650 or −0.700 V versus Ag/AgCl (within the limiting current regime) to the Pt working electrode will result in an observed current that is proportional to the PO_2 present in the sample (including whole blood). In the absence of any oxygen, the current at this applied voltage under amperometric conditions will be very near zero.

The outer gas-permeable membrane enables the Clark electrode to detect oxygen with very high selectivity over other easily reduced species that might be present in a given sample (e.g., metal ions, cystine). Indeed, only other gas species or highly lipophilic organic species will partition into and pass through such gas-permeable membranes. One type of interference in clinical samples is seen with certain anesthesia gases, such as nitrous oxide, halothane, and isoflurane. These species also (1) diffuse through the outer membrane of the sensor, (2) are electrochemically reduced at the platinum electrode, and (3) yield a false-positive value for the measurement of PO_2. However, optimized gas-permeable membrane materials and appropriate control of the applied potential to the cathode of the sensor have greatly reduced this problem in modern instruments. The outer gas-permeable membranes also help restrict the diffusion of analyte to the inner working electrode; hence the membrane can control the mass transport of analyte (D/δ term in Equation 18), such that in the presence or absence of sample convection, mass transport of oxygen to the surface of the platinum working electrode is essentially the same.

The basic design of the Clark amperometric PO_2 sensor has been extended to detect other gas species by altering

the applied voltage to the working electrode. For example, it is possible to detect nitric oxide (NO) with high selectivity using a similar gas electrode design in which the platinum is polarized at +0.900 versus Ag/AgCl to oxidize diffusing NO to nitrate at the platinum anode.[4] Such NO sensors have been used for a variety of biomedically important studies to deduce the amount of NO locally at or near the surface of various NO-producing cells.

Beyond amperometric devices, one specialized method for detecting trace concentrations of toxic metal ions in clinical samples is anodic stripping voltammetry (ASV). In ASV, a carbon working electrode is used (sometimes further coated with an Hg film), and the E_{appl} is first fixed at a very negative E_{appl} voltage so that all metal ions in the solution will be reduced to elemental metals (M°) within the mercury film and/or on the surface of the carbon. Then the E_{appl} is scanned more positive, and the reduced metals deposited in and/or on the surface of the working electrode are reoxidized, giving a large anodic current peak proportional to the concentration of metal ions in the original sample. The potential at which these peaks are observed indicates which metal is present, and the height of stripping peak current is directly proportional to the concentration of the metal ion in the original sample. Such ASV techniques have been used to detect the total concentration of Pb in whole blood samples, providing a rapid screening method for lead exposure and poisoning.[9]

Another biomedical example of modern voltammetry is a rapid scan cyclic voltammetric technique that has been used to quantify dopamine in brain tissue of freely moving animals.[17] In this application, oxidation of dopamine to a quinone species at an implanted microcarbon electrode (at approximately +0.600 V vs. Ag/AgCl) yields peak currents proportional to dopamine concentrations. The electrode has been used to measure this neurotransmitter in different regions of the brain or in a fixed location.

Voltammetric/amperometric techniques are applied to detect a wide range of species; however, the selectivity offered for measurements in complex clinical samples—where many species can be electroactive—is rather limited. For example, as stated in the previous discussion relevant to the Clark oxygen sensor, in the absence of the gas-permeable membrane, other species that are reduced at or near the same E_{appl} as oxygen would cause significant interference.

To greatly expand the range of analytes detected by voltammetric/amperometric methods, electrochemical techniques have been used as highly sensitive detectors for modern high-performance liquid chromatographic (HPLC) systems (see Chapter 12). In liquid chromatography with electrochemical detection (LC-EC), eluting solutes are detected by flow-through electrodes (usually carbon or mercury) designed to have extremely low dead volumes (Figure 10-8). These electrodes are operated in amperometric or voltammetric modes (with high scan speeds), and several electrodes are able to be operated simultaneously in series or in parallel flow arrangements to gain additional selectivity. For example, homocysteine has been measured with (1) the addition of reducing agents to a serum sample to generate free homocysteine, (2) precipitation of proteins in the sample (with trichloroacetic acid), and (3) separation of the serum components on a reversed phase octadecylsilane HPLC column. The eluting homocysteine is detected and measured with online electrochemical detection via homocysteine oxidation to the corresponding mercuric dithiolate complex.

Conductometry

Conductometry is an electrochemical technique used to determine the quantity of an analyte present in a mixture by measuring its effect on the electrical conductivity of the mixture. It is the measure of the ability of ions in solution to carry current under the influence of a potential difference. In a conductometric cell, an electrical potential is applied between two inert metal electrodes. An alternating potential with a frequency between 100 and 3000 Hz is used to prevent concentration polarization of the electrodes. A decrease in solution resistance results in an increase in conductance, and more current is passed between the electrodes. The resulting current flow is also alternating. The current is directly proportional to solution conductance. Conductance is considered the inverse of resistance and may be expressed in units of ohm^{-1} (siemens). In clinical analysis, conductometry is frequently used to measure the volume fraction of erythrocytes in whole blood (hematocrit) and serves as the transduction mechanism for some biosensors.

Erythrocytes act as electrical insulators because of their lipid-based membrane composition. This phenomenon was first used in the 1940s to measure hematocrit by conductivity and is used today to measure hematocrit on multianalyte instruments for clinical analysis. In addition, Na^+ and K^+ concentrations are usually measured in conjunction with hematocrit on systems designed for clinical analysis, and they are used to correct for the background conductivity of the plasma.

Conductivity-based hematocrit measurements have limitations. For example, abnormal protein concentrations will change plasma conductivity and interfere with the measurement. Low protein concentrations resulting from dilution of blood with protein-free electrolyte solutions during cardiopulmonary bypass surgery will result in erroneously low hematocrit values by conductivity. Preanalytical variables, such as insufficient mixing of the sample, will also lead to errors. Hemoglobin is the preferred analyte to monitor blood loss and the need for transfusion during trauma and surgery. However, the electrochemical measurement of hematocrit in conjunction with blood gases and electrolytes remains in use

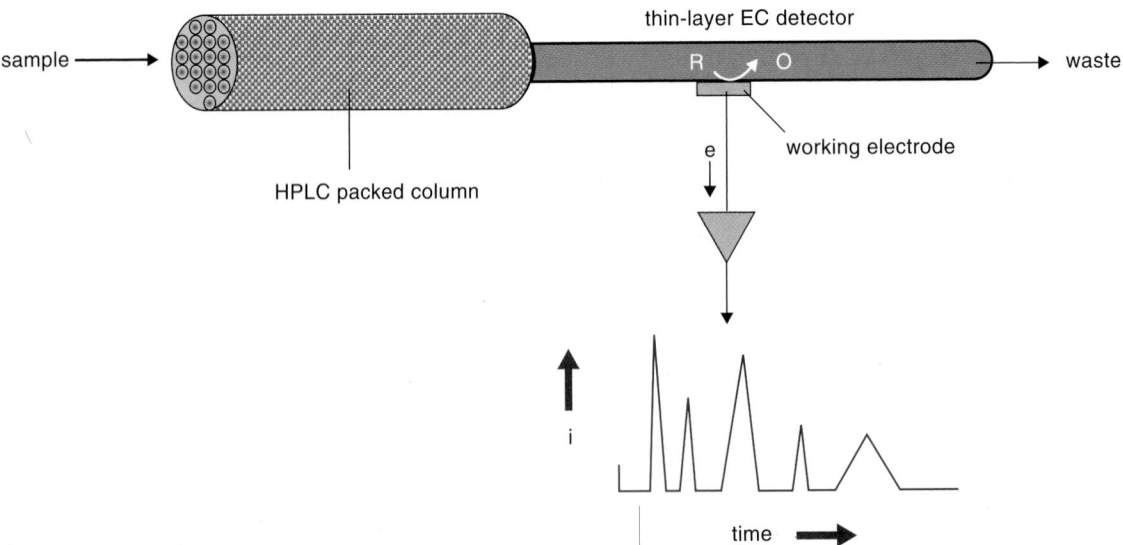

Figure 10-8 Schematic of liquid chromatography with electrochemical detection (LC-EC) system, with electrochemical detector monitoring the elution of analytes from an high-performance liquid chromatographic (HPLC) column by their oxidation or reduction (shown here as an example) at a suitable thin-layer working electrode.

mainly because of simplicity and convenience, despite some limitations.

Another clinical application of conductance is seen in electronic counting of blood cells in suspension. Termed the *Coulter principle,* it relies on the fact that the conductivity of blood cells is lower than that of a salt solution used as a suspension medium.[6] The cell suspension is forced to flow through a tiny orifice. Two electrodes are placed on either side of the orifice, and a constant current is established between the electrodes. Each time a cell passes through the orifice, resistance increases; this causes a spike in the electrical potential difference between electrodes. The pulses are then amplified and counted.

Coulometry

Coulometry measures the electrical charge passing between two electrodes in an electrochemical cell. The amount of charge passing between the electrodes is directly proportional to oxidation or reduction of an electroactive substance at one of the electrodes. The number of coulombs transferred in this process is related to the absolute amount of electroactive substance by Faraday's law:

$$Q = n \times N \times F \tag{22}$$

where

Q = the amount of charge passing through the cell (unit: C = coulomb = ampere • second);

n = the number of electrons transferred in the oxidation or reduction reaction;

N = the amount of substance reduced or oxidized in moles; and

F = the Faraday constant (96,487 coulombs/mole).

Measurement of current is related to charge as the amount of charge passed per unit of time (ampere = coulomb/s). Coulometry is used in clinical applications for the determination of chloride in serum or plasma and as the mode of transduction in certain types of biosensors.

Commercial coulometric titrators have been developed for determining chloride in blood, plasma, or serum. A constant current is applied between a silver wire (anode) and a platinum wire (cathode). At the anode, Ag is oxidized to Ag^+. At the cathode, H^+ is reduced to hydrogen gas. At a constant applied current, the number of coulombs passed between the anode and the cathode is directly proportional to time (coulombs = amperes × seconds). Thus the absolute number of silver ions produced at the anode may be calculated from the length of time that current passes through it. In the presence of Cl^-, Ag^+ ions formed are precipitated as $AgCl_{(solid)}$ and the amount of free Ag^+ in solution is low. When all Cl^- ions have been complexed, a sudden increase in the concentration of Ag^+ in solution is noted. The excess Ag^+ is sensed amperometrically at a second Ag electrode, polarized at negative potential. The excess Ag^+ is reduced to Ag, producing a current. When this current exceeds a certain value, the titration

is stopped. The absolute number of Cl^- ions present in the sample is calculated from the time during which titration with Ag^+ was in progress. Knowing the volumetric amount of serum or plasma sample originally used, it is possible to calculate the concentration of Cl^- in the sample. Coulometric titration is one of the most accurate electrochemical techniques because the method measures the absolute amount of electroactive substance in the sample. Coulometry is considered the gold standard for determining chloride in serum or plasma. However, the method is subject to interference from anions in the sample with affinity for Ag^+ greater than chloride, such as bromide.

Optical Chemical Sensors

An **optode** is an optical sensor used in analytical instruments to measure (1) pH, (2) blood gases, and (3) electrolytes. Optodes provide certain advantages over electrodes, including (1) ease of miniaturization, (2) less electronic noise (no transduction wires), (3) long-term stability using ratiometric-type measurements at multiple wavelengths, and (4) no need for a separate reference electrode. These advantages initially promoted the development of optical sensor technology for design of intravascular blood gas sensors. However, the same basic sensing principles have been used in clinical chemistry instrumentation designed for more classical in vitro measurements on discrete samples. With such systems, light is passed to and from the sensing site by optical fibers or simply by appropriate positioning of light sources (light-emitting diodes [LEDs]), filters, and photodetectors to monitor absorbance (by reflectance), fluorescence, or phosphorescence (Figure 10-9).

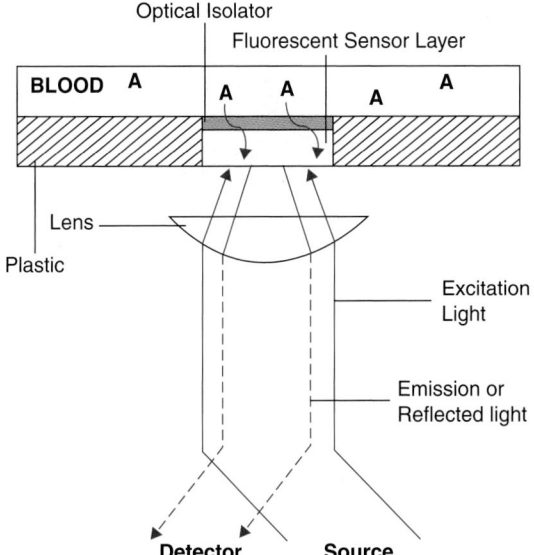

Figure 10-9 General design for an in vitro optical sensor to detect a given analyte (*A*) in blood. Polymer film contains dye that changes spectral properties in proportion to the amount of analyte in the sample phase. The example shown is used for sensing film that changes luminescence (fluorescence or phosphorescence).

Basic Concepts

Optical sensors devised for PO_2 measurements are typically based on the immobilization of certain organic dyes, such as (1) pyrene, (2) diphenylphenanthrene, (3) phenanthrene, (4) fluoranthene, and (5) metal ligand complexes (such as ruthenium[II] tris[dipyridine] and Pt and Pd metalloporphyrins) within hydrophobic polymer films (e.g., silicone rubber) in which oxygen is very soluble. The fluorescence or phosphorescence of such species at a given wavelength is often quenched in the presence of paramagnetic species, including molecular oxygen. In the case of embedded fluorescent dyes, the intensity of the emitted fluorescence of such films will decrease in proportion to the partial pressure of O_2 of the sample in contact with the polymer film in accordance with the Stern-Volmer equation for quenching:

$$\frac{I_0}{I_{PO_2}} = kPO_2 + 1 \qquad (23)$$

where

I_0 = fluorescence intensity in the absence of oxygen;
I_{PO_2} = fluorescence intensity at a given partial pressure of PO_2; and
k = quenching constant for the particular fluorophore used.

As indicated, the relationship between the ratio I_0/I_{PO_2} and the PO_2 in the sample phase is linear. Also, the larger the quenching constant, the greater is the degree of quenching for the given fluorophore. However, it is important that the quenching constant is in a range that will yield linear Stern-Volmer behavior over the physiologically relevant range of PO_2 in blood.

Phosphorescence intensity or phosphorescence lifetime measurements of immobilized metal ligand complexes have also been employed to measure pH, blood gases, or electrolytes. Sensors based on changes in luminescent lifetime offer the inherent advantage of being insensitive to perturbations in the optical pathlength and the amount of active dye present in the sensing layer.

Optical pH sensors require immobilization of appropriate pH indicators within thin layers of hydrophilic polymers (e.g., hydrogels) because equilibrium access of protons to the indicator is essential. Fluorescein, 8-hydroxy-1,2,6-pyrene trisulfonate (HPTS), and phenol red have been used as indicators. The absorbance or fluorescence of the protonated or deprotonated form of the dye is used for sensing purposes. One problem with respect to using immobilized indicators for accurate physiological pH measurements is the effect of ionic strength on the pKa of the indicator. Because optical sensors measure the concentration of protonated or deprotonated dye as an indirect measure of hydrogen ion activity, variations in the ionic strength of the physiological sample have been known to influence the accuracy of pH measurement.

Applications

Optical sensors suitable for the determination of PCO_2 employ optical pH transducers (with immobilized indicators) as inner transducers in an arrangement quite similar to the classic Stow-Severinghaus–style electrochemical sensor design (see Figure 10-3). The addition of bicarbonate salt within the pH-sensing hydrogel layer creates the required electrolyte film layer, which varies in pH depending on the partial pressure of PCO_2 in equilibrium with the film. The optical pH sensor is covered by an outer gas-permeable hydrophobic film (e.g., silicone rubber) to prevent proton access while allowing CO_2 equilibration with the pH-sensing layer. As the partial pressure of PCO_2 in the sample increases, the pH of the bicarbonate layer decreases, and the corresponding decrease in the concentration of the deprotonated form of the indicator (or increase in the concentration of the protonated form) is sensed optically.

Two approaches have been used to sense electrolyte ions optically in physiological samples. One method employs many of the same lipophilic ionophores developed for polymer membrane–type ion-selective electrodes (see Figure 10-2). These species are doped into very thin hydrophobic polymeric films along with a lipophilic pH indicator. In the case of cation ionophores (e.g., valinomycin for sensing potassium), when cations from the sample are extracted by the ionophore into the thin film, the pH indicator (RH) loses a proton to the sample phase to maintain charge neutrality within the organic film (yielding R^-). This results in a change in the optical absorption or fluorescence spectrum of the polymer layer. If the thickness of the films is kept <10 μm, equilibrium response times on the order of <1 minute have been achieved. The main limitation of this design is that the pH of the sample phase influences the overall extraction equilibrium for ions into the film. Thus simultaneous and independent measurement of sample pH is required, or buffered dilution and/or pH control of the sample phase are necessary to obtain accurate measurements of electrolytes.

A second method used to sense electrolyte ions consists of immobilizing a cation and/or anion recognition agent within a hydrogel matrix similar to the pH sensors described previously. The recognition agent in this case is not usually lipophilic; therefore it must be covalently anchored to the hydrogel so that it does not leach into the sample phase. The agent is designed so that selective cation or anion binding alters the absorbance or fluorescence spectrum of the species within the hydrogel. Typically, this is achieved by linking ion recognition and chromophoric properties within a single organic molecule. Such ion sensors have been employed successfully in at least one commercial blood gas–electrolyte analyzer using an array of sensors of the generic design similar to that illustrated in Figure 10-9.

Biosensors

A **biosensor** is a specific type of chemical sensor that consists of a biological recognition element and a physicochemical transducer, often an electrochemical[18] or optical device. The biological element is capable of recognizing the presence and activity and/or concentration of a specific analyte in solution. The recognition may involve a *biocatalytic reaction*

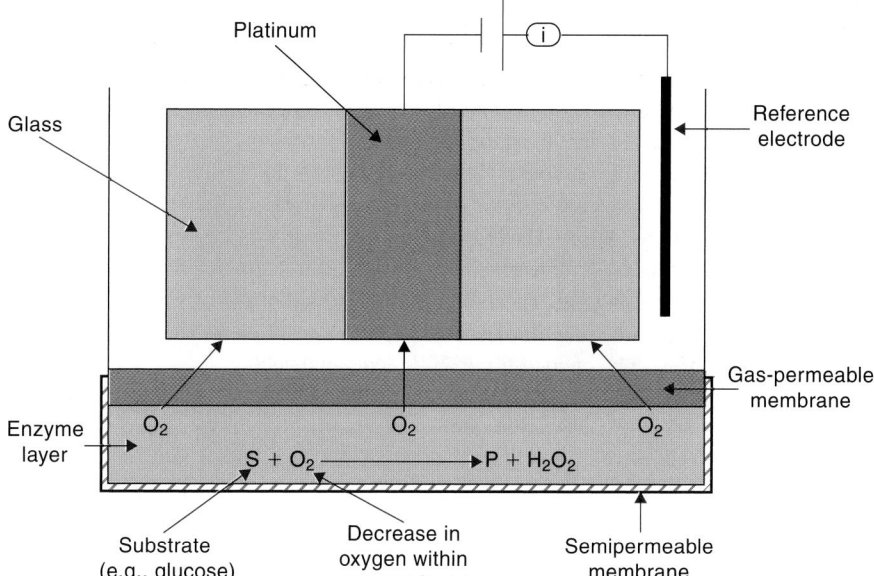

Figure 10-10 Illustration of an enzyme electrode prepared using oxidase enzyme immobilized at the surface of an amperometric PO_2 sensor. An increase in substrate concentration S reduces the amount of oxygen present at the surface of the sensor.

(enzyme-based biosensor) or a binding process (affinity-based biosensor), when the recognition element is, for example, (1) an antibody, (2) a DNA segment, or (3) a cell receptor. The interaction of the recognition element with a target analyte results in a measurable change in a solution property locally at the surface of the device, such as formation of a product or consumption of a reactant. The transducer then converts the change in solution property into an electrical signal. The mode of transduction may be one of several, including electrochemical or optical, and may involve the measurement of mass or heat. The present discussion will be limited to biosensors based on electrochemical and optical modes of transduction because they compose the majority of biosensors used for clinical applications.

Enzyme-Based Biosensors With Amperometric Detection

Enzyme-based biosensors based on electrochemical transducers, specifically, amperometric electrodes, are widely used for clinical analyses and are the most frequently cited in the literature. In 1962 Clark and Lyons developed an enzyme electrode for glucose that coupled a PO_2 electrode with a glucose oxidase catalyzed reaction. A decrease in PO_2, resulting from the action of glucose oxidase on glucose, was proportional to the glucose concentration of the sample. Within this device, a solution of glucose oxidase was physically entrapped between the gas-permeable membrane of the PO_2 electrode and an outer semi-permeable membrane (see Figure 10-10, general design). The outer membrane allowed substrate (glucose) and oxygen from the sample to pass, but not proteins and other macromolecules.

If the polarizing voltage of the PO_2 electrode is reversed, making the platinum electrode positive (anode) relative to the Ag/AgCl reference electrode, and if the gas-permeable membrane is replaced with a hydrophilic membrane containing the immobilized enzyme, it is possible to oxidize the H_2O_2

produced by the glucose oxidase reaction. The steady state current produced is directly proportional to the concentration of glucose in the sample.

In practice, a sufficiently high voltage (overpotential) is applied to the platinum anode to drive the oxidation of the hydrogen peroxide. An applied voltage of +0.7 volt or greater (relative to Ag/AgCl) is typically used. Figure 10-11 illustrates this basic hydrogen peroxide detection design, which is suitable for use in devising clinically useful sensors for glucose and for a host of other substrates for which suitable oxidase enzymes generate hydrogen peroxide (e.g., lactate).

Immobilization of enzymes in the early biosensors was a simple entrapment method behind a membrane of low-molecular-weight cutoff, and this approach is still used in some commercial applications. Many other schemes for enzyme immobilization for biosensor development have been suggested. Most common are (1) cross-linking of the enzyme with an inert protein, such as bovine serum albumin (BSA), using glutaraldehyde, (2) simple adsorption of enzyme to electrode surfaces, and (3) covalent binding of enzymes to insoluble carriers, such as nylon or glass. Another immobilization technique involves bulk modification of an electrode material, mixing enzymes with carbon paste that serves as both the enzyme immobilization matrix and the electroactive surface.

One of the first biosensor-based systems for the measurement of glucose in blood was commercialized by Yellow Springs Instruments, Inc. (YSI), Yellow Springs, Ohio, in 1975; it used the amperometric detection of H_2O_2 as the measurement principle (see Figure 10-11). Dependence of the measured glucose value on the oxygen concentration in the sample was a problem because significantly less than the stoichiometric amount of dissolved oxygen is present in blood to support the glucose oxidase reaction and produce a linear relationship of signal with glucose concentration found in blood. This is especially true at high concentrations of glucose found in samples from diabetic patients (>500 mg/dL). This problem with

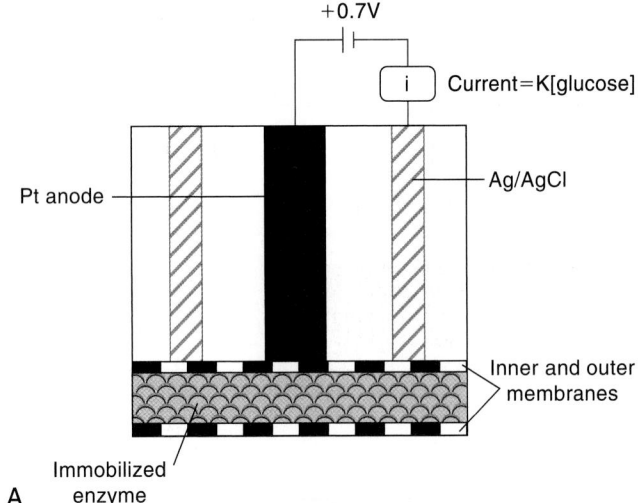

A

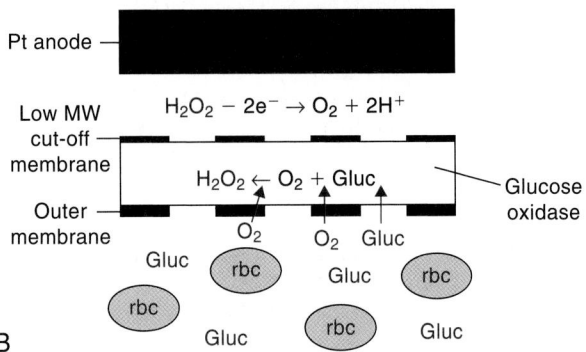

B

Figure 10-11 Design of amperometric enzyme electrode based on anodic detection of hydrogen peroxide generated from an oxidase enzymatic reaction (e.g., glucose oxidase) **(A)**, and expanded view of the sensing surface showing the different membranes and electrochemical processes that yield the anodic current proportional to the substrate concentration in the sample **(B)**. *(From Meyerhoff M. New in vitro analytical approaches for clinical chemistry measurements in critical care,* Clin Chem *1990;36:1570.)*

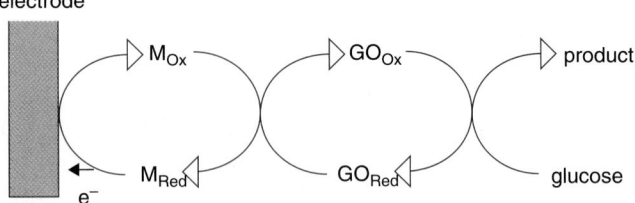

Figure 10-12 Scheme showing the use of electroactive mediator in the design of an amperometric enzyme electrode. The mediator accepts electrons directly from the enzyme and is oxidized at the surface of the working electrode, creating a more oxidized mediator to continue this process. *(From D'Orazio P. Electrochemistry. In: Lewandrowski, K, ed. Clinical chemistry laboratory management and clinical correlations. Philadelphia: Lippincott Williams & Wilkins, 2002:464.)*

the YSI design was resolved by diluting the sample and calibration solutions by at least 1:10 with buffer, thereby fixing the oxygen concentration in both the calibrator and the sample at a comparable concentration.

The problem of oxygen limitation for biosensors based on oxidase enzymes has been resolved by (1) designing semipermeable membranes that restrict the diffusion of the primary analyte (substrate) to the enzyme layer, (2) avoiding saturation of the enzyme, and (3) keeping the ratio of oxygen to analyte always in excess of 1. This extends the linearity of response to analyte concentrations substantially higher than the K_m of the enzyme and reduces the signal dependence on oxygen. Outer track-etched polycarbonate membranes are commonly used, as are membranes of poly(vinyl chloride), polyurethane, and silicone emulsions. Another approach has been to use an oxygen-rich electrode material as a reservoir of oxygen to support the bioreaction. A fluorocarbon (Kel-F oil) has been used to formulate a carbon paste electrode to act both as a source of oxygen and as the working electrode.[20]

Electron acceptors other than oxygen also have been used in the glucose oxidase reaction and have completely eliminated any dependence of the amperometric response on oxygen concentration of the sample. The electron acceptor, usually co-immobilized with the enzyme, transports electrons to the anode surface, where it is reoxidized, resulting in a cyclic reaction mechanism (Figure 10-12). Acceptors with electron transfer kinetics (little or no overpotential) more favorable than that of oxygen allow operation of the sensor at lower applied potentials (+0.2 V vs. Ag/AgCl or lower) than are typically used for the oxidation of H_2O_2. This approach not only eliminates dependency of the reaction rate on oxygen, it also serves to reduce the contribution from oxidizable interfering substances (e.g., uric acid, ascorbic acid, acetaminophen) to the sensor response. Examples of acceptors that have been used include (1) quinones, (2) conductive organic salts, such as tetrathiafulvalene-tetracyanoquinodimethane (TTF-TCNQ), and (3) ferricyanide and ferrocene derivatives.

Another technique that can be used to decrease interferences from easily oxidized species in a blood sample when traditional H_2O_2 electrochemical detection is used employs selectively permeable membranes in proximity to the electrode surface that allow transport of H_2O_2 to the electrode surface, but it rejects the interfering substances on the basis of size exclusion (see Figure 10-11, *B*). An example is a low-molecular-weight cutoff membrane, such as cellulose acetate, which is used in many commercial amperometric biosensors. Also used are electropolymerized films, such as poly(phenylenediamine) formed in situ, to reject interfering substances on the basis of size.[8] Another approach employed in a commercial application involves using a second correcting electrode, identical to the working electrode but without enzyme, sensitive only to the presence of oxidizable interfering substances. The resulting differential signal is proportional to the concentration of analyte.

A novel approach used to eliminate electroactive interfering substances in a commercially available glucose sensor consists of directly "wiring" the redox center of the enzyme glucose oxidase to a metallic, amperometric electrode using an osmium (III/IV)-based redox hydrogel.[15] The osmium sites effectively facilitate transfer of electrons directly from the entrapped enzyme to the metallic electrode, without the need for oxygen. This approach allows the operating potential of the electrode to be dramatically lowered to +0.2 V versus SCE (saturated calomel reference electrode), where currents resulting from electro-oxidation of possible interferences such as (1) ascorbate, (2) urate, (3) acetaminophen, and (4) L-cysteine are negligible.

Substitution of other oxoreductase enzymes for glucose oxidase allows amperometric biosensors for other substrates of clinical interest to be constructed. For example, sensors have been developed to measure (1) blood lactate, (2) cholesterol, (3) pyruvate, (4) alanine, (5) glutamate, and (6) glutamine. In addition, by using a multiple enzyme cascade, an amperometric biosensor for creatinine has been developed.

Enzyme-Based Potentiometric and Conductometric Biosensors

Ion-selective electrodes also have been used as transducers in potentiometric biosensors. An example is a biosensor for urea (blood urea nitrogen [BUN]) that is based on a poly(vinyl chloride) membrane ISE for ammonium ion (Figure 10-13). The enzyme urease is immobilized at the surface of the ammonium selective ISE based on the antibiotic nonactin (see structure of ionophore in Figure 10-2) and catalyzes the hydrolysis of urea to NH_3 and CO_2. The ammonia produced dissolves to form NH_4^+, which is sensed by the ISE. The signal generated by the NH_4^+ produced is proportional to the logarithm of the concentration of urea in the sample. The response may be steady state or transient. Typically, correction for background potassium is required because the nonactin ionophore has limited selectivity for ammonium over potassium ($K_{NH4/K}$ = 0.1). Potassium is measured simultaneously with urea and is used to correct the output of the urea sensor using the Nicolsky-Eisenman equation (Equation 11).

The above approach for measurement of urea using an enzyme-based potentiometric biosensor assumes that the turnover of urea to ammonium at steady state provides a constant ratio of ammonium ions to urea, independent of concentration. This is rarely the case, especially at higher substrate concentrations resulting in a nonlinear sensor response. The linearity of the sensor is also limited by the fact that hydrolysis of urea produces a local alkaline pH in the vicinity of the ammonium-sensing membrane, partially converting NH_4^+ to NH_3 (pKa = 9.3). Ammonia (NH_3) is not sensed by the ISE. The degree of nonlinearity may be reduced by placement of a semi-permeable membrane between enzyme and sample to restrict diffusion of urea to the immobilized enzyme layer.

A change in solution conductivity has also been used as a transduction mechanism in enzyme-based biosensors. Examples include the measurement of (1) glucose, (2) creatinine, and (3) acetaminophen using interdigitated electrodes.[7] Practical applications of conductometric biosensors are few because of the variable ionic background of clinical samples and the requirement to measure small conductivity changes in a medium with high ionic strength. A commercial system used to measure urea in serum, plasma, and urine is a BUN analyzer based on the enzyme urease. Dissolution of the products to NH_4^+ and HCO_3^- produces a change in sample

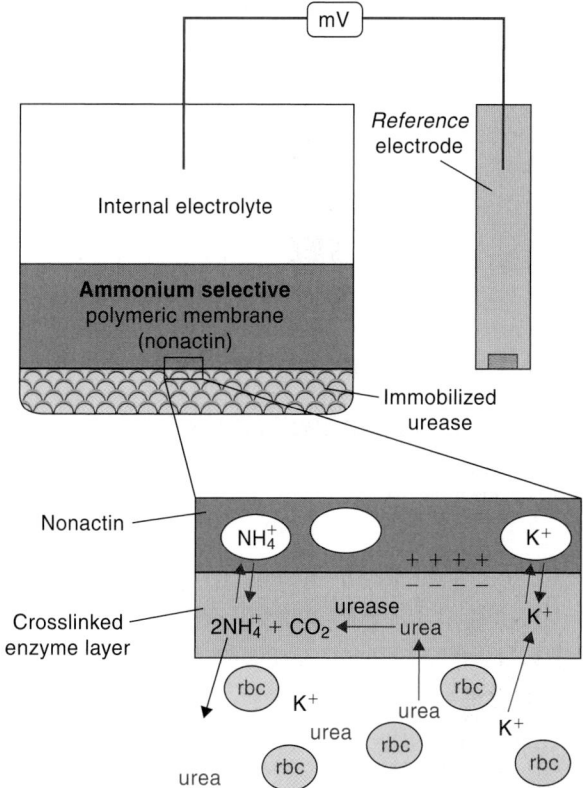

Figure 10-13 Potentiometric enzyme electrode for determination of blood urea based on the urease enzyme immobilized on the surface of an ammonium ion–selective polymeric membrane electrode.

conductivity. The initial rate of change in conductivity is measured to compensate for the background conductivity of the sample. This approach is limited to the measurement of analytes at relatively high concentrations because of small changes in conductivity produced by low concentrations of analyte.

Enzyme-Based Biosensors With Optical Detection

Optical sensors with immobilized enzymes and indicator dyes have been developed for the measurement of glucose and other substrates of clinical interest. These biosensors rely on measurements of pH or oxygen by (1) absorbance, (2) reflectance, (3) fluorescence, and (4) luminescence, coupled with an enzyme-catalyzed reaction. Enzyme immobilization methods resemble those used to construct electrochemical biosensors, including (1) physical entrapment or encapsulation in a gel matrix, (2) physical adsorption onto substrates, and (3) covalent binding to or absorption on an insoluble support. Using an example based on an optode for PO_2, a sensitive indicator is co-immobilized with an oxidase enzyme at the end of a fiber optic probe. The probe is used to monitor fluorescence of the indicator. Quenching of fluorescence of the indicator by O_2 is followed. A decrease in PO_2 resulting from a substrate reaction catalyzed by the enzyme will result in less quenching of the indicator and a fluorescent signal directly proportional to the concentration of the substrate. In an example of an optical biosensor probe for glucose, an oxygen-sensitive cationic dye $Ru[phen]_3^{2+}$ is immobilized along with glucose oxidase on the surface of an optical fiber.[14] A decrease in PO_2 arising from the enzyme-catalyzed oxidation of glucose results in an increase in luminescence intensity of the ruthenium tris (phenanthrene).

Similar optical biosensors have been prepared for other analytes. For example, a cholesterol optical biosensor has been devised that is based on fluorescence quenching of an oxygen-sensitive dye coupled to consumption of oxygen resulting from the enzyme-catalyzed oxidation of cholesterol by the enzyme cholesterol oxidase.[19] Serum bilirubin has been detected using bilirubin oxidase, co-immobilized with a ruthenium dye, on an optical fiber.[11] The bilirubin sensor (1) exhibited a lower detection limit of 10 μmol/L, (2) had a linear range up to 30 mmol/L, and (3) exhibited a typical reproducibility of 3% (coefficient of variation [CV]).

The pH change resulting from enzyme-catalyzed reactions has also been measured optically. The dye fluorescein is often used as a pH-sensitive indicator to construct such sensors. The protonated form of fluorescein does not fluoresce, but the conjugate base strongly fluoresces at 530 nm when excited at 490 nm. Using glucose oxidase as the enzyme, a pH optode has been employed to follow the formation of glucuronic acid. A disadvantage of optical sensors based on pH changes is that they are strongly dependent on the pH and buffer capacity of the sample. Moreover, the working range of the sensor is determined by the pKa of the indicator, at 6.8 to 7.2 for fluorescein, depending on the ionic strength of the sample matrix. A pH-sensitive indicator may also be used to follow enzymatic reactions that produce ammonia (e.g., urease action on urea).

Affinity Sensors

Affinity sensors are a special class of biosensors in which the immobilized biological recognition element is (1) a binding protein, (2) an antibody (immunosensors), or (3) an oligonucleotide (e.g., DNA, RNA, aptamers) that has high binding affinity and high specificity toward a clinically important analyte. Such sensors have been developed as alternatives to conventional binding assays to enhance the speed and convenience of a wide range of assays that would be typically run on sophisticated immunoassay analyzers. Ideally, direct binding of the immobilized species to its target in a clinical sample should yield a sensor signal proportional to the concentration of the analyte. However, "direct" sensing at analyte concentrations that would cover the full range of clinical applications is very difficult to achieve. Further, high affinity of such binding reactions, required to achieve optimal sensitivity, limits the reversibility of such devices. Affinity sensors based on electrochemical, optical, or other transduction modes are typically single-use devices, thus obviating the need for some type of regeneration step (pH change, etc.) to dissociate the tight binding between the recognition element and the target.

The number of research reports related to affinity biosensors continues to increase. However, commercialization has lagged behind research output, and movement of these types of biosensors from the research laboratory to the clinical laboratory has been slow. Affinity biosensors with promise of clinical utility are typically based on labeled reagents, such as enzymes, fluorophores, and electrochemical tags; hence they function more like traditional binding/immunoassays, except that one recognition element is immobilized on the surface of a suitable electrode or another type of transducer. For example, electrochemical oxygen sensors have been employed to perform heterogeneous enzyme immunoassays (sandwich or competitive type), using catalase as a labeling enzyme (catalyzes $H_2O_2 \rightarrow 2H^+$ and O_2) and immobilizing capture antibodies on the outer surface of the gas-permeable membrane. After binding equilibration and washing steps, the amount of bound enzyme is detected by adding the substrate and following the increase in current generation caused by local production of oxygen near the surface of the sensor.

Affinity Sensors for DNA Analysis Using Fluorescent Labels

Affinity-type sensors based on oligonucleotide binding represent perhaps the most promising application of affinity sensors to clinical chemistry. Fluorescent labels were the first to be used in an early commercial biosensor for DNA analysis (the GeneChip, introduced in 1996). High-density oligonucleotide arrays are formed on glass substrates. Target DNA is isolated and amplified using the polymerase chain reaction (PCR), while a fluorescent label is incorporated. The sample is incubated on the array, and detection of hybridization of labeled DNA to its complementary strands takes place by monitoring light emitted by the fluorescent labels. The primary application of the device has been for DNA sequencing, so the focus has been primarily on increasing the density of the DNA arrays. Applications of the device continue to expand with a variety of arrays developed for gene expression and whole genomic analysis related to (1) cancer, (2) inflammatory disease, (3) infectious disease, and (4) diabetes.

Affinity Sensors for DNA Analysis Using Electrochemical Labels

DNA sensors in which a segment of DNA complementary to a target strand is immobilized on a suitable electrochemical sensor have been demonstrated. These devices operate in direct (based on electrochemical oxidation of guanine in target DNA) (Figure 10-14, *A*) or indirect (with exogenous electrochemical markers/labels, see later and Figure 10-14, *B*) transduction modes. Although most of the proposed electrochemical DNA biosensors require amplification methods, such as PCR, to multiply small amounts of DNA into measurable quantities, some are sensitive enough to eliminate the need for target amplification. Nanotechnology has been proposed, in the indirect format, for signal amplification. For example, a capture probe DNA is immobilized on a gold electrode. Reporter probes with electrostatically bound ruthenium complexes $[Ru(NH_3)_6]^{3+}$ are loaded onto gold nanoparticles (AuNP) and are capable of hybridizing with one of two sequences on target DNA. The other sequence on the target DNA is capable of hybridizing with the immobilized capture probe. Hybridization events on the electrode surface bring multiple reporter probes for each AuNP. Electroactive $[Ru(NH_3)_6]^{3+}$ is reduced at the electrode surface, and the coulometric signal is proportional to the concentration of target DNA[21]. A commercial example of electrochemical

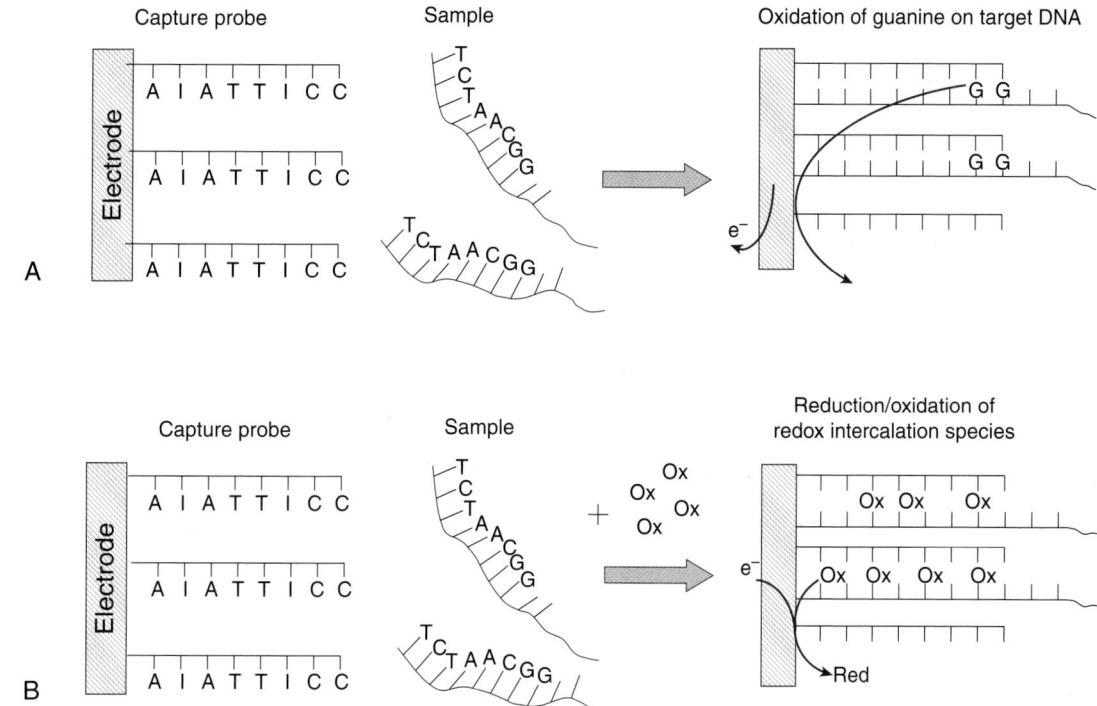

Figure 10-14 Examples of DNA biosensor configurations: **(A)** direct electro-oxidation detection of guanosine bases in target DNA after hybridization with immobilized capture probe on electrode surface; **(B)** electrochemical detection of hybridization using exogenous redox species that intercalate into a hybridized complex between the immobilized capture DNA probe and the target DNA.

DNA sensing, along with AuNP probes without need for PCR amplification, is the Verigene system (Nanosphere, Northbrook, IL), which is capable of detecting single-nucleotide polymorphisms related to common genetic disorders, such as (1) thrombophilia, (2) alterations of folate metabolism, (3) cystic fibrosis, and (4) hemochromatosis.

Another example of an electrochemical "gene" sensor array uses electrochemical probes that are selectively inserted into hybridized DNA duplexes. In one approach, after the immobilized capture of oligo anchored to the electrode surface is allowed to bind the target sequence, hybridization is detected by exposing the surface of the electrode to an exogenous electroactive species (Co[III]tris-phenanthroline, ruthenium complexes, etc.) that intercalates within the duplex, but not to single-stranded DNA. After unbound electroactive species are removed by washing, the presence of hybridization is readily detected by voltammetry, scanning the potential of the underlying electrode to oxidize or reduce any intercalated electroactive species, with the current detected being proportional to the number of duplex DNA species on the surface of the electrode.

Review Questions

1. Ion-selective electrodes measure electrical potential difference across a membrane using the principles of:
   a. coulometry.
   b. potentiometry.
   c. amperometry.
   d. conductivity.

2. An optical sensor used in analytical instruments to measure pH, blood gases, and electrolytes is referred to as a(n):
   a. potientiometer.
   b. optode.
   c. affinity-type sensor.
   d. coulometer.

3. Voltammetry/amperometry measurements are based on which of the following electrochemical cell types?
   a. Ion-selective electrode cells
   b. Galvanic electrochemical cells
   c. Electromotive force cells
   d. Electrolytic electrochemical cells

4. An affinity-based biosensor is one in which:
   a. the biological element recognizes the analyte on the basis of its binding to an immobilized substance.
   b. the fluorescence of a solution is coupled to an enzyme-catalyzed reaction.
   c. the biological element reacts with an ion-selective electrode that is used as a potentiometric transducer.
   d. an electron acceptor is used to form a colored reaction product.

5. A voltmeter that measures the potential across an electrochemical cell (between the two electrodes) is referred to as a:
   a. conductometer.
   b. amperometer.
   c. direct-reading potentiometer.
   d. redox meter.

6. Membrane potentials caused by the permeability of certain types of membranes to selected anions or cations are measured by which type of electrode?
   a. Ion-selective electrode
   b. Saturated calomel electrode
   c. Platinum electrode
   d. Gas-sensing electrode

7. The maximum difference in potential between the two electrodes in an electrochemical cell obtained with the current at zero is the definition of:
   a. electrical potential.
   b. electromotive force.
   c. electrochemical gradient.
   d. Nernst equation.

8. In this type of measurement, a constant current is applied to a solution, and a substance in that solution is changed to a different state through oxidation or reduction. The time it takes for this to occur is measured. This electrochemical technique is called:
   a. amperometry.
   b. voltammetry.
   c. potentiometry.
   d. coulometry.

9. The measurement of ions by direct potentiometry provides a value for the concentration of free, unbound ion in solution that is called the ionic:
   a. force.
   b. potential.
   c. activity.
   d. action.

10. The predominant class of potentiometric electrodes used in the clinical laboratory is the:
    a. gas-sensing electrode.
    b. glass membrane electrode.
    c. coulometric electrode.
    d. polymer membrane ion-selective electrode.

References

1. Apple FS, Koch DD, Graves S, et al. Relationship between direct potentiometric and flame photometric measurement of sodium in blood. Clin Chem 1982;28:1931–5.
2. Astrup P, Severinghaus JW. The history of blood gases, acids and bases. Copenhagen: Munksgaard, 1986.
3. Bates RG. Determination of pH: theory and practice. New York: John Wiley & Sons, 1973.
4. Bedioui F, Villeneuve N. Electrochemical nitric oxide sensors for biological samples: principle, selected examples and applications. Electroanalysis 2003;15:5–18.
5. Bijster P, Vader HL, Vink CLJ. Influence of erythrocytes on direct potentiometric determination of sodium and potassium. Ann Clin Biochem 1983;20:116–20.
6. Coulter WH. Means for counting particles suspended in a fluid. US Patent 2,656,508, Oct 20, 1953. Washington DC: US Patent Office.
7. Cullen D, Sethi R, Lowe C. A multi-analyte miniature conductance biosensor. Anal Chim Acta 1990;231:33–40.
8. Emr S, Yacynych A. Use of polymer films in amperometric biosensors. Electroanalysis 1995;7:913–23.
9. Feldman BJ, Oserioh JD, Hata BH, et al. Determination of lead in blood by square wave anodic stripping voltammetry at a carbon disk ultramicroelectrode. Anal Chem 1994;66:1983–7.
10. Lee HJ, Yoon IJ, Yoo CL, et al. Potentiometric evaluation of solvent polymeric carbonate-selective membranes based on molecular tweezer-type neutral carriers. Anal Chem 2000;72:4694–9.
11. Li X, Rosenweig Z. A fiber-optic sensor for rapid analysis of bilirubin in serum. Anal Chim Acta 1997;353:263–73.
12. Ma SC, Meyerhoff ME, Yang V. Heparin-responsive electrochemical sensor: a preliminary report. Anal Chem 1992;64:694–7.
13. Mathison S, Bakker E. Effect of transmembrane electrolyte diffusion on the detection limit of carrier-based potentiometric ion sensors. Anal Chem 1998;70:303–9.
14. Moreno-Bondi MC, Wolfbeis OS, Leiner MJP, et al. Oxygen optode for use in a fiber-optic glucose biosensor. Anal Chem 1990;62:2377–80.
15. Ohara TJ, Rajagopalan R, Heller A. "Wired" enzyme electrodes for amperometric determination of glucose or lactate in the presence of interfering substances. Anal Chem 1994;66:2451–7.
16. Pioda LA, Simon W, Bosshard HR, et al. Determination of potassium ion concentration in serum using a highly selective liquid-membrane electrode. Clin Chim Acta 1970;29:289–93.
17. Robinson DL, Venton BJ, Helen MLAV, et al. Detecting sub-second dopamine release with fast-scan voltammetry in freely moving rats. Clin Chem 2003;49:1763–73.
18. Thevenot DR, Toth K, Durst RA, et al. Electrochemical biosensors: recommended definitions and classifications. Biosen Bioelectron 2001;16:121–31.
19. Trettnak W, Wolfbeis OS. A fiber-optic cholesterol biosensor with an oxygen optode as the transducer. Anal Biochem 1990;184:124–7.
20. Wang J, Lu F. Oxygen rich oxidase enzyme electrodes for operation in oxygen-free solutions. J Am Chem Soc 1998;120:1048–50.
21. Zhang J, Song SP, Wang LH, et al. A gold nanoparticle-based chrono-coulometric DNA sensor for amplified detection of DNA. Nat Protoc 2007;2:2888–95.

Electrophoresis

Lindsay A.L. Bazydlo, Ph.D., and James P. Landers, Ph.D.

Objectives

1. Define the following:

Agarose	Electroendosmosis
Ampholyte	Electrophoresis
Amphoteric	Electrophoretic mobility
Blot/blotting	Polyacrylamide
Densitometry	Wick flow

2. State the theory of electrophoresis.
3. List and describe the components of an electrophoresis system, including buffers, support media, separation techniques, stains, and detection methods; quantify the individual fractions of a scanned gel when given total protein value.
4. Identify how each of the following affects electrophoresis: size and shape of molecule, heat and current produced by the power supply, buffer pH, specific type of gel used, and specimen appearance.
5. Describe and compare the following types of electrophoretic techniques, including clinical uses, system components, and detection methods:

Capillary	Microchip
Disc	Two-dimensional
Isoelectric focusing	Zone

6. Compare Southern, Northern, and Western blotting, including technical relations to electrophoresis, laboratory uses, and techniques.
7. State three advantages of capillary electrophoresis over conventional electrophoresis.
8. Explain how the following technical aspects affect the performance of the electrophoresis process: endomosis, buffer and stain integrity, sample type or appearance, and overapplication or underapplication of the sample; evaluate an electrophoresis pattern and identify problems.

Key Words and Definitions

Ampholyte A molecule that is positively or negatively charged on the basis of the pH of the solution in which it resides; proteins, because they contain many ionizable amino and carboxyl groups, behave as ampholytes in solution and are considered amphoteric.

Capillary electrophoresis A method in which the classic techniques of electrophoresis are carried out in a small-bore, fused silica capillary tube coated with a polymeric covering.

Densitometry A measuring technique that uses an optical system to scan and quantify electrophoretic fractions separated on a gel or other medium.

Electrophoresis The migration of charged solutes or particles within a liquid medium under the influence of an electrical field.

Electrophoretic mobility (µ) The rate of migration (cm/s) of a charged solute in an electrical field, expressed per unit field strength (volts/cm).

Electropherogram A densitometric display of protein zones on a support material after separation and staining.

Endosmosis (electroendosmotic flow) Preferential movement of water in one direction through an electrophoresis medium due to selective binding of one type of charge on the surface of the medium.

Isoelectric focusing An electrophoretic technique that separates amphoteric compounds within a medium that possesses a stable pH gradient.

Isoelectric point (pI) The pH at which a molecule has no net charge and will not migrate during electrophoresis.

Microchip electrophoresis An electrophoretic technique whereby separation is conducted in fluidic channels on a microchip and detection occurs through laser-induced fluorescence.

Wick flow Movement of water from the buffer reservoirs toward the center of an electrophoresis gel or strip to replace water lost by evaporation.

Electrophoresis is a versatile and powerful analytical technique that is capable of separating and analyzing a diverse range of ionized analytes. This chapter discusses (1) basic concepts and definitions, (2) theory, (3) description and types of electrophoresis, including capillary and microchip electrophoresis, and (4) their applications in the routine clinical laboratory, as well as in the developing fields of genomics and proteomics.

Basic Concepts and Definitions

Electrophoresis is a comprehensive term that refers to the migration of charged solutes or particles within a liquid medium under the influence of an electrical field. *Iontophoresis* is a similar term that applies only to the migration of small ions. *Zone electrophoresis* is the technique most commonly used in clinical applications. With this technique, charged molecules migrate as zones, usually in a porous supporting medium such as agarose gel film, after the sample is mixed with a buffer solution. It generates an **electropherogram,** a display of protein zones, each sharply separated from neighboring zones, on the support material. Protein zones are visualized when the support medium is stained with a protein-specific stain; then the medium is dried and zones are quantified in a densitometer. The support medium is dried and is kept as a permanent record.

Theory of Electrophoresis

In an electrophoresis system, ionized chemical species that have an electrical charge move toward the cathode (negative electrode) or the anode (positive electrode). Positive ions (cations) migrate toward the cathode, and negative ions (anions) migrate toward the anode (Figure 11-1). An **ampholyte** molecule (also called a *zwitterion*) contains both positive and negative charges, depending on the functional groups present in the molecule and the pH of the liquid in which they reside. The **isoelectric point (pI)** of an ampholyte molecule is the pH at which such a molecule has no electrical charge and does not migrate within an electrical field. Electrochemically, an ampholyte molecule takes on a positive charge in a solution that is more acidic than its pI and migrates toward the cathode. In a more alkaline solution, an ampholyte molecule is negatively ionized and migrates toward the anode. Because proteins contain many ionizable amino ($-NH_2$) and carboxyl ($-COOH$) groups, they behave as ampholytes in solution.

The rate of migration is dependent on factors such as (1) the net electrical charge of the molecule, (2) the size and shape of the molecule, (3) electrical field strength, (4) properties of the supporting medium, and (5) the temperature of operation. **Electrophoretic mobility (μ)** is defined as the rate of migration (cm/s) per unit field strength (volts/cm). Equation 1 expresses electrophoretic mobility and is derived from two formulas: one expressing the driving force of the electrical field on the ion and the other expressing the retarding force caused by frictional resistance of the medium.[5]

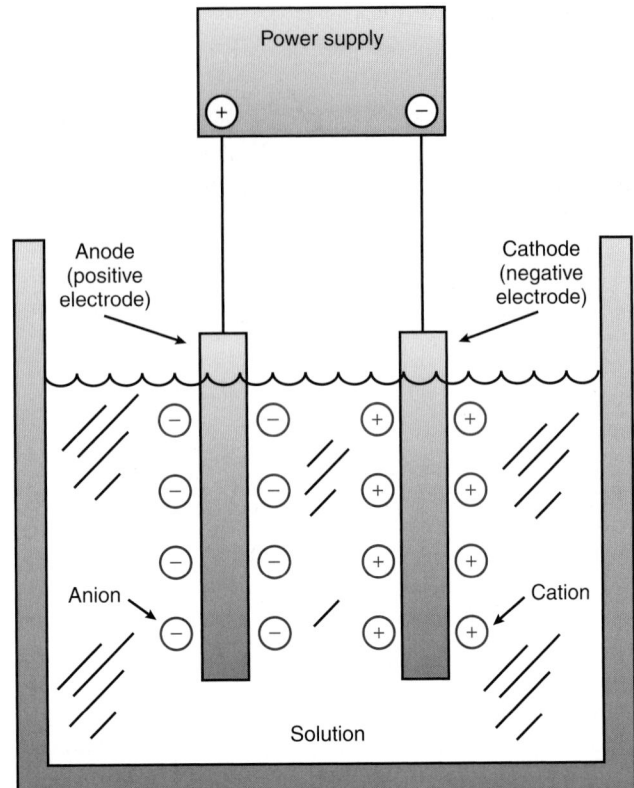

Figure 11-1 Movement of cations and anions within an electrical field.

$$\mu = \frac{Q}{6\pi r \eta} \tag{1}$$

where

μ = electrophoretic mobility in $cm^2/(V)(s)$;
Q = the net charge on the ion;
r = the ionic radius of the solute; and
η = the viscosity of the buffer solution in which migration is occurring.

Thus electrophoretic mobility is directly proportional to net charge and inversely proportional to molecular size and viscosity of the electrophoresis medium.

Other factors that affect mobility include endosmotic flow (which will be discussed in a later section of this chapter) and **wick flow.** The latter is a result of the electrophoretic process that generates heat, causing evaporation of solvent from the electrophoretic support. This drying effect causes buffer to rise into the electrophoresis support from both buffer compartments. This flow of buffer from both directions is called *wick flow,* and it affects protein migration and hence mobility.

Description of Technique

Topics discussed in this section include (1) electrophoresis instrumentation, (2) reagents, and (3) a general procedure.

Instrumentation and Reagents

A schematic diagram of a conventional electrophoresis system is shown in Figure 11-2. Two buffer chambers (1) with baffle plates contain the buffer used in the process. Each buffer box contains an electrode (2) made of platinum or carbon, the polarity of which is determined by the mode of connection to the power supply. The electrophoresis support (3) on which separation takes place may contact the buffer directly or by means of wicks (4). The entire apparatus is covered (5) to minimize evaporation and protect the system and is powered by a direct current power supply.

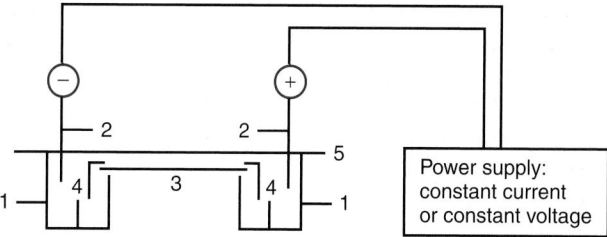

Figure 11-2 A schematic diagram of a typical electrophoresis apparatus showing two buffer chambers with baffle plates (1), electrodes (2), electrophoretic support (3), wicks (4), cover (5), and power supply.

Power Supplies

The function of a power supply in an electrophoretic process is to supply electrical power. Commercially available power supplies allow operation under conditions of (1) constant current, (2) constant voltage, or (3) constant power, all of which are adjustable. The flow of current through a medium that offers electrical resistance is associated with production of Joule heat:

$$\text{Heat} = (E)\ (I)\ (t) \qquad (2)$$

where

E = electromotive force (EMF) in volts (V);
I = current in amperes (A); and
t = time in seconds (s).

Heat evolved during electrophoresis increases the conductance of the system (decreases resistance). With constant-voltage power sources, the resultant rise in current, which is due to the increase in thermal agitation of all dissolved ions, causes an increase in both the migration rate of the protein and the rate of evaporation of water from the stationary support medium. The water loss causes an increase in ion concentration and further decreases resistance (R). To minimize these effects on migration rate, it is best to use a constant-current power supply. According to Ohm's law:

$$E = (I)\ (R) \qquad (3)$$

Therefore, if R is decreased, the applied EMF also decreases (current remains constant). This in turn decreases the heat effect and keeps the migration rate relatively constant.

For **isoelectric focusing** (IEF), a power supply capable of constant power is recommended because both current and voltage change as separation occurs during performance of this technique. **Capillary electrophoresis** (CE) systems (discussed later in this chapter) use power supplies capable of providing voltages in the kilovolt range. Pulsed-power or pulsed-field techniques periodically change the orientation of the applied field relative to the direction of migration by alternately applying power to different pairs of electrodes or electrode arrays. During each cycle, molecules must reorient themselves to the new field direction to fit through the pores in the gel before migration continues. Because reorientation time depends on molecular size, net migration becomes a function of the frequency of field alteration. This permits separation of very large molecules such as DNA fragments

that are not resolved by the relatively small pores in agarose or polyacrylamide gels.[12]

Buffers

The buffer serves as a multifunctional component of the electrophoretic process as it (1) carries the applied current, (2) establishes the pH at which electrophoresis is performed, and (3) determines the electrical charge on the solute. The buffer's ionic strength influences (1) the conductance of the support, (2) the thickness of the ionic cloud (buffer and nonbuffer ions) surrounding a charged molecule, (3) the rate of its migration, and (4) the sharpness of the electrophoretic zones. With increasing buffer concentration, the ionic cloud increases in size, and the molecule becomes hindered in its movement. High ionic strength buffers yield sharper band separations but also produce increased Joule heat as the result of increased current levels—an effect that leads to denaturation of heat-labile proteins.

Ionic strength (also denoted by the symbol μ) is computed according to the following:

$$\mu = 0.5 \sum c_i\ z_i^2 \qquad (4)$$

where

c_i = ion concentration in mol/L; and
z_i = the charge on the ion.

The ionic strength of an electrolyte (buffer) composed of monovalent ions is equal to its molarity (mol/L). The ionic strength of a 1 mol/L electrolyte solution with one monovalent and one divalent ion is 3 mol/L, and for a doubly divalent electrolyte, it is 4 mol/L.

Support Media

The support medium provides the matrix in which separation takes place. Various types of support media are used in electrophoresis and vary from pure buffer solutions in a capillary to insoluble gels (e.g., sheets, slabs, or columns of starch, agarose, or polyacrylamide) or membranes of cellulose acetate. Gels are cast in a solution of the same buffer to be used in the procedure and may be used in a horizontal or vertical orientation. In either case, maximum resolution is achieved if the sample is applied within a very fine starting zone. Separation is based on differences in charge-to-mass ratio of the proteins and, depending on the pore size of the medium, possibly molecular size.

Starch Gel and Cellulose Acetate

Starch gel was the first material to be used as a support medium for electrophoresis. It was used to separate macromolecules on the basis of both surface charge and molecular size. Because preparation of a reproducible starch gel is difficult, this medium is now rarely used in the clinical laboratory. Cellulose acetate membranes are dry, opaque, brittle films made by treating cellulose with acetic anhydride. Because they need to be soaked in buffer to soften them before use and also need to be cleared before scanning for densitometry, they are seldom used in routine clinical applications. Currently, agarose and polyacrylamide gels are the support media of choice for electrophoresis.

Agarose

Agarose is a purified, essentially neutral fraction of agar obtained by separating agarose from agaropectin, a more highly charged fraction caused by acidic sulfate and carboxylic side groups. It is used in agarose gel electrophoresis (AGE) for the separation of a variety of analytes including (1) serum, urine, or CSF proteins, (2) hemoglobin variants, (3) isoenzymes, and (4) lipoproteins. Because the pore size in agarose gel is large enough for all proteins to pass through unimpeded, separation is based only on the charge-to-mass ratio of the protein. Advantages of agarose gel include its lower affinity for proteins and its native clarity after drying, which permits excellent densitometric examination. It is essentially free of ionizable groups and so exhibits little **endosmosis** (discussed later in this chapter).

Most routine procedures for AGE today are carried out on commercially produced, prepackaged microzone gels. Sample is applied by means of a thin plastic template with small slots corresponding to sample application points in manual procedures or a comb applicator if an automated system is used. The template is placed on the agarose surface, and 5- to 7-μL samples are placed on each slot. After sample is allowed to diffuse into the agarose for 5 minutes, any excess is removed by blotting, and the template is removed. An AGE separation for most routine serum applications requires an electrophoresis time of 20 to 30 minutes.

Operationally, 0.5 to 1.0 g of agarose/dL of buffer provides a gel with suitable strength and good migration properties for proteins and DNA fragments in the range of 0.5 to 20.0 kbp (kilobase pairs). Smaller DNA fragments may be resolved with special grades of agarose. Because all nucleic acids have essentially the same charge-to-mass ratios, separation is based primarily on molecular size and in part on molecular form, both of which determine how fast the molecule or fragment migrates through the pores of the gel. Smaller DNA fragments have migration rates in agarose that are inversely proportional to the logs of their molecular weights, but this relationship decreases as their fragment size increases. Fragments larger than 50 to 100 kbp migrate at the same rate through agarose

and require an alternative technique such as pulse-field electrophoresis for separation.

Polyacrylamide

Polyacrylamide is a polymer that is prepared by heating acrylamide with a variety of catalysts, with or without cross-linking agents. Polyacrylamide gel is (1) thermostable, (2) transparent, (3) strong, and (4) relatively chemically inert. Furthermore, these gels are uncharged, thus eliminating endosmosis, and they are prepared in a variety of pore sizes. As compared with agarose gel, the average pore size in a typical 7.5% polyacrylamide gel is about 5 nm (50 Å)—large enough to allow most serum proteins to migrate unimpeded—but proteins with a molecular radius and/or length that exceeds critical limits will be more or less impeded in their migration. Some of these proteins are (1) fibrinogen, (2) β_1-lipoprotein, (3) α_2-macroglobulin, and (4) γ-globulins. With polyacrylamide, proteins are separated on the basis of both charge-to-mass ratio and molecular size—a phenomenon referred to as *molecular sieving*. Because of the potential carcinogenic character of acrylamide, appropriate caution must be exercised when this material is handled if gels are prepared manually.

When used for the separation of nucleic acids, polyacrylamide is capable of resolving DNA molecules that differ by as little as 2% in length (1 bp in 50 bp). It accommodates a larger amount of sample (up to 10 μg) in a single sample slot, and, compared with DNA from agarose, the DNA recovered from a polyacrylamide gel is extremely pure, containing no inhibitors. Polyacrylamide is most useful for mixtures of smaller DNA fragments and is able to resolve fragments smaller than 1 kbp; however, its small pore size prevents supercoiled DNA from entering the gel.

Automated Systems

Because of increased volume of testing, primarily for serum proteins, many laboratories are converting to automated systems for electrophoresis. These systems provide (1) automated sample and reagent application, (2) electrophoretic separation, (3) staining of analytes, and (4) drying of a variety of gel sizes. They are capable of processing 10 to 100 samples simultaneously. Most capillary systems have autosampling capability for sequentially processing specimens and some permit simultaneous processing of multiple samples with the use of multiple capillaries. Newer microchip-based analyzers significantly miniaturize and increase the speed of the process for separating proteins, nucleic acids, or even entire cells. These advances substantially reduce the labor component associated with this technique.

Description of a Conventional Electrophoretic Procedure

General operations performed in conventional electrophoresis include (1) separation, (2) staining detection, and (3) quantification. In addition, several electrophoretic "blotting" techniques have been developed. Following here is a description of the details associated with a general electrophoretic separation.

Separation

To perform an electrophoretic separation, a hydrated support material, such as a precast microzone agarose or polyacrylamide gel, is blotted to remove excess buffer and then is placed into the electrophoresis chamber. Care should be taken that the gel has neither excess liquid nor bubbles on it. Next, the sample is added to the support material, and it is placed in contact with buffer previously added to the electrode chambers. Electrophoresis is conducted for a determined length of time under conditions of constant voltage or constant current.

Staining Detection

When electrophoresis is completed, the support is removed from the electrophoresis cell and is rapidly dried or placed in a fixative to prevent diffusion of sample components. It is then stained to allow visualization of the individual protein zones. After a washing step to remove excess dye, the support is dried.

Stains used to visualize the separated protein fractions are listed in Table 11-1 and differ according to type of application. The amount of dye taken up by the sample is affected by many factors such as the type of protein and the degree of its denaturation by fixing agents. Most commercial methods for serum protein electrophoresis use Amido Black B or members of the Coomassie Brilliant Blue series of dyes for staining. Isoenzymes are typically visualized by incubating the gel in contact with a solution of substrate, which is linked structurally or chemically to a dye, before fixing. Silver nitrate or silver diamine has been used to stain proteins and polypeptides with sensitivity 10- to 100-fold greater than that of dyes used for the same purpose.[14] Selective fixing and staining of protein subclasses also has been achieved by combining a stain molecule with an antiglobulin, as is done in immunofixation.

TABLE 11-1	Suggested Wavelengths for Quantification of Protein Zones by Direct Densitometry

Separation Type	Dye	Nominal Wavelength, nm
Serum proteins in general	Amido Black (Naphthol Blue Black)	640
	Coomassie Brilliant Blue G-250 (Brilliant Blue G)	595
	Coomassie Brilliant Blue R-250 (Brilliant Blue R)	560
	Ponceau S	520
Isoenzymes ormazan	Nitrotetrazolium Blue (as the formazan)	570
Lipoprotein zones	Fat Red 7B (Sudan Red 7B)	540
	Oil Red O	520
	Sudan Black B	600
DNA fragments	Ethidium bromide (fluorescent)	254 (Ex) 590 (Em)
CSF proteins	Silver nitrate	—

CSF, Cerebrospinal fluid.

Detection and Quantification

Once the steps of electrophoretic separation and staining are complete, it is possible to quantify the individual zones as a percentage of the total or as absolute concentration by direct **densitometry**, if the total protein concentration is known. In the densitometer, the gel (or other medium) is moved past a measuring optical system, and the absorbance of each fraction is displayed on a recorder chart or on an electronic display. Typically, the area under each peak is automatically integrated. Reliable quantification of stained zones using densitometry requires (1) light of an appropriate wavelength, (2) a linear response from the instrument, and (3) a transparent background in the strip being scanned. The response linearity may be verified with a neutral density filter designed with separated or adjacent zones of density, which increase in a linear fashion and have expected absorbance values. Recording the pattern of absorbance obtained for each zone checks the (1) optical, (2) mechanical, and (3) electrical functions of the densitometer.

Useful features generally found in a densitometer include (1) the ability to scan gels 25 to 100 mm in length; (2) automatic gain control, which adjusts the most intense peak of an electropherogram to full scale; (3) automatic background zeroing, which selects the lowest point in the electropherogram as baseline so that minor peaks are not lost or "cut off"; (4) variable wavelength control over the range of 400 to 700 nm; (5) variable slits to allow adjustment of the beam size; (6) an integrating device with both automatic and manual selection of cut points between peaks; (7) automatic indexing—a feature that advances the electrophoresis strip from one sample channel to the next; and (8) the ability to measure ultraviolet fluorescence.

Other desirable features of an electrophoretic instrument and densitometer include (1) computerized integration and printout, (2) built-in diagnostics for instrument troubleshooting, (3) choice of one of several scanning speeds, and (4) ability to measure in the reflectance mode. Models with a separate personal computer for data processing permit (1) storage and reformatting of data, if desired, and (2) reprinting or delayed transmission to a host computer.

Modern DNA analysis techniques, which may produce several dozen bands of DNA fragments of different length, require a type of densitometer referred to as a *flat bed scanner* or a *digital image analyzer.*[3] These instruments use ultrasensitive charge-coupled device (CCD) detectors or cameras, have resolution of up to 1200 dots per inch, and are capable of scanning and storing digitized light intensity readings from large areas.

In addition to scanning by densitometry, electrophoresis gels are now being analyzed by mass spectrometers to (1) determine the molecular weights of proteins, (2) determine the cleavage products of proteins,[11] and (3) perform peptide sequencing.[4]

Types of Electrophoresis

The original moving boundary electrophoresis system devised by Tiselius in 1937 separated serum proteins into only five component mixtures: albumin, α_1-, α_2-, β-, and γ-globulins, with the α_1 fraction incompletely separated from albumin.

Modern techniques use different media in different physical formats and a variety of instrumental configurations to achieve much better separations than those obtained by Tiselius. The following section describes several different techniques used for the separation of various analytes.

Zone Electrophoresis

Zone electrophoresis techniques produce zones of proteins that are heterogeneous and physically separated from one another, as shown in Figure 11-3. They are classified according to the type and structure of support materials used and are commonly referred to as (1) *agarose gel electrophoresis* (AGE), (2) *cellulose acetate electrophoresis* (CAE), and (3) *polyacrylamide gel electrophoresis* (PAGE).

Slab Gel Electrophoresis

Traditional methods that use a rectangular gel regardless of thickness are referred to collectively by the term *slab gel electrophoresis*. Its main advantage is its ability to simultaneously separate several samples in one run. Starch, agarose (AGE), and polyacrylamide (PAGE) media have been used in this format. It is the primary method used in clinical chemistry laboratories for separation of various classes of serum or cerebrospinal fluid (CSF) proteins and DNA or RNA fragments. Gels (usually agarose) may be cast on a sheet of plastic backing or completely encased within a plastic walled cell, which allows horizontal or vertical electrophoresis and submersion for cooling, if necessary.

Slab gels may be cast with additives such as (1) ampholytes, which create a pH gradient (see "Isoelectric Focusing Electrophoresis [IEF]"), or (2) sodium dodecyl sulfate (SDS), which denatures proteins (see "Two-Dimensional [2D] Electrophoresis"). In addition to conventional serum proteins, applications include separation of (1) isoenzymes, (2) lipoproteins, (3) hemoglobins, and (4) fragments of DNA and RNA. One-dimensional separations of the last two often involve the addition of a mixture of known fragment size markers, referred to as a *ladder*, to one lane to enable size identification of sample fragments.

Disc Electrophoresis

Protein electrophoresis using agarose gel yields only five zones, namely, (1) albumin, (2) α_1-, (3) α_2-, (4) β-, and (5) γ-globulins, although some subfractionation of the α_2- and β-globulins is possible with high-resolution gels. Because the pore size in a polyacrylamide gel is controlled by the percent composition of the polyacrylamide and is much smaller than that found in agarose gel, these gels may yield 20 or more fractions and are widely used to study individual proteins in serum, especially genetic variants and isoenzymes.

With PAGE, samples are separated in individual gels prepared in open-ended glass tubes (referred to as *rod PAGE*), which form a bridge between two buffer reservoirs. Although precast gel tubes are now commercially available, the original technique involved a three-gel system consisting of a small-pore separating gel, a larger-pore spacer gel, and a thin layer of large-pore monomer solution containing about 3 µL of serum. The different compositions caused *discontinuities* in the electrophoretic matrix and gave the technique its original name, *disc electrophoresis*. In this system, when electrophoresis begins, all protein ions migrate easily through the large-pore gels (which do not impede movement of most proteins in serum) and stack up on the separation gel in a very thin zone. This process improves resolution and concentrates protein components at the border (or starting zone) so that preconcentration of specimens with low protein content (e.g., CSF) may not be necessary. Separation then takes place in the bottom separation gel with retardation of some proteins caused by the molecular sieve phenomenon.

Isoelectric Focusing Electrophoresis

Isoelectric focusing electrophoresis (IEF) separates amphoteric compounds such as proteins with increased resolution in a medium possessing a stable pH gradient. The protein migrates to a zone in the medium where the pH of the gel matches the protein's pI. At this point, the charge of the protein becomes zero, and its migration ceases. Figure 11-4 illustrates the procedure and shows electrophoretic conditions before

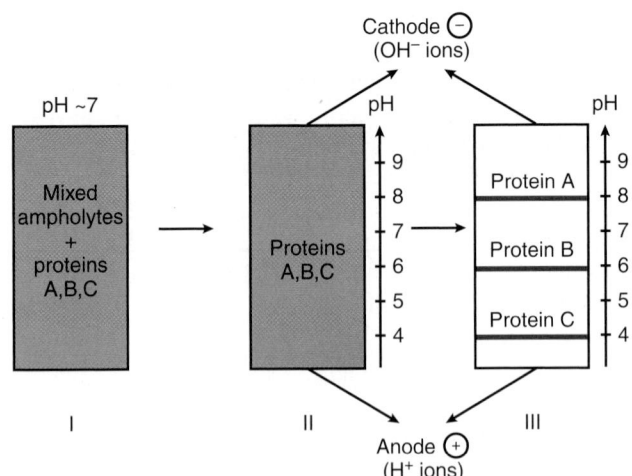

Figure 11-4 Schematic of an isoelectric focusing (IEF) procedure. *I,* A homogeneous mixture of carrier ampholytes, pH range 3 to 10, to which proteins A, B, and C with pI 8, 6, and 4, respectively, were added. *II,* Current is applied and the carrier ampholytes rapidly migrate to the pH zones where net charge is zero (the isoelectric point [pI] value). *III,* The proteins A, B, and C migrate more slowly to their respective pI zones, where migration ceases. The high buffering capacity of the carrier ampholytes creates stable pH zones in which each protein may reach its pI.

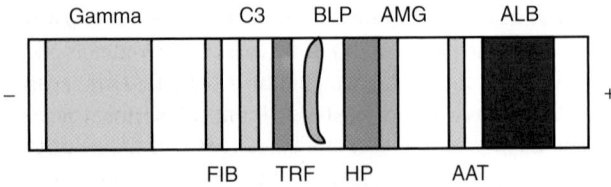

Figure 11-3 A simplified schematic drawing of a protein pattern from the serum of a subject with haptoglobin type 2-1 (separation by polyacrylamide gel electrophoresis [PAGE]). Some zones contain more than the one protein shown, as demonstrated by immunological techniques. *AAT,* α_1-antitrypsin; *ALB,* albumin; *AMG,* α_2-macroglobulin; *BLP,* β-lipoprotein; *C3,* complement 3; *FIB,* fibrinogen; *gamma,* γ-globulin; *HP,* haptoglobin; *TRF,* transferrin.

and after current is applied. The protein zones are very sharp because the region associated with a given pH is very narrow. Normal diffusion is counteracted because the protein acquires a charge as it migrates from its pI position and subsequently migrates back because of electrophoretic forces. Proteins that differ in their pI values by only 0.02 pH units have been separated by IEF.

The pH gradient is created with carrier ampholytes, a group of amphoteric polyaminocarboxylic acids that have slight differences in pKa values and molecular weights of 300 to 1000 Da. Mixtures of 50 to 100 different compounds are added to the medium and create a "natural pH gradient" when the individual ampholytes reach their pI values during electrophoresis. Narrow buffered zones are established with stable but slightly different pHs, through which the slower-moving proteins migrate and stop at their individual pIs. Because carrier ampholytes are generally used in relatively high concentrations, a high-voltage power source (up to 2000 V) is necessary. As a result, the electrophoretic matrix must be cooled. IEF is widely used in neonatal screening programs to test for variant hemoglobins.

Two-Dimensional (2D) Electrophoresis

Two-dimensional (2D) electrophoresis is extensively used to (1) study families of proteins, (2) search for genetic or disease-based differences, and (3) study the protein content of cells of various types.[8] This technique uses charge-dependent IEF electrophoresis in the first dimension and molecular weight–dependent electrophoresis in the second dimension. The first-dimension electrophoresis is carried out in a large-pore medium, such as agarose gel or large-pore polyacrylamide gel. Ampholytes are added to yield a pH gradient. The second dimension is often polyacrylamide in a linear or gradient format. This type of electrophoresis achieves the highest resolving power for separation of DNA fragments. With this application, normal AGE is carried out in the first dimension and ethidium bromide is added to the gel for the second dimension to open the fragments and cause changes in their electrophoretic mobility.

The 2D electrophoresis method of O'Farrell uses rod PAGE-IEF for the first dimension and incorporates ampholytes that cover a pH range of 3 to 10 units. The gel is extruded from the gel tube at the end of electrophoresis and is placed in contact with a thin polyacrylamide gradient gel slab that incorporates SDS. Separated proteins may be detected by using a variety of techniques, including (1) staining with Coomassie dyes, (2) silver stain, (3) radiography (exposure of photographic film to emissions of isotopically labeled polypeptides), or (4) fluorographic analysis (X-ray film exposed to tritium-labeled polypeptides in the presence of a scintillator). The latter two methods are 100 to 1000 times more sensitive than the use of Coomassie dyes.

Analytical and preparative 2D electrophoresis provides high-resolution techniques for protein separation, which are the methods of choice when complex samples need to be arrayed for characterization, as in **proteomics**.[1]

Newer developments in proteomics combine analytical techniques to achieve 2D separation by linking, for example, liquid IEF with nonporous silica reversed-phase, high-performance liquid chromatography (HPLC; see Chapter 12) and by detecting intact proteins by electrospray ionization and time of flight mass spectrometry[4] (see Chapter 13).

Blotting Techniques

In 1975, Edward Southern developed a technique that is widely used to detect fragments of DNA. This technique, known as *Southern blotting,* first requires electrophoretic separation of DNA or DNA fragments by AGE. Next a strip of nitrocellulose or a nylon membrane is laid over the agarose gel, and the DNA or DNA fragments are transferred or "blotted" onto it by (1) capillary blotting, (2) electroblotting, or (3) vacuum blotting. They are then detected and identified by hybridization with a labeled complementary nucleic acid probe. This technique is widely used in molecular biology for (1) identifying a particular DNA sequence; (2) determining the presence, position, and number of copies of a gene in a genome; and (3) typing DNA.

Northern and Western blotting techniques, named by analogy to Southern blotting, were subsequently developed to separate and detect ribonucleic acid (RNA) and proteins, respectively. Northern blotting is carried out identically to Southern blotting, except that a labeled RNA probe is used for hybridization. Western blotting is used to (1) separate, (2) detect, and (3) identify one or more proteins in a complex mixture. It involves first separating the individual proteins in polyacrylamide gel and then transferring or "blotting" them onto an overlying strip of nitrocellulose or a nylon membrane by electroblotting. The strip or membrane is then reacted with a reagent that contains an antibody raised against the protein of interest. (See Chapter 15 for further details and applications of this technique.)

Capillary Electrophoresis

In capillary electrophoresis (CE), the classic techniques of electrophoresis are carried out in a small-bore, fused silica capillary tube typically coated with a thin (exterior) polymeric covering (polyimide). For example, the outer diameter of the capillary tubing used to make such tubes typically ranges from 180 to 375 μm, the inner diameter from 20 to 180 μm, and the total length from 20 cm up to several meters. This capillary tube serves as a capillary electrophoretic chamber that is connected to a detector at its terminal end[16] and, via buffer reservoirs, to a high-voltage power supply (Figure 11-5). The main advantage of CE comes from efficient heat dissipation, which permits the application of voltages in the range of 25 to 30 kV. This enhances separation efficiency and reduces separation time in some cases to less than 1 minute.[9] Sample volumes are kept in the picoliter-to-nanoliter range to minimize distortions in the applied field caused by the presence of sample.

Buffers for CE

As with conventional electrophoresis, the choice of a buffer is critical for obtaining successful separation with CE. In practice, it is critical to select a buffer that (1) does not interfere with the ability to detect the analytes of interest, (2) maintains

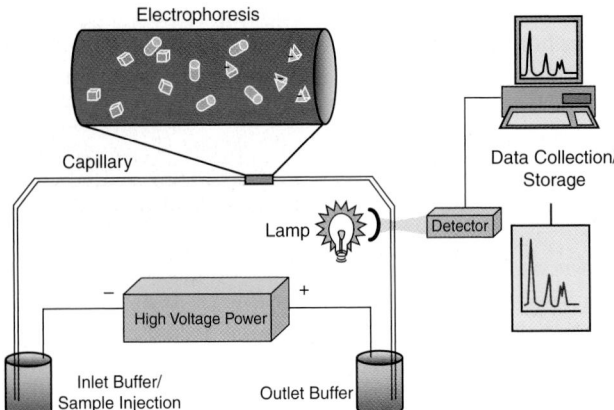

Figure 11-5 Schematic for capillary electrophoresis (CE) instrumentation.

solubility of the analytes, (3) maintains buffering capacity through the analysis, and (4) produces the desired separation. For low-pH buffers, (1) phosphate, (2) acetate, (3) formate, and (4) citrate have commonly been used effectively. For buffers in the basic pH range, (1) Tris, (2) Tricine, (3) borate, and (4) CAP (*N*-cyclohexyl-3-aminopropanesulfonic acid) buffers are used.

Ionic strength is an important variable that has been known to have adverse effects (both positive and negative) on electrophoretic separation, mainly because high ionic strength buffers generate excessive Joule heat. Although capillary thermostatting (inherent dissipation combined with active cooling) is very effective, the current (Joule heat) associated with buffer concentrations greater than 100 mmol/L may overcome capillary thermostatting at higher applied voltages. One exception to this rule is borate buffer, a classic CE buffer that generates relatively low current (and therefore, Joule heat) in high applied fields. Consequently, in the pH 7 to 9 range, 500 mmol/L borate is the buffer of choice for CE separations.

Sample Injection

To perform a CE separation, sample volumes of 1 to 50 nL are injected into the capillary chamber by *hydrodynamic injection* or *electrokinetic injection*. With hydrodynamic injection, an aliquot of sample is introduced by applying positive pressure to the sample inlet vial. Alternatively, gravity may be used by raising the inlet vial (or lowering the outlet reservoir) to allow siphoning to occur. The volume of sample loaded is governed by a number of parameters, including (but not restricted to) (1) the inner diameter of the capillary, (2) buffer viscosity, (3) applied pressure, (4) temperature, and (5) time. With electrokinetic (EK) injection, an aliquot of a sample is introduced by applying a voltage between a sample vial and the outlet buffer reservoir for a timed interval. The magnitude of the voltage is dependent on the analyte and buffer system used but typically involves field strength 3 to 5 times lower than that used for separation. It is important to note that although hydrodynamic methods introduce a sample representative of the bulk specimen, EK injection favors those analytes that have higher electrophoretic mobility; thus it is consider a "biased"

injection mode. With either mode, to maintain high separation efficiency, the length of the sample plug should remain at <2% of the total capillary length.

Detection

The detection modes that have been designed for HPLC are equally applicable to CE. For example, ultraviolet-visible photometers are widely used as detectors to monitor CE separations.[13] However, as opposed to being distinct from flow cells in liquid chromatography (LC) systems, the inner diameter of the capillary tube (20 to 100 µm) defines the optical pathlength (OPL) for detection. Because optical detection is governed by Beer's law, the 20 to 100 µm inner diameter (i.d.) of the capillary limits ultraviolet–visible spectroscopy (UV-Vis) absorbance detection to 10^{-6} to 10^{-8} mol/L. In addition to OPL constraints, when nanoliter volumes are injected, the mass of analyte injected is extremely small. More sensitive optical techniques that have been used with CE include (1) fluorescence, (2) refractive index, (3) chemiluminescence, and (4) laser-induced fluorescence (LIF), which is the most sensitive method and is capable of detection limits of 10^{-18} to 10^{-21} mol/L.

In addition to the use of sensitive detectors, techniques have been developed to preconcentrate the sample. One of the simplest techniques used for this involves inducing a "stacking" effect with the sample components—something that is easily accomplished by exploiting ionic strength differences between the sample matrix and the separation buffer.[2] This can be done because sample ions have decreased electrophoretic mobility in a higher conductivity environment. When voltage is applied to the system, sample ions in the sample plug instantaneously accelerate toward the adjacent separation buffer zone. Upon crossing the boundary, the higher conductivity environment induces a decrease in electrophoretic velocity and subsequent "stacking" of the sample components into a smaller buffer zone than was seen in the original sample plug. Within a short time, the ionic strength gradient dissipates and the charged analyte molecules begin to move from the "stacked" sample zone toward the cathode. Stacking is used with hydrostatic or EK injection and typically yields a tenfold enhancement in sample concentration and hence lower limits of detection.

An alternative approach to stacking is a "focusing" technique that is based on pH differences between the sample plug and the separation buffer. This has been shown to be very useful for analysis of peptides, mainly because of their relative stability over a wide pH range.[10]

Modes of Operation

CE is capable of multiple modes of operation, including (1) capillary zone electrophoresis, (2) capillary gel electrophoresis, and (3) capillary IEF..

Capillary zone electrophoresis (CZE), the simplest form of CE, is unique as a result of its ability to electrophoretically resolve analytes in the absence of a separation medium (polymer, ampholytes). The power of the CZE mode is its ability to resolve charged species electrophoretically without a sieving matrix; it is broadly applicable to a spectrum of analytes, including (1) proteins,[17] (2) peptides, (3) amino acids, and (4) other small molecules such as drugs and ions.[15] A submode of CZE is *capillary ion electrophoresis,* which refers to analysis of inorganic ions by CZE, particularly when indirect detection is used. With this mode of detection, a strongly absorbing ion is added to the running electrolyte and is monitored at a wavelength that provides constant, high background absorbance. As solute ions move into their discrete zones during the electrophoretic process, they displace the indirect detection agent; this produces a decrease in background absorbance as the zone passes through the detector.

Micellar electrokinetic chromatography (MEKC) is a hybrid of electrophoresis and chromatography but is distinct from capillary electrokinetic chromatography (CEC), where the capillary is actually filled with a solid phase. MEKC is an unusually effective electrophoretic technique because it can be used for the separation of neutral and charged solutes. Separation of neutral species is accomplished by the use of micelles formed by additives in the separation buffer (e.g., SDS). Differential interaction of analytes with micelles provides separation that is based on chromatography, whereas the application of an electrical field provides electrophoretic separation of charged analytes and flow.

Capillary gel electrophoresis (CGE) is directly comparable with traditional slab or tube gel electrophoresis because the separation mechanisms are identical.[6] Size separation is achieved with a suitable polymer that is loaded into the capillary, used for one separation, and then replaced. Separation is size-based for DNA- and SDS-saturated proteins and requires a gel because they contain mass-to-charge ratios that do not vary. A variety of polymeric matrices have been defined for both DNA (e.g., polyacrylamide and cellulosic materials) and protein analysis (e.g., dextran-based matrices). One of the requirements that often accompany this type of analysis is that electro-osmotic flow must be reduced. This is accomplished by (1) covalently, (2) adsorptively, or (3) dynamically coating the surface.

Capillary IEF (cIEF) is comparable with tube IEF and is governed by the same principles and procedures. It differs from conventional IEF in that it is carried out using a free solution of ampholytes or a precast gel. As is expected with a CE mode, and unlike conventional IEF, the focused zones migrate past the online detector during or after the focusing process.

Microchip Electrophoresis

Microchip electrophoresis platforms were first developed in the 1990s.[7] Subsequent developments by numerous laboratories have advanced analytical microchip technology to the point where it functions as an alternative platform to CE. Similar in principle to CE, microchips differ from capillaries in that the (1) separation channels, (2) sample injection channels, and (3) reservoirs are fabricated into the same planar substrate using photolithographic processes employed by the microelectronics industry. Additionally, (1) sample preparation and/or precolumn or postcolumn reactors, (2) detectors, and (3) excitation sources have been integrated into the chips.

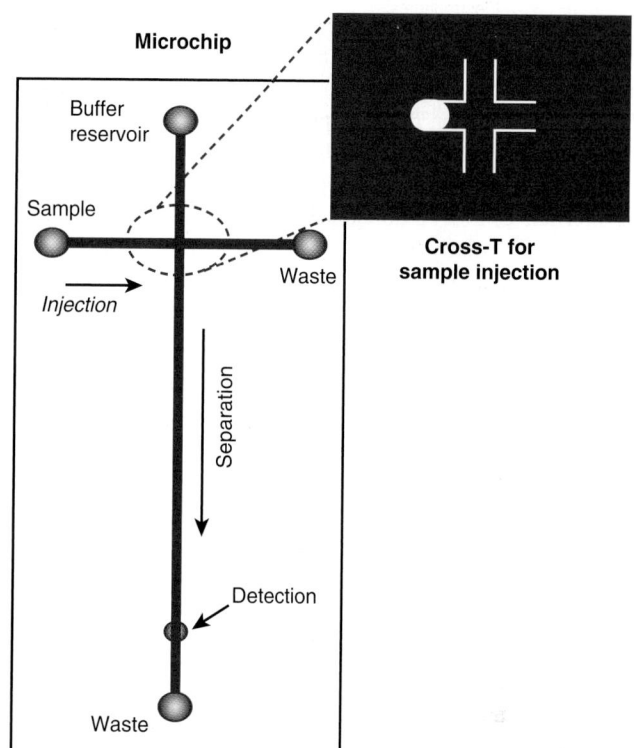

Figure 11-6 Simple cross-T microstructure design on chips used for electrophoretic separation.

The classic cross-T design of a single-channel microchip (Figure 11-6) involves a short (injection) channel that intersects a longer (separation) channel with reservoirs at the ends of each of these channels. The cross-T design is important for injecting sample volumes an order of magnitude smaller in the chip system than in the capillary system. This is accomplished through EK sample injection by applying a field of several hundred volts across the sample and sample waste reservoirs, thereby inducing migration of 50 to 500 pL of sample into the injection cross. A higher voltage (1 to 4 kV) is then applied to the separation channel, which induces separation of the analyte zones before they reach the detection window downstream.

In the same manner that optical detection is conducted in a capillary system, it is accomplished on a single channel in a microchip. For example, UV-Vis absorbance detection has been used but is more difficult than in CE because the substrates used to fabricate the chips often are not as "pure" as the fused silica used in capillaries, or they may have different spectral properties. Consequently, detection occurs primarily through LIF because this is easily implemented with the planar configuration of the microchip. Detection limits for fluorescein-like fluors have been easily demonstrated at the 10^{-11} mol/L level of detection and have been pushed as low as 10^{-13} mol/L—a mass detection limit of a few hundred molecules. This allows for detection, for example, of polymerase chain reaction (PCR)-amplified DNA fragments at a level that competes with ^{32}P-autoradiography from Southern blots.[6] Typical microchip separation times are around 50 to 200 seconds. In the clinical diagnostic arena, the main analytes of interest for extrapolation to the microchip platform are proteins and DNA.

As a result of the large number of fluorescent intercalators that have been incorporated into double-stranded (ds) DNA and the excellent detection sensitivity that results from LIF, DNA separations on microchips have developed more rapidly than protein separations. This has accelerated the rate at which capillary and microchip electrophoresis methods have emerged as alternatives to traditional slab gel electrophoresis for DNA analysis, particularly for sequencing applications. This is signified by sequencing of the human genome using CE.

Technical Considerations

Several technical aspects of the electrophoretic process have to be considered to obtain acceptable performance. They include (1) electroendosmosis, (2) handling of buffers and stain solutions, (3) sampling considerations, and (4) a number of problems commonly encountered in performing electrophoresis.

Endosmosis or Electroendosmotic Flow

Certain electrophoretic support media in contact with water take on a negative charge as the result of adsorption of hydroxyl ions. These ions become fixed to the surface and are rendered immobile. Positive ions in solution cluster about the fixed negative charge sites, forming an ionic cloud of mostly positive ions. The number of negative ions associated with this ionic cloud increases with increasing distance from the fixed negative charge sites until eventually positive and negative ions are present in equal concentrations (Figure 11-7).

When current is applied to such a system, charges attached to the immobile support remain fixed, but the cloud of ions in solution is free to move to the electrode of opposite polarity. Because these ions are highly hydrated, their movement causes movement of the solvent as well. This phenomenon, referred to as *endosmosis,* causes preferential movement of water in one direction. Macromolecules in solution that would otherwise move in the opposite direction to this flow may remain immobile or may even be swept back toward the opposite pole if they are insufficiently charged. In electrophoretic media in which surface charges are minimal (starch gel, purified agarose, and polyacrylamide gel), endosmosis is also minimal. Because the inner surface of a glass capillary contains many such charged groups, endosmosis is very strong and is actually the primary driving force for migration in CE systems.

Buffers and Stain Solutions

Buffers are good culture media for the growth of microorganisms and should be refrigerated when not in use. Moreover, a cold buffer improves resolution and reduces evaporation from the electrophoretic support. Buffer used in a small-volume apparatus should be discarded after each run because of pH changes caused by the electrolysis of water that accompanies electrophoresis. If volumes used are larger than 100 mL, buffer from both reservoirs may be combined, mixed, stored at 4 °C, and reused for four subsequent electrophoretic runs.

A typical stain solution may be used several times. The stain or substrate reagent, in the case of isoenzymes, may be considered faulty whenever protein zones appear too lightly stained. Stain solution must be stored tightly covered to prevent evaporation.

Sampling

Because albumin in serum is about 10 times more concentrated than the α_1-globulins, the amount of serum applied should avoid overloading with albumin while adequately quantifying α_1-globulin. Typical amounts of serum applied in agarose gel electrophoresis are 0.6 to 2.0 μL, depending on the test requirements. If procedures call for multiple applications, as in isoenzyme analysis, concern about albumin overloading is no longer a factor. Urine specimens require 50- to 100-fold concentration for adequate sensitivity, and CSF may or may not require concentration, depending on the staining approach used.

Maintaining a Healthy Capillary

Capillary preparation and maintenance play a critical role in attaining reproducible results with CE. When a new capillary is used or a change is made to a new separation buffer, the capillary must be adequately equilibrated with the separation buffer—a process termed *conditioning.* Equilibration is particularly important when a phosphate-containing buffer is involved. For acceptable reproducibility, a phosphate-containing buffer should be equilibrated in the capillary a minimum of 4 hours before use. As with any untreated silica surface, ionized silanol groups are ideal for interaction with charged analytes, particularly peptides and proteins in neutral/basic pH buffers. Hence, after each separation, the capillary surface must be "regenerated" or "reconditioned" by the cleansing of any material adsorbed onto the wall. This is accomplished by following each run with

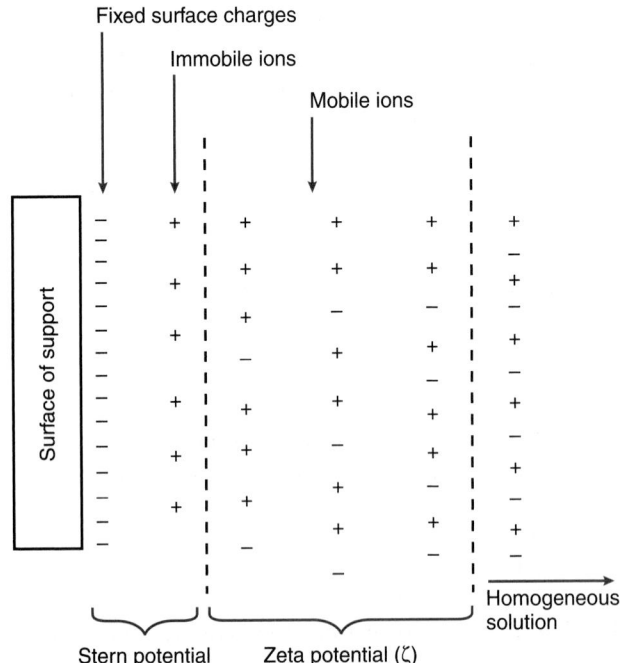

Figure 11-7 Distribution of + and − ions around the surface of an electrophoretic support. Fixed on the surface of the solid is a layer of − ions. (These may be + ions under suitable conditions.) A second layer of + ions is attracted to the surface. Extending farther from the surface of the solid is homogeneous solution.

a 3 to 5 column volume rinse with 100 mmol/L NaOH, then by flushing with 5 to 8 column volumes of fresh separation buffer.

Common Problems

The following problems may be encountered when slab gel electrophoresis is performed:

1. *Discontinuities* in sample application may be due to dirty applicators, which are best cleaned by agitating in water followed by gently pressing the applicators against absorbent paper. Caution must be used, and it is inadvisable to clean wires or combs by manual wiping.
2. *Unequal migration* of samples across the width of the gel may be due to dirty electrodes causing uneven application of the electrical field or to uneven wetting of the gel.
3. *Distorted protein zones* may be due to (1) bent applicators, (2) incorporation of an air bubble during sample application, (3) overapplication of sample, or (4) excessive drying of the electrophoretic support before or during electrophoresis.
4. *Irregularities* (other than broken zones) in sample application may be due to excessively wet agarose gels. Parts of the applied samples may look washed out.
5. *Unusual bands* are usually artifacts that may be easily recognized. Hemolyzed samples are frequent causes of an increased β-globulin (where free hemoglobin migrates) or an unusual band between the α_2- and β-globulins as the result of a hemoglobin-haptoglobin complex. A band at the starting point may be fibrinogen, and the sample should be verified as being serum before this band is reported as an abnormal protein. Split α_1, α_2-, and β-globulin bands are not unusual and should not be considered errors. In some samples, the α_1- and β-lipoproteins may migrate ahead of their normal positions and appear as an atypical band. Occasionally, a split albumin zone is observed in *bis*-albuminemia, but a grossly widened albumin zone may be due to certain medications that are albumin bound.

   Atypical bands in an isoenzyme pattern may be the result of binding by an immunoglobulin. An irregular but sharp protein zone at the starting point that lacks the regular, somewhat diffuse appearance of proteins may actually be denatured protein resulting from deteriorated serum. When one is faced with an unusual band anywhere in a serum protein pattern, the possibility that it is a true paraprotein (see Chapter 18 for further details) must always be considered. Finally, it is good laboratory practice to include a control serum with each electrophoretic run to evaluate its quality and that of the densitometer.

Review Questions

1. The isoelectric point of an amino acid or protein is defined as the:
   a. ability of the amino acid or protein to carry both positive and negative charges.
   b. pH at which the amino acid or protein has a negative charge.
   c. pH at which a molecule has no net charge.
   d. point on an electrophoretic gel at which that specific protein migrates.

2. The term *amphoteric* means:
   a. the pH at which a protein has no net charge.
   b. that a protein will have a negative charge at a high pH.
   c. that a protein has both positive and negative charges because of its side chains.
   d. the positive electrode.

3. Unequal migration of samples down the gel in an electrophoresis assay is an interference usually caused by:
   a. dirty electrodes causing uneven application of the electrical field.
   b. dirty pipette tips or applicators.
   c. too much sample being applied.
   d. inappropriate binding of immunoglobulins to other proteins in a sample.

4. In serum protein electrophoresis, the greater the charge of a molecule:
   a. the slower it will migrate.
   b. the faster it will migrate.
   c. the less migration rate will be affected.

5. Serum protein electrophoresis is what kind of basic technique?
   a. Immunoassay
   b. Standardization
   c. Qualitative technique
   d. Separation

6. Specimens with very low protein content sometimes require preconcentration before they are loaded onto an electrophoretic gel. An electrophoretic technique that *does not* require this concentration step is:
   a. disc electrophoresis.
   b. capillary electrophoresis.
   c. zone electrophoresis.
   d. two-dimensional gel electrophoresis.

7. What optical measuring technique allows for the scanning and quantification of electrophoretic fractions separated on a support medium?
   a. Spectrophotometry
   b. Chromatography
   c. Densitometry
   d. Nephelometry

8. A Southern blot is used to detect fragments of:
   a. RNA.
   b. protein.
   c. agarose.
   d. DNA.

9. A 1% agarose gel is best suited for separating DNA fragments in which one of the following size ranges:
   a. 500 bp (0.5 kbp) to 20 kbp
   b. 50 to 100 kbp
   c. 100 to 500 kbp
   d. larger than 500 kbp

10. The component of an electrophoresis system in which separation takes place is the:
    a. stain.
    b. support medium.
    c. densitometer.
    d. zone.

References

1. Anderson NL, Anderson NG. The human plasma proteome: history, character, and diagnostic prospects. Mol Cell Pro 2002;1;845–67.
2. Chien RL, Burgi DS. Field amplified sample injection in high-performance capillary electrophoresis. J Chromatogr 1991;559:141–52.
3. Horgan G, Glasbey CA. Uses of digital image analysis in electrophoresis. Electrophoresis 1995;16:298–305.
4. Jensen ON, Wilm M, Shevchenko A, et al. Peptide sequencing of 2-DE gel isolated proteins by nanoelectrospray tandem mass spectrometry. Methods Mol Biol 1999;112:571–88.
5. Karcher RE, Landers JP. Electrophoresis. In: Burtis CA, Ashwood ER, Bruns DE, eds: Tietz textbook of clinical chemistry, 4th edition. Philadelphia: WB Saunders, 2006:121–40.
6. Landers JP. Molecular diagnostics on electrophoretic microchips. Anal Chem 2003;75:2919–27.
7. Manz A, Graber N, Widmer HM. Miniaturized total chemical analysis systems: a novel concept for chemical sensing. Sens Actuators 1990;B1:244–8.
8. Molloy MP. Two-dimensional electrophoresis of membrane proteins using immobilized pH gradients. Anal Biochem 2000;280:1–10.
9. Nelson RJ, Burgi DS. Temperature control in capillary electrophoresis. In: Landers JP, ed. Handbook of capillary electrophoresis. Boca Raton: CRC Press, 1994:549–62.
10. Oda RP, Bush VJ, Landers JP. Clinical applications of capillary electrophoresis. In: Landers JP, ed. Handbook of capillary electrophoresis, 2nd edition. Boca Raton: CRC Press, 1997:639–73.
11. Ogorzalek RR, Loo JA, Andrews PC. Obtaining molecular weights of proteins and their cleavage products by directly combining gel electrophoresis with mass spectrometry. Methods Mol Biol 1999;112:473–85.
12. O'Reilly MJ, Kinnon C. The technique of pulsed field gel electrophoresis and its impact on molecular immunology. J Immunol Methods 1990;131:1–31.
13. Pentoney SL Jr, Sweedler JV. Optical detection techniques for capillary electrophoresis. In: Landers JP, ed. Handbook of capillary electrophoresis, 2nd edition. Boca Raton: CRC Press, 1997:379–423.
14. Rabilloud T. A comparison between low background silver diamine and silver nitrate protein stains. Electrophoresis 1992;13:429–39.
15. St. Claire RL III. Capillary electrophoresis. Anal Chem 1996;68:569–86.
16. Viskari P, Landers JP. Unconventional detection methods for microfluidic devices. Electrophoresis 2006;27:1797–810.
17. Wang C, Fang X, Lee CS. Recent advances in capillary electrophoresis-based proteomic techniques for biomarker discovery. Methods Mol Biol. 2013;984:1–12.

Chromatography*

Glen L. Hortin, M.D., Ph.D., and Carl A. Burtis, Ph.D.

Objectives

1. Define the following:

Chromatography	Resolution
Column chromatography	Retention factor
Derivatization	Retention time
Mobile phase	Stationary phase
Planar chromatography	

2. Evaluate a chromatogram to determine resolution; list four ways to improve resolution.
3. State the need for extraction or precipitation processing of clinical specimens before chromatographic separation.
4. Describe the following types of chromatographic separation mechanisms, including the principles of separation, by stating the stationary and mobile phases and listing the clinical applications, if any, of each:

Ion exchange	Steric exclusion
Partition	Affinity
Adsorption	

5. Explain the principle of thin-layer chromatography, including mobile and stationary phases, and its use in a clinical laboratory.
6. Calculate retention factor and identify compounds using the retention factor obtained from a planar chromatography procedure.
7. State the basic method of gas chromatography; list the mobile and stationary phases and the two gases commonly used in this technique.
8. Summarize the components of a gas chromatograph.
9. Describe the two types of chromatographic columns used for gas chromatography; state the function of the injector and the importance of temperature.
10. List and describe five detectors used in gas chromatography, including the advantages and disadvantages of each.
11. State the basic method of liquid chromatography; list the mobile and stationary phases.
12. Summarize the components of a high-pressure liquid chromatograph.
13. State the function and type of injector used in HPLC and the importance of the flow cell in detection.
14. Differentiate between the following four types of particulate column packings used in HPLC:

Bonded phase packings	Chiral packings
Polymeric packings	Restricted access packings

15. Describe three types of detectors that are used in HPLC.
16. Explain the need for sample extraction and derivatization used in sample preparation for HPLC.
17. Discuss analyte identification and quantification in chromatography, including retention time, the need for and comparison with an internal standard, and the need for increased chromatographic efficiency for low-concentration analytes.

Key Words and Definitions

Adsorption chromatography A separation mechanism based on the differential adsorption of analytes on the surface of a stationary phase and using hydrogen bonding and hydrophobic interactions as the forces behind the separation.

Affinity chromatography A separation mechanism in which one component of a specifically matched pair (such as antigen/antibody or hormone/receptor) is immobilized in a stationary phase and is used to capture the other component of the pair that is in the mobile phase.

Chromatogram A plot of detector response used in column chromatography to the presence of analyte in the mobile phase as a function of time or mobile phase volume.

*The authors gratefully acknowledge the original contributions of Drs. Larry D. Bowers, M. David Ullman, and Bruce A. Goldberger, on which portions of this chapter are based.

Key Words and Definitions—cont'd

Chromatography A group of separation techniques that separate analytes by differential distribution between a stationary phase and a mobile phase.

Column chromatography A separation method in which the stationary phase is packed into a tube or is coated onto the inner surface of the tube.

Column packing Particulate matter packed into a column used for chromatographic techniques.

Derivatization Labeling of or chemical addition to an analyte performed to increase the column retention or detectability of that analyte.

Detector A device that responds to the presence of analyte in the mobile phase, the magnitude of which is used to identify and quantify analytes; universal units detect most analytes and selective devices detect only analytes with specific properties.

Gas chromatography (GC) Column chromatography in which the mobile phase is a gas.

High-performance liquid chromatography (HPLC) Liquid chromatography that uses columns containing small particles of stationary phase and requiring high pressure to push the mobile phase past the stationary phase.

Ion-exchange chromatography A separation mechanism that is based on the exchange of ions between a charged stationary phase and oppositely charged ions in the mobile phase.

Liquid chromatography (LC) Column chromatography using a liquid mobile phase.

Mobile phase A gas or a liquid that flows in a chromatographic system and carries the sample past the stationary phase.

Partition chromatography A separation mechanism that is based on the differential distribution of solutes between two immiscible liquids.

Planar chromatography A separation technique in which the stationary phase is on a thin support such as paper or a glass plate.

Resolution A measure of the separation of two adjacent chromatographic peaks; resolution equals the difference in retention time for two components divided by the average of their peak widths.

Retention time The time interval between specimen injection and solute reaching the detector; retention time helps identify and quantify analyte.

Reversed-phase chromatography: A partitioning type of chromatography in which the mobile phase is polar relative to the nonpolar stationary phase.

Size-exclusion chromatography A separation mechanism that separates solutes on the basis of the molecular size of the solutes in a solution.

Stationary phase A solid or a liquid phase that interacts with components of the mobile phase.

Diverse forms of chromatography are used in the clinical laboratory for separating and quantifying a variety of clinically relevant analytes.[9] This chapter describes (1) basic concepts, (2) separation mechanisms, (3) specific chromatographic and detection techniques, (4) extraction techniques, and (5) qualitative and quantitative analyses.

Basic Concepts

Chromatography is a physical process whereby the components (solutes/analytes) of a sample mixture are separated as a result of their differential distribution between stationary and mobile phases.[14,15] During this process, the mobile phase carries the sample through a (1) bed, (2) layer, or (3) column containing the stationary phase. As the mobile phase flows past the stationary phase, the solutes may (1) reside only in the stationary phase (no migration), (2) reside only in the mobile phase (migration with the mobile phase), or (3) distribute between the two phases (differential migration). Those solutes with greater affinity for the stationary phase reside in the stationary phase and migrate more slowly than those with less affinity. Those with less affinity reside mostly in the mobile phase and migrate faster. Thus, the lower-affinity solutes separate from solutes having greater affinities for the stationary phase. Strongly bound solutes subsequently are displaced from the stationary phase by changing the physical or chemical nature

of the mobile phase. In this chapter, the term *chromatograph* is used as a verb and as a noun. As a verb, it means to separate by the process of chromatography. As a noun, it refers to the assembly of components that are necessary to effect a chromatographic separation.

Forms

Planar and column are the two basic forms of chromatography (Figure 12-1). In **planar chromatography**, the **stationary phase** is coated on a sheet of paper (paper chromatography) or is bound to a solid surface (thin-layer chromatography [TLC]).

In **column chromatography**, the stationary phase may consist of a particle of pure silica or polymer, or it may be coated onto or chemically bonded to these support particles. The stationary phase may be "packed" into a tube, or it may be coated onto the inner surface of the tube. The technique is termed **gas chromatography** (GC) or **liquid chromatography** (LC), depending on whether the mobile phase involves a gas or a liquid.

Operationally the instrument used to perform a GC or LC separation is known as either a *gas* or *liquid chromatograph*. When the stationary phase in LC consists of small-diameter particles, the technique is **high-performance liquid chromatography** (HPLC). When a gas or liquid chromatograph is connected to a mass spectrometer, the combined or "hyphenated/hybrid" techniques are **gas chromatography-mass**

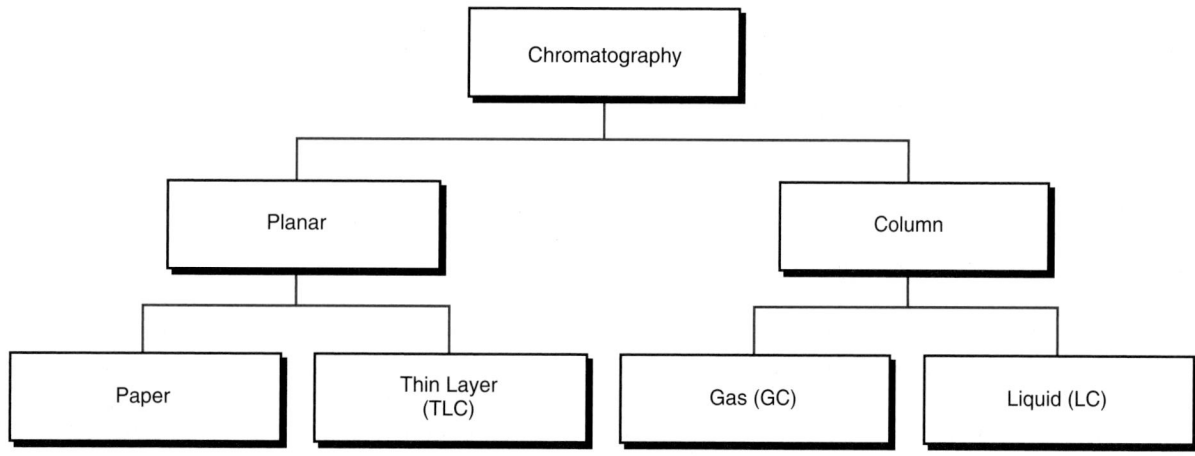

Figure 12-1 Forms of chromatography.

spectrometry (GCMS) and **liquid chromatography-mass spectrometry** (LCMS).

Detector Response

In analytical GC and LC, the **mobile phase**, or eluent, exits from the column and passes through a **detector** that produces an electronic signal that is plotted as a function of (1) time, (2) distance, or (3) volume. The resulting graphical display is a **chromatogram** (Figure 12-2). The **retention time** or volume is the time or volume when a solute exits the column and passes through the detector. The data represented by the chromatogram are used to help identify and quantify the solute(s). Because eluting solutes are displayed graphically as a series of peaks, they are frequently referred to as *chromatographic peaks*. These peaks are described in terms of peak (1) retention time or volume, (2) width, (3) height, and (4) area. In planar chromatography, the separated zones are detected by their natural colors or are visualized through chemical modification that produces colored "spots" or "bands" that are used qualitatively to identify various analytes or to quantify them.

Resolution

Resolution (R_s) is a measure of chromatographic separation; it requires that two peaks have different elution times for the peak centers and sufficiently narrow bandwidth to eliminate or minimize overlap (Figure 12-3),[9] and it is expressed mathematically as follows:

$$R_S = \frac{V_r(B) - V_r(A)}{\left[\dfrac{w(A) + w(B)}{2}\right]} \quad (1)$$

where
$V_r(A)$ = retention volume for solute A;
$V_r(B)$ = retention volume for solute B;
$w(A)$ = bandwidth (units of volume) measured at base for solute A; and
$w(B)$ = bandwidths (units of volume) measured at base for solute B.

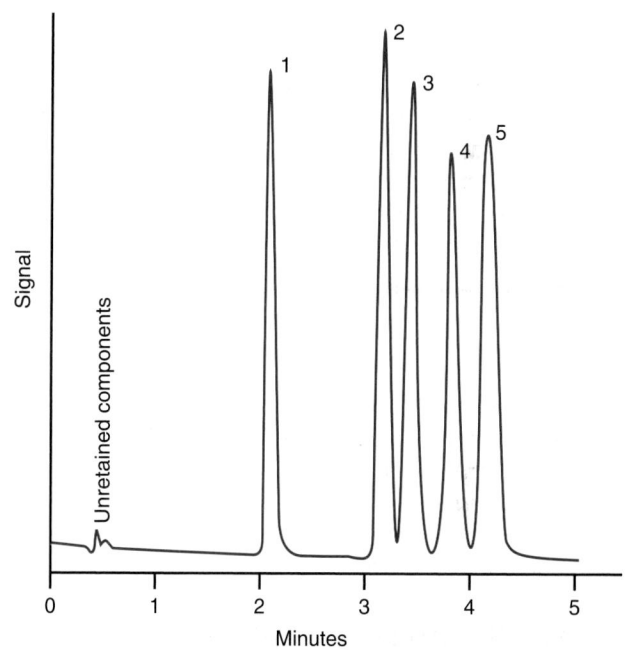

Column: C18, 3μ, 0.46 × 10 cm
Eluent: Isocratic, 0.025 M phosphate
Buffer: pH 3.0 in 25% acetonitrile
Flow rate: 2 mL/min
Detection: 215 nm, 0.1 AUFS

Compounds: 1. Doxepin
2. Desipramine
3. Imipramine
4. Nortriptyline
5. Amitriptyline

Figure 12-2 Chromatogram from an HPLC reversed-phase separation of tricyclic antidepressants with the use of a UV photometer detector set at 215 nm. Signal is displayed at 0.1 AUFS. *AUFS*, Absorbance units full scale; *HPLC*, high-performance liquid chromatography; *UV*, ultraviolet. *(Courtesy Vydac/The Separations Group, Hesperia, Calif.)*

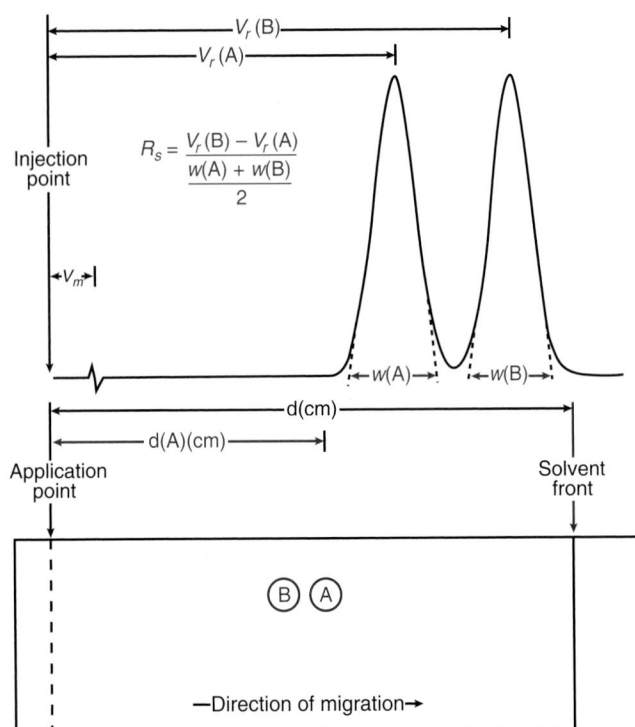

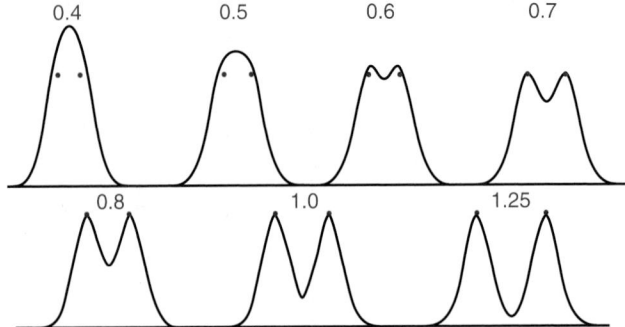

Figure 12-4 Separation of chromatographic peaks present in a 1:1 ratio as a function of resolution (R_S). *(From Snyder LR. A rapid approach to selecting the best experimental conditions for high-speed liquid column chromatography. Part I. Estimating initial sample resolution required by a given problem, J Chrom Sci 1972;10:202.)*

Figure 12-3 Schematic diagram of a chromatogram obtained from a column and open-bed chromatograph (planar). In open-bed chromatography *(bottom)*, strongly retained compounds (B) move more slowly than less strongly retained compounds. In column chromatography *(top)*, compound B is eluted later than compound A, again because of stronger retention. *A*, Solute A; *B*, solute B; *d(A)*, distance traveled by solute A; R_S, resolution; V_m, volume between injector and detectors; $V_r(A)$, retention volume for solute A; $V_r(B)$, retention volume for solute B; *w(A)*, bandwidth (units of volume) measured at base for solute A; *w(B)*, bandwidth (units of volume) measured at base for solute B.

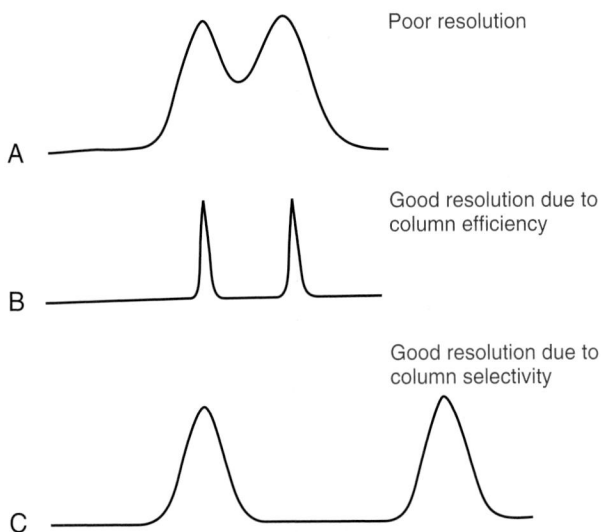

Figure 12-5 Effects of selectivity and efficiency on chromatographic resolution. **A,** Poor resolution. **B,** Good resolution caused by column efficiency. **C,** Good resolution caused by column selectivity. *(From Johnson EL, Stevenson R. Basic liquid chromatography, Palo Alto, Calif: Varian Associates, 1978.)*

Resolution also is expressed in terms of time, with $Vr(A)$ and $Vr(B)$ being replaced with retention times $tr(A)$ and $tr(B)$, and $w(A)$ and $w(B)$ being expressed in units of time.

Incomplete separation occurs when the calculated value for R_s is less than 0.8, whereas baseline separation is obtained when R_s is greater than 1.25 (Figure 12-4). As demonstrated in Figure 12-5, when R_s is unacceptable for a given separation, it is improved through a change in (1) the column retention factor *(k')*, (2) column efficiency *(N)*, or (3) column selectivity *(a)*. The retention factor describes the distribution of solutes between stationary and mobile phases. Column efficiency accounts for the ease of physical interaction between solute molecules and **column-packing** material. Selectivity characterizes the specific chemical affinity between solute molecules and column packing. Thus by rearranging Equation 1 and expressing the parameters in terms of retention, efficiency, and selectivity, resolution also is expressed as:

$$R_S = \left(\frac{k'}{k'+1} \right) \times \frac{\sqrt{N}}{4} \times \left(\frac{\alpha - 1}{\alpha} \right) \quad (2)$$

where

k' = retention or capacity factor (a thermodynamic term);
N = number of theoretical plates (a kinetic term representing column efficiency); and
α = "alpha" the selectivity factor (a thermodynamic term).

Selectivity and efficiency are important chromatographic parameters that are varied to affect the degree of resolution of a given separation. For example, enhanced resolution is achieved by changing the selectivity of separation by altering factors such as (1) the composition of the mobile phase, (2) the stationary phase, or (3) temperature. Alternatively, improved resolution is achieved by enhancing column efficiency by (1) using smaller particles, (2) changing flow rate, (3) using a longer column, and (4) minimizing the so-called dead volume. This latter term refers to the volume of tubing, connectors, and other spaces without a stationary phase packing. The dead

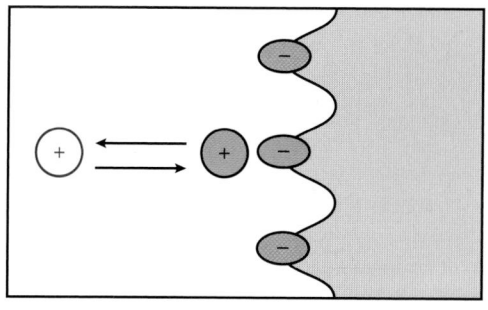

Ion-exchange chromatography

Separation is based on exchange of ions between surface and eluents.

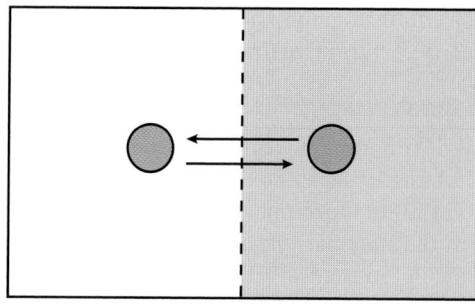

Partition chromatography

Separation is based on solute partitioning between two liquid phases.

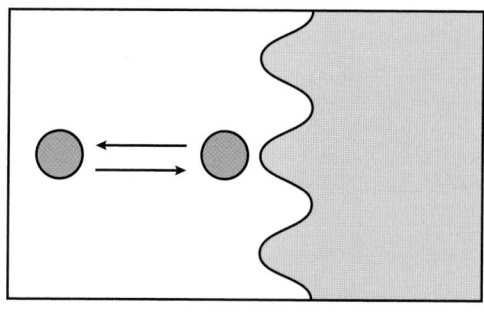

Adsorption chromatography

Separation is due to a series of adsorption/desorption steps.

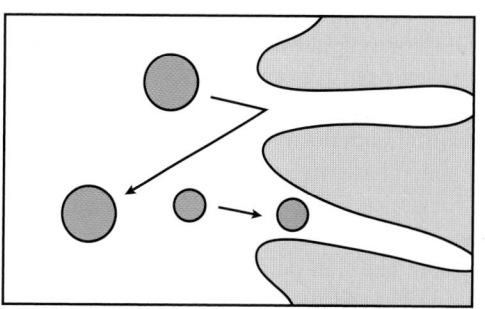

Size-exclusion chromatography

Separation is based on molecular size.

Figure 12-6 Examples of separation mechanisms used in chromatography. *(Courtesy James K. Hardy, Akron, Ohio [http://ull.chemistry.uakron.edu/accessed August 6, 2013].)*

volume serves as a mixing space where solute distributes into a larger volume, which degrades a separation.

Column efficiency is often described as the number of theoretical plates (N) per column length. An increase in N represents improved chromatographic efficiency and sharper peaks. Efficiency is often expressed as the number of theoretical plates per column length (N/L).*

The efficiency and the number of theoretical plates for a column are directly related to the column length, but usually a tradeoff of longer analysis times for longer columns occurs.

Separation Mechanisms

Chromatographic separations are classified by the process s used to separate the solutes. These include (1) ion-exchange, (2) partition, (3) adsorption, (4) size-exclusion, and (5) affinity mechanisms.

*Column efficiency also is expressed as the height equivalent of a theoretical plate (HETP) where HETP = L/N. In theory, a theoretical plate is equivalent to the length of a column necessary to allow one equilibration of the solute to occur between stationary and mobile phases. To increase the efficiency of a column, the number of theoretical plates is increased. In practice, this typically is accomplished by increasing the length of the column.

Ion-Exchange Chromatography

Ion-exchange chromatography is based on an exchange of ions between a charged stationary phase and ions of the opposite charge in the mobile phase (Figure 12-6). Cation-exchange particles contain negatively charged functional groups such as (1) carboxyl, (2) phosphate, or (3) sulfonate ions. These groups bind positively charged components (cations) in the mobile phase. Anion-exchange particles contain positively charged groups such as primary, tertiary, or quaternary amines that bind negatively charged components (anions) in the mobile phase. Ionic interactions are strong interactions, and displacement of ions bound to the stationary phase depends on competition by other ions in the mobile phase. The retention of components by the stationary phase is adjusted by changing the ionic strength or pH of the mobile phase. Retention is decreased by higher ionic strength (high salt concentration) or by adjustment of pH to decrease the charge of analytes or the stationary phase. Ion-exchange chromatography has several clinical applications, including the separation of (1) amino acids, (2) glycated hemoglobin, (3) hemoglobin variants, and (4) oligonucleotides.[3] Extraction with small ion-exchange columns is often used as a preparative rather than an analytical technique to isolate nucleic acids from blood or other specimens for molecular analysis. Another important application of ion-exchange chromatography is the removal of inorganic ions from aqueous mixtures (see Chapter 8).

Partition Chromatography

The differential distribution of solutes between two immiscible liquids is the basis for separation by **partition chromatography** (see Figure 12-6). Operationally, one of the immiscible liquids serves as the stationary phase. To prepare this phase, a thin film of the liquid is adsorbed or is chemically bonded onto the surface of support particles or onto the inner wall of a capillary column. Separation is based on differences in the relative solubility of solute molecules between stationary and mobile phases. Reversed-phase chromatography is a highly versatile technique that is widely used for the analysis of analytes of clinical relevance.[9]

Partition chromatography is classified as gas-liquid chromatography (GLC) or as liquid-liquid chromatography (LLC). LLC is further categorized as normal phase or reversed phase. For normal-phase LLC, a polar liquid is used as the stationary phase and a relatively nonpolar solvent or solvent mixture is used as the mobile phase. In **reversed-phase chromatography,** the stationary phase is nonpolar, and the mobile phase is relatively polar.

Ion-suppression and ion-pair chromatography are two forms of reversed-phase chromatography that are used to separate ionic solutes. With ion-suppression chromatography, the ionic character of a weakly acidic or basic analyte is neutralized or "suppressed" through modification of the mobile phase pH. The suppressed analyte thus has the properties of a neutral species and is separated by reversed-phase chromatography. In ion-pair chromatography, a counter ion—opposite in charge to that of the analyte—is added to the mobile phase, where it forms ion pairs with ionic analytes, displaces the usual base pairs, and neutralizes the analyte ion(s). These ion pairs then are separated by reversed-phase chromatography.

Hydrophilic interaction chromatography (or hydrophilic interaction liquid **chromatography,** HILIC) is a version of partition chromatography wherein analytes elute in order of increasing polarity. This mode of separation is used extensively for separation of biological, organic, and inorganic molecules by differences in polarity. Its utility has increased because of the simplified sample preparation for biological samples.

Adsorption Chromatography

The basis of separation by **adsorption chromatography** is differential adsorption of solutes on the surface of the stationary phase (see Figure 12-6). Hydrogen bonding and hydrophobic interactions[6] are the forces that mediate separations. In this type of chromatography, retention depends on the surface area of the stationary phase and the affinity of the solutes for the stationary phase. In GC, this mode is used to separate low-molecular-weight compounds (e.g., methyl, ethyl, isopropyl alcohols) and compounds that are normally gases at room temperature.

Size-Exclusion Chromatography

Size-exclusion chromatography, also known as (1) *gel-filtration,* (2) *gel-permeation,* (3) *steric-exclusion,* (4) *molecular-exclusion,*

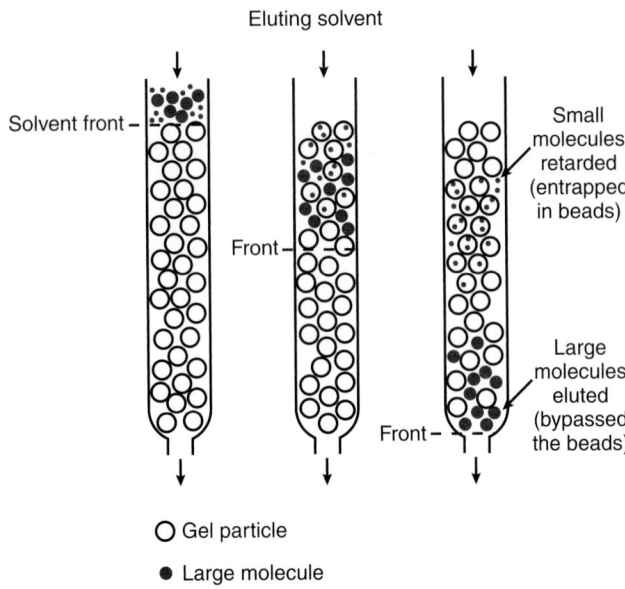

Figure 12-7 Schematic representation of gel-filtration column chromatography. *(Modified from Bennett TP. Graphic biochemistry, vol 1. Chemistry of biological molecules. New York: Macmillan, 1968.)*

or (5) *molecular-sieve chromatography,* separates solutes on the basis of their molecular size in solution (see Figure 12-6). This technique is commonly used in a preparative mode to separate large molecules such as proteins and nucleic acids from small molecules such as salts or oligonucleotides. The latter application may be performed in small spin columns where elution is driven by spinning in a centrifuge.

A variety of materials are used as stationary phases for size-exclusion chromatography, including (1) cross-linked dextran, (2) polyacrylamide, (3) agarose, (4) polystyrene-divinylbenzene, and (5) porous glass. Beads of these materials have pores that allow small molecules to enter and to be retained to a greater extent than large molecules that are excluded from pores (Figure 12-7). Large molecules elute before small molecules. The goal is to select a stationary phase with minimal adsorption of analytes that acts purely by steric exclusion. All solutes should be eluted by a mobile phase volume equal to the column volume. Salt may be added to the mobile phase to suppress ionic interactions with the stationary phase. Stationary phases are available in a variety of pore sizes, and the appropriate pore size must be selected for the molecules of interest. Separations by this technique have low resolution unless there is a large difference in molecular weights—usually twofold or more.

Affinity Chromatography

In **affinity chromatography,**[18] one component of highly specific molecular interaction pairs, such as (1) enzyme-inhibitor, (2) hormone-receptor, (3) antigen-antibody, or (4) aptamer-ligand, is immobilized in a stationary phase and is used to capture molecules from the mobile phase.[8,11] The affinity interactions usually are quite strong, allowing the stationary

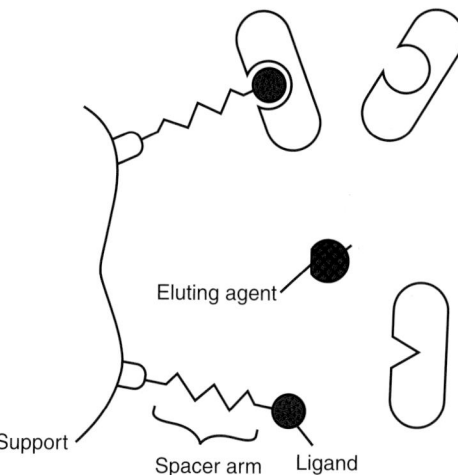

Figure 12-8 Principle of affinity chromatography. The analyte (enzyme, antibody, antigen, tissue receptor, etc.) binds to the support-bound ligand. Subsequently, it is eluted with a general eluent (such as a chaotropic agent), pH change, or a biospecific eluent (such as an inhibitor or a substrate).

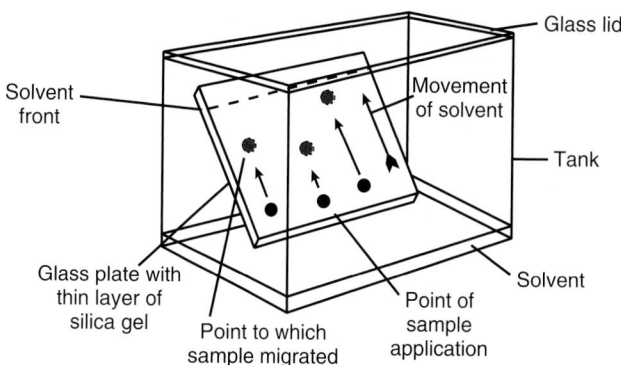

Figure 12-9 Illustration of planar chromatography (also known as *thin-layer chromatography* [TLC]). The solvent moves up the thin layer of adsorbent by capillary action. *(Modified from Bennett TP. Graphic biochemistry, vol 1. Chemistry of biological molecules, New York: Macmillan, 1968.)*

phase to be washed extensively by the mobile phase to remove all nonbound components, while bound components are retained. Some affinity separations, such as antibody-antigen interactions, offer great specificity. Immunoaffinity chromatography, often in a lateral flow format, is applied in (1) pregnancy tests, (2) rapid microbial antigen tests, and (3) a wide range of other clinical tests. Column chromatographic applications of affinity chromatography often entail a stepwise elution with a change in the composition of the mobile phase, as described in the caption of Figure 12-8. Elution is achieved by adding an excess of competing ligand or by changing the mobile phase to conditions where affinity is lost, for example, by extreme changes in pH or by addition of high concentrations of chaotropic agents, such as urea or guanidine.

Chiral chromatography is a variant of affinity chromatography in which the stationary phase contains a single enantiomer of a chiral compound.[1,17,31] In this type of chromatography, two enantiomers of a compound in the mobile phase bind with different affinity to the chiral stationary phase and therefore exit the column at different times.

Planar Chromatography

In planar chromatography, the stationary phase is coated on a sheet of paper (paper chromatography) or is bound to a solid surface (thin-layer chromatography). In TLC the stationary phase, a thin layer of particles of a material such as silica gel is spread uniformly on a glass plate or a plastic or aluminum sheet.[21] When the thin layer consists of particles of small diameter (4.5 μm), the technique is known as *high-performance thin-layer chromatography* (HPTLC).[19]

In paper chromatography, the stationary phase consists of a layer of water or a polar solvent coated onto the fibers of a sheet of paper. Separation is normal-phase partition chromatography between the nonpolar mobile phase and the polar stationary phase.

In TLC, the sample is applied as a small spot or band near the bottom edge of the plate. Then, the plate is placed in a closed tank containing the mobile phase, which migrates up the plate by capillary action (Figure 12-9). After the mobile phase travels a desired distance, the plate is removed from the tank and is dried. Solutes are visualized directly if they are colored or fluorescent by eliciting a chemical reaction to yield a visible product, or by performing autoradiography for radioactive compounds.

A solute's migration in TLC or PC is expressed as an R_f value, the ratio of solute migration to solvent front migration:

$$R_f = \frac{\text{distance from application point to solute center}}{\text{distance from application point to mobile phase front}} \quad (3)$$

Many stationary phases are available for TLC, including (1) silica, (2) cellulose, (3) alumina, and (4) alkyl-bonded silica particles for reversed-phase chromatography. TLC and PC have been used for clinical applications such as (1) identification of drugs in urine, (2) analysis of amino acids or glycosaminoglycans in urine, and (3) analysis of lipids in amniotic fluids. Use of TLC and PC in the clinical laboratory has been declining because of the introduction of more automated, reproducible, and quantitative column chromatographic methods. Manual methods for TLC tend to be less quantitative and more labor intensive and technique dependent, although TLC does offer the advantages of simplicity and low cost for equipment.

A popular type of planar chromatography used in the clinical laboratory is lateral flow affinity chromatography, which uses a membrane such as nitrocellulose as the stationary phase with one or more zones of immobilized antibody or antigen. Using a pregnancy test as an example, a urine or serum specimen is applied to one end of the membrane and serves as the mobile phase. Human chorionic gonadotropin (hCG) in the mobile phase is captured by specific antibodies immobilized in small zones on the membrane. Detection of bound hCG is achieved by binding of colored particles coupled to antibody versus hCG. If hCG is present, the antibody-conjugated

TABLE 12-1   Forms of Chromatography

Types of Chromatography	Subtypes	Stationary Phase	Mobile Phase
Gas chromatography (GC)	Gas-solid chromatography (GSC)	Solid particles or capillary wall	Gas
Performed as column chromatography	Gas-liquid chromatography (GLC)	Liquid immobilized on particles or capillary wall	Gas
Liquid chromatography (LC)	Partition chromatography	Liquid immobilized on a surface	Immiscible liquid
Is performed as planar chromatography	Gel filtration	Porous solid with defined pore size	Liquid
or as column chromatography with packed or capillary columns. High-	Ion-exchange	Solid containing charged groups on its surface	Liquid with salts
performance liquid chromatography (HPLC) uses columns at high	Adsorption	Solid with a surface that adsorbs analytes	Liquid
pressures	Affinity	Solid with immobilized capture molecules with high specificity	Liquid suitable for affinity interaction

particles forms a visible zone. If no hCG is present, the particles do not concentrate in the detection zone. This sandwich-type format can be used to detect antigens such as proteins that are large enough to have sites for binding of two different antibodies. Detection of specific antibodies is achieved with analogous sandwich-type assays using capture and detection antigens. Small molecules, such as drugs of abuse, are too small to accommodate binding of two antibodies for a sandwich-type assay. Therefore, small antigens are detected by competitive inhibition of binding of labeled antibody to an antigen immobilized in the stationary phase.

A new type of chromatography is known as **overpressured layer chromatography (OPLC),** which is a separation technique that combines the advantages of conventional TLC/HPTLC with those of **HPLC.**[27] It employs a pressurized ultramicro (UM) chamber as a closed adsorbent layer chamber. This enables the use of a special chromatoplate and a pump to increase and optimize the mobile phase flow velocity through an optimal development distance in an adsorbent layer. This new system exploits the unique advantages of a planar-layer system for detection, isolation, and identification of new (1) antimicrobials, (2) antineoplastics, (3) biopesticides, and (4) other biologically active substances, as well as for the study of fundamental biochemical reactions and mechanisms.

Column Chromatography

In column chromatography, the stationary phase is coated onto or is chemically bonded to support particles that are then "packed" into a tube, or the stationary phase is coated onto the inner surface of a tube. GC and LC are two categories of column chromatography (Table 12-1). A third category, supercritical fluid chromatography,[7] which uses pressurized carbon dioxide as solvent is used only rarely for clinical applications and will not be discussed here.

Multiple factors determine which type of chromatography is best suited for a specific application. GC usually provides higher resolution as much longer columns and higher linear flow rates are used because of the lower viscosity of a gas versus a liquid. GC usually is the method of choice for volatile components. The main factor limiting the application of GC, however, is the volatility of analytes. Because of their lack of

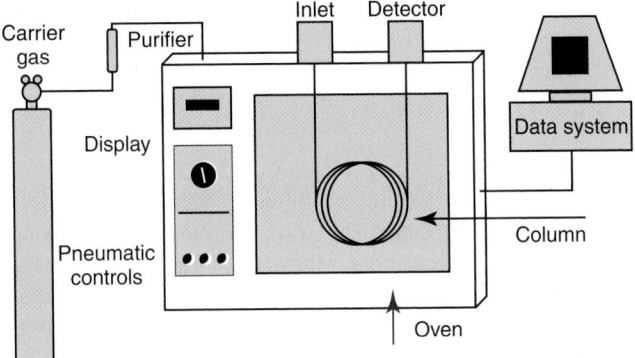

Figure 12-10 Schematic diagram of a gas chromatograph.

volatility, large molecules such as (1) peptides, (2) proteins, (3) nucleic acids, and (4) large polymers usually are analyzed by LC. Lower-molecular-weight analytes are analyzed by GC after chemical derivatization to increase their volatility.

Gas Chromatography

In GC, a gas mobile phase, or carrier gas, is used to carry a mixture of volatile solutes through a column containing the stationary phase, which usually is a nonvolatile liquid coated or bonded to particles or the inner surface of a capillary.[4,14] Less frequently, gas-solid chromatography is performed using a solid stationary phase, which directly adsorbs analytes to its surface. The mobile phase, or *carrier gas*, is typically an inert gas, such as (1) nitrogen, (2) helium, or (3) argon. Separation of analytes is based on differential partitioning into the stationary phase. In general, more volatile components have a higher vapor pressure and spend more resident time in the gas phase. The carrier gas carries analytes to a detector in the order of their elution. Analytes are identified qualitatively by their retention times or by mass spectra (see Chapter 13). The magnitude of detector responses is used to quantify analytes.

Instrumentation

A basic gas chromatograph (Figure 12-10) consists of the following:

1. A supply of carrier gas and flow controller.
2. An injector or injection port to introduce samples into the system.

3. A chromatographic column to separate the analytes.
4. A column oven to heat the column.
5. A detector that responds to solute/analyte concentration.
6. A computer to control the system and to process data.

Carrier Gas Supply and Flow Control

A constant flow of carrier gas is required for column efficiency and reproducibility. Use of temperature gradients requires sophisticated control of the carrier gas flow rate and pressure during a chromatographic run. The pressure required to maintain a constant flow varies as carrier gas viscosity changes with temperature. The flow rate of carrier gas depends on column diameter. Packed columns require a flow rate from 10 to 60 mL/min, but smaller-diameter capillary columns use flow rates of 1 to 2 mL/min.

The carrier gas used depends on the type of column and detector. Hydrogen and helium are the carrier gases of choice with capillary columns. Only high-purity hydrogen and helium are used as carrier gas impurities (1) harm the column, (2) decrease the performance of some detectors, and (3) adversely affect quantification. For packed columns, the most frequently used carrier gas is nitrogen, which is used with (1) flame ionization (FID), (2) electron capture (ECD), or (3) thermal conductivity (TCD) detectors. Helium also is used with FIDs and TCDs, and nitrogen-argon-methane mixtures are used with ECD. Carrier gases should be pure and dry. Molecular sieve beds and specialized inline traps are used to remove water, hydrocarbon, or oxygen from the carrier gas.

Injector

Samples are injected by a manual syringe or an automated injector. To introduce an aliquot of sample into the column, an injection needle passes through a septum into an injection port in the flow path of the carrier gas. Some volatile components such as alcohols are injected as a gas phase by headspace sampling of closed specimen vials. For most methods, however, specimens are dissolved in a volatile solvent. With packed columns, specimen volumes of about 1 to 10 μL are injected. The volatile solvent and analytes are "flash-vaporized" by maintaining the injection port at a higher temperature than the column, and the vaporized specimen is swept into the column by the carrier gas. Capillary columns have low sample capacities that often require split injections, in which only a small portion of the vaporized sample enters the column, versus the splitless mode, in which all of the sample enters the column.

Injectors are a potential source of problems with GC such as septum leaks and adsorption of components from the sample onto the septum during injection. Decomposition products will form on the heated septum, yielding spurious "ghost" peaks in chromatograms. To minimize this problem, the septum usually is coated with Teflon, and the inner surface of the septum is purged continuously with the carrier gas that is vented before it passes into the column. Most commercial injectors are equipped with continuous-purge capabilities. The septum needs periodic replacement.

Temperature-programmable injectors are available that allow injection of larger volumes of specimen, up to 100 microliters or more. The sample is injected at a temperature slightly higher than the boiling point of the solvent. Most of the sample components condense on glass wool or on fused silica wool packed into the injector inlet, while the solvent is removed. Then, the injector is rapidly heated to vaporize analytes, which flow into the column. Injection of a larger volume of specimen improves the limit of detection for some analyses.

Chromatographic Column

Packed and capillary are two types of columns used in GC. Packed columns are filled with uncoated support particles (gas solid chromatography/GSC) or, more often, with particles coated or chemically bonded with a nonvolatile stationary phase (gas liquid chromatography/GLC). These particles range (1) from 1 to 4 mm in internal diameter (ID), (2) from 1 mm or more in length, and (3) are fabricated from glass or stainless steel. Longer columns are more efficient but require increased carrier gas pressures and analysis time. Although narrow columns are more efficient, wider columns have increased sample capacities. Fast GC is a type of GC in which high-speed separations are achieved using short lengths of conventional columns.

Capillary columns, also known as *wall-coated open tubular columns,* are fabricated by coating the inner wall of a fused-silica tube with a thin film of liquid phase. These columns range from 0.1 to 0.5 mm in ID and from 10 to 150 mm in length. The ultrapure fused silica capillary tubing used in such columns is very fragile. To physically strengthen the tubing, a thin outside coating of polyimide or aluminum is added; this improves column durability. Capillary columns are very efficient but have low sample capacities.

In addition to packed and capillary columns, progress has been made in the development of micro-GC columns on silicon chips.

Temperature Control

GC requires careful control of (1) column, (2) injector, and (3) detector temperatures. Column temperature is controlled by placing the column in an oven or directly by providing resistive heating. Injector and detector temperatures usually are controlled by resistive heaters. Depending on the application, the column temperature is maintained constant (isothermal operation) during the chromatographic run or is varied as a function of time (temperature-programmed or temperature-gradient operation, which is used for most clinical applications). With temperature programming, more volatile analytes elute first, followed by those with higher boiling points. Consequently a complex mixture of analytes with a wide range of volatility is separated into sharper chromatographic peaks and more rapidly than with isothermal operation. The upper temperature limit of operation depends on the stability of the analytes and of the column coating.

Detectors

A variety of detectors are used for GC; the most commonly used types are listed in Table 12-2. These include universal units that detect most analytes and selective devices that detect

TABLE 12-2 | Examples of Detectors Used for Gas Chromatography

Type of Detector	Principle of Operation	Selectivity	Limit of Detection	Comments
Thermal conductance (TCD)	Measures thermal conductivity change in carrier gas on elution of compounds	Universal	<400 pg propane/mL He	Lower detection sensitivity
Flame ionization (FID)	CHNO + heat → CHNO$^+$ + e$^-$; electrons collected for detection	Hydrocarbon	10 to 100 pg CHO	Commonly used in clinical labs
Thermionic selective (TSD; NPD)	Alkaline bead selectively ionizes N- or P-containing compounds	N, P	0.4 to 10 pg N, 0.1 to 1.0 pg P	Offers higher sensitivity than FID
Electron capture (ECD)	e$^-$ + R + N$_2$ → Re$^-$ + N$_2$; analytes capture excess electrons	Electronegative atoms such as Cl, F, Br, and I	0.05 to 1.0 pg Cl$^-$-containing compounds	Analytes may be derivatized to add Fl or Cl
Mass spectrometer (MS)	Ionization of analytes by electrons; ions are separated according to mass/charge ratio	Highly selective, analyte must be ionizable	1 ng scanning 10 pg for selected ion monitoring (SIM)	Provides qualitative and quantitative information
Photoionization (PID)	CHNO + photon → CHNO$^+$ + e$^-$; detect electron	Hydrocarbon	1 to 10 pg CHO	May be seen as improvement on FID

CHNO, Carbon, hydrogen, nitrogen, and oxygen-containing compounds; *CHO*, carbon, hydrogen, and oxygen-containing compound; *NPD*, nitrogen-phosphorus detector.

only analytes with specific properties. Sometimes, two or more detectors are placed in a series to enhance analytical specificity and sensitivity. Mass spectrometers also are used as detectors for GC and are very useful for identifying analytes and increasing the specificity of analysis (see Chapter 13).

Note: When two columns or detectors are placed in series, the technique is known as *two-dimensional gas chromatography*.[16,26] With these systems, solutes that are insufficiently separated in the first column are introduced ("heart-cut") to a second, different column.[26] This enables analysis with a level of separation that is not attained in conventional single-column analysis.

Flame Ionization Detector. The FID is the most commonly used detector for clinical analysis. Its advantages include (1) simplicity, (2) reliability, (3) versatility, (4) sensitivity, and (5) ease of operation. During operation, the column effluent is mixed with hydrogen and air, and the eluting compounds are burned by a flame. About one molecule in 10,000 releases an electron, which is detected by a collector electrode positioned above the flame. The magnitude of the generated signal relates to the mass of carbon material delivered to the detector.

Thermionic Selective Detector. The TSD, also known as the *nitrogen-phosphorus detector* (NPD), is a modification of the FID, in which an alkaline bead is heated electrically in the area above the flame. The presence of alkaline atoms in the flame increases the signal of nitrogen-containing compounds by a factor of 15 and that of phosphorus-containing compounds by a factor of 300.

Photoionization Detector. With a PID, the energy for ionization is provided by an intense UV lamp rather than by a flame. The PID has a lower limit of detection than the FID because it produces a more stable signal with less baseline "noise."

Thermal Conductivity Detector. The TCD is based on the principle that addition of a compound to a gas alters its thermal conductance. TCD detects all compounds with little selectivity but is less sensitive than most other types of detectors.

Electron Capture Detector. An ECD is used for detecting electron-absorbing components such as halogenated elements—fluorine, chlorine, bromine, and iodine. It uses a radioactive beta particle (electron) emitter in conjunction with a so-called "makeup gas" flowing through the detector chamber. An ECD is often used as a detector for capillary GC. Because not all compounds contain halogenated functional groups, derivatization with reagents containing polychlorinated or polyfluorinated moieties is a common practice used with an ECD.

Computer/Controller

An automated GC is computer controlled, with the computer functioning both as a process controller and as a data processor. For example, as a process controller, the computer regulates various parameters such as (1) carrier gas composition and flow rate; (2) column backpressure; (3) column and detector temperatures; (4) sample injection, detector selection, and operation; and (5) the various timing steps that command the operation of the system. For data processing, the computer monitors signals generated by the system's detectors and commands the acquisition and storage of data at specified time intervals. The area, or height, of each chromatographic peak is determined from the stored data, and this information is used to compute the analyte concentration represented by each peak. Available algorithms for this computation include those based on calibration curves or conversion factors from internal or external calibration (described later). If desired, a complete report is prepared and printed for each chromatographic run. Alternatively, data are stored to be recalled and reprocessed, using different integration parameters.

Practical Considerations

Two examples of separation of volatile components by GC are shown in Figure 12-11. The figure provides examples of separation parameters that may be varied in GC. The examples use packed columns 30 m in length with 4 minutes required to complete an analysis. HPLC columns by comparison are usually about 100 times shorter—about 30 cm in length.

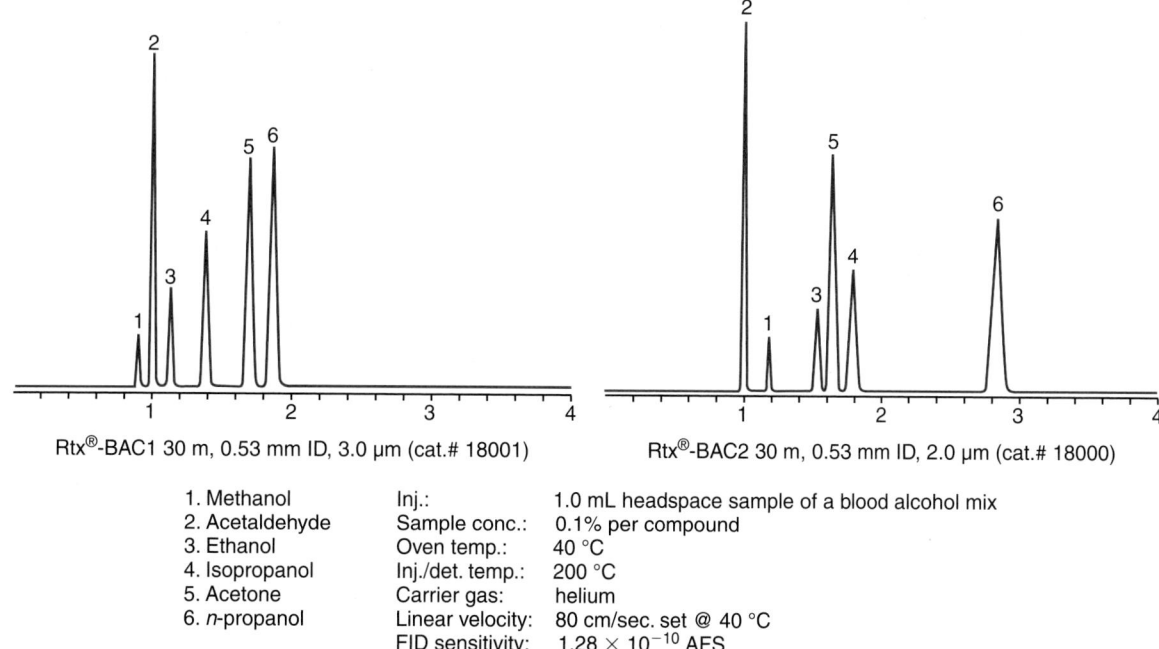

Rtx®-BAC1 30 m, 0.53 mm ID, 3.0 µm (cat.# 18001)   Rtx®-BAC2 30 m, 0.53 mm ID, 2.0 µm (cat.# 18000)

1. Methanol	Inj.:	1.0 mL headspace sample of a blood alcohol mix
2. Acetaldehyde	Sample conc.:	0.1% per compound
3. Ethanol	Oven temp.:	40 °C
4. Isopropanol	Inj./det. temp.:	200 °C
5. Acetone	Carrier gas:	helium
6. *n*-propanol	Linear velocity:	80 cm/sec. set @ 40 °C
	FID sensitivity:	1.28×10^{-10} AFS

Figure 12-11 Gas chromatography (GC) of alcohols by headspace sampling using two types of packed columns. The horizontal axis shows minutes. Note that analyte retention and order of elution (the specificity) are affected by the stationary phase. *(Courtesy Restek Corporation, Bellefonte, Pa.)*

Methods for sample preparation affect the practical application of GC to separate and quantify biological compounds. For example, nonvolatile compounds, such as proteins and inorganic salts, build up in a GC if injected. Extraction with an organic solvent such as dichloromethane or ethyl acetate is one means of recovering many analytes free of proteins and inorganic salts. Solid-phase extraction with small chromatographic columns is an alternative preparative step before specimen injection. The volatility of compounds often is a limiting factor in the application of GC. Many compounds, such as amino acids and sugars, are not sufficiently volatile to be analyzed by GC. Chemical modification or **derivatization** of such compounds, however, increases their volatility for GC analysis. Chemical reactions used to increase volatility include (1) acylation, (2) silylation, (3) esterification, and (4) oximation. In addition to increasing solute volatility, derivatization enhances the specificity and sensitivity of particular assays. For example, the use of a chiral reagent to derivatize amphetamine allows separation of the D- and L-isomers with a standard GC column. In practice, enhanced detection sensitivity is achieved by preparing pentafluoropropyl derivatives for use with ECD.

Liquid Chromatography

Separation by LC is based on the differential distribution of the solutes between a liquid mobile phase and a stationary phase. As discussed earlier, when particles of small diameter are used as the stationary-phase support, the technique is referred to as *high-performance liquid chromatography* (HPLC).[25] Because relatively high pressures are required to pump liquids through HPLC columns, the technique also has been referred to as *high-pressure liquid chromatography*. In the clinical laboratory, HPLC is the most widely used form of LC.

Instrumentation

A basic liquid chromatograph (Figure 12-12) consists of the following elements[13]:

1. A solvent reservoir to hold the mobile phase.
2. One or more pumps to force the liquid mobile phase through the system.
3. An injector to introduce an aliquot of sample into the column.
4. A chromatographic column to separate the solutes.
5. A column oven to maintain constant column temperature.
6. Online detector(s) to detect analytes as they elute from the column.
7. A computer to control the system and to process data.

Solvent Reservoir

In their simplest forms, the reservoirs are glass bottles or flasks into which "feed lines" to the pump are inserted. To remove particles from solvents, inline filters are placed on the inlets of the feed lines. Prepared buffers or solutions should be filtered before they are added to solvent reservoirs. Dissolved gases are removed by vacuum degassing or purging with helium in the solvent reservoir or by use of an inline vacuum degasser that has a gas-permeable membrane. Failure to remove dissolved gases may result in the formation of bubbles in detectors, resulting in unstable baseline signals. The components of the mobile phase are selected on the basis of the mode of chromatographic separation and the type of detector used. Methanol and acetonitrile are liquids commonly used in mobile

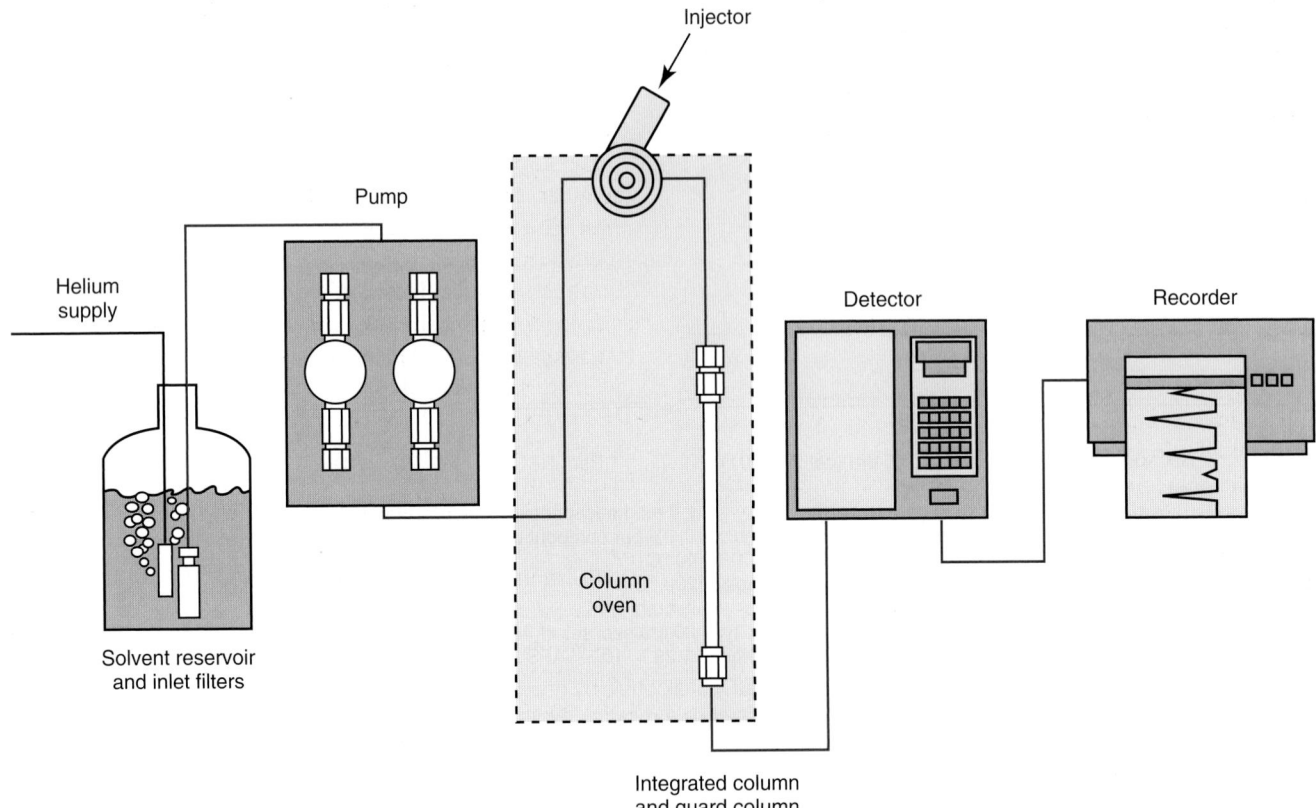

Figure 12-12 Schematic diagram of a liquid chromatograph.

phases for reversed-phase separations because of their low viscosity and low optical absorbance in the ultraviolet spectrum. High-purity solvents are required.

Pump

Pumps for HPLC must deliver a constant flow of solvent at pressures up to 6000 pounds per square inch (psi). Some applications have required higher pressures up to 15,000 psi, which have been referred to as *ultrahigh-performance liquid chromatography* (UHPLC or UPLC[R]).[29,32] Operation at higher pressures requires use of (1) pumps, (2) columns, and (3) other components specifically designed for higher pressures.

In practice, pumps used with HPLC must deliver a constant flow with low pulsation. Column life and the baseline stability of detectors are often adversely affected by pulsatile flow. Pressure sensors detect excessive increases in pressure that would cause pump failure and shut down the pump before damage to the pump occurs. Dual-piston reciprocating pumps are commonly used. In operation, an asymmetrical cam drives two pistons into and out of pumping chambers. The reciprocating action of the pump creates pulsatile flow that is smoothed by mechanical or electronic pulse dampers. For isocratic separations that use a solvent of constant composition (Figure 12-13), a single pump is needed. Gradient elution (see Figure 12-13) requires either mixing two or more solvents at low pressure using a proportioning valve before the pump inlet, or changing the flow rate of two pumps that are delivering differing solvents to a mixing chamber. In the latter case, solvent composition is controlled by changing the flow rate of the

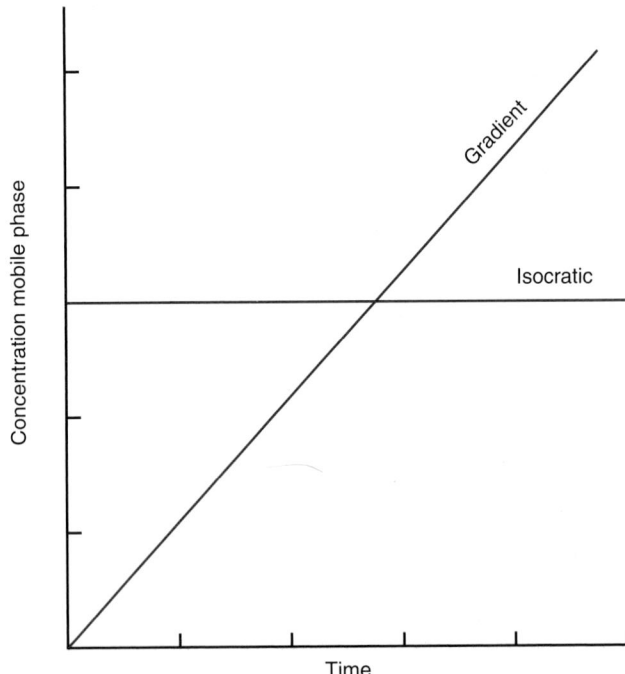

Figure 12-13 Examples of isocratic and gradient elution in LC. *LC,* Liquid chromatography.

two pumps. Solvent mixing is accomplished by static mixing produced by merging of two flowing solvents or by dynamic mixing with a magnetic stirrer. Solvent composition may be changed in a linear fashion or at various programmable rates. It is important for gradients to be highly reproducible. For some

TABLE 12-3 Internal Diameters (ID) of Columns Used in HPLC

Column Terminology	Column ID, mm	Optimal Flow Rate
Standard	4.6	1.25 mL/min
	4.0	1.0 mL/min
Narrow bore	3.0	0.6 mL/min
	2.0	200 µL/min
Microbore/capillary	1.0	50 µL/min
	0.5	12 µL/min
	0.1	0.5 µL/min

applications, such as amino acid analysis by cation-exchange chromatography, a step gradient is used with multiple changes in mobile phase made with a switching valve. Isocratic separations provide the advantage of simplicity. Gradient elution is useful for separating complex mixtures with widely varying affinity for the stationary phase. At the completion of a gradient, additional time is required to reequilibrate the system to initial mobile phase conditions before the next injection.

Injector

The first step of an LC separation is the introduction of an aliquot of sample into the column via an injector. The most widely used type of injector is the fixed-loop injector, which is switched into or out of the flow path by manual or automated injection. In the inject mode, the loop is switched into the flow path, and the sample is carried downstream and into the column. The loop continues as part of the flow path until it is switched back to the fill position. Important characteristics of injection systems include their (1) reproducibility, (2) amount of carryover, and (3) range of injected volumes. Some automated injectors have the capability of injecting multiple aliquots or of mixing a sample and a reagent before injection to attain derivatization reactions.

Chromatographic Columns

Both packed and capillary columns are used in LC, and there is great diversity in sizes of columns and types of column packing.[28] Advances in column technology have improved the (1) selectivity, (2) stability, and (3) reproducibility of LC analytical columns and the materials used to pack or coat the inner walls of such columns.[9]

Column Dimensions. Modern column technology has produced columns in different dimensions with the tendency toward smaller internal volumes prevailing for analytical, especially hyphenated, techniques (see Chapter 13). For use in the clinical laboratory, most analytical HPLC columns are fabricated from tubes made of 316 stainless steel that have IDs ranging from 0.3 mm to 5 mm and lengths from 50 mm to 250 mm (Table 12-3). Column end fittings, which have zero dead volume and frits to retain the support particles, are used to connect the column to the injector on the inlet end and the detector on the outlet end. Generally, lower detection limits are achieved with columns having smaller IDs. These smaller ID columns are manufactured from narrow-bore (approximately

2.1 mm ID) and microbore (approximately 1.0 mm ID) tubes. In addition to providing improved efficiency, columns with smaller IDs use decreased volumes in the mobile phase. For example, a 2-mm-ID column requires much less solvent than a 4.6-mm-ID column (see Table 12-3).

Capillary columns used in LC are constructed by coating the inner wall of a fused silica tube with a thin film of liquid phase. These columns vary from 0.1 to 0.5 mm in ID and from 10 to 50 cm in length.

A guard column commonly is placed before the analytical column. A guard column is packed with the same or similar stationary phase as the analytical column. It collects particulate matter and any strongly retained components from the sample and, thus, extends the life of the expensive analytical column. The guard column is replaced periodically because buildup of particulate matter and impurities on a column causes (1) increased back-pressure, (2) increased background, and (3) lower performance.

Column Stationary Phase. The type of stationary phase in the column is the major determinant of selectivity and resolution of LC separations.[2] The typical physical form of the stationary phase usually consists of a packed bed of small particles or a monolithic porous rod.

Particulate Column Packings. Particulate packings have diameters ranging from 1.8 to 10 µm. In general, the smaller the diameter of the particle, the more efficient is the column. Because the operating backpressure of an LC column is inversely proportional to the square of the particle diameter, relatively high pressures are required to pump liquids through HPLC columns. Historically, separations by HPLC commonly used particles about 5 µm in diameter, but a trend toward the use of progressively smaller particles of less than 2 µm in diameter has been noted. The use of columns with small-diameter particles has led to a new generation of HPLC systems with pressure limits up to about 1000 bar (15,000 psi), which is about twofold to threefold higher than in earlier HPLC systems. Most solid phases are porous, and pore size is another important parameter of particles. The pore size influences the surface area of particles and the access of analytes to the full surface area. Separation of small molecules often uses particles with small pore sizes in the range of about 6 to 12 nm (60 to 120 Å). Particles with smaller pores have a greater number of pores and a greater surface area. Larger molecules, such as (1) proteins, (2) nucleic acids, and (3) large peptides, are too large to access these small pores, and wide-pore particles (15 to 50 nm) are needed for analysis of these macromolecules. Nonporous particles also are available, but these particles have the drawbacks of low surface area and capacity. In general, retention of analytes is increased by higher surface area and higher carbon load (see next page).

Types of particulate packings include (1) bonded phase, (2) polymeric, (3) chiral, and (4) restricted access materials.

Bonded Phase Packings. With this type of packing, the stationary phase is bonded chemically to the surface of silica particles through a silica ester or a silicone polymeric linkage that is relatively chemically stable. Bonded phase packings are available for a variety of chromatographic applications, including (1) ion-exchange, (2) normal-phase, and (3) reversed-phase chromatography. In normal-phase HPLC, the functional groups of the stationary phase are polar relative to those of the mobile phase, which usually consists of nonpolar solvents, such as hexane. Examples of polar functional groups for normal-phase HPLC packings are (1) silanol, (2) amino, and (3) nitrile groups. Reversed-phase HPLC uses a nonpolar stationary phase. The most popular reversed-phase packing is the octadecyl or C18 (a straight aliphatic chain with 18 carbons) type, also sometimes called *octadecyl silica* or *ODS* columns. Reversed-phase column retention and selectivity characteristics also are altered via attachment of other groups, such as (1) octyl, (2) phenyl, (3) butyl, or (4) cyanopropyl, to the silica. Retention is also affected by the number of immobilized groups, often identified as the *percent carbon load,* and by chemical blocking of silanol groups on the surface of silica particles, which is often referred to as *endcapping.* Blocking of the hydroxyl groups on silica increases the stability of silica and decreases the effects of the hydroxyl groups on chromatography. The hydroxyl groups have weak ion-exchange properties that cause tailing of basic compounds. For this reason, endcapping sometimes is referred to as *base deactivation.* Because of variations in carbon load and endcapping chemistries, packings with the same type of bound stationary phase, such as ODS, may have differing chromatographic properties.

Polymeric Packings. Carbon particles that have been converted to graphite by a process known as *graphitization* or mixed copolymers are routinely used as polymeric packing (e.g., polystyrene-divinylbenzene) or further derivatized with ion-exchange or C4, C8, or C18 functional groups. Columns filled with these packings feature levels of performance comparable with those of silica-based columns and are stable from pH 2 to 13. Silica particles usually have decreased stability above pH 7.

Chiral Packings. Chiral packings are used to separate enantiomers, which are mirror-image forms of the same compound.[17,20] The chiral stationary phases are prepared by attaching a suitable chiral compound to the surface of an achiral support such as silica gel, which creates a chiral stationary phase (CSP).[1] Many common chiral stationary phases are based on oligosaccharides such as cellulose or cyclodextrin (in particular with β-cyclodextrin, a seven–sugar ring molecule). As with all chromatographic methods, various stationary phases are particularly suited to specific types of analytes. In the clinical laboratory, this type of packing is used to separate and quantify drug and amino acid enantiomers.

Restricted Access Packings. With this type of packing, the outer surfaces of the support particles are protected by a hydrophilic network. Smaller solutes, such as drugs, pass through the network into the pores, which are coated with hydrophobic stationary phase. Large protein molecules are denied access to the inner core and pass through the column. Columns filled with restricted access packing allow the direct injection of biological samples with high protein concentrations, which bypasses sample preparation and improves analytical accuracy.

Monolithic Columns. A monolithic column is one that is cast as a continuous homogeneous matrix ("just like concrete in a mold"). Such columns have bimodal pore structures with large pores (approximately 2 μm in diameter) that create high pore density, and smaller ones (approximately 13 nm in diameter) that create a large internal surface area. They have been found to be capable of efficient fast separations, as they allow higher flow rates than particulate columns at reasonable backpressures. In addition, they are capable of fast mass transfer and have high binding capacity. The lower back pressure provides highly reproducible column characteristics because many of the factors that degrade particulate columns are eliminated (e.g., packing down, channeling). The monolithic rods are encased in inert polytetrafluoroethylene (PTFE) tubing and are housed in stainless steel tubes. The inert tubing eliminates void volumes at the stainless steel tube/monolithic rod interface, thus improving resolution. Two additional advantages of these columns are that they are able to be used with mobile phase flow gradients (e.g., increasing flow rate at the end of a separation), and several columns may be coupled in a series to improve resolution with little increase in flow backpressure. Capillary monolithic columns also are available.

Of clinical interest, monolithic columns are being used to perform reversed-phase separations of peptides and proteins.

Column Heaters/Chillers

Control of column temperature is a factor in the reproducibility and efficiency of LC separations However, unlike GC separations, where temperature gradients are employed, in LC separations, a constant column temperature is maintained. It is achieved using a variety of techniques such as (1) column chambers, (2) water jackets, (3) temperature-controlled blankets, or (4) heating/cooling blocks. In addition, operation at high flow rates might require a heater/exchanger, usually a coil of tubing with good heat exchange properties, placed before the column inlet.

Detectors

Many different types of detectors have been used as monitors in liquid chromatographs (Table 12-4). Examples include (1) photometric or spectrophotometric, (2) fluorometric, (3) electrochemical, and (4) mass spectrometric detectors.

A key and integral component of such detectors is the flow cell through which the eluate from the chromatographic column passes. Dissolved analytes are detected and an electronic signal generated.

Operationally, detectors are used individually or are linked in series.[5] In addition, postcolumn reactors have been interposed between the column and the detector to perform a chemical reaction such as the reaction of ninhydrin with amino acids to generate products with a stronger and more specific signal.

Photometers and Spectrophotometers. UV and visible photometers and spectrophotometers measure the radiant energy absorbed by compounds as they elute from the chromatographic column (see Chapter 9). These detectors operate in the radiant energy regions of 190 to 400 nm and 400 to 700 nm, respectively. The devices are versatile and detect many

TABLE 12-4	Examples of Detectors Used in High-Performance Liquid Chromatography			
Type of Detector	**Principle of Operation**	**Range of Application**	**Detection Limit**	**Comments**
Spectrophotometer	Measures absorbance of light at a single wavelength	Diverse	<1 ng	Analytes must absorb light or must be derivatized
Spectrophotometer (diode array)	Measures absorbance of light at many wavelengths	Diverse	<1 ng	Detector provides complete spectra
Electrochemical	Measures current flow from oxidation/reduction reactions	Selective	pg to ng	Analytes must undergo oxidation or reduction
Fluorometer	Measures fluorescence at specific excitation and emission wavelengths	Very selective	pg to ng	Analyte must fluoresce or must be derivatized
Refractometer	Measures change in refractive index	Universal	μg	Offers relatively low sensitivity
Mass spectrometer (often a tandem mass spectrometer)	Detects ions after separation according to mass. Provides qualitative information	Diverse, limited only by ability to ionize analytes	pg to ng	Analytes must form ions. Can analyze multiple analytes simultaneously

solutes because most aromatic compounds are detected in the ultraviolet region from 250 to 300 nm, and many other compounds are detectable in the ultraviolet region from 190 to 220 nm, where amide, carboxylic acids, and many other groups have substantial absorbance.

These detectors operate at a fixed wavelength or at variable wavelengths. Most fixed-wavelength UV instruments use the intense 254-nm resonance line produced by a mercury arc lamp. This type of detector is extremely sensitive and is capable of operation at 0.005 absorbance unit full scale (AUFS). To provide fixed-wavelength detectors with greater flexibility, other less intense resonance lines of the mercury lamp are used. Alternatively, a phosphor is placed between the lamp and the flow cell, and the emitted fluorescence resulting from the 254-nm excitation is used as the light source. This latter approach is used in the dual-wavelength photometers that operate at two fixed wavelengths (e.g., 254 nm and 280 nm). The intense 214-nm or 229-nm resonance lines of a zinc or cadmium arc lamp, respectively, have been used for detection at lower wavelengths, where more compounds have strong absorbance.

The second type of photometric instrument is the variable-wavelength detector. It operates at a wavelength selected from a given wavelength range. Thus the detector is "tuned" to operate at the absorbance maximum for a given analyte or set of analytes; this greatly enhances the applicability and selectivity of the detector. Another advantage of this detector is its ability to operate at lower wavelengths (e.g., 190 nm). Because more compounds (e.g., cholesterol) absorb at lower wavelengths, this capability enhances the versatility of the detector. At lower wavelengths, however, many solvents absorb UV light and cannot be used as mobile phases. Fortunately, acetonitrile and methanol, two widely used solvents in reversed-phase chromatography, have low UV absorptions at 200 nm.

Diode arrays also are used as HPLC detectors because they rapidly yield spectral data over the entire wavelength range of 190 to 600 nanometers in about 10 milliseconds. Such detectors have been helpful in the identification of drugs in urine and serum.

In practice, when a photometric detector is used, it is necessary to use (1) solvents, (2) ion pairing agents, and (3) buffers with low absorbance at wavelengths of interest to maintain a low background signal. Solvents such as (1) water, (2) acetonitrile, (3) methanol, (4) isopropanol, and (5) hexane allow ultraviolet detection down to wavelengths of 200 nm, as do phosphate buffers. Many other solvents and buffers have substantial absorbance in the ultraviolet region that may limit ultraviolet detection. A problem with the operation of photometric detectors is the outgassing that occurs in the solvent as it exits from the high pressure of the column and into the low-pressure flow cell of the detector. Because these detectors are very sensitive, they detect these bubbles as noise that degrades the signal-to-noise ratio of the detector. Effective degassing of solvents and maintenance of some backpressure across the detector help to minimize bubble formation.

Fluorometers. As discussed in Chapter 9, fluorescence occurs when a molecule absorbs light at one wavelength and reemits light at a longer wavelength. Online fluorometers are used in liquid chromatographs to detect fluorescing compounds as they elute from the column. Fluorescence detectors generally are more sensitive than photometric ones. In addition, precolumn or postcolumn reactors have been used to chemically tag a compound with a fluorescent label for subsequent detection. For example, amino acids and other primary amines often are labeled with a dansyl or fluorescamine tag, followed by HPLC separation and fluorometric detection. Most fluorometers used with liquid chromatographs are relatively simple in design and are extremely selective and sensitive for compounds fluorescing within the detector's operating wavelength range. Deuterium and xenon arc lamps or lasers have been used as light sources in such detectors.

Electrochemical Detectors. In amperometric electrochemical detectors (see Chapter 10), an electroactive analyte enters the flow cell, where it is oxidized or reduced at an electrode surface under a constant potential. Electroactive compounds of clinical interest conveniently analyzed by HPLC with electrochemical detection include the urinary catecholamines (see Chapter 26). In addition, it is possible to add electrochemically active tags (e.g., bromine) to compounds such as unsaturated fatty acids or prostaglandins.

Coulometric detectors are also used. When placed in a series, such detectors are used to detect and quantify co-eluting compounds that differ in their half-wave potentials (the potential at half-signal maximum) by at least 60 mV. These detectors are extremely selective and sensitive, with wide linear response ranges. They are used in the clinical laboratory for analysis of (1) metanephrines, (2) vanillylmandelic acid, (3) homovanillic acid, and (4) 5-hydroxyindoleacetic acid in human urine. The high specificity allows analysis without extensive sample preparation.

Mass Spectrometers.[30] When a gas or liquid chromatograph is connected to a mass spectrometer (see Chapter 13), the combined techniques are referred to as gas chromatography–mass spectrometry (GCMS) and liquid chromatography–mass spectrometry (LCMS).[12,23,24]

A critical element in linking an HPLC to a mass spectrometer is the interface between them. For example, the interface has the challenging task of removing solvent molecules and transferring components from a liquid solution into a charged form in vacuum for analysis by the mass spectrometer. Therefore, all buffers used for chromatography need to be volatile to avoid overloading and contaminating the interface. In addition, a switching valve often is used to divert salts and other unretained components that elute early in the HPLC separation to waste. The switching valve then directs later parts of the HPLC run to the mass spectrometer. Several different ionization techniques, including (1) electrospray, (2) chemical ionization, and (3) photoionization, are discussed in greater detail in Chapter 13

System Controller and Data System

As with GC, computers provide system control and data processing functions for HPLC.[22] For example, the system controller manages (1) sample injections, (2) solvent delivery, (3) temperature control, (4) and detectors; it also provides an auditable record of analyst, method, calibration, controls, and specimens. Data systems take the thousands of data points from an individual run and identify a set of peaks with parameters such as (1) retention times, (2) peak areas, (3) peak heights, and (4) peak widths. Comparison of these parameters with those generated from reference materials yields identification of peaks and quantitative values. Software for data analysis becomes more critical as data streams become larger, such as from diode array and mass spectrometric detection, and multiple components are analyzed in a single run; libraries of spectra or other databases are searched for identification of compounds, peptides, or nucleic acid sequences.

Practical Considerations

Several techniques affect the practical application of HPLC in the clinical laboratory, including those used to prepare samples and mobile phases.

Sample Preparation

Sample preparation is an important step in HPLC analysis and includes procedures for (1) sample concentration by extraction, (2) purification, and (3) derivatization.[24] Particulate matter should be removed from specimens by high-speed centrifugation or by filtration. Solid phase extraction also serves as a means of filtration to remove particulate matter.

Sample Extraction and Precipitation. Before chromatographic separations are performed, many clinical specimens require some processing by extraction or precipitation steps before they undergo analysis.[10] Reasons to process such specimens include (1) removal of interfering binding proteins, (2) removal of components that precipitate or decrease the efficiency of chromatography, (3) concentration of specimens to a smaller volume, and (4) removal of water and salts. Methods used to precipitate proteins from blood or serum include addition of organic solvents, acids such as trichloroacetic acid, or high concentrations of salt. Precipitated proteins are removed by centrifugation or filtration. An aliquot of the resultant supernatant or filtrate is then chromatographically analyzed. Use of an immiscible solvent such as ethyl acetate or hexane extracts hydrophobic compounds such as (1) triglycerides, (2) carotene, (3) vitamin E, or (4) hydrophobic drugs and leaves most water, salts, and proteins that may interfere with analysis or derivatization. Also, use of volatile organic solvents allows for concentration of nonvolatile components by evaporation.

Use of solid-phase extraction, which is essentially a preparative chromatographic separation with stepwise elution of components, is increasing. Solid phase extraction is performed manually or robotically in a variety of formats, including (1) short columns, (2) 96-well plates with very short chromatographic beds at the bottom of wells, and (3) pipette tips packed with chromatographic media. Online solid phase extraction has been added to some HPLC systems with direct elution of analytes from the extraction column into the analytical column. Solid phase extractions use a variety of types of stationary phases, such as (1) ion-exchange, (2) reversed-phase, (3) affinity, and (4) normal phase. Common applications of solid phase extraction include extraction of drugs from urine or fat-soluble vitamins such as 25-hydroxyvitamin D from serum for chromatographic analysis. Most methods used for analysis of nucleic acids require an extraction step to recover DNA or RNA before analysis is begun.

Sample Derivatization. Some analytes need to be chemically derivatized before or after chromatographic separation to increase their column retention or detectability. For example, in automated amino acid analyzers, eluted amino acids are reacted with ninhydrin in a postcolumn reactor; this provides greater specificity and sensitivity in detecting amino acids. Other examples include labeling of amino acids or other primary amines with dansyl or fluorescamine tags in a precolumn or postcolumn reactor followed by fluorometric detection.

Preparation of Mobile Phase. In preparing the mobile phase, dissolved gases in the solvent need to be removed, and the solvent must be free of particulate matter. Mobile phases should be prepared from HPLC-grade solvents free of particulate matter. Any solutions prepared in the laboratory should be passed through a filter with approximately 0.5 micron pore size.

Qualitative and Quantitative Analyses

Chromatography is basically a separation technique. In practice, however, it is used both for identifying analytes and for performing quantitative analyses.

Analyte Identification

The retention time or volume or the distance traveled on a plate by a compound is often used for identification by comparison versus a reference standard.

In planar chromatography, reference compounds are chromatographed simultaneously with the unknown sample. Tentative identification is made by comparison of the migration distances and the detection characteristics of reference compounds with those of unknown analytes. If the R_f (see Equation 3) of the unknown analyte and that of the reference compound do not match, the compounds are judged to be different. If they match, the compounds are presumed to be identical. More than one compound may have the same R_f in a particular chromatographic system; therefore, the presumptive identification is often confirmed by other techniques such as use of (1) specific spray reagents, (2) antibody complexation, or (3) isolation of the compound, followed by chemical and/or instrumental analysis. Software is available for compound identification by library searching of ultraviolet (UV) spectra based on corrected R_f values.[9]

In column chromatography, analytes are identified by their detector response and retention times. Usually, a set of standards is run to identify the retention times of analytes. Identification of the same analytes in patient specimens in subsequent runs then depends on maintenance of highly consistent performance by the system. An internal standard may be added to specimens to check on consistency of retention times. In GC, (1) irregular gas flow, (2) leaks in the system, (3) changes in temperature control, or (4) degradation of the stationary phase may lead to problems with stable retention times. In LC, (1) changes in solvent (such as from refilling the solvent reservoir with fresh solvent), (2) irregular flow rate, (3) variation in gradient formation, (4) liquid leaks in the system, (5) degradation of columns with extended use, (6) changing to a new column, or (7) erratic temperature control may lead to variable retention times. Multiple components often have identical retention times. This problem may be addressed by using detectors with greater specificity, such as mass spectrometers that allow identification of multiple components eluting at the same time. Multiple detectors may be connected in series that assist with identification by their different specificities.[5] In LC, fluorometric or electrochemical detection often provides considerable specificity, or postcolumn reactors may selectively detect a specific class of compounds such as amino acids. In analysis of physiological specimens by column chromatography, unexpected interfering materials occasionally may arise from (1) medications, (2) diet, (3) herbal preparations, (4) unusual physiological states, or (5) specimen contamination. The frequency of such interference depends to some degree on the specificity of the chromatography and detection methods. Use of detection methods such as tandem mass spectrometry with very high specificity tends to decrease problems with interference.

Analyte Quantification

The electronic signals generated by the detector(s) are also used to produce quantitative information. Both external and internal calibrating techniques have been used. With external calibration, reference solutions containing known quantities of analytes are analyzed in a separate run to establish detector responses per amount of analyte (Figure 12-14). A calibration curve of (1) peak height, (2) peak area, or (3) spot density versus calibrator concentration is constructed and used to calculate the concentration of the analyte in the samples. With internal calibration, also called *internal standardization,* reference solutions of known analyte concentrations are prepared, and a constant amount of a different compound, the internal standard, is added to each reference solution and to each sample (Figure 12-15). A calibration curve is established for the ratio of detector response of the analyte versus the internal standard, and this calibration curve is applied to ratios of signal from analyte versus internal standard in patient specimens. Use of an internal standard is particularly useful when additional steps are involved, such as extractions with incomplete recovery of specimen. The internal standard helps correct for incomplete recovery. Internal

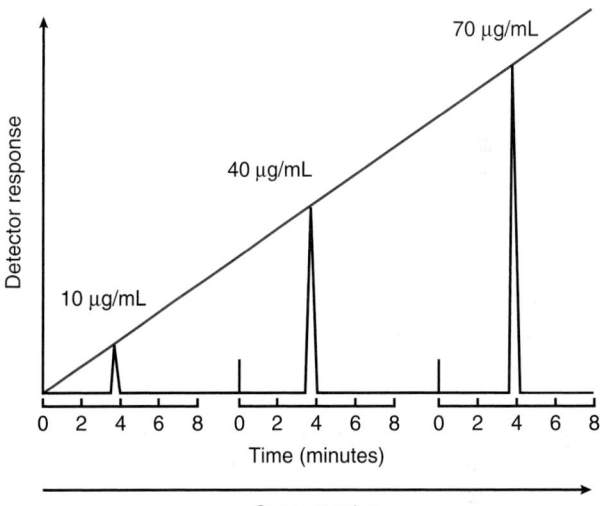

Figure 12-14 The use of external calibrators in the production of a calibration plot. *(From Krull I, Swartz M. Quantitation in method validation. LC-GC 1998;16:1084-90.)*

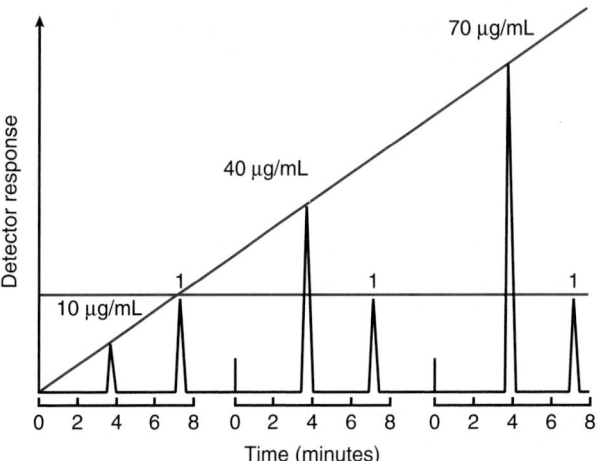

Figure 12-15 The use of internal calibrators in the production of a calibration plot (with peak 1 as the internal standard). *(From Krull I, Swartz M. Quantitation in method validation. LC-GC 1998;16:1084-90.)*

standards also are important in quantitation by mass spectrometry because the efficiency of ionization of analytes in the interface between HPLC and the mass spectrometer may vary. Ideally, in mass spectrometry, the internal standard has the same chromatographic retention and physical properties as the analyte. This often may be accomplished by using internal standards that have the identical chemical structure but substitute stable isotopes for hydrogen, carbon, or nitrogen.

Some important analytical characteristics of quantitative analysis include (1) limits of detection, (2) limits of quantification, (3) precision of analysis, and (4) carryover. Another important characteristic to establish is the analytical measuring range, which usually will extend from the limit of quantification on the low end to the upper limit of the measuring range. The response of many detectors is subject to saturation and nonlinearity of responses at very high concentrations. Also, in some cases, chromatographic systems may be overloaded by very high analyte concentrations. A range of high analyte concentrations should be tested to verify the highest concentration at which acceptable performance is achieved (the upper limit of the measuring range). Specimens with concentrations above that level should be diluted into an appropriate concentration range before analysis.

For analytes present in low concentrations, the major challenge often is to extend limits of quantification to low enough values. In general, the analytical limit of detection is improved by (1) increasing chromatographic efficiency (obtaining taller and sharper peaks), (2) increasing the amount of specimen loaded (possibly through extraction or the preconcentration step), (3) using smaller-diameter columns that elute the analytes in a smaller volume of solvent (with higher analyte concentration), and (4) appropriately selecting detectors and detector parameters such as wavelength of detection.

Review Questions

1. To be analyzed by gas chromatography, a compound must:
   a. be volatile or be made volatile.
   b. not be volatile.
   c. be water soluble.
   d. contain a nitrogen atom.
2. Which of the following statements concerning chromatography is *correct*?
   a. High-performance liquid chromatography (HPLC) involves the use of support particles coated on a piece of paper or glass.
   b. In affinity chromatography, a hormone can bind to its receptor that is coated on glass or resin beads.
   c. Thin-layer chromatography (TLC) is considered to be a quantitative type of chromatography.
   d. Ion-exchange chromatography uses the principle that particles compete for binding sites in the stationary phase.
3. The most commonly used detector for clinical lab analysis of analytes after gas chromatography (GC) is a:
   a. photoionization detector.
   b. thermionic selective detector.
   c. mass spectrometer.
   d. flame ionization detector.
4. Spotting a specimen on a silica-coated glass plate and calculating the retention factor (R_f) for migrated substances in a sample is referred to as TLC. What type of chromatography is this?
   a. Column chromatography
   b. Affinity chromatography
   c. Planar chromatography
   d. Liquid chromatography
5. Some point-of-care tests use chromatography as a processing step in the assay. In point-of-care pregnancy testing, for example, the stationary phase is nitrocellulose paper and the hCG antigen is present in a urine sample, which is considered the mobile phase. The antigen in the mobile phase binds with an antibody in the stationary phase. This is an example of planar chromatography using which of the following as the separation mechanism?
   a. Partition
   b. Ion exchange
   c. Affinity
   d. Steric exclusion (size)
6. A highly sensitive, specific, and quantatitive chromatographic method that uses pressure to push sample and solvent through a packed column is:
   a. TLC.
   b. GC.
   c. HPLC.
   d. Ion-exchange chromatography.
7. In column chromatography, unknown analytes are identified as they pass through the detector. Comparison of the _____ of unknown analytes with that of the internal standard is the method used for unknown identification.
   a. retention time
   b. retention factor
   c. resolution
   d. fluorescence
8. Which component of a gas chromatograph introduces an aliquot of sample to be analyzed into the column?
   a. Pipette
   b. Aliquotter
   c. Sample extractor
   d. Injector
9. Which phase of chromatography carries the sample?
   a. Stationary phase
   b. Mobile phase
   c. Retention phase
   d. Column phase
10. The component of a liquid chromatograph that is integral in passing the eluate from the chromatographic column into the detector is the:
    a. injector.
    b. diode array.
    c. flow cell.
    d. retainer.

References

1. Bhushan R, Brückner H. Use of Marfey's reagent and analogs for chiral amino acid analysis: assessment and applications to natural products and biological systems. Chromatogr B Analyt Technol Biomed Life Sci 2011;879:3148–61.

2. Carr PW, Stoll DR, Wang X. Perspectives on recent advances in the speed of high-performance liquid chromatography. Anal Chem 2011;83:1890–900.

3. Cook K, Thayer J. Advantages of ion-exchange chromatography for oligonucleotide analysis. Bioanalysis 2011;3:1109–20.

4. Eiceman GA, Gardea-Torresdey J, Overton E, et al. Gas chromatography. Anal Chem 2002;74:22771–80.

5. Gao M, Qi D, Zhang P, Deng C, Zhang X. Development of multidimensional liquid chromatography and application in proteomic analysis. Expert Rev Proteomics 2010;7:665–78.

6. Grumbach ES, Wagrowski-Diehl DM, Mazzeo JR, et al. Hydrophilic interaction chromatography using silica columns for the retention of polar analytes and enhanced ESI-MS sensitivity. LCGC Magazine 2004;27:October.

7. Guiochon G, Tarafder A. Fundamental challenges and opportunities for preparative supercritical fluid chromatography. J Chromatogr A 2011;1218:1037–114.

8. Hage DS, Anguizola J, Barnaby O, et al. Characterization of drug interactions with serum proteins by using high-performance affinity chromatography. Curr Drug Metab 2011;12:313–28.

9. Hortin GL, Goldberger BA. Chromatography and extraction. In: Burtis CA, Ashwood ER, Bruns DE, eds. Tietz textbook of clinical chemistry and molecular diagnostics, 5th edition. Philadelphia: WB Saunders, 2012:307–28.

10. Hyotylainenen T. Critical evaluation of sample pretreatment techniques. Anal Bioanal Chem 2009;394:743–58.

11. Kalmbach R, Paul L, Selhub J. Determination of unmetabolized folic acid in human plasma using affinity HPLC. Am J Clin Nutr 2011;94:343S–7S.

12. Kortz L, Helmschrodt C, Ceglarek U. Fast liquid chromatography combined with mass spectrometry for the analysis of metabolites and proteins in human body fluids. Anal Bioanal Chem 2011;399:2635–44.

13. Lavrik NV, Taylor LT, Sepaniak MJ. Nanotechnology and chip level systems for pressure driven liquid chromatography and emerging analytical separation techniques: a review. Anal Chim Acta 2011;694:6–20.

14. McNair HM, Miller JM. Basic gas chromatography, 2nd edition. Malden Mass: Wiley Interscience, 2009.

15. Miller JM. Chromatography: concepts and contrasts, 2nd edition. Malden, Mass: Wiley Interscience, 2009.

16. Mitrevski B, Wynne P, Marriott PJ. Comprehensive two-dimensional gas chromatography applied to illicit drug analysis. Anal Bioanal Chem 2011;401:2361–71.

17. Nic M, Jirat J, Kosata B, eds. Chirality: IUPAC compendium of chemical terminology (online edition). doi:10.1351/goldbook.C01058.

18. Roque AC, Lowe CR. Affinity chromatography: history, perspectives, limitations, and prospects. Methods Mol Biol 2008;421:1–21.

19. Poole SK, Poole CF. High performance stationary phases for planar chromatography. J Chromatogr A 2011;1218:2648–60.

20. Schmid MG, Gübitz G. Enantioseparation by chromatographic and electromigration techniques using ligand-exchange as chiral separation principle. Anal Bioanal Chem 2011;400:2305–16.

21. Sherma J. Planar chromatography. Anal Chem 2008;80:4235–57.

22. Shou WZ, Zhang J. Recent development in software and automation tools for high-throughput discovery bioanalysis. Bioanalysis 2012;4:1097–109.

23. Shushan B. A review of clinical diagnostic application of liquid chromatography-tandem mass spectrometry. Mass Spectrom Rev 2010;29:930–44.

24. Singleton C. Recent advances in bioanalytical sample preparation for LC-MS analysis. Bioanalysis 2012;4:1123–40.

25. Tao D, Zhang L, Shan Y, et al. Recent advances in micro-scale and nano-scale high-performance liquid-phase chromatography for proteome research. Anal Bioanal Chem 2011;399:229–41.

26. Tranchida PQ, Sciarrone D, Dugo P, et al. Heart-cutting multidimensional gas chromatography: a review of recent evolution, applications, and future prospects. Anal Chim Acta 2012;716:66–75.

27. Tyihák E, Mincsovics E, Móricz AM. Overpressured layer chromatography: from the pressurized ultramicro chamber to BioArena system. J Chromatogr A 2012;1232:3–18.

28. Unger KK, Liapis AI. Adsorbents and columns in analytical high-performance liquid chromatography: a perspective with regard to development and understanding. J Sep Sci 2012;35:1201–12.

29. Varma D, Jansen SA, Ganti S. Chromatography with higher pressure, smaller particles, and higher temperature: a bioanalytical perspective. Bioanalysis 2010;2:2019–34.

30. Vogeser M, Seger C. Pitfalls associated with the use of liquid chromatography-tandem mass spectrometry in the clinical laboratory. Clin Chem 2010;56:1234–44.

31. Ward TJ. Chiral separations. Anal Chem 2008;80:4363–72.

32. Wu N, Clausen AM. Fundamentals and practical aspects of ultra-high pressure liquid chromatography for fast separations. J Sep Sci 2007;30:1167–82.

CHAPTER

13   Mass Spectrometry*

Alan L. Rockwood, Ph.D., D.A.B.C.C., Thomas M. Annesley, Ph.D., and Nicholas E. Sherman, Ph.D.

Objectives

1. Define the following terms:

Base peak	Molecular ion
Ion trap	Product/Fragment ion
Mass analysis	Proteomics
Mass spectrometry	Time of flight (TOF)
Mass-to-charge ratio (*m/z*)	

2. List the applications of mass spectrometry analysis.
3. Describe a generic mass spectrometer, including principle of operation, components, and functions of these components.
4. For the following ionization methods, state the principle and specific uses of each type:

Electron	Atmospheric pressure chemical
Chemical	Inductively coupled plasma (ICP)
Electrospray	Matrix-assisted laser desorption/ ionization (MALDI)

5. For the following types of mass spectrometers, state the principle of operation, and list the designs, specialized components, and laboratory uses of each:
   - Beam-type
   - Trapping-type
   - Tandem
6. List three types of electron multiplier detectors and state the principle of this type of detection.
7. Describe the instrumentation and the principles of the techniques involved and state the clinical applications of each of the following:

Gas chromatography-mass spectrometry	MALDI-TOF
Liquid chromatography-mass spectrometry	ICP-mass spectrometry

8. Explain the role of mass spectrometry in the field of proteomics.

Key Words and Definitions

Base peak The ion with the highest abundance in the mass spectrum; it is assigned a relative abundance of 100%.

Electrospray ionization A commonly used technique in which a sample is ionized at atmospheric pressure before introduction into the mass analyzer.

Extracted ion profile The sum of ions over a limited *m/z* ranged displayed as a function of time.

Fragment ion An ion formed by dissociation of a molecular ion, by convention often limited to fragmentation prior to mass analysis.

Gas chromatography–mass spectrometry (GC-MS) A combined technique in which a mixture of analytes is separated into individual components by gas chromatography, followed by the ionization of the separated compounds in the ion source of a mass spectrometer.

Ion An atom that has acquired an electrical charge by losing or gaining one or more electrons.

Ionization The production of an ion from a neutral atom or molecule using various techniques including but not limited to chemical ionization or electrospray ionization; ionization is required for all mass spectrometry techniques.

Ion trap A component of a trapping-type mass spectrometer where ions are held in a spatially confined region of space using, for example, a magnetic or electrostatic field; manipulation of the traps allows *m/z* measurements to be performed.

Isotope A variant of a chemical element; each variant differs in the number of neutrons in the nucleus and therefore in atomic weight from other isotopes of the same element.

*The authors gratefully acknowledge the original contributions by Larry D. Bowers, upon which portions of this chapter are based. We also wish to acknowledge technical assistance by Jacquelyn McCowen-Rose and Martha Fowles and helpful suggestions from N. Leigh Anderson, Julianne C. Botelho, Pierre Chaurand, David K. Crockett, Ulrich Eigner, Steven A. Hofstadler, Andrew N. Hoofnagle, Gary H. Kruppa, Mark M. Kushnir, Donald Mason, Michael Morris, Maria M. Ospina, and Hubert W. Vesper.

Key Words and Definitions—cont'd

Isotope dilution mass spectrometry (IDMS) An analytical technique used to quantify a compound relative to an isotopic species of known or fixed concentration using isotopically labeled internal standards.

Liquid chromatography–mass spectrometry (LC-MS) An analytical process that uses a liquid chromatograph coupled to a mass spectrometer.

MALDI Acronym for matrix-assisted laser desorption/ionization. It is a soft ionization technique that allows the analysis of biomolecules and large organic molecules which tend to be fragile and fragment when ionized by more conventional ionization methods.

Mass analysis The process by which a mixture of ionic species is identified according to the mass-to-charge *(m/z)* ratios (ions).

Mass spectrometer An analytical instrument that first ionizes a target molecule and then separates and measures the mass-to-charge *(m/z)* ratio of these molecules or their fragments; this instrument interfaces with other instruments including but not limited to a second mass spectrometer or a gas chromatograph.

Mass spectrometry Study of matter through the formation of gas-phase ions that are characterized using mass spectrometers by their mass, charge, structure, and/or physico-chemical properties.

Mass spectrum A plot of the relative abundance of each ion plotted as a function of its mass-to-charge *(m/z)* ratio.

Mass-to-charge ratio *(m/z)* The quantity formed by dividing the mass of an ion by its charge.

Product ion A fragment ion formed when a molecular ion breaks into smaller pieces; in a tandem mass spectrometer, the fragmentation process takes place after ions have been separated by the *m/z* value in a first stage of mass spectrometry.

Proteomics The identification and quantification of proteins and their posttranslational modifications in a given system or systems.

Selected ion monitoring (SIM) A MS technique where only specified ions of interest are monitored.

Skimmer A cone with a central orifice that is designed to intercept the center of a spray or jet expansion so as to sample the central portion of the expansion.

Tandem mass spectrometer A mass spectrometer capable of successive separation of ions in an ion beam according to *m/z* value (tandem in space) or separation of a set of trapped ions in an ion trap according to *m/z* value (tandem in time).

Torr A non-SI unit of pressure with the ratio of 760 to 1 standard atmosphere, chosen to be roughly equal to the fluid pressure exerted by a millimeter of mercury. For example, a pressure of 1 torr is approximately equal to 1 mm of mercury.

Total ion chromatogram (TIC) The sum of all ions produced displayed as a function of time.

Mass spectrometry (MS) is a powerful qualitative and quantitative analytical technique that is used to measure a wide variety of clinically relevant analytes. When MS is coupled with **gas** or **liquid** chromatographs (see Chapter 12), the resultant analyzers have expanded analytical capabilities and widespread clinical applications. In addition, because of its ability to identify and quantify proteins, MS is a key analytical tool that is used in the emerging field of **proteomics**. This chapter begins with a discussion of the basic concepts and definitions of MS, which is followed by discussions of MS instrumentation and clinical applications.

Basic Concepts and Definitions

A **mass spectrometer** is an analytical instrument that first ionizes a target molecule and then separates and measures the **mass-to-charge ratio** *(m/z)* of the molecule or its fragments. Although mass spectrometers do not measure molecular mass, for historical reasons the mass-to-charge ratio is often loosely referred to as "mass." **Mass analysis** is the process by which a mixture of ionic species is identified according to the *m/z* ratios of the ions.[23] This analysis may be qualitative, or it may be both qualitative and quantitative. Mass spectrometry is extremely useful for identifying compounds and determining the elemental composition and structure of both inorganic and organic compounds, as well as for performing quantitative analysis of selected compounds.

A **mass spectrum** is represented by the relative abundance of each **ion** plotted as a function of its *m/z* ratio (Figure 13-1). Often, each ion has a single charge (z = 1), in which case the *m/z* ratio is equal to the mass. The unfragmented ion of the original molecule is called the *molecular ion*. **Fragment ions** are formed when a molecular ion breaks into smaller pieces. The ion with the highest abundance in the mass spectrum is assigned a relative value of 100% and is called the **base peak**. The base peak may be the molecular ion or a fragment ion. When this relative abundance scale is used, instrument-dependent variability in the mass spectrum is minimized, and it is then possible to compare the mass spectrum with spectra obtained on other instruments. Because the fragmentation of ions at specific bonds depends on their chemical nature, it is often possible to determine the structure of an analyte from the pattern of fragments in the mass spectrum.

In addition, the pattern of relative abundances among the fragment ions of a given compound is often unique to that compound, much as human fingerprints are unique for each individual. Computer-based libraries of spectra take advantage of this and are available to assist in identification of the analyte(s) from mass spectra.

Fragmentation of ions also takes place in a **tandem mass spectrometer.** Unlike fragment ions produced before mass analysis (e.g., in an ion source), the fragmentation process takes place after ions have been separated by the *m/z* value in a first stage of mass spectrometry. These fragment ions are more commonly known as **product ions.**

The mass spectrometer is considered to be a "universal detector" because all compounds have mass, and in theory it is possible to ionize and detect all compounds in a mass spectrometer. When interfaced with a liquid or a gas chromatograph, the mass spectrometer provides structural information and/or highly specific detection of individual analytes as they elute from a chromatography column. Depending on the operating characteristics of the mass spectrometer and the chromatographic peak width, several mass spectral scans are typically acquired across the peak. The sum of all ions produced is displayed as a function of time to yield a **total ion chromatogram** (TIC). It is possible to program the data

system to display the sum of ions over a restricted mass range rather than the full mass range. The resultant display is called an **extracted ion profile.** Both TICs and extracted ion profiles represent chromatograms, with signal intensity plotted as a function of time. Retention times are then measured and peak heights or peak areas integrated for use in quantitative analysis.

When only a few analytes are of interest for quantitative analysis and their mass spectrum is known, the mass spectrometer is programmed to monitor only those ions of interest. This selective detection technique is known as **selected ion monitoring** (SIM). The mass spectrometer cycles repeatedly through a table of selected *m/z* values, monitoring the abundance of each for a short time. SIM is typically employed in chromatographic applications of mass spectrometry. The time slice for each *m/z* value in this multiplexing scheme is typically selected to be short compared with the chromatographic time scale. Consequently, SIM provides an approximation of continuous and simultaneous monitoring of ions of all selected *m/z* values. Because SIM focuses on a limited number of ions, more ion signal is collected for each selected *m/z* compared with scanning of the full mass spectrum. This increases the signal-to-noise ratio of the analyte and improves the lower limit of detection. In general, an unknown is considered identified if the relative abundances of three or four ions agree within ±20% of those from a reference compound.

Mass spectra of most chemical compounds contain a series of peaks, most often differing by approximately one *m/z* unit, with the differing masses of the peaks attributed to the presence of atoms of different elemental **isotopes** in the molecule. These peaks are commonly referred to as isotope peaks or isotopic peaks. For example, the mass spectrum of $C_2H_7O^+$ consists primarily of three isotope peaks at nominal *m/z* values of 47, 48, and 49 with relative abundances of 100%, 2.4%, and 0.2%, respectively. The higher isotope peaks of $C_2H_7O^+$ contain contributions from ^{12}C, ^{13}C, ^1H, ^2H, ^{16}O, ^{17}O, and ^{18}O in various combinations. For example, the *m/z* 48 peak of $C_2H_7O^+$ is composed of $^{12}C^{13}C^1H_7^{16}O^+$, $^{12}C_2^1H_6^2H^{16}O^+$, and $^{12}C_2^1H_7^{17}O^+$. Calculation of isotopic patterns is often very challenging, particularly for high-molecular-weight compounds, and various methods that are used to meet this challenge have been discussed in the literature.[19]

It is possible to isotopically label molecules by artificially substituting atoms of a selected isotope for the naturally occurring isotopic atoms in specified portions of the molecule. Because of the mass difference compared with the masses of naturally occurring isotopic peaks in a mass spectrum, a labeled molecule is separated in the mass spectrometer from an unlabeled molecule and its abundance measured separately. **Isotope dilution mass spectrometry** takes advantage of this feature by spiking a specific concentration of labeled internal standard into a sample and basing a quantitative analysis on the ratio of abundance of the analyte to abundance of the internal standard in the mass spectrum.

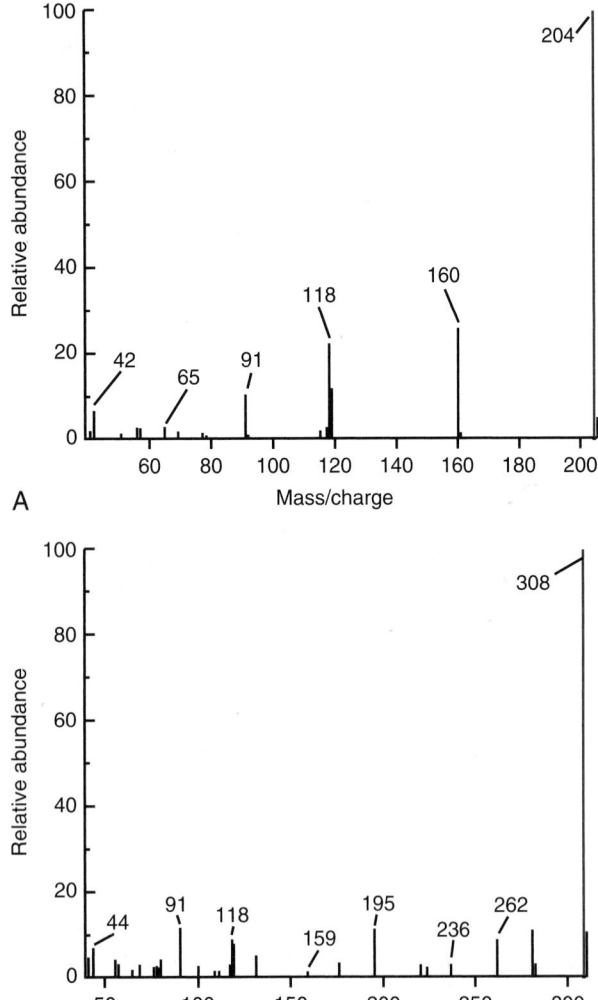

Figure 13-1 Mass spectrum of the **(A)** pentafluoropropionyl and **(B)** carbethoxyhexafluorobutyryl derivatives of D-methamphetamine.

Instrumentation

A mass spectrometer consists of an (1) ion source, (2) vacuum system, (3) mass analyzer, (4) detector, and (5) computer (Figure 13-2). In most cases, a chromatograph is also included as a sample introduction device.

Ion Source

All MS techniques require an **ionization** step in which an ion is produced from a neutral atom or molecule. Many approaches have been used to form ions in both high-vacuum and near–atmospheric pressure conditions. Electron ionization (EI) and chemical ionization (CI) are ionization techniques that are used when gas phase molecules are introduced directly into the analyzer from a gas chromatograph. The ionization methods used most frequently when a high-performance liquid chromatograph is interfaced with a mass spectrometer (HPLC-MS) include (1) **electrospray ionization** (ESI)[7] and (2) atmospheric pressure chemical ionization (APCI). Other ionization techniques include (1) atmospheric pressure photoionization (APPI),[18] (2) inductively coupled plasma (ICP),[2] and (3) matrix-assisted laser desorption/ionization (**MALDI**).[11]

Electron Ionization

In EI, gas phase molecules are bombarded by electrons emitted from a heated filament and attracted to a collector electrode (Figure 13-3). This process must occur in a vacuum to prevent both filament oxidation and collisional attenuation of the electron beam. Electrons are emitted from a hot filament by thermionic emission, accelerated through a potential difference of ≈70 volts, and directed toward a vaporized sample. These electrons have enough kinetic energy that the collision of an electron with most organic molecules ejects an electron from the analyte molecule and produces a *radical* cation, which is a chemical species that is both an ion and a radical.[23] In most cases, this radical ion then undergoes unimolecular rearrangement and fragmentation to produce a another cation and a radical:

$$AB^{+*} \rightarrow A^+ + B^*$$

As determined by their chemical stability, the relative proportions of molecular ion and various fragment ions are reasonably reproducible. Positive ions are repelled or drawn out of the ionization chamber by an electrical field. The cations then are electrostatically focused and are introduced into the mass analyzer. The mass spectral pattern, in most cases dominated by fragment ions, is often used much like a fingerprint to identify compounds by comparison with mass spectral libraries.

Chemical Ionization

Chemical ionization (CI) is a "soft" ionization technique, meaning that relatively little fragmentation is produced during the ionization process. A proton is transferred to, or abstracted from, a gas phase analyte by a reagent gas molecule. Typical reagent gases are (1) methane, (2) ammonia, (3) isobutane, and (4) water. The reagent gas is directed into a special CI source, so the source pressure is increased to about 0.1 torr; most of this pressure is attributable to the reagent gas. An electron beam ionizes the reagent gas and produces reactive species, often as a result of a cascade of ion molecule reactions, such

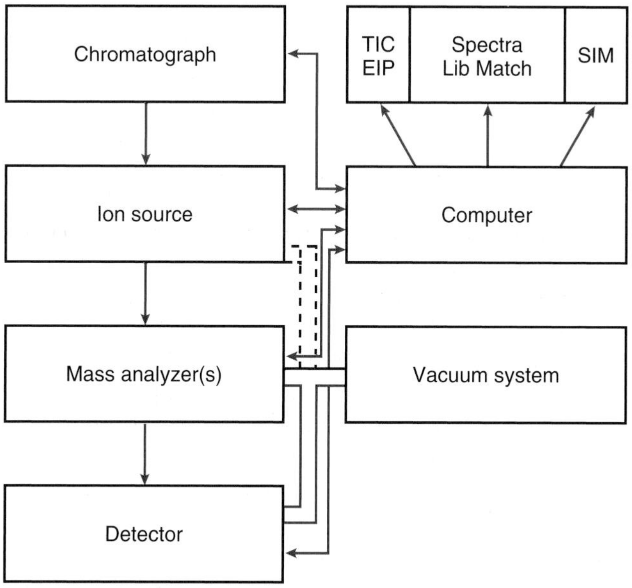

Figure 13-2 Block diagram of the components of a chromatograph-mass spectrometer system. The mass analyzer and the detector are always under vacuum. The ion source may be under vacuum or under near-atmospheric pressure conditions, depending on the ionization mode. The computer system is an integral part of data acquisition and output.

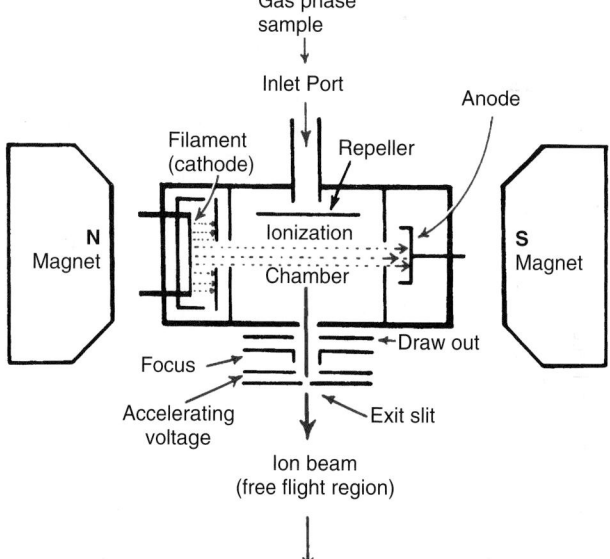

Figure 13-3 Electron impact ion source. The small magnets are used to collimate a dense electron beam, which is drawn from a heated filament placed at a negative potential. The electron beam is positioned in front of a repeller, which is at a slight positive potential compared with the ion source. The repeller sends any positively charged fragment ions toward the opening at the front of the ion source. The accelerating plates strongly attract the positively charged fragment ions.

as (in the case of methane reagent gas) proton transfer reactions to form CH_5^+, followed by proton transfer from CH_5^+ to the analyte molecule. This is a low-energy process, so relatively little fragmentation occurs. This process is advantageous for analyte molecular mass determination and for quantification.

Another variation of CI, negative ion electron capture CI, has become popular for quantification of drugs, such as benzodiazepines. Negative ion formation occurs when thermalized electrons are captured by an electronegative substituent, such as chlorine or fluorine on the analyte. Thus the number of compounds undergoing negative ionization is small, and background signal (noise) is decreased. When applicable, negative ion CI has acceptable limits of detection.

Electrospray Ionization

Electrospray ionization (ESI) is a technique in which a sample is ionized at atmospheric pressure before it is introduced into the mass analyzer.[25] The sample, typically an HPLC effluent, is passed through a narrow metal or fused silica capillary to which 1.5 to 5 kV voltage has been applied (Figure 13-4, A). Electrostatic forces on the liquid result in the expulsion of charged droplets from the tip of the capillary. In a typical electrospray ion source design, a coaxial nebulizing gas helps nebulize the liquid and direct the charged droplets toward a counter electrode. The droplets evaporate as they migrate through the atmospheric pressure region, expelling smaller droplets. The proton adduct of the molecule, which may be associated with solvent molecules, is "desolvated" to form "bare" ions, which then pass through apertures in a sampling cone and in one or more extraction **skimmers** before entering the mass analyzer. These devices are extraction cones that have a central

orifice that is designed to intercept the center of a spray or jet expansion so as to sample the central portion of the expansion.

Electrospray ionization is largely dependent on solution phase chemistry. Basic compounds, because they are easily protonated, tend to be efficiently detected in positive ion mode. Less commonly, rather than being formed by proton adduction, the ion is formed by adduction of some other positively charged ion, such as an ammonium ion or an alkali metal ion. In some cases, the ion may arise from a built-in charge of the analyte, such as a quaternary ammonium compound like choline. Occasionally, ionization occurs via electrochemical reactions in the ESI ion source. Acidic compounds, which readily lose a proton to become negatively charged ions in solution, tend to be efficiently detected in negative ion mode.

One unique feature of ESI is the production of multiple charged ions from some compounds, particularly from peptides and proteins. It is common to observe approximately one charge for every $\approx$10 amino acid residues in a protein. For example, because a molecule of mass 20,000 yields up to 20 charges, it is detected at m/z 1000 (20,000/20) with a lower resolution and less expensive analyzer. This greatly extends the accessible molecular weight range of such an instrument. In most cases where multiple charging occurs, a series of charge states are observed in the same mass spectrum (e.g., 19 charges, 20 charges, 21 charges). These appear at a series of m/z values (e.g., 1052.6, 1000, 952.4). In most cases, charging is produced by proton adduction, and peaks are observed at $m/z = (M+n)/n$, where M is the molecular weight and n is the charge (which equals the number of protons attached).

It should be noted that Figure 13-4, A, shows the probe as it is being directed toward the sampling cone of the mass

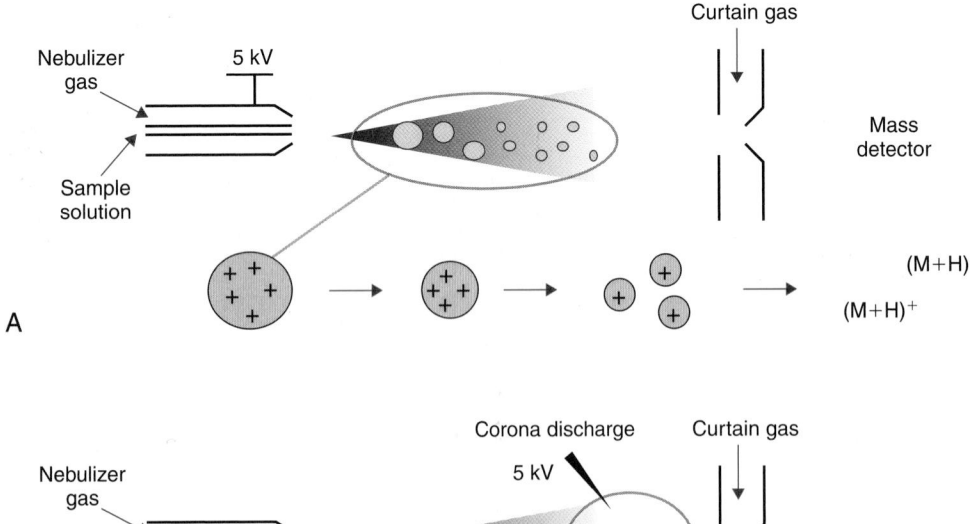

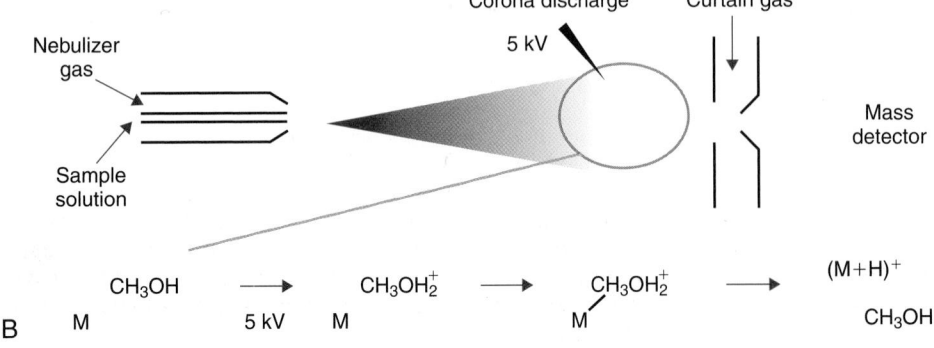

Figure 13-4 Schematics of **(A)** electrospray and **(B)** atmospheric pressure chemical ionization sources. Note the different points where ionization occurs, as described in the text.

detector. To enhance performance and minimize contamination of the mass detector, modern hardware configurations have been used to offset the probe and/or the mass detector relative to the sampling cone.

Atmospheric Pressure Chemical Ionization

APCI is similar to ESI as it (1) takes place at atmospheric pressure, (2) involves nebulization and desolvation, and (3) uses the same sample and extraction cones as ESI. Taken together, APCI and ESI represent most clinical mass spectrometry applications. The major difference between APCI and ESI lies in the mode of ionization (Figure 13-4, *B*). In APCI, no voltage is applied to the inlet capillary. Instead, a separate corona discharge needle is used to emit a cloud of electrons that ionize compounds after a series of ion molecule reactions, much as in CI, but with solvent molecules such as water and methanol serving as reagent molecules rather than ammonia or methane, as in CI. Products of these secondary reactions may contain clusters of solvent and analyte molecules, so a heated transfer tube or a countercurrent flow of a gas, such as nitrogen, is used to decluster the ions. As with ESI, relatively little fragmentation is seen, and APCI is used for quantitative analysis or for tandem MS.

Atmospheric Pressure Photoionization

APPI provides a complementary approach to ESI or APCI and is considered more universal across the polarity scale. It differs from APCI primarily in two respects. First, it replaces the corona discharge needle with an ultraviolet (UV) lamp (typically a 10 eV krypton discharge lamp) to generate gas phase ions via photoionization. Second, it usually includes an additional reagent gas that is easily ionized, such as toluene. As with APCI and CI, once the primary ions are produced (e.g., from toluene), they undergo a series of ion-molecule reactions that eventually result in the ionization of analyte molecules. Compared with ESI, the techniques of APPI and APCI tend to be more useful for less polar molecules, such as many steroids.

Inductively Coupled Plasma

Similar to ESI and APCI, ICP is an atmospheric pressure ionization method. However, unlike most atmospheric pressure ionization methods, which are "soft" and produce little fragmentation, ICP is the ultimate in "hard" ionization, typically leading to complete atomization of the sample during ionization. Consequently, its primary use is for elemental analysis. In the clinical laboratory, it is particularly useful for trace metal and heavy metal analysis in tissue or body fluids. ICP is extremely sensitive (e.g., parts per trillion) and is capable of extremely widedynamic ranges. The sample is typically prepared by acid digestion, and the liquid digest is introduced into the ion source via a nebulizer fed by a peristaltic pump. The nebulized sample is transmitted into hot plasma generated at atmospheric pressure by inductively coupling power into the plasma using a high-powered, radio frequency (RF) generator. A small orifice samples the plasma, and ions are transmitted to the mass analyzer through a series of differential pumping stages.

ICP-MS is comparatively free from most types of interference. However, some interferences, such as small polyatomics formed in the torch via ion-molecule reactions, cause problems. For example, ArO^+ interferes with iron at *m/z* 56. One solution to this problem is the dynamic reaction cell, which consists of a moderate pressure gas placed before the *m/z* analyzer. A reactant gas, such as NH_3, is directed into the reaction cell, where it reacts with polyatomic interferences and removes them before introduction into the mass analyzer.

Matrix-Assisted Laser Desorption/Ionization

The term *matrix-assisted laser desorption/ionization* (MALDI) was introduced in 1985 to describe a new soft ionization technique.[11] As currently used, the analyte is dissolved in a solution of *matrix,* which is a low-molecular-weight UV-absorbing compound. This solution is placed on a target that is then introduced into the mass spectrometer. The matrix-to-analyte ratio is generally around 1000 to 1. As the volatile solvents evaporate, the matrix compound crystallizes and incorporates analyte molecules. Figure 13-5 illustrates the use of a UV laser to vaporize small amounts of matrix and analyte into a plume of ions that is directed into a mass analyzer. MALDI is usually coupled with a time-of-flight (TOF) mass analyzer because MALDI produces discrete, pulsed-ion packets. This pulsed nature is well matched to the requirements of a TOF-MS analyser. Currently the most significant application of MALDI in the clinical laboratory is its use for bacterial identification.[4]

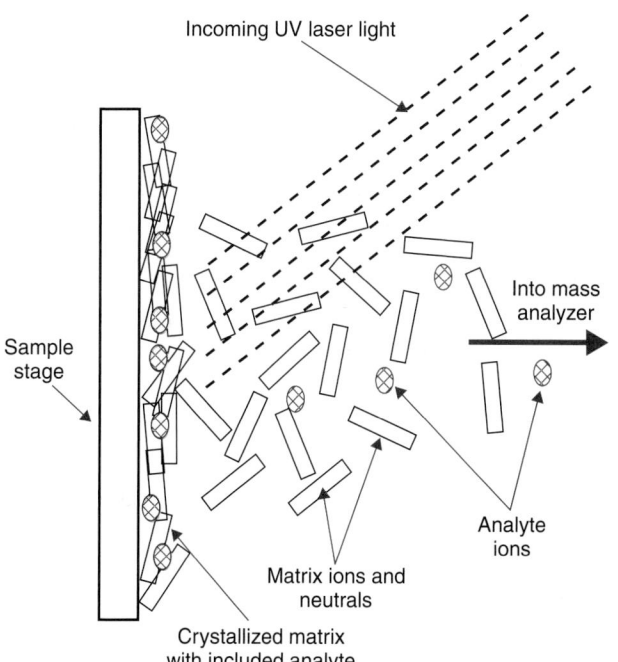

Figure 13-5 A generic view of the process of matrix-assisted laser desorption ionization. Co-crystallized matrix and analyte molecules are irradiated with an ultraviolet (UV) laser. The laser vaporizes the matrix, producing a plume of matrix ions, analyte ions, and neutrals. Gas phase ions are directed into a mass analyzer.

Vacuum System

With the exception of certain ion trap mass spectrometers, ion separation in a mass analyzer requires that the ions do not collide with any other molecules during interaction with magnetic or electrical fields. This requires the use of a vacuum from 10^{-3} to 10^{-9} **torr**, depending on the mass analyzer type. To reach this level of vacuum, a mass spectrometer uses both a mechanical vacuum and an efficient high-vacuum pump. During operation, the mechanical vacuum pump evacuates the system to a pressure at which the high-vacuum pump is then effective. A diffusion pump is the least expensive and most reliable high-vacuum pump. Turbomolecular pumps and cryopumps are also used on mass analyzers, and turbomolecular pumps have largely replaced diffusion pumps in currently marketed mass spectrometers. The high-vacuum pumps require routine maintenance for optimal operation.

Units used to express the levels of vacuum obtained include the *pascal* and *torr*. The pascal (symbol: *Pa*) is the SI derived unit of pressure. It is a measure of force per unit area, defined as 1 N/m^2. The torr is a unit of pressure defined as exactly 1/760 of a standard atmosphere, which in turn is defined as exactly 101325 pascals. Thus 1 torr is exactly $101325/760 \approx 133.3$ pascals.

Mass Analyzers, Ion Detectors, and Tandem Mass Spectrometers

Mass spectrometers measure m/z and not molecular mass. This has a fundamental impact on the physical operating principles of mass spectrometers and influences all aspects of (1) instrumentation design, (2) operation, and (3) interpretation of results. Most important, a peak in a mass spectrum will fall at an m/z that corresponds to a fraction of the molecular weight of the detected species if it is a multiply charged ion.

General Classes of Mass Spectrometers

Mass spectrometers are broadly classified as (1) beam-type or (2) trapping-type instruments. In a beam-type instrument, the ions make one trip through the instrument and then strike the detector, where they are destructively detected. The entire process, from the time an ion enters the analyzer until the time it is detected, generally takes microseconds to milliseconds.

In a trapping-type analyzer, ions are held in a spatially confined region of space by a combination of magnetic, electrostatic, and/or RF electrical fields. The trapping fields are manipulated in ways that allow m/z measurements to be performed. Trapping times vary from a small fraction of a second to minutes, although most clinical applications are seen at the low end of this range.

Beam-Type Designs

Beam-type mass spectrometers include (1) quadrupole, (2) magnetic sector, and (3) time-of-flight (TOF) instruments. It is convenient to categorize beam-type instruments into two broad categories: those that produce a mass spectrum by scanning the m/z range over a period of time (quadrupole and magnetic sector) and those that acquire successive instantaneous snapshots of the mass spectrum (TOF). This categorization is not definitive as certain instrument designs have been adapted to either scanning or nonscanning operation. Nevertheless, the categorization is a useful one because it covers most of the currently available instruments, and because scanning and nonscanning instruments are adapted for different optimal usages.

Quadrupole. Quadrupole mass spectrometers are sometimes known as *quadrupole mass filters* (QMFs). Analytically, they are currently the most widely used mass spectrometers and have displaced magnetic sector mass spectrometers as the standard instrument. Although these instruments lag behind magnetic sector instruments in terms of (1) limits of detection, (2) higher mass capabilities, (3) resolution, and (4) mass accuracy, they offer an attractive and practical mix of features, including (1) ease of use, (2) flexibility, (3) adequate performance for most applications, (4) relatively low cost, (5) noncritical site requirements, and (6) highly developed software systems.

A quadrupole mass spectrometer consists of four parallel electrically conductive rods arranged in a square array (Figure 13-6). The four rods enclose a long channel through which the ion beam passes. The beam enters near the axis at one end of the array, passes through the array in a direction generally parallel to the axis, and exits the far end of the array. The ion beam entering the quadrupole array may contain a mixture of ions of various m/z values, but only ions of a very narrow m/z range (typically $\Delta m/z < 1$) are successfully transported through the device to reach the detector. Ions outside this narrow range are ejected radially. The $\Delta m/z$ range represents a passband, analogous to the bandwidth of an interference filter in optics, which is why quadrupole mass spectrometers are often referred to as "mass filters" rather than "mass spectrometers."

Quadrupole mass spectrometers rely on a superposition of RF and direct current (DC) potentials applied to the quadrupole rods. DC voltages are applied to the electrodes in a quadrupolar pattern. For example, a positive DC potential is

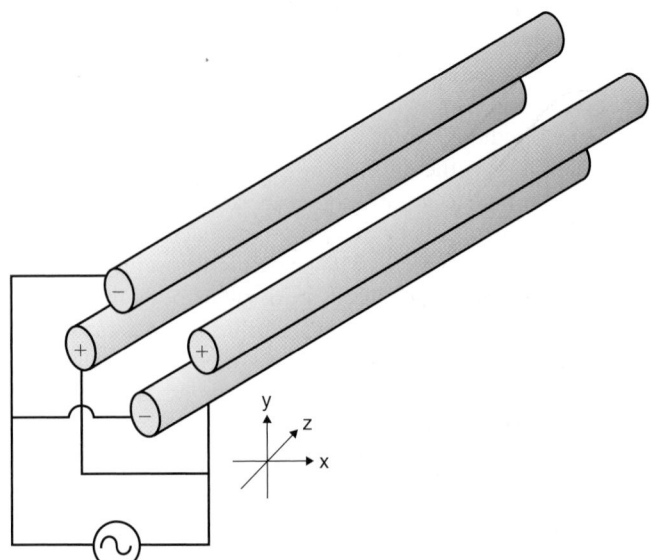

Figure 13-6 Diagram of quadrupole mass filter, including the RF part of the voltages applied to the quadrupole rods.

applied to electrodes 1 and 3, as indicated in Figure 13-7, and an equivalent negative DC potential is applied to electrodes 2 and 4. The DC potentials are relatively small, of the order of a few volts. Superimposed on the DC potentials are the RF potentials, also applied in a quadrupolar fashion. The RF potentials range up to the kilovolt range, and frequency is of the order of 1 MHz. The frequency is typically fixed to a highly stable value.

The device may be operated in a *selected ion mode* (SIM) mode or in a scanning mode. In an SIM mode, both DC and RF voltages are set. This in turn sets both the center of the passband and the width of the passband. For example, the mass spectrometer may be set to pass ions of m/z 363 ± 0.5. Both the center m/z and the $\Delta m/z$ are adjusted by the appropriate choice of DC and RF.

The combination of lower and upper m/z limits establishes a passband ($\Delta m/z$) and ultimately a resolution [$(m/z)/(\Delta m/z)$]. Generally, quadrupole instruments are limited to a resolution of several thousand, which is sufficient to achieve isotopic resolution for singly charged ions of m/z as high as several thousand. However, technical advances have enabled quadrupole mass spectrometers to achieve resolutions exceeding 10,000. The benefits of high resolution include reduction of interferences. In addition, high resolution, combined with high accuracy electronics, has enabled the measurement of "accurate masses" using quadrupole instruments. Accurate mass measurements are useful for confirmation of a chemical formula. Because of their lesser size and cost and relative simplicity of operation in comparison with magnetic sector analyzers, QMFs commonly are interfaced with both gas and liquid chromatographs.

Magnetic Sectors. Because magnetic sector mass spectrometers are rarely used in the clinical laboratory, they are mentioned here mainly for historical purposes. For a good introduction to magnetic sector technology, refer to the third edition of *Tietz Textbook of Clinical Chemistry.*

Time of Flight. TOF mass spectrometry (TOF-MS) is a nonscanning technique whereby a full mass spectrum is acquired as a snapshot rather than by sweeping through a sequential series of m/z values. TOF mass spectrometers are widely used and offer a number of advantages, including (1) a nearly unlimited m/z range, (2) high acquisition speed, (3) high mass accuracy, (4) moderately high resolution, (5) very sensitive, (6) absence of peak skew in the mass spectrum, and (7) reasonable cost. They are well adapted to pulsed ionization sources, which is an advantage in some applications, particularly with MALDI and related techniques.

Modern TOF mass spectrometers produce single-digit parts per million (ppm) mass accuracy. This allows TOF measurements to confirm the molecular formula of a compound. TOF mass spectrometers are conceptually simple to understand as they are based on the fact that a lighter ion travels faster than a heavier ion, provided that both have the same kinetic energy. A TOF-MS resembles a long pipe. Ions are created or injected at the source end of the pipe and are then accelerated by a potential of several kilovolts. They travel down the flight tube and strike the detector at the far end of the flight tube. The time it takes to traverse the tube is known as the *flight time*, which is related to the m/z of the ion.

The flight time for an ion of mass m and kinetic energy E to travel a distance L in a region free of electrical fields is given by:

$$t = L\left(\frac{m}{2E}\right)^{1/2}$$

A sample calculation for an ion of molecular weight 200 Da (3.32×10^{-25} kg) with a kinetic energy of 10 keV (1.60×10^{-15} J), traveling through a distance of 1 m, yields a flight time of 10.18 ms, and an ion of molecular weight 201 takes just 25 ns longer. To accurately capture such transitory signals, the data recording system must operate on a $\approx$1 ns time scale. Advances in signal processing electronics have made this practical at relatively modest cost, and this has been a major factor in the rise in popularity of TOF-MS.

TOF is inherently a pulsed technique, and it couples readily to pulsed ionization methods, with MALDI being the most common example. MALDI-TOF makes its biggest impact in the area of protein and peptide and bacterial identification. TOF is also used with continuous ion sources such as ESI with orthogonal injection from the ion source and application of a voltage pulse to a repeller to start the TOF process.

Another area where TOF-MS excels is high-mass analysis because its mass range is nearly unlimited. In MALDI-TOF, for example, it is not unusual to detect proteins with molecular weights exceeding 100,000 Da. TOF is also employed with ESI and EI ion sources. For technical reasons, ESI-TOF and EI-TOF instruments differ considerably in design from MALDI-TOF instruments, so TOF instruments are generally single-purpose instruments, as ion sources generally are not interchangeable between the different types of TOF instruments. Capability for high-mass analysis is expected to increase in importance as clinical laboratories gradually embrace proteomic-based diagnostic methods.

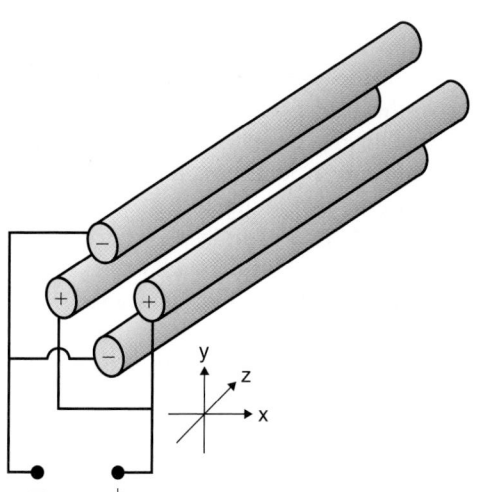

Figure 13-7 Direct current (DC) voltages applied to quadrupole rod assembly.

Absence of peak skew is another advantage of TOF-MS when it is used as a chromatographic detector. Peak skew is a distortion of the relative abundances of peaks in different parts of a mass spectrum, and this in turn distorts the shape of chromatograms derived from the mass spectral data. It arises from an interaction between the scanning function of the instrument and the changing concentrations of analytes over the chromatographic peak. TOF-MS instruments are essentially free of this artefact.

Trapping-Mass Spectrometers

In contrast to beam-type designs, these mass spectrometers are based on the trapping of ions to capture and hold ions for an extended time in a small region of space. Trapping times vary from a fraction of a second to minutes. The division between scanning and nonscanning instruments has less meaning for ion-trapping instruments than for beam-type instruments. The main practical difference between scanning and nonscanning instruments is related to peak skew, as discussed in the previous section on TOF. In terms of producing skewed spectra, trapping devices are more similar to nonscanning instruments, such as TOF (no skew), than to scanning instruments. This is so because the sample is captured in an instant and then is analyzed at leisure. Because the sample is captured in an instant, no skewing of the spectra occurs, regardless of whether the m/z analysis is performed by a scanning procedure or by a nonscanning procedure.

Classes of ion traps include (1) quadrupole **ion traps** (QITs), which rely on RF fields to provide ion trapping; (2) linear ion traps, which are closely related to QITs in their operating principles; (3) ion cyclotron resonance (ICR) mass spectrometers, which rely on a combination of magnetic fields and electrostatic fields for trapping; and (4) orbitrap mass spectrometers, which use a static electrical field and rely on orbital dynamics for trapping. Of these, we will briefly describe quadrupole and linear ion traps.

Quadrupole Ion Trap. QITs are used primarily as gas chromatography (GC) or HPLC detectors. They are (1) relatively compact, (2) inexpensive, (3) versatile, (4) excellent for exploratory studies, (5) useful for structural characterization and (6) useful for sample identification.

Operation of the QIT is based on the same physical principle that serves as the basis for the quadrupole mass spectrometer, as described previously. Both devices make use of the ability of RF fields to confine ions. However, the RF field of an ion trap is designed to trap ions in three dimensions rather than to allow the ions to pass through as in a QMF, which confines ions in only two dimensions.

A diagram of an ion trap mass spectrometer is shown in Figure 13-8. The trap is quite small—only a few centimeters in length. In practice, ions are trapped to be manipulated so they are dissociated into characteristic fragments and ejected to generate a mass spectrum.

Although QITs and QMFs were described at approximately the same time, the QMF initially achieved greater popularity as an analytical device. Later, two major discoveries changed the usage of the QIT. First, it was found that inclusion in the

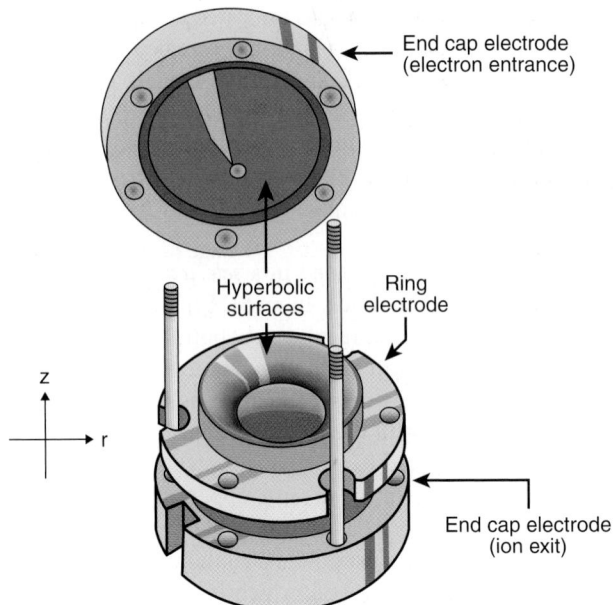

Figure 13-8 Diagram of quadrupole ion trap.

trap of a higher pressure (10^{-3} torr) of low-molecular-weight gas improved mass resolution and lowered detection limits. Second, the development of the mass-selective ejection, or mass instability scan function, improved QIT scanning. With no DC voltage and low RF voltage, ions of all m/z are stored in the QIT field. When the RF voltage is increased, ions of increasing m/z become axially unstable and leave the QIT sequentially by m/z. Ions leaving the QIT through one end cap are detected by an external electron multiplier. In addition, a lower limit of detection is obtained with QIT with the use of an axial modulation waveform to the end cap electrodes. This oscillating voltage improves the efficiency of ion ejection from the trap and improves mass resolution.

In addition to the oscillating voltage mode of operation, the QIT is capable of operation in other modes. For example, the QIT is also operated in a mass-selective storage mode that involves selecting RF and DC conditions such that only ions of one mass are stored in the QIT at any time.

The ability to apply customized waveforms to the QIT makes it one of the most versatile of mass spectrometers, rivaled only by the ICR mass spectrometer. This is most strongly evident in tandem mass spectrometry (MS/MS and related techniques), which will be discussed separately. It should be noted here, however, that multiple-stage MS/MS experiments (MS/MS/MS..., or MS^n) are readily performed in ion traps.

The ability to store ions also provides other distinct advantages. When the mass-selective ejection scan approach is used, mass resolution on the QIT is inversely proportional to the scan rate. With slowing of the scan rate, mass resolution similar to that achieved in magnetic sector instruments has been accomplished. For example, this technique has been used to determine the charge state of multiply charged protein ions generated by ESI.

The QIT also shares some advantages with TOF-MS. In particular, ion trap mass spectrometry is very sensitive.

Furthermore, sampling is decoupled from scanning, so no mass spectral peak skewing is seen in GC-MS and HPLC-MS.

Linear Ion Trap. The linear ion trap is an RF ion trap that is based on a modified linear QMF. Rather than serving as a pass-through device, as in a normal linear QMF, electrostatic fields are applied to the ends to prevent ions from exiting the device. After they are trapped, ions are manipulated in many of the same ways as in a QIT. An advantage of the linear quadrupole trap is that it generally has a higher dynamic range than a QIT. Commercial triple quadrupole mass spectrometers are available in which the third quadrupole is modified so it can function either as a QMF or as a linear trap.

Tandem Mass Spectrometers

Tandem mass spectrometry, or mass spectrometry/mass spectrometry (MS/MS), has become an important technique in clinical and analytical laboratories because it is a highly selective detection technique used for quantitative analysis of routine samples. However, it is also excellent for structural characterization and compound identification and therefore is useful for exploratory work, even when a final assay may be based on a different technology, such as an immunoassay. When coupled with the added selectivity of an HPLC, interferences in a well-designed MS/MS assay (and particularly an HPLC-MS/MS assay) are relatively uncommon. Because of its (1) low interference rate, (2) low consumable cost (as with most MS methods), and (3) high sample throughput rates, more and more clinical laboratories are purchasing and using tandem mass spectrometers.

The physical principle of tandem mass spectrometers is best understood by considering beam-type instruments—magnetic sectors and quadrupole mass spectrometers. Two mass spectrometers are arranged sequentially, with a "collision cell" placed between the two instruments. The first instrument is used to select ions of a particular *m/z*, called *precursor ions* or *parent ions*. The precursor ion is directed into the collision cell, where ions collide with background gas molecules and are broken into smaller ions, called *product ions* or *daughter ions*. The second mass spectrometer acquires the mass spectrum of the product ions.

The key to the high selectivity of MS/MS is that it characterizes a compound by two physical properties—precursor ion mass and product ion mass—rather than by a single property. If combined with chromatographic separation, the retention time is then added to the characterization, and the analytes are characterized by three physical properties; this eliminates most potential interferences.

As illustrated in Figure 13-9, a variety of scan functions are possible with tandem mass spectrometers. A *product ion scan* involves setting the first mass spectrometer, MS1, to select a given *m/z* and scanning through the full mass spectrum of product ions. This scan function is often used for structural characterization. A *precursor ion scan* reverses this relationship, with the second mass spectrometer, MS2, set to select a specific product ion, and MS1 is scanned through the spectrum. Peaks in the precursor ion scan are indicative of which parent ions produce a specific product ion—a capability that

is often used to analyze for specific classes of compounds. A *constant neutral loss* scan consists of scanning both mass spectrometers synchronously, with a constant offset between the two mass analyzers. This scan function is selective for ions that lose a neutral fragment of a specific mass corresponding to the constant offset between the two mass spectrometers. A *multiple reaction monitoring* (MRM) scan is not actually a scan function but is rather a method of jumping cyclically through a table of precursor/product ion pairs. It is the tandem mass spectrometry analogue to SIM in single-stage mass spectrometry.

As with single-stage mass spectrometers, tandem mass spectrometers are roughly categorized as beam-type and trapping instruments. The most popular beam-type instrument is the triple quadrupole. In this instrument, the first quadrupole (Q1) functions as MS1, and the third quadrupole (Q3) functions as MS2. Between these two quadrupoles is another quadrupole, Q2, which functions as the collision cell rather than as a QMF.

Another technological development in tandem mass spectrometry is the combination of two TOF mass spectrometers, TOF/TOF. These instruments are highly sensitive, have excellent throughput for MALDI-MS/MS, and are especially well suited for proteomics research. However, they are unable to perform true precursor ion scans or constant neutral loss scans.

So-called hybrid mass spectrometers include a combination of two different types of mass spectrometers in a tandem arrangement. One popular approach is the combination of a quadrupole for MS1 and a TOF for MS2. As with TOF/TOF, these instruments are presently used mainly for proteomics research. They are unable to perform true precursor ion scans or constant neutral loss scans.

Detectors

With the exception of an ICR-MS, nearly all mass spectrometers use electron multipliers for ion detection. Classes of electron multipliers include (1) discrete dynode multipliers; (2) continuous dynode electron multipliers (CDEMs), also known as *channel electron multipliers* (CEMs); and (3) microchannel plate (MCP) electron multipliers, also known as *multichannel plate electron multipliers*. Although they are different in detail, all three work by using a similar multiplication process—sometimes referred to as an *avalanche* or *cascade process*—that is repeated through a chain of dynodes, numbering between 12 and 24 for most designs. The multiplication process typically produces a gain of 10^4 to 10^8, where the generation of one electron at the first dynode produces a pulse of 10^4 to 10^8 electrons at the end of the cascade. The duration of the pulse is very short—typically less than 10 nanoseconds.

An additional detector used in mass spectrometers is the Faraday cup. This detector collects the ion current directly without going through a multiplication step. The Faraday cup is used when the ion abundance is so high that it would saturate the output of an electron multiplier. The Faraday cup is most commonly used with ICP-MS when signals are high enough to saturate an electron multiplier.

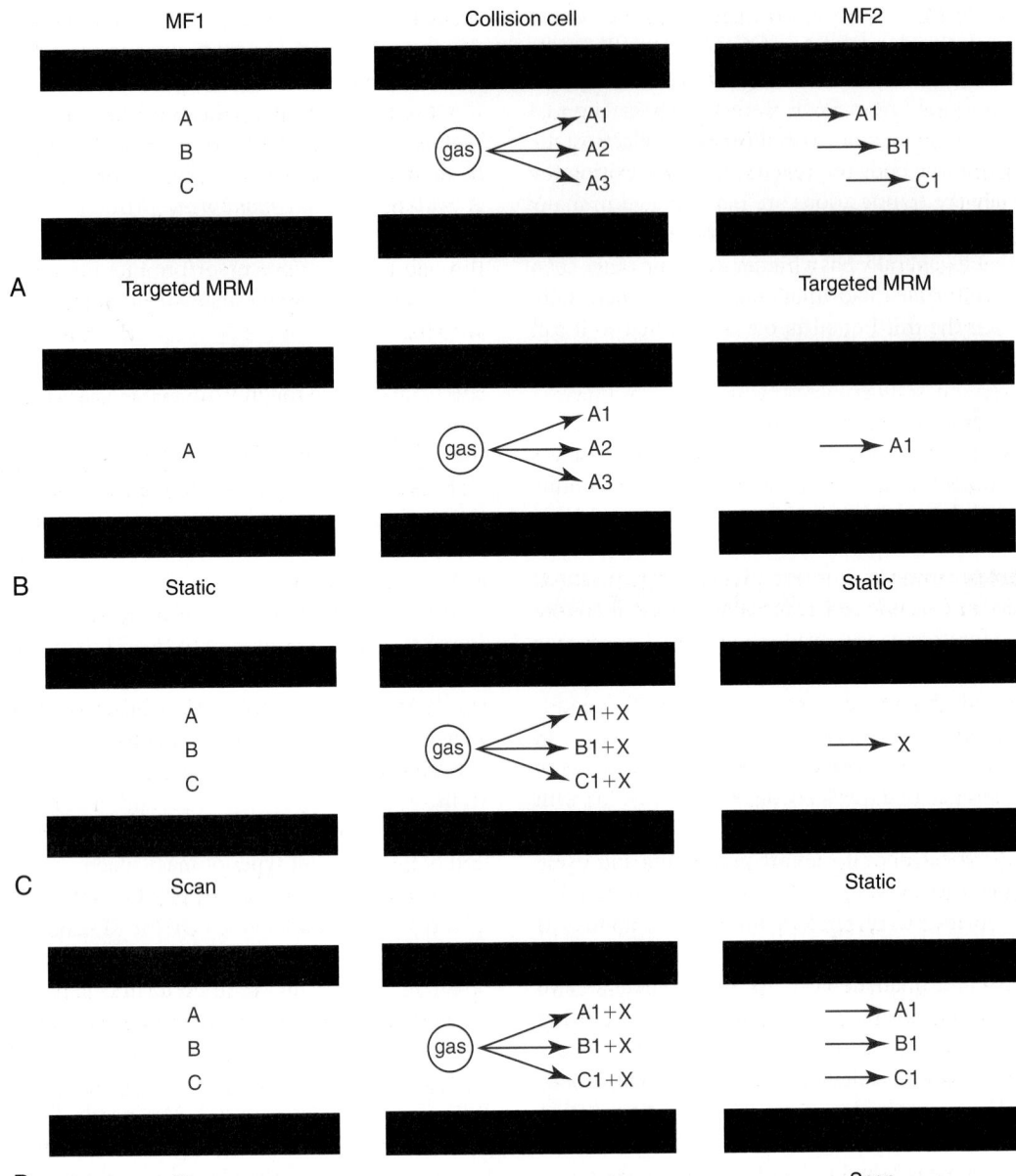

Figure 13-9 Scan modes in mass spectrometry/mass spectrometry (MS/MS). **A,** Multiple reaction monitoring (MRM), where *A, B, C, A1, B1,* and *C1* are ions. Monitoring of MS/MS transitions *A → A1, B → B1,* and *B → C1* is multiplexed. For simplicity, only the dissociation of *A* is shown in a collision cell in the figure. **B,** MRM of a single compound, where only one MS/MS transition is monitored. **C,** Precursor ion scan, where *A, B, C,* and *X* are all ions. The second mass filter (MF2) is fixed to monitor the mass-to-charge ratio *(m/z)* corresponding to ionic species *X,* and the first mass filter (MF1) is scanned through a range of *m/z* values. **D,** Constant neutral loss scan, where *X* is uncharged and *A, B, C, A1, B1,* and *C1* are ions. The two mass filters are scanned with a constant *m/z* offset between the two, corresponding to the mass of *X.*

Computer and Software

In modern mass spectrometers, the raw signal produced by the instrument is digitized, and the digital signal is recorded and processed by computers and their resident software. Because of their (1) mass resolution capabilities, (2) scanning functions, (3) ability to automatically switch from positive to negative ionization modes, and (4) speed with which multiple *m/z* signals are monitored, modern MS instruments generate immense quantities of raw data. Thus, their operation requires the use sophisticated computers and software programs.

For example, in toxicology laboratories, one important function of the data system is library searching to assist in compound identification. Several commercial libraries are available, including the (1) Wiley Registry of Mass Spectral Data (http://www.wiley.com/WileyCDA/; accessed on August 9, 2013), (2) the U.S. National Institute of Standards and

Technology (NIST) Mass Spectral Database (http://www.nist.gov/srd/nist1a.cfm/; accessed on August 9, 2013), and the (3) Pfleger, Maurer, Weber drug libraries.[1] In addition, many institutions and laboratories generate their own libraries. Important factors in the utility of using such libraries include (1) the quality and quantity of available spectra, (2) the search algorithm, and (3) whether condensed or full spectra are searched. Several library search algorithms are available; the most popular are probability-based matching and the dot product matching approach modified by the NIST. Both approaches allow assessment of match quality between observed spectra and library spectra.

The computer and software are also used to (1) integrate the signal from the mass spectrometer (usually in the form of integrated mass chromatograms), (2) generate calibration curves, (3) calculate concentration from calibration curves, (4) generate reports, and (5) perform other functions.

Clinical Applications

Mass spectrometers coupled with gas and liquid chromatographs (GC-MS and LC-MS) result in versatile analytical instruments that combine the separation power of chromatographs with the exquisite specificity and low detection limits of a mass spectrometer. Such instruments are powerful analytical tools that are used by clinical laboratories to identify and quantify organic analytes. For example, they provide structural and quantitative information on individual analytes as they elute from a chromatographic column. These coupled techniques are very sensitive, requiring only (1) nanogram, (2) pictogram, or (3) even lower quantities of an analyte for analysis. For example, one method used for analysis of estradiol using 250 μL of sample has a limit of quantitation of 1 pg/mL, corresponding to quantitation of 0.25 pg absolute.[15]

MALDI-TOF mass spectrometers and ICP ionization techniques have also enhanced the analytical capabilities of mass spectrometers. MALDI-TOF mass spectrometers have been used mainly for discovery rather than for routine analysis of patient samples. An important application of MS is its use as the primary analytical tool for discovery in the rapidly developing and expanding field of proteomics. In addition, MALDI is being used to identify bacteria.[4]

Gas Chromatography-Mass Spectrometry

Gas chromatography-mass spectrometry (GC-MS) has been used for several decades for the analysis of biological compounds. For example, it is used by the NIST as a definitive method of qualifying standard reference materials and assigning certified values to many clinical analytes (see Chapter 8). One of the most common applications of GC-MS consists of drug testing for clinical or forensic purposes. Many drugs have relatively small molecular weights and are sufficiently volatile for analysis by GC. Electron ionization with full-scan mass detection is the most widely used approach for comprehensive drug screening. Identification of unknown compounds is achieved by comparison of their full mass spectrum with a mass spectral library or database. Numerous state and federal agencies mandate that only GC-MS be used to confirm the presence of drugs in samples presumptively found to be positive by immunochemical analyses.

GC-MS has many applications beyond drug testing. For example, (1) xenobiotic compounds, (2) anabolic steroids, (3) pesticides, (4) pollutants, and (5) inborn errors of metabolism all have been analyzed by GC-MS.[13]

An important limitation of GC-MS is the requirement that compounds be sufficiently volatile to allow transfer from the solid phase to the mobile carrier gas and thus elution from the analytical column to the detector, which in this case is a mass spectrometer. Thus, many biological compounds need to be derivatized before they are amenable to analysis by GC-MS.

Liquid Chromatography-Mass Spectrometry

Compared with gas chromatographs, it is more difficult to interface liquid chromatographs with mass spectrometers because the analytes are dissolved in a liquid rather than a gas. This causes difficulties for the vacuum pumping system of the mass spectrometer. As discussed previously, several interface techniques have been developed for coupling a liquid chromatograph to a mass spectrometer, which has allowed HPLC-MS and HPLC-MS/MS to be successfully applied to a wide variety of compounds. In theory, as long as a compound is dissolved in a liquid, it is possible to introduce it into an HPLC-MS system. Thus, polar and nonpolar analytes and large molecular weight compounds, such as proteins, are analyzed using this technique.

An important area in which HPLC-MS/MS is used clinically is screening and confirmation of genetic disorders and inborn errors of metabolism.[8] Also, the ability to analyze multiple compounds in a single analytical run makes this technique an efficient tool for screening purposes. For example, electrospray tandem MS has become the recognized reference method for carnitine and acylcarnitine analysis to identify organic acidemias and fatty acid oxidation defects. It is also an excellent tool for analysis of amino acids, which then is used to diagnose various inborn errors of metabolism. In the case of carnitine and amino acid analysis, these compounds vary in their polarity, which creates problems with consistency of response factors. To address this, some procedures employ a butyl ester derivatization of the carboxyl group to force cationic character upon the amino acids, thus yielding similar ionization efficiencies for these compounds. Assays for acylcarnitines and amino acids that do not require derivatization have been described.[9,26] Other clinically relevant compounds that are amenable to HPLC-MS analysis include (1) immunosuppressants, (2) antiretrovirals, (3) biogenic amines, (4) methylmalonic acid, and (5) many steroid hormones.[3,5,14,21]

An important class of clinical applications relies on tandem mass spectrometry alone, without chromatographic separation. One method of expanded newborn screening uses butyl derivatization of acylcarnitines and amino acids, which subsequently are detected by tandem mass spectrometry. Acylcarnitines are selectively detected using an m/z 85 precursor ion scan, and amino acids are selectively detected using a 102 Da neutral loss scan.

MALDI-TOF Mass Spectrometry

MALDI-TOF has been used to analyze a large number of different classes of compounds. Its use generally falls into one of three broad categories: (1) detection of a specific compound(s), (2) identification of a protein(s) (Figure 13-10), or (3) identification of an organism. A requirement for small molecule detection by MALDI is that the molecule must (1) co-crystallize with the matrix (and not react), (2) be able to be desorbed back out of the matrix, and (3) form an ion or an adduct that is then detected.

MALDI-TOF also has been used to identify organisms such as bacteria.[4] A method has been described that attempts to identify bacteria by fingerprinting proteins that were extracted using gentle conditions.[24] The basis of this technique is that different bacteria should express unique proteins in the 2 to 20 kDa mass range, allowing classification according to the protein mass fingerprint. Historically, major problems included lack of actual protein mass information for various bacteria and lack of investigation into different strains of the same bacteria.[17] The protein mass fingerprints must be catalogued for each bacterium and determined to be completely reproducible for a given extraction method.

ICP Mass Spectrometry

ICP-MS is used for the determination of trace elements in many types of samples. However, it is known that the toxicity of an element may depend on the organic or inorganic state in which the element is present. In these cases it is more important to ascertain the concentrations of toxic species rather than the total concentration of the element. To extend the utility of this technique, GC and HPLC systems are now being coupled with ICP-MS to separate individual elemental species before ICP-MS analysis.[17]

Proteomics

The past 20 years has seen tremendous progress in genomics, with hundreds of genomes sequenced. However, this information has often failed to provide vast new understanding into cellular function—mainly because of the myriad changes that occur in the proteins produced from the genome throughout the life cycle of a cell. In the mid-1990s, MS came to the forefront of analytical techniques used to study proteins, and the term *proteomics* was coined. Proteomics encompasses knowledge of the (1) structure (identification), (2) function, and (3) quantitative expression of all proteins in the biochemical or biological contexts of all organisms.[12] Obtaining this knowledge is a challenging task, as every gene has potentially 100 or more distinct chemical protein isoforms. In addition, many other molecules (metals, lipids, etc.) interact with proteins in a noncovalent fashion. Therefore in a genome, such as human, a repertoire of millions of "proteins" may require identification and quantification.

Increasingly, much proteomic research has been devoted to analysis of complex mixtures of proteins from clinical samples. Currently, both instrumentation and analysis software are not sufficiently advanced to easily identify/quantify all of the proteins, including modifications, in these truly complex mixtures. As a result, much emphasis has been placed on

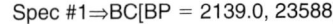

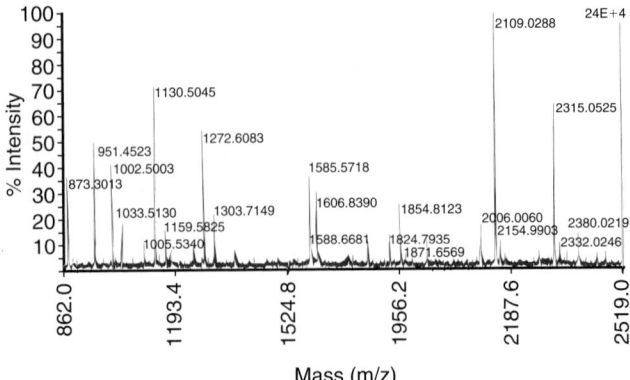

Figure 13-10 An example of a matrix-assisted laser desorption/ionization–time of flight (MALDI-TOF) spectrum showing peptides generated in a tryptic digest of a spot cored from a two-dimensional (2D) sodium dodecyl sulfate (SDS)-polyacrylamide gel electrophoresis (PAGE) gel.

separation methods for proteins and/or peptides, including (1) subcellular fractionation, (2) multidimensional chromatography, and (3) affinity labeling and/or purification. Through combinations of these approaches and with analysis by mass spectrometry many thousand "protein species" have been identified in a complex mixture.[10] In practice, MS/MS is used to obtain partial sequence information, followed by matching of this information with protein databases. The current state of proteomics is addressed in numerous papers every month in journals ranging from *Proteomics* to *Clinical Chemistry*. Although an exhaustive listing is impossible, several review or opinion references can serve as good starting points for exploration into the rapidly changing world of proteomics.[6,16,20,22]

Review Questions

1. Which of the following classes of mass spectrometers involves ions making a single trip through the instrument and then striking a detector where they are destructively detected?
   a. Trapping type
   b. Beam type
   c. Mass-selective ejection type
   d. Ion-cyclotron resonance type

2. In mass spectrometry, the sum of all ions produced is displayed as a function of time to yield a(n):
   a. product ion.
   b. extracted ion profile.
   c. mass spectrum.
   d. total ion chromatogram.

3. Which type of ionization technique uses an electron beam to ionize the reagent gas and produce a reactive species as a result of ion-molecule reactions?
   a. Electron
   b. Chemical
   c. Electrospray
   d. Inductively coupled plasma

4. Inductively coupled plasma mass spectrometry is typically used for:
   a. determination of trace elements.
   b. identification of a protein.
   c. drug identification.
   d. isotopic labeling of molecules.
5. The most widely used ionization approach coupled with gas chromatography and used for comprehensive drug screening is:
   a. electrospray ionization.
   b. chemical ionization.
   c. MALDI.
   d. electron ionization.
6. Currently, the most widely used mass spectrometer, which is flexible, easy to use, and of relatively low cost, is the:
   a. quadrupole mass spectrometer.
   b. time-of-flight instrument.
   c. magnetic sector mass spectrometer.
   d. linear ion trap mass spectrometer.

References

1. Aebi B, Bernhard W. Advances in the use of mass spectral libraries for forensic toxicology. J Anal Toxicol 2002;26:149–56.
2. Bonnefoy C. Menudier A, Moesch C, et al. Validation of the determination of lead in whole blood by ICP-MS. J Anal Atomic Spectr 2002;17:1161–5.
3. Ceglarek U, Lembcke J, Fiedler GM, et al. Rapid simultaneous quantification of immunosuppressants in transplant patients by turbulent flow chromatography combined with tandem mass spectrometry. Clin Chim Acta 2004;346:181–90.
4. Cherkaoui A, Hibbs J, Emonet S, et al. Comparison of two matrix-assisted laser desorption ionization-time of flight mass spectrometry methods with conventional phenotypic identification for routine identification of bacteria to the species level. J Clin Microbiol 2010;48:1169–75.
5. Colombo S, Beguin A, Telenti A, et al. Intracellular measurements of anti-HIV drugs indinavir, amprenavir, saquinavir, ritonavir, nelfinavir, lopinavir, atazanavir, efavirenz and nevirapine in peripheral blood mononuclear cells by liquid chromatography coupled to tandem mass spectrometry. J Chromatogr B Analyt Technol Biomed Life Sci 2005;819:259–76.
6. Dunn MJ. Proteomics clinical applications reviews 2012. Proteomics Clin Appl 2012;6:3–5.
7. Fenn J. Electrospray wings for molecular elephants (Nobel lecture). Angew Chem Int Ed Engl 2003; 25:3871–94.
8. Garg U, Dasouki M. Expanded newborn screening of inherited metabolic disorders by tandem mass spectrometry: clinical and laboratory aspects. Clin Biochem 2006;39:315–32.
9. Ghoshal AK, Guo T, Soukhova N, et al. Rapid measurement of plasma acylcarnitines by liquid chromatography-tandem mass spectrometry without derivatization. Clin Chim Acta 2005; 358:104–12.
10. Hoofnagle AN, Becker JO, Oda MN, et al. Multiple-reaction monitoring-mass spectrometric assays can accurately measure the relative protein abundance in complex mixtures. Clin Chem 2012;58:777–81.
11. Karas M, Bachmann DFH. Influence of the wavelength in high-irradiance ultraviolet laser desorption mass spectrometry of organic molecules. Anal Chem 1985;57:2935–9.
12. Kenyon GL, DeMarini DM, Fuchs E, et al. Defining the mandate of proteomics in the post-genomics era: workshop report. Mol Cell Proteomics 2002;1:763–80.
13. Kuhara T. Gas chromatographic-mass spectrometric urinary metabolome analysis to study mutations of inborn errors of metabolism. Mass Spectrom Rev 2005; 24:814–27.
14. Kushnir MM, Urry FM, Frank EL, et al. Analysis of catecholamines in urine by positive-ion electrospray tandem mass spectrometry. Clin Chem 2002; 48:323–31.
15. Kushnir MM, Rockwood AL, Yue B, et al. High sensitivity measurement of estrone and estradiol in serum and plasma using LC-MS/MS. Methods Mol Biol 2010;603:219–28.
16. Lin D, Tabb DL, Yates JR 3rd. Large-scale protein identification using mass spectrometry. Biochim Biophys Acta 2003;1646:1–10.
17. Mandal BK, Ogra Y, Suzuki KT. Speciation of arsenic in human nail and hair from arsenic-affected area by HPLC-inductively coupled argon plasma mass spectrometry. Toxicol Appl Pharmacol 2003;189:73–83.
18. Robb DB, Covey TR, Bruins AP. Atmospheric pressure photoionization: an ionization method for liquid chromatography—mass spectrometry. Anal Chem 2000;72:3653–9.
19. Rockwood A, Palmblad M. Mass spectrometry data analysis in proteomics, 2nd edition. New York: Springer Science + Business Media; 2013.
20. Romijn EP, Krijgsveld J, Heck AJ. Recent liquid chromatographic-(tandem) mass spectrometric applications in proteomics. J Chromatogr A 2003;1000:589–608.
21. Schmedes A, Brandslund I. Analysis of methylmalonic acid in plasma by liquid chromatography-tandem mass spectrometry. Clin Chem 2006;52:754–7.
22. Tao WA, Aebersold R. Advances in quantitative proteomics via stable isotope tagging and mass spectrometry. Curr Opin Biotechnol 2003;14:110–8.
23. Todd J. Recommendations for nomenclature and symbolism for mass spectroscopy. Pure Appl Chem 1991;63:1541–66.
24. Wang Z, Dunlop K, Long SR, Li L. Mass spectrometric methods for generation of protein mass database used for bacterial identification. Anal Chem 2002;74:3174–82.
25. Whitehouse CM, Dreyer RN, Yamashita M, et al. Electrospray interface for liquid chromatographs and mass spectrometers. Anal Chem 1985;57:675–9.
26. Zoppa M, Gallo L, Zacchello F, et al. Method for the quantification of underivatized amino acids on dry blood spots from newborn screening by HPLC-ESI-MS/MS. J Chromatogr B Analyt Technol Biomed Life Sci 2006;831:267–73.

CHAPTER

14

Enzyme and Rate Analyses*

Renze Bais, Ph.D., F.F.Sc. (R.C.P.A.), and Mauro Panteghini, M.D.

Objectives

1. Define the following terms:

Activator	Inhibition (reversible/
Active site	irreversible/antibody)
Apoenzyme	International unit
Catalyst	Isoenzyme
Coenzyme	Isoform
Denaturation	Katal
Enzyme	K_m
First- and zero-order	Substrate
kinetics	V_{max}
Holoenzyme	

2. State how enzymes are classified in the IUB system.

3. List and describe the four components of enzyme structure.

4. Describe completely the active site of an enzyme, including the size of the site, the location within the enzyme structure, the binding involved between site and substrate, and the specificity of the site for the substrate.

5. Explain the genetic origins of isoenzymes, including the difference between the formation of allozymes and the formation of hybrid isoenzymes, isoenzyme tissue localization, and changes in isoenzyme distribution in relation to development and disease.

6. List six nongenetic changes that produce enzyme isoforms.

7. State how enzyme activity is described with international units and SI-derived units.

8. Describe the effects that the following factors have on an enzyme-catalyzed reaction:

Enzyme concentration	Reaction temperature
Substrate concentration	Inhibitors
in single- and two-	Activators
substrate reactions	Coenzymes
pH	

9. Compare first-order with zero-order enzyme reaction kinetics with regard to dependence on substrate or enzyme concentration and how the reaction rate and kinetics vary with time.

10. Express the Michaelis-Menten curve using an equation; describe each component of the equation, and draw and label a Michaelis-Menten curve.

11. Express how V_{max} is calculated using a reciprocal form of the Michaelis-Menten equation; draw and label a Lineweaver-Burk plot.

12. Describe a consecutive enzymatic reaction and its analytical use; state the need for the primary reaction in this assay to be rate limiting.

13. Compare competitive, noncompetitive, and uncompetitive inhibitors, including the effect on reaction velocity and the location of attachment to the enzyme; using a Lineweaver-Burk plot, illustrate how each of the three types affects enzymatic reaction rate.

14. Compare fixed-time and continuous-monitoring methods of enzyme reaction rate measurement, including advantages and limitations.

15. Describe the self-indicating reaction used for substrate measurement.

16. Define optimization and standardization of enzyme reaction rates, including how these are performed in the laboratory and issues associated with each.

17. List the uses and advantages of immunoassays to measure enzyme mass concentration.

18. Describe the following enzyme methods used to measure metabolites, give examples of enzymes used in this measurement, and state the limitations, if any, of each method:

Equilibrium method	Bisubstrate reaction
Kinetic method	Enzyme immunoassay
Two-point kinetic method	

19. Give an example of how an immobilized enzyme is used in measurement techniques such as potentiometry and polarography.

20. List and describe five analytical techniques used to measure isoenzymes or isoforms; state the principle of selective chemical inactivation.

*The authors gratefully acknowledge the original contributions by Drs. A. Ralph Henderson and Donald W. Moss, upon which portions of this chapter are based.

Key Words and Definitions

Activator Small molecule or ion that increases the rate of an enzyme-catalyzed reaction by promoting formation of the most active state of the enzyme or of other reactants such as the substrate.

Active center/Active site That part of an enzyme formed by the tertiary structure at which the noncovalent binding of substrate occurs to form the intermediate enzyme/substrate complex.

Biomarker In medicine, a biomarker is a biological compound that is used as an indicator of a particular disease state or some other physiological state of an organism.

Catalyst A substance that modifies and increases the rate of a chemical reaction without being permanently changed or consumed; an enzyme is a protein catalyst of biological origin.

Clinical enzymology The branch of medical science that deals with the biochemical nature and activity of enzymes of clinical relevance.

Coenzyme A small molecule (some contain structures derived from vitamins) that is required for some enzyme-catalyzed reactions to occur; is temporarily or permanently bound to the enzyme.

Enzyme A protein with catalytic properties.

First-order kinetics In an enzymatic reaction, as more substrate is consumed, the reaction rate declines and becomes dependent on substrate concentration; this is a phase of first-order dependence on substrate concentration when the rate of the reaction is proportional to the concentration of substrate or when the enzyme concentration is fixed and the substrate concentration is varied.

Inhibitor A substance that reduces the rate of an enzymatic reaction and is classified as reversible or irreversible.

International unit The quantity of enzyme that catalyzes one micromole of substrate per minute.

Isoenzyme A form of an enzyme that originates at the level of the gene that encodes the structure of the enzyme protein and that is distinguished by certain physical properties.

Isoform A form of an enzyme that is modified by post-translational processing.

Katal The quantity of an enzyme that catalyzes a reaction rate of one mole of substrate per second.

Lineweaver-Burk plot A plot of the reciprocal of the velocity of an enzyme catalyzed reaction (ordinate; y-axis) against the reciprocal of the substrate concentration (abscissa; x-axis).

Michaelis-Menten constant (K_m) A constant for a given enzyme acting under given conditions; the experimentally determined substrate concentration at which the enzymatic reaction velocity equals ½ of the maximum velocity of the enzymatic reaction.

Product The substance produced by the enzyme catalyzed conversion of a substrate

Substrate A reactant in an enzyme-catalyzed reaction that binds to the active center of an enzyme

Zero-order kinetics In an enzymatic reaction, when the reaction rate is constant at maximum value, the reaction rate depends only on enzyme concentration and is independent of substrate concentration; the rate of reaction is proportional to the zero power of the substrate concentration.

Enzymes are proteins with catalytic properties; **clinical enzymology** is the application of the science of enzymes to the diagnosis and treatment of disease. In medicine, a **biomarker** is a biological compound that is used as an indicator of a particular disease state or some other physiological state of an organism. As such, enzymes are the original clinical biomarkers.[28] The principles of clinical enzymology will be introduced and discussed in this chapter, as will information on how enzymes are measured and how they are used as analytical reagents in various types of rate analysis. Individual topics include (1) basic principles, (2) enzyme kinetics, (3) analytical enzymology, and (4) rate analyses.

Basic Principles

This section begins with a presentation of enzyme nomenclature, which is followed by a discussion of enzymes as proteins and **catalysts**.

Enzyme Nomenclature

Historically, individual enzymes were identified using the name of the substrate or group upon which they act and then adding the suffix -ase. For example, the enzyme hydrolyzing urea was ure*ase*. Later, the type of reaction involved was

also identified, as in (1) carbonic anhydrase, (2) D-amino acid oxidase, and (3) succinate dehydrogenase. In addition, some enzymes had been given empirical names such as trypsin.

Because this combination of trivial common names and semi-systematic names was found to be inadequate, in 1955 the International Union of Biochemistry (IUB) appointed an Enzyme Commission (EC) to study the problem of enzyme nomenclature. Its subsequent recommendations, with periodic updating, provide a rational and practical basis for identifying all enzymes now known and enzymes that will be discovered in the future (http://www.chem.qmw.ac.uk/iubmb/enzyme/; accessed August 6. 2013).[14]

With the IUB system, a systematic and trivial name is provided for each enzyme. The systematic name describes the nature of the reaction catalyzed and is associated with a unique numerical code. The trivial or practical name, which may be identical to the systematic name but is often a simplification of it, is suitable for everyday use. The unique numerical designation for each enzyme consists of four numbers, separated by periods (e.g., 2.2.8.11), and is prefixed by the letters *EC*, denoting *Enzyme Commission*. The first number defines the class to which the enzyme belongs. All enzymes are assigned to one of six classes, characterized by the type of reaction they catalyze: they are (1) oxidoreductases, (2) transferases, (3) hydrolases,

(4) lyases, (5) isomerases, and (6) ligases. The next two numbers indicate the subclass and the sub-subclass to which the enzyme is assigned. For example, these may differentiate the amino-transferring subclass from the phosphate-transferring category, or the ethanol acceptor sub-subclass from that accepting acyl groups. The last number is the specific serial number given to each enzyme within its sub-subclass.

Several readily accessible databases contain comprehensive lists of enzymes, their classification, and other information. These include BRENDA (http://www.brenda-enzymes.org/index.php4; accessed August 6, 2013), ExPASy (http://www.expasy.org/; accessed August 6, 2013), and ExplorEnz (http://www.enzyme-database.org/; accessed August 6, 2013). Table 14-1 lists some selected enzymes of clinical interest, identified by (1) trivial, (2) abbreviated, and (3) systematic names and (4) code numbers.

Although it is not recommended by the EC, it is a common and convenient practice to use capital letter abbreviations for the names of certain enzymes, such as ALT (formerly GPT) for alanine aminotransferase, AST for aspartate aminotransferase, LD for lactate dehydrogenase, and CK for creatine kinase (see Table 14-1).

Enzymes as Proteins

All enzyme molecules have (1) primary, (2) secondary, (3) tertiary, and (4) quaternary structures. The *primary* structure, the linear sequence of amino acids linked through their α-carboxyl and α-amino groups by peptide bonds, is specific for each type of enzyme molecule (see Chapter 18). *Secondary* structure refers to the conformation of limited segments of the polypeptide chain such as (1) α-helices, (2) β-pleated sheets, (3) random coils, and (4) β-turns. The arrangement of secondary structural elements and amino acid side chain interactions that defines the three-dimensional structure of the folded

protein is referred to as its *tertiary* structure. In many cases, biological activity, such as the catalytic activity of enzymes, requires two or more folded polypeptide chains (subunits) to associate to form a functional molecule. The arrangement of these subunits defines the *quaternary* structure. The subunits may be copies of the same polypeptide chain, or they may represent distinct polypeptides.

The application of physical methods, such as X-ray crystallography and multidimensional nuclear magnetic resonance (NMR), has provided structural insights upon which enzyme mechanisms have been built. Furthermore, the tools of molecular biology, such as molecular cloning, have enabled the purification and characterization of enzymes that previously were available only in minute amounts. Molecular biology also enables the (1) manipulation of the amino acid sequence of enzymes, (2) site-directed mutagenesis (substituting one amino acid residue for another) and (3) deletion mutagenesis (eliminating sections of the primary structure). This has enabled the identification of chemical groups that participate in ligand binding and in specific chemical steps during catalysis.

In general, no feature of primary structures, such as repetition of particular amino acid sequences, is common to all enzyme molecules. However, considerable homologies of sequence are found between enzymes that appear to share a common evolutionary origin, such as the proteases trypsin and chymotrypsin, and similarities of sequence are even more marked among the members of a family of isoenzymes. The amino acid sequence in the immediate neighborhood of the **active center** of the enzyme (discussed later) is often closely similar in enzymes of related function (e.g., the *serine proteases* are so called because all of them have this amino acid in the active center).

Enzyme molecules differ in the proportions of secondary structures they contain. Regarding tertiary structure, different

---

TABLE 14-1   Enzyme Commission (EC) Numbers, Systematic and Trivial Names, and Frequently Adopted Abbreviations of Enzymes of Major Clinical Importance

EC Number	Systematic Name	Trivial Name	Abbreviation
1.1.1.27	L-Lactate: NAD⁺ oxidoreductase	Lactate dehydrogenase	LD
1.1.1.49	D-Glucose-6-phosphate: NADP⁺ oxidoreductase	Glucose-6-phosphate dehydrogenase	
1.4.1.3	L-Glutamate: NAD(P)⁺ oxidoreductase (deaminating)	Glutamate dehydrogenase	GLD
2.3.2.2	(γ-Glutamyl)-peptide: amino acid γ-glutamyltransferase	γ-Glutamyltransferase	GGT
2.6.1.1	L-Aspartate: 2-oxoglutarate aminotransferase	Aspartate aminotransferase (transaminase)	AST
2.6.1.2	L-Alanine: 2-oxoglutarate aminotransferase	Alanine aminotransferase (transaminase)	ALT
2.7.3.2	ATP: creatine N-phosphotransferase	Creatine kinase	CK
3.1.1.3	Triacylglycerol acylhydrolase	Lipase	LPS
3.1.1.7	Acetylcholine acetylhydrolase	Acetylcholinesterase, true cholinesterase, choline esterase I	—
3.1.1.8	Acylcholine acylhydrolase	Pseudocholinesterase, butyryl cholinesterase, choline esterase II (serum cholinesterase)	CHE
3.1.3.1	Orthophosphoric-monoester phosphohydrolase (alkaline optimum)	Alkaline phosphatase	ALP
3.1.3.2	Orthophosphoric-monoester phosphohydrolase (acid optimum)	Acid phosphatase	ACP
3.1.3.5	5′-Ribonucleotide phosphohydrolase	5′-Nucleotidase	NTP
3.2.1.1	1,4-α-D-Glucan glucanohydrolase	Amylase	AMY
3.4.21.4		Trypsin	TRY
4.1.2.13	D-Fructose-1,6-bisphosphate D-glyceraldehyde-3-phosphate-lyase	Aldolase	ALD

types of enzyme molecules are as individually characteristic as their primary structures; however, some common features can be seen. For example, enzyme molecules are roughly globular in overall shape, with a preponderance of polar amino acid side chains on the outside of the molecule and nonpolar side chains in the interior. These ionizable residues in contact with the surrounding medium are responsible for many of the properties of the enzyme. In addition, covalent disulfide bridges link different parts of the polypeptide chains in some enzyme molecules. The biological activity of a protein molecule depends generally on the integrity of its structure, and any condition that changes the shape of the protein is generally accompanied by loss of activity through a process known as *denaturation*. If the process of denaturation is minimal, it may be reversed with the recovery of enzyme activity upon removal of the denaturing agent. However, prolonged or severe denaturing conditions typically results in irreversible loss of activity. Denaturing conditions include (1) elevated temperatures, (2) extremes of pH, (3) changes in ionic strength, and (4) chemical additions. Heat inactivation of most enzymes takes place at an appreciable rate at room temperature and in most cases becomes almost instantaneous above 60 °C. The polymerases are an exception; they retain activity at temperatures as high as 90 °C—a property that has been used in the polymerase chain reaction (see Chapter 48). Low temperatures are used to preserve enzyme activity, especially in aqueous solutions such as serum. Extremes of pH also cause unfolding of enzyme molecular structures and, except for a few exceptions, should be avoided when enzyme samples are preserved. Addition of chemicals, such as urea and detergents, disrupts hydrogen bonds and hydrophobic interactions so that exposure of enzymes to strong solutions of these reagents results in inactivation.

Specificity and the Active Center

With the exception of enzymes such as (1) proteases, (2) nucleases, (3) amylases and (4) polymersases which act on macromolecular substrates, enzyme molecules are considerably larger than the molecules of their substrates. Consideration of the structure of an enzyme's active site and of its relationship to the structures of the enzyme's substrate(s) in its ground and transition states is necessary to understand the rate enhancement and specificity of the chemical reactions performed by the enzyme. The active site of an enzyme will vary between enzymes, but some general conditions apply[5]:

1. The active site of an enzyme is relatively small compared with the total volume of the enzyme molecule because its structure may involve less than 5% of the total amino acids in the molecule.
2. Active sites of enzymes are three-dimensional structures that are formed as a result of the overall tertiary structure of the protein. This occurs when the amino acids and cofactors in the active site of an enzyme are spatially structured in an exact three-dimensional relationship with respect to one another and to the structure of the substrate molecule.
3. Typically, the attraction between the molecules of the enzyme and its substrate molecules is noncovalent binding.

Physical forces used in this type of binding include (1) hydrogen bonding, (2) electrostatic and hydrophobic interactions, and (3) van der Waals forces.

4. Active sites of enzymes typically are noted in clefts and crevices in the protein. This excludes bulk solvent and reduces the catalytic activity of the enzyme.
5. The specificity of substrate binding is a function of the exact special arrangement of atoms in the enzyme active site, which complements the structure of the substrate molecule.

Isoenzymes and Other Multiple Forms of Enzymes

An **isoenzyme** is defined as "one of a group of related enzymes catalyzing the same reaction but having different molecular structures and characterized by varying physical, biochemical, and immunologic properties." However, the IUB recommends that use of the term isoenzyme be restricted to forms that originate at the level of the genes that encode the structures of the enzyme proteins in question.[4]

Isoenzymes may occur within a single organ or even within a single type of cell. The forms are distinguished on the basis of differences in various physical properties, such as electrophoretic mobility and resistance to chemical or thermal inactivation. They often have significant quantifiable differences in catalytic properties, but all forms of a particular enzyme retain the ability to catalyze its characteristic reaction.

The existence of multiple forms of enzymes in human tissue has important implications in the study of human disease. Identifying the presence in different organs of isoenzymes with distinctive properties facilitates our understanding of organ-specific patterns of metabolism, but genetically determined variations in enzyme structure between individuals account for such characteristics as differences in sensitivity to drugs and differences in metabolism (see Chapter 48), which manifest as hereditary metabolic diseases. For diagnostic enzymology, the existence of multiple forms of enzymes, whether as the result of genetic or nongenetic causes, provides opportunities to increase the diagnostic specificity and sensitivity of enzyme assays in body fluid samples.

Similar to other proteins, enzymes usually elicit the production of antibodies when they are injected into animals of a species other than those in which they originate. Even small structural differences between closely similar molecules, such as the members of a family of isoenzymes, are often sufficient to render them antigenically distinct, allowing antibodies to be produced that are specific to a single type of molecule. The availability of enzyme-specific antisera is responsible for a wide range of methods in enzyme analysis, some of which—such as immunoassay—do not depend on the catalytic activity of the enzyme molecules. The availability of immunochemical methods has been particularly important in the analysis of isoenzyme mixtures. Many commercial immunoassays now use monoclonal antibodies to increase specificity.

Genetic Origins of Enzyme Variants

True isoenzymes result from the existence of more than one gene locus coding for the structure of the enzyme protein.

Many human enzymes (perhaps more than one-third) are known to be determined by more than one structural gene locus. Genes at different loci have undergone differential modifications during the course of evolution, so that enzyme proteins coded by them no longer have identical structures but are considered isoenzymes.

The multiple genes that determine a particular group of isoenzymes are not necessarily closely linked on one chromosome. For example, the structural genes that code for human salivary and pancreatic amylases are located on chromosome 1, whereas the genes that code for cytoplasmic and mitochondrial malate dehydrogenase are carried on chromosomes 2 and 7, respectively. Among the enzymes of clinical importance that exist as isoenzymes because of the presence of multiple-gene loci are lactate dehydrogenase, creatine kinase, α-amylase, and some forms of alkaline phosphatase.

Biochemically, some enzymes are present in molecular forms that differ from one individual to another because of the existence of alternative alleles that are inherited according to mendelian laws. These give rise to gene products with the same function, and isoenzymes that result from the existence of allelic genes are termed *allozymes*. The proportion of human gene loci subject to allelic variation is considerable, and the probability that individual human beings will differ to some degree in their isoenzyme patterns is correspondingly high.

The number of allelic variants and the frequency with which particular variants occur within the population vary considerably from one enzyme to another. For example, mutations at either of the two principal loci that determine human lactate dehydrogenase are extremely rare, but a high incidence of mutant alleles occurs at the single locus that determines the structure of placental alkaline phosphatase. More than 400 mutations in the glucose-6-phosphate dehydrogenase gene have now been identified on the X chromosome (up-to-date genetic information on this and other enzymes is available from the Online Mendelian Inheritance in Man [OMIM] database at http://www.ncbi.nlm.nih.gov/Omim/; accessed August 6, 2013). Some of these alleles are extremely rare, whereas others occur with appreciable frequency in particular populations or geographical locations. When isoenzymes, because of variation at a single locus, occur with appreciable frequency in a human population, the population is said to be *polymorphic* with respect to the isoenzymes in question.

Another category of multiple molecular forms arises when enzymes are oligomeric and consists of molecules made up of subunits. The association of different types of subunits in various combinations gives rise to a range of active enzyme molecules. When the subunits are derived from different structural genes—multiple loci or multiple alleles—the hybrid molecules so formed are called *hybrid isoenzymes*. The ability to form hybrid isoenzymes is evidence of considerable structural similarities between the different subunits. Hybrid isoenzymes are formed in vitro, but they are also formed in vivo in cells in which different types of constituent subunits are present in the same subcellular compartment.

The number of different hybrid isoenzymes that are formed from two nonidentical protomers depends on the number

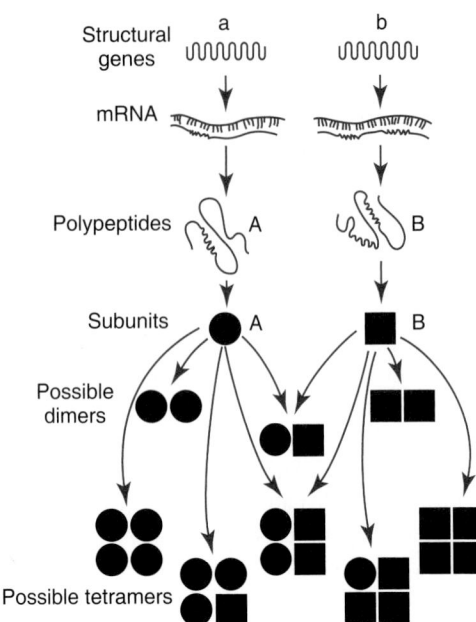

Figure 14-1 Diagram showing the origin of isoenzymes, assuming the existence of two distinct gene loci. When the active enzymes are polymers that contain more than one subunit, hybrid isoenzymes consisting of mixtures of different subunits may be formed. One such isoenzyme can be formed in the case of a dimeric enzyme, such as creatine kinase, and three if the enzyme is a tetramer (e.g., lactate dehydrogenase). In both cases, two homopolymeric isoenzymes can also exist. *(From Moss DW. Isoenzyme analysis. London: The Chemical Society, 1979. Reprinted by permission of The Royal Society of Chemistry.)*

of subunits in the complete enzyme molecule. For a dimeric enzyme, one mixed dimer (hybrid isoenzyme) is formed. If the enzyme is a tetramer, three heteropolymeric isoenzymes may be formed (Figure 14-1). Examples of hybrid isoenzymes include the mixed MB dimer of creatine kinase and the three hybrid isoenzymes—LD-2, LD-3, and LD-4—of lactate dehydrogenase.

Nongenetic Causes of Multiple Forms of Enzymes

Post-translational modifications of enzyme molecules give rise to multiple forms known as **isoforms** (Figure 14-2). For example, serum isoforms of creatine kinase are formed as part of the normal clearance process of the cell. Human myocardial and skeletal muscle tissues have the CK-MM and CK-MB isoenzymes, which are modified upon release into the circulation. This modification is due to sequential removal of the C-terminal amino acid, lysine, by the action of carboxypeptidase (see Chapter 19 for additional details).

Modifications that affect nonprotein components of enzyme molecules may lead to molecular heterogeneity. Many enzymes are glycoproteins, and variations in carbohydrate side chains are a common cause of nonhomogeneity of preparations of these enzymes. Some carbohydrate moieties, notably *N*-acetylneuraminic acid (sialic acid), are strongly ionized and consequently have a profound effect on some properties of enzyme molecules. For example, removal of terminal sialic

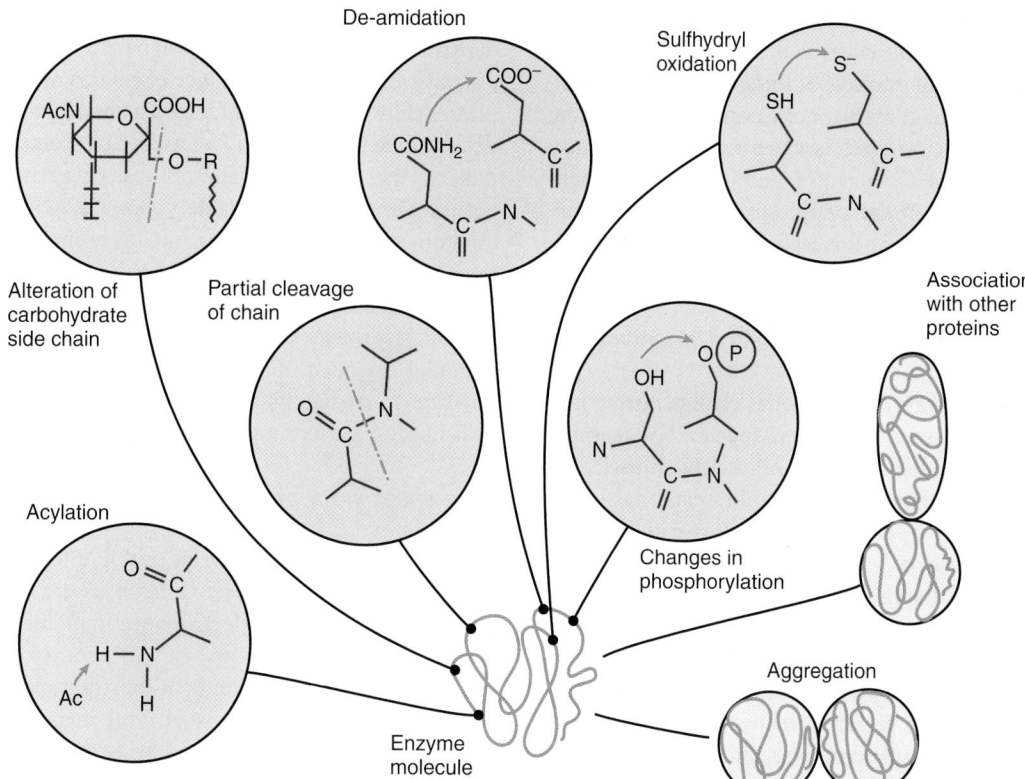

Figure 14-2 Nongenetic modifications that may give rise to multiple forms of enzymes. *(From Moss DW. Isoenzymes. London: Chapman & Hall, 1982.)*

acid groups from human liver and/or bone alkaline phosphatase with neuraminidase greatly reduces the electrophoretic heterogeneity of the enzyme.

Aggregation of enzyme molecules with each other or with nonenzymatic proteins may give rise to multiple forms that are separated by techniques that depend on differences in molecular size. For example, four catalytically active cholinesterase components with molecular weights ranging from about 80,000 to 340,000 are found in most sera, with the heaviest component, C_4, contributing most of the enzyme activity. Other enzyme forms are also occasionally present, but it appears that the principal serum cholinesterase fraction is attributed to different states of aggregation of a single monomer.

A specific form of interaction between enzymatic and nonenzymatic proteins is the cause of unusual enzyme components noted when some samples of human plasma are fractionated by electrophoresis or chromatography. These components are the result of the combination of apparently normal enzyme or isoenzyme molecules with plasma immunoglobulins. The enzyme/protein complexes *(macrocomplexes)* thus formed may themselves be heterogeneous. Since the identification of *macroamylase,* the first such enzyme/immunoglobulin complex to be identified, similar complexes have been observed involving (1) lactate dehydrogenase, (2) creatine kinase, (3) alkaline phosphatase, and (4) other enzymes.

A single polypeptide chain in theory exists in an infinite number of different conformations. However, one specific conformation generally appears to be the most stable for any given sequence of amino acids, and this conformation is assumed by the chain as it is synthesized within the cell. Thus, the primary structure of the polypeptide chain also determines its three-dimensional secondary and tertiary structures. It is conceivable that in some cases, several alternative conformations ("conformers") of a single chain that are almost equally stable may be present, and therefore these alternative forms may coexist. This possibility was first suggested to account for the heterogeneity noted in preparations of cytoplasmic and mitochondrial isoenzymes of malate dehydrogenase and has also been proposed as an explanation for the multiple electrophoretic zones of erythrocyte acid phosphatase. However, no multiple-enzyme forms have been shown unequivocally to be due to conformational isomerism.

Distribution of Isoenzymes and Other Multiple Forms of Enzymes

The existence of multiple-gene loci and the isoenzymes derived from them has presumably conferred an evolutionary advantage on the species and has thus become part of its normal metabolic pattern. Some of these adaptations are related to the division of function between and within different types of specialized cells and tissues. Thus, the distribution of isoenzymes is not uniform throughout the body, and wide variations in the activities of different isoenzymes are found at the organ, cellular, and subcellular levels. Tissue-specific differences are also found in the distributions of some multiple forms of enzymes that are not due to the existence of multiple-gene loci. The tissue-specific distribution of isoenzymes and other multiple forms of enzymes serves as the basis for organ-specific diagnosis through isoenzyme measurements.

A particularly striking example of local expression of multiple-gene loci is provided by distinct isoenzymes that occur exclusively in specific subcellular organelles. Differences between mitochondrial isoenzymes and their functionally analogous counterparts in the cytoplasm have been demonstrated in several cases (e.g., for aspartate aminotransferase and malate dehydrogenase).

Changes in Isoenzyme Distribution During Development and Disease

The patterns of several sets of isoenzymes change during normal development in tissues from many species. For example, during the embryonic development of skeletal muscle, the proportions of the electrophoretically more cathodal isoenzymes—both LD and CK—progressively increase in this tissue until approximately the sixth month of intrauterine life, when the pattern resembles that of differentiated muscle.

The liver also shows characteristic changes in the patterns of several isoenzymes during embryogenesis. In early fetal development, three aldolase isoenzymes—A, B, and C— together with various hybrid tetramers, are detected in extracts of liver. However, at birth, as in the adult liver, aldolase B is the predominant isoenzyme. Striking changes in the distribution of isoenzymes of alcohol dehydrogenase also occur in human liver during prenatal development.

Changes in isoenzyme patterns during development result from changes in the relative activities of gene loci within developing cells of a particular type (e.g., muscle cells). Other alterations in the balance of isoenzymes within the whole organism may derive from changes in the number or activity of cells that contain large amounts of a characteristic isoenzyme. An example of this is the increased number and activity of the osteoblasts, which are responsible for mineralization of the skeleton between the early postnatal period and the beginning of the third decade of life. An excess of ALP from active osteoblasts enters the circulation, where its presence is recognized by its characteristic properties, and where it elevates the total serum ALP activity of young people to above that of skeletally mature adults. ALP from the liver also contributes to the total activity of this enzyme in the plasma of healthy people, and the amount of this isoenzyme in plasma shows a small, progressive increase with age. The reason for the latter age-dependent change is not known, but it may result from increased synthesis of the isoenzyme by hepatocytes in response to continuing exposure to inducing factors.

Certain diseases, such as the progressive muscular dystrophies, appear to involve failure of the affected tissues to mature normally or to maintain a normal state. Cancer cells show progressive loss of the structure and metabolism of the healthy cells from which they arise. Therefore, the pattern of isoenzymes of mature, differentiated tissue may be lost or modified if normal differentiation is arrested or reversed, and many examples of isoenzyme changes accompanying such processes have been reported.

Reemergence of fetal patterns of isoenzyme distribution is a feature of malignant transformation in many tissues. This phenomenon was first studied extensively in the case of lactate dehydrogenase isoenzymes. Malignant tumors in general show a significant shift in the balance of isoenzymes toward electrophoretically more cathodal forms such as LD-4 and LD-5. The decline in activity of the LD-1 and LD-2 isoenzymes results in patterns that are reminiscent of those occurring in embryonic tissues. Tumors of (1) prostate, (2) cervix, (3) breast, (4) brain, (5) stomach, (6) colon, (7) rectum, (8) bronchus, and (9) lymph nodes are among those that show this transformation. In contrast, comparatively benign gliomas show a relative increase in anionic isoenzymes. A relative increase in the proportion of cathodal isoenzymes of LD has also been observed in tissue adjacent to malignant tumors (e.g., the colon), although the cells in these regions are morphologically normal.

Differences in Properties Between Multiple Forms of Enzymes

Structural differences between multiple forms of an enzyme give rise to greater or lesser differences in (1) physicochemical properties, such as electrophoretic mobility, resistance to inactivation, and solubility, or (2) catalytic characteristics, such as the ratio of reaction with substrate analogs or response to **inhibitors**. Methods of isoenzyme analysis have therefore been designed to investigate a wide range of catalytic and structural properties of enzyme molecules.[12,27]

Techniques of molecular biology, such as gene cloning and sequencing, have revolutionized the investigation of the primary structures of isoenzymes. Differences in primary structures between isoenzymes, whether derived from multiple-gene loci or from different alleles, are now known to exist in a growing number of cases. Furthermore, many questions have been answered about whether multiple-enzyme forms represented true (genetically determined) isoenzymes or arose from post-translational modification.

Isoenzymes caused by the existence of multiple-gene loci usually differ quantitatively in catalytic properties. These differences may be manifested in such characteristics as (1) molecular activity, (2) *Km* values for substrates, (3) sensitivity to various inhibitors, and (4) relative rates of activity with substrate analogs underscoring the biological importance of isoenzymatic variation. In contrast, multiple-enzyme forms that arise by such post-translational modifications as aggregation usually have similar catalytic properties.

Multilocus isoenzymes usually differ in terms of antigenic specificity, although these differences may be less pronounced among isoenzymes that have emerged relatively recently in evolutionary history and are still closely related in structure. Immunological cross-reaction is not uncommon among multilocus isoenzymes. Multiple-enzyme forms caused by post-synthetic modification frequently have common antigenic determinants. Isoenzymes derived from allelic genes (allozymes) are often antigenically similar, even to the extent that they may cross-react with antisera to the common isoenzyme even when a mutation has abolished enzyme activity altogether. The capacity for detecting differences between antigenically similar isoenzyme molecules depends on the extent of monoclonal antibody specificity.

Differences in resistance to denaturation by treatment with (1) heat, (2) concentrated urea solutions, and (3) detergents are commonly found between true isoenzymes, whether these are the products of multiple loci or multiple alleles. Other multiple forms of enzymes often do not differ or differ only slightly in this respect. The most commonly exploited difference between isoenzymes is the difference in net molecular charge that results from altered amino acid compositions of the molecules; this forms the basis of separation by (1) zone electrophoresis, (2) ion-exchange chromatography, and (3) isoelectric focusing. Separation methods that depend on differences in molecular size, such as gel filtration, do not distinguish between the small size differences that often exist between true isoenzyme molecules but are important in the detection of multiple forms that involve aggregation or association of enzyme molecules with other proteins.

Enzymes as Catalysts

A catalyst is a substance that modifies and increases the rate of a particular chemical reaction without being consumed or permanently altered. Enzymes are protein catalysts of biological origin. Metabolism is a coordinated series of chemical reactions that occur within a living cell to provide energy and accomplish biosynthesis. The process is regarded as an integrated series of enzymatic reactions and some diseases as a derangement of the normal pattern of metabolism. Apart from these fundamental considerations, it is the remarkable properties of enzymes that make them such sensitive indicators of pathological change.

Because of their catalytic activity, a given number of enzyme molecules convert an enormous number of substrate molecules to products within a short time. This property is used to measure changes in quantities of enzymes in the bloodstream, although the amount of enzyme protein released from damaged cells is small compared with the total quantity of nonenzymatic proteins in blood. Thus a change in the quantity of a particular enzyme is recognized by its characteristic effect on a given chemical reaction.

Units for Expressing Enzyme Activity

When enzymes are measured by their catalytic activities, the results of such determinations are expressed in terms of the concentration of the number of activity units present in a convenient volume or mass of specimen. The unit of activity is the measure of the rate at which the reaction proceeds (e.g., the quantity of **substrate** consumed or **product** formed in a chosen unit of time). In clinical enzymology, the activity of an enzyme is generally reported in terms of unit of volume, such as activity per 100 mL or per liter of serum or per 1.0 mL of packed erythrocytes. Because the rate of the reaction depends on experimental parameters, such as (1) pH, (2) type of buffer, (3) temperature, (4) nature of substrate, (5) ionic strength, (6) concentration of **activators**, and (7) other variables, these parameters must be specified in the definition of the unit.

To standardize how enzyme activities are expressed, the EC proposed that the unit of enzyme activity should be defined as the quantity of enzyme that catalyzes the reaction of 1 μmol

of substrate per minute, and that this unit should be termed the **international unit** (U). Catalytic concentration is to be expressed in terms of U/L or kU/L, whichever gives the more convenient numerical value. In this chapter, the symbol U is used to denote the international unit. In those instances in which some uncertainty exists as to the exact nature of the substrate, or when difficulty is encountered in calculating the number of micromoles that are reacting (as with macromolecules such as starch, protein, and complex lipids), the unit is expressed in terms of the chemical group or residue measured in the following reaction (e.g., glucose units, amino acid units formed).

The International System of Units (SI)-derived unit for catalytic activity is the **katal**, defined as moles converted per second. The name *katal* became the official SI-derived unit in 1999, with Resolution 12 of the 21st French Conférence Général des Poids et Mesures (CGPM), on the recommendation of the International Federation of Clinical Chemistry and Laboratory Medicine (IFCC). Both the International Union of Pure and Applied Chemistry (IUPAC) and the IUB now recommend that enzyme activity be expressed in moles per second, and that the enzyme concentration be expressed in terms of katals per liter (kat/L).[9] Thus, 1 U = 10^{-6} mol/60 s = 16.7 × 10^{-9} mol/s, or 1.0 nkat/L = 0.06 U/L.

Enzyme Kinetics

The Enzyme/Substrate Complex

Enzymes act through the formation of an enzyme/substrate (*ES*) complex, in which a molecule of substrate is bound to the *active center* of the enzyme molecule. The binding process transforms the substrate molecule to its activated state, with the energy required for this transformation provided by the free energy of binding of *S* to *E*. Therefore, activation takes place without the addition of external energy, so that the energy barrier to the reaction is lowered and the breakdown to products is accelerated (Figure 14-3). The ES complex breaks down to give the reaction products *(P)* and the free enzyme *(E)*:

$$E + S \rightleftharpoons ES \rightarrow P + E \qquad (1)$$

All reactions catalyzed by enzymes are in theory reversible. However, in practice, the reaction is usually found to be more rapid in one direction than in another, so that an equilibrium is reached in which the product of the forward or the backward reaction predominates, sometimes so markedly that the reaction is virtually irreversible.

If the product of the reaction in one direction is removed as it is formed (e.g., because it is the substrate of a second enzyme present in the reaction mixture), the equilibrium of the first enzymatic process will be displaced, so that the reaction will proceed to completion in that direction. Reaction sequences in which the product of one enzyme-catalyzed reaction becomes the substrate of the next enzyme and so on, often through many stages, are characteristic of biological processes. In the laboratory also, several enzymatic reactions may be linked

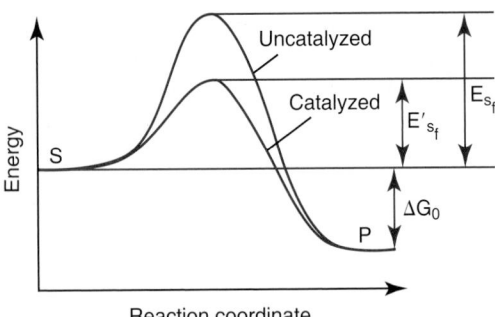

Figure 14-3 Activation energy barrier and reaction course, with and without enzyme catalysis. E_{Sf} is the activation energy for the forward reaction (S → P) in the absence of a catalyst, and E'_{Sf} is the activation energy in the presence of a catalyst. ΔG_0 is the change in free energy for the reaction.

together to provide a means of measuring the activity of the first enzyme or the concentration of the initial substrate in the chain. For example, the activity of CK is usually measured by a series of linked reactions, and the concentration of glucose is determined by consecutive reactions catalyzed by hexokinase and glucose-6-phosphate dehydrogenase.

When a secondary enzyme-catalyzed reaction, known as an *indicator reaction,* is used to determine the activity of a different enzyme, the primary reaction catalyzed by the enzyme to be determined must be the rate-limiting step. Conditions are chosen to ensure that the rate of reaction catalyzed by the indicator enzyme is directly proportional to the rate of product formation in the first reaction.

Factors Governing the Rate of Enzyme-Catalyzed Reactions

Factors that affect the rate of enzyme-catalyzed reactions include enzyme and substrate concentration, pH, temperature, and the presence of inhibitors, activators, coenzymes, and prosthetic groups.

Enzyme Concentration

The simplest enzymatically catalyzed reaction for converting substrate S into product P with the intermediate formation of an ES complex is as follows:

$$E_f + S \underset{k_{-1}}{\overset{k_1}{\rightleftharpoons}} ES \xrightarrow{k_2} E_f + P \qquad (2)$$

where

E_f = free enzyme;
k_1 = rate constant for the association of the complex;
k_1 = rate constant for the dissociation of the complex;
ES = enzyme/substrate complex;
k_2 = rate constant for breakdown of ES to E_f and P; and
P = product.

Michaelis and Menten assumed that equilibrium is attained rapidly among E, S, and ES, with the effect of product formation (ES → P) on the concentration of ES being negligible. In addition, the formation of product is written as an irreversible process because no product is present in the solution

under initial conditions. Therefore the overall rate of the reaction under otherwise constant conditions is proportional to the concentration of the ES complex.

Provided that an excess of free substrate molecules is present, addition of more enzyme molecules to the reaction system increases the concentration of the ES complex and thus the overall rate of reaction. This accounts for the observation that the rate of reaction is generally proportional to the amount of enzyme present in the system and is the basis for the quantitative determination of enzymes by measurement of reaction rates. Reaction conditions are selected to ensure that the observed reaction rate (enzyme activity) is proportional to enzyme concentration over as wide a range as possible.

Substrate Concentration

In addition to explaining the dependence of reaction rate on enzyme concentration under conditions in which excess substrate is present, the formation of an ES complex accounts for the hyperbolic relationship between reaction velocity and substrate concentration (Figure 14-4, *A*).

Single-Substrate Reactions

If the enzyme concentration is held constant and the substrate concentration varied, the rate of reaction is almost directly proportional to the substrate concentration at low values of the latter. Under these conditions the rate of the reaction is proportional and dependent on the substrate concentration, a situation termed **first order**. At low concentrations of substrate, only a fraction of the enzyme is associated with substrate, and the rate observed reflects the low concentration of the *ES* complex. At high substrate concentrations, the reaction rate is known as **zero order** and is independent of substrate concentration. With a zero-order reaction, the entire enzyme is bound to substrate, and a much higher rate of reaction is obtained. Moreover, because the entire enzyme is present in the form of the complex, no further increase in complex concentration and no further increment in reaction rate are possible. The maximum possible velocity for the reaction has been reached.

The significance of substrate rate curves was first emphasized by Michaelis and Menten, and such curves are referred to as Michaelis-Menten plots. A typical Michaelis-Menten curve (Figure 14-4, *A,* is described by the equation[*]

$$v = \frac{V_{max}[S]}{K_m + [S]} \qquad (3)$$

where V_{max} is the velocity that the observed value of the velocity (v) approaches at high values of substrate ([S]). It increases with increasing enzyme concentration. K_m, the Michaelis-Menten constant, is the substrate concentration at which $v = V_{max}/2$, and it is a constant for a given enzyme acting

---

[*]A derivation of this equation is found in Bais R, Panteghini M. Principles of clinical enzymology. In: Burtis CA, Ashwood ER, Bruns DE, eds, Tietz textbook of clinical chemistry and molecular diagnostics. 5th ed. St Louis: Saunders, 2012:355-77.

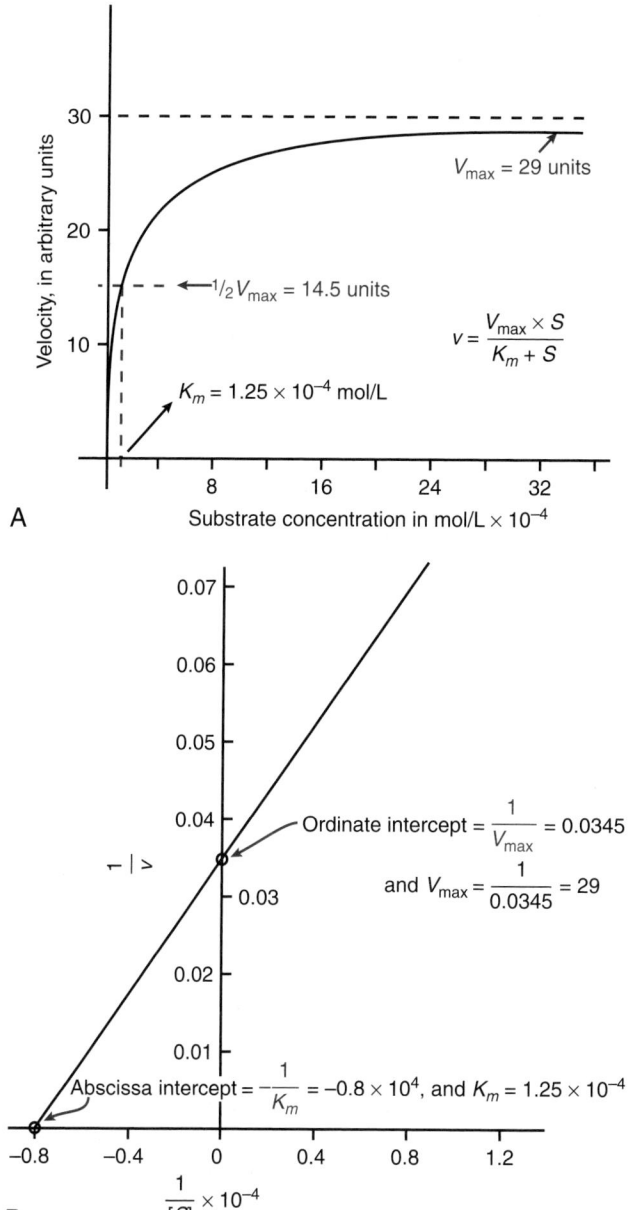

Figure 14-4 A, Michaelis-Menten curve relating the velocity (rate) of an enzyme-catalyzed reaction to substrate concentration. The value of K_m is given by the substrate concentration at which one-half of the maximum velocity is obtained. **B,** Lineweaver-Burk transformation of the curve in **(A)**, with $1/v$ plotted on the ordinate (y-axis), and $1/[S]$ on the abscissa (x-axis). The indicated intercepts permit calculation of V_{max} and K_m.

substrate, so the calculated value of V_{max} cannot be achieved in practice. In the past it was common practice to transform the **Michaelis-Menten equation** (2) into one of several reciprocal forms, and either $1/v$ was plotted against $1/[S]$, or $[S]/v$ was plotted against $[S]$.

$$\frac{1}{v} = \left(\frac{K_m}{V_{max}} \times \frac{1}{[S]} \right) + \frac{1}{V_{max}} \qquad (4)$$

This equation, when plotted, gives a straight line, with intercepts at $1/V_{max}$ on the ordinate and $-1/K_m$ on the abscissa. The graph on which the plots are made is known as the **Lineweaver-Burk plot** (Figure 14-4, *B*).

It is now routine practice to determine kinetic constants such as K_m and V_{max} using a software package. A large number of such packages are available; however, these vary from specialized routines for kinetic simulations or for data fitting to general mathematical, statistical, or graphical packages. These packages are free (public domain, shareware, or free license) or are commercially available. An example of the free software is the ENCORA 1.2 freeware package available from R.J.W. Slats and colleagues at the Delft University of Technology (http://www.tnw.tudelft.nl/en/about-faculty/departments/biotechnology/research/download-centre/encora/; accessed August 8, 2013), which was developed for an enzymatic kinetic parameter fitting using progressive curve analysis. DynaFit is an example of a commercially available routine (http://www.biokin.com/dynafit/; accessed August 8, 2013) that performs nonlinear least-squares regression of chemical kinetic, enzyme kinetic, or ligand receptor binding data. The data can be initial reaction velocities for different concentrations of varied species (e.g., inhibitor concentration vs. velocity), or reaction progress curves (e.g., time vs. absorbance). SigmaPlot 11 is another example of commercially available software that will compute and plot enzyme kinetic data (http://www.sigmaplot.com/products/sigmaplot/enzyme-mod.php/; accessed August 8, 2013).

When setting up methods of enzyme assay, it is necessary to (1) explore the relationship between reaction velocity and substrate concentration over a wide range, (2) determine K_m, and (3) detect any inhibition at high substrate concentrations. Zero-order kinetics is maintained if the substrate is present in large excess (i.e., concentrations of at least 10 and preferably 100 times that of the value of K_m). When $[S] = 10 \times K_m$, v is approximately 91% of the theoretical V_{max}. The K_m values for most enzymes are on the order of 10^{-5} to 10^{-3} mol/L; therefore substrate concentrations are usually chosen to be in the range of 0.001 to 0.10 mol/L. On occasion, the optimal concentrations of substrate cannot be used (e.g., when the substrate has limited solubility, when the concentration of a given substrate inhibits the activity of another enzyme needed in a coupled reaction system).

Two-Substrate Reactions

Most enzymes catalyze reactions with two or more interacting substrates symbolized by the following equation:

$$\text{Substrate 1} + \text{Substrate 2} \overset{E}{\rightleftarrows} \text{Product 1} + \text{Product 2} \qquad (5)$$
$$\quad S_1 \qquad\qquad S_2 \qquad\qquad\quad P_1 \qquad\qquad P_2$$

under given conditions. If an equilibrium is set up between enzyme and substrate, K_m is the equilibrium constant of this reaction. However, the symbol K_S (substrate constant) is used if this meaning is intended, and K_m is reserved for the experimentally determined value of $[S]$ at which at which the reaction proceeds at one half of its maximum velocity ($v = V_{max}/2$).

Although it is straightforward to set up an experiment to determine the variation of v with $[S]$, the exact value of V_{max} is not easily determined from hyperbolic curves. Furthermore, many enzymes deviate from ideal behavior at high substrate concentrations and indeed may be inhibited by excess

Among the bisubstrate reactions important in clinical enzymology are the reactions catalyzed by dehydrogenases—in which the second substrate is a specific coenzyme, such as reduced nicotinamide-adenine dinucleotide (NADH) or reduced NAD phosphate (NADPH)—or by aminotransferases. The concentrations of both substrates affect the rates of two-substrate reactions. Values of K_m and V_{max} for each substrate are derived from experiments in which the concentration of the first substrate is held at saturating levels while the concentration of the second substrate is varied, and vice versa.

In practice, the choice of substrate concentrations is limited by such considerations as the solubility of the substrates, the viscosity and high initial absorbance of concentrated solutions, and the relative costs of the reagents. Furthermore, the selection of appropriate substrate concentrations is only one of the factors to be considered in formulating an optimal assay system for the measurement of activity of a specific enzyme. Critical choices must also be made with respect to other, frequently interdependent factors that affect reaction rate, such as the concentrations of activators and the nature and pH of the buffer system. The traditional empirical approach to optimization has been replaced by newer techniques of simplex co-optimization and response surface methodology.[16] As an example, this technique has been used to determine optimal conditions for the IFCC-recommended method for amylase.[18]

Consecutive Enzymatic Reactions

As discussed previously, an enzymatic reaction is usually found to be more rapid in one direction than in the other, so that the reaction is virtually irreversible. If the product of the reaction in one direction is removed as it is formed, the equilibrium of the first enzymatic process is displaced, so that the reaction may continue to completion in that direction. Reaction sequences in which the product of one enzyme-catalyzed reaction becomes the substrate of another enzyme, often through many stages, are characteristic of metabolic processes. Analytically, several enzymatic reactions also may be linked together to provide a means of measuring the activity of the first enzyme or the concentration of the initial substrate in the chain. For example, the activity of creatine kinase is usually measured by a series of linked reactions, and glucose can be determined by consecutive reactions catalyzed by hexokinase and glucose-6-phosphate dehydrogenase.

When a linked enzyme assay, known as an *indicator reaction*, is used to determine the activity of a different enzyme, it is essential that the primary reaction be the rate-limiting step. For example, in the determination of aspartate aminotransferase activity, the indicator reaction is the reduction of the oxaloacetate formed in the aminotransferase reaction to malate by malate dehydrogenase and NADH. The activity of the indicator enzyme must be sufficient to ensure the virtually instantaneous removal of the product of the first reaction, to prevent significant reversal of the first reaction. The measured enzyme is typically acting under conditions of saturation with respect to its substrate; however, the concentration of the substrate of the indicator enzyme (i.e., the product of the first reaction) remains in the region of the Michaelis-Menten curve in which

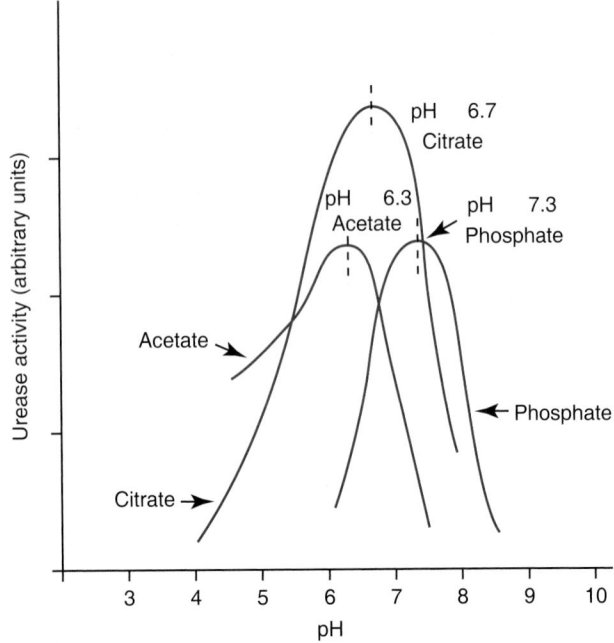

Figure 14-5 The pH activity curves for urease show the effects of buffer species on pH optimum. *(Modified from Howell SF, Sumner JB. The specific effects of buffers upon urease activity, J Biol Chem 1934;104:619.)*

v is directly proportional to [S]. Therefore the rate of reaction catalyzed by the indicator enzyme is directly proportional to the rate of product formation in the first reaction.

During a lag period that occurs after the start of the first reaction, the concentration of its product reaches a steady state. Because the rate of the second reaction depends on the activity of the indicator enzyme and on the concentration of its substrate (the product of the primary reaction), the duration of the lag period is reduced by increasing the concentration of the indicator enzyme, thus lowering the steady state concentration of the product of the primary reaction.

Effect of pH

The rate of enzyme-catalyzed reactions typically shows marked dependence on pH (Figure 14-5). Many of the enzymes in blood plasma show maximum activity in vitro in the pH range from 7 to 8. However, activity has been observed at pH values as low as 1.5 (pepsin) and as high as 10.5 (ALP). The optimal pH for a given forward reaction may be different from the optimal pH for the corresponding reverse reaction. The form of the pH dependence curve is the result of a number of separate effects, including ionization of the substrate and the extent of dissociation of certain key amino acid side chains in the protein molecule, both at the active center and elsewhere in the molecule. Both pH and ionic environment will also have an effect on the three-dimensional conformation of the protein and therefore on enzyme activity to such an extent that enzymes may be irreversibly denatured at extreme values of pH.

The pronounced effects of pH on enzyme reactions emphasize the need to control this variable by means of adequate buffer solutions. Enzyme assays should be carried out at the pH of optimal activity. In addition, the buffer system must be capable of counteracting the effect of adding the specimen (e.g., serum itself is a powerful buffer) to the assay system, as well as the effects of acids or bases formed during the reaction. Because buffers have their maximum buffering capacity close to their pK_a values, whenever possible a buffer system should be chosen with a pK_a value within 1 pH unit of the desired pH of the assay. Interaction between buffer ions and other components of the assay system (e.g., activating metal ions) may eliminate certain buffers from consideration.

Temperature

The rate of an enzymatic reaction is proportional to its reaction temperature. However, an increase in the rate of the catalyzed reaction is not the only effect of increasing temperature on an enzymatic reaction. In theory, the initial rate of reaction measured instantaneously will increase with rising temperature. In practice, however, a finite time is needed to allow the components of the reaction mixture, including the enzyme solution, to reach temperature equilibrium and to permit the formation of a measurable amount of the product. During this period, the enzyme is undergoing thermal inactivation and denaturation—a process that has a very large temperature coefficient for most enzymes and thus becomes virtually instantaneous at temperatures of 60 °C to 70 °C. The counteracting effects of the increased rate of the catalyzed reaction and more rapid enzyme inactivation as the temperature increases account for the existence of an apparent *optimal temperature* for enzyme activity (Figure 14-6).

As stated earlier, at some critical temperature, an enzyme will undergo thermal inactivation influenced by a number of factors. These include (1) presence of substrate and its concentration, (2) pH, and (3) nature and ionic strength of the buffer. In general, storage of serum samples at low temperatures is necessary to minimize loss of enzyme activity while awaiting analysis, although repeated freezing and thawing should be avoided. However, individual enzymes vary in their stability characteristics, and appropriate storage conditions vary correspondingly. Amylase, for example, is stable at room temperature (22 °C to 25 °C) for 24 hours, whereas acid phosphatase is exceedingly unstable, even when refrigerated, unless kept at a pH below 6.0. ALP exhibits an unusual property: the tendency for the activity of frozen, partially purified preparations of the enzyme to increase after thawing over a period of 24 hours or longer. This effect is shared by reconstituted, lyophilized preparations of the enzyme and affects their use for quality control purposes. A few enzymes are inactivated at refrigerator temperatures; an example is the liver-type isoenzyme of lactate dehydrogenase, LD-5, which appears to be less stable at lower temperatures. As a result, sera for lactate dehydrogenase determinations should be kept at room temperature and should not be refrigerated.

Historically, the choice of temperature for the assay of enzymes of clinical importance was the subject of extensive debate. However, 37 °C is now the accepted measuring temperature for enzymes in the clinical laboratory. Reference methods for several clinically relevant enzymes have been developed at 37 °C.[14-26] In practice, accurate temperature

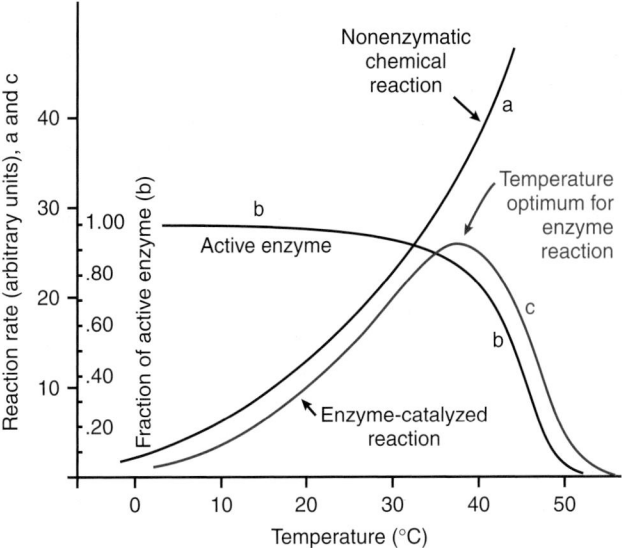

Figure 14-6 Schematic diagram showing effects of temperature on rates of non–enzyme-catalyzed and enzyme-catalyzed reactions.

control to within ±0.1 °C during the enzymatic reaction is essential.

Inhibitors and Activators

The rates of enzymatic reactions are often affected by substances other than the enzyme or the substrate. These modifiers may be inhibitors because their presence reduces the reaction rate, or they may be activators because they increase the rate of reaction. Activators and inhibitors are usually small molecules (compared with the enzyme itself) or even ions. They vary in specificity, ranging from modifiers that exert similar effects on a wide range of different enzymatic reactions at one extreme to substances that affect only a single reaction. Reagents, such as strong acids or multivalent anions and cations that denature or precipitate proteins, destroy enzyme activity and thus may be regarded as extreme examples of nonspecific enzyme inhibitors. These effects usually are not included in discussions of enzyme inhibition, although they have obvious practical implications in the treatment and storage of specimens in which enzyme activity is to be measured. The activity of some enzymes depends on the presence of particular chemical groups, such as reduced sulfhydryl (–SH) groups, in the active center. Reagents that alter these groups (e.g., oxidants of SH groups) therefore act as general inhibitors of such enzymes.

Some phenomena of enzyme activation or inhibition are caused by interactions between the modifier and a nonenzymatic component of the reaction system, such as the substrate (e.g., Mg^{2+} combining with ATP to form MgATP, the required substrate for the creatine kinase reaction). In most cases, however, the modifier combines with the enzyme itself in a manner analogous to the combination of enzyme and substrate.

Inhibition of Enzyme Activity

Inhibitors are classified as reversible or irreversible.

Reversible Inhibition. Reversible inhibition is characterized by the existence of equilibrium between enzyme, E, and inhibitor, I:

$$E + I \rightleftarrows EI \qquad (6)$$

The equilibrium constant of the reaction, K_i (the *inhibitor constant*), is a measure of the affinity of the inhibitor for the enzyme, just as K_m generally reflects the affinity of the enzyme for its substrate.

A *competitive* inhibitor is usually a structural analog of the substrate that combines with the free enzyme and competes with the normal substrate for binding at the active site. The actual rate of the reaction is strictly dependent on the relative concentrations of substrate and inhibitor.

Competitive inhibition is responsible for the inhibition of some enzymes by excess substrate caused by competition between substrate molecules for a single binding site. In two-substrate reactions, high concentrations of the second substrate may compete with binding of the first substrate. For example, aspartate aminotransferase is inhibited by excess concentrations of the substrate 2-oxoglutarate, and this inhibition is competitive with respect to L-aspartate. Therefore, to maintain a given velocity at high 2-oxoglutarate concentrations, the concentration of L-aspartate has to be increased to a value above that needed at lower concentrations of 2-oxoglutarate.

Competitive inhibition also contributes to the reduction in the rate of an enzymatic reaction over time. For example, a rate reduction occurs because increasing concentrations of reaction products tend to drive the reaction backward, if it is freely reversible. A product may itself be an inhibitor of the forward reaction, so even if the reaction is not readily reversible, it proceeds against a rising concentration of inhibitor. A familiar example of *product inhibition* is the release of the competitive inhibitor, inorganic phosphate, by the action of ALP on its substrates. In this case, both organic phosphates and inorganic phosphates bind to the active center of the enzyme with similar affinities (e.g., K_m and K_i are of the same order of magnitude).

Product inhibition is a cause of nonlinearity of reaction progress curves during fixed-time methods of enzyme assay. For example, oxaloacetate produced by the action of aspartate aminotransferase inhibits the enzyme, particularly the mitochondrial isoenzyme. The inhibitory product may be removed as it is formed by a coupled enzymatic reaction: Malate dehydrogenase converts the oxaloacetate to malate and at the same time oxidizes NADH to NAD$^+$.

Competitive inhibition by metal ions occurs when two metal ions compete for the same binding site on the enzyme. Sodium and lithium are potent inhibitors of pyruvate kinase, for which potassium is an obligatory activator.

A *noncompetitive* inhibitor is usually structurally different from the substrate. It is assumed to bind at a site on the enzyme molecule that is different from the substrate-binding site; thus, there is no competition between inhibitor and substrate, and a ternary enzyme/substrate/inhibitor (ESI) complex is formed. Attachment of the inhibitor to the enzyme does not alter the affinity of the enzyme for its substrate (i.e., K_m is unaltered), but the ESI complex does not break down to yield products. Because the substrate does not compete with the inhibitor for binding sites on the enzyme molecule, increasing the substrate concentration does not overcome the effect of a noncompetitive inhibitor. Thus, V_{max} is reduced in the presence of such an inhibitor, whereas K_m is not altered, as the Lineweaver-Burk plot shows (Figure 14-7).

Uncompetitive inhibition is produced by a combination of the inhibitor with the ES complex. It is more common in two-substrate reactions, in which a ternary ESI complex is formed after the first substrate has combined with the enzyme. In uncompetitive inhibition, parallel lines are obtained when plots of $1/v$ against $1/[S]$ with and without the inhibitor are compared (see Figure 14-7), that is, both K_m and V_{max} are decreased.

Irreversible Inhibition. Irreversible inhibitors inactivate the enzyme molecule by covalently and permanently modifying a functional group required for catalysis. The effect of an irreversible inhibitor is progressive with time and becomes complete when the amount of inhibitor present exceeds the total amount of enzyme. The rate of the reaction between enzyme and inhibitor is expressed as the fraction of enzyme activity that is inhibited in a fixed time by a given concentration of inhibitor. The velocity constant of the reaction of the inhibitor with the enzyme is a measure of the effectiveness of the inhibitor.

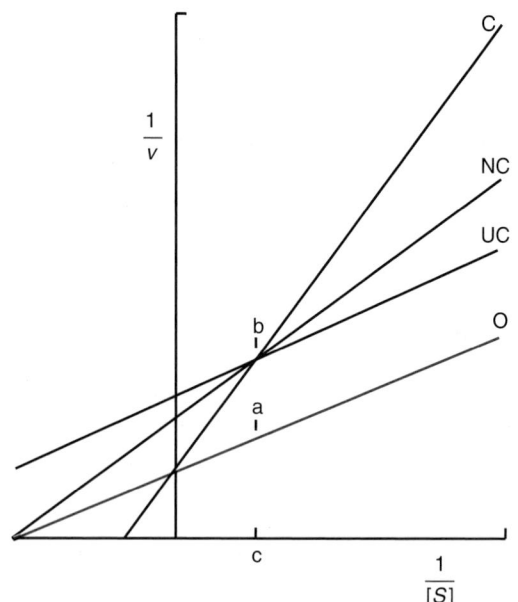

Figure 14-7 Effects of different types of inhibitors on the double-reciprocal plot of $1/v$ against $1/[S]$. Each of the inhibitors has been assumed to reduce the activity of the enzyme by the same amount, represented by the change in $1/v$ from *a* to *b* at a substrate concentration of *c*. Line *O* is the plot for enzyme without inhibitor, *C* with a competitive inhibitor, *NC* with a noncompetitive inhibitor, and *UC* with an uncompetitive inhibitor. *(From Moss DW. Measurement of enzymes. In: Hearse DJ, de Leiris J, eds. Enzymes in cardiology: diagnosis and research. New York: John Wiley & Sons Inc., 1979. Reprinted by permission of John Wiley & Sons, Inc.)*

Irreversible inhibitors have been useful in mapping active sites by covalently modifying different types of functional groups in the enzyme molecule to establish whether such groups are necessary for catalytic activity.

A physiologically important category of irreversible enzyme inhibition is exemplified by various trypsin inhibitors. These are proteins that bind to trypsin irreversibly, nullifying its proteolytic activity. One such inhibitor is present in the α_1-globulin fraction of serum proteins; others are found in soybeans and lima beans. Similar proteolysis inhibitors present in plasma prevent the accumulation of excess thrombin and other coagulation enzymes, thus keeping the coagulation process under control.

Inhibition by Antibodies. The combination of enzyme molecules with specific antibodies often has no effect on catalytic activity, which is retained by the enzyme/antibody complex.[2] However, in some cases, the reaction of the enzyme and the antibody reduces or even abolishes enzymatic activity. The most probable explanation for this type of inhibition is that the antibody molecule restricts access of the substrate molecules to the active center by steric hindrance or, in extreme cases, completely masks the substrate-binding site. However, it appears that some examples of enzyme inhibition by combination with antibodies are caused by a conformational change induced in the enzyme molecule.

Inhibition of the activity of an enzyme molecule labeled with a hapten (e.g., morphine) as a result of combination with a specific antibody forms the basis for a homogeneous enzyme immunoassay See Chapter 15 for additional details.

Enzyme Activation

Activators increase the rates of enzyme-catalyzed reactions by promoting formation of the most active state of the enzyme itself or of other reactants, such as the substrate. This generalization covers a wide variety of mechanisms of activation. For example, many enzymes contain metal ions as an integral part of their structure (e.g., zinc in ALP and carboxypeptidase A). Removal of divalent metal ions by treatment with an appropriate quantity of ethylenediaminetetraacetic acid (EDTA) solution is accompanied by conformational changes and inactivation of the enzyme. The enzyme often is reactivated by dialysis against a solution of the appropriate metal ion or simply by addition of the ion to the reaction mixture.

When the activator ion is an essential part of the functional enzyme molecule, it is usually incorporated quite firmly into the enzyme molecule. Therefore it is not usually necessary to add the activator to reaction mixtures, and an excess of the ion may even have an inhibitory effect. However, in some cases, the activating ion is attached only weakly or transiently to the enzyme (or its substrate) during catalysis. Enzyme samples therefore may be deficient in the ion, so that addition of the ion increases the reaction rate or indeed may be essential for the reaction to take place. For example, all phosphate transfer enzymes (kinases), such as creatine kinase, require the essential presence of Mg^{2+} ions. Other common activating cations are Mn^{2+}, Fe^{2+}, Ca^{2+}, Zn^{2+}, and K^+. More rarely, anions may act as activators. For example, amylase functions at its maximal rate only if Cl^- or other monovalent anions, such as Br^- or NO_3^-, are present.[11] Some enzymes require the obligate presence of two activating ions. K^+ and Mg^{2+} are essential for the activity of pyruvate kinase, and both Mg^{2+} and Zn^{2+} are required for ALP activity.

Coenzymes and Prosthetic Groups

Coenzymes are generally more complex molecules than activators, although they are smaller molecules than the enzyme proteins themselves. Some compounds, such as the dinucleotides NAD and NADP, are classified as coenzymes even though they are specific substrates in two-substrate reactions. Their effects on the rate of reaction follow the Michaelis-Menten pattern of dependence on substrate concentration. The structures of these two coenzymes are identical, except for the presence of an additional phosphate group in NADP; nevertheless, individual dehydrogenases, for which these coenzymes are substrates, are predominantly or even absolutely specific for one or the other form.

Coenzymes, such as NAD and NADP, are bound only momentarily to the enzyme during the course of the reaction, as is the case for substrates in general. Therefore no reaction takes place unless the appropriate coenzyme is present in solution (e.g., when it is added to the reaction mixture in the assay of dehydrogenase activity). In contrast to these entirely soluble coenzymes, some coenzymes are more or less permanently bound to the enzyme molecules, where they form part of the active center and undergo cycles of chemical change during the reaction. When bound, the coenzyme is known as a *prosthetic group*.

An active *holoenzyme* results from the combination of the inactive *apoenzyme* with the *prosthetic group*. An example of a prosthetic group is pyridoxal-5′-phosphate (P-5′-P), a component of AST and ALT. The P-5′-P prosthetic group undergoes a cycle of conversion of the pyridoxal moiety to pyridoxamine and back again during the transfer of an amino group from an amino acid to an oxo-acid. Prosthetic groups, such as activators with a structural role, do not usually have to be added to elicit the full catalytic activity of the enzyme unless previous treatment has caused the prosthetic group to be lost from some enzyme molecules. However, both normal and pathological serum samples contain appreciable quantities of apo-aminotransferases, which are converted to active holoenzymes through a suitable period of incubation with P-5′-P.

Study of the formulas of coenzyme and prosthetic groups reveals that many contain structures derived from the vitamins (see Chapter 27). Thus, the nicotinamide portion of NAD and NADP derives from the vitamin niacin, whereas the P-5′-P prosthetic group of the aminotransferases is a derivative of pyridoxine, vitamin B_6. Other derivatives of the B-group vitamins also participate in enzymatic reactions.

Analytical Enzymology

Analytically, the clinical laboratorian is concerned with measuring the activity or mass in serum or plasma of enzymes that are predominantly intracellular and that are physiologically present in the serum in low concentrations only. By measuring changes in the quantities of these enzymes in disease, it is possible to infer the location and nature of pathological changes in tissues of the body.

Measurement of Reaction Rates

The rate of an enzyme-catalyzed reaction is directly proportional to the amount of active enzyme present in the system. Consequently, determination of the rate of reaction under defined and controlled conditions provides a measure of the amount of enzyme in a sample, such as serum.

Determination of reaction rate involves the kinetic measurement of the amount of change produced within a defined time interval.[6,30] Both *fixed-time* and *continuous-monitoring* methods are used to measure reaction rates. In the fixed-time method, the amount of change produced by the enzyme is measured after the reaction is stopped at the end of a fixed time interval. With the continuous-monitoring method, the progress of the reaction is monitored continuously. These two methods have different advantages and limitations. To appreciate them, it is necessary to consider the way in which the rate of an enzymatic reaction varies with time.

The progress of an enzyme reaction is monitored by measuring in time the decreasing concentration of the substrate or the increasing concentration of the products. Measurement of product formation is preferable, as determination of the increase in the concentration of a substance above an initially zero or low concentration has less analytical uncertainty than measurement of a decline from an initially high concentration.

At the moment when the enzyme and the substrate are mixed, the rate of the reaction is zero. The rate then typically rises rapidly to a maximum value, which remains constant for a period of time (Figure 14-8). During the period of constant reaction rate, the rate depends only on enzyme concentration and is completely independent of substrate concentration. The reaction is said to follow zero-order kinetics because its rate is proportional to the zero power of the substrate concentration. Ultimately, however, as more substrate is consumed, the reaction rate declines and enters a phase of first-order dependence on substrate concentration. Other factors that contribute to the decline in reaction rate include (1) accumulation of products that may be inhibitory, (2) the growing importance of the reverse reaction, and (3) enzyme denaturation. Although it is possible to compare the rates of reaction produced by different amounts of an enzyme under first-order conditions, it is obviously easier to standardize such comparisons when the enzyme concentration is the only variable that influences the reaction rate. Therefore, enzyme assays are usually made under conditions that are initially saturating with respect to substrate concentration. The rate of reaction during the zero-order phase is determined by measuring the product formed during a fixed period of incubation where the rate remains constant. This is illustrated in Figure 14-9. Measurement of reaction rates at any portion of curve A yields results that are identical to the true *initial rate*. However, curve B deviates from linearity over its entire course, and rates fall off with time. From curve C, correct results are obtained only if the rate is measured along

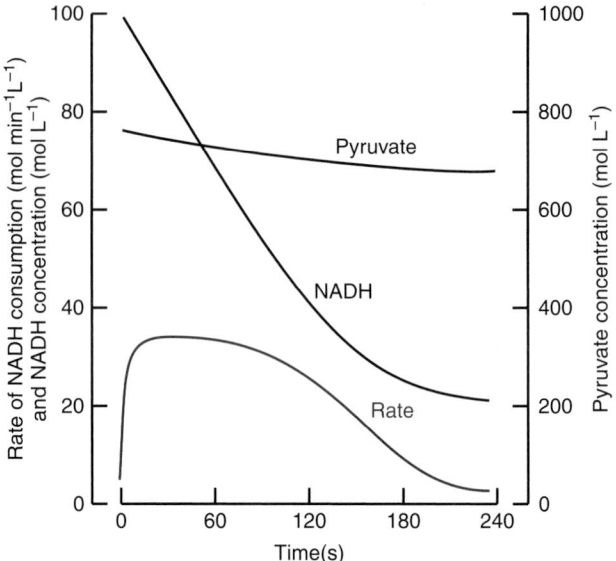

Figure 14-8 Changes in substrate concentrations and rates of reaction during an assay of lactate dehydrogenase activity at 37 °C in phosphate buffer, with pyruvate and NADH as substrates. This reaction is followed by observation of the fall in absorbance at 340 nm as NADH is oxidized to NAD^+. The rate of reaction rises rapidly to a maximum value, from which it declines only slightly until about half the NADH has been used up. During this phase of the reaction, the rate is essentially zero order with respect to substrate concentration. At the point at which the rate falls below about 90% of its maximum value, NADH concentration is approximately $10 \times K_m$. The K_m for NADH is on the order of 5×10^{-6} mol/L, whereas for pyruvate it is 9×10^{-5} mol/L. Thus an initial pyruvate concentration approximately 10 times that of NADH is used. (Concentrations per liter of reaction mixture are given.) *(From Moss DW. Measurement of enzymes. In: Hearse DJ, de Leiris J, eds. Enzymes in cardiology: diagnosis and research. New York: John Wiley & Sons Inc., 1979. Reprinted by permission of John Wiley & Sons, Inc.)*

segment II. Incorrect results are obtained if the rate is measured during phase I (the lag phase) or during phase III.

Careful selection of reaction conditions, such as the concentrations of substrates and cofactors, improves the reaction progress curves, eliminating lag phases and prolonging the period of linearity so that fixed-time methods of analysis become feasible. Improvements in optical techniques, leading to more reliable and sensitive measurement of product formation, have also allowed the duration of incubation to be shortened compared with older assays. This has resulted in a corresponding increase in the interval over which enzyme activity is measured. Nevertheless, an upper limit of activity exists in all fixed-time methods, above which progress curves will no longer be linear. The upper limit of activity that is acceptable in the unmodified method is chosen so that samples with activities below it are presumed with a high degree of certainty to yield linear progress curves; alternatively, if the limit is set too low, many samples will be reanalyzed unnecessarily. Samples that are above the limit should ideally be reassayed by shortening the incubation period until a constant reaction rate is obtained. However, this is difficult or impossible with some

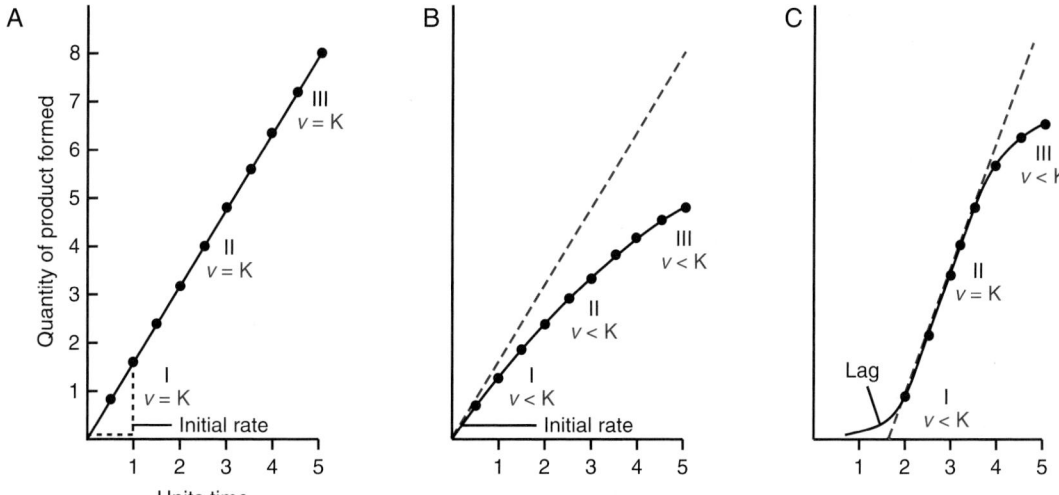

Figure 14-9 Forms of graphs showing changes in enzyme reaction rate as a function of time. In **A,** the rate is constant during the entire run, and rates calculated as *I, II,* and *III* will be identical to the initial rate. In **B,** the rate falls off continuously; rates calculated at *I, II,* and *III* will be different and less than the true initial rate. In **C,** a measurement at *II* will be representative of the maximum rate, but at *I* (lag period) and *III* (substrate depletion), it will be less than at *II.*

automated methods, in which the duration of incubation is fixed by the configuration of the apparatus. It then becomes necessary to dilute the specimen; however, dilution may not always result in a proportional change in activity.

The initial rate of reaction theoretically increases without limit as enzyme concentration increases, as long as no other factor, such as substrate concentration, becomes limiting. In practice, the reaction rate becomes so rapid at high enzyme activities that it is impossible to measure the initial rate of reaction, even with continuous-monitoring methods. Therefore, an upper limit of activity that is measurable without modification of the assay procedure exists even in continuous-monitoring methods, but this limit is usually much higher than that applied in corresponding fixed-time methods. Fewer samples therefore require special treatment. Furthermore, continuous monitoring allows identification of the appropriate zero-order portion of the progress curve for each sample and identification of samples that require special treatment. Continuous-monitoring methods provide a decisive advantage in enzyme assay and should be used whenever possible.

Measurement of Substrates

The amount of substrate transformed into products during an enzyme-catalyzed reaction can be measured with any appropriate analytical method, such as (1) spectrophotometry, (2) fluorometry, or (3) chemiluminescence (see Chapter 9).[10,17] For example, *self-indicating* reactions are particularly valuable, as they allow continuous monitoring. Important examples of self-indicating reactions include determination of dehydrogenase activity by monitoring the change in absorbance at 339 (340) nm of the coenzyme NADH or NADPH during oxidation or reduction, and measurement of ALP activity by generation of the yellow *p*-nitrophenolate ion from the

substrate *p*-nitrophenyl phosphate in alkaline solution. These indicator reactions are so versatile that coupled reactions are frequently used to provide an observable optical change accompanying a primary reaction in which such a change is not present.

Optimization, Standardization, and Quality Control

To measure enzyme activity reliably, all factors that affect the reaction rate—other than the concentration of active enzyme—need to be optimized and rigidly controlled. Furthermore, because the reaction velocity is at or near its maximum under optimal conditions, a larger analytical signal is obtained that is measured more reliably. Much effort therefore has been devoted to determining optimal conditions for measuring the activities of enzymes of clinical importance.

Optimization

Optimization of reaction conditions for enzyme assays traditionally has been carried out by varying a single factor and studying its effect on the reaction rate, then repeating the experiment with a second factor and so on, until the effects of all variables have been tested. An optimal combination of variables is selected on the basis of these experiments, and the validity of the chosen conditions is verified. Not only is this approach labor intensive, it also is difficult to adapt in situations in which the effects of different variables are interdependent, as is frequently the case in enzyme analysis. This traditional empirical approach to optimization has been replaced by newer techniques of simplex co-optimization and response surface methodology.[16]

Standardization

Despite substantial effort and the development of reference procedures, considerable variability of results between

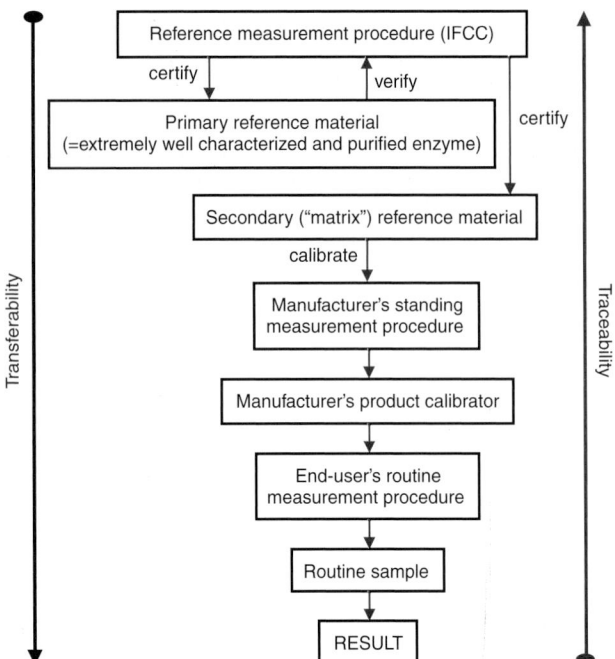

Figure 14-10 The proposed reference system for enzyme measurement showing the traceability of the laboratory result to the reference measurement procedure. *(From Panteghini M, Ceriotti F, Schumann G, et al. Establishing a reference system in clinical enzymology. Clin Chem Lab Med 2001;39:795-800. Reprinted with permission of Walter de Gruyter.)*

laboratories is still observed.[7,31] Consequently, current enzyme standardization efforts are focused on the development of a system that allows comparability of test results, independent of the measurement method. To achieve this, a "reference measurement system" based on the concepts of metrological traceability and on the hierarchy of analytical methods has been proposed.[8,15,32] A reference procedure and certified reference materials form the basis of the metrological traceability chain (Figure 14-10).[1,3] As part of this hierarchy, reference procedures at 37 °C for the most common enzymes have been developed, and reference laboratories are now available (http://www.bipm.org/jctlm/; accessed August 7, 2013) to perform enzyme measurements at an appropriately high metrological level.[18-26]

Reference procedures set standards of accuracy against which the relative performance of methods intended for routine use is judged. The reference procedure is used to assign a certified value to the reference material. Provided that its commutability is proven, this certified material is then used by manufacturers to assign values to commercial calibrators, resulting in traceability of the value obtained in the laboratory.

Several studies have demonstrated that it is possible to produce enzyme preparations with reproducible properties and purity and with assured stability. These may be derived from animal sources in which the enzymes closely resemble their human counterparts, although new possibilities have been created by gene transfer and recombinant techniques.

For a reference system to be capable of standardizing the results of different assays of a given enzyme activity, some conditions must be satisfied.[13] First, the reference procedure used to assign the value of the reference material and the routine method(s) to be calibrated must have identical specificities for the analyte enzyme, isoenzyme, or isoform under study. Second, the properties of the calibrator material must be the same as or closely similar to those of the analyte enzyme in its natural matrix, must be "commutable—substituted or interchanged," and must be capable of being exchanged for another or for something else that is equivalent to human serum samples for that particular method.

Quality Control

The application of quality control programs is as essential in enzyme analysis as it is in other forms of clinical analysis if the results obtained are to be useful in diagnosis and treatment.

Lyophilized and liquid preparations containing various enzymes are available from commercial sources; these have a useful function in quality control.

Measurement of Enzyme Mass Concentration

Many immunoassays have been developed for human enzymes and isoenzymes that measure protein mass instead of catalytic activity. To develop such assays, purified enzyme protein has to be prepared to (1) act as a calibrator, (2) be labeled, and (3) be used to raise the enzyme-specific antibody. These methods identify all molecules with the antigenic determinants necessary for recognition by the antibody, so that inactive enzyme molecules that are immunologically unaltered are measured along with active molecules. This has been found to be significant in the determination of some digestive enzymes, such as trypsin, when inactive precursors and inhibitors of catalytic activity are present in plasma. In most cases, however, no degradation or changes in the active enzyme occur in blood; therefore the clinical equivalence of the different measurement approaches is obtained.

Immunoassays typically are not used for determination of total activities for the more important diagnostic enzymes, as these assays generally cannot compete with automated measurements of catalytic activity in terms of (1) speed, (2) precision, and (3) cost. Furthermore, several enzyme activities in serum are caused by mixtures of immunologically distinct forms, so an assay using a single type of antibody usually determines only one of the enzyme forms. However, this disadvantage in the determination of total enzyme activity becomes a marked advantage in the measurement of specific isoenzymes and isoforms, and immunological methods have assumed great importance in isoenzyme analysis for diagnostic purposes.

Enzymes as Analytical Reagents

Enzymes are used as analytical reagents for the measurement of several metabolites and substrates and in immunoassays to detect and quantify immunological reactions.

Measurement of Metabolites

The use of enzymes as analytical reagents to measure metabolites frequently offers the advantage of great specificity for the substance being determined. This high specificity typically removes the need for preliminary separation or purification stages, so the analysis is carried out directly on complex mixtures such as serum. Uricase (urate oxidase), urease, and glucose oxidase are examples of highly specific enzymes used in clinically important assays for the measurement of (1) uric acid, (2) urea, and (3) glucose, specifically in biological fluids. However, high specificity is not always achieved in practice; knowledge of the substrate specificities of reagent enzymes is therefore essential to allow possible interferences with the assay to be anticipated and corrected. Coupled reactions are often used to construct an enzymatic analytical system that is used to determine a particular compound. An example of this is the determination of glucose by the hexokinase reaction. Hexokinase converts sugars other than glucose to their 6-phosphate esters. However, the indicator reaction used to monitor this change is catalyzed by glucose-6-phosphate dehydrogenase—an enzyme that is highly specific for its substrate—so the overall process is highly specific for glucose. In practice, both equilibrium and kinetic (rate) methods have been developed that use enzymes as reagents.[29]

Equilibrium Methods

Most assays used to determine the amount of a substance enzymatically are allowed to continue to completion, so that all substrate has been converted into a measurable product. These methods are called *end point* or, more correctly, *equilibrium* methods, because the reaction ceases when equilibrium is reached. Reactions in which the equilibrium point corresponds virtually to complete conversion of the substrate are obviously preferable for this type of analysis. However, an unfavorable equilibrium is often displaced in the desired direction by additional enzymatic or nonenzymatic reactions that convert or "trap" a product of the first reaction (e.g., in measuring lactate with lactate dehydrogenase, the pyruvate formed is trapped by the addition of hydrazine, with which it forms an irreversible hydrazone).

Kinetic Methods

First-order or pseudo–first-order reactions are the most important reactions for the kinetic determination of substrate concentration. For any first-order reaction, the substrate concentration $[S]$ at a given time t after the start of the reaction is given by

$$[S] = [S_0] \times e^{-kt} \tag{7}$$

where $[S_0]$ is the initial substrate concentration, e is the base of the natural log, and k is the rate constant.

The change in substrate concentration $\Delta[S]$ over a fixed time interval, t_1 to t_2, is related to $[S_0]$ by the equation

$$[S_0] = \frac{-\Delta[S]}{e^{-kt_1} - e^{kt_2}} \tag{8}$$

which demonstrates that the change in substrate concentration over a fixed time interval is directly proportional to its initial concentration. This is a general property of first-order reactions.

For an enzymatic reaction, first-order kinetics is followed when $[S]$ is small compared with K_m. Thus,

$$v = \frac{V_{max}}{K_m} \times [S] \tag{9}$$

or

$$v = k[S] \tag{10}$$

Methods in which some property related to substrate concentration such as (1) absorbance, (2) fluorescence, and (3) chemiluminescence is measured at two fixed times during the course of the reaction are known as *two-point* kinetic methods. Theoretically, they are most accurate for the enzymatic determination of substrates. However, these methods are technically more demanding than equilibrium methods, and all factors that affect reaction rate, such as (1) pH, (2) temperature, and (3) amount of enzyme, must be kept constant from one assay to the next, as must the timing of the two measurements. These conditions are readily achieved in automatic analyzers. A reference solution of the analyte (substrate) is used for calibration. To ensure first-order reaction conditions, the substrate concentration must be low compared with the K_m (i.e., on the order of less than $0.2 \times K_m$). Enzymes with high K_m values therefore are preferred for kinetic analysis to obtain a wider usable range of substrate concentrations.

Immunoassay

In enzyme immunoassay, first, enzyme-labeled antibodies or antigens are allowed to react with ligand; then an enzyme substrate is added. Enzymes such as (1) ALP, (2) horseradish peroxidase, (3) glucose-6-phosphate dehydrogenase, and (4) β-galactosidase have all been used as enzyme labels. A modification of this method is the enzyme-linked immunoabsorbent assay (ELISA), in which one of the reaction components is bound to a solid phase surface. With this technique, an aliquot of sample is allowed to interact with the solid phase antibody. After washing, a second antibody labeled with enzyme is added to form an Ab/Ag/Ab enzyme complex. Excess free enzyme–labeled antibody is then washed away, and the substrate is added; the conversion of substrate is proportional to the quantity of antigen. In immunoassays, it is not the specificity of labeled enzymes that is important, but their sensitivity.

Analytical Applications of Immobilized Enzymes

For some types of enzymatic analyses, enzyme consumption is reduced by the use of immobilized enzymes that are reused for several analyses. Immobilized enzymes have been chemically bonded to adsorbents, such as (1) microcrystalline cellulose, (2) diethylaminoethyl (DEAE) cellulose,

(3) carboxymethyl cellulose, and (4) agarose. Chemical groups such as (1) diazo, (2) triazine, and (3) azide are used to join the enzyme protein to the insoluble matrix, forming particles in contact with the substrate solution or a surface in contact with substrate solution, such as a membrane or a coating on the inner surface of a vessel holding the substrate solution. Among the enzymes available in such an immobilized form are (1) urease, (2) hexokinase, (3) α-amylase, (4) glucose oxidase, (5) trypsin, and (6) leucine aminopeptidase. Stability to heat and other forms of inactivation is considerably increased compared with enzymes in solution. Immobilized proteolytic enzymes are not subject to autodigestion. However, some properties of the enzyme, such as its K_m or its pH optimum, may be altered.

Electrochemical techniques, such as (1) potentiometry, (2) polarography, and (3) microcalorimetry, have been chosen to exploit the benefits of immobilized enzymes (see Chapter 10). Enzymes incorporated into membranes form a part of enzyme electrodes. The surface of an ion-sensitive electrode is coated with a layer of porous gel in which an enzyme has been polymerized. When the electrode is immersed in a solution of the appropriate substrate, the action of the enzyme produces ions to which the electrode is sensitive. For example, an oxygen electrode coated with a layer containing glucose oxidase has been used to determine glucose from the amount of oxygen consumed in the reaction. Urea has been estimated by the combination of a selective ammonium ion–sensitive electrode and a urease membrane.

Measurement of Isoenzymes and Isoforms

Various analytical techniques have been used to measure isoenzymes or isoforms. They include (1) electrophoresis (see Chapter 11), (2) chromatography (see Chapter 12), (3) chemical inactivation, and (4) differences in catalytic properties, but the most common routine methods are now based on (5) immunochemical assays.

Immunochemical methods of isoenzyme analysis are particularly applicable to isoenzymes derived from multiple gene loci, because they are usually most clearly antigenically distinct. However, the greater discriminating power of monoclonal antibodies has potentially brought all multiple forms of an enzyme within the scope of immunochemical analysis. Some of these methods make use of catalytic activity of the isoenzymes. For example, residual activity may be measured after reaction with antiserum. Radioimmunoassays, in which isoenzyme labeled with a radioactive tracer competes with unlabeled isoenzyme for antibody-binding sites, have also been applied to isoenzyme measurement. These methods do not depend on the catalytic activity of the isoenzyme being determined. However, with the development of automated immunoassay systems, the most common routine methods for measuring isoenzymes, such as CK-MB, are solid phase ELISAs.

The selection and application of various methods of isoenzyme analysis in clinical enzymology are discussed in Chapter 19 in relation to specific isoenzyme systems.

Review Questions

1. The Michaelis-Menten constant is:
   a. V_{max}.
   b. K_m.
   c. $1/v$.
   d. [S].

2. The "active center" of an enzyme is:
   a. the protein part of an enzyme without the cofactor necessary for catalysis.
   b. that part of an enzyme that diminishes the rate of a chemical reaction.
   c. a site other than the substratebinding site.
   d. that part of an enzyme at which substrate binding occurs.

3. Which statement(s) below is (are) *correct*?
   a. Apoenzyme + Prosthetic group = Holoenzyme
   b. An enzyme without the prosthetic group attached is referred to as an *apoenzyme*.
   c. A prosthetic group is a coenzyme permanently bound to an enzyme molecule.
   d. All of the above statements are correct.

4. The graph on which the plot of 1/velocity versus 1/substrate concentration is illustrated is referred to as a:
   a. rate plot.
   b. Lineweaver-Burk plot.
   c. maximum velocity plot.
   d. Michaelis-Menten plot.

5. An enzyme assay during which a single measurement is taken at the termination of the enzymatic reaction is referred to as a:
   a. fixed-time assay.
   b. terminator assay.
   c. kinetic assay.
   d. continuous-monitoring assay.

6. A reactant in a catalysis reaction that binds to the enzyme's active site is the:
   a. enzyme.
   b. product.
   c. substrate.
   d. coenzyme.

7. Every enzymatic reaction follows specific kinetics as it proceeds from enzyme + substrate to product + enzyme. As substrate is consumed, the reaction rate decreases and becomes *directly proportional to the amount of substrate* that is present in low concentration. This is referred to as:
   a. V_{max}.
   b. K_m.
   c. first-order kinetics.
   d. zero-order kinetics.

8. An international unit (U) of enzyme activity is the amount of enzyme that will catalyze the reaction of:
   a. one micromole of substrate per minute.
   b. one mole of substrate per second.
   c. one micromole of enzyme per hour.
   d. one millimole of substrate per minute.

9. In an analytical enzymatic measurement of substrate, an enzyme reaction is accompanied by a change in absorbance of one component of the assay system. If this change is continuously monitored while it is occurring, the reaction is referred to as a(n):
   a. fixed-time reaction.
   b. end point assay.
   c. rate-limiting reaction.
   d. self-indicating reaction.

10. The most widely used method of isoenzyme analysis that allows the best discrimination between antigenically distinct isoenzymes derived from multiple-gene loci is:
    a. electrophoresis.
    b. an immunochemical method.
    c. chemical inactivation.
    d. chromatography.

References

1. Armbruster D, Miller RR; The Joint Committee for Traceability in Laboratory Medicine (JCTLM). A global approach to promote the standardisation of clinical laboratory test results. Clin Biochem Rev 2007; 28:105–14.
2. Bais R, Huxtable A, Edwards JB. Human prostatic acid phosphatase: properties of the native enzyme and the enzyme-antibody complex. Ann Clin Biochem 1983;20:374–80.
3. Canalias F, Camprubí S, Sánchez M, et al. Metrological traceability of values for catalytic concentration of enzymes assigned to a calibration material. Clin Chem Lab Med 2006;44:333–9.
4. Commission on Biochemical Nomenclature. I. Nomenclature of multiple forms of enzymes. J Biol Chem 1977;252:5939–41.
5. Copeland RA. Enzymes: a practical introduction to structure, mechanism, and data analysis. Basel: VCH Publishers, 1996.
6. Harris TK, Keshwani MM. Measurement of enzyme activity. Methods Enzymol 2009;463:57–71.
7. Infusino I, Bonora R, Panteghini M. Traceability in clinical enzymology. Clin Biochem Rev 2007;28:155–61.
8. Infusino I, Schumann G, Ceriotti F, et al. Standardization in clinical enzymology: a challenge for the theory of metrological traceability. Clin Chem Lab Med 2010;48:301–7.
9. IUPAC Commission on Quantities and Units and IFCC Expert Panel on Quantities and Units. Approved recommendations (1978): quantities and units in clinical chemistry. Clin Chim Acta 1979;96:157F–83F.
10. Marquette CA, Blum LJ. Chemiluminescent enzyme immunoassays: a review of bioanalytical applications. Bioanalysis 2009;1:1259–69.
11. Maurus R, Begum A, Kuo HH, et al. Structural and mechanistic studies of chloride induced activation of human pancreatic alpha-amylase. Protein Sci 2005;14:743–55.
12. Moss DW. Isoenzyme analysis. London: The Chemical Society, 1979.
13. Moss DW. Enzyme reference materials: their place in diagnostic enzymology. Ann Biol Clin 1994;52:143–6.
14. Nomenclature Committee, I.E. Recommendations of the Nomenclature Committee of IUB on the nomenclature and classification of enzymes (1978). New York: Academic Press, 1979.
15. Panteghini M, Ceriotti F, Schumann G, et al. Establishing a reference system in clinical enzymology. Clin Chem Lab Med 2001;39:795–800.
16. Rautela GS, Snee RD, Miller WK. Response-surface co-optimization of reaction conditions in clinical chemical methods. Clin Chem 1979; 25:1954–64.
17. Roda A, Guardigli M. Analytical chemiluminescence and bioluminescence: latest achievements and new horizons. Ann Clin Biochem 2010;47:189–94.
18. Schumann G, Aoki R, Ferrero CA, et al. IFCC primary reference procedures for the measurement of catalytic activity concentrations of enzymes at 37°C. Part 8: reference procedure for the measurement of catalytic concentration of α-amylase. Clin Chem Lab Med 2006;44:1146–55.
19. Schumann G, Bonora R, Ceriotti F, et al. IFCC primary reference procedures for the measurement of catalytic activity concentrations of enzymes at 37°C. Part 2: reference procedure for the measurement of catalytic concentration of creatine kinase. Clin Chem Lab Med 2002;40:635–42.
20. Schumann G, Bonora R, Ceriotti F, et al. IFCC primary reference procedures for the measurement of catalytic activity concentrations of enzymes at 37°C. Part 3: reference procedure for the measurement of catalytic concentration of lactate dehydrogenase. Clin Chem Lab Med 2002;40:643–8.
21. Schumann G, Bonora R, Ceriotti F, et al. IFCC primary reference procedures for the measurement of catalytic activity concentrations of enzymes at 37°C. International Federation of Clinical Chemistry and Laboratory Medicine. Part 4: reference procedure for the measurement of catalytic concentration of alanine aminotransferase. Clin Chem Lab Med 2002;40:718–24.
22. Schumann G, Bonora R, Ceriotti F, et al. IFCC primary reference procedures for the measurement of catalytic activity concentrations of enzymes at 37°C. International Federation of Clinical Chemistry and Laboratory Medicine. Part 5: reference procedure for the measurement of catalytic concentration of aspartate aminotransferase. Clin Chem Lab Med 2002;40:725–33.
23. Schumann G, Bonora R, Ceriotti F, et al. IFCC primary reference procedures for the measurement of catalytic activity concentrations of enzymes at 37°C. International Federation of Clinical Chemistry and Laboratory Medicine. Part 6: reference procedure for the measurement of catalytic concentration of γ-glutamyltransferase. Clin Chem Lab Med 2002;40:734–8.
24. Schumann G, Klauke R, Canalias F, et al. IFCC primary reference procedures for the measurement of catalytic activity concentrations of enzymes at 37°C. International Federation of Clinical Chemistry and Laboratory Medicine. Part 9. Reference procedure for the measurement of catalytic concentration of alkaline phosphatase. Clin Chem Lab Med 2011;49:1439–46
25. Siekmann L, Bonora R, Burtis CA, et al. IFCC primary reference procedures for the measurement of catalytic activity concentrations of enzymes at 37°C. Part 1: the concept of reference procedures for the measurement of catalytic activity concentrations of enzymes. Clin Chem Lab Med 2002;40:631–4.
26. Siekmann L, Bonora R, Burtis CA, et al. IFCC primary reference procedures for the measurement of catalytic activity concentrations of enzymes at 37°C. International Federation of Clinical Chemistry and Laboratory Medicine. Part 7: certification of four reference materials for the determination of enzymatic activity of gamma-glutamyltransferase, lactate dehydrogenase, alanine aminotransferase and creatine kinase accord. Clin Chem Lab Med 2002;40:739–45.
27. Stein M, Gabdoulline RR, Wade RC. Calculating enzyme kinetic parameters from protein structures. Biochem Soc Trans 2008;36:51–4.
28. Strimbu J, Tavle JA. What are biomarkers? Curr Opin HIV AIDS 2010;5:463–6.
29. Tiffany TO, Jansen JM, Burtis CA, et al. Enzymatic kinetic rate and end-point analyses of substrate using a GeMSAEC Fast Analyzer. Clin Chem 1972;18:829–40.
30. Uttamchandani M, Moochhala S. Microarray-based enzyme profiling: recent advances and applications. [Review] Biointerphases 2010;5:FA24–31.
31. Vesper HW, Thienpont LM. Traceability in laboratory medicine. Clin Chem 2009;55:1067–75.
32. Wu AH. Standardization of assays for clinically important enzymes that have high biologic variation: what is all the fuss about? Clin Chem Lab Med 2010;48:299–300.

Immunochemical Techniques*

*L.J. Kricka, D. Phil., F.A.C.B., C.Chem., F.R.S.C., F.R.C.Path.
and J.Y. Park, M.D., Ph.D., F.C.A.P*

Objectives

1. Define the following:

Affinity	Immunoassay
Antibody	Immunogen
Antigen	Monoclonal antibody
Avidity	Polyclonal antiserum
Hapten	Sandwich immunoassay

2. Diagram, label and state the function of the components of an IgG antibody molecule.
3. List three binding forces that act to produce antigen/antibody binding.
4. Explain how the following factors affect antigen/antibody binding:

Addition of a linear polymer	Mechanism of reaction
Ion species	Precipitin reaction

5. For each of the following qualitative immunochemical techniques, state the principle and clinical use:

Immunoelectrophoresis	Passive gel immunodiffusion
Immunofixation	Western blotting

6. For each of the following quantitative immunochemical techniques, state the principle and clinical use:

Electroimmunoassay	Radial immunodiffusion
Nephelometry	Turbidimetry

7. List five nonisotopic labels used in a labeled immunochemical assay and provide one example of each type of label.
8. Compare the following types of assays, including procedure, assay components, and uses in the clinical laboratory: competitive with noncompetitive immunoassays and heterogeneous with homogeneous immunoassays.
9. For each of the following immunochemical techniques, state the principle, the components of each assay, the type of assay and the clinical uses:

Cloned enzyme donor immunoassay	Fluoroimmunoassay
Enzyme immunoassay	Immunocytochemistry
Enzyme-linked immunosorbent assay	Nanoparticle immunoassay
Enzyme-multiplied immunoassay	Simultaneous multianalyte immunoassay

10. State what is meant by the phrase "simplified immunoassay"; provide two examples of this type of assay used in a clinical setting.
11. Evaluate issues that can affect patient results when an immunoassay is used.

Key Words and Definitions

Affinity Energy of interaction of a single antibody-combining site and its corresponding epitope on the antigen.

Antibody Immunoglobulin (Ig) class of molecule (e.g., IgA, IgG, IgM) that binds specifically to an antigen or hapten.

Antigen Any material capable of reacting with an antibody without necessarily being capable of inducing antibody formation.

Avidity Overall strength of binding of antibody and antigen; includes the sum of the binding affinities of all individual combining sites on the antibody.

Competitive immunoassay An immunoassay in which all reactants are simultaneously or sequentially mixed together and unlabeled antigen competes with labeled antigen for binding sites on the antibody; no separation step is included in this assay.

Dot blotting A blotting technique in which the biomolecules to be detected are applied directly on a membrane as dots.

Hapten A chemically defined determinant that, when conjugated to an immunogenic carrier, stimulates the synthesis of antibody specific for the hapten.

*The author gratefully acknowledges the original contributions of Dr. Gregory Buffone, on which portions of this chapter are based.

Key Words and Definitions—cont'd

Heterogeneous immunoassay An immunochemical reaction in which it is assumed that the formation of the antigen/antibody complex occurs more quickly than the breakdown of the complex into antigen and antibody; in this assay, the antigen is labeled and separation of the free from the bound labeled antigen is required.

Homogeneous immunoassay An immunochemical reaction in which the activity of the label attached to the antigen is modulated directly by antibody binding; this assay does not require a separation.

Hook effect A phenomenon occurring with certain mmunoassays due to very high concentrations of a particular analyte; it results in a false negative result. The hook effect mostly affects one-step immunometric assays.

Immunoassay An assay based on the reaction of an antigen with an antibody specific for the antigen.

Immunogen A substance capable of inducing an immune response.

Label Any substance with a measurable property attached to an antigen, antibody, or binding substance.

Noncompetitive immunoassay An immunoassay in which a capture antibody is bound to a surface with subsequent antigen binding followed by the addition of a second labeled antibody that reacts with the initial antigen/antibody complex.

Ouchterlony technique A technique in which both antigen and antibody are allowed to diffuse to each other in a gel in a precipitation reaction.

Northern blotting Membrane-based assay in which molecules of RNA are separated by electrophoresis, which is followed by transfer to a membrane and probing with a labeled antibody.

Radial immunodiffusion an immunodiffusion technique used to determine the quantity of an antigen by measuring the diameters of circles of precipitin complexes surrounding samples of the antigen.

Western blotting Membrane-based assay in which proteins are separated by electrophoresis, which is followed by transfer to a membrane and probing with a labeled antibody.

Immunochemical reactions form the basis for sensitive and specific clinical assays known as **immunoassays**.[1,2,7,10] In a typical immunoassay, an antibody is used as a reagent to detect the analyte of interest. The exquisite specificity and high affinity of antibodies for specific antigens, coupled with the unique ability of antibodies to cross-link antigens, allows for the identification and quantification of specific substances by a variety of methods. Many of these assays are now automated. The principles of the methods most commonly used in the laboratory are discussed in this chapter.

Basic Concepts and Definitions

An **antigen** is any material capable of reacting with an antibody. With immunoassay, the antigen is the analyte of clinical interest that is being measured. **Antibodies** are immunoglobulins that bind specifically to a wide array of natural and synthetic antigens, such as (1) proteins, (2) carbohydrates, (3) nucleic acids, (4) lipids, and (5) other molecules. Analytically, immunoglobulin G (IgG) is the most prevalent immunochemical reagent in use. It is a glycoprotein that has a molecular weight (MW) of 158,000 Da and is composed of two duplex chains, with each set composed of a heavy (γ) and a light (λ or κ) chain joined by disulfide bonds (Figure 15-1). Interchain disulfide bonds hold the duplex chains together and create a symmetrical molecule. The variable amino acid sequence at the amino terminal end of each chain determines the antigenic specificity of the particular antibody. Each unique amino acid sequence is a product of a single plasma cell line or clone, and each plasma cell line produces antibodies with single specificities. A complex antigen elicits a multiplicity of antibodies with different specificities derived from different cell lines. An antibody developed in this manner is termed *polyclonal* and

exhibits diverse specificities in its reactivity with the immunogen. Each unique region of the molecular antigen that binds a complementary antibody is termed an *epitope* (antigenic determinant).

An **immunogen** is a protein or a substance coupled to a carrier, usually a protein. Introduction of an immunogen into a foreign host induces the formation of an antibody. A **hapten** is a chemically defined determinant that by itself will not stimulate an immune response. However, when conjugated to an immunogenic carrier, the conjugated molecule stimulates the synthesis of antibody specific for the hapten. Some general properties required for immunogenicity include the following:

1. Areas of structural stability within the molecule
2. Randomness of structure
3. Minimum MW of 4000 to 5000 Da
4. Ability to be metabolized (a necessary but insufficient criterion for some classes of antigens)
5. Accessibility of a particular immunogenic configuration to the antibody-forming mechanism
6. Structurally foreign quality

The strength or energy of interaction between the antibody and the antigen is described in two terms. **Affinity** refers to the thermodynamic quantity defining the energy of interaction of a single antibody-combining site and its corresponding epitope on the antigen. **Avidity** refers to the overall strength of the binding of antibody and antigen and includes the sum of the binding affinities of all individual combining sites on the antibody. Thus affinity is a property of the substance bound (antigen), and avidity is a property of the binder (antibody).

Polyclonal antiserum is produced in a normal animal host in response to immunogen administration. In contrast, a *monoclonal antibody* is the product of a single clone or plasma cell line rather than a heterogeneous mixture of antibodies

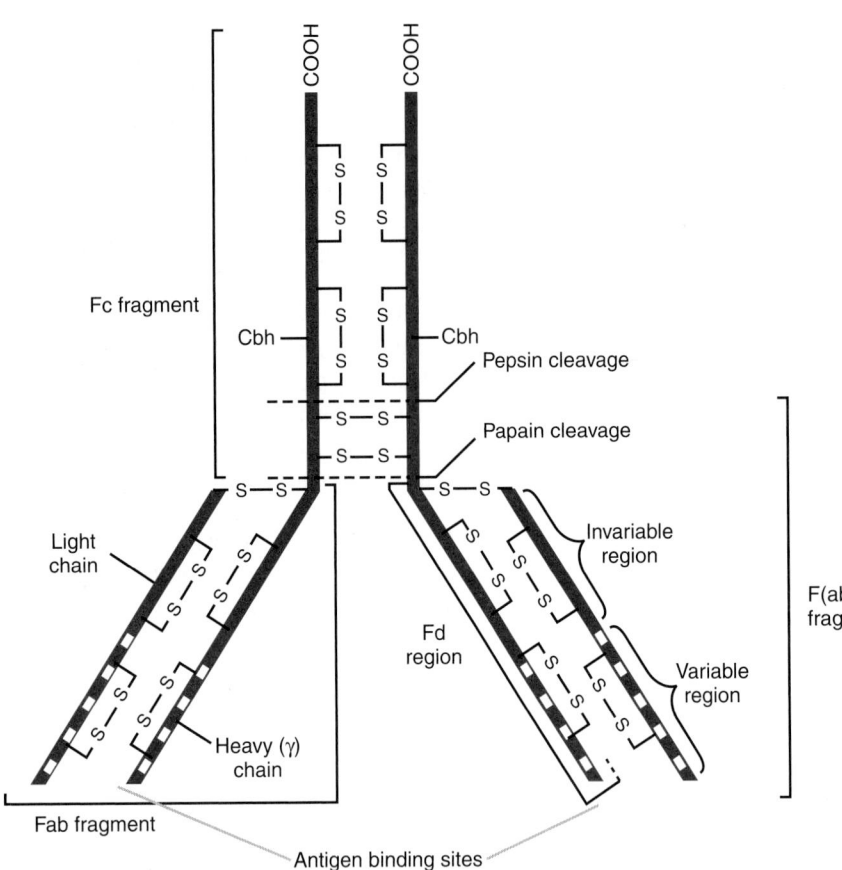

Figure 15-1 Schematic diagram of IgG (immunoglobulin G) antibody molecule showing carbohydrate (Cbh), disulfide bonds (SS), and major fragments produced by proteolytic enzyme treatment (F[ab']$_2$, Fc, Fab, Fd).

produced by many cell clones in response to immunization. Monoclonal antibodies now are used widely as reagents in immunoassay techniques.[3] The usual method of production of monoclonal antibodies involves fusing of sensitized lymphocytes from the spleens or lymph nodes of immunized mice with a murine myeloma cell line from tissue culture (an immortal B-cell line). The murine myeloma cell lines most commonly used are deficient in the enzyme hypoxanthine guanine phosphoribosyl transferase (HGPRT) and therefore do not synthesize purine bases from thymidine and hypoxanthine in the presence of aminopterin. After the fusion, the cells are placed into a selection medium containing hypoxanthine, aminopterin, and thymidine (HAT medium) to grow selectively fused hybrid cell lines. The fused hybrid cells will survive in a HAT medium because the cells combine the immortality of the myeloma cell with the genetic material of the spleen cell necessary for synthesis of HGPRT. Colonies arising from the fused cells then are screened for antibody production, and those cell lines secreting antibody of the desired specificity are cloned in subcultures. Thus a single clonal line is then isolated that produces an antibody with a specificity for a single antigen epitope and with a single binding energy or affinity.

Monoclonal antibodies provide an analytical advantage in that two different antibody specificities are used in a single assay. For example, a solid phase antibody specific for a unique epitope and another labeled antibody specific for a different epitope are reacted with antigen in a single incubation step. This combination eliminates (1) the two-step sequential

addition of antigen and labeled antibody to the solid phase, (2) one incubation step, and (3) one washing step, which would be necessary when polyclonal antibodies binding to both sites are used. However, the unique ability of a monoclonal antibody to react with a single epitope on a multivalent antigen results in an inability of most monoclonal antibodies to cross-link and precipitate macromolecular antigens. Thus monoclonal antibodies are not applicable for all immunoassays in the clinical laboratory, especially those that use traditional precipitin methods.

Phage-display technology is a different in vitro approach for the production of antibodies that mimic the immune system.[11] Through this process, genes coding for the heavy and light chain variable domains of immunoglobulin isolated from lymphocytes are amplified by the polymerase chain reaction (PCR) and ligated into a filamentous bacteriophage vector to form combinatorial libraries of V_H and V_L genes. Individual *bacteriophages* display copies of a specific antibody on their surface, and the phage library then is screened for antibody of defined specificity through the use of immobilized antigen ("panning"). This technique mimics immune selection, and antibodies with different binding specificities are isolated. Through this process, large libraries displaying more than 10^{12} antibodies have been formed.

Antigen-Antibody Binding

In this section, several of the factors that affect the binding of antigens and antibodies are discussed.

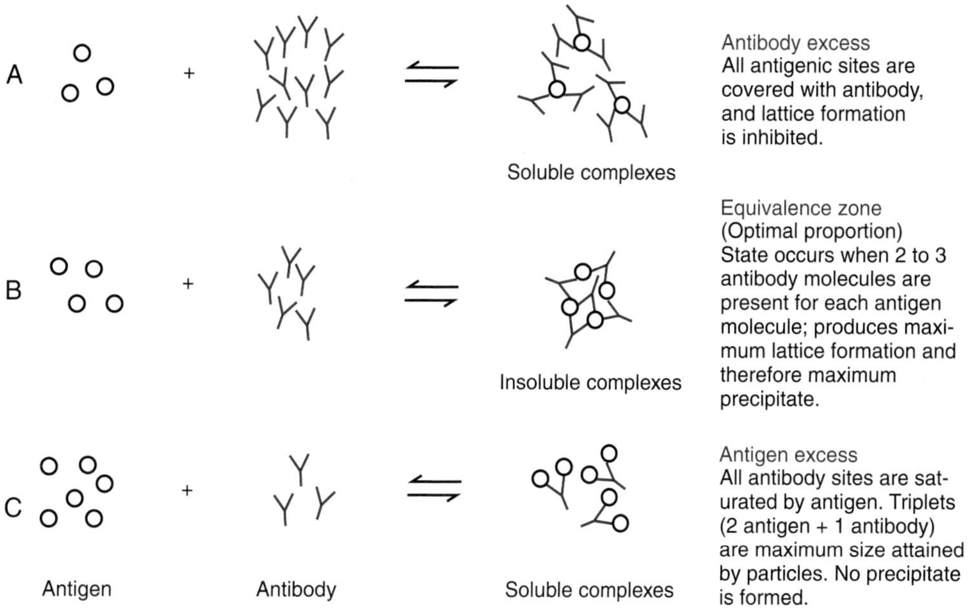

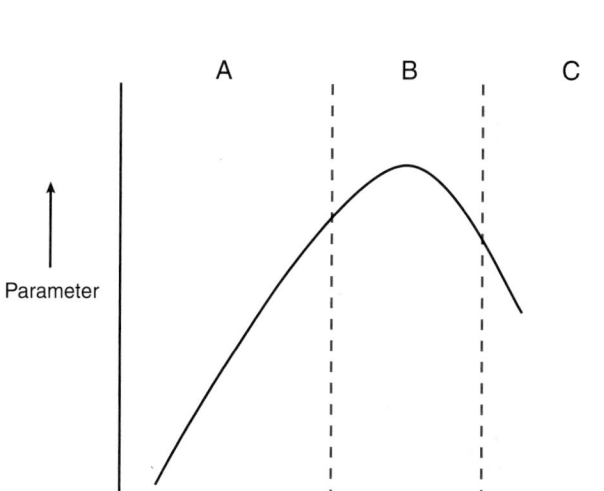

Antibody excess
All antigenic sites are covered with antibody, and lattice formation is inhibited.

Soluble complexes

Equivalence zone
(Optimal proportion)
State occurs when 2 to 3 antibody molecules are present for each antigen molecule; produces maximum lattice formation and therefore maximum precipitate.

Insoluble complexes

Antigen excess
All antibody sites are saturated by antigen. Triplets (2 antigen + 1 antibody) are maximum size attained by particles. No precipitate is formed.

Soluble complexes

Figure 15-2 Schematic diagram for precipitin reaction. **A,** Antibody excess. **B,** Equivalence zone. **C,** Antigen excess.

Antigen   Antibody

Binding Forces

Several forces act cooperatively to produce antigen-antibody binding. The three major contributing forces are (1) electrostatic van der Waals–London dipole-dipole interactions, (2) hydrophobic interactions, and (3) ionic coulombic bonding (primarily between COO^- and NH_4^+ groups on the antigen and the antibody).

Reaction Mechanism

The binding of antigen to antibody is not static but is an equilibrium reaction that proceeds in three phases. The initial reaction (phase 1) of a multivalent antigen (Ag_n) and a bivalent antibody (Ab) occurs very rapidly in comparison with subsequent growth of the complexes (phase 2) and is depicted by the following equation:

$$Ag_n + Ab \underset{k_{-1}}{\overset{k_1}{\rightleftharpoons}} Ag_n Ab \underset{k_{-2}}{\overset{k_2}{\rightleftharpoons}} Ag_a Ab_b \qquad (1)$$

where $k_1 >>> k_2$, n is the number of epitopes per molecule, and a and b are the numbers of antigen and antibody molecules per complex. Phase 3 of the reaction involves the precipitation of the complex after a critical size is reached. The speed of these reactions depends on electrolyte concentration, pH, and temperature, as well as on antigen and antibody types and the binding affinity of the antibody.

Precipitin Reaction

If the number of antibody combining sites [Ab] is significantly greater than the number of antigen binding sites [Ag], then antigen binding sites are quickly saturated by antibody before cross-linking occurs, and the formation of small antigen/antibody complexes of the composition AgAb results (Figure 15-2, A). For the case in which antibody is in moderate excess ([Ab] > [Ag]), the probability of cross-linking of Ag by Ab is more likely, hence large complex formation is favored (Figure 15-2, B).

Figure 15-3 Schematic diagram of precipitin curve illustrating different antigen concentration zones. **A,** Antibody excess. **B,** Equivalence. **C,** Antigen excess. The parameter measured may be the quantity of protein precipitated, light scattering, or another measurable parameter. Antibody concentration is held constant in this example.

In the case in which [Ag] is in great excess, large complexes are less probable, and the theoretical minimum size of complexes is Ag_2Ab (Figure 15-2, C).

This model describes the results observed when antigens and antibodies are mixed in various concentration ratios. The curve shown in Figure 15-3 is a schematic diagram of the classic precipitin curve. Although the concentration of total antibody is constant, the concentration of free antibody, $[Ab]_f$, and of free antigen, $[Ag]_f$, varies for any given Ag/Ab ratio. A low Ag/Ab ratio exists in Figure 15-3, A (zone of antibody excess). Under these conditions, $[Ab]_f$ exists in solution, but $[Ag]_f$ does not. As total antigen increases, the size of the immune complexes increases up to equivalence (Figure 15-3, B), where little or no $[Ab]_f$ or $[Ag]_f$ exists. This is the zone of equivalence, and it is the optimal combining ratio for cross-linking in the particular system under examination. As Ag/Ab increases (Figure 15-3, *C*), the immune complex size decreases and $[Ag]_f$ increases (zone of antigen excess).

Chemical Factors

Chemical factors that influence antibody-antigen binding include ionic species, ionic strength, and polymeric molecules.

Ion Species and Ionic Strength Effects

Cationic salts produce inhibition of the binding of antibody with a cationic hapten. The order of inhibition by various cations is $Cs^+ > Rb^+ > NH_4^+ > K^+ > Na^+ > Li^+$. This order corresponds to the decreasing ionic radius and the increasing radius of hydration. For anionic haptens and anionic salts, the order of inhibition of binding is $CNS^- > NO_3^- > I^- > Br^- > Cl^- > F^-$, again in the order of decreasing ionic radius and increasing radius of hydration.

Polymer Effect

The addition of a linear polymer to a mixture of antigen and antibody causes a significant increase in the rate of immune complex growth and enhances the precipitation of immune complex, especially with low-avidity antibody. Numerous polymer species, such as (1) dextran (a high-molecular-weight polymer of D-glucose), (2) polyvinyl alcohol, and (3) polyethylene glycol 6000 (PEG or Carbowax), have been used in immunochemical methods. The most desirable characteristics of the polymer are high (1) molecular weight, (2) degree of linearity (minimum branching), and (3) aqueous solubility. PEG 6000 has these characteristics and is particularly useful in immunochemical methods at concentrations of 3 to 5 g/dL.

Qualitative Methods

Immunochemical techniques used for qualitative purposes include (1) passive gel diffusion, (2) immunoelectrophoresis (IEP), and (3) western blotting.

Passive Gel Diffusion

Many qualitative and quantitative immunochemical methods are performed in semisolid media, such as agar or agarose. This practice stabilizes the diffusion process with regard to mixing caused by vibration or convection and allows visualization of precipitin bands for qualitative and quantitative evaluation of the reaction. Antigen/antibody ratio, salt concentration, and polymer enhancement have the same influence on the antigen-antibody reaction in gels as they have on reactions in solution.

If the matrix does not interact with the molecular species under investigation, passive diffusion of reactants in a semisolid matrix is described by Fick's equation

$$\frac{dQ}{dt} = -DA\frac{dc}{dx} \qquad (2)$$

where

dQ = amount of diffusing substance that passes through area A during time t;

dt = change in time;

dC/dx = concentration gradient; and

D = diffusion coefficient.

The diffusion coefficient, D, is a direct function of temperature; it is inversely proportional to the hydrated molecular volume of the diffusing species. The ratio dQ/dt is a function of dC/dx, the concentration gradient. The amount of diffusing species transferred from the origin to a distant point (over the migration distance) is dependent on the length of time diffusion is allowed to occur.

The initial concentrations of antigen and antibody are critical. Each molecule in the system achieves a unique concentration gradient with time. When the leading fronts of antigen and antibody diffusion overlap, the reaction begins, but formation of a precipitin line does not occur until moderate antibody excess is achieved. A precipitin band may form and be dissolved many times by incoming antigen before equilibrium is established and the position of the precipitin band is stabilized.

Simple diffusion and double diffusion are the two basic approaches used for qualitative applications of passive diffusion. In simple diffusion, a concentration gradient is established for only a single reactant. This approach, which is called *single immunodiffusion,* usually depends on diffusion of an antigen into agar impregnated with antibody. A quantitative technique based on this principle is called **radial immunodiffusion** (RID).

In the second approach, which is called *double diffusion,* a concentration gradient is established for both antigen and antibody (Figure 15-4). This approach is known as the **Ouchterlony technique.** In practice, it permits direct comparison of two or more test materials and provides a simple and direct method by which to determine whether antigens in the test specimens are (1) identical, (2) cross-reactive, or (3) nonidentical.

Immunoelectrophoresis

Immunoelectrophoresis (IEP) is an analytical technique that combines separation of antigens by electrophoresis with immunodiffusion against an antiserum. It is used in a clinical laboratory to separate and identify the various protein species contained in a common solution, such as serum or spinal fluid. This technique has been used extensively for the study of antigen mixtures and for the evaluation of human gammopathies. Proteins in the serum are separated according to their electrophoretic mobility (Figure 15-5). After electrophoresis, an antiserum against the protein of interest is placed in a trough parallel and adjacent to the electrophoresed sample. Simultaneous diffusion of the antigen from the separated sample and of antibody from the trough results in the formation of precipitin arcs with shapes and positions characteristic of the individual separated proteins in the specimen.

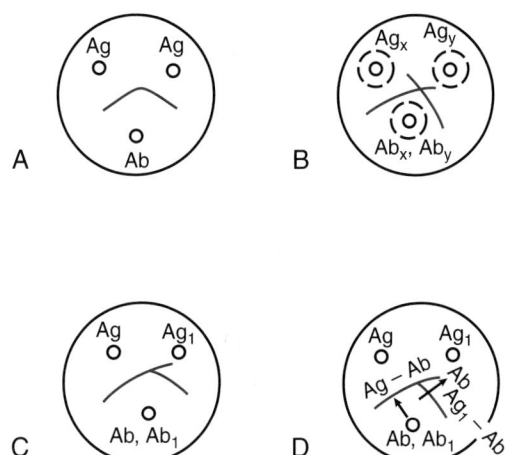

Figure 15-4 Double immunodiffusion in two dimensions by the Ouchterlony technique. Sample is placed in each Ag circular well. Antibodies or serum is placed in each Ab circular well. At the completion of the reaction, the antigen/antibody complex is visualized as a precipitated line. **A,** Reaction of identity; a single continuous line of precipitation is noted. The two samples have the same antigen(s) recognized by the antibody placed in the Ab circular well; the samples are antigenically identical. **B,** Reaction of nonidentity; two lines briefly overlap but appear to be independent. The two samples Ag_x and Ag_y are different antigens that react with their respective antibodies Ab_x and Ab_y; no cross-reaction is seen. **C,** Reaction of partial identity; two lines partially join and a "spur" is formed. The two samples have some epitopes that overlap, but complete identity does not occur. **D,** Scheme for spur formation. *Ab,* Antibody; *Ag,* antigen.

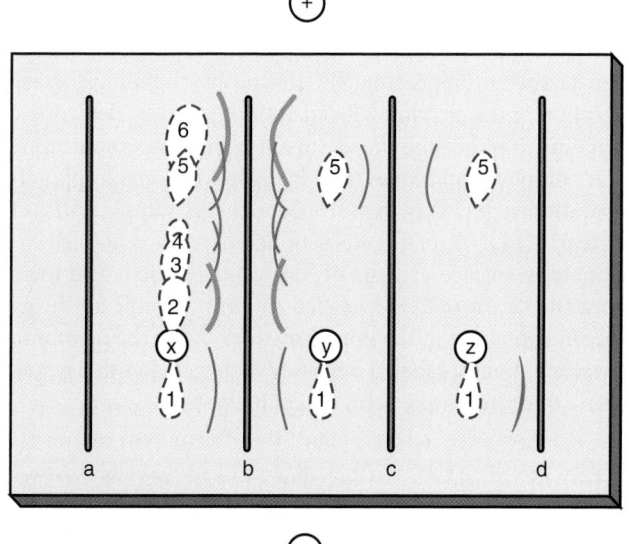

Figure 15-5 Configuration for immunoelectrophoresis. Sample wells are punched in the agar/agarose (x, y, z), sample is applied, and electrophoresis is carried out to separate the proteins in the sample. Antiserum is loaded into the troughs, and the gel is incubated in a moist chamber at 4 °C for 24 to 72 hours. Track *x* represents the shape of the protein zones after electrophoresis; tracks *y* and *z* show the reaction of proteins 5 and 1 with their specific antisera in troughs *c* and *d*. Antiserum against proteins 1 through 6 is present in trough *b*.

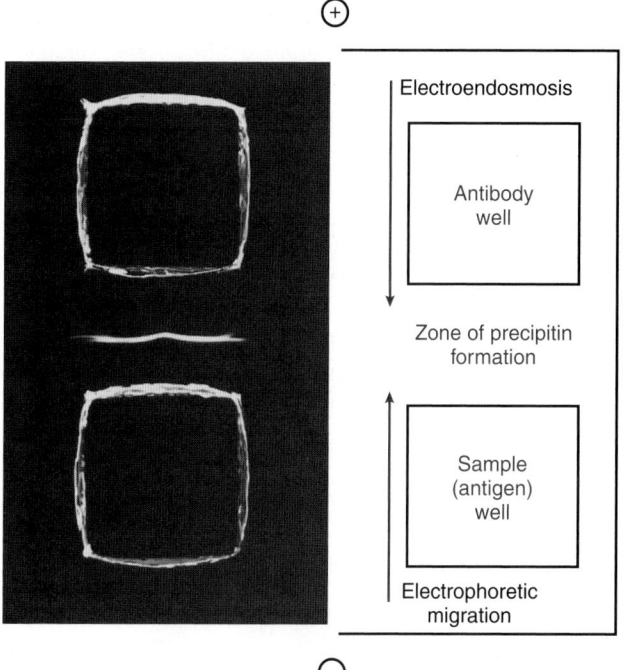

Figure 15-6 Counter immunoelectrophoresis showing a positive reaction between anti-*Haemophilus influenzae B (upper well)* and a cerebrospinal fluid (CSF) sample containing *H. influenzae B (lower well).*

In the clinical laboratory, this procedure has been applied to the evaluation of human myeloma proteins. However, the method gradually is being replaced by immunofixation electrophoresis, particularly in the study of protein antigens and their split products and in the evaluation of myeloma.

Crossed immunoelectrophoresis (CRIE, also known as *two-dimensional immunoelectrophoresis*) is a variation of IEP wherein electrophoresis is also used in the second dimension to drive the antigen into a gel containing antibodies specific for the antigens of interest.[5] In practice, CRIE is more sensitive and produces higher resolution than is possible with IEP. In counter immunoelectrophoresis (CIE), two parallel lines of wells are punched in the agar. One row is filled with antigen solution, and the opposing row is filled with antibody solution (Figure 15-6). Voltage is applied across the gel, causing antigen and antibody to move toward each other at a faster rate. A precipitin line is formed where they meet. This qualitative information is used to identify the antigen and is provided within 1 to 2 hours. CIE has found application in the detection of bacterial antigens in (1) blood, (2) urine, and (3) cerebrospinal fluid.

Immunofixation (IF) has gained widespread acceptance as an immunochemical method used to identify proteins. With this technique, electrophoresis is first performed in agarose gel to separate the proteins in the mixture. Subsequently, antiserum spread directly on the gel causes the protein(s) of interest to precipitate. The immune precipitate is trapped within the gel matrix, and all other nonprecipitated proteins are then removed by washing of the gel. The gel then is stained for identification of the proteins. In practice, however, CRIE is more

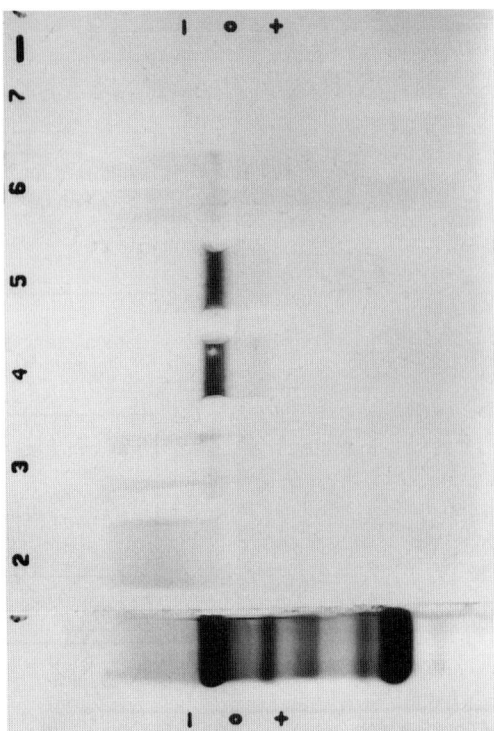

Figure 15-7 Immunofixation of a serum containing an immuno-globulin (Ig)M kappa paraprotein. *Lane 1,* Serum electrophoresis stained for protein; *lane 2,* Anti-IgG, Fc piece-specific; *lane 3,* Anti-IgA, α-chain–specific; *lane 4,* Anti-IgM, α-chain–specific; *lane 5,* Anti-κ light chain; *lane 6,* Anti-λ light chain. *(Courtesy Katherine Bayer, Philadelphia.)*

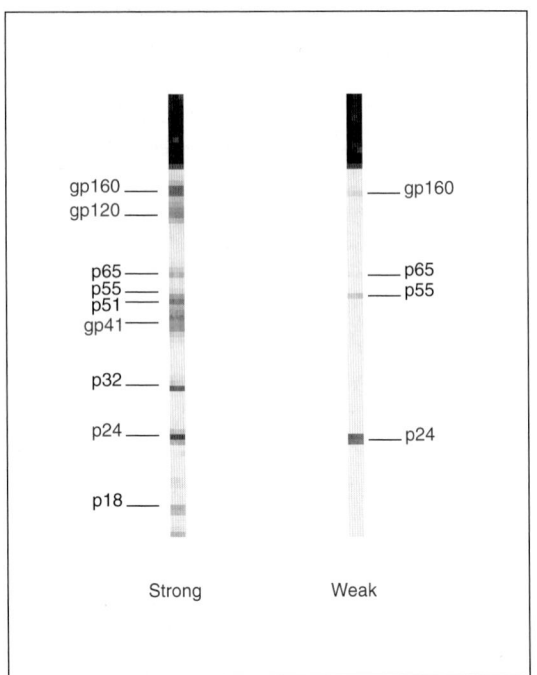

Figure 15-8 Blot analysis of serum samples strongly positive and weakly positive for human immunodeficiency virus (HIV)-1 antibody. Core proteins (GAG, group-specific antigens) p18, p24, and p55; polymerase (POL) p32, p51, and p65; and envelope proteins (ENV) gp41, gp120, and gp160. *(Courtesy Bio-Rad Laboratories Diagnostics Group, Hercules, Calif.)*

sensitive than IF in terms of limits of detection, and it demonstrates improved resolution. In addition, proteins of closely related or identical electrophoretic mobility are distinguished better by CRIE because in IF they appear as a single band. The utility of IF, which now is used widely for the evaluation of myeloma proteins, is illustrated in Figure 15-7.

Blotting

The previously discussed techniques use direct examination of immunoprecipitation of the protein(s) in the gel. However, certain media, such as polyacrylamide, do not lend themselves to direct immunoprecipitation, nor does sufficient antigen concentration always exist to produce an immunoprecipitate that is retained in the gel during subsequent processing. Under these circumstances, the technique of **Western blotting** is used. This technique involves an electrophoresis step, followed by transfer of the separated proteins onto an overlying strip of nitrocellulose or nylon membrane by a process called *electro-blotting*. Once the proteins are fixed to the membrane, they are detected with antibody probes labeled with molecules such as enzymes. With the use of such probes, the limits of detection are 10 to 100 times lower than the values obtained through direct immunoprecipitation and staining of proteins. This technique is analogous to *Southern blotting* (electrophoresed DNA blotted onto a membrane) and **Northern blotting** (electrophoresed RNA blotted onto a membrane).

An example of a blotting analysis for human immunodeficiency virus type 1 (HIV-1) antibodies is shown in Figure 15-8. When applied to antigen assays, concentrations of antigen as low as 500 ng/mL or 2.5 ng per band in the gel have been detected. The detection limit of the technique is lowered even farther to approximately 100 pg by chemiluminescent detection of the enzyme-labeled antibody and by detection of light emission through the use of X-ray or photographic film.[4]

A simpler technique that bypasses the electrophoretic separation step is known as **dot blotting**. A sample of the (1) protein, (2) DNA, or (3) RNA to be analyzed is applied to a membrane surface as a small "dot" and is dried. The membrane then is exposed to a labeled antibody specific for the test antigen contained in the dotted mixture. After the membrane is washed, bound-labeled antibody is detected with a photometric or chemiluminescent detection system.

Quantitative Methods

Immunochemical techniques have been used to develop quantitative methods and include (1) radial diffusion and electroimmunoassays, (2) turbidimetric and nephelometric assays, and (3) labeled immunochemical assays.

Radial Immunodiffusion (RID) and Electroimmunoassay

Radial immunodiffusion (RID) and electroimmunoassay are commonly used for quantitative immunochemical measurements. RID is a passive diffusion method in which

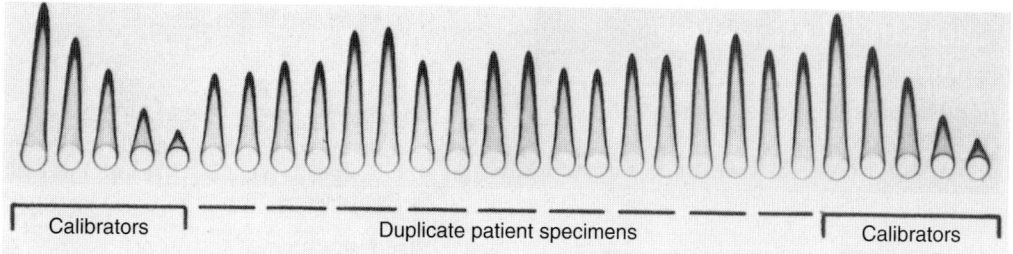

Figure 15-9 Rocket immunoelectrophoresis of human serum albumin. Patient samples were applied in duplicate. Calibrators were placed at opposite ends of the plate.

a concentration gradient is established for a single reactant, usually the antigen. The antibody is dispersed uniformly in the gel matrix. Antigen is allowed to diffuse from a well into the gel until antibody excess exists and immune precipitation occurs; a well-defined ring of precipitation around the well indicates the presence of antigen. The ring diameter continues to increase until equilibrium is reached. Calibrators are run simultaneous with the sample, and a calibration curve of ring area or diameter versus concentration is generated.

Electroimmunoassay (known as the "rocket" technique) is a type of immunoassay wherein a single concentration gradient is established for the antigen, and an applied voltage is used to drive the antigen from the application well into a homogeneous suspension of antibody in the gel (Figure 15-9). This process produces a unidirectional migration of antigen and results in a lowered limit of detection. The height of the resulting rocket-shaped precipitin line is proportional to the antigen concentration. Quantification is achieved through the processing of aliquots of calibrators and samples on the same plate Concentrations of the samples are subsequently estimated by comparing the height of the rockets obtained from the samples with a calibration curve generated from the heights of the rockets obtained from the calibrators. The calibration curve is linear only over a narrow concentration span; consequently, samples may have to be diluted or concentrated as necessary.

Turbidimetric and Nephelometric Assays

Turbidimetry and nephelometry are convenient techniques used to measure the rate of formation of immune complexes in vitro. Instrumental principles for these methods are described in Chapter 9. Studies have shown that the reaction between antigen and antibody begins within milliseconds and continues for hours. The performance of both types of assays has been improved significantly by increases in the reaction rate attained by the addition of water-soluble linear polymers.

Both turbidimetric and nephelometric immunochemical methods using rate and pseudoequilibrium protocols have been described for (1) proteins, (2) antigens, and (3) haptens. In rate assays, measurements usually are made early in the reaction because the largest change (dI_s/dt) in intensity of scattered light (I_s) with respect to time is attained during this time interval. For pseudoequilibrium assays, waiting 30 to 60 minutes is necessary so that the dI_s/dt is small relative to the time required to make the necessary measurements.

(*Note:* Such assays are termed *pseudoequilibrium* rather than *equilibrium* because true equilibrium is not reached within the time allowed for these assays.)

Nephelometric methods in general are more sensitive than turbidimetric assays and have a lower limit of detection of approximately 1 to 10 mg/L for a serum protein. Lower limits of detection are attained in fluids such as cerebrospinal fluid and urine because of their lower lipid and protein concentrations, which result in a higher signal-to-noise ratio. In addition, for low-molecular-weight proteins such as myoglobin (MW 17,800 Da), limits of detection have been lowered through a latex-enhanced procedure based on antibody-coated latex beads.

Nephelometric and turbidimetric assays have also been applied to the measurement of drugs (haptens) with the use of inhibition techniques. To make the reagent, the drug of interest is attached to a carrier molecule, such as bovine serum albumin. The hapten-bound albumin then competes with free hapten (drug introduced in the sample) for antihapten-antibody. In the presence of free hapten, immune complex formation is decreased because more antibody sites are saturated; thus light scattering is decreased. The decrease in light scattering is related to the concentration of free hapten. Both kinetic and pseudoequilibrium methods have been described. In the absence of free hapten, bound hapten-albumin reacts with available antihapten-antibody sites to form cross-linked immune complexes with high light-scattering abilities.

Labeled Immunochemical Assays

The previously discussed methods rely on examination of the immune complex formation as an index of antigen-antibody reaction. As demonstrated in equation (1), the overall reaction occurs in sequential phases, and only the final phase consists of formation of the immune complex. However, initial binding of antibody and antigen has been used with antigens and antibodies that have **labels** to develop many sensitive and specific immunochemical assays. The reaction describing this initial binding and the kinetic constant for the overall reaction are shown in equations (3a) and (3b), respectively.

$$Ab + Ag \underset{k_{-1}}{\overset{k_1}{\rightleftharpoons}} AbAg \tag{3a}$$

$$K = \frac{[AbAg]}{[Ab][Ag]} \tag{3b}$$

TABLE 15-1	Labels Used for Nonisotopic Immunoassay
Chemiluminescent	Acridinium ester, sulfonyl acridinium ester, isoluminol
Cofactor	Adenosine triphosphate, flavin adenine dinucleotide
Enzyme	Alkaline phosphatase, marine bacterial luciferase, β-galactosidase, firefly luciferase, glucose oxidase, glucose-6-phosphate dehydrogenase, horseradish peroxidase, lysozyme, malate dehydrogenase, microperoxidase, urease, xanthine oxidase
Fluorophore	Europium chelate, fluorescein, phycoerythrin, terbium chelate
Free radical	Nitroxide
Inhibitor	Methotrexate
Metal	Gold sol, selenium sol, silver sol
Particle	Bacteriophage, erythrocyte, latex bead, liposome, quantum dot
Phosphor	Up-converting lanthanide-containing nanoparticle
Polynucleotide	DNA
Substrate	Galactosyl-umbelliferone

where

k_1 = rate constant for the forward reaction;
k_{-1} = rate constant for the reverse reaction; and
K = equilibrium constant for the overall reaction.

As predicted from the law of mass action, the concentrations of Ab, Ag, and Ab:Ag are dependent on the magnitude of k_1 and k_{-1}. For polyclonal antiserum, the average avidity of the antibody populations determines K, and the magnitude of k_1 in comparison with k_{-1} determines the ultimate limit of detection attainable with a given antibody population.

Types of Labels

In the decade following the pioneering developments of Yalow and Berson,[12] all immunoassays used radioactive labels in competitive assays. Since the introduction of enzyme immunoassays in the 1970s, sophisticated assays with nonisotopic labels (Table 15-1)[7] have been developed.

Methodological Principles

To capitalize on the exquisite specificity and enhanced sensitivity of immunochemical assays, various methodological principles have been applied in their development. These include competitive and noncompetitive reaction formats and different processing schemes for performing assays.

Competitive Versus Noncompetitive Reaction Formats

As shown in Figure 15-10, the two major types of reaction formats used in immunochemical assays are termed *competitive* (limited reagent assays) and *noncompetitive* (excess reagent, two-site, or sandwich assays).

Competitive Immunoassays. In a competitive immunochemical assay, all reactants are simultaneously or sequentially mixed together. In the simultaneous approach, labeled antigen

Competitive (limited reagent)

Simultaneous

Ab + Ag + Ag–L $\rightleftharpoons$ Ab:Ag + Ab:Ag–L
(free)   (bound)

Sequential

Step 1 Ab + Ag $\underset{k_{-1}}{\overset{k_1}{\rightleftharpoons}}$ Ab:Ag + Ab

Step 2 Ab:Ag + Ab + Ag–L $\rightleftharpoons$ Ab:Ag + Ab:Ag–L + Ag–L

Noncompetitive (excess reagent, two-site, sandwich)

▨–Ab $\xrightarrow{+\ Ag}$ ▨–Ab:Ag $\xrightarrow{+\ Ab–L}$ ▨–Ab:Ag:Ab–L

Figure 15-10 Immunoassay designs. *Ab,* Antibody; *Ag,* antigen; *k_1,* forward rate constant; *k_{-1},* reverse rate constant; *L,* label.

(Ag*) and unlabeled antigen (Ag) compete to bind with the antibody. In such a system, the avidity of the antibody for labeled and unlabeled antigen must be the same. Under these conditions, the probability of the antibody binding the labeled antigen is inversely proportional to the concentration of unlabeled antigen, hence bound label is inversely proportional to the concentration of unlabeled antigen.

In a sequential competitive assay, unlabeled antigen is mixed with excess antibody and binding allowed to reach equilibrium (Figure 15-10, *step 1*). Labeled antigen is then added sequentially (Figure 15-10, *step 2*) and allowed to equilibrate. After separation, the bound label is measured and is used to calculate the unlabeled antigen concentration. With this two-step method, a larger fraction of unlabeled antigen is bound by the antibody than that fraction in the simultaneous assay, especially at low antigen concentrations. Consequently, a twofold to fourfold lowering of the detection limit is seen in a sequential immunoassay, compared with that in a simultaneous assay, provided $k_1 \gg k_{-1}$. This improvement in detection limit results from an increase in AgAb binding (and thus a decrease in Ag* binding), which is favored by the sequential addition of Ag and Ag*. If $k_1 \geq k_{-1}$, dissociation of AgAb becomes more probable, resulting in increased competition between Ag* and Ag. A typical immunochemical binding curve is shown in Figure 15-11.

Noncompetitive Immunoassays. In a typical noncompetitive assay, the "capture" antibody is first passively adsorbed or covalently bound to the surface of a solid phase. Next, the antigen from the sample is allowed to react and is captured by the solid phase antibody. Other proteins then are washed away, and a labeled antibody (conjugate) is added that reacts with the bound antigen through a second and distinct epitope. After additional washing to remove the excess unbound labeled antibody, the bound label is measured, and its concentration or activity is directly proportional to the concentration of antigen.

In noncompetitive assays, either polyclonal or monoclonal, antibodies are used as capture and labeled antibodies. If monoclonal antibodies with specificity for distinct epitopes

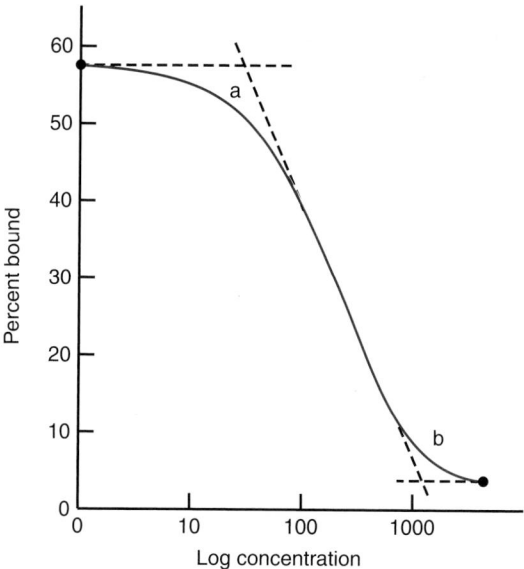

Figure 15-11 Schematic diagram of the dose-response curve for a typical immunoassay. The analytically useful portion of the curve is bracketed by points *a* and *b*.

are used, simultaneous incubation of the sample and the conjugate with the capture antibody is possible, thus simplifying the assay protocol.

Noncompetitive immunoassays are performed in simultaneous or sequential mode. In the simultaneous mode, a high concentration of analyte saturates both capture and labeled antibodies. Under these conditions, the analyte is present in such high concentrations that it reacts simultaneously with the capture and labeled antibodies, reducing the number of complexes formed and producing a falsely low result. Thus the calibration curve of the assay exhibits a "**hook effect**," in which the assay response drops off at high analyte concentrations in assays for analytes for which the normal pathological concentration range is very wide. For example, assays for chorionic gonadotropin (CG) and alpha fetoprotein (AFP) are particularly prone to this problem. Dilutions of a sample usually are reanalyzed to check for this type of analytical interference. In practice, the hook effect is eliminated if a sequential assay format is adopted and the concentrations of capture and labeled antibody are sufficiently high to cover analyte concentrations over the entire analytical range of the assay.

Heterogeneous Versus Homogeneous Immunochemical Assays
Immunochemical assays that require separation of the free from the bound label are termed **heterogeneous immunoassays**. **Homogeneous immunoassays** do not require separation.

Heterogeneous Immunoassays. Heterogeneous immunoassays implicitly assume that $k_1 \gg k_{-1}$, and several physical separation techniques (Box 15-1) are used to separate the free, labeled (Ag^*) from the bound, labeled antigen ($Ag^*{:}Ab$).

Precipitation of the bound, labeled antigen ($Ag^*{:}Ab$) from the reaction mixture is achieved chemically or immunologically. Chemically, a protein-precipitating chemical, such as $(NH_4)_2SO_4$, is added. Immunologically, a second,

"precipitating" antibody is added. In liquid phase adsorption, the free antigen is adsorbed onto particles of activated charcoal or dextran-coated charcoal that are added directly to the reaction mixture. The particles of charcoal and the adsorbed antigen then are removed by allowing the particles to settle or by performing centrifugation.

Solid phase adsorption is a widely used separation technique. With this method, binding and competition of labeled and unlabeled antigens for the binding sites of the antibody occur on the surface of a solid support. On the surface of this support, the capture antibody is attached by physical adsorption or by covalent bonding. Several different types of solid support are used, including (1) the inner surface of plastic tubes or wells of microtiter plates and (2) the outer surface of insoluble materials, such as cellulose or magnetic latex beads or particles.

Homogeneous Immunoassays. Homogeneous immunoassays do not require separation of bound and free labeled antibody or antigen.[8] In this type of assay, the activity of the label attached to the antigen is modulated directly by antibody binding. The magnitude of the modulation is proportional to the concentration of the antigen or antibody being measured. Consequently, it is necessary only to incubate the sample containing the analyte antigen with the labeled antigen and antibody and then directly measure the activity of the label "in place," making these assays technically easier and faster.

Immunoassay Calibration
Calibration of an immunoassay involves performing an assay of a series of calibrators with known values and fitting a straight line or curve to the resulting data to link the signal to concentration over the assayed range. This dose-response curve is then used to determine the concentration of analyte in the sample. Joining successive points in a calibration curve is usually achieved by means of an appropriate mathematical equation. Several curve-fitting methods are in use. Interpolation methods join successive points by straight lines (linear

TABLE 15-2	Detection Limits for Isotopic and Nonisotopic Immunoassay Labels	

Label	Detection Limit in Zeptomoles* (10^{-21} moles)	Method
Alkaline phosphatase	50,000	Photometry
	300	Time-resolved fluorescence
	100	Fluorescence
	10	Enzyme cascade
	1	Chemiluminescence
β-D-galactosidase	5000	Chemiluminescence
	1000	Fluorescence
Europium chelate	10,000	Time-resolved fluorescence
Glucose-6-phosphate dehydrogenase	1,000	Chemiluminescence
^{3}H	1,000,000	Scintillation
Horseradish	2,000,000	Photometry
peroxidase	1	Chemiluminescence
^{125}I	1000	Scintillation
Ruthenium (II) tris(bipyridyl)	20†	Electrochemiluminescence

*One zeptomole = 10^{-3} attomoles or 10^{-6} femtomoles.
†Personal communication.

interpolation) or curved lines (curvilinear interpolation). When the latter approach is used, a cubic polynomial (y = a + bx + cx$_2$ + dx$_3$) links the response (y) to the calibrator concentration (x), and the best fit is attained through a series of recalculations (iterations) that smooth the joints between the curves linking successive points on the curve. The resulting equation is called a *spline function*. Empirical curve-fitting methods use different mathematical models, including (1) hyperbolic, (2) polynomial, and (3) log-logit and its variants (e.g., four-parameter log-logistic), to calculate a curve to fit the calibration data.

It should be appreciated that a source of error with all curve-fitting methods is the uncertainty of the shape of the curve between successive calibrators and the imprecision in the measurement of each calibrator. Imprecision may not be constant over the concentration range represented by the calibrators, and in this case the response variable is termed *heteroscedastic*.

Analytical Detection Limits

The analytical limits of detection of competitive immunoassays are determined principally by the affinity of the antibody. Calculations have indicated that a lower limit of detection of 10 fmol/L (i.e., 600,000 molecules of analyte in a typical sample volume of 100 μL) is possible in a competitive assay when an antibody with an affinity of 10^{12} mol/L is used.

For noncompetitive immunoassays, the ability of the detector to measure the label determines the detection limit of an assay. Table 15-2 illustrates the detection limits for noncompetitive immunoassays when isotopic and nonisotopic labels are used. A radioactive label, such as ^{125}I, has low specific activity (7.5 million labels necessary for detection of 1 disintegration/s) compared with enzyme labels and chemiluminescent and fluorescent labels. Enzyme labels provide an amplification (each enzyme label producing many detectable

product molecules), and the detection limit for an enzyme is lowered if the conventional photometric detection is replaced with chemiluminescent or bioluminescent detection. The combination of amplification and an ultrasensitive detection reaction makes noncompetitive chemiluminescent enzyme immunoassays among the most sensitive types of immunoassays. Fluorescent labels also have high specific activity; a single high–quantum-yield fluorophore is capable of producing 100 million photons/s. In practice, several factors degrade the detection limit of an immunoassay. These include (1) background signal from the detector, (2) assay reagents, and (3) nonspecific binding of the labeled reagent.

Secondary labels such as biotin are used to introduce amplification into an immunoassay. The binding constant of the biotin/avidin complex is extremely high (10^{15} mol/L). This high binding allows for the design of immunoassay systems that are even more sensitive than the simple antibody systems. Such a biotin/avidin system uses a biotin-labeled first antibody. Biotin is attached to the antibody in relatively high proportion without loss of immunoreactivity of the antibody. When an avidin-conjugated label is added, a complex of Ag:Abbiotin:avidin label is formed. Further amplification is achieved by a biotin:avidin:biotin linkage because the binding ratio of biotin:avidin is 4:1 (e.g., Ag:Ab-biotin:avidin:[3 biotin labels]). If the label is an enzyme, large numbers of enzyme molecules in the complete complex provide a large increase in enzymatic activity, coupled with the small amount of antigen being determined, and the antigen assay is correspondingly more sensitive. Other tactics that have been used to lower the analytical detection limits of immunoassays include the use of streptavidin-thyroglobulin conjugates and macromolecular complexes of multiple-label thyroglobulin and streptavidin-thyroglobulin. With these reagents, thyroglobulin acts as a carrier for multiple labels (e.g., Eu^{3+}), and amplification factors of several thousand are achieved.

BOX 15-2 Examples of Other Nonisotopic Immunoassays

Bioluminescent Immunoassays

Native or recombinant apoaequorin (from the bioluminescent jellyfish *Aequorea*) is used as the label. It is activated by reaction with coelenterazine, and light emission at 469 nm is triggered by reaction with calcium ions (calcium chloride).

Erenna Immunoassay

The Erenna Immunoassay System uses a modified microparticle-based sandwich immunoassay and single-molecule counting technology. It integrates capillary flow, laser-induced fluorescence, a highly sensitive detection optics module, and a 384-well plate format for sample analysis.

Fluorescence Excitation Transfer Immunoassay

Homogeneous competitive assay in which a fluorophore (donor)-labeled antigen competes with an antigen in the sample for binding sites on an antibody labeled with a fluorescent dye (acceptor). The fluorescence of the donor is quenched when it is bound to the acceptor-labeled antibody.

Immuno-PCR

Heterogeneous immunoassay in which a piece of single- or double-stranded DNA is used as a label for an antibody in a sandwich assay. Bound DNA label is amplified using the polymerase chain reaction (PCR). The amplified DNA product is separated by gel electrophoresis and is quantitated by densitometric scanning of an ethidium-stained gel.

Nanotechnology-Based Assays

A variety of immunoassays employ nanoparticles, spheres, or tubes as solid phases.

Luminescent Oxygen Channeling Immunoassay (LOCI)

Homogeneous sandwich immunoassay in which an antigen links an antibody-coated sensitizer dye-loaded particle (250 nm diameter) and an antibody-coated particle (250 nm diameter) loaded with a mixture of a precursor of a chemiluminescent compound and a fluorophore. Irradiation produces singlet oxygen at the surface of the sensitizer dye–loaded particle. This diffuses ("channels") to the other particle held in close proximity by the immunochemical reaction between antigen and antibodies on the particles. The singlet oxygen reacts with the chemiluminescent compound precursor in the particle to form a chemiluminescent dioxane, which then decomposes to emit light via a fluorophore-sensitized mechanism. No signal is obtained from precursor fluorophore-loaded particles that are not linked via immunological reaction with an antigen.

Phosphor Immunoassay

Heterogeneous immunoassay in which an up-converting phosphor nanoparticle is used as a label. The nanoparticle (200 to 400 nm diameter) is a crystalline lanthanide oxysulfide. It absorbs two or more photons of infrared light (980 nm) and produces light emission at a shorter wavelength (anti-Stokes shift). The phosphorescence is not influenced by reaction conditions (e.g., temperature, buffer), and no up-converted signal from biological components is present in the sample (low background). Multiplexing is possible because different types of particles produce different wavelengths of phosphorescence (e.g., yttrium/erbium oxysulfides are green [550 nm], yttrium/thulium oxysulfide particles are blue [475 nm]).

Quantum Dot Immunoassay

Heterogeneous immunoassay in which a nanometer-sized (<10 nm) semiconductor quantum dot is used as a label. A quantum dot is a highly fluorescent nanocrystal composed of CdSe, CdS, ZnSe, InP, or InAs or a layer of ZnS or CdS on, for example, a CdSe core. Multiplexing is possible with these labels because the emission properties can be modulated by changing the size and composition of the nanocrystal (e.g., CdS emits blue light, InP emits red light).

Solid Phase, Light-Scattering Immunoassay

Indium spheres are coated on glass to measure an antibody binding to an antigen. Binding of antibodies to antigens increases dielectrical layer thickness, which produces a greater degree of scatter than in areas where only an antigen is bound. Quantitation is achieved by densitometry.

Surface Effect Immunoassay

An antibody is immobilized on the surface of a waveguide (quartz, glass, or plastic slide, or a gold- or silver-coated prism), and binding of an antigen is measured directly by total internal reflection fluorescence, surface plasmon resonance, or attenuated total reflection.

Examples of Labeled Immunoassays

Specific examples of different types of labeled immunoassays are discussed in the following section. Others are described in Box 15-2.

Radioimmunoassay

Radioimmunoassays (RIAs) were developed in the 1960s and used radioactive isotopes of iodine, ^{125}I and ^{131}I, and tritium (^3H) as labels.[12] Combinations of labels (e.g., ^{57}Co, ^{125}I) have been used for simultaneous assays (e.g., vitamin B_{12} and folate). In practice, competition between radiolabeled and unlabeled antigen or antibody in an antigen-antibody reaction is used to analytically determine the concentration of the unlabeled antigen or antibody. It takes advantage of the specificity of the antigen-antibody interaction and the ability to measure very low quantities of radioactive elements. RIAs have been used to determine the concentration of antibodies or any antigen against which a specific antibody is produced. When used to measure the concentration of an antigen, RIA requires that the antigen be available in a pure form and be labeled with a radioactive isotope. An alternative assay design uses labeled antibody (e.g., immunoradiometric assay [IRMA]) and does not require purified antigen because the antigen need not be labeled. This obviates potential problems that may be caused by iodination of labile antigens. Antibodies are more stable proteins and are easier to label without damage to the function of the protein.

Nonseparation RIAs have also been developed that are based on the modulation of a tritium or ^{125}I label by microparticles loaded with a scintillant.[6] These scintillation proximity assays have found routine application in high-throughput screening assays used for drug discovery.

Although they were once popular, the use of RIAs in clinical laboratories has declined primarily because of concerns over safe handling and disposal of radioactive reagents and waste.

Enzyme Immunoassay

Enzyme immunoassay (EIA) uses the catalytic properties of enzymes to detect and quantify immunological reactions. Enzymes such as (1) alkaline phosphatase (ALP), (2) horseradish peroxidase (HRP), (3) glucose-6-dehydrogenase (G6D), and (4) β-galactosidase are commonly used as labels in EIA.

Various detection systems have been used to monitor EIAs. Assays that produce compounds that are monitored photometrically are widely used and have been automated. EIAs that use fluorogenic or chemiluminogenic substrates are also popular because their measurement is inherently sensitive. Enzyme cascade reactions have been applied to the detection of enzyme labels in EIA; the principle of a cascade assay for ALP is illustrated in Figure 15-12. The advantage of such an assay is that it combines the amplification properties of two enzymes—the ALP label and the alcohol dehydrogenase in the assay reagent, thereby producing an extremely sensitive assay (see Table 15-2).

Examples of EIA include (1) enzyme-linked immunosorbent assay (ELISA), (2) enzyme-multiplied immunoassay technique (EMIT), and (3) cloned enzyme donor immunoassay (CEDIA).

Enzyme-Linked Immunosorbent Assay. ELISA is a heterogeneous EIA technique. With this type of assay, one of the reaction components is attached to the surface of a solid phase, such as that of a microtiter well. This attachment may consist of nonspecific adsorption or chemical or immunochemical bonding and facilitates separation of bound and free labeled reactants. Typically, with ELISA, an aliquot of sample or calibrator containing the antigen to be measured is added to and allowed to bind with a solid phase antibody. After the solid phase has been washed, an enzyme-labeled antibody different from the bound antibody is added and forms a "sandwich complex" of solid phase–Ab:Ag:Ab enzyme. Excess (unbound) antibody then is washed away, and enzyme substrate is added. The enzyme label then catalyzes the conversion of substrate to product(s), the amount of which is proportional to the quantity of antigen in the sample. Antibodies in a sample also are quantified through the use of an ELISA procedure in which antigen instead of antibody is bound to a solid phase, and the second reagent is an enzyme-labeled antibody specific for the analyte antibody. For example, in a microtiter plate format, ELISA assays have been used extensively for detection of antibodies to viruses and parasites in serum or whole blood. In addition, enzyme conjugates coupled with substrates that produce visible products have been used to develop ELISA-type assays with results that are interpreted visually. Such assays have been very useful in (1) screening, (2) point-of-care, and (3) home testing applications.

Enzyme-Multiplied Immunoassay Technique. EMIT is a homogeneous EIA (Figure 15-13).[8] Because it does not require a separation step, an EMIT assay is simple to perform and has been used to develop a wide variety of (1) drug, (2) hormone, and (3) metabolite assays. EMIT-type assays are automated easily and are included in the repertoire of the most automated clinical and immunoassay analyzers.

With the EMIT technique, the antibody against the analyte (1) drug, (2) hormone, or (3) metabolite is added together with substrate to the patient's sample. Binding of the antibody and the analyte then occurs. An aliquot of the enzyme conjugate of the analyte drug, hormone, or metabolite then is added as a second reagent; the enzyme-analyte conjugate then binds with the excess analyte antibody, forming an antigen/antibody complex.

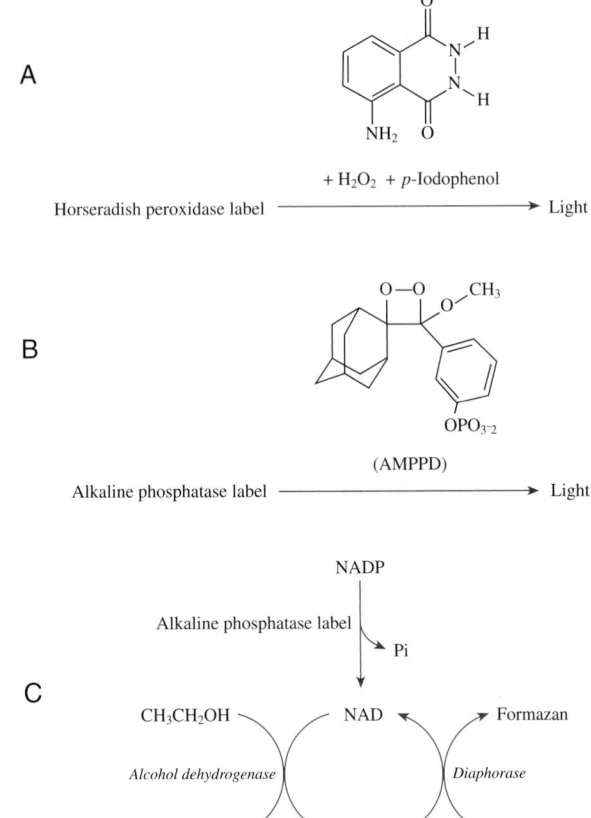

Figure 15-12 Ultrasensitive assays for horseradish peroxidase and alkaline phosphatase labels. **A,** Chemiluminescent assay for horseradish peroxidase label using luminol. **B,** Chemiluminescent assay for an alkaline phosphatase label using AMPPD (disodium 3-(4-methoxyspiro[1,2-dioxetane-3,2′-tricyclo[3.3.1.1]-decan]4-yl)phenyl phosphate). **C,** Photometric assay for an alkaline phosphatase label using a cascade detection reaction. *INT,* p-Iodonitrotetrazolium violet.

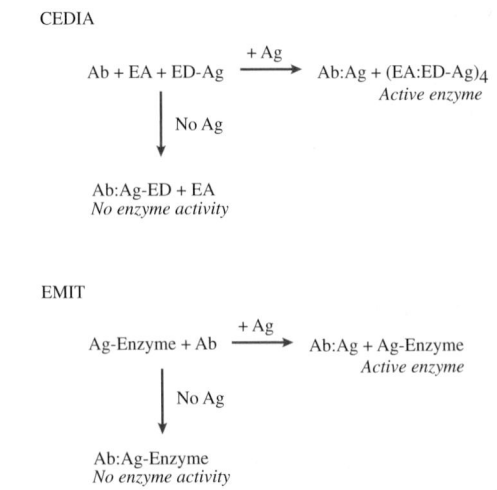

Figure 15-13 Cloned enzyme donor immunoassay and enzyme-multiplied immunoassay technique for homogeneous immunoassays. *Ab,* Antibody; *Ag,* antigen; *EA,* enzyme acceptor; *ED,* enzyme donor; *SP,* scintillant-filled microparticle.

TABLE 15-3 Properties of Fluorescent Labels

Fluorophore	Excitation, nm	Emission, nm	Fluorescence Quantum Yield*	Lifetime, ns
Fluorescein isothiocyanate	492	520	0.0-0.85	4.5
Europium (β-naphthoyl trifluoroacetone)	340	590,613	—	500,000
Lucifer yellow VS	430	540	—	—
Phycobiliprotein	550-620	580-660	0.5-0.98	—
Rhodamine B isothiocyanate	550	585	0.0-0.7	3.0
Umbelliferone	380	450	—	—

*Fluorescence quantum yield: fraction of molecules that emit a photon.

This binding of the analyte antibody with the enzyme-analyte conjugate affects the enzyme and alters its activity. The relative change in enzyme activity is proportional to the analyte concentration in the patient's sample. Concentration of the analyte is calculated from a calibration curve prepared by analysis of calibrators that contain known quantities of analyte.

Cloned Enzyme Donor Immunoassay. CEDIA is a second type of homogeneous EIA (see Figure 15-13). It was the first EIA designed and developed through the use of genetic engineering techniques.[7] With this technique, inactive fragments (the enzyme donor and acceptor) of β-galactosidase are prepared by manipulation of the Z gene of the *lac* operon of *Escherichia coli*. These two fragments spontaneously reassemble to form active enzyme even if the enzyme donor is attached to an antigen. However, binding of an antibody to the enzyme donor-antigen conjugate inhibits reassembly, thereby blocking the formation of active enzyme. Thus competition between antigen and the enzyme donor-antigen conjugate for a fixed amount of antibody in the presence of the enzyme acceptor modulates the measured enzyme activity. High concentrations of antigen produce the least inhibition of enzyme activity; low concentrations, the greatest.

Fluoroimmunoassay

Fluoroimmunoassay (FIA) uses a fluorescent molecule as an indicator label to detect and quantify immunological reactions. Examples of fluorophores used as labels in FIA and their properties are listed in Table 15-3. An early problem with FIA was that background fluorescence from within the sample limited its utility. This problem has been overcome by the use of time-resolved immunoassay techniques that use chelates of rare earth (lanthanide) elements as labels (see Chapter 9). These techniques are based on the fact that fluorescent emissions from lanthanide chelates such as (1) europium, (2) terbium, (3) samarium have long lives (>1 μs) compared with the typical background fluorescence encountered in biological specimens. In a time-resolved FIA, a europium chelate label is excited by a pulse of excitation light (0.5 μs), and the long-lived fluorescence emission from the label is measured after a delay (400 to 800 μs); by this time, any short-lived background signal has decayed.

Fluorescent polarization immunoassay is a type of homogeneous FIA that is used widely (Figure 15-14). With this

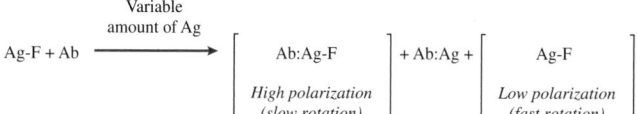

Figure 15-14 Homogeneous polarization fluoroimmunoassay. *Ab*, Antibody; *Ag*, antigen; *F*, fluorescein.

technique, the polarization of the fluorescence from a fluorescein-antigen conjugate is determined by its rate of rotation during the lifetime of the excited state in solution. A small, rapidly rotating fluorescein-antigen conjugate has a low degree of polarization; however, binding to a large antibody molecule slows the rate of rotation and increases the degree of polarization. Thus binding to antibody modulates polarization. The change in polarization is measured and related to antigen concentration.

Another type of nonseparation FIA uses a multilayer device to eliminate the need for separation of bound and free fractions. The device consists of two agarose layers separated by an opaque layer of iron oxide. Sample is added to the upper (10 μm) layer and diffuses through the iron oxide (10 μm) layer to the thin (1 μm) signal layer, which contains antibody:antigen/rhodamine complexes. Antigen-rhodamine conjugate is displaced from the signal layer by antigen within the sample and diffuses into the upper layer. Residual bound antigen-rhodamine conjugate in the signal layer is measured by front surface fluorometry. Displaced free conjugate does not contribute to the signal because it is shielded from the fluorescence excitation light by the iron oxide layer. As listed in Box 15-2, many other types of homogeneous FIAs have been developed.

Chemiluminescent Immunoassay

Chemiluminescence is the light emission produced during a chemical reaction (see Chapter 9). In a chemiluminescent immunoassay, a chemiluminescent molecule is used as an indicator label to detect and quantify immunological reactions. Acridinium esters are examples of chemiluminescent labels. Oxidation of an acridinium ester by alkaline hydrogen peroxide in the presence of a detergent (e.g., Triton X-100) produces a rapid flash of light at 429 nm. Acridinium esters are high–specific activity labels (detection limit for the label being 800 zeptomoles) that have been used to label both antibodies and haptens (Figure 15-15, *A*).

A

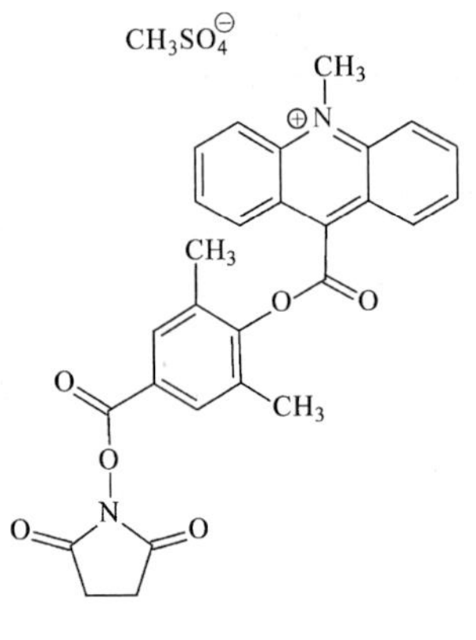

B

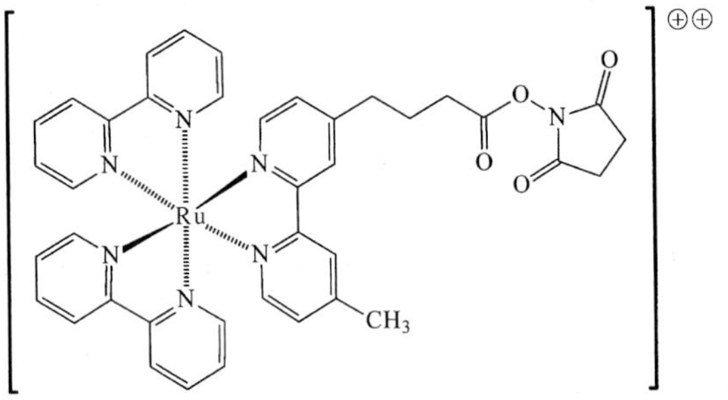

Figure 15-15 Luminescent labels. **A,** Chemiluminescent acridinium ester label. **B,** Electrochemiluminescent ruthenium (II) tris(bipyridyl) NHS (*N*-hydroxysuccinimide) ester label. (*A, From Law S-J, Miller T, Piran U, et al: Novel poly-substituted aryl acridinium esters and their use in immunoassay. J Biolum Chemilum 1989;4:88-98.*)

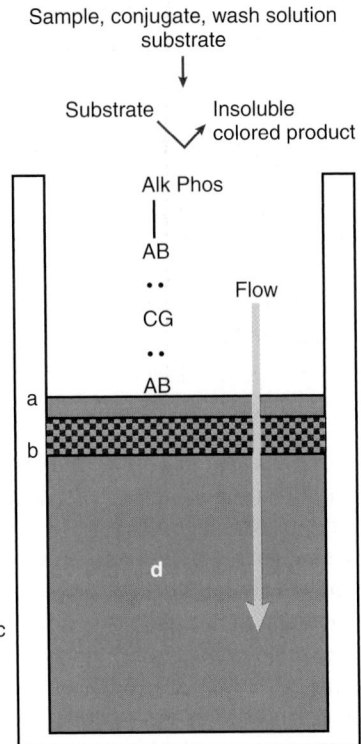

Figure 15-16 ICON immunoassay device illustrating immobilized antibody membrane *(a)*, separating membrane *(b)*, container *(c)*, and adsorbent pad *(d)*. *AB,* Monoclonal antibody to CG; *Alk Phos,* alkaline phosphatase; *CG,* human chorionic gonadotropin.

Electrochemiluminescence Immunoassay

In an electrochemiluminescence immunoassay, an electrochemiluminescence molecule, such as ruthenium, is used as an indicator label in competitive and sandwich immunoassays. In such assays, ruthenium (II) tris(bipyridyl) (Figure 15-15, *B*) undergoes an electrochemiluminescent reaction (620 nm) with tripropylamine at an electrode surface. With this label, various assays have been developed in a flow cell, with magnetic beads as the solid phase. Beads are captured at the electrode surface, and unbound label is washed from the cell by a wash buffer. Label bound to the bead undergoes an electrochemiluminescent reaction, and the light emission is measured by an adjacent photomultiplier tube.

Simplified Immunoassays

The integration of technical advances made in molecular immunology with those made in the material and processing sciences has resulted in the development of several "simplified" immunoassays for use in physicians' offices or in the home (see Chapter 17). Early efforts were directed toward pregnancy and fertility testing and were based on agglutination and inhibition of agglutination using labeled red blood cells or latex particles in a slide format. Subsequently, sandwich immunoassays have been adapted for similar applications. For example, as listed in the package insert, the ICON II pregnancy test (Beckman

Coulter, Fullerton, Calif) is an operationally simple and sensitive assay for human chorionic gonadotropin (CG) that has a lower limit of detectiony of 10 mIU/mL for serum and 20 mIU/mL for urine. As shown in Figure 15-16, the ICON II test is a sandwich EIA device that uses a murine monoclonal antibody, which is immobilized onto the surface of a microporous nylon membrane located on top of an adsorbent pad. The pad functions as a capillary pump to draw liquid through the membrane. To perform an analysis, an aliquot of urine is added to the surface of the membrane; CG is removed as liquid is drawn through it, resulting in the removal of CG in the sample by its binding to the capture antibody on the membrane. Next, a matched murine monoclonal anti-CG antibody ALP conjugate is added and is allowed to drain into the adsorbent pad. Wash solution is then added, followed by an indoxyl phosphate substrate. Bound conjugate converts this to an insoluble indigo dye, which appears as a discrete blue spot. The second generation of the ICON test includes two additional control zones. An immobilized anti-ALP zone acts as a procedural control; it binds the ALP conjugate and appears as a blue spot. A further zone contains an immobilized irrelevant murine monoclonal antibody; this detects the presence of heterophile antibodies in samples, particularly human antimouse antibodies. These mimic antigen and bridge the capture and conjugated mouse antibodies, thus yielding what appears to be a positive result.

Other point-of-care testing (POCT) devices require only the addition of sample, simplifying the assay protocol and minimizing possible malfunction resulting from operator error. The TestPack Plus (Iverness Medical International, Cranfield, United Kingdom) is a one-step pregnancy test that illustrates the general principles of the new devices. It uses colloidal selenium particles (160 nm in diameter) labeled with monoclonal anti-α-CG antibody, which is red and is easily visible. Sample (urine) is applied to the sample well and soaks into a glass fiber pad containing the conjugate. Any CG in the urine sample combines with the selenium-labeled antibody, and the mixture migrates along a nitrocellulose track to a region where a line of polyclonal anti-CG antibody and an orthogonal line of anti-α-CG:CG complex have been immobilized. The complex captures unreacted selenium-labeled anti-α-CG to form a minus sign visible in the viewing window. If CG was present in the urine sample, then the selenium-labeled anti-α-CG:CG complexes bind to the immobilized polyclonal anti-CG, and a plus sign is formed, denoting a positive result. The remainder of the reaction mixture migrates to the end of the track and reacts with a Quinaldine red pH indicator in an "end-of-assay" window to signal that the flow in the device has functioned correctly. Variants of this type of device use antibody-coated beads loaded with blue dye and include a microspectrophotometer that reads the blue line and displays on a built-in LCD screen a result of "Pregnant" or "Not pregnant" based on the intensity of the blue line (e.g., Clearblue Digital Pregnancy Test; SPD Swiss Precision Diagnostics GmbH, Geneva, Switzerland).

Nanoparticle Immunoassay

In one type of highly sensitive nanoparticle immunoassay, the conjugate is a gold nanoparticle that is coated with both capture antibody and hundreds of carrier-oligonucleotides hybridized to its complementary oligonucleotide (biobarcodes). Isolated complexes (magnetic particle-capture antibody:antigen:capture antibody-gold nanoparticle-carrier oligonucleotides) are heated to release the biobarcode oligonucleotides from the carrier oligonucleotides attached to the gold nanoparticles. The biobarcodes are then captured by an oligonucleotide immobilized on a slide surface, and the captured biobarcode is hybridized to a gold nanoparticle (13 nm in diameter) labeled detection probe. A final amplification procedure deposits silver (silver decoration) onto the gold nanoparticle labels attached to the detection probes and the silver-decorated gold nanoparticles detected by light scattering.

Simultaneous Multianalyte Immunoassays

Types of simultaneous multianalyte immunoassays in which two or more analytes are detected in a single assay are becoming increasingly popular both for routine immunoassays and in proteomic research. Two different strategies have been developed on the basis of discrete reaction zones (planar arrays or sets of microbeads) or combinations of different labels.[9]

For example, the Afinion AS100 Analyze is a POCT device (Alere, Waltham, Mass) that measures simultaneously several clinically-related analytes. For example, in the Alere Toxicology drug screen, discrete test zones are placed on a small piece of nylon membrane. Each test zone is composed of antibodies to a specific drug immobilized onto the membrane surface. This zone captures free gold sol-drug conjugate from the sample antidrug:antibody gold conjugate reaction mixture and appears as a purple band. A variant of this strategy uses small pieces of glass or plastic, onto which is spotted an array of capture antibody or antigen for different tests (e.g., antigen arrays for antinuclear antibody [ANA] testing). Yet another strategy uses combinations of distinguishable microbeads (e.g., Luminex beads have a unique fluorescent signature) in which each type of bead is coated with a different capture antibody or antigen. A panel of reagent beads is mixed with the sample and fluorescent detection reagents. Fluorescent measurements identify the different beads (via their fluorescence signature) and quantitate the signal caused by the captured analyte. The benefit of this approach consists of work simplification because all of the tests are performed simultaneously on the same array or in the same tube in the case of microbead-based assays.

Combinations of distinguishable labels, such as europium (613 nm, emission lifetime of 730 µs) and samarium (643 nm, emission lifetime of 50 µs) chelates, serve as the basis for quantitative simultaneous immunoassays. These two chelates have different fluorescence emission maxima and different fluorescence decay times and thus are distinguished easily from measurements at 613 nm, delay time 0.4 ms (europium), and 643 nm, delay time 0.05 µs (samarium). Two examples of clinically useful combined assays using these differences in fluorescence wavelengths and delay times are combined free and bound prostate-specific antigen and combined myoglobin and carbonic anhydrase III.

Protein Microarrays

Arrays of hundreds or thousands of micrometer-sized dots of antigens or antibodies immobilized on the surface of a glass or plastic chip are emerging as an important tool in genomic studies and in assessment of protein-protein interactions.[9] This format facilitates simultaneous multianalyte immunoassays using, for example, enzyme- or fluorophore-labeled conjugates. The arrays are made by printing or spotting 1-nL drops of protein solutions onto a flat surface, such as a glass microscope slide. In a typical sandwich assay, the array on the surface of the slide is incubated with sample and then with conjugate. Bound conjugate is detected using chemiluminescence or fluorescein using a scanning device. The pattern of the signal provides information on the presence and quantities of individual analytes in the sample or the reactivity of a single analyte with the range of proteins arrayed on the surface of the slide.

Interferences

A particular problem that has been recognized for sandwich immunoassays is an interference caused by circulating human antibodies that react with animal immunoglobulins, particularly human antimouse antibodies (HAMAs). This type of antibody causes positive or negative interferences in two-site antibody-based sandwich assays that use mouse monoclonal capture antibody reagents. HAMAs cause false positive interference by bridging between a mouse immunoglobulin capture antibody and a mouse immunoglobulin conjugate, thus mimicking the specific analyte. A false negative result is thought to be caused by HAMA reacting with one of the assay reagents (immobilized antibody or the conjugate) and preventing formation of the sandwich with specific analyte.

HAMAs often are present in the blood of patients who have received mouse monoclonal antibody imaging or therapeutic agents. They also occur because of exposure to mouse antigens (e.g., as a result of handling mice). Nonimmune mouse serum usually is included in mouse monoclonal antibody-based immunoassays to complex HAMAs. However, despite this precaution, reactivity leading to false positive or false negative results still is encountered. The presence of HAMAs and other antianimal antibodies is uncovered by dilution experiments because samples containing antianimal antibodies do not give proportional results. Reanalysis of a sample after incubation with an animal protein or serum (e.g., mouse IgG, mouse serum for HAMA) can also reveal and confirm an interference.

Other Immunochemical Techniques

Other analytical methods of clinical interest that employ antibodies include cytochemical and agglutination assays.

Immunocytochemistry

Labeled antibody reagents are used as specific probes for protein and peptide antigens to examine single cells for synthetic capability and for specific markers for identification of various cell lines. Immunochemistry has been expanded rapidly by immunoenzymatic methods, such as HRP-labeled (immunoperoxidase) assays. Enzyme labels provide several advantages over fluorescent labels. First, they permit the use of fixed tissues (unembedded or embedded in paraffin), which provides excellent preservation of cell morphology and eliminates the problem of autofluorescence from tissue. Second, immunoperoxidase stains are permanent, and only a standard light microscope is needed to identify labeled features. Immunoperoxidase methods also are applicable in electron microscopy.

Immunochemical Agglutination Assays

Agglutination is the "clumping" together in suspension of antigen-bearing cells, microorganisms, or particles in the presence of specific antibodies, also known as *agglutinins*. Assays based on agglutination have been used for many years for the qualitative and quantitative measurement of antigens and antibodies. The visible clumping of particulates, such as cells and latex particles, is used to indicate the primary reaction of antigen and antibody. Agglutination methods require (1) stable and uniform particulates, (2) pure antigen, and (3) specific antibody. IgM antibodies are more likely to produce complete agglutination than are IgG antibodies because of the size and valence of the IgM molecule. Therefore when only IgG antibodies are

involved, the use of chemical enhancement or an antiglobulin-agglutination method may be necessary. As with all immunochemical reactions in which aggregation is the measured end point, the ratio of antigen to antibody is critical. Extremes in antigen or antibody concentration inhibit aggregation.

Hemagglutination describes an agglutination reaction in which the antigen is located on an erythrocyte. Erythrocytes are good passive carriers of antigen; they also are coated easily with foreign proteins and are easily obtained and stored. Direct testing of erythrocytes for blood group, Rh, and other antigenic types is used widely in blood banks. Specific antisera, such as anti-A, anti-C, and anti-Kell, are used to detect such antigens on the erythrocyte surface. In indirect or passive hemagglutination, the erythrocytes are used as particulate carriers of foreign antigen (and in some tests, of antibody); this technique has wide applications. Other materials available in the form of fine particles, such as latex, have been used as antigen carriers, but they are more difficult to coat, standardize, and store. In a related variation of this technique, known as *hemagglutination inhibition*, the ability of antigens, haptens, or other substances to inhibit specifically hemagglutination of sensitized (coated) cells by antibody is determined.

In general, agglutination methods are quite sensitive but not as quantitative as the other immunochemical methods discussed previously. Nonisotopic immunoassays, especially EIAs, are as convenient as agglutination reactions and therefore are replacing agglutination methods in many laboratories.

Review Questions

1. The component of an immunoassay that determines the analytical sensitivity and specificity of the reaction is the:
   a. labeled antigen.
   b. antigen.
   c. immunochemical label.
   d. antibody.
2. The energy of interaction of a single antibody-combining site and its corresponding epitope on the antigen is referred to as:
   a. sensitivity.
   b. specificity.
   c. immunogenicity.
   d. affinity.
3. The type of immunochemical assay that requires separation of the free label from the bound labeled substance is the:
   a. homogeneous assay.
   b. heterogeneous assay.
   c. competitive assay.
   d. simplified immunoassay.
4. An example of a simultaneous multianalyte immunoassay would be a(n):
   a. counter immunoelectrophoresis for myeloma proteins.
   b. nephelometric assessment of spinal fluid proteins.
   c. antigen array for antinuclear antibody testing.
   d. sandwich immunoassay using multiple antibodies.

5. An example of a qualitative immunochemical technique would be:
   a. immunoelectrophoresis.
   b. enzyme-multiplied immunoassay technique.
   c. radial immunodiffusion.
   d. nephelometry.

6. The addition of a linear polymer such as dextran to a mixture of antigen and antibody causes_____ in the rate of immune complex formation and precipitation.
   a. a decrease
   b. an increase
   c. no change

7. Transferring electrophoretically separated proteins into a strip of nylon membrane by electro-blotting is the second step in:
   a. radial immunodiffusion.
   b. enzyme-linked immunosorbent assay.
   c. western blotting.
   d. immunofixation.

8. In a two-site antibody-based sandwich immunoassay, the presence of human antimouse antibodies produces a false negative result by:
   a. binding a mouse immunoglobulin capture antibody and the mouse immunoglobulin conjugate to form a bridge.
   b. mimicking the specific analyte being assessed.
   c. binding to the mouse monoclonal capture antibody reagents.
   d. reacting with one of the assay reagents to prevent formation of the sandwich.

9. An immunoassay procedure that involves the coating of a solid phase with antibody or antigen is:
   a. enzyme-multiplied immunoassay technique (EMIT).
   b. enzyme immunoassay.
   c. enzyme-linked immunosorbent assay (ELISA).
   d. affinity immunoassay.

10. The immunoglobulin most often used in immunochemical assays is:
    a. IgG.
    b. IgA.
    c. IgM.
    d. IgE.

References

1. Diamandis EP, Christopoulos TK. Immunoassay. San Diego: Academic Press, 1996.
2. Gosling JP. Immunoassays: a practical approach. Oxford: Oxford Press, 2000.
3. Kohler G, Milstein C. Continuous cultures of fused cells secreting antibody of predefined specificity. Nature 1975;256:495–7.
4. Kricka LJ. Chemiluminescent and bioluminescent techniques. Clin Chem 1991;37:1472–81.
5. Laurell CB. Antigen-antibody crossed electrophoresis. Anal Biochem 1965;10:358–61.
6. Picardo M, Hughes KT. Scintillation proximity assays. In: Devlin JP, ed. High throughput screening. New York: Marcel Dekker, 1997:307–16.
7. Price CP, Newman DJ, eds. Principles and practice of immunoassay, 2nd edition. New York: Stockton Press, 1997.
8. Rubenstein KE, Schneider RS, Ullman EF. "Homogeneous" enzyme immunoassay: new immunochemical technique. Biochem Biophys Res Commun 1972;47:846–51.
9. Schena M. Protein microarrays. Sudbury, Mass: Jones and Bartlett, 2005.
10. Wild D, ed. The immunoassay handbook, 3rd edition. San Diego: Elsevier, 2005.
11. Winter G. Synthetic human antibodies and a strategy for protein engineering. FEBS Lett 1998;430:92–4.
12. Yalow RS, Berson SA. Assay of plasma insulin in human subjects by immunological methods. Nature 1959;184:1648–69.

James C. Boyd, M.D., and Charles D. Hawker, Ph.D., M.B.A., F.A.C.B.

Objectives

1. Define the following terms:

Automation	Integrated automation
Carry-over	Multiple/single-channel analysis
Closed-system analyzer	Open-system analyzer
Continuous-flow analysis	Random-access analysis
Discrete analysis	Unit operations
Instrument cluster	

2. List four benefits of automation use in the clinical laboratory.
3. Describe the steps involved in the completion of an automated analysis; state the problems encountered in each step and how these are resolved.
4. Compare the following analyzer configurations with regard to specimen and reagent handling and processing:

Random-access	Continuous-flow
Sequential	Multiple-channel
Discrete	Single-channel

5. State five advantages of the use of bar-coded labels to identify a specimen.
6. State the benefit of using whole blood in an automated assay system.
7. Compare an "open" versus a "closed" automated analyzer with regard to reagent usage.
8. Describe six measurement approaches that are used with automated chemistry analyzers.
9. List and describe the three main data processing functions performed by a computer in an automated analyzer.
10. Describe two types of automated specimen processing operations.
11. List and describe the considerations that must be evaluated when an automated laboratory system is selected.
12. List the problems encountered when automated laboratory processes are used and integrated, including during specimen identification, specimen delivery, reagent identification, and the chemical reactant phases.

Key Words and Definitions

Automation The process whereby an analytical instrument performs many tests with only minimal involvement of an analyst; also defined as the controlled operation of an apparatus, process, or system by mechanical or electronic devices without human intervention.

Batch analysis Type of analysis in which many specimens are grouped in the same analytical session.

Carry-over The transport of a quantity of analyte or reagent from one specimen reaction into and contaminating a subsequent one.

Continuous-flow analysis Type of analysis in which each specimen in a batch passes through the same continuous stream at the same rate and is subjected to the same analytical reactions.

Discrete analysis Type of analysis in which the sample is aspirated into the sample probe and then is delivered, often with reagent, through the same orifice into a reaction cup or another container.

Multiple-channel analysis Type of analysis in which each specimen is subjected to multiple analytical processes so that a set of test results is obtained on a single specimen; similar to random-access analysis.

Parallel analysis Type of analysis in which all specimens are subjected to a series of analytical processes at the same time and in a parallel fashion.

Random-access analysis The most common configuration of an automated analyser, in which analyses are performed on a collection of specimens sequentially and each specimen is analyzed for a different selection of tests.

Sequential analysis Type of analysis in which each specimen in a batch enters the analytical process one after another, and each result or set of results emerges in the same order as the specimens are entered.

Single-channel analysis Type of analysis in which each specimen is subjected to a single process so that only results for a single analyte are produced; similar to batch analysis.

Throughput The number of specimens processed by an analyzer during a given period of time, or the rate at which an analytical system processes specimens.

Workstation A clinical laboratory workstation dedicated to a defined task and contains appropriate laboratory instrumentation to carry out that task.

The term **automation** has been applied in clinical chemistry to describe the process whereby an analytical instrument performs many tests with only minimal involvement of an analyst. The availability of automated instruments enables laboratories to process much larger workloads without comparable increases in staff. The evolution of automation in the clinical laboratory has paralleled that in the manufacturing industry, progressing from fixed automation, whereby an instrument performs a repetitive task by itself, to programmable automation, which allows the instrument to perform a variety of different tasks. *Intelligent automation* also has been introduced into some individual instruments or systems to allow them to self-monitor and respond appropriately to changing conditions.

One benefit of automation is a reduction in the variability of results and errors of analysis through elimination of tasks that are repetitive and monotonous for most individuals. The improved reproducibility gained by automation has led to a significant improvement in the quality of laboratory tests.

Many small laboratories now have consolidated into larger, more efficient entities in response to market trends involving cost reduction. The drive to automate these mega-laboratories has led to new avenues in laboratory automation. No longer is automation being used simply to assist the laboratory technologist in test performance; it now includes (1) processing and transport of specimens, (2) loading of specimens into automated analyzers, and (3) assessing the results of the tests performed. We believe that automating these additional functions is crucial to the future prosperity of the clinical laboratory.[1,3]

This chapter discusses the principles that apply to automation of the individual steps of the analytical process—both in individual analyzers and in the integration of automation throughout the clinical laboratory.

Basic Concepts

Automated analyzers generally incorporate mechanized versions of basic manual laboratory techniques and procedures. However, modern instrumentation is packaged in a wide variety of configurations. The most common configuration is the *random-access analyzer*. In **random-access analysis**, analyses are performed on a collection of specimens sequentially, with each specimen analyzed for a different selection of tests. The tests performed with random-access analyzers are selected through the use of different vials of (1) liquid reagents, (2) reagent packs, or (3) reagent tablets, depending on the analyzer. This approach permits measurement of variable numbers and types of analytes in each specimen. Profiles or groups of tests are defined for a specimen at the time the tests to be performed are entered into the analyzer (1) via a keyboard or touchscreen, (2) by instruction from a laboratory information system in conjunction with bar coding on the specimen tube, or (3) by operator selection of appropriate reagent packs.

Historically, other *analyzer configurations* used include continuous-flow, and centrifugal analyzers. Continuous-flow analyzers were the first automated analyzers used in clinical laboratories. Initially, these analyzers were used in a

---

BOX 16-1 Unit Operations in an Analytical Process

- Specimen identification
- Specimen preparation
- Specimen delivery
- Specimen loading and aspiration
- Specimen processing
- Sample introduction and internal transport
- Reagent handling and storage
- Reagent delivery
- Chemical reaction phase
- Measurement approaches
- Signal processing, data handling, and process control

---

single-channel analysis configuration to carry out a **sequential analysis** of each specimen. Subsequently, **multiple-channel analysis** versions were developed in which analysis of each specimen was performed on every channel in parallel. Results from nonrequested tests in the test profile were discarded as necessary after the analysis was complete. Inflexibility in the menu of tests that could be performed on these analyzers eventually led to their replacement in the marketplace by more versatile configurations.

Centrifugal analyzers use discrete pipetting to load *aliquots* of specimens and reagents sequentially into discrete chambers in a rotor, with the specimens subsequently analyzed in parallel (**parallel analysis**). Such analyzers are operated in a multiple-specimen/single-chemistry mode or in a single-specimen/multiple-chemistry mode.

Automation of Analytical Processes

The following individual steps required to complete an analysis often are referred to collectively as *unit operations* (Box 16-1). These operations are described individually in this section, and examples are provided that demonstrate how they have been automated in terms of operational and analytical performance. With most automated systems, these steps usually are performed sequentially, but with some instruments, they may occur in parallel.

Specimen Identification

Typically the identifying link (identifier) between patient and specimen is confirmed at the patient's bedside, and maintenance of this connection throughout (1) transport of the specimen to the laboratory, (2) subsequent specimen analysis, and (3) preparation of a report is essential. Several technologies are available for automatic identification and data collection purposes (Box 16-2). In practice, automatic identification consists of only those technologies that electronically detect a unique characteristic or a unique data string associated with a physical object. For example, identifiers such as (1) serial number, (2) part number, (3) manufacturer, and (4) assigned patient number have been used to identify an object or a patient through electronic data processing. In the clinical laboratory, labeling with a bar code has become the technology of choice for purposes of automatic identification.

- Bar coding
- Optical character recognition
- Magnetic stripe and magnetic ink character recognition
- Voice identification
- Radio frequency identification
- Touch screens
- Light pens
- Hand print tablets
- Optical mark readers
- Smart cards

Labeling

With many laboratory information systems, electronic entry of a test order in the laboratory or at a nursing station for a uniquely identified patient generates a specimen label bearing a unique laboratory accession number. A record is established that remains incomplete until a result (or a set of results) is entered into the computer against the accession number. The unique label is affixed to the specimen collection tube when the blood is drawn. Proper alignment of the label on the collection tube is critical for subsequent specimen processing when bar-coded labels are used. Arrival of the specimen to the laboratory is recorded by a computerized log-in procedure. With other systems, the specimen is labeled at the patient's bedside, patient identification and collection information is added, and the labeled specimen is sent to the laboratory along with a requisition form. Once in the laboratory, it is assigned a computer accession number as part of the log-in procedure.

After accessioning, specimens begin to undergo technical handling processes. For those processes that require physical removal of serum from the original tube, secondary labels bearing essential information from the original label must be affixed to any secondary tubes created. Some automated analyzers sample directly from the original collection tube while simultaneously reading the accession number from the bar-coded label on the tube. Secondary bar-coded labels, if necessary, may be generated at the time of accessioning or, with some analyzers, by a built-in printer that is activated when the analyzer is programmed.

Many methods are used to achieve secondary labeling when bar-coded labels are not available. A number may be handwritten on the specimen cup, or a coded label may be affixed to the original tube or to a specimen cup. Label numbers may require correlation with a manually prepared or computer-generated work or load list. The load list usually records accession numbers in sequence along with the physical positions of cups or tubes in the loading zone of the analyzer. This loading zone may consist of (1) a revolving tray or turntable, (2) a mechanical belt, or (3) a rack or a set of racks by which specimens are delivered in a predetermined order to the sample aspiration station of the analyzer.

For those analyzers that do not automatically link specimen identity and sample aspiration, the sequence of results produced must be linked manually with the sequence of entry of specimens. Some analyzers print out or transmit to a host computer each result or set of results from a specimen either through the position of the specimen in the loading zone or by the accession number programmed to that position.

Bar Coding

A major advance in the automation of specimen identification in the clinical laboratory is the incorporation of bar coding technology into analytical systems. In practice, a bar-coded label (often generated by the laboratory information system and bearing the sample accession number) is placed onto the specimen container and is subsequently "read" by one or more bar code readers placed at key positions in the analytical sequence. The resultant identifying and ancillary information is then transferred to and processed by the system software. Initiating bar code identification at a patient's bedside ensures greater integrity of the specimen's identity in an analyzer. Systems that transfer information concerning a patient's identity to blood tubes at the patient's bedside are now commercially avaiailble.

Unequivocal positive identification of each specimen is achieved by analyzers that contain bar code readers. Advantages of the use of coded labels include the following:

1. Elimination of work lists for the system.
2. Avoidance of mistakes in placement of the tubes into the analyzer or during sampling.
3. Analysis of specimens in random sequence.
4. Avoidance of possible tube mix-up when serum must be transferred to a secondary container.

The Clinical Laboratory and Standards Institute (CLSI) Standard AUTO02-A2 specifies that the bar code symbology that should be used in clinical laboratories for laboratory automation systems and for sample handling in automated instrumentation is Code 128.[6] The standard notes that the bar code symbologies Code 39, Codabar, NW7, and Interleaved 2 of 5 all should have been replaced by Code 128 by December 31, 2003.

Identification Errors

Many opportunities arise for the mismatch of specimens and results. Risks begin at the bedside and are compounded with each processing step that a specimen undergoes between collection from the patient and analysis by the instrument. The risks are particularly great when hand transcription is invoked for accessioning and labeling and relabeling, and for the creation of load lists. An incorrect accession number, one in which the digits are transposed, or a load list with transposed accession numbers may cause test results to be attributed to the wrong patient. An additional hazard exists when specimens must be inserted into certain positions in the loading zone as defined by a load list. Human misreading of specimen labels or loading lists may cause misplacement of specimens, calibrators, or controls. Automatic reading of bar-coded labels reduces the error rate from 1 in 300 characters (for human entry) to about 1 in 1 million characters.

Specimen Delivery

Several methods are used to deliver specimens to the laboratory, including (1) courier service, (2) pneumatic tube systems, (3) electric track vehicles, and (4) mobile robots.

Courier Service

Historically, couriers have been used to transport specimens from collection sites to the laboratory and between laboratories. Courier service, although generally reliable, has its drawbacks. Delivery is a batch process, and couriers usually service a given pickup point only at specified times. Arrangements for immediate pickup are possible but add costs to the analytical process and delay reporting of results. In addition, the risk of specimen breakage or loss is greater when specimens are handled manually.

Pneumatic Tube Systems

Pneumatic tube systems provide rapid specimen transportation and are reliable when installed as point-to-point services. However, when switching mechanisms are introduced to allow carriers (the bullet-shaped containers used to hold specimens) to be sent to various locations, mechanical problems in the switching process have been known to cause misrouting of carriers. In addition, close attention to the design of the pneumatic tube system is necessary to prevent hemolysis of the specimen. Avoidance of sudden accelerations and decelerations and the use of proper packing material inside the carriers will minimize hemolysis.

Electric Track Vehicles

Electric track vehicles have a larger carrying capacity than pneumatic tube systems and are not associated with problems such as damage to specimens caused by acceleration and/or deceleration forces. Some systems maintain the carrier in an upright position by using a gimbal (a device that permits a body to incline freely in any direction or suspends it so that it will remain level when its support is tipped), which enables the carrier to move both vertically and horizontally on an installed electric track. The larger carrying capacity of containers allows them to hold dry ice or refrigerated gel packs along with the specimens if desired.

Mobile Robots

Mobile robots from several vendors have been used successfully to transport laboratory specimens both within the laboratory and outside the central laboratory.[16] These robots are easily adapted to carry specimen containers of various sizes and shapes and are reprogrammable with changes in laboratory geometry. In addition, in a busy laboratory setting, delivery of specimens to lab benches by a mobile robot is usually more frequent than human pickup and has been shown to be cost-effective. Inexpensive models follow a line on the floor, whereas others use more sophisticated guidance systems. Limitations include the need to batch specimens (**batch analysis**) for greater efficiency and, in most cases, the requirement that laboratory personnel place specimens onto or remove specimens from the mobile robot at each stopping place.

Specimen Preparation

The (1) clotting of blood in specimen collection tubes, (2) their subsequent centrifugation, and (3) transfer of serum to secondary tubes require a finite time to complete. This process, if performed manually, delays the preparation of a specimen for analysis. To eliminate such delays in specimen preparation, various automated approaches have been developed.

Use of Whole Blood for Analysis

When whole blood is used in an assay system, specimen preparation time essentially is eliminated. Automated or semi-automated ion-selective electrodes, which measure ion activity in whole blood rather than ion concentration, have been incorporated into automated systems to provide certain test results within minutes of drawing a specimen. This approach now is used commonly for assays of electrolytes and some other common analytes. Another approach involves manual or automated application of whole blood to dry reagent films and visual or instrumental observation of a quantitative change (see Chapter 17).

Automation of Specimen Preparation

Several manufacturers have developed fully automated specimen preparation systems. (These systems will be described in later sections of this chapter.)

Specimen Loading and Aspiration

In most situations the specimen for automatic analysis is serum or plasma. Many analyzers sample directly from primary collection tubes of various sizes. With such analyzers, the collection tubes most frequently used contain separator material that forms a barrier between supernatant and cells (see Chapter 6).

Many analyzers also sample from cups or tubes filled with aliquots from the original specimen tubes. Often the design of the sampling cup is unique for a particular analyzer. Sample cups are designed to minimize dead volume—the excess amount of sample that must be present in a cup to permit aspiration of the full volume required for testing. Their shape should, even without a cap, minimize evaporation, and they should be made of inert material that does not interact with the analytes being measured.

Specimens may undergo other forms of degradation in addition to evaporation. Specimens that contain thermolabile constituents may undergo degradation of such analytes if held at ambient temperatures. Other constituents, such as bilirubin, are photolabile. Thermolability is minimized when both specimens and calibrators are held in a refrigerated loading zone. Photodegradation is reduced by the use of semi-opaque cups and by placement of smoke-colored or orange plastic covers over the specimen cups.

The loading zone of an analyzer is the area in which specimens are held inside the instrument before they are analyzed. The holding area may be a circular tray, a rack or series of racks built into a cassette, or a serpentine chain of containers into which individual tubes are inserted. When specimens are not identified automatically, they must be presented to the sampling device in the correct sequence, as specified by a loading list. The sampling mechanism determines the exact volume of sample removed from the specimen.

With many analyzers, specimens for a subsequent run may be prepared on a separate tray while one run is already in progress. This process permits machine operation and human actions to proceed in parallel for optimal efficiency. With other analyzers, specimens may be added continuously by the operator as they become available. A desirable feature of any automated analyzer is the ability to insert new specimens ahead of specimens already in place in the loading zone. This feature allows for the rapid analysis of specimens with high medical priority. With bar-coded specimens in random-access analyzers, it is possible for the operator to easily reposition specimens within the loading zone. When specimen identification is tied to a loading list, however, insertion or repositioning of specimens must be accompanied by revision of the loading list.

Transmission of infectious diseases by automated equipment is a matter of concern in clinical laboratories. The method of transmission by equipment primarily involves splatter of serum or blood from rapidly moving specimen probes during the acquisition of samples. The use of level sensors, which restrict the penetration of sample probes into specimens and provide smoother motion control, greatly reduces splatter.

Because the potential for contamination exists when the stoppers of primary containers are opened or "popped" to decant serum into specimen cups, several firms have developed closed-container sampling systems for use in their automated hematology and chemistry analyzers. With these systems, the specimen probe passes through a hollow needle that initially penetrates the primary container's rubber stopper. This configuration prevents damage to or plugging of the specimen probe, while allowing the level sensor (used to reduce carry-over and detect short sample) to remain active. After the specimen probe is withdrawn, the outer hollow needle is withdrawn so that the stopper reseals and no specimen escapes.

Specimen Processing

Automation of some analytical procedures requires the capability to remove proteins and other interferents from specimens and to separate free and bound fractions of heterogeneous immunoassays.

Removal of Protein and Other Interferents

The removal of proteins and other interferents from specimens is sometimes necessary to ensure the specificity of an analytical method. Procedures used to remove proteins and other interferents from specimens include (1) dialysis, (2) column chromatography, and (3) filtration.[2]

Separations in Immunoassay Systems

Automation of some immunoassay procedures requires the separation of free and bound fractions of heterogeneous immunoassays. To achieve this separation step, several automated immunoassay analyzers use bound antibodies or proteins in a solid-phase format. Through this approach, binding of antigens and antibodies occurs on a solid surface to which the antibodies or other reactive proteins have been adsorbed

or chemically bonded. Different types of solid phases are used, including (1) beads, (2) coated tubes, (3) microtiter plates, (4) magnetic and nonmagnetic microparticles, and (5) fiber matrices. Additional details on automated systems that use various solid phases are found in books by Wild[17] and Price and Newman.[15]

Sample Introduction and Internal Transport

The method used to introduce the sample into the analyzer and to provide its subsequent transport within the analyzer is the major difference between continuous-flow and discrete systems. With continuous-flow systems, the sample is aspirated through the sample probe into a stream of flowing liquid, from which it is transported to analytical stations in the instrument. In **discrete analysis,** an aliquot of the sample is aspirated into the sample probe and then is delivered, often with reagent, through the same orifice into an individual reaction cup or another container. Carry-over is a potential problem with both types of systems.

Continuous-Flow Analyzers

Of historical note, the Technicon Instruments Corporation (Tarrytown, New York) pioneered the use of peristaltic pumps and plastic tubing to advance the sample and reagents in **continuous-flow analysis.** Although these types of analyzers are no longer used owing to inflexibility in the test menu as outlined previously, the peristaltic pump still is used in some analyzers with ion-selective electrodes. Peristaltic pumps trap a "slug" of fluid between two rollers that occlude the tubing. As the rollers travel over the tubing, the trapped fluid is pushed forward and, as the leading roller lifts from the tubing, is added to the fluid.

Discrete Processing Systems

Positive–liquid displacement pipettes are used for sampling in most discrete automated systems in which (1) specimens, (2) calibrators, and (3) controls are delivered by a single pipette to the next stage in the analytical process.

A positive-displacement pipette may be designed for one of two operational modes: (1) to dispense only an aliquot of aspirated sample into the reaction receptacle, or (2) to flush out the aliquot together with diluent. Both systems use a plastic or glass syringe with a plunger, the tip of which usually is made of Teflon.

Pipettes may be categorized as (1) fixed-, (2) variable-, or (3) selectable-volume (see Chapter 9). Selectable-volume pipettes allow the selection of a limited number of predetermined volumes. In general, pipettes with selectable volumes are used in systems that allow many different applications, whereas fixed-volume pipettes usually are used for samples and reagents in instruments dedicated to the performance of only a small variety of tests.

Carry-over

Carry-over is defined as the transport of a quantity of analyte or reagent from one specimen reaction into a subsequent one. Because it erroneously affects the analytical results obtained from the subsequent reaction, carry-over needs to be minimized. Most manufacturers of discrete systems reduce carry-over by setting an adequate flush-to-specimen ratio and incorporating wash stations for the sample probe. As much as a 4:1 ratio of flush to specimen may be needed to limit carry-over to less than 1%, although advances in materials and in dispenser velocity control have permitted lower ratios. Appropriate choices of (1) sample probe material, (2) geometry, and (3) surface conditions also will reduce carry-over.

With some systems, carry-over has been reduced by flushing the internal and external surfaces of the sample probe with copious amounts of diluent. The outside of the sample probe in other instruments is wiped clean to prevent transfer of a portion of the previous specimen into the next specimen cup. In discrete systems with disposable reaction vessels and measuring cuvets, carry-over is caused by the pipetting system. In instruments with reusable cuvets or flow cells, carry-over may arise at each point through which samples pass sequentially. Disposable sample-probe tips eliminate both the contamination of one sample by another inside the probe and the carry-over of one specimen into the specimen in the next cup. Because a new pipette tip is used for each pipetting, carry-over is eliminated completely.

In practice, reduction of carry-over is a stricter requirement for automated analyzers that perform immunoassays, as some analytes have a wide range of concentrations. For example, the concentrations of chorionic gonadotropin vary over a wide range. Some systems use extra steps, such as additional washes, or an additional washing device to reduce carry-over to acceptable limits. Because extra steps reduce the overall **throughput**, additional rinsing functions are initiated (by computer operator selection) only for assays like chorionic gonadotropin that have large clinical measurement ranges.

Reagent Handling and Storage

Many automated systems use liquid reagents stored in plastic or glass containers. For those analyzers in which a working inventory of reagents is maintained in the system, the volumes of reagents stored depend on the number of tests to be performed between cycles of restocking reagents. Whenever possible, manufacturers use single reagents for test procedures, although two or more reagents may be required for some tests. Some analyzers use reagents in dry tablet form. Others use reagent-impregnated slides or strips. Still others rely entirely on electrodes to react with specimens.

For many analyzers in which specimens are not processed continuously, reagents are stored in laboratory refrigerators and are introduced into the instruments as required. In larger systems, sections of the reagent storage compartments are maintained at 4 °C to 10 °C. Refrigerated storage for reagents also is provided in most immunoassay systems. Many of the reagents delivered in liquid form by the manufacturers of these systems are stable for 2 to 12 months.

Reagent Identification

Labels on reagent containers include information such as (1) reagent identification, (2) volume of the contents or number of tests for which the contents of the container are to be used, (3) expiration date, and (4) lot number. Many reagent containers carry bar codes that contain some or all of this information, and the manufacturer is able to retrieve any pertinent information when necessary.

Other advantages of using reagent bar codes include (1) facilitation of inventory management, (2) ability to insert reagent containers in random sequence, and (3) ability to automatically dispense a particular volume of liquid reagent. Furthermore, when a bar code reader is coupled with a level-sensing system on the reagent probe, the operator is alerted as to whether a sufficient quantity of reagent exists to complete a workload.

In immunoassay systems, a bar code on a reagent container contains key information about (multiple) calibrators, such as the definition of a calibration curve algorithm and values of curve constants defined at the time of reagent manufacture. Accompanying calibrator materials provided in their own bar-coded tubes at the time of manufacture ensure that calibration functions are integrated properly into the analysis.

Open Versus Closed Systems

Automated analyzers are classified as "open" or "closed." With an open analyzer, the operator is able to change the parameters related to an analysis and prepare "in-house" reagents or use reagents from a variety of suppliers. Such analyzers usually have considerable flexibility and are adapted readily to new methods and analytes.

A closed-system analyzer requires the reagent to be in a unique container or format provided by the manufacturer. In general, liquid reagents for open systems are less expensive than the proprietary components required for closed analyzers. Yet closed systems contain a hidden cost advantage because reconstitution or preparation of reagents for use does not require a technologist's time. The variability arising from reconstitution of dry reagents has been overcome by the use of predispensed liquid reagents or the provision of premeasured liquids. Liquid reagents for some open systems now are approaching the longer stability that has characterized many closed systems. Most immunoassay systems are closed, as are most systems that have been developed for point-of-care applications (see Chapter 17).

Reagent Delivery

Liquid reagents are acquired and are delivered to mixing and reaction chambers by pumps (through tubes) or by positive-displacement syringe devices. In a few high-throughput automated analyzers, reagents and diluent are drawn from bulk containers through tubes, and the sample from the specimen cup is drawn through the aspirating probe.

Syringe devices for reagent and sample delivery are common to many automated systems. They are usually positive-displacement devices, and the volume of reagents they deliver is programmable. For those analyzers in which more than one reagent is acquired and dispensed by the same syringe, washing or flushing of the probe is essential to prevent reagent carry-over.

Chemical Reaction Phase

Sample and reagents react in the chemical reaction phase. Factors that are important in this phase include (1) the vessel in which the reaction occurs, (2) the cuvet in which the reaction is monitored, (3) the timing of the reaction(s), (4) mixing and transport of reactants, and (5) thermal conditioning of fluids. As discussed previously, separation of bound and unbound fractions is a fifth issue for some immunoassay systems.

Type of Reaction Vessel and Cuvet

In a continuous-flow system, each specimen passes through the same continuous stream and is subjected to the same analytical reactions as every other specimen and at the same rate. In such systems, the reaction occurs within the tube that serves as both a flow container and a cuvet.

In discrete systems, each specimen in a batch has its own physical and chemical space, separate from every other specimen. Discrete analyzers use individual (disposable or reusable) reaction vessels transported through the system after sample and reagent have been dispensed, or they use a stationary reaction chamber. In some discrete systems, reaction vessels are discarded after each use. The use of disposable cuvets has simplified automation and has eliminated carry-over in the cuvets and the maintenance of flow cells. Disposable cuvets became possible through the development of improved plastics (notably acrylic and polyvinyl chloride) and manufacturing technology.

In other instruments, reaction vessels are reused. The time before reusable cuvet/reaction vessels must be replaced depends on their composition (e.g., 1 month for plastic, 2 years for standard glass vessels). Pyrex glass vessels usually are not replaced unless physically damaged.

The typical cleaning sequence of a reusable cuvet/reaction vessel involves aspiration of the reaction mixture from the cuvet at an in situ wash station. A detergent, alkaline, or acid wash solution then is dispensed repeatedly into and aspirated from the cuvet. The cuvet is rinsed several times with deionized water and is dried by vacuum or pressurized air.

Dry reagent systems, which use slides of multilayer films or impregnated fiber strips, eliminate the need for dispensing and mixing of liquid reagents. Nevertheless, these instruments still require a mechanism to maintain a stable temperature and provide accurate positioning of the reaction unit for optical measurements.

Timing of Reactions

The time allowed for a reaction to occur depends on a variety of factors. In some analyzers, reaction time depends on (1) the rate of transport of reaction mixture through the system to the measurement station, (2) on timed events of reagent addition (or activation) relative to measurement, or (3) on both. In discrete random-access analyzers, samples and reagents are added to a cuvet in a timed sequence, and detector signals are measured at intervals to follow the course of each reaction. Usually, the total read time for a reaction in these systems is constrained to a maximum value defined by the manufacturer, but it may be programmed to be shorter.

Mixing of Reactants

Various techniques are used to mix reactants. In a discrete system, these include:

1. Forceful dispensing.
2. Magnetic stirring.
3. Vigorous lateral displacement.
4. A rotating paddle.
5. The use of ultrasonic energy.

Continuous-flow analyzers rely on the tumbling action of the stream in a mixing coil. Dry reagent systems obviate the need for mixing because the serum completely interacts with the dry chemicals as it flows through the matrix of the reaction unit. However, regardless of the technique used, mixing is a difficult process to automate.

Thermal Regulation

Thermal regulation requires the establishment of a controlled-temperature environment in close contact with the reaction container and efficient heat transfer from the environment to the reaction mixture. Devices used to control temperature include (1) air baths, (2) water baths, and (3) contact with warm plates.

Measurement Approaches

Automated chemistry analyzers use a variety of optical measurement devices including (1) photometers (2) spectrophotometers, (3) reflectance photometers, (4) fluorometers, and (5) luminometers. Immunoassay systems use reaction schemes that produce (1) fluorescence, (2) chemiluminescence, and (3) electrochemiluminescence to enhance sensitivity. Ion-selective electrodes and other electrochemical techniques also are used widely.

Photometry/Spectrophotometry

Measurement of absorbance requires the following three basic components (see Chapter 9):

1. An optical source.
2. A means of spectral isolation.
3. A detector.

Optical Source

Optical sources used in automated systems include (1) tungsten lamps, (2) quartz-halogen lamps, (3) deuterium lamps, (4) mercury lamps, (5) xenon lamps, and (6) lasers. In the quartz-halogen lamp, low-pressure halogen vapor such as iodine, bromine is enclosed in a fused silica envelope in which a tungsten filament serves as an incandescent light source. The spectrum produced includes wavelengths from approximately 300 to 700 nm.

Spectral Isolation

In automated systems, spectral isolation commonly is achieved with interference filters. Typical interference filters have peak transmissions of 30% to 80% and bandwidths of 5 to 15 nm (see Chapter 9). In several multitest analyzers, filters are mounted in a filter wheel, and the appropriate filter is moved into place under command of the system's computer.

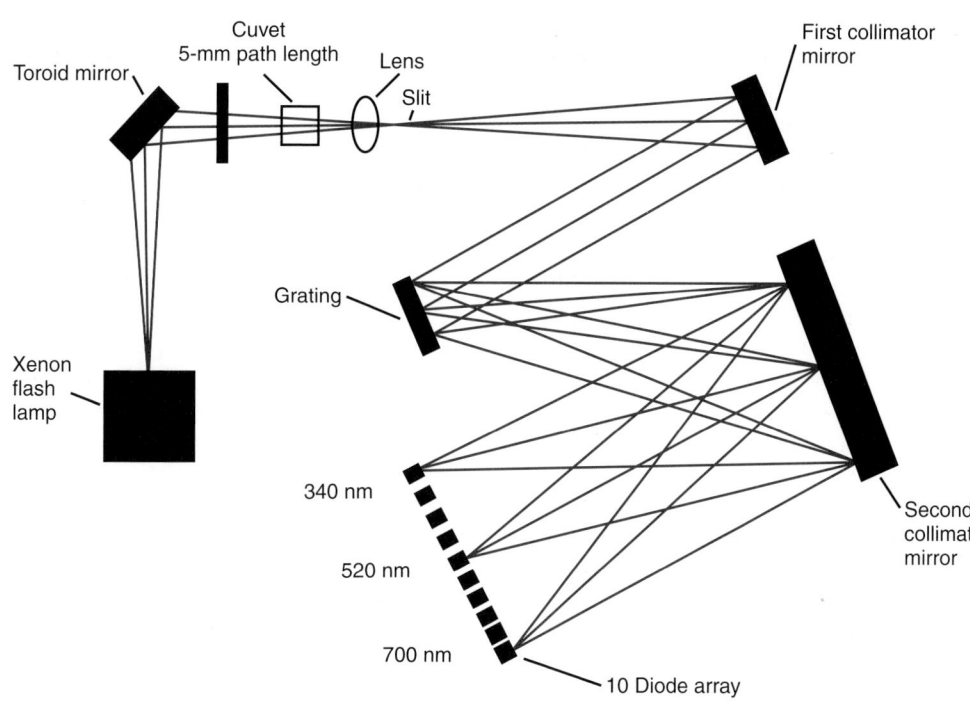

Figure 16-1 Use of a diode array in the SYNCHRON CX7 monochromator reduces requirements for moving parts. For simplicity, ray traces for only three wavelengths are shown. *(Courtesy Beckman Coulter, Inc.; www.beckmancoulter.com.)*

Monochromators with movable gratings and slits provide a continuous choice of wavelengths. They offer great flexibility and are suited especially for the development of new assays. However, because relatively few wavelengths are required for analyses in routine analyzers, many manufacturers use a stationary, holographically ruled grating, coupled with a stationary photodiode array, to isolate the spectrum. These two elements are coupled with fiber-optic light guides to transfer the passage of light energy through cuvets at locations convenient for mechanization. Use of these passive elements enhances the reliability of a system because no moving parts are required for spectral isolation (Figure 16-1).

Photometric Detectors

Photodiodes are used as detectors in many automated systems, either as individual components or in multiples as an array. Photomultiplier tubes are required in many immunoassay systems to provide a high signal-to-noise ratio and fast detector response times for fluorescent and chemiluminescent measurements.

Proper alignment of cuvets with the light path(s) is important in both automated and manual analyzers. In addition, stray energy and internal reflections must be kept to acceptable levels. When the light path is not perpendicular to the cuvet, inaccuracy and imprecision may occur, particularly in kinetic analyses.

Reflectance Photometry

In reflectance photometry, diffuse reflected light is measured. The reflected light results from illumination with diffused light of a reaction mixture in a carrier or from the diffusion of light by a reaction mixture in an illuminated carrier. The intensity of the reflected light from the reagent carrier is compared with that reflected from a reference surface. As the intensity of reflected light is nonlinear with concentration of the analyte, mathematical algorithms commonly are used to linearize the relation of reflectance to concentration.[2]

Fluorometry

Fluorescence is the emission of electromagnetic radiation by a species that has absorbed exciting radiation from an outside source. Intensity of emitted (fluorescent) light is directly proportional to the concentration of the excited species (see Chapter 9).

Fluorometry is used widely for automated immunoassay. It is approximately 1000 times more sensitive than comparable absorbance spectrophotometry, but background interference due to fluorescence of native serum is a major problem. This interference is minimized by (1) careful design of the filters used for spectral isolation, (2) selection of a fluorophor with an emission spectrum distinct from those of interfering compounds, or (3) the use of time- or phase-resolved fluorometry (see Chapter 9).

Different optical configurations are represented in different manufacturers' equipment. Right-angle fluorescence measurement is one of the common approaches, with emitted light passing through the emission interference filter to a photomultiplier tube. In fluorescence polarization, the light source takes the form of polarized light. The change in the degree of polarized light emitted by a fluorescent molecule is then measured (see Chapters 9 and 15).

Turbidimetry and Nephelometry

Turbidimetry and nephelometry are optical techniques that are applicable particularly to methods used to measure precipitate formation in antigen-antibody reactions (see Chapter 15). These techniques are used to measure plasma proteins and to perform therapeutic drug monitoring.

Chemiluminescence and Bioluminescence

Chemiluminescence and bioluminescence differ from fluorometry in that the excitation event is caused by a chemical or electrochemical reaction, not by photoluminescence (see Chapter 9). Applications of chemiluminescence and bioluminescence have increased significantly with the development of automated instrumentation and several new reagent systems. Because of their attamole-to-zeptomole lower limits of detection, chemiluminescence and bioluminescence reactions have been used widely as direct and indicator labels in the development of immunoassays.

Electrochemical

A variety of electrochemical methods have been incorporated into automated systems. The most widely used electrochemical approach involves ion-selective electrodes. These electrodes have replaced flame photometry in the determination of sodium and potassium. Electrochemical detectors also have been used for the measurement of other electrolytes and for indirect application in the analysis of several other serum constituents (see Chapter 10). The relationship between ion activity and the concentration of ions in the specimens must be established with calibrating solutions, and such electrodes need to be recalibrated frequently to compensate for alterations in electrode response.

Peristaltic pumps are used to move the sample into chambers containing fixed sample and reference electrodes. The electrodes must remain in contact with the specimen from 7 to 45 seconds to reach steady-state conditions. The most common arrangement is to provide electrodes to assay (1) sodium, (2) potassium, and (3) chloride. Because specimens and calibrators usually flow past a group of electrodes, results for all analytes are reported for most systems. Ion-selective electrode capability also has been incorporated into medium-sized and large automated analyzers as integrated three- and four-parameter modules; this incorporation has increased throughput of these systems as several results are produced in parallel.

Signal Processing, Data Handling, and Process Control

The interfacing and integration of computers into automated analyzers and analytical systems have had a major impact on the acquisition and processing of analytical data. Analog signals from detectors are converted to digital forms by analog-to-digital converters at a rate of 10^3 to 10^5 conversions per second. The computer and resident software then process the digital data into useful and meaningful output. Data processing has allowed automation of such procedures as nonisotopic immunoassays and reflectance spectrometry because computer algorithms readily transform complex, nonlinear standard responses into linear calibration curves. Several functions performed by integrated computers in automated analyzers are listed in Box 16-3. Additional functions include the following:

1. *Computer control of the electromechanical operation of the analyzer,* ensuring that all functions are performed uniformly, in a repeatable manner, and in the correct sequence.

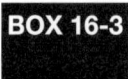

BOX 16-3   Signal and Data Processing Functions Performed by Computers of Automated Analyzers

Data Acquisition and Calculation

Acquisition of response signal and signal averaging

Subtraction of blank response

Correction of response of unknown for interferences (e.g., Allen-type corrections)

Linear regression for determining slope ($\Delta A/\Delta t$) of rate reactions; ($\Delta A/\Delta C$) of absorbance/concentration relation; ($\Delta R/\Delta C$) of any response parameter to concentration

Statistics (mean, SD, CV) on patient or control values

Mathematical transformation of nonlinear relations to linear counterpart

Mathematical transformation of results to alternative reporting units

Monitoring

Test for fit of data to linearity criteria for calibration curves or rate reactions

Test of patient result against reference interval criteria

Test of control result against criteria of a quality control standard of performance

Test of moving average of patient results against quality criteria for detecting assay drift

Display

Display of specimens currently being analyzed, tests ordered on each specimen, and expected times of completion

Accumulation of sets of patient results

Collation of results for patient-oriented printout

Warning messages provided to alert operator to instrument malfunction, need for maintenance, or unusual clinical situation

Quality control charts provided for operator review

Troubleshooting flow charts provided to assist operator

CV, Coefficient of variation; *SD,* standard deviation.

Such control of the automated equipment, calculation of results, and monitoring of operation contribute to the increased reproducibility of results.

2. *Computer acquisition, processing, and storage of operational data from the analyzers.* Built-in computers monitor instrument functions for correct execution and react to improper function by recording the site and nature of the malfunction.

3. *Computer interfacing with the instrument operator.* Diagnostic computer messages to the user describing the site and type of problem enable quick identification of problems and prompt correction. Graphical displays provide detailed and interactive troubleshooting guidance to instrument operators and visual display of the status of each specimen and associated quality control data. Output data are flagged by comparison with pre-set criteria and are displayed for the operator's evaluation and assessment. Such information may specify that (1) linearity of a reaction has been exceeded, (2) a reaction is nonlinear, (3) substrate exhaustion has occurred, (4) absorbance of a reagent is too high or too low, or (5) baseline drift is excessive. Operators may reprogram certain functions of the analyzer (e.g., the timing interval for a kinetic reaction and set point of the reaction temperature); enter certain values, such as calibrator

concentrations; display stored information in raw or processed form; or define the format of printed output through simple interaction with the computer software.

4. *Computer facilitation of communication with mainframe computers.* Typical interfaces in the past have used serial Recommended Standard 232 (RS-232) connections to permit interactive communication between computer systems in the modern laboratory analyzer and the Laboratory Information System (LIS). More recently, instrument manufacturers have been developing ethernet interfaces for networked connections with TCP/IP (Transmission Control Protocol/Internet Protocol).

5. *Computer integration of the monitoring functions of one or more analyzers with a single workstation.* Typically, the workstation (1) serves as the point of interaction with the instrument operator, (2) accepts test orders, (3) monitors the testing process, (4) assists with analysis of process quality, and (5) provides facilities for review and verification of test results. The workstation is usually directly interfaced with the LIS host, accepting downloaded test orders and uploading test results. Most workstations have facilities to (1) display Levy-Jennings quality control charts, (2) monitor the progress of each test order, and (3) troubleshoot the analyzers. They may also provide facilities to assist with the review of completed test results. Some workstations have rule-based software, which allows the operator to program rules for autoverification of test results.

Integrated Automation for the Clinical Laboratory

Considerable progress has been made in integrating the individual steps of the analytical process into analytical systems. Consequently, advanced analytical systems are now available from multiple vendors for automated (1) chemistry, (2) hematology, (3) immunoassay, (4) coagulation, (5) microbiology, and (6) nucleic acid testing, which provide efficient and cost-effective operation with a minimum of operator input. In addition, clinical laboratories are automating their preanalytical and postanalytical operations.

Some manufacturers have developed stand-alone "front-end" automation systems, which (1) sort, (2) centrifuge, (3) decap, (4) aliquot, and (5) label tubes. Although they require manual transport of the tubes to the analytical areas, these systems have automated steps in specimen processing. More advanced automation systems provide options such as (1) conveyors to transport specimens, (2) direct sampling interfaces to the laboratory's higher-volume analyzers, and (3) refrigerated storage and retrieval systems.[16]

Large-scale automation of the laboratory includes an automated specimen processing area where specimens are (1) identified, (2) labeled, (3) scheduled for analysis, (4) centrifuged, and (5) sorted. After specimens are processed, automated specimen conveyor devices transport the sorted specimens to appropriate workstations in the laboratory, where they are analyzed without human intervention. Rule-based expert system software (1) assists with the review of laboratory results by automatically releasing results that have no associated problems and (2) identifies any problematic results to be brought to the attention of trained medical technologists. All specimens are catalogued after analysis and are stored in a central storage facility, available for automated retrieval if necessary. As previously discussed, particularly important aspects of large-scale automation projects are the approaches used to process and transport specimens and the overall integration of automated components into a smoothly functioning whole.

Workstations

The task of integrating laboratory automation begins with the laboratory **workstation**. In general, a clinical laboratory workstation is usually dedicated to a defined task and contains appropriate laboratory instrumentation to carry out that task. Frequently, the workstation in the modern laboratory is defined in terms of the automated analyzer that is being used. Current laboratory instruments and systems are highly developed for stand-alone operation and fit into the workstation concept. Movement of specimens into and out of the workstation is accomplished by manual transport, and the instrument operator activities are largely independent of those at other workstations. On a typical instrument, the instrument operator follows a manufacturer-recommended sequence of (1) calibration, (2) quality control, and (3) daily maintenance activities, and (4) uses the instrument's front-panel functions to introduce specimens for analysis. If the analyzer has a bidirectional interface with an LIS and bar code–reading capabilities, information regarding which assays should be run on each specimen is downloaded from the LIS, and the instrument operator simply loads bar code–labeled specimens into the specimen input area. The built-in diagnostics supplied in most modern analyzers provide sufficient "intelligence" in the analyzer that the operator is able to "walk away" from the instrument for short periods, confident of its reliable operation. Nevertheless, the operator needs to attend periodically to (1) performing instrument operation, (2) replenishing reagents, (3) evaluating instrument diagnostic messages, and (4) introducing new specimens into the specimen input tray.

Instrument Clusters

To reduce labor costs, instrument manufacturers are developing approaches that will allow a single technologist to simultaneously control and monitor the functions of several instruments. Initially, such workstations were configured with *clusters* of identical instruments, such as (1) chemistry, (2) immunochemistry, or (3) hematology analyzers. More advanced instrument clusters may incorporate both chemistry and immunoassay analyzers from the same vendor, and a possible extension of this concept is the development of clusters of unlike instruments that cross traditional laboratory disciplines. An example might be a cluster of chemistry and hematology analyzers.

A cluster of analyzers has its own central control module (a PC) with software designed to assist the technologist in monitoring the functions of each analyzer and to aid in the review of laboratory results generated by the cluster. Access to the many front-panel functions of each analyzer is provided by the interface between the analyzer and the central control module. Thus, the technologist loads specimens onto each instrument in the cluster and then monitors subsequent instrument operation and reviews the results at the central workstation. By incorporating the activities of what would be *several* workstations in most current laboratories into a *single* integrated workstation, this approach shows promise in saving laboratory manpower.

Work Cells

Another extension of the instrument cluster concept is the addition of robotic specimen handling and preparation. A robotic system is used to carry out various specimen preparation steps, such as checks of specimen adequacy, and will (1) centrifuge, (2) aliquot, (3) label, (4) transport, and (5) store specimens. The robotic system is then responsible for introducing specimens into the appropriate analyzer, allowing the technologist to assume primarily a monitoring role. An interface between the central control module and the robot controller (or combining these functions in a single computer) allows the activities of the robotic cluster to be fully coordinated.

Automated Specimen Transport

Different approaches have been developed to transport and manipulate specimens within the laboratory.[10,11]

Conveyor Belts

Conveyor belts have been used in the laboratory to transport specimens from one clinical laboratory workstation to another. Ordinary industrial conveyor belts have been used successfully when only transportation is required. However, when conveyors have been integrated with other robotic systems to automate preanalytical and/or postanalytical functions, this technology has had difficulty in handling the large variety of specimen containers found in the clinical laboratory. To increase the variety of types of specimen containers that are carried on a conveyor belt system, specimens are placed into specially designed carriers that fit on the conveyor belt line. Sometimes known as "pucks" or "racks" (depending on whether they carry individual specimens or groups of specimens), the carriers have receptacles for variously sized tubes, generally ranging from 13 × 75 mm to 16 × 100 mm—sizes that are consistent with the CLSI Standard AUTO01-A.[5]

Transfer of specimens from the conveyor belt to the laboratory workstation has been implemented in various ways. For example, many manufacturers have equipped their laboratory instruments with devices to obtain specimens from conveyor belt systems. In practice, the automation system requires a device that stops the tube in the exact location required by the analyzer and verifies and transfers the tube's bar code identification to the analyzer. In another example, a specialized robotic system is required to remove the tube from its carrier and place it in the analyzer's rack or carousel.

Robot Arms

Robotic arms are capable of performing highly complex clinical assays.[15] Cartesian, cylindrical, and articulating robotic devices are available commercially (Figure 16-2). Robots, by virtue of their operational flexibility, enable the rapid reconfiguration of systems for new and varying protocols. This ability (1) enhances versatility and safety, (2) improves precision and productivity, and (3) reduces errors due to human mismatch of specimen identity.

Cartesian systems currently are the most common form of robotics used in laboratories. These systems are built into programmable pipette stations and provide flexible pipetting routines to suit varied protocols.

Automated Specimen Processing

Although the manual operations carried out in a specimen processing area look simple, considerable complexity underlies them. Consequently, specimen processing has been one of the most difficult areas of the clinical laboratory to automate. It has been approached in various ways using both integrated and modular approaches, which are discussed later. Each specimen passing through a specimen processing area has to undergo a series of operations, beginning with (1) receiving the specimen, (2) inspecting it for appropriateness (labeling, container type, temperature, and quantity of specimen), (3) logging onto the LIS, (4) labeling the specimen with an accession number, and (5) separating urgent and stat specimens

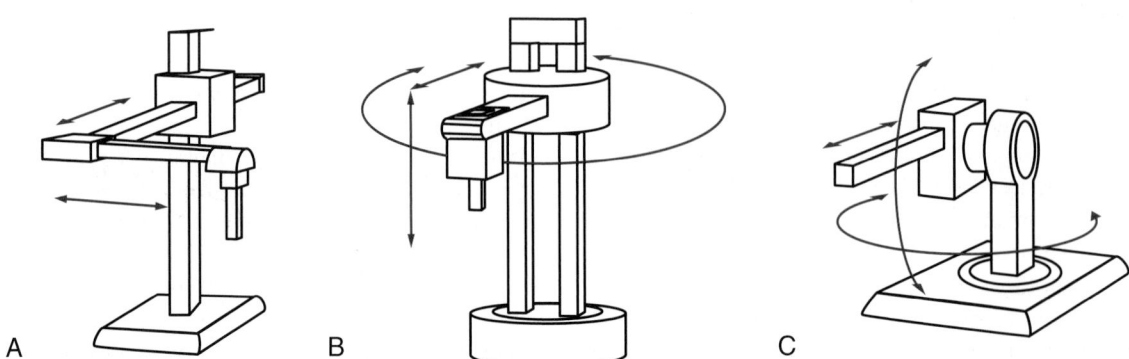

Figure 16-2 Three basic configurations of robotic devices that have applications in the clinical laboratory. **A,** Cartesian. **B,** Cylindrical. **C,** Articulating (polar) or jointed. *(Modified from Journal of the International Federation of Clinical Chemistry 1992;4:175.)*

from routine specimens. Also, specimens have to be sorted for centrifugation, aliquoted, or otherwise prepared for the appropriate laboratory station.

Stand-alone Specimen Processing Systems

An example of a stand-alone specimen processing system is shown in Figure 16-3. Similar systems place processed specimens into racks that are transported manually to the testing areas, with some exceptions. Some of these are about the size of a large automated analyzer, and others may be a little larger. They may be a good choice for laboratories (1) with daily workloads of 500 to 2500 specimens, (2) with space limitations, or (3) that desire an upgrade path and ease of use with different analyzers from different vendors. Some laboratories may choose to use multiples of a stand-alone specimen processing system to automate archiving and preanalytical specimen processing.

These systems will (1) receive incoming specimens, (2) sort, (3) decap, (4) aliquot, and (5) label aliquot specimen containers with bar codes. All are interfaced to the laboratory's LIS. Some systems even include automated centrifugation. Several of the systems sort into instrument-specific racks for analyzers from a number of different vendors. In addition to sorting for particular analyzers or laboratory sections, some users apply these systems to aliquot and sort reference or "send-out" testing, saving considerable time in locating the original specimens after testing in their own laboratory.

Integrated and Modular Automation Systems

Several manufacturers offer integrated or modular automation systems for specimen processing that provide additional functionality. In addition to the functions described in the preceding section, these systems typically add (1) conveyor transport, (2) interfacing to automated analyzers, (3) more sophisticated process control, and, in some cases, (4) a specimen storage and retrieval system. All systems are of modular design, allowing the customer to choose which modules/features should be included. Some systems use an open design, which permits interfaces to analyzers from a variety of vendors, whereas other systems are of a closed design and are interfaced only to the vendor's own or a limited number of analyzers. It should be noted that closed systems typically do not have process control software that is independent of the instruments or system, but rather, the automation process control is integrated to work with the vendor's analyzers. An example of one integrated automation system is shown in Figure 16-4.

To achieve maximum effectiveness of an automation system, process control software should be able to read the specimen's identification (ID) bar code and obtain information from the laboratory's LIS about specimen type and ordered tests. It should then determine the processes the specimen requires and the exact route or course of action needed for each specimen. The software should be able to (1) calculate the number of aliquots and the proper volume for each, depending on the tests requested, (2) route the specimens to analyzers, (3) recap the specimens, and (4) retain the specimens for automatic recall. In addition, the software should be able to monitor analyzers for in-control production status and automatically make decisions if a test is not available. Specimen integrity checking should be automatic; rules-based decisions should monitor specimen quality and enable these decisions. Finally, most process control software should include (1) "autoverification," which consists of validating analyzer results by making rules-based decisions that flag exceptions for technologist review, and (2) "autoretrieval" of specimens for repeat, reflex, and dilution testing.

Although most of these systems are restricted to handling specific types of specimen containers, they are capable of processing much of the daily workload of a large clinical laboratory. Although a few laboratories with daily workloads as low as 600 to 800 specimen tubes have justified these systems

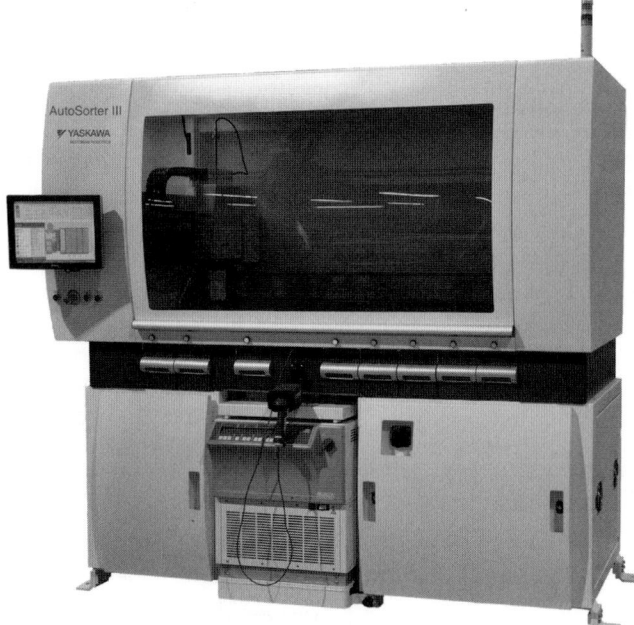

Figure 16-3 The Yaskawa AutoSorter III work cell uses two cartesian robots to perform automated centrifugation, decapping, and sorting into analyzer-specific racks selected by the customer with a maximum throughput of 800 tubes per hour. *(Courtesy Yaskawa America, Inc., Motoman Robotics Division, West Carrollton, OH; www.motoman.com.)*

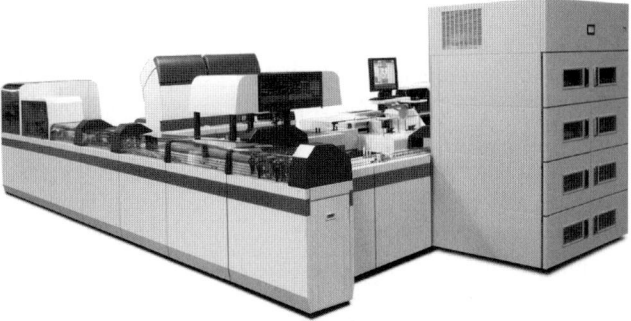

Figure 16-4 Beckman Coulter Power Express System. The system design includes preanalytical, connected, and analytical for all disciplines and postanalytical processing. *(Courtesy Beckman Coulter, Inc.; www.beckmancoulter.com.)*

because of a shortage of technical help, these systems typically are designed for laboratories with workloads of 1000 to 10,000 specimens per day. In addition to process control software and the ability to be interfaced to the laboratory's LIS, each of these systems incorporates some or all of the following components:

1. *Specimen input area.* A holding area where bar code–labeled specimens are introduced into the system.
2. *Bar code reading stations.* In most systems, the bar codes on specimens are read at the time the specimen is placed in a carrier or puck, which usually has its own ID in the automated system. The automated system then routes the carrier or puck to the correct destination, saving repeated reading of the specimen bar code.
3. *Transport system.* Segments of a conveyor belt line that move specimens to the appropriate location.
4. *High-level device to sort or route specimens.* A device that separates specimens by type (such as by tube height) or by order code and passes them to the transport system or to a system using racks. A high-level sorter is often used to separate specimens that require centrifugation or other processing steps from specimens that do not, or to route specimens into completely different pathways within the total automation system.[10,11]
5. *Automated centrifuge.* An area of the specimen processor in which specimens requiring centrifugation are removed from the conveyor belt, introduced into a centrifuge that is automatically balanced, centrifuged (refrigerated or at room temperature), and then removed from the centrifuge and placed back on the transport system.
6. *Level detection and evaluation of specimen adequacy (specimen integrity).* An area in which sensors are used to evaluate the volume of specimen in each specimen container and to look for the presence of hemolysis, lipemia, or icterus.
7. *Decapper station.* An area or device in the automated system in which specimen caps or stoppers are automatically removed and discarded into a waste container.
8. *Recapper station.* An area or device in the automated system in which specimen tubes are automatically recapped with new stoppers or covered with an air-tight closure.
9. *Aliquoter.* Aspirates appropriately sized aliquots from each original specimen container and places them into bar-coded secondary specimen containers for sorting and transport to multiple analytical workstations.
10. *Interface to automated analyzer.* A direct physical connection to an automated analyzer that permits the analyzer's sampling probe to aspirate directly from an open specimen container while the container is still on the conveyor, or that may robotically lift the container from the conveyor and place it into the analyzer. Some automation systems interface only to their own brand of analyzers or to a limited number of systems, whereas other automation systems use a so-called open design that complies with CLSI standards and permits interfaces to a variety of automated analyzers.
11. *Sorter.* An automated sorter used to sort specimens not going to a conveyor-interfaced analyzer or workstation.

Such a sorter typically sorts into 30 to 100 different sort groups in racks or carriers. In some systems, the racks are specific to certain analyzers for convenience.

12. *Take-out stations.* Temporary storage areas for specimens before or after analysis. The take-out station may be the same as the sorter described earlier, where specimens are sorted for manual delivery. However, it may also serve as a holding area (stockyard) for specimens awaiting autoverification of results in case a repeat test is required.
13. *Storage and retrieval system.* This unit may serve the same function as the take-out station or stockyard—that of holding specimens after analysis in case a specimen is necessary for a repeat test, but it has one major difference. These units are typically refrigerated and hold many more specimens (3000 to 30,000) than the typical take-out station or stockyard. Depending on daily workloads, the laboratory may be able to retain up to 1 week of specimens for possible repeat or additional tests. Specimen containers are loaded and retrieved with a robot.

Automated Specimen Sorting

Several approaches have been used to automatically sort specimens, including (1) a conveyor belt, (2) automated sorter using racks, and (3) stand-alone sorters. Selecting the correct one of these approaches is an extremely important determinant of the overall scheme of automation in any particular laboratory.[10,11]

Integration With a Conveyor System

Three types of conveyor sorting systems have been used. One type uses a continuous loop in which all specimens follow the loop and go past each workstation or analyzer. Specimens are sampled directly by the analytical instrument while on the conveyor, or a robot attached to the workstation removes selected specimens from the conveyor for analysis (Figure 16-5). This approach offers the advantage that it does not require that specimens be aliquoted because specimens pass by all workstations at which tests are performed. However, the continuous loop also has some disadvantages, as specimen throughput is often limited by the slowest direct sampling analyzer on the loop. Exceptions include systems that use bypass

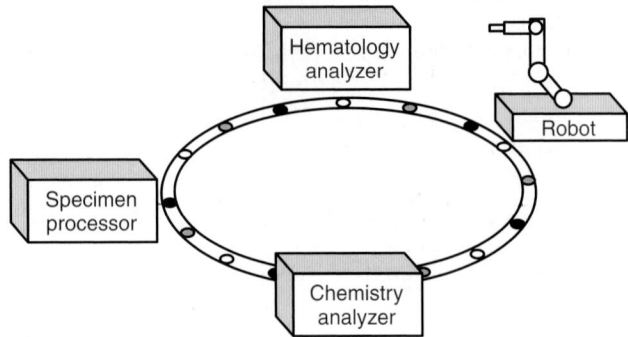

Figure 16-5 Direct sampling from a conveyor track in a loop configuration eliminates the need for separate equipment to sort specimens but may limit the rate of specimen movement on the track to the sampling speed of the slowest workstation. *(From Boyd JC, Felder RA, Savory J. Robotics and the changing face of the clinical laboratory. Clin Chem 1996;42:1901-10.)*

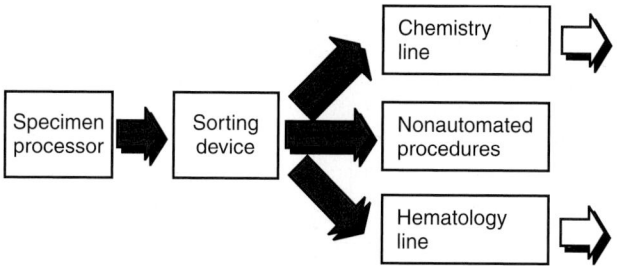

Figure 16-6 Sorting of laboratory specimens before introduction to an automated specimen conveyor system simplifies the design and construction of the conveyor. *(From Boyd JC, Felder RA, Savory J. Robotics and the changing face of the clinical laboratory. Clin Chem 1996;42:1901-10.)*

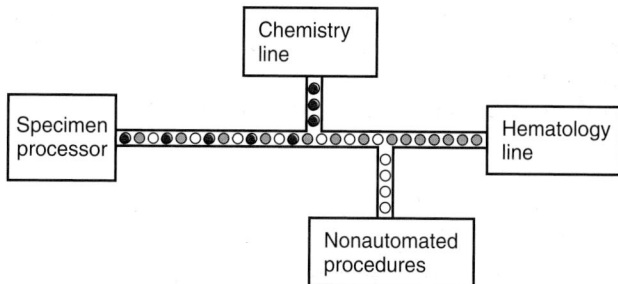

Figure 16-7 Use of the conveyor system to sort specimens dynamically during specimen transport eliminates the requirement for separate equipment to sort specimens but requires a more sophisticated conveyor system with numerous bar code–reading stations and gates to direct specimens to the appropriate workstation. *(From Boyd JC, Felder RA, Savory J. Robotics and the changing face of the clinical laboratory. Clin Chem 1996;42:1901-10.)*

tracks to enable specimens to bypass stations to get to their correct destinations. It should also be noted that if specimens are removed from their carriers on the line for testing, a system of queuing empty carriers is required to return the tubes to the conveyor.

In a second approach, some automated processing conveyor systems sort specimens into groups according to their destination in the laboratory, such as for hematology or chemistry tests. Downstream from the sorter, separated specimens are routed down a dedicated conveyor line (Figure 16-6). This method follows the approach used in most manual specimen processing areas. The extent of specimen transport via conveyor depends on the activities to be included. For example, these designs may include (1) a centrifuge and aliquoter, (2) an interfaced chemistry or immunochemistry analyzers, (3) an additional sorter, (4) a take-out station, and even (5) a refrigerated storage and retrieval station at the end of the chemistry line. The hematology line may lead directly to hematology and coagulation analyzers and to an automated slide preparation machine.

In the third approach, the sorter is integral to the conveyor system, and specimens are sorted as they are transported (Figure 16-7). The advantages of this approach are that a dedicated specimen sorter is not necessary in the specimen processing system, and that with appropriate specimen transport, the requirement for specimen aliquots may be avoided.

Automated Sorting Into Racks

Some sorters are designed to sort the specimens into racks for transfer to particular laboratory sections or analyzers, as described previously. These systems sort the aliquot and original tubes into racks for manual transport to analyzers or laboratory sections. In some cases, the racks may be specific for a specific analyzer, eliminating additional handling of tubes.

Automated Specimen Storage and Retrieval

Automated capability to store and retrieve specimens on demand is an important aspect of automated specimen delivery systems. A few of the integrated systems described earlier offer specimen storage and retrieval modules as options in their systems. These robotic modules store specimens refrigerated in specific locations that are logged into a database maintained by the specimen delivery system. When a user requests

retrieval of a specific specimen, the robot is given commands to retrieve the specimen from the appropriate archived location and to route the specimen to the requested station using the specimen transportation system. Some large reference laboratories have adapted large storage systems commonly used in other industries for use in their own settings.

Practical Considerations

In this section the practical considerations that influence a laboratory's decision to automate part or all of its operations are discussed.

Evaluation of Requirements

Any consideration of total or modular laboratory automation should start with an evaluation of requirements.[16] Such an evaluation begins with mapping of the current laboratory work flow from the arrival of patient specimens through completion of testing and reporting of results. Box 16-4 lists potential work flow steps that should be mapped. Mapping of material (specimen) flows and data flows is directly related to process flow and will assist the laboratory in determining process steps that (1) are bottlenecks, (2) waste labor, and (3) are prone to error.[13] Work-flow mapping thus enables the laboratory to better identify what steps should be considered for automation.

Some laboratorians use 80% as a "rule of thumb" in guiding decisions about automation. Clinical laboratories have many (1) exceptional tests, (2) specimen containers, and (3) handling situations. Nevertheless, if 80% of the specimen containers and handling situations can be standardized and automated, the laboratory will achieve a dramatic reduction in labor and costs, which should be sufficient to justify the investment in automation and the planning and evaluation time involved.

Once the laboratory's workflow has been mapped and its requirements have been identified, alternative solutions are next considered. Vendors are invited to make presentations and to host visits of the laboratory management team at other laboratories where the vendors have successful installations.

BOX 16-4 — Clinical Laboratory Steps for Workflow Mapping

Unpacking from transport containers
Presorting
Temperature preservation
Order entry
Document management (requisitions, etc.)
Labeling
Sorting
Centrifugation
Labeling of aliquot tubes
Pouring of aliquots
More sorting
Delivery to laboratory sections
More sorting
Preparing work lists
Decapping
Labeling analyzer-specific tubes for specimens
Pouring or pipetting analyzer-specific specimens
Loading tubes onto analyzers
Performing tests (steps such as extraction, centrifugation, precipitation, dilution, etc., are not specifically listed)
Unloading analyzers
Recapping
Data manipulations (calculations)
Result review and verification
Reporting results
Delivering specimens to archival storage system
Archival storage of specimens
Reflexive testing
Repeat testing, diluting, if necessary
Additional physician-ordered testing
Specimen retrieval for additional or repeat testing
Disposal of expired specimens

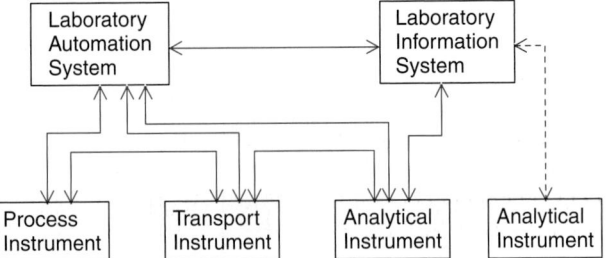

Figure 16-8 Functional Control Model of CLSI AUTO03-A Standard. The solid lines and arrows depict logical information flows supported by the standard. The dotted lines and arrows show logical information flows permitted, but not supported, by the standard. *(Clinical and Laboratory Standards Institute. Laboratory automation: communications with automated clinical laboratory systems, instruments, devices, and information systems. CLSI Approved standard AUTO03-A2. 2nd edition. Wayne, PA: Clinical and Laboratory Standards Institute, 2009. Figure reproduced with permission of CLSI.)*

It is important at this stage to focus on the requirements identified by the workflow mapping and not allow the vendor to try to sell equipment that may not be necessary.

Problems of Integration

Building a highly integrated laboratory generates many potential problems. Because it is unlikely that a laboratory will use only the equipment of a single equipment manufacturer, integration of instruments and robotic devices from different manufacturers typically is necessary. Decisions must be made concerning which device will be the master controller and which vendor will develop the software that provides overall control of the automation scheme. In addition, individuals or firms that will be responsible for configuration of the automation to the geometry and production schedule of the laboratory must be recruited and trained. Although industrial automation schemes have been developed to solve many of these problems, experience in using these approaches in the very different operating environment of a clinical laboratory is insufficient.

The reader is referred to the CLSI standard AUTO03-A2, which is described in the following section and in particular to the functional control model, which describes the relationships between the LIS, the Laboratory Automation System (LAS), and various devices. In this model, and throughout the series of CLSI automation standards,[5-7] the term LAS represents the computer system that controls the automation system, not the actual automation hardware. Most often, it is the LAS that provides the requisite process control software to support automation. The functional control model, which is depicted in Figure 16-8, supports analytical instruments that may be physically attached to the automation system and analyzers that may not be attached but are still interfaced to the LIS. This model does not give dominance to the LIS or the LAS but rather allows essential information flows in either direction to make the most efficient use of the strengths of each system.

Device Integration

One objective of developing an integrated laboratory is to link laboratory instruments and devices into an automated system to maximize the number of functions automated. Automatic specimen introduction requires the development of mechanical interfaces between each laboratory analyzer and devices such as (1) conveyor belts, (2) mobile robots, or (3) robot arms. Enhancements to electronic interfaces for laboratory instruments are necessary to allow (1) remote computer control of front-panel functions, (2) notification of instrument status information, and (3) coordination of the distribution of specimens between instruments. Most existing LIS interfaces with laboratory analyzers provide only the ability to download accession numbers and the tests requested on each specimen and to upload the results generated by the analyzer.

Process Controllers and Software

Process controllers provide computer integration of the many decision-making tasks that occur in the daily activity of a laboratory. Consequently, process control software is needed to coordinate the overall activities of the laboratory. To integrate the various devices in the laboratory, communications with a master controller device need to be established. In addition, communication is needed between (1) the LIS computer,

(2) the LAS computer (that provides process control), (3) laboratory analyzers, and (4) specimen conveyor and specimen manipulation devices, such as automated centrifuges, aliquoters, decappers, etc. The distribution of tasks must be carefully specified when such a communications network is developed.

Other Areas of Automation

In addition to the automated devices described previously, a variety of instruments and processes have been automated and used in the clinical laboratory. They include (1) urine analyzers, (2) cell counters, (3) nucleic acid analyzers, (4) microtiter plate systems, (5) automated pipetting stations, and (6) point-of-care testing analyzers.

Urine Analyzers

Many of the same analytical principles are used for the quantification of serum and urine constituents. It is more difficult, however, to automate testing of urine than serum because of the broad range of concentrations of many urine constituents. This requires a low limit of detection to measure low concentrations, as well as expanded linearity to permit measurement of high concentrations without dilution. This requirement, together with the relatively low demand for urine tests compared with that for serum tests, has restricted the development of analyzers designed specifically for urine constituents. Nevertheless, selected urine analyses are performed on the available analyzers in some institutions.[9]

Cell Counters

Analyzers that perform a complete blood count have been automated through the use of the "Coulter principle," which is based on (1) cell conductivity, (2) light scatter, and (3) flow cytometry. Individual blood cells are analyzed by application of one or more of these techniques. The Coulter principle is based on changes in electrical impedance produced by nonconductive particles suspended in an electrolyte as they pass through a small aperture between electrodes. In the sensing zone of the aperture, the volume of electrolyte displaced by the particle (cell) is measured as a change in voltage that is proportional to the volume of the particle. With careful control of the quantity of electrolyte drawn through the aperture, several thousand particles per second are counted and sized individually. Cells identified by their size include (1) red blood cells, (2) white blood cells, and (3) platelets. Alternating current in the radio frequency range short-circuits the bipolar lipid layer of the cell membrane, allowing energy to penetrate the cell. Information about intracellular structure, including chemical composition and nuclear volume, is collected by this technique.

Flow cytometry typically uses cells stained with a supravital or fluorescent dye that travel in suspension one by one past a laser light source (unstained cells also are measured.) Scattered light and emitted light are collected in front of the light source and at right angles, respectively. Information derived through measurement of light scatter when a cell is struck by the laser beam is then used to estimate (1) cell shape, (2) cell size, (3) cellular granularity, (4) nuclear lobularity, and (5) cell surface structure. Some cell counters classify white cells using the Coulter principle, cell conductivity, and light scattering of unstained cells to differentiate cell types, whereas other cell counters use multiple flow cytometry channels or a combination of (1) flow cytometry, (2) cell conductivity, and (3) light scattering.

Nucleic Acid Analyzers

Automation of the analysis of nucleic acids developed rapidly as an outgrowth of the Human Genome Project.[12] Several manufacturers have developed automation to assist with the isolation of nucleic acids and with analysis of nucleic acids using several amplification schemes and nucleic acid sequencing. Many of these techniques have been miniaturized using chip technology.[4,14] Microfluidic chip-based approaches hold promise for reducing analysis time and reagent consumption, as well as for reducing the costs associated with robotics and laboratory apparatus needed for the macroscale approaches.

Microtiter Plate Systems

Microtiter plate systems are commonly used in immunoassays and nucleic acid analyses. As used for enzyme-linked immunosorbent assays (ELISAs), microtiter plates usually are made of polystyrene and consist of 48 or 96 wells coated with antibody specific for the antigen of interest. After incubation of serum in the microtiter plate well, the well is washed to remove unbound antigen, and a second antibody with conjugated indicator enzyme is added. After a second incubation period, the well is washed to remove the unbound conjugate. An absorbance-producing product is developed by the addition of enzyme substrate, and the reaction is terminated at a specific time. With the development of automated pipetting stations, the liquid handling steps required for microtiter plate assays have been fully automated to make microtiter plate assays a viable technology for carrying out large numbers of immunoassays. Automated pipetting stations have a cartesian robot with a pipette fixed to the end of a probe that moves about a rectangular space. The probe is capable of moving in the X, Y, and Z axes. Liquids may be aspirated and dispensed in any location within the rectangular space.

Automated Pipetting Stations

Pipetting stations may be used to automate an analytical procedure for which an automated analyzer does not exist or cannot be cost justified. Most pipetting robots (1) are relatively easy to program, (2) rarely malfunction, and (3) are capable of delivering aliquots of liquids with extreme precision and accuracy. Multiple-channel pipetting robots allow parallel processing of specimens with 8- or 12-channel probes to handle microtiter plates.

POCT Analyzers

Point-of-care testing (POCT) is a rapidly growing component of laboratory testing.[8] Many of the analyzers developed for this type of testing have been automated (see Chapter 17).

1. Which type of specimen label has resulted in a reduction in preanalytical specimen identification errors and is used extensively in automated specimen identification?
   a. Social Security numbers stamped on all individual specimen containers
   b. Hospital identification numbers written on tubes of blood
   c. Labels containing bar codes that are unique identifiers
   d. Medical accounting numbers written on the lids of all containers

2. The transport of a quantity of analyte or reagent from one specimen reaction into a subsequent one is referred to as:
   a. carry-over.
   b. misdelivery.
   c. indiscrete handling.
   d. batching.

3. A type of analysis in which each specimen is subjected to multiple analytical processes so that a set of test results is obtained on a single specimen is:
   a. batch analysis.
   b. discrete analysis.
   c. sequential analysis.
   d. multiple-channel analysis.

4. In an automated chemistry analyzer, one measurement technique that is commonly used measures diffuse reflected light. This measurement approach is called:
   a. fluorometry.
   b. reflectance photometry.
   c. chemiluminescence.
   d. potentiometry.

5. One serious issue with the use of accelerating/decelerating pneumatic tube systems to deliver specimens to the laboratory is the occurrence of:
   a. hemolysis.
   b. specimen volume loss.
   c. specimen breakage.
   d. clot formation.

6. The initial step in the evaluation of laboratory automation is:
   a. assessment of the integrative ability of several pieces of instrumentation.
   b. determination of which device will be the master controller.
   c. mapping of laboratory work flow.
   d. determining the correct type of process controller required.

7. The most widely used automated type of electrochemical system incorporated into a chemistry analyzer involves:
   a. fluorometry.
   b. nephelometry.
   c. chemiluminescence.
   d. ion-selective electrodes.

8. Elimination or reduction of specimen preparation time occurs when which of the following specimen types is used in a chemistry assay system?
   a. Serum
   b. Whole blood
   c. Urine
   d. Plasma

9. One of the most important benefits of the use of automated systems in a laboratory is the:
   a. reduction of result variability and analysis errors.
   b. need for specialized training for users of a system.
   c. reduction of the workforce required.
   d. ability of the system to choose which type of analysis will be done without user input.

10. The process whereby an analytical instrument performs many tests with only minimal involvement of an analyst is referred to as:
    a. batch analysis.
    b. discrete analysis
    c. automation.
    d. throughput rate.

References

1. Boyd J. Tech. Sight. Robotic laboratory automation. Science 2002;295(5554):517–8.
2. Boyd JC, Hawker CD. Automation in the clinical laboratory. In: Burtis CA, Ashwood ER, Bruns DE, eds. Tietz textbook of clinical chemistry and molecular diagnostics, 5th ed. Philadelphia: Saunders/Elsevier, 2012:469–85.
3. Boyd JC, Felder RA. Preanalytical automation in the clinical laboratory. In: Ward-Cook KM, Lehmann CA, Schoeff LE, Williams RH, eds. Clinical diagnostic technology: the total testing process. Volume 1. The preanalytical phase. Washington, DC: AACC Press, 2002:107–29.
4. Cheng J, Fortina P, Surrey S, Kricka LJ, Wilding P. Microchip-based devices for molecular diagnosis of genetic diseases. Mol Diagn 1996;1:183–200.
5. Clinical and Laboratory Standards Institute. Laboratory automation: specimen container/specimen carrier. CLSI Approved Standard AUTO01-A. Wayne, PA: Clinical and Laboratory Standards Institute, 2000.
6. Clinical and Laboratory Standards Institute. Laboratory automation: bar codes for specimen container identification. CLSI Approved Standard Second Edition AUTO02–A2. Wayne, PA: Clinical and Laboratory Standards Institute, 2005.
7. Clinical and Laboratory Standards Institute. Laboratory automation: communications with automated clinical laboratory systems, instruments, devices, and information systems. CLSI Approved Standard AUTO03-A2, 2nd edition. Wayne, PA: Clinical and Laboratory Standards Institute, 2009.
8. Giuliano KK, Grant ME. Blood analysis at the point of care: issues in application for use in critically ill patients. AACN Clin Issues 2002;13:204–20.
9. Guder WG, Ceriotti F, Bonini P. Urinalysis—challenges by new medical needs and advanced technologies. Clin Chem Lab Med 1998;36:907.
10. Hawker CD, Garr SB, Hamilton LT, Penrose JR, Ashwood ER, Weiss RL. Automated transport and sorting system in a large reference laboratory: Part 1. Evaluation of needs and alternatives and development of a plan. Clin Chem 2002;48:1751–60.
11. Hawker CD, Roberts WL, Garr SB, et al. Automated transport and sorting system in a large reference laboratory: Part 2. Implementation of the system and performance measures over three years. Clin Chem 2002;48:1761–7.

12. Jaklevic JM, Garner HR, Miller GA. Instrumentation for the genome project. Annu Rev Biomed Eng 1999;1:649–78.

13. Middleton S, Mountain P. Process control and on-line optimization. In: Kost GJ, ed. Handbook of clinical automation, robotics, and optimization. New York: John Wiley & Sons, 1996:515–40.

14. Paegel BM, Blazej RG, Mathies RA. Microfluidic devices for DNA sequencing: sample preparation and electrophoretic analysis. Curr Opin Biotechnol 2003;14:42–50.

15. Price CP, Newman DJ, eds. Principles and practice of immunoassay, 2nd edition. New York: Stockton Press, 1997.

16. Sasaki M, Kageoka T, Ogura K, et al. Total laboratory automation in Japan: past, present, and the future. Clin Chim Acta 1998;278:217–27.

17. Wild DG. The immunoassay handbook, 3rd edition. New York, NY: Elsevier, 2005.

Point-of-Care Instrumentation

Christopher P. Price, Ph.D., F.R.C.Path., and Andrew St. John, Ph.D., F.F.Sc. (R.C.P.A.)

Objectives

1. Define the following terms:

Biosensor	Recognition element
Connectivity	Sensor
Informatics	Transducer
Point-of-care testing	

2. List five advantages of the use of point-of-care testing (POCT).
3. List five requirements of point-of-care testing devices.
4. List the eight key components of a point-of-care testing device.
5. Compare the following in vitro point-of-care testing devices, including design, reaction principles used with each type, examples of each device, result interpretation, and clinical applications:

Single-use qualitative strip or cartridge and/or strip	Multiple-use cartridge
	Bench top systems
Single-use quantitative cartridge or strip tests with a monitoring device	

6. Describe in vivo, ex vivo, and minimally invasive point-of-care-testing devices, including analytical principles, and provide a clinical application of each.
7. Given an analyte, draw an example of an immunostrip format used in a point-of-care testing device and label the components.
8. State the need for and benefits of standardized connectivity for point-of-care testing devices linked to a laboratory information system; state the purpose of the Connectivity Industry Consortium.
9. List and explain the eight steps involved in implementing and managing a point-of-care testing service; list the elements of a training program necessary for POCT personnel.
10. List three quality control methods used with a point-of-care test; state the issues that involve performance of conventional quality control methods on certain POCT devices.

Key Words and Definitions

Biosensor A sensor design in a point-of-care testing device that has a biological or biochemical component as the recognition element.

Chemosensor A sensor design in a point-of-care testing device that detects intrinsic properties of an analyte or that is combined with a transducing element to detect signals produced by the analyte binding to some indicator.

Clinical Laboratory Improvement Amendments of 1988 (CLIA-88) United States federal regulatory standards that apply to all clinical laboratory testing performed on humans in the United States, except clinical trials and basic research.

Connectivity In a clinical laboratory, the linking of an analytical device via an electronic interface to a laboratory information system computer.

Dipsticks Single- or multi-pad measurement devices that quantify from one to several analytes.

Immunostrip (immunosensor) A point-of-care device in which the recognition element is an antibody that binds to the analyte; the binding event is typically detected by an optical mechanism.

Informatics In a clinical sense, the design, management, and study of systems that store and communicate medical information; in the clinical laboratory, this refers to the communication and management of information related to laboratory testing and test interpretation.

Operator interface The part of a device that the operator is required to use for the device to work (e.g., switch on a reader, entry of a patient or sample identification, calibration of the device).

Point-of-care testing (POCT) A mode of testing in which the analysis is performed at a site closer to the patient than the conventional laboratory.

Reaction cell The location in a point-of-care testing device where the analytical reaction takes place.

Recognition element A chemosensor with a transducing element that recognizes the analyte to be measured and produces a signal.

Sensor A component of a point-of-care testing device that identifies a signal produced by the presence of an analyte.

Transducing element A component of a point-of-care testing device such as a chemical indicator or a binding molecule that recognizes the analyte of interest and produces an electrical or optical signal.

Waived test A test that (1) employs methodologies that are so simple and accurate as to render the likelihood of erroneous results negligible; (2) poses no reasonable risk of harm to the patient if the test is performed incorrectly and (3) has been cleared by the Food and Drug Administration for home use. (http://www.aafp.org/; accessed August 13, 2013)

Point-of-care testing (POCT) is a method of clinical laboratory testing in which the analysis is performed at the site close to where healthcare is provided to the patient. Other terms used to describe POCT have included (1) "bed side," (2) "near patient," (3) "physician's office," (4) "extra-laboratory," (5) "decentralized,"(6) "off site," (7) "ancillary," (8) "alternative site" and (9) "unit-use" testing. POCT is performed in a number of different clinical settings (Box 17-1).[10-12] Its main advantages are (1) reduced *turnaround time* (TAT), (2) reduced risk of error in the testing process (e.g., order being lost, sample being lost, result being lost), (3) reduced risk of a disconnection between the process of testing and clinical decision making (Figure 17-1), and (4) improved health outcomes (Box 17-2).

The following sections of this chapter will describe the technology available for POCT and the organizational factors that complement the technology in delivering reliable healthcare.

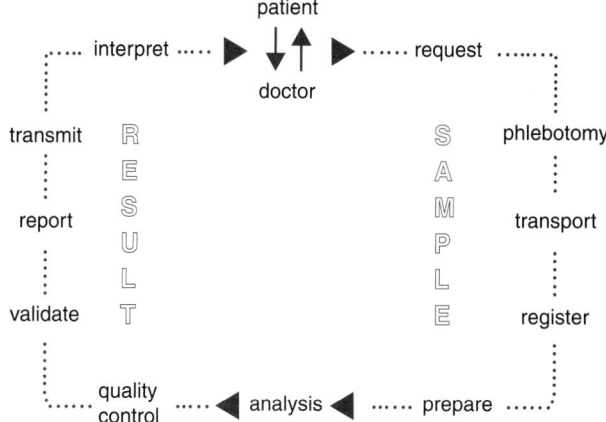

Figure 17-1 A schematic representation of the key steps in requesting, delivering, and using a diagnostic test result.

Analytical and Technological Considerations

Miniaturization has been a long-term trend in clinical diagnostics instrumentation that has resulted in the evolution of POCT devices that measure (1) electrolytes, (2) blood gases, and (3) other *analytes*. It has led to the development of dry, stable reagents in disposable unit-dose devices. Although the throughput of tests for these devices is low, the time required to produce the results is usually short. In addition, these devices are often small enough to be portable, further enhancing the possibility of "bringing tests closer to the patient."

Topics to be discussed in this section include (1) instrument requirements, (2) instrument and **operator interface** design, (3) examples of POCT devices, and (4) the role of **informatics**. Readers requiring additional information are referred to more comprehensive texts[8,9,11,12] or to the vendors of POCT devices.

Requirements

Characteristics and requirements of POCT devices are listed in Box 17-3.

BOX 17-2 Advantages of Point-of-Care Testing

Reduced turnaround time (TAT) of test results
Improved patient management
Reduction in the administrative work associated with test requesting
Minimization of delays during sample collection and sample requirement(s)
Reduction in the time delay resulting from transport of the sample to the testing laboratory
Reduction in the time delay resulting from having to log in (register) the sample
Reduction in the time delay that results from entry of a sample into a complex testing facility
Reduction in process errors
Opportunity for more informed discussion with the patient

BOX 17-1 Environments for Which Point-of-Care Testing Might Be Employed

Primary Care
Home
Community pharmacist
Health center (general practice, primary care)
Retail clinic
Workplace clinic
Physician's office and community clinic
Diagnostic and treatment center
Paramedical support vehicle (ambulance, helicopter, aircraft)

Secondary and Tertiary Care
Emergency room
Admissions unit
Ambulatory diagnostic and treatment center
Operating room
Intensive care unit
Ward
Outpatient clinic

BOX 17-3 Characteristics/Requirements of a Point-of-Care Testing Analyzer

Reduced errors and enhanced patient care
Results produced in a rapid and timely manner (typically within a minute)
Portable instruments with consumable reagent cartridges
Capability of performing direct specimen analysis on whole blood and urine (nonprocessed samples)
Simple operating procedures (typically a one- or two-step operating protocol)
Flexible test menus
Quantitative results with accuracy and precision comparable with those of the central laboratory
Built-in/integrated calibration and quality control
Ambient storage temperature for reagents
Results provided as hard copy, stored, and available for transmission
Low instrument cost
Service by exchange
Built-in regulatory record keeping

Modified from Maclin E, Mahoney WC. Point-of-care testing technology. J Clin Ligand Assay 1995;18:21-33.

TABLE 17-1	Classification of Types of Point-of-Care Testing Instruments or Devices	
Type of Technology	**Analytical Principle**	**Analytes**
Single-use, qualitative or semi-quantitative cartridge/strip tests	Reflectance	Urine and blood chemistry
	Lateral-flow or flow-through immunoassays	Infectious disease agents, cardiac markers, hCG
Single-use quantitative cartridge/strip tests with a reader device	Reflectance	Glucose
	Electrochemistry	Glucose
	Reflectance	Blood chemistry
	Light scattering/optical motion	Coagulation
	Lateral-flow, flow-through, or solid phase immunoassays	Cardiac markers, drugs, CRP, allergy and fertility tests
	Immunoturbidimetry	HbA_{1c}, urine albumin
	Spectrophotometry	Blood chemistry
	Electrochemistry	pH, blood gases, electrolytes, metabolites
	Fluorescence, electrochemistry with PCR	Infectious agents
Multiple-use quantitative cartridge/bench top devices	Electrochemistry	pH, blood gases, electrolytes, metabolites
	Fluorescence	pH, blood gases, electrolytes, metabolites
	Multiwavelength spectrophotometry	Hemoglobin species, bilirubin
	Time-resolved fluorescence	Cardiac markers, drugs, CRP
	Electrical impedance	Complete blood count

CRP, C-reactive protein; *HbA*$_{1c}$, glycosylated hemoglobin; *hCG*, human chorionic gonadotropin; *PCR*, polymerase chain reaction.

Design

Great diversity is evident in the devices used for POCT (Table 17-1). This breadth of technology encompasses a large range of analytes, and many devices use the same analytical principles as those found in conventional laboratory analysers. The key components of POCT device design include (1) the operator interface, (2) bar code identification systems, (3) sample and reagent delivery mechanisms, (4) the **reaction cell**, (5) **sensors**, (6) control and communications systems, (7) data management and storage, and (8) manufacturing requirements. The main objectives of the design are to (1) enable the required reaction to take place that facilitates recognition of the analyte of interest, (2) ensure reliable performance of the device over a specified period of time, and (3) minimize the risk of error associated with use of the device—as well as within a wide range of environmental settings (e.g., temperature, humidity).

Operator Interface

The operator or user interface for a POCT device should (1) require minimal operator interaction, (2) guide the user through the operation, (3) indicate whether any key steps have not been completed correctly, and (4) identify the operator, the patient, and the test to be measured. Advances in information technology and consumer electronics have had a major impact in this area. Other forms of user interface include (1) keypads, (2) bar code readers, and (3) possibly a printer. In some devices, the display is the only means of showing the result, but with the development of mobile telephone and computing technology, displays are rapidly becoming more sophisticated, with touch screens used for many different functions.

Bar Code Identification Systems

Many POCT devices incorporate linear and two dimensional bar codes for a number of purposes. These include (1) identifying the reagent package to the system, (2) incorporating factory calibration data, and (3) programming the instrument to process a particular test or group of tests. In addition to the linear bar codes, two dimensional codes are also used as they have the capability of storing more information than the linear ones. Such codes consist of black square dots arranged in a square grid on a white background, which is read by an imaging device and processed. Information is then extracted from patterns present in both horizontal and vertical components of the image. Some POCT devices use magnetic strips for similar purposes. Other functions of a bar code reader that are of growing importance are to identify both the operator and the patient sample to the system. This provides traceability to the person who performed the test, and it links the results to the correct patient. The latter has assumed increasing importance as part of the focus on patient safety.

Sample

Sample access and delivery of the sample to the (1) actual sensing component of the strip, (2) cassette, (3) cartridge, or (4) fluidic cell are key interactions of the user with the device; in some cases, removal of the sample may also require user intervention. Ideally, after the sample has been added, there should be no further need for operator intervention,[14] and devices are now available that minimize the degree of interaction to the point where a closed tube has simply to be placed in a holder and the instrument automatically performs all other functions.[11]

Reaction Cell

The design of the location where the analytical reaction takes place varies from a simple porous pad to a cell or surface within a chamber. However, to simplify the user interface, it is often necessary to design complexity into the reaction chamber. Advances in fluidics and fabricating techniques have been basic to the development of POCT devices.[7] As analytical reactions have increased in complexity, more reaction cells/zones have been added. Thus in the case of molecular tests, different reaction zones may be required for DNA extraction, the amplification reaction, and probe detection; in these situations, it may be necessary to remove some of the reaction constituents downstream from each zone before the next reaction zone is reached. Reaction temperature requirements may be different for each reaction zone.

Sensors

Much of the focus on POCT devices has involved the advances in sensor design.[16] Various sensor designs have been developed, and both **chemosensors** and **biosensors** may be included (Figure 17-2). Examples of chemosensors include simple ones where the analyte has an intrinsic property, such as fluorescence, that is detected directly with a fluorometer. A popular version of chemosensors includes the addition of a **transducing element** such as a chemical indicator or a binding molecule that recognizes the analyte to be measured and produces a signal, usually electrical or optical. A biosensor has a biological or biochemical component as the **recognition element**. Enzymes are the most common biological element used, followed by antibodies; transduction typically occurs via an optical or electrical signal, although the use of antibody and nucleotide recognition elements is increasing.

Control and Communications Systems

Even the smallest device has a control subsystem that coordinates all the other systems and ensures that all required processes for an analysis take place in the correct order. Operations that require control include (1) insertion or removal of the strip, cartridge, cassette, or reagent; (2) temperature control; (3) sample injection or aspiration; (4) sample detection; (5) reagent addition—especially in a fluid-based system; (6) mixing; (7) timing of the detection process; and (8) waste removal. Fluid movement is often accomplished by mechanical means through pumps or centrifugation, and by fluidic properties, such as surface tension; the latter is often a critical element in the design of simple strip tests and microfabricated systems.[7]

Data Management and Storage

Information technology (IT) is also crucial to POCT devices. IT includes data management of calibration curve data, as well as quality control (QC) limits and patient results. With some systems, data transfer and management take place when the meter or the reader is linked to a small bench top device called a *docking station*. These and other devices include communication protocols that allow data to be transferred to other data

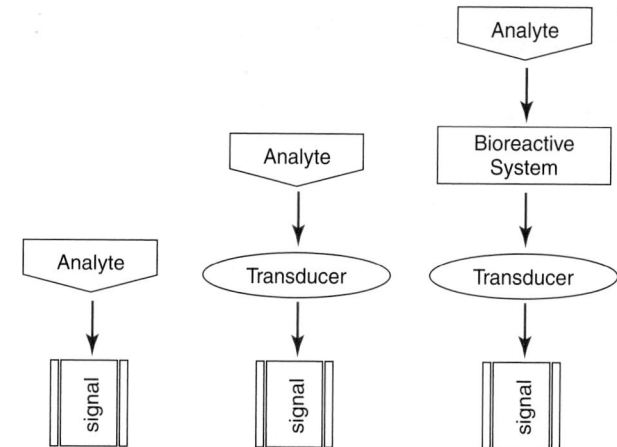

Figure 17-2 Diagram showing the key types of sensor technology used in point-of-care testing (POCT) instruments.

management systems, to electronic medical records, and to other mobile computing devices.[4,5,15]

Manufacturing of POCT Devices

Because many POCT devices are used only once and then are discarded, the reproducibility of manufacture is a key requirement, so that consistent performance extends across a large number of strips or devices. The manufacturing process includes steps that are taken to ensure that the devices are reproducible and that they remain stable during transit and storage for a stated period of time.[1]

Examples of POCT Devices

POCT devices are classified as (1) in vitro, (2) in vivo, (3) ex vivo, or (4) minimally invasive.

In Vitro Devices

The diversity of in vitro POCT technology and the range of analytes make it difficult to devise a simple classification that avoids overlap between various technologies. For the purposes of highlighting key or novel POCT technologies, the following discussion classifies various devices largely according to size and complexity: (1) single-use qualitative or semi-quantitative cartridge and/or strip tests, (2) single-use semi-quantitative or fully quantitative cartridge and/or strip tests with a monitoring device, and (3) multiple-use cartridge and bench top systems.

Single-use Qualitative Strip or Cartridge and/or Strip Devices

Many devices fall into this category, including (1) single- or multi-pad urine tests (**dipsticks**) that are read visually; (2) more complex strips that use light reflectance for measurement; and (3) fabricated cassettes or cartridges that incorporate techniques such as immunochromatography and are used as immunosensors.

Dipsticks. Dipsticks are single- or multi-pad measurement devices that are used to quantify up to 10 different urine analytes using reflectance technology.[11] These devices are relatively simple in construction and are composed of a pad of porous material, such as cellulose, that is impregnated with reagent and then dried.[19]

Complex Strips. More complex pads are composed of several layers, the uppermost of which is a semi-permeable membrane that prevents red cells from entering the matrix. With these devices, a critical operator factor is the need to cover the whole pad with the sample. In addition, because the reactions often do not proceed to completion, it is necessary to time the period between placing the sample on the pad and comparing the resulting color with a color chart. Development of these single-stick devices involves the inclusion of two pads, which are used for measurement of (1) different concentrations of the same analyte, such as hemoglobin and glucose[11,19] and

(2) both albumin and creatinine (semi-quantitative) to obtain an albumin/creatinine ratio.[11] A chromatographic device has also been developed for the quantitative measurement of cholesterol, which does not require the use of any instrumentation.[11] Table 17-2 lists some of the tests performed by single- or multi-pad dipsticks and the chemistry used for the analysis.

Immunostrips. Immunostrips are biosensors in which the recognition agent is an antibody that binds to the analyte. Detection of the binding event or signal transducer is usually accomplished via an optical mechanism, either reflectance or fluorescence spectrophotometry. Immunosensors usually use solid phase technologies in conjunction with (1) flow-through, (2) lateral-flow, or (3) immunochromatography processes. In the flow-through format, a heterogeneous immunoassay takes place in a porous matrix cell that acts as the solid phase. In lateral flow, the separation stage takes place as the sample passes along the porous matrix. [20]

A typical immunoassay format is seen in a flow-through device that has an antibody covalently coupled to the surface of a porous matrix. When the patient sample is added to the matrix, the analyte of interest binds to the antibody. Addition of a second labeled antibody forms a sandwich and traps the label at the position of the first antibody.[12] If the label consists of gold sol particles or colored latex, it is directly visualized or quantified by reflectance spectrophotometry in a separate reader. Another important feature of this type of technology is the incorporation of a built-in quality monitor that indicates positive if all reagents have been stored and the device is operated correctly. In all these different formats, uniform and predictable flow of the sample through or along the solid phase matrix is a major determinant of the reproducibility of the technique. Therefore the choice of matrix and how it interacts with the sample are of particular importance, and advances in the understanding of solid phase and surface chemistry technology have made a major contribution to the development of immunosensors.[11] An example of this technology is shown in Figure 17-3. In this device, the blood sample is added and first flows through a glass fiber fleece, which separates plasma

TABLE 17-2	Examples of Single or Multi-pad Stick Tests	
Test	**Sample**	**Chemistry**
Acetaminophen	Whole blood	Acyl dehydrogenase
Alanine aminotransferase	Whole blood	Alanine/glutamate
Albumin	Whole blood, urine	Dye binding
Cholesterol	Whole blood	Cholesterol oxidase
Creatinine	Whole blood, urine	Copper complexation
Glucose	Whole blood	Glucose oxidase
Lactate	Whole blood	Lactate dehydrogenase
Uric acid	Whole blood	Uricase
Alcohol	Urine	Alcohol dehydrogenase
Bilirubin	Urine	2,4-Dichloroaniline
Hemoglobin	Urine	Peroxidase activity
Leukocyte esterase	Urine	Pyrrole amino ester hydrolysis
Ketones	Urine	Sodium nitroprusside reaction
Nitrite	Urine	p-Arsanilic acid reaction
pH	Urine	Double indicator principle
Protein	Urine	Protein error of indicators
Specific gravity	Urine	Polyacid pH change
Urobilinogen	Urine	Ehrlich's reaction

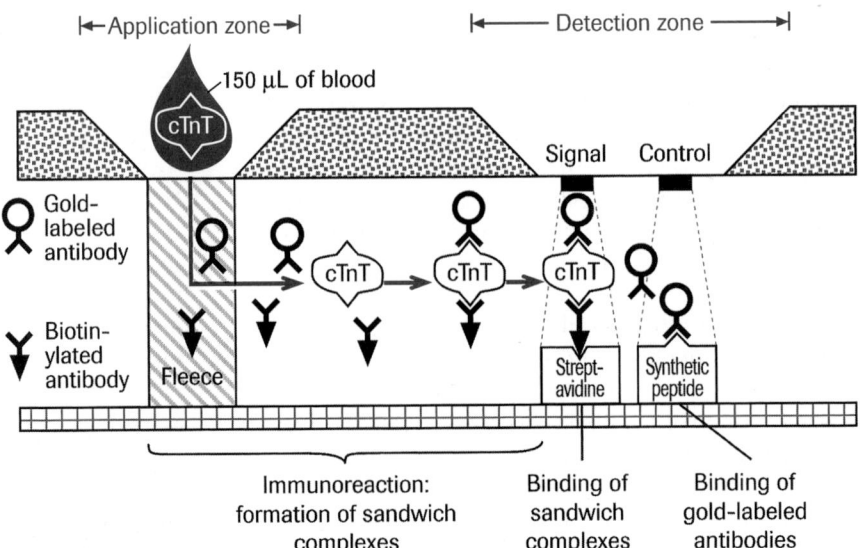

Figure 17-3 Schematic diagram of a lateral-flow immunoassay for troponin T. *(Courtesy Roche Diagnostics, Mannheim, Germany.)*

from whole blood. Simultaneously, two monoclonal antihuman cardiac troponin T (cTnT) antibodies, one conjugated to biotin and one labeled with gold particles, bind to the troponin T in the sample. The antibody/troponin complex then flows in a lateral direction along the cellulose nitrate test strip until it reaches the capture zone, which contains streptavidin bound to a solid phase. The biotin in the antibody/troponin complex binds to the streptavidin and immobilizes the complex. The complex is then visualized as a purple band by the gold particles attached to one of the antibodies. The unreacted gold-labeled antibody moves farther down the strip, where it is captured by a zone containing a synthetic peptide consisting of the epitope of human cTnT and is visualized as a separate but similar colored band. The presence of this second band serves as an important quality indicator because it shows that the sample has flowed along the test strip and the device has performed correctly.

Single-use Quantitative Cartridge and Strip Tests With a Monitoring Device

The availability of small, compact detectors is a result of advances in modern electronics and miniaturization. An integral part of many of these instruments is a charge-coupled device (CCD) camera that is a multichannel light detector, similar to a photomultiplier tube in a spectrophotometer, but detects much lower levels of light. For example, the Roche Cardiac Reader contains a CCD that quantitates separate lateral-flow immunoassay strips for measurement of (1) troponin T, (2) myoglobin, and (3) D-dimer.

Glucose Measurement. Clinically, POCT is most frequently used to measure glucose. These devices are biosensors because they all use an enzyme such as (1) glucose oxidase (GO), (2) hexokinase (HK), or (3) glucose dehydrogenase (GDH) as the recognition agent with photometric (reflectance) and electrochemical detection.

In general, all modern glucose strips are a form of what is called *thick-film* technology in that the film is composed of several layers, each having a specific function. When blood is added to a strip, both water and glucose pass into the film or analytical layer; for some photometric systems, erythrocytes must be excluded. These processes are achieved by what is called the separating layer that contains various components, including (1) glass fibers, (2) fleeces, (3) membranes, and (4) special latex formulations. In photometric systems, a spreading layer is important for the fast homogeneous distribution of the sample, whereas electrochemical strips use capillary fill systems. The support layer is usually a thin plastic material that in the case of reflectance-based strips may also have reflective properties. Additional reflectance properties have been achieved through inclusion of substances such as (1) titanium oxide, (2) barium sulfate, and (3) zinc oxide.

With systems that measure reflectance, the relationship between reflectance and the glucose concentration is described by the Kubelka-Munk equation:

$$C\alpha\frac{K}{S} = \frac{(1-R)^2}{2R}$$

where C is the analyte concentration, K is the absorption coefficient, S is the scattering coefficient, and R is the percent of reflectance. In practice, glucose strips are produced in large batches, and, after extensive quality assurance procedures, each batch is given a code that is stored in a magnetic strip on the underside of each test strip. This code describes the performance of the batch, including the calibrating relationship between the photometric or electrochemical signal and the concentration of glucose. In current practice, strips that do not require coding have become more commonplace.

Since their introduction, a steady stream of innovation in the development of glucose meters has been seen, with the goal of making the devices smaller and easier to use with less risk of error and reducing interference from other compounds and effects. The latter includes other (1) reducing substances, (2) low sample oxygen tension, and (3) extremes of hematocrit. A major step in this development process was the use of ferrocene and its derivatives as immobilized mediators in the construction of an electrochemical glucose strip (Figure 17-4). This is composed of an Ag-AgCl reference electrode and a carbon-based active electrode, both manufactured using screen printing technology, with ferrocene or its derivatives contained in the printing ink. The sample is placed in the sample observation window, and the hydrophilic layer serves to direct the sample over the reagent layer. The conversion of glucose is accompanied by reduction of ferrocene and the release of electrons (see Figure 17-4). The introduction of electrochemical technology has facilitated the production of smaller meters that use nonwipe strips. Such meters have less need (1) to clean the instrument optics, (2) produce test results more rapidly, and (3) require smaller sample volumes. Some of these features are now available with photometric glucose meters.

Other Applications. Several immunosensor-based POCT devices have been developed that are capable of measuring a panel of analytes, such as (1) cardiac markers, (2) allergy tests, (3) fertility tests, and (4) drugs of abuse. In these devices, a mixture of antibodies is immobilized at the origin, and complementary antibodies for the various analytes are immobilized

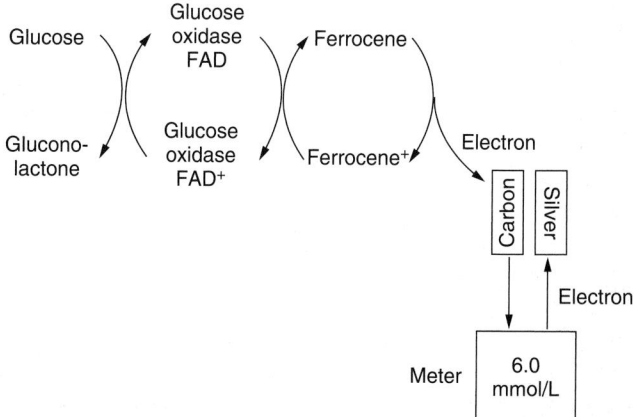

Figure 17-4 Schematic diagram of the reactions taking place in a MediSense electrochemical glucose strip. *(Modified from Henning TP, Cunningham TP. Biosensors for personal diabetes management. In: Ramsay G ed. Commercial biosensors. New York: John Wiley & Sons, 1998:3-46.)*

at varying positions along the porous strip. In the case of drugs of abuse, devices are designed such that positive responses are obtained only when the concentration is above a precalibrated cutoff value.[11]

In contrast to the thick-film technology already described, single-use sensors have been constructed using *thin-film* technology, the most common commercial example being the i-STAT analyser (http://www.abbottpointofcare.com/; accessed August 13, 2013). This handheld blood gas device measures (1) electrolytes, (2) glucose, (3) creatinine, (4) certain coagulation parameters, and (5) cardiac markers. In thin-film sensors, electrodes are wafer structures constructed with thin metal oxide film using microfabrication techniques. The result consists of small, single-use cartridges containing an array of electrochemical sensors that operate in conjunction with a handheld analyzer. Because the sensor layer is very thin, blood permeates this layer quickly, and the sensor cartridge is used immediately after it is unwrapped from its packing. This provides an advantage over some thick-film sensors that require an equilibration or wet-up time before they are used to measure blood samples. A disadvantage of thin-film technology is that manufacturing costs are high because of the need for special clean air facilities. Thus more recently, technology to measure blood gases and related parameters has been devised using less costly smart card technology, where sensors and internal fluidics are incorporated into credit card–sized devices manufactured on a 35-mm tape-on-reel format. This technology is used in conjunction with a handheld analyzer that also has been used for immunoassay measurement.[11]

A number of single-use, quantitative POCT devices are available that employ a cassette or cartridge design rather than lateral-flow strips. One such device separates plasma from red cells, after which the plasma reacts with pads of dry reagents for analytes such as (1) glucose, (2) cholesterol, or (3) triglycerides. The resultant change in absorbance is then measured by a small photometer. Several cassette-based systems have been developed for measurement of hemoglobin. In one such system, (1) red cells are lysed in a minicuvet, (2) hemoglobin is converted to methemoglobin, and (3) methemoglobin is measured at 570 nm; turbidity is corrected for by an additional measurement at 880 nm.

Another type of cartridge design uses a light-scattering immunoassay to measure glycated hemoglobin, together with a photometric assay for total hemoglobin. The cartridge is a relatively complex structure that contains antigen-coated latex particles, antibodies to HbA_{1c}, and lysing reagents that are mixed after the sample is added. Measurement takes place when the cartridge is placed into a temperature-controlled reader, and the analytical performance is sufficient for quantitative monitoring of glycemic control. The size of the device allows it to be used in diabetes clinics, where it is also used for measurement of urinary albumin and creatinine.

POCT devices for monitoring anticoagulant therapy have also been developed for use in clinics or by the patient at home. Historically, early systems used magnets to detect the decrease in sample flow or movement that results from the

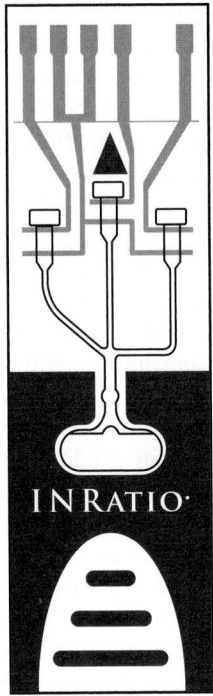

Figure 17-5 Alere INRatio® 2 PT/INR Test Strip. *(Used with permission from Alere.)*

clotting process, but this required careful timing and a large blood sample, while an alternative technology used optical sensors to monitor the decrease in sample speed as the clot forms. Speckle detection technology whereby an intensity pattern produced by the mutual interference of a set of wavefronts has also been used to measure (1) prothrombin time (PT), (2) activated partial thromboplastin time (APTT), and (3) activated clotting time (ACT). With this approach, the instrument contains an infrared light source that directs a coherent light beam onto the oscillating sample. Movement of red cells in the blood results in refraction of the light to produce an interference or "speckle" pattern that is recorded by the photodetector. This "speckle" pattern changes when the capillary flow slows as the sample clots. The time it takes for this to happen is a measure of the clotting time. Newer detection technologies that have been widely adopted for measurement of the international normalized ratio (INR) in the home and clinic use electrochemical measurements. With the Alere device (http://www.hemosenseinratio.com/; accessed August 13, 2013), clotting is detected by a change in impedance (Figure 17-5), and with a CoaguChek® XS system (www.Roche.com/; accessed August 13, 2013), a change in current is detected. Both devices incorporate built-in QC systems that are activated when a patient sample is placed on the strip.[11]

It should be noted that the sizes of some of the single-use, cartridge-based systems are comparable with certain of the bench top systems. In addition, some of the multiple-use devices incorporate on-board centrifugation. Other small analyzers are used at point-of-care but require preliminary centrifugation of the sample.

Multiple-use Cartridge and Bench Top Systems

Many of the POCT devices in this category are used for critical care testing in locations such as (1) the intensive care unit, (2) the surgical suite, and (3) the emergency room (see Box 17-1). Some of these devices use thick-film sensors or electrodes in strips to measure (1) glucose, (2) lactate, (3) urea, (4) blood gases , and (5) electrolytes incorporating the same technology described previously, but differ in that the sensors are designed to be reusable. They are manufactured from thick films of paste and inks using screen printing techniques to produce individual or multiple sensors. The sensors have been incorporated with reagents and calibrators into a single cartridge or pack, which is placed in the body of a small to medium-sized portable critical care analyzer. Each pack contains reagents sufficient to measure a certain number of samples during a certain time period, after which it is relatively simple to replace.

Other key developments for devices include liquid calibration systems that use a combination of aqueous base solutions and conductance measurements to calibrate the pH and PCO_2 electrodes, with oxygen being calibrated with an oxygen-free solution and room air. In addition, automated QC packages are integrated into these analyzers to ensure that QC samples are analyzed at regular intervals. These comprise packs or bottles of QC material that are contained within the instrument and are sampled at predetermined intervals, with onboard software interpreting the results and generating alerts, if necessary. Such devices have the capability to be remotely monitored and programmed to respond to problems with instruments located long distances from the central laboratory.

Critical care POCT instruments are also available for measuring various hemoglobin species and for performing CO-oximetry determinations. The latter rely upon multiwavelength spectrophotometry, where light absorption by hemolyzed blood is measured at up to 60 or more wavelengths to determine the concentration of the five hemoglobin species. One manufacturer has extended multiwavelength spectrophotometry to measure bilirubin directly in whole blood.[11]

Bench top devices are also available to perform complete blood counts (CBCs) using analytical principles similar to those used with laboratory-based devices. In addition, single-use cartridge technology is now available to provide full white cell differentiation. Immunoassay measurements are now available in a compact device for use in clinics and similar locations. One such device uses dry-coated reagents and time-resolved fluorescence for detection. Results are produced within 20 minutes, and the assay menu includes (1) C-reactive protein (CRP), (2) human chorionic gonadotropin (hCG), and (3) cardiac markers.[11]

In Vivo, Ex Vivo, or Minimally Invasive and
Noninvasive Devices

Although most POCT devices are used for in vitro applications, a smaller group is classified as (1) in vivo, (2) ex vivo, or (3) minimally invasive (Table 17-3). In vivo or continuous monitoring applications are those in which the sensing device is inserted into the bloodstream and is used to measure blood

TABLE 17-3	Types of Ex Vivo and Noninvasive Point-of-Care Testing Technology	
Type of Technology	**Analytical Principle**	**Analytes**
In vivo	Optical fluorescence	pH, blood gases
	Electrochemistry	Subcutaneous glucose
Ex vivo	Optical fluorescence	pH, blood gases
	Electrochemistry	pH, blood gases, electrolytes, glucose
Noninvasive	Electrochemistry/ iontophoresis	Transcutaneous glucose
	Multiwavelength spectrophotometry	Bilirubin

gases and glucose using optical or electrochemical technology. Electrochemical sensors are also used in an ex vivo application for the same parameters, the difference being that the sensors are actually external to the body but are present in a closed loop of blood that leaves the body and is then returned downstream from the sensing device. The major application for *minimally invasive devices* is primarily glucose, such as the Medtronic continuous glucose monitoring system (www.medtronicdiabetes.com/; accessed August 14, 2013), by which glucose measurements in interstitial fluid are transmitted back to a monitor linked to an insulin pump.[11]

For noninvasive testing, several POCT devices are available for the transcutaneous measurement of bilirubin in newborn babies.[12]

Informatics and POCT

Most analytical devices used in clinical laboratories are directly linked or connected via an electronic interface to a laboratory information system (LIS). In this progression, many different informatic functions are used, including electronic transfer of data from the analyzers to the LIS and ultimately into a patient's electronic medical record. This provides healthcare professionals with (1) quick, (2) accurate, and (3) appropriate access to the patient's medical history and information.

Considerable effort has been expended to incorporate these informatic processes into POCT devices because of the vital importance of capturing analytical data in a patient's medical record to avoid the errors associated with manual transcription of data. Newer POCT devices have addressed this problem by incorporating the prerequisite hardware and software into their design, and in the last decade so-called **connectivity** standards have been introduced, which facilitate linking of devices to information management systems. Previously, interfacing was very difficult because of multiple proprietary interfaces, but through the efforts of the POCT industry and a Connectivity Industry Consortium (CIC), a set of seamless—"plug and play"—point-of-care communication standards have been developed and subsequently incorporated into a Clinical Laboratory and Standards Institute (CLSI) standard called POCT01-A2.[4] Adherence to these connectivity standards ensures that POCT devices meet critical user requirements, such as (1) bidirectionality,

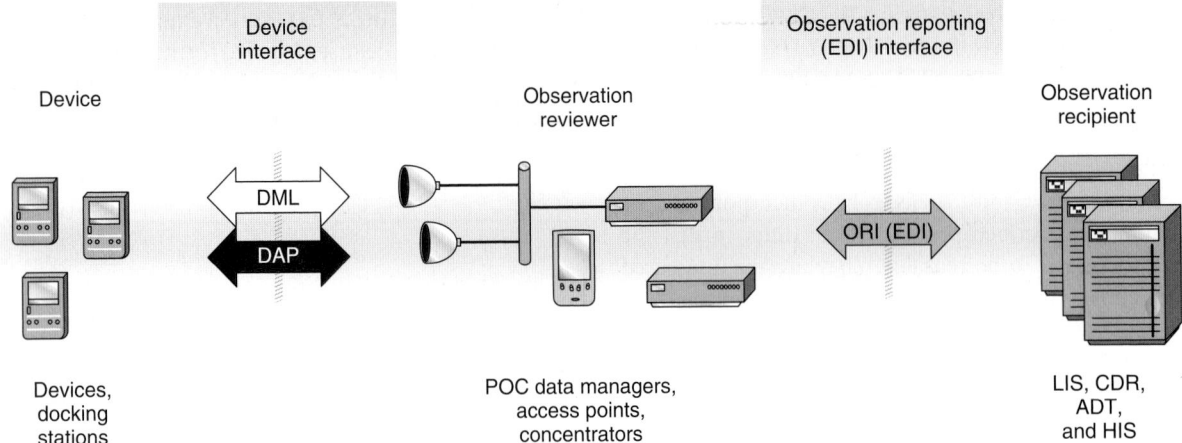

Figure 17-6 Schematic diagram of the interfaces between POCT devices and information systems. *(Modified from Clinical and Laboratory Standards Institute/NCCLS. Point-of-care connectivity: approved Standard CLSI . Approved standard POCT1-A2. Wayne, PA: Clinical and Laboratory Standards Institute, 2006.)*

(2) device connection commonality, (3) commercial software intraoperability, (4) security, and (5) QC and/or regulatory compliance.

Description of Connectivity Standards

The CIC connectivity standards are represented simply as the two interfaces between the POCT devices and information systems (Figure 17-6). The device interface passes patient results and QC information between the POCT instrument and devices, such as (1) docking stations, (2) concentrators, (3) terminal servers, and (4) point-of-care data managers. The latter have to be linked to a variety of information systems via the observation reporting interface or the electronic data interface for transmission of ordering information and patient results.

Benefits of POCT Connectivity

Currently, one of the most important benefits of connectivity is that it facilitates the transfer and capture of patient POCT and quality-related data into permanent medical records. In addition, innovations in the area of POCT quality are facilitated by the ability to easily link devices to networks and to those who are ultimately responsible for the device. The potential benefits of POCT connectivity and what users should look for in POCT01-A2[4] compliant devices are described in a CLSI document (POCT02-A[5]. Examples of these benefits are shown in the software products of several POCT device manufacturers, which allow central laboratories to monitor their instruments in remote locations. In conjunction with network technology, remote control software not only allows monitoring of the performance of the device but also enables those responsible for the instrument to carry out some service procedures or even shut the instrument down completely if required. The ability to interface devices more easily with other information systems should enable the development of applications that add value to patient data, such as the use of decision support software to assist with interpretation and other tele-health-care applications.

Implementation and Management Considerations

The (1) implementation, (2) management, and (3) maintenance of a POCT service in a healthcare facility require the necessary planning, oversight, and inventory control and assurance of the reliability of results through adequate training and QC. Consequently, a number of factors must be considered (Box 17-4).

Establishment of Need

As with general laboratory testing, the decision to implement a POCT service requires (1) establishment of need, (2) consideration of the clinical, operational, and economic benefits, and (3) examination of the costs and changes to the clinical process involved.

Addressing the questions listed in Box 17-5 is useful in establishing the requirement for a POCT service.[13] Answering these questions facilitates identification of the test itself and should also explain why the current service is not meeting the needs of the patient, the clinician, or the healthcare provider.

A risk assessment should be conducted that will focus primarily on the procedures and processes that have to be put in place to ensure continued high quality of service. Issues of concern that need to be addressed when such an assessment is conducted are listed in Box 17-6.

Organization and Implementation of a POCT Coordinating Committee

When organizing and implementing a POCT service, it is important to consult with all involved parties. It is recommended that a POCT coordinating committee be established first. Such a committee is charged with managing the whole process of delivering a high-quality POCT service. The committee should consist of representatives of those who use the service and those who deliver the service, together with a representative of the organization's

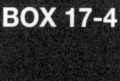

BOX 17-4 Factors That Need to Be Considered in the Implementation, Management, and Maintenance of a POCT Service

Establishing need
Organizing and implementing a coordinating committee
Establishing a POCT testing policy and accountability
Procuring equipment and performing its evaluation
Training and certifying operators
Establishing a QC, quality assurance, and audit policy
Ensuring documentation
Establishing accreditation and regulation of POCT policy

BOX 17-5 Assessing the Need for a Point-of-Care Testing Service

Which tests are required?
What TAT is required?
What clinical question is being asked when this test is requested?
What clinical decision is likely to be made upon receipt of the result?
What action is likely to be taken upon receipt of the result?
What outcome should be expected from the action taken?
Why isn't the laboratory able to deliver the required service?
Will POCT provide the required accuracy and precision of the result?
Is staff available to perform the test?
Are adequate facilities available in which to perform the test and store the equipment and reagents?
Will you abide by the organization's POCT policy?
Are operational benefits associated with this POCT strategy?
Are economic benefits derived from this POCT strategy?
Will a change in practice be required to deliver these benefits?
Is it feasible to deliver the changes in practice that might be required?

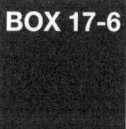

BOX 17-6 Issues of Concern When a Risk Assessment Is Performed for Consideration of Implementing a POCT Service

Robustness of the POCT device
Quality of the results produced
Competence of the operator of the device
Effectiveness of the process of transmitting results to the caregiver
Competence of the caregiver in interpreting the results provided
Procedures in place to ensure that an accurate record of the results is kept
Identification of what practice changes may have to be made to deliver the benefits that have been identified
Determination of how the staff will be retrained if appropriate
Determination of how the changes in practice will be implemented

management system, (2) part of its clinical governance policy, and (3) required for accreditation purposes.[10] The elements of a POCT policy are listed in Box 17-7.

Equipment Procurement and Evaluation

After the requirement, the coordination committee, and the policy have been established, the next stage in the process is equipment procurement. This involves first identifying candidate POCT equipment that has the prerequisite analytical and operational capabilities to meet the clinical requirements of a POCT service. As discussed in Chapter 2 and in a CLSI protocol,[3] the performance characteristics of these devices are then determined and compared. In addition, performance requirements of the operator have to be identified and the potential for operator error determined. Independent validation of these analytical and operational characteristics is obtained from (1) the manufacturer, (2) published evaluations performed by government agencies, and (3) reports in the peer-reviewed literature. When performance data are reviewed, particular attention should be paid to the precision and accuracy of measurement, including the concordance between results produced by the POCT device and by a routine laboratory method, because patients are likely to be managed using both analytical systems. This concordance may be difficult to assess, and it may be necessary to seek endorsements from current users of the systems and possibly to conduct some form of internal trial.

An economic assessment of the planned POCT service, including the costs of consumables and servicing, should also be completed. This is likely to be a comparative exercise between the various point-of-care systems under consideration. Any comparison of costs with the laboratory service will only be emphasizing the cost per test, which will not give an accurate assessment of the cost utility of the system. However, it is helpful at this point to have a good assessment of the relative staff costs associated with different systems because these are likely to be key features in the decision-making process. It is probable that the chosen system will be operated by staff already performing a wide range of other duties involving the care of patients, and therefore the amount of time required to operate the device may be critical.

management team. Users will include (1) physicians, (2) physician assistants, (3) family nurse practitioners, (4) nurses, (5) other healthcare providers, and (6) patients. The providers should include at least one representative from the laboratory and those involved in the use of other diagnostic and therapeutic equipment close to the patient. Typically a laboratory professional will chair such a committee because it is the laboratory that will provide the necessary backup if a service failure should occur; furthermore, the laboratory professional will have received training and developed expertise with the analytical issues that are likely to arise. It is recommended that the committee report to the medical director. The committee should designate members who will take responsibility for overseeing the training and accreditation of all POCT operators, as well as for QC and quality assurance. The work of the committee should be governed by the organization's policy on POCT.[13]

POCT Policy and Accountability

Implementation of a POCT service requires a POCT policy that establishes all of the procedures required to ensure the delivery of a high-quality service, together with the responsibility and accountability of all staff associated with the POCT. This may be (1) part of the organization's total *quality*

BOX 17-7 Elements of a Point-of-Care Testing Policy

Catalog Information Review Time
- Approved by
- Original distribution
- Related policies
- Further information
- Policy replaces

Introduction/Background
- Definition
- Accreditation of services
- Audit of services

Laboratory Services in the Organization—Location
- Logistics
- Policy on diagnostic testing

Management of POCT—Committee and Accountability
- Officers
- Committee members
- Terms of reference
- Responsibilities
- Meetings

Equipment and Consumable Procurement—Criteria for Procurement
- Process of procurement

Standard Operating Procedures
- Training and certification of staff—training
- Certification
- Recertification

Quality Control and Quality Assurance Procedures
- Documentation and review

Health and Safety Procedures

Bibliography

BOX 17-8 The Main Elements of a Point-of-Care Testing Training Program

Understanding the Context of the Test—Pathophysiological Context
- Clinical requirement for the test
- Action taken on basis of result
- Nature of test and method used

Patient Preparation Required—Relevance of Diurnal Variation
- Relevance of drug therapy

Sample Requirement and Specimen Collection

Preparation of Analytical Device—Machine and/or Consumables

Performance of Test

Performance of Quality Control

Documentation of Test Result and Quality Control Result

Reporting of Test Result to Appropriate Personnel

Interpretation of Result and Sources of Advice

Health and Safety Issues (e.g., disposal of sample and test device, cleaning of machine and test area)

After the comparison data have been obtained, tabulated, and interpreted, a POCT device is selected. The laboratory professional then conducts a short evaluation of the equipment to become familiar with the system. This evaluation will help to determine the content of the training routine that will have to be subsequently developed and whether troubleshooting of problems is required. Such an evaluation should document the concordance between results generated with the device and those provided by the laboratory. All of this information should then be recorded in a logbook associated with the equipment. In addition, the organization may (1) wish to undertake some form of safety check, (2) give the device some form of local code, and (3) enter the code into the local equipment register.

Training and Certification

The confidence of (1) the clinician, (2) the caregiver, and (3) the patient in the results generated by a POCT device depends on the performance and robustness of the instrument and the competence of the operator. Many of the agencies involved in the regulation of healthcare delivery now require that all personnel associated with the delivery of diagnostic results demonstrate their competence through a process of regulation, and this applies equally to POCT personnel. Typically,

those healthcare professionals involved in POCT will not have received training in the use of analytical devices as part of their core professional training but may be called upon to operate a number of complex pieces of equipment.

The elements of a training program are listed in Box 17-8. In practice, the extent of this program will vary according to how well the complexity of the analytical method has been engineered into the device. Such a program is tailored to meet the needs of the individual and the organization. The program may include (1) formal presentation to groups or on a one-to-one basis, (2) self-directed learning using agreed documentation, or (3) computer-aided learning. For example, several of the current models of blood gas and electrolyte analyzers have onboard computer-aided training modules. Whatever the training strategy employed, it is important to document the satisfactory completion of training and that the individual has been tested and found competent through a combination of questions concerned with understanding and practically demonstrating the skills gained. The latter is achieved by performing tests on a series of QC materials and repeat testing samples that have recently been analyzed (parallel testing). Finally the operator should be observed through the whole procedure involved in the POCT on a minimum of three occasions.

Competence is maintained on a long-term basis through regular practice of skills and continuing education, and it is important to build these features into any education and training program. Regular review of performance in QC and quality assurance programs will provide a means of monitoring and overseeing the competence of operators. However, this is not always sufficient, particularly when operators are employed on irregular shifts or may not always be called upon to perform POCT. In this latter situation, it may be necessary to create specific arrangements by which individuals can undertake tests on QC material. The error log may highlight when problems are arising. However, it is important to encourage an open approach to the assessment of competence so that operators themselves seek help if they believe that problems are occurring. Such an open approach should be supported with audit and performance review meetings where problems are aired and developments discussed. The regular assessment of competence should be built into a formal program for recertification that will be a requirement of most accreditation programs.[13]

Quality Control, Quality Assurance, and Audit

QC and quality assurance programs provide a formal means of monitoring the quality of a service (see Chapter 7). The internal QC program gives a relatively short-term view and typically compares current performance with that of the previous analysis. External quality assurance is a longer-term process that addresses other issues surrounding the quality of the result. Thus, quality assurance compares the testing performance of different sites and/or different pieces of equipment or methods.[11] An audit is a more retrospective form of analysis of performance that takes a more complete view of the entire process. However, the foundation for ensuring good quality remains a successful training and certification scheme.

Classically, quantitative internal QC involves the analysis of a sample for which the analyte concentration is known and the mean and range of results quoted for the method used. Several challenges are associated with the classical approach to POCT. The first concern to be considered is the frequency of testing—Should a QC sample be analyzed every time that (1) a sample is analyzed, (2) a new operator uses the system, (3) a new lot number of reagents is used, or (4) the system is recalibrated? No consistent agreement has determined the correct approach, and one probably has to be guided by the reproducibility and overall analytical performance of the system. The approach used is also influenced by local circumstances, such as the number and competence of the operators and the frequency with which the system is used. For a bench top and/or multitest analyzer, at least one QC sample should be run a minimum of once per shift—three times a day. Some critical care analyzers are programmed to perform a QC check at intervals set by those responsible for the device.

For single-use POCT disposable devices, this strategy does not completely monitor the quality of the test system. For example, when conventional QC material is analyzed on a unit-use or single-test POCT system, only that testing unit is monitored. Thus it is impossible to test every unit with control material because by definition these are single-test systems, and it is not possible to analyze both control material and a patient sample with the single unit. Under these circumstances, greater dependence is placed on the manufacturing reproducibility of the devices to ensure a good quality service. A 2010 CLSI guideline reports quality management procedures for POCT.[6]

In practice, the user may wish to continue with a QC testing strategy that is similar to that applied for multiuse devices, namely, analyzing a minimum of one QC sample per run during each shift. If testing is infrequent, another approach would be to analyze a QC sample whenever a change is made to the testing system, such as when a different batch of testing materials is used or a different operator is performing the testing.

Other QC approaches may be used, but many do not test the whole process. For example, the use of a plastic surrogate reflectance pad as a QC sample will only test the performance of the reflectance meter and does not test the process of sample addition, etc. Similarly, some forms of electronic internal QC do not test the sampling technique but simply the functionality of the cassette and the docking station.[11]

External quality assurance or proficiency testing is a systematic approach to QC monitoring by which standardized samples are analyzed by one or more laboratories to determine the capability of each participant. With this approach, the operator has no knowledge of the analyte concentration, and therefore it is considered closer to a "real testing situation." The results are transmitted to a central authority, who then prepares a report and returns a copy to each participating laboratory. The report will identify the range of results obtained for the complete group of participants and may be classified according to the different methods used by participants in the scheme. The scheme may encompass both laboratory and POCT users, which provides an opportunity to compare results with laboratory-based methods. In practice, external quality assurance or proficiency testing is used in POCT to determine and document long-term performance and the concordance of results between the POCT service and an organization's central laboratory. It is also possible to operate an external quality assurance scheme within a hospital or organizational setting; such a scheme would and should be run by qualified laboratory personnel. This provides the opportunity to compare the results being reported by the laboratory and by other POCT sites within the same organization. This is important when patients are managed in several departments—or when machines break down and samples are taken to other sites for testing. When deteriorating or poor performance is identified in one of these schemes, it is important to document the problem, and then provide and document a solution. It may be necessary as part of this exercise to review some of the patient's notes to ensure that incorrect results have not been reported and inappropriate clinical actions taken. In addition, if the solution highlights a vulnerable feature of the process overall or for one particular operator, a process of retraining must be instituted.

Maintenance and Inventory Control

Implementation and maintenance of a POCT service requires that a supply of devices be maintained at all times and a formal program for doing so employed. The key points in this process are to (1) adhere to the recommended storage conditions, (2) be aware of the stated shelf life of the consumables, and (3) ensure that stocks are released in time for any preanalytical preparation to be accommodated (e.g., thawing). When multiple sites are using the same materials, a central purchasing, supply, and inventory control system should be implemented. This will gain the benefit derived from bulk purchasing and will ensure that individual systems are not supplied unknowingly with different batches of consumables.

The complexity in the maintenance of reusable devices will vary from system to system, but clear guidelines will be available from the manufacturer and should be adhered to rigorously. Issues that usually require particular vigilance include (1) expiration dates, (2) biocontamination, (3) electrical safety, (4) maintenance of optics, and (5) inadvertent use of inappropriate consumables.

Documentation

Documentation of all aspects of a POCT service is essential and it is critically important to keep an accurate record of (1) test requests, (2) results, and (3) actions taken, as an absolute minimum. Some of the prior issues associated with documentation are now being resolved with the advent of (1) the patient electronic record, (2) electronic requesting, and (3) better connectivity of POCT instrumentation to information systems and the patient record (see earlier discussion). The documentation should extend from the standard operating procedure(s) for the POCT systems to records of training and certification of operators and internal QC and quality assurance, together with error logs and any corrective action taken.

Accreditation and Regulation of POCT

The features of the organization and management of POCT described previously are the same as those associated with the accreditation of any diagnostic services.[2] Accreditation of POCT should be part of the overall accreditation of laboratory medicine services, or indeed part of the accreditation of the full clinical service, as has been the case in many countries, including the United States and the United Kingdom, for a number of years. For example, the U.S. Congress passed the **Clinical Laboratory Improvement Amendments of 1988 (CLIA-88)**, which established quality standards for all laboratory testing to ensure (1) accuracy, (2) reliability, and (3) timeliness of patient test results, regardless of where the test was performed. The final CLIA regulations were published in the *Federal Register* on February 28, 1992. These requirements are based on the complexity of the test, not on the type of laboratory in which the testing is performed. The CLIA regulations list three testing categories: (1) waived, (2) moderate complexity, and (3) high complexity. Of importance to a discussion of POCT is the "waived" category, with a **waived test** defined as a "simple laboratory examination and procedure that have an insignificant risk of an erroneous result" (http://www.cms.gov/; accessed on August 14, 2013). Many POC tests have been categorized as "waived." In addition, CLIA legislation in the United States stipulates that all POCT must meet certain minimum standards.[17,18] In the United States, (1) the Centers for Medicare & Medicaid Services, (2) the Joint Commission, and (3) the College of American Pathologists are responsible for inspecting sites. Each is committed to ensuring compliance with testing regulations for POCT.[8]

Review Questions

1. Are the results obtained from a point-of-care test (POCT) device qualitative, quantitative, or semi-quantitative, or can they be all of these?
   a. Qualitative only
   b. Quantitative only
   c. Semi-quantitative only
   d. All of the above result types can be obtained from a point-of-care test device.

2. Which of the following is *not* considered an advantage of POCT?
   a. Reduced need for quality control
   b. Reduced turnaround time
   c. Reduced length of time between test results and clinical decisions
   d. Improved health outcomes

3. The most frequently tested analyte that is measured by a point-of-care device is:
   a. arterial blood pH.
   b. glucose.
   c. hemoglobin.
   d. a cardiac marker.

4. One of the benefits for the lab regarding POC testing is a reduction in *controllable* preanalytical variables and errors. An example of one of these types of variables would be:
   a. not having to run controls.
   b. not performing preventive maintenance on the equipment.
   c. obtaining blood in the wrong type of tube.
   d. the individual's age.

5. With regard to point-of-care testing, examining a urine specimen for the presence (not a specific concentration) of a drug metabolite would likely be performed using a:
   a. single-use quantitative test cartridge.
   b. single-use qualitative test cartridge.
   c. multiple-use test cartridge.
   d. continuous monitoring device.

6. The most common biological recognition element used as a biosensor in a point-of-care device is a(n):
   a. antibody.
   b. antigen.
   c. hormone.
   d. enzyme.

7. To perform quality control on a new lot of multiuse point-of-care devices that are used infrequently, a minimum of one control sample per lot is sufficient to test the whole assay process.
   a. True
   b. False

8. A systematic, long-term approach to quality control of POCT devices that is sometimes referred to as "external" quality control involves enrollment in a proficiency testing program. This type of QC testing involves:
   a. analysis of unknown samples as a sort of test to determine the capability of participants in the program.
   b. testing of a plastic reflectance pad in some POCT devices to test the performance of the reflectance meter.
   c. a standardized program that asks questions of the operators of the POCT.
   d. analysis of the external parts of a POC testing device such as the reagent delivery system.

References

1. Attia UM, Marson S, Alcock JR. Micro-injection moulding of polymer microfluidic devices. Microfluidics and Nanofluidics 2009;7:1–29.
2. Burnett D. Accreditation and point-of-care testing. Ann Clin Biochem 2000;37:241–3.
3. Clinical and Laboratory Standards Institute. Evaluation of precision performance of clinical chemistry devices, 2nd edition. CLSI Document EP05-A2. Wayne, PA: CLSI, 2004.
4. Clinical and Laboratory Standards Institute. Point-of-care connectivity: approved standard, 2nd edition. CLSI Document POCT01-A2. Wayne, PA: CLSI, 2006.
5. Clinical and Laboratory Standards Institute. Implementation guide of POCT01 for healthcare providers: approved guideline, 2nd edition. CLSI Document POCT02-A. Wayne, PA: CLSI, 2008.
6. Clinical and Laboratory Standards Institute. Quality management: approaches to reducing errors at the Point-of-Care. Approved guideline. CLSI Document POCT07-A. Wayne, PA: CLSI, 2010.
7. Khandurina J, Guttman A. Bioanalysis in microfluidic devices. J Chromatogr A 2002;943:159–83.
8. Kost GJ, ed. Principles and practice of point-of-care testing. Philadelphia: Lippincott Williams & Wilkins, 2002.
9. Nichols JH, ed. NACB laboratory medicine practice guidelines: evidence-based practice for point-of-care testing. Washington, DC: AACC Press, 2006. http://www.aacc.org/AACC/members/nacb/LMPG/ (accessed on December 11, 2012).
10. Price CP. Point of care testing. BMJ 2001;322:1285–8.
11 Price CP, St John A, Kricka LJ, eds. Point-of-care testing, 3rd edition. Washington, DC: AACC Press, 2010.
12. Price CP, St John A. Point-of-care testing. In: Burtis CA, Ashwood ER, Bruns DE, eds. Tietz textbook of clinical chemistry and molecular diagnostics, 5th edition. St Louis: Saunders, 2012:487–505.
13. Price CP, St John A. Point-of-care testing: making innovation work for patient-centred care. Washington, DC: AACC Press, 2012.
14. Reid PP, Compton WD, Grossman JH, Fanjiang G, eds. National Academy of Engineering and Institute of Medicine. Building a better delivery system. Washington, DC: National Academies Press, 2005.
15. Savage GT, van der Reis L. A Dutch and American commentary on IT in healthcare: roundtable discussion on IT and innovations in healthcare. Adv Health Care Mgmt 2012;12:61–74.
16. Turner APF ed Biosensors: fundamentals and applications. Oxford: Oxford University Press, 1987.
17. U.S. Department of Health and Human Services. Medicare, Medicaid and CLIA programs: regulations implementing the Clinical Laboratory Improvement Amendments of 1988 (CLIA). Final rule. Federal Register 1992;57:7002–186.
18. U.S. Department of Health and Human Services. Medicare, Medicaid and CLIA programs: regulations implementing the Clinical Laboratory Improvement Amendments of 1988 (CLIA) and Clinical Laboratory Act program fee collection. Federal Register 1993;58:5215–37.
19. Walter B. Dry reagent chemistries. Anal Chem 1983;55:A498–A514.
20. Wong R, Tse H. Lateral flow immunoassay. New York: Humana Press, 2009.

CHAPTER 18

Amino Acids, Peptides, and Proteins*

Glen L. Hortin, M.D., Ph.D.

Objectives

1. Define the following terms:

   Acute-phase reaction; acute-phase reactant

   Ampholyte

   Amyloid

   Bence-Jones proteins

   Complement protein

   Cryoglobulin

   Essential amino acid

   Globulin

   Immunoglobulin

   Isoelectric point

   Paraprotein

   Peptide

   Peptide bond

   Protein

   Proteinuria

2. Diagram and describe the basic chemical structures of an amino acid and a peptide bond.

3. Explain the metabolism of amino acids and proteins, including sites of formation and breakdown.

4. Describe amino acid and protein analyses, including specimen requirements and quantitative analytical techniques.

5. List the following with regard to proteins:

   Physiological functions

   Structural elements

   Physical properties

6. Explain the principle of serum protein electrophoresis, including a description of properties needed for separation, staining methods, separation techniques, and immunofixation electrophoresis.

7. State the utility and problems of using mass spectrometry and MALDI in the assessment of proteins.

8. Compare plasma and serum with regard to protein concentration.

9. State the formula for calculating globulin concentration; calculate globulin concentration when given appropriate information.

10. List the acute-phase response proteins and the negative acute-phase response proteins.

11. Classify the following plasma proteins as to their function, globulin class (if any), and clinical significance and explain how they are affected by disease, including but not limited to, liver, gastrointestinal, and kidney disease:

    Prealbumin

    Retinol-binding protein

    Albumin

    HDL, LDL

    α_1-Antitrypsin

    α-Fetoprotein

    Haptoglobin

    Ceruloplasmin

    Transferrin

    C-reactive protein

12. Discuss the complement proteins, including their clinical significance, abundance, pathway involvement, and disease associations.

13. List the immunoglobulin classes. Describe their biochemistry, function, and clinical significance, and explain how they are affected by disease, including multiple myeloma, macroglobulinemia, and lymphoid tumors; discuss free immunoglobulin light chains, including their function, clinical importance, and presence in urine.

14. Explain the presence of protein in urine and describe four types of proteinuria; describe how protein is analyzed in urine.

15. Explain the presence of protein in CSF and the significance of increased CSF protein.

16. Analyze and solve case studies related to amino acids and proteins, including analytical problems, disorders of metabolism, and other disorders.

---

*The author gratefully acknowledges the previous contributions of A. Myron Johnson, Robert H. Christenson Hassan, M.E. Azzazy, Lawrence M. Silverman, and Elizabeth M. Rohlfs, on which portions of this chapter are based.

Key Words and Definitions

Acute-phase response Body's response to injury or inflammation.

Acute poststreptococcal glomerulonephritis (APSGN) Inflammation of the kidney glomeruli, following a streptococcal infection; also called postinfectious glomerulonephritis.

Amino acid An organic compound containing both amino (–NH$_2$) and carboxyl (–COOH) functional groups.

Aminoaciduria An excess of amino acids in the urine.

Amyloidosis A metabolic disease characterized by abnormal deposits of amyloid in the body.

Bence-Jones proteins Small light chains of immunoglobulin found in the urine.

Complement system Complex system of proteins found in blood that combines with antibodies to destroy pathogenic bacteria and other foreign cells.

Essential amino acids Amino acids that are not synthesized by humans and therefore are essential dietary constituents for maintaining health or growth.

Globulin Proteins that precipitate in water and redissolve when the salt concentration is raised.

Hereditary angioedema (HAE) Genetic disorder characterized by recurrent episodes of severe swelling.

Immunoglobulins A family of proteins also known as *antibodies* that contain highly specific antigen-binding sites consisting of two identical heavy (H) chains encoded on chromosome 14 and two identical light (L) chains encoded on chromosome 2.

Inborn error of metabolism Genetically determined biochemical disorder in which a specific enzyme defect causes a metabolic block in the individual at birth or in later life.

Isoelectric focusing An equilibrium technique that is used to separate charge variants of proteins and is applied to analysis of certain genetic variants of proteins.

Kwashiorkor A form of protein-energy malnutrition produced by severe protein deficiency.

Marasmus A form of protein-energy malnutrition predominantly due to prolonged severe caloric deficit.

Monoclonal gammopathy of undetermined significance (MGUS) A condition in which a paraprotein is found in an individual's blood.

Multiple myeloma A cancer in which antibody-producing plasma cells grow in an uncontrolled and malignant manner.

Paraprotein A monoclonal immunoglobulin produced in excessive amounts in disorders such as multiple myeloma.

Paroxysmal nocturnal hemoglobinuria (PNH) Disease of the blood characterized by complement-induced intravascular hemolytic anemia, red colored urine and thrombosis.

Peptide A compound consisting of two or more amino acids linked in a chain via peptide bonds.

Peptide bond The amide bond formed between the carboxyl group of one amino acid and the amino group of another.

Plasma proteins Proteins present in blood, including carrier proteins, fibrinogen and other coagulation factors, complement components, immunoglobulins, enzyme inhibitors, and many others; most are found in other body fluids but in lower concentrations.

Protein A polymer of amino acids linked by peptide bonds with a specific sequence that folds into a defined structure; any of a group of complex organic compounds that contain carbon, hydrogen, oxygen, nitrogen, and usually sulfur (the characteristic element being nitrogen).

Proteome The total complement of proteins expressed by the genetic material of an organism under a given set of environmental conditions.

Side chain A chemical group that is attached to a core part of the molecule.

Systemic lupus erythematosus (SLE or lupus) A condition that can affect any part of the body.

Waldenström's macroglobulinemia A chronic cancer of the immune system characterized by hyperviscosity, or thickening, of the blood.

Amino acids, **peptides**, and **proteins** play crucial roles in virtually all biological processes, with amino acids being the basic building block of proteins. In humans, more than 20,000 genes encode peptides and proteins that have diverse structures and functions (www.genome.gov/; accessed August 27, 2013). This chapter includes discussions of (1) amino acids and their analyses, (2) major proteins in biological fluids, and (3) analytical techniques used to analyze proteins.

Amino Acids

Amino acids serve as the basic structural units of peptides and proteins; they also have diverse roles in metabolism and neurotransmission. [3] Measurement of amino acids in physiological fluids assists with studies of metabolism and the diagnosis of pathological and inherited disorders (see Chapter 45).

Basic Biochemistry

Amino acids are organic compounds that contain both an amino group (–NH$_2$) and a carboxyl group (–COOH). Those that occur in proteins are α–amino acids that are also known as 2-Oxo amino acids. Structurally, the amino group is in the position to the carboxyl group that have the general formula RCH(NH$_2$)COOH, wherein R has varying structures that are often referred to as the side chain. This side chain plays a key role in maintaining nitrogen balance in mammals.

α-carbon atom

Technically, proline is an imino acid not an amino acid, but it is usually grouped with amino acids. Amino acids in physiological fluids also include β-amino acids, such as β-alanine, and γ-amino acids, such as the neurotransmitter γ-aminobutyric acid. Table 18-1 lists the 21 amino acids that are incorporated by ribosomes into proteins with a sequence specified by messenger RNA. Most proteins contain 20 of the 21 amino acids. Selenocysteine is an uncommon amino acid that is incorporated into only a few proteins, where it usually serves as an important residue at catalytic sites of enzymes. With the exception of glycine, all α-amino acids are asymmetrical about the α-carbon, and four different groups are linked to this carbon. Most α-amino acids in humans, including all of the amino acids incorporated into proteins, have the L-configuration.

Acid-Base Properties

The acid-base properties of amino acids depend on the amino and carboxyl groups attached to the α-carbon and present on any ionizable groups included in the side chains (R). In the physiological pH range of near 7.4, the carboxyl group of an amino acid is dissociated and the amino group protonated, as follows:

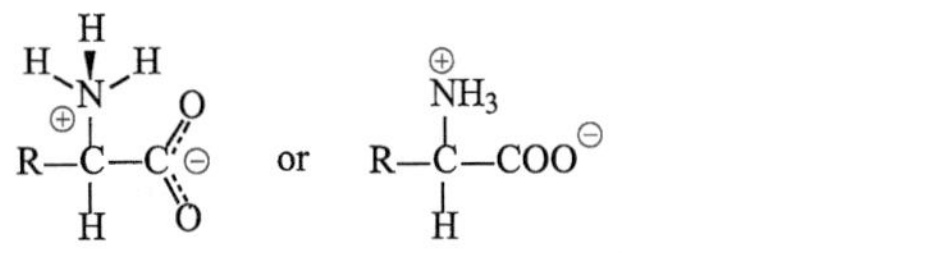

At neutral pH, there is zero net charge as the negative and positive charge balance in what sometimes is termed an *ampholyte or zwitterion* (see Chapter 11). At low pH, an amino acid has a net positive charge, with both its amino and carboxyl groups protonated ($-NH_3$ and $-COOH$). At high pH, amino acids have a net negative charge, with both amino and carboxyl groups deprotonated. The amino $-NH_3$ is also deprotonated:

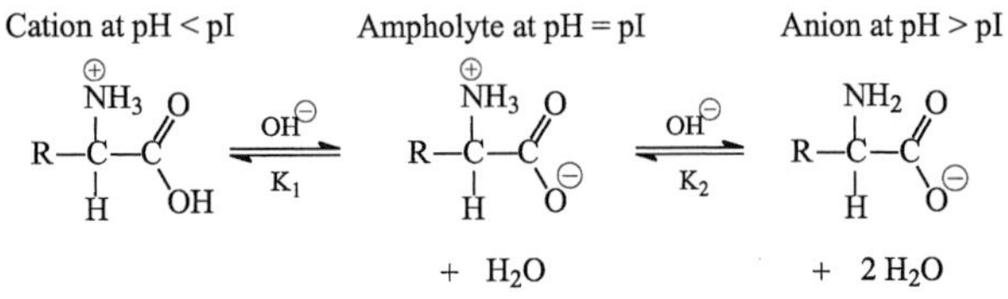

The dissociation constants for the carboxyl group, K_1, and the amino group, K_2, usually are expressed as pK_1 and pK_2, where $pK = -\log K$, in a manner analogous to the notation for pH. A pK is the pH at which equal quantities of the protonated and deprotonated forms of an ionizable group are present. The *isoelectric point*, pI, is the pH at which a molecule has a net charge of 0. The isoelectric point of a neutral amino acid is the midpoint between the pK's of its amino and carboxyl groups

TABLE 18-1			Amino Acids Incorporated Into Protein: Their Properties and Structures	
Name and Abbreviation	**HI**	**MW**	**Structure at pH 6 to 7**	**Comments**
Neutral Amino Acids				
Alanine Ala, A	1.8	89.09	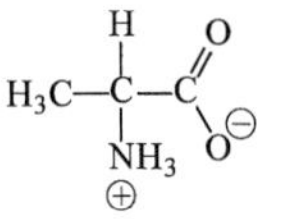	Important metabolic substrate in alanine cycle; substrate for ALT
Leucine Leu, L	3.8	131.17	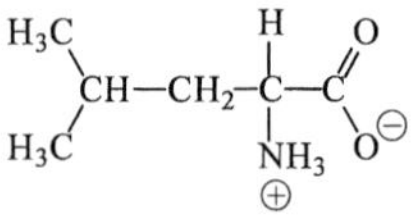	Essential; branched-chain R group; ketogenic; metabolism is faulty in maple syrup urine disease
Isoleucine Ile, I	4.5	131.17	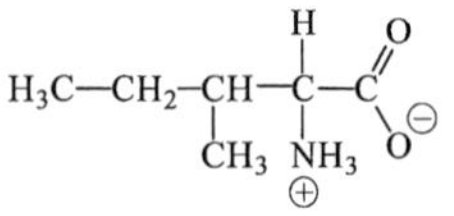	Essential; partly ketogenic; see Leucine above
Valine Val, V	4.2	117.17	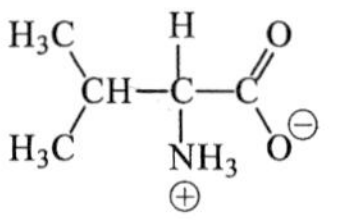	Essential; partly ketogenic; see Leucine above
Proline Pro, P	1.6	115.13	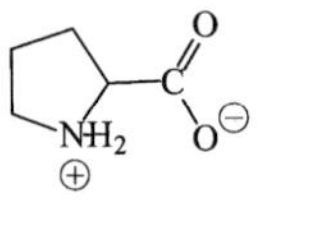	Has α-imino rather than α-amino; high content in collagens and can be hydroxylated to hydroxyproline; destabilizes α-helical structures
Methionine Met, M	1.9	149.18	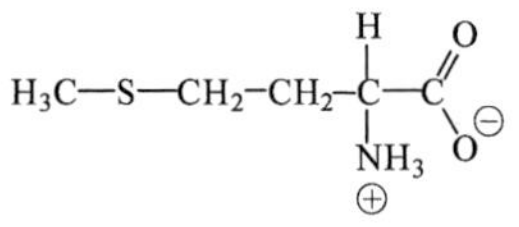	Essential; important as donor of methyl groups; provides sulfur for other sulfur-containing compounds
Phenylalanine Phe, F	2.8	165.19	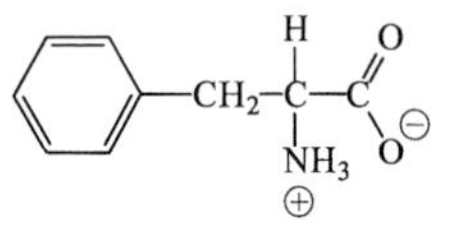	Essential; elevated concentrations in phenylketonuria as conversion to Tyr is impaired

TABLE 18-1	Amino Acids Incorporated Into Protein: Their Properties and Structures—cont'd

Name and Abbreviation	HI	MW	Structure at pH 6 to 7	Comments
Neutral Amino Acids—cont'd				
Tryptophan Trp, W	−0.9	204.22		Essential; metabolites in carcinoid disease; contains indole ring; precursor of serotonin, melatonin
Glycine Gly, G	−0.4	75.07		No stereoisomer; used in biosynthesis of purines and porphyrins; transfer to bile acids, hippurates, and other conjugates
Serine Ser, S	−0.8	105.09		Source of one-carbon groups for folates; can undergo post-translational addition of phosphate, sugars
Threonine Thr, T	−0.7	119.12		Essential; can undergo post-translational addition of phosphate or sugars
Cysteine Cys, C	2.5	118.16		Sulfhydryl group in active sites of some enzymes; forms disulfides; homocysteine is homologue with side chain one carbon longer
Selenocysteine Sec, U		168.05		Active form of selenium; found in some enzymes involved in oxidation reduction reactions; formed on a specific transfer RNA
Tyrosine Tyr, Y	−1.3	181.19		Usually nonessential; intermediate in synthesis of catecholamines, thyroxine, and melanin; functional phenolic group
Glutamine Gln, Q	−3.5	146.15		Transport form of ammonia; supplies nitrogen atoms used in purine and pyrimidine biosynthesis
Asparagine Asn, N	−3.5	132.12		Attachment site of oligosaccharides in Asn-Xxx-(Ser or Thr) sequences
Acidic Amino Acids				
Aspartic acid Asp, D	−3.5	133.10		Precursor for pyrimidine and purine biosynthesis; a substrate in urea cycle
Glutamic acid Glu, E	−3.5	147.13		Transport form of ammonia γ-glutamyl transfer from glutathione; a neurotransmitter
Basic Amino Acids				
Lysine Lys, K	−3.9	146.19		Essential; side chain has an additional amino group
Arginine Arg, R	−4.5	174.20		Involved in urea synthesis; side chain has a guanidinium group
Histidine His, H	−3.2	155.16		The imidazole group has a pK near physiological pH, so charge can vary with physiological pH change

*A higher value for hydropathy index (HI) indicates greater hydrophobicity of amino acid side chains.

TABLE 18-2   Ionization Constants of Ionizable Groups in Free Amino Acids and in Proteins*

Ionizing Group		Range of pK Values	
		Free Amino Acids	Proteins
Principal carboxyl = pK_1	$-C{\overset{O}{\underset{O^{\ominus}}{\big\|}}}$	1.7-2.6	3.0-3.2
α-Amino = pK_2	$-\overset{\oplus}{N}H_3$	9.0-10.8	7.6-8.4
Second carboxyls of Glu and Asp	$-C{\overset{O}{\underset{O^{\ominus}}{\big\|}}}$	3.8-4.3	3.0-4.5
Imidazole nitrogen of His	$\overset{\oplus}{N}H$	6.0	6.0-7.0
Sulfhydryl of Cys	$-SH$	8.3	9.1-10.8
Phenolic hydroxyl of Tyr	$-OH$	10.1	9.2-9.8
ε-Amino of Lys	$-\overset{\oplus}{N}H_3$	10.5	9.4-10.6
Guanidinium group of Arg	$-NH-C{\overset{NH_2}{\underset{\underset{\oplus}{NH_2}}{\diagup}}}$	12.5	11.5-12.6

*The pK value for the primary carboxyl varies from 1.71 for Cys to 2.63 for Thr. The pK for the α-amino group varies from 8.95 for Lys to 10.78 for Cys. In protein chains, the local environment modifies the pK for any given ionizable group. The amino acid symbols are listed in Table 18-1.

($pI = \frac{1}{2}[pK_1 = pK_2]$). Amino acids also contain several different ionizable groups on their side chains. Table 18-2 lists pK values for various ionizable groups of amino acids. The exact pK values for different groups vary slightly in different amino acids, depending on neighboring groups; in proteins, even greater variation often results from the effects of neighboring amino acids.

Influence of R Groups

The R groups of individual amino acids provide considerable variation in structure and physical properties. Side chains may be (1) acidic, (2) basic, or (3) neutral and vary in size and hydrophobicity. The hydropathy index listed in Table 18-1 is an index of the water solubility of the side chains. Amino acids with charged groups or polar groups like hydroxyl or amide groups in their side chains have high water solubility and low hydropathy. Amino acids with aliphatic or aromatic side chains tend to have low water solubility and high hydropathy. The differing charge and properties of amino acids serve as a basis for their chromatographic separation.

Amino Acid Metabolism

Amino acids are synthesized from α-ketoacids, and later are transaminated from another amino acid, usually glutamate. They participate in many metabolic pathways, in addition to serving as substrates for protein synthesis (see Chapter 37).

Dietary protein usually serves as the primary source of amino acids for protein synthesis. The adult daily requirement for protein intake is about 0.8 g/kg body weight, and demand is higher during (1) growth, (2) pregnancy, (3) lactation, (4) states of protein loss, and (5) many disease states with increased protein breakdown. Endogenous protein turnover serves as another source of free amino acids. In the absence of protein uptake, breakdown of muscle protein serves as a source of amino acids. Eight amino acids used for protein synthesis—(1) isoleucine, (2) leucine, (3) lysine, (4) methionine, (5) phenylalanine, (6) threonine, (7) tryptophan, and (8) valine—are not synthesized by humans and, thus, are considered to be **essential amino acids.** Meat, milk, eggs, and fish contain a full range of essential amino acids. Gelatin is deficient in tryptophan. Individual plant sources may be deficient in (1) lysine, (2) methionine, or (3) tryptophan.

Dietary supply of amino acids has important clinical implications. A diet with adequate calories but low protein intake has been known to lead to **kwashiorkor** (malnutrition due to protein deficiency) with (1) decreased serum albumin, (2) edema, (3) ascites, (4) growth failure, (5) immune deficiency, and (6) apathy. Deficiency of both calories and protein (protein-calorie malnutrition), also termed **marasmus** causes generalized muscle wasting but less edema when compared with kwashiorkor. Inadequate protein nutrition is frequently a problem for (1) surgical, (2) burn, or (3) trauma patients in a catabolic state and for those with decreased food intake. Adequate nutrition is important for immune function and tissue repair. In kidney disease, high protein intake appears to be harmful, and protein restriction has been used as a therapeutic intervention to slow the progress of kidney disease.

Amino acids are important intermediates in many metabolic pathways, including (1) the urea cycle for converting ammonia to urea, (2) the alanine cycle for transferring nitrogen and energy sources from muscle to liver, (3) ammonia generation in the kidney from glutamine and glutamic acid, and (4) glutathione formation to maintain a reducing intracellular environment. Amino acids are precursors for many hormones and signaling molecules, such as (1) thyroid hormones, (2) catecholamines, (3) serotonin, (4) nitric oxide, (5) melatonin, and (6) hydrogen sulfide. Serine is a major source of one-carbon units transferred by tetrahydrofolic acid for purine synthesis and conversion of homocysteine to methionine. Amino acid precursors for purine and pyrimidine synthesis include (1) glycine, (2) aspartic acid, (3) glutamine, and (4) serine. Methionine serves as a methyl donor for many reactions after activation as *S*-adenosylmethionine. Several amino acids participate in conjugation reactions that serve as excretory pathways and generate products such as glycine or taurine conjugates of bile acids. Cysteine and glutathione form mercapturates with reactive compounds as a protective mechanism. The liver is a very active site in amino acid metabolism and synthesis, as outlined in Figure 18-1. The liver is the primary site for the urea cycle and for uptake of amino acids from the circulation and conversion to a fuel source via transamination. The liver is also a primary source of many of the major plasma proteins in the circulation.

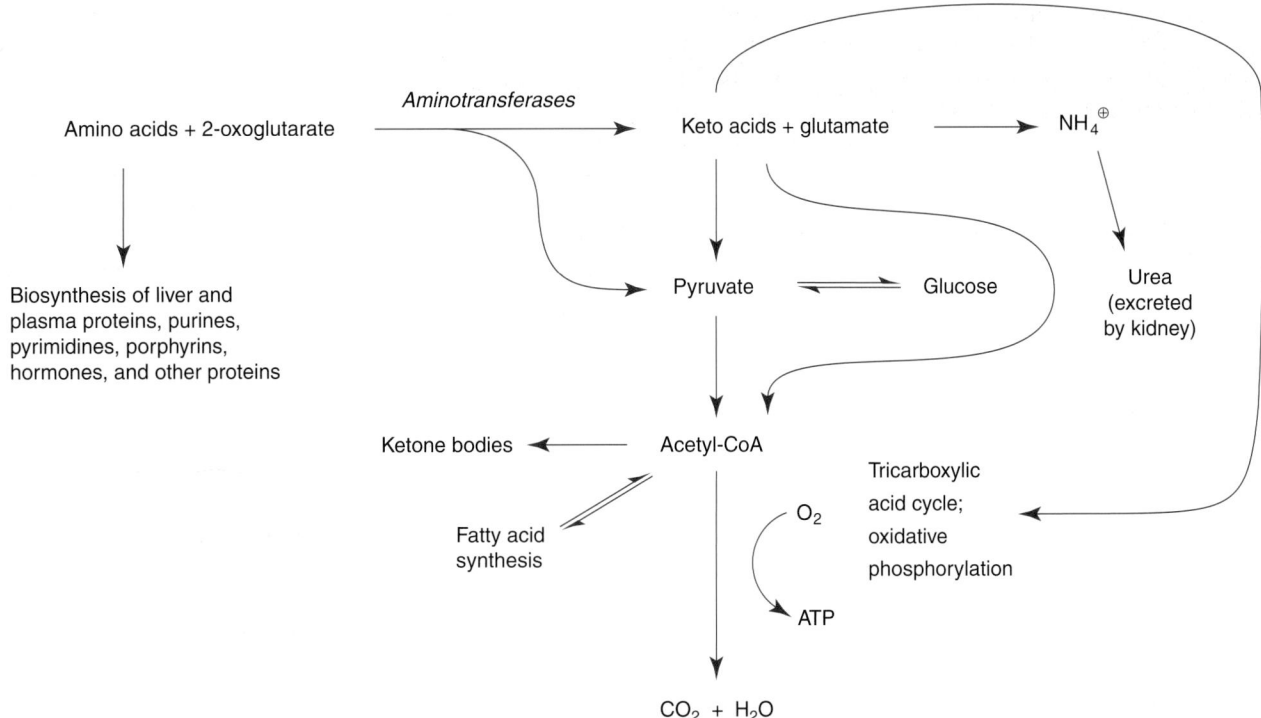

Figure 18-1 A generalized scheme of amino acid metabolism in the liver.

Clinical Implications

Disorders of amino acid metabolism have been assessed by analysis of amino acids in plasma or urine. Increased urinary excretion of amino acids may be primary or secondary. Primary disease is due to an inherited enzyme defect. **Inborn errors of metabolism** are described in Chapter 45. The defect may be located in the pathway by which a specific amino acid is metabolized or in a transport system for an amino acid. Secondary aminoaciduria is due to disease of an organ, such as the liver, which is an active site of amino acid metabolism, or generalized renal tubular dysfunction.

Analysis of Amino Acids

Amino acid concentrations usually are assessed in (1) plasma, (2) urine, or (3) cerebrospinal fluid. Plasma amino acid concentrations vary during the day by about 30%; therefore, it is preferable to collect specimens at the same time during the day if changes are to be monitored. Amino acid concentrations are highest in midafternoon and lowest in early morning. Plasma amino acid concentrations are high during the first days of life, especially in premature neonates, but they tend to be low in infants with birth weight low for gestational age; malnutrition due to placental insufficiency is the cause. Maternal values are low in the first half of pregnancy.

Amino acids are freely filtered through the glomerular membranes of kidneys, but most amino acids are reabsorbed in kidney tubules by saturable transport systems (see Chapters 21 and 35). Increased urinary excretion of one or more amino acids occurs as the result of (1) excessive plasma concentration of an amino acid overwhelming the tubular reuptake (overflow

aminoaciduria), (2) tubular injury, or (3) a defect in a reuptake system for an amino acid. Urinary excretion of amino acids varies with age. For example, infants, particularly premature infants, have a generalized aminoaciduria caused by immature reuptake systems. During pregnancy, the renal threshold for many compounds including amino acids is decreased, resulting in increased **aminoaciduria**. In healthy adults, (1) glycine is the most abundant amino acid, followed by (2) histidine, (3) taurine, (4) glutamine, (5) serine, and (6) alanine.

Specimen Requirements

For diagnosis of an inherited disorder of amino acid metabolism, care must be taken to obtain valid and representative samples. For example, individuals should follow a normal diet for 2 to 3 days before collection. Testing for some disorders during newborn screening, such as for phenylketonuria, has been known to fail to detect the disorder if the newborn has had no dietary intake. Blood and urine specimens should be collected simultaneously. Use of heparinized plasma is preferable to use of serum and other anticoagulants. Screening tests for newborns commonly are collected as dried blood spots on filter paper. Because some drugs administered to the mother before she gives birth or to the infant interfere with specimens, all medications should be noted. Most amino acids are stable in blood specimens, except for glutamine, which undergoes cyclization to form pyroglutamic acid (5-oxoproline) with release of ammonia. Specimens should be processed rapidly and frozen rapidly to preserve glutamine. Homocysteine is gradually released from blood cells, so that plasma needs to be separated from whole blood rapidly to obtain accurate homocysteine measurements. Before analysis, most procedures for analyzing amino acids entail removal of proteins by precipitation or by ultrafiltration. This yields good recovery of most amino acids. Recovery of tryptophan may vary as the result of protein binding, and substantial amounts of cysteine, homocysteine, and thiol-containing peptides are linked via disulfide bonds to proteins. Recovery of total cysteine and homocysteine requires reduction of specimens before protein removal.

Screening Tests

Historically, a variety of methods have been used to screen newborns for disorders of amino acids in body fluids. These have included thin-layer chromatography (TLC) and the Guthrie test. Currently, newborn screening is widely performed on dried blood spots through liquid chromatography–tandem mass spectrometry (see Chapter 45).

Quantitative Tests

Screening tests yield some false-positive or indeterminate results, particularly during screening for relatively rare disorders, such as inherited disorders of amino acid metabolism. Confirmatory diagnostic testing is required on plasma or urine specimens collected for quantitative analysis. Monitoring of patients requires similar quantitative analysis. Also, newborn screening of blood spots may not detect some disorders, such as disorders of urinary amino acid transport.

For many years, quantitative clinical analysis of amino acids was performed mainly by ion exchange chromatography with postcolumn reaction with ninhydrin to generate a product detected by a photometer.

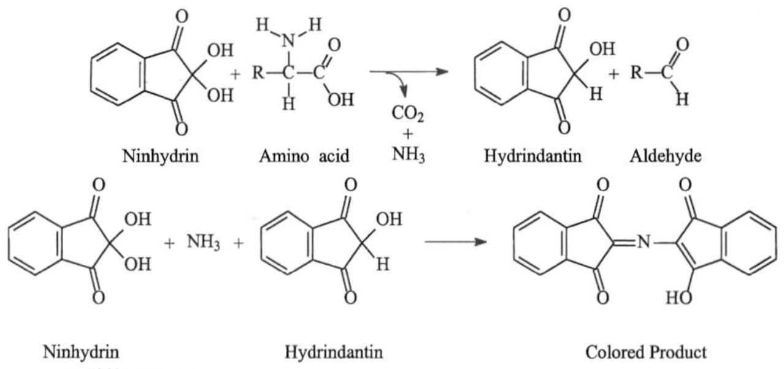

In addition to the ion exchange chromatography/ninhydrin system, a number of other techniques are used, including (1) liquid chromatography–tandem mass spectrometry (LC-MS/MS), (2) reversed-phase high-performance liquid chromatography, (3) capillary electrophoresis (CE), and (4) gas chromatography (GC). These procedures usually employ chemical derivatization of amino acids before analysis. Some advantages of these methods versus the ion exchange method include higher throughput and greater analytical specificity. Currently, the main clinical use of amino acid analysis is detection and monitoring of inherited disorders. Selective quantification of plasma homocysteine is the only exception; the plasma concentration of it has been determined by selective (1) enzyme assays, (2) immunoassays, and (3) chromatographic assays.

These measurements have been used as a marker for deficiency of folic acid or vitamin B_{12} and as a marker associated with increased risk for cardiovascular disease.

Peptides and Proteins

Humans have more than 20,000 genes encoding proteins that serve as major structural elements and as the machinery of life. The total complement of proteins present at a time in a cell or cell type is known as its **proteome**, and the study of such large-scale data sets defines the field of proteomics, named by analogy to the related field of genomics.[4] Diverse functions of proteins include (1) serving as structural components, (2) facilitating catalysis of chemical reactions, including synthesis of DNA, RNA, and proteins, (3) generating energy through electron transfer, (4) producing motility through contractile elements, (5) serving as ion channels and pumps, (6) acting as carrier molecules, (7) effecting immune defense, (8) serving as receptors, hormones, and cytokines for intercellular communication, and (9) constituting signaling networks for intracellular communication. To perform all of these functions, proteins must have great structural diversity. Diversity from the primary genetic sequence encoding proteins is compounded by (1) variable splicing of messenger RNA, (2) somatic recombination and mutation of selected genes such as those for antibodies, (3) proteolytic processing, and (4) numerous post-translational modifications of proteins.

Basic Biochemistry

Proteins are polymers of amino acids that are linked covalently through an amide linkage that is referred to as the **peptide bond**. This bond is formed when the α-amino group of one amino acid is linked covalently with the α-carboxyl of a second amino acid (with loss of water) by the protein biosynthetic machinery, as follows:

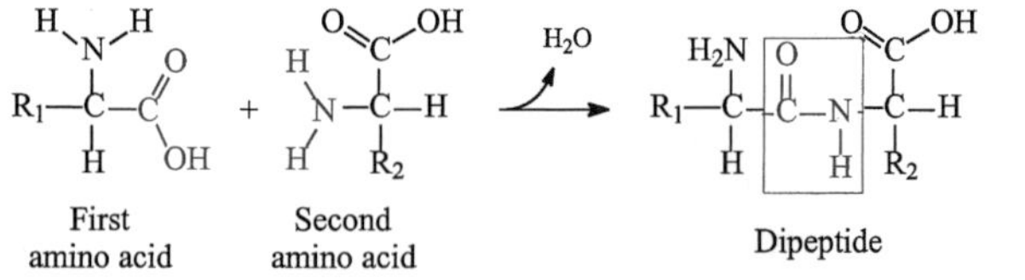

The peptide bond is described by the structure in the enclosed area. The amino acid with the free amino group in the peptide is termed the *N-terminal residue* and the amino acid with the free carboxyl group is termed the *C-terminal residue*. Protein synthesis begins with the N-terminal residue and peptides are named from the N-terminal residue. Alanylglycine, for example, is a peptide with alanine as the N-terminal residue and glycine as the C-terminal residue.

Short chains of linked amino acids are designated as (1) dipeptides, (2) tripeptides, (3) tetrapeptides, or (4) pentapeptides according to the number of amino acids. Chains of up to five residues are called oligopeptides. Longer chains (6 to 30 residues) are referred to as polypeptides. When the number of amino acids linked together exceeds 40 or more, the chain is referred to as a *protein*. The different side chains found in amino acids provide peptides and proteins with great diversity in both structure and function. Most peptides in the body, other than a few short peptides such as glutathione, are synthesized as larger precursor proteins, and the peptides are generated by proteolytic cleavage of the precursor.

Structure

The structure of peptides and proteins consists of four elements:

1. *Primary structure* is the sequence of amino acids in a peptide or protein. Post-translational modifications add to diversity.
2. *Secondary structure* is the specific organization of segments of the polypeptide backbone into structures that are termed (1) α-*helix, (2),* β-*sheet* and (3) β-*turn. Random coil* refers to segments that lack these structures.
3. *Tertiary structure* refers to the folding of the chain of amino acids into a three-dimensional structure. This structure may be stabilized by disulfide bonds between cysteine residues. Hydrophobic amino acids tend to fold into the interior, and charged and polar amino acids reside on the surface of the protein. *Denaturation* refers to the unfolding of proteins and the disruption of secondary and tertiary structures that occur with (1) increased temperature, (2) extremes of pH, (3) organic solvents, and (4) detergents or agents that disrupt hydrogen bonds. Extensive denaturation of proteins leads to irreversible loss of structure and function, and the protein may aggregate or precipitate.
4. *Quaternary structure* refers to the association of multiple peptide chains. Examples include (1) creatine kinase with two subunits, (2) lactate dehydrogenase with four subunits and (3) hemoglobin with four subunits.

In addition, ligands and prosthetic groups, such as heme in hemoglobin and cytochromes and lipids in lipoproteins, serve as additional structural elements. Proteins without their associated ligands are often referred to as apoproteins (e.g., apotransferrin without iron, apolipoproteins without lipid).

Many proteins are organized as a chain of smaller structural units or domains analogous to a string of beads. Similar domains are found in different proteins, but diversity in structure is achieved by assembly of domains in different combinations and three-dimensional configurations. Proteins have a variety of shapes, ranging from compact globular proteins that are nearly spherical to highly elongated fibrous proteins. Many proteins belong to families of homologous proteins that arose from duplication of ancestral genes. Examples of protein families in humans include the serpin (originally from serine proteinase inhibitor) superfamily with 36 members, including α_1-antitrypsin, α_1-antichymotrypsin, and antithrombin III, and the albumin family with three members, including albumin and α-fetoprotein.

Properties

Proteins have varying physical properties that are used for separation and analysis:

1. *Molecular size.* Proteins have varying molecular sizes. It is possible to separate proteins from small molecules by dialysis or ultrafiltration. Proteins of varying size are separated by (1) gel filtration chromatography, (2) gradient pore gel electrophoresis, or (3) ultracentrifugation. The size of most proteins increases substantially when they are denatured. Polyacrylamide gel electrophoresis[6] in the presence of the denaturing detergent sodium dodecyl sulfate is a high-resolution technique for separating proteins and estimating their molecular weight. Mass spectrometry separates peptides and proteins by their molecular mass.
2. *Differential solubility.* Protein solubility is affected by (1) pH, (2) ionic strength, (3) temperature, and (4) the dielectric constant of the solvent. Varying (1) pH, (2) salt concentration, or (3) concentration of an organic solvent like ethyl alcohol, are techniques used to selectively precipitate proteins. This has been used as a preparative technique for albumin and for some globulins.
3. *Electrical charge.* The variable charge and isoelectric points of proteins enable their separation by electrophoresis, **isoelectric focusing**, and ion exchange chromatography.
4. *Differential adsorption.* Liquid chromatography is performed in a variety of stationary phases. Reversed-phase chromatography serves as a valuable tool for separating peptides, but some proteins may precipitate or denature in the organic solvents typically used in this technique. Reversed-phase chromatography separates polypeptides and other molecules on the basis of their affinity for a hydrophobic stationary phase.
5. *Specific molecular interactions.* Highly specific molecular interactions such as binding of (1) an antibody with antigen, (2) a receptor with its ligand, or (3) an enzyme with a selective inhibitor or substrate have been used to bind a protein or a peptide to a stationary phase, while other proteins and peptides are removed. This is usually termed affinity chromatography. Affinity purification of antibodies or proteins may be used as a preparative technique to prepare specific antibodies or proteins as assay components. Affinity capture is a step in many immunoassay methods.
6. *Density.* Density gradient ultracentrifugation is used to separate some protein complexes that have a different density when compared with most proteins. This applies mainly to lipoproteins that have lower density as the result of a high content of lipid (refer to Chapter 23 on lipids and lipoproteins).

Analysis of Proteins

Analysis of proteins includes both qualitative and quantitative analysis.

Quantitative analysis employs a variety of approaches, including (1) physical methods, such as (a) dye binding, (b) direct absorbance measurements, (c) measurement of protein ligands such as lipids or metal ions, (d) selective precipitation, and (e) mass spectrometry; (2) activity measurements for components such as binding protein, protease inhibitors, complement factors, and coagulation factors; and (3) immunoassays. Qualitative analysis of proteins reveals changes in the structure of proteins through techniques such as

(1) electrophoresis, (2) chromatography, (3) genetic analysis, (4) functional assays (coupled with quantitative analysis to identify changes in specific activity), and (5) mass spectrometry.

Measurement of Total Protein Concentration

Measurement of the concentration of protein in solution simply by drying the solution and weighing the residue is a simple technique, but it is inaccurate because of (1) salts, (2) adsorbed water, and (3) other impurities such as carbohydrates or lipids that may remain after drying. Development of reference materials for specific proteins is a challenging task that usually requires extensive purification of the protein and assignment of values by weight or amino acid composition analysis after hydrolysis of the protein. Reference materials are then used to assign values to calibrators for specific assays. Calibration of assays for measuring the total protein content of mixtures may rely on calibration with a single purified protein such as albumin or with a representative mixture of proteins with an assigned calibrator value.

A variety of other methods are used to determine the total protein content of solutions, including the (1) Kjeldahl, (2) biuret, (3) direct spectrophotometric, (4) Folin-Ciocalteu (Lowry), (5) dye-binding, (6) refractometric, and (7) turbidimetric methods.

Kjeldahl Method

In the Kjeldahl method, the sample is digested with acid to convert nitrogen in the protein to ammonium ion, and the ammonium ion is measured. The ammonia nitrogen value is multiplied by a factor of 6.25 (to correct for the average nitrogen content of protein) to calculate total protein. This method is reproducible but (1) time-consuming, (2) inconvenient, and (3) impractical for routine use. Kjeldahl determination, however, still remains a means by which reference materials are characterized and validated. Nitrogen from small compounds such as urea also is measured, so that a precipitation step may be required.

Biuret Method

Under alkaline conditions, Cu^{2+} ions complex with peptide bonds in proteins. Binding shifts the absorption spectrum of Cu^{2+} ions to shorter wavelengths, leading to a color change from blue to violet that has been termed the *biuret reaction*. The absorbance change from the protein addition is measured spectrophotometrically at a wavelength of approximately 540 nm. The biuret reagent also usually contains tartrate salts to maintain the solubility of Cu^{2+} ions and iodide as an antioxidant. The absorbance change produced is approximately the same for each peptide bond in a polypeptide chain, except for bonds containing proline. Therefore, the absorbance is proportional to the number of peptide bonds and the amount of protein present in the reaction system, unless an unusual content of proline is present. A variety of (1) small compounds, (2) amino acids, (3) dipeptides, and (4) any peptide without proline react to some degree with the biuret reagent. Only the peptide component of glycoproteins reacts. The biuret method has moderate sensitivity and is useful for solutions with high protein concentrations such as serum or plasma. Analysis of serum has been known to be affected slightly by the presence of bilirubin or lipemia, so that a fasting specimen is preferred. Biuret based assays are commonly calibrated with reference solutions of albumin.

Direct Photometric Methods

The absorbance of ultraviolet (UV) light at 200 to 225 nm and 270 to 290 nm has been used to measure the protein content of biological samples. Absorbance of UV light at 280 nm depends primarily on the aromatic rings of tyrosine and tryptophan. Accuracy and specificity suffer from the variable content of these amino acids among individual proteins in a mixture and from the presence in body fluids of (1) free tyrosine, (2) free tryptophan, (3) uric acid, and (4) bilirubin, all of which also absorb light near 280 nm. Peptide bonds are responsible chiefly for UV absorption between 200 and 225 nm (70% at A_{205}); specific absorption by proteins at 200 to 225 nm is 10 to 30 times greater than at 280 nm. Measurement of protein concentration by this method may require removal of low-molecular-weight molecules before absorbance measurements are performed. Absorbance measurements have been used to assess the concentrations of purified proteins with a known extinction coefficient (absorbance per concentration). Also, absorbance measurements are often used to monitor protein and peptide elution in liquid chromatography and protein migration in capillary electrophoresis.

Dye-Binding Methods

Dye-binding methods depend on shifts in the absorbance spectra of dyes when they bind to proteins. Variable binding of dyes to different proteins is a limitation of such methods. Also, calibration with a protein mixture may be difficult to define consistently. Calibration with a pure protein such as albumin may not simulate binding to proteins in complex mixtures such as serum. With use of the dye Coomassie brilliant blue, **immunoglobulins** often give only 60% of the response of an equal concentration of albumin or transferrin. This dye binds peptide chains under acidic conditions, with increased absorbance at 595 nm. Dye-binding methods offer good sensitivity and low interference from small compounds. Assays using the dye pyrogallol red are used for analysis of protein concentrations in dilute fluids such as urine and cerebrospinal fluid.

Folin-Ciocalteu (Lowry) Method

This method is largely of historical interest. It responds to tyrosine and tryptophan content of proteins and was extensively used in the past as a sensitive method for total protein determination.

Refractometry

Refractometry (measurement of refractive index) has been used to rapidly assess high concentrations of protein. Accuracy decreases at protein concentrations <3.5 g/dL, at which salts, glucose, and other low-molecular-weight compounds begin to contribution more to refractive index. Refractometry is used in clinical laboratories more often to assess total solutes in urine specimens than to determine total protein.

Turbidimetric and Nephelometric Methods

Because of their speed and ease, nephelometric and turbidimetric methods are widely used to assay high-abundance proteins (see Chapter 9).

These techniques assess the formation of aggregates when a reagent is added to lower protein solubility or when an antibody is added to a protein. Turbidimetry measures changes in absorbance caused by the formation of aggregates. Many different reagents have been used to aggregate protein for turbidimetric assays, including (1) trichloroacetic acid, (2) sulfosalicylic acid, (3) sulfosalicylic acid combined with sodium sulfate, or (4) benzethonium chloride and (5) benzalkonium salts under alkaline conditions. These reagents form a fine precipitate of uniform, insoluble protein particles, which scatter incident light. Nephelometry measures the light reflected at an angle by the aggregates.

Precipitation methods sometimes have been used qualitatively to assess whether increased protein is present in urine that may be missed by urine dipsticks, which detect mainly albumin.

Analytically, turbidimetric and nephelometric measurements may be performed as an end point (equilibrium) method or as a kinetic (rate) method. Protein and antibodies must be in approximate equivalence for large aggregates to form. If large antigen or antibody excess is present, formation of aggregates is impaired, and falsely low values may be obtained. Limits of detection of turbidimetric and nephelometric assays are improved by the use of particle-enhanced assays, which use antibodies coupled to particles. One limitation of these direct optical methods is that turbid specimens such as lipemic sera may interfere with measurements. Some turbid specimens may need to be cleared of lipids or particulate material by high-speed centrifugation to enable accurate analysis.

Calibration of Total Protein Methods

Bovine or human albumin is used routinely to calibrate biuret methods, which react nearly equivalently with the peptide content of most proteins. Albumin (1) is available in high purity, (2) is highly soluble and stable, (3) is well characterized, and (4) contains no carbohydrate. Calibration of precipitation and dye-binding methods often uses a serum pool, with a normal albumin-to-globulin ratio. The total protein concentration of the calibrator is assigned using a biuret or Kjeldahl method. In sulfosalicylic acid precipitation methods, albumin provides about 2.5 times the turbidity that serum globulins do. When trichloroacetic acid precipitation is used, the difference between albumin and globulins is lessened.

Reference Intervals

The total protein concentration of serum obtained from healthy ambulatory adults is about 6.4 to 8.3 g/dL, and for adults at bed rest, 6.0 to 7.8 g/dL. Plasma usually contains a protein concentration about 0.3 g/dL higher (unless diluted with a volume of liquid anticoagulant such as citrate solution) because fibrinogen is removed from plasma when it is clotted to form serum. The reference intervals for neonates and young children and for adults over age 60 are slightly lower.

Electrophoretic Techniques

Electrophoresis is used in clinical laboratories to study and measure qualitative and quantitative changes in the protein content of biological fluids, including serum, urine, and CSF (see Chapter 11). Common electrophoretic techniques for serum include the use of zone electrophoresis on cellulose acetate or agarose gel and the use of capillary zone electrophoresis. The mobility of proteins in zone electrophoresis depends on the ratio of charge to size, so it is a good technique for detecting protein variants that differ in charge. Isoelectric focusing is an equilibrium technique that is useful for separating charge variants of proteins; it has been applied to analysis of genetic variants of proteins such as α_1-antitrypsin and hemoglobin and to analysis of immunoglobulin (Ig) in cerebrospinal fluid. Basic principles of electrophoresis and specialized techniques such as two-dimensional (2D) electrophoresis and blotting techniques are described in Chapter 11.

Serum Protein Electrophoresis

Electrophoretic analysis of serum or plasma typically is performed in clinical laboratories by zone electrophoresis on supports such as sheets of agarose gel or cellulose acetate or in an open capillary tube. In zone electrophoresis, the supports have minimal interaction with the proteins, and proteins migrate according to the ratio of their charge to hydrodynamic size (resistance to migration in the fluid). Usually, serum electrophoresis is performed at pH 8.6 in a low ionic strength buffer. A narrow zone of specimen is added, and a current is applied. Proteins with a negative charge at pH 8.6 move toward the anode (positive pole), and proteins with a positive charge move toward the cathode (negative pole). After electrophoretic separation, proteins on a solid support are stained with dyes such as (1) amido black, (2) Ponceau S, or (3) Coomassie brilliant blue. The intensity of staining individual bands of protein generally is proportional to the amount of protein in a band, although glycoproteins and lipoproteins tend to stain less intensely with commonly used protein stains. Densitometry of the stained bands provides quantitative assessment of each band. Initial methods for serum protein electrophoresis separated serum into four bands, which, from the anodal end, were termed *albumin* and α-, β-, and γ-*globulins*. Later improvements in resolution further resolved the α- and β-globulins, each into two components (α_1 and α_2 and β_1 and β_2). Plasma proteins historically were classified according to their mobility on zone electrophoresis. This classification still is often applied to individual proteins and to the naming of proteins. Table 18-3 lists a number of plasma proteins, together with their electrophoretic region.

Special fat stains are needed to visualize lipoproteins that migrate in bands of variable mobility in the (1) α_1-region (high-density lipoprotein [HDL]), (2) the α_2- or pre-β-region (very low-density lipoprotein), and (3) the β_1-region (low-density lipoprotein [LDL]), or that (4) remain at the origin (chylomicrons). Refer to Chapter 23 for a discussion of the lipoproteins

TABLE 18-3   Properties of Selected Plasma Proteins

Electrophoretic Region	Protein	Half-life	pI	MW (daltons)	Comments
	Retinol-binding protein (RBP)	12 h	4.9	21,000	Transports retinol (vitamin A); bound to prealbumin
	Prealbumin (Transthyretin)	48 h	4.7	54,980	Transports thyroid hormones, RBP
Albumin	Albumin	15-19 d	4.7-5.5	66,400	Transports fatty acids, bilirubin, and other compounds; maintains oncotic pressure
α_1	High-density lipoprotein (HDL)	About 5 d		180,000- 360,000	Density >1.063 g/dL; about half protein; apolipoprotein A-I is main protein
	α_1-Antitrypsin (AAT)	4 d	4.8	51,000	Protease inhibitor, especially elastase
	α_1-Acid glycoprotein (AAG, orosomucoid)	5 d	2.7-4	40,000	Binds steroid hormones and cationic drugs
	α_1-Fetoprotein (AFP)	3-6 d	4.8-5.2	69,000	Principal fetal protein; albumin analogue
α_2	Haptoglobin (Hp, HAP)	2 d	4.1 for Hp 1-1	85,000-840,000	Binds hemoglobin; reduced by hemolysis
	α_2-Macroglobulin (AMG)	5 d	5.4	720,000	General protease inhibitor
	Ceruloplasmin (CER)	4-5 d	4.4	132,000	Oxidizes iron to ferric state
β_1	Transferrin (Tf)	7 d	5.7	79,600	Transports iron
	C4	2-3 d	6.0-6.4	206,000	Complement factor
	Low-density lipoprotein (LDL)	About 3 d		About 3×10^6	Density 1.019-1.063 g/mL; about 20% protein; main protein is apolipoprotein B
β_2	C3	2-3 d	5.8	180,000	Complement factor
	β_2-Microglobulin (BMG)	2-5 h	5.8	11,800	Small component of HLA shed from cell surfaces
	IgA	6 d	5.2-6.6	160,000	Major secretory antibody
β-γ border	Fibrinogen	4 d	5.1-6.3	340,000	Forms fibrin clots
γ	IgG	24 d	5.0-9.5	$\approx$150,000	Most abundant antibody
	IgM	5 d	5.1-7.8	900,000	Antibody from primary response
	C-reactive protein (CRP)	20 h	6.2	$\approx$115,000	Nonspecific defense; binds phospholipid

that are major plasma proteins. Efficient visualization of some glycoproteins, such as α_1-acid glycoprotein, requires staining for carbohydrate sidechains.

Applications of capillary electrophoresis rely on direct spectrophotometric detection of proteins at a wavelength of about 200 to 225 nm, rather than staining of a solid support. Proteins migrate through the detector according to their electrophoretic mobility combined with electroendosmotic flow, which is generated by application of an electrical potential. Use of narrow-bore capillaries allows the use of very high voltages that speed separation. Detection of proteins by their ultraviolet absorbance yields better quantitative results and slightly different peak heights for different components than are produced by staining of gels. Low-molecular-weight compounds present in serum at high concentrations, such as radiocontrast dyes, potentially showing up as interfering peaks. Analysis of urine proteins by capillary electrophoresis generally requires some processing of specimens to concentrate proteins and to remove low-molecular-weight compounds that may interfere with analysis, because a smaller amount of protein and a larger number of low-molecular-weight solutes are present in urine.

Figure 18-2 shows comparisons of serum protein electrophoresis (SPE) separations on cellulose acetate and agarose gels with capillary zone electrophoresis (CZE). In this figure, the order of migration of components on the gels and in CZE is shown as reversed, and a marker is added to the CZE analysis to serve as an internal standard. Note that the CZE analysis was completed within 120 seconds. Albumin is the main component in each analysis of the specimen in row A, representing a normal profile. In row B, a second major peak is due to large amounts of a **paraprotein** in the γ-region. Row C shows patterns for a specimen with small amounts of a paraprotein in the γ-region.

The concentrations of many proteins are too low for them to be seen as distinct stained bands, or they are overshadowed by proteins of higher concentrations that migrate near them. However, from changes in intensity of the small number of major bands and in the overall distribution of proteins, it is often possible to interpret patterns as consistent with particular disease processes, such as (1) acute inflammation, (2) nephrotic syndrome, or (3) chronic inflammation. Some examples are shown in Figure 18-3, together with quantitative measurements of selected proteins. In practice, however, these disorders usually are assessed with the use of specific quantitative tests; the main current application of SPE is for the detection or quantification of monoclonal immunoglobulins that occur in disorders such as **multiple myeloma**. Monoclonal immunoglobulins usually appear as sharp bands in the γ- or β-region. They differ from normal immunoglobulins, which migrate as a diffuse zone, mainly in the γ-region, in terms of the sequence and charge heterogeneity of polyclonal immunoglobulins.

Immunofixation Electrophoresis

An example of immunofixation electrophoresis (IFE) is shown in Chapter 15 on immunochemical techniques. IFE relies on

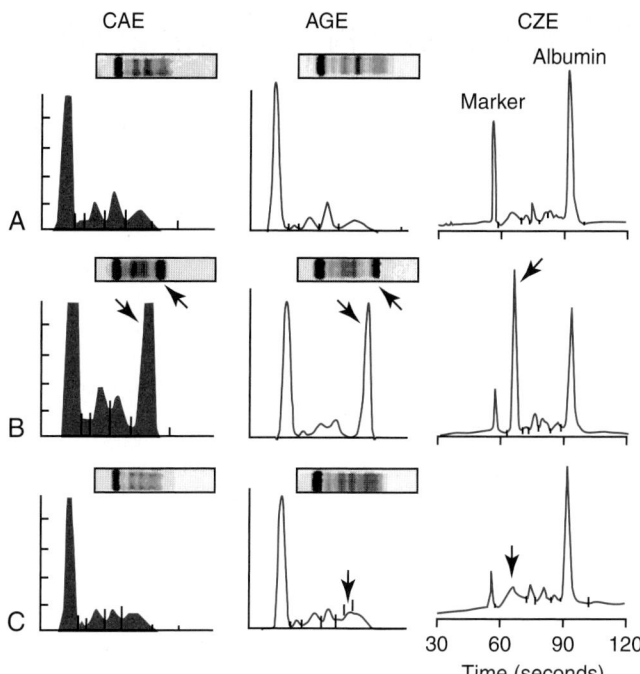

Figure 18-2 Rapid protein electrophoresis of serum protein; comparison with scanning densitometry profiles obtained from cellulose acetate (CAE) and agarose (AGE) electrophoresis. **A,** Normal serum. **B,** Patient serum containing a large M-protein. **C,** Patient serum containing a small monoclonal protein. *Arrows indicate the position of the monoclonal proteins. (From Karcher RE, Landers JP, Electrophoresis. In: Burtis CA, Ashwood ER, Bruns DE eds. Tietz textbook of clinical chemistry, 5th edition. Philadelphia: WB Saunders, 2012:299.)*

the application of specific antibodies directed against classes of immunoglobulin (IgG, IgM, IgA) or κ- and λ-light chains on top of several lanes of an agarose gel after separation of serum proteins. The antibodies form immune precipitates through complexation in the gel with their specific antigens. Other proteins that are not bound by antisera are washed out of the gel, and the remaining bands of immunoprecipitate are stained. Polyclonal immunoglobulins form diffuse bands. Monoclonal immunoglobulins form sharp bands, which react with only a single type of light chain and usually with antibody to a single class of Ig. Sometimes multiple dilutions of serum must be run to provide the right ratio of serum immunoglobulins to antiserum to form an immunoprecipitate in the gel. Antigen and antibody must be approximately equivalent to form an immunoprecipitate. IFE offers more sensitive detection of monoclonal components than is provided by SPE. It also demonstrates the monoclonal nature of immunoglobulins in a band (reactivity with only a single type of light chain and immunoglobulin class) and provides typing of the class of antibody.

Electrophoretic Separation of Urinary Proteins

The procedure for electrophoresis of urine on agarose gel is identical to that for serum, with the exception that usually urine specimens are concentrated about 100-fold before application. Concentration of specimens usually is performed by ultrafiltration, which retains proteins while removing water and low-molecular-weight compounds. Exceptions are specimens with high protein concentrations and procedures modified so by using more sensitive staining methods. Electrophoresis of urine is commonly used to detect the presence of free monoclonal immunoglobulin light chains (also sometimes termed *Bence-Jones proteins*) or other low-molecular-mass proteins typical of tubular proteinuria.

Mass Spectrometry

General principles of mass spectrometry (MS) are described in Chapter 13. MS relies on the separation of ions in an electrical field in a vacuum. Separations are independent of shape and are based purely on the mass-to-charge ratio (m/z). This is advantageous for proteins that have complex and varying shapes. The large size and multiple charge states of proteins pose some challenges in MS, however. When electrospray ionization (ESI) is used, small fluid droplets containing a single protein molecule are evaporated to leave an isolated protein ion, which usually is multiply charged, and different ions of the same protein have varying charge (varying z). Therefore, a purified protein yields multiple peaks separated according to their m/z, with multiple values of z. Many proteins also have heterogeneity in m because of variable modifications such as (1) phosphorylation, (2) glycosylation, (3) oxidation, and (4) deamidation. Therefore, many proteins yield a very complex pattern on ESI-MS, and dividing the ions into many peaks lowers the instrument's limit of detection. Analysis of proteins by ESI-MS poses a significant computational problem to "deconvolute" the pattern of multiple peaks into single peaks corresponding to the protein mass. This has been accomplished and variants in protein structure identified when the mixture is not too complex. An alternative approach in addressing the problem of protein heterogeneity and multiple charge states is to cut proteins into smaller peptides for analysis by MS. Fragmentation of proteins results in some loss of information about the intact protein structure, but peptides are suitable for highly precise qualitative analysis by ESI-MS. Two stages of MS with an intermediary fragmentation step (tandem MS or MS/MS) are used for rapid sequencing of peptides and identification of post-translational modifications. MS has served as a key tool for identifying the sites and structures of the wide range of post-translational modifications of proteins. MS also is used to identify changes in the primary sequence of proteins, although increasingly this is achieved by genetic analysis rather than by direct analysis of the protein.

Accurate quantitative analysis of protein-derived peptides is performed using appropriate internal standards. The quantitative analysis of peptides derived from proteins is being used increasingly as a method of assessing concentrations of proteins. For example, this approach has been used as a reference method for measuring hemoglobin A_{1c} and as a clinical assay for measuring thyroglobulin. Peptides in the circulation, such as C-peptide, are suitable for direct quantitative analysis using appropriate internal

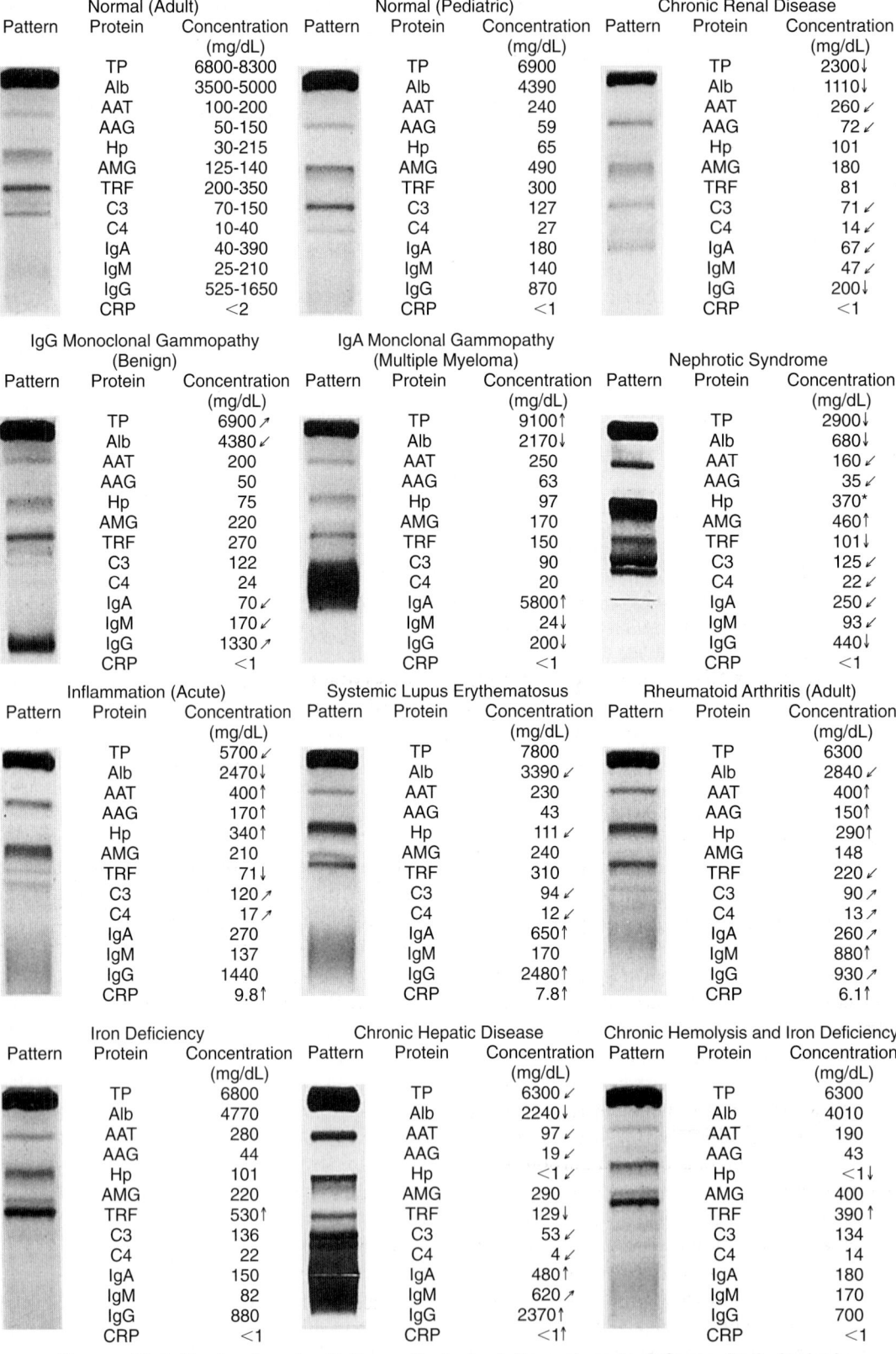

Figure 18-3 Electrophoretic Patterns Typical of Normal and of Some Pathological Conditions (Agarose Gel) Upward- and downward-pointing arrows indicate increase and decrease from the reference interval, respectively. Right- and left-slanting arrows indicate variation from normal to an increase and from normal to a decrease from the reference interval, respectively.

Normal (Adult)

Pattern	Protein	Concentration (mg/dL)
	TP	6800-8300
	Alb	3500-5000
	AAT	100-200
	AAG	50-150
	Hp	30-215
	AMG	125-140
	TRF	200-350
	C3	70-150
	C4	10-40
	IgA	40-390
	IgM	25-210
	IgG	525-1650
	CRP	<2

Normal (Pediatric)

Pattern	Protein	Concentration (mg/dL)
	TP	6900
	Alb	4390
	AAT	240
	AAG	59
	Hp	65
	AMG	490
	TRF	300
	C3	127
	C4	27
	IgA	180
	IgM	140
	IgG	870
	CRP	<1

Chronic Renal Disease

Pattern	Protein	Concentration (mg/dL)
	TP	2300↓
	Alb	1110↓
	AAT	260 ↙
	AAG	72 ↙
	Hp	101
	AMG	180
	TRF	81
	C3	71 ↙
	C4	14 ↙
	IgA	67 ↙
	IgM	47 ↙
	IgG	200↓
	CRP	<1

IgG Monoclonal Gammopathy (Benign)

Pattern	Protein	Concentration (mg/dL)
	TP	6900 ↗
	Alb	4380 ↙
	AAT	200
	AAG	50
	Hp	75
	AMG	220
	TRF	270
	C3	122
	C4	24
	IgA	70 ↙
	IgM	170 ↙
	IgG	1330 ↗
	CRP	<1

IgA Monclonal Gammopathy (Multiple Myeloma)

Pattern	Protein	Concentration (mg/dL)
	TP	9100↑
	Alb	2170↓
	AAT	250
	AAG	63
	Hp	97
	AMG	170
	TRF	150
	C3	90
	C4	20
	IgA	5800↑
	IgM	24↓
	IgG	200↓
	CRP	<1

Nephrotic Syndrome

Pattern	Protein	Concentration (mg/dL)
	TP	2900↓
	Alb	680↓
	AAT	160 ↙
	AAG	35 ↙
	Hp	370*
	AMG	460↑
	TRF	101↓
	C3	125 ↙
	C4	22 ↙
	IgA	250 ↙
	IgM	93 ↙
	IgG	440↓
	CRP	<1

Inflammation (Acute)

Pattern	Protein	Concentration (mg/dL)
	TP	5700 ↙
	Alb	2470↓
	AAT	400↑
	AAG	170↑
	Hp	340↑
	AMG	210
	TRF	71↓
	C3	120 ↗
	C4	17 ↗
	IgA	270
	IgM	137
	IgG	1440
	CRP	9.8↑

Systemic Lupus Erythematosus

Pattern	Protein	Concentration (mg/dL)
	TP	7800
	Alb	3390 ↙
	AAT	230
	AAG	43
	Hp	111 ↙
	AMG	240
	TRF	310
	C3	94 ↙
	C4	12 ↙
	IgA	650↑
	IgM	170
	IgG	2480↑
	CRP	7.8↑

Rheumatoid Arthritis (Adult)

Pattern	Protein	Concentration (mg/dL)
	TP	6300
	Alb	2840 ↙
	AAT	400↑
	AAG	150↑
	Hp	290↑
	AMG	148
	TRF	220 ↙
	C3	90 ↗
	C4	13 ↗
	IgA	260 ↗
	IgM	880↑
	IgG	930 ↗
	CRP	6.1↑

Iron Deficiency

Pattern	Protein	Concentration (mg/dL)
	TP	6800
	Alb	4770
	AAT	280
	AAG	44
	Hp	101
	AMG	220
	TRF	530↑
	C3	136
	C4	22
	IgA	150
	IgM	82
	IgG	880
	CRP	<1

Chronic Hepatic Disease

Pattern	Protein	Concentration (mg/dL)
	TP	6300 ↙
	Alb	2240↓
	AAT	97 ↙
	AAG	19 ↙
	Hp	<1 ↙
	AMG	290
	TRF	129↓
	C3	53 ↙
	C4	4 ↙
	IgA	480↑
	IgM	620 ↗
	IgG	2370↑
	CRP	<1↑

Chronic Hemolysis and Iron Deficiency

Pattern	Protein	Concentration (mg/dL)
	TP	6300
	Alb	4010
	AAT	190
	AAG	43
	Hp	<1↓
	AMG	400
	TRF	390 ↑
	C3	134
	C4	14
	IgA	180
	IgM	170
	IgG	700
	CRP	<1

standards. Accurate quantification by MS usually requires some type of internal standardization because efficiency of ionization and fragmentation (in tandem MS) of different components often is quite variable.

An alternative approach to MS analysis of proteins is matrix-assisted laser desorption ionization (MALDI). With this ionization technique, proteins are dried on a target plate, together with a light-absorbing compound that serves as the matrix. A pulse of light from a laser vaporizes some of the matrix, and energy is transferred to the protein, releasing individual protein ions from the surface. This is a relatively "soft" ionization technique, which generates ions without fragmenting large polypeptide chains; for proteins with non-covalently bound subunits, each subunit is released as an individual ion. An important aspect of MALDI ionization is that the ions produced, even for a large molecule such as a protein, usually acquire only a single charge, $z = 1$. Therefore, only a single main peak is obtained for each protein, and it is easy to calculate the mass (m) for m/z when $z = 1$. The challenge presented by proteins is that many mass spectrometers using quadrupoles or ion traps have an upper limit of analysis of 3000 or less for m/z and cannot analyze the large ions generated from proteins by MALDI. Analysis of proteins, then, requires use of a time-of-flight (TOF) mass spectrometer in the combined technique of MALDI-TOF-MS. TOF-MS measures how long an ion takes to move in an electrical field from the target plate to the detector. Light ions arrive faster than heavy ions, and with appropriate calibration, the masses of proteins are determined. This technique has been used to analyze proteins with a molecular weight of 100 kDa or more, although resolution declines for larger molecules. MALDI-TOF-MS is also used to analyze complex mixtures and to determine precisely the mass of small proteins and peptides; it has been used to examine the patterns of peptides and small proteins in biological fluids. The power of this approach has been widely applied in clinical laboratories for identification of bacteria that are isolated by culture techniques. Bacteria can be identified rapidly when the pattern of proteins from an individual colony is compared with an extensive database of patterns.

Plasma and Serum Proteins

As discussed in Chapter 6, plasma is the fluid portion of the blood in which the cells are suspended. It differs from serum in that it contains fibrinogen and related proteins that are removed from serum when blood clots. The major protein components in plasma are often considered collectively as the **plasma proteins**.[1] Many proteins have similar concentrations in serum and plasma. Serum has lower viscosity and about 5% lower total protein concentration owing mainly to loss of fibrinogen during clotting of plasma to form serum. Serum is depleted of fibrinogen and some coagulation factors, and increased numbers of some factors are released from platelets and peptides generated during coagulation. Serum and plasma are sometimes considered to consist of two fractions—albumin, which makes up slightly more than half of the

total protein, and the other proteins, which are classified as **globulins**. The concentration of globulins usually is calculated as follows:

$$\text{Globulins (g/dL)} = \text{Total protein (g/dL)} - \text{Albumin (g/dL)}$$

Globulins tend to be characterized as proteins that precipitate in water (such as dialysis of serum vs. water) and that redissolve when the salt concentration is raised. Proteins with this characteristic sometimes are termed *euglobulins*. Albumin remains soluble at low ionic strength. The solubility characteristics of globulins must be considered when serum or plasma is diluted extensively with water. Sometimes precipitation of protein may occur if water rather than saline is used for dilutions.

The most abundant plasma proteins are mainly proteins secreted by the liver or by B lymphocytes. Table 18-3 lists characteristics of a number of the major plasma proteins, organized according to their electrophoretic mobility in zone electrophoresis at pH 8.6. The reference intervals for several of these proteins are listed in Table 18-4 and are based on calibration with European Reference Material ERM-DA470.

For most clinical applications, quantitative changes in specific proteins are the major diagnostic indicator. In a few cases, qualitative changes assessed by techniques such as electrophoresis serve as diagnostic indicators. Plasma proteins are variably distributed between the intravascular space and the larger extravascular space. Large proteins are more likely to be retained in the intravascular space. Small proteins and peptides are distributed more evenly between intravascular and extravascular

TABLE 18-4	Interim Consensus Reference Intervals for 14 Plasma Proteins in Human Serum Referenced to ERM-DA470*	
Protein	**g/L**	**mg/dL**
α_1-Acid glycoprotein	0.5-1.2	50-120
Albumin	35-52	3500-5200
α_1-Antitrypsin	0.9-2.0	90-200
C3*	0.9-1.8[†]	90-180[†]
C4	0.1-0.4	10-40
Ceruloplasmin	0.2-0.6	20-60
C-reactive protein	<0.005	<0.5
Haptoglobin	0.3-2.0	30-200
IgA	0.7-4.0	70-400
IgG	7-16	700-1600
IgM	0.4-2.3	40-230
Prealbumin (transthyretin)	0.2-0.4	20-40
α_2-Macroglobulin	1.3-3.0	130-300
Transferrin	2.0-3.6	200-360

These reference intervals apply to adults between 20 and 60 years of age.

*ERM-DA470 (European Reference Material, Clinical [D] Proteins [A]) was formerly known as Certified Reference Material 470 (CRM 470).

[†]Values are slightly lower in fresh samples (assayed <8 h after draw).

From Dati F, Schumann G, Thomas L, et al. Consensus of a group of professional societies and diagnostic companies on guidelines for interim reference intervals for 14 proteins in serum based on the standardization against the IFCC/BCR/CAP reference material (CRM 470). Eur J Clin Chem Clin Biochem 1996; 34:517-20.

spaces. A slight redistribution of fluid is noted with movement from lying down to standing up. Consequently, plasma protein concentrations are slightly lower when collected from a patient who is lying down, because of the higher intravascular volume. If a tourniquet is applied for a prolonged time, a slight hemoconcentration is noted along with an increase in both cellular and protein components in the vein, while fluid passes into the extravascular space. The state of hydration of a patient may also slightly affect the concentration of all plasma proteins. Dehydration leads to increased protein concentration.

Several physiological and pathological factors, such as (1) nutritional status, (2) liver function, (3) physiological changes, and (4) therapeutic changes in steroid hormone concentrations, selectively affect the concentrations of subsets of plasma protein. One of the most important factors affecting clinical measurements of plasma protein concentrations in disease is the **acute-phase response** (APR). The APR is a systemic response to (1) infection, (2) tissue injury, or (3) inflammatory processes,[2] resulting in fever, increased white blood cell count, and changes in the concentration of many plasma proteins.* The proteins affected are known as acute-phase proteins (APPs). Proteins such as (1) α_1-antitrypsin, (2) α_1-acid glycoprotein, (3) haptoglobin, (4) ceruloplasmin, (5) C4, (6) C3, (7) fibrinogen, (8) C-reactive protein (CRP),[9] and (9) serum amyloid A show increased concentrations in response to an APR and are known as *positive APPs*. In extreme cases, concentrations of CRP and serum amyloid A have been known to increase up to 1000-fold from a low initial baseline value. The concentration of other plasma proteins, including (1) transthyretin, (2) albumin, and (3) transferrin, are decreased and they are known as *negative APPs*. Changes in plasma protein concentrations are triggered by interleukin-6 (IL-6) and other cytokines. Plasma concentrations of individual APR proteins change at different rates after the initial trigger. Procalcitonin is a rapidly responding APP that has been applied as an indicator of whether patients are at risk for bacterial infection. In practice, measurement of APPs assists in detection of inflammation, and sequential measurements of proteins such as CRP are used to monitor the progress of the inflammation or its response to treatment. Increased erythrocyte sedimentation rate (ESR) provides an alternative means of measuring inflammatory responses. Fibrinogen concentrations are considered to be a major determinant of ESR; therefore ESR probably reflects changes in fibrinogen concentration in the APR.

Chronic infection often yields a different pattern of plasma proteins than is seen in acute infection. In chronic infection, such as infection with hepatitis B or C and tuberculosis, immunoglobulins are often increased.

Concentrations of plasma proteins depend on their (1) rates of synthesis, (2) extracellular distribution, and (3) rates of clearance. Proteins and peptides substantially smaller than albumin are cleared from the circulation by glomerular filtration, unless they are bound to larger carriers, such as small apolipoproteins bound to lipoprotein particles or retinol-binding protein bound to prealbumin. Peptides and small proteins with half-lives of about 2 hours are cleared under conditions of normal kidney function, and they accumulate to higher concentrations in kidney failure. Examples of small proteins that accumulate in kidney failure are (1) β_2-microglobulin, (2) cystatin C, (3) Ig light chains, (4) complement factor D, and (5) retinol-binding protein. Some bioactive peptides in plasma, such as (1) insulin, (2) intact parathyroid hormone, and (3) kinins, have circulating half-lives of only a few minutes, indicating receptor-mediated clearance or degradation by peptidases. Proteins of the size of albumin or larger generally have a half-life with an upper limit of about 7 days as determined by pinocytosis (introduction of fluids into a cell) and degradation of proteins by cells. Two exceptions to this are albumin and IgG, which have a receptor-mediated process that recycles these proteins from pinocytotic vesicles. The recycling mechanism extends the half-lives of these proteins several-fold. Many proteins are subject to uptake by specific receptors or to degradation by proteolysis. Half-lives well under 7 days for a large protein suggest the presence of clearance mechanisms in addition to pinocytosis.

Individual Plasma Proteins

Prealbumin (Transthyretin) and Retinol-Binding Protein (RBP)

Prealbumin and retinol-binding protein (RBP) are transport proteins. RBP is bound to prealbumin, which was named for its electrophoretic mobility. In 1981, the term *transthyretin* was proposed for prealbumin to reflect its binding and transport of thyroid hormones and RBP. Both *prealbumin* and *transthyretin* are commonly used terms.

Biochemistry and Function

Prealbumin is a nonglycosylated protein (molecular mass, 55 kDa) composed of four identical subunits that associate to form a hollow core containing T_3- and T_4-binding sites. It binds and transports approximately 10% of both hormones. Prealbumin binding of one hormone molecule decreases the binding affinity of the second (a process known as negative cooperativity) so that only one site is normally occupied. Prealbumin is synthesized in the liver and to a lesser extent in the choroid plexus of the central nervous system, accounting for the relatively high concentration of prealbumin in CSF. Its synthesis is stimulated by (1) glucocorticosteroid hormones, (2) androgens, and (3) many nonsteroidal anti-inflammatory drugs (NSAIDs), including aspirin.

RBP is a small (21 kDa), monomeric transport protein for all-*trans*-retinol, the active form of vitamin A. RBP synthesis requires zinc, and retinol is required for its transport out of the Golgi apparatus. When circulating in the plasma, RBP is present in a 1:1 complex with prealbumin, slowing glomerular filtration of RBP. Uptake of retinol by target cells is followed by dissociation of the prealbumin/RBP complex and clearance of apoRBP (RBP without retinol) from the circulation by the kidneys. RBP is reabsorbed by the proximal renal tubular cells and catabolized. RBP has a usual half-life of only about 12 hours, but it is extended in renal failure.

---

*In 1992, the Consensus Conference Committee of the American College of Chest Physicians/Society of Critical Care Medicine produced and promulgated guidelines that recommend that the term "Systemic Inflammatory Response System (SIRS)" be used instead of "Acute Phase Reaction (APR)." Further information on this issue can be found in Chapter 27.

Clinical Significance

If vitamin A intake is adequate and renal function is normal, concentrations of prealbumin and RBP tend to rise and fall in parallel. Serum RBP is increased in chronic renal disease, including diabetic nephropathy, as the result of decreased renal clearance. Interest in RBP has been stimulated by recognition that it is synthesized by adipose tissue and that excretion of RBP may be increased, together with other products of fat cells such as leptin, in syndromes of insulin resistance. Concentrations of both prealbumin and RBP are increased with corticosteroid or NSAID therapy and in Hodgkin disease.

Decreased concentrations of RBP are seen primarily with (1) liver disease, (2) protein malnutrition, and (3) the APR. Zinc deficiency is characterized by low serum concentrations of both RBP and vitamin A. The short half-life of RBP allows its concentration to respond rapidly to changes in nutrition.

Prealbumin concentrations are often used as an indicator of protein nutrition because of its relatively short half-life and high proportion of essential amino acids. It responds much more rapidly to nutritional changes than do proteins such as albumin. Concentrations fall in (1) inflammation and malignancy (2) cirrhosis of the liver and (3) protein-losing diseases of the gut or kidneys. Prealbumin is a negative APP. Therefore, a sensitive APP such as CRP should be assayed along with prealbumin when concentrations are used to estimate nutritional status. History and physical examination are additional important aspects of nutritional assessment.

Several genetic variants of prealbumin have been described, some of which are associated with increased (familial euthyroid hyperthyroxinemia) or decreased T_3 and T_4 binding. Several variants aggregate to form amyloid fibrils in various tissues. These autosomal dominant hereditary amyloidoses can have various clinical presentations and sites of amyloid deposition, including the heart, the peripheral nerves, and the brain. Variants have been identified by mass spectrometry or by genetic analysis.

Laboratory Considerations

Prealbumin migrates as a minor band anodal to albumin on routine serum electrophoresis. Prealbumin and RBP usually are measured by immunoturbidimetric or immunonephelometric methods. The adult reference interval for RBP is 3.0 to 6.0 mg/dL, and for prealbumin, 20 to 40 mg/dL (see Table 18-4). On the basis of these reference intervals, approximately three times as many prealbumin molecules as RBP molecules have been identified, so that less than half of the prealbumin molecules are complexed with RBP.

Albumin

Albumin is a nonglycosylated protein of 585 amino acids with calculated molecular weight of 66,438 Da. It is the most abundant protein in plasma from midgestation until death, usually accounting for slightly more than one-half of plasma protein mass. Because of its high plasma concentration and medium size, albumin is the major contributor to colloidal oncotic pressure (COP) in the vascular space. This force helps to retain fluid within the vascular space, and albumin solutions sometimes have been infused to assist in maintaining intravascular volume. When albumin concentrations are decreased, the tendency for fluid to go into extravascular spaces and to produce edema is increased. Albumin is the major protein component of most extravascular body fluids, including (1) CSF, (2) interstitial fluid, (3) urine, and (4) amniotic fluid. Approximately 60% of the total body albumin is found in the extravascular space, although the concentration is higher in the vascular space (plasma concentration). Albumin is highly soluble in water because of its high abundance of charged amino acids. It has a net charge of about −12 at neutral pH. At normal concentrations, albumin contributes about 6 to 10 mmol/L to the anion gap. Low albumin concentrations contribute to a decreased anion gap.

Biochemistry and Function

Albumin is synthesized by the hepatic parenchymal cells. The synthetic reserve of the liver is substantial; in the nephrotic syndrome, the synthetic rate has been known to increase to threefold above normal. The synthesis of albumin is controlled primarily by COP and secondarily by protein intake. Catabolism occurs primarily by pinocytosis in all tissues, but albumin, together with IgG, has a half-life that is extended by about two- to fourfold because of the action of the neonatal IgG receptor that selectively recycles these two proteins from pinocytosed fluids. The usual half-life of albumin is 15 to 19 days. Most other plasma proteins have half-lives of 7 days or less. Albumin has multiple functions, including maintenance of COP and binding and transport of a large number of compounds, including (1) free fatty acids, (2) bilirubin, (3) calcium, (4) thyroid and steroid hormones, (5) drugs, and (6) thiol-containing compounds.

More than 80 genetic variants of albumin have been reported. Many variants have altered electrophoretic migration, resulting in so-called bisalbuminemia (two bands for albumin), for heterozygotes. Bound drugs and metabolites also may change the electrophoretic migration of albumin. A few variants have increased binding affinities for thyroxine (T_4). Affected individuals have increased serum T_4 but are euthyroid and have normal thyrotropin concentrations.

Clinical Significance

Increased concentrations of albumin are seen with dehydration or prolonged tourniquet time or with specimen evaporation before analysis. Therefore high albumin concentrations suggest problems with patient hydration or specimen handling. Decreased concentrations are seen in a multitude of clinical conditions.

Analbuminemia. Only about 20 families with this rare genetic deficiency have been reported. Individuals with analbuminemia have plasma albumin concentrations less than 0.5 g/L. Symptoms often are absent or consist of mild edema and dyslipidemia.

Inflammation. Albumin is a negative APP and acute inflammation and chronic inflammation are common causes of hypoalbuminemia. Inflammatory processes decrease plasma albumin by (1) increasing capillary permeability, allowing more albumin to enter the extravascular space, (2) decreasing hepatic synthesis of albumin in response to factors such as IL-6, (3) stimulating catabolism, and (4) slowing synthesis in response to COP contributions of positive APPs.

Hepatic Disease. The liver has synthetic capacity to maintain albumin concentration until parenchymal damage results in greater than 50% loss of function. Additional mechanisms may contribute to decreased albumin concentrations in many cases of liver disease, including (1) nutritional deficiency, (2) increased distribution into the extravascular space, and (3) direct inhibition of synthesis by toxins such as alcohol.

Urinary Loss. Normally, the glomerular filtration barrier efficiently prevents entry into the urinary ultrafiltrate by proteins the size of albumin or larger. Usually, only 1 to 2 g/d of albumin pass through the glomerular barrier, and 99.9% of albumin in the glomerular ultrafiltrate is taken up by the proximal tubules of the kidney, where it is degraded. Only about 10 mg/d of albumin is normally excreted in urine. Small increases in albumin excretion to >30 mg/d indicate early stages of glomerular or tubular injury and risk of progression to more severe kidney disease. This has been termed *microalbuminuria.* (*Note:* "micro" refers to excretion of small amounts, not a smaller form, of albumin). Nonpathological increases in urine albumin excretion sometimes are observed with postural changes, strenuous exercise, and fever. Collection of first or second voided urine specimens in the morning may minimize postural effects. Severe glomerular injury produces the nephrotic syndrome, which is characterized by excretion of >3.5 g/d of protein, which is mainly albumin. In the nephrotic syndrome, the kidney maintains some size selectivity. Concentrations less than 200 kDa of protein such as albumin generally are substantially decreased, even though hepatic production is increased. Concentrations of a few very large proteins, such as α_2-macroglobulin (AMG) and apolipoprotein B–containing lipoproteins, are increased.

Gastrointestinal Loss. Inflammatory disease of the intestinal tract is associated with increased gastrointestinal (GI) loss of albumin with, losses of albumin being as great as renal losses in the nephrotic syndrome.

Protein-Energy Malnutrition (Marasmus). Albumin concentrations help to detect and monitor protein nutritional status. Responses to dietary intake are slow because of the long half-life of albumin. The APR often has to be considered as a potential complicating factor in patients with low albumin concentrations.

Burn Injury. Patients with burn injury have been observed to experience severe loss of albumin from wounds. Severely decreased albumin concentrations with massive burn injuries probably are related to combined effects of epithelial losses, accelerated catabolism, and the APR.

Edema and Ascites. Edema and ascites usually are secondary to increased vascular permeability, rather than to hypoalbuminemia per se. Plasma albumin concentrations are decreased as a result of redistribution of albumin into extravascular spaces.

Laboratory Considerations

Most clinical laboratories assay albumin in plasma or serum samples using dye-binding methods, which rely on a shift in the absorption spectrum of dyes such as bromcresol green (BCG) or purple (BCP) upon albumin binding. The affinity of these dyes is higher for albumin than for other proteins, and partial specificity is provided for albumin. BCP generally is slightly more specific for albumin and yields lower values than BCG, particularly in patients with kidney disease. Albumin concentration is considered an important indicator of adequate nutrition in patients with kidney failure. Nutritional supplementation usually is recommended for patients with kidney failure and albumin <4 g/dL as determined by a BCG method. The dye-binding assays tend to have decreased accuracy when the serum protein pattern is abnormal. Immunoturbidimetry and nephelometry offer greater specificity and accuracy for albumin measurement, along with the lowered limits of detection needed for specimens with low albumin concentrations, such as urine and cerebrospinal fluid. Albumin concentrations can be calculated from densitometric scans of electrophoretic patterns, together with total protein measurements, but this approach usually is associated with lower accuracy and precision. Reference intervals are listed in Table 18-4.

High-Density Lipoprotein

High-density lipoprotein (HDL) formerly was termed α-*lipoprotein* on the basis of its electrophoretic mobility (see Chapter 23 for a more detailed discussion of lipoproteins), but it is not visualized satisfactorily by protein stains. It is characterized by high density (>1.063 g/mL) because of its content of about 50% protein and phospholipid as a major lipid component. Apolipoprotein A-I of 29 kDa is the major protein, although small amounts of many other proteins are present. High concentrations of HDL, usually measured as the cholesterol in HDL or as apolipoprotein A-I, lower the risk of cardiovascular disease. Apolipoprotein A-I is a negative APP that is considered to have anti-inflammatory properties. In inflammatory states, the composition of HDL may change as amounts of apolipoprotein A-I decline, and it may be replaced by serum amyloid A.

α₁-Acid Glycoprotein (AAG)

α_1-Acid glycoprotein (AAG), also known as *orosomucoid,* is a member of the lipocalin family of proteins that bind lipophilic substances. AAG actually consists of two proteins that are products of closely homologous genes, which differ in only 21 out of 183 amino acid residues.

Biochemistry and Function

AAG contains 183 amino acids and a total molecular mass of about 40 kDa, of which approximately 45% is carbohydrate, including about 12% sialic acid. The oligosaccharide structures and charge of AAG change slightly with inflammation, as do many proteins. It is synthesized mainly by hepatic parenchymal cells. Intact AAG has a half-life of about 3 days, but when sialic acid is lost from its oligosaccharides, it is cleared within a few minutes by hepatic asialoglycoprotein receptors.

AAG binds a variety of lipophilic hormones, such as progesterone, and basic drugs, including (1) propranolol, (2) quinidine, (3) chlorpromazine, (4) cocaine, and (5) benzodiazepines. Binding of drugs to AAG increases the plasma drug concentration while reducing the proportion of drug that is free and bioactive. Because AAG concentrations may change several-fold in the APR, interpretation of total drug concentrations for some drugs requires measurement of AAG or alternative measures of free rather than total drug concentrations.

Clinical Significance

AAG is a positive APP. Plasma concentrations often increase several-fold in APRs, especially in GI inflammatory disease and malignant neoplasms. Concentrations are increased by corticosteroids and by some NSAIDs. Estrogens (e.g., from pregnancy, from oral contraception) decrease synthesis of AAG. Concentrations also are low in protein-losing syndromes, such as nephrotic syndrome.

Laboratory Considerations

Although AAG is one of the highest-concentration proteins in the α_1-globulin region, on routine serum electrophoresis, it does not stain satisfactorily with protein stains because of its high CHO content. It is visualized with the use of periodic acid–Schiff or other carbohydrate stains. AAG usually is quantified by immunochemical methods, including turbidimetry and nephelometry. Reference intervals are listed in Table 18-4.

α_1-Antitrypsin

α_1-Antitrypsin (AAT) is a serpin (serine proteinase inhibitor) that inactivates serine proteases such as neutrophil elastase that are structurally related to trypsin.[10] Other serpins include (1) α_1-antichymotrypsin, (2) α_2-antiplasmin, (3) antithrombin III, and (4) C1 inhibitor.

Biochemistry and Function

AAT is synthesized primarily by hepatic parenchymal cells. On a molar basis, AAT is the highest-concentration protease inhibitor in plasma. It acts as a suicide substrate of serine proteases and remains covalently attached to the protease. The complex of AAT with proteases is removed from the circulation rapidly by specific receptors. Physiologically, it is the most important inhibitor of leukocyte elastase, as released by neutrophils. If a deficiency of AAT is present, unchecked action of the leukocyte elastase cleaves elastin, which is important for maintaining the architecture of lung tissue. Loss of elastin leads to emphysema. Smoking serves as a cofactor by stimulating inflammation and neutrophil infiltration in the lungs and by lowering AAT activity by oxidizing a methionine residue in AAT, which is the reactive site residue in the inhibitor.

At least 75 genetic variants of AAT are known, several of which are associated with low serum concentrations. The common wild phenotype is designated PiMM ("Pi" for protease inhibitor); the most common deficiency genotypes of clinical importance are PiZZ and SZ. Other genotypes include PiMZ and PiSS. In many populations, 10% or more of individuals are heterozygous for AAT variants. Most clinical disorders occur in individuals with two variant alleles. AAT deficiency is decreased by about 85% in individuals who are PiZZ and by about 63% for PiSZ. AAT variants have a disorder of protein folding that leads to intracellular aggregation and decreased secretion of AAT.

Clinical Significance

AAT concentrations are elevated by the APR and by estrogens (pregnancy, oral contraception). AAT concentrations are secondarily low in individuals with (1) neonatal respiratory distress syndrome, (2) severe pancreatitis, and (3) protein-losing disorders. Decreased AAT concentrations due to genetic deficiency are associated with high risk for developing basilar pulmonary emphysema (in contrast to the apical disease present in other forms of emphysema). Onset of disease is usually much earlier than for most other forms of emphysema, with changes beginning in the second to fourth decades of life in 90% of PiZZ individuals. The process is promoted by smoking. Severe genetic deficiency occurs with a frequency of about 1 in 3000.

Genetic deficiency of AAT also is associated with diseases of the liver, including (1) neonatal cholestasis, (2) cirrhosis, and (3) hepatocellular carcinoma. About 10% of infants with PiZZ or PiZnull genotypes have prolonged obstructive jaundice, and 2% progress to liver failure in childhood. Early histologic differentiation of cholestasis from AAT deficiency and biliary atresia is challenging. Liver disease with AAT variants is associated with risk for progression to hepatocellular carcinoma. Hepatic injury in AAT deficiency probably is related to intracellular aggregation of AAT variants.

Laboratory Considerations

Quantitative testing of AAT is recommended for patients with onset or family history of chronic obstructive pulmonary disease before age 45. AAT usually is quantified by immunoturbidimetry or immunonephelometry. Reference intervals for AAT are listed in Table 18-4. Phenotyping of AAT usually is performed by isoelectric focusing. Genotyping assays detect common variants of AAT.

AAT usually is the major constituent of the α_1-globulin band on routine clinical serum electrophoresis. AAG and α-lipoprotein also are included in the α_1-globulin band but do not stain well with peptide stains because of their high contents of CHO and lipid, respectively. Decreases in the α_1-band suggest a decrease in AAT or variants of AAT with altered mobility.

α-Fetoprotein

α-Fetoprotein (AFP) is the most abundant plasma protein in early embryonic life. AFP is homologous to albumin but differs in having about 4% carbohydrate. Its molecular mass is about 70 kDa. AFP usually is present at very low concentrations after the neonatal period, and highly sensitive immunoassays are required for analysis. The serum concentration of AFP serves as a tumor marker for hepatocellular and germ cell carcinoma (refer to Chapter 20 on tumor markers). Maternal serum concentrations are analyzed as indicators of fetal trisomy of chromosome 18 or 21 (refer to Chapter 44 for a description of testing in pregnancy).

Haptoglobin

Haptoglobin (Hp) is an α_2-glycoprotein that binds free hemoglobin (Hb). It is synthesized by the liver and consists of equal numbers of α- and β-subunits in variable proportions depending on genotype. Each $\alpha\beta$ pair in Hp binds an $\alpha\beta$ dimer from Hb.

Biochemistry and Function

Hp is synthesized as a single peptide chain by hepatocytes and is cleaved into α- and β-chains. Hp is polymorphic because of the variable occurrence of two types of α-chain—α^1 and α^2. Three Hp genotypes—designated Hp1-1, Hp 2-1, and Hp 2-2—result from the combination of two genes for α^1, one each for α^1 and α^2, or 2 α^2 genes. Hp 1-1 consists of two each of α- and β-chains with a total molecular weight of about 85 kDA, Hp 1-2 consists of multiple forms ranging from 85 kDa to 300 kDa, and Hp 2-2 has larger multimers ranging from 170 to 900 kDa.

Hp 1-1 genotype has a frequency of about 50% in some African and indigenous South American populations but less than 20% in most North American and Asian populations. The Hp 1-1 genotype is associated with decreased risk of cardiovascular disease that may be related to a (1) higher concentration, (2) Hb affinity, and (3) greater extracellular distribution. Hp/Hb complexes are rapidly bound by receptors on reticuloendothelial cells. Because Hp is removed from the circulation and is degraded after complexing with Hb, Hp concentration drops severely when intravascular hemolysis occurs, so that Hp measurement assists in identifying hemolytic disorders. Hp has a capacity to bind only about 1% of the Hb in red cells at usual hematocrits and Hp concentrations. Hemolysis of specimens during or after blood collection does not decrease amounts of Hp, so that Hp measurement sometimes helps to distinguish in vivo from in vitro hemolysis.

Binding of Hb by Hp prevents renal clearance of Hb and loss of iron, and hematuria will occur only after Hp is depleted. Hp binding of Hb also prevents toxic effects of Hb on kidney tubules. A consequence of Hp depletion in chronic hemolytic states, such as sickle cell disease, is that the plasma concentration of Hb increases, and the Hb acts as a scavenger of the physiologically important vasodilator, nitric oxide. Free Hb in the circulation therefore contributes to vascular disorders such as pulmonary hypertension.

Clinical Significance

Hp concentrations are increased by (1) glucocorticosteroids, (2) androgens, and (3) many NSAIDs. It is a weak and late-reacting APP. Hp concentrations are elevated in selective protein-losing syndromes, such as nephrotic syndrome, in individuals with the Hp 2-1 or 2-2 genotype, which produces Hp with a high molecular weight. Biliary obstruction in the absence of severe hepatocellular disease is associated with significantly increased Hp concentrations, and most forms of liver disease are associated with decreased amounts of Hp. Concentrations of Hp are low during pregnancy and are very low in the neonatal period. Reference intervals for Hp vary with genotype—57 to 227 mg/dL in Hp 1-1, 44 to 183 mg/dL in Hp2-1, and 38 to 150 mg/dL in Hp 2-2. The adult reference intervals for undefined genotypes are listed in Table 18-4.

Laboratory Considerations

Immunoturbidimetry and immunonephelometry usually are employed for clinical assays of Hp. Traditionally, Hp was measured by assaying peroxidase activity after serum was mixed with an excess of Hb, the so-called Hb-binding capacity (BC). On average, approximately 1 mg Hb is bound by 1.5 mg Hp. Hp and α_2-macroglobulin (AMG) constitute the major α_2-globulins on serum zone electrophoresis.

α_2-Macroglobulin

AMG is a major plasma proteinase inhibitor. Unlike AAT and most other proteinase inhibitors, it is a very large molecule (molecular mass, $\approx$725 kDa) that does not diffuse from the plasma space into extracellular fluids in significant amounts.

Biochemistry and Function

AMG inhibits many different classes of proteinases, including those with (1) serine, (2) cysteine, and (3) metal ions in their catalytic sites. AMG is homologous to complement components C3 and C4, and, like those proteins, it contains an internal thioester bond that is activated by proteolytic cleavage and reacts to bind covalently with proteases. Intact AMG has a half-life of several days, but it is cleared rapidly by a hepatic receptor when it is cleaved by a protease.

Clinical Significance

AMG is synthesized by the liver. Estrogen increases AMG concentrations, so that women of childbearing age demonstrate higher concentrations than men of the same age. Concentrations in infants and children are two to three times adult concentrations. High AMG concentrations in children may delay symptoms resulting from deficiency of antithrombin III or C1 inhibitor. AMG is not an APR in humans, and concentration stays fairly constant during the APR. AMG tends to increase in the nephrotic syndrome, while most other plasma proteins decrease; the liver increases synthesis of all proteins, but loss of proteins exceeds production, except for very large proteins, which still are retained by the impaired glomerular filtration barrier. Decreased plasma concentrations of AMG often are seen in individuals with severe acute pancreatitis or with advanced carcinoma of the prostate. Although genetic variants of AMG have been noted, they have no known clinical significance.

Laboratory Considerations

AMG and Hp together constitute the major α_2-globulins on serum zone electrophoresis. In the newborn period, and after in vivo hemolysis, AMG alone is the major contributor to this zone. AMG usually is quantified by immunoturbidimetry or immunonephelometry. The reference intervals for AMG are listed in Table 18-4.

Ceruloplasmin

Ceruloplasmin (Cp) is an α_2-globulin that contains approximately 95% of the total serum copper, giving Cp a blue color. When Cp concentrations are significantly elevated (e.g., during pregnancy) or the normal yellow pigments of plasma are decreased, plasma may have a greenish tint.

Biochemistry and Function

Cp is synthesized primarily by the liver. Copper is added to the peptide chain by an intracellular ATPase and is essential for the normal folding of the polypeptide chain. ApoCp synthesized in the absence of copper or the ATPase is degraded primarily intracellularly, and decreased amounts are released into the circulation.

The primary physiological role of Cp is catalysis of reduction and oxidation (redox) reactions. Cp is vitally important in regulating the ionic state of iron, oxidizing Fe^{2+} to Fe^{3+} (from the ferrous to the ferric states), thus permitting incorporation of the iron into transferrin. The copper in Cp serves as an electron receptor in this reaction, going from Cu^{2+} to Cu^+. In the absence of this reaction, iron cannot be mobilized efficiently from tissue stores into circulation on transferrin. Although Cp contains primarily plasma copper, albumin and transcuprein probably serve as the most important copper transport proteins.

Clinical Significance

Cp is a weak, late-reacting positive APP. Concentrations are increased significantly by estrogens, as in pregnancy or with the use of oral contraceptives. Primary genetic deficiency of Cp is rare and results in iron deposition in tissue, similar to hereditary hemochromatosis, because of impaired export of iron from tissues into transferrin. Individuals have normal tissue copper but increased tissue iron stores and decreased serum iron. Secondary deficiency of Cp due to decreased incorporation of Cu^{2+} into apoCp during synthesis is more common than primary deficiency. Secondary deficiency may be due to (1) dietary copper insufficiency (including malabsorption), (2) inability to transport Cu^{2+} from the GI epithelium into the circulation (as in Menkes disease), or (3) defective incorporation of Cu^{2+} into the developing Cp molecule (as in Wilson disease). Cp concentrations also may be low in cases of blood loss or GI or renal protein-losing syndromes. Dietary deficiency, secondary to nutritional copper deficiency, is associated with (1) neutropenia, (2) thrombocytopenia, (3) low serum iron, and hypochromic, normocytic, or microcytic (4) anemia that does not respond to iron therapy.

Wilson disease, or _hepatolenticular degeneration,_ differs from dietary deficiency in that total body copper is increased significantly and deposited in tissues, including the (1) hepatic parenchymal cells, (2) the brain, and (3) the periphery of the iris (resulting in the characteristic Kayser-Fleischer rings). Copper is absorbed from the diet and is transported to the liver, but the absence of a specific ATPase impairs incorporation of copper into Cp. Symptoms in individuals with Wilson disease usually begin in the second or third decade of life

and include (1) hepatitis, (2) neurological disorders, and (3) renal tubular dysfunction. Mutations that completely destroy the ATPase function may be associated with the onset of liver disease as early as 3 years of age. Treatment of Wilson disease aims to remove tissue copper through chelation with agents such as penicillamine or trientene and inhibition of dietary copper uptake with supplemental zinc.

Laboratory Considerations

Cp usually is measured by immunoturbidimetry or immunonephelometry. Cp functional activity is measured in oxidase assays. It is subject to oxidation and proteolysis during storage that may affect immunoreactivity. This lability poses problems with (1) calibrators, (2) control materials, and (3) patient samples. Serum or plasma should be separated from blood as soon as possible, and specimens should be refrigerated for up to 3 days or frozen at below −70 °C for prolonged storage. The adult reference intervals for Cp are listed in Table 18-4. Plasma concentrations of Cp are low at birth, increase to peak concentrations at 2 or 3 years of age, and decline slowly until adolescence, when adult concentrations are reached.

Transferrin

Transferrin (TRF), or siderophilin, is the major plasma transport protein for iron (see Chapter 28). TRF accounts for most of the total iron-binding capacity (TIBC) of plasma; one molecule binds two ferric ions that physiologically are generated by oxidation of ferrous ion by Cp. The $TRF-Fe^3$ complex then transports iron to cells for incorporation into cytochromes, Hb, and myoglobin, and to storage sites, such as the liver and the reticuloendothelial system. Virtually every cell type has surface receptors for TRF.

Biochemistry and Function

TRF is synthesized primarily in the liver and usually migrates in the β-region on routine clinical electrophoresis of serum. Plasma concentrations are regulated primarily by availability of iron, with plasma concentrations rising with iron deficiency and falling with adequacy of iron. As with albumin, about one-half of the TRF exists outside the vascular compartment in extracellular fluids.

Clinical Significance

Evaluation of plasma TRF concentrations aids in the differential diagnosis of anemia and in monitoring of treatment for iron deficiency anemia. In cases of iron deficiency, the TRF concentration is increased, but the protein has low saturation with iron. In anemia of chronic disease instead of deficiency of iron, TRF concentration may be normal or low, but the protein is highly saturated with iron. In iron-overload states, such as hereditary hemochromatosis, TRF concentration is normal, but iron saturation often exceeds 55%—considerably above reference values. Interpretation of serum iron and iron saturation is complicated by large diurnal variation. Serum iron concentration usually is highest in the morning and decreases markedly in the evening. Saturation >100% may be observed with parenteral iron infusion or with toxic overdoses of iron, for which high saturation may be a sign of severe overdose. High concentrations of TRF are present in pregnancy and during estrogen administration.

TRF is a negative APP, and low concentrations occur in inflammation or malignancy. Decreased synthesis occurs with chronic liver disease or protein malnutrition. Protein loss, such as that seen in the nephrotic syndrome or in protein-losing enteropathy, also causes low concentrations. In the rare disorder congenital atransferrinemia, a very low concentration of TRF is accompanied by iron overload and severe hypochromic anemia that is resistant to iron therapy.

Laboratory Considerations
The availability of simple photometric assays for TIBC, or the ability to calculate TIBC from assays of iron plus unsaturated iron binding capacity (UIBC) where TIBC = UIBC + iron, is used to estimate functional TRF. TIBC also is used to estimate TRF by the following equation:

$$TRF\ (mg/dL) = 0.70 \times TIBC\ (\mu g/dL)$$

or

$$TIBC = 1.43 \times Tf$$

TRF is more accurately quantified by immunochemical methods, including immunoturbidimetry and immunonephelometry, and these measurements have been used to calculate the TIBC. As was noted previously, TRF migrates in the β_1-region on routine serum electrophoresis, where it usually is the major component, but genetic variants may cause changes in mobility. Reference intervals are listed in Table 18-4.

Carbohydrate-deficient TRF (CDT) is a form of TRF that has decreased or absent glycosylation. CDT usually is a minor component of TRF (<2%), but amounts of CDT are often increased in congenital disorders of glycosylation that affect the glycosylation of many proteins. Amounts of CDT also are increased in individuals with chronic alcohol abuse, and quantitative analysis of CDT may serve as a marker for alcohol abuse. CDT migrates in the β_2-region during zone electrophoresis rather than in the usual β_1-region for TRF because of the lower negative charge. CDT is a major fraction of TRF in CSF, and it has been used as an indicator of whether clear fluids coming from the ear or nasal passages represent leakage of CSF. Electrophoretic analysis often has been used for this analysis, with the β_2-TRF band serving as a marker for CSF.

Low-Density Lipoprotein
Low-density lipoprotein (LDL) is often termed β-*lipoprotein* on the basis of its electrophoretic mobility. (Refer to Chapter 23 for a more extensive discussion of lipoproteins). LDL has a density between 1.019 and 1.063 g/mL when separated by density gradient ultracentrifugation. It consists of about 80% lipid and 20% protein. Cholesterol ester is the main lipid component, and apolipoprotein B is the main protein. Apolipoprotein B is a large protein of 500 kDa, which is very hydrophobic and inserts into the lipid particle similarly to an intrinsic membrane protein. Increases in LDL concentration confer increased risk of cardiovascular disease. Concentrations of LDL are assessed by calculation of LDL cholesterol that are based on other lipid measurements, direct quantification of LDL cholesterol, or quantification of apolipoprotein B. One apolipoprotein B is usually present per LDL particle, so that measurement of apolipoprotein B serves as a measure of the number of LDL particles.

β₂-Microglobulin
β_2-Microglobulin (BMG) is a low-molecular-mass (11.8 kDa) protein found on the cell surfaces of all nucleated cells; small amounts are shed into plasma.

Biochemistry and Function
BMG, the light or β-chain of the human leukocyte antigens (HLAs), consists of a single polypeptide chain with no carbohydrate. Some BMG is shed into the plasma, particularly by lymphocytes and tumor cells. The small size of BMG allows it to be filtered through the glomerular membrane, but typically less than 1% of the filtered BMG is excreted in the urine. The remainder of the BMG is reabsorbed and catabolized in the proximal tubules of the kidneys.

Clinical Significance
High plasma concentrations of BMG are present in individuals with (1) renal failure, (2) inflammation, and (3) neoplasms, especially those associated with B lymphocytes. Urinary BMG is used as a marker for renal tubular function. (See later section on urinary proteins.) Measurement of plasma BMG has been used as a staging criterion for multiple myeloma, with higher BMG representing more advanced disease. In patients with chronic lymphocytic leukemia, high BMG concentrations are a prognostic marker for decreased survival.

Rapid clearance of BMG typically keeps the plasma concentration low. The reference interval is 0.7 to 1.8 mg/L. However, the concentration increases substantially in renal failure, to concentrations of up to about 40 mg/L. BMG concentrations in patients with renal failure and efficiency of BMG clearance during dialysis treatment are clinically significant because BMG can deposit as amyloid, leading to systemic **amyloidosis** in many patients on long-term dialysis.[7]

Fibrinogen
Fibrinogen, the terminal component of the coagulation system, aggregates to form a fibrous network when it is cleaved by the protease thrombin. Maintaining adequate concentrations of fibrinogen is important for preventing bleeding. Fibrinogen is a positive APP.

Biochemistry and Function
Fibrinogen is a highly elongated protein that consists of six polypeptide chains joined by disulfide bonds. Two each of Aα-, Bβ-, and γ-chains are the products of separate genes. The total molecular mass is about 340 kDa. Removal of small A- and B-fibrinopeptides from the Aα- and Bβ-chains by thrombin causes fibrinogen to aggregate into long fibers of fibrin. Fibrin has binding sites for platelets, and other cells such as red cells become entrapped in the fibrous network of fibrin as

a clot forms. Contractile elements in platelets gradually cause the clot to retract (clot retraction) and to squeeze serum out of the clot. Fibrin monomers then slowly become covalently cross-linked by the action of a transglutaminase (coagulation factor XIIIa), which makes a clot firmer and more rigid.

Clinical Significance

Low plasma concentrations occur as the result of consumption from extensive bleeding or dysregulation of the coagulation system, such as disseminated intravascular coagulation. Functional disorders of fibrinogen (dysfibrinogenemia) may be seen with liver disease or as a rare inherited disorder. Fibrinogen is a positive APP. It is one of the major contributors to plasma viscosity because of its large size and highly elongated structure, and it accounts for the higher viscosity of plasma relative to serum (which has fibrinogen removed). High plasma concentrations of fibrinogen on a chronic basis are associated with increased risk of cardiovascular disease, which may relate to increased plasma viscosity or the increased tendency for thrombosis.

Laboratory Considerations

Fibrinogen typically is measured by functional clotting assays. It is also measured by immunoturbidimetric methods or by turbidimetric methods based on the addition of precipitating reagents. Plasma concentrations of fibrinogen are normally in the interval of about 150 to 350 mg/dL but vary slightly with the method of analysis. Fragments of fibrin generated by the protease plasmin, such as fibrin-degradation products or D-dimer, are measured as indicators of increased thrombosis, suggesting the presence of pulmonary embolism or venous thrombosis. If fibrinogen is not completely removed from serum, it may give a band on serum protein electrophoresis at the anodal end of the γ-region that is mistaken for a paraprotein. This may occur if the patient is receiving anticoagulation, or if the specimen is contaminated with an inhibitor of coagulation such as heparin. The pseudoparaprotein band from fibrinogen will not show any corresponding band on immunofixation electrophoresis, indicating that the band does not consist of immunoglobulins.

C-Reactive Protein

C-reactive protein (CRP) is a substance found in the sera of acutely ill individuals that is able to bind the cell wall C-polysaccharide of *Streptococcus pneumoniae*. It is an early positive APR and exhibits some of the most dramatic increases in concentration. It has been used extensively as a marker of inflammation.

Biochemistry and Function

CRP consists of five identical, nonglycosylated subunits of 23 kDa that associate to form a disc-shaped structure. Its pentameric structure leads to the family name *pentraxin* for CRP and related proteins. CRP is synthesized by the liver. Functions of CRP include protecting against foreign organisms and assisting in clearing tissue debris. CRP binds a variety of compounds in the presence of Ca^2: (1) polysaccharides present in many bacteria, fungi, and protozoans; (2) phosphorylcholine; (3) phosphatidylcholines, such as lecithin; and (4) polyanions, such as nucleic acids. In the absence of Ca^2, CRP binds polycations, such as histones. Complexation of CRP activates the classic complement pathway starting at C1q, thus initiating (1) opsonization, (2) phagocytosis, and (3) lysis of invading organisms, such as bacteria and viruses. CRP also helps to clear tissue debris from damaged tissue.

Clinical Significance

CRP is one of the strongest-reacting APPs, with plasma concentrations rising dramatically after (1) myocardial infarction, (2) stress, (3) trauma, (4) infection, (5) inflammation, (6) surgery, or (7) neoplastic proliferation. CRP begins to rise within 6 to 12 hours of the onset of any of these stimuli and usually peaks within 48 hours. CRP concentration may increase more than 1000-fold from a low initial baseline. Bacterial infection usually is a stronger stimulus than viral infection, and CRP has been used as a marker for bacterial infection in newborns. CRP measurements are used as an indicator of inflammatory processes, and they are used to assess the activity of disorders such as rheumatoid arthritis and Crohn disease. For unknown reasons, CRP responses to some inflammatory disorders such as systemic lupus erythematosus and ulcerative colitis are mild.

Epidemiological studies demonstrate that slightly increased serum CRP concentrations are associated with increased risk of cardiovascular disease. These slight increases in CRP may reflect low-grade chronic inflammation associated with atherosclerosis. This application of CRP requires assays with detection limits of about 1 mg/L, which often are referred to as *high-sensitivity CRP (hsCRP) assays*. CRP >2.0 mg/L has been suggested as an indicator of increased cardiovascular risk. Separate assays with a higher measuring range are commonly used to measure CRP in cases of infection or severe inflammation.

Laboratory Considerations

CRP is normally present in plasma at concentrations <5 mg/L. High concentrations of CRP in inflammatory states are measured with direct immunoturbidimetric or immunonephelometric assays using antibody to CRP. Assays to measure basal CRP in healthy subjects usually require different technologies to achieve lower detection limits; hsCRP assays include (1) particle-enhanced immunoturbidimetry or nephelometry, or (2) sandwich immunoassays with fluorescence or chemiluminescent detection. CRP migrates on cellulose acetate or agarose gel electrophoresis anywhere from the slow-γ- to mid-β-regions, depending on the calcium ion content of the buffer. Serum concentrations are too low to show as a stained band except in an extreme APR.

Complement Proteins

Complement is a complex system of proteins found in normal blood plasma that combines with antibodies to destroy pathogenic bacteria and other foreign cells. It helps or "complements" the ability of antibodies and phagocytic cells to clear pathogens from an organism. It consists of at least 20 proteins

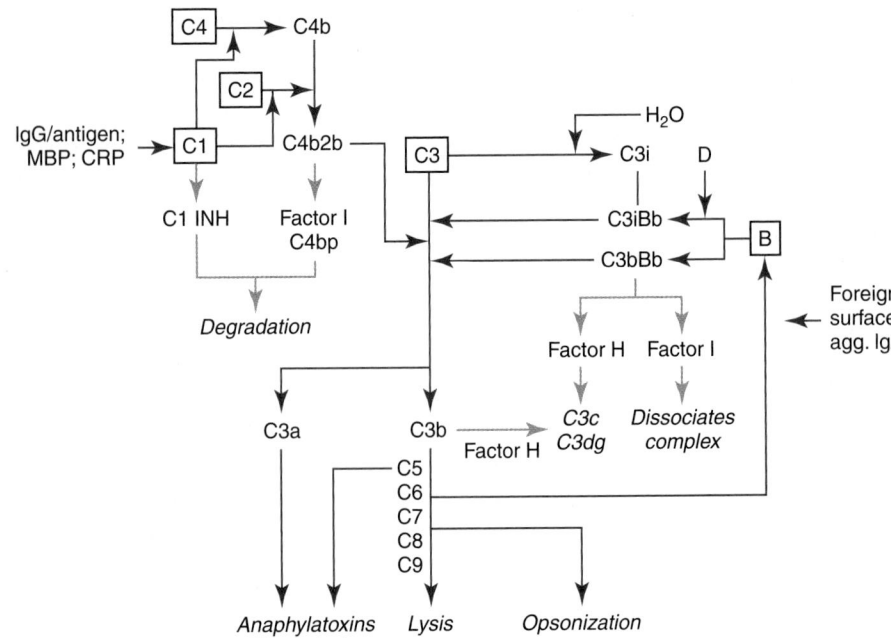

Figure 18-4 Overview of the Complement Cascades. Activation via the classical pathway and the lectin pathway is shown on the left and via the alternative pathway on the right. Gradual activation by spontaneous hydrolysis of C3 to C3i is shown at the center top. Direct activation of C3 by neutrophil and plasma proteases also may occur. The control mechanisms are shaded. *(Courtesy J.W. Whicher, with modifications.)*

in plasma and a number of cellular receptors and regulators on cell surfaces; some of the interactions of major components are diagrammed in Figure 18-4.[11] Complement proteins are divided into six groups by function:

1. The *classic pathway,* which includes C1, C4, C2, and C3 (in order of activation).
2. The *alternative pathway,* which includes C3, factors B and D, and properdin.
3. The *lectin pathway,* which includes mannan-binding protein (MBP), ficolins, and associated proteases.
4. The *membrane attack complex,* which includes C5 through C9 and inserts into cell membranes and lyses cells.
5. *Inhibitors and inactivators of the previous pathways,* including C1 inhibitor, factors H and I, and C4-binding protein (C4bp).
6. *Cellular receptors and regulators* for activated or cell-bound components.

The classic pathway is activated primarily by complexes of immunoglobulins with antigen or bacteria or other ligands with CRP (see Figure 18-4), whereas the alternative pathway is activated by (1) bacterial lipopolysaccharides, (2) cellular proteases, and (3) cobra venom. The lectin pathway is activated by binding of ficolins and MBP to mannose-rich oligosaccharides that are present in the cell walls of many microorganisms. Activation of the classic pathway through C3 also activates the alternative pathway, which amplifies the production of effector molecules. Other mechanisms also may activate the **complement system,** including the action of proteases released by leukocytes and other inflammatory cells. The common step involved is the activation of C3 to C3b.

A number of the complement components are proteases. Each of the three pathways of complement activation consists of a cascade of several protease zymogens, including C1r, C1s, C2, factor D, factor B, and MBP-associated serine protease-I and -II. Zymogens are activated by cleavage of preceding

factors in a pathway. Multiple factors act to control the protease activities. The protease inhibitor C1 inhibitor is an important regulator, as are the binding proteins factor H and C4bp and the protease factor I, which breaks down activated complement factors.

During activation, many complement components are cleaved by proteases into two fragments—in general, (1) one larger fragment that binds to various surfaces, such as bacterial membranes, plus (2) a smaller fragment that may become active in chemotaxis (movement or orientation of an organism or cell along a chemical concentration gradient) and vascular permeability. The larger fragments are designated by a lowercase "b," and the smaller fragments by a lowercase "a." The larger fragments may contain a binding site for cell membranes and immune complexes or a protease that then activates the next component(s). Thus, the active, cell-bound fragment of C3 is C3b, whereas the anaphylotoxin peptide C3a is released into the surrounding fluid. Inactivated fragments are designated by the letter "i" (e.g., C3bi). Both C4 and C3 contain an internal thioester bond that is activated by cleavage to C4b and C3b and that reacts to form a covalent bond with neighboring molecules such as components of a cell surface. Surface-bound C4b and C3b then direct further complement targeting to that site.

Activation of the (1) classic, (2) lectin, or (3) alternative pathways, with or without activation of the membrane attack complex, produces effector molecules that initiate inflammation and facilitate elimination of antigens by lysis (disintegration of a cell by rupture of the cell wall or membrane) or by phagocytosis (engulfing and ingestion of bacteria or other foreign bodies by phagocytes). The complement system is a major mediator of inflammation. Increased vascular permeability permits the passage of further antibody, complement, and phagocytes into the extravascular space, which helps kill and remove infectious agents and immune complexes.

Biochemistry and Function

Plasma complement components are synthesized mainly by the liver, although small quantities are synthesized by monocytes and other cell types. C3, the most abundant complement component, is a common component of the three pathways of complement activation. C3 is a large protein of about 180,000 Da that is homologous to C4, C5, and AMG. A reactive thioester bond in C3, C4, and AMG plays a central role in binding these proteins covalently to neighboring targets when they are activated. The thioester is not completely stable, and gradual hydrolysis of the thioester in C3 continuously generates small amounts of C3i in plasma, leading to a low rate of complement activation. Slow ongoing activation of complement factors would lead to accumulation of complement factors on cells such as red blood cells and might cause their lysis or clearance when factors are not present on cell surfaces to promote removal of complement bound to cell surfaces. A few of these factors include (1) decay-accelerating factor (DAF or CD55), (2) protectin (CD59), (3) membrane cofactor protein (MCP), and (4) complement receptor 1. Deficiencies of DAF and protectin result in increased red cell lysis in the disorder **paroxysmal nocturnal hematuria**, and demonstrate the important role of these proteins. Complement regulatory factors on cell surfaces help to prevent destruction of endogenous cells at the same time that nearby foreign cells are destroyed by complement. Plasma factors also help turn off complement activation. Factor H and C4bp are binding proteins for C4b and C3b that serve as cofactors in the cleavage of C4b and C3b by factor I and help to dissociate complexes of complement factors.

Clinical Significance

The clinical importance of the complement system is demonstrated by the disease associations present in inherited or secondary deficiencies of various components. Several complement proteins, notably C3 and C4, are increased in number after an APR; however, they are weak and late-reacting APPs. C1, C1 inhibitor, C3, C3 proactivator (factor B), and C4 are the components most often measured for clinical purposes because their concentrations are important in relatively common disease states, and because assays are available readily. Activity of the complete classic pathway, often termed *total hemolytic complement* or CH_{50} is measured by the extent of lysis of antibody-coated red cells or liposomes.

Both genetic variants and deficiencies of nearly each complement component have been described. Deficiencies in particular may be associated with disease. For example, genetic deficiency of C2 and C4 typically is associated with (1) autoimmune immune complex diseases such as **systemic lupus erythematosus** (SLE), (2) polymyositis, and (3) glomerulonephritis. Partial deficiency of C4 is common. Two closely related genes encode C4, so four alleles are present. About 10% of the population has a deficiency in two of the four alleles. In contrast, the rare deficiency of C3 is associated with infection, often severe, with encapsulated bacteria. Deficiency of any of the membrane complex components (C5 through C9) is associated with recurrent and severe neisserial infection. Heterozygous deficiency of C1 inhibitor results in **hereditary**

angioedema (HAE), with excessive activation of complement factors. HAE is characterized by recurrent attacks of (1) subcutaneous, (2) laryngeal, (3) bronchial, and (4) GI edema, which may be life threatening. Decreased C4 concentrations have been used to screen for the disorder; if C1 inhibitor concentrations are normal in individuals with clinical symptoms and decreased C4, functional assays should be performed. Some cases of HAE have adequate quantities of C1 inhibitor, but the protein has mutations that decrease activity. Genetic deficiency of MBP occurs in up to 5% of the population and may increase susceptibility to infection in infancy, when antibody concentrations are low. MBP deficiency appears to have little effect on adults, unless severe immunosuppression is present.

Secondary decreases in components occur as a result of consumption. The classic examples of this are depletion of C4 in HAE and of C3 and C4 in **acute poststreptococcal glomerulonephritis**. In diseases such as SLE and other disorders associated with formation of immune complexes, differentiation of genetic and secondary deficiency may require (1) family studies, (2) phenotyping, (3) DNA analysis, or (4) combinations of these.

Coagulation Proteins

The coagulation system is a complex system designed to prevent bleeding from injuries by forming blood clots. (For more detail on this process, the reader is directed to Chapter 59, Higgins RA, Kitchen S, Olson JD. Hemostasis In: Burtis CA, Ashwood ER, Bruns DE eds. Tietz textbook of clinical chemistry, 5th edition. Philadelphia: WB Saunders, 2012:2083-128.) This process requires careful regulation and balance between hemostasis (formation of clots where needed) and thrombosis (pathological clotting) leading to [1] venous thrombosis, [2] pulmonary emboli, [3] strokes, and [4] myocardial infarction. The coagulation system has been divided functionally into intrinsic and extrinsic pathways, which merge into a final common pathway, generating fibrin (see Figure 59-2; Higgins RA, Kitchen S, Olson JD. Hemostasis. In: Burtis CA, Ashwood ER, Bruns DE eds. Tietz textbook of clinical chemistry, 5th edition. Philadelphia: WB Saunders, 2012:2085). The intrinsic pathway is activated by negatively charged surfaces and is assessed by a clot-based assay, activated partial thromboplastin time (APTT). The intrinsic pathway is activated by tissue factor released by tissue injury and is assessed by prothrombin time (PT) clotting assays. The pathways are cascades of protease zymogens that are sequentially activated by factor V and factor VIII, which serve as cofactors to organize protease activity. Not shown on the pathway are inhibitors such as antithrombin III that help to prevent uncontrolled action of the proteases.

A number of clotting factors such as fibrinogen are consumed or entrapped in the clot during clotting of blood to form serum. Therefore, plasma for coagulation testing usually is collected with one part of 3.2% sodium citrate (109 mmol/L) as anticoagulant per nine parts of blood. Citrate inactivates coagulation by chelating calcium required for activity of coagulation factors. Clotting assays add back calcium and other activators of clotting and measure the time required to form a clot. Clotting assays are used to measure activity of complete pathways or of individual factors. Clotting assays are also frequently used to monitor the action of the anticoagulants Coumadin and heparin. Selective factors and inhibitors also are measured in direct enzyme activity assays with the use of selective chromogenic substrates. Chromogenic substrates have come into increased use to measure functional concentrations of low-molecular-weight heparin by determining the inhibition of factor Xa.

Coagulation factors are synthesized mainly by the liver. Fibrinogen, the most abundant factor, is described in a preceding section. Other factors are present at more than 10-fold lower concentrations and are not visualized as major bands on protein electrophoresis. Factor concentrations have been observed to be low as the result of (1) hereditary deficiencies, (2) consumption by active clotting, (3) liver disease, or (4) anticoagulant therapy. Some hereditary disorders lead to excessive bleeding, such as (1) hemophilia A, (2) factor VIII deficiency, (3) hemophilia B, and (4) factor IX deficiency. Others lead to risk of thrombosis, such as (1) factor V Leiden, (2) antithrombin III deficiency, and (3) protein C deficiency. Usually, specific factor concentrations are assessed by functional assays, with activity assessed as a percentage versus reference plasma. Liver disease has been known to result in lower factor concentrations that commonly are identified using the PT assay. This assay is also used to monitor the anticoagulant activity of Coumadin. Coumadin blocks a post-translational modification—the carboxylation of glutamic acid side chains to form γ-carboxyglutamic acid—of several coagulation factors (prothrombin and factors VII, IX, and X). Vitamin K is a cofactor in this reaction. Factors lacking γ-carboxyglutamic acid have a decreased ability to bind calcium and to function in the coagulation pathways. PT assay results are commonly reported in seconds and as an international normalized ratio (INR), which helps in standardizing results obtained with different batches of reagents.

Immunoglobulins

Immunoglobulins (antibodies) are a family of proteins that contain highly specific antigen-binding sites. Synthesis of immunoglobulins is stimulated by foreign immunogens, leading to immunoglobulins that selectively bind foreign molecules or organisms (see Chapter 15). Regulatory mechanisms usually suppress formation of autoantibodies against the body's own structures and failure of regulatory mechanisms and production of autoantibodies contributes to autoimmune disease. Each of five classes of Ig is characterized by sequence heterogeneity of antigen-binding sites that allows binding of a diverse variety of molecules with high specificity.

Basic Biochemistry and Function

All immunoglobulins include one or more basic units consisting of two identical heavy (H) chains encoded on chromosome 14 and two identical light (L) chains encoded on chromosome 2 (see Figure 15-1, Chapter 15, for a diagram of IgG structure) that are joined by disulfide bonds. Each of the four chains has a variable and one or more constant domains. Two variable domains, one from the light chain and one from the heavy chain, together form an antigen-binding site. Extensive diversity in the variable domains is generated by somatic recombination and mutation of the Ig genes. Constant domains of immunoglobulins have little sequence diversity, and these domains provide sites for complement activation and receptor binding, as well as a structure to hold the variable domains together to form antigen binding sites. Ig light chains usually are produced in slight excess of heavy chains and are of two types—kappa (κ) and lambda (λ)—defined by different constant domains. Each B lymphocyte or clone of B lymphocytes synthesizes Ig with a single type of light chain and a single set of variable domain sequences, which binds a specific antigen. Usually, about twice as many lymphocytes synthesize immunoglobulins containing κ-light chains as λ-light chains

Immunoglobulins are synthesized by cells of B-lymphocyte lineage. Immature B-lymphocytes have surface-bound IgM. Upon binding of a target antigen, immature B lymphocytes proliferate and develop into a clone of plasma cells. Secretion of IgM is the primary response to antigenic stimulation. With further maturation of plasma cells, splicing of heavy chain constant domains yields class switching as Ig production switches from IgM to IgG and IgA. Later exposure of B cells activates memory B cells, and this yields a more rapid and a larger secondary or anamnestic response with IgG secretion. As an example, initial vaccination may require two or more doses, and a single booster dose at a later time is adequate to generate a strong antibody response.

Individual Immunoglobulins

The five classes of immunoglobulins are (1) IgG, (2) IgM, (3) IgA, (4) IgD, and (5) IgE; they vary in the constant domains of their heavy chains.

Immunoglobulin G (IgG)

IgG is the most abundant class of Ig, making up 70% to 75% of total Ig. Of this amount, 65% is extravascular and 35% is found in plasma. IgG consists of two γ-heavy chains and two light chains. Its molecular weight is about 150 kDa, including about 3% carbohydrate from one oligosaccharide chain on each heavy chain. During zone electrophoresis, IgG migrates broadly in the γ- and slow β-regions as a result of heterogeneity of the IgG molecules.

IgG includes four subclasses—IgG_1, IgG_2, IgG_3, and IgG_4. Their circulating half-life is approximately 22 days, which is much longer than the half-life of most plasma proteins. IgG_1 and IgG_3 strongly activate complement via the classical pathway. IgG_2 weakly activates complement, and IgG_4 does not activate complement. Clustering of multiple IgG molecules is required to activate complement. IgG_1 and IgG_3 bind Fc receptors on phagocytic cells and cross the placenta via receptor-mediated active transport. IgG_1 is the major neonatal Ig, with concentrations similar to maternal concentrations. Transport of maternal IgG into the fetal circulation sometimes causes lysis of fetal red cells (hemolytic disease of the newborn) when the mother generates antibodies to fetal red cell antigens. Neonates have low production of Ig as the result of immaturity of their immune systems, and IgG concentrations fall early in infancy as maternally acquired Ig is cleared.

Immunoglobulin M

Immunoglobulin M (IgM) is produced at early stages of B-cell development. In the immature immune system of neonates, IgM is the major immunoglobulin synthesized. In adults, it accounts for only 5% to 10% of total circulating Ig. IgM as a membrane receptor molecule is monomeric, but most of the serum IgM is a pentamer, which contains five monomers, similar to IgG linked via disulfides to the small J chain. Plasma cell malignancies may secrete monomeric IgM, in addition to, or instead of, pentamers. The high molecular weight of IgM (970 kDa; –10% carbohydrate) prevents its ready passage into extravascular spaces. IgM is not transported across the placenta and, therefore, is not involved in hemolytic disease of neonates. It activates complement even more efficiently than IgG; binding of one IgM molecule may be adequate to activate complement. In rare hyper-IgM syndromes, class switching to IgG and IgA is deficient. Affected patients have deficiency of IgG and IgA and increased susceptibility to infection.

Immunoglobulin A

Approximately 10% to 15% of serum immunoglobulin is immunoglobulin A (IgA), which contains 10% carbohydrate and has a molecular weight of 160 kDa and a half-life of 6 days. Two subclasses have been identified—IgA$_1$ and IgA$_2$. In its monomeric form, its structure is similar to that of IgG, but 10% to 15% of IgA in serum is dimeric, particularly IgA$_2$, which is more resistant than IgA$_1$ to destruction by some pathogenic bacteria. On electrophoresis, IgA migrates near the junction of the β- and γ-regions, anodal to most IgG.

Secretory IgA is found in (1) tears, (2) sweat, (3) saliva, (4) milk, (5) colostrum, (6) gastrointestinal secretions, and (7) bronchial secretions. It has a molecular mass of 380 kDa and consists of two monomers of IgA—a secretory component (molecular mass, 70 kDa) and a J chain (15.6 kDa). It is synthesized mainly by plasma cells in the mucous membranes of the gut and bronchi and in the ductules of the lactating breast. The secretory component helps transport secretory IgA across mucosal epithelium and into secretions. Secretory IgA is more abundant than IgG in colostrum and milk and may help protect neonates from intestinal infection. IgA also activates complement by the alternative pathway, but the exact role of IgA in plasma is not clear.

Immunoglobulin D

Immunoglobulin D (IgD) accounts for less than 1% of plasma Ig. It is monomeric, contains about 12% carbohydrate, and has a molecular mass of 184 kDa. Its structure is similar to that of IgG. Like IgM, IgD can occur as a surface receptor for antigen on B lymphocytes, but its primary function is unknown.

Immunoglobulin E

Immunoglobulin E (IgE) is so rapidly and firmly bound to mast cells that only trace amounts of it are normally present in serum. IgE contains 15% carbohydrate and has a molecular mass of 188 kDa. Its structure is similar to that of IgG. IgE binds to mast cells via binding sites on its Fc region. When the antigen (allergen) cross-links two surface-bound IgE molecules, the mast cell is stimulated to release histamine and other vasoactive amines. These compounds increase vascular permeability and smooth muscle contraction, thereby mediating type 1 hypersensitivity reactions such as (1) hay fever, (2) asthma, (3) urticaria, and (4) eczema. A rare regulatory disorder, Job's syndrome, leads to increased production of IgE, eczema, and recurrent infection. IgE molecules specific for particular allergens are measured by sensitive immunoassays using immobilized allergens to capture specific IgEs. These assays help identify the triggers for allergic responses in different individuals. The total concentration of IgE may be increased in allergic disorders.

Free Immunoglobulin Light Chains

Light chains usually are synthesized in slight excess over quantities required for intact immunoglobulins. Consequently, small quantities of free light chains, representing only about 0.1% of total Ig, usually are present in serum or plasma. Amounts in plasma usually are kept low by rapid renal clearance of these small proteins. Free κ-light chains (23 kDa) are cleared about three times faster than free λ-light chains (which form a disulfide-linked dimer of 46 kDa), which have a usual half-life of 4 to 6 hours. Consequently, even though production of κ-light chains is about twice as great as that of λ-light chains, the plasma concentration of free λ-light chains usually is higher, except in renal failure. Free light chains are not functional, but immunoassays specific for free light chains, commonly measuring the ratio of free κ:free λ light chains, are very sensitive indicators of disorders of Ig synthesis such as multiple myeloma, where clones are synthesizing increased amounts of Ig with either κ- or λ-light chains. Because free light chains are cleared by the kidneys, urine provides a specimen proportionally enriched in free light chains relative to plasma, and analysis of urine provides more sensitive detection of monoclonal free light chains than analysis of serum.

Clinical Significance

Typically, serum contains a heterogeneous, polyclonal mixture of immunoglobulins, with varying amino acid sequences and binding specificities. Benign or malignant proliferation of one such clone produces a high concentration of a single monoclonal antibody, which may appear as a sharp, narrow band on protein electrophoresis. Unbalanced production of free light chains might also lead to a second band, representing a free light chain. If a few clones proliferate, several sharp bands (e.g., the oligoclonal bands seen in electrophoresis of CSF) may be noted in (1) demyelinating diseases such as multiple sclerosis, (2) serum following successful bone marrow transplantation, or (3) early response to such organisms as *Streptococcus pneumoniae*. Disease may be associated with a decrease or an increase in normal polyclonal immunoglobulins or with an increase in one or more monoclonal immunoglobulins.

Immunoglobulin Deficiency

Immune defense depends on four complex, interactive systems: (1) cell-mediated immunity (T lymphocytes), (2) antibodies (immunoglobulins), (3) the phagocytic system, and

(4) the complement system. The last two systems are nonspecific in that they have no immunological memory for the antigen. *Immunodeficiency* states may be the result of a deficiency of a single factor or of combinations affecting multiple systems and factors. Immunodeficiency results in increased susceptibility to infections that usually do not cause disease in people with normal immune systems.

Deficiency of IgG and other immunoglobulins may be secondary to protein loss or to depletion of B lymphocytes; primary deficiencies may result from genetic disorders. Infants have transient physiological IgG immunodeficiency, with a baseline concentration observed at about 3 months of age. Concentrations of maternal IgG, transferred across the placenta, rise rapidly in the fetus during the last half of pregnancy. After birth, concentrations of IgG gradually decline and then begin to rise as the infant slowly begins to produce IgG (Figure 18-5). A delay in IgG production may be associated with increased infection rates. Neonates who are particularly at risk include premature infants, who start with less maternal IgG and may have slower initiation of IgG synthesis. Monitoring of IgG concentrations is used to assess this problem. Rising serum IgM and salivary IgA concentrations at 6 weeks of age suggest a favorable prognosis. Contact of the neonate with environmental antigens normally causes B lymphocytes to begin to multiply and IgM concentrations to start to rise, followed weeks to months later by increased concentrations of IgA and IgG.

The diagnosis of an immunoglobulin deficiency state is clinically important because replacement therapy with IgG is possible. Selective deficiency of individual IgG subclasses is not rare, and deficiency of IgG$_2$ may confer slightly increased risk of infection by encapsulated bacteria. IgA deficiency occurs in about 1 in 500 whites and less frequently in Asian populations. IgA deficiency usually is not associated with severe infection, but risk of infection with *Giardia* or other non–life-threatening organisms may be increased. IgA deficiency may lead to false-negative assays for IgA autoantibodies that are indicators of celiac disease. IgA-deficient individuals have some risk of anaphylaxis if they receive blood products that contain IgA. A variety of uncommon genetic disorders are associated with decreased production of IgG, which leads to increased risk of pyogenic infection. Severe combined immunodeficiency is one example of a disorder in which IgG production is decreased.

Polyclonal Hyperimmunoglobulinemia

Polyclonal increases in plasma immunoglobulins constitute the normal response to infection. IgG response predominates in most autoimmune responses; IgA in (1) skin, (2) gut, (3) respiratory, and (4) renal infections; and IgM in primary viral infections and with bloodstream parasites, such as malaria. *Chronic bacterial infections* may cause an increase in serum concentration of all immunoglobulins. Selective changes in Ig concentrations assist in the differential diagnosis of liver disease and of intrauterine infection. In (1) *primary biliary cirrhosis,* the IgM concentration is greatly increased; (2) *chronic active hepatitis,* IgG and sometimes IgM are increased; and (3) *portal cirrhosis,* IgA and sometimes IgG are increased. In *intrauterine infection,* production of IgM by the fetus is increased, as is the IgM concentration in the umbilical cord blood.

Monoclonal Immunoglobulins (Paraproteins)

A single clone of plasma cells produces Ig molecules with a single amino acid sequence. If the clone expands greatly, the concentration of its monoclonal Ig in the patient's serum may produce a discrete band on electrophoresis, often referred to as an *M-spike* or *M-protein,* visible against the diffuse polyclonal background. These monoclonal immunoglobulins, termed *paraproteins,* may be (1) intact Ig, (2) polymers of Ig, (3) free light chains or heavy chains, or (4) fragments of immunoglobulins. About 60% of paraproteins are associated with plasma cell malignancies (multiple myeloma or solitary plasmacytoma), and approximately 15% are due to overproduction by B lymphocytes, mainly in lymph nodes of patients with (1) lymphomas, (2) chronic lymphocytic leukemia, (3) Waldenström's macroglobulinemia, or (4) heavy chain disease. Up to 25% of paraproteins are benign and have been termed **monoclonal gammopathy of undetermined significance** (MGUS). MGUS is characterized by (1) paraprotein concentrations <3 g/dL, (2) <10% clonal plasma cells in bone marrow,

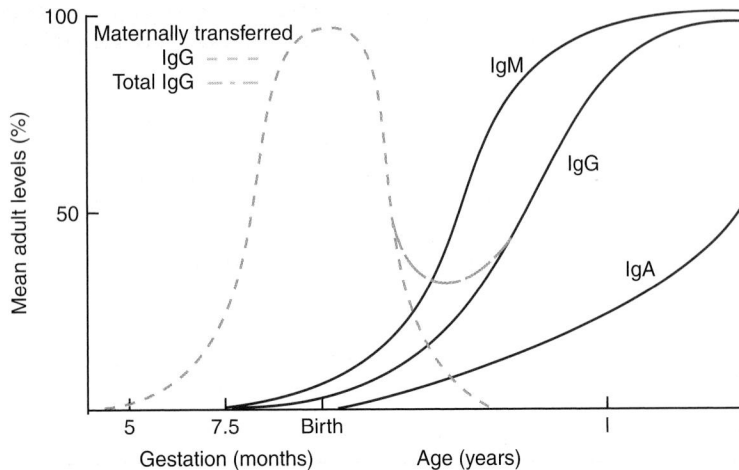

Figure 18-5 Serum immunoglobulin concentrations as percent of mean adult concentrations before birth and for the first year of life.

and (3) lack of evidence of paraprotein-related organ injury. The incidence of MGUS increases with age, with 1% incidence reported for people 50 to 70 years of age and 3% incidence for those over the age of 70. Occurrence of MGUS is associated with increased risk of progression to multiple myeloma that should be monitored. Multiple myeloma appears to be preceded in most cases by MGUS.

The primary clinical interest in identifying paraproteins involves the detection or monitoring of proliferative disorders of B lymphocytes. However, from the viewpoint of the laboratory, paraproteins also are significant as a potential, unpredictable interference with many assays. Paraproteins may aggregate or precipitate in a variety of photometric reactions and hematology analyzers. Occasionally, specimens with paraproteins form gels that plug sample probes and disable automated analyzers (see later section on cryoglobulins).

Many patients with paraproteins have nonspecific presentations such as (1) anemia, (2) low or high globulins, (3) hypercalcemia, or (4) infection. The concentration of polyclonal Ig often is decreased when a paraprotein is present, accounting for increased susceptibility to infection. Identification and typing of paraproteins in serum usually are based on protein electrophoresis and immunofixation electrophoresis of serum or urine,[5] as described in a later section. Analysis of urine is helpful mainly in identifying patients with monoclonal urinary light chains, which are sometimes referred to as Bence-Jones proteins. This term originally referred to a subset of free light chains in urine that precipitated upon heating to 50 °C to 60 °C and redissolved upon further heating to 90 °C to 100 °C. Introduction of capillary electrophoresis and assays for free light chains has led to several alternative approaches for detecting paraproteins. Serum protein electrophoresis combined with analysis of free light chains in serum appears to have a diagnostic yield similar to use of immunofixation electrophoresis. Analysis of free light chains tends to detect residual disease or recurrence at lower concentrations than does immunofixation. The prognosis of paraproteins generally depends on (1) the type of disorder producing the paraprotein, (2) the class of the paraprotein, and (3) its concentration. The concentration of paraprotein at the time of diagnosis usually correlates with the extent of disease. The rate of increase in concentration is indicative of expansion of the clone producing the paraprotein.

Multiple Myeloma. **Multiple myeloma** is a malignant neoplasm, usually of a single clone of plasma cells. The plasma cells usually proliferate diffusely throughout the bone marrow, but occasionally they form a solitary tumor called a *plasmacytoma*. Osteolytic bone lesions are produced, and the other bone marrow cells are reduced so that platelets, red cells, and neutrophils may be decreased. Normal plasma cells are inhibited; consequently, synthesis of other immunoglobulins is reduced, and recurrent infections may occur. The incidence of multiple myeloma is low in individuals younger than 60 years and increases with age. Patients may have local symptoms of a bone lesion, such as pain or fracture, but more often have nonspecific symptoms, such as (1) weight loss, (2) anemia, (3) hemorrhage, (4) repeated infections, or (5) renal failure. Significant diagnostic features include (1) detection of neoplastic plasma cells in bone marrow aspirates, (2) radiological findings of osteolytic lesions, and (3) identification of a paraprotein in serum or urine. All patients with suggestive symptoms should be screened for paraproteins; less than 1% of patients with multiple myeloma do not have detectable paraproteins. Table 18-5 lists the paraproteins that are associated with multiple myeloma and some of their characteristic findings.

Lymphoid Tumors. Lymphoid tumors such as lymphomas or chronic lymphocytic leukemias, arise from less mature stages in B-lymphocyte development. About one in five cases produce paraproteins, usually of the IgM class.

Waldenström's Macroglobulinemia (WM). Waldenström's macroglobulinemia is a malignant proliferation of plasmacytoid cells producing IgM. It differs from multiple myeloma in terms of (1) biology, (2) outcome, and (3) treatment. Clonal expansion in WM involves more immature B lymphocytes. IgM is a high-molecular-weight protein, and IgM paraproteins cause hyperviscosity that may require treatment by plasma exchange. Serum viscosity measurement helps to assess this problem. Monoclonal IgM also may behave as a cryoglobulin.

Heavy Chain Disease. Heavy chain disease is a rare disorder in which a free Ig heavy chain is produced. Heavy chains

TABLE 18-5	Monoclonal Immunoglobulins (Paraproteins) in Multiple Myeloma			
Plasma Paraprotein	Incidence (%)	Age of Occurrence (Mean)	Incidence of Light Chain Proteinuria (%)	Comments
IgG	50	65	60	Patients more susceptible to immunodeficiency; paraproteins reach highest concentrations
IgA	25	65	70	Tend to have hypercalcemia and amyloidosis; paraprotein often in β-region
Free Ig light chains (Bence-Jones)	20	56	100	Often renal failure; bone lesions; amyloidosis; poor prognosis
IgD	2	57	100	90% λ-type; often have amyloidosis, renal failure; poor prognosis
IgM	1	—	100	May have hyperviscosity
IgE	0.1	—	Most	—
Biclonal	1	—	—	—
None detected	<1	—	0	Usually decreased normal immunoglobulins

are shorter than usual and lack a segment that links them to light chains. The most common form is α-chain disease (the heavy chain of IgA), which may be associated with intestinal infiltration with clonal lymphocytes, possibly resulting in malabsorption.

Cryoglobulinemia. *Cryoglobulins* are serum proteins or protein complexes that precipitate at temperatures lower than normal core body temperature.[8] Precipitation of cryoglobulins in tissues results in vasculitis and ischemic injury to peripheral tissues at a lower temperature. Patients must be kept in a warm environment until treatment lowers cryoglobulin concentrations. Type I cryoglobulins consist of monoclonal immunoglobulins, often IgM. Occasionally, specimens with high paraprotein concentrations will gel, and the gel will plug sample probes of automated analyzers. Most cryoglobulin complexes consist of polyclonal immunoglobulins with a monoclonal Ig (type II cryoglobulin) or polyclonal immunoglobulins without a monoclonal component (type III). Polyclonal cryoglobulins often present with chronic infection, particularly with hepatitis C. Laboratory testing for cryoglobulins requires (1) transport, (2) clotting, and (3) centrifugation of specimens at temperatures near body temperature to avoid loss of cryoglobulins during clotting or centrifugation. For cryoglobulin analysis, serum usually is refrigerated for 7 days and centrifuged. Cryoglobulins precipitated in the cold should redissolve when warmed back to 37 °C, whereas cryofibrinogen will not redissolve when warmed. Unusual solubility properties of cryoglobulins and paraproteins may result in unpredictable interferences in photometric assays, and precipitated cryoglobulins may interfere with automated hematology analyzers.

Amyloidosis. Amyloidosis is a pathological process in which proteins are deposited in tissues as aggregates, termed amyloid, that form β-sheet structures. Depending on the site of deposition, amyloidosis has been observed to result in (1) kidney failure, (2) heart failure, (3) peripheral neuropathies, and (4) other disorders. The aggregates are stable filamentous structures resistant to proteolysis and normal clearance mechanisms, so they accumulate over time. Formation of amyloid occurs when production of (1) specific proteins, (2) genetic variants of proteins, or (3) fragments of proteins that are prone to aggregation is increased. At least 26 different proteins are identified as primary components of amyloid. Amyloidoses have often been classified according to sites or clinical presentation of tissue injury, but it may be more useful to classify amyloidosis according to the primary component in amyloid deposits. Amyloidosis cannot be diagnosed by analysis of plasma proteins because it is a process that occurs in tissues. Diagnosis is made by analysis of tissues obtained from (1) fat aspirates, (2) rectal biopsy specimens, or (3) biopsy specimens of affected tissues. The β-sheet structure of amyloid has characteristic staining with Congo red dye. Genetic variants of several proteins, including (1) prealbumin, (2) apolipoproteins A-I and A-II, (3) fibrinogen, (4) gelsolin, (5) cystatin C, and (6) other proteins, are associated with amyloidosis that has widely varying clinical presentation depending on the main site of amyloid deposition. Amyloidosis may be suspected if one of these protein variants is detected. Amyloidosis occurs as the result of increased concentrations of a number of proteins including (1) Ig light chain paraproteins (AL amyloidosis), (2) BMG in renal failure (Aβ2 amyloidosis), and (3) serum amyloid A (AA amyloidosis). The latter protein is increased up to 1000-fold in chronic inflammatory conditions such as (1) rheumatoid arthritis, (2) tuberculosis, (3) osteomyelitis, (4) renal and gastric carcinomas, and (5) Hodgkin lymphoma. Amyloid produced by serum amyloid A deposition accumulates gradually in a variety of tissues, including (1) kidney, (2) liver, and (4) spleen. Patients with chronic renal failure or chronic inflammatory states are at high risk for amyloidosis.

Proteins in Other Body Fluids

In addition to plasma, proteins of clinical interest are found in several other body fluids and tissues, including (1) urine, (2) CSF, (3) amniotic fluid, (4) saliva, (5) feces, and (6) pleural and peritoneal fluids.

Urinary Proteins

Urine usually represents a fluid with much lower protein concentration than plasma. Urine represents, in part, an ultrafiltrate of plasma, with most of the plasma proteins, particularly the larger proteins, removed by the combined action of glomerular filtration and tubular uptake of protein. The urinary epithelium adds a few proteins, such as Tamm-Horsfall protein, that are not present in plasma. Analysis of urinary proteins is performed mainly to diagnose kidney disease (see Chapter 35) or disorders with paraprotein production. Four basic causes of increased urinary protein excretion (proteinuria) are known: (1) glomerular injury, (2) tubular injury, (3) overflow proteinuria of low-molecular-weight proteins, and (4) postrenal proteinuria.

Glomerular Proteinuria. Glomerular proteinuria sometimes is referred to as *albuminuria,* because albumin is the major protein. Many disease processes produce glomerular injury, including (1) diabetes, (2) SLE, (3) IgA nephropathy, (4) various forms of glomerulonephritis, and (5) hepatitis and human immunodeficiency virus (HIV) infections. Urine dipsticks detect the markedly increased urinary protein excretion when major glomerular injury occurs. The dipstick test for protein relies on a pad coated with a pH indicator dye such as tetrabromphenol blue, together with a citrate buffer at pH 3. The dye changes color in the presence of protein with a lower detection limit of about 15 to 30 mg/dL. The test is more sensitive to albumin than globulins. Positive dipstick reactions for protein are often followed by quantitative assays for urine protein. A variety of methods are used, including pyrogallol red dye-binding assays and benzethonium chloride turbidity assays. Normal urinary protein excretion is <150 mg/d. Excretion of >1 g/d of protein usually indicates glomerular injury. Excretion of >3.5 g/d protein is a criterion for the nephrotic syndrome, which is also characterized by (1) hypoalbuminemia, (2) hypercholesterolemia, and (3) edema.

Early stages of glomerular injury are characterized by modestly increased urinary albumin excretion of 30 to 300 mg/d, also termed *microalbuminuria,* which is a risk factor for progression of kidney disease in diabetes. Urine albumin (often called *microalbumin*) assays usually rely on immunoturbidimetric or immunonephelometric methods to achieve adequate sensitivity and specificity. Because of the inconvenience and problems associated with collecting 24-hour urine specimens, urine albumin usually is measured on random urine specimens and expressed as a ratio versus creatinine to correct for the degree of urine dilution. A reference value of 30 mg albumin/g creatinine has often been used, although females tend to have slightly higher values because of their lower rates of creatinine excretion. For this reason, guidelines recommend using a reference value of 23 mg/g for males and 32 mg/g for females. Increased albumin excretion has been used as a staging criterion for chronic renal disease and is a risk factor for increased overall mortality.

Proteinuria due to pathological processes must be distinguished from *functional* or *benign proteinuria* that occurs with (1) exercise, (2) fever, and (3) exposure to cold. Protein excretion rates are less than 1 g/d. *Postural* or *orthostatic proteinuria,* associated with the upright position, is also a form of functional proteinuria, but excretion may exceed 1 g/d. Orthostatic proteinuria complicates assessment of otherwise symptomless patients. If transient, it is probably benign; persistence of proteinuria suggests underlying renal disease. Analysis of random urine specimens collected in the morning, such as the first voided specimen of the day, may minimize the effects of orthostatic proteinuria. In normal pregnancy, protein excretion may increase slightly (<300 mg/d). Urinary protein is tested in pregnancy as an indicator of preeclampsia, which is characterized by an increase in blood pressure and proteinuria >300 mg/d. Identification of preeclampsia is important in that it can progress to eclampsia, a severe hypertensive crisis in pregnancy.

Tubular Proteinuria. In tubular proteinuria, low-molecular-weight proteins appear in the urine as a result of decreased reabsorption by the proximal tubules. Tubular proteinuria may be caused by (1) hereditary disorders of tubular function such as Fanconi syndrome; (2) toxicity from compounds such as (a) aminoglycosides, (b) cyclosporine, (c) tacrolimus, (d) amphotericin B, (e) radiocontrast dyes, (f) cisplatin, and (g) ethylene glycol; (3) poisoning with heavy metals such as cadmium and lead; (4) ischemia due to obstruction of blood flow or decreased blood flow in shock or heart failure; or (5) toxicity from overload with proteins such as free Ig light chains, hemoglobin, or myoglobin. When tubular proteinuria occurs alone, albumin excretion may not increase sufficiently to give a positive dipstick reaction. More specific tests are required to detect simple tubular proteinuria. Agarose electrophoresis of urine from afflicted patients gives a characteristic pattern, with prominent α- and β-bands and a relatively faint albumin band. Electrophoretic methods use gradient pore gels or other methods that separate on the basis of size, such as sodium dodecyl sulfate polyacrylamide gel electrophoresis (SDS-PAGE).

Quantitative immunoassays for low-molecular-weight proteins such as BMG help identify increased excretion as an indicator of tubular injury in disorders such as poisoning with lead or other heavy metals. One problem with measurement of BMG is that it is unstable at a urine pH <6. For this reason, a variety of other low-molecular-weight proteins,

such as cystatin C and α_1-microglobulin, have been considered markers for tubular injury. Some proteins made by the tubules also are potential markers, including (1) *N*-acetyl-β-glucosaminidase (NAG), (2) kidney injury molecule-1 (KIM-1), and (3) neutrophil gelatinase-associated lipocalin (NGAL). Synthesis of the latter two markers is induced by tubular injury. These markers have not been widely used in clinical practice, but researchers are interested in finding better markers for acute kidney injury than serum creatinine, which responds by rising relatively slowly after kidney injury.

Overload Proteinuria. Overload proteinuria occurs when an increased load of small proteins filtered through the glomerulus exceed the tubular uptake capacity. Some examples of proteins causing overload proteinuria are (1) hemoglobin, (2) myoglobin, and (3) free Ig light chain paraproteins, when massive amounts of these proteins are released, respectively, by (1) red cell lysis, (2) muscle cell injury, and (3) multiple myeloma. Detection of light chains depends on electrophoretic and immunochemical testing. Hemoglobin or myoglobin confers a brown color to urine, and both yield positive reactions in the dipstick test for blood, which relies on the peroxidase activity of heme in hemoglobin or myoglobin. Muscle injury is identified by symptoms of muscle injury and high activities or concentrations of muscle markers such as creatine kinase and myoglobin in serum.

Postrenal Proteinuria. Postrenal proteinuria arises from (1) injury, (2) inflammation, or (3) malignancy of the lower urinary tract. Microscopic examination of urine may reveal inflammatory and malignant cells and bacteria; formed elements called *casts* that arise in kidney tubules help to distinguish whether a process is occurring in the kidneys or in the lower urinary tract.

Laboratory Considerations

Qualitative detection of excess protein in urine is most commonly achieved using dipstick tests, which are more sensitive to albumin than to most other plasma proteins. Therefore, dipsticks are excellent screening tests for major glomerular injury, but they are less useful for detecting tubular proteinuria or overload proteinuria from Ig light chains. Immunoassays for urine albumin detect glomerular injury at an earlier stage than assays for urine total protein or urine dipsticks.

Proteins in Cerebrospinal Fluid

CSF is the extracellular fluid around the brain and spinal column. CSF usually has total protein concentrations about 100-fold lower than those of plasma and a different protein composition. CSF for laboratory testing usually is obtained by a physician performing a spinal tap in the lumbar region.

Biochemistry and Function

CSF is secreted by the choroid plexuses, along the walls of the ventricles of the brain, and is reabsorbed into the blood through the arachnoid villi. CSF turnover normally is rapid, exchanging totally about four times per day. More than 80% of CSF protein originates from plasma by ultrafiltration and pinocytosis; the remainder is derived from intrathecal synthesis.

The protein concentration of CSF is lowest in ventricular fluid and is slightly higher along the spinal cord, where specimens usually are collected. Because CSF is mainly an ultrafiltrate of plasma, relatively small plasma proteins, such as (1) prealbumin, (2) albumin, and (3) transferrin, typically predominate. No protein with a size larger than that of IgG is present in sufficient amounts to be visible in electrophoretic patterns. The β_2-transferrin band represents carbohydrate-deficient transferrin (CDT).

Clinical Significance

Analysis of CSF proteins is performed mainly to determine whether permeability of the blood–brain barrier or intrathecal synthesis of immunoglobulins is increased.

Increased Permeability. Increased permeability of the blood–brain barrier may result from (1) a brain tumor, (2) intracerebral hemorrhage, (3) traumatic injury, or (4) inflammation associated with meningitis, encephalitis, or poliomyelitis. Among inflammatory processes, the greatest elevations in CSF total protein are seen in bacterial meningitis. Premature and full-term neonates have greater permeability and, as a result, considerably higher concentrations of total CSF protein (up to 130 mg/dL) when compared with healthy adults. Premature infants have CSF protein of up to 400 mg/dL.

Intrathecal Synthesis. Demonstration of increased intrathecal synthesis of immunoglobulins aids in the diagnosis of demyelinating diseases of the central nervous system (CNS). In multiple sclerosis, synthesis of immunoglobulins in the CNS is increased; the CSF concentration of immunoglobulins is increased, and the immunoglobulins have an oligoclonal pattern that is suggestive of multiple sclerosis.

Laboratory Considerations

Similar methods often are used to measure urine and CSF proteins. Common methods for measuring CSF protein include (1) pyrogallol red dye-binding assays, (2) benzethonium chloride turbidity assays, and (3) biuret assays. The reference interval for CSF total protein collected by lumbar puncture is 15 to 48 mg/dL. Elderly adults have slightly higher values—up to 60 mg/dL. The presence of blood in the CSF indicates contamination during collection or bleeding within the CNS.

The reference interval for albumin in lumbar CSF is 18 to 25 mg/dL. In normal CSF, individual IgA, IgD, and IgM values are less than 0.2 mg/dL. The reference interval for CSF IgG in adults is 0.8 to 4.2 mg/dL. Calculating the ratio of CSF albumin to serum albumin provides a measure of permeability of the blood–brain barrier; a ratio <9 indicates an intact barrier (where CSF albumin is measured in mg/dL and serum albumin is measured in g/dL). Calculations based on CSF IgG and albumin and on serum IgG and albumin provide estimates of rates of IgG synthesis in the CNS. Increased IgG synthesis, together with the finding of oligoclonal bands of Ig upon immunofixation electrophoresis or isoelectric focusing, supports the presence of an inflammatory process in the CNS such as multiple sclerosis. Because of the relatively low protein concentration of CSF, it must be concentrated before electrophoretic analysis, or high-sensitivity staining techniques must be used. Relatively high-resolution agarose zone gel electrophoresis or isoelectric focusing is required to achieve optimal detection of oligoclonal bands of Ig.

CSF is enriched in a number of proteins released by neural and glial cells. Active investigation is continuing to explore specific immunoassays of a number of CSF proteins as potential markers for traumatic or ischemic injury or for disease processes such as Alzheimer disease. The relatively large amounts of β_2-transferrin or prostaglandin D synthase (also known as β-trace) in CSF are sometimes used as a marker to determine whether clear fluid from the nasal or ear passages represent leakage of CSF.

Proteins in Amniotic Fluid

Amniotic fluid is analyzed for α-fetoprotein (AFP) and other analytes in antenatal screening for fetal defects (refer to Chapter 44 on disorders of pregnancy).

Proteins in Saliva and Oral Fluid

Saliva represents the fluid secreted by several salivary glands and has a very different protein composition than plasma, with amylase and small peptides representing the major components. Protein composition depends on the site and method of sampling saliva. Saliva is tested for secretory IgA in evaluation of possible immunological deficiency and for BMG in Sjögren syndrome. Oral fluid or crevicular fluid represents fluids released from the oral epithelium combined with saliva. Oral fluid is of interest because of the higher concentrations of immunoglobulins that allow it to be used as a test specimen for antibodies to infectious diseases such as HIV. Saliva is lacking in many of the hormone-binding proteins present in plasma; concentrations of hormones such as cortisol are much lower and are related to the concentrations of free hormone in plasma.

Proteins in Feces

Assay of feces for AAT is used sometimes in the diagnosis of gastrointestinal protein loss. Unlike most other plasma proteins, it is resistant to breakdown by proteolytic enzymes in the gut. Fecal AAT preferably is determined as clearance on a timed collection to determine an excretion rate corrected for the activity of serum AAT. For inflammatory bowel disease, it is useful to have markers of inflammation, as well as of increased permeability to plasma proteins. Fecal content of products secreted by white cells, such as lactoferrin and calprotectin, has been used as a measure of disease activity in inflammatory bowel disease.

Proteins in Peritoneal and Pleural Fluid

Pathological accumulations of fluid in the peritoneal (abdominal) and pleural (lung) cavities or elsewhere vary greatly in protein content. For example, they may be (1) *transudates* that represent ultrafiltrates with low protein concentrations relative to plasma and scant amounts of large proteins, or (2) *exudates* with relatively high protein concentrations resulting from increased vascular permeability related to tissue injury and inflammation. The distinction of transudates from exudates assists in diagnosing the cause of fluid accumulation. The major cause of pleural transudates is congestive heart failure. Pleural exudates occur with infection, pleuritis, pulmonary embolism, and cancer. The following criteria have been commonly applied to identify exudates in pleural fluid: (1) pleural fluid protein/serum protein >0.5, (2) pleural LDH/serum LDH >0.6, and (3) pleural fluid LDH >200 IU/L. Pleural fluid may be turbid because of the presence of numerous white cells, fibrin particles, or chylomicrons. Chylous effusion (containing chylomicrons) results from lymphatic obstruction related to cancer, surgery, trauma, or other causes. Lymphatics serve as the major route for chylomicrons from the intestine to the blood circulation via the thoracic duct. Entry of chylomicrons into the pleural space in cases of lymphatic obstruction, therefore, is related to dietary fat intake, and fasting lowers the fat content of chylous effusions. Chylomicrons in fluids may be identified by separation of an upper creamy layer upon standing or by triglyceride analysis.

For peritoneal fluid, determination of the serum-to-fluid albumin gradient is useful in distinguishing transudates from exudates (which often are related to infection or cancer). Usually, transudates have a serum albumin-to-fluid albumin gradient >1.1 g/dL. Exudates have a smaller gradient because of a breakdown in the vascular barrier.

Review Questions

1. A nonspecific response to inflammation that includes elevation of certain plasma proteins and decrease of others due to cytokine production is referred to as a(n):
   a. cytokine response.
   b. acute-phase response.
   c. reduction reaction.
   d. allergic reaction.

2. An ampholyte is a(n):
   a. protein that contains one or more prosthetic groups.
   b. organic compound that contains both amino and carboxyl functional groups.
   c. ionized molecule with balanced negative and positive charges.
   d. relatively short chain of amino acids.

3. The pH at which a molecule such as a protein has a net charge of zero is referred to as the:
   a. isoelectric point.
   b. dissociation constant.
   c. isoelectric focus point.
   d. solubility point.

4. A paraprotein is:
   a. immunoglobulin heavy chains.
   b. a sidechain of a protein.
   c. a prosthetic group.
   d. a monoclonal immunoglobulin.

5. In the biuret reaction for protein quantification:
   a. an increase in buffer pH causes protein to bind to a blue dye.
   b. copper ions complex with peptide bonds in proteins.
   c. a change in the refractive index of light is measured.
   d. protein is precipitated by the addition of an acid solution.

6. As a separation technique, serum protein electrophoresis depends on:
   a. the number of peptide bonds present in a protein molecule.
   b. the tertiary structure of the protein.
   c. the ratio of the protein's charge to hydrodynamic size.
   d. the affinity of the protein for the support medium.

7. Analyzing protein in cerebrospinal fluid is done to:
   a. asssess the permeability of the blood–brain barrier.
   b. determine the permeability of the glomerular membrane.
   c. determine the presence of fetal defects.
   d. diagnose gastrointestinal protein loss.

8. The plasma protein that serves to transport a large number of compounds including bilirubin, calcium, drugs and free fatty acids is:
   a. prealbumin.
   b. immunoglobulin G.
   c. haptoglobin.
   d. albumin.

9. Most proteins are synthesized:
   a. in the kidney juxtaglomerular cells.
   b. by the hepatic parenchymal cells.
   c. in the gastrointestinal tract.
   d. in cellular mitochondria.

10. A malignant neoplasm of a clone of plasma cells that diffuses throughout the bone marrow and that is diagnosed in part by identification of a paraprotein in blood or urine is referred to as:
    a. multiple myeloma.
    b. Bence-Jones protein.
    c. hypogammaglobulinemia.
    d. Wilson disease.

References

1. Craig WY, Ledue TB, Ritchie RF. Plasma proteins, clinical utility and interpretation. Scarborough, ME: Foundation for Blood Research, 2001.
2. Gabay C, Kushner I. Acute-phase proteins and other systemic responses to inflammation. N Engl J Med 1999;340:448–54.
3. Hortin GL. Amino acids, peptides, and proteins. In: Burtis CA, Ashwood ER, Bruns DE eds. Tietz textbook of clinical chemistry, 5th edition. Philadelphia: WB Saunders, 2012:509–63.
4. Hortin GL, Sviridov D, Anderson NL. High-abundance polypeptides of the human plasma proteome comprising the top 4 logs of polypeptide abundance. Clin Chem 2008;54:1608–16.
5. Katzmann JA, Kyle RA, Benson J, et al. Screening panels for detection of monoclonal gammopathies. Clin Chem 2009;55:1–6.
6. Keren DF. Protein electrophoresis in clinical diagnosis. Chicago: ASCP Press; 2012.
7. Pepys MB. Amyloidosis. Annu Rev Med 2006;57:223–41.
8. Ramos-Casals M, Stone JH, Cid MC, Bosch X. The cryoglobulinemias. Lancet 2012;379;348–60.
9. Ridker PM. C-reactive protein: eighty years from discovery to emergence as a major risk marker for cardiovascular disease. Clin Chem 2009;55:209–15.
10. Silverman EK, Sandhaus RA. Alpha1-antitrypsin deficiency. N Engl J Med 2009;360:2749–57.
11. Unsworth DJ. Complement deficiency and disease. J Clin Pathol 2008;61:1013–7.

Serum Enzymes

Mauro Panteghini, M.D., and Renze Bais, Ph.D., F.F.Sc. (R.C.P.A.)

Objectives

1. Define the following and give an example of each type:

   Hydrolase   Phosphotranferase
   Lyase   Transferase
   Oxidoreductase

2. List the factors that affect enzyme activity and appearance in blood.

3. For each of the following enzymes, state and describe the biochemistry, physiological actions (if known), tissue distribution, clinical significance, method of laboratory analysis, and possible analytical interferences:

   5′-Nucleotidase   Amylase
   Alanine aminotransferase   Aspartate aminotransferase
   Aldolase   Creatine kinase
   Alkaline phosphatase   γ-Glutamyltransferase

   Lactate dehydrogenase   Serum cholinesterase
   Lipase   Tartrate-resistant acid
                                phosphatase

4. List the isoenzymes, the clinical significance of the isoenzymes (if any), and methods of laboratory analysis used to assess the isoenzymes of each of the following:

   Alkaline phosphatase   Lactate dehydrogenase
   Amylase   Tartrate-resistant acid phosphatase
   Creatine kinase

5. Describe two serum enzymes that are related to future cardiovascular (CV) events, including tissue distribution, rationale for association with adverse CV events, and methods of laboratory analysis.

6. Assess and solve case studies involving serum enzymes and isoenzymes and the laboratory analysis of these.

Key Words and Definitions

Acid phosphatase All phosphatases with optimal activity below pH 7.0 that catalyze the cleavage of orthophosphate from orthophosphoric monoesters; most of the activity in serum is of a tartrate-resistant type.

Acute pancreatitis A sudden inflammation of the pancreas that is usually accompanied with severe upper abdominal pain.

Aldolase A lyase that catalyzes cleavage of fructose-1,6-disphosphate into dihydroxyacetone-phosphate and glyceraldehyde 3-phosphate in the glycolytic breakdown of glucose to lactate.

Alkaline phosphatase A hydrolase that catalyzes the alkaline hydrolysis of a large variety of naturally occurring and synthetic substrates.

α-Amylase An enzyme that catalyzes the hydrolysis of 1,4-alpha-glycosidic linkages in starch, glycogen, and related polysaccharides and oligosaccharides.

Aminotransferases A subclass of enzymes of the transferase class that catalyze the transfer of an amino group from a donor (generally an amino acid) to an acceptor (generally a 2-koxo acid). Most of these enzymes are pyridoxyl phosphate proteins. Alanine and aspartate aminotransferase are examples that are of significant clinical utility.

Apoenzyme The protein component of an enzyme.

Cholinesterase An enzyme of the hydrolase class that catalyzes the cleavage of the acyl group from various esters of choline, including acetylcholine, and some related compounds.

Cholecystitis A painful inflammation of the gallbladder.

Coenzyme An organic nonprotein molecule that binds with the protein molecule (apoenzyme) to form the active enzyme (holoenzyme).

Creatine kinase A dimeric transferase enzyme that catalyzes the reversible phosphorylation of creatine by ATP. CK has four forms: CK-MM, CK-MB, CK-BB, and mitochondrial CK.

γ-Glutamyltransferase A transferase enzyme that reversibly catalyzes the transfer of a glutamyl group from a glutamyl-peptide and an amino acid to a peptide and a glutamyl-amino acid.

Holoenzyme Active enzyme formed by combination of a coenzyme and an apoenzyme.

Isoenzyme A molecular form that originates at the level of the genes that encode the structures of the enzyme proteins in question.

Isoform An enzyme molecular form that has been post-translationally modified.

Lactate dehydrogenase An oxidoreductase enzyme that reversibly catalyzes the reduction of pyruvate to (L)-lactate, using NADH (reduced form of nicotinamide adenine dinucleotide) as an electron donor.

Key Words and Definitions—cont'd

Lipase A hydrolase that hydrolyzes glycerol esters of long-chain fatty acid.

Lipoprotein-associated phospholipase A_2 An enzyme member of the phospholipase A_2 superfamily that cleaves oxidized phosphatidylcholine components of lipoprotein particles.

Myeloperoxidase An enzyme that catalyzes the conversion of chloride anion and hydrogen peroxide to hypochlorite, a metal chlorinating oxidant with a potent microbicidal activity.

5′-Nucleotidase A phosphatase that acts only on nucleoside-5′-phosphates, such as adenosine-5′-phosphate (AMP), releasing inorganic phosphate.

Paget disease A chronic disorder that results in enlarged and deformed bones (also known as osteitis deformans, osteodystrophia deformans).

Prosthetic group A tightly-bound, non-peptide structure required for the activity of an enzyme.

Regan isoenzyme Isoenzyme of alkaline phosphatase that has been observed in the plasma of patients with malignant tumors.

The basic principles of Enzyme and Rate Analyses are discussed in Chapter 14. Individual enzymes of diagnostic utility are discussed in this chapter. To better clarify their clinical application, the individual enzymes are discussed relative to the organ in which they are clinically most important. However, overlap may occur for this classification, as the same enzyme may be used for investigating disease in different organs.

Basic Concepts

Injury to tissue releases cellular substances such as enzymes that are used as plasma markers of tissue damage. For a substance to serve as a biochemical marker of damage to a specific organ or tissue, it must arise predominantly from the organ or tissue of interest. Some enzymes are found predominantly in specialized tissue (e.g., **lipase** in the pancreas); others, more widely distributed, have tissue-specific **isoenzymes** or **isoforms** (e.g., the pancreatic isoenzyme of **α-amylase**) that are evaluated to enhance tissue and organ specificity.

In general, clinical laboratorians are principally concerned with changes in activity in the serum or plasma of enzymes that are predominantly intracellular and physiologically present in the blood at low activity concentrations only. Changes in the serum activities of these enzymes are used to infer the location and nature of pathological changes in tissues of the body. Therefore, an understanding of the factors that affect the rate of release of enzymes from their cells of origin and the rate at which they are cleared from the circulation is necessary to interpret correctly changes in activity that occur with disease.

Knowledge of the intracellular locations of enzymes assists in determining the nature and severity of a pathological process. For instance, a mild, reversible viral inflammation of the liver, such as a mild attack of viral hepatitis, is likely to increase only the permeability of the cell membrane, thereby allowing cytoplasmic enzymes to leak out into the blood. However, a severe attack causing cell necrosis also disrupts the mitochondrial membrane, and both cytoplasmic and mitochondrial enzymes are detected in the blood. The timing of the enzyme's diagnostic window is another important aspect to be considered when these markers are used to evaluate acute injury. The diagnostic window for an injury marker is defined as the interval of time after an episode of injury during which plasma concentrations of the marker are increased, thereby demonstrating the occurrence of injury.

The main enzymes of established clinical value, together with their tissues of origin and their major clinical applications, are listed in Table 19-1.

Muscle Enzymes

Enzymes in this category include **creatine kinase** and **aldolase**.

Creatine Kinase

Creatine kinase (CK) (EC 2.7.3.2; adenosine triphosphate:creatine N-phosphotransferase) is a dimeric enzyme (82 kDa)

TABLE 19-1 Distribution and Application of Clinically Important Enzymes

Enzyme	Principal Sources of Enzyme in Blood	Principal Clinical Applications
Alanine aminotransferase	Liver	Hepatic parenchymal disease
Alkaline phosphatase	Liver, bone, intestinal mucosa, placenta	Hepatobiliary disease, bone disease
Amylase	Salivary glands, pancreas	Pancreatic disease (pancreatic isoenzyme)
Aspartate aminotransferase	Heart, liver, skeletal muscle, erythrocytes	Hepatic parenchymal disease
Creatine kinase	Skeletal muscle, heart	Muscle disease
γ-Glutamyltransferase	Liver, pancreas, kidney	Hepatobiliary disease
Lactate dehydrogenase	Heart, erythrocytes, lymph nodes, skeletal muscle, liver	Hemolytic and megaloblastic anemias, leukemia and lymphoma, oncology
Lipase	Pancreas	Pancreatic disease

that catalyzes the reversible phosphorylation of creatine (Cr) by adenosine triphosphate (ATP).

TABLE 19-2	Approximate Concentrations of Tissue Creatine Kinase Activity (Expressed as Multiples of CK Activity Concentrations in Serum) and Cytoplasmic Isoenzyme Composition

| | | Isoenzymes, % | | |
Tissue	Relative CK Activity	CK-BB	CK-MB	CK-MM
Skeletal muscle (type I, slow twitch, or red fibers)	50,000	<1	3	97
Skeletal muscle (type II, fast twitch, or white fibers)	50,000	<1	1	99
Heart	10,000	<1	22	78
Brain	5,000	100	0	0
Smooth muscle				
Gastrointestinal tract	5,000	96	1	3
Urinary bladder	4,000	92	6	2

Physiologically, when muscle contracts, ATP is converted to adenosine diphosphate (ADP), and CK catalyzes the rephosphorylation of ADP to ATP using creatine phosphate (CrP) as the phosphorylation reservoir. Optimal pH values for the forward (Cr + ATP → ADP + CrP) and reverse (CrP + ADP → ATP + Cr) reactions are 9.0 and 6.7, respectively. Mg^{2+} is an obligate activating ion that forms complexes with ATP and ADP. The optimal concentration range for Mg^{2+} is narrow, and excess Mg^{2+} is inhibitory. Other inhibitors of CK activity include (1) Mn^{2+}, (2) Ca^{2+}, (3) Zn^{2+}, (4) Cu^{2+}, (5) iodoacetate, and (6) other sulfhydryl-binding reagents. The enzyme in serum is relatively unstable, and activity is lost as a result of sulfhydryl group oxidation at the active site of the enzyme. It is possible to partially restore activity by incubating the enzyme preparation with sulfhydryl compounds, such as (1) N-acetylcysteine, (2) dithiothreitol (Cleland reagent), and (3) glutathione.

Biochemistry

CK activity is greatest in striated muscle and heart tissue, which contain some 2500 and 550 U/g of protein, respectively. Other tissues, such as (1) brain, (2) gastrointestinal tract, and (3) urinary bladder, contain significantly less activity, and the liver and erythrocytes are essentially devoid of activity (Table 19-2).

CK is a dimer that is composed of two subunits, each with a molecular weight of about 40,000 Da. These subunits (B and M) are the products of loci on chromosomes 14 and 19, respectively. Because the active form of the enzyme is a dimer, only three different pairs of subunits can exist: BB (or CK-1), MB (or CK-2), and MM (or CK-3). The distribution of these isoenzymes in the various tissues of humans is shown in Table 19-2. All three of these isoenzyme species are found in the cytosol of the cell or are associated with myofibrillar structures. However, there exists a fourth form that differs from the others both immunologically and by electrophoretic mobility. This isoenzyme (CK-Mt) is located between the inner and outer membranes of mitochondria, and it constitutes, in the heart for example, up to 15% of total CK activity. The gene for CK-Mt is located on chromosome 15.

CK activity may also be found in macromolecular form—the so-called macro-CK. Macro-CK is found, often transiently, in the sera of up to 6% of hospitalized patients, but only a minor proportion of these have increased CK activities in serum. It exists in two forms: types 1 and 2. Type 1 is a complex of CK, typically CK-BB, and an immunoglobulin, often IgG. It is not of pathological significance, but it can be the cause of elevated CK results, causing diagnostic confusion and leading to unnecessary further investigation. Prevalence has been estimated as between 0.8% and 2.3%. Macro-CK type 2 is oligomeric CK-Mt, with a reported prevalence of between 0.5% and 2.6%. It is found predominantly in adults who are severely ill with malignancy or liver disease and in children who have notable tissue distress. The appearance of this isoenzyme in serum is usually associated with a poor prognosis. Macro-CK can interfere with the assay of CK-MB by some immunoinhibition methods.

Both M- and B-subunits have a C-terminal lysine residue, but only the former is hydrolyzed by the action of carboxypeptidases present in blood. Carboxypeptidases B (EC 3.4.17.2) and N (arginine carboxypeptidase; EC 3.4.17.3) sequentially hydrolyze the lysine residues from CK-MM to produce two CK-MM isoforms: $CK-MM_2$ (one lysine residue removed) and $CK-MM_1$ (both lysine residues removed). Loss of the positively charged lysine produces a more negatively charged CK molecule with greater anodic mobility at electrophoresis. Because CK-MB has only one M-subunit, the dimer coded by the M and B genes is named $CK-MB_2$, and the lysine-hydrolyzed dimer is named $CK-MB_1$.

Clinical Significance

Serum CK is increased in nearly all patients when (1) injury, (2) inflammation, or (3) necrosis of skeletal or heart muscle occurs.

Elevation of serum CK activity may be the only sign of subclinical neuromuscular disorders. Serum CK activity is greatly elevated in all types of muscular dystrophy. In progressive muscular dystrophy (particularly Duchenne sex-linked muscular dystrophy), enzyme activity in serum is highest in infancy and childhood and may be increased long before the disease is clinically apparent. Serum CK activity characteristically falls as patients get older and as the mass of functioning muscle diminishes with progression of the disease. About 50% to 80% of asymptomatic female carriers of Duchenne dystrophy show a threefold to sixfold increase in CK activity. High values of CK are noted in (1) viral myositis, (2) polymyositis, and (3) similar muscle diseases. However, in neurogenic muscle diseases, such as (1) myasthenia gravis, (2) multiple sclerosis, (3) poliomyelitis, and (4) Parkinsonism, serum enzyme activity is not increased.

In acute rhabdomyolysis due to crush injury, with severe muscle destruction, serum CK activities exceeding 200 times the upper reference limit (URL) may be found. If the CK remains below 5000 U/L (about 30 times the URL) during the first 3 days after the insult, the probability of developing acute renal failure appears to be low. Serum CK is also increased by other direct trauma to muscle, including intramuscular injection and surgical intervention. Finally, a number of drugs when given at pharmacologic doses increase serum CK activities. The drugs principally responsible are (1) statins, (2) fibrates, (3) antiretrovirals, and (4) angiotensin II receptor antagonists.

Changes in serum CK and its MB isoenzyme after acute myocardial infarction have been used for diagnosis for many years. However, it is now more advantageous to use more cardiac-specific nonenzymatic markers, such as cardiac troponin I or T.

During normal childbirth, a sixfold elevation in maternal total serum CK activity occurs. Surgical intervention during labor further increases the activity of CK in serum.

Methods for Determination of Creatine Kinase Activity

Currently, all commercial assays for total CK are based on the reverse reaction, which proceeds about six times faster than the forward reaction.

CK catalyzes the conversion of CrP to Cr with concomitant phosphorylation of ADP to ATP. The ATP produced is measured by hexokinase (HK)/glucose-6-phosphate dehydrogenase (G6PD) coupled reactions that ultimately convert $NADP^+$ (nicotinamide adenine dinucleotide phosphate) to NADPH (reduced form of NADP), which is monitored spectrophotometrically at 340 nm. The assay is optimized by adding (1) N-acetylcysteine to activate CK, (2) EDTA to bind Ca^{2+} and increase the stability of the reaction mixture, and (3) adenosine pentaphosphate (Ap_5A) in addition to AMP to inhibit adenylate kinase (AK). A reference procedure based on this reaction principle and on optimization was developed by the International Federation of Clinical Chemistry and Laboratory Medicine (IFCC) for the measurement of CK at 37 °C.[4]

Specimens for CK analysis include heparinized serum and heparinized plasma. Anticoagulants other than heparin should not be used in collection tubes because they inhibit CK activity. CK activity in serum is relatively unstable and is rapidly lost during storage. Average stabilities are less than 8 hours at room temperature, 48 hours at 4 °C, and 1 month at −20 °C. Therefore the serum specimen should be chilled to 4 °C if the serum is not analyzed immediately and should be stored at −80 °C if

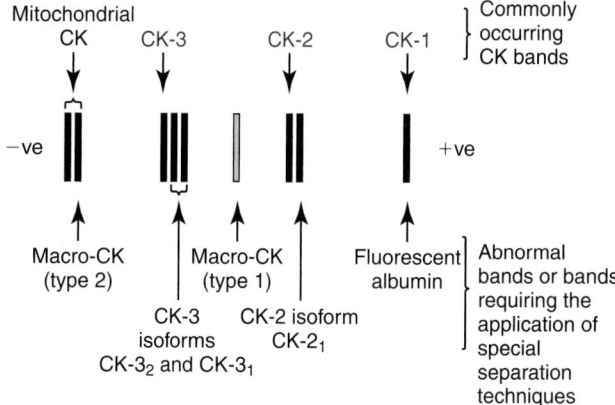

Figure 19-1 A diagrammatic representation of the electrophoretic pattern of CK isoenzymes (some of which are seen in blood only in disease) and some of the reported anomalous forms.

analysis is delayed for longer than 30 days. A moderate degree of hemolysis (<1 g/L hemoglobin) is tolerated because erythrocytes contain no CK activity. However, severely hemolyzed specimens are unsatisfactory because enzymes and intermediates (AK, ATP, and G6P/glucose-6-phosphate) liberated from the erythrocytes may affect the lag phase and side reactions occurring in the assay system.

Serum CK activity is subject to a number of physiological variations. It is influenced by (1) sex, (2) age, (3) race, (4) muscle mass, and (5) physical exercise. Men have higher values than women, and blacks have higher values than nonblacks. In white subjects, the reference interval was found to be 46 to 171 U/L for males and 34 to 145 U/L for females, when measured with an assay traceable to the IFCC 37 °C reference procedure.[4] Newborns generally have higher CK activity resulting from skeletal muscle trauma during birth.

Methods for Separation and Quantification of Creatine Kinase Isoenzymes

Electrophoretic methods are useful for separation of all CK isoenzymes. The isoenzyme bands are visualized by incubating the support (e.g., agarose, cellulose acetate) with a concentrated CK assay mixture using the reverse reaction. NADPH formed in this reaction is then detected by observing the bluish-white fluorescence after excitation by longwave (360 nm) ultraviolet light. NADPH may be quantified by fluorescent densitometry, which is capable of detecting bands of 2 to 5 U/L. The mobility of CK isoenzymes at pH 8.6 toward the anode is BB > MB > MM, with the MM remaining cathodic to the point of application. The discriminating power of electrophoresis also allows the detection of abnormal bands (Figure 19-1).

Immunochemical methods are applicable to the direct measurement of CK-MB. Immunoinhibition techniques measuring the catalytic activity of the B subunit of CK dimer were first introduced. These methods were limited in their use in that interference from CK-BB, macro-CKs, or CK-Mt led to low specificity. Furthermore, because the CK-B subunit accounts for one-half of CK-MB activity, the change in absorbance should be doubled to obtain CK-MB activity. This resulted in a significant decrease in the analytical sensitivity of the method.

The recommended approach is to measure concentrations of the CK-MB protein ("mass") by using immunoassays with monoclonal antibodies. Measurements use the "sandwich" technique, in which one antibody specifically recognizes only the MB dimer. The sandwich technique ensures that only CK-MB is estimated because neither CK-MM nor CK-BB reacts with both antibodies. Mass assays are very sensitive, with a lower limit of detection for CK-MB usually less than 1 µg/L. Other advantages include (1) sample stability; (2) noninterference with hemolysis, (3) anticoagulants, (4) other catalytic activity inhibitors, (5) full automation; and (6) fast turnaround time.

CK activity in the serum of healthy people is due almost exclusively to CK-MM activity (although small amounts of CK-MB may be present) and is the result of physiological turnover of muscle tissue. With CM-MB mass assays, the URL for males is 5.0 µg/L, with values for females being less than male values.

Aldolase

Aldolase (ALD) (EC 4.1.2.13; D-fructose-1,6-bisdiphosphate D-glyceraldehyde-3-phosphate-lyase) catalyzes the splitting of D-fructose-1,6-diphosphate to D-glyceraldehyde-3-phosphate (GLAP) and dihydroxyacetone-phosphate (DAP)—an important reaction in the glycolytic breakdown of glucose to lactate.

Serum ALD determinations have been of some clinical interest in diseases of skeletal muscle. Some researchers believe that increased ALD activity in combination with the CK/AST ratio is useful in distinguishing neuromuscular atrophies from myopathies. In general, however, measurement of ALD activity in the serum of subjects with suspected muscle disease does not add information to that available more readily from measurement of other enzymes, especially CK.

Liver Enzymes

Enzymes in this category include (1) alanine aminotransferase (2) aspartate aminotransferases, (3) **γ-glutamyltransferase**, (4) **alkaline phosphatase**, and (5) **5′-nucleotidase**.

Clinically, the most common alterations in liver enzyme activities are (1) hepatocellular damage (elevated aminotransaminase activities) and (2) cholestasis (elevated alkaline phosphatase, 5′-nucleotidase, and γ-glutamyltransferase activities).

Aminotransferases

The **aminotransferases** constitute a group of enzymes that catalyze the interconversion of amino acids to 2-oxo-acids by transfer of amino groups. **Aspartate aminotransferase (AST)** (EC 2.6.1.1; L-aspartate: 2-oxoglutarate aminotransferase) and **alanine aminotransferase (ALT)** (EC 2.6.1.2; L-alanine: 2-oxoglutarate aminotransferase) are examples of aminotransferases that are of clinical interest.

The 2-oxoglutarate/L-glutamate couple serves as one amino group acceptor and donor pair in all amino-transfer reactions; the specificity of the individual enzymes derives from the particular amino acid that serves as the other donor of an amino group. Thus AST catalyzes the following reaction:

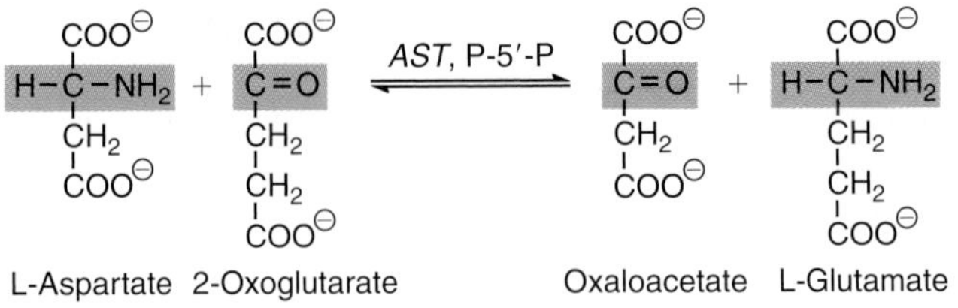

L-Aspartate · 2-Oxoglutarate · Oxaloacetate · L-Glutamate

ALT catalyzes the analogous reaction:

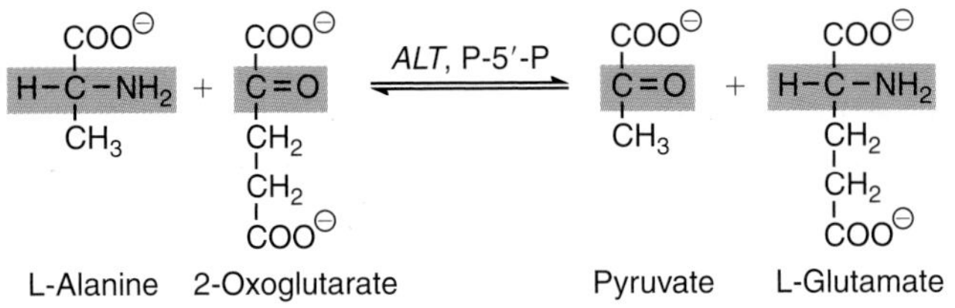

L-Alanine · 2-Oxoglutarate · Pyruvate · L-Glutamate

The reactions are reversible, but the equilibria of the AST and ALT reactions favor formation of aspartate and alanine, respectively.

Pyridoxal-5′-phosphate (P-5′-P) and its amino analogue, pyridoxamine-5′-phosphate, function as **coenzymes** in aminotransfer reactions. The P-5′-P is bound to the **apoenzyme** and serves as a true **prosthetic group**. P-5′-P bound to the apoenzyme accepts the amino group from the first substrate—aspartate or alanine—to form enzyme-bound pyridoxamine-5′-phosphate and the first reaction product, oxaloacetate or pyruvate, respectively. The coenzyme in amino form then transfers its amino group to the second substrate, 2-oxoglutarate, to form the second product, glutamate. P-5′-P is thus regenerated.

Both coenzyme-deficient apoenzymes and **holoenzymes** may be present in serum. Therefore, addition of P-5′-P under conditions that allow recombination with the enzymes usually produces an increase in aminotransferase activity. In accordance with the principle that all factors affecting the rate of reaction must be optimized and controlled, the addition of P-5′-P in aminotransferase methods ensures that all enzymatic activity is measured.

Biochemistry

Aminotransaminases are widely distributed throughout the body. AST is found primarily in the (1) heart, (2) liver, (3) skeletal muscle, and (4) kidney, whereas ALT is found primarily in the liver and kidney, with lesser amounts in heart and skeletal muscle (Table 19-3). ALT is exclusively cytoplasmic; however, both mitochondrial and cytoplasmic forms of AST are found in cells. These are genetically distinct isoenzymes with a dimeric structure composed of two identical polypeptide subunits of about 400 amino acid residues.

Clinical Significance

Liver disease is the most important cause of increased aminotransaminase activity in serum. In most types of liver disease, ALT activity is higher than that of AST. Exceptions may

TABLE 19-3	Aminotransferase Activities in Human Tissues, Relative to Serum as Unity	
	AST	**ALT**
Heart	7800	450
Liver	7100	2850
Skeletal muscle	5000	300
Kidneys	4500	1200
Pancreas	1400	130
Spleen	700	80
Lungs	500	45
Erythrocytes	15	7
Serum	1	1

From King J. Practical clinical enzymology. London: D. Van Nostrand Co. Ltd., 1965.

be seen, however, in (1) alcoholic hepatitis, (2) hepatic cirrhosis, and (3) liver neoplasia. In viral hepatitis and other forms of liver disease associated with acute hepatic necrosis, serum AST and ALT activities are elevated even before the clinical signs and symptoms of disease (such as jaundice) appear. Activities for both enzymes may reach values as high as 100 times the URL, although 10-fold to 40-fold elevations are most frequently encountered. The most efficient aminotransferase threshold for diagnosing acute liver injury lies at seven times the URL (clinical sensitivity and specificity >95%). Peak values of aminotransaminase activity occur between the 7th and 12th days; activities then gradually decrease, reaching physiological concentrations by the 3rd to 5th week if recovery is uneventful. Peak activities bear no relationship to prognosis and may fall with worsening of the patient's condition.

Persistence of increased ALT activity for longer than 6 months after an episode of acute hepatitis is used to diagnose chronic hepatitis. Most patients with chronic hepatitis have maximum ALT activities less than seven times the URL. The activity of ALT may be persistently normal in 15% to 50% of patients with chronic hepatitis C, but the likelihood of continuously normal ALT activity decreases with an increasing number of measurements. In patients with acute hepatitis C, the activity of ALT should be measured periodically over the next 1 to 2 years to determine if it becomes and stays normal. The clinical situation in toxic hepatitis is different from that in infectious hepatitis. In acetaminophen-induced hepatic injury, the peak of aminotransaminase activity is more than 85 times the URL in 90% of cases—a value rarely seen with acute viral hepatitis.

The activities of aminotransferases are also elevated in nonalcoholic fatty liver disease (NAFLD). This disease includes a spectrum of liver pathology, from simple steatosis to nonalcoholic steatohepatitis (NASH), in which inflammatory changes and focal necrosis may progress to (1) liver fibrosis, (2) cirrhosis, and (3) hepatic failure (see Chapter 37). NAFLD is now considered to be an additional feature of the "metabolic syndrome" with elevation of serum aminotransferase activities associated with (1) higher body mass index, (2) increased waist circumference, (3) elevated serum triglycerides, (4) elevated fasting insulin and (5) lower HDL cholesterol—all characteristic features of this syndrome.

Aminotransferase activities observed in cirrhosis vary with the status of the cirrhotic process and vary from the URL to four to five times higher, with an AST/ALT ratio (AAR) greater than 1. This appears to be attributable to a reduction in ALT production in a damaged liver, associated with reduced clearance of AST in advancing liver fibrosis. An AAR ≥1 has ≈90% positive predictive value for diagnosing the presence of advanced fibrosis in patients with chronic liver disease. Furthermore, the extent of elevation in the AAR has been known to reflect the grade of fibrosis in these patients.

Twofold to fivefold elevations of the activities of both enzymes occur in patients with primary or metastatic carcinoma of the liver, with the activity of AST usually higher than ALT activity, but their values are often within the reference interval in the early stages of malignant infiltration of the liver. Slight or moderate elevations in AST and ALT activities have been observed after administration of various medications, such as (1) nonsteroidal anti-inflammatory drugs, (2) antibiotics, (3) antiepileptic drugs, and (4) statins. Over-the-counter medications and herbal preparations are also implicated. In patients with (1) increased aminotransaminase activities, (2) negative viral markers, and (3) a negative history for drugs or alcohol ingestion. The diagnostic evaluation should include investigation of less common causes of chronic hepatic injury such as (1) hemochromatosis, (2) Wilson disease, (3) autoimmune hepatitis, (4) primary biliary cirrhosis, (5) sclerosing cholangitis, (6) celiac disease, and (7) α_1-antitrypsin deficiency.

Although serum activities of both AST and ALT become elevated whenever disease processes affect liver cell integrity, ALT is the more liver-specific enzyme. Serum elevations of ALT activity are rarely observed in conditions other than parenchymal liver disease. Thus the incremental benefit of determination of AST, in addition to ALT, may be limited.

After acute myocardial infarction, increased AST activity appears in serum (see Table 19-3). AST activity also is increased in progressive muscular dystrophy and dermatomyositis, although it is usually normal in other types of muscle disease, especially in those of neurogenic origin. Slight to moderate AST elevations are noted in hemolytic disease.

Several studies have described AST activities linked to immunoglobulins, or macro-AST. Typical findings include a persistent increase in serum AST activity in an asymptomatic patient, with absence of any demonstrable pathology in organs rich in AST. Increased AST activity reflects decreased clearance of the abnormal complex from plasma. Macro-AST has no known clinical relevance. However, identification is important to avoid unnecessary diagnostic procedures in these patients. The demonstration of macro-AST in serum is obtained by differential precipitation with polyethylene glycol (PEG) 6000 (see "Amylase" section later in this chapter).

Methods of Analysis

Continuous-monitoring methods are commonly used to measure aminotransaminase activity by coupling aminotransaminase reactions to specific dehydrogenase reactions. The oxo-acids formed in the aminotransaminase reaction are measured indirectly by enzymatic reduction to corresponding hydroxy acids, and the accompanying change in NADH concentration is monitored spectrophotometrically. Thus oxaloacetate, formed in the AST reaction, is reduced to malate in the presence of malate dehydrogenase (MD).

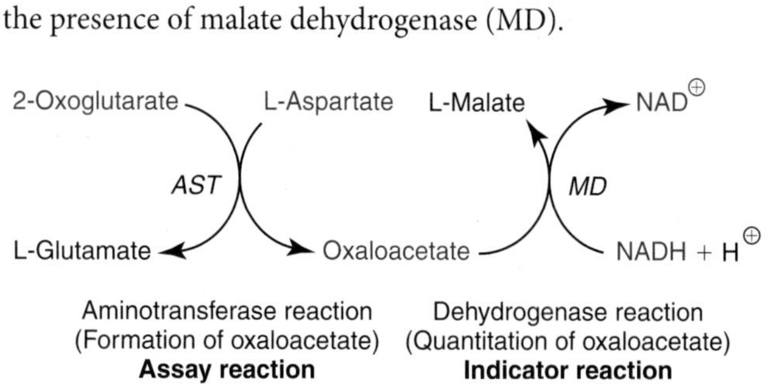

Aminotransferase reaction	Dehydrogenase reaction
(Formation of oxaloacetate)	(Quantitation of oxaloacetate)
Assay reaction	**Indicator reaction**

Pyruvate formed in the ALT reaction is reduced to lactate by **lactate dehydrogenase** (LD). The substrate, NADH, and an auxiliary enzyme, MD or LD, are present in sufficient quantities so that the reaction rate is limited only by the amounts of AST and ALT, respectively. As the reactions proceed, NADH is oxidized to NAD^+ (nicotinamide adenine dinucleotide). The disappearance of NADH is followed by measurement of the decrease in absorbance at 340 nm. The change in absorbance per minute (ΔA/min) is proportional to the micromoles of NADH oxidized and in turn to micromoles of substrate transformed per minute. A preliminary incubation period is necessary to ensure that NADH-dependent reduction of endogenous oxo-acids in the sample is completed before 2-oxoglutarate is added to start the aminotransaminase reaction. As has been mentioned, supplementation with P-5′-P ensures that all aminotransaminase activity of the sample is measured.

Primary IFCC reference procedures are available for the measurement of catalytic activity concentrations of AST and ALT at 37 °C.[13,14] To assure accuracy and comparability between laboratories, the manufacturer's product calibrator values and measurement results obtained with commercial systems in daily routine practice should be traceable to these reference measurement procedures.[4]

AST activity in serum is stable for up to 48 hours at 4 °C. Specimens need to be stored frozen if they are to be kept longer. ALT activity should be assayed on the day of sample collection because activity is lost at room temperature, at 4 °C, and at −25 °C. ALT stability is better maintained at −70 °C. Hemolyzed specimens should not be used, especially when AST is measured, because of the large amount of this enzyme present in red cells.

When assays traceable to the IFCC reference procedures are used, the AST URL for adults is 35 U/L, with no significant sex-related differences.[1] Conversely, a difference in ALT activities has been noted between adult males and females. Corresponding ALT URLs are 60 U/L and 42 U/L, respectively.[1] ALT does not reveal an age dependency during childhood, whereas serum AST activity in neonates and in children younger than 3 years old is twice that in adults.

γ-Glutamyltransferase

Peptidases catalyze the hydrolytic cleavage of peptides to form amino acids or smaller peptides. They constitute a broad group of enzymes of varied specificity, and some individual enzymes act as amino acid transferases and catalyze the transfer of amino acids from one peptide to another amino acid or peptide. γ-Glutamyltransferase (GGT) (EC 2.3.2.2; γ-glutamyl-peptide: amino acid γ-glutamyltransferase) catalyzes the transfer of the γ-glutamyl group from peptides and compounds to an acceptor. Substrates for GGT include (1) the γ-glutamyl acceptor, (2) some amino acid or peptide, or (3) even water, in which case simple hydrolysis takes place. The enzyme acts only on peptides or peptide-like compounds that contain a terminal glutamate residue joined to the remainder of the compound through the terminal (-γ-) carboxyl. Glycylglycine is five times more effective as an acceptor than is glycine or the tripeptide (gly-gly-gly). An example of a reaction catalyzed by the GGT is shown here:

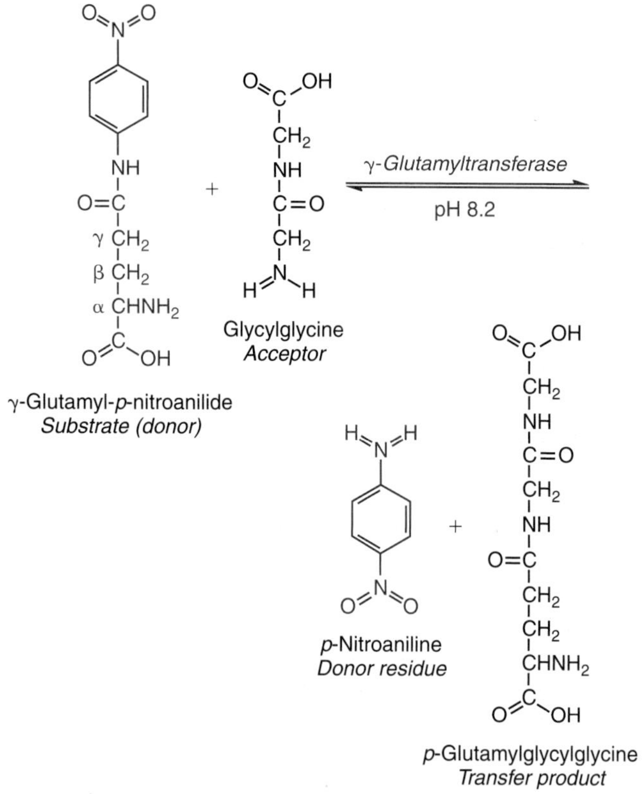

Biochemistry

GGT is present (in decreasing order of abundance) in (1) proximal renal tubule, (2) liver, (3) pancreas, and (4) intestine. The enzyme is present in cytoplasm (microsomes), but the larger fraction is located in the cell membrane and may transport amino acids and peptides into the cell across the cell membrane in the form of γ-glutamyl peptides. GGT is critical for the maintenance of adequate intracellular levels of reduced glutathione, a major antioxidant agent.

Clinical Significance

Even though renal tissue has the highest concentration of GGT, the enzyme present in serum appears to originate primarily from the hepatobiliary system. Thus, the activity of GGT is considered a sensitive indicator of the presence of hepatobiliary disease, but its usefulness is limited by lack of specificity. Similar to alkaline phosphatase, GGT activity is highest in cases of intrahepatic or post-hepatic biliary obstruction, reaching activities some 5 to 30 times the URL. High elevations of GGT activity are also observed in patients with primary or metastatic liver neoplasm. Moderate elevations occur in infectious hepatitis. Small increases in GGT activity are observed in more than 50% of patients with NAFLD, and similar but transient increases are noted in cases of drug intoxication. In acute and chronic pancreatitis and in some pancreatic malignancies (especially if associated with hepatobiliary obstruction), enzyme activity may be 5 to 15 times the URL.

Elevated activities of GGT also are found in the sera of patients with alcoholic hepatitis and in most sera from people who are heavy drinkers. Increased activities of the enzyme are also found in the serum of patients receiving anticonvulsant drugs such as phenytoin and phenobarbital. Such an increase in GGT activity in serum may reflect induction of new enzyme activity by the action of alcohol and drugs and/or their toxic effects on microsomal structures in liver cells.

Epidemiological studies have shown that serum GGT activity possesses an independent prognostic value for cardiovascular morbidity and mortality.

Methods of Analysis

Early GGT assays used L-γ-glutamyl-p-nitroanilide (GGPNA) as the substrate, with glycylglycine serving as the γ-glutamyl residue acceptor. The p-nitroaniline produced in the reaction is determined by its yellow color, which is measured at 405 nm. However, GGPNA has limited solubility in the reaction mixture. Therefore, with GGPNA, it is difficult to obtain saturating concentrations of substrate. Derivatives of GGPNA, in which various groups have been introduced into the benzene ring, have been used to increase solubility in water. The most useful of these substrates is L-γ-glutamyl-3-carboxy-4-nitroanilide, which is readily soluble in water and is split by GGT at a rate comparable with that observed with GGPNA. In the IFCC reference measurement procedure for GGT, L-γ-glutamyl-3-carboxy-4-nitroanilide serves as the substrate, with glycylglycine serving as an acceptor. Buffering is provided by glycylglycine itself. The temperature of the reaction is 37 °C, and the wavelength of measurement of the reaction product, 5-amino-2-nitrobenzoate, is 410 nm.

GGT activity is stable for at least 1 month at 4 °C and for 1 year at −20 °C. Nonhemolyzed serum is the preferred specimen, but EDTA plasma has also been used. Heparin may produce turbidity in the reaction mixture; citrate, oxalate, and fluoride depress GGT activity by 10% to 15%.

In adults, the URL for GGT activity in serum is 40 U/L for females and 70 U/L for males when measured with an assay traceable to the IFCC reference procedure.[1] Reference limits are approximately twofold higher in people of African ancestry. In normal full-term neonates, GGT activity at birth is approximately six to seven times the adult reference interval. The activity then declines, reaching adult values by the age of 5 to 7 months.

Alkaline Phosphatase

Alkaline phosphatase (ALP) [EC 3.1.3.1; orthophosphoric-monoester phosphohydrolase (alkaline optimum)] catalyzes the alkaline hydrolysis of a large variety of naturally occurring and synthetic substrates. Divalent ions, such as (1) Mg^{2+}, (2) Co^{2+}, and (3) Mn^{2+}, are activators of the enzyme, and Zn^{2+} is a constituent metal ion. Inhibitors of ALP activity include (1) phosphate, (2) borate, (3) oxalate, and (4) cyanide ions. Buffers for ALP assay are classified as (1) inert (carbonate and barbital), (2) inhibiting (glycine and propylamine), or (3) activating (2-amino-2-methyl-1-propanol [AMP], tris(hydroxymethyl) aminomethane [TRIS], and diethanolamine [DEA]).

Biochemistry

ALP activity is present in most organs of the body and is located in the (1) mucosa of the small intestine, (2) proximal convoluted tubules of the kidney, (3) bone (osteoblasts), (4) liver, and (5) placenta. Although the exact metabolic function of the enzyme is not yet understood, it appears that ALP is associated with lipid transport in the intestine and with the calcification process in bone.

ALP exists in multiple forms, some of which are true isoenzymes, encoded at separate genetic loci (Figure 19-2). Bone, liver, and kidney ALP forms share a common primary structure coded for by the same genetic locus, but they differ in carbohydrate content.

The ALP activity present in the sera of healthy adults originates mainly in the liver, with most of the rest coming from the skeleton. The respective contributions of these two forms to the total activity are age dependent. Minimal amounts of intestinal ALP may also be present, particularly in the sera of individuals of blood group B or O. Because intestinal ALP activity in serum may increase after a meal, ALP should be measured preferentially in fasting sera.

Clinical Significance

Clinically, serum ALP measurements are of particular value in the investigation of hepatobiliary disease and bone disease associated with increased osteoblastic activity.

Hepatobiliary Disease

The response of the liver to any form of biliary tree obstruction induces the synthesis of ALP by hepatocytes. Some of the newly formed enzyme enters the circulation to increase enzyme activity in serum. Elevation tends to be threefold greater in extrahepatic obstruction (e.g., by stone, by cancer of the head of the pancreas) than in intrahepatic obstruction and is greater the more complete the obstruction. Serum enzyme activities may reach 10 to 12 times the URL and usually return to normal on surgical removal of the obstruction. A similar increase is seen in patients with advanced primary liver cancer or widespread secondary hepatic metastases. Liver diseases that principally affect parenchymal cells, such as infectious hepatitis, typically show only moderately (less than threefold) increased or even normal serum ALP activities. Increases may also be seen as a consequence of a reaction to drug therapy. Intestinal ALP isoenzyme, an asialoglycoprotein normally

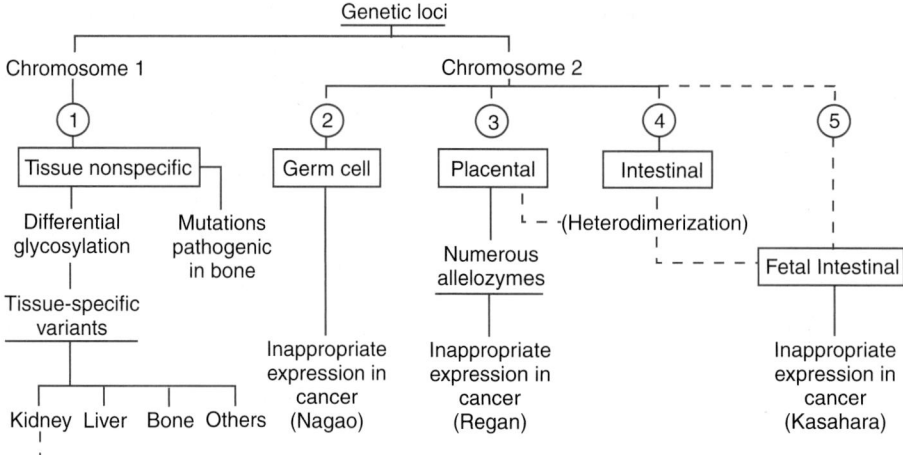

Figure 19-2 Identities, chromosomal assignments, and main physiological and pathological expression of genes encoding human alkaline phosphatases. The gene names (and gene symbols) are alkaline phosphatase, liver/bone/kidney *(ALPL)*; alkaline phosphatase, intestinal *(ALPI)*; alkaline phosphatase, placental *(ALPP)*; and alkaline phosphatase, placental-like 2 *(ALPPL2)*. *Broken lines* show two alternative proposed origins of the fetal intestinal alkaline phosphatase; the sequence of a cDNA is reportedly identical to that of adult intestinal alkaline phosphatase. All isoenzymes and isoforms are glycoproteins, thus imposing a further level of microheterogeneity. Different processes of cleavage or preservation of the membrane-anchoring domain can generate additional isoforms. *(Modified from Moss DW. Perspectives in alkaline phosphatase research. Clin Chem 1992;38:2486-92.)*

cleared by the hepatic asialoglycoprotein receptors, is often elevated in patients with liver cirrhosis.

Bone Disease

Bone ALP is produced by the osteoblast and has been demonstrated in matrix vesicles deposited as "buds" derived from the cell's membrane. The enzyme therefore is an excellent indicator of global bone formation activity. Genetic inability to produce tissue-nonspecific ALP, including bone isoform, a rare inherited disorder known as hypophosphatasia, results in severe bone disease and impaired bone growth.

Among the bone diseases, the highest concentrations of bone ALP are encountered in **Paget disease** (osteitis deformans) as a result of the action of osteoblastic cells as they try to rebuild bone that is being resorbed by uncontrolled activity of osteoclasts (see Chapter 39). Activities from 10 to 25 times the URL are not unusual with the increase reflecting the extent of disease. In vitamin D deficiency (osteomalacia and rickets), concentrations two to four times the URL may be observed. Primary hyperparathyroidism and secondary hyperparathyroidism are associated with slight to moderate elevations of bone ALP in serum, with the existence and degree of elevation reflecting the presence and extent of skeletal involvement. Very high enzyme concentrations are present in patients with osteogenic bone cancer. Bone ALP is slightly increased in osteoporosis, but osteoporotic individuals are not clearly distinguished from age-matched controls. Transient elevations of ALP may be found during healing of bone fractures. Physiological bone growth increases bone ALP in serum, and this accounts for the fact that in the sera of growing children, the enzyme concentration is 1.5 to 7 times that in healthy adult serum; the maximum is reached earlier in girls than in boys.

Other Conditions That Increase ALP

An increase in ALP activity of up to two to three times the URL is observed in women in the third trimester of pregnancy, and the additional enzyme is of placental origin. Reports have described a benign familial elevation in serum ALP activity due to increased concentrations of intestinal ALP. Transient, benign increases in serum ALP activity may be observed in infants and children, with changes often more than 10 times the URL. Increases in both liver and bone forms are seen. These changes seem to reflect a reduction in the removal of ALP from blood caused by transient modifications of enzyme glycosylation.

ALP forms essentially identical to the normal placental or germ cell isoenzymes appear in the sera of some patients with malignant disease. These carcinoplacental isoenzymes (e.g., **Regan isoenzyme**) result from derepression of the placental or placental-like 2 ALP genes. The presence of these isoenzymes is readily detected in serum by their stability at 65 °C. Tumors have also been found to produce ALPs that appear to be post-translationally modified forms of nonplacental isoenzymes.

Methods of Analysis for Total ALP Activity and Isoenzyme Content

The most popular of the chromogenic substrates for ALP is 4-nitrophenyl phosphate (usually abbreviated 4-NPP, or PNPP from the older name, *p*-nitrophenyl phosphate). This ester is colorless, but the final product is yellow at the pH of the reaction:

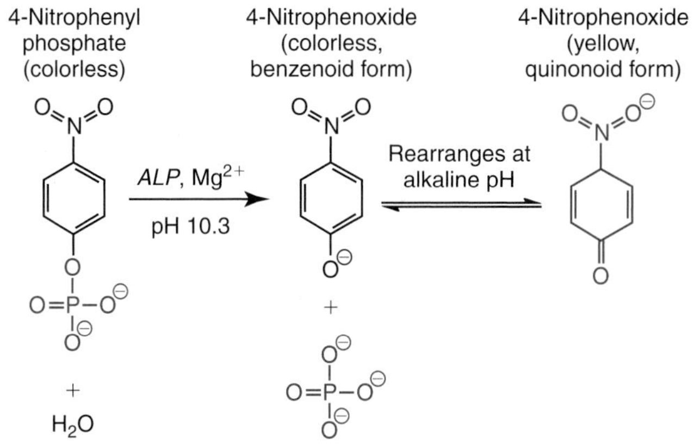

4-Nitrophenyl phosphate (colorless)   4-Nitrophenoxide (colorless, benzenoid form)   4-Nitrophenoxide (yellow, quinonoid form)

The enzyme reaction is continuously monitored by observing the rate of formation of the 4-nitrophenoxide ions at 405 nm. This reaction forms the basis of current methods of ALP assay. The liberated phosphate group is transferred to water, and the rate of phosphatase action is enhanced if certain amino alcohols are used as phosphate-accepting buffers. Among these activators are compounds such as (1) AMP, (2) DEA, (3) TRIS, and (4) N-methyl-d-glucamine (MEG). The IFCC-recommended procedure uses 4-NPP as the substrate and AMP as the phosphate-acceptor buffer.[15]

Serum or heparinized plasma, free of hemolysis, should be used. Complexing anticoagulants—such as citrate and EDTA—must be avoided because they bind cations, such as Mg^{2+} and Zn^{2+}, which are necessary cofactors for ALP activity measurement. Freshly collected serum samples should be kept at room temperature and assayed as soon as possible but preferably within 4 hours after collection. In sera stored at a refrigerated temperature, ALP activity increases slowly (2% per day); this is thought to be due to the reincorporation of the cations required for full activity. Frozen specimens should be thawed and kept at room temperature for 18 to 24 hours before measurement to achieve full enzyme reactivation.

ALP activities in serum vary with age. Children show higher ALP activity than healthy adults as a result of leakage of bone ALP from osteoblasts during bone growth. When assays that are traceable to the IFCC reference procedure were used, the ALP reference intervals (central 95th percentiles) for adult males and adult premenopausal females were 43 to 115 U/L and 33 to 98 U/L, respectively.[15]

Assays for ALP isoenzymes are needed when (1) the source of an elevated ALP activity in serum is not obvious and should be clarified; (2) the main clinical question is concerned with detecting the presence of liver or bone involvement; and (3) it is important to ascertain any modifications in the activity of osteoblasts to monitor disease activity and the effects of appropriate therapies in the case of bone disorders. Criteria that have been used to differentiate the isoenzymes and other multiple forms of ALP include (1) electrophoretic mobility; (2) stability to denaturation by heat or chemicals; (3) response to the presence of selected inhibitors; (4) affinity for specific lectins; and (5) immunochemical characteristics.

After electrophoresis, ALP zones are visualized by incubating the gel in a solution of buffered substrate. The liver ALP typically moves most rapidly toward the anode. Bone ALP, which typically gives a more diffuse zone than the liver form, has slightly reduced anodal mobility, although the two zones usually overlap to some extent. Intestinal ALP migrates more slowly than the bone enzyme, whereas the placental isoenzyme commonly appears as a discrete band overlying the diffuse bone fraction. An additional band, which is frequently present in the serum of patients with various hepatic diseases, contains a high-molecular-weight form of ALP but is strongly negatively charged. Therefore, it moves slowly into or may even fail to enter polyacrylamide gel, but it migrates more anodally than the main liver zone on nonsieving media, such as cellulose acetate. This form corresponds to the main liver form attached to the membrane moiety. Complexes between ALP and immunoglobulins, or macro-ALP, occur occasionally in serum, giving rise to abnormally migrating bands in the γ-globulin zone; however, they do not provide specific diagnostic information in the present state of knowledge.

In general, electrophoretic separation of bone and liver ALP forms is difficult because of structural similarity. To improve their separation, serum is pretreated for 15 minutes at 37 °C with neuraminidase to remove part of the terminal sialic acid residues. As the sialic acid residues of bone ALP are more readily attacked than those of liver ALP, the electrophoretic mobility of the bone form is reduced to a greater extent than that of liver ALP. The improved separation allows quantitative estimates to be made by densitometric scanning. Measurement of GGT, which is increased in liver disease but not in bone disease, may be a useful rapid alternative tool to distinguish between the two diseases as the explanation for increased serum ALP.

Overnight incubation of the serum sample with neuraminidase is used to confirm the presence of intestinal ALP. This treatment reduces the anodal mobility of all ALP isoenzymes except that of intestinal origin, which is neuraminidase resistant because terminal sialic acid residues are not present in the molecule.

Immunoassays for direct determination of bone ALP, which measure enzyme activity or mass concentration, are commercially available. Cross-reactivity with the liver isoform varies by 6% to 20%. Despite lack of complete specificity, immunoassays of bone ALP may offer some advantages in monitoring bone disease and the effects of appropriate therapies once the diagnosis of bone involvement has been established.

5′-Nucleotidase

5′-Nucleotidase (NTP) (EC 3.1.3.5; 5′-ribonucleotide phosphohydrolase) is a phosphatase that acts only on nucleoside-5′-phosphates, such as adenosine-5′-phosphate (AMP) and adenylic acid, releasing inorganic phosphate.

NTP is a glycoprotein that is widely distributed throughout the tissues of the body and is principally localized in the cytoplasmic membrane of the cells in which it occurs. Despite its ubiquitous distribution, serum NTP activities appear to reflect hepatobiliary disease with considerable specificity. NTP is increased in those hepatobiliary diseases characterized by interference with the secretion of bile. This may be due to extrahepatic causes (a stone or a tumor occluding the bile duct), or it may arise from intrahepatic conditions, such as cholestasis caused by malignant infiltration of the liver or biliary cirrhosis. When parenchymal cell damage is predominant, as in infectious hepatitis, serum NTP activity is only moderately elevated.

The assay of NTP activity has been considered of value as an addition to measurement of nonspecific total ALP in patients with suspected hepatobiliary disease, and abnormal NTP activity is routinely interpreted as evidence of hepatic origin of increased ALP activity in serum. However, approximately half of individuals in whom liver ALP activity is increased in serum may simultaneously show a normal NTP activity. Alternatively, increased NTP activity in the serum of patients with normal liver ALP activity is very often associated with the presence of liver disease. Thus the frequent dissociation of the two enzyme activities supports the usefulness of determining both (liver) ALP and NTP to enhance diagnostic efficiency in diseases of the liver.[7]

In a commercially available assay, serum NTP catalyzes the hydrolysis of inosine-5′-phosphate (IMP) to yield inosine, which is then converted to hypoxanthine by purine-nucleoside phosphorylase (EC 2.4.2.1). Hypoxanthine is oxidized to urate with xanthine oxidase (EC 1.2.3.2). Two moles of hydrogen peroxide are produced for each mole of hypoxanthine liberated and converted to uric acid. The formation rate of hydrogen peroxide is monitored by a spectrophotometer at 510 nm by the oxidation of a chromogenic system. The effect of ALPs on IMP is inhibited by β-glycerophosphate.

NTP activity in serum or plasma heparin is stable for at least 4 days at 4 °C and 4 months at −20 °C. The reference interval for NTP activity at 37 °C ranges from 3 to 9 U/L, with no sex-related differences.

Pancreatic Enzymes

The most commonly used serum biomarkers for investigation of pancreatic disease, and more specifically **acute pancreatitis**, are the digestive enzymes—(P-type) amylase and lipase. Pancreatic function and pathology are discussed in Chapter 38.

Amylase

Alpha-amylase (AMY) (EC 3.2.1.1; 1,4-α-d glucan glucano-hydrolase) catalyzes the hydrolysis of 1,4-α-glucosidic linkages in polysaccharides. Both straight-chain (linear) polyglucans (amylose) and branched polyglucans (amylopectin and glycogen) are hydrolyzed but at different rates. The enzyme does not attack the α-1,6-linkages at the branch points. AMYs are calcium metalloenzymes, with the calcium essential for functional integrity. However, full activity is displayed only in the presence of various anions, with chloride and bromide being the most effective activators. AMY in human serum has a moderately sharp pH optimum at 6.9 to 7.0.

Biochemistry

Amylases that occur normally in human plasma are small molecules with molecular weights varying from 54 to 62 kDa. The enzyme is small enough to pass through the glomeruli of the kidneys, and AMY is the only plasma enzyme physiologically found in urine. It is present in a number of organs and tissues. The greatest concentration is present in the salivary glands, which secrete a potent AMY (S-type) to initiate hydrolysis of starches while food is still in the mouth and esophagus. In the pancreas, the enzyme (P-type) is synthesized by acinar cells and then is secreted into the intestinal tract by way of the pancreatic duct system. AMY activity is also found in extracts from (1) ovaries, (2) fallopian tubes, (3) lungs, and (4) adipose tissue. Some tumors of lung and ovary may also contain considerable AMY activity (usually S-type). Ascitic and pleural fluids may contain AMY as a result of the presence of a tumor or pancreatitis.

The enzyme present in normal serum and urine is predominantly of pancreatic (P-AMY) and salivary gland (S-AMY) origin. These isoenzymes are products of two closely linked loci on chromosome 1. AMY isoenzymes also undergo posttranslational modification of (1) deamidation, (2) glycosylation, and (3) deglycosylation to form various isoforms, which have been separated in both serum and urine using isoelectric focusing or electrophoresis.

Clinical Significance

Total blood AMY activity is physiologically low and constant and is greatly increased in acute pancreatitis and salivary gland inflammation. In **acute pancreatitis**, a rise in serum AMY activity occurs within 5 to 8 hours of symptom onset. Activities typically return to normal by the third or fourth day. A fourfold to sixfold elevation in AMY activity above the URL is usual, with maximal concentrations attained in 12 to 72 hours. The magnitude of the AMY elevation is not related to the severity of pancreatic involvement; however, the greater the rise, the greater the probability of acute pancreatitis. The clinical specificity of total AMY for the diagnosis of acute pancreatitis is, however, low because increased values are also found in a number of acute intra-abdominal disorders and in several extrapancreatic conditions (Table 19-4).

Lack of specificity of total AMY measurement has resulted in the direct measurement of P-AMY instead of total enzyme activity for the differential diagnosis of patients with acute abdominal pain. When a decision limit of an activity equal to threefold the URL was applied, the clinical specificity of P-AMY for the diagnosis of acute pancreatitis was greater than 90%.[11] Sensitivity in late detection of this condition is also notably improved with P-AMY. P-AMY values remain elevated in 80% of patients with uncomplicated pancreatitis 1 week after onset, when only 30% still show increased total AMY activity.

Biliary tract diseases, such as **cholecystitis**, cause up to fourfold elevation in serum P-AMY activity as a result of primary or secondary pancreatic involvement. Other intra-abdominal events also lead to a significant increase in serum P-AMY activity. In renal insufficiency, serum AMY activity

TABLE 19-4 Causes of Hyperamylasemia

Pancreatic disease	Pancreatitis, any cause (P-AMY↑)*
	Pancreatic trauma (P-AMY↑)
Intra-abdominal diseases other than pancreatitis	Biliary tract disease (P-AMY↑)
	Intestinal obstruction (P-AMY↑)
	Mesenteric infarction (P-AMY↑)
	Perforated peptic ulcer (P-AMY↑)
	Gastritis, duodenitis (P-AMY↑)
	Ruptured aortic aneurysm
	Acute appendicitis (perforated)
	Peritonitis
	Trauma
Genitourinary disease	Ectopic, ruptured tubal pregnancy (S-AMY↑)
	Salpingitis (S-AMY↑)
	Ovarian malignancy (S-AMY↑)
	Renal insufficiency (Mixed)
Miscellaneous	Salivary gland lesions (S-AMY↑)
	Acute alcoholic abuse (S-AMY↑)
	Diabetic ketoacidosis (S-AMY↑)
	Macroamylasemia (S-AMY↑ or P-AMY↑)
	Septic shock (S-AMY↑)
	Cardiac surgery (S-AMY↑)
	Tumor (usually S-AMY↑)
	Drugs (usually S-AMY↑)

*Predominant isoenzyme type is shown in parentheses.
Mixed, Either or both isoenzymes may be present; *P-AMY,* pancreatic; *S-AMY,* salivary.

is increased in proportion to the extent of renal impairment (usually, no more than five times the URL). Hyperamylasemia (with an S-type isoenzyme mobility) may also occur in neoplastic diseases with elevations as high as 50 times the URL.

In 1% of the population, macroamylases are present in sera and may cause hyperamylasemia; these are complexes between ordinary AMY (usually S-type) and immunoglobulin (IgG or IgA). These macroamylases are not filtered through the glomeruli of the kidneys because of their large size (greater than 200 kDa) and are thus retained in the plasma, where their presence may increase AMY activity some twofold to eightfold above the URL. No clinical symptoms are associated with this disorder.

Methods of Analysis for Total and Pancreatic Amylase Activity

When hydrolyzed by AMY, small oligosaccharide substrates have been found to yield better defined products than do starches. Use of defined substrates in the AMY assay has improved the reaction stoichiometry and has led to more controlled and consistent hydrolysis conditions. Substrates used include (1) maltotetraose, (2) maltopentaose, and (3) 4-nitrophenyl (4-NP)-glycoside substrates prepared by bonding 4-NP to the reducing end of a defined oligosaccharide. If the oligosaccharide is maltoheptaose (G7), the substrate is then 4-NP-G7. AMY splits this substrate to produce free oligosaccharides (G5, G4, and G3) and 4-NP-G2, 4-NP-G3, and 4-NP-G4. Combined hydrolysis by AMY in the specimen and by the reagent α-glucosidase (EC 3.2.1.20; maltase) results in free NP production, which is detected by its absorbance at 405 nm.

$$5 \text{ ethylidene-4-NP-G}_7 + 5\,H_2O \xrightarrow{\alpha\text{-amylase}}$$
$$2 \text{ ethylidene-G}_5 + 2\text{ 4-NP-G}_2 +$$
$$2 \text{ ethylidene-G}_4 + 2\text{ 4-NP-G}_3 +$$
$$\text{ethylidene-G}_3 + 4\text{-NP-G}_4$$

$$2\text{ 4-NP-G}_2 + 2\text{ 4-NP-G}_3 + 10\,H_2O \xrightarrow{\alpha\text{-glucosidase}} 4\text{ 4-NP} + 10\,G$$

Historically, problems arose with use of the 4-NP-glycoside assay with regard to the poor stability of the reconstituted assay mixture, because of slow hydrolysis of the 4-NP-glycoside by α-glucosidase. This effect has been reduced by covalently linking a "blocking" group such as 4,6-ethylidene group the nonreducing end of the molecule. Such a substrate is known as an ethylidene-protected substrate (EPS). These substrates have shown a more advantageous hydrolysis pattern, thus increasing liberation of 4-NP. A novel-type α-glucosidase is also available (recombinant enzyme AGH-211) that completely hydrolyzes nitrophenylated substrates. As a result, cleavage of one α-glucosidic linkage by AMY results in the release of one molecule of 4-NP. The IFCC has optimized this method at 37 °C, recommending it as a reference measurement procedure for AMY.[12] The serum reference interval for the IFCC recommended method is 31 to 107 U/L.

With the exception of heparin, all common anticoagulants inhibit AMY activity because they chelate Ca^{2+}. Therefore, AMY assays should be performed only on serum or heparinized plasma. AMY is quite stable, and activity is fully retained during storage for 4 days at room temperature, for 2 weeks at −4 °C, for 1 year at −25 °C, and for 5 years at −75 °C.

Only methods based on selective S-AMY inhibition by monoclonal antibodies have shown sufficient (1) precision, (2) reliability, (3) practicability, and (4) analytical speed to be clinically useful for P-AMY determination. A double monoclonal antibody assay is commercially available that uses the synergistic action of two immunoinhibitory monoclonal antibodies to S-AMY. After S-AMY activity is inhibited by the addition of antibodies, uninhibited P-AMY activity is measured using EPS-4-NP-G7 as a substrate.[11] False-positive P-AMY results have been reported in subjects with macroamylasemia, in whom immunoglobulin complexed to AMY forms diminishes or voids the ability of monoclonal antibodies included in the test to efficiently inhibit S-AMY. Upon electrophoresis, macro-AMY usually forms a broad migrating band, different from the homogeneous bands that are produced by AMY isoenzymes present in serum. If electrophoretic separation is not available, precipitation of the macrocomplex by a PEG 6000 solution (240 g/L) represents an alternative. Residual AMY activity of less than 30% in the supernatant is indicative of macroamylasemia (Figure 19-3).

In healthy adults, P-AMY represents approximately 40% to 50% of total AMY activity in serum. When the immunoinhibition method is used at 37 °C, the reference interval for P-AMY activity in sera from adults was 13 to 53 U/L.[5]

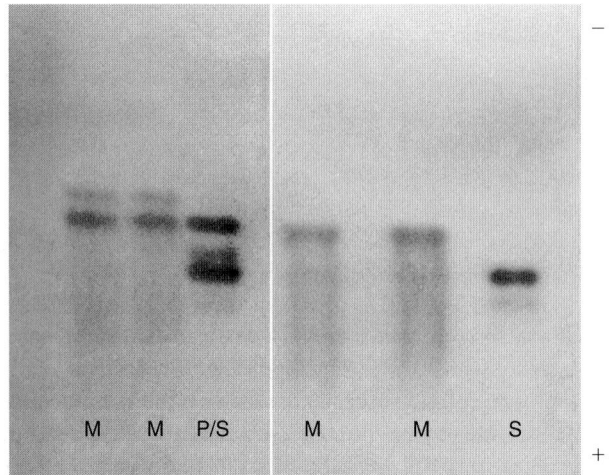

Figure 19-3 Demonstration of macroamylasemia by polyethylene glycol (PEG) 6000 solution. *P-AMY,* Pancreatic amylase.

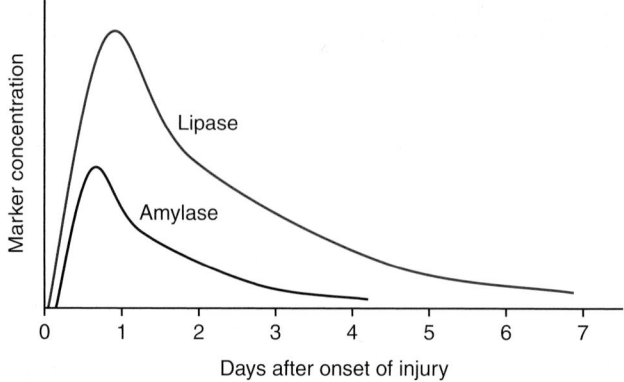

Figure 19-4 Time-dependent changes in serum amylase and lipase after acute pancreatitis.

Lipase

Human pancreatic **lipase** (LPS) (EC 3.1.1.3; triacylglycerol acylhydrolase) is a single-chain glycoprotein with a molecular weight of 48 kDa. The LPS gene resides on chromosome 10. For full catalytic activity and greatest specificity, the presence of bile salts and a cofactor called *colipase*, which is a small protein secreted by the pancreas, is required.

Biochemistry

Lipases hydrolyze glycerol esters of long-chain fatty acids.

$$
\begin{array}{l}
\text{H}_2\text{C—OFA(1)} \\
\text{HC—OFA(2)} \xrightarrow[\text{H}_2\text{O} \;\; \text{OH}^{\ominus}]{\textit{Lipase}}
\begin{array}{l}\text{H}_2\text{C—OH} \\ \text{HC—OFA(2)} \\ \text{H}_2\text{C—OFA(3)}\end{array} \xrightarrow[\text{H}_2\text{O} \;\; \text{OH}^{\ominus}]{\textit{Lipase}}
\begin{array}{l}\text{H}_2\text{C—OH} \\ \text{HC—OFA(2)} \\ \text{H}_2\text{C—OH}\end{array}
\end{array}
$$

Triglyceride   →   α,β-Diglyceride + FA(1)OH (Fatty acid I)   →   β-Monoglyceride + FA(3)OH (Fatty acid III)

Isomerization

Glycerol + FA(2)OH (Fatty acid II)   ←   α-Monoglyceride

$$\text{H}_2\text{C—OH} \atop \text{HC—OH} \atop \text{H}_2\text{C—OH} \xleftarrow[\text{H}_2\text{O} \;\; \text{OH}^{\ominus}]{\textit{Lipase}} \text{H}_2\text{C—OH} \atop \text{HC—OH} \atop \text{H}_2\text{C—OFA(2)}$$

Only ester bonds at carbons 1 and 3 (α-positions) are attacked, and products of the reaction include 2 moles of fatty acids and 1 mole of 2-acylglycerol (β-monoglyceride) per mole of substrate. The latter is resistant to hydrolysis, but it spontaneously isomerizes to the α-form (3-acylglycerol), which allows the third fatty acid to be split off but at a much slower rate.

LPS acts only when the substrate is present in an emulsified form at the interface between water and substrate. The rate of LPS action depends on the surface area of the dispersed substrate. Bile acids ensure that the surface of the dispersed substrate remains free of other proteins, including lipolytic enzymes, by lining the surface of the insoluble substrate and the aqueous medium.

Most LPS activity found in serum derives from the pancreas, but some is secreted by gastric and intestinal mucosa. The concentration of LPS in the pancreas is about 5000-fold greater than in other tissues, and the concentration gradient between pancreas and serum is ≈20,000-fold. LPS is a small enough molecule to be filtered through the glomerulus, but it is totally reabsorbed by the renal tubules and thus is not physiologically detected in urine.

Clinical Significance

LPS measurement of serum is used to diagnose acute pancreatitis. The clinical sensitivity is 80% to 100% depending on the selected diagnostic cutoff, and the clinical specificity is 80% to 100% depending on the mix of the patient population studied. After an attack of acute pancreatitis, serum LPS activity increases within 4 to 8 hours, peaks at about 24 hours, and decreases within 7 to 14 days. Elevations between 2 and 50 times the URL have been reported.

Acute pancreatitis is sometimes difficult to diagnose because it must be differentiated from other acute intra-abdominal disorders with similar clinical findings, such as (1) perforated gastric or duodenal ulcer, (2) intestinal obstruction, or (3) mesenteric vascular obstruction. In differential diagnosis, elevation of serum LPS activity to greater than 3 times the URL, in the absence of renal failure, is a more specific diagnostic finding than increases in serum AMY activity.[2] Furthermore, LPS concentrations remain elevated longer than those of AMY, which is another advantage over AMY measurement in patients with delayed presentation (Figure 19-4). Therefore, it is recommended that LPS should replace AMY as the initial diagnostic test for acute pancreatitis in the emergency department; obtaining both serum activities for both AMY and LPS is not warranted.

In patients with a reduced glomerular filtration rate, serum LPS activity is increased. Thus care should be exercised in interpretation of elevated serum LPS values in the presence of renal insufficiency.

Methods of Analysis

Many LPS methods have been described and have used both triglyceride and nontriglyceride substrates and (1) titrimetric, (2) turbidimetric, (3) spectrophotometric, (4) fluorometric, and (5) immunologic techniques. In general, long-chain triglyceride (and some diglyceride) substrates have demonstrated correlation of results with the clinical state that is superior to that seen with methods using other substrates.[9]

Numerous substrates and complex auxiliary and indicator systems have been used in spectrophotometric methods. Particularly, synthetic 1,2-O-dilauryl-rac-glycero-3-glutaric acid-(4-methyl-resorufin)-ester consisting of two glycerol ether bonds and one ester bond has been proposed, and assays based on its use are currently gaining widespread use. LPS hydrolyzes the ester bond in an alkaline medium to an unstable dicarbonic acid ester that spontaneously hydrolyzes to yield glutaric acid and methylresorufin; this is a bluish-purple chromophore with peak absorption at 580 nm.

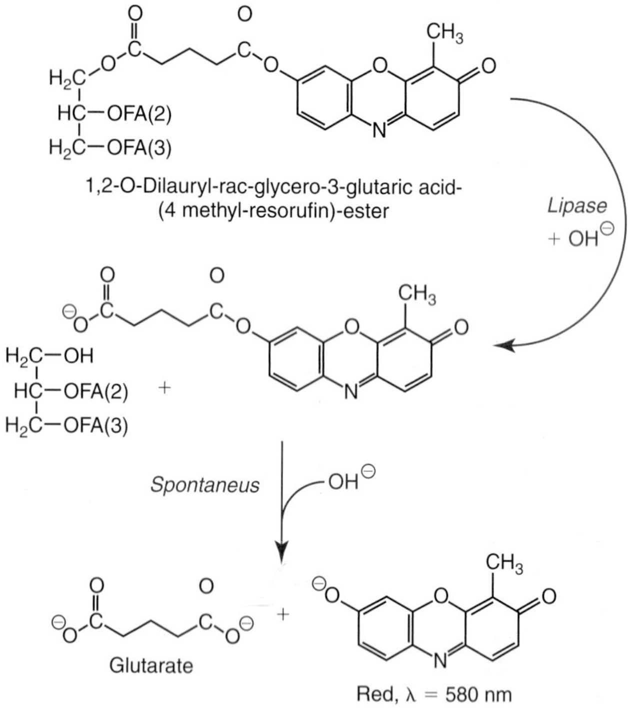

1,2-O-Dilauryl-rac-glycero-3-glutaric acid-(4 methyl-resorufin)-ester

Red, λ = 580 nm

The rate of methylresorufin formation is directly proportional to the LPS activity of the sample. The URL is 38 U/L at 37 °C, and no sex- or age-related differences have been noted.[10]

LPS activity in serum is stable at room temperature for 1 week; sera may be stored for 3 weeks in the refrigerator and for several years if frozen.

Other Clinically Important Enzymes

Lactate Dehydrogenase

Lactate dehydrogenase (LD) (EC 1.1.1.27; I-lactate: NAD$^+$ oxidoreductase) catalyzes the oxidation of L-lactate to pyruvate with the mediation of NAD$^+$ as a hydrogen acceptor.

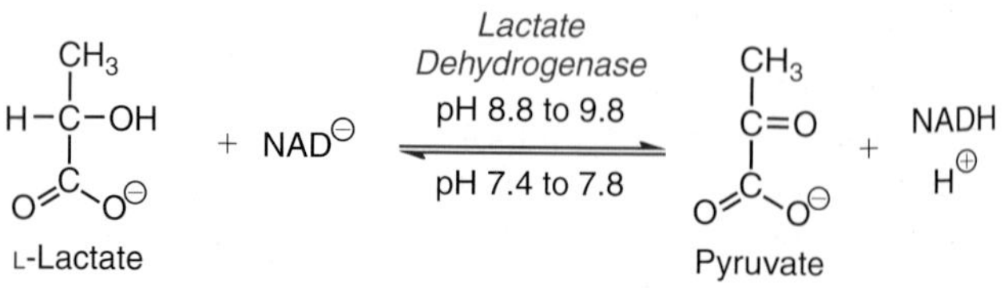

As indicated, the reaction is reversible, and the reaction equilibrium strongly favors the reduction of pyruvate to lactate (P → L)—the "reverse reaction." The optimal pH varies with the predominant isoenzymes in the sample and depends on the temperature and on substrate and buffer concentrations. Both pyruvate and lactate in excess inhibit LD activity, although the effect of pyruvate is greater. Substrate inhibition decreases with increases in pH. EDTA inhibits the enzyme, perhaps by binding Zn^{2+}.

Biochemistry

LD has a molecular weight of 134 kDa and is composed of four peptide chains of two types: M (or A) and H (or B), each under separate genetic control. The structures of LD-M and LD-H are determined by loci on human chromosomes 11 and 12, respectively. The subunit compositions of the five isoenzymes are listed in Box 19-1 in order of their decreasing anodal mobility in an alkaline medium.

A different, sixth LD isoenzyme, LD-X (also called LD$_C$), composed of four X (or C) subunits, is present in postpubertal human testes. A seventh LD, called LD-6, has been identified in the sera of severely ill patients.

LD activity is present in many cells of the body and is invariably found only in the cytoplasm of the cell. Different tissues show different isoenzyme composition. In the (1) heart, (2) kidneys, and (3) erythrocytes, the electrophoretically faster moving isoenzymes LD-1 and LD-2 predominate, whereas in liver and skeletal muscle, the more cathodal LD-4 and LD-5 isoenzymes predominate. However, skeletal muscle damage may result in anodic LD patterns. Isoenzymes of intermediate mobility account for LD activity from many sources such as (1) spleen, (2) lungs, (3) lymph nodes, (4) leukocytes, and (5) platelets.

Clinical Significance

Because of its wide tissue distribution, serum elevations in the activities of LD are seen in a variety of clinical conditions, including (1) myocardial infarction, (2) hepatitis, (3) hemolysis, and (4) disorders of the lung and muscle. Serum LD

BOX 19-1	Subunit Compositions of the Five Isoenzymes of LD in Order of Their Decreasing Anodal Mobility in an Alkaline Medium

LD-1 (HHHH; H$_4$)
LD-2 (HHHM; H$_3$M)
LD-3 (HHMM; H$_2$M$_2$)
LD-4 (HMMM; HM$_3$)
LD-5 (MMMM; M$_4$)

measurement is relevant, however, only in hematology and oncology.[3]

Hemolytic anemias significantly increase LD concentrations in serum. Marked elevations of LD activity—up to 50 times the URL—are observed in the megaloblastic anemias, usually resulting from deficiency of folate or vitamin B_{12}. These elevations rapidly return to normal after appropriate treatment. For monitoring purposes, LD is relevant in predicting disease activity in leukemia, as well as the survival rate (probability of survival) and duration in Hodgkin's disease and non-Hodgkin's lymphoma.

Patients with malignant disease often show increased LD activity in serum; up to 70% of patients with liver metastases and 20% to 60% of patients with other nonhepatic metastases (e.g., in lymph nodes) have elevated LD activity. Notably elevated activities of LD-1 are observed in germ cell tumors (≈60% of cases) such as seminoma of the testis and dysgerminoma of the ovary. The percentage of patients with increased amounts of LD depends on the stage of disease. LD appears to be a useful predictor of outcome in patients with (1) testicular tumor, (2) melanoma, and (3) small cell lung cancer.

Elevations in LD activity are observed in liver disease, but their clinical use in a liver profile appears limited and would not appear to add significantly to the use of the measurement of aminotransferase activities for this purpose.

Macro-LD, usually due to the formation of an autoantibody/enzyme complex that leads to a persistent increase in the amount of circulating enzyme, has been estimated to occur in <1 in 10,000 individuals. Documentation of a macro-LD by the presence of an abnormally migrating band at electrophoresis should be established in suspected individuals to avoid additional follow-up investigation or unnecessary treatment.

Methods of Analysis for Total Lactate Dehydrogenase Activity and Isoenzyme Content

Routine methods for quantitation of total LD activity use kinetic spectrophotometry to measure the interconversion of the coenzyme NAD^+ and NADH at 340 nm. Procedures employing the L → P reaction are recommended, as less dependence on NAD^+ and lactate concentrations and less contamination of NAD^+ with inhibiting products are observed compared with NADH. An L → P reference method has been developed by the IFCC as a reference procedure for LD at 37 °C.[16,17]

Serum is the preferred specimen for measuring LD activity. Plasma samples may be contaminated with platelets, which contain high concentrations of LD. Serum should be separated from the clot as soon as possible after the specimen has been obtained. Hemolyzed serum must not be used because erythrocytes contain 4000 times more LD activity than does serum. The different isoenzymes vary in their sensitivity to cold, and LD-4 and LD-5 are especially labile. Thus, serum specimens should be stored at room temperature, at which no loss of activity occurs for at least 3 days.

The reference interval for LD activity in adult white subjects, as determined at 37 °C with a procedure traceable to the IFCC reference method, is 125 to 220 U/L.[4] LD reference limits are higher in children, and a gradual decrease is noted over the whole childhood period.

Electrophoretic separation is the only procedure commercially available to demonstrate LD isoenzymes.

Cholinesterase

Two related enzymes have the ability to hydrolyze acetylcholine. One is acetylcholinesterase (EC 3.1.1.7; acetylcholine acetylhydrolase), which is called *true cholinesterase* or *choline esterase I*. True **cholinesterase** is found in (1) erythrocytes, (2) the lungs and spleen, (3) nerve endings, and (4) the gray matter of the brain. It is responsible for the prompt hydrolysis of acetylcholine released at the nerve endings to mediate transmission of the neural impulse across the synapse. Degradation of acetylcholine is required for depolarization of the nerve and repolarization in the next conduction event. The second cholinesterase is acylcholine acylhydrolase (EC 3.1.1.8; acylcholine acylhydrolase), also called *pseudocholinesterase, serum cholinesterase* (CHE), *butyrylcholinesterase,* or *choline esterase II.* It is found in (1) liver, (2) pancreas, (3) heart, (4) white matter of the brain, and (5) serum. Although its exact biological role is unknown, a physiological role for CHE in deactivation of octanoyl ghrelin, a hormone that stimulates feeding and promotes weight gain through its metabolic actions, has been proposed.

The type of reaction catalyzed by both cholinesterases is shown:

Biochemistry

CHE in normal sera is separated by electrophoresis into 7 to 12 bands. The forms of CHE differ in molecular size and appear to be aggregates of different numbers of the same basic unit. Of greater interest are the atypical (genetic) variants of the enzyme, characterized by diminished activity against acetylcholine and other substrates, which are found in the sera of a small fraction of apparently healthy people. The gene controlling the synthesis of CHE exists in many allelic forms. Four of the most common forms are designated as E^u, E^a, E^f and E^s These four allelic genes are combined to form one normal and nine abnormal genotypes. The normal, most common phenotype is designated as $E^u E^u$ or UU (u for *usual*). The gene E^a is referred to as the *atypical* gene; the sera of people homozygous for this gene ($E^a E^a = AA$) are only weakly active toward most substrates for CHE and demonstrate increased resistance to inhibition of enzyme activity by dibucaine. The E^f gene (f for *fluoride resistant*) gives rise to

a weakly active enzyme but with increased resistance to fluoride inhibition. The E^s gene (s for silent) is associated with the absence of enzyme or the presence of a protein with minimal or no catalytic activity. The variant enzymes (allelozymes) are less effective catalysts than the usual form; the affinity of the enzymes for the substrates is reduced (K_m is increased), and the affinity for competitive inhibitors, such as dibucaine or fluoride, is similarly decreased. This gives rise to the characteristic dibucaine- or fluoride-resistant properties of the genetic variants that are exploited in their characterization. Homozygous forms, AA and FF, are found in 0.3% to 0.5% of the white population; their incidence among blacks is even lower.

Clinical Significance

Measurements of CHE activity in serum are used (1) as a test of liver function, (2) as an indicator of possible insecticide poisoning, and (3) for the detection of patients with atypical forms of the enzyme who are at risk for prolonged responses to certain muscle relaxants used in surgical procedures.

In the absence of genetic causes or known inhibitors, any decrease in CHE activity reflects impaired synthesis of the enzyme by the liver. Serial measurement of CHE has been promoted as an indication of prognosis in patients with liver disease and for monitoring of liver function after liver transplantation.

Among the organic phosphorous compounds that inhibit cholinesterase activity are many insecticides, such as (1) parathion, (2) sarin, and (3) tetraethyl pyrophosphate. Workers in agriculture and in organic chemical industries may be subject to poisoning by inhalation of these materials or by direct contact with them. Both cholinesterases are inhibited, but the activity of CHE falls more rapidly than does that of the erythrocyte enzyme. A decrease in the erythrocyte enzyme is used as a measure of chronic exposure.

Succinyldicholine (suxamethonium) and mivacurium, drugs used in surgery as muscle relaxants, are hydrolyzed by CHE, and their pharmacologic effect normally persists only long enough to meet the needs of the surgical procedure. In patients with low enzyme activities or in those with a weakly active variant, destruction of the drug will not occur rapidly enough, and the patient may enter a period of prolonged paralysis of the respiratory muscles (apnea) requiring mechanical ventilation until the drug effects gradually wear off. The degree of drug sensitivity varies with the phenotype of the patient. Total CHE activity is highest in individuals who are homozygous for the usual allele and is progressively lower in (1) those who are heterozygous for the usual and a variant allele, (2) those who are homozygous or heterozygous for variant alleles, and (3) those in whom two "silent" alleles are paired and no activity is detected. Measurements of total CHE activity and determination of "dibucaine number" and "fluoride number" are needed to fully characterize CHE variants. The latter values indicate the percentage inhibition of enzyme activity toward specified substrates in the presence of standard concentrations of dibucaine or fluoride. Mutation genotyping may confirm CHE gene abnormalities.

Methods of Analysis

Many contemporary methods use acylthiocholine esters as substrates. Also, the iodide salts of (1) acetylthiocholine, (2) propionylthiocholine, (3) butyrylthiocholine, (4) benzoylthiocholine, and (5) succinylthiocholine have all been used. These latter substrates are hydrolyzed at approximately the same rate as choline esters, and the thiocholine formed is measured by reaction with chromogenic disulfide agents, such as 5,5′-dithio-bis(2-nitrobenzoate) (DTNB) (Ellman's reagent). The reaction of the thiocholine product with colorless DTNB forms colored 5-mercapto-2-nitro-benzoic acid, which is measured spectrophotometrically at 410 nm. Measuring CHE activity using succinyldithiocholine is the method of choice to diagnose succinylcholine sensitivity, which is purely based on the enzyme activity recorded in serum. This method is also well suited for other clinical applications of the test.[6]

Based on differences in sensitivity to inhibition by the local anesthetic dibucaine, a simple test was developed to classify the type of CHE as (1) usual, (2) intermediate, or (3) atypical ("dibucaine number"). Particularly, the usual CHE is inhibited by 80%, but atypical CHE is inhibited by only 20%. Subjects heterozygous for the normal and the atypical gene show about 60% inhibition of CHE. Molecular biological methods are used to identify various CHE genetic defects.

Serum is the sample of choice. Enzyme activity in serum is stable for several weeks if the specimen is stored under refrigeration, and for several years if stored at −20 °C.

When the succinyldithiocholine/DTNB method is used at 37 °C, the reference interval for healthy adults with the usual CHE genotype is 33 to 76 U/L for women and 40 to 78 U/L for men, respectively. The median activity in individuals with a heterozygous genotype is 22 U/L (range, 5 to 35 U/L), and for atypical homozygotes 1.5 U/L (range, 1 to 4 U/L). A significant CHE decrease ($\approx$30%) during pregnancy and early puerperium is explained by hemodilution.

Acid Phosphatase (Tartrate-Resistant 5b Isoform)

Under the name of **acid phosphatase** (ACP) (EC 3.1.3.2; orthophosphoric-monoester phosphohydrolase [acid optimum]), all phosphatases with optimal activity below a pH of 7.0 are categorized. ACP is present in lysosomes, which are organelles present in all cells with the possible exception of erythrocytes. Extralysosomal ACPs are also present in many cells. The greatest concentrations of ACP activity are seen in (1) prostate, (2) bone (osteoclasts), (3) spleen, (4) platelets, and (5) erythrocytes. The lysosomal and prostatic enzymes are strongly inhibited by dextrorotatory tartrate ions, whereas the erythrocyte and bone isoenzymes are not. Most of the physiologically low ACP activity of (unhemolyzed) serum is of a tartrate-resistant type (TR-ACP) and probably originates mainly in osteoclasts. Activities of this fraction are increased in growing children and pathologically in conditions of increased osteolysis and bone remodeling.

At least four ACP-determining genes have been identified and mapped. The erythrocyte ACP gene is located on chromosome 2; a further gene on chromosome 19 encodes the TR-ACP expressed in osteoclasts and other tissue macrophages, such as alveolar macrophages and Kupffer cells (type 5 ACP). Isoenzyme 5 consists of two structurally related isoforms that differ in terms of their carbohydrate content: TR-ACP 5a, which derives mainly from macrophages and dendritic cells, and type 5b, a more specific marker of osteoclastic activity. Genes that encode the tartrate-inhibited lysosomal and prostatic ACPs, mapped to chromosomes 11 and 13, respectively, exhibit considerable homology.

TR-ACP is a potentially useful marker of conditions with a marked osteolytic component. Elevations in serum TR-ACP activity occur in (1) Paget's disease, (2) hyperparathyroidism with skeletal involvement, and (3) the presence of malignant invasion of the bones by cancers. The activity of TR-ACP appears to show relatively small dynamic changes in comparison with other markers of bone resorption (e.g., those related to type I collagen metabolism). This may be attributable to the fact that the enzyme is released into the sealed osteoclast microenvironment, rather than directly into the circulation. Unlike blood concentrations of other markers of bone resorption (e.g., C-telopeptide of type I collagen), activity of TR-ACP is not affected by renal dysfunction. The only nonbone condition in which elevated activities of TR-ACP are found in serum is Gaucher's disease of the spleen, a lysosomal storage disorder. The hairy cells of hairy cell leukemia (leukemic reticuloendotheliosis) also express the osteoclast-type ACP, providing a useful histological marker. However, in this condition, the isoenzyme does not enter the plasma in increased amounts.

Immunoassays for serum TR-ACP have been developed that preferentially detect isoform 5b. One method uses a monoclonal antibody to bind serum TR-ACP in a solid phase format. After the capture, osteoclastic enzyme (type 5b) is specifically determined by measuring its activity at optimal pH 6.1. Another assay uses two monoclonal antibodies generated against purified bone TR-ACP 5b. One of the antibodies captures active intact isoform, while the second eliminates interference of inactive 5b fragments in serum. After the immunoreaction, the activity of bound TR-ACP 5b is measured.

Serum should be immediately separated from erythrocytes and stabilized by the addition of 50 µL of acetic acid (5 mol/L) per milliliter of serum to lower the pH to below 6.5. Under these conditions, TR-ACP activity is maintained at room temperature for several hours, for up to a week if the serum is refrigerated, and for 4 months if stored at −20 °C. Hemolyzed serum specimens are contaminated with considerable amounts of the erythrocyte tartrate-resistant isoenzyme and should be rejected.

Enzymes as Cardiovascular Risk Markers

Several cells typical for atherosclerotic plaque secrete enzyme molecules that mirror plaque destabilization and rupture. Their concentrations in the circulation have been shown to be associated with future cardiovascular (CV) events. Enzymes in this category include lipoprotein-associated phospholipase A_2 and myeloperoxidase.

Lipoprotein-Associated Phospholipase A_2

Lipoprotein-associated phospholipase A_2 (Lp-PLA$_2$) (EC 3.1.1.47; platelet-activating factor [PAF] acetylhydrolase), a 45.4 kDa monomeric protein, is a member of the phospholipase A_2 superfamily. It is produced mainly by (1) monocytes, (2) macrophages, (3) T lymphocytes, and (4) mast cells and has been found to be upregulated in atherosclerotic lesions, especially in complex plaque prone to rupture. Lp-PLA$_2$ displays proatherogenic properties by promoting modification of oxidized LDLs.

Several prospective epidemiologic studies have reported an association between increased plasma concentrations of Lp-PLA$_2$ and future coronary and cerebrovascular events. The strength of association varies and is generally modest (hazard ratios <2). However, because some controversy persists as to its independence from LDL cholesterol, no clear recommendation on the clinical usefulness of Lp-PLA$_2$ can be given until definitive data document its incremental value above and beyond traditional CV risk factors. A manual ELISA method for Lp-PLA$_2$ mass concentration has received U.S. Food and Drug Administration (FDA) clearance for use as an aid in CV risk prediction. An immunoturbidimetric method that uses the same monoclonal antibodies has become commercially available, allowing the assay to be run on automated chemistry analyzers. It has been recommended that an Lp-PLA$_2$ concentration >200 µg/L be used as the threshold for higher risk of CV events.

EDTA plasma is the recommended sample for measuring Lp-PLA$_2$. Average stabilities are up to 4 hours at ambient temperature, 12 hours at 4 °C, and 6 months at −20 °C.

Myeloperoxidase

Myeloperoxidase (MPO) (EC 1.11.1.7; donor, hydrogen peroxide oxidoreductase) is a member of the heme peroxidase superfamily. It is a tetrameric hemoprotein (molecular weight 144 kDa) consisting of a pair of heavy (57 kDa) and light (15 kDa) chains. It is stored in azurophilic granules of polymorphonuclear neutrophils and monocytes-macrophages; when released (typically with inflammation), it catalyzes the conversion of chloride anion and hydrogen peroxide to hypochlorite (HOCl), a metal ion–independent chlorinating oxidant that possesses potent microbicidal activity. Thus it has a role in host defense against pathogens.

It is surprising to note that MPO also may have a causative role in plaque destabilization through its ability to activate latent metalloproteinases (MMPs). Infiltrating macrophages and neutrophils participate in the transformation of stable coronary artery plaques to unstable lesions with a thin fibrous cap through secretion of MMPs and MPO, which degrade the collagen layer that protects atheromas from erosion or abrupt rupture. As a result, plaques that have been highly infiltrated with macrophages have a thin fibrous cap and are vulnerable to erosion or rupture, converting late-stage atherosclerosis into acute CV events.

Several epidemiologic studies indicate that MPO concentrations in plasma may be an important CV risk marker, especially in patients with unstable coronary artery disease. However, uncertainty continues regarding the additional benefits conferred by MPO beyond those of standard cardiac biomarkers such as troponin.[8] Increased MPO is not likely to be specific for cardiac disease, as activation of neutrophils and macrophages can occur in any (1) infectious, (2) inflammatory, or (3) infiltrative disease process.

MPO mass assays based on sandwich ELISA methods have been developed and are commercially available. One has been approved by the FDA for use in conjunction with (1) clinical history, (2) electrocardiography, and (3) other cardiac biomarkers to evaluate patients presenting with chest pain at risk of major adverse cardiac events. This assay has been licensed to three other companies and has been made suitable for automated platforms or point-of-care instruments.

MPO is reasonably stable, and EDTA is the preferred anticoagulant. MPO is continuously released from white blood cells in heparinized blood, and a spurious increase in MPO concentrations is noted when blood collection tubes are left standing at room temperature. Higher MPO concentrations also have been found in serum as the result of leakage of enzyme from leukocytes during coagulation.

An MPO concentration of 640 pmol/L, which was reported as the URL, is not influenced by sex or age.

Review Questions

1. The enzyme that demonstrates highest serum activity in intrahepatic biliary obstruction and is also elevated in primary liver neoplasm is:
   a. alkaline phosphatase (ALP).
   b. creatine kinase (CK).
   c. amylase (AMY).
   d. γ-glutamyltransferase (GGT).
2. Activity of which of the following isoenzymes of CK is highest in the serum of healthy individuals?
   a. CK-MM
   b. CK-MB
   c. CK-BB
   d. CK-Mt
3. The serum enzyme that demonstrates an increase in activity 4 to 8 hours after an attack of acute pancreatitis, peaks at 24 hours, and then returns to normal within a week is:
   a. AMY.
   b. lipase (LPS).
   c. ALP.
   d. serum cholinesterase (CHE).
4. Which of the following enzymes catalyzes the reaction of glutamate and pyruvate to form 2-oxoglutarate and an amino acid?
   a. ALP
   b. Aspartate aminotransferase (AST)
   c. Alanine aminotransferase (ALT)
   d. CK
5. In the laboratory measurement of ALP, a chromogenic assay forms the basis of almost all current methods used for ALP analysis. The substrate in this assay is:
   a. acid phosphatase.
   b. 4-nitrophenyl phosphate.

c. p-nitroaniline.
   d. succinyldithiocholine.
6. Measurement of decreased activity of which of the following enzymes is used to determine possible insecticide poisoning?
   a. CK
   b. ALP
   c. ALT
   d. CHE
7. Children have higher ALP activity than healthy adults because:
   a. ALP leaks from osteoblasts during normal bone growth.
   b. developing hepatocytes produce excess ALP during normal growth.
   c. striated muscle contains the greatest activity of ALP, and children are more energetic than adults with concomitant release of excess ALP from muscle.
   d. the presence of ALP in the pancreas is elevated during childhood.
8. The isoenzyme of amylase that is synthesized by acinar cells of the pancreas and that remains elevated in most individuals for at least one week after the onset of pancreatitis is:
   a. S-AMY.
   b. macro-AMY.
   c. P-AMY.
   d. G-AMY.
9. Which of the following enzymes demonstrates an increase in activity with progressive Duchenne muscular dystrophy, followed by a decrease as muscle mass decreases?
   a. ALP
   b. ALT
   c. CHE
   d. CK
10. The oxidoreductase that is increased significantly during megaloblastic anemia is:
    a. lactate dehydrogenase.
    b. CK.
    c. ALP.
    d. acid phosphatase.

References

1. Ceriotti F, Henny J, Queraltó J, et al. Common reference intervals for aspartate aminotransferase (AST), alanine aminotransferase (ALT) and γ-glutamyl transferase (GGT) in serum: results from an IFCC multicenter study. Clin Chem Lab Med 2010;48:1593–601.
2. Forsmark CE, Baillie J. AGA Institute technical review on acute pancreatitis. Gastroenterology 2007;132:2022–44.
3. Huijgen HJ, Sanders GT, Koster RW, et al. The clinical value of lactate dehydrogenase in serum: a quantitative review. Eur J Clin Chem Clin Biochem 1997;35:569–75.
4. Infusino I, Schumann G, Ceriotti F, Panteghini M. Standardization in clinical enzymology: a challenge for the theory of metrological traceability. Clin Chem Lab Med 2010;48:301–7.
5. Junge W, Wortmann W, Wilke B, et al. Development and evaluation of assays for the determination of total and pancreatic amylase at 37 °C according to the principle recommended by the IFCC. Clin Biochem 2001;34:607–15.

6. Mosca A, Bonora R, Ceriotti F, et al. Assay using succinyldithiocholine as substrate: the method of choice for the measurement of cholinesterase catalytic activity in serum to diagnose succinylcholine sensitivity. Clin Chem Lab Med 2003;41:317–22.

7. Pagani F, Panteghini M. 5′-Nucleotidase in the detection of increased activity of the liver form of alkaline phosphatase in serum. Clin Chem 2001;47:2046–8.

8. Panteghini M. Cardiac troponin: is this biomarker ready for the prime time? Scand J Clin Lab Invest 2010;70(Suppl 242):66–72.

9. Panteghini M. The never-ending search of an acceptable compromise for pancreatic lipase standardisation. Clin Chem Lab Med 2012;50:419–21.

10. Panteghini M, Bonora R, Pagani F. Measurement of pancreatic lipase activity in serum by a kinetic colorimetric assay using a new chromogenic substrate. Ann Clin Biochem 2001;38:365–70.

11. Panteghini M, Ceriotti F, Pagani F, et al; for the Italian Society of Clinical Biochemistry and Clinical Molecular Biology (SIBioC) Working Group on Enzymes. Recommendations for the routine use of pancreatic amylase measurement instead of total amylase for the diagnosis and monitoring of pancreatic pathology. Clin Chem Lab Med 2002;40:97–100.

12. Schumann G, Aoki R, Ferrero CA, et al. IFCC primary reference procedures for the measurement of catalytic activity concentrations of enzymes at 37 °C. Part 8. Reference procedure for the measurement of catalytic concentration of α-amylase. Clin Chem Lab Med 2006;44:1146–55.

13. Schumann G, Bonora R, Ceriotti F, et al. IFCC primary reference procedures for the measurement of catalytic activity concentrations of enzymes at 37 °C. Part 4. Reference procedure for the measurement of catalytic concentration of alanine aminotransferase. Clin Chem Lab Med 2002;40:718–24.

14. Schumann G, Bonora R, Ceriotti F, et al. IFCC primary reference procedures for the measurement of catalytic activity concentrations of enzymes at 37 °C. Part 5. Reference procedure for the measurement of catalytic concentration of aspartate aminotransferase. Clin Chem Lab Med 2002;40:725–33.

15. Schumann G, Klauke R, Canalias F, et al. IFCC primary reference procedures for the measurement of catalytic activity concentrations of enzymes at 37 °C. Part 9. Reference procedure for the measurement of catalytic concentration of alkaline phosphatase. Clin Chem Lab Med 2011;49:1439–46.

16. Schumann G, Bonora R, Ceriotti F, et al. IFCC primary reference procedures for the measurement of catalytic activity concentrations of enzymes at 37 degrees C. Part 3. Reference procedure for the measurement of catalytic concentration of lactate dehydrogenase. Clin Chem Lab Med 2002;40:643–8.

17. Siekmann L, Bonora R, Burtis CA, et al. IFCC primary reference procedures for the measurement of catalytic activity concentrations of enzymes at 37 degrees C. International Federation of Clinical Chemistry and Laboratory Medicine. Part 7. Certification of four reference materials for the determination of enzymatic activity of gamma-glutamyltransferase, lactate dehydrogenase, alanine aminotransferase and creatine kinase accord. Clin Chem Lab Med 2002;40:739–45.

Tumor Markers and Cancer Genes

Lori J. Sokoll, Ph.D., F.A.C.B., Alex J. Rai, Ph.D., D.A.B.C.C., F.A.C.B., and Daniel W. Chan, Ph.D., D.A.B.C.C., F.A.C.B.

Objectives

1. Define the following terms:

Cancer	Mucin
Carbohydrate-related marker	Oncofetal antigen
Carcinogen	Oncogene
Cathepsin	Proto-oncogene
Ectopic syndrome	Tumor marker
Metastasis	Tumor-suppressor gene
Microarray	

2. State the clinical utility of tumor marker assessment and list the properties of an ideal tumor marker; list the concerns associated with using tumor markers for cancer assessment.

3. For each of the following, state the purpose, the need for evaluation, and the way in which each is determined with regard to tumor marker analysis:

Marker distribution	Reference interval
Predictive value	Role in disease management

4. For each of the following classes of tumor markers, list examples and state the clinical applications, the specificity, and the analytical methodology used to assess each example:

Blood group antigens	Hormones
Carbohydrate marker	Oncofetal antigens
Circulating tumor cells	Proteins
Enzymes	Receptors
Genetic markers	

5. Compare oncogenes, proto-oncogenes, and tumor-suppressor genes in terms of normal function of these genes (if any), what cellular changes occur when the gene is altered, what diseases occur when the gene is altered, and how these genes are assessed in the clinical laboratory.

6. Evaluate and assess case studies related to tumor markers and tumor marker analysis.

Key Words and Definitions

Adenocarcinoma A carcinoma derived from glandular tissue.

Apha fetoprotein (AFP) A plasma protein produced by the fetal liver, yolk sac, and gastrointestinal tract; serum levels decline markedly by the age of one year but are again elevated in many hepatocellular carcinomas and teratocarcinomas and embryonal cell carcinomas.

Benign prostatic hyperplasia (BPH) A noncancerous enlargement of the prostate gland.

Blood group antigen Antigen containing a major carbohydrate component usually found on the surface of cells or secreted by cells.

Cancer A relative autonomous growth of tissue.

Cancer staging The process by which cancer is divided into groups of early and late disease; useful for prognosis and for guiding therapy.

Carbohydrate markers Carbohydrate-related tumor markers may be (1) antigens on the tumor cell surface or (2) secreted by the tumor cells.

Carcinoembryonic antigen (CEA) A glycoprotein secreted into the glycocalyx coating the luminal surface of gastrointestinal epithelia.

Carcinogen Any cancer-producing substance.

Carcinoma A malignant new growth made up of epithelial cells tending to infiltrate the surrounding tissues and give rise to metastases.

Chronic myelocytic leukemia (CML) Chronic leukemia characterized by granular leukocytes.

Cytokeratin One of the two types of keratin normally found in human tissue, constituting a group of proteins; these are normally found in keratin filaments.

Digital rectal examination (DRE) A technique used for the for early detection of prostate cancer. It is performed by inserting a gloved, lubricated finger into the rectum and feeling for abnormalities.

Ectopic syndrome Production of a hormone by nonendocrine cancerous tissue that normally does not produce the hormone (e.g., ACTH production by small-cell lung carcinoma).

Fluorescence in situ hybridization (FISH) An in situ hybridization technique in which DNA probes are labeled with fluorescent tags and hybridized to DNA to identify and localize specific sequences.

Key Words and Definitions—cont'd

Genetic Information Nondiscrimination Act of 2008 (GINA) Legislation enacted by the Congress of the United States that prohibits the use of genetic information in health insurance and employment.

Gleason Score A grading system used to help evaluate the prognosis of men with prostate cancer.

Glioma A malignant tumor of the glial tissue of the nervous system.

Immunoglobulin superfamily (IgSF) A large group of cell surface and soluble proteins that are involved in the recognition, binding, or adhesion processes of cells.

Lymphoma Any neoplastic disorder of the lymphoid tissue.

Medullary thyroid cancer (MTC) A slow-growing tumor associated with multiple endocrine neoplasia (MEN) syndromes.

Mesothelioma A tumor derived from mesothelial tissue (peritoneum, pleura, pericardium); both benign and malignant varieties exist. Malignant varieties are often the result of excessive exposure to asbestos.

Metastasis The spread of cancer from one part of the body to another.

Microarray-based genotyping A molecular technique used to simultaneously screen hundreds to thousands of genetic markers per individual.

Mucin A high-molecular-weight glycoprotein complex.

Multiple endocrine neoplasia (MEN) syndromes Three disorders affecting the thyroid and other hormonal (endocrine) glands.

Oncofetal antigen Protein produced during fetal life that decreases to low or undetectable levels after birth; reappears in some forms of cancer as the result of reactivation of genes in transformed malignant cells.

Oncogene A mutated normal cellular gene (proto-oncogene) that causes the malignant transformation of normal cells when activated.

Partin tables A statistical model developed by Alan W. Partin, M.D., Ph.D. at the Johns Hopkins University School of Medicine that show the probability that the cancer is confined to the prostate and likely to be cured with surgery.

Philadelphia chromosome An abnormality of chromosome 22 present in marrow cells of most patients with chronic granulocytic leukemia. It is generally a reciprocal translocation between chromosomes 9 and 22 that results in expression of a fusion gene (called *BCR-ABL*) that acts as an oncogene.

Prognosis A prediction of the future course and outcome of a patient's disease based on currently known indicators (e.g., age, sex, tumor stage, tumor marker level).

Receiver operating characteristic (ROC) curve A plot of sensitivity versus 1 minus specificity, or the true-positive rate versus the false-positive rate; it allows one to pinpoint the decision cut point at which optimal sensitivity and specificity can be achieved.

Survivin A protein that neutralizes caspase activity and thus inhibits apoptosis, expressed during the G_2/M phase of the cell cycle in many tumors but not in most normal differentiated adult tissues.

Tumor marker A substance produced by a tumor found in blood, body fluids, or tissue that may be used to predict the presence and size of the tumor and monitor its response to therapy.

Tumor-suppressor gene A gene involved in the regulation of cellular growth; loss of a tumor-suppressor gene has the potential to allow autonomous growth.

A **tumor marker** is a substance produced by a tumor or by the host in response to a tumor, which is used (1) to differentiate a tumor from normal tissue, or (2) to detect the presence of a tumor based on measurements in the blood or secretions.[3,12] Such substances are found in cells, tissues, or body fluids and are measured qualitatively or quantitatively by chemical, immunological, or molecular biological methods.

Morphologically, cancer tissue has been recognized by pathologists as resembling fetal tissue more than normal adult differentiated tissue. Tumors are graded according to their degree of differentiation as (1) well differentiated, (2) poorly differentiated, or (3) anaplastic (without form). Tumor markers are the biochemical or immunological counterparts of the differentiation state of the tumor. In general, some tumor markers represent re-expression of substances produced normally by embryogenically closely related tissue (Table 20-1).

Some tumor markers are associated with one type of cancer; others are seen in several cancer types. Many of the

TABLE 20-1 Expression of Oncodevelopmental Tumor Markers

Production of Tumor Markers by Various Tissues				
Marker	Normal Producing	Embryogenically Closely Related	Distantly Related	Unrelated
CEA	Colon	Stomach, liver, pancreas	Lung, breast	Lymphoma
AFP	Liver, yolk sac	Colon, stomach, pancreas	Lung	
CG	Placenta	Germinal tumors	Liver	Epidermal lung
Serotonin	Enteroendocrine	Adrenal carcinoid	Oat cell, lung	Epidermal lung

AFP, α-Fetoprotein; *CEA,* carcinoembryonic antigen; *CG,* human chorionic gonadotropin.
Modified from Sell S. Cancer markers. In: Moossa AR Schempff SC, Robson MC, eds. Comprehensive textbook of oncology, 2nd edition, volume 1. Baltimore: Williams & Wilkins, 1991:225-38.

better-known markers are also seen in noncancerous conditions. Consequently, these tumor markers are not diagnostic for cancer. However, it is thought that the concentration of tumor markers in blood reflects tumor activity and volume.

Clinically, an ideal tumor marker should be both specific for a given type of cancer and sensitive enough to detect small tumors for early diagnosis or during screening.[12] Unfortunately, few markers are specific for a single individual tumor (tumor-specific markers); most are found with different tumors of the same tissue type (tumor-associated markers). Tumor markers are present in greater quantities in cancer tissue or in blood from cancer patients than in benign tumors or in blood from healthy subjects. In practice, current tumor markers are most useful for evaluating the progression of disease after initial therapy and for monitoring subsequent treatment modalities.

This chapter begins with general discussions on (1) cancer, (2) clinical applications of tumor markers, (3) how the utility of tumor markers is evaluated, (4) clinical guidelines for the use of tumor markers,[1,10-13] and (5) how tumor markers are measured. Several clinically relevant tumor markers from each of these general categories are then discussed in detail: (1) enzymes, (2) hormones, (3) oncofetal antigens, (4) **carbohydrate markers**, (5) **blood group antigens**, (6) proteins, (7) receptors, and (8) genes and molecular tests.

Cancer

In 2013, the estimated number of new cancer cases (excluding skin cancer) was 1.66 million. Prostate cancer was the leader among men, and breast cancer was the leader in women, followed by cancer of the lung, colon-rectum, and bladder (men) or uterine corpus (women). After peak death rates from all cancers were reached in 1990 for men and 1991 for women, death rates decreased by 22.9% in men and by 15.3% in women from 1990/1991 to 2008. Death rate reductions in men from lung, prostate, and colorectal cancers accounted for 78% of the decrease, and in women breast and colorectal cancers accounted for 56% of the decrease. These trends support the conclusion that early detection and more effective treatment combined with prevention (e.g., decreasing smoking, improving diet) will reduce the mortality rate of cancer in the future.[6] The American Cancer Society (ACS) estimates that in 2013, 174,100 cancer deaths are expected to be caused by tobacco use, and one-third of cancer deaths will likely be related to (1) excess weight, (2) physical inactivity, and (3) poor nutrition.[2]

A simple definition of **cancer** is "a relatively autonomous growth of tissue." Other more detailed definitions exist and are continually being refined and new ones proposed. For example, the National Cancer Institute (http://www.cancer.gov/; accessed September 9, 2013) defines cancer as "a term used for diseases in which abnormal cells divide without control and are able to invade other tissues. Cancer cells can spread to other parts of the body through the blood and lymph systems." Common to all of the definitions is the concept of autonomous and abnormal cell growth. An understanding of the cause of this autonomous and abnormal growth would clearly facilitate the search for a cure.

Also of importance in the search for a cure to cancer is the determination of which **carcinogen** (any cancer producing agent) is responsible for any given cancer. For example, a carcinogen may be (1) physical (e.g., radiation), (2) chemical (e.g., a polycyclic hydrocarbon), or (3) biological (e.g., a virus). Exposure to such an agent may cause cancer by producing direct genotoxic effects on deoxyribonucleic acid (DNA) (e.g., as with radiation) or by increasing cell proliferation (e.g., by a hormone), or cancer may be caused in both ways (e.g., through the use of tobacco).

Advances in molecular genetics have resulted in a better understanding of the genesis of human cancer. The proliferation of normal cells is thought to be regulated by growth-promoting *oncogenes* and counterbalanced by growth-constraining **tumor-suppressor genes**. The development of cancer appears to involve the activation or the altered expression of oncogenes, or the loss or inactivation of a tumor-suppressor gene.

Early detection of cancer offers the best chance for cure, as the tumor is still small enough to be completely removed surgically. Unfortunately, most cancers do not produce symptoms until the tumors are too large to be removed surgically, or until cancerous cells have already spread to other tissue (metastasized).

Although other modes of therapy, such as administration of chemical toxins or irradiation, are effective in destroying most tumor cells, they usually are not curative. The few residual viable tumor cells are able to (1) proliferate, (2) develop resistance to further therapy, and (3) eventually cause death.

Clinical Applications

Potential uses of tumor markers are summarized in Table 20-2. In general, tumor markers may be used (1) for diagnosis, **prognosis**, and prediction; (2) for monitoring the effects of therapy; and (3) as targets for localization and therapy. Ideally, a tumor marker should be produced by tumor cells and should be detectable in body fluids. It should not be present in healthy people or in benign conditions. Therefore, it could be used in screening for the presence of cancer in asymptomatic individuals in the general population. Most tumor markers, however, are present in (1) normal, (2) benign, and (3) cancerous tissues and lack specificity. However, if the incidence of cancer is high among certain populations, screening could be feasible. An example is the use of α-fetoprotein (AFP) in screening for hepatocellular **carcinoma** in China and Alaska. Prostate-specific antigen (PSA) has been used in conjunction with **digital rectal examination (DRE)** for early detection of prostate cancer. Because of elevation of serum PSA in **benign prostatic hyperplasia (BPH)**, approaches such as PSA velocity and percent free PSA have been used to increase specificity of PSA and improve the detection of prostate cancer.

The clinical staging of cancer **cancer staging** is aided by quantification of the concentration of marker that is considered a reflection of the tumor burden. Marker concentration at the time of diagnosis may be used as a prognostic indicator of disease progression and patient survival. After successful initial treatment,

TABLE 20-2   Current Applications of Tumor Markers and Their Limitations

Application	Current Usefulness	Comments
Screening for cancer	Limited	1. For screening, you must have a marker that is elevated at early disease stages, when the disease is localized and potentially curable. Most circulating cancer markers (with the exception of PSA) are elevated notably only in the late stages of disease. Thus diagnostic sensitivity is usually low for early-stage disease. 2. With the exception of PSA, most cancer markers are not specific for a particular tissue, and elevations may be due to diseases of other tissue, including benign and inflammatory diseases. Thus diagnostic specificity may be low, leading to many false positives. In screening, there is a necessity for a definitive diagnostic method that will separate true positives from false positives. If this procedure is invasive (e.g., surgery) and/or expensive, patients will not accept it. 3. Screening, even if effective for early cancer diagnosis, must demonstrate benefit to the screened population in terms of survival or other clinical end points.
Diagnosing cancer	Limited	Same as above. Low diagnostic sensitivity and specificity. However, for selected subgroups of high-risk patients for whom the chance of cancer is high (high prevalence), tumor marker analysis may not aid the clinician in ordering more elaborate testing (e.g., imaging techniques, laparoscopic investigations).
Evaluating cancer prognosis	Limited	Most cancer markers have prognostic value, but their accuracy is not good enough to warrant specific therapeutic interventions. For example, higher preoperative concentrations of PSA are associated with capsular penetration, high Gleason score, positive surgical margins, and positive lymph node status, but the decision to treat with which of two different modalities (e.g., radical prostatectomy vs. nonsurgical approaches) cannot be made on the basis of tumor marker data alone. Same applies to many other cancers.
Predicting therapeutic response	Important	Despite the importance of using biomarkers in predicting response to specific therapies, very few known markers have such predictive power. These include the steroid hormone receptors for predicting response to antiestrogens and HERr-2/*neu* amplification for predicting response to Herceptin in breast cancer patients. More predictive markers are needed to individualize therapy and maximize clinical response.
Performing tumor staging	Limited	Same as for prognosis. The data are not good enough for accurate staging unless the value reflects tumor volume.
Detecting tumor recurrence or remission	Controversial	Despite the importance of using biomarkers to detect cancer relapse, current markers are limited by the following: 1. Lead time is short (weeks to a few months) and does not significantly affect outcome, even if therapy is instituted earlier. 2. Therapies for treating recurrent disease are not effective at present. 3. In certain groups of patients, biomarkers are not produced and do not detect relapses. 4. Sometimes biomarkers provide misleading information (e.g., clinical relapses occur without biomarker elevation, or biomarker is elevated nonspecifically, without progressive disease, leading to overtreatment or discontinuation of a current and successful treatment protocol).
Localizing tumor and directing radiotherapeutic agents	Limited	Only a few biomarkers are available for this application, and success is limited at present.
Monitoring the effectiveness of cancer therapy	Important	For patients with advanced disease who are treated with various modalities, it is important to know whether therapy works. In this regard, biomarkers usually provide information that is (1) readily interpretable, (2) more economical, (3) more sensitive, and (4) safer than radiological or invasive procedures. For certain cancers, this may facilitate increased enrollment of patients into therapeutic clinical trials.

Modified from Diamandis EP. Tumor markers: past, present, and future. In: Diamandis EP, Fritsche HA, Lilja H, et al, eds. Tumor markers: physiology, pathobiology, technology, and clinical application. Washington, DC: AACC Press, 2002:5.

such as surgery, the marker concentration should decrease. If the half-life after treatment is longer than the expected half-life, treatment has not been successful in removing the tumor. However, the magnitude of reduction may reflect the degree of success of treatment or the extent of disease involvement.

Targeted therapy in oncology is becoming more effective and is considered by many to be the therapeutic choice of the future. Tumor markers capable of guiding targeted therapy will improve therapeutic efficacy and will generate less toxicity. Examples in breast cancer are the estrogen and progesterone receptors for the selection of hormonal therapy, HER-2, and for the selection of breast cancer patients for trastuzumab (Herceptin) therapy; and Onco*type* DX (Genomic Health, Inc., Redwood City, Calif; http://www.genomichealth.com/; accessed on September 9, 2013) for the identification of patients who most likely will benefit from adjuvant tamoxifen or chemotherapy.

Most tumor marker concentrations correlate with effectiveness of treatment and responses to therapy. In breast cancer, the concentration of markers, such as CA 15-3 or CA 27.29, changes with treatment and with the clinical outcome of the patient. Concentrations usually (1) increase with progressive disease, (2) decrease with remission, and (3) do not change significantly with stable disease. In reality, tumor marker kinetics in the monitoring of cancer may be more complicated. Marker concentrations in response to treatment may show an initial delay before demonstrating the expected pattern of change.

In addition, antibodies to tumor markers labeled with a radioactive tag are used to localize the tumor masses (radioimmunoscintigraphy) or to provide direction for labeled antibodies to attack the tumor site. Examples include the use of radiolabeled antibodies to **carcinoembryonic antigen (CEA)** to localize colon tumors and the application of labeled antibodies against ferritin to target hepatocellular carcinoma. This approach is also used for treatment by allowing the antibody to bind to the tumor marker epitopes and kill the tumor cell with the dose of radioactivity.

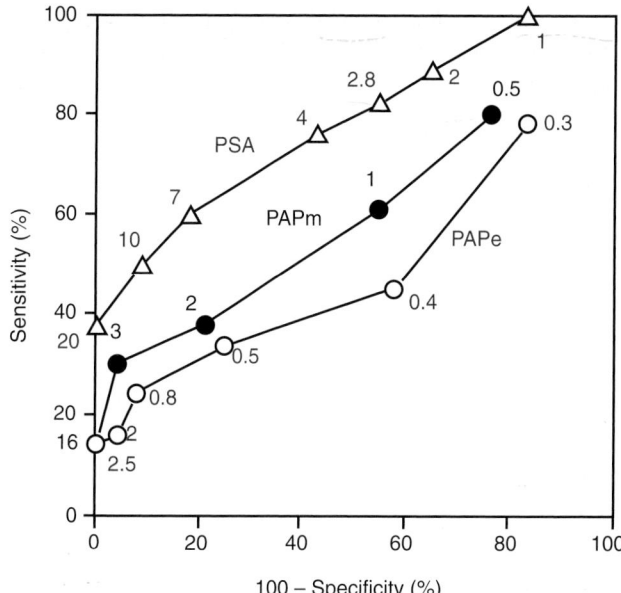

Figure 20-1 Receiver operating characteristic (ROC) curves for prostate-specific antigen (PSA), prostatic acid phosphatase by monoclonal immunoassay (PAPm), and enzymatic prostatic acid phosphatase (PAPe). Data for all 128 patients with prostatic disease are plotted, along with several quantitative decision cut points (as indicated in the figure) for each assay. Units are μg/L for PAPm and PSA, and U/L for PAPe. *(From Rock RC, Chan DW, Bruzek DJ, et al. Evaluation of a monoclonal immunoradiometric assay for prostate-specific antigen. Clin Chem 1987;33:2257-61.)*

Evaluating Clinical Utility

To evaluate the clinical usefulness of a tumor marker, it is necessary to (1) establish reference intervals, (2) calculate predictive values, (3) evaluate the distribution of marker concentrations, and (4) determine its role in disease management.

Reference Intervals

Reference intervals are obtained from a healthy population, preferably by using individuals of the same age and sex as those with the cancer of interest (see Chapter 5). In practice, reference intervals determined using healthy subjects are applicable to analytes with physiologically well-defined concentrations. However, for testing with relatively specific applications, such as the use of tumor markers in the diagnosis and management of cancer, a decision cut point may be more appropriate than the upper limit of the reference population. In most cases, using patients with benign disease as the nondisease group is more appropriate than using a healthy population. The decision cut point is determined using a predictive value model.

Predictive Value Models

The predictive value model includes the clinical sensitivity and specificity and the predictive value of a test (see Chapter 3). A useful approach to evaluating multiple tests for the same analyte or multiple markers for the same type of cancer is the **receiver operating characteristic (ROC)** curve. An example is shown in Figure 20-1.

Distribution of Markers

The distribution of tumor marker concentrations is usually shown as the percentage of patients with elevated concentrations as determined by using various cutoffs in (1) healthy, (2) benign, and (3) cancerous groups. When available, international staging criteria should be used to classify cancer patients. Diagnosis should be based on pathological findings.

In breast cancer, for example, normal women are used as the healthy population for comparison. Nonmalignant or benign groups are selected to include people with the most likely causes of marker elevation, including (1) benign liver disease, (2) breast disease, and (3) pregnancy. Non–breast metastatic cancer groups are selected to show the specificity of the marker by using (1) endometrial, (2) colon, (3) lung, (4) prostate, and (5) ovarian carcinoma, and (6) other patients.

Disease Management

Most tumor markers are used to monitor treatment and progression of cancer. Markers may be used to (1) determine the success of initial treatment (e.g., surgery, radiation), (2) detect the recurrence of cancer, and (3) monitor the effectiveness of the treatment modality.

When the effectiveness of cancer therapy is monitored, marker concentration should (1) increase with progression of cancer, (2) decrease with regression of cancer, and (3) remain constant in the presence of stable disease. With recurrence of cancer after successful initial treatment, the marker concentration may not fall within the expected time according to its half-life. It may fall to a steady concentration that is higher than normal, or it may fall within the reference interval of healthy individuals. A subsequent rise in the marker concentration suggests cancer recurrence.[1]

If therapy is given, changes in marker concentrations should reflect the clinical progression of the disease. "Progressive disease is defined by an increase in the marker concentration of at least 25%. Sampling should be repeated within 2 to 4 weeks for additional evidence. The sampling interval during therapy may depend on the type of tumor and should be related to clinical follow-up."

A decrease in marker concentration of at least 50% is indicative of partial remission, "with the concept that tumor load is related to the changes in serum tumor marker concentrations."

Clinical Guidelines

The diagnosis and staging of cancer involve a number of tools, including (1) physical examination, (2) imaging, and (3) laboratory studies. Application of these tools has resulted in several tumor markers that are used for (1) screening, (2) diagnosis, (3) staging, (4) prognosis, and (5) directing treatment modalities. However, not all tumor markers are appropriate for all uses, and not all cancers have established tumor markers. Therefore, each type of cancer and each tumor marker must be properly evaluated for use, and clinicians must be educated regarding proper use of tumor markers to conserve resources.

Several national and international groups have released guidelines on the selection and clinical use of tumor markers. These groups include the National Academy of Clinical Biochemistry (NACB), the European Group on Tumor Markers (EGTM), the American Cancer Society (ACS), the American Society for Clinical Oncology (ASCO), and others. Table 20-3 summarizes the recommendations of several of these groups and their websites.

Analytical Methods

Tumor markers are measured by a variety of analytical techniques, including enzyme assay (see Chapters 14 and 19); immunoassay (see Chapter 15); receptor assay and instrumental techniques such as chromatography (see Chapter 12); electrophoresis (see Chapter 11); mass spectrometry interfaced with liquid or gas chromatography (see Chapter 13); and microarrays.

Enzymes

Enzymes were one of the first groups of tumor markers identified. Their elevated activities were used to indicate the presence of cancer. Their measurement is relatively easy using spectrophotometric determination of enzymatic activities. With the introduction of radioimmunoassay (RIA) in the late 1950s, the mass of an enzyme could be measured as a protein antigen instead of its catalytic activity.

With few exceptions, an increase in the activity or mass of an enzyme or isoenzyme is not specific nor sensitive enough to be used to identify the type of cancer or the specific organs involved. Therefore, enzymes are most suitable as nonspecific tumor markers. Elevated enzymes may signal the presence of malignancy. Isoenzymes and multiple forms of enzymes may provide additional organ specificity.

Enzymes discussed in this chapter include (1) alkaline phosphatase, (2) lactate dehydrogenase, (3) neuron-specific

enolase, (4) prostatic acid phosphatase, (5) prostate-specific antigen, (6) the urokinase-plasminogen activator system, and (7) cathepsins.

Alkaline Phosphatase

(1) Liver, (2) bone, and (3) placenta are primary sources of alkaline phosphatase (ALP). The ALP in the sera of normal adults is derived primarily from the liver or biliary tract. Elevated ALP is seen in primary or secondary liver cancer. Quantification may be helpful in evaluating metastatic cancer with bone or liver involvement. Greatest elevations are seen in patients with osteoblastic lesions, such as those with prostatic cancer with bone metastases. Minimal elevations are seen in patients with osteolytic lesions, such as those with breast cancer with bone metastases.

In liver metastases, serum ALP shows a better correlation with the extent of liver involvement than do the results of other liver function tests. To determine the origin of elevated ALP, tests of other liver enzymes may be performed. Elevations in 5′-nucleotidase or γ-glutamyltransferase suggest that the elevated ALP is of liver origin. Determination of ALP isoenzymes may provide additional specificity. Other malignancies, such as (1) leukemia, (2) sarcoma, and (3) lymphoma complicated with hepatic infiltration, may also elevate alkaline phosphatase.

Placental alkaline phosphatase (PALP) is synthesized by the trophoblast and is elevated in the sera of pregnant women. PALP was first identified as the Regan isoenzyme in 1968 by Fishman and colleagues and was recognized as one of the first oncodevelopmental markers, along with α-fetoprotein and CEA. It is elevated in a variety of malignancies, including (1) ovarian, (2) lung, (3) trophoblastic, and (4) gastrointestinal cancers; as well as in (5) seminoma and (6) Hodgkin's disease.

Lactate Dehydrogenase

Lactate dehydrogenase (LD) is an enzyme in the glycolytic pathway that is released as the result of cell damage. Elevation of LD in malignancy is rather nonspecific. It has been demonstrated in a variety of cancers, including (1) liver cancer, (2) non-Hodgkin's lymphoma, (3) acute leukemia, (4) nonseminomatous germ cell testicular cancer, (5) seminoma, and (6) neuroblastoma; as well as in (7) other carcinomas, such as breast, colon, stomach, and lung cancer. Serum LD has been shown to correlate with tumor mass in solid tumors and provides a prognostic indicator for disease progression. Its value in monitoring of therapy, however, is limited. Serum markers are rarely considered for tumor staging; however, LD concentrations are used in the staging of testicular cancers and melanoma.

Neuron-Specific Enolase

Neuron-specific enolase (NSE) is the γ-subunit of the glycolytic enzyme phosphopyruvate hydrolase, which exists as a homodimer (γγ) and a heterodimer (αγ). The enzyme is found in neuronal tissue and in cells of the diffuse neuroendocrine system. NSE therefore is associated with tumors of neuroendocrine origin. NSE is released into the blood as a result

TABLE 20-3	Summary of Key Guideline Recommendations*			
Cancer Type	**NACB**	**ASCO**	**ACS**	**EGTM**
Breast	• ER and PR and HER-2 in all cancers for predicting response to therapy • CA 15-3/CA 27.29 and CEA for monitoring advanced disease • Tissue UPA/PAI-1 by ELISA for prognosis in node-negative breast cancer • Onco*type* DX for predicting recurrence in node-negative, ER-positive breast cancer patients receiving adjuvant tamoxifen	• Routine use of CA 15-3, CA 27.29, or CEA alone *not* recommended • Increasing CA 15-3, CA 27.29, and CEA may be used to suggest treatment failure • ER and PR determined for primary lesions. Steroid hormone receptors to be used to select patients for endocrine therapy • HER-2 overexpression or amplification in tissue may be used to select patients for Herceptin (trastuzumab) therapy • Tissue UPA/PAI-1 by ELISA for prognosis in node-negative breast cancer • Onco*type* DX for predicting recurrence/treatment response to tamoxifen in node-negative, ER-positive breast cancer	None	• Steroid receptors in tissue predicting response to hormone therapy • CEA and one *MUC1* gene–related protein in serum for prognosis, follow-up, and monitoring of therapy • HER-2/*neu* in tissue for predicting response to Herceptin (trastuzumab) in patients with advanced disease
Ovarian	CA 125 as an aid in diagnosis and for monitoring therapy, detecting recurrence, and determining prognosis	None	None	• CA 125 as an aid in diagnosis and prognosis, and in follow-up and monitoring of treatment • Risk of malignancy Index as an aid in diagnosis
Prostate	• PSA for early detection (with DRE), prognosis, and monitoring • % fPSA for PSA between 4 and 10 µg/L and negative DRE	None	PSA (DRE optional) screening and detection	• PSA for detection in symptomatic men • PSA in follow-up and monitoring of therapy
Germ cell	• AFP, CG, LD for diagnosis/case finding, staging/prognosis, recurrence, and monitoring of therapy in testicular tumors • AFP for differential diagnosis of NSGCT	None	None	• AFP, CG, LD, and PLAP† for case finding, staging, prognosis, follow-up, and monitoring of therapy • PLAP† for case finding
Colon	CEA for prognosis, postoperative surveillance, and monitoring of advanced disease	CEA for prognosis, detection of recurrence, and monitoring of therapy	None	CEA for prognosis and monitoring of therapy
Lung	CEA and CYFRA 21-1 in NSCLC and NSE and ProGRP in SCLC for differential diagnosis, postoperative surveillance, monitoring of therapy in advanced disease, and detection of recurrence; CYFRA 21-1 in NSCLC for prognosis	None	None	• NSE in SCLC, CYFRA 21-1, and SCC in NSCLC for differential diagnosis • CEA, CYFRA 21-1 in NSCLC, and NSE in SCLC for prognosis and for follow-up and monitoring of therapy

*"None" indicates that the relevant group has not yet considered this type of cancer.

†Placental alkaline phosphatase (PLAP) is used to monitor seminomas in nonsmokers only.

ACS, American Cancer Society; *ASCO,* American Society of Clinical Oncology; *EGTM,* European Group on Tumor Markers; *fPSA,* free PSA; *NACB,* National Academy of Clinical Biochemistry; *NSGCT,* nonseminomatous germ cell tumors; *tPSA,* total PSA.

From Sturgeon CM, Duffy MJ, Stenman UH, et al. National Academy of Clinical Biochemistry laboratory medicine practice guidelines for use of tumor markers in testicular, prostate, colorectal, breast, and ovarian cancers. Clin Chem 2008;54:e11-79; Harris L, Fritsche H, Mennel R, et al. American Society of Clinical Oncology 2007 update of recommendations for the use of tumor markers in breast cancer. J Clin Oncol 2007;25:5287-312; Locker GY, Hamilton S, Harris J, et al. ASCO 2006 update of recommendations for the use of tumor markers in gastrointestinal cancer. J Clin Oncol 2006;24:5313-27; Wolf AM, Wender RC, Etzioni RB, et al. American Cancer Society guideline for the early detection of prostate cancer: update 2010. CA Cancer J Clin 2010;60:70-98; http://www.egtm.eu/.

of cell lysis as opposed to secretion. NSE is also released into CSF with neuronal injury. NSE is found in tumors associated with neuroendocrine origin, including (1) small cell lung cancer (SCLC), (2) neuroblastoma, (3) pheochromocytoma, (4) carcinoid, (5) medullary carcinoma of the thyroid, (6) melanoma, and (7) pancreatic endocrine tumor.

Serum NSE concentrations have been measured by immunoassay. When a cutoff of 12.5 μg/mL is used, NSE has a clinical sensitivity of 80% in patients with SCLC and a clinical specificity of 80% to 90%. The NSE concentration appears to correlate with stage and provides a useful prognosis for disease progression. The value of NSE in detecting disease relapse has not been proved. Although the findings are mixed, NSE appears to be useful in monitoring chemotherapy and correlates with disease state. Immunostaining of tissue for NSE may provide the differential diagnosis between SCLC and other histological carcinoma types.

More than 90% of children with advanced neuroblastoma have been reported to have elevated serum concentrations of NSE. High concentrations of NSE are associated with poor prognosis, and concentrations seem to correlate with stage of disease.

Prostatic Acid Phosphatase

Prostatic acid phosphatase (PAP) used clinically has been replaced by PSA, as it not as sensitive as PSA for the detection of early cancer. Also, it is less likely to be elevated in BPH than is PSA. However, as an individual marker, PAP may be useful for disease management in the rare patient whose tumor does not secrete PSA, and it may prove useful when combined with other markers for improving prostate cancer detection or predicting recurrence after radical prostatectomy. The method of choice for the use of PAP is measurement of its enzymatic activity, although at present its mass is more commonly measured by immunoassay.

Prostate-Specific Antigen

Prostate-specific antigen (PSA) is a protein that is produced by the prostate gland. Functionally, PSA is a serine protease of the kallikrein family and has been widely used to screen men for prostate cancer. It is also used to monitor for recurrence after initial treatment and response to therapy.

Biochemistry

PSA is a single-chain glycoprotein that is 7% carbohydrate. It consists of 237 amino acid residues and four carbohydrate sidechains and has an MW of 28,430 Da. The complete gene encoding PSA, *KLK3*, has been sequenced and located on chromosome 19. It is produced exclusively by epithelial cells of the acini and ducts of the prostate gland. PSA is secreted into the lumina of the prostatic duct. In seminal fluid, PSA cleaves seminal vesicle–specific proteins into several low-molecular-weight proteins as part of the process of liquefaction of the seminal coagulum. Therefore, PSA possesses chymotrypsin-like and trypsin-like activity. The PSA promoter contains three androgen response elements and is activated by (1) androgens, (2) progestins, and (3) glucocorticoids.

Molecular Forms of Prostate-Specific Antigen

Most PSA is complexed with two protease inhibitors (1) α_1-antichymotrypsin (ACT) (MW, 100,000 Da) and (2) α_2-macroglobulin (AMG); a minor component is free PSA (MW, 28,430 Da). Most immunoassays measure both free and ACT-complexed PSA but not PSA-AMG, which is sterically inhibited. In human seminal fluid, approximately 60% to 70% of PSA is enzymatically active, and the remainder is inactive. Inactive forms of free PSA are composed of three distinct molecular forms: (1) BPSA, (2) pPSA, and (3) iPSA. BPSA is a degraded form of free PSA that contains two internal peptide bond cleavages at Lys 145 and Lys 183. In tissue, BPSA is relatively localized in the transition zone of the prostate and contributes to free PSA in BPH serum.

Physiological Properties

The metabolic clearance rate of PSA follows a two-compartment model, with initial half-lives of 1.2 and 0.75 hours for free PSA and total PSA and subsequent half-lives of 22 and 33 hours. Because of this relatively long half-life, at least 2 to 3 weeks may be necessary for the serum PSA to return to baseline concentrations after certain procedures, including (1) transrectal biopsy, (2) transurethral resection of the prostate, and (3) radical prostatectomy. Benign prostatic conditions, such as BPH and prostatitis, will also elevate PSA concentrations. Although the DRE typically causes no clinically important effects on serum PSA concentrations in most patients, in some it may lead to a twofold elevation. Inhibitors of 5α-reductase, such as finasteride, for the treatment of BPH cause a decrease in PSA concentrations of approximately 50%; therefore, results should be adjusted. Significant physiological variation in serum PSA concentrations (up to 30%) has been noted.

Clinical Applications

The measurement of PSA is used to detect and monitor treatment of prostate cancer.

Screening and Early Detection of Prostate Cancer

By itself, PSA testing is limited in the screening or detection of early prostate cancer. PSA is specific for prostatic tissue but not for prostatic cancer. Thus serum PSA is increased not only by prostate cancer but also by BPH and other conditions that affect the prostate. BPH is a common disease in men 50 years of age and older and studies have shown that PSA concentrations in patients with BPH are similar yet statistically different from those associated with early prostatic cancer. Unfortunately, the overlap of PSA concentrations between these two groups is so extensive, particularly between 4 and 10 μg/L, that selecting an optimum cutoff of PSA for the recommendation of a prostate biopsy is almost impossible. Results from the Prostate Cancer Prevention Trial showed the presence of prostate cancer over all ranges of PSA. The clinical sensitivity of PSA is 78% at the typically used cutoff of 4.0 μg/L. With lowering of the cutoff to 2.8 μg/L, sensitivity increases to 92%, whereas specificity decreases from 33% to 23%. Raising the cutoff to 8 μg/L improves the specificity to

90%. Cutoffs lower than 4 µg/L have been suggested by some, for example, the National Comprehensive Cancer Network (NCCN/ http://www.nccn.org/; accessed September 9, 2013)

In practice, the clinical utility of using serum PSA together with DRE is considered by many to be more accurate and sensitive than digital examination alone. However, DRE testing is considered optional according to recent guidelines promulgated by ACS.[9] Of note, the use of PSA measurements is now controversial with the recent recommendation against screening by the U.S. Preventive Services Task Force. The ACS emphasizes informed choice based on the use of decision-making tools and screening discussions between patients and physicians at age 50 for men at average risk with a 10-year life expectancy, and at earlier ages for men at high risk. Men at high risk include (1) black men and (2) men with a strong family history of prostate cancer. To improve the usefulness of PSA testing in detecting early prostate cancer (clinical sensitivity) and/or to spare unnecessary biopsies (clinical specificity), several approaches have been suggested.[11] One approach involves the use of age-adjusted reference intervals as follows: 0 to 2.5 µg/L for men aged 40 to 49 years, 0 to 3.5 µg/L for those 50 to 59 years, 0 to 4.5 µg/L for men 60 to 69 years, and 0 to 6.5 µg/L for those 70 to 79 years. With lowering of the upper limit of the reference interval, cancer will be detected more frequently in younger men, for whom potential cure by radical prostatectomy is most beneficial, although this may also allow improved detection of insignificant tumors. Increasing the upper limit for older men takes into account increases in PSA with aging due to BPH. However, 25% of men with a PSA between 2 and 4 µg/L may have cancer, similar to the 4 to 10 µg/L range; thus use of age-specific ranges may result in missed, clinically significant tumors in older men.

Another approach is to use PSA density (division of PSA concentration by prostatic volume as determined by transrectal ultrasonography) to account for increased PSA from larger prostates, as in men with BPH. Patients with PSA between 4 and 10 µg/L, a negative DRE result, and elevated PSA density (typical cutoff, 0.15) are at increased risk for prostate cancer. The third approach is to use PSA velocity (the rate of PSA increase as a function of time). It is recommended that velocity be calculated on the basis of at least three PSA results determined over at least 18 months. Increases in PSA in (1) health, (2) BPH, and (3) prostatic cancer appear to be different, with the highest rate (>0.75 µg/L/y) observed in patients with prostate cancer. Specificity is improved to 90% for BPH, and sensitivity is 72% for prostate cancer. The PSA velocity cutoff of 0.75 µg/L/y is recommended for men with a total PSA concentration of 4 to 10 µg/L; lower cutoffs of 0.35 to 0.4 µg/L/y are suggested when PSA concentrations are <4 µg/L.

An additional approach involves the use of molecular forms of PSA and free PSA. Percent free PSA, that is (free PSA/total PSA) × 100, has been used to improve the clinical sensitivity and specificity of detecting prostate cancer, particularly for patients in the diagnostic "gray" zone of PSA between 4 and 10 µg/L or between 2 and 20 µg/L.[8] Men with cancer have less circulating free PSA (≈10% to 30%) and more PSA bound to protease inhibitors (≈70% to 90%) compared with men without cancer. Percent free PSA results are interpreted by using a single cutoff or a continuum of values to determine the relative risk of prostate cancer in individual men. In biopsied men with a total PSA between 4 and 10 µg/L and a DRE nonsuspicious for cancer, sensitivity for cancer detection is 95% when a percent free PSA cutoff of ≤25% is used. If this same cutoff (>25%) is used, 20% of biopsied men with benign disease could be spared from biopsy. Percent free PSA may have particular usefulness in evaluating men who had a previous negative biopsy. A prostate health index that incorporates total, free, and [−2]proPSA has shown further improvement for prostate cancer detection in the 2 to 10 ng/mL PSA interval. Complexed PSA (cPSA) has also shown improved specificity over total PSA for prostate cancer detection in specific PSA subranges in a multicenter clinical trial.

Staging of Prostate Cancer

Concentrations of PSA has been found to correlate with clinical stages of prostate cancer PSA has also been found to correlate with (1) pathological stages of tumor extension and metastases, (2) cancer volume, and (3) cancer grade (Gleason score). Approximately 80% of men with PSA concentrations <4 µg/L at diagnosis have organ-confined disease; this decreases to 70% and 50% for PSA concentrations of 4 to 10 µg/L and >10 µg/L, respectively. Because significant overlap is seen in PSA concentrations among stages, PSA cannot be used to determine the pathological stage in a given individual. Therefore, PSA by itself should not be used to decide whether a patient has prostate cancer confined to the organ and therefore is a likely candidate for radical prostatectomy or other treatment, or for active surveillance. The concentration of PSA serves as a guide and is more useful in evaluating the presence of metastases. Patients with PSA concentrations less than 20 µg/L rarely have bone metastases. PSA contributes to the prediction of prostate cancer pathological stage as part of a nomogram (the **Partin tables**) that also includes clinical stage and biopsy **Gleason score**. Multivariate logistic regression is used to estimate (1) the probability of organ-confined disease, (2) extraprostatic extension, (3) seminal vesicle involvement, or (4) lymph node involvement.

Monitoring Treatment

The greatest clinical use of PSA involves monitoring of definitive treatment for prostate cancer. Such treatment includes (1) radical prostatectomy, (2) radiation therapy, and (3) antiandrogen therapy.

PSA is produced almost exclusively by prostatic tissue; thus after radical prostatectomy, the PSA concentration should fall to below the detection limit of the assay. This may require 2 to 3 weeks owing to the half-life of PSA. If the half-life is longer than usual, residual tumor may be present, although detectable PSA may also reflect benign prostatic tissue. Biochemical recurrence has been defined as two postprostatectomy PSA concentrations ≥0.2 µg/L. A cutoff of 0.4 µg/L is also used. Increasing PSA after radical prostatectomy is a strong indication of disease recurrence. The time between PSA concentration elevation and clinical evidence of recurrence (metastases) averages 8 years. PSA doubling time is also useful in assessing risk of progression to **metastasis**, with a low likelihood if the doubling time is greater than 10 to 15 months.

Unlike with surgery, normal prostatic tissue remains with external beam radiation treatment; therefore, PSA concentrations fall but do not become undetectable. The recent American Society for Therapeutic Radiology and Oncology (ASTRO) Phoenix guidelines (http://www.acr.org/; accessed September 9, 2013) define biochemical failure after radiotherapy, which also includes interstitial prostate brachytherapy, as a PSA rise of 2.0 μg/L or greater over the nadir.

Hormone therapy includes (1) bilateral orchiectomy, (2) treatment with luteinizing hormone–releasing hormone agonists, and (3) antiandrogen therapy. PSA testing is useful for predicting prognosis and monitoring treatment response to this type of therapy in patients with metastatic prostate cancer. The concentration of PSA is inversely proportional to the survival time and (1) increases with cancer progression, (2) decreases in remission, and (3) remains unchanged in stable disease. Androgen deprivation therapy may have a direct effect on PSA concentration that is independent of the antitumor effect. Production of PSA may be seen under the influence of androgenic hormones such as dihydrotestosterone. Thus PSA concentrations in patients who receive antiandrogen therapy may have a different meaning than they do in patients receiving other types of therapies.

Analytical Methods

Sandwich immunoassays using labels such as (1) enzymes, (2) fluorescence, or (3) chemiluminescence are used to measure PSA. Most of these assays are automated on commercially available immunoassay systems. Different assays and even the same assay with different lots of reagent, however, may produce different results. Such differences are due to (1) changes in assay calibration, (2) production lot variation, (3) assay reaction time, (4) reagent matrices, (5) assay limit of detection, and (6) imprecision. Antibodies may react with different PSA epitopes; therefore, some antibodies react dissimilarly with various molecular forms of PSA. Currently, most PSA assays are standardized to the Hybritech (Beckman Coulter, Inc., Brea, Calif; https://www.beckmancoulter.com/; accessed on September 9, 2013) PSA method or to standards introduced by the World Health Organization in 1999. The two international preparations consist of 100% free PSA (code 96/668) and 90% PSA/ACT complex, with 10% free PSA (code 96/670). Because of differences in the molar absorptivities used, PSA results from Hybritech standardized assays are approximately 20% higher than those obtained with WHO standardized assays.

One of the most valuable applications of PSA is the detection of residual or recurrent disease following radical prostatectomy. Traditionally, 0.1 μg/L has been used as the lower limit of detection, which was based on assay analytical characteristics as well as clinical need. Ultrasensitive PSA assays can be defined as those with a functional sensitivity (20% CV) of 0.01 μg/L or lower. One PSA assay has been labeled as a third-generation assay, and many automated assays now achieve limits of detection close to 0.001 μg/L.

Although cancer recurrence may be detected earlier, the effect on clinical management is unclear, and no assay has a specific FDA claim for earlier detection of recurrence.

Free PSA is not typically used as a single measurement but is expressed as a ratio or percentage of total PSA. Because of assay differences among manufacturers, total and free PSA should be measured in the same specimen using assays from the same diagnostics company. %fPSA is approved by the FDA as an aid in distinguishing prostate cancer from benign prostatic conditions in men aged 50 and older with a total PSA between 4 and 10 μg/L with a nonsuspicious DRE. The complexed PSA (cPSA) assay (Siemens Healthcare Diagnostics, Deerfield, Ill) measures PSA-ACT and other minor PSA complexes by rendering free PSA nonreactive with a free PSA-specific antibody. The two FDA intended uses are the same as for total PSA: (1) as an aid in the detection of prostate cancer in men aged 50 years or older in conjunction with DRE, and (2) for serial measurements to aid in the management of prostate cancer patients. A cPSA concentration of 3.2 μg/L is equivalent to a PSA cutoff of 4.0 μg/L, and a PSA threshold of 2.5 μg/L corresponds to a cPSA concentration of 2.2 μg/L.

The Urokinase-Plasminogen Activator System

The urokinase-plasminogen activator system consists of three main components: (1) the enzyme urokinase-plasminogen activator (uPA; a 53 kDa serine protease), (2) the uPA membrane-bound receptor (uPAR), and (3) the uPA inhibitors, PAI-1 and PAI-2.

The urokinase-plasminogen activator is produced as a single inactive polypeptide, which is activated by cleavage between lysine 158 and isoleucine 159. The cleavage is catalyzed by a number of proteases, including (1) cathepsin B, (2) cathepsin L, and (3) hK2. The active form of uPA consists of an A chain, which interacts with its cell surface receptor, uPAR, and a catalytically active B chain. The most thoroughly characterized activity of uPA is the conversion of plasminogen to active plasmin, which degrades extracellular matrix (ECM) components and activates matrix metalloproteinases (MMPs). These further degrade the ECM and activate and release specific growth factors (fibroblast growth factor [FGF]-2 and transforming growth factor [TGF]-β). The activity of uPA is controlled in vivo by two inhibitor molecules: PAI-1 and PAI-2. These not only act to inhibit uPA but also have a number of other functions, including (1) angiogenesis, (2) cell adhesion and migration, and (3) inhibition of apoptosis.

Historically, uPA was the first protease implicated in metastasis evaluated for prognostic value in humans. For example, breast cancer patients with high activity of uPA in their primary tumors have a poorer disease-free pattern than those patients with low uPA activity. The prognostic impact of uPA appears to be independent of other traditionally used markers, such as (1) axillary node status, (2) tumor size, (3) tumor grade, and (4) estrogen receptor (ER) status. In most studies, uPA is a more potent predictor of overall survival than tumor size, tumor grade, or ER status, and is equally powerful as nodal status. ASCO has recommended uPA/PAI, measured by ELISA on 300 mg of breast cancer tissue, to determine prognosis in newly diagnosed node-negative patients; concentrations of both markers may aid in determining the benefit of chemotherapeutic treatment.

uPA has been used as a prognostic marker in breast cancer and has demonstrated utility in colorectal cancer. Preliminary studies have implicated uPA as a prognostic marker in (1) ovarian, (2) renal, (3) hepatocellular, (4) pancreatic, (5) urinary, (6) bladder, (7) lung (adenocarcinoma), and (8) cervical cancers, as well as (9) **gliomas**. High concentrations of uPA also correlate with aggressive disease in both gastric and esophageal cancers. Thus uPA may be useful as a general prognostic marker in cancer.

The original assay developed for uPA measured its catalytic activity. This assay has been replaced by enzyme-linked immunosorbent assay (ELISA), and several research and commercially available kits have been developed for detection of uPA and PAI-1 in tumor tissue. Generally, increased concentrations of uPA, PAI-1, or both indicate poor prognosis. A uPA concentration below 3 ng/mg total tissue and a PAI-1 below 14 ng/mg total tissue have a notably better prognosis.

Cathepsins

Cathepsins are lysosomal protease enzymes; cathepsins (1) B, (2) D, and (3) L have been investigated for their role in tumor development and progression.

Similar to other proteases, cathepsins are synthesized as high-molecular-weight precursors that require processing for activation. For example, cathepsin B (CB) is a thiol-dependent protease normally found in lysosomes; it is activated by cathepsin D (CD) and matrix metalloproteinases. Activated CB in turn activates uPA and specific metalloproteinases. Cathepsin L (CL) is similar in specificity to CB; however, it shows little activity toward small molecular substrates. Cathepsin D, similar to CB, is a lysosomal protease; however, CD belongs to the aspartyl group of proteases.

Expression and localization of CB appear to be altered in tumors relative to normal tissue. In tumor tissue, CB is associated with the plasma membrane or is secreted. Increased expression has been demonstrated in (1) breast, (2) colorectal, (3) gastric, (4) lung, and (5) prostate carcinomas, as well as in (6) gliomas, (7) melanomas, and (8) osteoclastomas, suggesting a link with tumor development and/or progression. Altered localization of CB has been seen in various tumor tissues, such as (1) colon, (2) carcinoma, (3) thyroid cancer, (4) glioma, and (5) breast epithelial tumor. Altered expression and localization are thought to be involved in tissue invasion through ECM degradation and growth promotion. ECM degradation occurs through activation of CB and other proteases, such as MMPs and uPA. In addition to ECM degradation, CB releases growth factors such as (1) basic fibroblast growth factor (bFGF), (2) insulin-like growth factor-1 (IGF-1), (3) epidermal growth factor (EGF), and (4) TGF-β associated with the ECM.

A limited number of studies have associated high values of CB in multiple tumor types with aggressive disease. All, with one exception, are retrospective studies with low numbers of patients. In one large study ($N = 1500$ patients), CB was shown

to be an independent prognostic marker for both relapse-free and overall survival in breast cancer patients; however, it is not as good a marker as uPA. Most data related to the prognostic value of CD are in relation to breast cancer; however, its usefulness in (1) squamous cell carcinoma (SCC) of the head and neck, (2) hepatocellular carcinoma, and (3) gastric **adenocarcinoma** has been investigated in limited studies.

Cathepsin concentrations are generally measured in tissue extracts by ELISA or directly in the tissues by immunohistochemistry.

Hormones

With the introduction of specific RIA methods for a particular hormone 50 years ago, hormones were used as tumor markers to monitor the treatment of cancer patients. This application has proved more useful with the introduction and use of monoclonal antibody-based immunoassays.

The production of hormones in cancer involves two separate routes. First, the endocrine tissue that normally produces it produces excess amounts of a hormone. Second, a hormone may be produced at a distant site by a nonendocrine tissue that normally does not produce the hormone. The latter condition is called **ectopic syndrome**. For example, the production of adrenocorticotropic hormone (ACTH) is normotropic by the pituitary and is ectopic by the small cell of the lung. Consequently, elevation of a given hormone is not diagnostic of a specific tumor because a hormone may be produced by a variety of cancers.

Multiple endocrine neoplasia (MEN) syndromes (MEN-1, MEN-2A, and MEN-2B) are familial disorders inherited in an autosomal dominant fashion that are manifested by both benign and malignant tumors. Various polypeptide hormones, such as (1) ACTH, (2) calcitonin, (3) gastrin, (4) glucagon, (5) insulin, (6) secretin, and (7) vasoactive intestinal polypeptide, may be produced by the pancreatic islet cell, by pituitary tumors found in MEN-1, and by **medullary thyroid cancer** found in MEN-2A and -2B, as well as in familial medullary thyroid cancer (FMTC), a variant of MEN-2A. Examples of hormones that are used as tumor markers are listed in Table 20-4. Of these, (1) ACTH, (2) calcitonin, and (3) human chorionic gonadotropin (CG) are discussed in greater detail in the following section.

Adrenocorticotropic Hormone

ACTH is a polypeptide hormone with 39 amino acids and an MW of 4500 Da that is produced by corticotropic cells of the anterior pituitary gland (see Chapter 40). In 1928, a patient who had the signs and symptoms of what is now known to be cortisol excess was described as having a small cell carcinoma of the lung. A small number of these carcinomas have been known to produce pro-ACTH, the precursor to ACTH. This precursor has (1) an MW of 22,000 Da, (2) 5% bioactivity, and (3) most of the immunoactivity of ACTH. Traditional RIA assays measure precursors pro-ACTH and pro-opiomelanocortin (POMC), as well as the intact molecule and ACTH fragments that may be beneficial for detection of

TABLE 20-4 Hormones as Tumor Markers

Hormone	Type of Cancer
ACTH	Cushing syndrome, lung (small cell)
Antidiuretic hormone	Lung (small cell), adrenal cortex, pancreatic, duodenal
Bombesin	Lung (small cell)
Calcitonin	Medullary thyroid
Gastrin	Glucagonoma
Growth hormone	Pituitary adenoma, renal, lung
CG	Embryonal, choriocarcinoma, testicular (nonseminoma)
Human placental lactogen	Trophoblastic, gonads, lung, breast
Neurophysins	Lung (small cell)
Parathyroid hormone	Liver, renal, breast, lung, various
Prolactin	Pituitary adenoma, renal, lung
Vasoactive intestinal peptide	Pancreas, bronchogenic, pheochromocytoma, neuroblastoma

ectopic ACTH-producing tumors, whereas reactivity of the immunometric assay depends on the antibodies used and may measure ACTH as well as its precursors.

Elevated plasma concentrations of ACTH could be the result of pituitary or ectopic production. A high concentration of ACTH (>200 ng/L) is suggestive of ectopic origin. Failure of dexamethasone to suppress cortisol is also indicative of ectopic production. About half of the ectopic production of ACTH is a result of small cell carcinoma of the lung. Other conditions that elevate ACTH concentrations have been reported, including (1) pancreatic, (2) breast, (3) gastric, and (4) colon cancer, and benign conditions, such as (1) chronic obstructive pulmonary disease, (2) mental depression, (3) obesity, (4) hypertension, (5) diabetes mellitus, and (7) stress. The value of ACTH in monitoring therapy is still unknown.

Calcitonin

Calcitonin is a polypeptide with 32 amino acids and an MW of about 3400 Da; it is produced by the C cells of the thyroid (see Chapter 39). Normally, calcitonin is secreted in response to increased serum calcium. It inhibits the release of calcium from bone and thus lowers the serum calcium concentration. The serum half-life is about 12 minutes. The concentration in healthy individuals is less than 0.1 µg/L. An elevated concentration is usually associated with medullary carcinoma of the thyroid.

Approximately 75% of medullary thyroid cancer (MTC) cases are sporadic, and 25% are familial. Most familial MEN-2A, MEN-2B, and FMTC cases are the result of mutations of the *RET* proto-oncogene, a receptor tyrosine kinase, and almost all develop MTC. Calcitonin is most useful for diagnosing sporadic MTC or for identifying the index case in familial MTC; genetic testing has supplanted calcitonin for screening family members of the index case. Calcitonin is also used for monitoring MTC. Provocative testing with intravenous administration of calcium and/or pentagastrin produces increased calcitonin concentrations and is used to increase the sensitivity and specificity of MTC detection. Microscopic

or occult malignancy has been detected in patients who have a negative radioisotopic scan and normal thyroid glands on physical examination.

In practice, calcitonin concentrations appear to correlate with indicators of the extent of disease, such as tumor volume and tumor involvement in local and distant metastases. Calcitonin is useful for monitoring treatment and detecting the recurrence of disease.

Calcitonin concentrations are also elevated in some patients with carcinoid tumors and cancers of the (1) lung, (2) breast, (3) kidney, and (4) liver. The usefulness of calcitonin as a tumor marker in these malignancies, however, has not been proved. Calcitonin elevation has been reported in other nonmalignant conditions, such as (1) pulmonary disease, (2) pancreatitis, (3) hyperparathyroidism, (4) pernicious anemia, (5) Paget's disease of bone, and (6) pregnancy.

Human Chorionic Gonadotropin (CG) HCG

Elevated CG concentrations are seen in (1) pregnancy, (2) trophoblastic disease, and (3) germ cell tumors. CG is a useful tumor marker for tumors of the placenta (trophoblastic tumors) and for some tumors of the testes. It is also useful for diagnosing and monitoring pregnancy (see Chapter 44).

Biochemistry

Human chorionic gonadotropin is a glycoprotein secreted by the syncytiotrophoblastic cells of the healthy placenta. It consists of two dissimilar α- and β-subunits and has an MW of 45,000 Da. The α-subunit is common to several other hormones such as (1) luteinizing hormone (LH), (2) follicle-stimulating hormone (FSH), and (3) thyroid-stimulating hormone (TSH). The β-subunit is unique to CG, and the 28 to 30 amino acids making up the carboxyl terminal are antigenically distinct. Additional serum forms, including hyperglycosylated (CGh) and nicked CG (CGn) and the urine form CGβ core fragment (CGβcf), have relevant clinical utility.

Production of the two CG subunits is under separate genetic control. Trophoblastic tumors of placental and germ cell origin primarily produce intact CG, and differential production of the subunits, primarily the free β-subunit, has been observed in nontrophoblastic cancer patients. CG assays with a detection limit <2 IU/L, cross-reactivity with LH <2%, and equimolar recognition of CG and CGβ (or a separate assay for CGβ) are desired for tumor marker use.

Clinical Applications

Patients with trophoblastic tumors typically have elevated concentrations of CG (>1 million IU/L). They are also elevated in 70% of those with nonseminomatous testicular germ cell tumors and less frequently in those with seminoma. Elevated serum concentrations of CG are found in 45% to 60% of (1) biliary and (2) pancreatic cancers and in 10% to 30% of many other cancers, including (3) bladder, (4) renal, (5) prostate, (6) liver, (7) colorectal, (8) non–small cell lung, (9) breast, and (10) head and neck cancers, as well as (11) hematological malignancies. Most neuroendocrine tumors produce CGβ, and carcinoid tumors produce CGα. Elevations have also

TABLE 20-5 Oncofetal Antigens as Tumor Markers

Name	Nature	Type of Cancer
AFP	Glycoprotein, 70 kDa, 4% CHO	Hepatocellular, germ cell (nonseminoma)
Oncofetal antigen	80 kDa	Colon
Carcinofetal ferritin	Glycoprotein, 600 kDa	Liver
CEA	Glycoprotein, 22 kDa, 50% CHO	Colorectal, gastrointestinal, pancreatic, lung, breast
Pancreatic oncofetal	Glycoprotein, 40 kDa	Pancreatic
Squamous cell antigen	Glycoprotein, 44 to 48 kDa	Cervical, lung, skin, head and neck (squamous)
Tennessee antigen	Glycoprotein, 100 kDa	Colon, gastrointestinal, bladder
Tissue polypeptide antigen	Cytokeratins 8, 18, 19	Various (breast, colorectal, ovarian, bladder)

CHO, Carbohydrate.

been reported in benign conditions such as (1) cirrhosis, (2) duodenal ulcer, and (3) inflammatory bowel disease.

In practice, CG is most useful for monitoring treatment and progression of trophoblastic disease. Concentrations of CG correlate with tumor volume. A patient with an initial CG concentration greater than 400,000 IU/L is considered at high risk for treatment failure. After surgical removal of the tumor, CG concentration is expected to decline. The normal half-life of serum CG is about 12 to 20 hours. Slowly decreasing or persistent concentrations of CG may indicate the presence of residual disease. During chemotherapy, weekly CG measurement is recommended. After remission is achieved, yearly CG measurement is recommended to detect relapse. The detection limit of the assay is important, because any residual CG activity may indicate the presence of a tumor.

In addition to its usefulness in identifying patients with trophoblastic tumor, CG together with AFP also is useful in detecting nonseminomatous testicular tumor. Its concentrations correlate with tumor volume and disease prognosis. The hyperglycosylated form of CG may aid in the early detection of new or recurrent active trophoblastic malignancy and may discriminate quiescent gestational trophoblastic disease from active gestational trophoblastic neoplasia/choriocarcinoma. Because CG does not cross the blood-brain barrier, the normal cerebrospinal fluid-to-serum ratio is 1:60. Higher concentrations in cerebrospinal fluid may indicate metastases to the brain. Furthermore, response to therapy for patients with central nervous system metastasis may be observed by monitoring the CSF CG concentration.

Analytical Methods

Measurement of serum CG improved greatly in the 1970s as assay specificity was improved by use of an antibody to the β-subunit of CG that had little cross-reactivity with other glycoprotein hormones. Currently, most CG assays use an immunometric ("sandwich") format. An CG assay measures the intact (whole) molecule only when an antibody for the α-subunit and an antibody for the β-subunit are used in the immunometric format. A total β-CG assay measures both intact CG and free β-subunits. As a tumor marker, a total β-CG assay is preferred because many cancer patients produce notable amounts of free β-subunit. World Health Organization (WHO) international reference reagents (IRRs)

have been developed for CG isoforms, including (1) intact CG, (2) nicked CG, (3) CGβ, (4) nicked CGβ, (5) CGβcf, and (6) CGα. Studies with these preparations have indicated that varying specificity of these variants in commercial CG assays contributes to methodological differences. To date, none of the commercially available CG assays have been approved by the U.S. Food and Drug Administration (FDA) for use as a tumor marker assay. Heterophile antibodies and antianimal antibodies such as human antimouse antibodies (HAMAs) are known to cause false-positive or false-negative results in immunoassays, including those for CG. Urine CG testing, among other approaches, helps to distinguish true positives from assay interference.

Oncofetal Antigens

Oncofetal antigens are proteins produced during fetal life. These proteins are present in high concentration in the sera of fetuses and decrease to low concentrations or disappear after birth. In cancer patients, these proteins often reappear, revealing that certain genes are reactivated as the result of the malignant transformation of cells.

Discovery of the oncofetal antigens AFP and CEA in the 1960s revolutionized the modern era of tumor markers. Oncofetal antigens that have been used as tumor markers are listed in Table 20-5.

α-Fetoprotein

AFP is a marker for hepatocellular and germ cell (nonseminoma) carcinoma. AFP was found first in the sera of mice with liver cancer and later in the sera of humans with hepatocellular carcinoma. It is a glycoprotein with a molecular mass of 70 kDa. It consists of a single polypeptide chain and is 4% carbohydrate. AFP is synthesized in large quantities during embryonic development by the fetal yolk sac and liver. It is one of the major proteins in the fetal circulation, but its maximum concentration is about 10% that of albumin. AFP is closely related both genetically and structurally to albumin and has extensive homologies in amino acid sequence. As albumin synthesis increases during later fetal development, AFP concentrations in fetal serum begin to decline. They finally reach the trace concentrations found in normal adults 18 months after birth.

Clinical Applications

The serum AFP concentration is less than 10 µg/L in healthy adults. The use of AFP for detecting fetuses with neural tube defects is discussed in Chapter 45. In addition to pregnancy, elevated concentrations of serum AFP are associated with benign liver conditions, such as hepatitis and cirrhosis. Most patients with these benign diseases (95%) have AFP concentrations less than 200 µg/L.

Except in the pregnant patient, AFP concentrations greater than 1000 µg/L are indicative of cancer. At these concentrations of AFP, about half of hepatocellular carcinomas may be detected. However, because the serum concentration of AFP correlates with the size of the tumor, detection of hepatocellular carcinoma is more useful at earlier stages, when the tumor is small enough to be resectable (<5 cm), than when the tumor is large. To detect small tumors, the cutoff for AFP is typically set at a low concentration; a cutoff point of 10 to 20 µg/L has been recommended. However, at this concentration, hepatitis and cirrhosis must be considered as possible causes of elevation. Screening for hepatocellular carcinoma has been instituted in high-incidence areas, such as (1) Africa, (2) China, (3) Taiwan, (4) Japan, and (5) Alaska.

AFP is also useful for determining prognosis and for monitoring therapy for hepatocellular carcinoma. The concentration of AFP is a prognostic indicator of survival. Elevated AFP concentrations (>10 µg/L) and serum bilirubin concentrations greater than 2 mg/dL are associated with a decreased survival time.

Differential binding of AFP to the lectin LCA forms the basis of the AFP-L3% test for hepatocellular carcinoma that was cleared by the FDA for clinical use in 2005. Total AFP has been separated into three glycoforms: (1) AFP-L1, (2) AFP-L2, and (3) AFP-L3, based on reactivity to LCA. The L1 fraction of total AFP is present in patients with chronic hepatitis and liver cirrhosis, and it constitutes the majority of total AFP in nonmalignant liver disease. AFP-L1 has low reactivity with LCA. AFP-L2 is mostly derived from yolk sac tumors and has an intermediate affinity to LCA. AFP-L3 is produced by cancer cells and has an additional α-1-6-fucose residue attached at the reducing terminus of N-acetylglucosamine. AFP-L3% is calculated as the proportion of measured AFP-L3 to total AFP.

The AFP-L3% test is indicated for use in risk assessment for the development of hepatocellular carcinoma in patients who have chronic liver disease. A cutoff of 10% is used, and those patients with chronic liver disease and an elevated AFP-L3% have a sevenfold increased risk of developing hepatocellular carcinoma within 21 months. The test is useful for early detection, particularly in the AFP range of 20 to 200 µg/L, as has been shown in patients with hepatitis C–related cirrhosis. In practice, although AFP-L3% is useful in detection and prognosis, it typically is used only when AFP concentrations are elevated.

The AFP concentration is a good indicator for use in monitoring therapy and the change in clinical status. Elevated AFP concentration after surgery may indicate incomplete removal of the tumor or the presence of metastasis. Falling or rising AFP concentration after therapy may reveal the success or failure of the treatment regimen. A notable increase in AFP concentration in patients considered free of metastatic tumor may indicate the development of metastasis.

The combination of measuring the concentration of both AFP and CG is useful in classifying and staging germ cell tumors. Germ cell tumors may be predominantly one type of cell or may be a mixture of (1) seminoma, (2) yolk sac, (3) choriocarcinomatous elements (embryonal carcinoma), and (4) teratoma. Serum concentrations of AFP are elevated in yolk sac tumors, whereas CG is elevated in choriocarcinoma. Both are elevated in embryonal carcinoma. In seminomas, AFP is not elevated, whereas CG is elevated in 10% to 30% of patients who have syncytiotrophoblastic cells in the tumor. Neither marker is elevated in teratoma. One or both of the markers are elevated in about 90% of patients with nonseminomatous testicular tumor. Elevations were noted in less than 20% of patients with stage I disease, in 50% to 80% with stage II disease, and in 90% to 100% with stage III disease. These markers correlate with tumor volume and the prognosis of disease.

The combined use of these markers is useful in monitoring patients with germ cell tumors: elevation of either marker indicates recurrence of disease or development of metastasis. The success of chemotherapy can be assessed by calculating the decrease in concentration of both markers using the half-lives of AFP (5 days) and CG (12 to 20 hours).

Analytical Methods

Serum AFP is determined by immunometric assay on many automated immunoassay systems. A reference material for AFP (First WHO International Standard [IS]) is available from the National Institute for Biological Standards and Control (NIBSC/ http://www.nibsc.org/; accessed September 9, 2013) in the United Kingdom. AFP is reported primarily in units of ng/mL (µg/L) and kIU/L. One international unit (IU) of AFP is equivalent to 1.21 ng. A detection limit of 1 ng/mL is recommended for clinical use. AFP-L3% is measured using a microfluidics-based instrument that utilizes immunochemical and electrophoretic techniques. (Wako Diagnostics, Richmond, Va; http://www.wakodiagnostics.com/; accessed on September 9, 2013).

Carcinoembryonic Antigen   CEA

CEA is a marker for (1) colorectal, (2) gastrointestinal, (3) lung, and (4) breast carcinoma. CEA was discovered by Gold and Freeman in 1965 and was known initially as the Gold "antigen." Rabbits were immunized with extracts of human colon cancer tissue, and the resultant antisera were absorbed with extracts of normal human colon. Some antisera reacted with the tumor extracts but not with the extracts of normal tissue. The antigen, which was also found in embryonic tissue, was named *carcinoembryonic antigen.*

Biochemistry

CEA is a glycoprotein with a molecular mass of 150 to 300 kDa; it contains 45% to 55% carbohydrate. It is a single polypeptide chain consisting of 641 amino acids, with lysine in the N-terminal position. The heterogeneity of CEA has been demonstrated with the use of isoelectric focusing electrophoresis to separate the variants.

CEA consists of a large family of related cell surface glycoproteins. CEA proteins are encoded by about 10 genes located on chromosome 19. Up to 36 different glycoproteins have been identified in the CEA family. The major proteins are CEA and nonspecific cross-reacting antigen (NCA). The domain structures of (1) CEA, (2) NCA 50, and (3) the heavy chain of IgG are very similar. Thus, CEA is part of the **immunoglobulin gene "superfamily."**

Clinical Applications

CEA is elevated in a number of cancers at varying percentages, such as (1) colorectal—70%, (2) lung—45%, (3) gastric—50%, (4) breast—40%, (5) pancreatic—55%, (6) ovarian—25%, and (7) uterine—40% carcinomas.

CEA testing may be useful as an adjunct to clinical staging. Persistently elevated concentrations that are 5 to 10 times the upper reference limit strongly suggest the presence of colon cancer but may be associated with other cancers. In colon cancer, CEA concentrations correlate with the stage of disease. High pretreatment CEA concentrations are associated with greater likelihood of developing metastasis.

After successful initial therapy, CEA concentrations decline. During remission, CEA concentrations are stable. Rising CEA concentrations may indicate recurrence of disease. The lead time from CEA elevation to clinical recurrence is about 5 months. A repeat laparotomy is performed to confirm the relapse, which is detected in 90% of cases. In monitoring metastatic colon cancer, CEA is useful for following patients throughout therapy and the clinical course of the disease.

CEA is also useful for monitoring (1) breast, (2) lung, (3) gastric, and (4) pancreatic carcinomas. In breast cancer, elevated CEA is associated with metastatic disease. Early or localized breast cancer does not show CEA elevation and CEA is less sensitive than CA 15-3 and CA 27.29. CEA is most useful for monitoring metastatic breast cancer during therapy and for detecting the development of bone or lung metastasis. An increasing serum CEA concentration may reflect treatment failure when measurable disease is not present. In lung cancer, CEA determination is helpful in diagnosing non–small cell lung carcinoma (>65% of patients have elevated CEA) and in monitoring disease.

Analytical Methods

As with AFP, most assays use the immunometric format for determination of serum CEA. Polyclonal and monoclonal antibodies and combinations of the two types have been used in CEA immunoassays.

In the healthy population, the upper limit of CEA is about 3 µg/L for nonsmokers and 5 µg/L for smokers. Because the concentration of CEA measured is method dependent, values should always be compared by using the same method. When methods are changed, all patients who are being monitored should be tested in parallel with the use of both old and new methods. CEA may be elevated in patients with benign conditions, such as cirrhosis (45%), pulmonary emphysema (30%), rectal polyps (5%), benign breast disease (15%), and ulcerative colitis (15%).

Cytokeratins

The **cytokeratins** are a group of approximately 20 proteins that make up the cytoskeletal intermediate filaments of epithelial cells and cells of epithelial origin. The cytokeratins are divided into two groups: type 1 is smaller and acidic, and type 2 is larger and neutral to basic. As discussed below, clinically useful members of this family are (1) tissue polypeptide antigen (TPA), (2) tissue polypeptide-specific antigen (TPS), and (3) cytokeratin 19 fragments (CYFRA 21-1).

Tissue Polypeptide Antigen

The discovery of TPA preceded that of AFP and CEA, but TPA is not a specific tumor marker. It was found later that TPA could be identified by antibodies that react with cytokeratins 8, 18, and 19. TPA is produced by both normal and cancerous cells. Elevated serum concentrations of TPA are related to the proliferative activity and turnover of cells, allowing it to be used as a proliferation marker. In pregnancy, TPA increases throughout gestation. After pregnancy, the concentration returns to normal after 5 days. TPA is also elevated in inflammatory disease and in cancer; thus it is not useful for diagnosis. In monitoring of metastatic disease, TPA is useful when combined with CEA and CA 15-3 in breast cancer, with CEA and CA 19-9 in colon cancer, and with CA 125 in ovarian cancer. TPA may be helpful in the differentiation of cholangiocarcinoma (in which TPA concentration is elevated) from hepatocellular carcinoma (in which TPA is not elevated).

Tissue Polypeptide-Specific Antigen

TPS is an antigenic site on cytokeratin 18 that is specifically recognized by the M3 monoclonal antibody. This epitope has been proposed as a specific marker of cell proliferation and is detectable in serum with the use of a specific immunoassay. TPS appears to correlate with proliferation activity of lung tumors, irrespective of histology and tumor volume, and TPS concentrations increase with advancing stage. Elevated concentrations of TPS correlate with a poorer outcome.

CYFRA 21-1

CYFRA 21-1 is elevated in all types of lung cancer, although it is most sensitive for non–small cell lung cancer, primarily SCC. Concentrations of CYFRA 21-1 positively correlate with advancing stage and are useful in monitoring the disease course and in providing postsurgical follow-up. In non–small cell lung cancer patients, CYFRA 21-1 has been shown to independently correlate with (1) decreased survival, (2) nodal status, and (3) tumor stage. Blood concentrations are not affected by smoking status and may be increased in (1) renal failure, (2) liver cirrhosis, and (3) benign pulmonary disease. CYFRA 21-1 immunoassays use two monoclonal antibodies—BM 19.21 and KS 19.1—to detect cytokeratin 19 fragments.

TABLE 20-6 Mucin Tumor Markers

Name	Antigen and Source	Antibody	Type of Cancer
CA 125	Glycoprotein, >200 kDa, OVCA 433	OC 125	Ovarian, endometrial
Episialin (MUC1)			
• CA 15-3	Glycoprotein, 400 kDa, membrane-enriched BRCA	DF3 and 115D8	Breast, ovarian
• CA 549	High-MW glycoprotein	BC4E549, BC4N154	Breast, ovarian
• CA 27.29	High-MW glycoprotein	B27.29	Breast
MCA	350 kDa glycoprotein	b-12	Breast, ovarian
DU-PAN-2	Mucin, 1000 kDa peptide epitope	DU-PAN-2	Pancreatic, ovarian, gastrointestinal, lung

BRCA, Breast cancer.

TABLE 20-7 Blood Group Antigen–Related Cancer Markers

Name	Antigen and Source	Antibody	Type of Cancer
CA 19-9	Sialylated Le^{xa}, SW-1116 colon CA	19-9	Pancreatic, gastrointestinal, hepatic
CA 19-5	Le^a and sialylated Le^{ag}	19-5	Gastrointestinal, pancreatic, ovarian
CA 50	Sialylated Le^a and afucosyl form	C50	Pancreatic, gastrointestinal, colon
CA 72-4	Sialylated Tn	B27.3, cc49	Ovarian, breast, gastrointestinal, colon
CA 242	Sialylated CHO	C242	Gastrointestinal, pancreatic

CHO, Carbohydrate.

Squamous Cell Carcinoma Antigen (SCCA)

SCCA is a glycoprotein previously referred to as *tumor-associated antigen 4*. Subfractions of SCCA have been separated by isoelectric electrophoretic focusing into neutral and acidic fractions. Molecular weights range from 42,000 to 48,000 Da. Both malignant and nonmalignant squamous cells have been shown to contain the neutral fraction, whereas the acidic fraction is found mainly in malignant cells. The acidic fraction is the one released into the blood circulation.

SCCA is elevated in a variety of SCCs, including those of the (1) cervix, (2) lung, (3) skin, (4) head, (5) neck, (6) digestive tract, (7) ovaries, and (8) urogenital tract. In general, the concentration of SCCA is proportional to advancing stages of cancer. It is not useful for screening because only a small percentage of patients with early stages of cancer show elevated serum SCCA concentrations. High pretreatment SCCA concentrations appear to be associated with a poor prognosis. SCCA is useful in detecting recurrence of cancer and in monitoring treatment and disease progression.

Healthy, nonpregnant women have SCC antigen concentrations below 1.5 µg/L. Serum SCC antigen concentrations may be elevated (>1.5 µg/L) in certain benign conditions, including (1) pulmonary infection, (2) skin disease, (3) renal failure, and (4) liver disease. SCC antigen is also present in saliva, sweat, and respiratory secretions.

Carbohydrate Markers

Carbohydrate-related tumor markers may be (1) antigens on the tumor cell surface, or (2) secreted by the tumor cells. Monoclonal antibodies against these antigens have been developed. These markers have been found to be clinically useful as tumor markers and tend to be more specific than naturally secreted markers, such as enzymes and hormones. Biochemically, they are high-molecular-weight **mucins** (Table 20-6) or blood group antigens (Table 20-7).

Mucins

CA 15-3 and CA 27.29 assays detect a high-molecular-weight glycoprotein mucin expressed by the mammary epithelium known as *episialin;* thus they are used as markers for breast carcinoma. Episialin, also known as polymorphic epithelial mucin (PEM), is a product of the *MUC1* gene and is a transmembrane protein with a 69 amino acid cellular domain and an extracellular domain of 20 amino acid tandem repeats. In breast cancer, *MUC1* is upregulated and glycosylation is decreased and incomplete, exposing epitopes on the core polypeptide background. Assays for CA 15-3 and CA 27.29 use different antibodies that detect overlapping epitopes on the episialin molecule.

Mucins discussed in greater detail below include (1) CA 15-3, (2) CA 27.29, and (3) CA 125.

CA 15-3

CA 15-3 is detected by a murine monoclonal antibody (MAb) DF3 produced against a membrane-enriched extract of a human breast cancer metastatic to liver. The antibody binds in the tandem repeat region of the peptide core and is carbohydrate independent. Another monoclonal antibody, 115D8, was developed against the human milk fat globule membrane. This antibody does not bind in the tandem repeat region and is carbohydrate dependent.

In healthy subjects, the upper limit of CA 15-3 concentrations is 25 kU/L. When this cutoff is used, 5.5% of normal individuals, 23% of patients with primary breast cancer, and 69% of those with metastatic breast cancer have elevated

CA 15-3 concentrations. Elevated CA 15-3 concentrations are also found in other malignancies, including pancreatic (80%), lung (71%), breast (69%), ovarian (64%), colorectal (63%), and liver (28%) cancers. CA 15-3 is also reported to be elevated in benign disease, including benign liver disease (42%) and benign breast disease (16%).

CA 15-3 should not be used to diagnose primary breast cancer because the incidence of elevation is fairly low (23%). It is most useful in monitoring therapy and disease progression in metastatic breast cancer patients. A significant change of at least 25% correlates with disease progression in 90% of patients, and regression is noted in 78%. No change is correlated with disease stability in 60%.

Two antibodies are used in CA 15-3 immunoassays. The MAb 115D8 is attached to a solid support, whereas MAb DF3 is labeled. Assays using alternative antibodies against the same common antigen are also available for clinical use.

CA 27.29

CA 27.29 is recognized by a monoclonal antibody, B27.29, which is produced against an antigen in ascites of patients with metastatic breast carcinoma. It has been approved by the FDA for clinical use for detecting recurrent breast cancer in patients with stage II or stage III disease and for monitoring response to therapy in patients with stage IV (metastatic) disease. The assay provides similar information to that used for CA 15-3.

Immunoassays for CA 27.29 immunoassay have both competitive and sandwich formats that incorporate the B27.29 monoclonal antibody. Assays that use alternative antibodies against the same common antigen are also available for clinical use.

CA 125

CA 125 is a marker for monitoring ovarian cancer. It is a high-molecular-mass (>200 kDa) glycoprotein recognized by the monoclonal antibody OC 125. It contains 24% carbohydrate and is expressed by epithelial ovarian tumors and other pathological and normal tissues of müllerian duct origin. The molecule has been cloned and designated CA 125/MUC 16. Its physiological function is unknown.

Bast and associates developed the MAb OC 125 using a cell line (OVCA 433) from a patient with a serous papillary cystadenocarcinoma of the ovary. The OC 125 clone was selected for its reactivity with the OVCA 433 cell line and for its lack of reactivity with a B-lymphocyte line from the same patient.

Clinical Applications

The primary FDA-indicated use for CA 125 is to monitor response to therapy in patients with epithelial ovarian cancer. The second FDA-indicated use is to detect residual or recurrent disease in patients who have undergone first-line therapy and would be considered for second-look procedures. However, second-look laparotomy is now considered controversial except for use in clinical trials, or when surgical findings would alter disease management. In a healthy population, the upper limit of CA 125 is 35 kU/L. CA 125 is elevated in nonovarian carcinoma, including (1) endometrial, (2) pancreatic, (3) lung, (4) breast, (5) colorectal, and (6) other gastrointestinal tumors. Also, CA

125 is useful for determining the prognosis of patients with endometrial carcinoma. It is elevated in women in the follicular phase of the menstrual cycle and with benign conditions such as (1) cirrhosis, (2) hepatitis, (3) endometriosis, (4) pericarditis, and (5) early pregnancy. It cannot be used to differentiate ovarian cancer from other malignancies. CA 125 is not useful in screening asymptomatic populations for ovarian cancer, but screening is recommended in at-risk women with a family history of hereditary ovarian cancer, in conjunction with pelvic examination and ultrasound testing. Strategies to improve the clinical usefulness of CA 125 for screening/early detection of ovarian cancer to achieve needed high sensitivity and very high specificity include (1) combining with transvaginal sonography, (2) assessing changes in concentrations measured over time, and (3) using multimarker panels.

In ovarian carcinoma, CA 125 is elevated in (1) 50% of patients with stage I disease, (2) 90% with stage II, and (3) more than 90% with stages III and IV. The concentration of CA 125 correlates with tumor size and staging. CA 125 is also useful in differentiating benign from malignant disease in patients with palpable ovarian masses. This differentiation is important because surgical intervention for malignant ovarian masses is far more extensive than that for benign masses. A preoperative CA 125 concentration less than 65 kU/L is associated with a significantly greater 5-year survival rate (42%) when compared with a concentration greater than 65 kU/L (5%). Postoperative CA 125 concentrations and rate of decline are also predictors of survival. The half-life of CA 125 is normally 4.8 days. A group of patients with a CA 125 half-life of 22 days responded poorly to chemotherapy as compared with another group with a CA 125 half-life of 9 days.

After chemotherapy, CA 125 concentrations provide an indication of disease prognosis. A decrease in the CA 125 concentration by a factor of 10 after the first cycle of chemotherapy is indicative of response. Persistent elevation of CA 125 concentration after three cycles of chemotherapy indicates a poor prognosis.

Analytical Methods

An immunoradiometric assay for CA 125 was first developed that and manufactured by Centocor, Inc. (now Fujirebio Diagnostics, http://www.fdi.com/; accessed on September 9, 2013); it incorporated the OC 125 antibody for both capture and detection, allowing recognition of multiple CA 125 determinants. A second-generation assay (CA 125II) typically uses the monoclonal antibody, M11, as the capture antibody and OC 125 as the conjugate antibody. Other FDA-cleared assays for CA 125, which employ antibodies other than the OC 125 and M11 antibodies, are available on automated immunoassay platforms. Results from different assays are not interchangeable, and individual patients should be monitored with a single assay.

Other Ovarian Cancer Biomarkers

Human epididymis protein 4 (HE4) and OVA1 (Vermillion, Inc., Austin, Tex) are other ovarian cancer markers discussed in the following section.

HE4

The gene for HE4, *Homo sapiens* epididymis specific, *WFDC2*, was initially discovered with the use of microarrays to be overexpressed in epididymal tissue and later in ovarian cancer tissue.[7] Tumor expression is histologically dependent, with most serous and endometrioid tumors expressing HE4 and only 50% clear cell and 0% mucinous tumors. The protein is characterized as part of the four-disulfide core protein family and contains whey acid protein domains (WAPs). These proteins typically are secreted and are protease inhibitors, although this function has not been ascribed to HE4; its physiological role is unknown and studies have shown that HE4 is not specific for ovarian tumors.

At the HE4 cutoff of 150 pMol/L, covering 95% of healthy women, 79% of women with ovarian cancer have elevated concentrations. HE4 is elevated in other cancers, including (1) breast—13%, (2) endometrial—26%, (3) gastrointestinal—16%, and (4) lung—42%, as well as in (5) benign gynecological—7% and (6) other benign disease—24%. The assay is FDA cleared for monitoring recurrence or progressive disease in patients with epithelial ovarian cancer. Results comparing HE4 and CA 125 to distinguish women with ovarian cancer from normal women or those with benign processes appear to depend on the population studied, although combining the two markers may allow more accurate prediction of cancer than use of the individual markers. An algorithm incorporating HE4 and CA 125 has been reported to successfully classify women with a pelvic mass as at high or low likelihood for malignancy at the time of surgery. This algorithm was accurate in classifying a high percentage (93.8%) of women with cancer as high risk. The algorithm, termed the Risk of Malignancy Index (ROMA has been cleared for use by the FDA. HE4 may also have usefulness as a marker in endometrial cancer.

HE4 is measured by an enzyme immunoassay, with 2H5 as the capture antibody and 3D8 as the detector antibody (Fujirebio Diagnostics; http://www.fdi.com/; accessed on September 9, 2013). This assay is not recommended for patients with mucinous or germ cell ovarian cancer.

OVA1

Based on the proteomics biomarker discovery approach using mass spectrometry, Zhang and colleagues[14] identified several proteins that, when combined with CA 125, provide diagnostic value for ovarian cancer as the OVA1 test. It is considered the first in vitro diagnostic multivariate index assay proteomic diagnostic for cancer (Vermillion, Inc.; http://www.vermillion.com/; accessed on September 9, 2013). The OVA1 test is a qualitative serum test that combines five immunoassay results—(1) CA 125, (2) prealbumin (transthyretin), (3) apolipoprotein A1 (apo A1), (4) transferrin (Tfr), and (5) β2M (beta-2-microglobulin)—into a single numerical score. Its use is indicated for women who meet the following criteria: (1) older than age 18, (2) ovarian adnexal mass present for which surgery is planned, and (3) not yet referred to an oncologist. The OVA1 test is an aid in further assessment of the likelihood that malignancy is present when the physician's independent clinical and radiological evaluation does not indicate

malignancy. The addition of OVA1 to the presurgical clinical assessment improved the sensitivity of predicting malignancy from 72% to 92% for non–gynecological oncologist (GO) patients and from 78% to 99% for GO patients.

Blood Group Antigens

Blood group carbohydrates identified by monoclonal antibodies that have been used as markers of cancer are listed in Table 20-7. CA 19-9 (sialylated Le^{xa}) is an example of blood group antigens used frequently for clinical purposes. It is a marker for gastrointestinal cancers and is used primarily in patients with pancreatic carcinoma. CA 19-9 has been approved by the FDA for quantitative measurement in serum and as an aid in monitoring pancreatic cancer patients.

The CA 19-9 carbohydrate antigen is sialylated lacto-*N*-fucopenteose II ganglioside; it is a sialylated derivative of the Le^a blood group antigen denoted as Le^{xa}. Expression of the antigen requires the Lewis gene product, 1,4-fucosyl transferase. CA 19-9 is synthesized by (1) normal human pancreatic and biliary ductular cells and by (2) gastric, (3) colon, (4) endometrial, and (5) salivary epithelia. In serum, it exists as a mucin—a high-molecular-mass (200 to 1000 kDa) glycoprotein complex. Patients who are genotypically Le^{a-b-} (about 5%) do not express CA 19-9.

The CA 19-9 upper reference limit is 37 kU/L, as determined from the 99th percentile of healthy subjects. This cutoff discriminates between pancreatic cancer and benign pancreatic disease with clinical sensitivities of 69% to 93% and clinical specificities of 76% to 99%. Elevated CA 19-9 concentrations (>37 kU/L) are found in patients with (1) pancreatic—80%, (2) hepatobiliary—67%, (3) gastric—40% to 50%, (4) hepatocellular—30% to 50%, (5) colorectal—30%, and (6) breast—15% cancers. Some patients (10% to 20%) with pancreatitis and other benign gastrointestinal diseases have elevated concentrations up to 120 kU/L. CA 19-9 is useful in monitoring (1) pancreatic, (2) colorectal, and (3) gastric cancers. CA 19-9 concentrations correlate with pancreatic cancer staging. At a cutoff of 37 kU/L, 67% of patients with resectable and 87% of those with unresectable pancreatic cancers have elevated concentrations. When the cutoff is raised to 1000 kU/L, 35% of patients with unresectable tumors and only 5% of those with resectable tumors have elevated CA 19-9 concentrations. CA 19-9 is also useful for establishing prognosis for pancreatic cancer at initial diagnosis, as concentrations have independent predictive value for determination of resectability and of overall survival. Elevated or increasing concentrations have been known to indicate recurrence 1 to 7 months before it is detected by radiographs or clinical findings. Unfortunately, early detection of relapse may not be useful because of the lack of effective therapy for pancreatic cancer.

Most diagnostics companies have developed a CA 19-9 immunoassay. Typically, the CA 19-9 antibody is used as both the capture and the signal antibody. Considerable differences among value assays have been noted, and assay results are not interchangeable for individual patients.

Proteins

Several proteins that have tumor marker potential are listed in Table 20-8. Included in this group of tumor markers are proteins that are not enzymes or hormones and are not high in carbohydrate content.

Immunoglobulin

Monoclonal immunoglobulin has been used as a marker for multiple myeloma for more than 100 years. Monoclonal paraproteins appear as sharp bands in the globulin region of serum electrophoretic patterns. More than 95% of patients with multiple myeloma have such an electrophoretic pattern. Appearance of nonmalignant monoclonal immunoglobulins increases with age, reaching 5% in patients older than 75 years. These nonmalignant monoclonal bands are usually lower in concentration than malignant bands and are not associated with Bence-Jones protein. Bence-Jones protein is a free monoclonal immunoglobulin light chain in the urine. The concentration of monoclonal immunoglobulin at initial diagnosis is a prognostic indicator of disease progression. During treatment, the serum concentration of urinary Bence-Jones protein may reflect the success of therapy. Lower concentrations are associated with more favorable outcomes. Serum paraproteins are discussed in Chapter 18.

Bladder Cancer Markers

It is estimated that 600,000 Americans are currently affected by bladder cancer, and approximately 70,000 new cases will be diagnosed each year. Symptoms are (1) intermittent hematuria, (2) voiding problems and (3) dysuria. The most common type of bladder cancer, transitional cell carcinoma (TCC), is treated on the basis of the extent of tumor invasion. Carcinoma in situ (stage Tis) and superficial bladder cancers (stages Ta and T1) occur on the epithelial lining and do not invade the muscle layer. Stage Ta tumors are confined to the mucosa, and stage T1 tumors superficially invade the lamina propria. Stage T2 tumors extend into the muscle layer, and T3 tumors invade beyond the muscle layer. Stage T4 tumors have metastasized to local nodes or distant organs.

Urinary Bladder Tumor Markers

Bladder cancer is detected through cystoscopy or cytology of shed cells. Noncellular tumor antigens present in urine, such as (1) NMP22, (2) complement factor-H (CFH), and (3) fibronectin, are used in a complementary manner with cystoscopy and cytology. Other markers have been evaluated as markers for bladder cancer, including (1) telomerase, (2) cytokeratins, and (3) **survivin**.

Two bladder cancer–related cellular tests that are fluorescence based have been cleared by the FDA. ImmunoCyt (Scimedx Corporation, Denville, NJ; http://www.scimedx.com/; accessed on September 9, 2013) uses three fluorescently labeled monoclonal antibodies and microscopy to identify bladder cancer markers on cells found in urine. This test appears most useful with cytology in identifying low-grade tumors. UroVysion (Abbott Molecular, Abbott Park, Ill; http://www.abbottdiagnostics.com/; accessed on September 9, 2013), a **fluorescence in situ hybridization (FISH)** technique, uses fluorescently labeled probes to detect aneuploidy (abnormal number of chromosomes) of chromosomes 3, 7, and 17, and deletion of the 9p21 locus that contains the tumor suppressor p16, which is the most common alteration seen in urothelial carcinoma.

Nuclear Matrix Protein (NMP22)

Nuclear matrix proteins (NMPs) make up the internal structure of the nucleus. Their function has been associated with regulating key reactions in the nucleus, such as DNA replication and RNA synthesis. NMPs released by the cancer cell may be different from those in normal healthy cell. In a multicenter study of 90 patients with 33 pathologically confirmed TCCs of the urinary tract, 70% of 33 recurrences had urinary NMP greater than 10 U/mL. Among patients with NMP less than 10 U/mL, 86% had no malignancy at subsequent cystoscopy.

An ELISA for the measurement of an NMP, called *nuclear mitotic apparatus protein (NuMa)* in urine, has been approved by the FDA for the management of patients with TCC of the urinary tract, to aid in diagnosis of symptomatic patients or those with risk factors, and to identify patients with recurrent

TABLE 20-8 Proteins as Tumor Markers

Name	Nature	Type of Cancer
β_2-Microglobulin	11 kDa	Multiple myeloma, B-cell lymphoma, chronic lymphocytic leukemia, Waldenström's macroglobulinemia
C-peptide	3.6 kDa	Insulinoma
Ferritin	450 kDa iron-binding protein	Liver, lung, breast, leukemia
HER-2/*neu*	97 to 115 kDa, 20% CHO	Breast
Immunoglobulin	160 to 900 kDa, 3% to 12% CHO	Multiple myeloma, lymphomas
Melanoma-associated antigen	90 to 240 kDa	Melanoma
Pancreas-associated antigen	100 kDa, 20% CHO	Pancreatic, stomach
Pregnancy-specific protein 1	10 kDa, 30% CHO	Trophoblastic, germ cell
Pro-gastrin releasing peptide	Amino acid residues 31 to 98	Small cell lung
Prothrombin precursor	Des-γ-carboxy prothrombin	Hepatocellular
Soluble mesothelin-related peptides	Mesothelin/megakaryocyte potentiating factor peptides	Mesothelioma, ovarian
Tumor-associated trypsin inhibitor	6 kDa polypeptide	Lung, gastrointestinal, ovarian

CHO, Carbohydrate.

TCC. This test, which is called NMP22, is manufactured by Alere North America, Inc. (Princeton, NJ; http://www.alere.com/; accessed on September 9, 2013). A qualitative, immunochromatographic point-of-care version of the test is available as an aid in monitoring patients with a history of bladder cancer.

Bladder Tumor–Associated (BTA) Analytes

A qualitative, lateral flow immunoassay for BTA analytes in urine, termed the BTA *stat* test, detects the antigen human complement factor H–related protein (hCFHrp), which is a variant of human complement factor H (hCFH). It functions in the alternative complement pathway by interacting with complement factor C3b to prevent cell lysis. Bladder tumor–associated antigen may allow tumor cells to evade the host immune system. A multicenter trial compared the BTA *stat* test with voided urine cytology studies in 499 patients undergoing surveillance cystoscopy for recurrent bladder cancer. The BTA *stat* test identified 40% of patients with positive cystoscopy results, and cytology detected 17%. A positive test may result in a higher degree of suspicion for recurrence. A quantitative test in ELISA format, BTA TRAK, is also available. Both tests have FDA-approved indications for use as an aid in conjunction with cystoscopy in the management of bladder cancer patients.

Soluble Mesothelin-Related Peptides (SMRPs)

Mesothelioma is a rare cancer of the mesothelial surfaces of the pleural and peritoneal cavities or the pericardium that is linked to asbestos exposure. Mesothelin is a cell surface glycoprotein expressed on mesothelial cells, and mesothelin fragments, which are soluble mesothelin-related peptides, are found in the circulation of patients with mesothelial tumor. An ELISA assay has been developed (Mesomark, Fujirebio Diagnostics; http://www.fdi.com/; accessed on September 9, 2013) that measures serum soluble molecules related to the mesothelin/megakaryocyte potentiating factor (MPF) family of proteins recognized by the monoclonal antibody OV569. The assay also incorporates the 4H3 monoclonal antibody. This test is approved by the FDA under the Humanitarian Device Exemption, which is used for medical devices for diseases affecting fewer than 4000 individuals a year; demonstration of effectiveness is not required. It is intended as an aid in monitoring patients who have been diagnosed with epithelioid mesothelioma. A cutoff of 1.5 nmol/L was derived from the 99th percentile of healthy subjects. In addition to patients with mesothelioma (52%), approximately 10% to 15% of patients with other cancers, such as (1) ovarian, (2) lung, (3) colon, and (4) pancreatic cancers, may have elevations in SMRP compared with 5% of individuals exposed to asbestos. SMRP increases with increasing stage of malignant pleural mesothelioma. With the use of ROC analysis, an AUC of 0.81 was obtained to distinguish malignant pleural mesothelioma patients ($n = 90$) from asbestos-exposed individuals ($n = 66$) with clinical sensitivity, specificity, and accuracy of 60%, 89%, and 73%, respectively, at a cutoff of 1.9 nmol/L. The AUC for distinguishing malignant pleural mesothelioma from lung cancer ($n = 170$) was 0.82.

Des-γ-Carboxy Prothrombin (PIVKA-II)

Des-γ-carboxy prothrombin (DCP), also called PIVKA-II (proteins induced by vitamin K absence or antagonism II), is an abnormal form of prothrombin and a tumor marker for hepatocellular carcinoma. Prothrombin is a vitamin K–dependent coagulation factor produced in the liver that undergoes post-translational modification in which the 10 glutamic acid (glu) residues in the N-terminus are carboxylated to form γ-carboxy glutamic acid (gla) that is functional. The γ-glutamyl carboxylase requires vitamin K as a cofactor, and in cases of dietary deficiency or antagonism, such as by warfarin, DCP is produced. Obstructive jaundice with an effect on vitamin K may result in increased DCP. In hepatocellular carcinoma, gene expression of the enzyme is defective, resulting in DCP.

DCP is most commonly used clinically for (1) early detection, (2) monitoring, and (3) detecting recurrence in countries with a high prevalence of hepatocellular carcinoma, such as Japan. When an ELISA was used to compare patients with hepatocellular carcinoma versus those with cirrhosis or chronic hepatitis, sensitivity for detection was 48% and specificity 96%. DCP and AFP are independent markers, and in a case control study of patients with hepatocellular carcinoma or cirrhosis, clinical sensitivity for cancer detection in early-stage disease increased to 78% compared with 53% for AFP alone and 61% for DCP alone. DCP correlates with tumor size, although it is less sensitive for detecting (1) small tumors, (2) tumor stage, and (3) prognosis. In the United States, the Wako DCP assay (http://www.wakodiagnostics.com/; accessed September 9, 2013) has been FDA cleared as an aid in the risk assessment of patients with chronic liver disease for progression of hepatocellular carcinoma. When this assay was used in a prospective study of 334 patients with hepatitis C virus (HCV) cirrhosis, the relative risk of developing hepatocellular carcinoma was 5.7 with a cutoff of 7.5 µg/L.

S-100 Proteins

The S-100 proteins constitute a group of at least 19 related calcium-binding proteins. All contain two high-affinity and selective EF-hand calcium-binding domains. Their physiological role is uncertain; however, some members have been associated with cancer progression, namely, (1) S-100A4, (2) S-100A2, (3) S-100A6, and (4) S-100β. S-100A4 is normally expressed in selected immune cells, with faint expression in (1) keratinocytes, (2) melanocytes, and (3) Langerhans' cells. It is not expressed in (1) breast, (2) colon, (3) thyroid, (4) lung, (5) kidney, or (6) pancreas. Expression of S-100A4 in (1) breast cancer, (2) esophageal-squamous carcinoma, and (3) gastric cancer correlates with a worse outcome and more aggressive disease and was shown to be an independent marker of prognosis in multivariate analysis. Lack of expression in normal tissue and expression in cancer tissue make it an excellent candidate for routine histological use as a cancer marker.

S-100β is routinely used as a diagnostic histological marker of melanoma and melanoma metastases. Measurement of serum concentrations of S-100β has been investigated for monitoring disease recurrence. In the absence of melanoma, serum S-100β concentrations are normally undetectable;

however, with recurrent disease, S-100β concentrations rise. With the use of an immunoassay, clinical sensitivity and specificity of 0.29 and 0.93, respectively, with diagnostic accuracy of 0.84, were obtained when a cutoff of 0.12 µg/L was used. S-100β is a more sensitive and specific marker for recurrent melanoma that is able to detect recurrence earlier than LD or alkaline phosphatase (traditional markers of melanoma recurrence). An automated assay is available on the LIAISON analyzer (DiaSorin, Inc., Stillwater, Minn; http://www.diasorin.com/; accessed on September 9, 2013).

Thyroglobulin and Antibodies

Thyroglobulin (Tg) is produced by the thyroid gland as the precursor to thyroid hormone (see Chapter 42). The primary use of Tg measurement is for monitoring patients with a diagnosis of differentiated thyroid cancer after thyroid gland ablation. Approximately two-thirds of these patients have an elevated preoperative Tg concentration. An elevated preoperative concentration of Tg confirms the tumor's ability to secrete Tg and validates the use of postoperative measurement of Tg to monitor for tumor recurrence. Postoperatively, the most sensitive time to detect residual tumor or metastasis is after TSH stimulation. In well-differentiated tumors, a tenfold increase in Tg concentrations is seen after TSH stimulation.

Antithyroglobulin antibodies have been proposed to monitor residual disease and/or recurrence. Serial anti-Tg measurements may be an independent prognostic indicator of therapy because an increase in anti-Tg antibodies may suggest recurrence of the tumor.

Immunometric assays (IMAs) and RIAs are the two main methods used for measurement of Tg (see Chapter 42). IMA assays provide the advantage of having a shorter incubation time and have been automated; however, they suffer from greater interferences. The main interferants in both assays are antithyroglobulin antibodies, which typically cause an underestimation of Tg concentrations in the IMA. Antithyroglobulin antibodies have been measured directly in all patients; if both IMA and RIA are used to measure Tg, a discordant result suggests an interference from antithyroglobulin antibodies.

Chromogranins

Chromogranins are a family of proteins that are major components of the secretory granules of most neuroendocrine cells. The granin family consists of three members: (1) chromogranin A (CgA); (2) chromogranin B (CgB); and (3) secretogranin II, III, IV, and V. Chromogranins are found in neuroendocrine cells throughout the body, including the neuronal cells of the central and peripheral nervous systems. Intracellularly located chromogranins have been suggested to play a role in the regulation of secretory granules. In addition, secreted chromogranins are proteolytically processed to form bioactive peptides. Chromogranin A has been the best studied of the chromogranins, has been shown to be widely expressed by neuroendocrine tissue, and is co-secreted by neuroendocrine cells, along with peptide hormones and neuropeptides. This wide distribution and co-secretion make it an excellent histochemical and plasma marker of neuroendocrine tumors.

Both CgA and CgB are useful in detecting various neuroendocrine tumors, including (1) carcinoid tumor, (2) pheochromocytoma, and (3) neuroblastoma. In most cases, CgA is produced at higher concentrations than CgB; however, in some cases, CgB is positive when CgA is negative; therefore, it is recommended that both should be measured. In the case of carcinoid tumor, foregut and midgut tumors are normally functional tumors producing serotonin. CgA is as specific for the detection of both foregut and midgut carcinoid tumors. Also, the serotonin metabolite 5-hydroxyindoleacetic acid (5-HIAA) is the preferred marker in hindgut tumors, which commonly are nonfunctional. Although nonfunctional tumors have lost the ability to secrete serotonin, they retain the ability to secrete chromogranins. For detection of pheochromocytomas, CgA is at least as sensitive and specific as plasma catecholamines or urinary metanephrines.

CgA is measured by immunoassay. Depending on the assay, polyclonal or monoclonal antibodies are used. Care must be taken in choosing an assay, however, because CgA and the other chromogranins are heavily processed after release, which may render them nondetectable by the assay and may produce false-negative results. Therefore, an assay that recognizes both intact and processed molecules should be considered.

Receptors

Various receptors have found use as tumor markers. They include (1) estrogen, (2) progesterone, and (3) epidermal growth factor receptors.

Estrogen and Progesterone Receptors

Estrogen (ERs) and progesterone (PRs) receptors are used in tumor markers as indicators of breast cancer for hormonal therapy. Patients with positive estrogen and progesterone receptors tend to respond to hormonal treatment. Those with negative receptors will be treated using other therapies, such as chemotherapy. Hormone receptors also serve as prognostic factors in breast cancer. Patients positive for hormone receptors tend to have a better prognosis.

Estrogen receptors and progesterone receptors are members of the nuclear steroid hormone receptor family and are involved in hormone-directed transcriptional activation. The general structure of nuclear steroid hormone receptors, including ERs and PRs, consists of a large N-terminal domain containing (1) transcriptional activation domains, (2) a DNA-binding domain, (3) a hinge region, and (4) the hormone-binding domain at the C-terminus. Both ERs and PRs are present in a large protein complex, and upon hormone binding, some members of the complex dissociate, and the receptors bind to their respective response elements and activate transcription.

Both estrogen and progesterone have at least two separate receptors. Estrogen has ERα and ERβ, which are transcribed from separate genes. ERα and ERβ show 96% and 58% homology in their DNA- and hormone-binding domains, respectively, with a more divergent sequence in the N-terminal region. Two forms of PR—PR-A and PR-B—also have been identified; both are transcribed from the same gene. PR-A lacks the first 165 amino acids of PR-B.

ERs and PRs are found in target tissue cells, such as (1) uterus, (2) pituitary gland, (3) hypothalamus, and (4) breast, and appear to be involved in tumor development and progression. Furthermore, ER status and PR status correlate with both prognosis and treatment response. For example, measurement of ER content in breast tumor tissue is useful in determining the probability of hormonal therapy and as a prognostic indicator. In addition, ERs and PRs are routinely measured in all newly diagnosed breast cancers. Among patients with carcinoma of the breast, 60% have tumors that are ER positive. ER-positive tumors are seven to eight times more likely to respond to endocrine therapy, such as tamoxifen. Ninety-five percent of patients with ER-negative tumors fail to respond. The greater the ER content of the tumor, the higher the response rate to endocrine therapy. As a prognostic indicator, ER positivity suggests a better 5-year outcome; however, after 5 years, ER-negative tumors have a better prognosis.

The PR assay is a useful adjunct to the assay of ERs. Because PR synthesis appears to be dependent on estrogen action, measurement of PR activity provides confirmation that all steps of estrogen action are intact. Indeed, metastatic breast cancer patients with both ER- and PR-positive tumors have a response rate of 75% to endocrine therapy, whereas those with ER-positive and PR-negative tumors have a 40% response rate. In addition, only 25% of ER-negative/PR-positive patients respond to endocrine therapy, whereas less than 5% of ER-negative/PR-negative patients respond.

Immunohistochemistry assay is used to measure steroid hormone receptors in breast tumor tissue specimens. In practice, the reader should note that the (1) classical quantitative biochemical method, (2) multiple-point dextran-coated (DCC) titration assay, and (3) enzyme immunoassays are obsolete. They have been replaced with immunohistochemical assays as they are simple and less expensive and use small amounts of tissue. In 2010, ASCO and the College of American Pathologists (CAP) collaborated to develop guidelines for estrogen and progesterone receptor analysis by immunohistochemistry in an effort to standardize and improve the quality of testing among laboratories.

Epidermal Growth Factor Receptor

The epidermal growth factor receptor (EGFR) is a prototype of a family of tyrosine kinase receptors. Natural ligands for the EGFR include epidermal growth factor and transforming growth factor-α. In cancerous tissue, these growth factors promote growth in both a paracrine and an autocrine fashion.

Several compounds have been developed that inhibit EGFR signaling by blocking ligand binding or inhibiting tyrosine kinase activity. Also, mutations in the *EGFR* gene that are predictive of sensitivity to these drugs have been identified; the primary example is that of the *L858R* mutation in EGFR. This information is useful because it allows for the appropriate selection of therapy for a subset of patients, as demonstrated in individuals with non–small cell lung cancer. The tumors of some patients undergoing this therapy eventually become resistant to this medication. It is interesting to note that these resistant tumors are characterized by a different mutation in the EGFR—the *T790M* mutation.

EGFR is identified in tissue by immunohistochemistry and FISH. Detection of the EGFR protein (HER1) in EGFR-expressing cells by immunohistochemistry has been approved by the FDA for use as a companion diagnostic to aid in identifying colorectal cancer patients for treatment with the EGFR inhibitors cetuximab and panitumumab. A genetic test for the *KRAS* gene mutation to determine which advanced colorectal cancer patients have the wild-type gene (mutation negative) is also FDA approved. Individuals with wild-type *KRAS* tumors are much more likely to benefit from monoclonal antibody treatments targeting the EGFR pathway than individuals whose tumor carries mutated *KRAS*. This is because the K-ras protein is downstream of the EGFR protein in a signaling pathway. Thus, if K-ras protein is mutated such that it is constitutively activated, treatment that blocks EGFR will not be effective, as K-ras will continue to send a signal that promotes growth and proliferation.

Circulating Tumor

Circulating tumor cells are also used as tumor markers.

A majority of all cancers are derived from epithelial cells. Under appropriate conditions, these cells break from the primary tumor and shed into the circulation. These circulating tumor cells (CTCs) are very rare (approximately 1 CTC per 5 to 10 million red blood cells and lymphocytes), but techniques are available that make it possible to (1) capture, (2) enrich, and (3) count them. Consequently, their quantification has been demonstrated to be an independent predictor of overall survival and progression-free survival in patients suffering from metastatic (1) breast, (2) colon, and (3) prostate cancers. This technology, as applied using the Veridex CellSearch platform (Veridex LLC, Raritan, NJ; https://www.cellsearchctc.com/; accessed September 9, 2013), is FDA approved for these applications.

The assay uses a combination of positive and negative selection methods to isolate circulating epithelial cells from whole blood. This allows rapid assessment of therapeutic response and hence adjustment of therapy as needed. For patients not responding to a particular line of therapy, alternative regimens have been prescribed, or dosages adjusted as needed.

The greatest demonstration of the use of this technology is seen in breast cancer patients. In metastatic breast or prostate cancer, a CTC count of five or more cells per 7.5 mL of blood is associated with a poor prognosis and is predictive of shorter progression-free survival and overall survival. The same is true in metastatic colorectal cancer with a CTC count of three or more cells per 7.5 mL of blood.

Genetic and Molecular Markers

Cancerous growth is an inheritable characteristic of cells that is thought to be the outcome of genetic changes. Multiple genetic alterations may be necessary for the transformation of a cell from a healthy state to a cancerous one and, finally, for metastatic spread. Therefore, evaluation of chromosomal changes is now being used to establish cancer risk and to screen for cancer (see Chapters 47 and 49).

Classes of genes implicated in the development of cancer are (1) **oncogenes** (cell *activation* genes) and (2) tumor-suppressor genes (genes involved in the *recognition* and *repair* of damaged DNA; Table 20-9). Oncogenes are derived from proto-oncogenes that may be activated by dominant mutations, such as (1) point mutations, (2) insertions, (3) deletions, (4) translocations, or (5) inversions. Most oncogenes code for proteins that function at some stage of activation of cells for proliferation, and their activation leads to cell division. Many oncogenes are associated with hematological malignancies such as leukemia[5] and solid tumors. Tumor-suppressor genes, the other class of cancer-associated genes, have been isolated mostly from solid tumors. The oncogenicity of tumor-suppressor genes is derived from loss of the gene rather than from their activation, as with oncogenes. Deletion or monosomy (the presence of only one chromosome) may lead to loss of tumor suppressor genes. The major tumor suppressor gene, *p53*, functions to repair damaged DNA through apoptosis (programmed cell death). Repair is mediated by activation of the production of p21, which blocks the cell cycle in late G_1 to allow repair to take place. Loss of function of this gene caused by loss or mutation may result in an impaired DNA repair process, leading to the development of tumorigenesis.

Advances in technologies (both hardware and software), coupled with robust expansion of nucleotide and protein databases, have led to the development of new tools that allow the simultaneous interrogation of hundreds to thousands of variables simultaneously. In particular, microarray-based analyses are at the forefront of translation to clinical practice.

Oncogenes

Proto-oncogenes are normal cellular genes that are similar to tumor virus genes. Activation of proto-oncogenes is found to be associated with cancer. These genes code for products that are involved in normal cellular processes, such as growth factor signaling pathways. Overexpression of the oncogene will lead to abnormal cell growth, resulting in malignancy. Of the many proto-oncogenes recognized, only a few have been shown to be useful tumor markers. A detailed description of three representative oncogenes is presented next: (1) *RAS* genes, (2) *HER2,* and (3) *BCR/ABL*. Others are listed in Table 20-9.

RAS Genes

The *RAS* genes were first identified as being responsible for the tumorigenic properties of the Harvey (H-*ras*) and Kirsten (K-*ras*) sarcoma viruses, which produce tumors in animals, and they provided the first evidence that cellular counterparts in human cells might be involved in the development of human tumors. RAS proteins coded for by the *RAS* genes are located at the inner face of the plasma membrane, as well as

TABLE 20-9 Oncogenes and Tumor-Suppressor Genes

Oncogenes	Cellular Function	Representative Cancers*	Protein Function/Comments
RAS	Proliferation, cell growth	N-*ras:* AML, neuroblastoma K-*ras:* leukemia, lymphoma	GTP/GDP binding protein, p21
c-myc	Transcriptional regulation	B- and T- cell lymphoma, SCLC	Master transcriptional regulator: induces expression of ≈15% of all genes
HER2 (c-erbB2)	Receptor tyrosine kinase	Breast, ovarian, GI tumors	Plasma membrane receptor, p185; ligand binding induces dimerization
BCL2	Apoptosis	Leukemia, lymphoma	Two isoforms; antiapoptotic regulatory protein; higher protein levels in some cancers
BCR/ABL	Signal transduction protein	CML, RCC, GIST	Tyrosine kinase fusion protein resulting from Philadelphia chromosome reciprocal translocation, p185/p210

Tumor Suppressors	Cellular Function	Representative Cancers*	Chromosomal Locus
Rb	Cell cycle regulation	Retinoblastoma, osteosarcoma, SCLC	13q14
TP53	Transcriptional regulation, apoptosis	Breast, colorectal, lung, liver, renal, bladder, sarcoma	17p13
p21(WAF1/CIP1)	Cell cycle progression	Breast, pancreatic, and multiple cancers	6p21
APC	Cell-cell interaction	Colorectal	5q21
NF1	Proliferation and cell growth, negative regulator	von Recklinghausen's disease; colorectal, melanoma, neuroblastoma	17q
WT1	Transcriptional regulation	Wilms' tumor	11p13
nm23	Metastasis-related functions	(Multiple) metastatic human cancers	17q21
BRCA1/2	Transcriptional regulation, DNA repair	Breast cancer	BRCA1: 17q; BRCA2: 13q12.3
DCC	Membrane protein of IgG superfamily	Colorectal	18q21
PTEN	Lipid kinase	Glioblastoma, endometrial, prostate	10q23

*This list is not meant to be exhaustive but merely to provide representative examples.

in other internal cellular membranes. They bind to guanine nucleotides and function as molecular switches that regulate mitogenic signals from growth factors to the nucleus via signal transduction pathways. The ras proteins are activated in association with protein-tyrosine kinase receptors and are required for growth factor proliferation or differentiation of a number of cell types.

In oncology, the most important human RAS genes are *NRAS* and *KRAS*. The *NRAS* gene is found on the short arm of human chromosome 1. Changes in *NRAS* appear to be the critical step in carcinogenesis. The mutated *NRAS* gene is found in neuroblastomas and acute myeloid leukemia. In addition, it is present in (1) 95% of pancreatic cancers, (2) 40% of colon cancers, and (3) 30% of lung and bladder cancers, and in lower percentages in other tumors. The *KRAS* gene is on the short arm of chromosome 12. A single point mutation at codon 12 changes a coded amino acid from glycine to valine in the p21 protein. This mutation is by far the most frequently found in cancer, but other mutations have also been demonstrated, including those at codons 13 and 61. *KRAS* mutations appear to correlate with poor prognosis and shorter disease-free survival in patients with adenocarcinoma of the lung and endometrial carcinoma. Activated *ras* is detected by expression of the *RAS* gene product, p21, in cancer tissue. By immunohistochemistry, the *ras* protein is found not only in about 40% of colon cancers, but also in colon polyps believed to be premalignant. Higher relative intensity of staining for p21-*ras* may differentiate malignant from normal tissues or benign lesions in (1) breast, (2) pancreas, (3) stomach, (4) lung, (5) uterus, or (6) thyroid tissues. Expression in tissue appears to correlate with stage or grade of the tumor, but p21-*ras* may also be seen in some normal tissue, and other studies show no significant difference between benign and malignant tumors. Use of the p21 protein as a tumor marker in tissue or serum is not well established. Mutations of *RAS* oncogenes have been detected in DNA in the stool of symptomatic and asymptomatic patients with colorectal tumors, suggesting a novel, noninvasive paradigm for population screening. Several studies have underscored the importance of *KRAS* mutations in therapeutic regimen selection. Individuals with a diagnosis of metastatic colorectal cancer with wild-type *KRAS* tumors are much more likely to benefit from monoclonal antibody treatments targeting the EGFR pathway, such as cetuximab and panitumumab, than individuals whose tumor carries mutated *KRAS* (at codons 12 and 13). Thus, *KRAS* mutation testing is advocated in patients suffering from metastatic colorectal carcinoma who are candidates for anti-EGFR treatments. Further, if the tumor tests positive for mutation at codon 12 or 13, the patient should not receive anti-EGFR treatment.

HER2

The HER2/*neu* gene (also known as c-erbB-2, symbol *ERBB2*) is named for its association with neural tumors (*neu*). The *ERBB2* gene codes for a 185 kDa transmembrane protein expressed on epithelial cells and belongs to the EGF family of tyrosine kinase receptors. The EGF family includes four members: (1) *EGFR* (also known as *ErbB1/HER-1*), (2) *ERBB2*

(HER2 or HER2/*neu*), (3) *ERBB3*, and (4) *ERBB4*. Members of the EGF family of receptors have the same overall structure consisting of (1) an extracellular ligand-binding domain (ECD), (2) a single transmembrane domain, and (3) an intracellular tyrosine kinase domain. The extracellular domain undergoes proteolytic cleavage by metalloproteases, releasing the ECD (known as p105) into the blood, which is then detected. All are involved in (1) cell proliferation, (2) differentiation, and (3) survival. HER2 is normally expressed on the epithelia of numerous organs, including (1) lung, (2) bladder, (3) pancreas, (4) breast, and (5) prostate, and has been found to be elevated in cancer cells.

Amplification of *ERBB2* is found in (1) breast, (2) ovarian, and (3) gastrointestinal tumors. In breast cancer, it appears to be as useful a prognostic indicator of overall survival and tumor size as ER and PR expression, but not as good as the number of lymph nodes involved in metastases. Of the three oncogenes—*ERBB2*, *RAS*, and *MYC*—*ERBB2* has the strongest prognostic value in breast cancer. Herceptin treatment is administered only to those breast cancer patients who have HER2 amplification.

Measurement of the serum concentrations of the HER2 proteins is considered most useful in breast cancer, with some use in ovarian cancer patients. The assay is cleared by the FDA for use in follow-up and monitoring of patients with metastatic breast cancer with a HER-2 concentration >15 µg/L. Approximately 30% of patients have elevated concentrations. HER2 concentrations in breast cancer correlate with a worse prognosis and a shorter disease-free state. Elevated HER2 concentrations also correlate with (1) large tumor size, (2) lymph node positivity, and (3) a high grading score. Serum concentrations of HER2 may also be useful in monitoring the response of breast cancer patients to treatment.

Immunohistochemistry is used to detect increased tissue expression of the HER2 protein. FISH is used for detection of *HER2* gene amplification. ASCO and CAP have collaborated to develop comprehensive guidelines for HER2 testing. The ECD of HER2 in serum is detected by ELISA and automated immunoassay. Both assays use the same monoclonal antibodies, recognizing different epitopes of the ECD, which does not cross-react with any other member of the EGF family. It is important to note that no interference from the therapeutic monoclonal antibody, Herceptin, is noted with either assay.

BCR-ABL

Chronic myelogenous leukemia (CML) is a myeloproliferative disorder that results from the clonal expansion of a transformed multipotent hematopoietic stem cell. In approximately 90% of CML patients, the transforming event is the formation of the Philadelphia chromosome—a balanced translocation between chromosomes 9 and 22 [t(9;22)(q34;q11)] creating the *BCR-ABL* fusion gene. The protein derived from this fusion is a constitutively active cytoplasmic tyrosine kinase that activates several signaling pathways, leading to (1) uncontrolled growth, (2) inhibition of apoptosis, and (3) other aspects of neoplastic transformation.

Detection of the *BCR-ABL* gene is useful in diagnosing CML and in directing treatment. Once detected, several tactics are then used that target the *BCR-ABL* gene by oligonucleotides (antisense or ribozyme based) or the *BCR-ABL* kinase domain by the tyrosine kinase inhibitor STI571 (also known as Gleevec, or imatinib mesylate). For example, *BCR-ABL* detection by reverse transcription–polymerase chain reaction (RT-PCR) is useful in monitoring minimal residual disease in patients who have undergone bone marrow transplantation. In the subset of acute lymphoblastic leukemia patients who harbor the Philadelphia chromosome, a positive RT-PCR for the *BCR-ABL* gene carries much higher risk of relapse compared with a negative result. In CML patients after bone marrow transplantation, positive RT-PCR results at 6 to 12 months were associated with a 26-fold elevated risk of relapse, and a positive result at 3 months was not predictive of risk. Also, the amount of *BCR-ABL* transcript per μg of RNA correlated with risk of relapse; less than 1% of patients with fewer than 50 transcripts per μg of RNA relapsed, as did 72% of patients with more than 50 transcripts per μg of RNA.

Tumor-Suppressor Genes

Historically, evidence of tumor-suppressor genes was derived from the study of hybrid cells of normal and malignant cells that behaved in a typical manner. It was concluded that healthy cells contained a gene that suppressed the expression of malignancy. Reversion to malignancy occurred when the cultured cells lost normal chromosomes. The clinical usefulness of detection of mutations in tumor-suppressor genes lies not only in the diagnosis and prognosis of cancer, but also in the prediction of susceptibility when the mutation is carried in the germline, such as with the breast cancer genes *BRCA1* and *BRCA2*. Examples of tumor suppressors are (1) RB, (2) APC, and the (3) *BRCA1-2*. Additional tumor suppressors are listed in Table 20-9.

Retinoblastoma Gene

Retinoblastoma (RB) is a rare tumor of children that occurs both in families and sporadically. In Knudson's two-hit hypothesis, it is considered that in the inherited form of the tumor, one mutation is present in the germline and in all cells of the body, and the other mutational event occurs somatically in one of the cells of the developing retina. *RB* is a tumor-suppressor gene, as it suppresses DNA synthesis. Detection of mutations in RB is useful in determining the susceptibility of an individual to development of RB in the familial form, but it is not typically used as a tumor marker.

Adenomatous Polyposis Coli *(APC)* Gene

One of the first events in the putative steps of progression of precursor lesions to colon cancer is loss of the *APC* gene in premalignant polyps. The *APC* gene encodes a 300 kDa protein that may be truncated in cancer cells. The healthy function of the *APC* gene product is not known, but it interacts with proteins, such as α- and β-catenin, involved in cell-cell interactions in epithelial cells. This gene is mutated

in hereditary colorectal cancer syndromes—polyposis and nonpolyposis types. In the polyposis types, hundreds and even thousands or more benign tumors (polyps) arise before the development of cancer. Among nonpolyposis types, very few polyps are seen, but the elevated risk of cancer is essentially similar. The *APC* gene was detected by an interstitial deletion on chromosome 5q in a patient with hundreds of polyps. More than 80% of individuals with hereditary colorectal cancer have germline mutations in one of the *APC* alleles, including gross deletions or localized mutations. Hereditary forms of colorectal cancer are relatively uncommon, but somatic mutations appear to be of great importance in the development of nonhereditary colorectal cancers. More than 70% of colorectal tumors, regardless of size or histology, have a specific mutation in one of the two *APC* alleles, and mutation may be found in other types of tumors, including (1) breast, (2) esophageal, and (3) brain tumors. The usefulness of loss of the APC protein for diagnosis and prognosis is the subject of ongoing investigation. However, recent evidence suggests the importance of APC functional activity for prognostic purposes, as well as for directing therapy in colorectal cancer.

BRCA1 and *BRCA2*

A subset of breast cancer patients have been shown to have an inherited predisposition to developing breast and ovarian cancer that is inherited as an autosomal dominant trait. Two genetic loci have been identified (1): *BRCA1* on chromosome 17q, and (2) *BRCA2*, which localizes to 13q12-13. *BRCA1* encodes an 1863 amino acid protein that plays a role in transcriptional regulation and in DNA repair. *BRCA2* encodes a protein of 3418 amino acids that functions in DNA repair. The ability to detect mutations in *BRCA1* and *BRCA2* in the germline permits the identification of individuals in breast cancer families who carry the mutated gene.

It is estimated that as many as 1 in 200 women in the United States may have a germline mutation in the *BRCA1* gene. This has created an ethical dilemma for (1) physicians, (2) patients and their families, (3) insurance companies, and (4) health maintenance organizations, as it is now possible to predict that an individual who carries a mutation in one of these genes will develop breast and/or ovarian cancer. For example, carriers of a *BRCA1* gene mutation have an 85% risk of developing breast cancer and a 45% risk of developing ovarian cancer by the age of 85. This leads to the following questions

(1) What should be done if an otherwise healthy individual is shown to carry a *BRCA* gene mutation?
(2) Should such patients undergo preventive mastectomy or oophorectomy?
and
(3) Should insurance companies and healthcare maintenance organizations charge higher rates for carriers? This latter question has been answered with passage of the GINA legislation (**Genetic Information Nondiscriminatory Act**/ http://www.eeoc.gov/; accessed September 09, 2013) that prohibits discrimination based on genetic information.

Other Molecular Tests

Other molecular tests used to detect cancer include the (1) prostate cancer gene, or antigen 3 (PCA3), (2) single-nucleotide polymorphisms, and (3) cell-free nucleic acids.

Prostate Cancer Gene or Antigen 3 (PCA3)

Measurement of PCA3 mRNA in urine is a molecular test for prostate cancer. The PCA3 gene is also known as $PCA3^{DD3}$ or $DD3^{PCA3}$. PCA3 mRNA is noncoding, and its function is unknown. It is highly overexpressed in prostate cancer tissue compared with healthy or benign prostate tissue, which has low expression. Also, it is not detectable in healthy tissue or in tumors from (1) bladder, (2) testis, and (3) other organs. PCA3 score correlates with biopsy outcome in men undergoing a first or a repeat biopsy. Unlike PSA, PCA3 is independent of prostate volume, and PCA3 scores have been associated with both grade and extent of prostate cancer. Urine specimens for PCA3 are collected after digital rectal examination (DRE) to release prostate cells. PCA3 and PSA mRNA are quantitated using transcription-mediated nucleic acid amplification. The PCA3 mRNA copy number is normalized with the PSA mRNA housekeeping gene to generate the PCA3 score. The PCA3 assay (Hologic Gen-Probe PROGENSA; http://www.gen-probe.com/; accessed on September 9, 2013) was approved by the FDA in 2012 to help determine the need for a repeat prostate biopsy in men with a previous negative prostate biopsy result.

Single-Nucleotide Polymorphisms

The Human Genome Project identified all of the ≈25,000 transcriptional units in the human genome and determined the sequences of the 3 billion chemical base pairs that constitute human DNA (http://www.genome.gov/; accessed September 9, 2013). A byproduct of the sequencing effort was the identification of a very large number of single-nucleotide polymorphisms (SNPs; single nucleotides that differ between individuals and are inherited). These have been formalized and detailed through the efforts of the HapMap Project (http://hapmap.ncbi.nlm.nih.gov/; accessed September 9, 2013). This project is a partnership of scientists and funding agencies from Canada, China, Japan, Nigeria, the United Kingdom, and the United States to develop a public resource that will help researchers find genes associated with human disease and with response to pharmaceuticals. It has been estimated that it is possible to find one SNP in every ≈300 bases of human DNA. Most of these SNPs are present in introns, and only a relatively small number (approximately 60,000 of the 2,000,000 SNPs) are present within exons. Groups of SNPs (called *haplotypes*) are inherited together in blocks. Scientists are currently investigating SNPs in the hope of identifying characteristic SNPs or haplotypes that can be used for diagnostic purposes, or of determining future risk (predisposition) for developing certain diseases.

Cell-Free Nucleic Acids

Circulating DNA and RNA have been recognized since the 1970s, but it was not until the late 1980s that the neoplastic characteristics of DNA were recognized. Circulating DNA and RNA have been proposed as markers for certain types of cancer. To use circulating DNA as a cancer marker, a mechanism must differentiate normal DNA from neoplastic DNA. This is achieved by detecting mutations in circulating DNA that are present in cancer cells (e.g., *ras* mutations that occur in various cancers) (1) by performing microsatellite analysis of circulating DNA, (2) by detecting common cancer-causing chromosomal translocations, or (3) detecting epigenetic alterations of circulating DNA, such as altered methylation patterns. Cell-free nucleic acids have been detected in bronchial lavage fluid from lung cancer patients and in plasma from colorectal cancer patients.

Microarray-Based Markers

Microarray-based genotyping is a molecular technique used to simultaneously screen hundreds to thousands of markers per individual. It is a technology suited for applications requiring whole-genome coverage. It is associated with relatively low cost and consequently is a useful technique for large populations. The three early assays described next give a taste of the applications to cancer.

Roche Amplichip P450

The Amplichip P450 (Roche Molecular Diagnostics, http://molecular.roche.com/assays/; accessed on September 9, 2013) detects variations in P450 genes that are involved in the metabolism of many clinically prescribed drugs, including (1) β-blockers, (2) antidepressants, (3) antipsychotics, and (4) chemotherapeutic agents such as tamoxifen and cyclophosphamide.

Drugs that are metabolized through the cytochrome P450 2D6 pathway are inactivated or activated through enzymatic action of 2D6. One example is tamoxifen, which is used currently as the standard of care treatment for estrogen receptor–positive (ER+) breast cancer. Tamoxifen is a prodrug that undergoes a series of modifications leading to its activation. Clinically, endoxifen is the most important active metabolite and has been shown to have 50 to 100 times greater antitumor activity compared with tamoxifen in in vitro assays, along with higher affinity for the estrogen receptor. It is produced by the action of the cytochrome P450 2D6 enzyme in the liver.

Poor and intermediate metabolizers of 2D6 may experience suboptimal effects because of reduced endoxifen concentrations. In contrast, ultra-rapid metabolizers may experience toxic effects caused by high concentrations of the active metabolite.

Oncotype Dx

The Onco*type* Dx assay (Genomic Health Inc., Redwood City, Calif); (http://www.genomichealth.com/; accessed on September 9, 2013), determines the expression of 21 genes in breast tissue. I provides an assessment of the likelihood of response to chemotherapy and of recurrence within 10 years.

MammaPrint

The MammaPrint assay (Agendia, http://www.agendia.com/; accessed on September 9, 2013) is used to assess the risk of breast cancer recurrence. Assessment is performed on fresh frozen tumor tissue obtained during surgery, and samples are sent directly to Agendia Laboratories in The Netherlands. This assay measures the expression of 70 genes involved in important signal transduction pathways responsible for breast cancer metastasis.

Review Questions

1. Protein tumor markers found both in normal fetal tissue and in certain tumors are referred to as:
   a. embryonic proteins.
   b. tumor-associated antigens.
   c. oncogenes.
   d. oncofetal antigens.

2. Moderate elevation of which one of the following indicates normal pregnancy, while an extreme elevation is indicative of a trophoblastic tumor?
   a. CG
   b. HPL
   c. AFP
   d. PSA

3. Which of the following statements most correctly describes the usefulness of clinical laboratory assays for tumor markers?
   a. Tumor markers are useful in diagnosing asymptomatic patients for tumors.
   b. Tumor markers are useful for monitoring treatment.
   c. Tumor markers are diagnostic for cancer in all cases.
   d. Tumor markers are highly specific.

4. An example of a blood group antigen that may be elevated in pancreatic cancer is:
   a. CA 125.
   b. CA 15-3.
   c. CA 19-9.
   d. PSA.

5. A genetic tumor marker that, when mutated, loses its ability to stop cell division is referred to as a(n):
   a. tumor-suppressor gene.
   b. proto-oncogene.
   c. oncofetal antigen.
   d. repair process gene.

6. The greatest usefulness of a tumor marker is its:
   a. use in the evaluation of progression of disease after initial therapy.
   b. use in the diagnosis of the presence of a tissue-specific tumor in an asymptomatic individual.
   c. sensitivity and specificity in assessment of the presence of a tumor.
   d. diagnostic ability in all cases of cancer.

7. A *molecular* test for prostate cancer involves measurement of:
   a. circulating tumor cells specific for prostate.
   b. the cell-free nucleic acid that contains a methylated region of *PCA3*.
   c. elevated prostate-specific antigen in serum.
   d. *PCA3* in urine.

8. An elevated serum concentration of calcitonin is usually associated with:
   a. parathyroid gland tumors.
   b. medullary carcinoma of the thyroid.
   c. small cell lung carcinoma.
   d. trophoblastic tumors.

9. In an individual with a poorly differentiated tumor, the tissue of origin test measures, to determine the primary tumor site, is/are:
   a. gene expression of many genes compared with known tumor genes using microarrays
   b. immunoassay results using specific antibodies against many different cell surface receptors
   c. circulating tumor cell numbers
   d. risk percentage of the primary tumor site using a multivariate index assay

10. The primary FDA-indicated use for CA 125, a high-molecular-weight mucin, is for assessment of:
    a. human breast cancer that has become metastatic to liver.
    b. women with ovarian cancer and to distinguish them from normal women or those with benign processes.
    c. response to therapy in patients with epithelial ovarian cancer.
    d. metastatic cancer with bone or liver involvement.

References

1. Bonfrer JMG. Working group on tumor marker criteria (WGTMC). Tumour Biol 1990;11:287–8.
2. Cancer facts and figures 2012. Atlanta, Ga: American Cancer Society, 2012:1–66.
3. Diamandis EP, Fritsche HA, Lilja H, et al, eds. Tumor markers: physiology, pathobiology, technology and clinical applications. Washington, DC: AACC Press, 2002.
4. Esserman LJ, Thompson IM, Reid B. Overdiagnosis and Overtreatment in cancer: an opportunity for improvement. JAMA 2013;310:797–98
5. Goldman JM, Melo JV. Chronic myeloid leukemia—advances in biology and new approaches to treatment. N Engl J Med 2003;349:1451–64.
6. Hanahan D, Weinberg RA. Hallmarks of cancer: the next generation. Cell 2011;144:646–74.
7. Montagnana M, Danese E, Giudici S, et al. HE4 in ovarian cancer: from discovery to clinical application. Adv Clin Chem 2011;55:1–20.
8. Prensner JR, Rubin MA, Wei JT, Chinnaiyan AM. Beyond PSA: the next generation of prostate cancer biomarkers. Sci Transl Med 2012;4:1–11.
9. Smith RA, Cokkinides V, Brawley OW. Cancer screening in the United States, 2012: a review of current American Cancer Society guidelines and issues in cancer screening. CA Cancer J Clin 2012;62:129–42.
10. Sturgeon CM, Hoffman BR, Chan DW, et al; National Academy of Clinical Biochemistry. National Academy of Clinical Biochemistry laboratory medicine practice guidelines for use of tumor markers in clinical practice: quality requirements. Clin Chem 2008;54:e1–10.
11. Sturgeon CM, Duffy MJ, Stenman UH, et al; National Academy of Clinical Biochemistry. National Academy of Clinical Biochemistry laboratory medicine practice guidelines for use of tumor markers in testicular, prostate, colorectal, breast, and ovarian cancers. Clin Chem 2008;54:e11-79.
12. Sturgeon CM, Lai LC, Duffy MJ. Serum tumour markers: how to order and interpret them. BMJ 2009;339:852–8.
13. Sturgeon CM, Duffy MJ, Hofmann BR, et al; National Academy of Clinical Biochemistry. National Academy of Clinical Biochemistry laboratory medicine practice guidelines for use of tumor markers in liver, bladder, cervical, and gastric cancers. Clin Chem 2010;56:e1–48.
14. Zhang Z. Combining multiple biomarkers in clinical diagnostics—a review of methods and issues. In: Diamandis EP, Fritsche HA, Lilja H, et al, eds. Tumor markers: physiology, pathobiology, technology and clinical applications. Washington DC: AACC Press, 2002:133–9.

Kidney Function Tests—Creatinine, Urea, and Uric Acid

Edmund J. Lamb, Ph.D., F.R.C.Path., and Christopher P. Price, Ph.D., F.R.C.Path.

Objectives

1. Define the following:
   Creatinine   Uric acid
   Urea   Gout
2. Diagram the pathway that results in the formation of creatinine.
3. State the clinical usefulness of measuring serum and urine creatinine.
4. State the principle of the Jaffe reaction and list five interferences that affect this method.
5. List and describe three enzymatic assays used to measure creatinine in serum.
6. Describe "compensated assays" in relation to the measurement of creatinine.
7. Diagram the catabolic pathway that results in the formation of urea.
8. State the clinical usefulness of measuring serum urea; list the causes of increased and decreased serum urea.
9. Describe the urease approach for measuring urea in serum; list one interference that affects this method.
10. Convert serum urea nitrogen given in mg/dL to urea nitrogen in mmol/L.
11. Diagram the pathway that results in the formation of uric acid.
12. State the clinical usefulness of measuring serum uric acid.
13. List the causes of hyperuricemia; explain the pathogenesis of gout and urinary tract uric acid stones.
14. Compare and contrast primary and secondary gout.
15. List the causes of hypouricemia.
16. Describe the uricase method of measuring uric acid in serum; list two interferences that affect this method.

Key Words and Definitions

BUN (blood urea nitrogen) Obsolete term used to report results of a urea assay, particularly in the United States.

Creatinine A nonprotein nitrogen compound derived from the spontaneous hydrolysis of creatine or the cyclization of phosphocreatine; creatinine production is relatively constant, is related to muscle mass, and is used as a marker of the glomerular filtration rate of the kidneys.

Fanconi syndrome A rare recessive disorder characterized by pancytopenia, bone marrow hypoplasia, and patchy brown skin discoloration due to deposition of melanin, as well as multiple congenital anomalies of the musculoskeletal and genitourinary systems.

Gout A group of disorders of purine metabolism due to primary (inherited) or secondary causes such as chronic kidney disease.

Hyperuricemia An excess of uric acid or urates in the blood with many causes; it is a prerequisite for the development of gout and may lead to renal disease.

Hypouricemia Decreased uric acid concentration in the blood, secondary to a number of underlying conditions such as severe hepatocellular disease and defective renal tubular reabsorption.

Jaffe reaction The reaction of creatinine with alkaline picrate to form a colored compound; this creatinine assay is subject to numerous interferences.

Urea The major nitrogen-containing metabolic product of protein catabolism in humans.

Urease methods Enzymatic assays that initially involve the hydrolysis of urea by urease to generate ammonia, which is quantified by a variety of methods.

Uremia The entire constellation of signs and symptoms of chronic renal failure; also known as *azotemia*.

Uric acid A nitrogenous compound derived from the catabolism of purine nucleosides.

Uricase methods A group of enzymatic assays that initially involve oxidation of uric acid by uricase to eventually produce a chromogen that is spectrophotometrically measured to determine uric acid concentration.

Creatinine, urea, and uric acid are nonprotein nitrogenous metabolites that are cleared from the body by the kidney after glomerular filtration. Measurements of plasma or serum* concentrations of these metabolites are commonly used as indicators of kidney function and other conditions.

Creatinine

Creatinine (MW 113 Da) is the cyclic anhydride of creatine that is produced as the final product of decomposition of phosphocreatine. It is excreted in the urine; measurements of plasma creatinine and its renal clearance are used as diagnostic indicators of kidney function (see Chapter 35).

Biochemistry and Physiology

Creatine is synthesized in the (1) kidneys, (2) liver, and (3) pancreas by two enzymatically mediated reactions. In the first, transamidation of arginine and glycine forms guanidinoacetic acid. In the second reaction, methylation of guanidinoacetic acid occurs with S-adenosylmethionine as the methyl donor. Creatine is then transported in blood to other organs, such as muscle and brain, where it is phosphorylated to phosphocreatine, a high-energy compound.

Creatine + ATP →(Creatine kinase)→ Phosphocreatine + ADP

Creatine →(Spontaneous)→ H_2O + Creatinine

Phosphocreatine →(Spontaneous)→ P_i + Creatinine

Interconversion of phosphocreatine and creatine is a particular feature of the metabolic processes of muscle contraction. A proportion of the free creatine in muscle (thought to be between 1% and 2%/d) spontaneously and irreversibly converts to its anhydride waste product—creatinine. Thus the amount of creatinine produced each day is relatively constant and is related to the muscle mass. In health, the concentration of creatinine in the bloodstream is also relatively constant, although dietary meat intake may influence the value. Creatinine is present in all body fluids and secretions and is freely filtered by the glomerulus. Although it is not reabsorbed to any great extent by the renal tubules, a small but significant tubular secretion occurs.

*Concentrations of creatine, urea, and uric acid in serum and plasma are equivalent: "serum" has been used throughout this chapter.

Clinical Significance

Serum creatinine concentration is maintained within narrow limits predominantly by glomerular filtration. Consequently, both serum creatinine concentration and its renal clearance ("creatinine clearance") have been used as markers of the glomerular filtration rate (GFR). The application and limitations of these tests are discussed in Chapter 35.

Analytical Methodology

Serum creatinine is commonly measured using chemical or enzymatic methods.[5,9,11] Other methods, including isotope-dilution mass spectrometry (IDMS) and high-performance liquid chromatography (HPLC), have also been used. Most laboratories use adaptations of the same assay for measurements in both serum and urine.

Chemical Methods: The Jaffe Reaction

Most chemical methods used to measure creatinine are based on its reaction with alkaline picrate. As was first described by Jaffe in 1886, creatinine reacts with picrate ion in an alkaline medium to yield an orange-red complex.

A serious analytical problem with the **Jaffe reaction** is its lack of specificity for creatinine. For example, many compounds have been reported to produce a Jaffe-like chromogen, including (1) ascorbic acid, (2) blood-substitute products, (3) cephalosporins, (4) glucose, (5) guanidine, (6) ketone bodies, (7) protein, and (8) pyruvate. The degree of interference from these compounds is dependent on the specific reaction conditions chosen. The effects of ketones and ketoacids are probably of greatest significance clinically, although this determination is highly method dependent. Thus reports on acetoacetate interference vary from a negligible increase to an increase of 3.5 mg/dL (310 µmol/L) in the apparent creatinine concentration at an acetoacetate concentration of 8 mmol/L. Bilirubin is a negative interferant with the Jaffe reaction. The addition of buffering ions, such as borate and phosphate, together with surfactant, has been used to minimize the effects of this interference. In addition, ferricyanide—O'Leary method—has been added that oxidizes bilirubin to biliverdin, hence reducing its interference. Noncreatinine chromogens do not generally contribute to measured urinary creatinine concentration.

The greatest success in terms of common usage and specificity has been seen in the use of a kinetic measurement approach in combination with careful choice of reactant concentrations. In general, manual methods have traditionally been equilibrium methods, with 10 to 15 minutes allowed to complete the color development at room temperature. Kinetic assays have been developed to provide more (1) specific, (2) faster, and (3) automated analyses. Early studies of interferences in the kinetic methods identified two types of noncreatinine chromogens. In one group, the rate of adduct formation is very rapid, and such formation occurs in the first 20 seconds after mixing of the aliquots of reagent and sample. Acetoacetate is an example of this type of interferant. In the second group, the rate of adduct formation does not become significant until 80 to 100 seconds after mixing. The "window" between 20 and 80 seconds therefore was a period in which the rate signal that was being observed could be attributed predominantly to the creatinine-picrate reaction. Thus improvement of specificity in the kinetic assays was achieved by selecting times for rate measurements 20 to 80 seconds after initiation of the reaction (mixing). This approach has been implemented with various automated instruments, and kinetic assays are now widely used to measure creatinine concentrations in body fluids.

Extensive literature describes the choice of reactant concentrations and reading intervals, as well as the choice of wavelength and reaction temperature. Brief comments follow.

Picrate Concentration

The Jaffe reaction is pseudo first order with respect to picrate up to 30 mmol/L, and most methods employ a concentration between 3 and 16 mmol/L. At concentrations above 6 mmol/L, the rate of color development becomes nonlinear, so a two-point fixed interval rather than a multiple data point approach is required.

Hydroxide Concentration

The initial rate of reaction is pseudo first order with respect to hydroxide concentrations greater than 0.5 mmol/L. However, at 500 mmol/L, degradation of the Jaffe complex is increased. Furthermore, at hydroxide concentrations greater than 200 mmol/L, the blank absorbance is increased significantly.

Wavelength

Although the absorbance maximum of the Jaffe reaction is between 490 and 500 nm, improved method linearity and reduced blank values have been reported at other wavelengths, with the choice varying with hydroxide concentration.

Temperature

The rate of Jaffe complex formation and the absorptivity of the complex are temperature-dependent with measurable differences observed even between 25 °C and 37 °C. Consequently, temperature control is an important component of assay reproducibility.

"Compensation"

As a result of the reaction with noncreatinine chromogens, Jaffe methods often have historically overestimated true serum creatinine concentrations at physiological concentrations by up to 20% compared with HPLC or IDMS methods. In an attempt to adjust for this, some manufacturers have introduced so-called "compensated" Jaffe assays, in which a fixed concentration is automatically subtracted from each result. For example, Roche Diagnostics Ltd. (Lewes, Sussex, United Kingdom) has realigned its assays on the Cobas Integra and Hitachi systems by −0.20 mg/dL and −0.32 mg/dL (−18 and −28 μmol/L), respectively. Such assays produce lower results more closely aligned with IDMS reference measurement procedures at concentrations within the reference interval. However, the purveyors make an assumption that the noncreatinine chromogen interference is a constant between samples; this is clearly an oversimplification, especially when adult and pediatric samples are compared.

Enzymatic Methods

Enzymes from a number of metabolic pathways have been investigated for the enzymatic measurement of creatinine. All methods involve a multistep approach leading to a photometric equilibrium (Figure 21-1). Primarily three approaches may be used and are described in the following sections.

Creatininase

Creatininase (EC 3.5.2.10; creatinine amidohydrolase) catalyzes the conversion of creatinine to creatine. The creatine is then detected with a series of enzyme-mediated reactions involving (1) creatine kinase, (2) pyruvate kinase, and (3) lactate dehydrogenase, with monitoring of the decrease in absorbance at 340 nm (see Figure 21-1, *A*). Initiating the reaction with creatininase allows for the removal of endogenous creatine and pyruvate in a preincubation reaction. The kinetics of the reaction is analytically problematic, and 30-minute incubation is required to allow the reaction to reach equilibrium. This shortcoming has been overcome by a kinetic approach but with a further reduction in the ability of the method to detect creatinine. Consequently, this approach is not widely used.

Creatininase and Creatinase

An alternative approach has involved the use of creatinase (EC 3.5.3.3; creatine amidinohydrolase) that yields sarcosine and urea, with the former measured by further enzyme-mediated steps using sarcosine oxidase (EC 1.5.3.1). This produces (1) glycine, (2) formaldehyde, and (3) hydrogen peroxide (see Figure 21-1, *B*), and the latter is detected and measured by a variety of methods. Care must be taken, however, because of interference (e.g., by bilirubin) in the final reaction sequence. This problem has been minimized by adding potassium ferricyanide (with limited success) or bilirubin oxidase. The potential interference caused by ascorbic acid has been overcome by the inclusion of ascorbate oxidase (L-ascorbate:oxygen oxidoreductase; EC 1.10.3.3). The influence of endogenous intermediate creatine and urea has been minimized by adding a preincubation step and then initiating the reaction with creatininase. This system has been incorporated in a point-of-care testing device using polarographic detection. An alternative detection system involves measurement of the reduction of nicotinamide adenine dinucleotide by formaldehyde in the presence of formaldehyde dehydrogenase (see Figure 21-1, *C*).

Creatinine Deaminase

Creatinine deaminase (EC 3.5.4.21; creatinine imino-hydrolase) catalyzes the conversion of creatinine to *N*-methylhydantoin and ammonia. Early methods concentrated on the detection of ammonia using glutamate dehydrogenase or the Berthelot reaction. An alternative approach involves the enzyme *N*-methylhydantoin amidohydrolase (see Figure 21-1, *D*).

Dry Chemistry Systems

Several multilayer dry reagent methods have been described for the measurement of creatinine using enzyme-mediated reactions. An early "two-slide" approach employed creatinine deaminase, with the ammonia diffusing through a semipermeable and

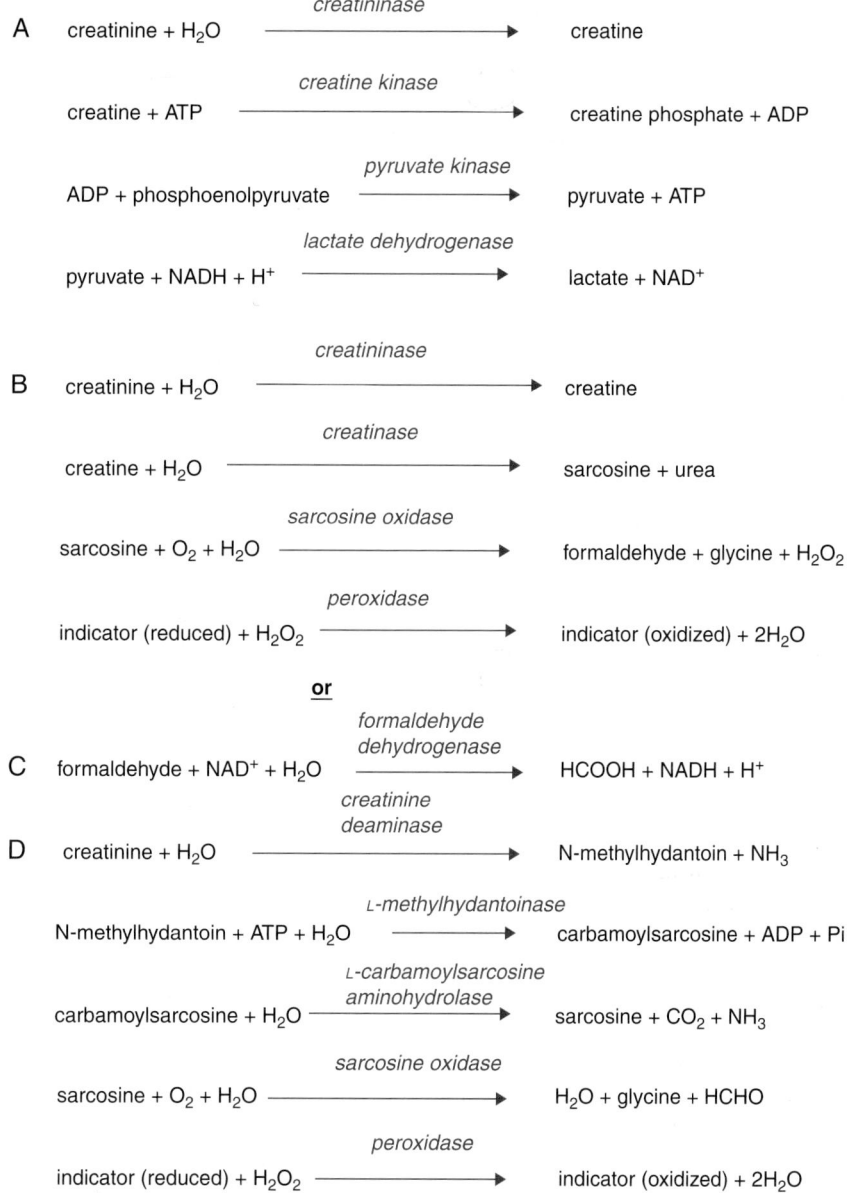

Figure 21-1 Determination of creatinine using a variety of enzymatic methods. For further details, see text.

optically opaque layer to react with bromophenol blue to give an increase in absorbance at 600 nm. A second multilayer film lacking the enzyme was used to quantitate endogenous ammonia, enabling blank correction. A later single-slide method used the creatininase-creatinase reaction sequence. Lidocaine metabolites have been reported to interfere with this method. The creatinine deaminase system described above has also been used and adapted for use as a point-of-care testing device (see Figure 21-1, *D*). In all cases, the color produced in the film is quantified by reflectance spectrophotometry.

Other Methods
A definitive method employing IDMS was described by Welch in 1986.[13] Gas chromatography–IDMS (GC-IDMS) is now accepted as the method of choice for establishing the true concentration of creatinine in serum because of its excellent specificity and low imprecision. Three GC-IDMS methods have been approved by the Joint Committee for Traceability in Laboratory Medicine (JCTLM) as reference measurement procedures for serum creatinine.[5] With these procedures, creatinine must be derivatized before GC analysis because of its polarity. In addition, a cation exchange cleanup step is necessary before GC analysis because creatine is derivatized into the same chemical species as creatinine.

Quality Issues and Preanalytical Considerations With Creatinine Methods
The method used for measurement of creatinine is complex by virtue of the number of variants of the Jaffe reaction and the introduction of enzymatic procedures that overcome the limitations of the former. Although enzymatic methods are more expensive, they are used in dry chemistry systems

(with their lower reagent requirement), including some point-of-care testing devices. Kinetic Jaffe approaches predominate in wet chemistry analytical systems. Any laboratorian assessing a new creatinine method (e.g., as part of an analyzer purchase) should review the data for that method on common interferences. Despite criticism of the Jaffe methods, adequate correlation has been noted invariably between them and enzymatic procedures, with differences likely to be due as much to calibration as to interference.

Creatinine in serum or urine is stable for at least 7 days at 4 °C, and serum creatinine is stable during long-term frozen storage (at −20 °C and below) and after repeated thawing and refreezing. However, it should be noted that delayed separation (beyond 14 hours) of serum from erythrocytes leads to a significant increase in apparent serum creatinine concentration using some kinetic Jaffe (but not enzymatic) assays. Creatinine concentration is increased in blood after meals containing cooked meat because of the conversion of creatine to creatinine; ideally, blood for serum creatinine measurement should be obtained in the fasting state. Clearly, this latter problem will affect both enzymatic and Jaffe creatinine methods.

Different methods for assaying serum creatinine have varying degrees of accuracy and imprecision. Mean within-individual biological variation for serum creatinine has been reported as 4.3%, indicating a desirable analytical performance goal of <2.2%. Intralaboratory imprecision at a concentration of 88 µmol/L varies between approximately 2.0% and 8.4%. [5] Clearly, many laboratories do not meet desirable and even minimum performance standards. Proficiency studies demonstrate that although between-laboratory coefficients of variation (CVs) of approximately 3% are achievable within method groups, overall between-laboratory agreement across methods is much poorer. Further, interlaboratory and within-laboratory agreement deteriorates as serum creatinine concentration nears the reference interval; the exponential relationship between serum creatinine and GFR means that imprecision at lower creatinine concentrations contributes to greater error in GFR estimation than is seen at higher creatinine concentrations.

Over the past decade, appreciation of chronic kidney disease (CKD) as a major public health issue[3,6,7] and of its identification with the use of GFR-estimating equations has led to increased focus on the measurement of creatinine. Creatinine-based estimates of GFR (see Chapter 35) will clearly vary, depending on how accurate the creatinine measurement is that is used in the calculation. The more a method overestimates "true" creatinine, the greater will be the underestimation of GFR, and vice versa. Standardized serum matrix reference materials (SRM 967) with established creatinine concentrations (0.80 mg/dL [71 µmol/L] and 4.00 mg/dL [354 µmol/L]) have been prepared by the National Institute of Standards of Technology (NIST) and have been included in a list of higher order reference materials by the JCTLM. The material was value-assigned with the use of mass spectrometry and was issued in 2007.[2] This material, in combination with GC-IDMS reference methodology, was used by reagent manufacturers to restandardize their methods,[8] and by the end of 2009, most clinical laboratory methods had calibration traceable to the reference measurement procedure and standard.[4]

Although undoubtedly desirable, it must be recognized that standardization is only one part of the problem. Standardization does not solve the problem of different reactivity with noncreatinine chromogens across different patient samples, which will be resolved only by the use of highly specific creatinine methods such as the enzymatic methods.

Reference Intervals

Reference intervals for serum creatinine are method dependent. A systematic review of creatinine reference intervals from methods whose calibration was traceable to the reference IDMS procedure proposed adult reference intervals of 0.72 to 1.18 mg/dL (64 to 104 µmol/L) in men and 0.55 to 1.02 mg/dL (49 to 90 µmol/L) in women.[1] These data were derived using an enzymatic (Roche Diagnostics Ltd.) assay. Reference interval data for children may be found in the same publication. Serum creatinine concentration in patients with untreated end-stage renal disease (ESRD) may exceed 11 mg/dL (1000 µmol/L).

Urinary creatinine excretion is higher in men (14 to 26 mg/kg/d, 124 to 230 µmol/kg/d) than in women (11 to 20 mg/kg/d, 97 to 177 µmol/kg/d). Creatinine excretion decreases with age. Typically, for a 70-kg man, creatinine excretion will decline from approximately 1640 to 1030 mg/d (14.5 to 9.1 mmol/d) with advancing age from 30 to 80 years. Measurement of urinary creatinine excretion has been found to be a useful indication of the completeness of a timed urine collection. In addition, creatinine excretion is often used as a method of normalizing the urinary excretion of analytes, that is, excretion of the test analyte (in millimoles or grams) is divided by the total amount of creatinine (in millimoles or grams) excreted in the same urine specimen. This method provides a rough correction for volume differences between patient specimens. Similarly, expressing the concentration of a substance as a ratio to the creatinine concentration is a useful method of adjusting for urinary concentration differences in random ("spot") urine samples.

Urea

Catabolism of proteins and amino acids results in the formation of **urea**, which is predominantly cleared from the body by the kidneys.

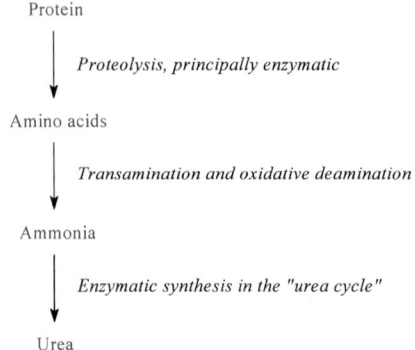

Biochemistry and Physiology

Urea is the major nitrogen-containing metabolic product of protein catabolism in humans, accounting for more than 75% of the nonprotein nitrogen eventually excreted. The biosynthesis of urea from amino acid nitrogen–derived ammonia is carried out exclusively by hepatic enzymes of the urea cycle. During the process of protein catabolism, amino acid nitrogen is converted to urea in the liver by the action of the so-called urea cycle enzymes (Figure 21-2).

More than 90% of urea is excreted through the kidneys, with losses through the gastrointestinal tract and skin accounting for most of the remaining minor fraction. Consequently, kidney disease is associated with accumulation of urea in blood. An increase in blood urea concentration characterizes the uremic (azotemic) state. Urea is neither actively reabsorbed nor secreted by the tubules but is filtered freely by the glomeruli. In a healthy kidney, 40% to 70% of the highly diffusible urea moves passively out of the renal tubule and into the interstitium, ultimately to re-enter blood. The back-diffusion of urea is also dependent on urine flow rate, with less entering the interstitium in high-flow states (e.g., pregnancy) and vice versa. Consequently, urea clearance generally underestimates GFR.

Clinical Significance

Measurement of blood and serum urea has been used for many years as an indicator of kidney function. However, it is now generally accepted that creatinine measurement provides better information in this respect. Serum and urinary urea measurement, however, may still provide useful clinical information in particular circumstances, and measurement of urea in dialysis fluids is widely used to assess the adequacy of renal replacement therapy. Several extrarenal factors influence the circulating urea concentration, limiting its value as a test of kidney function. For example, serum urea concentration is increased by (1) a high-protein diet, (2) increased protein catabolism, (3) reabsorption of blood proteins after gastrointestinal hemorrhage, (4) treatment with cortisol or its synthetic analogues, (5) dehydration, and with (6) decreased perfusion of the kidneys (e.g., heart failure). In these prerenal situations, the serum creatinine concentration may be within its reference interval. In obstructive postrenal conditions such as (1) malignancy, (2) nephrolithiasis, and (3) prostatism, both serum creatinine and urea concentrations will be increased, However, in these situations, a greater increase in serum urea than in creatinine is often seen because of increased back-diffusion. These considerations give rise to the principal clinical utility of serum urea, which lies in its measurement in conjunction with that of serum creatinine and subsequent calculation of the urea-to-creatinine ratio, which has been used as a crude discriminator between prerenal and postrenal **uremia**.

Measurement of urinary urea has little place in clinical diagnosis. However, it does provide a crude index of overall nitrogen balance and may be used as a guide to replacement in patients receiving parenteral nutrition. With an average protein diet, urinary excretion expressed as urea nitrogen is 12 to 20 g/d.

Although the term **blood urea nitrogen** (or **BUN**) continues to be used for ordering the serum urea test, this terminology is incorrect and obsolete because blood is rarely the sample that is analyzed for urea. The long-established habit of reporting and expressing results of a urea assay in units of urea nitrogen appears to be strongly entrenched in the United States, although the SI system recommends reporting of urea, expressed in mmol/L. Thus, students of clinical chemistry need to know the conversion factors for urea to urea nitrogen. Because 60 g (1 g MW) of urea contains 28 g (2 g atomic weight) of nitrogen, the factor is 0.467 for converting urea mass units to those of urea nitrogen, and 2.14 for converting urea nitrogen mass units to those of urea. The factor for converting urea nitrogen in mg/dL to urea in mmol/L is 0.357.

Analytical Methodology

Both chemical and enzymatic methods are used to quantify urea in body fluids.[12]

Chemical Methods

Most chemical methods for urea are based on the Fearon reaction, in which molecules of diacetyl condense with those of urea to form the chromogen diazine, which absorbs strongly at 540 nm. Because diacetyl is unstable, it is usually generated in the reaction system from diacetyl monoxime and acid. Although once widely used, the method has largely been superseded by enzymatic approaches.

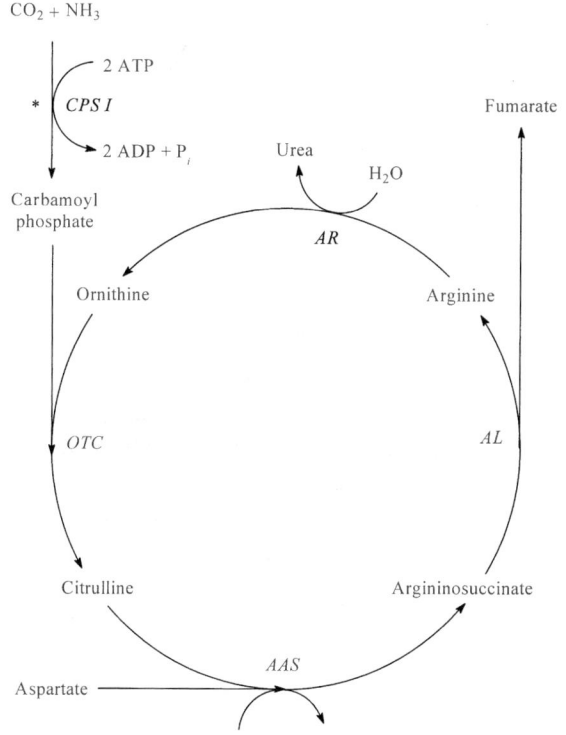

Figure 21-2 The urea cycle pathway. *N-acetylglutamate as a positive allosteric effector. *AAS*, Argininosuccinate synthetase; *ADP*, adenosine diphosphate; *AL*, argininosuccinate lyase; *AMP*, adenosine monophosphate; *AR*, arginase; *ATP*, adenosine triphosphate; *CPS I*, carbamoyl phosphate synthetase I; *OTC*, ornithine transcarbamylase; *P_i*, inorganic phosphate.

Enzymatic Methods

Enzymatic methods for the measurement of urea are based on preliminary hydrolysis of urea with **urease** (urea amidohydrolase, EC 3.5.1.5; main source jack bean meal) to generate ammonia, which is then quantified. This approach has been used in (1) equilibrium photometric, (2) kinetic photometric, (3) conductimetric, and (4) dry chemistry systems.

$$\underset{\text{Urea}}{\overset{\displaystyle H_2N}{\underset{\displaystyle H_2N}{\diagdown}}C{=}O} \; + \; 2\,H_2O \;\; \xrightarrow{\textit{Urease}} \;\; 2\,NH_4^{\oplus} \; + \; CO_3^{\ominus\ominus}$$

Spectrophotometric approaches to ammonia quantitation include the Berthelot reaction and the enzymatic assay with glutamate dehydrogenase (L-glutamate:NAD[P] oxidoreductase [deaminating], EC 1.4.1.3). This latter approach has been accepted as a reference method and has been adapted to many analytical platforms.

$$NH_4^{\oplus} + 2\text{-Oxoglutarate} \xrightarrow[\underset{+\,H^{\oplus}}{NADH \quad NAD^{\oplus}}]{\textit{Glutamate dehydrogenase}} Glutamate + H_2O$$

For serum assays, the reaction system contains urease, so that the addition of sample containing urea starts the reaction. A decrease in absorbance resulting from the glutamate dehydrogenase reaction is monitored at 340 nm. In another example of a coupled-enzyme assay system for urea, ammonia produced from urea by urease then reacts with glutamate and adenosine triphosphate in the presence of glutamine synthetase (EC 6.3.1.2). Adenosine diphosphate produced in this second enzymatic reaction is then measured in a third and fourth step using pyruvate kinase (EC 2.7.1.40) and pyruvate oxidase (EC 1.2.3.3), respectively, thus generating peroxide. In the final step, peroxide reacts with phenol and 4-aminophenazone, catalyzed by horseradish peroxidase (donor:hydrogen-peroxide oxidoreductase; EC 1.11.1.7), to yield a quinone-monoamine dye that is quantified spectrophotometrically.

Methods for the measurement of urea using dry chemistry systems have been described using the urease approach and a variety of detection methods. In one approach, a semipermeable membrane separates the first stage of the reaction involving urease, and ammonia is detected by using a simple pH indicator reaction. Urea has also been measured by means of a conductimetric method in which a sample and a urease-containing reagent are incubated in a conductivity cell with the rate of change of conductivity monitored as urea is converted to an ionic species. With a potentiometric approach, an ammonium ion-selective electrode is employed, and urease is immobilized on a membrane; this principle has been applied in some point-of-care testing devices.

The specificity of all methods is generally acceptable, particularly for the urease–glutamate dehydrogenase procedure; however, endogenous ammonia interference must be expected when the protocol employs the sample to initiate the reaction. This may be relevant in (2) aged samples, (2) some urines samples, and (3) particular metabolic disorders. Typically, within-run CVs of less than 3.0% with between-day values of less than 4.0% are achievable in the concentration range of 14 to 20 mg/dL (5.0 to 7.0 mmol/L). Given the high intrinsic biological variation of serum urea, this is well within desired standards of analytical performance.

Reference Intervals

The reference interval for blood urea nitrogen in healthy adults is 6 to 20 mg/dL (2.1 to 7.1 mmol/L). In adults older than 60 years of age, the reference interval is 8 to 23 mg/dL (2.9 to 8.2 mmol/L). Serum concentrations tend to be slightly lower in children and in pregnancy and slightly higher in males than in females. Serum urea concentrations in a patient with untreated ESRD typically reach 108 to 135 mg/dL (40 to 50 mmol/L).

Uric Acid

Uric acid is a nitrogenous compound (2,6,8-trihydroxypurine) that is present as the principal nitrogenous component of the excrement of reptiles and birds. It is found in small amounts in mammalian urine, and its salts occur in the joints in gout.

Biochemistry and Physiology

In humans, uric acid is the major product of catabolism of the purine nucleosides adenosine and guanosine (Figure 21-3). Purines from catabolism of dietary nucleic acid are converted to uric acid directly. The bulk of purines excreted as uric acid arise from degradation of endogenous nucleic acids. The daily synthesis rate of uric acid is approximately 400 mg. Dietary sources contribute another 300 mg. In men consuming a purine-free diet, the total body pool of exchangeable urate is estimated at 1200 mg. In women it is estimated to be 600 mg. By contrast, patients with gouty arthritis and tissue deposition of urate may have urate pools as large as 18,000 to 30,000 mg. Overproduction of uric acid may result from increased synthesis of purine precursors.

Renal handling of uric acid is complex and involves four sequential steps: (1) glomerular filtration of virtually all the uric acid in capillary plasma entering the glomerulus; (2) reabsorption in the proximal convoluted tubule of about 98% to 100% of filtered uric acid; (3) subsequent secretion of uric acid into the lumen in the distal portion of the proximal tubule; and (4) further reabsorption in the distal tubule. The net urinary excretion of uric acid is 6% to 12% of the amount filtered.

Clinical Significance

More than 20 inherited disorders of purine metabolism giving rise to both hyperuricemias and hypouricemias have been recognized to date. Most are very rare, and the diagnosis requires support from a specialist purine laboratory. Symptoms that should raise suspicion include (1) kidney failure or stones in a child or young adult, (2) "gravel" in an infant's diaper, (3) unexplained neurological problems in an infant, child, or adolescent, and (4) gout presenting in a man or woman younger than 30 years of age.

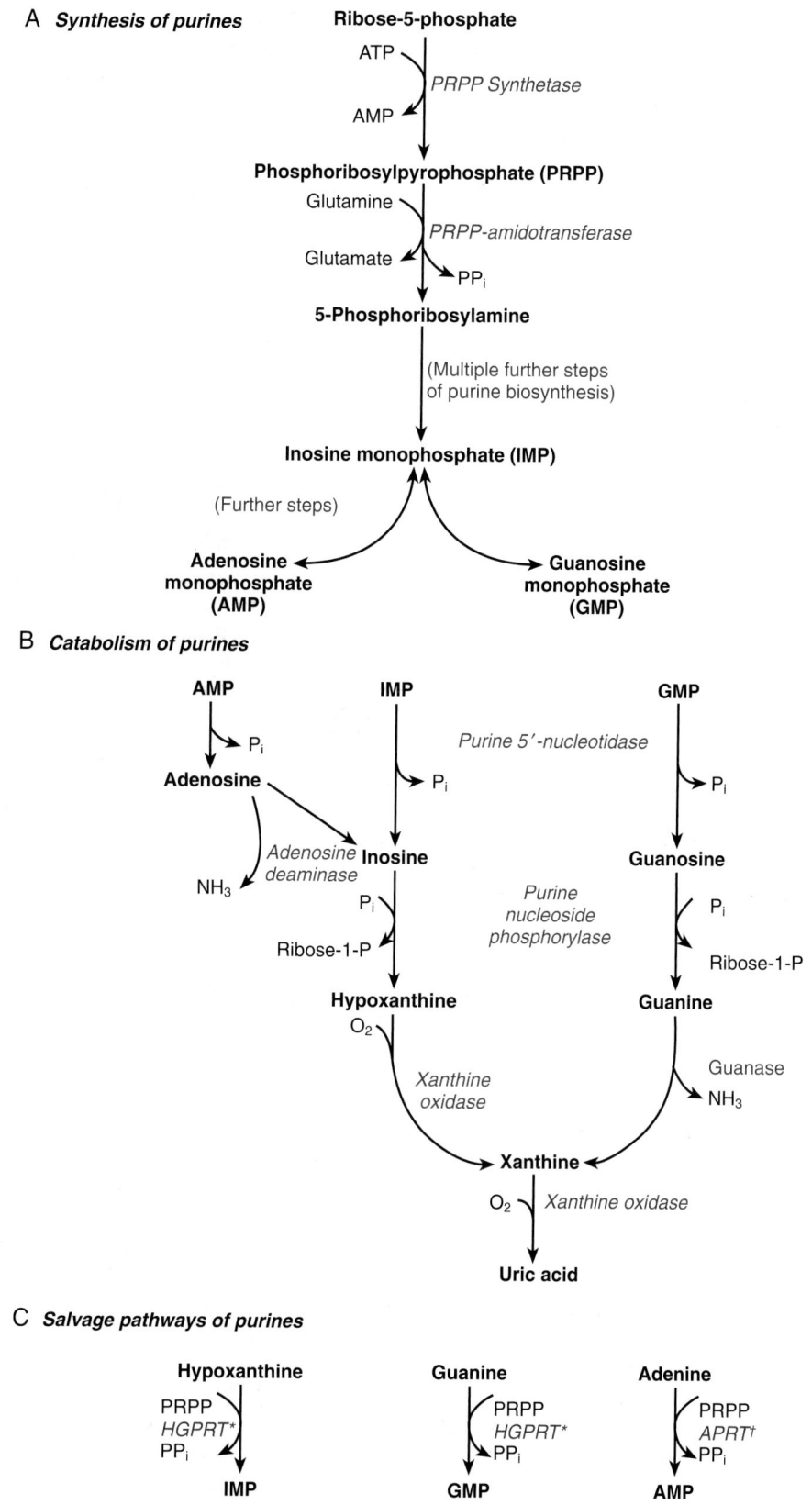

Figure 21-3 Metabolism of purines: **A,** synthesis; **B,** catabolism; and **C,** salvage pathways.

Hyperuricemia

Hyperuricemia is most commonly defined by serum uric acid concentrations greater than 7.0 mg/dL (0.42 mmol/L) in men or greater than 6.0 mg/dL (0.36 mmol/L) in women. The major causes of hyperuricemia are summarized in Box 21-1. Asymptomatic hyperuricemia is frequently detected through biochemical screening. Long-term follow-up of asymptomatic hyperuricemic patients is undertaken because many are at risk for kidney disease that may develop as a result of hyperuricemia and hyperuricuria; few of these patients ever develop the clinical syndrome of gout.

Serum uric acid is measured predominantly in the investigation and management of gout as a result of a primary hyperuricemia or of other conditions or treatments that give rise to secondary hyperuricemias.

Gout

Gout occurs when monosodium urate precipitates from supersaturated body fluids. The deposits of urate are responsible for the clinical signs and symptoms. Gouty arthritis may be associated with urate crystals in joint fluid and with deposits of crystals (tophi) in tissue surrounding the joint. These deposits also may occur in other soft tissue. Wherever they occur, they elicit an intense inflammatory response consisting of polymorphonuclear leukocytes and macrophages. The big toe (first metatarsophalangeal) joint is the classic site for gout. Gout is a condition characterized by occasional attacks and long periods of remission. It is important to appreciate that the serum uric acid concentration is often normal during an acute attack. Kidney disease associated with hyperuricemia may take one or more of several forms: (1) gouty nephropathy with urate deposition in renal parenchyma, (2) acute intratubular deposition of urate crystals, and (3) urate nephrolithiasis.

Gout is classified as primary or secondary. *Primary gout* is associated with "essential" hyperuricemia, which has a polygenic basis. In more than 99% of cases, the cause is uncertain, but the condition is probably due to a combination of (1) metabolic overproduction of purines (25% of patients have increased phosphoribosylpyrophosphate [PRPP]-amidotransferase [EC 2.4.2.14] activity), (2) decreased renal excretion (80% of patients show decreased renal tubular secretion of uric acid), and (3) increased dietary intake. Very rarely, primary gout is attributable to inherited defects of enzymes in the pathways of purine metabolism. The *Lesch-Nyhan syndrome* is characterized by complete deficiency of hypoxanthine-guanine phosphoribosyl transferase (HGPRT, EC 2.4.2.8), the major enzyme of the purine salvage pathways (see Figure 21-3). This X-linked genetic disorder is manifested clinically by (1) mental retardation, (2) abnormal muscle movements, and (3) behavioral problems (self-mutilation and pathological aggressiveness). Patients may present in the first weeks of life with (1) crystalluria, (2) acute kidney failure, (3) gout, (4) hyperuricemia, (5) hyperuricuria, and (6) greatly decreased activities of HGPRT in primarily erythrocytes and fibroblasts. Also, intracellular concentrations of PRPP and rates of purine synthesis are increased. Neurological symptoms of this syndrome may be related to decreased availability of purines to the developing brain, which has limited capacity for de novo purine synthesis. It relies therefore on the purine salvage pathways to supply it with most of the purine nucleotides that it requires. DNA technology has been applied to prenatal diagnosis in the first trimester using chorionic biopsy material. HGPRT assays on cultured fibroblasts obtained by amniocentesis may be used in the second trimester. Partial deficiency of HGPRT (severe X-linked gout) presents in adolescence or early adulthood as (1) early gout, (2) kidney failure, or (3) nephrolithiasis. Increased concentrations of intracellular PRPP with consequent increased uric acid concentrations have been known to occur as a result of mutations in PRPP synthetase (EC 2.7.6.1; PRPP synthetase superactivity), which is also inherited as an X-linked recessive trait. An autosomal dominant familial juvenile hyperuricemic nephropathy has also been recognized. Glucose-6-phosphatase deficiency leads to hyperuricemia as a result of both overproduction and underexcretion of uric acid.

Secondary gout is a result of hyperuricemia attributable to several identifiable causes. Renal retention of uric acid may occur in acute or chronic kidney disease of any type or as a consequence of administration of drugs. Diuretics, in particular, are implicated in the latter instance. Organic acidemia—caused by increased acetoacetate in diabetic ketoacidosis or by lactic acidosis—may interfere with tubular secretion of urate. Increased nucleic acid turnover and a consequent increase in catabolism of purines may be encountered in rapid proliferation of tumor cells and in massive destruction of tumor cells when therapy with certain chemotherapeutic agents is provided.

BOX 21-1   Causes of Hyperuricemia

Increased Formation

Primary

  Idiopathic
  Inherited metabolic disorders

Secondary

  Excess dietary purine intake
  Increased nucleic acid turnover (e.g., leukemia, myeloma, radiotherapy, chemotherapy, trauma)
  Psoriasis
  Altered ATP metabolism
  Tissue hypoxia
  Preeclampsia
  Alcohol

Decreased Excretion

Primary

  Idiopathic

Secondary

  Acute or chronic kidney disease
  Increased renal reabsorption
  Reduced secretion
  Lead poisoning
  Preeclampsia
  Organic acids (e.g., lactate, acetoacetate)
  Salicylate (low doses)
  Thiazide diuretics
  Trisomy 21 (Down syndrome)

Management of an acute attack of gout generally involves the use of nonsteroidal anti-inflammatory drugs (NSAIDs). Patients should be advised to avoid (1) foods that have high purine content (e.g., liver, kidneys, red meat, sardines) and (2) drugs that affect urate excretion (thiazide diuretics and salicylates). Specific pharmacological interventions include the use of uricosuric drugs (e.g., probenecid, sulfinpyrazone), which enhance renal excretion of uric acid by blocking carriers in the tubular cells that mediate reabsorption, or the xanthine oxidase inhibitor allopurinol. Measurement of urinary uric acid excretion facilitates selection of appropriate treatment in this context. Patients excreting less than 600 mg/d (3.6 mmol/d) of uric acid are candidates for treatment with uricosuric drugs, which are contraindicated in patients with urate stones or kidney failure. Conversely, patients excreting more than 600 mg/d (3.6 mmol/d) are candidates for treatment with allopurinol. The NSAIDs azapropazone and tiaprofenic acid have a uricosuric effect and so have a place in both long-term and short-term management of gout. For patients treated for gout, a target concentration of <6.0 mg/dL (<0.36 mmol/L) has been recommended.[14]

About one in five patients with clinical gout also has urinary tract uric acid stones. Although serum and urinary uric acid should be measured in stone formers, many uric acid stone formers do not demonstrate hyperuricuria or hyperuricemia. However, this may reflect the use of reference intervals derived in a purine-rich, westernized society. The cause of uric acid stone formation also involves the passage of persistent acid urine with loss of the postprandial alkaline tide. Undissociated uric acid (pK_a = 5.57) is relatively insoluble. Above pH 5.57, it exists predominantly as its more soluble urate ion, and at pH 7.0, it is greater than 10 times more soluble. Thus in patients with urinary pH persistently less than 6.0, normal urinary concentrations of uric acid will produce supersaturation. Thus measurement of urinary pH throughout the day is often useful. Pure uric acid stones account for approximately 8% of all urinary tract stones and, unlike many of the calcium-containing stones, are radiolucent. Allopurinol is the mainstay of treatment for uric acid stones. Hyperuricuria is also a risk factor for calcium stone formation. Consequently, attempts to increase urinary pH with potassium alkaline salts may be counterproductive as a result of increased calcium stone formation.

Hypouricemia

Hypouricemia is defined as a condition whereby serum urate concentrations are less than 2.0 mg/dL (0.12 mmol/L). It is much less common than hyperuricemia. It may be secondary to any of a number of underlying conditions. Examples include (1) severe hepatocellular disease with reduced purine synthesis or xanthine oxidase activity and (2) defective renal tubular reabsorption of uric acid. Defective reabsorption may be congenital, as in generalized **Fanconi syndrome**, or acquired. The reabsorption defect may be acquired acutely as a result of injection of radiopaque contrast media or chronically because of exposure to toxic agents. Overtreatment of patients with hyperuricemia with allopurinol or uricosuric drugs and

cancer chemotherapy with 6-mercaptopurine or azathioprine (inhibitors of de novo purine synthesis) may also cause hypouricemia. Very rarely, hypouricemia may occur as the result of an inherited metabolic defect. Hypouricemia in combination with xanthinuria is rarely encountered and suggests a deficiency of xanthine oxidase, either in isolation or as part of combined molybdenum cofactor deficiency (sulfite oxidase/xanthine oxidase deficiency).

Analytical Methodology

Common techniques for measuring uric acid in body fluids include (1) phosphotungstic acid (PTA), (2) uricase, and (3) HPLC-based methods.[10]

Phosphotungstic Acid Methods

These methods are based on the development of a blue reaction chromogen (tungsten blue) as PTA is reduced by urate in an alkaline medium. Absorbance of the chromogen in the reaction mixture is measured at wavelengths of 650 to 700 nm. PTA methods are subject to many interferences, and efforts to modify them have had little success in improving their specificity. *darker blue = ↑ uric acid*

Uricase Methods

Uricase methods are more specific than PTA approaches. Uricase ([urate:oxygen] oxidoreductase; EC 1.7.3.3; main sources *Aspergillus flavus*, *Candida utilis*, *Bacillus fastidiosus*, and hog liver) isused as a single step or as the initial step in oxidizing uric acid. Uricase acts on uric acid to produce allantoin, hydrogen peroxide, and carbon dioxide.

Uricase methods became feasible and popular as a result of the availability of high-quality, low-cost preparations of the bacterial enzyme. Preliminary precipitation of protein is not required. Generally, only (1) guanine, (2) xanthine, and (3) a few other structural analogs of uric acid act as alternative substrates, and then only at concentrations improbable in biological fluids.

The reaction is executed in either the kinetic or equilibrium mode with the decrease in absorbance measured with a spectrophotometer at 293 nm. This forms the basis of a proposed reference procedure but requires a high-quality spectrophotometer with a narrow bandpass, which is rarely included in automated analyzers. Most current enzymatic assays for uric acid in plasma involve a peroxidase system coupled with one of a number of oxygen acceptors to produce a chromogen. For example, one method measures hydrogen peroxide with the aid of horseradish peroxidase and an oxygen acceptor to yield a chromogen in the visible spectrum. Oxygen acceptors that have been used for this purpose include (1) 4-aminophenazone and a substituted phenol, (2) 3-methyl-1-benzothiazoline hydrazone (MBTH), 2,2′-azino-di-(3-ethyl-benzothiazoline)-6-sulfonate (ABTS), and (3) *o*-dianisidine.

Although many combinations of oxygen acceptor and phenol have been described, the choice should be guided by minimization of interference and sufficient absorbance to ensure a precise method. Use of a substituted phenol yielding a highly absorbing product helps to reduce potential interference by reducing the sample volume requirement. The major interferants that should be minimized are ascorbic acid and bilirubin. For example, some methods use ascorbate oxidase to eliminate ascorbic acid. Aminophenazone with a substituted phenol or with the addition of ferricyanide has been used to minimize bilirubin interference. It has also been shown that unknown metabolites in plasma of patients with kidney failure, thought to be phenolic compounds, will interfere by competing with the reagent phenol, resulting in low recovery of urate. A phenolic derivative has been used to minimize this interference, thereby generating a higher absorbing product and reducing the sample volume.

Devices that use uricase in a dry reagent format to measure uric acid have also been described. For example, a multilayer film system employs uricase and peroxidase separated by a semi-permeable membrane from a leuco dye that is oxidized to form a colored product. A cellulose matrix pad system employs uricase, peroxidase, and MBTH as oxygen acceptors. In addition, this method needs only a diluted plasma sample, which helps to reduce interferences. Ascorbic acid, however, is a significant interferant. A third system incorporates separation of plasma from red cells and uricase, peroxidase, and a substituted phenol to measure uric acid. All three systems employ a reflectance meter system to facilitate accurate and precise quantitation of the color change.

HPLC Methods

HPLC methods with ion exchange or reversed-phase columns have been used to separate and quantify uric acid. The column effluent is monitored at 293 nm to detect the eluting uric acid. (1) HPLC methods are specific, (2) mobile phases are simple, and (3) retention time for uric acid is less than 6 minutes. Because of these multiple attributes, HPLC has been used to develop reference methods for measuring uric acid. A proposed definitive method for the assay of uric acid in plasma uses IDMS.

Reference Intervals

When an enzymatic method is used, the reference interval for uric acid has been reported to be 3.5 to 7.2 mg/dL (0.208 to 0.428 mmol/L) for males and 2.6 to 6.0 mg/dL (0.155 to 0.357 mmol/L) for females. The concentration of serum uric acid increases gradually with age, rising about 10% between the ages of 20 and 60 years. A rise in women is noted after menopause, when uric acid reaches concentrations similar to those in men. During pregnancy, serum uric acid concentrations fall during the first trimester and until about 24 weeks of gestation. At that time, concentrations begin to rise and eventually exceed nonpregnant concentrations.

An alternative approach to the interpretation of serum uric acid concentrations is to consider the degree of hyperuricemia in relation to the risk of developing gout; men with plasma uric acid concentrations exceeding 9.0 mg/dL (0.540 mmol/L) are approximately 150 times more likely to have coexisting gouty arthritis than are men with uric acid concentrations less than 6.0 mg/dL (0.360 mmol/L).

Urinary uric acid excretion in individuals on a diet containing purines is 250 to 750 mg/d (1.5 to 4.5 mmol/d). Excretion may decrease by 20% to 25% on a purine-free diet to less than 400 mg/d.

Review Questions

1. The plasma concentration of creatinine is maintained within narrow limits predominantly by:
   a. the constant catabolism of purines.
   b. the constant rate of protein metabolism.
   c. the glomerular filtration rate.
   d. an individual's diet.
2. Symptoms of gout are caused by:
   a. decreased renal perfusion as in heart failure.
   b. precipitation of excessive uric acid in joints and the urinary tract.
   c. a low-protein diet.
   d. liver dysfunction as in hepatitis.
3. The main nitrogen-containing compound that accounts for more than 75% of excreted nonprotein nitrogen is:
   a. uric acid.
   b. creatinine.
   c. creatine.
   d. urea.
4. A deficiency of the enzyme xanthine oxidase due to severe hepatocellular disease will lead to:
   a. increased urea concentration.
   b. decreased creatinine concentration.
   c. hypouricemia.
   d. hyperuricemia.
5. During protein breakdown, the amino acid nitrogen groups are converted to urea through the urea cycle in which of the following?
   a. Liver
   b. Kidneys
   c. Heart
   d. GI tract
6. Compensated Jaffe assays for creatinine assessment:
   a. add a fixed value to the assay result to compensate for interferants.
   b. subtract a fixed value from each result to compensate for noncreatinine interference.
   c. use a special formula that involves body mass and urine production to "normalize" creatinine results.
   d. involve averaging of values to remove possible discrepancies between two samples obtained at different times of the day.

7. A value of 8.4 mg/dL of urea converts to what in mmol/L?
   a. 2.99
   b. 29.9
   c. 3.92
   d. 39.2

8. Ascorbic acid and bilirubin are interferants in which of the following assays?
   a. Jaffe reaction and uricase methods
   b. Jaffe reaction only
   c. Jaffe reaction, urease methods, and uricase methods
   d. Urease methods only

9. In the uricase method of uric acid measurement, the main interferants that must be minimized are:
   a. phenol and bilirubin.
   b. ascorbic acid and bilirubin.
   c. endogenous ammonia and oxidizing agents.
   d. ketone bodies and protein.

10. Uric acid is:
    a. the major product of protein catabolism.
    b. a derivative of muscle creatine.
    c. a metabolite of urinary nitrogen.
    d. the major product of purine catabolism.

References

1. Ceriotti F, Boyd JC, Klein G, et al. Reference intervals for serum creatinine concentrations: assessment of available data for global application. Clin Chem 2008;54:559–66.
2. Dodder NG, Tai SS, Sniegoski LT, et al. Certification of creatinine in a human serum reference material by GC-MS and LC-MS. Clin Chem 2007;53:1694–9.
3. Kidney Disease Improving Global Outcomes. KDIGO 2012 clinical practice guideline for the evaluation and management of chronic kidney disease. Kidney Int 2013;(Suppl 1).
4. Miller WG. Estimating glomerular filtration rate. Clin Chem Lab Med 2009;47:1017–9.
5. Myers GL, Miller WG, Coresh J, et al. Recommendations for improving serum creatinine measurement: a report from the Laboratory Working Group of the National Kidney Disease Education Program. Clin Chem 2006;52:5–18.
6. National Institute for Health and Clinical Excellence (NICE). Chronic kidney disease: national clinical guideline for early identification and management in adults in primary and secondary care. Clinical Guideline 2008;73.
7. National Kidney Foundation. K/DOQI clinical practice guidelines for chronic kidney disease: evaluation, classification, and stratification. Am J Kidney Dis 2002;39:S1–266.
8. Panteghini M, Myers GL, Miller WG, Greenberg N. The importance of metrological traceability on the validity of creatinine measurement as an index of renal function. Clin Chem Lab Med 2006;44:1287–92.
9. Perrone RD, Madias NE, Levey AS. Serum creatinine as an index of renal function: new insights into old concepts. Clin Chem 1992;38:1933–53.
10. Price CP, James DR. Analytical reviews in clinical biochemistry: the measurement of urate. Ann Clin Biochem 1988;25(Pt 5):484–98.
11. Spencer K. Analytical reviews in clinical biochemistry: the estimation of creatinine. Ann Clin Biochem 1986;23(Pt 1):1–25.
12. Taylor AJ, Vadgama P. Analytical reviews in clinical biochemistry: the estimation of urea. Ann Clin Biochem 1992;29 (Pt 3):245–64.
13. Welch MJ, Cohen A, Hertz HS, et al. Determination of serum creatinine by isotope dilution mass spectrometry as a candidate definitive method. Anal Chem 1986;58:1681–5.
14. Zhang W, Doherty M, Bardin T, et al. EULAR evidence based recommendations for gout. Part II. Management. Report of a task force of the EULAR Standing Committee for International Clinical Studies Including Therapeutics (ESCISIT). Ann Rheum Dis 2006;65:1312–24.

Carbohydrates

David B. Sacks, M.B., Ch.B., F.R.C.Path.

Objectives

1. Define the following:

Carbohydrate	Glycolysis
Gluconeogenesis	Glycoprotein
Glycogen	Hypoglycemia
Glycogen storage	Ketone
disease	Monosaccharide, disaccharide,
Glycogenesis	and polysaccharide
Glycogenolysis	

2. Provide two examples each of a monosaccharide, a disaccharide, and a polysaccharide; describe the chemical structure of each.
3. Summarize the regulation of glucose concentration in the blood, including two hormones involved in this process.
4. Explain the relationship between glucose, lactate, and pyruvate.
5. Discuss the brain's dependence on glucose, including how the brain is affected in a hypoglycemic state and the alternative energy source used.
6. State the blood glucose concentration at which hypoglycemia is typically diagnosed.
7. List three causes of fasting hypoglycemia and three causes of postprandial (nonfasting) hypoglycemia; describe the 72-hour fast test for diagnosing hypoglycemia.
8. List two causes of hypoglycemia in persons with type 1 diabetes.
9. Compare glucose values in fasting whole-blood, capillary, and venous blood specimens; state the reasons for the discrepant values.
10. State the effects of glycolysis on glucose in uncentrifuged blood; list two ways in which glycolysis can be inhibited.
11. Describe the hexokinase method for measurement of glucose in blood; state the specimen requirements and the principle of the reaction, and list the known interferences.
12. Describe the glucose oxidase method for measurement of glucose in blood; state the specimen requirements and the principle of the reaction, and list the known interferences.
13. Describe the chemical reaction used to assess lactate concentration in blood; describe the chemical reaction used to assess pyruvate concentrations in blood.
14. State the specimen collection and storage requirements for blood lactate and pyruvate analyses.
15. Analyze and resolve case studies regarding carbohydrate disorders; correlate the results of carbohydrate analysis with carbohydrate disorders.

Key Words and Definitions

Aldehyde An organic compound with a carbonyl group (a carbon atom double-bonded to an oxygen) at the end of the carbon chain bonded to hydrogen and an R group (usually an alkyl group).

Carbohydrate Aldehyde or ketone derivatives of polyhydroxy alcohols composed of carbon, hydrogen, and oxygen in a ratio of 1:2:1.

Cori cycle The mechanism by which lactate produced by muscles is carried to the liver, converted back to glucose via gluconeogenesis, and returned to the muscles.

Diabetes Control and Complications Trial (DCCT) A medical study of diabetic patients conducted in the United States and Canada in 1983-1993 by the National Institute of Diabetes and Digestive and Kidney Diseases (NIDDK).

Diabetes mellitus A group of metabolic disorders of carbohydrate metabolism in which glucose is underutilized, producing hyperglycemia.

Glucagon A protein hormone that maintains blood glucose concentration by increasing blood glucose through glycogenolysis.

Gucagonoma A type of islet cell tumor of the alpha cells of the pancreas that secretes glucagon; some are malignant.

Glucose A six-carbon monosaccharide derived from the breakdown of carbohydrates in the diet or in body stores; also can be endogenously synthesized from protein or the glycerol moiety of triglyceride.

Glycogen An extensively branched polysaccharide containing many glucose residues and found particularly in muscle and liver cells for glucose storage.

Glycogen storage disease A group of rare inborn errors of metabolism caused by defects in specific enzymes or transporters involved in the metabolism of glycogen.

Key Words and Definitions—cont'd

Hypoglycemia An abnormally diminished concentration of glucose in the blood.

Idiopathic postprandial syndrome Repeated occurrence of the clinical manifestations of hypoglycemia after meals.

Insulin A protein hormone from the pancreas that maintains blood glucose concentration by decreasing blood glucose through cellular uptake.

Ketone An organic compound that has a carbonyl group (carbon atom double-bonded to an oxygen atom) at any position other than at the end of the carbon chain.

Lactate An intermediary product in glucose metabolism that accumulates in the blood predominantly when tissue oxygenation is decreased, as during strenuous exercise; an increased blood lactate concentration is called *lactic acidosis.*

Oral glucose tolerance test (OGTT) The most common kind of glucose tolerance test in which glucose is ingested by a fasting patient and their concentration of plasma glucose measured over time.

Pyruvate An organic acid formed from glucose through glycolysis.

Stereoisomer One of a group of compounds differing only in the spatial arrangement of their atoms.

Whipple's triad A collection of three criteria suggesting a patient's symptoms result from hypoglycemia.

Carbohydrates, including sugar and starch, are widely distributed in plants and animals. They perform multiple functions, such as serving as structural components in RNA and DNA (ribose and deoxyribose sugars) and providing a source of energy (glucose). **Glucose** is derived from (1) the breakdown of carbohydrates in the diet (grains, starchy vegetables, and legumes) or in body stores (glycogen), and (2) endogenous synthesis from protein or from the glycerol moiety of triglycerides. When energy intake exceeds expenditure, the excess is converted to fat and glycogen for storage in adipose tissue and liver or muscle, respectively. When energy expenditure exceeds caloric intake, endogenous glucose formation occurs from the breakdown of carbohydrate stores and from noncarbohydrate sources (e.g., amino acids, lactate, glycerol).

The glucose concentration in the blood is maintained within a fairly narrow interval under diverse conditions (feeding, fasting, or severe exercise) by hormones such as (1) **insulin**, (2) **glucagon**, and (3) epinephrine. Measurement of glucose is one of the most commonly performed procedures in (1) hospital laboratories, (2) other healthcare chemistry laboratories, (3) point-of-care applications, and (4) home-use meters The most frequently encountered disorder of carbohydrate metabolism is high blood glucose concentration due to **diabetes mellitus**, which affects approximately 9% of the U.S. adult population. The incidence of **hypoglycemia** (low blood glucose) is unknown but is low (excluding patients who use exogenous insulin to control blood glucose).

Chemistry of Carbohydrates

Carbohydrates are **aldehyde** or **ketone** derivatives of polyhydroxy (more than one –OH group) alcohols or compounds that yield these derivatives on hydrolysis.

Monosaccharides

A monosaccharide is a simple sugar that consists of a single polyhydroxy aldehyde or ketone unit and is unable to be hydrolyzed to a simpler form. The backbone is made up of several carbon atoms. Sugars containing three, four, five, six, and seven carbon atoms are known as *trioses, tetroses, pentoses, hexoses,* and *heptoses,* respectively. One of the carbon atoms is double-bonded to an oxygen atom to form a carbonyl group. An aldehyde has the carbonyl group at the end of the carbon chain, whereas if the carbonyl group is at any other position, a ketone is formed (Figure 22-1). The simplest carbohydrate is glycol aldehyde, the aldehyde derivative of ethylene glycol. The aldehyde and ketone derivatives of glycerol are, respectively, glyceraldehyde and dihydroxyacetone (see Figure 22-1). Monosaccharides are termed *aldoses* and *ketoses* according to the position of the carbonyl group (Figure 22-2).

Compounds that are identical in composition and differ only in spatial configuration are called **stereoisomers**. The carbon atoms in the unbranched chain are numbered 1 to 6, as shown by the numbers at the left of the formula for D-glucose in Figure 22-2. The designation D- or L- refers to the position

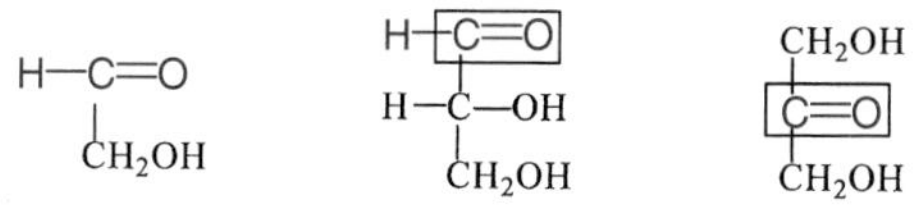

Glycol aldehyde | Glyceraldehyde (aldehyde) | Dihydroxyacetone (ketone)

Figure 22-1 Three-carbon carbohydrates.

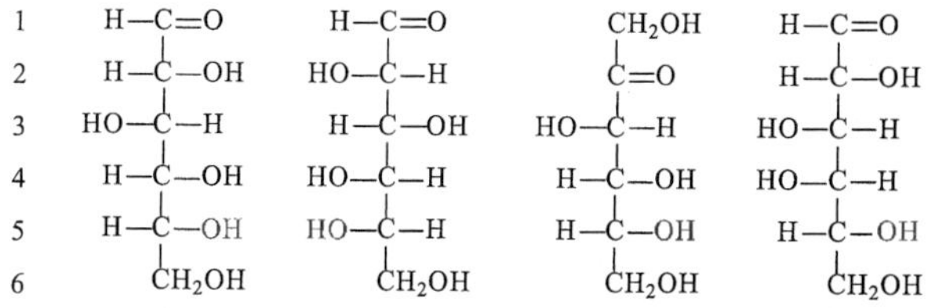

D-Glucose (Aldose) | L-Glucose (Aldose) | D-Fructose (Ketose) | D-Galactose (Aldose)

Figure 22-2 Typical six-carbon sugars.

of the hydroxyl group on the carbon atom adjacent to the last (bottom) CH$_2$OH group. In general, designations of D- and L- for a sugar molecule refer to the stereoisomeric forms of the highest-numbered asymmetrical carbon atom.[*] By convention, the D-sugars are written with the hydroxyl group on the right, and the L-sugars are written with the hydroxyl group on the left (see Figure 22-2). Most sugars in the human body are of the D-configuration. Several different structures exist, depending on the relative positions of the hydroxyl groups on the carbon atoms.

The formula for glucose can be written in the form of aldehyde or enol, a short-lived reactive species. Shift to the enol anion is favored in alkaline solution, as follows:

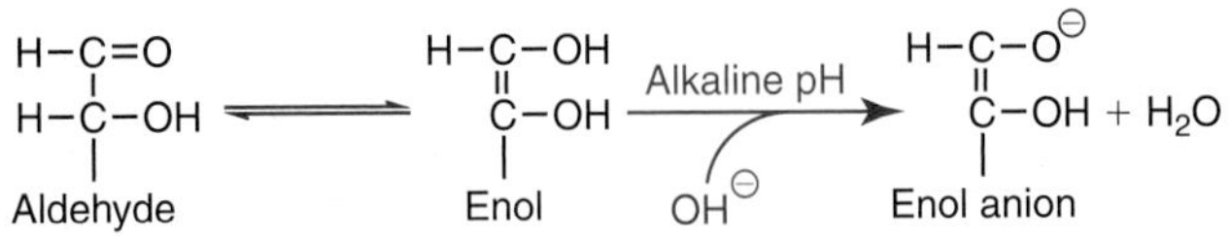

The presence of a double bond and a negative charge in the enol anion makes glucose an active reducing substance that is oxidized by relatively mild oxidizing agents, such as cupric (Cu2$^+$) and ferric (Fe3$^+$) ions. Glucose in hot alkaline solution readily reduces cupric ions to cuprous ions. The color change has been used as a presumptive indication for the presence of glucose; for many years, blood and urine glucose concentrations were measured using this approach. Some other sugars also reduce cupric ions in alkaline solution; these are collectively referred to as reducing *sugars*.

The aldehyde group reacts with the hydroxyl group on carbon 5, represented by a symmetrical ring structure and depicted by the Haworth formula, in which glucose is considered as having the same basic structure as pyran (Figure 22-3). In this formula, the plane of the ring is considered to be perpendicular to the plane of the paper, with the heavy lines pointing toward the reader. Hydroxyl groups in position 1 are then below the plane (α-configuration) or above the plane (β-configuration). A six-member ring sugar containing five carbons and one oxygen is a derivative of pyran and is called a *pyranose*. When linkage occurs with formation of a five-member ring containing four carbons and one oxygen, the sugar has the same basic structure as furan and is called a *furanose*. Fructose is shown in two cyclical forms. Fructopyranose is the configuration of the free sugar, and fructofuranose occurs whenever fructose exists in combination with disaccharides and polysaccharides, as in sucrose and inulin.

Disaccharides

Two monosaccharides join covalently by an *O*-glycosidic bond, with loss of a molecule of water, to form a disaccharide. The chemical bond between the sugars always involves the aldehyde or ketone group of one monosaccharide joined to an alcohol group (e.g., maltose) or an aldehyde or ketone group

(e.g., sucrose) of the other monosaccharide (Figure 22-4). The most common disaccharides are as follows:

Maltose = glucose + glucose
Lactose = glucose + galactose
Sucrose = glucose + fructose

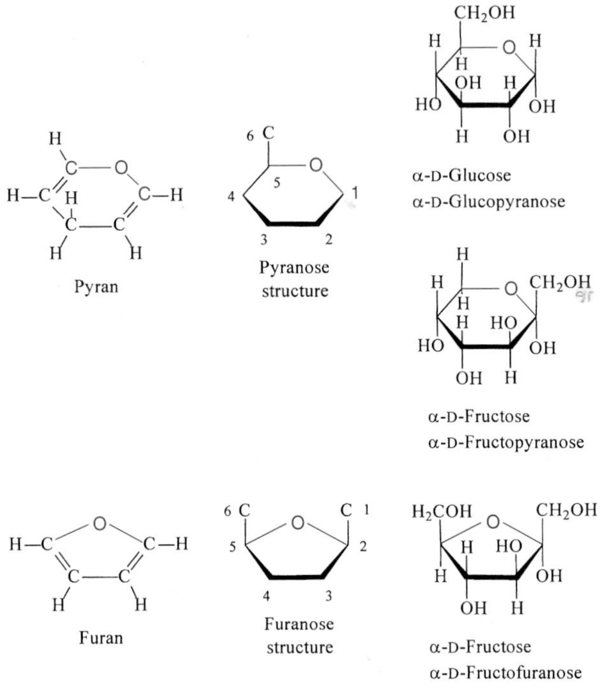

Figure 22-3 The Haworth formula for sugars.

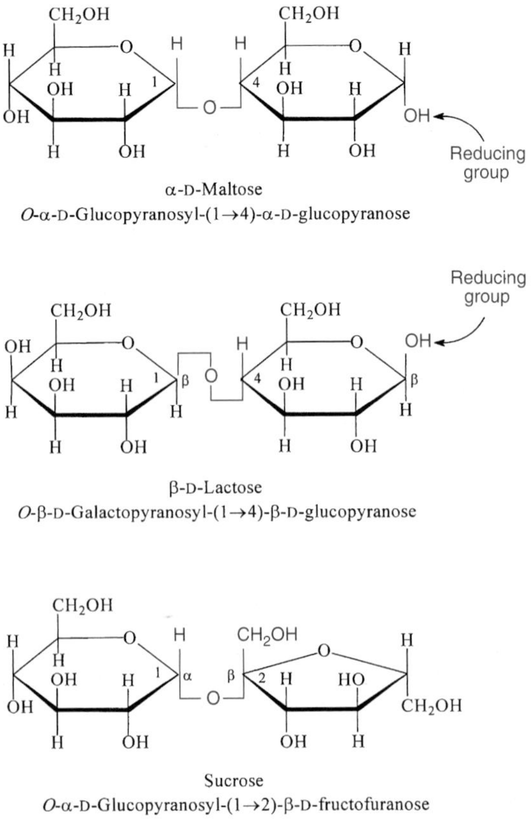

Figure 22-4 Structural formulas of disaccharides.

---

[*]Although the D and L designations are used in this chapter, readers should be aware that in the Cahn-Ingold-Prelog system, a series of rules determine configurations. In this new system, the symbols *R* and *S* are used to designate configurations.

If the linkage between two monosaccharides is between the aldehyde or ketone group of one molecule and a hydroxyl group of another molecule (as in maltose and lactose), one potentially free ketone or aldehyde group remains on the second monosaccharide. Consequently, the second glucose residue can be oxidized and is capable of existing in α- or β-pyranose form. Thus the disaccharide is a reducing sugar, but its reducing power is only approximately 40% of the reducing power of the two single monosaccharides added together. Alternatively, if the linkage between two monosaccharides involves the aldehyde or ketone groups of both molecules (as in sucrose), a nonreducing sugar is formed because no free aldehyde or ketone group remains.

Polysaccharides

The linkage of multiple monosaccharide units results in the formation of polysaccharides. The major storage carbohydrates are starch in plants and glycogen in animals, both of which form granules inside cells. Polysaccharides also provide structural support. For example, the polysaccharide cellulose is used by plants, whereas chitin is the principal component of the exoskeleton of arthropods (insects and crustacea).

Starch and Glycogen

Most starches are composed of a mixture of amyloses and amylopectins. Amylose consists of one long unbranched chain of glucose units linked together by α-1,4-linkages, with only the terminal aldehyde group free. In amylopectin, most of the units are joined by α-1,4-links, but α-1,6-glycosidic bonds also exist every 24 to 30 residues, producing sidechains. Amylopectin contains up to 1 million glucose residues. The structure of **glycogen** is similar to that of amylopectin, but branching is more extensive and is evident every 8 to 12 glucose residues. These branches enhance the solubility of glycogen and allow the glucose residues to be more readily mobilized. Glycogen is most abundant in the liver and also is found in skeletal muscle. The difference in structure between amylose and amylopectin is important in selection of the appropriate starch substrate for amylase determinations (see Chapter 19). The rate of hydrolysis is affected by structural differences in the starch.

Cellulose

Cellulose is an important structural polysaccharide in plants. It is an unbranched polymer of glucose residues joined by β-1,4-linkages. The β-configuration facilitates the formation of long straight chains, producing fibers of high tensile strength. The β-1,4-linkages are not hydrolyzed by α-amylases. Because humans do not have cellulases, they are unable to digest vegetable fiber.

Glycoproteins

Many integral membrane proteins have oligosaccharides covalently attached to the extracellular region, forming glycoproteins. In addition, most proteins that are secreted, such as (1) antibodies, (2) hormones, and (3) coagulation factors, are glycoproteins. The number of attached carbohydrate residues varies among proteins and constitutes 1% to 70% of the weight of the glycoprotein. The oligosaccharides are attached by O-glycosidic linkages to the sidechain oxygen of serine or threonine residues or by N-glycosidic linkages to the sidechain nitrogen of asparagine residues.

One of the biological functions of the carbohydrate chains is to regulate the life span of proteins. Loss of sialic acid residues from the ends of oligosaccharide chains on erythrocytes results in the removal of red blood cells from the circulation. Carbohydrates have also been implicated in cell-cell recognition, in secretion, and in targeting of proteins to specific subcellular domains.

Biochemistry and Physiology[6]

Glucose is the primary energy source for the human body. After absorption (see Chapter 38), the metabolism of all hexoses proceeds according to the body's requirements. This metabolism results in (1) energy production by conversion to carbon dioxide and water, (2) storage as glycogen in the liver or as triglyceride in adipose tissue, or (3) conversion to keto acids, amino acids, or protein.

The complete picture of intermediary metabolism of carbohydrates is complex and is interwoven with the metabolism of lipids and amino acids. For details, readers should consult a biochemistry textbook.

Regulation of Blood Glucose Concentration

The concentration of glucose in the blood is regulated by a complex interplay of multiple pathways that are modulated by several hormones. *Glycogenesis* is the name for the conversion of glucose to glycogen, the most important storage polysaccharide in liver and muscle. The reverse process, namely, the breakdown of glycogen to glucose and other intermediate products, is termed glycogenolysis. The formation of glucose from noncarbohydrate sources, such as (1) amino acids, (2) glycerol, or (3) lactate, is termed *gluconeogenesis*. The conversion of glucose or other hexoses into lactate or **pyruvate** is called *glycolysis*. Further oxidation to carbon dioxide and water occurs through the Krebs (citric acid) cycle and the mitochondrial electron transport chain coupled to oxidative phosphorylation, which generates the adenosine triphosphate (ATP) that provides chemical energy for many bodily processes. Oxidation of glucose to carbon dioxide and water also occurs through the hexose monophosphate shunt pathway, which produces the reduced form of nicotinamide-adenine dinucleotide phosphate (NADPH).

Hypoglycemia[4]

Hypoglycemia is a blood glucose concentration below the fasting value, but the definition of a specific limit is difficult. The most widely used cutoff is 50 mg/dL (2.75 mmol/L), but some authors suggest 60 mg/dL (3.50 mmol/L). A transient decline may occur 1.5 to 2 hours after a meal, and it is not uncommon for plasma glucose concentration as low as 50 mg/dL (2.75 mmol/L), to be observed 2 hours after ingestion of an oral glucose load. Similarly, extremely low fasting blood glucose values may be occasionally noted without symptoms or evidence of underlying disease. Hypoglycemia is rare in persons who do not have drug-treated diabetes mellitus.

Symptoms of hypoglycemia vary among individuals, and none is specific. Epinephrine produces the classic signs and symptoms of hypoglycemia, namely, (1) trembling, (2) sweating, (3) nausea, (4) rapid pulse, (5) light-headedness, (6) hunger, and (7) upper abdominal discomfort. These autonomic symptoms are nonspecific and may be noted in other conditions, such as (1) hyperthyroidism, (2) pheochromocytoma, or even (3) anxiety. Although controversial, some investigators have proposed that a rapid decrease in blood glucose concentrations may trigger the symptoms even though the blood glucose itself may not reach hypoglycemic values, whereas gradual onset to a similar glucose concentration may not produce symptoms.

The brain is completely dependent on blood glucose for energy production under physiological conditions, and approximately half of the glucose used in resting adults is found in the CNS. Very low concentrations of plasma glucose (<20 or 30 mg/dL (1.10-1.65 mmol/L) cause severe CNS dysfunction. During prolonged fasting or hypoglycemia, ketones may be used as an energy source. The broad spectrum of symptoms and signs of CNS dysfunction vary from (1) headache, (2) confusion, (3) blurred vision, (4) dizziness, (5) seizures, (6) loss of consciousness, and (6) even death. These symptoms are known as *neuroglycopenia*. Restoration of plasma glucose usually produces prompt recovery, but irreversible damage may occur.

The age of onset of hypoglycemia is a convenient way to classify the disorder, but some overlap occurs among the various groups. For example, some glycogen storage disorders may arise in the third decade of life, and hormone deficiencies may occur in childhood.

Hypoglycemia in Neonates and Infants

Neonatal blood glucose concentrations are much lower than those of adults (mean, <35 mg/dL/1.93 mmol/L) and decline shortly after birth when liver glycogen stores are depleted. Glucose concentrations as low as 30 mg/dL (1.65 mmol/L) in a term infant and 20 mg/dL 1.10 mmol/L in a premature infant may occur without clinical evidence of hypoglycemia. The more common causes of hypoglycemia in the neonatal period include (1) prematurity, (2) maternal diabetes, (3) gestational diabetes mellitus (GDM), and (4) maternal toxemia. Hyperglycemia in these cases is usually transient. Hypoglycemia with onset in early infancy is usually less transitory and may be due to inborn errors of metabolism or ketotic hypoglycemia; this type of hypoglycemia usually develops after fasting or a febrile illness.

Fasting Hypoglycemia in Adults

Hypoglycemia results from a decreased rate of hepatic glucose production or an increased rate of glucose use. Symptoms suggestive of hypoglycemia are fairly common, but hypoglycemic disorders are rare. However, true hypoglycemia usually indicates serious underlying disease and may be life threatening. An exact threshold for the establishment of hypoglycemia is not always possible, and values as low as 30 mg/dL (1.65 mmol/L) may be encountered in healthy, premenopausal women during the classic test—a 72-hour fast. Symptoms usually begin at plasma glucose concentrations below 55 mg/dL 3.03 mmol/L), and impairment of cerebral function begins when glucose is less than 50 mg/dL (2.75 mmol/L).

The 72-hour fast should be conducted in a hospital. During the fast, the patient should be allowed a liberal intake of calorie-free and caffeine-free fluids. Samples typically are drawn every 6 hours for analysis of plasma glucose, insulin, C-peptide, and proinsulin. When plasma glucose concentration is 60 mg/dL (3.30 mmol/L) or less, analyses are performed every 1 to 2 hours. The fast should be concluded when plasma glucose concentration falls to a predetermined concentration (such as 45 mg/dL/2.47 mmol/L or less) or the patient exhibits signs or symptoms of hypoglycemia, or after 72 hours. Most patients with true hypoglycemia show an abnormally low value within 12 hours of beginning a fast. Women exhibit significantly lower glucose concentrations than men. Low plasma glucose alone is not sufficient to establish the diagnosis, and the absence of signs or symptoms of hypoglycemia during the fast excludes the diagnosis of a hypoglycemic disorder as the cause of such symptoms.

More than 100 causes of hypoglycemia have been reported. Drugs are the most prevalent cause, and many widely used drugs, including (1) propranolol, (2) salicylates, and (3) disopyramide, produce hypoglycemia. Oral hypoglycemic agents, which have long half-lives (35 hours for chlorpropamide), are the most frequent cause of drug-induced hypoglycemia and may be directly measured in blood or urine. Surreptitious administration of insulin is detected by the discovery of low C-peptide concentrations with increased insulin concentrations.

Ethanol produces hypoglycemia by inhibiting gluconeogenesis, and this inhibition is aggravated by malnutrition (low glycogen stores) in individuals with chronic alcoholism. Individuals with hepatic failure (e.g., viral hepatitis, ingestions of toxins) have impaired gluconeogenesis or glycogen storage, which may result in hypoglycemia. Decreased hepatic glucose production requires dysfunction of more than 80% of the liver. Deficiencies of (1) growth hormone (especially with coexistent ACTH deficiency), (2) glucocorticoids, (3) thyroid hormone, or (4) glucagon may also produce hypoglycemia. Although a deficiency of glucocorticoids (e.g., Addison disease) is most consistently associated with hypoglycemia, most glucocorticoid-deficient adults are not hypoglycemic. Hormonal deficiency causes hypoglycemia in children more frequently than in adults.

Demonstration of a low plasma glucose concentration in the presence of a high plasma insulin value is highly suggestive of an insulin-producing pancreatic islet cell tumor. Because healthy people exhibit a wide range of insulin concentrations, absolute hyperinsulinemia occurs in less than 50% of individuals with insulinomas. Serum insulin concentrations inappropriately high for concurrent plasma glucose values denote autonomous insulin secretion. Provocative tests (glucagon, tolbutamide, or calcium) or suppression tests (infusion of insulin and measurement of C-peptide), although strongly recommended in the past, generally are not necessary.

Nonpancreatic neoplasms that cause hypoglycemia are rare, but, when present, they often are extremely large mesenchymal neoplasms. No single mechanism explains the hypoglycemia in all cases, but secretion of a precursor of insulin-like growth factor (IGF)-2 is the most commonly encountered finding. Glucose utilization is increased, especially in muscle, presumably reflecting activity of the hormone.

Hypoglycemia caused by septicemia should be relatively easy to diagnose. The mechanism is not well defined, but depleted glycogen stores, impaired gluconeogenesis, and increased peripheral use of glucose may all be contributing factors. Glucose tolerance is commonly depressed in individuals with renal disease, and hypoglycemia may occur in those with end-stage renal failure.

Some of the conditions that produce fasting hypoglycemia are readily apparent, but others require a lengthy diagnostic work-up. Once fasting hypoglycemia is demonstrated, specific tests should be performed to establish the underlying cause. The **oral glucose tolerance test (OGTT)** is not an appropriate study for evaluation of a patient suspected of having hypoglycemia.

Postprandial Hypoglycemia

Drugs, antibodies to insulin or the insulin receptor, inborn errors (e.g., fructose-1,6-diphosphatase deficiency), and *reactive hypoglycemia* (also referred to as *functional hypoglycemia*) produce hypoglycemia in the postprandial (fed) state. It has been proposed that for individuals with vague symptoms after food ingestion, the preferred terminology should be *idiopathic reactive hypoglycemia* or **idiopathic postprandial syndrome**.

At the Third International Symposium on Hypoglycemia, reactive hypoglycemia was defined as a "clinical disorder in which the patient has postprandial symptoms suggesting hypoglycemia that occur in everyday life and are accompanied by a blood glucose concentration less than 45 to 50 mg/dL (2.48-2.75 mmol/L) as determined by a specific glucose measurement on arterialized venous or capillary blood, respectively." Patients complain of autonomic symptoms that occur approximately 1 to 3 hours after eating and seem to obtain relief, lasting 30 to 45 minutes, by food intake. These symptoms are rarely due to low blood glucose concentrations. A 5- or 6-hour glucose tolerance test had been the standard procedure to establish the presence of postprandial hypoglycemia, but that has been discredited. Consequently, an *OGTT should not be used in the diagnosis of reactive hypoglycemia*.

Postprandial hypoglycemia is infrequent, and demonstration of hypoglycemia during spontaneously occurring symptomatic episodes is necessary to establish the diagnosis. If this is not possible, a 5-hour meal tolerance test (which simulates the composition of a normal diet) or a "hyperglucidic" (high glucose) breakfast test has been proposed.

The diagnosis of hypoglycemia has also been used to explain a wide variety of disorders that appear unrelated to blood glucose abnormalities. These nonspecific symptoms include (1) fatigue, (2) muscle spasms, (3) palpitations, (4) numbness,

(5) tingling, (6) pain, (7) sweating, (8) mental dullness, (9) sleepiness, (10) weakness, and (11) fainting. Behavioral abnormalities, poor school performance, and delinquency have been incorrectly attributed to low blood glucose concentrations. A diagnosis of hypoglycemia should not be made unless a patient meets the criteria of **Whipple's triad** of low blood glucose concentration. They are (1) symptoms known or likely to be caused by hypoglycemia, (2) low glucose measured when symptoms occur, and (3) relief of symptoms when glucose is increased to normal. Demonstration of normal plasma glucose concentration when the patient exhibits symptoms excludes the possibility of a hypoglycemic disorder.

Hypoglycemia in Diabetes Mellitus[9]

Hypoglycemia occurs frequently in individuals with type 1 or type 2 diabetes.[1] Patients using insulin experience approximately one to two episodes of symptomatic hypoglycemia per week, and severe hypoglycemia that requires assistance from others or is associated with loss of consciousness affects about 10% of this population per year. In patients practicing intensive insulin therapy (e.g., multiple injections, continuous subcutaneous insulin infusion), these figures are increased twofold to sixfold. The chief adverse event associated with intensive therapy in the **Diabetes Control and Complications Trial (DCCT)** was a threefold increase in the incidence of severe hypoglycemia.[5] Similarly, hypoglycemia occurs in patients with type 2 diabetes (caused by oral hypoglycemic agents or insulin) but is less frequent than in type 1 diabetes.[10] Pathophysiological mechanisms that contribute to hypoglycemia in patients with diabetes are (1) defective glucose counterregulation (ability to increase glucose, counter to the effect of insulin) and (2) unawareness of hypoglycemia.

Defective Glucose Counterregulation

Counterregulatory responses become impaired in patients with type 1 diabetes, increasing the risk of hypoglycemia. The secretion of glucagon in response to hypoglycemia is impaired by an unknown mechanism early in the course of type 1 diabetes. The secretory response of epinephrine to hypoglycemia becomes deficient later in the course of the disease. These defects are selective because other stimuli continue to elicit glucagon and epinephrine secretion. Glucose counterregulation does not appear to be notably defective in patients with type 2 diabetes.

Unawareness of Hypoglycemia

Up to 50% of patients with long-standing (longer than 30 years) type 1 diabetes do not experience neurogenic warning symptoms and are prone to more severe hypoglycemia. The mechanism is thought to be associated with a decreased epinephrine response to hypoglycemia. Intensively treated patients with type 1 diabetes require lower plasma glucose concentrations to elicit symptoms of hypoglycemia. Some authors have claimed that therapeutic use of human insulin rather than other insulins results in an increased incidence of unawareness of hypoglycemia, but analysis of 45 studies revealed no significant differences in hypoglycemic episodes among insulin species.

Lactate and Pyruvate

Lactic acid, an intermediary in carbohydrate metabolism, is predominantly derived from (1) white skeletal muscle, (2) brain, (3) skin, (4) renal medulla, and (5) erythrocytes. The blood lactate concentration depends on the rate of production in these tissues and the rate of metabolism in the liver and kidneys. The liver uses approximately 65% (75 g/d) of the total basal lactate produced, predominantly in gluconeogenesis. The **Cori cycle** is the conversion of glucose to **lactate** in the periphery and reconversion of lactate to glucose in the liver. Extrahepatic removal of lactate occurs by oxidation in red skeletal muscle and the renal cortex. A moderate increase in lactate production results in increased hepatic lactate clearance, but uptake by the liver is saturable when concentrations exceed 2 mmol/L. During strenuous exercise, for example, lactate concentrations may increase significantly, from an average concentration of about 0.9 to more than 20 mmol/L within 10 seconds. No concentration of lactate is uniformly accepted for the diagnosis of lactic acidosis, but lactate concentrations exceeding 5 mmol/L with pH less than 7.25 indicate significant lactic acidosis.

Lactic Acidosis[7]

Lactic acidosis occurs in two clinical settings: (1) type A (hypoxic), associated with decreased tissue oxygenation, such as shock, hypovolemia, and left ventricular failure; and (2) type B (metabolic), associated with (1) diseases such as (e.g., diabetes mellitus, neoplasia, liver disease), (2) drugs/toxins (e.g., ethanol, methanol, salicylates), or (3) inborn errors of metabolism. Lactic acidosis is not uncommon and occurs in approximately 1% of those admitted to the hospital. It has a mortality rate greater than 60%, which approaches 100% if hypotension also is present. Type A is much more common.

An uncommon but often undiagnosed cause of lactic acidosis is D-lactic acidosis. Absorption and accumulation of D-lactate from abnormal intestinal bacteria may cause systemic acidosis. This condition occurs after jejunoileal bypass surgery and manifests as altered mental status (from mild drowsiness to coma) with increased blood concentrations of D-lactate. Virtually all the commonly used laboratory assays for lactate use L-lactate dehydrogenase, which does not detect D-lactate. D-Lactate is also measured by gas-liquid chromatography or, enzymatically, with a specific D-lactate dehydrogenase.

Lactate in cerebrospinal fluid normally parallels blood concentrations. With biochemical alterations in the CNS, however, CSF lactate values change independently of blood values. Increased CSF concentrations are noted in individuals with (1) cerebrovascular accidents, (2) intracranial hemorrhage, (3) bacterial meningitis, (4) epilepsy, and (5) other CNS disorders.

Inborn Errors of Carbohydrate Metabolism

Deficiency or absence of an enzyme that participates in carbohydrate metabolism may result in accumulation of monosaccharides, which are measured in the urine. Techniques used to separate and identify these sugars include (1) fermentation, (2) optical rotation, (3) osazone formation with phenylhydrazine, (4) specific chemical tests, and (5) paper or thin-layer chromatography. The availability of glucose oxidase test strips, specific for glucose, has greatly simplified the differentiation of glucose from other reducing substances. For practical purposes, the only urinary sugars of clinical interest are glucose and galactose. Urine from infants and children should be tested by both the glucose oxidase and copper reduction tests to identify individuals with inborn errors of metabolism.

Glycogen Storage Disease

Glycogen, although present in most tissues, is stored predominantly in the liver and skeletal muscle. During fasting, liver glycogen is converted to glucose to provide energy for the whole body. In contrast, skeletal muscle lacks glucose-6-phosphatase, and muscle glycogen is used locally for energy. **Glycogen storage disease** is a generic name encompassing at least 10 rare inherited disorders of glycogen storage in tissues.[3] The different forms of glycogen storage disease are categorized by numerical type in the chronological sequence in which these defects were identified. Each form is due to a deficiency of a specific enzyme in glycogen metabolism, producing a quantitative or a qualitative defect of glycogen storage.

Because both the liver and skeletal muscle have the highest rates of glycogen metabolism, these structures are most affected. The liver forms (types I, III, IV, and VI) are marked by hepatomegaly (due to increased liver glycogen stores) and hypoglycemia (caused by inability to convert glycogen to glucose). Hypoglycemia is manifested by (1) autonomic clinical symptoms (sweating, shakiness, and a light-headed feeling), (2) growth retardation, and (3) laboratory findings of decreased insulin and increased glucagon concentrations in the blood. The muscle forms (types II, IIIa, V, and VII), in contrast, have mild symptoms that usually appear in young adulthood during strenuous exercise owing to the inability to provide energy for muscle contraction. Other muscle disorders may exhibit similar symptoms but are readily differentiated through evaluation of glycogen stores. The specific diagnosis of each type is made directly by demonstrating the enzyme defect in tissue.

Analytical Methodology

Analytical methods for measuring (1) glucose, (2) ketone bodies, (3) lactate, (4) pyruvate, (5) insulin, and (6) proinsulin are discussed in this section.

Measurement of Glucose in Body Fluids

Several methods are used to measure glucose in (1) blood, (2) serum, (3) plasma, and (4) urine. Current surveys conducted by the College of American Pathologists (CAP) demonstrate that all methods exhibit a coefficient of variation (CV) among laboratories that is less than or equal to 2.6% for glucose values on lyophilized serum.

Specimen Collection and Storage

In individuals with a normal hematocrit, fasting whole-blood glucose concentration is approximately 10% to 12% lower than plasma glucose. Although the glucose concentrations in the water phase of red blood cells and plasma are similar (the erythrocyte plasma membrane is freely permeable to glucose), the water content of plasma (93%) is approximately 11% greater than that of whole blood at a normal hematocrit. In most clinical laboratories, plasma or serum is used for most glucose determinations. However, methods for self-monitoring of glucose typically use whole-blood samples but may measure the glucose concentration in the plasma phase. During fasting, capillary blood glucose concentration is only 2 to 5 mg/dL higher than that of venous blood. After a glucose load, however, capillary blood glucose concentrations are 20 to 70 mg/dL (1.11 -3.89 mmol/L) (mean, ≈30 mg/dL/1.67 mmol/L; equivalent to 20% to 25%) higher than the concentrations in concurrently drawn venous blood samples.

Glycolysis decreases serum glucose by approximately 5% to 7% in 1 hour (5 to 10 mg/dL) in normal uncentrifuged coagulated blood at room temperature. The rate of in vitro glycolysis is higher in the presence of leukocytosis or bacterial contamination. In separated, nonhemolyzed sterile serum, the glucose concentration is generally stable as long as 8 hours at 25 °C and up to 72 hours at 4 °C; variable stability is observed with longer storage periods. Plasma, removed from the cells after moderate centrifugation, contains leukocytes that also metabolize glucose—although cell-free sterile plasma has no glycolytic activity.

Sodium fluoride or, less commonly, sodium iodoacetate, is used to inhibit glycolysis.[2] Fluoride ions prevent glycolysis by inhibiting enolase, an enzyme that requires Mg^{2+}. Inhibition is due to the formation of an ionic complex consisting of Mg^{2+}, inorganic phosphate, and fluoride ions; this complex interferes with the interaction of enzyme and substrate. Fluoride is also a weak anticoagulant because it binds calcium; however, clotting may occur after several hours, and it is therefore advisable to use a *combined fluoride-oxalate mixture,* such as 2 mg of potassium oxalate ($K_2C_2O_4$) and 2 mg of NaF/mL of blood, to prevent late clotting. Other anticoagulants such as (1) ethylenediaminetetraacetic acid, (2) citrate, or (3) heparin have also been used. Fluoride ions in high concentration inhibit the activity of urease and certain other enzymes; consequently the specimens may be unsuitable for determination of urea in procedures that require urease and for direct assay of some serum enzymes. $K_2C_2O_4$ causes loss of cell water, thereby diluting the plasma. Samples collected in these tubes therefore should not be used for measurement of other analytes.

Although fluoride has been widely used to inhibit glycolysis, the rate of decline in the first 1 to 2 hours after sample collection is not altered, and glycolysis may continue at a slower rate for up to 4 hours. Acidification of blood using citrate buffer inhibits in vitro glycolysis more effectively than fluoride.

To minimize glycolysis, the cells should be removed within minutes. Alternatively, the tube should be placed in an ice-water slurry and the cells separated within 30 minutes. Neither of these approaches is practical in routine analysis. It may not be necessary in routine analysis to use a fluoride-containing tube if plasma is separated from cells or if glucose is measured within 30 minutes of blood collection. However, inhibitors of glycolysis are necessary in patients with greatly increased leukocyte counts

because differences of up to 65 mg/dL (3.60 mmol/L) have been observed between glucose values with and without glycolytic inhibitors after 1 to 2 hours of contact with the blood cells.

CSF may be contaminated with bacteria or other cells and should be analyzed immediately for glucose. If a delay in measurement is unavoidable, the sample should be centrifuged and stored at 4 °C or −20 °C.

In 24-hour collections of urine, glucose may be preserved by adding 5 mL of glacial acetic acid to the container before starting the collection. The final pH of the urine is usually between 4 and 5, which inhibits bacterial activity. Other preservatives that have been proposed include 5 g of sodium benzoate per 24-hour specimen, or chlorhexidine and 0.1% sodium nitrate with 0.01% benzethonium chloride. These may be inadequate, and urine should be stored at 4 °C during collection. Urine samples may lose as much as 40% of their glucose after 24 hours at room temperature.

Measurement of Glucose in Blood

Hexokinase or glucose oxidase is widely used in assays to measure the concentration of glucose in body fluids.

Hexokinase Methods

Hexokinase (HK) methods are based on a coupled enzyme assay that uses HK and glucose-6-phosphate dehydrogenase (G-6-PD):

$$Glucose + ATP \xrightleftharpoons{Hexokinase} Glucose\text{-}6\text{-}phosphate + ADP$$

$$Glucose\text{-}6\text{-}phosphate \xrightleftharpoons{G\text{-}6\text{-}PD} 6\text{-}Phosphogluconate$$

$$NADP^{\oplus} \rightarrow NADPH + H^{\oplus}$$
$$(or\ NAD^{\oplus}) \quad (or\ NADH)$$

As indicated, glucose is first phosphorylated by ATP in the presence of HK and Mg^{2+}. The glucose-6-phosphate formed is oxidized by G6PD to 6-phosphogluconate in the presence of $NADP^+$ or NAD^+. The amount of reduced NADP (NADPH) or NADH produced is directly proportional to the amount of glucose in the sample and is measured by the increase in absorbance at 340 nm. $NADP^+$ is the cofactor when G6PD derived from yeast is used in the assay; NAD^+ is the cofactor when bacterial (*Leuconostoc mesenteroides*) G6PD is used. A reference method based on this principle has been developed and validated. In the reference method, serum or plasma is deproteinated by the addition of solutions of barium hydroxide and zinc sulfate. The clear supernatant is mixed with a reagent containing ATP, NAD^+, hexokinase, and G6PD, incubated at 25 °C until the reaction is complete and NADH is measured. Calibrators and blanks are carried through the entire procedure, including the deproteination step.

Although highly accurate and precise, the reference method is too exacting and time-consuming for routine use in a clinical laboratory. An alternative approach is to apply the reaction directly to serum or plasma and use a specimen blank to correct for interfering substances that absorb at 340 nm.

Serum or plasma may be used. NaF, with an anticoagulant such as (1) EDTA, (2) heparin, (3) oxalate, or (4) citrate, may be used. Hemolyzed specimens containing more than 0.5 g of hemoglobin/dL are unsatisfactory because phosphate esters and enzymes released from red blood cells interfere with the assay. Other sources of interference include drugs, bilirubin, and lipemia (triglycerides of 500 mg/dL or greater causing a positive interference).

Absorbances of sample or calibrator reaction mixtures are measured after the reactions have continued to completion (equilibrium reaction, "end-point" method) or at a fixed time after initiation of the reaction (fixed-time kinetics). In the equilibrium methods for glucose concentrations may be calculated directly, based on the molar absorptivity of NADPH or NADH, but inclusion of a set of calibrators is recommended to detect possible deterioration of enzymes, ATP, NADP$^+$, or NAD$^+$—all of which are unstable. Reagents may also contain substances that react with the coenzymes. The presence of these substances is evaluated by measurement of the increase in absorbance observed in a reagent blank. The highest calibrator provides a check on the linearity of the response and the adequacy of the enzyme reagent. The procedures typically show a linear relation between absorbance and glucose concentrations of 0 to 500 mg/dL (27.75 mmol/L). Serum or plasma samples with glucose concentrations that exceed 500 mg/dL (27.75 mmol/L) should be diluted (usually with isotonic saline) and re-assayed.

Also available are hexokinase procedures in which indicator reactions produce colored products, enabling absorbance measurements in the visible range. An oxidation reduction system containing phenazine methosulfate and a substituted tetrazolium compound, 2-(p-iodophenyl)-3-p-nitrophenyl-5-phenyltetrazolium chloride (INT), is reacted with NADPH formed in the reaction. The reduced INT is colored, with maximal absorbance at 520 nm.

Glucose Oxidase Methods

Glucose oxidase catalyzes the oxidation of glucose to gluconic acid and hydrogen peroxide:

$$\text{Glucose} + H_2O + O_2 \xrightarrow{\text{Glucose Oxidase}} \text{Gluconic acid} + 2\,H_2O_2$$

Addition of the enzyme peroxidase and a chromogenic oxygen acceptor, such as o-dianisidine, results in the formation of a colored compound that is measured:

$$o\text{-Dianisidine} + H_2O_2 \xrightarrow{\text{Peroxidase}} \text{Oxidized } o\text{-Dianisidine} + H_2O \quad \text{(Colored)}$$

Glucose oxidase is highly specific for β-D-glucose. Because 36% and 64% of glucose in solution are in the α- and β-forms, respectively, complete reaction requires mutarotation of the α-form to the β-form. Some commercial preparations of glucose oxidase contain an enzyme, mutarotase, that accelerates this reaction. Otherwise, extended incubation time allows spontaneous conversion.

The second step, involving peroxidase, is much less specific than the glucose oxidase reaction. Various substances, such as (1) uric acid, (2) ascorbic acid, (3) bilirubin, (4) hemoglobin, (5) tetracycline, and (6) glutathione, inhibit the reaction (presumably by competing with the chromogen for H_2O_2), producing lower values. Some glucose oxidase preparations contain catalase as a contaminant that decomposes peroxide and decreases the intensity of the final color obtained. Calibrators and unknowns should be simultaneously analyzed under conditions in which the rate of oxidation is proportional to the glucose concentration.

Glucose oxidase methods are suitable for measurement of glucose in CSF. Urine, however, contains high concentrations of substances (such as uric acid) that interfere with the peroxidase reaction, producing falsely low results. The glucose oxidase method therefore should not be used for urine. A method in which the urine is first pretreated with an ion exchange resin to remove interfering substances has been described.[8]

Some instruments use a polarographic oxygen electrode that measures the rate of oxygen consumption after the sample is added to a solution containing glucose oxidase. Because this measurement involves only the glucose oxidase reaction, interferences encountered in the peroxidase step are eliminated. To prevent formation of oxygen from H_2O_2 by catalase present in some preparations of glucose oxidase, H_2O_2 is removed by two additional reactions:

$$H_2O_2 + C_2H_5OH \xrightarrow{\text{Catalase}} CH_3CHO + 2\,H_2O$$
$$H_2O_2 + 2H^+ + 2I^- \xrightarrow{\text{Molybdate}} I_2 + 2\,H_2O$$

The latter reaction is effective even when catalase activity has diminished on storage of reagents. The procedure has been applied directly to (1) urine, (2) serum, (3) plasma, or (4) CSF. However, this approach should not be used for determination of glucose in whole blood because blood cells consume oxygen.

In dry, multilayer, slide automated systems, glucose is measured by a glucose oxidase procedure. A 10-μL sample of (1) serum, (2) plasma, (3) urine, or (4) CSF is placed on a porous film on top of the layer containing the reagents. Glucose diffuses through the film and reacts with the reagents to produce a colored end product or dye. The intensity of this dye is measured through a lower transparent film by reflectance spectrophotometry. Advantages include (1) small sample size, (2) no liquid reagents, and (3) improved stability on storage.

Glucose Dehydrogenase Method

The enzyme glucose dehydrogenase (β-D-glucose: NAD oxidoreductase, EC 1.1.1.47) catalyzes the oxidation of glucose to gluconolactone with concomitant reduction of NAD$^+$ to NADH. Mutarotase is added to shorten the time necessary to reach equilibrium. The amount of NADH generated is proportional to the glucose concentration. The reaction appears to be (1) highly specific for glucose, (2) shows no interference from common anticoagulants and substances normally found in serum, and (3) provides results in close agreement with hexokinase procedures. The glucose dehydrogenase procedure is not widely used in the United States, except in a glucose meter.

Measurement of Glucose in Urine

A method for the examination of urine for glucose is rapid, inexpensive, and noninvasive and has been used to screen large numbers of samples.[8] Monitoring of urine glucose lacks sensitivity and specificity and provides no information about blood glucose concentrations below the renal threshold (usually 180 mg/dL/9.99 mmol/L). Older screening tests detect all sugars that reduce copper and produce a chromagen. Unfortunately, these tests also react with reducing substances other than glucose. Qualitative, quantitative, and semi-quantitative methods are widely available for measuring glucose in urine and have essentially replaced the nonspecific tests in adults. Note that a reducing sugar method other than an enzymatic method for glucose must be used when neonates or infants are screened for inborn errors of metabolism that result in the appearance of reducing sugars other than glucose (e.g., galactose, fructose) in the urine.

Qualitative Method for Measurement of Total Reducing Substances

Benedict qualitative reagent contains cupric ion complexed to citrate in alkaline solution. Reducing substances convert cupric to cuprous ions, forming yellow cuprous hydroxide or red cuprous oxide. A convenient adaptation of the procedure is marketed in tablet form (Bayer Corporation CLINITEST Reagent Tablets).

Semi-quantitative Measurement of Glucose in Urine

Paper test strips are commercially available from several manufacturers. All use the glucose-specific enzyme glucose oxidase in a chromogenic assay. Dyes used include o-tolidine and. Tetramethylbenzidine (TMB) with the intensity of the color developed proportional to the concentration of glucose in the urine sample. A typical cutoff is a glucose concentration of 100 mg/dL (5.55 mmol/L) with an upper limit of detection of 250 mg/dL/13.8 mmol/L).

When using these strips, false positive results may be produced by contamination of urine with H_2O_2 or a strong oxidizing agent, such as hypochlorite (bleach). False negative results may occur with large quantities of reducing substances, such as (1) ketones, (2) ascorbic acid, and (3) salicylates. For routine examinations, a negative result by the strip test is usually interpreted to mean that the urine specimen is negative for glucose.

Other strip tests have been designed for the semi-quantitative estimation of both glucose and ketone bodies.

Quantitative Methods for Determination of Glucose in Urine

Applications of various procedures for quantitative determination of glucose in urine were previously discussed in the section on the determination of glucose in body fluids. Hexokinase or glucose dehydrogenase procedures are recommended for greatest accuracy and specificity. Glucose oxidase procedures that depend only on the consumption of oxygen or the production of H_2O_2 are also reliable. Glucose oxidase procedures that include the H_2O_2-peroxidase reaction are not used for urine.

Reference Intervals

Although glucose is assayed by several different analytical procedures, reference intervals do not vary significantly among methods. The following values are representative of glucose assays:

Sample Reference Intervals for Fasting Glucose	
Plasma/Serum	
Adults	74 to 100 mg/dL (4.1 to 5.5 mmol/L)
Children	60 to 100 mg/dL (3.5 to 5.5 mmol/L)
Premature neonates	20 to 60 mg/dL (1.1 to 3.3 mmol/L)
Term neonates	30 to 60 mg/dL (1.7 to 3.3 mmol/L)
Whole blood	65 to 95 mg/dL (3.6 to 5.3 mmol/L)
CSF	40 to 70 mg/dL (60% of plasma value) (2.2 to 3.9 mmol/L)
Urine	
24 hour	1 to 15 mg/dL (0.1 to 0.8 mmol/L)

No sex difference exists. Plasma glucose concentrations increase with age—fasting glucose concentrations increase approximately 2 mg/dL (0.11 mmol/L) per decade; postprandial concentrations increase by 4 mg/dL (0.22 mmol/L) per decade; and concentrations after a glucose challenge increase by 8 to 13 mg/dL (0.44- 0.72) per decade.

CSF glucose concentrations should be approximately 60% of the plasma concentrations and must always be compared with concurrently measured plasma glucose for adequate clinical interpretation.

Lactate and Pyruvate

Measurement of pyruvate is useful in the evaluation of patients with inborn errors of metabolism who have increased serum lactate concentrations. A lactate-to-pyruvate ratio of less than 25 suggests a defect in gluconeogenesis, whereas an increased ratio (<35) indicates reduced intracellular conditions found in hypoxia. Inborn errors associated with an increased lactate-to-pyruvate ratio include pyruvate carboxylase deficiency and defects in oxidative phosphorylation. Pyruvate is also measured in clinical studies evaluating reperfusion after myocardial ischemia.

Determination of Lactate in Whole Blood

Lactate is oxidized to pyruvate by lactate dehydrogenase in the presence of NAD^+. The NADH formed in this reaction is measured spectrophotometrically at 340 nm and serves as a measure of the lactate concentration:

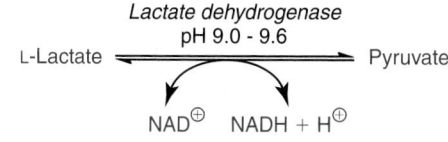

The equilibrium of the reaction typically lies far to the left. However, by buffering the pH between 9.0 and 9.6, adding an excess of NAD⁺, and trapping the reaction product pyruvate with hydrazine, the equilibrium is shifted to the right. Pyruvate can also be removed through reaction with L-glutamate in the presence of alanine aminotransferase.

Because of its high specificity and simplicity, the enzymatic method is the method of choice for the measurement of lactate, although other methods such as gas chromatography have been used.

Specimen Collection and Storage

Careful techniques are necessary to prevent changes in lactate concentration while blood is drawn and afterward. Patients should be fasting and at complete rest for at least 2 hours to allow lactate concentrations to reach steady state.

Venous specimens should be obtained without the use of a tourniquet or immediately after the tourniquet has been applied. Alternatively, the tourniquet should be removed after the puncture has been performed, and the blood should be allowed to flow for several minutes before the sample is withdrawn. Arterial blood sampling, which prevents these potential pitfalls, may also be used. Patients should avoid exercise of the hand or arm immediately before and during the procedure.

Both venous and arterial blood may be collected in heparinized syringes and immediately delivered into a premeasured amount of chilled protein precipitant, such as (1) trichloroacetic, (2) metaphosphoric, or (3) perchloric acid. The clear supernatant, after centrifugation, is stable at 4 °C for as long as 8 days. Meticulous attention to sample preparation is required. If blood is not preserved as directed, lactate rapidly increases in blood as a result of glycolysis. Increases may be as great as 20% within 3 minutes and 70% within 30 minutes at 25 °C. Specimens collected as described in this section are also suitable for determination of pyruvate.

If plasma is required as specimen, blood should be collected in a tube containing 10 mg of NaF and 2 mg of K₂C₂O₄ per milliliter of blood. Ideally, the specimen should be immediately cooled and the cells separated within 15 minutes, but reasonable stability of volunteers' lactate is seen at room temperature for 30 minutes in whole blood with NaF. Once the plasma is separated from the cells, lactate is stable.

Reference Intervals

The reference intervals for lactate are:

Specimen	Lactate	
	mmol/L	mg/dL
Venous Blood		
At rest	0.5 to 1.3	5 to 12
In hospital	0.9 to 1.7	8 to 15
Arterial Blood		
At rest	0.36 to 0.75	3 to 7
In hospital	0.36 to 1.25	3 to 11

Individuals in the hospital exhibit a wider range of values. Lactic acidosis occurs with blood lactate concentrations exceeding 5 mmol/L (45 mg/dL). Severe exercise dramatically increases lactate concentrations, and even movement of leg muscles by individuals at bed rest may result in significant increases. Plasma values are about 7% higher than those in whole blood, although differences depend on the procedure used. CSF values are usually similar to blood concentrations but may change independently in CNS disorders. Normal 24-hour urine output of lactate is 5.5 to 22 mmol/d.

Determination of Pyruvate in Whole Blood

The reaction involved in the determination of pyruvate is essentially the reverse of the reaction used in the lactate procedure:

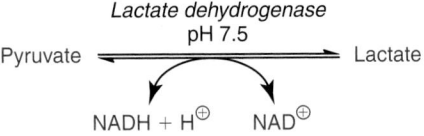

At about pH 7.5, the equilibrium constant strongly favors the reaction to the right. The method is very specific, and (1) 2-oxoglutarate, (2) oxaloacetate, (3) acetoacetate, and (4) β-hydroxybutyrate do not interfere as with photometric methods. Pyruvate is extremely unstable in blood, more so than lactate; immediate use of a chilled protein precipitant is recommended.

Fasting venous blood, drawn when the individual is at rest, has a pyruvate concentration of 0.03 to 0.10 mmol/L (0.3-0.9 mg/dL). Arterial blood contains 0.02 to 0.08 mmol/L (0.2-0.7 mg/dL). Values for CSF are 0.06 to 0.19 mmol/L (0.5-1.7 mg/dL). Urine output of pyruvate is 1 mmol/d or less. Few clinical indications warrant the measurement of blood or urine pyruvate concentrations.

Glucagon

Extremely high concentrations of glucagon are present in individuals with a **glucagonoma**, which are tumors of the α-cells of the pancreas. Individuals with this type of tumor frequently experience (1) weight loss, (2) necrolytic migratory erythema, (3) diabetes mellitus, (4) stomatitis, and (5) diarrhea. Most tumors have metastasized at the time of diagnosis. Low glucagon concentrations are associated with chronic pancreatitis and long-term sulfonylurea therapy.

A standard preparation, WHO Glucagon International Standard (69/194), is available to manufacturers of reagent sets (kits) for use in assigning values to calibrators.

Fasting plasma concentrations of glucagon vary from 20 to 52 pmol/L (70 to 180 ng/L). Values up to 500 times the upper reference limit may be found in individuals with autonomously secreting α-cell neoplasms.

Review Questions

1. The formation of glucose from noncarbohydrate sources occurs mostly in the liver and is referred to as:
   a. gluconeogenesis.
   b. glycogenesis.
   c. glycolysis.
   d. glycogenolysis.

2. Which of the following hormones decreases blood glucose?
   a. Epinephrine
   b. Glucagon
   c. Cortisol
   d. Insulin

3. Which anticoagulant is considered the best for serum glucose analysis because it inhibits glycolysis?
   a. Sodium oxalate
   b. EDTA
   c. Sodium fluoride
   d. Heparin

4. An example of a disaccharide is:
   a. glucose.
   b. starch.
   c. lactose.
   d. fructose.

5. The conversion of glucose into its storage form is referred to as:
   a. glycogenesis.
   b. glycolysis.
   c. glycogenolysis.
   d. glyconeogenesis.

6. Which of the following statements concerning carbohydrates is *incorrect*?
   a. Individuals diagnosed with type 1 diabetes mellitus can display hypoglycemic symptoms because of the impairment of glucagon secretion.
   b. Ethanol produces hypoglycemia by inhibiting gluconeogenesis.
   c. Monosaccharides are formed from the breakdown of starches and disaccharides within the small intestine.
   d. The brain functions normally with a low concentration of plasma glucose (<20 to 30 mg/dL).

7. The formation of 6-phosphogluconate with concomitant production of NADH is the final step in which of the following coupled-enzyme assays for glucose?
   a. Hexokinase method
   b. Glucose oxidase method
   c. Glucose dehydrogenase method
   d. Polarographic method

8. The typical cause of an inborn error of carbohydrate metabolism is:
   a. lack of insulin production.
   b. glucagonoma.
   c. absence of an enzyme involved in carbohydrate metabolism.
   d. chronic alcoholism with hepatic failure.

9. The most widely used cutoff blood glucose concentration that indicates hypoglycemia is:
   a. 100 mg/dL.
   b. 75 mg/dL.
   c. 50 mg/dL.
   d. 25 mg/dL.

10. Deficiency of a specific enzyme involved in glycogen metabolism will produce some type of:
    a. glycogen storage disease.
    b. lactic acidosis.
    c. insulin deficiency.
    d. glycolysis.

References

1. American Diabetes Association. Standards of medical care in diabetes—2012. Diabetes Care 2012;35(Suppl 1):S11–63.
2. Chan AY, Swaminathan R, Cockram CS. Effectiveness of sodium fluoride as a preservative of glucose in blood. Clin Chem 1989;35:315–7
3. Chen Y-T, Burchell A. Glycogen storage diseases. In: Scriver AL, Beaudet AL, Sly WS, Valle D, eds. The metabolic and molecular bases of inherited disease, 7th edition. New York: McGraw-Hill, 1995:935–65.
4. Cryer PE, Fisher JN, Shamoon H. Hypoglycemia. Diabetes Care 1994;17:734–55.
5. DCCT. The effect of intensive treatment of diabetes on the development and progression of long-term complications in insulin-dependent diabetes mellitus. N Engl J Med 1993;329:977–86.
6. Gerich JE. Physiology of glucose homeostasis. Diabetes Obes Metab 2000;2:345–50.
7. Robinson BH. Lactic acidemia (disorders of pyruvate carboxylase, pyruvate dehydrogenase). In: Shriver CR, Beaudet AL, Sly WS, et al, eds. The metabolic and molecular bases of inherited disease. New York: McGraw-Hill, 1995:1479–99.
8. Sacks DB. Carbohydrates. In: Burtis C, Ashwood E, Bruns D, eds. Tietz textbook of clinical chemistry and molecular diagnostics, 5th edition. St Louis: Saunders, 2012:709–30.
9. Sacks DB, Arnold M, Bakris GL, et al. Guidelines and recommendations for laboratory analysis in the diagnosis and management of diabetes mellitus. Clin Chem 2011;57:e1–47.
10. U.K.Prospective Diabetes Study (UKPDS) Group. Intensive blood-glucose control with sulphonylureas or insulin compared with conventional treatment and risk of complications in patients with type 2 diabetes (UKPDS 33). Lancet 1998;352:837–53.

Lipids, Lipoproteins, Apolipoproteins, and Other Cardiac Risk Factors*

Alan T. Remaley, M.D., Ph.D., Nader Rifai, Ph.D., and G. Russell Warnick, M.S., M.B.A.

Objectives

1. Define the following terms:

Apolipoprotein	Lipid
Atherosclerosis	Lipoprotein
Cholesterol	Lipoprotein lipase
Cholesterol ester	Phospholipid
Emulsification	Prostaglandin
Fatty acid	Sphingolipid
Glycerol	Triglyceride
Ketone bodies	

2. List and describe the six classes of lipids based on chemical structure and function.

3. Discuss the metabolism of cholesterol, fatty acids, and triglycerides, including biochemical structure, synthesis, esterification, absorption, and catabolism.

4. Compare and contrast the six lipoprotein classes on the basis of their characteristics, functions, and clinical significance; list the apolipoproteins that are carried by these lipoproteins and their functions.

5. Describe the exogenous, endogenous, intracellular-cholesterol transport, and reverse-cholesterol transport pathways of lipoprotein metabolism, including the following:

Function	Enzymes involved
Lipoproteins and apolipoproteins involved	Cells/cellular components and organs involved

6. State the effects that the following disorders have on lipid metabolism, lipoproteins, apolipoproteins, and laboratory lipid values, and state the genetic defect, if any:

Uncontrolled diabetes mellitus	Familial combined hyperlipidemia
Lipoprotein lipase deficiency	Familial hypertriglyceridemia

Type V hyperlipoproteinemia	Familial defective apolipoprotein B-100
Dysbetalipoproteinemia	Hypoalphalipoproteinemia disorders
Familial hypercholesterolemia	

7. List five major risk factors for coronary heart disease; describe how lipoprotein disorders are managed in adults and children, including therapeutic lifestyle changes and use of pharmacological agents.

8. List five specific causes of secondary hyperlipidemia/dyslipoproteinemia, including examples of exogenous, endocrine, storage, and renal disorders.

9. Diagram the typical enzymatic procedures used in the laboratory to measure cholesterol and triglyceride; state specimen requirements and describe current assays used to assess the following analytes:

HDL	Apolipoprotein A-I and B-100
LDL	Lipoprotein(a)

10. State the uses for and the calculation of the Friedewald formula; calculate LDL cholesterol using this formula when given appropriate information.

11. Describe high-sensitivity CRP and state its usefulness in predicting coronary heart disease events; state the laboratory technique used to detect hsCRP.

12. Analyze and solve case studies related to disorders of lipids and lipoproteins.

*The authors gratefully acknowledge the contributions by Drs. John Albers and Paul Bachorik, on which portions of this chapter are based. Additional portions have been adapted from Rifai N, Kwiterovich PO Jr. Disorders of lipid and lipoprotein metabolism in children and adolescents. In: Soldin SJ, Rifai N, Hick JMB, eds. *Biochemical basis of pediatric diseases*, 3rd edition. Washington, DC: AACC Press, 1998.

Key Words and Definitions

Acylglycerol (glycerol ester) A three-carbon alcohol that contains a hydroxyl group on each of its carbons and is classified by the number of fatty acyl groups present; triglycerides are the predominant form of glycerol ester in plasma.

Apolipoproteins The major protein components of lipoproteins.

Atherosclerosis A pathogenic process that is the underlying cause of the common cardiovascular disorders of (1) myocardial infarction, (2) cerebrovascular disease, and (3) peripheral vascular disease.

Cholesterol A steroid alcohol with 27 carbon atoms that are arranged in a tetracyclical sterane ring system, with a C-H side chain and a polar hydroxyl group on its A-ring, making it an amphipathic molecule.

Coronary heart disease A narrowing of the small blood vessels that supply blood and oxygen to the heart.

Fatty acid Any straight-chain monocarboxylic acid with an alkyl chain generally classed as saturated fatty acids with no double bonds; monounsaturated fatty acids with one double bond; and polyunsaturated fatty acids—those with multiple double bonds.

Lipids A class of compounds that are soluble in organic solvents but are nearly insoluble in water and that contain nonpolar carbon-hydrogen bonds.

Lipoproteins Spherical particles involved in the transport of lipids with nonpolar neutral lipids (triglycerides and cholesterol esters) in their core and more polar amphipathic lipids (phospholipids and free cholesterol) at their surface.

Lipoprotein(a) A lipoprotein structurally similar to low-density lipoprotein but containing a carbohydrate-rich protein and that carries only a relatively small fraction of total cholesterol; it is considered particularly pro-atherogenic.

Phospholipid A polar amphipathic lipid located on the surface of a lipoprotein; phospholipids are also found at the aqueous interface of biological membranes.

Prostaglandin Any of a group of compounds derived from unsaturated 20-carbon fatty acids (primarily arachidonic acid) via the cyclo-oxygenase pathway; these compounds are involved in a number of physiological processes.

Triglyceride A glycerol ester consisting of three molecules of fatty acid esterified to glycerol and constituting 95% of tissue storage fat.

Lipids have important roles in virtually all aspects of life, including (1) serving as hormones, (2) serving as an energy source, (3) assisting digestion, and (4) acting as structural components in cell membranes. In addition, lipids and **lipoproteins**, the particles that transport lipids in the blood, are intimately involved in the development of **atherosclerosis**—a common disorder that occurs when fat, cholesterol, and other substances build up in the walls of arteries and form hard structures called *plaques*. It is a pathogenic process that is the underlying cause of the common cardiovascular disorders of (1) myocardial infarction, (2) cerebrovascular disease, and (3) peripheral vascular disease. In this chapter, the basic biochemistry, clinical significance, and laboratory analysis of each of the major lipid and lipoprotein classes and other cardiovascular risk factors are discussed.

Basic Lipids[1,12]

The term lipid applies to a class of compounds that are soluble in organic solvents but nearly insoluble in water. Lipids primarily contain nonpolar carbon-hydrogen (C-H) bonds and often yield fatty acids and/or complex alcohols after hydrolysis. Some lipids also contain charged or polar groups, which makes these lipids amphipathic with affinity for both water and organic solvents, such as lipids like phospholipids, which are found at the aqueous interface of biological membranes. **Phospholipids** are a class of lipids that are a major component of all cell membranes, as they can form lipid bilayers. Most phospholipids contain a diglyceride, a phosphate group, and a simple organic molecule such as choline; one exception to this rule is sphingomyelin, which is derived from sphingosine instead of glycerol. Overall, lipids are broadly subdivided into six groups on the basis of their chemical structure, namely, (1) cholesterol, (2) **fatty acids,** (3) **acylglycerols,** (4) sphingolipids, (5) **prostaglandins,** and (6) terpenes.

Cholesterol

Cholesterol is found almost exclusively in animals and is a key membrane component of all cells. It is a steroid alcohol with 27 carbon atoms that are arranged in a tetracyclical sterane ring system, with a C-H sidechain (Figure 23-1). Although it is relatively hydrophobic, cholesterol does contain a polar hydroxyl (OH) group on its A-ring (see Figure 23-1), thus

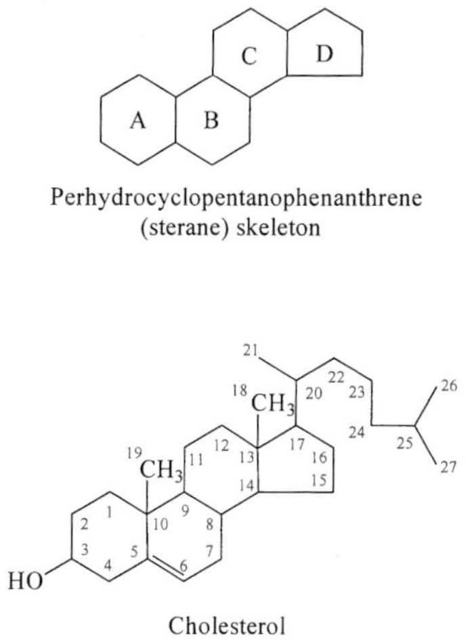

Perhydrocyclopentanophenanthrene
(sterane) skeleton

Cholesterol

Figure 23-1 Structure of cholesterol.

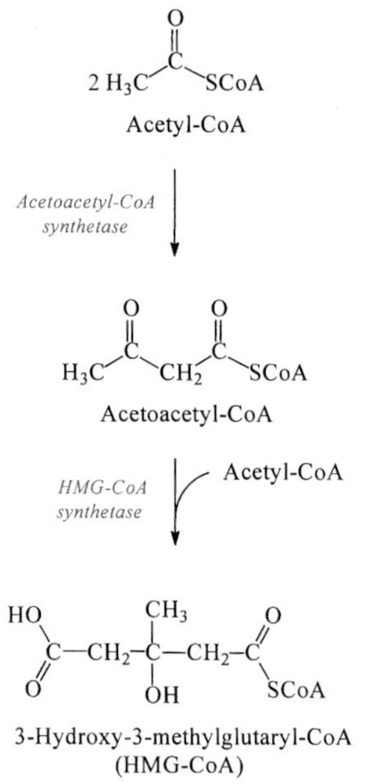

Figure 23-2 Cholesterol biosynthesis (stage 1).

making it amphipathic (i.e., possessing both hydrophilic and lipophilic properties) and accounting for its ability to insert into cell membranes.

Cholesterol Absorption

The average Western diet contains approximately 300 to 450 mg of cholesterol per day, which is derived mostly from animal and dairy products, but only 30% to 60% of it is absorbed. Any dietary esterified cholesterol that contains a fatty acid attached to the hydroxyl group on the A-ring is rapidly hydrolyzed in the intestine to free cholesterol and fatty acids by cholesterol esterases secreted from the pancreas and the small intestine.

Before it is absorbed, cholesterol is first solubilized through a process called *emulsification,* which involves the formation of mixed micelles that contain (1) unesterified cholesterol, (2) fatty acids, (3) monoglycerides, (4) phospholipids, and (5) conjugated bile acids. Bile acids, by acting as detergents, are the most critical factor in micelle formation. Increased amounts of fat favor the absorption of cholesterol by the formation of

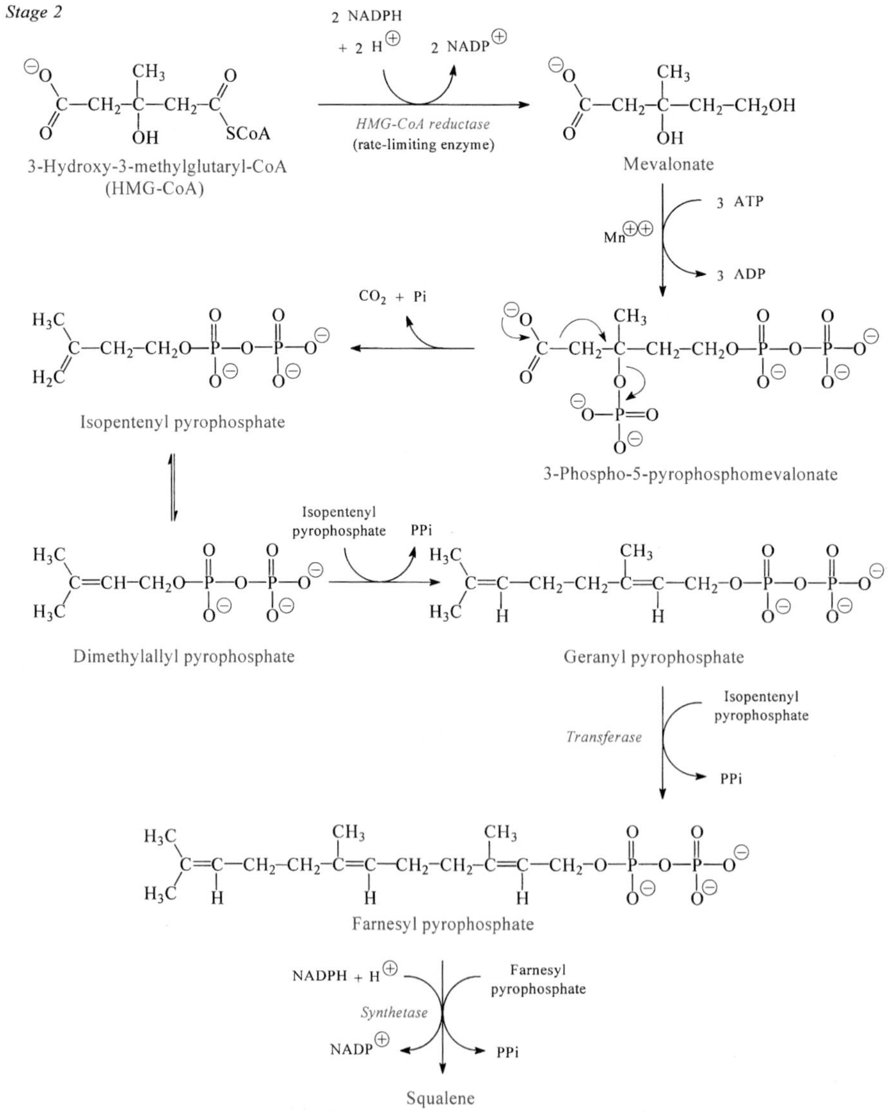

Figure 23-3 Cholesterol biosynthesis (stage 2).

more micelles. Most cholesterol absorption occurs in the middle jejunum and the terminal ileum of the small intestine and is mediated by the enterocyte protein, NPC1L1 (Niemann-Pick C1-like 1), which is the target for the drug ezetimibe, which blocks cholesterol absorption. Once cholesterol enters the intestinal mucosal cell, it is packaged with **triglycerides,** *phospholipids,* and a large protein called **apolipoprotein (apo)** *B-48* into large lipoprotein particles called *chylomicrons.* Chylomicrons are secreted into the lymph and eventually enter the circulation, where they deliver the absorbed dietary lipid to the liver and peripheral tissues.

Cholesterol Synthesis

Cholesterol is synthesized by all cells in the body, but particularly by the liver and the intestine. Cholesterol biosynthesis occurs in three stages. In the first stage (Figure 23-2), acetyl-coenzyme A (CoA), a key metabolic intermediate, forms the six-carbon thioester 3-hydroxy-3-methyl-glutaryl (HMG)-CoA. In the second stage (Figure 23-3), HMG-CoA is reduced to mevalonate and then is decarboxylated to a series of five-carbon isoprene units. These isoprene units are condensed to form first a 10-carbon (geranyl pyrophosphate) and then a 15-carbon intermediate (farnesyl pyrophosphate). Two of these C_{15} molecules then combine to produce the final product of the second stage, squalene, a 30-carbon acyclic hydrocarbon. The second stage is important because it contains the step involving the microsomal enzyme HMG-CoA reductase, which is the rate-limiting enzyme in cholesterol biosynthesis; it is inhibited by statins, the most effective class of current cholesterol-lowering drugs. The third stage (Figure 23-4) occurs in the endoplasmic reticulum, with many of the intermediate products bound to a specific carrier protein. In a series of oxidation-decarboxylation reactions, a number of sidechains are removed from the tetracyclical sterane ring structure to form the 27-carbon molecule of cholesterol.

Cholesterol Esterification

Cholesterol is esterified to a fatty acid to form a cholesteryl ester by two different enzymes. In cells, excess cholesterol is esterified by acylcholesterol acyltransferase (ACAT) (Figure 23-5), which helps reduce the cytotoxicity of excess free cholesterol. Once esterified, cholesteryl esters are stored in intracellular lipid drops. Cholesteryl esters also are formed in the circulation by the action of a plasma enzyme called lecithin cholesterol acyltransferase (LCAT), which is bound to lipoproteins, particularly high-density lipoproteins (HDL). The reaction involves the transfer of a fatty acid from the second carbon position of phosphatidylcholine (lecithin) to cholesterol (see Figure 23-5). Cholesteryl esters account for about 70% of the total cholesterol in plasma. Once cholesterol is esterified, it loses its free hydroxyl group and becomes much more hydrophobic, moving from the surface of lipoprotein particles to the hydrophobic core.

Cholesterol Catabolism

Except for specialized endocrine cells that use cholesterol for the synthesis of steroid hormones, most peripheral cells have limited ability to further catabolize cholesterol. Cholesteryl esters are hydrolyzed to free cholesterol by various lipases in all cells, but thereafter, cholesterol has to be returned to the liver to undergo any further catabolism. Approximately one-third of the daily production of

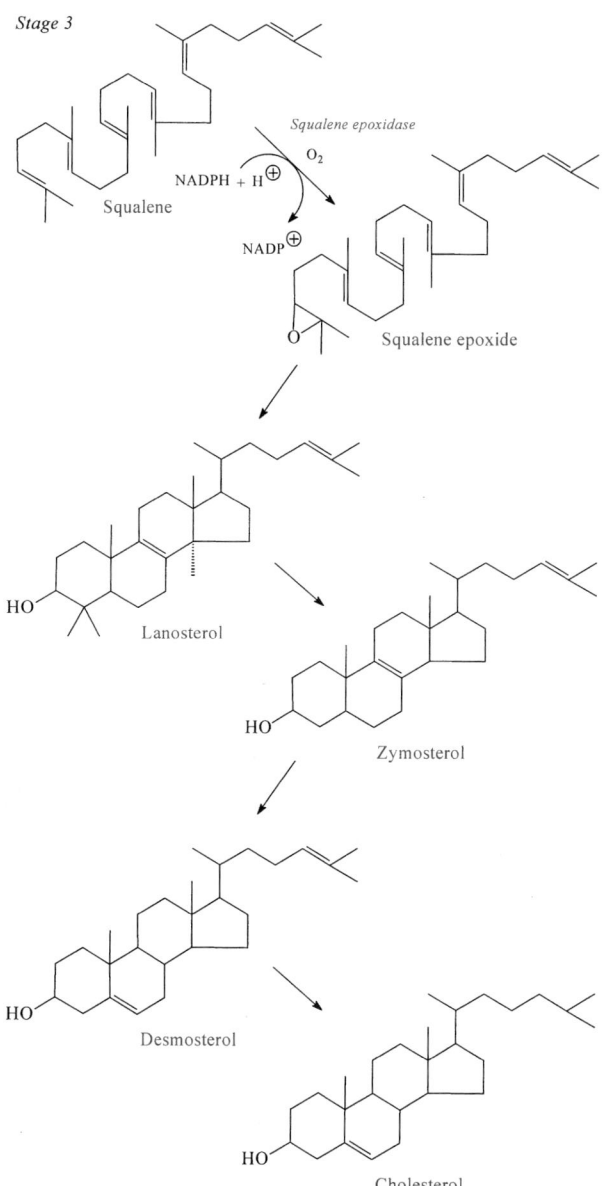

Figure 23-4 Cholesterol biosynthesis (stage 3).

Intracellular:

$$\text{Fatty acid} + \text{CoASH} \xrightarrow{\textit{Acyl-CoA synthetase}} \text{Acyl-CoA}$$

ATP   PPi + AMP

$$\text{Acyl-CoA} + \text{cholesterol} \xrightarrow{\textit{ACAT}} \text{Cholesterol ester} + \text{CoASH}$$

Intravascular:

$$\text{Lecithin} + \text{cholesterol} \xrightarrow{\textit{LCAT}} \text{Cholesterol ester} + \text{lysolecithin}$$

Figure 23-5 Intracellular and intravascular esterification of cholesterol mediated by acylcholesterol acyltransferase (ACAT) and lecithin cholesterol acyltransferase (LCAT), respectively.

cholesterol, or about 400 mg/day, is converted in the liver into bile acids (Figure 23-6). About 90% of these bile acids are reabsorbed in the lower third of the ileum and are returned to the liver by the enterohepatic circulation. Bile acids that enter the large intestine are partially deconjugated by bacterial enzymes to secondary bile acids. Cholic acid is converted, for example, to deoxycholic acid, and chenodeoxycholic acid is converted to lithocholic acid.

Not all cholesterol delivered to the liver is converted to bile salts. Much of it is resecreted into the circulation on lipoproteins, and the remainder is directly excreted into the bile unchanged, where it is solubilized into mixed micelles by bile acids and phospholipids. When the amount of cholesterol in bile exceeds the capacity of these solubilizing agents, it is possible for cholesterol to precipitate and form gallstones.

Fatty Acids

RCOOH is the general chemical formula for a fatty acid, where "R" is an alkyl chain. Fatty acid chain lengths vary and are commonly classified as short-chain (2 to 4 carbon atoms), medium-chain (6 to 10 carbon atoms), or long-chain (12 to 26 carbon atoms) fatty acids. Those of importance in human nutrition and metabolism are included in the long-chain class and contain an even number of carbon atoms.

Fatty acids are further classified according to their degree of saturation. Saturated fatty acids have no double bonds (C=C) between their carbon atoms; monounsaturated fatty acids contain one double bond; and polyunsaturated fatty acids contain multiple double bonds (Figure 23-7). The double bonds in polyunsaturated fatty acids are usually three carbon atoms apart. Fatty acids from fish, such as

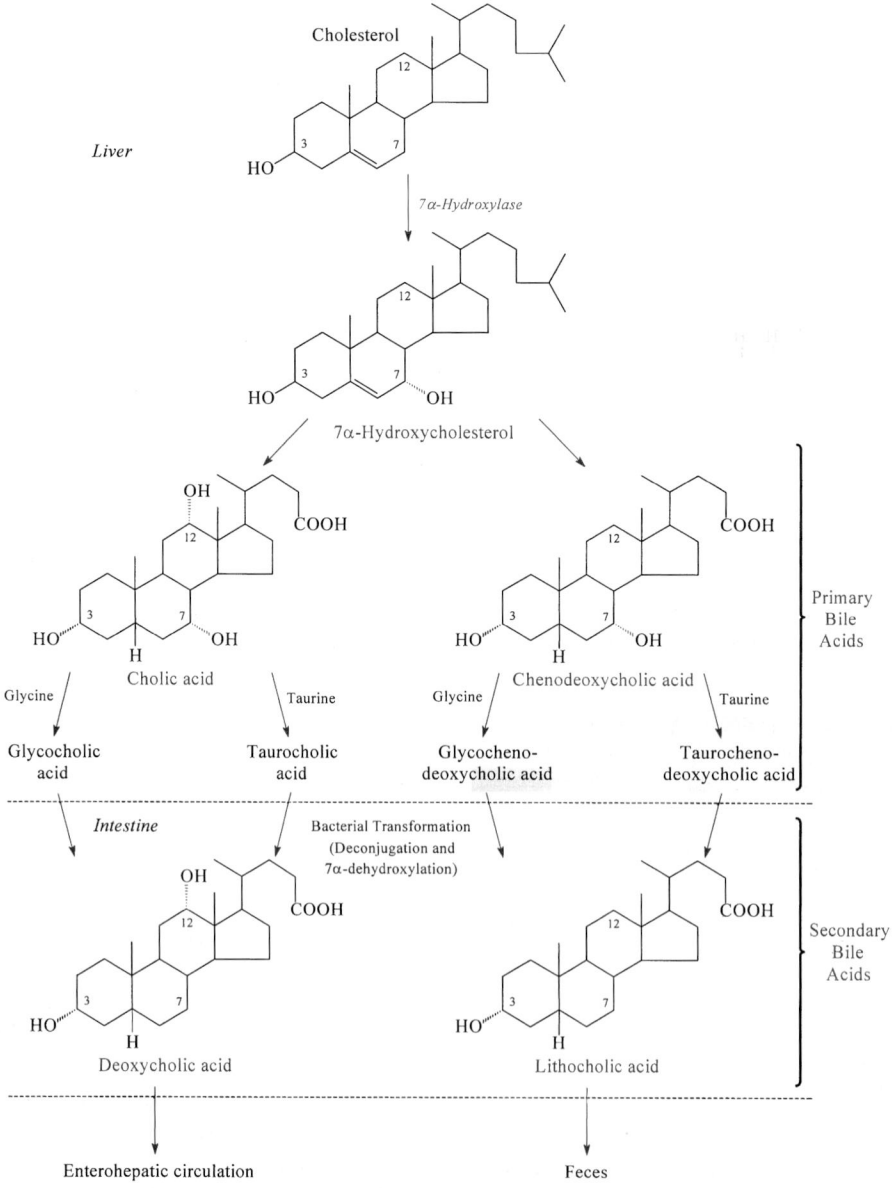

Figure 23-6 Bile acid synthesis.

salmon, possess up to six unsaturated double bonds and usually are more than 20 carbon atoms long. Unsaturated fatty acids are prone to oxidation by the nonenzymatic reaction of oxygen with their double bonds. Numbering of the carbon atoms in fatty acids is done from the carboxyl terminal end (Δ-numbering system) or from the methyl terminal end (η- or ω-numbering system; Table 23-1). In addition, carbon atoms may be labeled with Greek symbols, with α being adjacent to the carboxyl group and ω being farthest away. In the Δ-system, fatty acids are abbreviated according to the (1) number of carbon atoms, (2) number of double bonds, and (3) position(s) of double bond(s). For example, linoleic acid would be written as $C_{18}:2^{9,12}$ and contains 18 carbons and two unsaturated bonds between carbons 9 and 10 and carbons 12 and 13. When the η- or ω-system is used, linoleic acid would be abbreviated as $C_{18}:2n-6$, where only the first carbon forming the unsaturated pair is written. The *Geneva* or *systematic* classification, which is based on their chemical names, is a third common nomenclature system for fatty acids (see Table 23-1).

In saturated fatty acids, the chain is extended and flexible; the carbon atoms rotate freely around their longitudinal axis. Unsaturated fatty acids, however, have fixed 30° bends in their chains at each double bond. Depending on the plane in which this bend occurs, the *cis* or the *trans* isomer is produced. In mammals, all naturally occurring unsaturated fatty acids are of the *cis* variety. *Trans* fatty acids in our diet result primarily from catalytic hydrogenation in which unsaturated double bonds are chemically reduced to raise their melting point. This process is used to "harden" or solidify fats in the manufacture of certain foods, such as margarine.

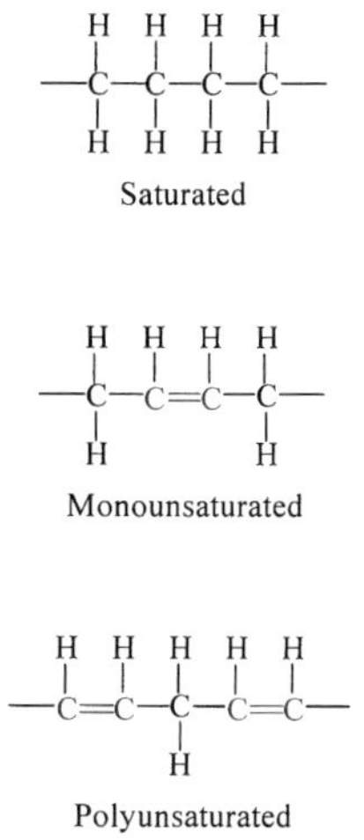

Most fatty acids are also synthesized by the body except for essential fatty acids such as linoleic acid ($C_{18}:2^{9,12}$), which is made only by plants. Linoleic acid is also converted to arachidonic acid, which is a precursor for prostaglandin synthesis.

Fatty acids exist in the circulation in an unesterified or free state, the latter primarily bound to albumin, or in various esterified forms, such as triglycerides, phospholipids, or cholesteryl esters. The free fatty acid carboxyl group has a pK_a of approximately 4.8; thus free fatty acid molecules exist primarily in their ionized forms. The normal concentration of free fatty acids in human plasma is 0.3 to 1.1 mmol/L (8 to 31 mg/dL) and is very sensitive to physiological energy demands and the availability of alternative forms of metabolic fuel, such as glucose.

Figure 23-7 Saturated and unsaturated fatty acids.

Fatty Acid Catabolism

Fatty acids are catabolized in the mitochondria and produce energy by a series of reactions known as β-oxidation. This process is repeated to shorten the fatty acid chain by two carbon atoms at a time from the carboxy terminal end of the molecule. For example, one mole of palmitic acid (C_{16}) is converted to eight moles of acetyl-CoA. Acetyl-CoA does not normally accumulate in the cell but is condensed enzymatically with oxaloacetate, derived largely from carbohydrate metabolism (Figure 23-8), to yield citrate, a major component of the tricarboxylic acid cycle (Krebs cycle). The Krebs cycle is a common pathway for the final oxidation of nearly all metabolic fuels, whether derived from carbohydrate, fat, or protein, and ultimately results in the production of adenosine triphosphate (ATP), the main energy storage molecule in the body. Triglycerides contain three fatty acid molecules and are, therefore, a relatively efficient storage form of metabolic energy. Furthermore, energy storage by triglycerides is efficient in terms of space because it does not require any water for hydration, unlike carbohydrates.

Ketone Formation

During prolonged starvation, or when carbohydrate metabolism is impaired, as in uncontrolled diabetes mellitus, the formation of acetyl-CoA exceeds the supply of oxaloacetate. The resulting acetyl-CoA excess is diverted to an alternative pathway in the mitochondria for the formation of (1) acetoacetic acid, (2) β-hydroxybutyric acid, and (3) acetone—the three compounds known collectively as *ketone bodies* (Figure 23-9). Ketosis, therefore, develops from excessive production of acetyl-CoA, as the body attempts to obtain necessary energy from stored fat in the

TABLE 23-1	Fatty Acids Commonly Found in Human Tissue		
Common Name	**Systematic Name**	**D-Numbering**	**h-(ω) Numbering**
Lauric	Dodecanoic	12:0	12:0
Myristic	Tetradecanoic	14:0	14:0
Palmitic	Hexadecanoic	16:0	16:0
Palmitoleic	9-Hexadecanoic	$16:1^9$	16:1n-7
Stearic	Octadecanoic	18:0	18:0
Oleic	9-Octadecanoic	$18:1^9$	18:1n-9
Linoleic*	9,12-Octadecadienoic	$18:2^{9,12}$	18:2n-6
Linolenic*	9,12,15-Octadecatrienoic	$18:3^{9,12,15}$	18:3n-3
Arachidic	Eicosanoic	20:0	20:0
Arachidonic	5,8,11,14-Eicosatetraenoic	$20:4^{5,8,11,14}$	20:4n-6

*Essential fatty acids.

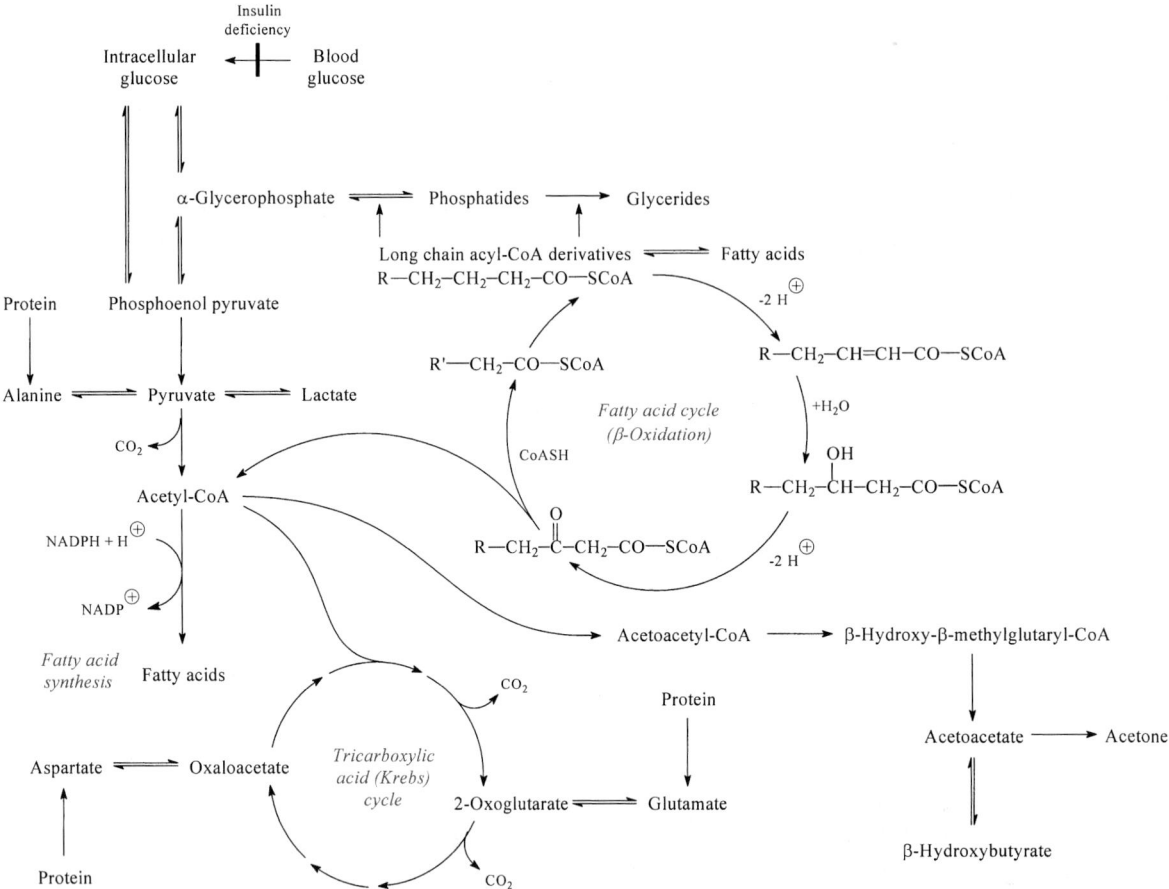

Figure 23-8 Metabolic relations among intermediates of carbohydrate, fat, and protein metabolism. Note that acetyl-CoA is produced from both carbohydrate and fat. The gluco-genic amino acids, derived from protein metabolism, enter glycolytic paths as α-keto acids. Ketogenic amino acids enter as acetyl-CoA.

absence of an adequate supply of carbohydrate metabolites (see Chapter 22).

Acylglycerols (Glycerol Esters)

Glycerol is a three-carbon alcohol that contains a hydroxyl group on each of its carbon atoms (Figure 23-10).

$$
\begin{array}{c}
\alpha \quad H-C-OH \\
\beta \quad H-C-OH \\
\alpha' \quad H-C-OH
\end{array}
$$

The two terminal carbon atoms in the glycerol molecule are chemically equivalent and are designated α and α′. The center carbon is labeled β. A common alternative labeling system uses the numeral 1 for the α-carbon, 2 for the β-carbon, and 3 for the α′-carbon. The class of acylglycerol is determined by the number of fatty acyl groups present: (1) one fatty acid—monoacylglycerols (monoglycerides); (2) two fatty acids—diacylglycerols (diglycerides); and (3) three fatty acids—triacylglycerols (triglycerides). For example, 1-monoglyceride indicates that a fatty acid is attached to the α-carbon. This numbering system applies to all acylglycerols, including the phosphoglycerides (Figure 23-11).

Triglycerides constitute 95% of tissue storage fat and are the predominant form of glyceryl esters found in plasma. The fatty acid residues found in (1) monoglycerides, (2) diglycerides, or (3) triglycerides vary considerably and usually include different combinations of long-chain fatty acids (see Table 23-1). In general, triglycerides from plant sources, such as corn, sunflower, and safflower, tend to be enriched in unsaturated fatty acids and are liquid oils at room temperature. Triglycerides from animals, especially ruminants, tend to have saturated acids and are solids at room temperature.

Dietary triglycerides are digested in the duodenum and are absorbed in the proximal ileum. Through the action of pancreatic and intestinal lipases and in the presence of bile acids, they are first hydrolyzed to glycerol, monoglycerides, and fatty acids. After absorption, these components of tri-glycerides are reassembled as triglycerides in the intestinal epithelial cells and then are packaged with cholesterol and apo B-48 to form chylomicrons. Chylomicrons are secreted into the lymphatic system and eventually reach the circula-tion. Triglycerides are the main metabolic fuel carried by

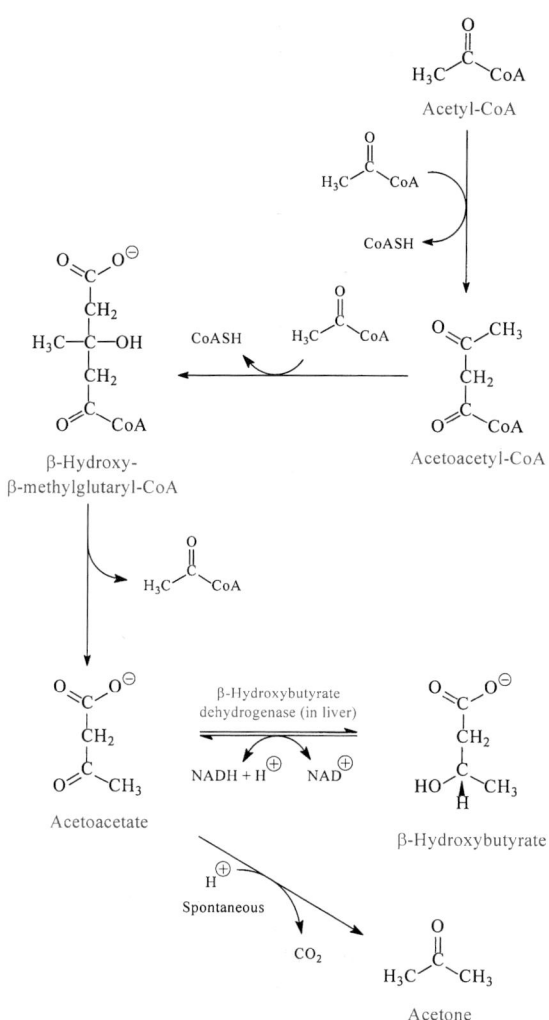

Figure 23-9 Formation of ketone bodies.

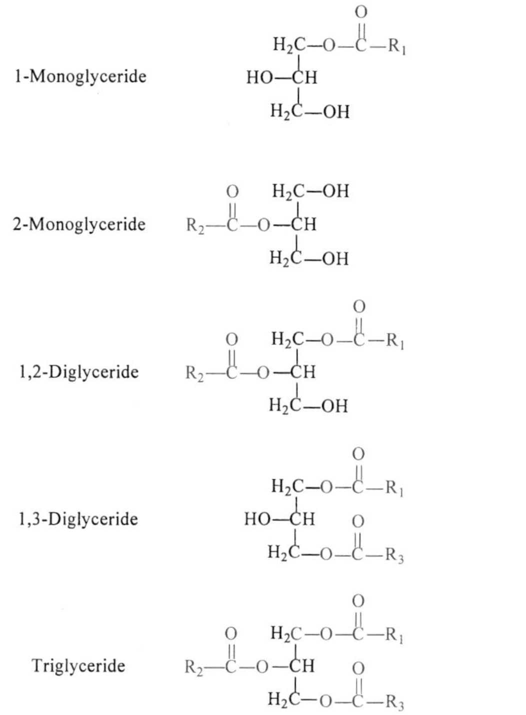

1-Monoglyceride

2-Monoglyceride

1,2-Diglyceride

1,3-Diglyceride

Triglyceride

Figure 23-10 Structure and classification of glycerol esters (acylglycerols). R_1, R_2, and R_3 are fatty acids of varying chain length.

Phosphatidic acid
$A = —H$

Phosphatidylethanolamine*
$A = —CH_2CH_2\overset{\oplus}{N}H_3$

Phosphatidylcholine (lecithin)
$A = —CH_2CH_2\overset{\oplus}{N}(CH_3)_3$

Phosphatidylserine*
$A = —CH_2\overset{\oplus}{CH}NH_3$
$\qquad\qquad\underset{COO^{\ominus}}{|}$

Phosphatidylinositol*
$A =$

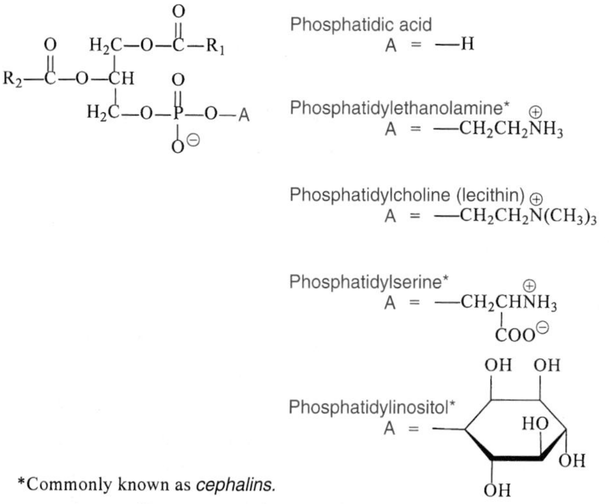

*Commonly known as *cephalins.*

Figure 23-11 Structures of phosphoglycerides and common alcohol groups associated with them. R_1 and R_2 are fatty acids of varying carbon atom lengths.

chylomicrons; they are delivered to the liver and peripheral cells after they have been hydrolyzed to fatty acids by lipases.

Another major class of acylglycerols includes those containing phosphoric acid at the third (α') carbon atom, which are referred to as *phosphoglycerides* (see Figure 23-11). In their simplest form, the A group consists of a hydrogen atom and the molecule is called *diacylphosphoglyceride*. Usually, the A group is in alcohol, such as (1) choline, (2) serine, (3) inositol, or (4) ethanolamine. If the A group is choline, for example, the molecule is referred to as *phosphatidylcholine* (lecithin). As the types of fatty acid residues R_1 and R_2 are varied, numerous types of phospholipids are formed. These phosphoglycerides are named according to the fatty acid acyl esters attached at C-1 and C-2 of the glycerol. Saturated fatty acids are typically esterified to the C-1 position, whereas polyunsaturated fatty acids are often attached to the C-2 position. In inner mitochondrial membranes, more complex phosphoglycerides, known as *cardiolipins,* are found. They are derived from two phosphoglyceride molecules joined by a glycerol bridge.

Sphingolipids

Sphingolipids make up a fourth class of lipids derived from the amino alcohol sphingosine (Figure 23-12). This dihydric 18-carbon alcohol contains an amino group at C-17. A fatty acid containing 18 or more carbon atoms is attached to the amino group through an amide linkage to form a *ceramide*. This is an intermediate structure in the formation of (1) sphingomyelin, (2) galactosylceramide,

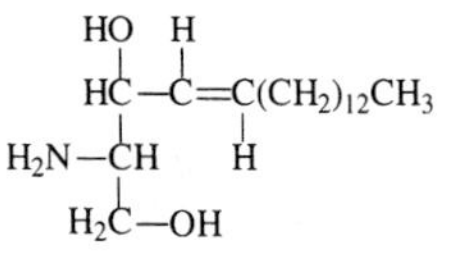

HO H
HC—C=C(CH₂)₁₂CH₃
H₂N—CH H
H₂C—OH

Sphingosine

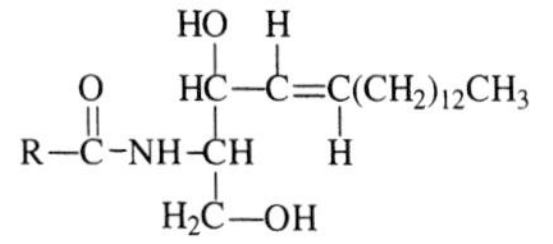

O   HO H
‖   HC—C=C(CH₂)₁₂CH₃
R—C—NH-CH H
H₂C—OH

Ceramide

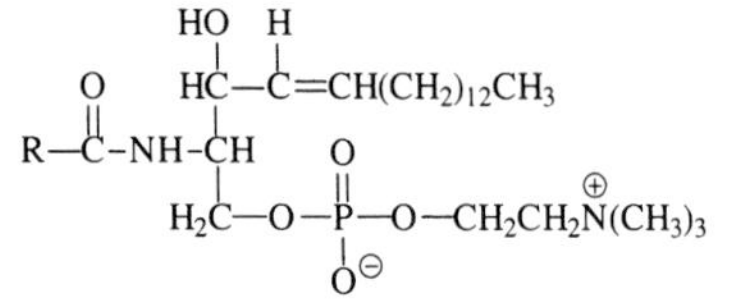

O   HO H
‖   HC—C=CH(CH₂)₁₂CH₃
R—C—NH-CH   O
H₂C—O—P—O—CH₂CH₂N(CH₃)₃
O⊖

Sphingomyelin

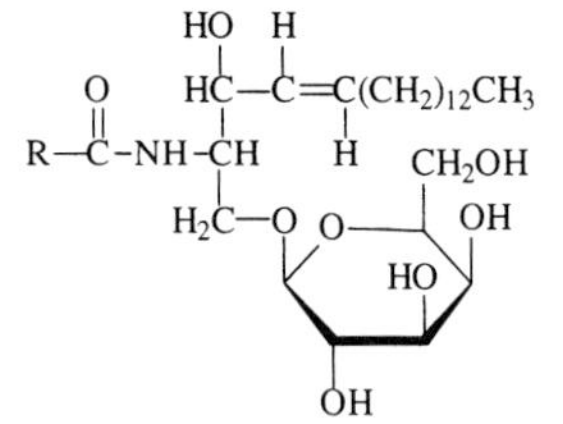

O   HO H
‖   HC—C=C(CH₂)₁₂CH₃
R—C—NH-CH H CH₂OH
H₂C—O O   OH
HO

OH

Galactosylceramide

O   HO H
‖   HC—C=C(CH₂)₁₂CH₃
R—C—NH-CH H CH₂OH
H₂C—O O
HO

OH

OH

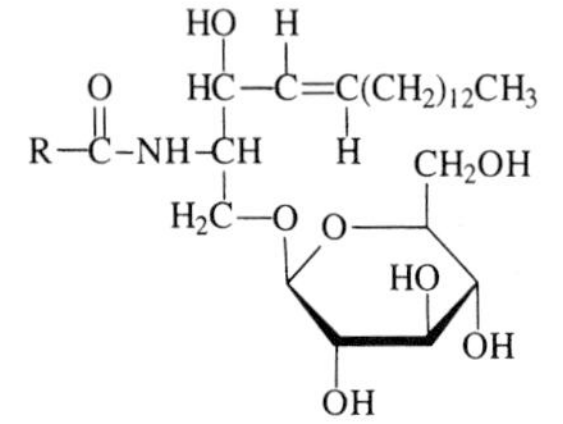

Glucosylceramide

Figure 23-12 Structures of sphingolipids.

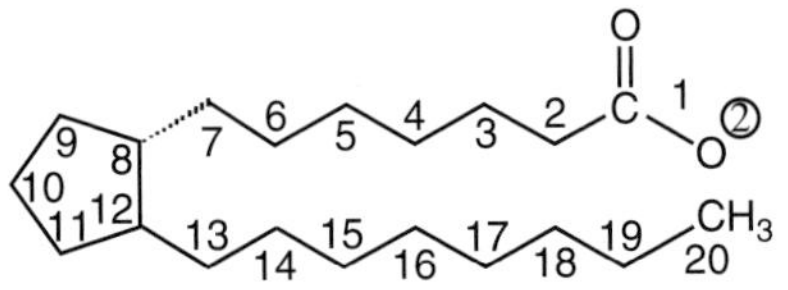

and (3) glucosylceramide (see Figure 23-12). In addition, the sugar-containing ceramides have a sulfate group that is usually attached to the 2-position of the galactose residue to form the sulfatides. The glycosyl ceramides have additional monosaccharide moieties, such as (1) galactose, (2) *N*-acetylgalactosamine, and (3) *N*-acetylneuraminic acid, to form complex globosides and gangliosides. Gangliosides are especially abundant in the membranes of the gray matter of the brain, whereas glycosphingolipids have a more general role in cellular interactions and serve as a source of blood group and tumor antigens.

Prostaglandins

Prostaglandins and related compounds, such as thromboxanes and leukotrienes, are derivatives of fatty acids, primarily arachidonate. These bioactive lipids exert diverse physiological actions (Table 23-2) at concentrations as low as 1 µg/L.

TABLE 23-2	Prostaglandin-Mediated Effects
Site of Action	**Physiological Response**
Arterial smooth muscle	Alters blood pressure
Uterine muscle	Induces labor, therapeutic abortion
Lower gastrointestinal tract	Increases motility
Bronchial smooth muscle	Causes bronchospasm
Platelets	Increase coagulability
Capillaries	Increase permeability
Stomach	Enhances gastric acid secretion
Adipose tissue	Inhibits triglyceride lipolysis

The prostaglandins are a series of C_{20} unsaturated fatty acids that contain a cyclopentane ring; the parent fatty acid has been given the trivial name *prostanoic acid*. By convention, prostaglandins are abbreviated *PG*, with the class designated by a capital letter (A, B, E, F, G, H, and I), followed by a number and, in some cases, a Greek letter (Figure 23-13). The number after the capital letter is usually written as a subscript and is used to designate the number of unsaturated bonds in the PG sidechains and not within the ring structure itself. Sixteen naturally occurring prostaglandins have been described (Table 23-3), but only seven, along with two thromboxanes, are commonly found in the body. These are termed *primary prostaglandins*.

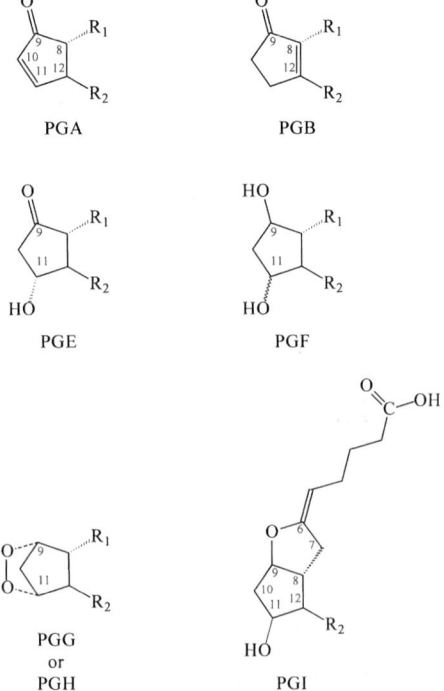

Figure 23-13 Major prostaglandin classes (series). R_1 and R_2 are prostaglandin sidechains.

TABLE 23-3	Naturally Occurring Prostaglandins (PGs)
Primary PG	**Other PGs**
PGE_1	PGA_1
$PGF_{1\alpha}$	PGA_2
PGE_2	$19\alpha\text{-OHPGA}_1$
$PGF_{2\alpha}$	$19\alpha\text{-OHPGA}_2$
PGG_2	PGB_1
PGH_2	PGB_2
PGI_2	$19\alpha\text{-OHPGB}_2$
Thromboxane A_2	PGE_3
Thromnane B_2	$PGF_{3\alpha}$

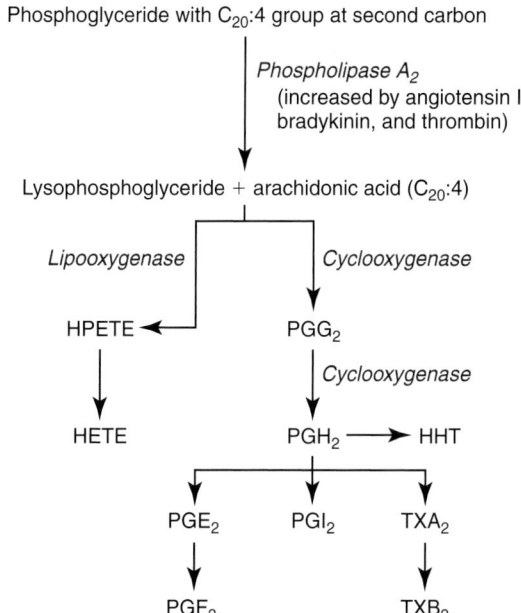

Figure 23-14 Synthesis of prostaglandins from an arachidonic precursor. *HPETE, HETE, HHT,* 12-L-Hydroxy-5,8,10-heptadecatrienoic acid; *PG,* prostaglandin; *TX,* thromboxane.

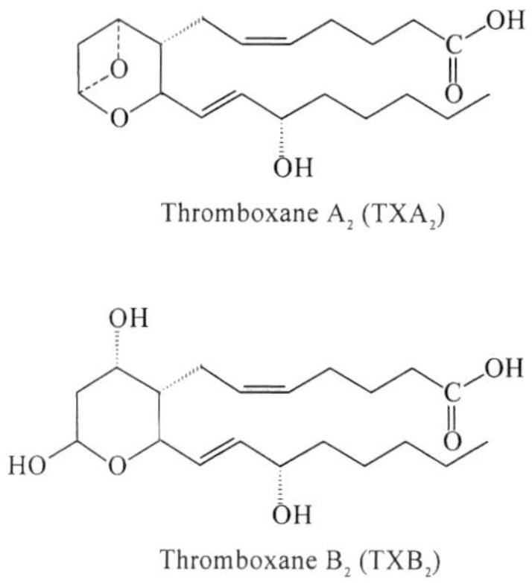

Although prostaglandins have hormone-like action, they are different from conventional hormones in that they are synthesized at the site of action and are made in almost all tissues. Linoleic acid ($C_{18}:2^{9,12}$) is the precursor of two of the three 20-carbon fatty acids that form prostaglandins; linolenic acid ($C_{18}:2^{9,12,15}$) is the other precursor. Both of these fatty acids are considered essential because they are not synthesized in the body and therefore must be present in the diet. Once formed, prostaglandins have short-lived effects and are catabolized within seconds. Inactivation of prostaglandin appears to be mediated by two enzymes: 15α-hydroxy-prostaglandin dehydrogenase and Δ^{13}-prostaglandin reductase. Prostaglandins are not stored, but the precursor C_{20} fatty acids are present in tissue attached to the C-2 position of phosphoglycerides. When prostaglandin synthesis is stimulated, the C_{20} precursor is hydrolyzed from phospholipids by phospholipase A_2. Release of the C_{20} fatty acid appears to be the rate-limiting step in prostaglandin synthesis and is stimulated by various mediators, such as bradykinin, thrombin, or angiotensin II.

Once released, arachidonic acid follows one of two pathways. The lipoxygenase route produces 12-L-hydroperoxy-5,8,10,14 eicosatetraenoic acid (HPETE); HPETE spontaneously decomposes to 12-L-hydroxy-5,8,10,14 eicosatetraenoic acid (HETE) (Figure 23-14). The alternative pathway is mediated by cyclo-oxygenase (COX) to produce the endoperoxides PGG_2 and PGH_2. Nonsteroidal anti-inflammatory drugs (NSAIDs, such as aspirin, ibuprofen, naproxen, and indomethacin) inhibit the COX enzymes, thereby decreasing prostaglandin synthesis.

PGI_2, or prostacyclin, is derived from arachidonic acid (see Figure 23-13) in the vascular endothelium. It has a powerful vasodilatory action, especially on the coronary arteries, and inhibits platelet aggregation. Thromboxane A_2 is synthesized from arachidonic acid but is also produced by platelets. It has the opposite effect of prostacyclin because it stimulates the contraction of arterial smooth muscle and enhances platelet aggregation. It has a half-life of about 30 seconds and is rapidly converted to its inactive metabolite, thromboxane B_2. Thromboxanes are slightly different in structure from the other prostaglandins in that they contain six-sided rings of five carbon atoms and one oxygen atom (Figure 23-15).

Thromboxane A_2 (TXA_2)

Thromboxane B_2 (TXB_2)

Figure 23-15 Structures of thromboxanes.

Terpenes

Terpenes are polymers of the five-carbon isoprene unit and include vitamins A, E, and K and the dolichols, which play important roles in protein glycation.

Lipoproteins[1,5,7]

Lipids synthesized in the liver and in the intestine are transported in the plasma in macromolecular complexes known as lipoproteins. Lipoproteins are typically spherical particles with nonpolar neutral lipids (triglycerides and cholesterol esters) in their core and more polar amphipathic lipids (phospholipids and free cholesterol) at their surface (Figure 23-16). They also contain one or more specific proteins, called *apolipoproteins,* on their surface.

Classification

Lipoproteins have different physical and chemical properties (Table 23-4) because they contain different proportions of lipids and proteins (Table 23-5). Traditionally, lipoproteins have been categorized on the basis of differences in their hydrated densities, as determined by ultracentrifugation.

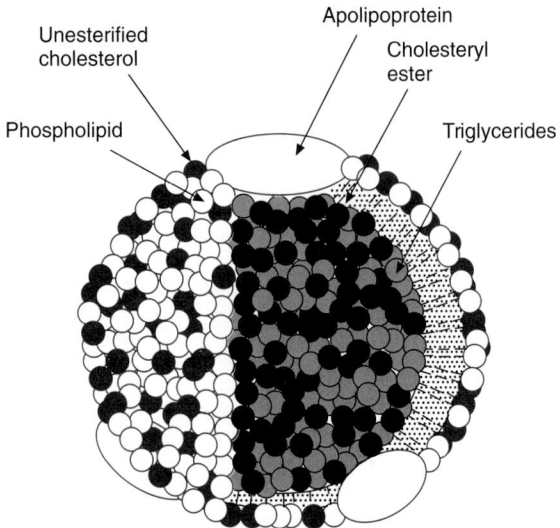

Figure 23-16 Structure of a typical lipoprotein particle.

These categories include (1) chylomicrons, (2) very-low density lipoprotein (VLDL), (3) intermediate-density lipoprotein (IDL), (4) low-density lipoprotein (LDL), (5) high-density lipoprotein (HDL), and (6) **lipoprotein(a)** [Lp(a)]. In general, the larger lipoproteins contain more core lipids, triglycerides, and cholesteryl esters and are lighter in density and contain a smaller percentage of protein. In the fasting state, most plasma triglycerides are present in VLDL, but 2 to 6 hours after a meal, most triglycerides are transported on chylomicrons. LDL carries about 70% of total plasma cholesterol but very little triglyceride (see Table 23-5). HDL typically contains about 20% to 30% of plasma cholesterol.

Lp(a) is a distinct class of lipoprotein (Table 23-6) that is structurally related to LDL because both lipoproteins possess one molecule of apo B-100 per particle with similar lipid compositions. Unlike LDL, Lp(a) also contains a carbohydrate-rich protein [apo(a)], which is covalently bound to the apo B-100 through a disulfide linkage. Apo(a) exhibits a significant sequence homology with plasminogen and a high degree of variation in polypeptide chain length (Figure 23-17). Apo(a) contains a tandem array of a protein motif called a *kringle domain* with different-sized apo(a) molecules (polymorphisms) reflecting the inclusion of variable numbers of kringle 4 type 2 domains.

Lipoproteins have been electrophoretically separated, and this forms the basis for their nomenclature. For example,

TABLE 23-4   Characteristics of Human Plasma Lipoproteins

Variable	Chylomicron	VLDL	IDL	LDL	HDL	Lp(a)
Density (g/mL)	<0.95	0.95-1.006	1.006-1.019	1.019-1.063	1.063-1.210	1.040-1.130
Electrophoretic mobility	Origin	Pre-beta	Between beta and pre-beta	Beta	Alpha	Pre-beta
Molecular weight (Da)	$0.4\text{-}30 \times 10^9$	$5\text{-}10 \times 10^6$	$3.9\text{-}4.8 \times 10^6$	2.75×10^6	$1.8\text{-}3.6 \times 10^5$	$2.9\text{-}3.7 \times 10^6$
Diameter (nm)	>70	26-70	22-24	19-23	4-10	26-30
Lipid:lipoprotein ratio	99:1	90:10	85:15	80:20	50:50	75:26-64:36
Major lipids	Exogenous	Endogenous	Endogenous, cholesteryl esters	Cholesteryl esters	Phospholipids	Cholesteryl esters, Phospholipids
Major proteins	A-I	B-100	B-100	B-100	A-I	(a)
	B-48	C-I	E	—	A-II	B-100
	C-I	C-II	—	—	—	—
	C-II	C-III	—	—	—	—
	C-III	E	—	—	—	—

HDL, High-density lipoprotein; *IDL*, intermediate-density lipoprotein; *LDL*, low-density lipoprotein; *Lp(a)*, lipoprotein(a); *VLDL*, very low-density lipoprotein.

TABLE 23-5   Chemical Composition (%) of Human Plasma Lipoproteins

		Surface Components		Core Lipids	
Core Lipid Esters	Cholesterol	Phospholipids	Apolipoproteins	Triglycerides	Cholesteryl
Chylomicrons	2	7	2	86	3
VLDL	7	18	8	55	12
IDL	9	19	19	23	29
LDL	8	22	22	6	42
HDL₂	5	33	40	5	17
HDL₃	4	25	55	3	13

Surface components and core lipids given as percentage of dry mass.
HDL, High-density lipoprotein; *HDL₂*, HDL syndrome 2; *HDL₃*, HDL syndrome 3; *IDL*, intermediate-density lipoprotein; *LDL*, low-density lipoprotein; *VLDL*, very low-density lipoprotein.
From Havel RJ, Kane JP. Introduction: structure and metabolism of plasma lipoproteins. In: Scriver CR, Beaudet AL, Sly WS, Valle D, eds. The metabolic and molecular bases of inherited diseases, 7th edition, volume II. New York: McGraw-Hill, 1995:1841-50. Reproduced with permission of The McGraw-Hill Companies.

TABLE 23-6	Classification* and Properties of Major Human Plasma Apolipoproteins			
Apolipoprotein	Molecular Weight (Da)	Chromosomal Location	Function	Lipoprotein Carrier(s)
Apo A-I	29,016	11	Cofactor LCAT	Chylomicron, HDL
Apo A-II	17,414	1	Not known	HDL
Apo A-IV	44,465	11	Activation of LCAT	Chylomicron, HDL
Apo B-100	512,723	2	Secretion of triglycerides from liver binding protein to LDL receptor	VLDL, IDL, LDL
Apo B-48	240,800	2	Secretion of triglycerides from intestine	Chylomicron
Apo C-I	6630	19	Activation of LCAT	Chylomicron, VLDL, HDL
Apo C-II	8900	19	Cofactor LPL	Chylomicron, VLDL, HDL
Apo C-III	8800	11	Inhibition of apo C-II activation of LPL	Chylomicron, VLDL, HDL
Apo E	34,145	19	Facilitation of uptake of chylomicron remnant and IDL	Chylomicron, VLDL, HDL
Apo(a)	187,000-662,000	6	Unknown	Lp(a)

*Both Roman and Arabic numerals are used to label the individual classifications. In this chapter, Roman symbols are used.
HDL, High-density lipoprotein; *IDL*, intermediate-density lipoprotein; *LCAT*, lecithin cholesterol acyltransferase; *LDL*, low-density lipoprotein; *Lp(a)*, lipoprotein(a); *LPL*, lipoprotein lipase; *VLDL*, very low-density lipoprotein.

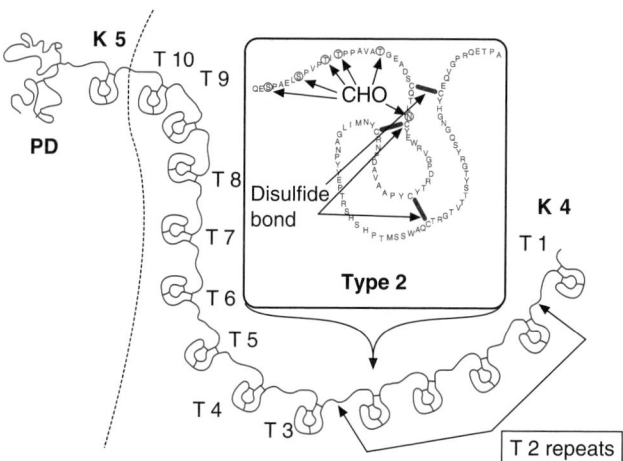

Figure 23-17   Structure of lipoprotein(a).

at pH 8.6, HDL migrates with the α-globulins, LDL with the β-globulins, and VLDL and Lp(a) between the α- and β-globulins, in the pre–β-globulin region. IDL forms a broad band between β- and pre–β-globulins. Chylomicrons remain at the application point. Traditionally, lipoprotein classes were referred to by their electrophoretic locations as pre–β-lipoprotein, VLDL; β-lipoprotein, LDL; and α-lipoprotein, HDL. Electrophoresis provided the foundation for an early original phenotypical classification system (Types 1 to 5) for familial dyslipidemias.

Apolipoproteins

Apolipoproteins are the major protein components of lipoproteins (see Table 23-6). Each class of lipoprotein carries several apolipoproteins in differing proportions. Apo A-I is the major protein in HDL. Apo B-100 is the main protein on LDL and Lp(a), and apo B-48, which is produced from apo B-100 messenger RNA (mRNA) by an RNA editing process,

is found on chylomicrons. Both apo B-100 and apo B-48 are found at one molecule per particle, are firmly bound, and do not exchange between particles, as the other apolipoproteins do. Apolipoproteins perform the following major functions: (1) modulate the activity of enzymes that act on lipoproteins, (2) maintain the structural integrity of the lipoprotein complex, and (3) facilitate the uptake of lipoprotein by acting as ligands for specific cell-surface receptors. Most apolipoproteins contain amphipathic helices, which are α-helices with one face containing hydrophobic amino acids and the other face containing polar or charged amino acids. This feature enables apolipoproteins to bind to lipids and still interact with the surrounding aqueous environment.

Metabolism of Lipoproteins[1,5,7]

Lipoprotein metabolism is commonly divided into (1) exogenous, (2) endogenous, (3) intracellular-cholesterol transport, and (4) reverse-cholesterol transport pathways.

Exogenous Pathway

The role of the exogenous pathway—transport of dietary lipids from the intestine to the liver and peripheral cells—is largely mediated by chylomicrons (Figure 23-18). Nascent chylomicrons, which are 90% triglcyerides by mass, are first assembled by the microsomal transfer protein (MTP) in the endoplasmic reticulum of enterocytes by combining triglycerides and other lipids with apo B-48. Chylomicrons are secreted into the lymph and, after entering the circulation, acquire from HDL additional apolipoproteins, such as apo E and apo C-II. Apo E is a ligand for uptake by the liver, whereas C-II is a potent activator of lipoprotein lipase (LPL), which is attached to the luminal surface of endothelial cells and rapidly hydrolyzes the triglycerides on chylomicrons to free fatty acids. Liberated fatty acids combine with albumin and are taken up by muscle cells as an energy

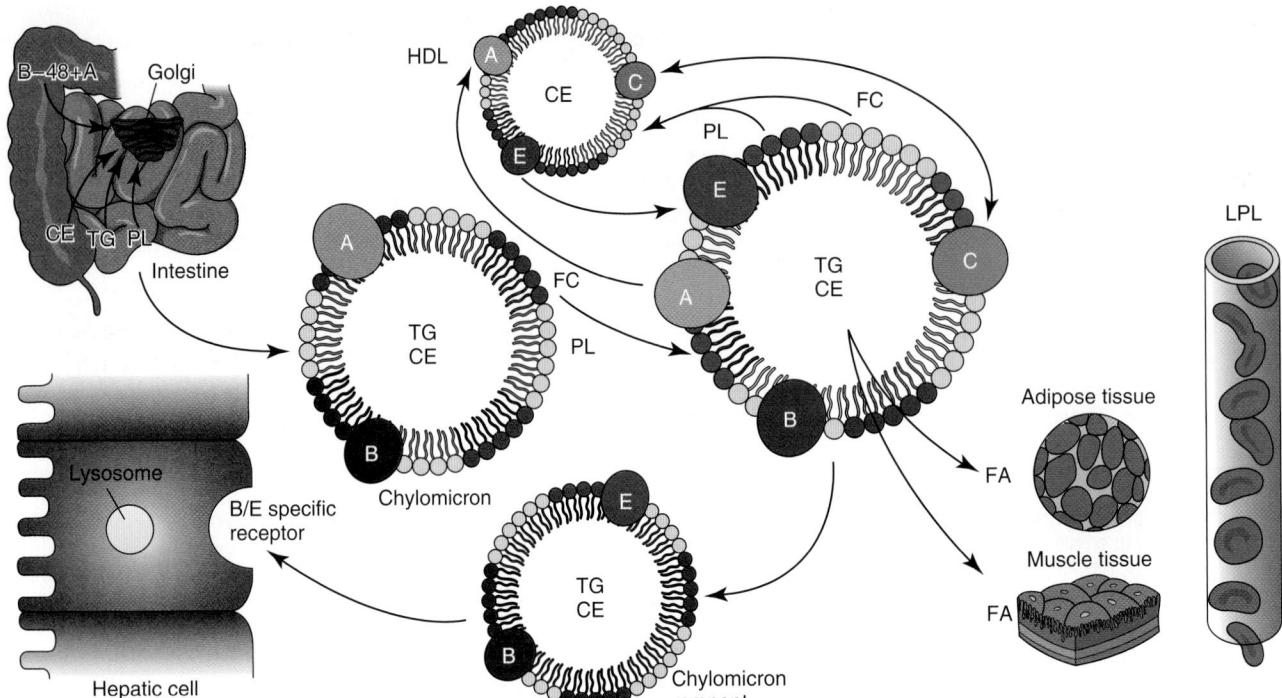

Figure 23-18 Exogenous lipoprotein metabolism pathway. *A*, Apolipoprotein A-I; *B*, apolipoprotein B-48; *C*, apolipoprotein C-II; *CE*, cholesterol ester; *E*, apolipoprotein E; *FA*, fatty acid; *FC*, free cholesterol; *HDL*, high-density lipoprotein; *LPL*, lipoprotein lipase; *PL*, phospholipid; *TG*, triglyceride. *(From Rifai N. Lipoproteins and apolipoproteins: composition, metabolism, and association with coronary heart disease. Arch Pathol Lab Med 1986;110:694-701. Copyright 1986, American Medical Association.)*

source or by adipose cells for energy storage as triglycerides. As a consequence of lipolysis, chylomicrons are transformed into smaller chylomicron remnant particles, which are rapidly removed by the liver.

Endogenous Pathway

The function of the endogenous pathway is to transfer hepatically derived lipids, especially triglycerides, to peripheral cells for energy metabolism. It is mediated by the apo B-100–containing lipoproteins (Figure 23-19). Hepatically derived lipids represent lipids that were synthesized by the liver or dietary lipids that were transferred to the liver by the exogenous pathway. VLDL, which contains approximately 55% triglcycerides by mass and includes one molecule of apo B-100, is the principal apo B–containing lipoprotein that is secreted by the liver. As it does on chylomicrons, the apo C-II present on the surface of VLDL activates LPL on endothelial cells. This leads to hydrolysis of VLDL triglycerides and release of free fatty acids, which are taken up by cells. The progressive lipolysis of triglycerides from the core of VLDL transforms it to IDL and eventually to LDL. The triglycerides on LDL is further depleted by the cholesterol ester transfer protein (CETP), which removes from LDL and exchanges it for cholesteryl esters from HDL. Although almost all cells express the LDL receptor, most LDL is eventually returned to the liver via the LDL receptor, which recognizes apo B-100. Cholesterol returned to the liver is (1) reused for the secretion

of lipoproteins, (2) used in the production of bile salts, or (3) excreted directly into the bile.

Intracellular-Cholesterol Transport Pathway

The intracellular-cholesterol transport pathway maintains cellular homeostasis of cholesterol. Although cholesterol is a necessary and critical component of all cell membranes, excess cholesterol will alter the biophysical properties of membranes and eventually will become toxic to the cell. Besides through biosynthesis, all cells receive cholesterol via uptake of extracellular lipoproteins by cell surface receptors, such as the LDL receptor (Figure 23-20). Most lipoprotein receptors deliver intact lipoprotein particles to lysosomes, where they are degraded. Cholesteryl esters are converted to free cholesterol by lysosomal acid lipase. Because most cells do not catabolize cholesterol further, any cholesterol delivered to the cell is (1) used for membrane biogenesis, (2) stored in intracellular lipid drops after reesterification by ACAT, or (3) removed from the cell by the reverse-cholesterol transport pathway. In addition, cells have a complex mechanism involving both transcriptional and posttranscriptional regulation, so that any excess intracellular cholesterol will inhibit cholesterol biosynthesis and expression of the LDL receptor.

Reverse-Cholesterol Transport Pathway

The function of the reverse-cholesterol transport pathway is to remove excess cellular cholesterol from peripheral cells and

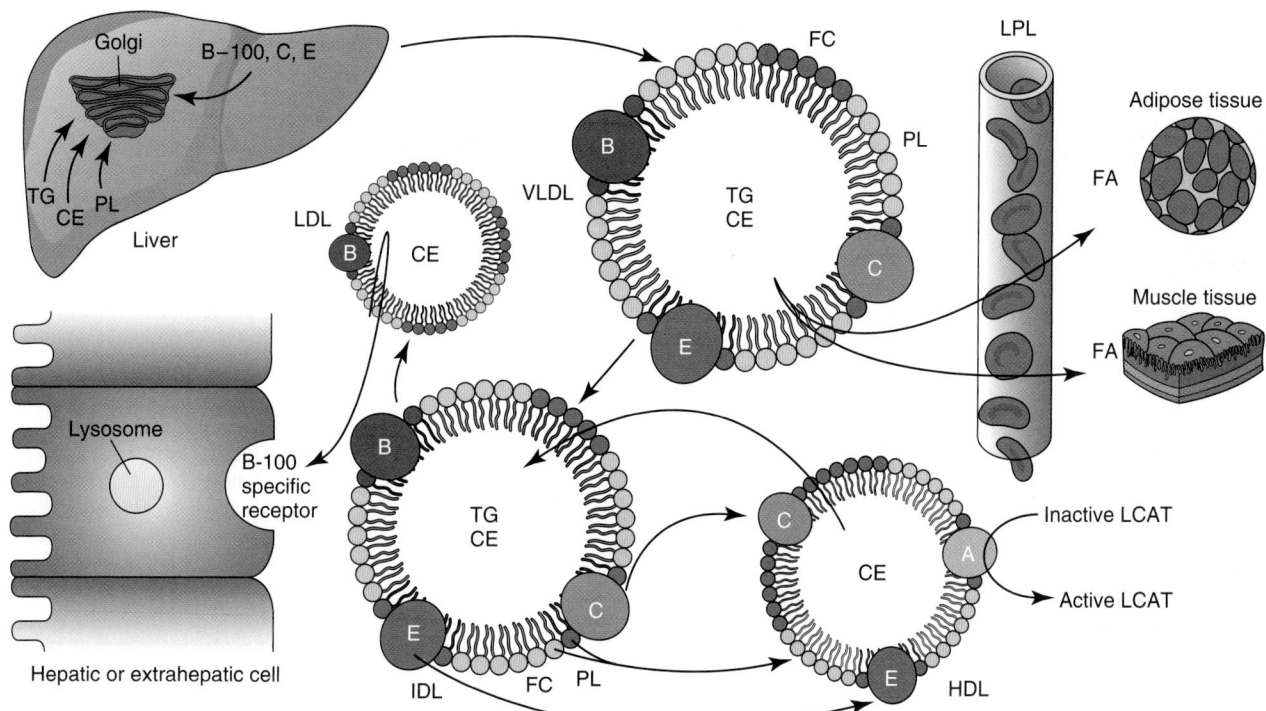

Figure 23-19 Endogenous lipoprotein metabolism pathway. *A,* Apolipoprotein A-I; *B,* apolipoprotein B-100; *C,* apolipoprotein C-II; *CE,* cholesterol ester; *E,* apolipoprotein E; *FA,* fatty acid; *FC,* free cholesterol; *HDL,* high-density lipoprotein; *IDL,* intermediate-density lipoprotein; *LCAT,* lecithin cholesterol acyltransferase; *LDL,* low-density lipoprotein; *LPL,* lipoprotein lipase; *PL,* phospholipid; *TG,* triglyceride; *VLDL,* very low-density lipoprotein. *(From Rifai N. Lipoproteins and apolipoproteins: composition, metabolism, and association with coronary heart disease. Arch Pathol Lab Med 1986;110:694-701. Copyright 1986, American Medical Association.)*

return it to the liver for excretion. This process is largely mediated by HDL (Figure 23-21). Cholesterol is actively pumped out of cells by the ABCA1 transporter onto lipid-poor apo A-I, which binds to cells. This process results in the formation of disc-shaped nascent HDL, which is made in the liver and in the intestine. Discoidal HDL interacts with ABCA1 in peripheral cells, such as macrophages, and removes additional cholesterol. LCAT, which esterifies cholesterol on HDL, plays a key role in reverse-cholesterol transport, because cholesteryl esters are much more hydrophobic than cholesterol and remain trapped in the core of HDL until they are removed by the liver. The esterification of cholesterol on HDL converts the disc-shaped nascent HDL to spherical HDL. Spherical HDL, the main form of HDL in the circulation, acts as an extracellular acceptor for cholesterol that may be removed from cells by other mechanisms.

In the next stage of the reverse-cholesterol transport pathway, the liver selectively removes cholesteryl esters from the lipid-rich spherical HDL via binding of the HDL to the SR-BI receptor and lets the lipid-depleted HDL return to the circulation for additional rounds of cholesterol removal from peripheral cells. CETP also plays an important role in this pathway because a significant fraction of cholesterol that is removed from cells by HDL is transferred as cholesteryl esters onto LDL by CETP and is eventually removed from the circulation by hepatic LDL receptors.

Clinical Significance[4,6,9]

The clinical significance of lipids is primarily associated with their contribution to **coronary heart disease (CHD)** and various lipoprotein disorders. CHD is a disease in which plaque builds up inside the coronary arteries that supply oxygen-rich blood to heart muscle. Numerous studies have established that when total cholesterol and LDL cholesterol (LDL-C) concentrations are high, the incidence and prevalence of CHD are also high. In contrast to LDL-C, increased HDL cholesterol (HDL-C) concentrations have been shown to be protective for CHD in both epidemiological and clinical trial studies. Because atherosclerosis begins at an early age and can take decades to manifest clinically, measurement of plasma lipids and lipoproteins is a valuable means of identifying individuals at risk for CHD and determining the most appropriate therapy.

Genetic Disorders of Lipoprotein Metabolism

Most patients with dyslipidemia do not have a single readily identifiable genetic mutation. Because of the complexity of lipoprotein metabolism, a multitude of environmental factors and common genetic polymorphisms that vary in importance, depending on the individual, probably account for most cases of hypercholesterolemia. Many secondary causes of dyslipidemia are a consequence of relatively common disorders or conditions (Table 23-7). Although rare, established genetic causes

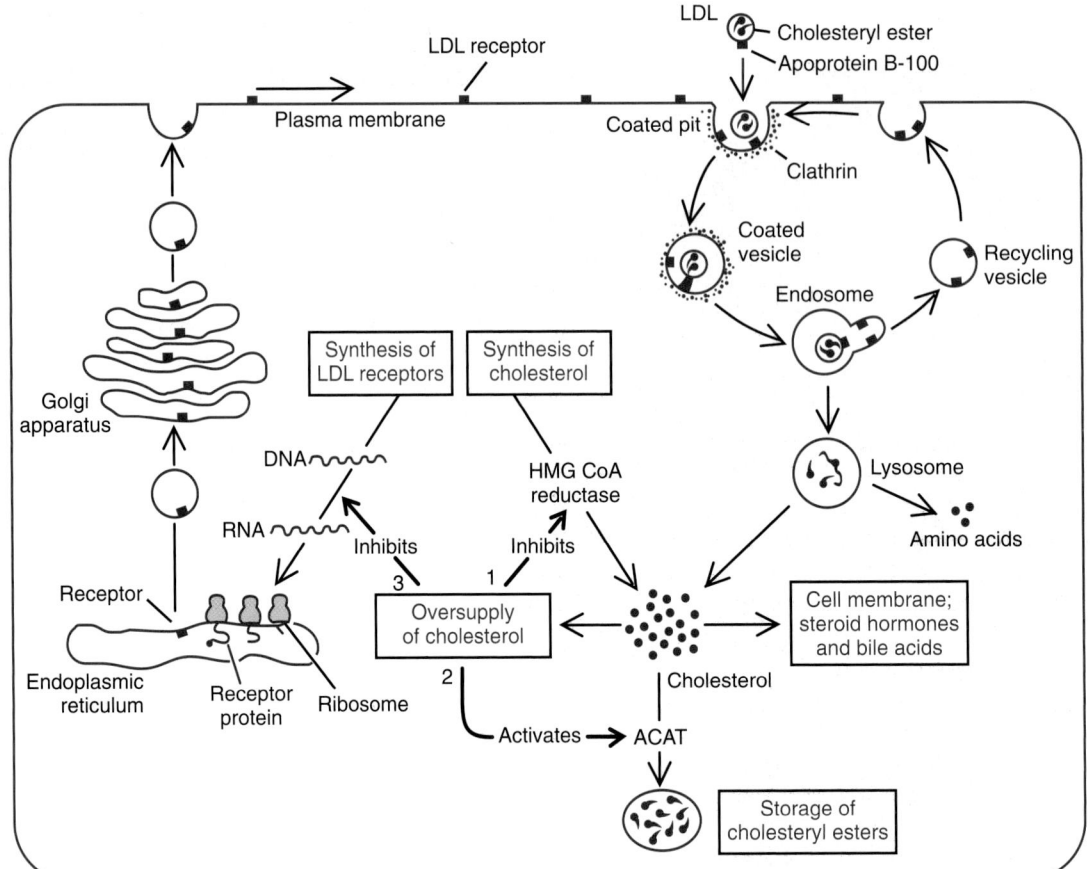

Figure 23-20 Intracellular-cholesterol transport pathway. *ACAT,* Acyl-CoA cholesterol acyl-transferase; *HMG-CoA reductase,* 3-hydroxy-3-methylglutaryl coenzyme A reductase; *LDL,* low-density lipoprotein. Because of the presence of apolipoprotein B-100 on its surface, the LDL particle is recognized by a specific LDL receptor in a coated pit and is taken into the cell in a coated vesicle *(top right).* Coated vesicles fuse together to form an endosome. The acidic environment of the endosome causes the LDL particle to dissociate from the receptors, which return to the cell surface. The LDL particles are taken to a lysosome, where apolipoprotein B-100 is broken down into amino acids and cholesterol ester is converted to free cholesterol for cellular requirements. The cellular cholesterol concentration is self-regulated. Oversupply of cholesterol will lead to (1) a decreased rate of cholesterol synthesis by inhibiting HMG-CoA reductase, (2) increased storage of cholesteryl esters by activating ACAT, and (3) inhibition of the synthesis of new LDL receptors by suppressing the transcription of the receptor gene into mRNA. *(From Brown MS, Goldstein JL. How LDL receptors influence cholesterol and atherosclerosis. Sci Am 1984;251:58-66. Copyright 1984 by Scientific American, Inc. All rights reserved.)*

of dyslipidemia have been identified and are illustrative of the role of lipid metabolism in the development of atherosclerosis.

Deficiency in Lipoprotein Lipase Activity

Deficient lipoprotein lipase activity due to mutations in the *LPL* gene is a rare autosomal recessive disorder characterized by hyperchylomicronemia (type I pattern),[*] with triglyceride concentrations reaching as high as 10,000 mg/dL (113 mmol/L). LPL is critical for the hydrolysis of triglycerides on chylomicrons and their subsequent conversion to chylomicron

remnants. This disorder is often first diagnosed in childhood, usually after recurrent episodes of severe abdominal pain and repeated attacks of pancreatitis. Eruptive xanthomas (a skin condition in which certain fats build up under the surface of the skin) and lipemia retinalis (a condition that occurs in patients when their plasma triglyceride concentrations exceed 2000 and 4000 mg/dL [22.6 to 45.2 mmol/L]) may be seen. The concentration of triglycerides often shows great fluctuation in response to diet and other factors that are not well understood. Individuals with this disorder are not predisposed to atherosclerotic disease, most likely because the chylomicron particles are too large to enter the vessel wall. The diagnosis is made by determination of LPL activity in plasma collected after heparin is injected into patients to release the LPL that is

---

[*]Both Roman and Arabic numerals are used to denote the individual conditions, but most often, Roman numerals are used. In this chapter, Roman symbols are used.

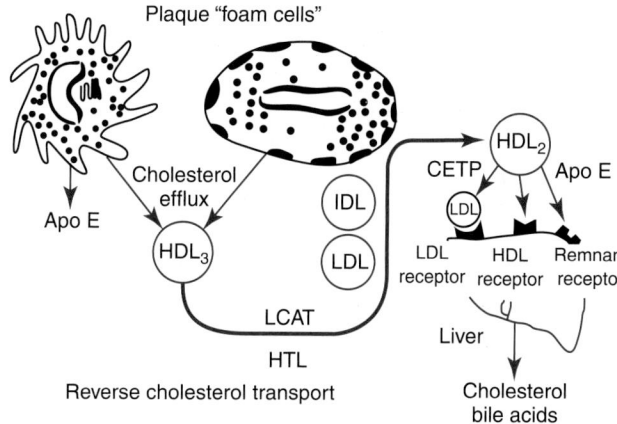

Figure 23-21 Reverse-cholesterol transport pathway. *ABCA1,* ATP binding cassette transporter A1; *ABCG1,* ATP binding cassette transporter G1; *APOA-1,* apolipoprotein A-1; *CETP,* cholesteryl ester transfer protein; *HDL,* high-density lipoprotein; *LCAT,* lecithin cholesterol acyltransferase; *LDL,* low-density lipoprotein; *LDL-R,* LDL-receptor; *SR-B1,* scavenger receptor B-1. After formation in the liver and intestine, nascent discoidal HDL removes cholesterol from peripheral cells by the ABCA1 transporter. Additional cholesterol can also be removed by HDL by the ABCG1 transporter and by a passive diffusion mechanism. LCAT esterifies the cholesterol content of HDL to prevent it from reentering the cells. Cholesterol esters are delivered to the liver by the SR-B1 receptor or by the LDL-R after transfer to LDL by CETP.

bound to heparin sulfates and other glycosaminoglycans on the surface of endothelial cells.

Mutations in apo C-II, the main activator of LPL, also result in impairment of chylomicron catabolism, although this usually is less severe than with *LPL* gene mutations. The diagnosis of this rare autosomal recessive condition is made by demonstrating low LPL activity in post-heparin plasma that is restored after the addition of apo C-II to the LPL assay mixture.

Familial Combined Hyperlipidemia

Familial combined hyperlipidemia (FCHL) accounts for as many as 10% to 15% of individuals with premature CHD. Families with FCHL often have increased plasma concentrations of total and LDL-C (type IIa) or triglyceride (type IV), or both (type IIb). Lipoprotein patterns also vary within an individual over time. In all cases, apo B-100 concentrations are increased because of overproduction. LDL particles in these patients tend to be small and dense because of a decreased lipid-to-protein ratio. LDL-C is usually only modestly increased to about 190 mg/dL (2.14 mmol/L), which is less than what is typically observed in heterozygous familial hypercholesterolemia (FH) (350 mg/dL; 3.95 mmol/L). The concentration of triglycerides usually is between 200 and 400 mg/dL (2.26 and 4.52 mmol/L) but may be significantly higher. The underlying genetic basis of FCHL is not known; it is mostly likely a polygenetic disorder.

Familial Hypertriglyceridemia

Familial hypertriglyceridemia (FHTG) is characterized by a moderate increase in serum triglycerides. Overproduction

TABLE 23-7	**Causes of Secondary Hyperlipidemia and Dyslipoproteinemia**
Disorder	**Cause**
Exogenous	Drugs: corticosteroids, isotretinoin (Accutane), thiazides, anticonvulsants, β-blockers, anabolic steroids, certain oral contraceptives
	Alcohol
	Obesity
Endocrine and metabolic	Acute intermittent porphyria
	Diabetes mellitus
	Hypopituitarism
	Hypothyroidism
	Lipodystrophy
	Pregnancy
Storage disease	Cystine storage disease
	Gaucher disease
	Glycogen storage disease
	Juvenile Tay-Sachs disease
	Niemann-Pick disease
	Tay-Sachs disease
Renal	Chronic renal failure
	Hemolytic-uremic syndrome
	Nephrotic syndrome
Hepatic	Benign recurrent intrahepatic cholestasis
	Congenital biliary atresia
Acute and transient	Burns
	Hepatitis
	Acute trauma (surgery)
	Myocardial infarction
	Bacterial and viral infections
Others	Anorexia nervosa
	Starvation
	Idiopathic hypercalcemia
	Klinefelter syndrome
	Progeria (Hutchinson-Gilford syndrome)
	Systemic lupus erythematosus
	Werner syndrome

of large VLDL particles with abnormally high triglyceride content is thought to be responsible for this disorder, but decreased lipolysis is sometimes a contributory factor. Because of the hypertriglyceridemia, plasma HDL-C is often notably decreased. This disorder is inherited in an autosomal dominant pattern with delayed expression, but it is a polygenic disorder with an estimated frequency in the population of about 1 in 500.

Type V Hyperlipoproteinemia

Type V hyperlipoproteinemia is characterized by an increase in both chylomicrons and VLDL and typically presents in adults. Although its exact cause is unknown, it appears to be associated with increased production and/or decreased removal of VLDL. The activity of LPL in these individuals may be normal or low, and the plasma concentration of apo C-II is normal. Clinical presentations include (1) eruptive xanthomas, (2) lipemia retinalis, (3) pancreatitis, and (4) abnormal glucose tolerance. Most of these patients have a modestly increased risk of cardiovascular disease.

Dysbetalipoproteinemia (Type III)

Dysbetalipoproteinemia, also called *type III hyperlipoproteinemia,* is caused by a defect in the removal of lipoprotein remnants from both chylomicrons and VLDL. Apo E present on the surface of lipoprotein remnant particles interacts with specific hepatic receptors and facilitates the removal of these particles. Apo E exists in three common polymorphisms or variants, designated E_2, E_3, and E_4. Some individuals with dysbetalipoproteinemia are homozygous for the apo E_2 isoform, which does not efficiently bind to hepatic remnant receptors, thus leading to accumulation of remnant particles. Although rare, genetic mutations in the *APOE* gene have been associated with the disorder. The remnant particles that accumulate are enriched in cholesterol, have a density less than 1.006 g/mL, and are commonly referred to as β-VLDL, or floating β-lipoprotein. Dysbetalipoproteinemia has a late onset and may manifest in patients with a secondary cause of dyslipidemia or obesity. The most distinctive clinical feature of dysbetalipoproteinemia is the presence of palmar xanthomas—yellow fat deposits in the creases of the palms. Tuberous and tuberoeruptive xanthomas may occur but are not unique to this syndrome. Premature atherosclerosis commonly develops, particularly in the lower extremities. The incidence of dysbetalipoproteinemia is approximately 0.1% in the general population. Apo E_2 homozygosity, however, is seen in about 1% of the population in North America; thus the occurrence of defective alleles is necessary but is not sufficient to produce the disorder.

Familial Hypercholesterolemia

FH is caused by defects in the LDL receptor pathway, which binds and removes LDL from the circulation. LDL thus accumulates in the plasma, resulting in its increased deposition in the skin, tendons, and arteries, where it causes atherosclerosis. LDL particles tend to be larger and carry increased amounts of cholesterol. Triglyceride concentration may be normal or only slightly increased, and HDL-C concentration is slightly decreased. Most of these patients have gene defects in the LDL receptor gene (*LDLR*). Less commonly, defects in two other genes, *RHOA* (formerly called *ARH-1*) and *PCSK9*, which code for proteins involved in internalization or processing of the LDL receptor, may cause FH. Mutations in the LDL receptor gene (*LDLR*) and in *PCSK9* are inherited in an autosomal co-dominant pattern. Homozygous FH patients are severely affected, whereas heterozygotes usually have a milder phenotype but are still clinically affected. Defects in *RHOA* are inherited in an autosomal recessive pattern.

Heterozygous FH due to mutations in the LDL receptor gene is one of the most common genetic disorders, with an estimated incidence of 1 in 500 in the United States. The mean plasma LDL-C in children and adult heterozygotes is usually two to three times that of normal individuals, whereas LDL-C of homozygotes is usually fourfold to sixfold above normal. In heterozygotes, xanthomas appear toward the end of the second decade of life, and clinical manifestations of atherosclerotic disease often are noted during the fourth decade. In homozygotes, cutaneous xanthomas often develop by 4 years of age, if they are not already present at birth. Left untreated, death from myocardial infarction generally occurs in homozygotes before the end of the second or third decade of life.

Familial Defective Apolipoprotein B-100

Familial defective apo B-100 is the result of mutations in the gene *APOB*, which reduce its affinity for the LDL receptor. LDL-C is increased, but triglycerides and HDL-C are usually within reference intervals. Like those with FH, these individuals have an increased incidence of CHD. Clinical differentiation between this disorder and heterozygous FH is sometimes difficult, but management of the two disorders is similar. The frequency of this mutation is 1:500 to 1:600 in hypercholesterolemic individuals from populations of European descent, but it is very rare in non-Europeans.

Hypoalphalipoproteinemia

Hypoalphalipoproteinemia, or low HDL-C, is caused by several genetic defects and is often but not always associated with an increased incidence of CHD. Mutations or deletions of the *APOA1* gene are a rare cause of hypoalphalipoproteinemia. LCAT deficiency is also associated with low HDL. These patients often have cloudy corneas as a result of infiltration of lipid, as well as glomerulosclerosis because of the production of abnormal lipoprotein particles that become trapped in the glomerulus.

Tangier disease is a rare autosomal recessive disorder that is associated with a notable reduction in HDL. The major clinical signs of Tangier disease are (1) hyperplastic orange tonsils, (2) splenomegaly, and (3) peripheral neuropathy. Deposition of cholesteryl esters is increased in various tissues of the body, particularly macrophages, which form foam cells. Tangier disease is caused by mutations in the *ABCA1* gene for the ABCA1 transporter, which mediates the first step of the reverse-cholesterol transport pathway—efflux of cholesterol from cells (see Figure 23-20).

Adult Management of Lipoprotein Disorders[4,13]

The initial diagnosis of a dyslipoproteinemia and determination of the best treatment approach for a patient have been based largely on measurements of (1) total cholesterol, (2) triglyceride, (3) HDL-C, and (4) LDL-C; this is commonly referred to as a *lipid panel.* Lipid and lipoprotein test results, however, must be interpreted in the context of a medical history if the risk for developing CHD is to be established. Medical history and other laboratory test results are also important for determining whether a dyslipoproteinemia is the result of a primary lipoprotein disorder or is a consequence of one or more of the secondary causes of hyperlipidemia (see Table 23-7), which, if present, should also be addressed. In contrast to most other laboratory tests, hypercholesterolemia is defined on the basis of findings from epidemiological studies that were used to establish a desirable concentration for reducing CHD risk (Table 23-8), rather than a reference study of normal

TABLE 23-8	Adult Treatment Panel (ATP) III Classification of LDL, Total, and HDL Cholesterol (mg/dL)	
LDL cholesterol	<100	Optimum
	100-129	Near or above optimum
	130-159	Borderline high
	160-189	High
	≥190	Very high
Total cholesterol	<200	Desirable
	200-239	Borderline high
	≥240	High
HDL cholesterol	<40	Low
	≥60	High

HDL, High-density lipoprotein; *LDL,* low-density lipoprotein.
Modified from executive summary of the Third Report of the National Cholesterol Education Program (NCEP) Expert Panel on Detection, Evaluation, and Treatment of High Blood Cholesterol in Adults (Adult Treatment Panel III). JAMA 2001;285:2486-97.

BOX 23-1	Major Risk Factors (Exclusive of LDL Cholesterol)

- Cigarette smoking
- Hypertension (blood pressure ≥140/90 mm Hg or on antihypertensive medication)
- Low HDL cholesterol (<40 mg/dL)*
- Family history of premature CHD (CHD in male first-degree relative <55 years; CHD in female first-degree relative <65 years)
- Age (men ≥45 years; women ≥55 years)

Modified from executive summary of the Third Report of the National Cholesterol Education Program (NCEP) Expert Panel on Detection, Evaluation, and Treatment of High Blood Cholesterol in Adults (Adult Treatment Panel III). JAMA 2001;285:2486-97.

*HDL cholesterol ≥60 mg/dL counts as a "negative" risk factor; its presence removes one risk factor from the total count.
HDL, High-density lipoprotein; *LDL,* low-density lipoprotein.

individuals.[†] Cholesterol screening is recommended every 5 years for all adults over 20 years of age and should involve measurements of fasting (1) total cholesterol, (2) triglyceride, (3) HDL-C, and (4) calculated or measured LDL-C. If a fasting sample is not available initially, then only total cholesterol and HDL-C should be considered.

Next, an assessment should be made of the risk for CHD. This is based on clinical evidence of existing CHD or the presence of conditions that are closely associated with CHD, such as (1) symptomatic carotid artery disease, (2) peripheral vascular disease, and (3) abdominal aortic aneurysm, which are called *CHD risk equivalents.* Risk assessment for CHD is also based on the presence of known risk factors for CHD, such as (1) hypertension, (2) smoking, and (3) family history (Box 23-1). Low HDL-C is considered a risk factor, whereas high HDL-C is considered a negative risk factor.

[†]Several tables of population distributions of lipids have been published in Remaly AT, Rifai N, Warnick GR. Lipids, lipoproteins, apolipoproteins, and other cardiovascular risk factors. In: Burtis CA, Ashwood ER, Bruns DE, eds. Tietz fundamentals of clinical chemistry and molecular diagnostics, 5th edition. Philadelphia: Saunders, 2012:751-754.

BOX 23-2	Therapeutic Life-Style Changes for the Prevention of CHD

- Diet
  - Saturated fat <7% of calories, cholesterol <200 mg/day
  - Consider increased viscous (soluble) fiber (10 to 25 g/day) and plant stanols/sterols (2 g/day) as therapeutic options to enhance LDL lowering
- Weight management
- Increased physical activity

Modified from executive summary of the Third Report of the National Cholesterol Educational Program (NCEP) Expert Panel on Detection, Evaluation, and Treatment of High Blood Cholesterol in Adults (Adult Treatment Panel III). JAMA 2001;285:2486-97.

Therapeutic life-style changes (Box 23-2) serve as the cornerstone of therapy for lipid disorders. The concentration of LDL-C is used both to decide the most appropriate therapy and to monitor the effectiveness of treatment. Adult treatment guidelines for hypercholesterolemia are illustrated in Table 23-9. Note that aggressiveness of treatment depends on the risk category of the patient and his or her starting LDL-C concentration. Patients at highest risk for CHD (10-year risk >20%) and those who already have clinical evidence of CHD or a CHD risk equivalent have the lowest LDL-C treatment threshold and the lowest LDL-C target goal. Ideally, for such patients, LDL-C should be below 100 mg/dL (2.59 mmol/L) after therapy; this will likely involve some type of drug treatment. Patients in an intermediate risk category (10-year risk <20%) have a higher concentration for their LDL-C target goal and, in some cases, depending on their starting LDL-C, may be treated only by therapeutic life-style changes. For patients in the lowest risk category (0 to 1 risk factors), desirable LDL-C is <160 mg/dL (4.14 mmol/L), and drug therapy should be considered only if initial LDL-C is above 190 mg/dL (2.15 mmol/L). Specific recommendations have been put forth for the frequency of monitoring lipids and lipoprotein tests, and for when drug therapy should be tried for patients who do not reach their LDL-C target treatment goals with just therapeutic life-style changes.

Increased triglycerides and low HDL-C are considered conditions that independently alter the risk for CHD and may alter the recommended treatment. In both cases, however, the primary goal of therapy should be to lower LDL-C and secondarily to improve the increased triglycerides or low HDL, if these conditions persist after LDL-C is lowered. Each patient at risk for CHD should also be assessed for the presence of metabolic syndrome and should be treated for underlying causes and associated symptoms. Other newly developed lipoprotein tests, such as (1) Lp(a), (2) remnant lipoproteins, and (3) small dense LDL, and other markers, such as (4) C-reactive protein (CRP), and (5) homocysteine, may also be valuable in CHD risk stratification, particularly for patients who are at borderline or intermediate risk, based on conventional lipid and lipoprotein tests.

A wide variety of pharmacological agents for cholesterol lowering in adults are prescribed individually or in

TABLE 23-9   LDL Cholesterol Goals and Cut Points for Therapeutic Life-Style Changes (TLC) and Drug Therapy in Different Risk Categories

Risk Category	LDL Goal (mg/dL)	LDL Concentration at Which to Initiate Therapeutic Life-Style Changes (mg/dL)	LDL Concentration at Which to Consider Drug Therapy (mg/dL)
CHD or CHD risk equivalents (10-year risk >20%)	<100	≥100	≥300 (100-129; drug optional)
2+ risk factors (10-year risk ≤20%)	<130	≥130	10-year risk 10%-20%: ≥130 10-year risk <10%: ≥160
0-1 risk factor (10-year risk <10%)	<160	≥160	≥190 (160-189; LDL-lowering drug optional)

CHD, Coronary heart disease; *LDL,* low-density lipoprotein.
Modified from executive summary of the third report of the National Cholesterol Education Program (NCEP) Expert Panel on Detection, Evaluation, and Treatment of High Blood Cholesterol in Adults (Adult Treatment Panel III). JAMA 2001;285:2486-97.

combination to lower LDL-C, including (1) bile acid–binding resins (cholestyramine and colestipol), (2) niacin, (3) gemfibrozil, (4) ezetimibe, and (5) HMG-CoA reductase inhibitors (e.g., atorvastatin, fluvastatin, lovastatin, pravastatin, rosuvastatin, simvastatin, pitavastatin); agents in the latter group have been found to reduce LDL-C by as much as 40%. Some of these drugs are better tolerated by individual patients than others; all have demonstrated long-term safety in adults and have been shown to decrease CHD risk. Niacin has been the most effective therapy for raising HDL-C, but the value of raising HDL-C has been called into question by trials of the CETP inhibitors, which dramatically increase HDL-C but have not decreased CHD events.

Management of Lipoprotein Disorders in Pediatrics[9,13]

Because the process of atherosclerosis begins in children, and CHD risk factors that start in childhood, such as obesity and dyslipidemia, often persist into adulthood, it is important to identify children at risk for CHD, with the expectation that early intervention will be the most effective way to prevent future disease. This goal has to be tempered by the concern that unlike in adults, clinical studies supporting the long-term effectiveness and safety of any type of therapy, particularly the use of lipid-lowering medications in children, are limited.

The 2011 guidelines for cardiovascular health and risk reduction in the pediatric population from the National Heart, Lung and Blood Institute (NHLBI) are integrated guidelines that make age-specific recommendations on the multiple risk factors that contribute to CHD. They are aimed at primary care physicians and other health professionals who treat children. They provide guidance not only on the diagnosis and management of dyslipidemias but also on how to monitor (1) family history, (2) tobacco exposure, (3) degree of physical activity, (4) diet, (5) growth charts, (6) blood pressure, and (7) diabetes, as well as (8) how to educate children and parents on healthy lifestyles.

Previous guidelines did not recommend universal lipid testing and instead relied upon identifying children at risk on the basis of family history of CHD or dyslipidemia. Although family history integrates (1) genetic, (2) behavioral, and (3) environmental factors, it is often inadequate and has been shown to miss as many as half of children at risk for CHD. Current guidelines recommend universal lipid screening between ages 9 and 11, and then later between 18 and 21 years of age. Age 9 to 11 was chosen because lipids often change after puberty, and because this is the age at which children with severe lipid disorders should first be considered as possible candidates for drug therapy. Age 18 to 21 was chosen as a second time to screen because some lipid disorders do not become manifest until late teenage years or young adulthood, and because after this point in time, many individuals may not participate in lipid screening until many years later, when advanced disease has already developed. Because it is more convenient, particularly for young children, it is recommended that a nonfasting sample be analyzed to determine non–HDL-C. It is simply calculated as total cholesterol minus HDL-C and has been shown in both children and adults to be just as effective as LDL-C as a CHD risk marker. For other ages, lipid testing is recommended on a fasting sample, only if children have a strong family history of CHD and/or have a parent with a dyslipidemia or a condition that puts them at high risk for CHD, such as diabetes.

As in adult guidelines, recommended interventions are calibrated to the degree of CHD risk; and life-style changes, such as low-fat diet and increasing physical activity, are recommended first for all patients (Figure 23-22). If, after a 3-month period, life-style changes prove ineffective in reaching the LDL-C target goal, which varies depending on the overall risk, then drug treatment with a statin and/or a bile acid sequestrant should be considered for children 10 years of age or older. All children, even those younger than age 10, who present with a marked increase in serum lipids (LDL-C >250 mg/dL [6.46 mmol/L]) may have a genetic lipid disorder, should be referred to a lipid specialist, and may require additional types of drugs or other treatment approaches, such as LDL apheresis in the case of FH. Because of the high prevalence of obesity in the pediatric population, the most common pattern of dyslipidemia in children consists of (1) a moderate to severe increase in triglycerides, (2) a mild increase in LDL-C, and (3) decreased HDL-C. In general,

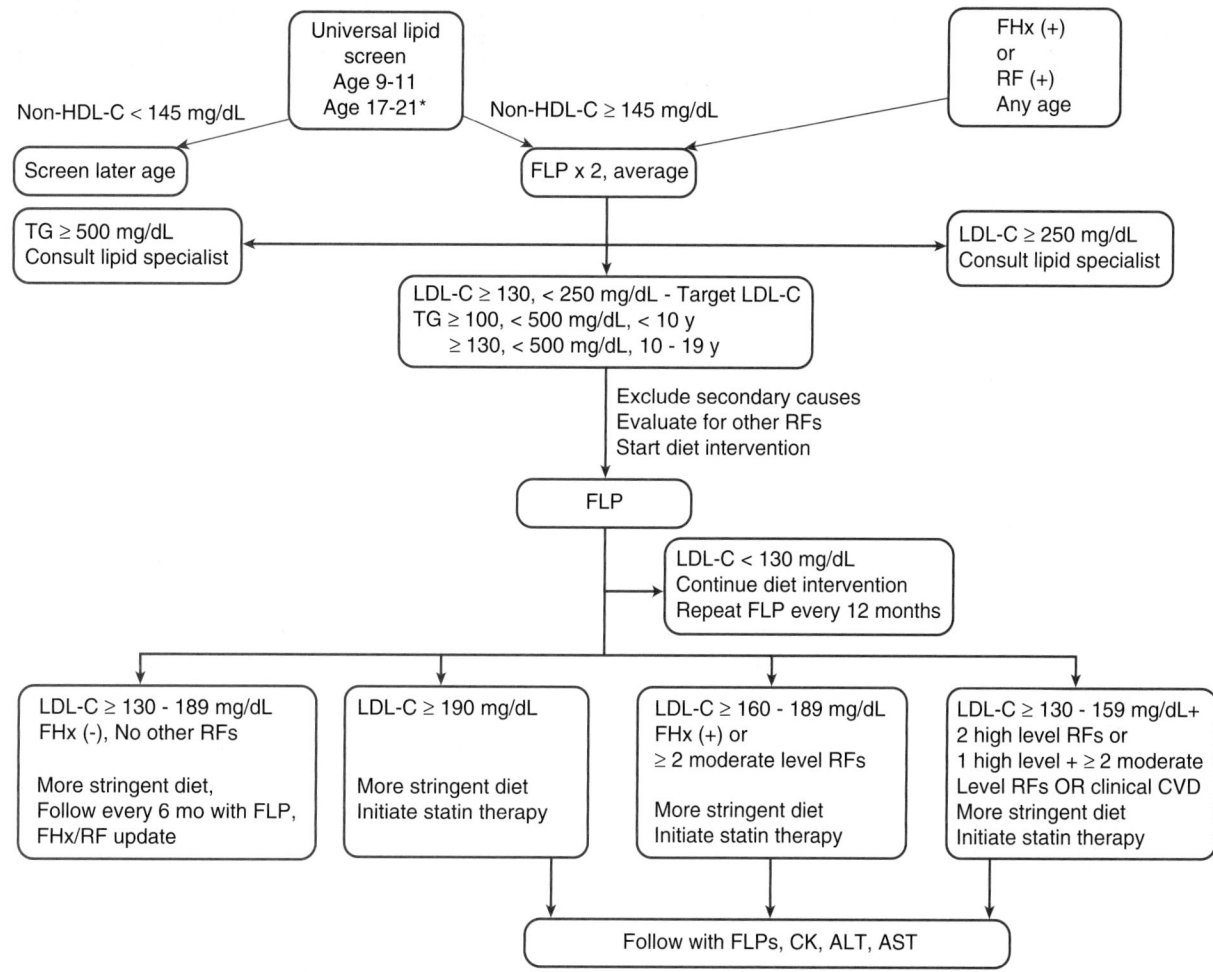

Figure 23-22 Algorithm for assessment of coronary heart disease (CHD) risk in children based on lipid screening. *(Modified from Expert Panel on Integrated Guidelines for Cardiovascular Health and Risk Reduction in Children and Adolescents. Summary report. Pediatrics 2011;128:S1-S44.)* *For ages 19 to 21, non–HDL-C ≥190 mg/dL is the recommended cut point. *FHx(+),* Positive family history; *RF,* risk factor; *FLP,* fasting lipid profile. Other positive risk factors or risk equivalents for cardiovascular disease include RF(+). *ALT,* Alanine aminotransferase; *AST,* aspartate aminotransferase; *CK,* creatine kinase.

patients respond well to changes in diet and weight loss and often do not require drug therapy. Children who present with a marked increase in triglycerides to over 500 mg/dL (>5.65 mmol/L) may have a primary genetic defect, such as LPL deficiency, are at risk for pancreatitis, and should be seen by a lipid specialist. It is recommended that children treated with lipid-lowering drugs start with the lowest possible dose; when placed on statins, hepatic transaminases and creatine kinase should be measured to monitor for hepatic and muscle toxicity. Decisions about placing a child on a lipid-lowering drug should be based on an average of at least two fasting serum lipid profiles that are at least 2 weeks apart but no more than 3 months apart.

Analysis of Lipids, Lipoproteins, and Apolipoproteins[2,3,8,10,12]

As risk-related cutoff points (see Table 23-9) were developed, much effort has gone into improvement and standardization

TABLE 23-10	National Cholesterol Education Program Recommendations for Analytical Performance of Lipid and Lipoprotein Measurements

		Consistent With	
	Total Error (%)	Bias (%)	CV (%)
Cholesterol	8.9	≤±3	≤3
Triglycerides	≤15	≤±5	≤5
HDL cholesterol	≤13	≤±5	≤4
LDL cholesterol	≤12	≤±4	≤4

CV, Coefficient of variation; *HDL,* high-density lipoprotein; *LDL,* low-density lipoprotein.

of lipid and lipoprotein assays to ensure their proper performance (Table 23-10) and to ensure comparability of test results between different methods and different clinical laboratories, thus reducing misclassification of patients' CHD risk.

Cholesterol Assays

Enzymatic methods have become the assays of choice for the routine measurement of cholesterol. A commonly used three-step procedure is shown below. Enzyme reagents are mixed with serum or plasma and are incubated under controlled conditions for color development; absorbance is measured in the visible portion of the spectrum, generally at about 500 nm. The reagents typically use a bacterial cholesteryl ester hydrolase to cleave cholesteryl esters:

$$\text{Cholesteryl ester} + H_2O \xrightarrow{\text{Cholesteryl ester hydrolase}} \text{cholesterol} + \text{fatty acid} \quad (1)$$

The 3-OH group of cholesterol is then oxidized to a ketone in an oxygen-requiring reaction catalyzed by cholesterol oxidase:

$$\text{Cholesterol} + O_2 \xrightarrow{\text{Cholesterol oxidase}} \text{choles-4-en-3-one} + H_2O_2 \quad (2)$$

H_2O_2 is measured in a peroxidase-catalyzed reaction that forms a colored dye:

$$\text{H}_2\text{O}_2 + \text{phenol} + \text{4-aminoantipyrine} \\ \xrightarrow{\text{Peroxidase}} \text{quinoneimine dye} + 2\,H_2O \quad (3)$$

Enzymatic methods are subject to interference from other colored compounds or from those that compete with the oxidation reaction, such as (1) bilirubin, (2) ascorbic acid, and (3) hemoglobin. Assays are usually linear up to about 600 to 700 mg/dL (15.54 to 18.13 mmol/L).

Triglycerides

Triglycerides are also routinely measured with enzyme reagents. Several different enzyme sequences have been used. With all of these methods, the first step is the lipase-catalyzed hydrolysis of triglycerides to glycerol and fatty acids.

$$\text{Triglyceride} + 3\,H_2O \xrightarrow{\text{Lipase}} \text{glycerol} + 3 \text{ fatty acids} \quad (4)$$

Glycerol is then phosphorylated in an ATP-requiring reaction catalyzed by glycerokinase:

$$\text{Glycerol} + \text{ATP} \\ \xrightarrow{\text{Glycerokinase}} \text{glycerophospate} \\ + \text{adenosine diphosphate (ADP)} \quad (5)$$

With the most commonly used methods, glycerophosphate is oxidized to dihydroxyacetone and H_2O_2 in a glycerophosphate oxidase–catalyzed reaction:

$$\text{Glycerophosphate} + O_2 \\ \xrightarrow{\text{Glycerophosphate oxidase}} \text{dihydroxyacetone} + H_2O_2 \quad (6)$$

and H_2O_2 formed in the reaction is measured as described in reaction (3).

Enzymatic triglyceride methods are fairly specific in that they do not detect glucose or phospholipids. They are linear in the concentration range up to about 700 mg/dL (7.91 mmol/L) and, when automated, are operated with coefficients of variation in the range of approximately 2% to 3%. Because glycerol is a product of normal metabolic processes, it is present in serum. Thus the measured quantity of triglycerides in serum is overestimated slightly, if not corrected for endogenous glycerol. In healthy individuals, endogenous glycerol represents the equivalent of less than 10 mg/dL (0.11 mmol/L) of triglyceride; therefore the error due to glycerol is not usually clinically significant. Some laboratories employ an alternative triglyceride assay, in which the endogenous glycerol is first "blanked out" by adjustment of the calibrators to compensate for an average bias or by enzymatic consumption of glycerol in a prereaction step before triglycerides are measured.

High-Density Lipoprotein Cholesterol

The concentration of cholesterol associated with HDL is determined after the non-HDL lipoproteins are physically removed or effectively masked.

Traditionally, non-HDL lipoproteins—VLDL, IDL, Lp(a), LDL, and chylomicrons—were precipitated with polyanions. Polyanions react with positively charged groups on lipoproteins, and this interaction is further facilitated in the presence of divalent cations, such as magnesium, to create a precipitate. The precipitate is removed by centrifuging for at least 45,000 g-minutes, and cholesterol is measured enzymatically in the supernatant. Several polyanion-divalent cation combinations have been used, including (1) heparin sulfate-MnCl₂, (2) dextran sulfate–MgCl₂, and (3) phosphotungstate-MgCl₂. HDL-C assays are considered inaccurate in samples containing triglyceride concentrations above 400 mg/dL (4.52 mmol/L). To minimize this problem, such samples are pretreated to remove or reduce interference by triglyceride-rich lipoproteins, which do not fully precipitate. Techniques used to pretreat samples include (1) centrifugation, (2) filtration, and (3) dilution. The preferred anticoagulant for lipoprotein measurements is ethylenediaminetetraacetic acid (EDTA) because it inhibits the oxidation of lipids and the proteolysis of apolipoproteins. However, it causes a slight dilution of about 3% when compared with lipoprotein measurements on serum, upon which current cut points are based.

Direct HDL-C assays, also known as *homogeneous assays*, are most commonly used to measure HDL-C. In contrast to precipitation-based assays, no physical separation of HDL from non-HDL fractions occurs. Instead, HDL-C is selectively measured by effective masking or promoting the consumption of cholesterol from non-HDL fractions so that it does not react with the enzymes used to measure cholesterol on HDL. This is achieved by a variety of methods, depending on the type of assay. For example, some assays involve the use of antibodies or various polymers or complexing agents, such as cyclodextrin, that shield the cholesterol in the non-HDL fractions from reacting with cholesterol-measuring enzymes. Some assays depend on modifications of cholesteryl esterase and cholesterol oxidase that make them more selective for HDL-C. Finally, some assays use a blanking step that enzymatically consumes cholesterol from non-HDL fractions. Unlike with the other HDL-C assays, no sample pretreatment step is performed with direct assays and thus they can be fully automated. However, these assays sometimes show relatively poor performance compared with reference methods on dyslipidemic samples, particularly those with high triglycerides.

Low-Density Lipoprotein Cholesterol

Until recently, LDL-C was determined indirectly. In the most widely used indirect method, (1) total cholesterol, (2) triglycerides, and (3) HDL-C are measured in a fasting sample, and LDL-C is calculated from the primary measurements by the empirical *Friedewald equation:*

$$\text{LDL Cholesterol} = [\text{Total cholesterol}] - [\text{HDL Cholesterol}] - [\text{Triglyceride}]/5 \quad (7)$$

where all concentrations are given in milligrams per deciliter. Triglycerides/2.22 is used when LDL-C is expressed in millimoles per liter. The factor (triglycerides)/5 is an estimate of the VLDL cholesterol concentration and is based on the average ratio of triglycerides to cholesterol in VLDL.

In practice, the Friedewald equation should not be used (1) in samples that have triglyceride concentrations above 400 mg/dL (4.52 mmol/L), (2) in samples that contain significant quantities of chylomicrons (nonfasting specimen), or (3) in patients with dysbetalipoproteinemia. In these cases, the factor (triglyceride)/5 does not provide an accurate estimate of VLDL cholesterol, and this leads to large errors in calculated LDL-C. As with HDL-C, several methods are now used for the direct measurement of LDL-C. In general, these assays yield results similar to those obtained by calculating LDL-C and performing the β-quantification reference method, which is based on ultracentrifugation, but performance may not be as good on high-triglyceride samples. Evidence suggests that different direct assays may not be specific and may include some of the other apo B–containing lipoproteins or may miss some LDL subfractions, such as the more atherogenic small, dense LDLs.

Measurement of Apolipoproteins

Immunoturbidimetric and immunonephelometric assays are typically used in measuring apo A-I and apo B-100. Alternatively, more sensitive techniques, such as enzyme-linked immunosorbent assay (ELISA) and radioimmunoassay (RIA), are usually more suitable for apolipoproteins that are present in significantly lower concentrations, such as apo C-I and apo C-II. Considerable effort has been expended in the past to standardize apo A-I and B-100 measurements, leading to significant improvement in the overall performance of these assays. Immunoassays for total apo E are not commonly done, but genotyping of apo E is used to identify the apo E_4 isoform, which is associated with increased cholesterol and risk for Alzheimer's disease.

Lipoprotein(a)

Although Lp(a) particles typically carry only a relatively small fraction of total cholesterol, these lipoprotein particles are particularly pro-atherogenic. Therefore, Lp(a) is often measured in individuals with a normal lipid panel but with a history of premature cardiovascular disease and/or a strong family history of cardiovascular disease. Turbidimetric, nephelometric, RIA, and ELISA methods are all currently used for Lp(a) measurement. Most of these assays, except for ELISA, are based on the use of polyclonal antibodies. Sandwich-type ELISAs are usually based on the use of a combination of monoclonal and polyclonal antibodies to apo B and apo(a). The immunoreactivity of antibodies directed to the repeat kringle 4 type 2 domain in apo(a) makes some Lp(a) assays vary as a function of apo(a) size. These assays tend to underestimate apo(a) concentration in samples with apo(a) of smaller size than the apo(a) present in the assay calibrator, and to overestimate the apo(a) concentration in samples with larger apo(a). Traditionally, Lp(a) concentrations have been reported in terms of total Lp(a) particle mass, or, alternatively, in terms of Lp(a) protein. If the purpose is to provide Lp(a) values that are independent of apo(a) size, it is recommended that the Lp(a) assay use antibodies directed to an apo(a) domain other than kringle 4 type 2, or to the apo B-100 component of Lp(a). This would allow the values to be expressed in nanomoles per liter. At present, Lp(a) measurements are not well standardized, but a value of about 30 mg/dL of total Lp(a) particle mass has traditionally been used as a cutoff, above which increased concentrations of Lp(a) are associated with increased risk of CHD. Because Lp(a) values vary among ethnic groups, reference values ideally should be population based. For example, African Americans in general have significantly higher Lp(a) concentrations than Caucasians.

Sources of Variation and Bias in Test Measurement

Concentrations of various lipoproteins and their constituent parts—lipids and apolipoproteins—vary within individuals (see Chapter 6). Analytical variations for such measurements are relatively small—generally about 2% to 3% coefficients of variation (CVs) for cholesterol and —but some direct measurements of LDL-C and HDL-C do not meet National Cholesterol Education Program (NCEP) guidelines for analytical performance (see Table 23-10) on dyslipidemic samples. In contrast, physiological variations are much larger and contribute to the vast majority of overall variation in lipid and lipoprotein concentrations.[14] For this reason, a patient's usual lipid or lipoprotein concentration is not reliably established from a single measurement, and the NCEP Laboratory Standardization Panel has made several specific recommendations for reducing the effects of preanalytical factors and specimen-processing procedures on lipid and lipoprotein testing.

Advanced Testing for Risk of Cardiovascular Disease[2,11]

Despite the strong association of lipid concentrations with CHD risk, it has been long recognized that half of all myocardial infarctions occur among individuals with a normal lipid panel. Consequently, a wide variety of alternative or emerging biochemical markers and assays have been identified for possible use in better assessing cardiovascular risk. Some are based on lipids, such as LDL-P and HDL-P, which represent measurement of LDL and HDL particle number, respectively, and are performed by nuclear magnetic resonance (NMR). Some studies have shown that these tests may be superior to LDL-C and HDL-C as cardiovascular biomarkers, but findings are inconsistent. Other alternative tests are based on factors besides lipids that contribute to the development of atherosclerosis, such as plasma concentration of the amino acid homocysteine. At this time, no consensus has been reached on how most of these alternative tests are best utilized, but many studies now support the use of high-sensitivity C-reactive protein (hsCRP), a marker for inflammation, particularly for patients at intermediate risk of cardiovascular disease.

High-Sensitivity C-Reactive Protein

CRP was discovered in 1930 and was subsequently shown to be an acute-phase reactant. It is routinely monitored as an indication of infection and autoimmune disease (see Chapter 18).

Numerous epidemiological studies have demonstrated that increased serum CRP concentrations are positively associated with risk of future CHD events. These findings support the hypothesis that (1) inflammation, (2) atherothrombosis, (3) diabetes, and (4) hypertension are interrelated and share common pathogenic mechanisms.

Prospective epidemiological studies have shown that a single hsCRP measurement is a strong predictor of (1) myocardial infarction, (2) stroke, (3) peripheral vascular disease, and (4) sudden cardiac death, even in individuals with no history of heart disease. It has also been shown in prospective studies that hsCRP can be used to more accurately classify patients at intermediate risk of CHD. National guidelines for the measurement of hsCRP as a marker of CHD risk have been issued jointly by the American Heart Association and the Centers for Disease Control and Prevention (AHA/CDC). The Canadian Cardiovascular Society guidelines included hsCRP in the risk assessment of CHD and as a secondary target for treatment. An algorithm for the assessment of CHD risk that employs both hsCRP and LDL-C is shown in Figure 23-23.

Several pharmacological agents that have demonstrated cardioprotective ability, such as aspirin and statins, lower the risk of CHD that is associated with increased hsCRP concentration. In a large primary prevention trial, the reduction in risk of future myocardial infarction associated with assignment to aspirin was 56% among those with baseline hsCRP concentrations in the highest quartile and declined proportionately with hsCRP values in the lowest quartile. This suggests that aspirin may prevent ischemic events through anti-inflammatory and antiplatelet effects. All statin drugs have been shown to reduce hsCRP. Data from JUPITER, a randomized clinical trial of statin and placebo in individuals with high hsCRP but low LDL-C, show great benefit from statin therapy in terms of reducing cardiovascular events.

Methods have been developed to detect the low concentrations of hsCRP required for prediction of vascular risk. Of various techniques used to lower the limits of detection of CRP assays, the most successful approach has been to amplify the light-scattering properties of the antigen-antibody complex by covalently coupling latex particles to a specific antibody—a procedure that is easily automated on standard laboratory instrumentation. Many commercial hsCRP assays with low detection limits (<0.3 mg/L) are available, some with within-laboratory analytical imprecision of <10%.

Although it is an acute-phase reactant, hsCRP exhibits a relatively low degree of intraindividual variability in clinically stable patients. The AHA/CDC panel recommends two hsCRP measurements taken 2 or more weeks apart, with the average value used to estimate vascular risk. Furthermore, because hsCRP values are unaffected by food intake and exhibit almost no circadian variation, fasting specimens are not required.

Data from several large U.S. and European cohorts indicate that the distribution of circulating hsCRP concentrations appears comparable among men and women not using postmenopausal hormone replacement therapy (HRT), with the 50th percentile for both genders seen at about 1.5 mg/L. Concentrations of hsCRP are higher in women who use oral HRT than in women who do not. Reference values of <1, 1 to 3, and >3 mg/L, which correspond to approximate tertiles of the CRP distribution in healthy adults, are recommended by the AHA/CDC panel for classification of individuals into low, moderate, and high cardiovascular risk groups in primary prevention settings.

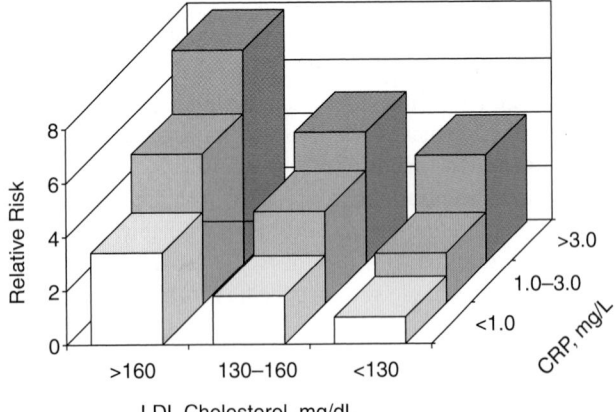

Figure 23-23 Algorithm for assessment of coronary heart disease (CHD) risk employing C-reactive protein (CRP) and low-density lipoprotein (LDL) cholesterol. *(From Rifai N, Ridker PM. Population distributions of C-reactive protein in apparently healthy men and women in the United States: implication for clinical interpretation. Clin Chem 2003;49:666-9.)*

Review Questions

1. Which of the following formulas shows the correct calculation for indirectly measuring LDL-C (Friedewald's formula)?
   a. LDL-C = HDL-C + (Triglyceride/5)
   b. LDL-C = Total cholesterol – (HDL-C) – (Triglyceride/5)
   c. LDL-C = Total cholesterol + HDL-C + (Triglyceride/5)
   d. LDL-C = HDL-C – (Triglyceride/5)

2. The protein component of a lipoprotein is referred to as a(n):
   a. terpene.
   b. apolipoprotein.
   c. prostaglandin.
   d. phospholipid.

3. The lipoprotein that contains a carbohydrate-rich protein covalently bound to apo B-100 and a special protein motif called the "kringle" domain is:
   a. LDL.
   b. HDL.
   c. chylomicron.
   d. lipoprotein(a).

4. What lipoprotein transports mostly cholesteryl esters through the blood?
   a. LDL
   b. VLDL
   c. Chylomicrons
   d. Lipoprotein(a)

5. The enzyme that is critical for hydrolysis of triglycerides on chylomicrons for their conversion to chylomicron remnants is:
   a. cholesterol oxidase.
   b. glycerol kinase
   c. lipoprotein lipase.
   d. HMG-CoA reductase.

6. The rate-limiting enzyme in cholesterol biosynthesis that is inhibited by statin drugs is:
   a. cholesterol oxidase.
   b. glycerol kinase
   c. lipoprotein lipase.
   d. HMG-CoA reductase.

7. Which of the following lipid metabolic pathways has a role in transferring hepatically derived lipids, particularly triglyceride, to peripheral cells for energy metabolism?
   a. Exogenous pathway
   b. Endogenous pathway
   c. Intracellular-cholesterol transport pathway
   d. Reverse-cholesterol transport pathway

8. The formation of mixed micelles containing unesterified cholesterol, fatty acids, monoglycerides, phospholipids, and bile acids is referred to as:
   a. emulsification.
   b. denaturation.
   c. esterification.
   d. saturation.

9. With regard to lipids, a carboxyl (−COOH) with a long sidechain (R) containing an even number of carbon atoms that is important in human nutrition and metabolism is a type of lipid referred to as a(n):
   a. acylglycerol.
   b. ester.
   c. fatty acid.
   d. terpene.

10. In the laboratory analysis of triglycerides, the initial step in all methods is:
    a. phosphorylation of glycerol catalyzed by glycerokinase.
    b. oxidation of cholesterol by cholesterol oxidase.
    c. hydrolysis of triglyceride by lipase.
    d. reduction of phenol and H_2O_2 by peroxidase.

References

1. Biggerstaff KD, Wooten JS. Understanding lipoproteins as transporters of cholesterol and other lipids. Adv Physiol Educ 2004;28:105–6.
2. Davidson MH, Ballantyne CM, Jacobson TA, Bittner VA, Braun LT, Brown AS, et al. Clinical utility of inflammatory markers and advanced lipoprotein testing: advice from an expert panel of lipid specialists. J Clin Lipidol 2011;5:338–67.
3. Demacker PN. Laboratory-based assessment of plasma lipids and lipoproteins for the classification of familial hypercholesterolemic and hypertriglyceridemic states. Semin Vasc Med 2004;4:13–22.
4. Expert Panel on Integrated Guidelines for Cardiovascular Health and Risk Reduction in Children and Adolescents: summary report. Pediatrics 2011;128:S1–S44
5. Havel RJ, Kane JP. Introduction: structure and metabolism of plasma lipoproteins. In: Scriver CR, Beaudet AL, Sly WS, Valle D, eds. The metabolic and molecular bases of inherited diseases, 8th edition. New York: McGraw-Hill, 2001:2705–16.
6. Huxley R, Lewington S, Clarke R. Cholesterol, coronary heart disease and stroke: a review of published evidence from observational studies and randomized controlled trials. Semin Vasc Med 2002;2:315–23.
7. Mahley RW, Innerarity TL, Rall SC Jr, Weisgraber KH. Plasma lipoproteins: apolipoprotein structure and function. J Lipid Res 1984;25:1277–94.
8. Marcovina SM, Koschinsky ML, Albers JJ, Skarlatos S. Report of the National Heart, Lung, and Blood Institute Workshop on Lipoprotein(a) and Cardiovascular Disease: recent advances and future directions. Clin Chem 2003;49:1785–96.
9. National Cholesterol Education Program (NCEP) Expert Panel on Detection, Evaluation, and Treatment of High Blood Cholesterol in Adults (Adult Treatment Panel III). Third report of the National Cholesterol Education Program (NCEP) Expert Panel on Detection, Evaluation, and Treatment of High Blood Cholesterol in Adults (Adult Treatment Panel III): final report. Circulation 2002;106:3143–421.
10. Recommendations on lipoprotein measurement: from the Working Group on Lipoprotein Measurement. Bethesda, MD: National Cholesterol Education Program, NIH/NHLBI NIH Publication, 1995:95–3044.
11. Ridker P, Rifai N, eds. C-reactive protein and cardiovascular disease. St Laurent, Canada: MediEdition, 2006.
12. Rifai N, Dominiczak M, Warnick GR, eds. Handbook of lipoprotein testing, 2nd edition. Washington, DC: AACC Press, 2000.
13. Toth PP. Drug treatment of hyperlipidaemia: a guide to the rational use of lipid-lowering drugs. Drugs 2010;70:1363–79.
14. Vesper HW, Wilson PW, Rifai N. A message from the laboratory community to the National Cholesterol Education Program Adult Treatment Panel IV. Clin Chem 2012;58:523–7.

CHAPTER

24   Electrolytes and Blood Gases

Mitchell G. Scott, Ph.D., Vicky A. LeGrys, Ph.D., Dr.A., M.T.(A.S.C.P.), C.L.S.(N.C.A.), and Emily I. Schindler, M.D., Ph.D.

Objectives

1. Define the following terms:

Anion	Oxygen dissociation curve
Blood gas	Oxygen saturation
Cation	P_{50}
Colligative property	pH
Ion-selective electrode	Partial pressure
Electrolyte	Pulse oximetry/
Electrolyte exclusion effect	Co-oximetry
FO_2Hb	SO_2
Osmolality	Sweat chloride test

2. For each of the following electrolytes, state and describe the biochemistry, physiological functions, localization, clinical significance, method of laboratory analysis and possible analytical interferences:

Bicarbonate	Potassium
Chloride	Sodium

3. Compare direct and indirect ion-selective electrode testing, including uses of and interferences in each method.

4. Discuss the measurement of sweat chloride, including reasons for performing, details of the three phases of testing, critical issues in each phase, and specimen requirements.

5. Describe the following methods of electrolyte/blood gas determination, including specific electrolyte(s) assessed with each, the principle of the method, specimen requirements, and possible interferences:

Coulometry-amperometry	Sweat testing
Osmometry	Tonometry
Potentiometry	

6. List and describe the four colligative properties of a solution, including the relationship of each property to the addition of solute; state and calculate the formula for urine and plasma osmolality determination.

7. State the formula that demonstrates the relationship between total concentration of CO_2, bicarbonate, and hydrogen ion concentration.

8. State the Henderson-Hasselbalch equation and explain each of its components; characterize its application in blood gas measurements.

9. List the three essential properties of arterial blood required for adequate oxygen delivery to tissues; state the normal arterio-venous difference interval in PO_2.

10. State and explain the three approaches to determining oxygen saturation; state and calculate the formula for determining hemoglobin oxygen saturation given the concentrations of oxyhemoglobin and deoxyhemoglobin.

11. List and describe three causes of decreased arterial FO_2Hb; list and describe one cause of decreased PO_2.

12. For blood gas determinations, describe each of the following:

Specimen requirements	Collection technique
Preferred anticoagulant	Specimen transport

13. List the analytical problems that arise in the analysis of pH, PO_2, and PCO_2 with inappropriate specimen collection or transport techniques

14. Diagram a generic blood gas analyzer; state and describe the methods or calculations used to measure pH, PO_2, and PCO_2, including noninvasive and continuous monitoring methods; describe two types of controls used for blood gas analysis.

15. Assess and solve case studies involving electrolyte and blood gas analysis.

Key Words and Definitions

Anemic hypoxia Hypoxia (a reduced supply of oxygen to the tissues) resulting from a decrease in amount of hemoglobin or number of erythrocytes in the blood.

Blood gases PCO_2 and PO_2 (partial pressures of carbon dioxide and oxygen), usually in whole blood.

Colligative properties Properties of solutions that depend on the number of particles in the solution; examples include (1) osmotic pressure, (2) boiling point elevation, (3) freezing point depression, and (4) vapor pressure lowering.

Key Words and Definitions—cont'd

Cystic fibrosis (CF) Inherited disorder of a transmembrane conductance regulator protein (CFTR) that leads to chronic pancreatic and obstructive pulmonary disease.

Cystic fibrosis transmembrane conductance regulator (CFTR) A transmembrane protein produced by the *CFTR* gene.

Electrolytes Charged low-molecular-mass molecules present in plasma and cytosol, usually ions of (1) sodium, (2) potassium, (3) calcium, (4) magnesium, (5) chloride, (6) bicarbonate, (7) phosphate, (8) sulfate, and (9) lactate.

Electrolyte exclusion effect Electrolytes are excluded from the fraction of total plasma volume that is occupied by solids, which leads to underestimation of electrolyte concentration by some methods.

Hemoglobin (Hb) An oxygen-carrying, heme-containing protein abundant in red blood cells.

Henderson-Hasselbalch equation Equation that defines the relationship between pH, bicarbonate, and the partial pressure of dissolved carbon dioxide gas:

$$pH = pK' + \log \frac{cHCO_3^-}{(\alpha + PCO_3)}$$

Ion-selective electrode (ISE) A type of special-purpose, potentiometric electrode consisting of a membrane selectively permeable to a single ionic species. The potential produced at the membrane–sample solution interface is proportional to the logarithm of the ionic activity or concentration.

Osmolal gap A difference between the observed and calculated osmolalities in serum analysis. The calculated osmolar values include sodium concentration multiplied by 1.86, plus glucose and blood urea nitrogen, plus 9.

Osmometry Technique for measuring the concentration of dissolved solute particles in a solution.

Osmotic pressure The pressure required to stop osmosis through a semipermeable membrane between a solution and pure solvent.

Oximetry A technique used to determine the oxygen saturation of arterial blood.

Oxygen dissociation curve The sigmoidal curve obtained when SO_2 of blood is plotted against PO_2.

Oxygen saturation (SO_2) The fraction (percentage) of functional hemoglobin that is saturated with oxygen.

Oxyhemoglobin An hemoglobin that contains bound O_2.

P_{50} PO_2 for a given blood sample at which the hemoglobin of the blood is half saturated with O_2; P_{50} reflects the affinity of hemoglobin for O_2.

Partial pressure The substance (mole) fraction of gas times the total pressure; i.e., the partial pressure of oxygen, PO_2, is the fraction of oxygen gas times the barometric pressure.

pH The negative logarithm of hydrogen ion activity.

Pilocarpine iontophoresis Noninvasive method that uses electricity to force the drug pilocarpine into the skin for the purpose of inducing sweating at the site.

Point-of-care testing (POCT) Clinical testing that occurs next to the patient, usually with a handheld device and an unprocessed specimen collected immediately before testing.

Sweat chloride The concentration of chloride in sweat; increased sweat chloride is characteristic of cystic fibrosis.

Water homeostasis The body process that maintains a balance of water intake and output.

Maintenance of **water homeostasis** is paramount to life for all organisms. In humans, the maintenance of water homeostasis is primarily a function of the four major **electrolytes**: Na⁺, K⁺, Cl⁻, and HCO₃⁻. These electrolytes also have a role in acid-base balance and muscle function, as well as serving as cofactors for enzymes. Abnormal electrolyte concentrations may be the cause or the consequence of a variety of medical disorders. Because of their physiological and clinical interrelationships, this chapter discusses determination of (1) **electrolytes**, (2) **osmolality**, (3) sweat testing, (4) **blood gases** and **pH**, and (5) blood oxygenation.

Electrolytes

Electrolytes may be classified as anions, negatively charged ions that move toward an anode, or cations, positively charged ions that move toward a cathode. Important physiological electrolytes include Na⁺, K⁺, Ca²⁺, Mg²⁺, Cl⁻, HCO₃⁻, H₂PO₄⁻, and HPO₄²⁻. The major electrolytes (Na⁺, K⁺, Cl⁻, HCO₃⁻) occur primarily as free ions, whereas significant amounts (>40%) of Ca²⁺, Mg²⁺, and trace elements are bound by proteins, mainly albumin. Determination of body fluid concentrations of the four major electrolytes (Na⁺, K⁺, Cl⁻, and HCO₃⁻) is commonly referred to as an "electrolyte profile."

Specimens for Electrolyte Determination

Serum and plasma are the specimens typically analyzed for their electrolyte content. Capillary blood is another sample commonly analyzed. Heparinized whole blood arterial or venous specimens obtained for blood gas and pH determinations may also be used with direct **ion-selective electrodes (ISEs)**. Differences in values between serum and plasma and between arterial and venous samples have been documented, but only the difference between serum and plasma K⁺ is considered clinically significant. Heparin, either the lithium or ammonium salt, is required if plasma or whole blood is assayed. Use of plasma or whole blood provides the advantage of shortening turnaround time because it is not necessary to wait for the blood to clot. Furthermore, plasma or whole blood provides a distinct advantage in determining K⁺ concentrations, which are invariably higher in serum depending on platelet count.[13] Grossly lipemic blood can be a source of analytical error (see "Electrolyte Exclusion Effect," later in this chapter), with some methods requiring ultracentrifugation of lipemic serum or plasma before analysis. Hemolysis of red blood cells will cause erroneously high K^+ results. In addition, unhemolyzed specimens that are not promptly processed may have increased K^+ concentrations because of K^+ leakage from red blood cells when whole blood is stored at 4 °C.

Collection of urine specimens for Na^+, K^+, or Cl^- assays should be done without the addition of preservatives. Other types of specimens used for electrolyte assays include (1) body fluid aspirates, (2) feces, (3) gastrointestinal fluid, and (4) sweat samples.

Sodium

Sodium is the major cation of extracellular fluid. Because it represents approximately 90% of the ≈154 mmol of inorganic cations per liter of plasma, Na^+ is responsible for almost one-half the osmotic strength of plasma. The daily diet of the adult male in the United States contains 3 to 6 g (90 to 250 mmol) of Na^+ (7 to 14 g of NaCl), which is nearly completely absorbed from the GI tract.[3] The body requires only 1 to 2 mmol/d, and the excess is excreted by the kidneys, which are the ultimate regulators of the amount of Na^+ (and thus water) in the body. The processes by which the kidneys regulate sodium balance are discussed in detail in Chapter 35.

Specimens

For sodium analysis, (1) serum, (2) plasma, and (3) urine specimens may be stored at 4 °C or may be frozen. Erythrocytes contain only one-tenth of the Na^+ present in plasma, so hemolysis does not cause significant errors in serum or plasma Na^+ values. Lipemic samples should be ultracentrifuged and the infranatant analyzed unless a direct ISE is used (see "Electrolyte Exclusion Effect").

Determination of Sodium in Body Fluids

Sodium may be determined (1) by atomic absorption spectrophotometry (AAS), (2) electrochemically with an Na^+-ISE, or (3) spectrophotometrically. Today, ISE methods are by far the most common. Because sodium and potassium are routinely assayed together, methods for their analysis are described together later in this chapter.

Reference Intervals

A typical reference interval for serum Na^+ is 136 to 145 mmol/L. The interval for premature newborns at 48 hours is 128 to 148 mmol/L, and the value for umbilical cord blood from full-term newborns is ≈127 mmol/L. Urinary sodium excretion varies with dietary intake, but for an adult male on an average diet containing 7 to 14 g of NaCl per day, an interval of 120 to 240 mmol/d is typical. A large diurnal variation in Na^+ excretion has been noted, with the rate of Na^+ excretion during the night being only 20% of the peak rate during the day.

Potassium

Potassium is the major intracellular cation. In tissue cells, its average concentration is 150 mmol/L, and in erythrocytes, the concentration is 105 mmol/L. High intracellular concentrations are maintained by the Na^+, K^+ adenosine triphosphate (ATP)ase pump, which is fueled by oxidative energy and continually transports K^+ into the cell against a concentration gradient. Diffusion of K^+ out of the cell into the extracellular fluid (ECF) and plasma occurs whenever pump activity is decreased.[10] The importance of these considerations for sample integrity in analysis of K^+ is discussed later. The body requirement for K^+ is satisfied by an average dietary intake of 2.4 to 4.4 g/d (60 to 120 mmol/d). Potassium absorbed from the gastrointestinal tract is rapidly distributed, and a small amount is taken up by cells, with most excreted by the kidneys.

Specimens

Comments made earlier on specimens for Na^+ analysis are generally applicable to those for K^+ analysis. However, potassium concentrations in plasma and whole blood are 0.1 to 0.7 mmol/L lower than those in serum, and most reference intervals for serum K^+ are 0.2 to 0.5 mmol/L higher than those for plasma K^+. The extent of this difference depends on the platelet count, because additional K^+ in serum is primarily a result of platelet rupture during coagulation.[13] This variability in the amount of additional K^+ in serum makes plasma the specimen of choice and emphasizes the necessity of noting on reports whether serum or plasma was assayed and using the appropriate reference interval.

Specimens for determining K^+ concentrations in serum or plasma must be collected by methods that minimize hemolysis because release of K^+ from as few as 0.5% of erythrocytes will increase K^+ values by 0.5 mmol/L. An increase in K^+ of 0.6% has been estimated for every 10 mg/dL of plasma **hemoglobin (Hb)** caused by hemolysis.[3] Therefore it is imperative that any visible hemolysis be noted with reported K^+ values with a comment that results are falsely elevated. Whenever hemolysis is suspected, a portion of the specimen should be centrifuged and visually inspected.

Preanalytical errors that are clinically significant have been observed for K^+ determinations when blood samples are not processed in a timely manner expediently. If a whole blood specimen is maintained at 4 °C versus 25 °C before separation, glycolysis is inhibited, and the energy-dependent Na^+, K^+-ATPase will not maintain the Na^+/K^+ gradient. An increase in plasma K^+ will occur as a result of K^+ leakage from erythrocytes and other cells.

The opposite effect, namely, a falsely decreased K^+ value, has been observed when an unseparated sample is stored at 37 °C because glycolysis occurs and K^+ shifts intracellularly. Even at room temperature, leukocytosis will initially cause falsely decreased K^+ concentrations. For reliable K^+ determinations, it is recommended to (1) collect blood with heparin, (2) maintain it near 25 °C, and (3) separate the plasma within minutes by high-speed centrifugation without cooling. In practical terms, separation within 1 hour when samples are maintained at room temperature is unlikely to introduce great error.

Finally, skeletal muscle activity causes K^+ ions to move from muscle cells into plasma that results in a marked elevation in plasma K^+ values, such as when an upper arm tourniquet is not released before the beginning of blood draw after a patient clenches his fist repeatedly.[8]

Reference Intervals

Reported reference intervals for serum vary from 3.5 to 5.1 mmol/L for adults and from 3.7 to 5.9 for newborns. For plasma, a frequently cited interval is 3.4 to 4.8 mmol/L for adults. Cerebrospinal fluid concentrations are ≈70% those of plasma. Urinary excretion of K^+ varies with dietary intake, but a typical interval observed in an average diet is 40 to 90 mmol/d. Fecal excretion has been reported as 18.2 ± 2.5 mmol/d, but in severe diarrhea, gastrointestinal loss may be as much as 60 mmol/d.

Methods for the Determination of Sodium and Potassium

Ion-selective electrodes and spectrophotometric assays are the techniques of choice to measure sodium and potassium.

Ion-Selective Electrodes

Analyzers connected to ISEs usually contain Na^+ electrodes with glass membranes and K^+ electrodes with liquid ion exchange membranes that incorporate valinomycin. These are potentiometric devices (see Chapter 10) that determine the change in electromotive force (E, potential) in a circuit between a measurement electrode (the ISE) and a reference electrode, as the selected ion interacts with the membrane of the ISE. Operationally, the measuring system is calibrated by the introduction of calibrator solutions containing defined amounts of Na^+ and K^+. The potentials of the calibrators are determined, and the $\Delta E/\Delta$ log concentration responses are stored in microprocessor memory as a comparison for calculating unknown concentration when E of the unknown is measured. Frequent calibration, initiated by the user or by microprocessor-controlled uptake of sample from a reservoir of the calibrator, is typical of most current ISE systems. Some instruments, particularly **point-of-care testing (POCT)** devices and many blood gas analyzers, are designed to measure Na^+ and K^+ in whole blood.

Both indirect and direct methods are used with ISE electrodes. With indirect ISE methods, the sample is introduced into the measurement chamber after mixing with a large volume of diluent. Indirect ISE methods are used most commonly on today's automated, high-throughput clinical chemistry systems. With direct ISE methods, the sample is presented to the electrodes without dilution. This approach became possible with the miniaturization of electrodes. Direct ISEs are most common in blood gas analyzers and point-of-care devices in which whole blood is directly presented to the electrodes.

Errors observed in the use of ISEs are due to (1) lack of selectivity, (2) repeated protein coating of the ion-sensitive membranes, or (3) contamination of the membrane or salt bridge by ions that compete or react with the selected ion and thus alter the electrode response.

Spectrophotometric Methods

Spectrophotometric methods fall into two categories: (1) those based on enzyme activation, and (2) those that detect the spectral shift produced when Na^+ or K^+ binds to a macrocyclic chromophore. The high cost of reagents for these methods and the fact that few problems are associated with ISE methods have resulted in small "niche" use of these methods, primarily with smaller instruments used in physicians' offices or clinics.

Electrolyte Exclusion Effect[1]

The electrolyte exclusion effect describes the exclusion of electrolytes from the fraction of the total plasma volume that is occupied by solids. The volume of total solids (primarily protein and lipid) in an aliquot of plasma is approximately 7%, so that ≈93% of plasma volume is actually water. The main electrolytes (Na^+, K^+, Cl^-, and HCO_3^-) are confined to the water phase. When a fixed volume of total plasma (e.g., 10 μL) is pipetted for dilution before indirect ISE analysis, only 9.3 μL of plasma water that contains the electrolytes is added to the diluent. Thus a concentration of Na^+ determined by indirect ISE to be 140 mmol/L is the concentration in the total plasma volume, *not* in the plasma water volume. In fact, if the plasma contains 93% water, the concentration of Na^+ in plasma water is [140 × (100/93)], or 150 mmol/L. This negative "error" in plasma electrolyte analysis has been recognized for many years. Even though it is the electrolyte concentration in plasma water that is physiological (the Na^+ concentration of normal saline is indeed 150 mmol/L), it was assumed that the volume fraction of water in plasma is sufficiently constant that this difference could be ignored. In fact, all electrolyte reference intervals are based on this assumption and actually reflect concentrations in total plasma volume, not in water volume. Indeed, virtually all concentrations measured in the clinical chemistry laboratory are related to the total sample volume rather than to the water volume. This electrolyte exclusion effect becomes problematic when pathophysiological conditions are present that alter the plasma water volume, such as hyperlipidemia or hyperproteinemia. In these settings, falsely low electrolyte values are obtained whenever samples are diluted before analysis, as with an indirect ISE method (Figure 24-1).[1]

It is the dilution of total plasma volume and the assumption that plasma water volume is constant that render the indirect ISE the method subject to the electrolyte exclusion effect. Direct ISE methods still determine the concentration relative to activity but do not require sample dilution. Because no dilution occurs, activity is directly proportional to the concentration in the water phase, not the concentration in the total volume. To ensure that results from direct ISEs are equivalent to those from indirect ISEs, most direct ISE methods actually operate in what is commonly referred to as the "flame mode."* In this mode, the directly measured concentration in plasma water is multiplied by the average water volume fraction of plasma (0.93). Although the latter may vary widely, as long as the activity of the specific ion is constant, the concentration of the ion in the water phase

---

*In the "flame mode", results were obtained with the traditional technique of flame photometry. Results for these analytes were expressed in terms of substance concentration. In current practice, the technique of flame photometry is no longer used in clinical laboratories.

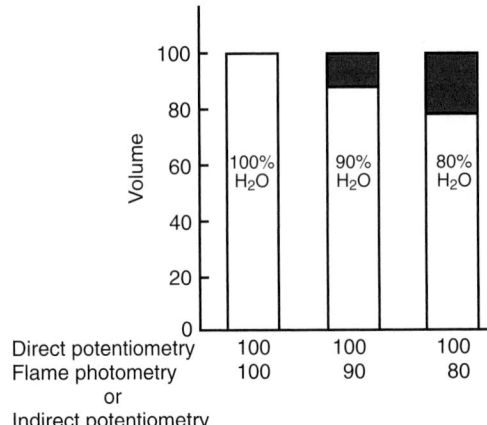

Figure 24-1 Predicted influence of water content on sodium measurements for a 100 mmol/L NaCl solution by direct ion-selective electrode (ISE) versus flame emission photometry or indirect ISE. *Red areas* represent nonaqueous volumes, which could consist of lipids, proteins, or even a slurry of latex or sand particles. *(Adapted from Apple FS, Koch DD, Graves S, Ladenson JH. Relationship between direct-potentiometric and flame-photometric measurement of sodium in blood. Clin Chem 1982;28:1931-5.)*

TABLE 24-1	Methods Measuring Concentration in the Whole Sample Volume and Thus Subject to Electrolyte Exclusion Effect
Method	**Analytes**
Atomic absorption spectrometry	Ca^{2+}, Mg^{2+}, and others
Amperometry/coulometry	Cl^-
Indirect potentiometry	Na^+, K^+, Ca^{2+}, Cl^-

TABLE 24-2	Methods Measuring Activity, Molality, or Concentration in the Water Phase and Thus Not Subject to Electrolyte Exclusion Effect
Method	**Analytes**
ISEs with *undiluted* sample	H^+ (pH), Na^+, K^+, Ca^{2+}, Cl^-, Li^+
Gas electrodes	CO_2 (PCO_2), O_2 (PO_2)
	HCO_3^- (calculated from pH and PCO_2)
Freezing point depression	H_2O (osmolality)

ISE, Ion-selective electrode.

becomes independent of the relative proportions of water and total solids if the ion is not bound by proteins. Therefore direct ISE methods are free of electrolyte exclusion effects.

Most clinical chemists and physicians have reached the conclusion that direct ISE methods for electrolyte analysis are the methods of choice. However, it is clear that results from direct methods will continue to be converted to total plasma volume concentrations by use of the "flame mode," and indeed this is the recommendation of the Clinical Laboratory and Standard Institute (CLSI). Table 24-1 and Table 24-2 summarize methods that are and are not subject to electrolyte exclusion effects, respectively.

Chloride

Chloride is the major extracellular anion; like Na^+, it is significantly involved in the maintenance of (1) water distribution, (2) osmotic pressure, and (3) anion-cation balance in the ECF. In contrast to its high ECF concentrations ($\approx$103 mmol/L), the concentration of Cl^- in the intracellular fluid of erythrocytes is 45 to 54 mmol/L, and only 1 mmol/L in the intracellular fluid in most other tissue cells. Chloride ions are almost completely absorbed from the intestinal tract and excreted by the kidneys.

Specimens

Chloride most often is measured in (1) serum. (2) plasma, (3) urine, or (4) sweat. Even gross hemolysis does not significantly alter serum or plasma Cl^- concentration because the erythrocyte concentration of Cl^- is approximately half that of plasma. Because very little Cl^- is protein bound, change in posture or stasis, or the use of tourniquets, has little effect on its plasma concentration.

Methods for Determination of Chloride in Body Fluids

Historically, chloride was measured in body fluids and solids by mercurimetric titration and spectrophotometric methods.

As these methods are no longer used, coulometric-amperometric titration and ISEs are now the methods of choice

Coulometric-Amperometric Titration

Reactions in coulometric-amperometric determinations of Cl^- depend on the generation of Ag^+ from a silver electrode at a constant rate and on the reaction of $Ag+$ with Cl^- in the sample to form insoluble silver chloride (AgCl):

$$Ag^+ + Cl^- \rightarrow AgCl$$

After the stoichiometric point is reached, excess Ag^+ in the mixture triggers shutdown of the Ag^+ generation system. A timing device records elapsed time between the start and stop of Ag^+ generation. Because the time interval is proportional to the amount of Cl^- in the sample, the concentration of Cl^- is then calculated. Applications of the coulometric-amperometric principle (often called the Cotlove chloridometer technique) are the most precise methods for measuring Cl^- over the entire range of concentrations found in body fluids.

Ion-Selective Electrode Methods

Solvent polymeric membranes that incorporate quaternary ammonium salt anion exchangers, such as tri-*n*-octylpropylammonium chloride decanol, are used to construct Cl^--selective electrodes in clinical analyzers. Although they are by far the most common methods of measuring Cl^- in clinical laboratories, these electrodes often suffer from membrane instability and lot-to-lot inconsistency in terms of selectivity for other anions. Anions that tend to be problematic include other halides and organic anions, such as SCN^-, which are particularly problematic because of their ability to solubilize in the polymeric organic membrane of these electrodes.

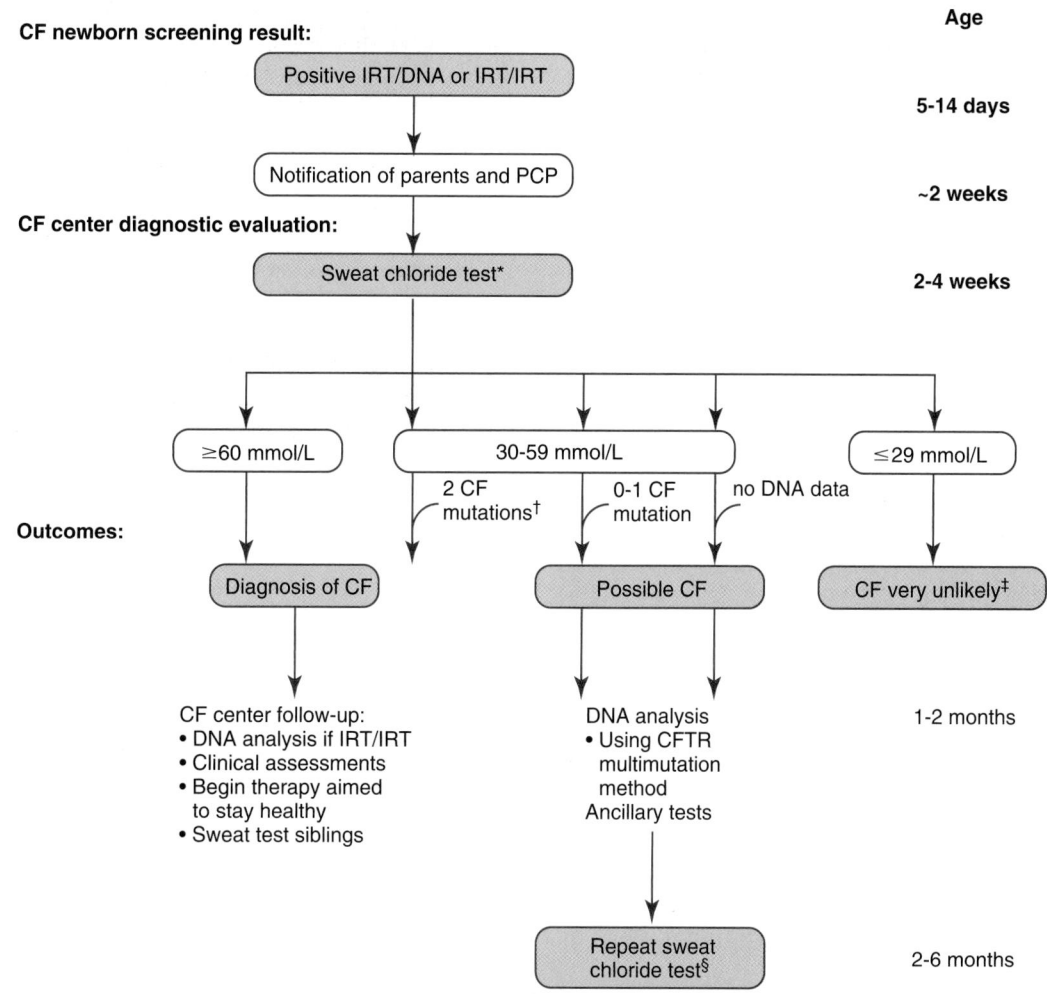

CF newborn screening result:

Positive IRT/DNA or IRT/IRT — 5-14 days

Notification of parents and PCP — ~2 weeks

CF center diagnostic evaluation:

Sweat chloride test* — 2-4 weeks

≥60 mmol/L   30-59 mmol/L   ≤29 mmol/L

2 CF mutations†   0-1 CF mutation   no DNA data

Outcomes:

Diagnosis of CF   Possible CF   CF very unlikely‡

CF center follow-up:
• DNA analysis if IRT/IRT
• Clinical assessments
• Begin therapy aimed to stay healthy
• Sweat test siblings

DNA analysis
• Using CFTR multimutation method
Ancillary tests

1-2 months

Repeat sweat chloride test§ — 2-6 months

*If the baby is at least 2 kg and more than 36 weeks gestation at birth, perform bilateral sweat sampling/analysis with either Gibson-Cooke or Macroduct® method; repeat as soon as possible if sweat quantity is less than 75 mg or 15 μl, respectively.

†CF mutation refers to a CFTR mutant allele known to cause CF disease.

‡The disease is very unlikely; however, if there are 2 CF mutations in trans, CF may be diagnosed.

§After a repeat sweat test, further evaluation depends on the results as implied above.

Figure 24-2 Diagnostic algorithm for cystic fibrosis (CF) after newborn screening. *(From Farrell PM, Rosenstein BJ, White TB, et al; Cystic Fibrosis Foundation. Guidelines for diagnosis of cystic fibrosis in newborns through older adults: Cystic Fibrosis Foundation consensus report. J Pediatr 2008;153:S4-S14.)*

Reference Intervals

Reported reference intervals for Cl⁻ in serum or plasma vary from 98 to 107 mmol/L to 100 to 108 mmol/L. Serum values vary little during the day. Spinal fluid Cl⁻ concentrations are ≈15% higher than those in serum. Urinary excretion of Cl⁻ varies with dietary intake, but an interval of 110 to 250 mmol/d is typical.

Measurement of Sweat Chloride (Sweat Testing)

Analysis of sweat for increased chloride concentration is used to confirm the diagnosis of **cystic fibrosis (CF)**. CF is the most common lethal genetic disorder of the Caucasian population, with a wide spectrum of clinical presentations, including chronic obstructive pulmonary disease and pancreatic insufficiency. CF is caused by a defect in the **cystic fibrosis transmembrane conductance regulator protein (CFTR)**, a protein that normally regulates electrolyte transport across epithelial membranes. More than 1500 mutations of CFTR have been identified. Although direct mutational analysis is available, it is not informative in all cases, and a quantitative **sweat chloride** test remains the standard for diagnostic testing. In an effort to standardize testing, the CLSI developed the guidelines document C34-A3.[5]

Sweat testing is often performed in conjunction with newborn screening programs (Figure 24-2). Newborn screening for CF occurs throughout the United States and the world.

Most newborn screening protocols begin with an immunore-active trypsinogen assay (IRT) from a dried blood spot and are followed by a second IRT or DNA testing.[7] Infants with a positive newborn screening test are referred for a quantitative sweat chloride test, which has resulted in an increase in the number of sweat tests performed on individuals younger than 2 months of age.

The sweat test is performed in three phases: (1) sweat stimulation by **pilocarpine iontophoresis**, (2) collection of the sweat, and (3) qualitative or quantitative analysis of sweat chloride, sodium, or conductivity.

Sweat Stimulation and Collection

Because of transient increases in sweat electrolytes shortly after birth, individuals should be at least 48 hours old before a sweat chloride test is performed. The child should be (1) physiologically and nutritionally stable, (2) thoroughly hydrated, and (3) free of acute illness. The skin should be free of cuts, rashes, and inflammation to avoid contamination of the sweat sample with serous fluid. For example, sweat testing never should be performed over an area of eczema.

Stimulation. To stimulate sweat, localized sweating is produced by pilocarpine iontophoresis into an area of the skin. Iontophoresis uses a small electrical current to deliver pilocarpine into the sweat glands from the positive electrode, while an electrolyte solution at the negative electrode completes the circuit. *Note:* Although the Occupational Safety and Health Administration (OSHA) does not list sweat as potentially infectious, laboratory personnel should practice the same universal precautions they would use with any other body fluid.

Collection. After iontophoresis, sweat is collected onto (1) preweighed gauze pads, (2) filter paper, (3) Macroduct coils,[11] or (4) Nanoduct conductivity sensor cells using techniques to minimize evaporation and contamination. If sweat is collected onto gauze or filter paper, the electrodes usually are made of copper and are slightly smaller than the stimulation and collection area. The composition of the electrolyte solution should be selected to avoid contamination with the sweat sample. Before collection is performed, the gauze or filter paper used for sweat collection should be placed into a weighing vial with a secure sealing lid, and the vial labeled and weighed with an analytical balance. For a detailed procedure for stimulation and collection, the reader should refer to the CLSI document C34-A3.[5]

Alternatively for sweat stimulation, the electrodes and the current source are integrated, as they are in the Wescor Macroduct and Nanoduct systems (http://www.wescor.com/; accessed September 30, 2015), which use gel reagents containing pilocarpine. In the Macroduct system, sweat is collected in a disposable microbore-tubing coil collector.[11] After sufficient sweat has been collected, the sweat is transferred from the coil into a sealable microsample cup. The Nanoduct system employs an integrated conductivity cell sensor in the single-use collection device.

Critical Issues Associated With Sweat Stimulation and Collection. During collection, the analyst must (1) avoid evaporation and contamination of the sample, (2) collect a sufficient amount of sample, and (3) minimize skin reactions. Determination of and adherence to a minimum sweat weight or volume are critical to obtain valid sweat testing results. The requirement for a minimum amount ensures an appropriate sweat rate and sweat electrolyte concentration and is independent of the instrument used to measure sweat electrolytes. Unfortunately, many laboratorians misunderstand the necessity of collecting the correct volume, leading to false-positive and false-negative sweat tests, which have significant implications for patient care.

Sweat electrolyte concentration is related to sweat rate. At low sweat rates, sweat electrolyte concentration decreases and the opportunity for sample evaporation increases. To ensure a valid result, the average sweat rate should exceed $1 \text{ g/m}^2/\text{min}$. To standardize and simplify the collection process, the size of the (1) electrodes, (2) reagent pads, and (3) collection material must be approximately the same. Insufficient samples must not be pooled for analysis.

When the acceptable rate is applied to the parameters described in the CLSI document, the minimum acceptable sample for analysis from a single site with use of 2 × 2-inch gauze or filter paper for stimulation and collection is 75 mg of sweat collected within 30 minutes. When the collection process deviates from standard parameters, the minimum acceptable sweat volume or weight changes, and sweat should be collected for only 30 minutes. If the collection time exceeds 30 minutes, the requirement for the amount of sweat needed to ensure adequate stimulation must increase. Extending the collection time allows additional opportunity for sweat evaporation and, practically, does not significantly increase the sweat yield.

Acquiring the minimum sample should not be a problem with most patients if the the CLSI[5] and the manufacturer's recommendations are followed. On average, the percentage of insufficient samples should not exceed 5% for patients older than 3 months of age and 10% for patients 3 months of age or younger.[5,12] If the laboratory collects sweat from two sites (bilateral testing), the test is considered QNS (quantity not sufficient) only when both sites are inadequate. Insufficient sweat samples result from several factors, such as (1) age, (2) race, (3) skin condition, and (4) hydration status. Also, collecting an adequate amount of sweat is more challenging in patients younger than 1 month of age.[12] For this reason, it is recommended that sweat testing in asymptomatic individuals be performed when the infant (1) is at least 2 weeks of age, (2) was more than 36 weeks' gestation at birth, and (3) weighs more than 2 kg.[5,12] If an adequate sweat sample is not obtained, the test should be repeated as soon as is practical.

Burns to the patient's skin after iontophoresis are extremely rare but have occurred at either electrode. If the burn occurs at the site of pilocarpine stimulation, sweat should not be collected.

Qualitative Tests

A qualitative sweat test represents a screening test for CF. Individuals who have positive or borderline results should then undergo quantitative sweat chloride testing. Examples of screening tests include Wescor Sweat-Chek and Nanoduct for conductivity. Screening tests may or may not measure the amount of sweat collected and may report a result as positive, negative, or borderline or give an actual concentration of sweat analytes. Although a variety of systems are used for sweat testing, problems have been documented for several methods, making them inappropriate for clinical use. For example, older conductivity analyzers using unheated collection cups and direct application chloride electrodes are not recommended as diagnostic procedures because problems have been reported with (1) sample evaporation, (2) condensation, and (3) the ability to quantify sweat samples adequately.

The Cystic Fibrosis Foundation has approved the Wescor Macroduct Sweat-Chek for screening at clinical sites, such as community hospitals, using the criterion that an individual who has a sweat conductivity of 50 mmol/L or greater should be referred to an accredited CF care center for a quantitative sweat chloride test. Note that sweat conductivity methods produce values that are approximately 15 mmol/L higher than those associated with sweat chloride concentration. Because of this difference, laboratories should not report conductivity results as if they were chloride results. In addition to conductivity results (in mmol/L), the report should include sweat conductivity reference intervals.

Quantitative Tests

The diagnosis of CF includes a quantitative measurement of sweat chloride, which consists of (1) collection of sweat into gauze, filter paper, or Macroduct coils; (2) evaluation of the amount collected in weight (milligrams) or volume (microliters); and (3) subsequent measurement of the sweat chloride concentration.[9] In general, chloride concentration is determined by coulometric titration with a chloridometer. If a laboratory chooses to quantify sweat chloride with an automated analyzer that employs an ISE, these methods must be validated systematically for accuracy, precision, and lower limit of detection. For any given method, the lower limit of the analytical measurement range for sweat chloride on unadulterated sweat should be less than or equal to 10 mmol/L.

Reference Intervals for Sweat Chloride

Reference intervals for sweat chloride must be stratified by patient age.[9]

Infants

For infants 6 months of age or younger, the following reference intervals are recommended.[9]

≤29 mmol/L: CF unlikely
30 to 59 mmol/L: intermediate
≥60 mmol/L: indicative of CF

However, as data continue to be generated from newborn screening programs, these reference intervals may have to be adjusted.

Beyond Infancy

For individuals older than 6 months, the following reference intervals are recommended[9]:

≤39 mmol/L: CF unlikely
40 to 59 mmol/L: intermediate chance of CF
≥60 mmol/L: indicative of CF

A healthy sweat chloride concentration alone is insufficient to rule out the diagnosis; it should be interpreted in light of the clinical picture and with the knowledge that "normal" concentrations have been associated with CF. Several mutations of the CF gene are associated with intermediate or normal sweat chloride concentrations.

Quality Assurance

Laboratories that provide high-quality sweat testing should (1) select appropriate methods, (2) have sufficient testing volumes to ensure familiarity with the test, and (3) limit testing personnel to a small number of well-trained individuals. To monitor the accuracy and precision of the analytical process, two concentrations of controls should be performed daily when patient samples are analyzed. Sweat chloride concentrations greater than 160 mmol/L are not physiologically possible and represent specimen contamination or analytical error. An important part of a quality assurance plan includes method validation and external validation of sweat analysis accuracy through participation in proficiency testing, such as that offered by the College of American Pathology (CAP). The reader is referred to reference 12 for additional suggestions on developing a robust quality assurance program for sweat chloride testing and techniques to minimize QNS collections.

Bicarbonate (Total Carbon Dioxide)

Total carbon dioxide is measured in the clinical laboratory by (1) acidification of a serum or plasma sample and measurement of carbon dioxide released by the process or (2) alkalinization and measurement of total bicarbonate.

Specimens

The same sample types used for Na^+ or K^+ may be assayed. Given a specimen in a vacuum draw tube, the concentration of total CO_2 is most accurately determined when the assay is done as promptly as possible after collection and centrifugation of the blood in the unopened tube. Ambient air contains far less CO_2 than does plasma, and dissolved CO_2 will escape from the specimen into the air, with a consequent decrease in the CO_2 value of up to 4 to 5 mmol/L in the course of 1 hour.

Methods for Determination of Serum or Plasma Total Carbon Dioxide

Methods used for total CO_2 measurement with today's automated instruments may be electrode based or enzymatic. With indirect electrode-based methods, the amount of released gaseous CO_2 after acidification is determined by a PCO_2 electrode. Direct ISE methods for total CO_2 are no longer common on automated analyzers because of problems with specificity. With enzymatic methods for CO_2, the specimen is first alkalinized to convert all CO_2 and carbonic acid to HCO_3^-. The enzymatic reactions lead to decreased absorbance of NADH at 340 nm that is proportional to the total CO_2 content.

Phosphoenolpyruvate + HCO_3^- → *Phosphoenolpyruvate carboxylase* → Oxaloacetate + P_i

Oxaloacetate → (*Malate dehydrogenase*, NADH + H^+ → NAD$^+$) → Malate

Reference Intervals

The reference interval for total carbon dioxide in healthy adults is 22 to 30 mmol/L but is method dependent.

Principles of Osmotic Pressure and Osmosis

Osmometry is a technique for measuring the concentration of solute particles that contribute to the osmotic pressure of a solution. **Osmotic pressure** governs the movement of solvent (water in biological systems) across membranes that separate two solutions. Different membranes vary in pore size and thus in their ability to select molecules of different size and shape. Examples of biologically important selective membranes are those enclosing the glomeruli of the kidney and capillary vessels that are permeable to water and to essentially all small molecules and ions, but not to larger protein molecules. Differences in the concentrations of osmotically active molecules that are unable to cross a membrane cause those molecules that are able to cross the membrane to move to establish an osmotic equilibrium. This movement of solute and permeable ions exerts osmotic pressure.

Colligative Properties

In addition to increasing osmotic pressure when the solute is added to the solvent, the vapor pressure of the solution is lowered below that of the pure solvent. As a result of the change in vapor pressure, the boiling point of the solution is raised above and the freezing point of the solution is lowered below that of the pure solvent. These four properties of solutions—(1) increased osmotic pressure, (2) lowered vapor pressure, (3) increased boiling point, and (4) decreased freezing point—are called **colligative properties**. All are directly related to the total number of solute particles per mass of solvent. The term osmolality expresses concentrations relative to *mass* of the solvent (1 osmolal solution is defined to contain 1 Osmol/kg H_2O), whereas the term osmolarity

expresses concentrations per volume of solution (1 osmolar solution is defined to contain 1 Osmol/L solution). Osmolality (Osmol/kg H_2O) is a thermodynamically more exact expression because solution concentrations expressed on a weight basis are temperature independent, whereas those based on volume vary with temperature. Although the term osmolarity is often used in the medical literature, osmolality is what the clinical laboratory measures.

An electrolyte in solution dissociates into two (in the case of NaCl) or three (in the case of $CaCl_2$) particles; therefore the colligative effects of such solutions are multiplied by the number of dissociated ions formed per molecule. However, because of incomplete electrolyte dissociation and associations between solute and solvent molecules, many solutions do not behave in the ideal case, and a 1-molal solution may give an osmotic pressure lower than is theoretically expected. The osmotic activity coefficient is a factor used to correct for deviation from the "ideal" behavior of the system:

$$\text{Osmolality} = \frac{\text{osmol}}{\text{Kg H}_2\text{O}} = \phi n C$$

where Φ = osmotic coefficient, n = number of particles into which each molecule in the solution potentially dissociates, and C = molality in mol/kg H_2O.

Glucose has an osmotic coefficient of 1.00, whereas the Φ for sodium chloride is 0.93 at the concentrations found in serum—thus the derivation of 1.86 × Na$^+$ (mmol) in the formula to calculate plasma osmolality (NaCl potentially contributes two osmotically active particles × 0.93 = 1.86). Ethanol has an osmotic coefficient of 0.83. The total osmolality or osmotic pressure of a solution is equal to the sum of the osmotic pressures or osmolalities of all solute species present. The electrolytes Na$^+$, Cl$^-$, and HCO_3^-, which are present in relatively high concentrations, make the greatest contributions to serum osmolality. Nonelectrolytes such as glucose and urea, which are present normally at lower molal concentrations, contribute less, and serum proteins contribute less than 0.5% of the total serum osmolality.

Determination of Plasma and Urine Osmolality

Determination of plasma and urine osmolality is useful in the assessment of electrolyte and acid-base disorders. The major osmotic substances in normal plasma are Na$^+$, Cl$^-$, glucose, and urea; thus expected plasma osmolality is calculated from the following empirical equation:

$$\begin{aligned}
\text{mOsmol/kg} = {} & 1.86\,[\text{Na}^+\,(\text{mmol/L})] \\
& + \text{glucose [mmol/L]} \\
& + \text{urea [mmol/L]} \\
& + 9
\end{aligned}$$

or

$$\begin{aligned}
\text{mOsmol/kg} = {} & 1.86\,[\text{Na}^+\,(\text{mmol/L})] \\
& + \text{glucose [mg/dL]/18} \\
& + \text{urea N[mg/dL]/2.8} \\
& + 9
\end{aligned}$$

The 9 mOsmol/kg added to the previous equation represents the contributions of other osmotically active substances in plasma, such as (1) K^+, (2) Ca^{2+}, and (3) proteins, and 1.86 is $2 \times$ the osmotic coefficient of Na^+, reflecting the contributions of both Na^+ and Cl^-. The reference interval for plasma osmolality is 275 to 300 mOsmol/kg. Comparison of measured osmolality versus calculated osmolality reveals the presence of an **osmolal gap**, which is used to detect the presence of exogenous osmotic substances.

Theoretically, any of the four colligative properties discussed previously—(1) vapor pressure, (2) boiling point, (3) freezing point, and (4) osmotic pressure—could serve as a basis for the measurement of osmolality. However, freezing point depression is most commonly used in clinical laboratories because of its simplicity. Furthermore, freezing point depression, unlike vapor pressure, is independent of changes in ambient temperature.

Freezing Point Depression Osmometer

The components of a freezing point depression osmometer include the following:

1. A thermostatically controlled cooling bath or block maintained at $-7\,°C$.
2. A rapid stir mechanism to initiate ("seed") freezing of the sample.
3. A thermistor probe connected to a circuit to measure the temperature of the sample.
4. A light-emitting diode (LED) display that indicates the time course of the freezing curve and the final result.

During analysis, the following steps occur. The sample, in which the thermistor probe and the stirring wire are centered, is lowered into the bath and, with gentle stirring, is supercooled to a temperature several degrees below its freezing point ($-7\,°C$). When the LED display indicates that sufficient super-cooling has occurred, the sample is raised to a point above the liquid in the cooling bath, and the wire stirrer is changed from a gentle rate of stir to a momentary vigorous amplitude, which initiates freezing of the super-cooled solution. This freezing occurs only to the slush stage, with about 2% to 3% of the solvent solidifying. The released heat of fusion initially warms the solution, and then the temperature plateaus and remains stationary, indicating the equilibrium temperature at which both freezing and thawing of the solution are occurring. An example of the calculation used to obtain osmolality is as follows: If the observed freezing point is $-0.53\,°C$, then

$$\text{Mosmol/kg H}_2\text{O} = \frac{-0.53}{-1.86} \times 1000 = 2.85$$

where $-1.86\,°C$ is the molal freezing point depression of pure water.

Vapor Pressure Osmometer

Another type of osmometer is the vapor pressure osmometer. However, osmolality measurement with these instruments is related directly not to a change in vapor pressure (in millimeters of mercury) but to the decrease in dew point temperature of the pure solvent (water) caused by the decrease in vapor pressure of the solvent by the solutes.

An important clinical difference between the vapor pressure technique and the freezing point depression osmometer is the failure of the former to include in its measurement of total osmolality any volatile solutes present in the serum. Substances such as (1) ethanol, (2) methanol, and (3) isopropanol are volatile and thus escape from the solution and increase the vapor pressure instead of lowering the vapor pressure of the solvent (water). This makes the use of vapor pressure osmometers impractical for identifying osmolal gaps in acid-base disturbances (see Chapter 36), and use of this type of osmometer is not recommended for most clinical laboratories.

Blood Gases and pH

Clinical management of respiratory and metabolic disorders often depends on rapid, accurate measurements of oxygen and carbon dioxide gas in blood. Determination of blood gases also plays an important part in the detection of acid-base imbalances. Details of the pathophysiology of blood gases in relation to respiration and acid-base disorders are discussed in detail in Chapter 36. Nomenclature for this area of analysis has been recommended by the CLSI,[6] but alternative nomenclatures exist and are in common use; these are summarized in Box 24-1.

Behavior of Gases

Determination of gas pressures in expired air or blood depends on the application of certain physical principles (Table 24-3). The **partial pressure** (tension) of a gas dissolved in blood is by definition equal to the partial pressure of the gas in an imaginary ideal gas phase in equilibrium with the blood. At equilibrium, the partial pressure of a gas is the same in erythrocytes and plasma, so that the partial pressure of a gas is the same in whole blood and plasma. The partial pressure of a gas in a gas mixture is defined as the substance fraction of gas (mole fraction) times the total pressure.

Various spaces where gases are present include the ambient environment (room air), the bronchial tree and alveoli of the patient, and the measuring chamber of a laboratory instrument. In all these spaces, atmospheric (barometric) pressure, $P(Amb)$, is the prevailing pressure, and partial pressures of each of the gases present in these spaces must add up to the value of $P(Amb)$, which will vary with altitude and barometric pressure. Scientific convention reduces measurements of gas volume made at $P(Amb)$ to *Standard Temperature* (0 °C, or 273.16 K) and *Pressure* (760 mm Hg, or 101.325 kPa) for *Dry* gas (STPD) to make experimental data transferable. However, in blood gas work, the standard is that measurements of partial pressure are always made at *Body Temperature* (usually 37 °C), at $P(Amb)$, and in the presence of *Saturated* water vapor (SVP) the $PH_2O = 47$ mm Hg.

BOX 24-1	Conversion Factors, Prefixes, Symbols, and Descriptors Used in Discussions of Gases Measured in Blood and Expired Air[*]

Conversion Factors

1 mm Hg = 0.133 kPa

1 kPa = 7.5 mm Hg

  kPa: 1 kilopascal = 1000 pascal. The pascal is the SI derived unit of pressure; it equals 1 Newton/m².

General Prefixes

P: partial pressure or tension

  Usage: PO_2, PCO_2, PH_2O

  Alternative: pO_2

S: saturation fraction

  Usage: SO_2

  Alternative: sO_2

c: substance concentration

  Usage: ctO_2 for concentration of total O_2

  Usage: $ctCO_2$ for concentration of total CO_2

  Usage: $cHCO_3^-$ for concentration of bicarbonate

d: dissolved gas, used with substance concentration *(c)*

t: total, used with substance concentration *(c)*, thus

$$ctCO_2 = HCO_3^- + cdCO_2$$

Specimen origin is indicated by lowercase letters. Whole blood and plasma are distinguished by capital letters.

a: arterial   B: blood

v: venous   P: plasma

c: capillary

  Usage: $PO_2(aB)$, for partial pressure of O_2 in arterial blood

Prefixes Associated With External Respiration

V: volume of air or blood (unit, L)

V̇: volume rate (unit, L/min)

F: substance fraction, also called *mole fraction*

E: expired air

I: inspired air

A: alveolar air

  Usage: V̇(A) means alveolar ventilation; V̇(B) cardiac output; $FO_2(I)$ fraction of O_2 in inspired air; $PO_2(A)$ partial pressure of O_2 in alveolar air; and $PCO_2(E)$ partial pressure of CO_2 in expired air.

Other Descriptors

BTPS: *B*ody *T*emperature (37 °C or 310.16 K) and ambient *P*ressure, fully *S*aturated (PH_2O = 47 mm Hg or 6.25 kPa)

STPD: *S*tandard *T*emperature (0 °C or 273.16 K) and standard *P*ressure (760 mm Hg or 101.08 kPa) of *D*ry gas

  Amb: ambient atmosphere (unit is atm, atmosphere)

  B: barometric (atmospheric)

  BTPS: usage: *P*(amb), *P*(Amb)

  SVP: *S*aturated *V*apor *P*ressure, the vapor pressure of water. SVPT means SVP at a specified temperature (e.g., $SVP_{37 °C}$ = 47 mm Hg; PH_2O[saturated])

  ATPS: *A*mbient *T*emperature and *P*ressure, *S*aturated with water vapor

From Maas AH. IFCC reference methods for measurement of pH, gases and electrolytes in blood: reference materials. Eur J Clin Chem Clin Biochem 1991;29:253-61.

[*]This list is not complete but is presented to facilitate interpretation of terms used in the text and to illustrate various forms that may be encountered in the literature.

TABLE 24-3	Physical Principles Applied in Blood Gas Measurements	
Boyle's law: The volume of an ideal gas at a constant temperature varies inversely with the pressure exerted to contain it.		$V \propto 1/P$
Charles' (Gay-Lussac's) law: The volume of an ideal gas at a constant pressure varies directly with its absolute temperature.		$V \propto T$
Avogadro's hypothesis: Equal volumes of different ideal gases at the same temperature and pressure contain the same number of molecules.		$n_i/V_i = n_j/V_j$
Dalton's law: The total pressure exerted by a mixture of ideal gases is the sum of the partial pressure of each of the gases in the mixture.		$P = \Sigma P_i$
Henry's law: The amount of a sparingly soluble gas dissolved in a liquid is proportional to the partial pressure of the gas over the liquid.		$c = \alpha \times P$

Boyle's and Charles' laws and Avogadro's hypothesis are combined in what is called the general gas equation:

$$P = \frac{nRT}{V}$$

where

P = pressure in units of millimeters of mercury (mm Hg) or kilopascals (kPa)

V = volume in liters in which an ideal gas is contained

T = temperature in degrees kelvin (0 °C = 273.16 K)

n = number of moles of gas, and

R = gas constant.

The SI unit of *P* is the pascal (Pa). Pressure, *P* (or *p*), may mean total pressure, as in the expression *P*(Amb) for the mixture of gases in ambient air, or partial pressure in arterial blood, as in $PO_2(aB)$.

Dalton's law (see Table 24-3) may be written for room air as follows:

$$P(Amb) = PO_2 + PCO_2 + PN_2 + PH_2O + PX$$

where *PX* is that of any other gas in the air sample. However, for gases in solution, Dalton's law does not apply, as the sum of partial pressures of all dissolved gases may be lower than, equal to, or higher than the measured pressure of the solution. Dalton's law of partial pressures remains important, however, for calibration and control of the measuring devices. Consider a calibrator gas certified to contain 15% O_2 (L/L or mol/mol) and 5% CO_2, with the remainder being N_2. This mixture, after saturation with water vapor at 37 °C (to mimic a patient's blood or alveolar air), is introduced into a blood gas instrument's measuring chamber (held at 37 °C to mimic a patient's body temperature) for the purpose of calibrating the instrument for subsequent measurement of gases in patients' samples. If the local barometric pressure, *P*(Amb), on this occasion is 747 mm Hg, then humidified calibrator gas is present in the chamber at ambient, barometric pressure, such that

$$P(Amb) = 747 \text{ mm Hg} = PO_2 + PCO_2 + PN_2 + PH_2O$$

To set the instrument to the PO_2 and PCO_2 of the calibrator gas, we first must account for PH_2O at 37 °C, which is equal to the SVP of water, 47 mm Hg. Therefore,

$$P(Amb) - PCO_2 = PO_2 + PCO_2 + PN_2$$
$$747 - 47 = 700 \text{ mm Hg}$$

If $P(Amb)$ corrected for PH_2O represents the sum of partial pressures for the dry gases whose mole fractions we know, it is possible to calculate the exact PO_2 and PCO_2 values for the calibrator gas.

The law of partial pressure is also applied in defining gas mixtures used to determine $PO_2(0.5)$ or P_{50} and other derived quantities, and to control instrumentation with tonometered samples. *Henry's law* predicts the amount of dissolved gas in a liquid in contact with a gaseous phase (see Table 24-3).

The coefficient for O_2 in blood, αO_2, is 0.00140 (mol/L)/mm Hg (the corresponding coefficient for the volume-volume relationship is 31 μL/L/mm Hg). Therefore when arterial PO_2 is normal (≈100 mm Hg), the concentration of dissolved O_2 in arterial blood, cdO_2, is 0.140 mmol/L, which is a very small proportion of the ctO_2 content in blood (≈9 mmol/L), the bulk of which is O_2 bound by hemoglobin. Increasing the O_2 fraction of inspired air to 100% or increasing the pressure of inspired air, as in a hyperbaric chamber, forces more O_2 into a solution. Prediction of concentrations of cdO_2 in these therapies is useful because tissue oxygenation by dissolved O_2 becomes increasingly important when hemoglobin-mediated O_2 delivery is impaired. The $cdCO_2$ is similarly calculated as αCO_2 at 37 °C in plasma = 0.0306 mmol/L/mm Hg.

Application of the Henderson-Hasselbalch Equation in Blood Gas Measurements

Carbon dioxide and water react to form carbonic acid, which in turn dissociates to hydrogen ions and HCO_3^-.

$$CO_2 + H_2O \underset{}{\overset{K_{hydration}}{\rightleftharpoons}} H_2CO_3 \underset{}{\overset{K_{dissociation}}{\rightleftharpoons}} H^{\oplus} + HCO_3^{\ominus}$$

Thus the (1) total concentration of CO_2 ($ctCO_2$), (2) concentration of bicarbonate (HCO_3^-), (3) concentration of dissolved CO_2 ($cdCO_2$), and (4) H^+ ion concentration (cH^+) are interrelated. In the classical 1908 formulation, Henderson, using concentrations for (1) bicarbonate, (2) CO_2, and (3) H^+, and assuming the concentration of water to be constant, incorporated the constant K' with a value of 4.68×10^{-7}, and thus a pK' of 6.33 at 37 °C:

$$K' = \frac{cH^+ \times cHCO_3^-}{cdCO_3^-}$$

The concentration of dissolved CO_2 includes the small amount of undissociated (dissolved) carbonic acid. It is expressed as $cdCO_2 = \alpha \times PCO_2$, where α is the solubility coefficient for CO_2. $cHCO_3^-$ then represents $ctCO_2 - cdCO_2$, which includes carbonic acid. The "bicarbonate" concentration by this definition includes undissociated sodium

bicarbonate, carbonate ($NaCO_3$), and carbamate (carbamino-CO_2; $RCNHCOO^-$), which are present in exceedingly small amounts in plasma. If the Henderson equation is rearranged and $cdCO_2$ is replaced by $\alpha \times PCO_2$, the following equation results:

$$cH^+ = K' \times \frac{\alpha \times PCO_2}{cHCO_3^-}$$

In 1916, Hasselbalch showed that a logarithmic transformation of the equation was a more useful form and used the symbols pH ($= -\log cH^+$) and pK' ($= -\log K'$). pH is defined as the negative log of the *activity* of H+ ($aH+$), which is the entity actually measured with pH meters. The resulting **Henderson-Hasselbalch equation** becomes

$$pH = pK' + \log \frac{cCHO_3^-}{\alpha \times PCO_2}$$

or

$$pH = pK' + \log \frac{ctCO_2 - \alpha \times PCO_2}{\alpha \times PCO_2}$$

K' is the apparent overall (combined) dissociation constant for carbonic acid. It is *apparent* because concentrations are used rather than activities and *overall* because both the $cdCO_2$ and the concentration of carbonic acid are used. K' depends not only on the temperature but also on the ionic strength of the solution.

When pK' and α for normal plasma at 37 °C are inserted, the Henderson-Hasselbalch equation takes the following form:

$$pH = 6.103 + \log \frac{cHCO_3^-}{0.0306 \times PCO_2}$$

where PCO_2 is measured in millimeters.

Therefore, by measuring any two of the four parameters—(1) PCO_2 or $cdCO_2$, (2) pH, (3) $ctCO_2$, and (4) $cHCO_3^-$—and by using the Henderson-Hasselbalch equation with the above values for pK' and α, the other two parameters may be calculated.

Oxygen in Blood

The total O_2 content (ctO_2) of a blood sample is the sum of the concentrations of hemoglobin-bound O_2 and of dissolved O_2. At a blood ctO_2 of 9 mmol/L, the O_2 associated with hemoglobin as **oxyhemoglobin** (O_2Hb) is 8.86 mmol/L. The O_2Hb is defined as erythrocyte hemoglobin with O_2 reversibly bound to Fe^{2+} of its heme group. Each mole of hemoglobin-Fe^{2+} binds 1 mol of O_2.

Thus 1 g of hemoglobin is capable of binding 1.39 mL (0.062 mmol) of O_2 at STPD (Standard Temperature and Pressure, Dry). This value is referred to as the specific O_2-binding capacity of hemoglobin A (Hb A, the normal adult gene product). Hb A reversibly binds O_2 at its heme moiety. Forms of hemoglobin that are not capable of reversibly binding O_2 include (1) methemoglobin (MetHb), (2) carboxyhemoglobin (COHb), (3) sulfhemoglobin (SulfHb), and (4) cyanmethemoglobin. Because of chemical alterations of their heme moiety (see Chapter 28), these chemically altered hemoglobins are collectively termed *dyshemoglobins*.

Uptake of O_2 by the blood in the lungs is governed primarily by the PO_2 of alveolar air and by the ability of O_2 to diffuse freely across the alveolar membrane into the blood. At the PO_2 normally present in alveolar air ($\approx$102 mm Hg) and with a normal membrane and normal hemoglobin A, more than 95% of hemoglobin will bind O_2. At a PO_2 >110 mm Hg, more than 98% of normal hemoglobin A binds O_2. When all hemoglobin is saturated with O_2, a further increase in the PO_2 of alveolar air simply increases the concentration of dO_2 in the arterial blood. Delivery of O_2 by the blood to the tissue is governed by the large gradient between PO_2 of the arterial blood and that of the tissue cells and by the dissociation of O_2 from Hb in the erythrocytes at the lower PO_2 of the blood-tissue cell interface.

The following properties of arterial blood are essential to ensure adequate O_2 delivery to the tissue:
1. Arterial PO_2 must be sufficiently high ($\approx$90 mm Hg) to create a diffusion gradient from the arterial blood to the tissue cells. Low arterial PO_2 (hypoxemia) results in tissue O_2 starvation (hypoxia).
2. The O_2-binding capacity of the blood must be normal. Decreased Hb concentration will cause so-called anemic hypoxia.
3. The hemoglobin must be able to bind O_2 in the lungs yet release it at the tissue, as the affinity of hemoglobin for O_2 must be normal. Too great an affinity of hemoglobin for O_2 may cause "affinity-based" tissue hypoxia, in which O_2 is not released at the capillary-tissue interface.

The PO_2 at the venous end of the capillaries should stay around 38 mm Hg; thus the normal arteriovenous difference in PO_2 is 50 to 60 mm Hg.

Hemoglobin Oxygen Saturation

At least three different approaches are known for determining oxygen "saturation," and although each is distinct, they are often used interchangeably. They include (1) hemoglobin oxygen saturation (SO_2), (2) fractional oxyhemoglobin (FO_2Hb), and (3) estimated oxygen saturation (O_2Sat). Each has been defined in a CLSI document.[6]

Before the factors that affect Hb affinity for O_2 are discussed, it is important to first define the concept of hemoglobin **oxygen saturation (SO_2):**

$$SO_2 = \frac{\text{Oxygen Content}}{\text{Oxygen Capacity}}$$

This is the fraction (percentage) of functional hemoglobin that is saturated with oxygen and is essentially an indirect means of estimating the PO_2. Spectrophotometric methods are used to determine O_2Hb and HHb, and SO_2 is calculated according to

$$SO_2 = \frac{cO_2Hb}{cO_2Hb + cHHb}$$

where cO_2Hb is the concentration of oxyhemoglobin, $cHHb$ is the concentration of deoxyhemoglobin, and the sum of oxyhemoglobin and deoxyhemoglobin represents all hemoglobin capable of reversibly binding O_2. SO_2 is usually expressed as a percent.

SO_2 most often is determined by simple pulse **oximetry**, a spectrophotometric approach that determines oxyhemoglobin and reduced hemoglobin (HHb) but not COHb, MetHb, or SulfHb. It should be noted that use of SO_2 in the initial evaluation of a patient with dyshemoglobins or other abnormal hemoglobins can be misleading. For instance, in a comatose patient with 15% COHb, the SO_2 by simple pulse oximetry might read 0.95, whereas the fraction of oxyhemoglobin in reality would be only 0.80. Thus it seems reasonable to assess for the presence of dyshemoglobins before SO_2 is used for clinical purposes. The reference interval for SO_2 from healthy adults is 0.94 to 0.98 (94% to 98%).

Another expression of oxygen "saturation" is fractional oxyhemoglobin (FO_2Hb), which is calculated as

$$FO_2Hb = (cO_2Hb/cHHb + cCOHb + cMethHb + cSulHb)$$

This value requires determination of all hemoglobin species and is performed on a co-oximeter present in many modern blood gas analyzers. These instruments prepare a hemolysate from whole blood by sonication, and by spectrophotometry they determine the total amount of hemoglobin and the percent of each of the aforementioned species. Because each species of hemoglobin has its own absorbance pattern, an onboard microprocessor calculates the percentage of each one. The reference interval for FO_2Hb is 0.90 to 0.95 (90% to 95%).

Finally, the microprocessors of many blood gas instruments are capable of estimating the oxygen saturation from measured (1) pH, (2) PO_2, and (3) hemoglobin with the use of empirical equations. This value should be clearly referred to as estimated oxygen saturation, but it frequently is reported as and referred to as "O_2Sat." Calculated values such as "O_2Sat" should be interpreted with reservation because the algorithm assumes (1) normal O_2, (2) normal affinity of the hemoglobin, (3) normal 2,3-diphosphoglycerol (2,3-DPG) concentrations, and (4) the absence of dyshemoglobins.

Decreases in arterial FO_2Hb may indicate a low arterial PO_2 or an impaired ability of hemoglobin to bind O_2. Decreases in PO_2 indicate a reduced ability of O_2 to diffuse from alveolar air into the blood. Decreases in the concentration of total hemoglobin can result from a decreased number of erythrocytes that contain a normal concentration of hemoglobin (normochromic anemia) or a decreased mean cell concentration of hemoglobin in the erythrocytes (hypochromic anemia). Decreased FO_2Hb hemoglobin also occurs as a result of poisonings that convert part of the hemoglobin into the species COHb, MetHb, SulfHb, or cyanmethemoglobin, which cannot properly bind or exchange O_2.

The oxygen concentration of blood (ctO_2) is the sum of O_2 bound to hemoglobin and cdO_2. Blood gas analyzers determine ctO_2 by the following calculation:

$$ctO_2 \, (mL/dL) = FO_2Hb \times bO_2 \times ctHb \, (g/dL) + (\alpha O_2) \times (PO_2)$$

where bO_2 equals 1.39 mL/g Hb and α, the solubility coefficient of O_2 at 37 °C, and STPD = 0.00140 (mmol/L)/mm Hg. Note that this calculation is based on FO_2Hb and $ctHb$. If SO_2 is used, it is necessary to use the effective hemoglobin concentration by subtracting the concentration of any dyshemoglobins present from the concentration of $ctHb$.

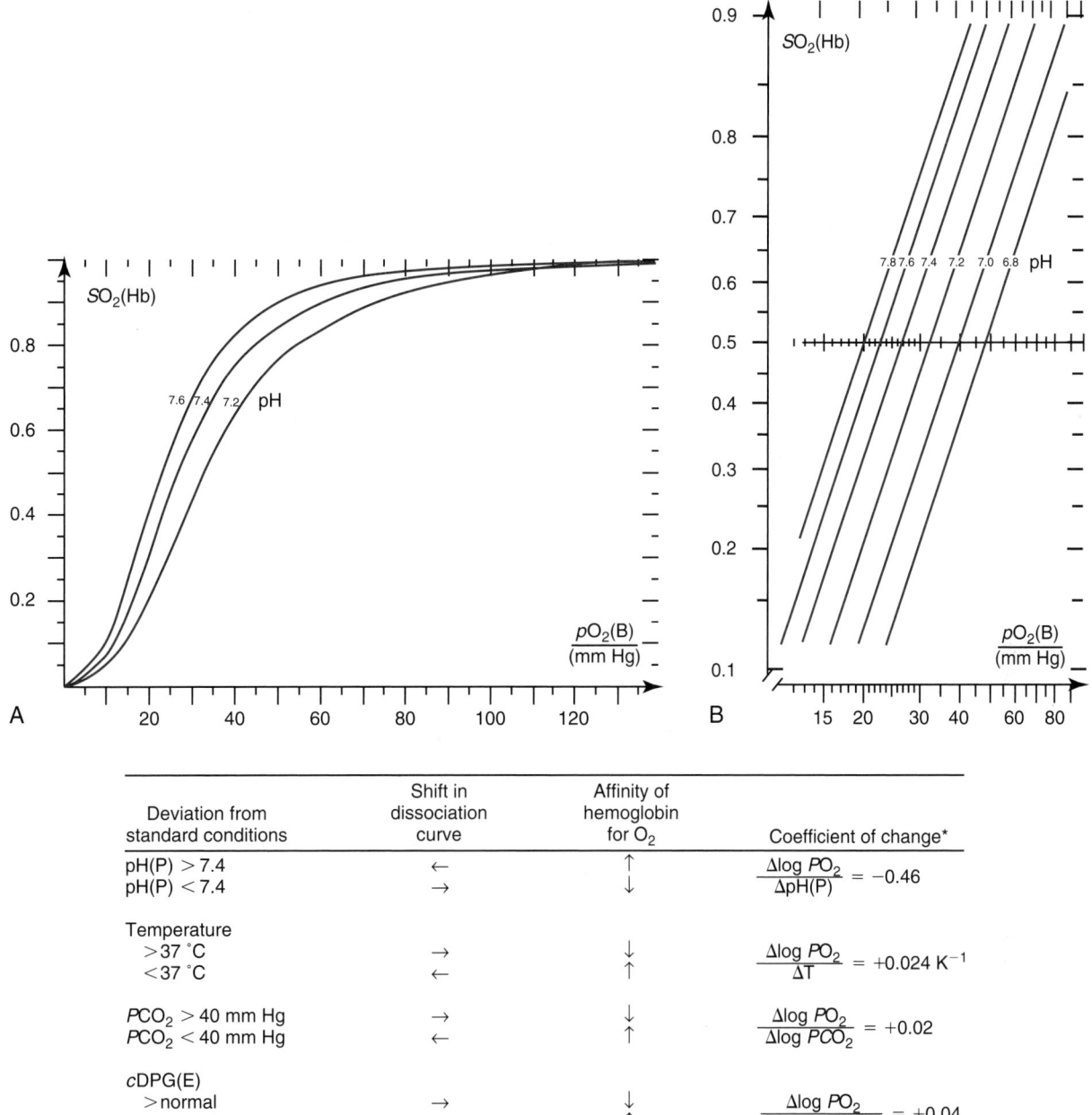

Figure 24-3 A, Oxygen dissociation curves for human blood with different plasma pH but constant PCO_2 of 40 mm Hg, a 2,3-diphosphoglycerol (2,3-DPG) concentration in erythrocytes of 5.0 mmol/L, and temperature at 37 °C. **B,** A Hill plot. Conditions are the same as in (A). The coefficients given in this chart form the basis for the correction of measured PO_2. **C,** The effect of pH(P) to shift the dissociation curve is called the *Bohr effect.*

Deviation from standard conditions	Shift in dissociation curve	Affinity of hemoglobin for O_2	Coefficient of change*
pH(P) > 7.4	←	↑	$\dfrac{\Delta \log PO_2}{\Delta pH(P)} = -0.46$
pH(P) < 7.4	→	↓	
Temperature			
>37 °C	→	↓	$\dfrac{\Delta \log PO_2}{\Delta T} = +0.024\ K^{-1}$
<37 °C	←	↑	
PCO_2 > 40 mm Hg	→	↓	$\dfrac{\Delta \log PO_2}{\Delta \log PCO_2} = +0.02$
PCO_2 < 40 mm Hg	←	↑	
cDPG(E)			
>normal	→	↓	$\dfrac{\Delta \log PO_2}{\Delta(cDPG(E)/c^*)} = +0.04$
<normal	←	↑	

Hemoglobin-Oxygen Dissociation

The degree of association or dissociation of O_2 with hemoglobin is determined by PO_2 and the affinity of hemoglobin for O_2. When the SO_2 of blood is determined over a range of PO_2 and is plotted against PO_2, a sigmoidal curve called the **oxygen dissociation curve** is obtained. The *shape* of the curve is affected by the increasing efficiency with which HHb molecules bind more O_2 once some O_2 has been bound (cooperativity; see also Chapter 28). The location of the curve relative to the PO_2 required to achieve a particular concentration of SO_2 in the blood is a function of the affinity of hemoglobin for O_2.

The affinity of hemoglobin for O_2 depends on the following five factors: (1) temperature, (2) pH, (3) PCO_2, (4) concentration of 2,3-DPG, and (5) the presence of minor hemoglobins such as COHb and metHb. The graph in Figure 24-3 shows the effect of plasma pH on the O_2 dissociation curve (the Bohr effect). Similar graphs can be constructed for variations in PCO_2, 2,3-DPG, and temperature.

Determination of P_{50}

P_{50} is defined as the PO_2 at which the hemoglobin of the blood is half saturated with O_2. The measured value of P_{50} differs from the standard value of P_{50} by an amount determined by the extent that (1) pH differs from 7.40, (2) PCO_2 differs from 40 mm Hg, (3) temperature differs from 37 °C, and (4) 2,3-DPG differs from 5.0 mmol/L. The value of P_{50} therefore becomes a measure of change in hemoglobin affinity because of the factors that affect it.

Reference Intervals

The P_{50} reference interval for adults, measured at 37 °C and corrected to a pH of 7.4, is 25 to 29 mm Hg. For newborn infants, the interval is 18 to 24 mm Hg because of the presence of Hb F.

Clinical Significance

Increased values for P_{50} indicate displacement of the O_2 dissociation curve to the right because of decreased affinity of the hemoglobin for O_2. The chief causes are (1) hyperthermia, (2) acidemia, (3) hypercapnia, (4) high concentrations of 2,3-DPG, and (5) the presence of a hemoglobin variant with decreased O_2 affinity. Low values for P_{50} signify displacement of the O_2 dissociation curve to the left because of increased affinity of hemoglobin. The main causes are (1) hypothermia, (2) acute alkalemia, (3) hypocapnia, (4) low concentrations of 2,3-DPG, and (5) a hemoglobin variant.

Tonometry

Tonometry is the process of exposing a sample to a gas phase in such a way that each gas in the gaseous phase partitions to an equilibrium between liquid and gas. Equilibration by tonometry uses gases of known fractional composition, humidified at 37 °C, to give a saturated water vapor pressure of 47 mm Hg. The PCO_2 or PO_2 of such gases is calculated according to Dalton's law (see earlier section on behavior of gases). Tonometry is used to treat blood samples for various special studies that are rarely requested in most hospital settings and to prepare quality control material in whole blood. Direct determination of P_{50} and of standard bicarbonate are two applications of tonometry.

Determination of PCO_2, PO_2, and pH

The instruments used for determination of PCO_2, PO_2, and pH are highly automated. Proper specimen collection and handling are critical for accurate determinations.

Specimens

Whole blood is the most likely specimen for a clinical laboratory to receive for gas analysis. Differences in measured blood gas values between arterial and venous blood are most pronounced for PO_2. In fact, PO_2 is the only clinical reason for arterial collections. PO_2 is generally ≈60 mm Hg lower in venous blood after O_2 is released in the capillaries, whereas PCO_2 is 2 to 8 mm Hg higher in venous blood. pH generally is only 0.02 to 0.05 pH units lower in a venous sample.

Arterial and venous specimens are best collected anaerobically with lyophilized heparin anticoagulant in 1- to 3-mL sterile syringes. Although in theory, glass syringes are preferred to prevent gas exchange through the syringe wall, most blood gas syringes today are plastic, and the gas exchange that occurs within 1 hour is trivial. Lyophilized heparin is preferable to liquid heparin because liquid heparin, which has atmospheric PO_2 and PCO_2 values, dilutes the sample, and the effect is greatest when the syringe is not completely filled.

For an anaerobic collection, the blood is not exposed to atmospheric air. The PCO_2 of air is about 0.25 mm Hg; this is much less than that of blood (≈40 mm Hg). Thus the CO_2 content and the PCO_2 of blood exposed to air will decrease, and blood pH, which is a function of PCO_2, will rise. The PO_2 of atmospheric air (≈155 mm Hg) is ≈60 mm Hg higher than that of arterial blood and ≈100 mm Hg higher than that of venous blood. Therefore blood from patients breathing room air that is exposed to atmospheric air gains O_2, and blood with PO_2 >150 mm Hg, as occurs in patients undergoing O_2 therapy, loses O_2. Blood can also be exposed to air simply from the air in the needle and in the syringe hub dead space.

Arterialized capillary blood is sometimes an acceptable alternative to arterial blood when an arterial cannula is not available, or when repeated arterial puncture must be prevented. Freely flowing cutaneous blood originates in the arterioles and corresponds closely to arterial blood in composition. The first blood drop to appear should be wiped away, and subsequent free-forming drops should be taken up in a capillary collection tube containing lyophilized heparin. Only free-flowing blood provides a satisfactory sample, and taking up the drops as soon as they form minimizes aerobic exposure.

Transport and analysis of specimens should be prompt. However, delayed analysis of up to 1 hour will have a minimal effect on reported values from most samples. The pH of freshly drawn blood decreases on standing at a rate of 0.04 to 0.08 pH unit/h at 37 °C, 0.02 to 0.03/h at 22 °C, and <0.01/h at 4 °C. The decrease in pH is accompanied by a corresponding decrease in glucose and an equivalent increase in lactate. PCO_2 increases by ≈5 mm Hg/h at 37 °C, by 1 mm Hg/h at 22 °C, and by only ≈0.5 mm Hg/h at 2 °C to 4 °C. The primary cause of these changes is glycolysis by leukocytes, platelets, and reticulocytes. In freshly drawn blood with a normal PO_2 that is maintained anaerobically, cell respiration causes PO_2 to decrease at a rate of ≈2 mm Hg/h at room temperature and 5 to 10 mm Hg/h at 37 °C. Adverse effects of glycolysis and respiration on pH, $ctCO_2$, PO_2, and PCO_2 of blood are best prevented by analysis within 30 minutes after collection. The small changes in values that are to be expected with delays in analysis are true **only** when the white blood cell count (WBC) is normal or is only slightly elevated. Glycolysis and the resulting effects on pH, PO_2, and PCO_2 increase dramatically with markedly elevated WBC, as occurs in leukemia.

Instrumentation

A schematic diagram characteristic of a typical instrument is shown in Figure 24-4. Operation of a traditional blood gas instrument begins with the operator presenting a blood specimen at the sample probe. The sample is taken through the probe by a peristaltic pump that loads the chamber with 60 to 150 μL of the sample. The sample then resides in the chamber long

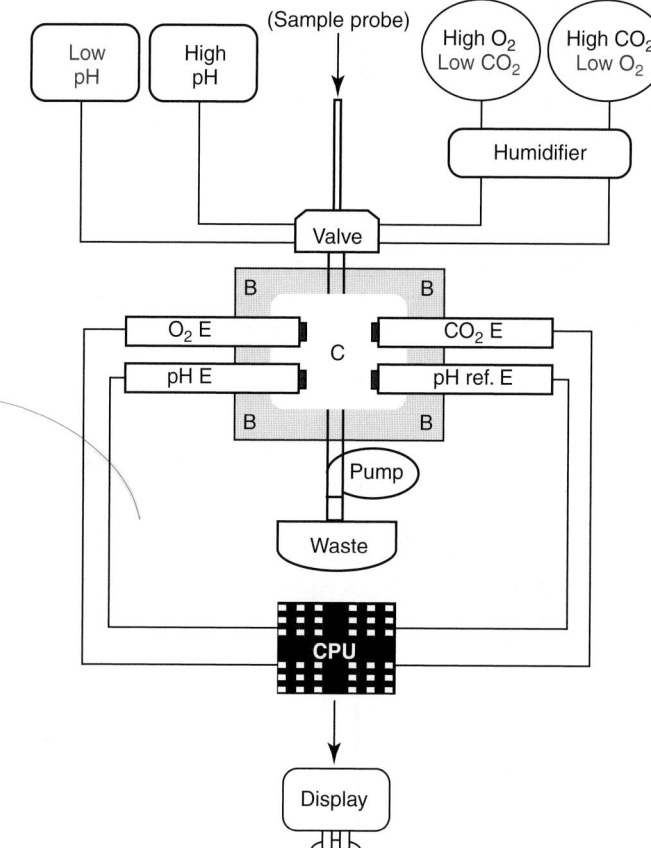

Figure 24-4 Diagram of blood gas instrumentation. *B,* Constant temperature bath at 37 °C. *CPU,* computer. *E (electrodes),* pH, and gas standards are shown at top of diagram.

enough to allow thermal equilibration and completion of measurements. On completion of measurement, the pump pushes the sample to waste, while output is made available on a display, a printed tape, and often a laboratory information system.

Because electrodes are not stable over long periods of time, frequent calibration of pH, PCO_2, and PO_2 is required. Most modern instruments are designed to be self-calibrating with microprocessor-controlled timed intervals of calibration.

Other instruments perform point-of-care or bedside testing. Almost all manufacturers now produce small, portable, stand-alone, easy-to-operate instruments designed for "satellite lab" operations; several handheld devices that use disposable electrodes are also available.

Electrodes
The tip of the pH-measuring electrode typically used in blood gas analyzers is made of H^+-sensitive glass, and, aside from miniaturization, most pH-measuring and reference electrodes differ little from those of free-standing pH meters. The membrane of the PCO_2 electrode usually consists of Teflon or silicone rubber that is approximately 25 μm thick. The electrolyte solution is a thin film containing sodium bicarbonate at 0.005 mol/L and sodium chloride (NaCl) at 0.1 mol/L saturated with AgCl. A spacer of nylon net or cellophane lies between the solution and the H^+-sensitive glass of the measuring element proper. As CO_2 diffuses from the sample into the

electrolyte solution, the slight rise in $[H^+]$ from its hydration reaction is measured as ΔpH by an especially sensitive potentiometer and is transformed electronically to Δlog PCO_2. The membrane of a PO_2 electrode in a standard blood gas analyzer is usually ≈20-μm-thick polypropylene. The electrolyte solution is a thin film of phosphate buffer saturated with AgCl but also containing potassium chloride (KCl); it is in contact with the polarized platinum cathode and the Ag/AgCl anode. As O_2 diffuses into the electrolyte, it reacts with the cathode to cause current to flow; the generated current is measured.

Maintenance of Instrumentation
Sophistication of contemporary equipment and availability of high-quality calibrator materials have made reliable and accurate determination of blood pH and gases primarily a matter of (1) meticulous maintenance, (2) adherence to the manufacturer's recommended procedures, (3) control of the equipment and (4) proper collection and handling of specimens. The frequency with which maintenance should be scheduled is in direct proportion to the volume of analyses performed in the laboratory. The manufacturer's suggested schedule should be considered a minimum guideline, with reliance on experience to indicate maintenance frequency.

Quality Assurance and Quality Control
Elements of good quality assurance of blood gas and pH measurements include (1) proper maintenance of the instrument, (2) use of control materials, (3) verification of electrode linearity, (4) checking of barometer accuracy, and (5) accurate measurement of temperature.

External quality assurance (proficiency testing) mandated by federal law in the United States (Clinical Laboratory Improvement Amendments [CLIA] '88) has assumed new importance for quality control of blood gas analysis. These rules became effective in January 1991, and set criteria for satisfactory interlaboratory performance are as follows: (1) pH, target value ± 0.04; (2) PO_2, target value ± 3 SD; and (3) PCO_2, target value ± 8% or ± 5 mm Hg, whichever is greater.

Newer analyzers, particularly the smaller satellite laboratory and point-of-care instruments, frequently have an "auto quality control (QC)" feature or use "electronic QCs." Auto QC consists of onboard QC material that is automatically analyzed by the instrument at designated intervals that fulfill regulatory requirements. Electronic QC, which is most common in devices with disposable electrode cartridges, consists of cartridges that verify the electronic specifications of the instruments.

Blood-Based and Fluorocarbon-Based Control Materials
Commercial blood-based control material usually consists of tanned human erythrocytes suspended in buffered medium and sealed in vials with a gas mixture of known O_2 and CO_2 content. Nonblood fluorocarbon materials with O_2-carrying properties similar to those of blood are also available. Unopened, these types of control materials have a long shelf life in the refrigerator (e.g., 20 to 28 days for tanned erythrocytes and even longer for the others).

Aqueous Fluid Control Materials

These materials consist of a buffered medium sealed in vials with gas mixtures; the fluid is equilibrated with the gas by vigorous shaking by hand immediately before the vial is opened, and a sample is admitted to the instrument. Disadvantages of aqueous controls stem from their dissimilarity to blood. Lower viscosity and surface tension confer different washout characteristics and impair their ability to reflect clogging. Greater electrical conductivity reduces their effectiveness in detecting inadequate grounding, and lower thermal coefficients make them slower to detect failures of temperature control. These disadvantages are most apparent with respect to PO_2, for which a fluorocarbon-based matrix is superior. Nevertheless, aqueous commercial controls are far and away the most common QC materials used for blood gas analysis.

Reference Intervals

Reference intervals for arterial blood PO_2, SO_2, PCO_2, and pH are listed in Chapter 50. Values for PO_2 and PCO_2 will decrease with increasing altitude, but compensatory mechanisms keep pH values the same. The P_{50} corrected to pH 7.40 is 18 to 24 mm Hg for newborns and 24 to 29 mm Hg for adults. PCO_2 values decrease with altitude above sea level at a rate of 3 mm Hg/km (5 mm Hg/mile). A physiological change occurs with change in posture; PCO_2 is 2 to 4 mm Hg higher for a sitting or standing person than for one in the supine position. During pregnancy, PCO_2 falls gradually to a mean of about 28 mm Hg just before term.

Temperature Control and Correction

In the Henderson-Hasselbalch equation, pK' and α are used as constants for a temperature of 37 °C. The temperature-controlled sample chamber of an instrument is specified to be 37 ± 0.1 °C. The body temperature of a febrile patient may be elevated to 40 °C to 41 °C, or a patient may be made hypothermic for some surgeries and have a temperature as low as 23 °C. Most blood gas instruments are able to calculate temperature-corrected pH and PCO_2. Correction of pH and PCO_2 to the actual temperature of the patient is usually omitted in states of hyperthermia. However, significant disagreement exists with respect to hypothermic states. Two basic strategies are used by anesthetists in managing hypothermic patients. With the pH-stat method, the measured pH is corrected to the actual body temperature of the patient and then is maintained as close to 7.4 as possible by introducing 3% to 5% CO_2 into the inhaled ventilator gas. Alternatively, with the α-stat strategy, uncorrected values are used to keep pH and PCO_2 close to the 37 °C reference value. In practice, the α-stat method is used, primarily because it is technically easier to perform.

---

†A technique in which arterial carbon dioxide tension and pH are maintained at 5.3 kPa (40 mm Hg) and 7.40 when measured at +37 °C. When a patient is cooled down, the pH value will increase, and if measured at the patient's temperature, the PCO_2 value and the PO_2 value will decrease with lowering of the temperature.

Continuous and Noninvasive Monitoring of Blood Gases

Pulse oximeters that continuously monitor SO_2Hb are common and are generally reliable. Transcutaneous monitoring of PCO_2 and PO_2 is a noninvasive continuous monitoring approach that has particular value and general success in neonatal and pediatric care. Transcutaneous monitoring of PO_2 will sometimes vary widely depending on whether the site of application reflects arterial, capillary, or venous blood flow. However, because little difference is noted between arterial and venous PCO_2, transcutaneous monitoring of PCO_2 is less problematic, and pulse oximeters often serve as a surrogate for PO_2.

Review Questions

1. Hemolysis of a plasma sample will most likely affect which of the following, and why?
   a. Sodium; it is present in equal amounts both intracellularly and extracellularly
   b. Glucose; it moves out of cells into plasma
   c. Insulin; it is the major intracellular anion and is present in high amounts in RBCs
   d. Potassium; it is localized mainly within cells, particularly RBCs

2. Which of the following equations is the correct Henderson-Hasselbalch equation?
   a. $pK' = pH + \log [cHCO_3]/[cH_2CO_3]$
   b. $pK' = pH + \log [cH_2CO_3]/[cHCO_3]$
   c. $pH = pK' + \log [cHCO_3]/[c H_2CO_3]$
   d. $pH = pK' + \log [c H_2CO_3]/[cHCO_3]$

3. Oxygen is transported in blood in two forms. Which of the following is the most prevalent method of transport?
   a. As carboxyhemoglobin
   b. Dissolved in body fluid
   c. Attached to carbon dioxide
   d. As oxyhemoglobin

4. The major extracellular anion is
   a. sodium
   b. potassium.
   c. chloride.
   d. carbon dioxide.

5. Circulating levels of sodium are ultimately regulated by which of the following?
   a. Kidneys
   b. Diet
   c. Gastrointestinal tract
   d. Hemoglobin saturation

6. The correct formula for calculating the SO_2% (oxygen saturation) of arterial blood is which of the following?
   a. ([oxyhemoglobin + deoxyhemoglobin]/oxyhemoglobin) × 100
   b. (oxyhemoglobin/[oxyhemoglobin + deoxyhemoglobin]) × 100
   c. (deoxyhemoglobin/[oxyhemoglobin + deoxyhemoglobin]) × 100
   d. (oxyhemoglobin/deoxyhemoglobin) × 100

7. Which of the following are causes of decreased PO_2?
   a. Elevated RBC count
   b. Defective alveoli in the lungs
   c. Increased hemoglobin concentration
   d. All of the above are correct

8. The oxygen dissociation curve is a graphic plot of
   a. the number of circulating erythrocytes.
   b. the normality of the hemoglobin structure.
   c. oxygen saturation of hemoglobin at a specific PO_2.
   d. the pressure of O_2 at 50 g/dL of hemoglobin.

9. If solute is added to pure solvent, the colligative properties of that solution are altered. The freezing point of a solution is beyond that of pure solvent when solute is added to solvent.
   a. lowered
   b. raised
   c. not changed

10. In the body, total CO_2, hydrogen ion, and HCO_3^- concentrations are interrelated. This can be illustrated by a formula. Fill in the blanks (a, b, and c) to correctly complete this formula:

$$a + H_2O \rightleftharpoons b \rightleftharpoons HCO_3 + c$$

   a. $a = CO_2$; $b = H$; $c = H_2CO_3$
   b. $a = H_2CO_3$; $b = CO_2$; $c = H$
   c. $a = H$; $b = H_2CO_3$; $c = CO_2$
   d. $a = CO_2$; $b = H_2CO_3$; $c = H$

References

1. Apple FS, Koch DD, Graves S, Ladenson JH. Relationship between direct-potentiometric and flame-photometric measurement of sodium in blood. Clin Chem 1982;28:1931–5.
2. Bisson J, Younker J. Correcting arterial blood gases for temperature: (when) is it clinically significant? Nurs Crit Care 2006;11:232–8.
3. Brydon WG, Roberts LB. The effect of haemolysis on the determination of plasma constituents. Clin Chim Acta 1972;41:435–8.
4. Clinical and Functional Translation of CFTR (CFTR2). Toronto, Ontario, Canada: US CF Foundation, Johns Hopkins University, The Hospital for Sick Children. www.cftr2.org (accessed on November 7, 2012).
5. CLSI (Clinical and Laboratory Standards Institute). Sweat testing: sample collection and quantitative chloride analysis: approved guideline, 3rd edition. C34–A3. Wayne, Pa: CLSI, 2009.
6. CLSI (Clinical and Laboratory Standards Institute). Blood gas and pH analysis and related measurements. C46–A2. Wayne, Pa: CLSI, 2009.
7. CLSI (Clinical and Laboratory Standards Institute). Newborn screening for cystic fibrosis: approved guideline, 1st edition. ILA35-A (New code: NB505-A). Wayne, Pa: CLSI, 2011.
8. Don BR, Sebastian A, Cheitlin M, Christiansen M, Schambelan M. Pseudohyperkalemia caused by fist clenching during phlebotomy. N Engl J Med 1990;322:1290–2.
9. Farrell, P, Rosenstein B, White T, Accurso F, Castellani C, Cutting G. Guidelines for diagnosis of cystic fibrosis in newborns through older adults: Cystic Fibrosis Foundation Consensus Report. J Pediatr 2008;153:S4–S14.
10. Graber M, Subramani K, Corish D, Schwab A. Thrombocytosis elevates serum potassium. Am J Kidney Dis 1988;12:116–20.
11. Hammond KB, Turcios NL, Gibson LE. Clinical evaluation of the mac-roduct sweat collection system and conductivity analyzer in the diagnosis of cystic fibrosis. J Pediatr 1994;124:255–60.
12. LeGrys VA, McColley S, Zhanhai L, Farrell P. The need for quality improvement in sweat testing infants following newborn screening for cystic fibrosis. J Pediatr 2010;157:1035–7.
13. Nijsten MW, de Smet BJ, Dofferhoff AS. Pseudohyperkalemia and platelet counts. N Engl J Med 1991;325:1107.

Hormones*

Michael Kleerekoper, M.D., F.A.C.B., F.A.C.P., M.A.C.E.

Objectives

1. Define the following:

Amino acid–related hormone	Hormone
Autocrine system	Incretin
Calcitriol	Paracrine system
Endocrine system	Protein hormone
Endocrinology	Steroid hormone

2. Describe the three classifications of hormones; include examples of each, chemical structures, characteristics, half-life, and tissues of origin.
3. List and describe three physiological functions of hormones; include the role of hormones in each category and give examples of hormones in each category.
4. Compare the two types of receptor-hormone interactions; include examples of each type, postreceptor actions, and the specific effects that each type of interaction produces in a cell.
5. Provide examples of feedback mechanisms in the endocrine system.
6. List and describe four techniques used to assess hormones; include basic principles, specimen requirements, and an advantage of each technique.

Key Words and Definitions

Adenohypophysis The anterior glandular lobe of the pituitary gland.

Adenylate cyclase An enzyme of the lyase class that catalyzes the formation of 3′,5′-cyclic adenosine monophosphate (cAMP) from ATP.

Autocrine A mode of hormone action in which a cell secretes a hormone that binds to autocrine receptors on that same cell, leading to changes in the cell.

Circadian rhythms Rhythmic repetition of certain phenomena in living organisms at about the same time each day.

Cyclic adenosine monophosphate (cAMP) A cyclic nucleotide that serves as an intracellular and, in some cases, extracellular "second messenger" mediating the action of many peptide or amine hormones.

Endocrine system The system of glands that release their secretions (hormones) directly into the circulatory system. In addition to the endocrine glands, included are the chromaffin and the neurosecretory systems.

Endocrinology The scientific study of the function and pathology of the endocrine glands.

First messenger A factor or hormone that binds to a receptor on the external surface of a cell and sets off a series of reactions that eventually convert a precursor into a second messenger.

Gonadotropin Any hormone that stimulates the gonads.

G-proteins Guanine nucleotide-binding proteins (G-proteins) are a family of proteins involved in transmitting chemical signals outside the cell, and causing changes inside the cell. They communicate signals from many hormones, neurotransmitters, and other signaling factors.

G-protein–coupled receptors (GPCR) A large superfamily of membrane receptors whose intracellular effects are mediated by G proteins.

Half-life In endocrinology, the time required for a hormone to fall to half its original concentration in the specified fluid or blood.

Homeostasis The maintenance of equilibrium of internal body functions in response to external changes.

Hormone A chemical substance that has a specific regulatory effect on the activity of a certain organ or organs on cell types.

Incretin Any of various gastrointestinal hormones and factors that act as potent stimulators of insulin secretion, such as gastric inhibitory polypeptide.

Neurohypophysis The posterior lobe of the pituitary gland, making up the neural portion that secretes various hormones.

Paracrine A type of hormone function in which hormone synthesized in and released from endocrine cells binds to its receptor in nearby cells of a different type and affects their function.

*The author gratefully acknowledges the original contribution by Dr. Ronald J. Whitley on which portions of this chapter are based.

Phospholipase C Any esterase that catalyzes the hydrolysis of the phosphoric ester bond of a membrane phospholipid, generating a phosphorylated alcohol and diacylglycerol.

Pituitary gland A small oval gland attached to the base of the vertebrate brain and consisting of an anterior and a posterior lobe (also known as the *hypophysis* and the *pituitary body*).

Receptor A molecular structure within a cell or on the surface characterized by (1) selective binding of a specific substance and (2) a specific physiological effect that accompanies the binding; examples include (1) cell surface receptors for peptide hormones, neurotransmitters, antigens, complement fragments and immunoglobulins, and (2) cytoplasmic receptors for steroid hormones.

Second messenger Any of several classes of intracellular signals that translate electrical or chemical messages from the environment (first messengers) into cellular responses.

Zinc finger protein Any of a class of nucleic acid–binding proteins that also contain one or more zinc-binding domains (tandemly repeated, highly conserved stretches of 28 nucleotides).

A **hormone** is a chemical substance produced in the body by (1) an organ, (2) cells of an organ, or (3) scattered cells that has a specific regulatory effect on the activity of an organ or organs.[15] Hormones are produced at one site in the body (Figure 25-1) and exert their action(s) at distant sites through what is called the (1) **endocrine system**. It is increasingly recognized that many hormones exert actions locally on nearby cells through what is termed (2) **paracrine** action. Finally, some hormones exert their action on the cells of origin, through (3) **autocrine** action. Examples of the classic endocrine hormones include (1) insulin, (2) thyroxine, and (3) cortisol. Neurotransmitters and neurohormones are examples of the paracrine system, and certain growth factors that stimulate synthesis and secretion of true hormones from the same cell are examples of an autocrine system.

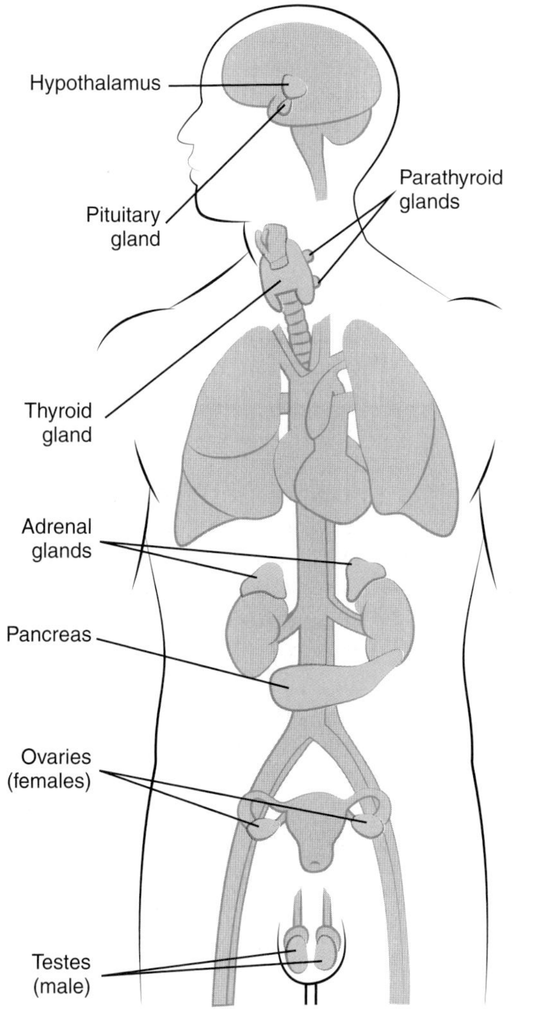

Table 25-1 lists hormones that are commonly measured in clinical practice plus a few others to illustrate concepts. Biochemical, clinical, and analytical information for specific hormones are presented in Chapters 33 and 40 through 44.

Classification

Hormones are classified chemically as (1) polypeptides or proteins, (2) steroids, or (3) derivatives of amino acids.

Polypeptide or Protein Hormones

Examples of polypeptide or protein hormones include (1) adrenocorticotropic hormone (ACTH), (2) insulin, and (3) parathyroid hormone (PTH). They are generally water soluble and circulate freely in plasma as the whole molecule or as active or inactive fragments. The **half-life** of these hormones in plasma is short (≤10 to 30 minutes), and wide fluctuations in their concentration may be seen in several physiological and pathological circumstances. These hormones initiate their response by binding to cell membrane **receptors** (on or in the membrane) and exciting a "**second messenger**" system, which continues the specific actions of these hormones.

Steroid Hormones

Steroid hormones such as cortisol and estrogen are hydrophobic and insoluble in water. These hormones circulate in plasma, reversibly bound to transport proteins with only a small fraction free, or unbound, and available to exert physiological action.[5,8,17] The half-life of steroid hormones is 30 to 90 minutes. Free steroid hormones, being hydrophobic, enter the cell by passive diffusion and bind with intracellular receptors in the cytoplasm or the nucleus.[3]

Amino Acid–Related Hormones

Thyroxine and catecholamine are examples of hormones that are derived from amino acids; they are water soluble and

Figure 25-1 Location of the endocrine glands in humans.

Labels: Hypothalamus, Pituitary gland, Thyroid gland, Adrenal glands, Pancreas, Ovaries (females), Testes (male), Parathyroid glands

TABLE 25-1 Major Hormones and Frequently Measured Hormone Precursors and Cytokines

Endocrine Organ and Hormone	Chemical Nature of Hormone	Major Sites of Action	Principal Actions
Hypothalamus			
Thyrotropin-releasing hormone (TRH)	Peptide (3aa,* Glu-His-Pro)	Anterior pituitary	Release of TSH and prolactin (PRL)
Gonadotropin-releasing hormone (GnRH) or luteinizing hormone-releasing hormone (LH-RH)	Peptide (10aa)	Anterior pituitary	Release of LH and FSH
Corticotropin-releasing hormone (CRH)	Peptide (41aa)	Anterior pituitary	Release of ACTH and β-lipotropic hormone (LPH)
Growth hormone-releasing hormone (GH-RH)	Peptides (40, 44aa)	Anterior pituitary	Release of growth hormone (GH)
Somatostatin† (SS) or growth hormone-inhibiting hormone (GH-IH)	Peptides (14, 28aa)	Anterior pituitary	Suppression of secretion of many hormones (e.g., GH, TSH, gastrin, vasoactive intestinal polypeptide [VIP], gastric inhibitory polypeptide [GIP], secretin, motilin, glucagon, and insulin)
Prolactin-releasing peptide	Peptide (20aa)	Anterior pituitary	Release of PRL
Prolactin-releasing/inhibiting factor	Dopamine	Anterior pituitary	Suppression of synthesis and secretion of PRL
Anterior Pituitary Lobe			
Thyrotropin or thyroid-stimulating hormone (TSH)	Glycoprotein, heterodimer‡ (α, 92aa; β, 112aa)	Thyroid gland	Stimulation of thyroid hormone formation and secretion
Follicle-stimulating hormone (FSH)	Glycoprotein, heterodimer‡ (α, 92aa; β, 117aa)	Ovary	Growth of follicles with LH, secretion of estrogens, and ovulation
		Testis	Development of seminiferous tubules; spermatogenesis
Luteinizing hormone (LH)	Glycoprotein, heterodimer‡ (α, 92aa; β, 121aa)	Ovary	Ovulation; formation of corpora lutea; secretion of progesterone
		Testis	Stimulation of interstitial tissue; secretion of androgens
PRL	Peptide (199aa)	Mammary gland	Proliferation of mammary gland; initiation of milk secretion; antagonist of insulin action
Growth hormone (GH) or somatotropin	Peptide (191aa)	Liver	Production of IGF-1 (promoting growth)
		Liver and peripheral tissues	Anti-insulin and anabolic effects
Corticotropin or adrenocorticotropin (ACTH)	Peptide (39aa)	Adrenal cortex	Stimulation of adrenocortical steroid formation and secretion
β-Endorphin (β-END)‡§	Peptide (31aa)	Brain	Endogenous opiate; raising of pain threshold and influence on extrapyramidal motor activity
Chorionic gonadotropin (CG) or choriogonadotropin	Glycoprotein, heterodimer‡ (α, 92aa; β, 145aa)		
α-Melanocyte-stimulating hormone (α-MSH)	Peptide (13aa)	Skin	Dispersion of pigment granules, darkening of skin
Leu-enkephalin (LEK)†§ and met-enkephalin (MEK)†§	Peptide (5aa)	Brain	Same as β-endorphin
Posterior Pituitary Lobe			
Vasopressin or ADH	Peptide (9aa)	Arterioles renal tubules	Elevation of blood pressure; water reabsorption
Oxytocin	Peptide (9aa)	Smooth muscles (uterus, mammary gland)	Contraction; action in parturition and in sperm transport; ejection of milk
Pineal Gland			
Serotonin or 5-hydroxytryptamine (5-HT)	Indoleamine	Cardiovascular, respiratory, and gastrointestinal systems; brain	Neurotransmitter; stimulation or inhibition of various smooth muscles and nerves
Melatonin	Indoleamine	Hypothalamus	Suppression of gonadotropin and GH secretion; induction of sleep
Thyroid Gland			
Thyroxine (T_4) and triiodothyronine (T_3)	Iodoamino acids	General body tissue	Stimulation of oxygen consumption and metabolic rate of tissue
Calcitonin or thyrocalcitonin	Peptide (32aa)	Skeleton	Uncertain in humans

TABLE 25-1 Major Hormones and Frequently Measured Hormone Precursors and Cytokines—cont'd

Endocrine Organ and Hormone	Chemical Nature of Hormone	Major Sites of Action	Principal Actions
Parathyroid Gland			
Parathyroid hormone (PTH) or parathyrin	Peptide (84aa)	Kidney	Increased calcium reabsorption, inhibited phosphate reabsorption; increased production of 1,25-dihydroxycholecalciferol
		Skeleton	Increased bone resorption
Adrenal Cortex			
Aldosterone	Steroid	Kidney	Salt and water balance
Androstenedione¶¶	Steroid	Hormone precursor	Conversion to estrogens and testosterone
Cortisol	Steroid	Many	Metabolism of carbohydrates, proteins, and fats; anti-inflammatory effects; others
Dehydroepiandrosterone (DHEA) and dehydroepiandrostenedione sulfate (DHEAS)	Steroids	Hormone precursors	Conversion to estrogens and testosterone
17-Hydroxyprogesterone	Steroid	Hormone precursor	Conversion to cortisol
Adrenal Medulla			
Norepinephrine and epinephrine	Aromatic amines	Sympathetic receptors	Stimulation of sympathetic nervous system
Epinephrine		Liver and muscle, adipose tissue	Glycogenolysis / Lipolysis
Ovary			
Activin A	Peptides¶ 2 β_A-subunits	Pituitary, ovarian follicle	Stimulation of release of FSH; enhanced FSH action; inhibition of androgen production by theca cells
Activin B	Peptides¶ 2 β_B-subunits beta	See activin A above	See activin A above
DHEA and DHEAS	Steroids	Hormone precursors	Conversion to androstenedione
Estrogens	Phenolic steroids	Female accessory sex organs	Development of secondary sex characteristics
		Bone	Control of skeletal maturation, etc.
Follistatin	Peptides (288aa, 315aa)	Pituitary, ovarian follicles	Inhibition of FSH synthesis and secretion by binding of activin
Inhibin A	Peptide (α-subunit and β_A-subunit)	Hypothalamus, ovarian follicle	Inhibition of FSH secretion; stimulation of theca cell androgen production
Inhibin B	Peptide (α-subunit and β_B-subunit)	See inhibin A above	See inhibin A above
Progesterone	Steroid	Female accessory reproductive structure	Preparation of the uterus for ovum implantation, maintenance of pregnancy
Relaxin	Peptide**	Uterus	Inhibition of myometrial contraction
Testis			
Inhibin B	See above	Anterior pituitary, hypothalamus	Control of LH and FSH secretion
Testosterone	Steroid	Male accessory sex organs	Development of secondary sex characteristics, maturation, and normal function
Placenta			
Estrogens	See above	See above	See above
Progesterone	See above	See above	See above
Relaxin	See above	See above	See above
Chorionic gonadotropin (CG) or choriogonadotropin	Glycoprotein, heterodimer‡ (α, 92aa; β, 145aa)	Same as LH	Same as LH; prolongation of corpus luteal function
Placental growth hormone (GH-V)	Peptides (22 and 26 kDa)	Same as GH	Same as GH
Chorionic somatomammotropin (CS) or placental lactogen (PL)	Peptide (191aa)	Same as PRL	Same as PRL
Pancreas			
Amylin	Peptide (37aa)	Pancreas	Inhibition of glucagon and insulin secretion
Glucagon	Peptide (29aa)	Liver	Glycogenolysis
Insulin	Peptide††	Liver, fat, muscle	Regulation of carbohydrate metabolism; lipogenesis

Continued

TABLE 25-1   Major Hormones and Frequently Measured Hormone Precursors and Cytokines—cont'd

Endocrine Organ and Hormone	Chemical Nature of Hormone	Major Sites of Action	Principal Actions
Pancreas—cont'd			
Pancreatic polypeptide (PP)	Peptide (36aa)	Gastrointestinal tract	Increased gut motility and gastric emptying; inhibition of gallbladder contraction
Somatostatin (SS)§	Peptide (14aa)	Pancreas	Inhibition of secretion of insulin, glucagon
Gastrointestinal Tract			
Gastrin§	Peptide (17aa)	Stomach	Secretion of gastric acid, gastric mucosal growth
Ghrelin§ (GHRP)	Peptide (28aa)	Anterior pituitary	Secretion of GH
Secretin	Peptide (27aa)	Pancreas	Secretion of pancreatic bicarbonate and digestive enzymes
Cholecystokinin-pancreozymin (CCK-PZ)§	Peptide (33aa)	Gallbladder and pancreas	Stimulation of gallbladder contraction and secretion of pancreatic enzymes
Motilin	Peptide (22aa)	Gastrointestinal tract	Stimulation of gastrointestinal motility
VIP§	Peptide (28aa)	Gastrointestinal tract	Neurotransmitter; relaxation of smooth muscles of gut and of circulation; increased release of hormones and secretion of water and electrolytes from pancreas and gut
Gastric inhibitory peptide (GIP)	Peptide (42aa)	Gastrointestinal tract	Inhibition of gastric secretion and motility; increase in insulin secretion
Glucagon-like peptide-1	Peptide (30-31aa)	Gastrointestinal tract	Increased insulin and decreased glucagon secretion; inhibition of gastric emptying
Bombesin§	Peptide (14aa)	Gastrointestinal tract	Stimulation of release of various hormones and pancreatic enzymes, smooth muscle contractions and hypothermia, changes in cardiovascular and renal function
Neurotensin§	Peptide (13aa)	Gastrointestinal tract and hypothalamus	Uncertain
Substance P (SP)§	Peptide (11aa)	Gastrointestinal tract and brain	Sensory neurotransmitter, analgesic; increase in contraction of gastrointestinal smooth muscle; potent vasoactive hormone; promotion of salivation, increased release of histamine
Kidney			
1,25-$(OH)_2$ cholecalciferol	Sterol	Intestine	Facilitation of absorption of calcium and phosphorus; increase in bone resorption in conjunction with PTH
		Bone	
		Kidney	Increase in reabsorption of filtered calcium
Erythropoietin	Peptide (165aa)	Bone marrow	Stimulation of red cell formation
Renin-angiotensin-aldosterone system	Peptides (renin, 297aa; Ang I, 10aa; Ang II, 8aa, produced from Ang I by angiotensin-converting enzyme)	Renin (from kidney) catalyzes hydrolysis of angiotensinogen (from liver, 485aa) to Ang I in the intravascular space	Increased blood pressure and stimulation of secretion of aldosterone (see adrenal) by Ang II
Liver			
IGF-1, formerly called somatomedin	Peptide (70aa)	Most cells	Stimulation of cellular and linear growth
IGF-2	Peptide (67aa)	Most cells	Insulin-like activity
Thymus			
Thymosin and thymopoietin	Peptides (28, 49aa)	Lymphocytes	Maturation of T lymphocytes
Heart			
Atrial natriuretic peptide (ANP, atriopeptin)	Peptide with an intrachain disulfide bond (28aa)	Vascular, renal, and adrenal tissues	Regulation of blood volume and blood pressure
B-type natriuretic peptide (BNP)	Peptide with an intrachain disulfide bond (32aa)	Vascular, renal, and adrenal tissues	Regulation of blood volume and blood pressure

TABLE 25-1	Major Hormones and Frequently Measured Hormone Precursors and Cytokines—cont'd		
Endocrine Organ and Hormone	**Chemical Nature of Hormone**	**Major Sites of Action**	**Principal Actions**
Adipose Tissue			
Adiponectin	Peptide oligomers of 30-kDa subunits	Muscle Liver	Increased fatty acid oxidation Suppression of glucose formation
Leptin	Peptide (167aa)	Hypothalamus	Inhibition of appetite, stimulation of metabolism
Resistin	Peptide (94aa)	Liver	Insulin resistance
Multiple Cell Types			
Estrogens	See above	See above	See above
Galanin	Peptide (30aa)	Brain, pancreas, GI tract	Regulation of food intake, memory, and cognition; inhibition of endocrine and exocrine secretions of pancreas; delayed gastric emptying; prolonged colonic transport times
Parathyroid hormone-related peptide (PTH-RP)	Peptides (139, 141, 173aa)	Kidney, bone	Physiological function conjectural; PTH-like actions; tumor marker
Growth factors (e.g., epidermal growth factor, fibroblast growth factor, transforming growth factor family, platelet-derived growth factor, nerve growth factors)	Peptides	Many	Stimulation of cellular growth
Monocytes/Lymphocytes/Macrophages			
Cytokines (e.g., interleukins 1 to 18, tumor necrosis factor, interferons)	Peptides	Many	Stimulation or inhibition of cellular growth; other

*aa, Amino acid residues.
†Also produced by gastrointestinal tract and pancreas.
‡Glycoprotein hormones composed of two dissimilar peptides. The α-chains are similar in structure or identical; the β-chains differ among hormones and confer specificity.
§Androstenedione is also produced in the ovary and testis.
¶Two chains linked by two disulfide bonds: α, 24aa; β, 29aa.
**Also produced in the brain.
††Two chains linked by two disulfide bonds: α, 21aa; β, 30aa.
¶¶Each activin and inhibin is found in multiple forms.

circulate in plasma bound to proteins (thyroxine) or free (catecholamines). Thyroxine binds avidly to three binding proteins and has a half-life of about 7 to 10 days in the circulation; free and unbound catecholamines such as epinephrine have a very short half-life of a minute or less. Like the water-soluble peptide and protein hormones, these hormones interact with membrane-associated receptors and use a second messenger system.

Release and Action of Hormones

The physiological functions of hormones have been broadly categorized into those that (1) affect growth and development, (2) exert homeostatic control of metabolic pathways, and (3) regulate the production, use, and storage of energy. The descriptions that follow illustrate examples of these functions and mechanisms of control of hormone secretion.

Growth and Development

Normal growth and development of the whole human organism are dependent on the complex integrative function of many hormones, including (1) gonadal steroids (estrogenic and androgenic), (2) growth hormone, (3) cortisol, and (4) thyroxine. Also, several **pituitary** hormones are responsible specifically for the growth and development of endocrine glands themselves, and thus are responsible for control of synthesis and secretion of

other hormones. Those other hormones provide negative feedback on secretion of the pituitary hormones. Other regulators of secretion of the pituitary hormones include **circadian rhythms** and a hypothalamic pulse generator that controls the pulsatile secretion of gonadotropins. Examples of hormones of the anterior pituitary gland (**adenohypophysis**) include the following:

- **Gonadotropins** (such as luteinizing hormone [LH] and follicle-stimulating hormone [FSH]) regulate the (1) development, (2) growth, and (3) function of the ovary and testis (see Chapter 43). Ovarian and testicular hormones in turn regulate (1) pubertal growth, (2) development and maintenance of secondary sex characteristics, (3) growth, (4) development, (5) maintenance of the skeleton and muscles, and (6) distribution of body fat
- ACTH regulates growth of the adrenal glands and synthesis and secretion of adrenal gland hormones (see Chapters 40 and 41)
- Thyroid-stimulating hormone (TSH) regulates growth of the thyroid gland and iodination of amino acids to produce the thyroid hormones triiodothyronine and thyroxine (see Chapter 42)[1]

Homeostatic Control of Metabolic Pathways

Homeostasis is defined as the ability or tendency of an organism or cell to maintain internal equilibrium by adjusting its physiological processes. Hormones are key to this maintainance, and the metabolic pathways under hormonal control are diverse and complex. The following important examples illustrate the feedback control of hormone secretion, which is critical for homeostasis:

- *Regulation of blood glucose:* In response to a glucose load (as with feeding), insulin is promptly released from the pancreas, which regulates the dispersal of glucose into cells (fat, muscle, liver, and brain) for the metabolism necessary to produce energy from glucose (see Chapter 33). As circulating glucose concentrations return to preload concentrations, insulin secretion slows. Several counter-regulatory hormones come into play to further regulate this process to ensure that blood glucose concentrations do not become too low. These include (1) glucagon, (2) cortisol, (3) epinephrine, and (4) growth hormone. In addition, attention has focused on a group of gastrointestinal hormones termed incretins (see Chapter 33) that are released during eating and stimulate insulin secretion from the pancreas in advance of any measurable increase in blood glucose. Incretins also affect the rate of absorption of nutrients from the gut by slowing down the rate of gastric emptying. Another mechanism by which incretins have a role in the regulation of blood glucose is by delaying release of the counter-regulatory hormone glucagon from the α-cells of the pancreatic islets. The most studied incretins are glucagon-like peptide-1 (GLP-1) and gastric inhibitory peptide (GIP).

- *Regulation of serum calcium* (see Chapter 39): The calcium-sensing receptor (CaSR) on the parathyroid gland recognizes the circulating concentration of ionized calcium, which, in turn, regulates the synthesis and secretion of PTH. For example, when ionized calcium concentrations fall, PTH synthesis and secretion are stimulated. This additional PTH will attempt to return the serum ionized calcium concentration to the previous level. PTH acts by enhancing renal tubular reabsorption of calcium and calcium efflux from the skeleton. PTH also catalyzes the synthesis of the renal hormone calcitriol (1,25-dihydroxy-vitamin D), which acts on the gut to increase intestinal absorption of calcium. These very rapid responses of PTH and calcitriol quickly restore ionized calcium to concentrations at which the CaSR is no longer activated, and PTH and calcitriol synthesis and secretion return to basal rates.

- *Water and electrolyte metabolism:* The metabolism of water and electrolytes is regulated by (1) aldosterone from the adrenal gland, (2) renin from the kidney, and (3) vasopressin (antidiuretic hormone [ADH]) from the posterior pituitary gland (**neurohypophysis;** see Chapters 35, 40, and 41).

Regulation of the Production, Use, and Storage of Energy

Under normal conditions, regulation of energy (1) production, (2) use, and (3) storage is under tight hormonal control. More energy is required under several conditions such as (1) exercise, (2) starvation, (3) infection, (4) trauma, or (5) emotional stress. In such conditions, many hormones act to control not only circulating levels of nutrients but also the metabolism of these nutrients into necessary energy. This very complex activity, which involves hormones from different organs, as already alluded to in the preceding section, is under neurological control, with numerous neuroendocrine hormones participating actively in this integrative metabolic process. This affects most organs in the body and modulates, for example, (1) heart rate, (2) sweating, (3) fertility, and (4) reproduction.

Role of Hormone Receptors

The "unique" or specific action of a hormone on its target tissue is a function of the interaction between the hormone and its receptor. As discussed previously, several types of hormone-receptor interactions occur.[3,5,8,17] The hormone-receptor complex provides the very high specificity of the action of the hormone, allowing the target tissue to accumulate the hormone from among all the molecules to which it is exposed. This is essential because hormones generally circulate in picomolar or nanomolar concentrations (10^{-9} to 10^{-12} mol/L).

Hormone receptors may be on the cell surface or may be intracellular within the cytoplasm or nucleus.

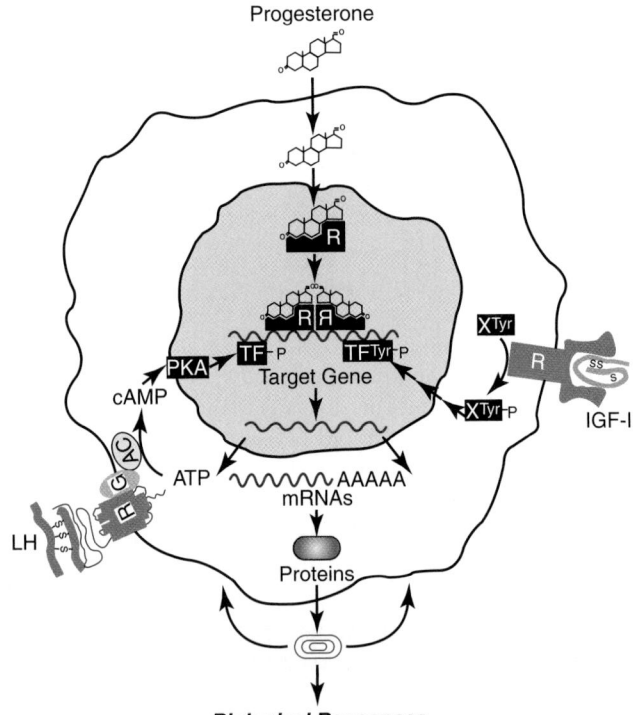

Figure 25-2 Hormonal signaling by cell surface and intracellular receptors. Receptors for the water-soluble polypeptide hormones, luteinizing hormone (LH), and insulin-like growth factor (IGF)-1, are integral membrane proteins located at the cell surface. They bind the hormone using extracellular sequences and transduce a signal through the generation of second messengers—cyclic adenosine monophosphate (cAMP) for the LH receptor and tyrosine-phosphorylated substrates for the IGF-1 receptor. Although effects on gene expression are indicated, direct effects on cellular proteins (e.g., ion channels) are also observed. In contrast, the receptor for the lipophilic steroid hormone progesterone resides in the cell nucleus. It binds the hormone and becomes activated and capable of directly modulating target gene transcription. *R,* Receptor molecule; *Tf,* transcription factor. *(From Conn PM, Melmed S. Textbook of endocrinology. Towanta NJ: Humana Press, 1997.)*

Cell Surface Receptors

Peptide hormones bind to cell surface receptors, and the conformational change resulting from this binding activates an effector system, which, in turn, is responsible for the downstream actions of the hormone (Figure 25-2).[11,12] For most peptide hormones, the intracellular effector that is activated by the hormone-receptor interaction is a specific **G-protein** (guanyl-nucleotide–binding protein),[4,10,13,18] and such receptors are called **G-protein–coupled receptors** (GPCRs; Figure 25-3). The major structural classes of GPCRs have been identified, each containing receptors for specific subsets of hormones. Group I, the largest group, contains receptors for many peptide hormones and catecholamines. Group II contains receptors for gastrointestinal hormones such as (1) secretin, (2) glucagons, and (3) vasoactive intestinal polypeptide. Group III contains the CaSR and the glutamate receptor. Stimulation of a G-protein initiates the intracellular processes of signal transduction that characterize the specific action of the hormone. G-proteins are composed of α-, β-, and γ-subunits and are classified according to the α-subunits, of which 20 have been identified to date. Some G-proteins (G$_S$ type) stimulate the enzyme adenylate cyclase to produce the second messenger cAMP; other G proteins (G$_i$ type) inhibit adenylate cyclase.

The classes of GPCRs and G-proteins briefly described in this section provide some insight into the mechanisms responsible for the specificity of hormone action. Some nonpeptide hormones also use cell surface receptors.

Intracellular Receptors

Lipid-soluble hormones such as progesterone (see Figure 25-2) are transported in plasma bound to carrier proteins, with only a small fraction of the hormone present in the free or unbound state. The free hormone enters the cell via passive diffusion and binds to intracellular receptors. The receptors may be in the cytoplasm or, more often, the nucleus, and may move between subcellular compartments (see Figure 25-2). These receptors are characterized by (1) a hormone-binding domain, (2) a deoxyribonucleic acid (DNA)-binding domain, and (3) an amino-terminal variable domain. Just as the interaction of protein or polypeptide hormones with cell surface receptors changes the conformation of the receptor protein, the binding of a lipid-soluble hormone with its specific hormone-binding domain on the intracellular receptor changes the molecular conformation of the intracellular receptor. This conformational change, or activation of the receptor, enables the hormone-receptor complex to bind to specific regulatory DNA sequences of a target gene or genes, permitting control of specific gene expression (see Figure 25-2).[7]

Postreceptor Actions of Hormones

Cell surface and intracellular receptors have different mechanisms of action within cells.

Cell Surface Receptors

Once GPCRs are occupied by a hormone, G-protein subunits begin a cascade of activation of specific enzymes that

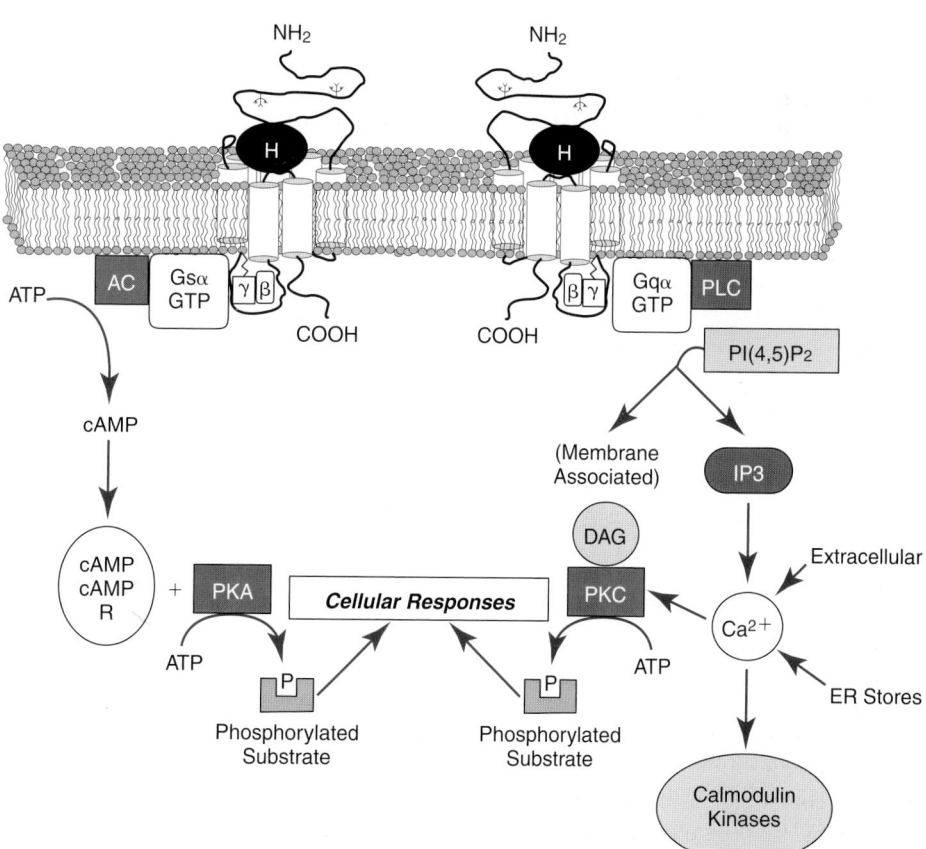

Figure 25-3 Signal transduction by cell surface receptors that are coupled to G-proteins. Two seven-transmembrane domains, coupled to different G-proteins (G$_S$ and G$_q$), are shown. Activation of G$_S$ leads to stimulation of the effector enzyme adenylate cyclase and production of a cyclic adenosine monophosphate (cAMP) second messenger, causing activation of protein kinase A (PKA) and the initiation of potential phosphorylation cascades. Activation of G$_q$ leads to stimulation of the effector enzyme phospholipase C-β and the production of inositol 1,4,5-trisphosphate (IP$_3$) and diacylglycerol (DAG) second messengers, one effect of which is to activate protein kinase C (PKC) and initiate a potential phosphorylation cascade. *(From Conn PM, Melmed S, eds. Textbook of endocrinology. Towanta NJ: Humana Press, 1997.)*

G-Protein–Coupled Receptor (GPCR) Superfamily

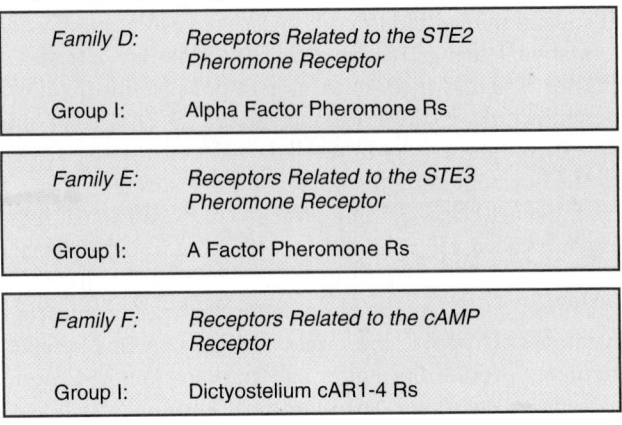

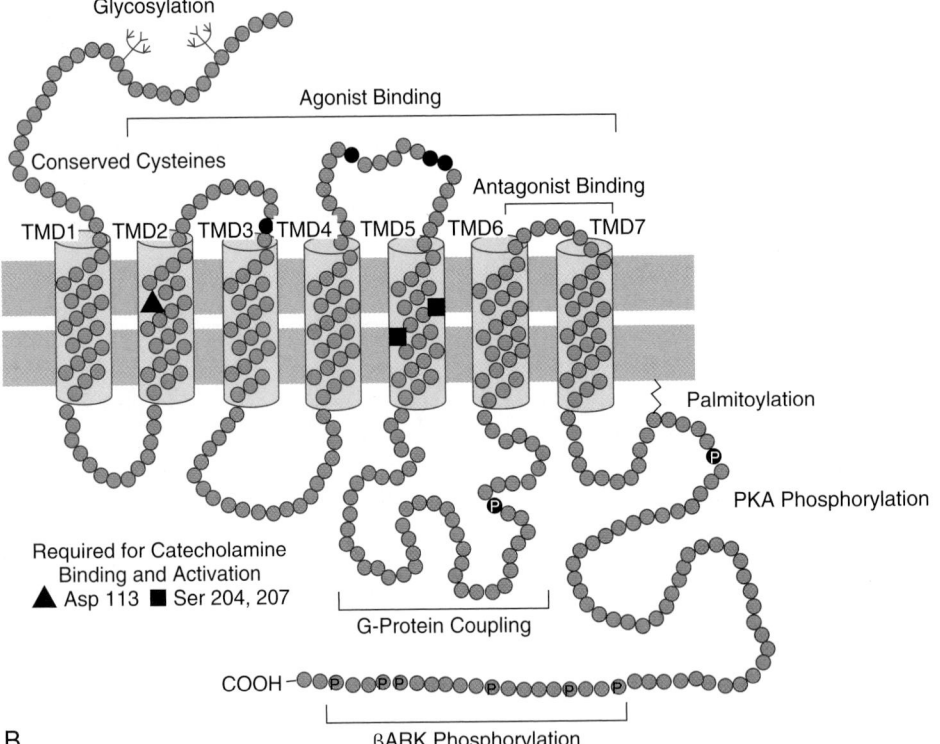

Figure 25-4 A, G protein–doubled receptor super family. **B,** Signaling by G_S. The α-, β-, and γ-subunits of G_s are shown. The α-subunit, when bound to guanosine triphosphate (GTP), activates adenylyl cyclase, which catalyzes the formation of cAMP from ATP. Then cAMP binds to the regulatory subunit (R) of protein kinase A (PKA, cAMP-dependent protein kinase), releasing the PKA catalytic subunit (C), thus leading to phosphorylation of target proteins.

generate molecules that serve as second messengers to affect the hormone response. The best known of these are (1) **adenylyl cyclase**, which generates **cyclic adenosine monophosphate (cAMP)**, and (2) **phospholipase C**, which generates both inositol 1,4,5-trisphosphate (IP_3) and diacylglycerol

(see Figure 25-3). The production of second messengers and the subsequent magnitude of the effect of the hormone are functions of the amount of hormone bound to the GPCR. The binding of a small number of hormone molecules on the cell surface leads to the production of many molecules of the second messenger, thus amplifying the signal sent by the hormone (which is considered the **first messenger**).

cAMP-dependent protein kinases (PKAs) are a family of enzymes that, in the presence of cAMP, phosphorylate a number of intracellular enzymes and other proteins to activate or inactivate the function of these enzymes and proteins. This process regulates their function. As a further means of regulating hormone action, these cAMP-dependent kinases consist of two catalytic and two regulatory subunits (C and R, respectively, in Figure 25-4). The regulatory subunits exist as a dimer (pair of subunits) that binds two molecules of cAMP. This binding releases the catalytic subunits, which then are active as phosphorylating enzymes, acting on serine and threonine residues in target proteins.

Phospholipase C (see Figure 25-3) acts on inositol phospholipids within the cell membrane to produce IP_3, which opens up ion channels to facilitate entry of (1) calcium into the cytoplasm, where it acts as a messenger, and (2) diacylglycerol, which modulates protein kinase C activity.

The insulin receptor represents a somewhat different class of cell surface receptors that contain intrinsic hormone-activated tyrosine kinase activity, that is, an activity to add phosphates to tyrosine residues in specific proteins. They do not otherwise involve a second messenger.[16] The insulin receptor, the prototype of this type of receptor, consists of two α- and two β-subunits joined by disulfide bridges. The extracellular hormone-binding domains are the α-subunits, and the β-subunits are intracellular. They contain an ATP-binding site and a catalytic kinase domain through which tyrosine kinase is activated immediately upon binding of insulin to the receptor.

Because hormones largely serve a regulatory function, of necessity many self-limiting steps are included in the previous processes. Without these self-limiting processes, hormone action would continue unabated. Cessation of hormone action of cAMP involves the inactivation of G-protein stimulation of adenylate cyclase by guanosine triphosphatase (GTPase) (Figure 25-5). In the absence of hormone interaction with the GPCR (basal or unstimulated state), G_s is bound to guanosine diphosphate (GDP). Once the hormone is bound to the receptor, GDP is released from G_s and is replaced by GTP, and the G_s-GTP complex activates adenylate cyclase. The G_s-GTP complex is inactivated by GTPase, restoring the G_s-GDP state, which cannot stimulate formation of cAMP until further hormone binding to the GPCR takes place. Within a few minutes (or less) of hormone-GPCR interaction and initiation of hormone action, the receptor is phosphorylated by protein kinase A and protein kinase C. This phosphorylation of the hormone receptor permits internalization of the complex from the cell surface into the cytoplasm. There, dephosphorylation occurs, permitting degradation of the hormone and recycling of the GPCR to its original transmembrane location, awaiting coupling with more hormone. In addition, one of the proteins that is phosphorylated and activated by PKA is an enzyme that breaks down cAMP, thus removing the key activator of PKA.

Intracellular Receptors

As previously noted, lipid-soluble hormones bind to the hormone-binding domain of cytosolic or nuclear receptors.[11,12]

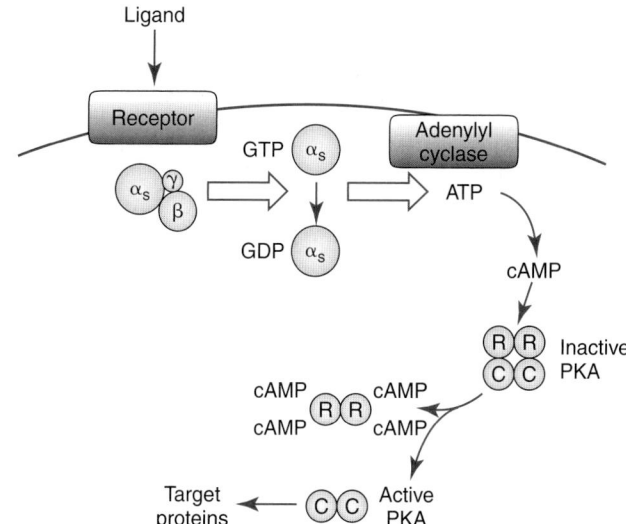

Figure 25-5 The G-protein cycle. The α-, β-, and γ-subunits of G_s are shown. The α-subunit, when bound to GTP, activates the effector molecule (such as adenylyl cyclase). GTP then is hydrolyzed to GDP, stopping activation of the effector molecule and leading to re-formation of the GDP-bound state of the G-protein.

This results in a conformational change that enables the hormone-receptor complex to bind to specific regulatory DNA sequences in the 5′ end of the target gene.[7] The binding specificity of the (hormone-bound) receptor for specific regions of DNA of the target gene is determined by **zinc finger protein** structures in the receptor's DNA-binding domain. It is the binding of the hormone-receptor complex to DNA regulatory elements that enhances or represses gene transcription. The messenger ribonucleic acid (RNA) that is enhanced or diminished by hormone-receptor binding to the target gene regulates the synthesis of specific proteins that mediate the hormone's physiological actions. The system is further regulated by the presence or absence of co-activators or co-repressors of gene expression. In addition, many actions of hormones that bind to intracellular receptors are rapid and do not depend on synthesis of protein, suggesting that these hormone-receptor complexes exert actions by mechanisms different from binding to DNA.

From these descriptions, it is possible for one to deduce both the complexity and the specificity of hormone action, in terms of an "on and/or off" concept and in terms of an "effect size" concept.

Measurements of Hormones and Related Analytes

Hormones are measured by a variety of analytical techniques, including (1) bioassay, (2) receptor assay, (3) immunoassay, and (4) instrumental techniques such as mass spectrometry interfaced with liquid or gas chromatography. A general overview of these techniques is given here with more detailed discussions found in Chapters 9 to 15. Also, analytical details for individual hormones using such techniques are found in the discussion of individual hormones in Chapters 40 through 43.

Bioassay Techniques

Bioassays are based on observations of physiological responses specific for the hormone being measured. In vivo bioassays usually involve the injection of test materials (such as blood or urine from a patient) into suitably prepared animals. Target gland responses such as growth or steroidogenesis are then measured. In vitro bioassays involve the incubation of (1) tissue, (2) membranes, (3) dispersed cells, or (4) permanent cell lines in a defined culture medium, with subsequent measurement of an appropriate hormone response. Most in vitro bioassays measure responses proximal or distal to a second messenger such as stimulation of cAMP formation. Bioassays, however, tend to be imprecise and are rarely necessary in clinical medicine.

Receptor-Based Assays

Receptor assays depend on the in vitro interaction of a hormone with its biological receptor. In this type of assay, unlabeled hormone displaces trace amounts of labeled hormone from receptor sites. A second approach is to measure a response, such as production of cAMP, when a test sample is added to a preparation that includes the receptor and necessary cofactors. In general, receptor assays are simpler to perform and are more sensitive than bioassays. Receptor assays also provide an advantage over immunoassays in that they reflect the biological function of a hormone, namely, the capacity to combine with specific receptor sites. By contrast, immunoassays may measure (1) active hormone, (2) inactive prohormone, (3) hormone polymer, and (4) metabolites when all share a common antigenic determinant or set of determinants. In general, receptor assays are not as sensitive as immunoassays, and enzymes in the biological specimen may degrade the receptor or destroy the labeled tracer. The added complexity and lability of receptor preparations also contribute to the limited application of these assays in the routine clinical laboratory.

Immunoassay Techniques

Immunoassays employing antibodies are widely used to quantify hormones (see Chapter 15). Currently labeled antibody (immunometric) assays with nonisotopic labels are the method of choice for measuring most hormones, especially peptides and proteins. Immunometric assays use saturating concentrations of two or more antibodies (often monoclonal) that are prepared against different epitopes of the protein molecule. One of the two antibodies is usually attached to a solid-phase separation system and extracts the hormone from the serum specimen. The second ("detection") antibody is linked to a signal molecule or "label". When the second antibody binds to the hormone, a "sandwich" is formed in which the hormone is in the middle, with an antibody on each side. At this point the whole sandwich is attached to the solid phase (such as plastic). When more hormone is present, more

labeled antibody is able to be bound. After washing away unbound labeled antibody, the label or signal that remains attached to the solid phase is then measured to quantify the bound hormone.

Instrumental Techniques

Mass spectrometers (see Chapter 13) coupled with gas and liquid chromatographs (see Chapter 12) are powerful qualitative and quantitative analytical tools that are widely used to measure hormones.[2,6,9,14] Technical advancements in mass spectrometry have resulted in the development of matrix-assisted laser desorption/ionization (MALDI) and electrospray ionization techniques that allow sequencing of peptides and mass determination of picomole quantities of analytes.

Compared with older methods, mass spectrometry offers greater analytical (1) sensitivity, (2) accuracy, and (3) speed, and allows simultaneous determination of multiple hormones related to a clinical condition.[14] Mass spectrometric methods are widely available to measure small molecules such as cortisol and, increasingly are used to measure even large peptide hormones and hormone precursors such as thyroglobulin.

Specimen Requirements

As seen from the brief descriptions of hormone action given previously and amplified in the hormone-specific chapters, particular attention must be paid to the clinical material sent to the laboratory for assay. Some hormones (such as insulin) are directly affected by intake of nutrients and others (such as cortisol) are affected by time of day. In many clinical circumstances, the metabolic environment plays a crucial role in hormone production, and it is essential to obtain a simultaneous sample for measurements of both the hormone and the molecule(s) regulated by that hormone. An isolated measurement of plasma insulin without concurrent knowledge of the plasma glucose, or measurement of parathyroid hormone independent of serum calcium, is of little value. For example, PTH concentrations in plasma should be very low when plasma calcium is high; failure of PTH to be suppressed is a sign of an overactive parathyroid gland.

When a patient is evaluated for possible hormone deficiency or hormone excess, it is often necessary to perform a stimulation or suppression test. Most hormone assays are performed on plasma or serum, and many are performed on urine samples, usually a 24-hour collection. Increasingly, saliva has become a convenient body fluid for hormone analysis, particularly for hormones secreted in a diurnal rhythm such as cortisol. Unlike blood sampling, patients are provided with salivary collection material such that they are able to provide to the laboratory specimens collected at multiple times during the day or at unusual (but biologically very relevant) times such as 21:00 (11:00 PM)—a commonly used time for obtaining a specimen for measurement of cortisol.

Review Questions

1. Steroid hormones, by binding specific nuclear receptors, have a direct effect on:
   a. enzyme phosphorylation.
   b. gene expression.
   c. cAMP formation.
   d DNA replication.

2. When a protein hormone binds a cell membrane receptor, the classical result is:
   a. phosphorylation of intracellular enzymes.
   b. inhibition of mRNA within the cell nucleus.
   c. replication of DNA and division of the cell.
   d. glycosylation of intracellular proteins.

3. An example of an amino acid–related hormone would be:
   a. testosterone.
   b. thyroid hormone.
   c. growth hormone.
   d. prostaglandin.

4. Which of the following hormones is classified as a polypeptide?
   a. Cortisol
   b. Estrogen
   c. Adrenocorticotropic hormone
   d. Thyroid hormone

5. The type of hormone assay that best reflects hormone functionality as opposed to quantification of the hormone itself is the:
   a. receptor-based assay.
   b. mass spectrometry–based assays.
   c. bioassay technique.
   d. liquid chromatography.

6. A hormone released from the pancreas in response to a glucose load that is involved in cellular energy production is considered to be involved in:
   a. modification of the response to stress.
   b. synthesis of milk proteins.
   c. promotion of bone development and growth
   d. homeostatic control of metabolism.

7. Which of the following is a characteristic of steroid hormones?
   a. Account for the majority of hormones
   b. Circulate freely
   c. Water soluble
   d. Long half-life in the circulation

References

1. Brent GA. The molecular basis of thyroid hormone action. N Engl J Med 1994;331:847–53.
2. Chace DH. Mass spectrometry in the clinical laboratory. Chem Rev 2001;101:445–77.
3. Edwards DP. The role of coactivators and corepressors in the biology and mechanism of action of steroid hormone receptors. J Mammary Gland Biol Neoplasia 2000;5:307–24.
4. Farfel Z, Bourne HR, Iiri T. The expanding spectrum of G protein disease. N Engl J Med 1999;340:1012–20.
5. Funder JW. Mineralocorticoids, glucocorticoids, receptors and response elements. Science 1993;259:1132–3.
6. Giese RW. Measurement of endogenous estrogens: analytical challenges and recent advances. J Chromatogr A 2003;1000:401–12.
7. Glass CK. Differential recognition of target genes by nuclear receptor monomers, dimers, and heterodimers. Endocr Rev 1994;15:391–407.
8. Klinge CM. Estrogen receptor interaction with estrogen response elements. Nucleic Acids Res 2001;29:2905–19.
9. Lagerstedt SA, O'Kane DJ. Measurement of plasma free metanephrine and normetanephrine by liquid chromatography-tandem mass spectrometry for diagnosis of pheochromocytoma. Clin Chem 2004;50:603–11.
10. Lefkowitz RJ. G proteins in medicine. N Engl J Med 1995;332:186–7.
11. Mangelsdorf DJ, Thummel C, Beato M, Herrlich P, Schutz G, Umesono K, et al. The nuclear receptor superfamily: the second decade. Cell 1995;83:835–9.
12. McKenna NJ, Lanz RB, O'Malley BW. Nuclear receptor coregulators: cellular and molecular biology. Endocr Rev 1999;20:321–44.
13. Neer EJ. Heterotrimeric G proteins: organizers of transmembrane signals. Cell 1995;80:249–57.
14. Nelson RE, Grebe SK, O'Kane DJ, Singh RJ. Liquid chromatography-tandem mass spectrometry assay for simultaneous measurement of estradiol and estrone in human plasma. Clin Chem 2004;50:373–84.
15. Newman WA. Dorland's illustrated medical dictionary, 30th edition. Philadelphia, Pa: WB Saunders, 2003.
16. Olefsky JM. The insulin receptor: a multifunctional protein. Diabetes 1990;39:1009–16.
17. Pike AC, Brzozowski AM, Hubbard RE. A structural biologist's view of the oestrogen receptor. J Steroid Biochem Mol Biol 2000;74:261–8.
18. Vaughan M. Signaling by heterotrimeric G proteins: minireview series. J Biol Chem 1998;273:667–713.

26 Catecholamines and Serotonin

Graeme Eisenhofer, Ph.D., Thomas G. Rosano, Ph.D., D.A.B.F.T., D.A.B.C.C., and Ronald J. Whitley, Ph.D., F.A.C.B., D.A.B.C.C

Objectives

1. Define the following terms:

5-HIAA	Metanephrine
Carcinoid	Neuroblastoma
Carcinoid syndrome	Normetanephrine
Catecholamine	Paraganglioma
Gastroenteropancreatic neuroendocrine tumor	Pheochromocytoma
	Serotonin
Homovanillic acid	

2. Discuss the following biogenic amines, including function and clinical relevance, synthesis, metabolism, and storage and release:

Norepinephrine	Serotonin
Epinephrine	Melatonin
Dopamine	

3. List the clinically relevant metabolites of the biogenic amines listed in Objective 2 above.

4. State the clinical significance and function of the catecholamines and serotonin in each of the following systems:

Central nervous system	Peripheral dopaminergic system
Sympathetic nervous system	
Adrenal medullary system	Enteric nervous system

5. Compare pheochromocytoma and neuroblastoma, including causes, symptoms, organ(s) and/or cell type involved, and laboratory evaluation of each; describe the clonidine suppression test and the results obtained when pheochromocytoma is present.

6. Explain the laboratory values obtained for serotonin and 5-HIAA in the assessment of a gastroenteropancreatic tumor and the carcinoid syndrome.

7. Describe the collection techniques used to obtain specimens for catecholamine, metanephrine, and serotonin analysis.

8. Describe how diet interferes with serotonin analysis; state how tricyclic antidepressants interfere in the measurement of catecholamines.

9. List the laboratory methods used to analyze metanephrines, catecholamines, serotonin, and 5-HIAA.

10. Analyze and solve case studies related to catecholamine and serotonin disorders using descriptions of symptoms and results of laboratory analyses.

Key Words and Definitions

Carcinoid syndrome A syndrome due to carcinoid tumors and characterized by attacks of severe cyanotic flushing of the skin—lasting from minutes to days—and by diarrheal watery stools, bronchoconstrictive attacks, sudden drops in blood pressure, edema, and ascites. Symptoms are caused by secretion from the tumor of serotonin, prostaglandins, and other biologically active substances.

Carcinoid tumor A yellow circumscribed tumor arising from enterochromaffin cells, usually in the small intestine, appendix, stomach, or colon, and less commonly in the bronchus; sometimes used alone to refer to the gastrointestinal tumor (called also *argentaffinoma*).

Catecholamine One of a group of biogenic amines having a sympathomimetic action, the aromatic portion of whose molecule is catechol, and the aliphatic portion an amine; examples include dopamine, norepinephrine, and epinephrine.

Catecholamine metabolites Products of catecholamine metabolism, such as dihydroxyphenylacetic acid, methoxytyramine, homovanillic acid, dihydroxyphenylglycol, methoxyhydroxyphenylglycol, normetanephrine, metanephrine, and vanillylmandelic acid.

Catechol-O-methyltransferase (COMT) An enzyme that degrades catecholamines.

Chromaffin cell Neuroendocrine cell derived from embryonic neural crest found in the medulla of the adrenal gland and in other ganglia of the sympathetic nervous system; so-named because of the presence of cytoplasmic granules that give a brownish reaction with chromium salts.

Key Words and Definitions — cont'd

3,4-Dihydroxyphenylglycol (DHPG) The metabolite produced within the peripheral sympathetic or central nervous system noradrenergic nerves by deamination of norepinephrine (can also be formed from epinephrine); *O*-methylated to methoxyhydroxyphenylglycol in extraneuronal tissues.

L-Dopa An amino acid—3,4-dihydroxyphenylalanine—produced by oxidation of tyrosine by tyrosine hydroxylase; the precursor of dopamine and an intermediate product in the biosynthesis of norepinephrine, epinephrine. Can also be formed in melanocytes by the actions of tyrosinase as part of the production of melanin.

Dopamine A catecholamine formed in the body by the decarboxylation of L-dopa; an intermediate product in the synthesis of norepinephrine; acts as a neurotransmitter in the central nervous system, produced peripherally and acts on peripheral receptors.

Enteric nervous system (ENS) An independent and integrated system of neurons and supporting cells.

Epinephrine (adrenaline) A catecholamine hormone secreted by the adrenal medulla.

Gastroenteropancreatic neuroendocrine tumor (GEP-NET) Encompasses neuroendocrine tumors of the digestive system and pancreas but also covers neuroendocrine pulmonary tumors and includes carcinoid tumorss.

Homovanillic acid (HVA) A product of dopamine metabolism; elevated urinary concentrations are used to diagnose neuroblastoma.

5-Hydroxyindoleacetic acid (5-HIAA) A metabolite of serotonin (5-hydroxytryptamine) that is excreted in large amounts by patients with carcinoid tumors.

Melatonin A hormone synthesized by the pineal gland in many species of animals; its secretion increases during exposure to light.

(MEN) Multiple endocrine neoplasia A group of rare genetic disorders characterized by hyperplasia and hyperfunction of two or more components of the endocrine system.

Metanephrine A catecholamine metabolite resulting from *O*-methylation of epinephrine; formed mainly within adrenal chromaffin cells; excreted mainly in the urine as a sulfate-conjugated metabolite; measurements of the free and conjugated metabolites provide useful tests for diagnosis of pheochromocytoma.

Methoxyhydroxyphenylglycol (MHPG) A metabolite of epinephrine and norepinephrine formed primarily from *O*-methylation of dihydroxyphenylglycol and in smaller amounts from deamination of normetanephrine and metanephrine; found in brain, blood, CSF, and urine, where its concentrations can be used to measure catecholamine turnover.

Neuroblastoma A sarcoma consisting of malignant neuroblasts, usually arising in the autonomic nervous system (sympathicoblastoma) or in the adrenal medulla; considered a type of neuroepithelial tumor that affects mostly infants and children up to 10 years of age.

Neuroendocrine tumors (NET) Neoplasms that arise from cells of the endocrine and peripheral nervous systems, most commonly in the digestive tract, but also found in the lung, pancreas, pituitary, thyroid, and other tissues.

Neurofibromatosis 1 (NF1) An autosomal dominant disorder due to mutation in the *NF1* gene.

Norepinephrine (noradrenaline) A major neurotransmitter produced by some brain neurons and peripheral sympathetic nerves that acts on α- and β_1-adrenergic receptors; produced in the adrenal chromaffin cells as a precursor for epinephrine.

Normetanephrine An *O*-methylated metabolite of norepinephrine produced in extraneuronal cells and the adrenal medulla; excreted in the urine largely as a sulfate-conjugated metabolite; measurements of free and conjugated metabolites provide useful tests for diagnosis of pheochromocytoma.

Paraganglioma A tumor of the tissue composing the paraganglia.

Parkinson disease A slowly progressive disorder affecting the basal ganglia, usually occurring in late life, with an average age of onset of 60 years.

Pheochromocytoma A usually benign, well-encapsulated, lobular, vascular tumor of chromaffin tissue of the adrenal medulla or sympathetic paraganglia.

Serotonin (5-hydroxytryptamine) A monoamine vasoconstrictor synthesized in the intestinal enterochromaffin cells or in central or peripheral neurons; found in high concentrations in many body tissues, including intestinal mucosa, pineal body, and central nervous system.

Vanillylmandelic acid (VMA) The main end-product of norepinephrine and epinephrine metabolism excreted in the urine; formed primarily in the liver from oxidation of methoxyhydroxyphenylglycol.

Catecholamines and serotonin are biogenic amines that facilitate neuronal or hormonal signaling for a wide range of physiological processes. The naturally occurring catecholamines, **dopamine** and **norepinephrine (noradrenaline)**, function as neurotransmitters in the brain and peripheral sympathetic nerves, whereas **epinephrine (adrenaline)** functions as a hormone released by the adrenal medulla. Catecholamines are critical in maintaining the body's homeostasis and in responding to acute and chronic stress through orchestration of (1) cardiovascular, (2) metabolic, (3) glandular, and (4) visceral organ activities.[4] **Serotonin (5-hydroxytryptamine)** also serves as a neurotransmitter in the brain and as a modulator of vascular and gastrointestinal functions in the periphery. Abnormal production of catecholamines or serotonin may occur in a number of neuroendocrine tumors, where clinical signs and symptoms reflect the pharmacological properties of the secreted amines. Clinical measurement of the biogenic amines or of their metabolites aids in tumor detection and monitoring, and analytical advances have produced sensitive and specific laboratory methods for clinical practice.[13,14]

Chemistry, Biosynthesis, Release, and Metabolism

Chemistry

The catecholamines—dopamine, norepinephrine (noradrenaline), and epinephrine (adrenaline)—are phenylethylamines with hydroxyl groups on positions three and four of the benzene ring and an ethylamine sidechain on position one (Figure 26-1). Hydroxyl and methyl substitutions on the ethylamine sidechain distinguish the individual catecholamines in terms of both structure and function. The catecholamines demonstrate varying degrees of alkaline instability in biological fluids, and their dihydroxybenzene or catechol structure is sensitive to oxidative formation of quinones in the presence of air and light. Serotonin with its indoleamine structure is distinct from the catecholamines but is an important naturally occurring biogenic amine. **Melatonin** is the principal indoleamine produced from serotonin by the pineal gland.

Biosynthesis

The rate-limiting step in catecholamine biosynthesis involves conversion of tyrosine to **3,4-dihydroxyphenylalanine (L-dopa)** by the enzyme tyrosine hydroxylase (Figure 26-2).[4] A related enzyme, tryptophan hydroxylase, catalyzes conversion of tryptophan to 5-hydroxytryptophan in the first step of serotonin synthesis. Tissue sources of catecholamines are principally dependent on the presence of tyrosine hydroxylase, which is largely confined to dopaminergic and noradrenergic neurons of the central nervous system and to the sympathetic and adrenal medullary systems in peripheral tissues.[4] Similarly, sources of serotonin are largely dependent on the presence of tryptophan hydroxylase in central nervous system serotonergic neurons, the pineal gland, and some peripheral endocrine tissue, particularly enterochromaffin cells of the digestive tract.[7] Platelets also contain large amounts of serotonin synthesized in enterochromaffin cells of the gastrointestinal tract.

Conversion of L-dopa to dopamine and 5-hydroxytryptophan to serotonin is catalyzed by aromatic-L-amino acid

decarboxylase (see Figure 26-2), an enzyme with a wide tissue distribution and broad substrate specificity for aromatic amino acids. The dopamine and serotonin formed in the cytoplasm by aromatic-L-amino acid decarboxylase are transported into vesicular secretory granules, where the amines are concentrated and stored ready for exocytotic release as the principal neurotransmitters of central nervous system dopaminergic and serotonergic neurons. The dopamine formed in noradrenergic neurons and **chromaffin cells** is further converted to norepinephrine by dopamine β-hydroxylase, an enzyme specifically located in secretory granules. The additional presence of phenylethanolamine N-methyltransferase in adrenal medullary chromaffin cells leads to further conversion of norepinephrine to epinephrine.

Melatonin is synthesized from serotonin in the pineal gland by two highly specific enzymes; the first step is catalyzed by serotonin-N-acetyltransferase and the second by hydroxyindole-O-methyltransferase.

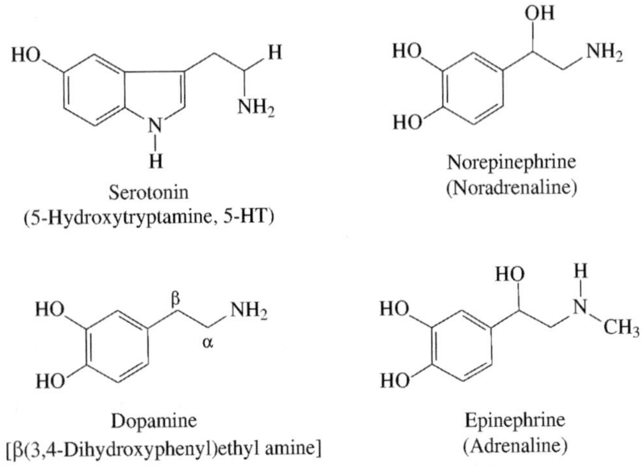

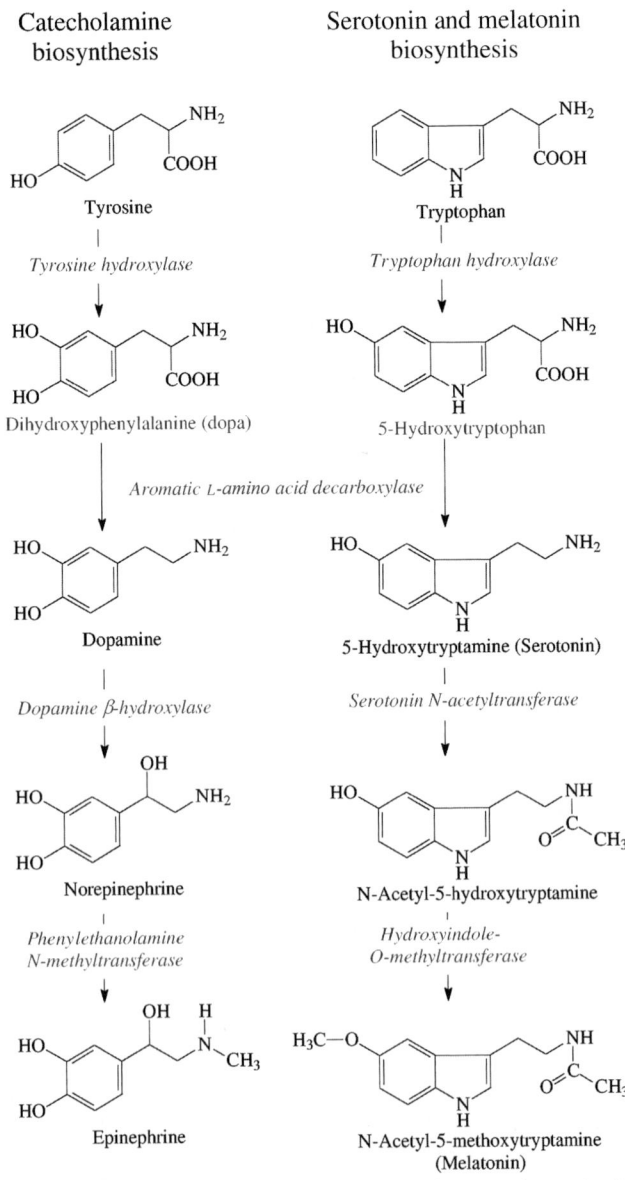

Figure 26-2 Biosynthesis of catecholamines and serotonin, and metabolism of serotonin to melatonin.

Figure 26-1 Chemical structures of the catecholamines and serotonin.

Storage and Release

Monoamines stored in secretory granules exist in a highly dynamic equilibrium with the surrounding cytoplasm, with passive outward leakage of monoamines into the cytoplasm counterbalanced by inward active transport under the control of vesicular monoamine transporters (Figure 26-3).[2] Monoamines share the acid environment of the secretory granule matrix with ATP, peptides, and proteins, the best known of which are the chromogranins. The chromogranins are common components of monoamine-containing secretory granules. Their widespread presence among endocrine tissues has led to their measurement in plasma as useful, albeit relatively nonspecific, markers of neuroendocrine tumors (see Chapter 20).

Monoamines are released from secretory vesicles into the extracellular space through the process of exocytosis. This event is stimulated by an influx of calcium, primarily controlled in neurons by nerve impulse–mediated membrane depolarization, and in adrenal medullary cells by acetylcholine released from innervating splanchnic nerves. Neuronal release may also occur by calcium-independent nonexocytotic processes involving increased loss of monoamines from storage vesicles into the cytoplasm and reversal of normal inward carrier-mediated transport to outward transport of monoamines into the extracellular environment. Examples of this process include the release of catecholamines induced by tyramine and amphetamine.

Uptake and Metabolism

Because the enzymes responsible for metabolism of catecholamines have intracellular locations, the primary mechanism limiting the duration of action of catecholamines in the extracellular space is uptake by active transport (see Figure 26-3).[2] Uptake is facilitated by transporters that belong to two families of proteins with mainly neuronal or extraneuronal locations. Neuronal monoamine transporters provide the principal mechanism for rapid termination of the signal in neuronal transmission, whereas transporters at extraneuronal locations are more important for limiting the spread of the signal and for clearance of catecholamines from the bloodstream. Of the norepinephrine released by sympathetic nerves, about 90% is removed back into nerves by neuronal uptake, 5% is removed by extraneuronal uptake, and 5% escapes these processes to enter the bloodstream. In contrast, of epinephrine released directly into the bloodstream from the adrenals, about 90% is removed by extraneuronal monoamine uptake.

In addition to terminating the actions of released monoamines, plasma membrane monoamine transporters function in sequence with vesicular monoamine transporters to recycle catecholamines for rerelease (see Figure 26-3).[2,4] Thus, most of the norepinephrine released and recaptured by sympathetic nerves is sequestered back into secretory granules by vesicular monoamine transporters, thereby reducing the requirements for synthesis of new transmitter. Plasma membrane monoamine transporters also function as part of metabolizing systems, requiring the additional actions of enzymes for irreversible inactivation of the released amines.

Catecholamines undergo metabolism by multiple pathways involving differing series of several enzymes with differing expression in various cells and tissues (Figure 26-4).[2] Most metabolism occurs within the same cells in which catecholamines are synthesized and is dependent on leakage of amines from secretory granules into the cytoplasm. In sympathetic nerves, the presence of monoamine oxidase (MAO) leads to conversion of norepinephrine to **3,4-dihydroxyphenylglycol (DHPG)**. This is then largely metabolized by **catechol-O-methyltransferase (COMT)** in extraneuronal tissues to **3-methoxy-4-hydroxyphenylglycol (MHPG)**. **Vanillylmandelic acid (VMA)**, the primary end-product of norepinephrine and epinephrine metabolism, is produced almost exclusively in the liver. This process is dependent on the hepatic localization of alcohol dehydrogenase, an enzyme required for conversion of MHPG to VMA.

In adrenal chromaffin cells, the additional presence of COMT leads to metabolism of norepinephrine to **normetanephrine** and of epinephrine to **metanephrine** (see Figure 26-4).[2] Because the intraneuronal deamination pathway far predominates over the extraneuronal O-methylation pathway, normetanephrine and metanephrine represent relatively minor products of catecholamine metabolism. As a consequence, the

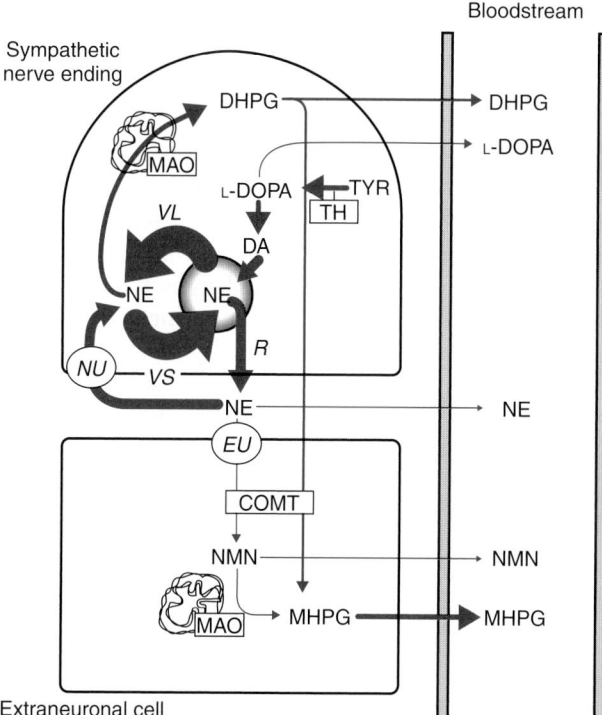

Figure 26-3 Schematic diagram illustrating the dynamics of synthesis, exocytotic release *(R)*, neuronal reuptake *(NU)*, extraneuronal uptake *(EU)*, vesicular leakage *(VL)*, vesicular sequestration *(VS)*, and metabolism of norepinephrine *(NE)* in sympathetic nerve endings in relation to extraneuronal tissue and the bloodstream. Relative magnitudes of the various processes are reflected by the relative sizes of arrows. *COMT,* Catechol-O-methyltransferase; *DA,* dopamine; *DHPG,* 3,4-dihydroxyphenylglycol; *L-dopa,* 3,4-dihydroxyphenylalanine; *MAO,* monoamine oxidase; *MHPG,* 3-methoxy-4-hydroxyphenylglycol; *NMN,* normetanephrine; *TH,* tyrosine hydroxylase; *TYR,* tyrosine.

adrenal medulla represents the single largest tissue source of normetanephrine and metanephrine, accounting for 24% to 40% of the former and more than 90% of the latter. The metanephrine and normetanephrine produced in the adrenal medulla or in extraneuronal tissues—the former from catecholamines leaking from secretory granules and the latter from

catecholamines released from sympathoadrenal sources—may be deaminated to MHPG and then converted to VMA in the liver or may be sulfate-conjugated by a sulfotransferase enzyme expressed mainly in the gastrointestinal tissues.

Serotonin is not a substrate for COMT; it follows simpler pathways of metabolism than those for catecholamines. Serotonin is deaminated to **5-hydroxyindoleacetic acid (5-HIAA)**, the major urinary excretion product of serotonin metabolism.

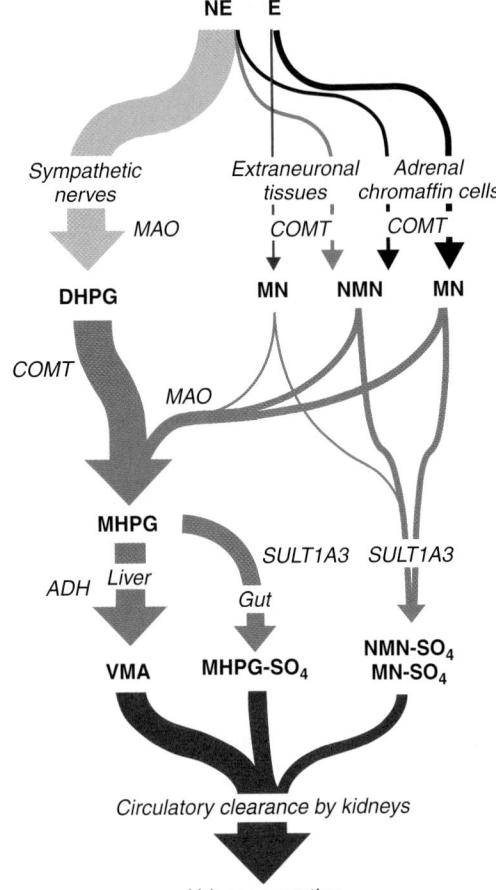

Figure 26-4 Schematic diagram showing the main pathways for metabolism of the norepinephrine and epinephrine derived from sympathoneuronal or adrenal medullary sources. Deamination in sympathetic nerves *(pink)* is the major pathway of catecholamine metabolism and involves intraneuronal deamination of norepinephrine leaking from storage granules, or of norepinephrine recaptured after release by sympathetic nerves. Metabolism in adrenal chromaffin cells *(black)* involves O-methylation of catecholamines leaking from storage granules into the cytoplasm of adrenal medullary cells. The extraneuronal pathway *(light red)* is a relatively minor pathway of metabolism of catecholamines released from sympathetic nerves or the adrenal medulla, but it is important for further processing of metabolites produced in sympathetic nerves and adrenal chromaffin cells. The free metanephrines produced in extraneuronal tissues or adrenal chromaffin cells are further metabolized by deamination or sulfate conjugation. *ADH,* Alcohol dehydrogenase; *COMT,* catechol-O-methyltransferase; *DHPG,* 3,4-dihydroxyphenylglycol; *E,* epinephrine; *MAO,* monoamine oxidase; *MHPG,* 3-methoxy-4-hydroxyphenylglycol; *MHPG-SO₄,* 3-methoxy-4-hydroxyphenylglycol sulfate; *MN,* metanephrine; *MN-SO₄,* metanephrine-sulfate; *NE,* norepinephrine; *NMN,* normetanephrine; *NMN-SO₄,* normetanephrine-sulfate; *SULT1A3,* phenolsulfotransferase type 1A3; *VMA,* vanillylmandelic acid.

Physiology of Catecholamine and Serotonin Systems

Catecholamines and serotonin regulate physiological events at the cellular level through interaction with families of cell surface receptors.[4,6,16] Norepinephrine and epinephrine act on two broad classes of adrenergic receptors: α- and β-adrenoceptor families. Dopamine transmits signals primarily by interaction with a large family of dopamine receptors. An even larger family of serotonergic receptor subtypes has been identified by histological and molecular techniques. The major physiological effects of catecholamines and serotonin are explained in part by these diverse receptor interactions that occur in function-specific locations throughout the vasculature and organ systems of the body.

Central Nervous System

Norepinephrine, dopamine, and serotonin are produced primarily in regions of the brainstem by neurons with projections to other areas of the brain or spinal cord.[16] About half of the norepinephrine in the brain is produced in norepinephrine-producing neurons in the lower brainstem that send diffuse axonal projections throughout the brain as high as the cerebral cortex. They also send descending fibers to the spinal cord, where they synapse with preganglionic sympathetic neurons that communicate with the peripheral sympathetic nervous system. The norepinephrine-producing neurons of the brainstem participate in regulating the activity of the sympathetic nervous system and the overall state of attention and vigilance.

Dopamine produced in dopaminergic neurons has functions and shows distributions that are notably different from those of norepinephrine. Dopamine in the brain influences reward-seeking behavior and is important for initiation and maintenance of movement. Disturbances in dopamine production and release in the brain are therefore involved in drug-dependency states and are central to the movement disorder that characterizes **Parkinson disease.**[4] Dopamine neurotransmission is also involved in processing sensory signals and in regulating hormonal release. Dopaminergic neurons in the retina and olfactory bulb have ultrashort projections that transmit signals within these neuronal centers for vision and smell. Dopamine neurons in the hypothalamus have regulatory influences on release of several hormones of the pituitary gland.

Serotonin, like norepinephrine, is produced by small clusters of neurons in the brainstem regions, but it serves a diverse range of behavioral and physiological functions. Physiological and behavioral processes influenced by this serotonergic system include (1) memory, (2) learning, (3) feeding behavior, (4) sleep patterns, (5) thermoregulation, (6) pain modulation, (7) cardiovascular function, and (8) hypothalamic regulation of pituitary hormones.

Sympathetic Nervous System

Sympathetic nerve transmission operates below the level of consciousness in controlling the physiological function of many organs and tissues of the body (Figure 26-5).[6] The sympathetic nervous system plays a particularly important role in regulating cardiovascular function in response to (1) postural, (2) exertional, (3) thermal, and (4) mental stress. With sympathetic activation, (1) heart rate is increased, (2) peripheral arterioles are constricted, (3) skeletal arterioles are dilated, and (4) blood pressure is elevated. Sympathetic signals work in balance with the parasympathetic portion of the autonomic nervous system to maintain a stable internal environment.

Efferent or outgoing signals from the central nervous system are transmitted by preganglionic, cholinergic, sympathetic neurons that exit the spinal cord and converge on sympathetic ganglia along the spinal column or in visceral ganglia (see Figure 26-5). The terminal branches of the postganglionic

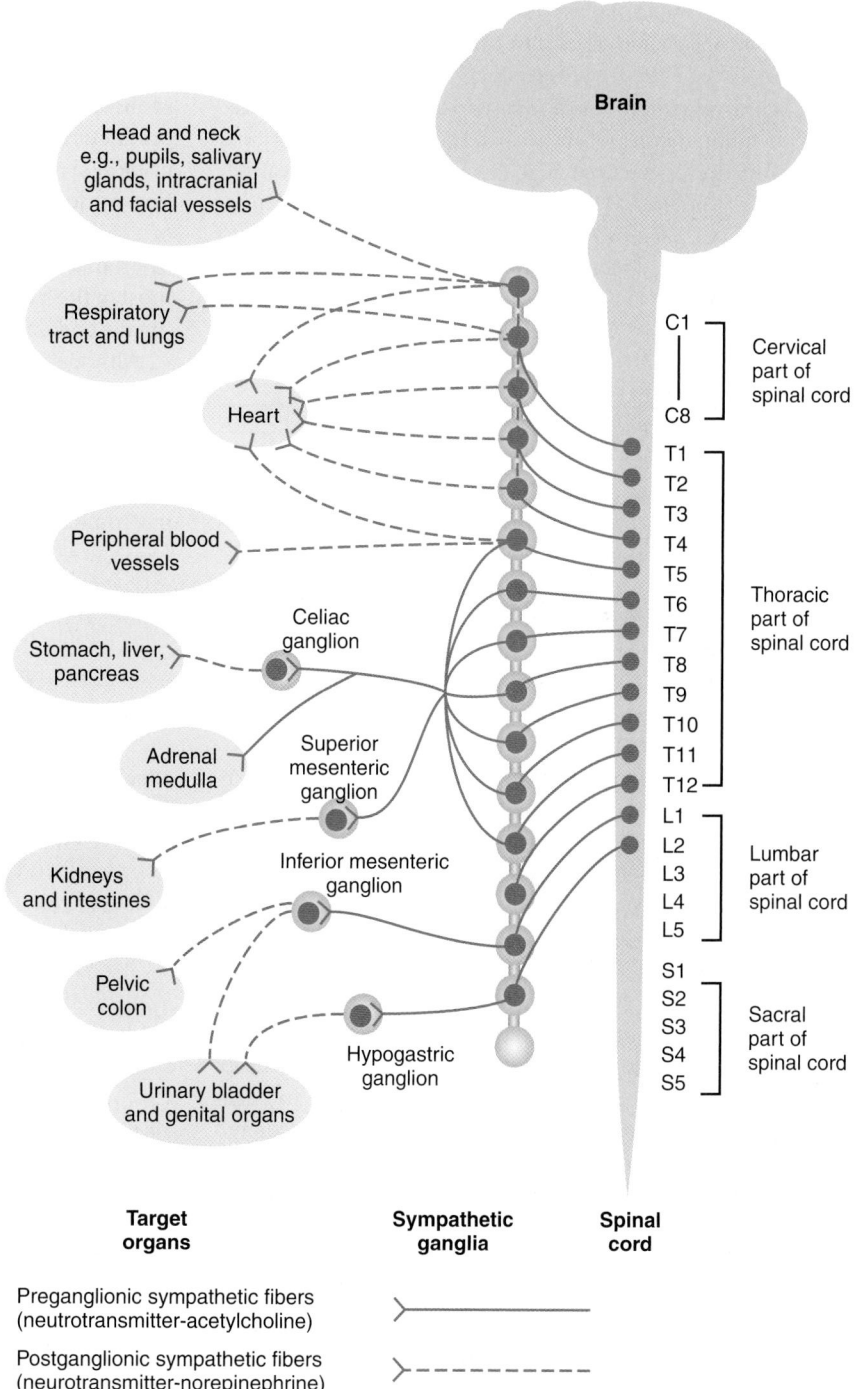

Figure 26-5 Schematic diagram of sympathetic division of the autonomic nervous system. Preganglionic cholinergic fibers *(solid lines)* from the spinal cord project to the paravertebral sympathetic chain, visceral peripheral ganglia, and the adrenal medulla, whereas postganglionic noradrenergic fibers *(dashed lines)* project from sympathetic ganglia to sympathetically innervated target organs. About 5% to 10% of the norepinephrine released from sympathetic nerves innervating target organs escapes neuronal and extraneuronal uptake to enter the bloodstream. This contrasts with epinephrine, which functions as a circulating hormone and is released directly from the adrenal medulla into the bloodstream. Most of the catecholamines entering the bloodstream are removed by extraneuronal uptake processes and are metabolized (e.g., in the liver), so that only small proportions are excreted in the urine.

fibers that project from these ganglia into target organs have varicosities that form a rich ground plexus for synaptic contact with a large number of effector cells in glands and muscle fibers. Most sympathetic postganglionic nerves liberate norepinephrine as their neurotransmitter. In limited locations, sympathetic nerve endings release acetylcholine. Sympathetic fibers that release acetylcholine innervate sweat glands and the adrenal medulla, the latter stimulating release of epinephrine from chromaffin cells.

Plasma and urinary norepinephrine are derived primarily from postganglionic sympathetic neurons with little contribution from the central nervous system or from hormonal release by the adrenal medulla.[4] Because of intervening neuronal and extraneuronal removal processes, the amount of norepinephrine that escapes into the bloodstream represents less than 10% of the total norepinephrine released by sympathetic nerves. Alterations in release and plasma concentrations of norepinephrine occur in response to physiological and pathological states, such as (1) exercise, (2) overeating, (3) low salt intake, (4) upright position, (5) mental stress, and (6) aging, all of which increase sympathetic outflow.[4] Increased plasma concentrations of norepinephrine are also found in disorders such as cardiac failure, hypertension, and depression.

Adrenal Medullary System

The human adrenal glands overlie the superior poles of the kidneys (see Chapter 41). Each gland consists of an outer cortex and a thin inner central medulla containing chromaffin cells. A characteristic feature of adrenal medullary chromaffin cells is the presence of numerous catecholamine storage granules. These granules turn brown when exposed to (1) potassium bichromate solutions, (2) ammoniacal silver nitrate, or (3) osmium tetroxide because of the oxidation and polymerization of epinephrine and norepinephrine. This process is known as the chromaffin reaction, hence the terms chromaffin cells and chromaffin granules.

Although often considered a part of the sympathetic nervous system, the adrenal medulla produces and secretes epinephrine with different functions from the norepinephrine secreted by sympathetic nerves.[4] The adrenal medulla and the sympathetic nerves are regulated separately, often in divergent directions in response to different forms of stress. Epinephrine is secreted from adrenal chromaffin cells directly into the bloodstream to act on cells distant from sites of release. Epinephrine and norepinephrine have overlapping but different potencies of effect on α- and β-adrenoceptors. The proximity of sites of norepinephrine and epinephrine release to adrenoceptors determines differences in adrenoceptor-mediated responses to the two catecholamines. Because of the factors mentioned earlier, epinephrine exerts its effects on different populations of adrenoceptors than those affected by norepinephrine. Epinephrine released from the adrenal glands is more important as a metabolic hormone than as a hemodynamic regulatory hormone. In particular, epinephrine stimulates (1) lipolysis, (2) ketogenesis, (3) thermogenesis, and (4) glycolysis. It also raises plasma glucose concentrations by stimulating glycogenolysis and gluconeogenesis. Epinephrine also has potent effects on pulmonary function, causing dilation of airways.

Peripheral Dopaminergic System

Dopamine is usually thought of as a neurotransmitter in the brain or as an intermediate in the production of norepinephrine and epinephrine in peripheral tissues. The contribution of the brain to plasma concentrations and urinary excretion of dopamine metabolites is, however, relatively minor, and dopamine produced in sympathetic nerves and the adrenal medulla is mainly converted to norepinephrine. Most circulating and urinary dopamine and dopamine metabolites are therefore derived from other sources (Figure 26-6).[2]

In the kidneys, dopamine functions as an autocrine or paracrine effector substance contributing to the regulation of sodium excretion.[4] Unlike neuronal catecholamine systems, production of dopamine in the kidneys is largely independent of local synthesis of L-dopa by tyrosine hydroxylase. Production of dopamine in the kidneys depends mainly on uptake of L-dopa from the circulation and conversion to dopamine by aromatic amino acid decarboxylase (see Figure 26-6). Thus most of the free dopamine excreted in urine derives from renal uptake and decarboxylation of circulating L-dopa.

Although the kidneys represent the major source of urinary free dopamine, this source does not account for the much larger quantities of excreted dopamine metabolites, such as **homovanillic acid (HVA)** and dopamine sulfate. Substantial proportions of these metabolites are produced in the gastrointestinal tract, where dopamine appears to function as

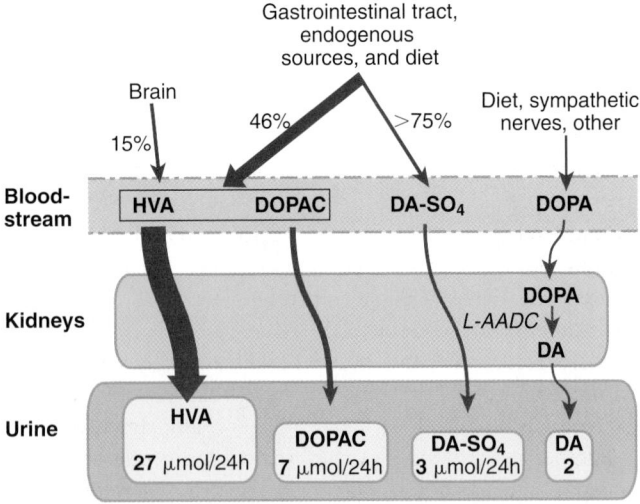

Figure 26-6 Schematic diagram illustrating the main plasma and urinary sources of dopamine (DA) and the principal metabolites of dopamine, homovanillic acid (HVA), dihydroxyphenylacetic acid (DOPAC), and dopamine sulfate (DA-SO$_4$). The brain makes a relatively minor contribution, whereas dopamine synthesized in the gastrointestinal tract or derived from the diet contributes substantially to dopamine metabolites in the bloodstream and urine. This contrasts with the free dopamine excreted in urine, which is derived almost entirely from renal extraction of circulating dihydroxyphenylalanine (DOPA) and local decarboxylation to dopamine by L-aromatic amino acid decarboxylase (L-AADC).

an enteric neuromodulator or as a paracrine or autocrine substance.[2,4] However, unlike in the kidneys, where dopamine is produced mainly from circulating L-dopa, in the gastrointestinal tract, production of dopamine requires the presence of tyrosine hydroxylase or other sources of L-dopa.

Consumption of food increases plasma concentrations of (1) L-dopa, (2) dopamine, and (3) dopamine metabolites, particularly dopamine sulfate, indicating that dietary constituents may represent an important source of peripheral dopamine (see Figure 26-6).[4] It is now clear that dopamine sulfate is produced mainly in the gastrointestinal tract from both dietary and locally synthesized dopamine. This is consistent with findings that the gastrointestinal tract contains high concentrations of the specific sulfotransferase enzyme responsible for sulfate conjugation of catecholamines and **catecholamine metabolites**.

Enteric Nervous System

The **enteric nervous system (ENS)** is defined as an independent and integrated system of neurons and supporting cells located in the (1) gastrointestinal tract, (2) gallbladder, and (3) pancreas.[5] The ENS is composed of two networks or plexuses of intrinsic neurons: the myenteric plexus and the submucous plexus. Both are embedded in the wall of the gut and extend from the esophagus to the anus. These networks contain more than 100 million (1) sensory neurons, (2) interneurons, and (3) motor neurons. The myenteric plexus lies between the longitudinal and circular layers of intestinal smooth muscle and controls propulsive movements (peristalsis). The submucous plexus innervates (1) glandular epithelium, (2) intestinal endocrine cells, and (3) submucosal blood vessels. This network (1) senses the environment within the lumen, (2) regulates local blood flow, and (3) controls epithelial cell secretion.

The ENS is connected to the central nervous system by extrinsic parasympathetic and sympathetic motor neurons, and by spinal and vagal sensory neurons. Through these bidirectional connections, the ENS is monitored and modified.[5] Despite the presence of these extrinsic nerve connections, the ENS functions autonomously in some intestinal regions. Neural transmission within the ENS is controlled by a large variety of neurotransmitters and neuromodulatory peptides, such as (1) serotonin, (2) norepinephrine, (3) acetylcholine, (4) ATP, and (5) nitric oxide. Serotonin acts as a local paracrine molecule, participating in mucosal sensory transduction. More than 95% of the body's serotonin is produced within the gastrointestinal tract, and most is synthesized and stored in enterochromaffin cells in the gut mucosa.[7] Intrinsic sensory neurons activated by serotonin stimulate peristaltic reflex and secretion, whereas extrinsic sensory neurons initiate bowel sensations such as (1) nausea, (2) vomiting, (3) abdominal pain, and (4) bloating. The paracrine actions of serotonin are terminated by uptake into epithelial cells by the same serotonin transporter used in serotonergic neurons.

Clinical Applications

Measurements of (1) catecholamines, (2) serotonin, and (3) their metabolites are used in investigations of a range of pathophysiological processes. Measurements of the amines and their metabolites are directed primarily at the diagnosis of neuroendocrine tumors. Catecholamine-producing neuroendocrine tumors include (1) **pheochromocytomas**, (2) **paragangliomas**, and (3) **neuroblastomas**, whereas serotonin-producing tumors are typically **carcinoid tumors**.

Pheochromocytoma and Paraganglioma

Catecholamine-producing tumors that derive from chromaffin cells may occur within the adrenal glands, where they are referred to as pheochromocytomas, or at extra-adrenal sites, where the tumors are termed paragangliomas.[8] Paragangliomas derived from extra-adrenal sympathetic chromaffin tissue usually produce significant quantities of catecholamines—and are commonly referred to as extra-adrenal pheochromocytomas. Pheochromocytomas are rare, with an annual detection rate of 2 to 5 per million. Autopsy studies, indicating prevalences of 0.05% to 0.1%, suggest that most of the tumors remain undetected and contribute to premature death.

The presence of a pheochromocytoma is usually suspected because of signs and symptoms that reflect the biological effects of catecholamines released by the tumor.[12] Hypertension, the most common sign, can be sustained or paroxysmal. Symptoms include (1) headache, (2) palpitations, (3) diaphoresis (excessive sweating), (4) pallor, (5) nausea, (6) attacks of anxiety, and (7) generalized weakness. Among patients tested because of such signs and symptoms, the pretest prevalence of tumors is low—usually less than 1%.

Patients with a higher risk for pheochromocytoma include those with (1) a hereditary predisposition to the tumor, (2) a previous history of the tumor, or (3) the incidental finding of an adrenal mass during routine abdominal imaging procedures.[8] In such patients, testing may be carried out independently of the presence of signs and symptoms. See Box 26-1 for a summary of the key points of pheochromocytomas.

Advances in understanding catecholamine metabolism have changed the approach to biochemical diagnosis of pheochromocytoma, concentrating now on measurements of metanephrines rather than their precursor catecholamines.[3,8] This has followed several observations, including findings that adrenal medullary cells and pheochromocytoma tumor cells contain COMT, the enzyme that converts catecholamines to their O-methylated metabolites.[2]

Normally, most norepinephrine is metabolized by deamination within sympathetic nerves, so that O-methylation represents a minor pathway of catecholamine metabolism. In patients with pheochromocytoma, intratumoral O-methylation becomes a dominant pathway of catecholamine metabolism. Consequently, the presence of the tumor leads to relatively large increases in production of O-methylated metabolites, compared with minor increases in deaminated metabolites. The metanephrines are produced continuously as a result of ongoing leakage of catecholamines from chromaffin granule stores into the cell cytoplasm; in contrast, catecholamines are often released episodically or in relatively low quantities compared with metanephrines.

BOX 26-1 Pheochromocytoma and Paraganglioma Key Points

Biology
- Rare tumors of mainly adrenal chromaffin cells that produce, store, metabolize, and secrete catecholamines, usually with a predominance of norepinephrine over epinephrine
- Those developing from extra-adrenal sympathetic chromaffin tissue—termed *paragangliomas*—usually produce near exclusively norepinephrine and very rarely predominantly dopamine

Presentation
- Tumor usually suspected because of signs and symptoms of catecholamine excess (e.g., hypertension, palpitations, headaches, excessive sweatiness) or the incidental finding of an adrenal mass during routine imaging procedures for unrelated medical conditions
- Most pheochromocytomas are benign; 15% of adrenal tumors and 35% of extra-adrenal tumors are malignant
- At least 30% of pheochromocytomas have a hereditary basis, resulting from mutations of ten genes identified to date
- Less than 1% of patients tested because of signs and symptoms have the tumor (low pretest prevalence), but the prevalence is higher among patients with identified mutations of disease-causing genes or those with an incidental adrenal mass; thus testing in these patients is recommended independently of the presence of signs and symptoms

Biochemical Diagnosis
- Biochemical diagnosis based on evidence of excess production of catecholamines, best determined from measurements of metanephrines in urine or plasma
- Because secretion of catecholamines by tumors is episodic, but metabolism to metanephrines within tumors is continuous, measurements of plasma or urinary fractionated metanephrines provide more reliable diagnostic tests for the tumor than measurements of catecholamines (metanephrines increased in >97% and catecholamines in 69% to 92% of patients with pheochromocytomas)

Numerous independent studies have now confirmed that the measurements of plasma metanephrines are very sensitive. This has led to the recommendation that measurements of either plasma or urinary fractionated metanephrines should always be used during initial work-up of a patient with a suspected pheochromocytoma.[3] Negative results of these tests virtually exclude a pheochromocytoma. Exceptions include small (<1 cm) tumors encountered during routine screening and tumors that do not synthesize norepinephrine and epinephrine. Among the latter, tumors that produce only dopamine may be detected by measurements of plasma or urinary methoxytyramine, the O-methylated metabolite of dopamine.[3] Measurements of plasma dopamine also are useful, whereas urinary dopamine is largely derived from renal extraction and decarboxylation of L-dopa and therefore provides a relatively insensitive and nonspecific test for detection of a dopamine-producing tumor (see Figure 26-6).

Plasma or urinary fractionated metanephrines are usually elevated sufficiently to conclusively establish the presence of most cases of pheochromocytoma.[12] However, in about 20% of patients with the tumor, increases are smaller. Such true-positive results are difficult to distinguish from the larger proportion of false-positive results. Additional biochemical

testing is then necessary. Before further biochemical testing is initiated, consideration should be given to eliminating possible causes of false-positive results. These may occur because of (1) inappropriate sampling conditions (e.g., blood sampling without a preceding 30-minute period of supine rest), (2) medications such as tricyclic antidepressants, or (3) clinical conditions that increase sympathetic outflow.

When biochemical testing continues to yield equivocal results, the clonidine suppression test may be useful for further confirming or excluding a pheochromocytoma.[12] As originally introduced, this test was designed to distinguish patients with increases in plasma catecholamines caused by pheochromocytoma from those with increases caused by sympathetic activation. By activating α_2-adrenoceptors in the brain and on sympathetic nerve endings, clonidine suppresses norepinephrine release by sympathetic nerves. Decreases in elevated plasma norepinephrine after clonidine therefore suggest sympathetic activation, whereas lack of decrease suggests a pheochromocytoma. The test has subsequently been shown to be useful for distinguishing increases in plasma normetanephrine due to a pheochromocytoma from those due to sympathetic activation.

Most pheochromocytomas are sporadic, but as many as 30% to 40% have a hereditary basis.[3] Hereditary forms of the tumor result from mutations of ten disease-causing genes identified to date. Pheochromocytomas occur at a relatively low prevalence in about 1% of patients with **neurofibromatosis type 1 (NF1)**. Risk for the other nine currently known hereditary conditions is higher. Pheochromocytomas in multiple endocrine neoplasia type 2 (**MEN 2**) result from mutations of the *ret* proto-oncogene, which also predisposes to medullary thyroid cancer. In von Hippel-Lindau syndrome (VHL), family-specific mutations of the VHL tumor suppressor gene determine the varied clinical presentation of tumors, which, in addition to pheochromocytomas and paragangliomas, include (1) retinal angiomas, (2) central nervous system hemangioblastomas, and (3) tumors in the kidneys, pancreas, and testis. Familial paragangliomas and pheochromocytomas may occur secondary to mutations of genes for four subunits of succinate dehydrogenase (*SDHA, SDHB, SDHC,* and *SDHD*). Mutations of genes encoding the SDH complex assembly factor 2 (*SDHAF2*), transmembrane protein 127 (*TMEM127*), and MYC-associated factor X (*MAX*) represent other recently identified tumor susceptibility genes.

Mutations of the different tumor susceptibility genes have been found to give rise to distinct catecholamine metabolite profiles.[3] Tumors in patients with MEN 2 and NF1 are almost always confined to the adrenals and are characterized by increases in plasma-free metanephrine, indicating epinephrine production. In contrast, tumors in patients with *VHL, SDHD,* and *SDHB* mutations, including those at adrenal locations, are characterized by increases in plasma or urinary normetanephrine without increases in metanephrine. Increases in methoxytyramine, the metabolite of dopamine, are additionally present in up to 70% of patients with mutations of *SDHD* and *SDHB* genes. In some patients, methoxytyramine represents the only metabolite increased.

The distinct mutation-dependent biochemical profiles are useful for stratifying patients for genetic testing and are important to consider during routine screening of tumors.[3] For mutations that confer a high risk of disease, such screening is generally recommended at yearly intervals and should include biochemical testing for evidence of excess catecholamine production individualized according to the expected biochemical profile of the tumor.

Although most often benign, about 10% of pheochromocytomas and 35% of paragangliomas eventually metastasize.[3,12] The risk of malignancy is particularly high in patients with *SDHB* mutations. Tumors in such patients typically produce low quantities of catecholamines and are much larger at diagnosis than tumors in other patients. This fact, along with their typically extra-adrenal location, explains their higher predisposition to malignancy.

Diagnosis of malignant pheochromocytoma on the basis of histopathological features is not possible and instead requires evidence of metastatic lesions in (1) liver, (2) lungs, (3) lymphatic nodes, and (4) bones. All patients with a previous history of tumor are at risk for recurrent or malignant disease and should undergo periodic tumor screening. Measurements of plasma methoxytyramine appear to serve as a promising new biomarker for malignant pheochromocytoma and therefore should be considered as part of biochemical testing in patients tested as a result of past history of the disease.[3]

Neuroblastoma

Neuroblastomas are neoplasms that derive from primordial neural crest cells of the sympathetic nervous system.[9] Neuroblastomas are almost exclusively a pediatric cancer, accounting for approximately 7% of all childhood neoplasms; they are the most common malignancies in the first year of life. The incidence of neuroblastoma is approximately 10 cases per million children. A vast majority of neuroblastomas develop sporadically. Activating mutations in the tyrosine kinase domain of the anaplastic lymphoma kinase oncogene account for most cases of hereditary neuroblastoma and may occur as somatic mutations in 5% to 15% of sporadic cases. Mutations of *paired-like homeobox 2b (PHOX2B)*, also known as *neuroblastoma Phox (NBPhox)*, account for other cases of hereditary neuroblastoma.

Most neuroblastomas are intra-abdominal, arising in the adrenal gland or in the upper abdomen. Less frequent locations include chest, neck, and pelvis. About 60% are extra-adrenal. Metastases in disseminated neuroblastomas may involve (1) bone marrow, (2) bone, (3) lymph nodes, (4) liver, and, less frequently, (5) skin, (6) testis, and (7) intracranial structures.

The biological behavior of a neuroblastoma varies from regression or maturation to an aggressive course with an unfavorable outcome.[9] Neuroblastomas are most notable for a subset of cases with complete regression or maturation to ganglioneuroma, a benign neoplasm. Most clinically diagnosed tumors, however, are aggressive and have an unfavorable outcome. This highly variable clinical outcome underlies a need for diagnostic markers to stratify patients for therapeutic intervention. Age at diagnosis serves as a primary criterion for stratification; infants younger than 18 months have a more

---

BOX 26-2   Neuroblastoma Key Points

Biology
- Tumors occurring almost exclusively in children that develop from primitive neural crest cells of the sympathoadrenal system, with about 60% derived from extra-adrenal sympathetic tissue and 40% from the adrenals
- Biological behavior of tumors is highly variable, with some tumors spontaneously regressing but most (60%) having an aggressive course with disseminated malignant disease and an unfavorable outcome

Presentation
- Neuroblastomas produce variable amounts of dopamine and norepinephrine but show a poor capacity for storage and release of catecholamines. Consequently, the tumors rarely produce signs and symptoms of catecholamine excess
- Suspicion of disease is usually based on palpation of a mass, space-occupying complications of the tumor, or effects of bone marrow involvement
- Hereditary causes of neuroblastomas are rare; most neuroblastomas occur sporadically

Biochemical Diagnosis
- Biochemical diagnosis based on overproduction of dopamine and norepinephrine, but because the tumors have poorly developed machinery for catecholamine storage and release, diagnosis depends mainly on measurements of catecholamine metabolites
- Measurements of urinary VMA and HVA represent the most widely used tests but in a large prospective screening study were shown to detect only 73% of tumors

---

favorable outcome than older children.[9] Beyond this, stratification for therapeutic intervention considers (1) clinical stage of the disease (localized vs. disseminated), (2) histopathological features, and (3) consideration of v-myc myelocytomatosis viral related oncogene *(MYCN)* expression status.

Somatic mutations of the α-thalassemia/MR, X-linked *(ATRX)* gene have recently emerged as defining a subset of older children with an indolent, but nevertheless chronic and progressive, course of disease.[1] Unfortunately, the overall incidence of metastatic neuroblastoma at the time of diagnosis is approximately 60%, and the need for earlier detection of children with the progressive disseminating tumor remains a diagnostic challenge. See Box 26-2 for a summary of the key points of neuroblastomas.

Hypertension and signs and symptoms of catecholamine excess are uncommon in neuroblastoma; this appears to reflect inefficient storage of catecholamines, leading to their intracellular metabolism and release as mainly inactive metabolites. Patients commonly present with a tumor mass and clinical signs from compression effects on neighboring structures or hematological abnormalities from bone marrow involvement.

Laboratory evidence of a functional catecholamine-producing tumor is important in the clinical evaluation when a neuroblastoma is suspected.[15] Catecholamine and metabolite secretion patterns, however, may differ markedly among patients with the tumor. Neuroblastoma tumor cells have the capacity to synthesize dopamine and norepinephrine, but lack phenylethanolamine *N*-methyltransferase and consequently do not produce epinephrine. Because of variability in catecholamine production and metabolism, no single reliable marker of catecholamine overproduction has been identified. Combinations of catecholamines and metabolites are therefore often measured in the diagnostic evaluation of neuroblastoma.

HVA and VMA, produced, respectively, from dopamine and norepinephrine, are most widely used for diagnosis of a neuroblastoma. A small diurnal variation in HVA and VMA excretion and a positive correlation between random and 24-hour urine test results allow the convenient use of random urine specimens, with results expressed as the ratio of catecholamine metabolites to creatinine excretion. Clinical sensitivity in the range of 90% has been reported by some centers for urinary HVA and VMA testing. However, others have reported a lower rate of neuroblastoma detection. In a large neuroblastoma screening program, in which the population with negative screening results was tracked for occurrence of neuroblastoma, an elevation in VMA, HVA, or both acid metabolites detected only 73% of the tumors.[15] Diagnostic sensitivity of these measurements in screening programs is therefore limited and in particular appears to miss patients with aggressive disease diagnosed at a later age. Consequently, screening programs have been generally unsuccessful in reducing the rate of metastatic neuroblastoma.

Additional markers of catecholamine overproduction have been employed to improve the detection of neuroblastomas. Plasma measurements of dopamine and L-dopa, the amino acid precursor of dopamine, may have clinical value and allow the alternate use of plasma. Measurement of O-methylated metabolites, especially normetanephrine, has also been studied. When urinary (1) normetanephrine, (2) metanephrine, (3) methoxytyramine, (4) dopamine, (5) norepinephrine, (6) VMA, and (7) HVA concentrations were measured, clinical sensitivity for detection of neuroblastomas was reported at 97% to 100%. Nevertheless, a low incidence of biochemically negative tumors must be considered in the interpretation of negative test results.

Some evidence suggests that the pattern of catecholamine metabolism is associated with important biological and genetic prognostic factors in neuroblastoma. Immature metabolic patterns in neuroblastoma tumor tissue are based on higher excretion of dopamine or HVA relative to norepinephrine or VMA. A high ratio of HVA/VMA, dopamine/VMA, or dopamine/norepinephrine indicates a relative deficiency in β-hydroxylation with a reduction in tumor cell conversion of dopamine to norepinephrine. The immature metabolic pattern is suggested to be associated with aggressive tumor behavior and other unfavorable prognostic factors, but the clinical application of such metabolic patterns has not been established.

Finally, clinical specificity in detecting neuroblastoma with catecholamine and metabolite measurements may be influenced by the choice of (1) laboratory methods, (2) dietary interference, and (3) other catecholamine overproduction conditions. Significant advances in the analytical specificity of laboratory methods have reduced many of the exogenous sources of interference. Histopathology remains the ultimate diagnostic criterion for distinguishing neuroblastoma from pheochromocytoma or other catecholamine-producing neurogenic tumors, such as ganglioneuroma and ganglioneuroblastoma.

Gastroenteropancreatic Neuroendocrine and Carcinoid Tumors

Gastroenteropancreatic neuroendocrine tumors (GEP-NET), including classical **carcinoid tumors**, are derived from a variety of neuroendocrine cell types, in particular, enterochromaffin cells.[10] These tumors are widely distributed in the body and are highly heterogeneous in their clinical presentation. The usual carcinoid tumor is solid and yellow-tan in appearance. Tumor cells exhibit a monotonous morphology, with pink granular cytoplasm and round nuclei with infrequent mitoses. Most of these neuroendocrine tumors are recognized by their reactions to silver stains and to neuroendocrine cell markers, such as chromogranin and neuron-specific enolase.

The tumors are traditionally classified according to their presumed origin from the embryonic (1) foregut (bronchus, lung, stomach, duodenum, and pancreas), (2) midgut (ileum, jejunum, appendix, and proximal colon), or (3) hindgut (rectum and distal colon).[10] The most common sites for these tumors are (1) bronchus or lung—33%, (2) ileum or jejunum—20%, (3) rectum—10%, and (4) appendix—8%. The annual incidence of clinically significant gastroenteropancreatic tumor is estimated at 2.5 to 5 cases per 100,000 persons. These tumors may develop in all age groups but appear most frequently in adults; a mean age of 63 has been reported for tumors of the small intestine and respiratory tract. Clinically, most patients are asymptomatic until metastases are present. Bowel obstruction and abdominal pain are the most frequent presenting symptoms.

Gastroenteropancreatic neuroendocrine tumors show aggressive malignant behavior depending on (1) origin, (2) depth of penetration, and (3) size of the primary tumor. Most rectal carcinomas are found incidentally at endoscopy. They are often smaller than 1 cm and have a low rate of metastasis, even though they may show extensive local spread. Carcinoids of the appendix are seen in about 1 in every 300 appendectomies. Almost all measure less than 1 cm, and distant metastasis is rare. By contrast, 90% of intestinal neuroendocrine tumors that penetrate halfway through the muscle wall will have spread to lymph nodes and distant sites at the time of diagnosis. More than 70% of these tumors 1 to 2 cm in diameter metastasize to the liver. Fortunately, most grow slowly, and patients may live for many years. See Box 26-3 for a summary of the key points of carcinoid tumors and gastroenteropancreatic neuroendocrine tumors.

As with normal gut endocrine cells, gastroenteropancreatic neuroendocrine tumors (1) synthesize, (2) store, and (3) release a variety of hormones and biogenic amines.[7,11] One of the best characterized of these substances in **carcinoid syndrome** is serotonin. These tumors also produce and secrete other biologically active substances, including (1) histamine, (2) kallikrein, (3) bradykinins, (4) tachykinins, (5) prostaglandins, (6) dopamine, (7) norepinephrine, and (8) peptide hormones. Production of these substances varies in relation to the tissue origin of the tumor. Midgut neuroendocrine tumors

Gastroenteropancreatic and Carcinoid Tumor Key Points

Biology
- Neuroendocrine tumors derived from enterochromaffin cells of the gastrointestinal and respiratory tracts
- Usually develop as small tumors (<2 cm) with slow growth but with propensity to metastasize
- Synthesize, store, and release a variety of peptide hormones and biogenic amines, including serotonin

Presentation
- Bowel obstruction and abdominal pain
- Symptoms related to secretion of vasoactive amines and peptides resulting in carcinoid syndrome (flushing, diarrhea, bronchoconstriction, and right-sided heart failure); relatively uncommon and usually occurring only after development of metastases

Biochemical Diagnosis
- Biochemical diagnosis of carcinoids depends mainly on measurements of serotonin, serotonin metabolites (5-HIAA), and the serotonin precursor (5-HTP) in urine, plasma, whole blood, and platelets
- False-positive results are a common problem resulting from dietary influences

release large quantities of serotonin, whereas tumors derived from the foregut secrete primarily 5-hydroxytryptophan (5-HTP) (a serotonin precursor) and histamine, rather than serotonin. Primary hindgut neuroendocrine tumors usually show no secretory activity. Pancreatic neuroendocrine tumors are capable of producing (1) gastrin, (2) insulin, (3) glucagon, and (4) vasoactive intestinal peptide (VIP).

Secretion of vasoactive substances into the systemic circulation plays an important role in development of the carcinoid syndrome. The fully developed syndrome associated with humoral manifestations of these tumors is striking but uncommon, usually occurring only after metastasis to the liver and release of these substances directly into the systemic circulation. The classic clinical presentation of the carcinoid syndrome includes pronounced (1) flushing (especially on the face and neck), (2) diarrhea, (3) bronchoconstriction, and (4) eventual right-sided valvular heart failure. Overproduction of serotonin is found in 90% to 100% of patients with the carcinoid syndrome and is thought to be responsible for diarrhea through its known effects on gut motility and fluid secretion.

Clinical laboratory evaluation of the carcinoid syndrome relies on measurements of serotonin and its metabolites in body fluids and tissue.[7] In patients with the typical carcinoid syndrome, 5-HTP is converted to serotonin and is stored in tumor secretory granules and in platelets. A small amount of serotonin remains in plasma, but most is converted to 5-HIAA, which is excreted in urine. These patients have increased blood and platelet serotonin concentrations and increased urinary 5-HIAA excretion. However, some foregut neuroendocrine tumors lack aromatic L-amino acid decarboxylase and secrete 5-HTP rather than serotonin into the bloodstream. Patients with these tumors have normal serotonin concentrations in blood and in platelets, but urinary amounts are increased because 5-HTP is converted to serotonin in the kidney; urinary 5-HIAA may be slightly elevated.

Patients with serotonin-producing carcinoid tumors usually have striking increases in urinary 5-HIAA excretion (at least tenfold), but occasionally elevations are smaller. False-positive elevations have been known to occur if the patient ingests a wide range of serotonin-rich foods or medications. Conversely, alcohol, aspirin, and other drugs suppress 5-HIAA concentrations. Patients should avoid these agents during 24-hour urine collections. Fasting plasma 5-HIAA has been proposed as a convenient replacement for urine collections.

Most physicians rely on measurement of 5-HIAA to diagnose carcinoid syndrome. But when a patient strongly suspected for carcinoid syndrome shows normal or borderline increases in urinary 5-HIAA, documentation of elevated serotonin concentrations in whole blood or platelets may help establish the diagnosis. Measurement of the concentration of platelet serotonin has been reported to be a more sensitive assay than that for urinary 5-HIAA for detecting carcinoids that produce small or moderate amounts of serotonin, such as foregut and hindgut carcinoids and midgut carcinoids with low tumor volume. Also, platelet serotonin concentrations are not affected by the patient's diet. Platelets can be saturated at high serotonin secretion rates, however, and 5-HIAA is often preferred for monitoring high serotonin production. Measurements of chromogranin A provide an important complement to measurements of serotonin and 5-HIAA and are particularly useful for many gastroenteropancreatic neuroendocrine tumors that do not produce appreciable amounts of serotonin.[11]

Analytical Methodology

In clinical practice, laboratory determinations of (1) catecholamines, (2) serotonin, and (3) their metabolites in biological fluids are performed primarily for diagnosis and follow-up of patients with catecholamine- or serotonin-producing tumors.[3,7,13,14] In accordance with changes in recommended clinical procedures, most laboratories now offer measurements of urinary or plasma metanephrines (normetanephrine and metanephrine) as primary tests for diagnosis of pheochromocytoma and paraganglioma. Liquid chromatography with tandem mass spectrometry (LC-MS/MS) is increasingly becoming the method of choice for these measurements (Figure 26-7). Measurements of catecholamines, usually in urine and less frequently in plasma, are also employed at some medical centers as secondary tests. Measurements of urinary VMA are of declining importance. For detection of neuroblastoma, urinary HVA and VMA remain the most commonly ordered biochemical tests in clinical practice, but other catecholamine metabolites and dopamine are also measured. Diagnostic evaluation of patients with carcinoid tumor routinely involves measurement of 5-HIAA; measurement of serotonin in platelets and urine has also been advocated.

Collection and Storage of Samples

The conditions under which plasma or urine samples are collected is crucial to the reliability and interpretation of test

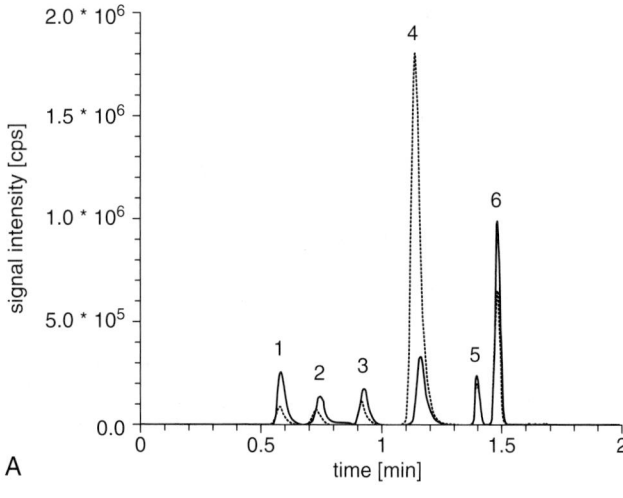

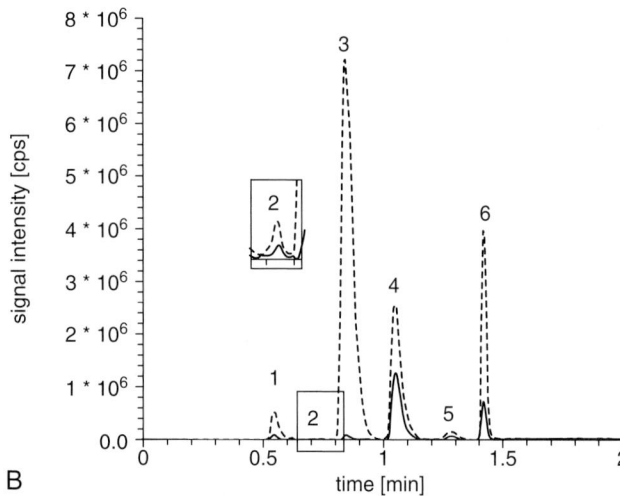

Figure 26-7 Chromatograms obtained by LC-MS/MS for simultaneous measurement of urinary catecholamines and their free O-methylated derivatives for a calibrator **(A)** and extracted urine samples of two patients **(B)**. Chromatographic peaks are shown for norepinephrine (1), epinephrine (2), normetanephrine (3), dopamine (4), metanephrine (5), and 3-methoxytyramine (6), with respective concentrations in the calibrator **(A)** of 59.1, 54.6, 54.6, 65.3, 50.7, and 59.8 nmol/L. For the calibrator, internal standards are shown by a *dotted line*. Patient sample–derived chromatograms **(B)** represent urinary output of catecholamines and their O-methylated metabolites from a patient with confirmed pheochromocytoma *(dashed line)* and a patient without pheochromocytoma. Note the much larger signal intensity (peak height) for normetanephrine (3) in the patient with than without pheochromocytoma.

results.[3,12] Some clinicians prefer 24-hour collection of urine to blood sampling because the former avoids the rigid sampling conditions associated with blood catecholamine collection (e.g., samples should be taken after supine rest) and is more convenient for clinical staff to implement. However, 24-hour urine collections are often difficult and inconvenient for patients. The reliability of the collection timing is frequently in doubt. Plasma metanephrines are not as readily influenced by the trauma of phlebotomy as catecholamines, but the conditions of blood sampling still require consideration to minimize

false-positive test results. It remains preferable to take blood with patients in the supine position and fasting. For urine collection, the influences of diet and sympathoadrenal activation associated with physical activity or changes in posture are not as easily controlled as they are for blood collections. Spot or overnight urine collection with correction for differences in duration of collection using urinary creatinine excretion provides an alternative to 24-hour urine collection that may overcome some of these problems.

For measurements of urinary metanephrines, no preservatives are required, whereas for catecholamines, samples are best preserved with hydrochloric acid to maintain urine acid. For storage over protracted periods, aliquots are best kept frozen at −80 °C to minimize auto-oxidation and deconjugation. Blood samples for both metanephrines and catecholamines are best collected into tubes containing heparin or ethylenediaminetetraacetic acid (EDTA) as an anticoagulant and stored on ice before centrifugation at 4 °C, with separation of plasma for further storage at −80 °C.

Whole blood measurement of serotonin is popular because time-consuming isolation of platelets is not required. For whole blood serotonin, venous blood is (1) drawn into a tube containing potassium EDTA as an anticoagulant, (2) gently mixed and placed on ice, and (3) transferred to a storage tube. An aliquot of blood is then removed for a platelet count. Blood serotonin samples are stored frozen at −20 °C, preferably within 2 hours after collection.

Platelet-rich plasma samples are prepared from whole blood by low-speed centrifugation. To prevent lowering of serotonin concentration, platelet-rich plasma is prepared within 1 hour after the blood is collected and placed on ice. Plasma and pellets are stored frozen at −20 °C and are analyzed within 1 to 2 weeks after collection.

Twenty-four-hour urine samples for serotonin and 5-HIAA are collected in 2-L brown polypropylene bottles, each of which contains 250 mg of sodium metabisulfite and EDTA as preservatives. Samples are acidified to pH 4 with acetic acid before freezing. Most important, the specimen should be refrigerated during collection.

Interferences from and Influences of Diet and Drugs

Dietary constituents or drugs may cause direct analytical interference in assays or influence the physiological processes that determine plasma and urinary concentrations of monoamines and monoamine metabolites. In the former circumstances, interference is highly variable depending on the particular measurement method used. In the latter circumstances, interference is usually of a more general nature and independent of the measurement method.

Development of new drugs, variations in assay techniques, and continuing improvements in analytical procedures make it difficult to identify which directly interfering medications should be avoided for a given analytical test. For modern mass spectrometric–based detection methods, however, such interferences are rarely a problem compared with electrochemical and spectrophotometric detection methods.

More readily identifiable and generalized sources of interference that are independent of the particular assay method tend to be associated with drugs that have primary actions on monoamine systems. Because these systems serve as important therapeutic targets, such drugs represent a relatively common source of false-positive results. Tricyclic antidepressants are a major source of false-positive results for measurements of norepinephrine and normetanephrine; this is a result of the primary actions of these agents to inhibit monoamine reuptake. Other medications that cause significant interference but are less commonly encountered during testing for pheochromocytoma include (1) L-dopa, (2) Sinemet, (3) α-methyldopa (Aldomet), and (4) MAO inhibitors.

Dietary interference is sometimes particularly troublesome for measurements of serotonin metabolites, requiring detailed dietary instruction for these patients.[7] Dietary sources of 5-hydroxyindoles such as (1) walnuts, (2) bananas, (3) avocados, (4) eggplants, (5) pineapples, (6) plums, and (7) tomatoes should be restricted 3 to 4 days before and during urine collection. If possible, patients should abstain from all known medications that may cause an apparent increase, such as (1) glycerol (2) guaiacolate, (3) mephenesin, (4) phenacetin, and (5) acetaminophen, or decrease in 5-HIAA, including (1) methenamine, (2) phenothiazine tranquilizers, (3) homogentisic acid, (4) acetic acid, and (5) levodopa. Measurements of methoxytyramine are subject to influences of dietary catecholamines.[2] For plasma measurements, an overnight fast is sufficient to avoid such influences.

Reference Intervals

Use of appropriately matched reference populations is important for effective screening for monoamine-producing tumors among different populations of patients. Urinary and plasma catecholamines and metanephrines vary with age and have different intervals in hospitalized patients compared with normotensive healthy volunteers and in males compared with females. Also, quantities of catecholamines and metanephrines in 24-hour urine specimens and plasma are non-normally distributed, necessitating nonparametric methods to establish reference intervals or logarithmic transformation to normalize before parametric analyses (Figure 26-8). Because of variations in methods of analysis and subsequent analytical test results, any laboratory establishing measurements of monoamines or metabolites for diagnostic purposes should validate its own reference intervals in line with current standards in clinical practice.

Urinary and Plasma Fractionated Metanephrines

The metanephrines, normetanephrine and metanephrine, and the O-methylated metabolite of dopamine, methoxytyramine, are present in plasma and urine in free and sulfate- or glucuronide-conjugated forms.[3,13] Plasma concentrations of the conjugates are 20- to 30-fold higher than those of the free metabolites, reflecting more rapid circulatory clearance of free than conjugated metabolites. Clearance of free metabolites occurs by active uptake into tissues followed by deamination or conjugation. The conjugated metabolites so produced are cleared relatively slowly by renal extraction and elimination in the urine. Metanephrines in urine are therefore routinely measured after acid hydrolysis and represent mainly conjugated metabolites, whereas metanephrines in plasma are usually measured in the free form.

Measurements of metanephrines in urine and plasma are now widely performed in many laboratories by LC-MS/MS (see Figure 26-7).[3] Such methods offer advantages of (1) short chromatographic run times, (2) high sample throughput, and (3) elimination of drug interference that render obsolete earlier methods, which used liquid chromatography with electrochemical detection (LC-EC). A sample preparation step, usually employing ion exchange chromatography, remains a requirement; however, this is accomplished more simply for LC-MS/MS than for LC-EC methods, with some methods allowing on-line sample purification.

Immunoassay measurements of plasma and urine metanephrines are used by some laboratories, particularly when sample throughput is not high enough to justify the expense of LC-MS/MS instrumentation. Nevertheless, immunoassay methods suffer from relatively poor accuracy and precision and are not recommended for routine clinical use.[3]

Urinary and Plasma Catecholamines

LC-EC methods are still commonly used for measurement of plasma catecholamines, whereas mass spectrometric methods are increasingly used for measurement of urinary catecholamines.[13,14] The most common extraction procedure employed for LC-EC measurement of plasma catecholamines involves alumina extraction (Figure 26-9). For urinary catecholamines, the alumina extraction procedure may be combined with or without a cation exchange step. Boric acid gels provide an alternate approach for selective adsorption of catecholamines. For LC-MS/MS methods, more simple methods of extraction are used, such as 96-well–based ion exchange chromatographic procedures, but with final elution of analytes from extraction columns under acid conditions rather than basic conditions commonly used for metanephrines. When appropriate exchange resins are used, an advantage of these methods over those previously used for preparation of samples for LC-EC is that catecholamines and metanephrines are purified and measured together by LC-MS/MS.

Urinary Vanillylmandelic Acid and Homovanillic Acid

Vanillylmandelic acid (VMA) is the major end-product of norepinephrine and epinephrine metabolism, whereas HVA is the major end-product of dopamine metabolism. Both metabolites are excreted in urine in relatively high amounts, making their analysis relatively simple. VMA in contrast to HVA is not significantly conjugated. Nevertheless, because large amounts of HVA are also present in urine in the free form, both metabolites are commonly measured without a hydrolysis step. Compared with metanephrines and catecholamines, measurements of VMA and HVA have limited value for diagnosis of pheochromocytoma but are commonly used for diagnosis of neuroblastoma.

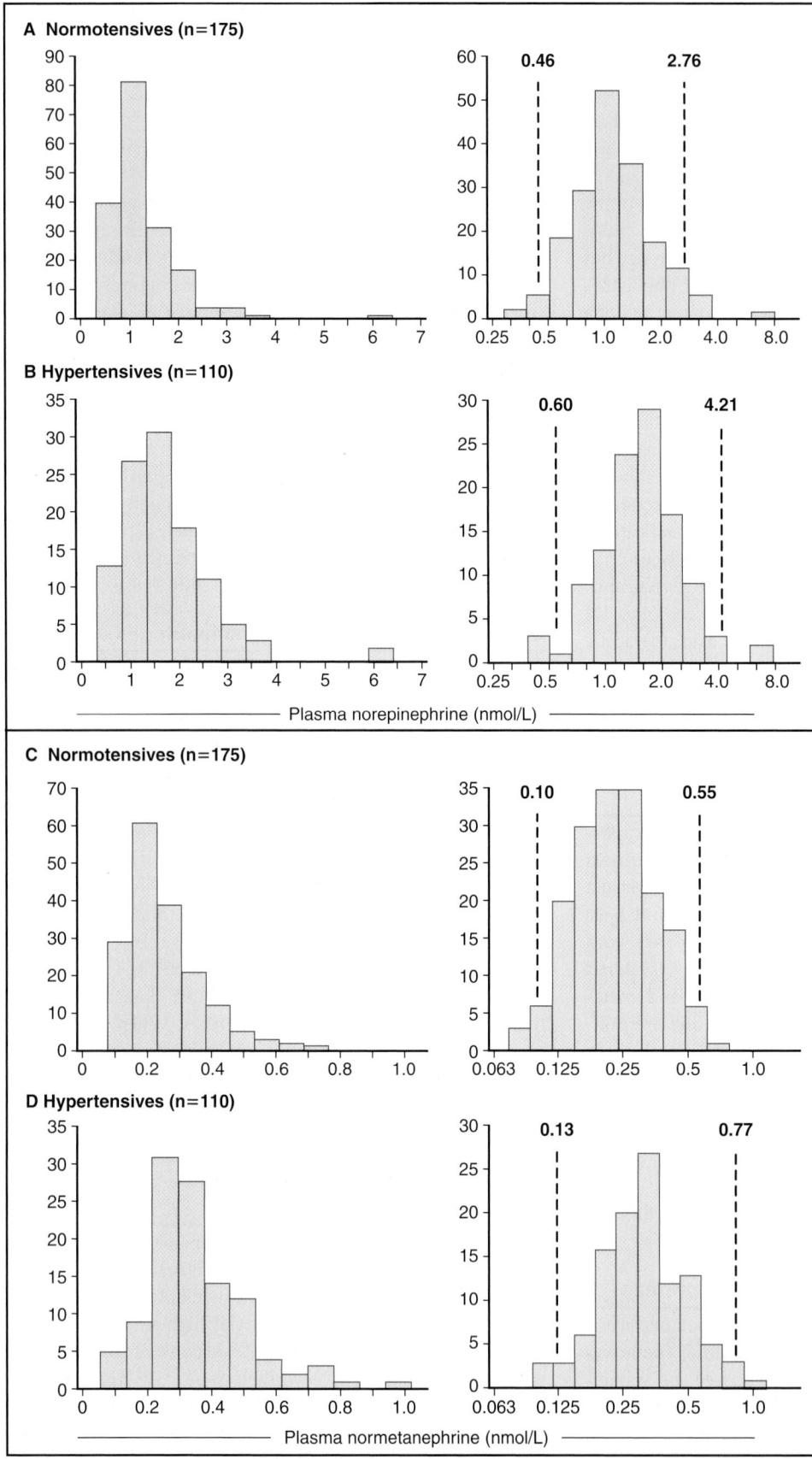

Figure 26-8 Frequency distributions for plasma norepinephrine (**A** and **B**) and plasma-free normetanephrine (**C** and **D**) in healthy normotensive volunteers (**A** and **C**) compared with patients with essential hypertension (**B** and **D**). Distributions shown in the panels on the right have been normalized by logarithmic transformation. The 95% confidence intervals (indicated by *vertical dashed lines*) were estimated using normalized distributions. Note that distributions in hypertensive individuals show a shift to higher plasma concentrations compared with distributions in normotensive individuals, with correspondingly higher lower and upper reference limits.

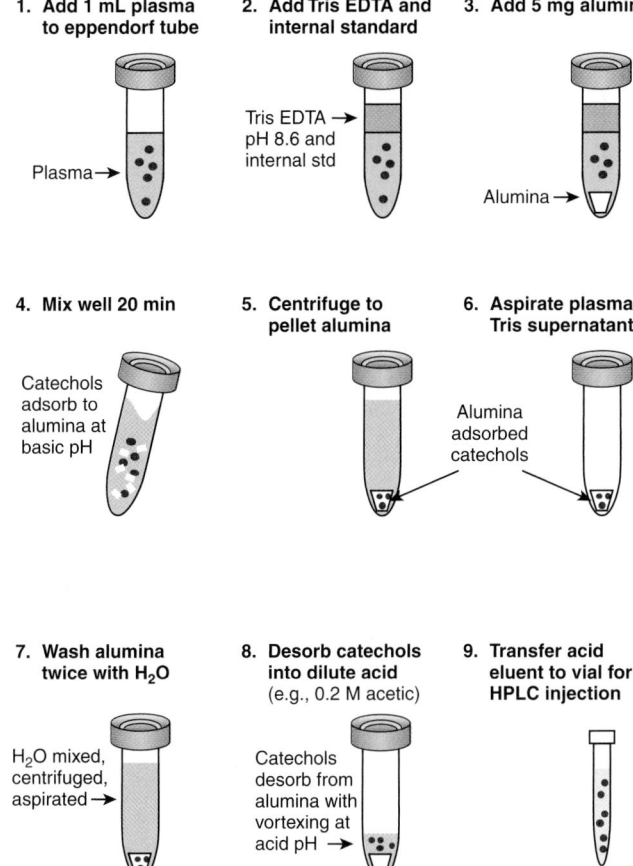

1. **Add 1 mL plasma to eppendorf tube**

Plasma →

2. **Add Tris EDTA and internal standard**

Tris EDTA → pH 8.6 and internal std

3. **Add 5 mg alumina**

Alumina →

4. **Mix well 20 min**

Catechols adsorb to alumina at basic pH

5. **Centrifuge to pellet alumina**

Alumina adsorbed catechols

6. **Aspirate plasma Tris supernatant**

7. **Wash alumina twice with H₂O**

H₂O mixed, centrifuged, aspirated →

8. **Desorb catechols into dilute acid** (e.g., 0.2 M acetic)

Catechols desorb from alumina with vortexing at acid pH →

9. **Transfer acid eluent to vial for HPLC injection**

Figure 26-9 Procedure for alumina extraction of plasma catecholamines. In addition to extraction of the catecholamines (norepinephrine, epinephrine, and dopamine), this procedure allows extraction of other catechols, including 3,4-dihydroxyphenylglycol (the deaminated metabolite of norepinephrine and epinephrine), 3,4-dihydroxyphenylacetic acid (the deaminated metabolite of dopamine), and L-dopa, the precursor of dopamine.

Spectrophotometric methods for determination of VMA and HVA have been superseded by gas or liquid chromatography–based methods, employing today mainly mass spectrometric detection.[13,14] Mass spectrometric methods are highly specific and, along with combined measurements of VMA and HVA, allow with some methods additional measurement of 5-HIAA. Gas chromatography–based methods typically employ extraction of urinary analytes into an organic phase followed by derivatization of analytes in the dried down residue. Sample preparation is simpler still for LC-MS/MS methods, some of which involve only dilution of urine in a suitable injection vehicle.

Serotonin and 5-Hydroxyindoleacetic Acid

Analyses of serotonin, its deaminated acid metabolite, and 5-HIAA and its precursor, 5-hydroxytryptophan (5-HTP), provide important biomarkers for diagnosis of carcinoid tumor.[7] Typically, circulating serotonin is almost entirely confined to platelets, so that measurements are usually performed in (1) whole blood, (2) platelet-rich plasma, or (3) isolated platelet pellets. With sensitive analytical instruments, measurements are possible in platelet-free plasma, which has been proposed as an alternative matrix, useful for detection of serotonin-producing neoplasms at locations where venous outflow does not empty into the portal circulation.

Measurements of urinary serotonin are of less importance because the serotonin in this matrix reflects primarily clearance of plasma-free serotonin and renal decarboxylation of circulating 5-HTP. Nevertheless, urinary measurement is helpful in identifying tumors deficient in aromatic amino acid decarboxylase that produce substantial amounts of 5-HTP, which consequently shows up in urine as serotonin. Such tumors may be more directly detected by measurement of circulating 5-HTP.

Measurements of 5-HIAA are most commonly carried out in urine. As an end-product of serotonin production, 5-HIAA better reflects tumor burden than serotonin. Measurements in plasma after an overnight fast have been advocated as more reliable because they avoid the confounding influence of dietary serotonin.

Liquid chromatography with fluorometric or electrochemical detection remains the most frequently used method for measurements of the concentrations of serotonin and 5-HIAA. Usually these techniques have been developed for measuring serotonin and 5-HIAA separately, but some methods allow for simultaneous measurement of catecholamine and indoleamine acid metabolites (i.e., 5-HIAA, VMA, and HVA). This is usually dependent on differences in analyte chemistry (e.g., amine vs. carboxylic acid), which define the required sample purification procedure and the purified analyte that is detected. For detection of high concentrations of serotonin, as in platelet-rich plasma, simple methods of deproteinization of samples with perchloric acid or trichloroacetic acid before direct injection onto the high-performance liquid chromatography (HPLC) column are used.

Most HPLC assays for serotonin and 5-HIAA employ octadecylsilyl (C18) reversed-phase columns, although strong cation exchange columns have been used for serotonin. The chromatography is usually performed with an isocratic mobile phase at an acid pH that contains an organic modifier and perhaps an ion-pair reagent for serotonin measurements. As with catecholamines, serotonin is protonated in the pH range of 3 to 6, and addition of an anionic ion-pair reagent creates an uncharged conjugate, which enhances the affinity of serotonin for the hydrophobic stationary phase.

For measurement of very small amounts of serotonin or for specialized projects, HPLC with amperometric or coulometric detection is often favored over fluorometric detection. To increase their lower limit of detection, some HPLC procedures incorporate precolumn derivatization with fluorescent and chemiluminescent reagents, thereby achieving detection limits in the femtomole range. Electrochemical detection using amperometric or coulometric measurement is preferred for specific measurement of small quantities of 5-HIAA. Some HPLC systems use fluorometric detection, with or without derivatization, for a less demanding measurement of 5-HIAA.

As with measurements of metanephrines and catecholamines, use of mass spectrometric–based methods of quantification of serotonin and 5-HIAA is increasing. With these methods, sample clean-up procedures are simpler, enabling online sample purification.

Review Questions

1. The urinary metabolite measured as an indicator of norepinephrine synthesis is:
   a. dopamine.
   b. homovanillic acid (HVA).
   c. serotonin.
   d. vanillylmandelic acid (VMA).

2. False-positive elevations of 5-hydroxyindoleacetic acid (5-HIAA) in urine can occur if:
   a. an individual is a chronic alcoholic.
   b. a patient is receiving aspirin therapy.
   c. an individual has recently eaten fruit, such as bananas, kiwis, and plums.
   d. a patient is currently using tricyclic antidepressants.

3. The two urine metabolites that are most widely used for diagnosis of neuroblastoma are:
   a. HVA and VMA.
   b. VMA and 5-HIAA.
   c. HVA and 5-HIAA.
   d. dopamine and epinephrine.

4. Midgut neuroendocrine tumors release which of the following substances in large quantity when compared with tumors derived from other developmental gut components?
   a. 5-Hydroxytryptophan
   b. Serotonin
   c. Epinephrine
   d. Dopamine

5. The method most frequently used for measuring 5-HIAA in urine to detect serotonin production is:
   a. nephelometry.
   b. mass spectrometry.
   c. liquid chromatography.
   d. ion exchange chromatography.

6. Although a 24-hour urine collection is often considered a better specimen for catecholamine analysis, blood samples can be used. Specimen requirements include:
   a. collection in no anticoagulant and immediate freezing of the specimen at −80 °C.
   b. collection in potassium EDTA with preparation of a platelet-rich plasma sample.
   c. collection in sodium oxalate from a fasting upright individual.
   d. collection in heparin or EDTA anticoagulant from a fasting supine individual.

7. A catecholamine-producing tumor derived from the chromaffin cells of the adrenal medulla is referred to as a:
   a. neuroblastoma.
   b. pheochromocytoma.
   c. paraganglioma.
   d. gastroenteropancreatic neuroendocrine tumor.

8. True or false: More than 95% of the serotonin in the body is produced within the gastrointestinal tract.
   a. True
   b. False

9. Chromaffin cells are located in the___ and are responsible for synthesis of ___.
   a. kidney; renin
   b. brain; dopamine
   c. adrenal gland; epinephrine
   d. gut; serotonin

10. Epinephrine is also called:
    a. noradrenaline.
    b. adrenaline.
    c. metanephrine.
    d. serotonin.

References

1. Cheung NK, Zhang J, Lu C, Parker M, Bahrami A, Tickoo SK, et al. St Jude Children's Research Hospital–Washington University Pediatric Cancer Genome Project. Association of age at diagnosis and genetic mutations in patients with neuroblastoma. JAMA 2012;307:1062–71.
2. Eisenhofer G, Kopin IJ, Goldstein DS. Catecholamine metabolism: a contemporary view with implications for physiology and medicine. Pharmacol Rev 2004;56:331–49.
3. Eisenhofer G, Tischler AS, de Krijger RR. Diagnostic tests and biomarkers for pheochromocytoma and extra-adrenal paraganglioma: from routine laboratory methods to disease stratification. Endocr Pathol 2012;23:4–14.
4. Goldstein DS. Catecholamines 101. Clin Auton Res 2010;20:331–52.
5. Goyal RK, Hirano I. The enteric nervous system. N Engl J Med 1996;334:1106–15.
6. Hoffman BB, Taylor P. Neurotransmission: the autonomic and somatic motor nervous system. In: Hardman JG, Limbird LE, Gilman AG, eds. Goodman and Gilman's the pharmacological basis of therapeutics, 10th edition. New York: McGraw-Hill, 2001:115–53.
7. Kema IP, de Vries EG, Muskiet FA. Clinical chemistry of serotonin and metabolites. J Chromatogr B Biomed Sci Appl 2000;747:33–48.
8. Lenders JW, Eisenhofer G, Mannelli M, Pacak K. Phaeochromocytoma. Lancet 2005;366:665–75.
9. Maris JM. Recent advances in neuroblastoma. N Engl J Med. 2010;362:2202–11.
10. Oberg K. Neuroendocrine tumors of the digestive tract: impact of new classifications and new agents on therapeutic approaches. Curr Opin Oncol 2012;24:433–40.
11. Oberg K. Circulating biomarkers in gastroenteropancreatic neuroendocrine tumours. Endocr Relat Cancer 2011;18(Suppl 1):S17–25.
12. Pacak K, Eisenhofer G, Lenders JWM. Pheochromocytoma: diagnosis, localization and treatment, 1st edition. Oxford: Wiley-Blackwell, 2007.
13. Peaston RT, Weinkove C. Measurement of catecholamines and their metabolites. Ann Clin Biochem 2004; 41:17–38.
14. Rosano TG, Swift TA, Hayes LW. Advances in catecholamine and metabolite measurements for diagnosis of pheochromocytoma. Clin Chem 1991;37:1854–67.
15. Schilling FH, Spix C, Berthold F, Erttmann R, Fehse N, Hero B, et al. Neuroblastoma screening at one year of age. N Engl J Med 2002;346:1047–53.
16. von Bohlen und Halbach O, Dermietzel R. Neurotransmitters and neuromodulators. Handbook of receptors and biological effects. Darmstadt, Germany: FRG, 2002.

Vitamins, Trace Elements, and Nutritional Assessment*

*Alan Shenkin, Ph.D., F.R.C.P., F.R.C.Path., and
Norman B. Roberts, M.Sc., Ph.D., C.Chem.*

Objectives

1. Define the following:

Beriberi	Scurvy
Chemical speciation	Speciation methods
Hypervitaminosis	Trace element
Hypovitaminosis	Ultratrace element
Pellagra	Vitamer
Pernicious anemia	Vitamin

2. Classify the vitamins discussed in this chapter according to their water or fat solubility; discuss what these terms mean in relation to vitamin physiology.
3. State the chemical names of each vitamin discussed in this chapter.
4. Summarize the physiological roles of each vitamin discussed in this chapter.
5. Describe the symptoms of toxicity and deficiency, if any, for each vitamin discussed in this chapter; state the names of the specific disorders related to deficiency of vitamin B_{12}, C, niacin, and thiamine.
6. List the most common method of laboratory analysis for each vitamin discussed in this chapter.
7. Analyze and solve case study problems related to vitamin deficiency or toxicity.

8. State what is meant when an element is considered "essential."
9. Correlate the importance of trace elements passing from a charged ionized form to the uncharged form with the role that each element exerts in its respective metalloprotein.
10. List eight essential trace elements and summarize the physiological functions and clinical significance of each listed element.
11. Describe instrumental methods used in the analysis of trace elements; list two of these methods and their principles.
12. Outline appropriate specimen collection procedures and possible preanalytical variables associated with to trace element analysis.
13. List and describe two deficiency disorders of the following trace elements: chromium, copper, manganese, selenium, and zinc; list and describe at least one genetic disorder that affects each of the following: copper, zinc, and iron.
14. Appraise the possible roles of the following elements in human physiology, including function and clinical significance: boron, silicon, vanadium.
15. Analyze and solve case study problems related to trace element deficiency.

Key Words and Definitions

Acrodermatitis enteropathica A hereditary disorder due to defective zinc uptake.

Acute phase reaction (APR) A response of the body to inflammation that results in an increase or decrease in the plasma concentrations of a class of proteins known as acute phase reactants.

Apoenzyme A protein moiety of an enzyme that requires a coenzyme.

Avitaminosis A disease condition, described as a deficiency syndrome, that results from lack of a vitamin.

Beriberi A disease caused by a deficiency of thiamine (vitamin B_1) and characterized by polyneuritis, cardiac pathology, and edema.

*The authors gratefully acknowledge the original contributions of Donald B. McCormick, Harry L. Green, George G. Klee, David B. Milne, Gordon S. Fell, David Lyons, and Malcolm Baines, on which portions of this chapter are based. The authors are also grateful for the assistance of Juha and Leila Risteli in revising the "Vitamin C" section.

Key Words and Definitions—cont'd

Chemical speciation Refers to the molecular form of atoms of an element or a cluster of atoms of different elements in a given matrix.

Coenzyme A diffusible, heat-stable substance or organic molecule (sometimes derived from a vitamin) of low molecular weight that, when combined with an inactive protein called an *apoenzyme*, forms an active compound or a complete enzyme called a *holoenzyme*, which functions catalytically in an enzyme system.

Cofactor A natural reactant, usually a metal ion or a coenzyme, that is required in an enzyme-catalyzed reaction.

Essential nutrients Nutrients (proteins, minerals, carbohydrates, lipids, vitamins) necessary for growth, normal functioning, and maintenance of life; they must be supplied by food because they cannot be synthesized by the body.

Estimated average requirement (EAR) The daily intake of a specific nutrient estimated to meet the requirement in 50% of healthy people in an age- and gender-specific group. The EAR is used to calculate the recommended dietary allowance.

Gucose tolerance factor A biologically active complex of chromium and nicotinic acid that facilitates the reaction of insulin with receptor sites on tissues.

Hartnup disease An inborn error of metabolism characterized by a massive aminoaciduria involving a group of neutral monoaminomonocarboxylic amino acids sharing a common renal reabsorption mechanism.

Hemorrhagic disease of newborn A self-limited hemorrhagic disorder of the first days of life, caused by a deficiency of the vitamin K–dependent blood coagulation factors II, VII, IX, and X.

Holoenzyme The functional (i.e., catalytically active) compound formed by the combination of an apoenzyme with its appropriate coenzyme.

Hypervitaminosis An unhealthy condition resulting from excessive amounts of a vitamin.

Hypovitaminosis An unhealthy condition resulting from too little of a vitamin; interchangeable with avitaminosis.

Kashin–Beck disease (KBD) A chronic, endemic osteochondropathy (disease of the bone).

Keshan disease A fatal, congestive cardiomyopathy caused by deficiency of essential trace elements in the diet.

Megaloblastic anemia Any anemia characterized by megaloblasts in the bone marrow, such as pernicious anemia.

Menkes disease An X-linked recessive disorder of copper metabolism caused by mutations in the *ATP7A* gene (locus: Xq12-q13), which encodes a copper transporter.

Nutriture The status of the body in relation to nutrition, generally or with regard to a specific nutrient such as a trace element.

Pellagra A clinical deficiency syndrome due to deficiency of niacin (or failure to convert tryptophan to niacin) and characterized by dermatitis, inflammation of mucous membranes, diarrhea, and psychic disturbances.

Pernicious anemia A deficiency in the production of red blood cells through a lack of vitamin B_{12}.

Recommended dietary allowance (RDA) The amount of nutrient and calorie intake per day considered necessary for maintenance of good health, calculated for males and females of various ages and recommended by the Food and Nutrition Board of the U.S. National Research Council. Popularly called *recommended daily allowance*.

Scurvy A condition due to deficiency of ascorbic acid (vitamin C) in the diet.

Systemic inflammatory response syndrome (SIRS) The systemic inflammatory response to a wide variety of severe clinical insults.

Speciation methods Techniques used to separate the chemical complexes of individual elements present in any particular medium.

Superoxide dismutase An enzyme of the oxidoreductase class that catalyzes the reduction of superoxide anions to hydrogen peroxide, protecting cells against dangerous levels of superoxide (oxygen).

Total parenteral nutrition (TPN) The practice of feeding a person intravenously, circumventing the gut.

Trace elements Inorganic molecules found in human and animal tissues in milligram per kilogram amounts or less.

Ultratrace elements Inorganic molecules found in human and animal tissues in microgram per kilogram amounts or less.

Vitamer Term used to describe any of a number of compounds that possess a given vitamin activity.

Vitamin An essential organic micronutrient that must be supplied exogenously and in many cases is the precursor to a metabolically derived coenzyme.

Wilson disease A rare, progressive, autosomal recessive disease due to a defect in metabolism of copper.

Zinc finger A finger-shaped fold in a protein that is created by the binding of specific amino acids in the protein to a zinc atom. Zinc-finger proteins regulate the expression of genes as well as nucleic acid recognition, reverse transcription, and virus assembly.

Adequate supplies of **vitamins** and **trace elements** are **essential nutrients** and critical for maintaining the health and development of humans (http://www.iom.edu/; accessed October 2, 2013).[1, 2-8,12] Table 27-1 summarizes the **recommended dietary allowance (RDA)** in the United States and population reference intakes from the European community for vitamins and trace elements. The consequences of an inadequate intake of trace elements are shown in Figure 27-1.

Vitamins

Historically, vitamin groups bear an Arabic subscript number following the letter either to designate structural and functional similarity (e.g., A_1 [retinol] and A_2 [3-dehydroretinol]) or to indicate the approximate order in which they are identified as members of the so-called B-complex (e.g., B_1 [thiamine] and B_2 [riboflavin]). Common chemical names are also used. These often reflect the presence of (1) some specific atom (thiamine), (2) a prime functional group (pyridoxamine), or (3) even a larger portion of the molecular structure (phylloquinone). Parts of some names reflect functional properties (cholecalciferol).

Another classification pertains to the relative solubility of vitamins. Those of the *fat-soluble* group (A, D, E, and K) are more soluble in organic solvents, whereas B-complex group vitamins and vitamin C are *water soluble*. This general separation based on solubility is useful not just for purposes of noting gross physical properties but also as a reminder that fat-soluble vitamins are (1) absorbed, (2) transported, and

(3) stored for longer periods of time. Most water-soluble vitamins are retained less and excreted more in the urine. In general, water-soluble vitamins function as **coenzymes** for several important enzymatic reactions in both mammals and microorganisms. By contrast, fat-soluble vitamins generally do not function as coenzymes and are rarely used by microorganisms.

Thirteen known vitamins and vitameric groups essential to humans are individually discussed below and are listed in Table 27-2.

Vitamin A

Vitamin A serves many important functions in the body; its role in vision is of particular significance.

Chemistry

Vitamin A is the nutritional term for the group of compounds with a 20-carbon structure containing a methyl-substituted cyclohexenyl ring (β-ionone ring) and an isoprenoid sidechain (Figure 27-2), with (1) a hydroxyl group (retinol), (2) an aldehyde group (retinal), (3) a carboxylic acid group (retinoic acid), or (4) an ester group (retinyl ester) at the terminal C15. Retinol, the principal vitamin A **vitamer,** will oxidize reversibly to retinal—which shares all the biological activity of retinol—or will further oxidize to retinoic acid, which shows some of its biological activity. The principal storage forms of vitamin A are retinyl esters, particularly palmitate. Included in the vitamin A family are some dietary carotenoids (C40 polyisoprenoid compounds) that are classified as provitamin A because they

TABLE 27-1	Oral and Intravenous Micronutrient Intakes for Adults[15]			
	RDA (USA)	**PRI (Europe)**	**Amount in 2000 kcal Tube-Feed**	**IV Intake**
Vitamins				
A µg	900	700	1000-2160	1000
D µg	5-15	0-10	8.5-14.6	5
E mg	15	0.4/g PUFA	20-64	10
K µg	120	100-200	150	
Thiamine mg	1.2	1.1	1.4-3.4	6
Riboflavin mg	1.3	1.6	2-6	3.6
Pyridoxine mg	1.3	1.5	2-13.8	6
Niacin mg	16	18	18-45	40
Folate µg	400	200	340-880	600
B_{12} µg	2	1.4	3-15	5
Pantothenic acid µg	5*	3-12†	7-20	15
Biotin µg	30*	15-100	100-660	60
Ascorbic acid mg	90	45	100-300	200
Trace Elements				
Zinc mg	11	9.5	13-36	3.2-6.5
Copper mg	0.9	1.1	2-3.4	0.3-1.3
Selenium µg	55	55	30-130	40-100
Chromium µg	25	30-200	10-20	
Molybdenum µg	45*	74-240	19	
Manganese mg	2-3*	1-10†	2.4-8	0.05-0.2

Reference intakes for infants and children are age and weight dependent.
PRI, Population reference intake (Europe); *PUFA,* polyunsaturated fatty acids; *RDA,* recommended dietary allowance (United States).
*Adequate intake.
†Acceptable range.

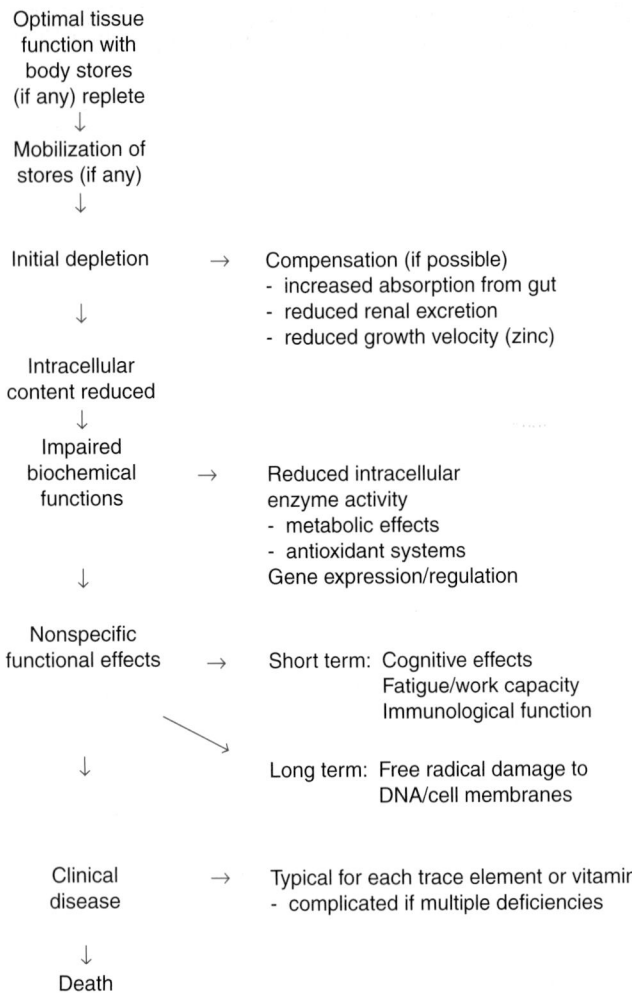

Optimal tissue
function with
body stores
(if any) replete
↓
Mobilization of
stores (if any)
↓
Initial depletion   →   Compensation (if possible)
                            - increased absorption from gut
  ↓   - reduced renal excretion
                            - reduced growth velocity (zinc)
Intracellular
content reduced
  ↓
Impaired
biochemical   →   Reduced intracellular
functions   enzyme activity
                       - metabolic effects
                       - antioxidant systems
  ↓   Gene expression/regulation

Nonspecific
functional effects →   Short term: Cognitive effects
                                     Fatigue/work capacity
                                     Immunological function

  ↓   Long term: Free radical damage to
                                     DNA/cell membranes

Clinical   →   Typical for each trace element or vitamin
disease   - complicated if multiple deficiencies
  ↓
Death

Figure 27-1 Consequences of inadequate mineral or trace element intake. *(From Shenkin A, Allwood MC. Trace elements and vitamins in adult intravenous nutrition. In: Rombeau JL, Rolandelli RH, editors. Clinical nutrition: parenteral nutrition. Philadelphia: WB Saunders, 2001:60–79.)*

are cleaved biologically to yield retinol. Examples include (1) α-carotene, (2) β-carotene, and (3) β-cryptoxanthin. Vitamin A compounds are yellowish oils or low-melting-point solids (depending on isomeric purity) that are practically insoluble in water but are soluble in organic solvents and mineral oil.

Dietary Sources

Preformed vitamin A is obtained from (1) liver, (2) other organ meats, (3) fish oils, (4) full cream milk, (5) butter, and (6) fortified margarines. The provitamin A carotenoids are obtained from yellow to orange pigment fruits and vegetables and from green leafy vegetables. The U.S. National Health and Nutrition Examination Survey (NHANES)-II indicated that approximately 25% of the vitamin A requirement was provided by carotenoids and about 75% by preformed retinol.

Absorption, Transport, Metabolism, and Excretion

Preformed vitamin A, most often in the form of retinyl ester, or carotenoids are subject to emulsification before being transported into the intestinal cell. There the retinyl esters are moved across the mucosal membrane and are hydrolyzed to retinol within the cell to be reesterified by cellular retinol-binding protein II and packaged into chylomicrons. These enter the mesenteric lymphatic system and pass into the systemic circulation.

Carotenoids, also in micellar form, are absorbed into the duodenal mucosal cells by passive diffusion. The efficiency of absorption of carotenoids is much less than for vitamin A. Once inside the mucosal cell, β-carotene is converted primarily to retinal by the enzyme β-carotene-15,15′-dioxygenase, and the retinal is converted by retinal reductase to retinol and is esterified. The newly synthesized retinyl esters then pass with chylomicrons via the lymphatic system to the liver, where uptake by parenchymal cells again involves hydrolysis. In the liver, retinol is bound with retinol-binding protein (RBP; MW ≈21,000 Da) and transthyretin (thyroxine-binding prealbumin) (MW ≈55,000 Da) in a 1:1:1 complex of sufficient size to prevent loss by glomerular filtration. Delivery of retinol to the tissue is controlled by the availability of the vitamin A protein complex in the circulation, although this control mechanism will be bypassed with large doses of retinol. Excretion of vitamin A occurs via the feces and urine, usually after conjugation or oxidation.

Functions

Vitamin A has a significant function in vision. All-*trans*-retinol is the predominant circulating form of vitamin A, and cells of the retina isomerize it to the 11-*cis* alcohol that is reversibly dehydrogenated to 11-*cis* retinal. This sterically hindered geometrical isomer of the aldehyde combines as a lysyl-linked Schiff base with suitable proteins such as opsin to generate photosensitive pigments such as rhodopsin. Illumination of such pigments causes photoisomerization and release of all-*trans*-retinal and the protein—a process that couples the large conformational change to ion flux and optic nerve transmission. The all-*trans*-retinal is isomerized to the 11-*cis* isomer, which again combines with the liberated protein to reconstitute the photo pigment in a visual cycle, as shown in Figure 27-3.

Other functions of vitamin A include its role in (1) reproduction, (2) growth, (3) embryonic development, and (4) immune function. In normal growth and in maintenance of the integrity of epithelial cells, retinoic acid acts through the activation of retinoic acid receptors (RARs) and retinoid X receptors (RXRs) in the nucleus to regulate various genes that encode for (1) structural proteins, (2) enzymes, (3) extracellular matrix proteins, and (4) RBP and receptors. Retinol, its metabolites, and synthetic retinoids provide protective effects against the development of certain types of cancer by (1) blocking tumor promotion, (2) inhibiting proliferation, (3) inducing apoptosis, (4) inducing differentiation, or (5) combining these actions. Some caution is required, however, regarding the use of vitamin A or β-carotene supplements because they appear to be of no benefit in reducing the incidence of gastrointestinal cancer and indeed may increase the incidence of lung cancer and mortality in certain other cancers.

TABLE 27-2	**Human Vitamin Requirements**			
Common Name	**Trivial Chemical Name**	**General Roles**	**Symptoms of Deficiency or Disease**	**Direct and Indirect Assays**
Fat Soluble				
Vitamin A	Retinol, retinal, retinoic acid	Vision, growth, reproduction	Nyctalopia, xerophthalmia, keratomalacia	Photometric, HPLC, fluorometric, RIA
Vitamins D_2, D_3	Ergocalciferol, cholecalciferol	Modulation of Ca^{2+} metabolism, calcification of bone and teeth	Rickets (young), osteomalacia (adult)	CPB, HPLC, RIA
Vitamin E	Tocopherols, tocotrienols	Antioxidant for unsaturated lipids, neurological and reproductive functions	Lipid peroxidation, including red blood cell fragility, hemolytic anemia (premature, newborn)	Photometric, HPLC, erythrocyte hemolysis
Vitamins K_1, K_2	Phylloquinones, menaquinones	Blood clotting, osteocalcins	Increased clotting time, RIA time, hemorrhagic disease (infant)	HPLC, prothrombin (abnormal prothrombin, PIVKA test)
Water Soluble				
Vitamin B_1	Thiamine	Carbohydrate metabolism, nervous function	Beriberi, Wernicke-Korsakoff syndrome	Fluorometric, transketolase, HPLC
Vitamin B_2	Riboflavin	Oxidation reduction reactions	Angular stomatitis, dermatitis, photophobia	Fluorometric, HPLC, glutathione reductase
Vitamin B_6	Pyridoxine, pyridoxal, pyridoxamine	Amino acid, phospholipid, and glycogen metabolism	Epileptiform convulsions, dermatitis, hypochromic anemia	HPLC, aspartate transaminase, urine pyridoxic acid
Niacin	Nicotinic acid, nicotinamide	Oxidation reduction reactions	Pellagra	Fluorometric, HPLC, niacinamide nicotinamide coenzymes
Folic acid	Pteroylglutamic acid	Nucleic acid and amino acid biosynthesis	Megaloblastic anemia, neural tube defects	CPB, microbiological, homocysteine
Vitamin B_{12}	Cyanocobalamin	Amino acid and branched chain keto acid metabolism	Pernicious and megaloblastic anemia, neuropathy	CPB, microbiological, RIA, methylmalonate
Biotin	—	Carboxylation reactions	Dermatitis	Microbiological, CPB, carboxylases, avidin binding
Pantothenic acid	—	General metabolism, acetyl and acyl transfer	Burning feet syndrome	Microbiological, RIA, CPB/HPLC
Vitamin C	Ascorbic acid	Connective tissue formation, antioxidant	Scurvy	Photometric, HPLC, enzymatic

CPB, Competitive protein binding; *HPLC*, high-performance liquid chromatography; *PIVKA test*, proteins induced by or involved in vitamin K antagonism or absence; *RIA*, radioimmunoassay.

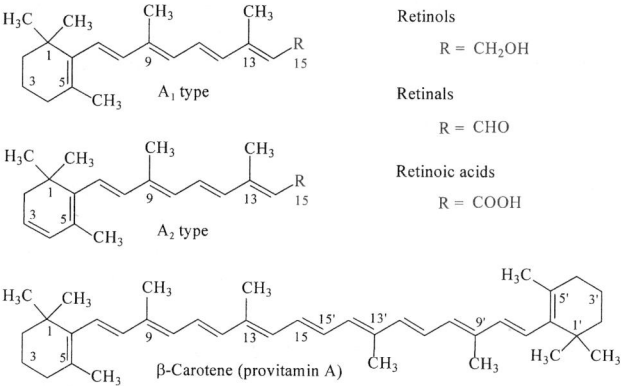

Figure 27-2 Vitaminic forms of A_1, A_2, and β-carotene.

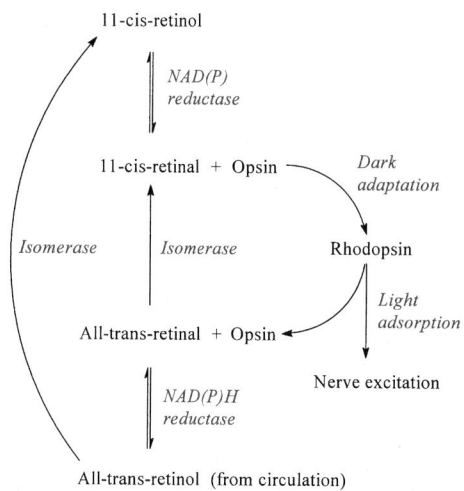

Figure 27-3 Participation of A vitamers in the visual cycle.

Requirements and Reference Nutrient Intakes[6,11]

Past studies suggest that intakes of retinol of 500 to 600 µg/d are required. For example, the Food and Nutrition Board of the U.S. Institute of Medicine recommends the retinol activity equivalent (RAE) as the basis of calculation of retinol intake. With this system, a ratio equivalence of 1:12:24 is recommended (12 µg β-carotene or 24 µg mixed carotenoids has the same biological activity as 1 µg retinol). With this system, current RDAs for vitamin A are 900 µg RAE for men 19 years and older and 700 µg RAE for women, with increased allowances for pregnancy and lactation.

Deficiency

Vitamin A deficiency primarily affects infants and children, and its prevalence is subject to World Health Organization (WHO) surveillance. Risk factors include (1) poverty, (2) low birth weight, (3) poor sanitation, (4) malnutrition, (5) infection, and (6) parasitism. Because hepatic accumulation of vitamin A occurs during the last trimester of pregnancy, preterm infants are relatively vitamin A deficient at birth. Providing a daily oral intake of vitamin A that meets the RDA of 400 µg RAE is therefore important. Infants with birth weights less than 1500 g (those under 30 weeks' gestation) have virtually no hepatic vitamin A stores and are at risk of vitamin A deficiency. Fat malabsorption, particularly caused by celiac disease or chronic pancreatitis, and protein-energy malnutrition predispose to vitamin A deficiency. Liver disease diminishes RBP synthesis, and ethanol abuse leads both to hepatic injury and to competition with retinol for alcohol dehydrogenase, which is necessary for the oxidation of retinol to retinal and retinoic acid. Vitamin A deficiency may lead to anemia, although the exact mechanism is not known.

The clinical features of vitamin A deficiency include degenerative changes in eyes and skin and poor dark adaptation (night blindness [nyctalopia]). More serious effects of deficiency are *xerophthalmia,* in which the conjunctiva becomes dry with small gray plaques with foamy surfaces (Bitot spots), and keratomalacia, which causes ulceration and necrosis of the cornea. Usually, associated skin changes include (1) dryness, (2) roughness, (3) papular eruptions, and (4) follicular hyperkeratosis.

Toxicity

Although vitamin A metabolism is tightly regulated, toxic effects of **hypervitaminosis** A have occurred as a result of ingestion of excess vitamin or as a side effect of inappropriate therapy. Hypervitaminosis A occurs (1) after liver storage of retinol and its esters exceeds 3000 µg/g tissue, (2) after more than 30,000 µg/d is ingested for months or years, or (3) when plasma vitamin A concentrations exceed 140 µg/dL (4.9 µmol/L). Acute toxicity from a single massive dose is rare. Chronic toxicity from moderately high doses taken for protracted periods is characterized by (1) bone and joint pain, (2) hair loss, (3) dryness and fissures of the lips, (4) anorexia, (5) benign intracranial hypertension, (6) weight loss, and (7) hepatomegaly.

Epidemiological and experimental evidence indicates that high vitamin A intake in humans, acting via 13-*cis*-retinoic acid, is teratogenic. The Food and Nutrition Board of the U.S. Institute of Medicine has recommended a tolerable upper intake concentration of 3000 µg/d of preformed vitamin A for men and lower concentrations for (1) women of child-bearing age, (2) infants, (3) children, and (4) adolescents. Carotenemia results from chronic excessive intake of carotene-rich foods, principally carrots. This condition, in which yellowing of the skin is observed, is benign because the excess carotene is deposited rather than converted to vitamin A.

Laboratory Assessment of Status

Measurement of the plasma concentration of vitamin A is widely used to assess vitamin A status. However, it is not an ideal indicator because vitamin A does not decline until liver stores become critically depleted. This is thought to occur at a concentration of approximately 20 µg/g of liver tissue. Early chemical methods, such as the Carr-Price and Neeld-Pearson methods, have largely been replaced by high-performance liquid chromatography (HPLC) methods. Both normal-phase and reverse-phase techniques have been used with (1) photometric, (2) electrochemical, or (3) mass spectrometric detectors.

As retinol circulates in plasma as a 1:1:1 complex with RBP and transthyretin, both of these hepatically produced proteins have been measured as an indicator of vitamin A status. RBP may be measured by nephelometry, but its circulating concentration may be affected by inadequate dietary (1) protein, (2) energy, or (3) zinc, all of which are necessary for RBP synthesis. Another confounding factor in the assessment of vitamin A status is the effect of the acute-phase response. Both RBP and transthyretin are negative acute-phase proteins, thus inflammatory changes will result in a transient fall in proteins and in plasma retinol. To distinguish inflammatory from nutritional causes of reduced plasma retinol concentrations, it is necessary to measure an acute-phase protein, such as C-reactive protein (CRP).

Reference Intervals

Guidance reference intervals for plasma vitamin A include the following: (1) 20 to 40 µg/dL (0.70 to 1.40 µmol/L) for 1- to 6-year-old children; (2) 26 to 49 µg/dL (0.91 to 1.71 µmol/L) for 7- to 12-year-old children; (3) 26 to 72 µg/dL (0.91 to 2.51 µmol/L) for 13- to 19-year-old adolescents; and (4) 30 to 80 µg/dL (1.05 to 2.80 µmol/L) for adults. Values above 30 µg/dL (1.05 µmol/L) are associated with appreciable reserves in the liver and correlate well with vitamin A intake. Within the reference interval, values for men are generally about 20% higher than those for women. The reference interval for plasma β-carotene is 10 to 85 µg/dL (0.19 to 1.58 µmol/L). Elevated concentrations are found in hypothyroid patients, in whom conversion to vitamin A is decreased, and in patients with hyperlipidemia associated with diabetes mellitus. The reference interval for plasma RBP is 3 to 6 mg/dL.

Vitamin D

Vitamin D plays an essential role as a hormone in the control of calcium and phosphorus metabolism (see Chapter 39).

Vitamin E

Vitamin E is an antioxidant that acts as a scavenger for molecular oxygen and free radicals and has a role in cellular respiration.

Chemistry

Vitamin E is the nutritional term for the group of naturally occurring tocopherols and tocotrienols that have biological activity similar to RRR-α-tocopherol (formerly D-α-tocopherol). Also note that RRR refers to its three stereo centers located at the 2, 4, and 8 positions of the tocopherol chain. The Greek letter prefixes α, β, γ, and δ indicate the presence or absence of methyl groups at positions 5 and 7 (Figure 27-4). Tocopherols and tocotrienols are (1) viscous oils at room temperature, (2) soluble in fat solvents, and (3) insoluble in aqueous solutions. Also, tocopherol and tocotrienols are stable to acid and heat in the absence of oxygen but labile to oxygen in alkaline solutions and to ultraviolet light.

Dietary Sources

The principal sources of dietary vitamin E are (1) oils and fats, particularly wheat germ oil and sunflower oil, (2) grains, and (3) nuts. Meats, fruits, and vegetables contribute little vitamin E. γ-Tocopherol is the major form of vitamin E in many plant seeds in the U.S. diet, but it is present at only one-quarter to one-tenth the concentration of α-tocopherol in human plasma.

Absorption, Transport, Metabolism, and Excretion

In the presence of bile, vitamin E is absorbed from the small intestine. Most forms of vitamin E are absorbed nonselectively and are secreted in chylomicron particles, which are then transported to the peripheral tissue (mainly adipose tissue) with the aid of lipoprotein lipase. The liver takes up the chylomicron remnants where the α-tocopherol is incorporated into very low-density lipoprotein (VLDL). Vitamin E is excreted via the bile and in the urine as tocopheronic acid and its β-glucuronide conjugate.

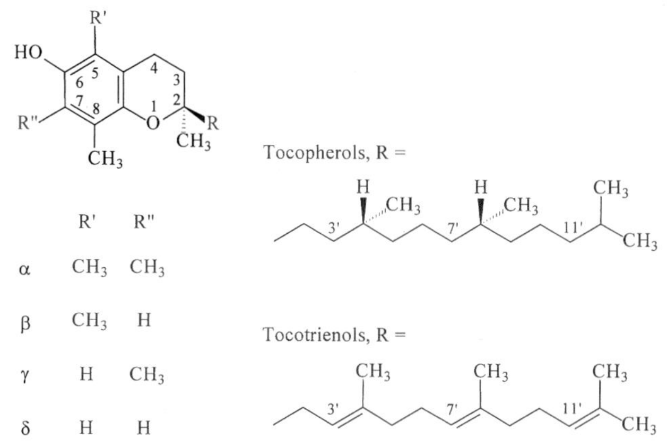

Figure 27-4 Vitaminic forms of vitamin E.

Functions

Vitamin E is considered necessary for (1) neurological and reproductive functions, (2) protection of the red cell from hemolysis, (3) prevention of retinopathy in premature infants, and (4) inhibition of free-radical chain reactions of lipid peroxidation. The latter occurs mainly within the polyunsaturated fatty acids of membrane phospholipids. Tocopherols and tocotrienols inhibit lipid peroxidation largely because they scavenge lipid peroxyl radicals faster than the radical reacts with adjacent fatty acid sidechains or membrane proteins. The resultant tocopheryl or tocotrienyl radicals then react with further peroxyl radicals to produce tocopherones (nonradicals), or are regenerated by transfer of an electron to ascorbate to form the ascorbyl radical. Thus, vitamins E and C act synergistically to reduce lipid peroxidation (Figure 27-5). Many epidemiological surveys have shown an association between reduced vitamin E intake (and other dietary factors) and an increase in the incidence of chronic disease, particularly cardiovascular disease and cancer. However, most studies on supplementation have failed to show any benefit.

Requirements and Reference Nutrient Intakes[6]

The daily requirement for vitamin E is related to the cellular polyunsaturated fatty acid content. The minimum adult requirement for vitamin E is thought to be approximately 3 to 4 mg/d for those who ingest a diet containing the minimum requirement of essential fatty acids. However, in the year 2000, the U.S. Food and Nutrition Board increased the RDA for vitamin E for adults from 10 to 15 mg/d. Most European reference intakes are related to polyunsaturated fatty acid intake. Another departure in the newer recommendations was that the daily requirement must be met by RRR-α-tocopherol alone, as the other forms of vitamin E are not converted to α-tocopherol and are poorly recognized by the α-tocopherol transfer protein in the liver.

Deficiency

Premature and low birth weight infants are particularly susceptible to development of vitamin E deficiency because placental transfer is poor and infants have limited adipose tissue. Signs of deficiency include (1) irritability, (2) edema, and (3) hemolytic anemia. In general, symptoms of vitamin E deficiency are rare in children and adults, although deficiency has occurred in some conditions. Fat malabsorption states, such as cystic fibrosis and chronic cholestasis in children, have been known to cause neuropathy and hemolytic anemia, as does the genetic disorder abetalipoproteinemia (within which vitamin E is transported).

Toxicity

Excess vitamin E intake is usually achieved only by dietary supplementation and may cause deficiency of fat-soluble vitamins D and K by competitive absorption. A comprehensive review of the tolerance and safety of vitamin E suggested that intakes up to 3000 mg/d were safe. Reversible side effects of (1) gastrointestinal symptoms, (2) increased creatinuria, and (3) impaired blood coagulation have been observed at intakes of 1000 to 3000 mg/d. The U.S. Food and Nutrition Board has

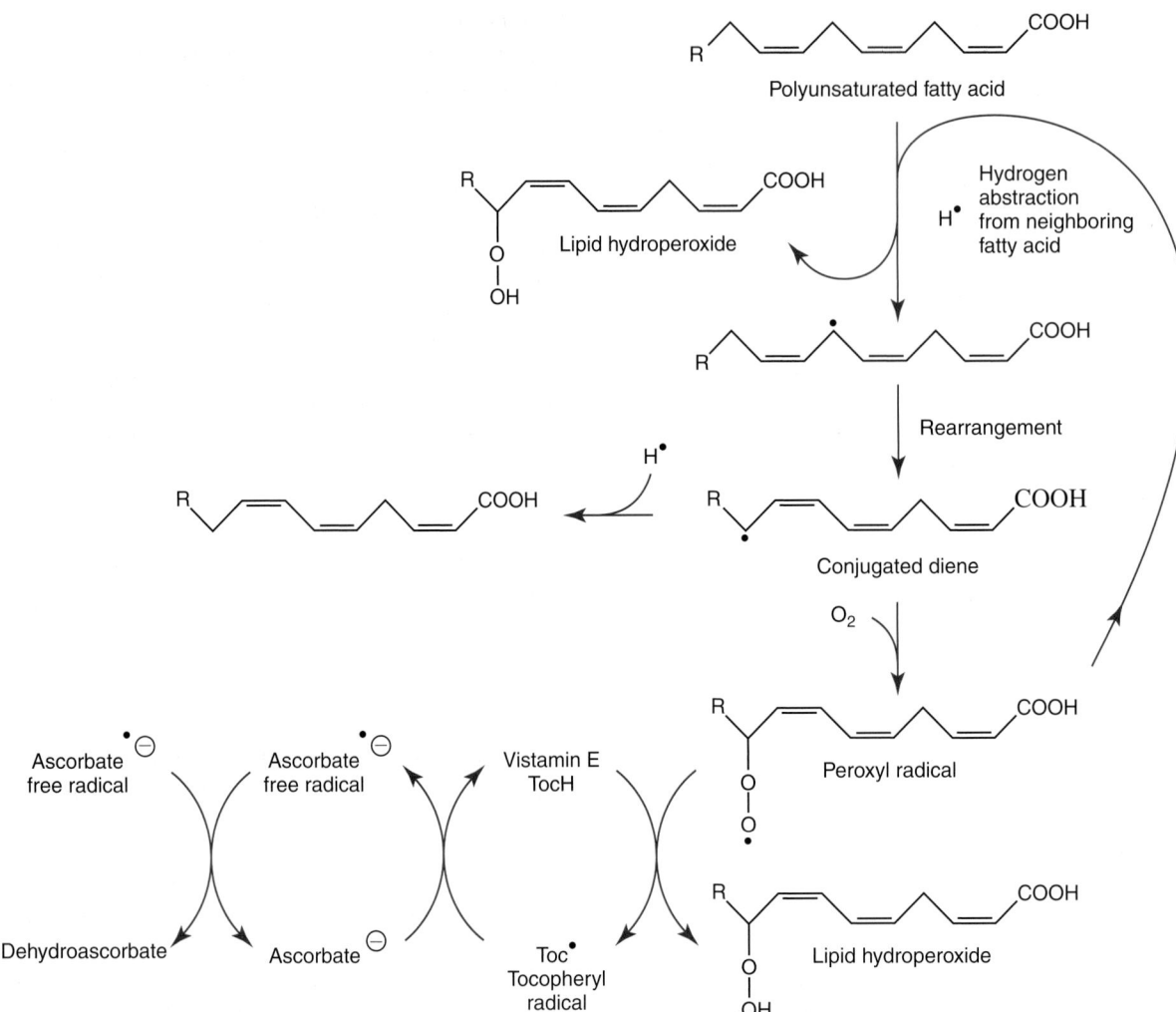

Figure 27-5 Synergistic action of vitamin E and ascorbate in radical chain breaking.

recommended a tolerable upper limit of 1000 mg/d of vitamin E for adults 19 years of age and older.

Laboratory Assessment of Status[11]

HPLC is presently the method of choice to quantify tocopherols in serum. α- and γ-Tocopherols are the principal vitamers seen, although others are detected with minor modifications to the analytical conditions. Thin-layer and gas-liquid chromatography methods have been used to separate the tocopherols and the tocotrienols.

Reference Intervals

Guidance reference intervals for serum or plasma (heparin) vitamin E are (1) 0.1 to 0.5 mg/dL (2.3 to 11.6 µmol/L) for premature neonates; (2) 0.3 to 0.9 mg/dL (7 to 21 µmol/L) for children (1 to 12 years); (3) 0.6 to 1.0 mg/dL (14 to 23 µmol/L) for adolescents; and (4) 0.5 to 1.8 mg/dL (12 to 42 µmol/L) for adults.

Vitamin K

Vitamin K promotes clotting of the blood and is required for the conversion of several clotting factors and prothrombin; it is a topic of growing interest in bone metabolism.

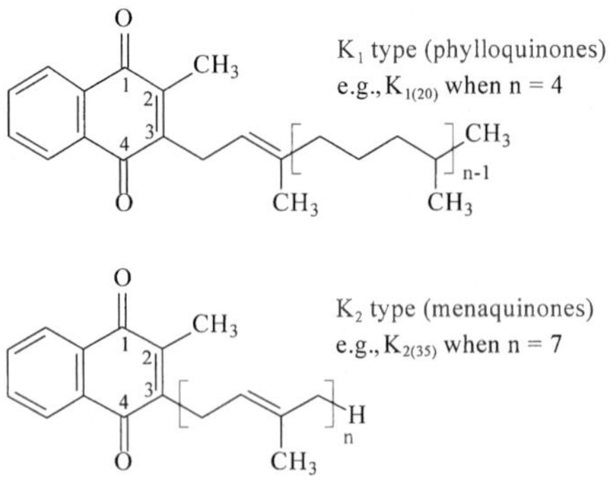

Figure 27-6 Vitaminic forms of vitamin K.

Chemistry

Compounds in the vitamin K series are 2-methyl-1,4-naphthoquinones, which are substituted with sidechains at carbon 3. The two principal natural classes of vitamin K are the *phylloquinones* (K_1 type) synthesized in plants and the menaquinones (K_2 type) of bacterial origin (Figure 27-6). Several synthetic analogues and derivatives have been used in human nutrition. Most relate to or are derived from menadione (K_3), which lacks a sidechain substituent at position 3 but is converted to

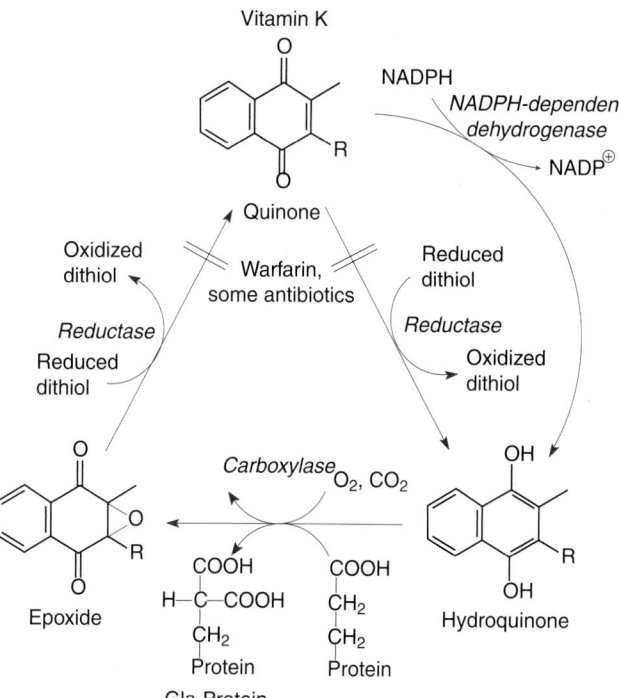

Vitamin K

Quinone

Oxidized dithiol

Warfarin, some antibiotics

Reduced dithiol

Reductase
Reduced dithiol

Reductase
Oxidized dithiol

NADPH

NADPH-dependent dehydrogenase

NADP⊕

Epoxide

Carboxylase O_2, CO_2

Hydroquinone

COOH
H–C–COOH
CH_2
Protein

COOH
CH_2
CH_2
Protein

Gla-Protein

Figure 27-7 Metabolic cycling of vitamin K, the effect of warfarin, and the formation of Gla proteins.

menaquinone (MK). They are destroyed by alkaline solutions and reducing agents and are sensitive to ultraviolet light.

Dietary Sources

The main dietary sources of phylloquinones are (1) green vegetables, (2) margarines, and (3) plant oils. Menaquinones are obtained from (1) cheese, (2) other milk products, and (3) eggs.

Absorption, Transport, Metabolism, and Excretion

Absorption of natural vitamin K from the small intestine into the lymphatic system is facilitated by bile. Efficiency of absorption varies from 15% to 65%. Vitamins K_1 and K_2 are bound to chylomicrons for transport from mucosal cells to the liver. Menadione (K_3) is more rapidly and completely absorbed from the gut before it enters the portal blood. In the liver, intracellular distribution occurs mostly in the microsomal fraction. Release of vitamin K to the bloodstream allows association with circulating β-lipoproteins for transport to other tissue.

Within metabolically active and vitamin K–using tissue, especially liver, a microsomal vitamin K cycle exists (Figure 27-7). The vitamin (quinone) is normally reduced by a thiol-sensitive flavoprotein system to the hydroquinone, which then couples to oxygen and carbon dioxide to form the Gla protein (e.g., prothrombin). The 2,3-epoxide of vitamin K that is subsequently formed is reduced to the starting vitamin K quinones—a process that is antagonized by such vitamin K antagonists as warfarin. Only traces of urinary metabolites of vitamins K_1 and K_2 appear in urine. A considerable portion of vitamin K_3 is conjugated to form β-glucuronide and sulfate esters, which are excreted.

Functions

The essential and most thoroughly defined role of vitamin K is that of a dietary antihemorrhagic factor. Vitamin K–dependent carboxylase converts specific glutamyl residues in target proteins to γ-carboxyglutamyl (Gla) residues. This γ-carboxylation increases the affinity of these proteins for calcium. Vitamin K is also needed for formation of the Gla proteins (1) prothrombin (factor II), (2) proconvertin (factor VII), (3) plasma thromboplastin component (factor IX), and (4) Stuart factor (factor X). These, together with two other hemostatic vitamin K–dependent proteins, proteins C and S and Ca^{2+}, initiate a process to form thrombin, which then catalyzes the conversion of fibrinogen to a fibrin clot.

Proteins that contain γ-carboxyglutamyl are also abundant in bone tissue; osteocalcin accounts for up to 80% of the total γ-carboxyglutamyl content of mature bone. A further major Gla protein, matrix Gla protein (MGP)—which contain five residues of γ-carboxyglutamic acid—is found in (1) vascular smooth muscle, (2) bone, and many soft tissues such as (3) heart, (4) kidney, and (5) lungs. It is thought that MGP accumulates at sites of calcification, including calcified aortic valves and bone, and is a potent inhibitor of calcification.

Requirements and Reference Nutrient Intakes[6]

Although the human gut bacteria synthesize large quantities of menaquinones, absorption of these compounds has been difficult to demonstrate, however, dietary restriction of vitamin K does lead to evidence of inadequacy. Dietary reference intakes for vitamin K have recently been revised by the Food and Nutrition Board of the U.S. Institute of Medicine to 120 µg/d for men over 18 years of age and 90 µg/d for women, including those pregnant or lactating. Dietary intake of phylloquinone in North American and most European populations studied has been estimated at around 150 µg/d for those older than 55 years of age and around 80 µg/d for younger individuals.

Deficiency

Although vitamin K deficiency is uncommon in the adult, risk is increased in fat malabsorption states such as (1) bile duct obstruction, (2) cystic fibrosis, (3) chronic pancreatitis, and (4) liver disease. Risk is also increased by the use of drugs that interfere with vitamin K metabolism, such as the coumarin anticoagulants (e.g., warfarin) and some antibiotics (e.g., cephalosporin). Defective blood coagulation and demonstration of abnormal noncarboxylated prothrombin are at present the only well-established signs of vitamin K deficiency.

Hemorrhagic disease of the newborn results from (1) poor placental transfer of vitamin K, (2) hepatic immaturity leading to inadequate synthesis of coagulation proteins, and (3) low vitamin K content in early breast milk. Prothrombin concentrations in the newborn during this period are only about 25% of adult concentrations. Severe diarrhea and antibiotics used to suppress diarrhea exacerbate the situation, so that when prothrombin concentrations drop to below 5% of the adult concentration, bleeding has been seen to occur. This condition is prevented by prophylactic administration of 0.5

to 1.0 mg of phylloquinone intramuscularly, or 2.0 mg given orally, immediately after birth.

Toxicity

The use of high doses of naturally occurring vitamin K (K_1 and K_2) appears to have no harmful effect; however, menadione (K_3) treatment can lead to the formation of erythrocyte cytoplasmic inclusions, known as Heinz bodies, as well as hemolytic anemia.

Laboratory Assessment of Status[11]

Because of its relatively low plasma concentration (approximately 50 times lower than vitamin D and at least one thousand times lower than vitamins A or E), vitamin K has long presented an analytical challenge. Consequently, vitamin K status has traditionally been assessed by functional methods, primarily by noting its effect on clotting time. Prothrombin time (PT) is assessed by adding to recalcified plasma a portion of tissue thromboplastin and measuring clotting time against a normal control sample. In vitamin K deficiency, PT may rise to above 30 seconds (normal, 10 to 14 seconds). Attempts at cross-laboratory standardization have led to the introduction of the international normalized ratio (INR), whereby the PT is expressed as a fraction of the control time.

Assays based on reduced activity of vitamin K, such as immunoassay for undercarboxylated plasma prothrombin and osteocalcin, are more sensitive but are not widely used.

Direct measurement of plasma phylloquinone is probably the best indicator of vitamin K status and has been shown to correlate well with intake. HPLC methods typically require 0.5 to 2.0 mL of serum or plasma and involve (1) protein precipitation and lipid extraction (often into hexane), (2) solvent evaporation, (3) preparative LC (to isolate vitamin K from other lipids), (4) reevaporation of the vitamin K–rich fraction, (5) dilution in the mobile phase, and (6) HPLC with electrochemical or fluorometric detection, often after postcolumn reduction. Typical between-batch imprecision values are 11% to 18% (coefficient of variation [CV]), with limits of detection lower than 50 pmol/L.

Reference Interval

A guidance reference interval for plasma vitamin K is 0.13 to 1.19 ng/mL (0.29 to 2.64 nmol/L).

Vitamin B₁—Thiamine

Vitamin B₁—also known as thiamine—forms the coenzyme thiamine pyrophosphate (TPP). It is required for the essential decarboxylation reactions catalyzed by the pyruvate and 2-oxoglutarate complexes.

Chemistry

The structure of *thiamine* (3-[4-amino-2-methyl-pyrimidyl-5-methyl]-4-methyl-5-[β-hydroxyethyl]thiazole) is that of a pyrimidine ring, bearing an amino group and linked by a methylene bridge to a thiazole ring (Figure 27-8). Thiazole has a primary alcohol sidechain at C5, which is phosphorylated in vivo to produce thiamine phosphate esters,

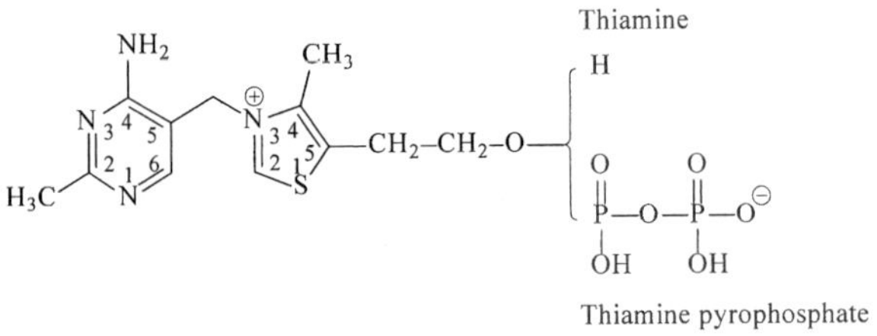

Figure 27-8 Thiamine and the pyrophosphate coenzyme.

the most common of which is TPP (also known as thiamine diphosphate, cocarboxylase). Monophosphate and triphosphate esters also occur.

Dietary Sources

Small quantities of thiamine and its phosphates are present in most plant and animal tissue, but the most abundant sources are unrefined cereal grains. Enrichment of flour and derived food products, particularly breakfast cereals, has considerably increased the availability of this vitamin.

Absorption, Transport, Metabolism, and Excretion

Thiamine absorption occurs primarily in the proximal small intestine. The absorbed thiamine undergoes intracellular phosphorylation, mainly to the pyrophosphate, but at the serosal membrane side 90% of the transferred thiamine is present in free form. Thiamine is carried by the portal blood to the liver. Free vitamin occurs in the plasma, but TPP is the primary cellular component. Approximately 30 mg is stored in the body: 80% as pyrophosphate, 10% as triphosphate, and the rest as thiamine and its monophosphate. The three tissue enzymes known to participate in the formation of phosphate esters are (1) thiaminokinase, (2) TPP-ATP phosphoryl-transferase (cytosolic 5′-adenylic kinase), and (3) thiamine triphosphatase.

About half of the body stores are found in (1) skeletal muscle, with much of the remainder in the (2) heart, (3) liver, (4) kidneys, and (5) nervous tissue (including the brain, which contains most of the triphosphate). The estimated half-life of thiamine is 9.5 to 18.5 days.

Functions

Thiamine is required by the body as the TPP in two general types of reaction: (1) oxidative decarboxylation of 2-oxo acids catalyzed by dehydrogenase complexes and (2) formation of 2-ketols (ketoses) as catalyzed by transketolase. TPP functions as the Mg^{2+}coordinated coenzyme for the so-called active aldehyde and transfers in multienzyme dehydrogenase complexes that affect decarboxylative conversion of 2-oxo acids to acyl-coenzyme A (acyl-CoA) derivatives, such as pyruvate dehydrogenase and 2-oxoglutarate dehydrogenase. These are often localized in the mitochondria, where efficient use in the Krebs tricarboxylic acid (citric acid) cycle follows.

Transketolase is a TPP-dependent enzyme found in the cytosol of many tissues, especially liver and blood cells, in which principal carbohydrate pathways exist. In the pentose phosphate pathway, which additionally supplies reduced NADPH necessary for biosynthetic reactions, this enzyme catalyzes the reversible transfer of a glycoaldehyde moiety from the first two carbons of a donor ketose phosphate to the aldehyde carbon of an aldose phosphate.

Requirements and Reference Nutrient Intakes[2]

As thiamine is necessary for the metabolism of carbohydrates, fats, and alcohol, a direct correlation of need with the amount of metabolizable food intake is evident. The requirement is increased under situations in which metabolism is increased, such as in normal conditions of (1) increased muscular activity, (2) pregnancy, and (3) lactation, or in abnormal cases of (1) protracted fever, (2) post trauma, and (3) hyperthyroidism. Clinical signs of deficiency in adults are prevented by intakes of thiamine above 0.15 to 0.2 mg/1000 kcal, but 0.35 to 0.4 mg/1000 kcal may be closer to the amount necessary to maintain urinary excretion and TPP-dependent erythrocyte transketolase activity within reference intervals. The current RDA is 1.2 mg/d for adult males and 1.1 mg/d for adult females. Additional requirements are recommended for pregnancy and lactation.

Deficiency

Beriberi is a disease that results from thiamine deficiency. Clinical signs of thiamine deficiency primarily involve the nervous and cardiovascular systems. In the adult, symptoms most frequently observed are (1) mental confusion, (2) anorexia, (3) muscular weakness, (4) ataxia, (5) peripheral paralysis, (6) ophthalmoplegia, (7) edema (wet beriberi), (8) muscle wasting (dry beriberi), (9) tachycardia, and (10) an enlarged heart. In infants, symptoms appear suddenly and severely, often involving cardiac failure and cyanosis.

Thiamine deficiency occurs because of (1) inadequate intake caused by diets largely dependent on milled, non-enriched grains, such as rice and wheat, or (2) ingestion of raw fish containing microbial thiaminases. Chronic alcoholism often leads to thiamine deficiency caused by (1) reduced intake, (2) impaired absorption, and (3) reduced storage and may lead clinically to the Wernicke-Korsakoff syndrome. Other at-risk groups include (1) those receiving **total parenteral nutrition (TPN)** without adequate thiamine supplementation, (2) elderly patients taking diuretics, and (3) patients undergoing long-term renal dialysis.

Toxicity

No reports have described adverse effects resulting from consumption of excess thiamine from food and supplements (supplements of 50 mg/d are widely available without prescription).

Laboratory Assessment of Status[11]

Because the basic biological function of thiamine is to act as the pyrophosphate **cofactor** in a number of enzyme systems, two differing approaches to assessment of status are used. In one approach, the analyte, free or phosphorylated, is measured directly in a suitable body fluid or tissue. In the other approach, its properties as an enzymatic cofactor are exploited in a functional assay. Both approaches have associated advantages and disadvantages, each supplying some, but not all, of the information necessary for full assessment of thiamine adequacy. In clinical practice, direct measurement is now used more frequently.

The most commonly used enzyme for the functional assay is transketolase, and several methods are available for its measurement. With the Brin procedure, activities of holo forms and apo forms of transketolase in erythrocyte hemolysates are measured before and after the addition of TPP. The transketolase activation test consists of two tests: one a measurement of basal activity, and the other assesses the degree to which basal activity is increased by exogenous TTP; each may be influenced by different factors. Evidence suggests that chronic deficiency states of thiamine may decrease the synthesis of the **apoenzyme.** In comparison studies against erythrocyte TPP concentrations, better correlations were obtained with basal activity rather than with the activation coefficient.

Direct measurement of circulating thiamine concentrations may be made in (1) plasma, (2) erythrocytes, or (3) whole blood. The plasma (or serum) concentration is thought to reflect recent intake and involves mainly unphosphorylated thiamine at low concentrations (around 10 to 20 nmol/L). Because the erythrocyte contains approximately 80% of the total thiamine content of whole blood, mainly as the pyrophosphate, and erythrocyte thiamine stores deplete at a similar rate to other major organs, HPLC measurement of TPP in erythrocytes is a good indicator of body stores. Typical HPLC methods include (1) a protein precipitation step, (2) precolumn or postcolumn formation of the fluorophore thiochrome, usually with alkaline ferricyanide, (3) isocratic separation, and (4) fluorometric measurement. Whole blood samples may be analyzed in a manner similar to that used for washed erythrocytes.

Reference Intervals

Guidance reference intervals for erythrocyte transketolase activity include the following: 0.75 to 1.30 U/g Hb (48.4 to 83.9 kU/mol Hb) for percent TPP effect (activation), 0% to 15% normal, 16% to 25% marginally deficient, and >25% severely deficient with clinical signs. For direct TPP concentration measurements, typical intervals are 173 to 293 nmol/L erythrocytes and 90 to 140 nmol/L whole blood.

Vitamin B$_2$—Riboflavin

Vitamin B$_2$, also known as riboflavin, is an essential component of flavin adenine dinucleotide (FAD) and flavin mononucleotide (FMN)—coenzymes that are involved in many redox reactions.

Chemistry

Vitamin B$_2$ refers to riboflavin and its related metabolites, which act as cofactors to several reduction oxidation enzymes. The parent compound, riboflavin (7,8-dimethyl-10-[1′-D-ribityl]isoalloxazine), is a yellow fluorescent compound. Its major physiological role is to act as a precursor for FMN (riboflavin-5′-phosphate) and FAD. FMN is formed from riboflavin by flavokinase-catalyzed phosphorylation, and FAD

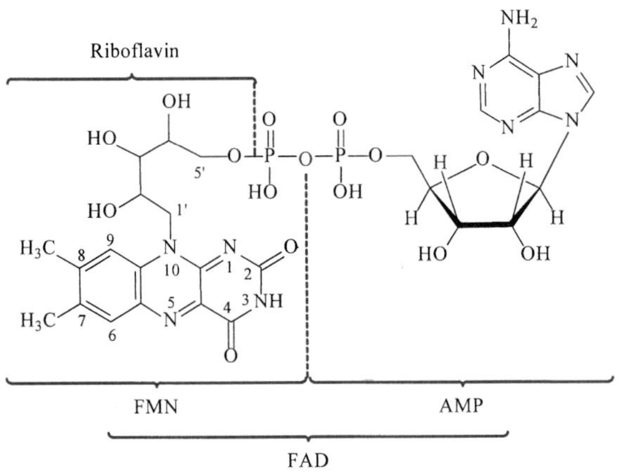

Figure 27-9 Riboflavin and FMN as components of FAD.

is formed from FMN and ATP by the action of FAD synthetase (Figure 27-9). Flavins are stable during exposure to heat but are decomposed by light.

Dietary Sources
Rich sources of coenzyme forms of the vitamin are (1) liver, (2) kidney, and (3) heart. Many (4) vegetables are also good sources, as is (5) milk, but cereals are rather low in flavin content. However, current practices of fortification and enrichment of cereal products have made them significant contributors to the daily requirement.

Absorption, Transport, Metabolism, and Excretion
Most dietary riboflavin is consumed as a complex of food protein with the coenzymes FMN and FAD. These coenzymes are released from noncovalent attachment to proteins by gastric acidification. The vitamin is primarily absorbed in the proximal small intestine by a saturable transport system that is rapid and proportional to intake before reaching a plateau at doses near 27 mg riboflavin per day. Bile salts appear to facilitate the uptake. The transport of flavins in human blood involves loose binding to albumin and tight binding to a number of globulins, particularly immunoglobulins. Uptake of riboflavin into the cells of organs is a process that requires a specific carrier at physiological concentrations. At higher concentrations, uptake occurs by passive diffusion.

Conversion of riboflavin to coenzymes occurs within the cellular cytoplasm of most tissue, but particularly in (1) small intestine, (2) liver, (3) heart, and (4) kidney. The obligatory first step is ATP-dependent phosphorylation of the vitamin catalyzed by flavokinase. The FMN product is complexed with specific apoenzymes to form several functional flavoproteins, but the larger quantity is further converted to FAD in a second ATP-dependent reaction catalyzed by FAD synthetase (pyrophosphorylase). Because little storage of riboflavin occurs, urinary excretion reflects dietary intake.

Functions
The riboflavin coenzymes are capable of both one- and two-electron transfer processes and play a pivotal role in coupling two-electron oxidation of most organic substrates to the one-electron

transfer of the respiratory chain. Additionally, flavoproteins catalyze (1) dehydrogenation reactions, (2) hydroxylations, (3) oxidative decarboxylations, (4) deoxygenations, and (5) reductions of oxygen to hydrogen peroxide. Other major functions of riboflavin include drug metabolism in conjunction with the cytochrome P$_{450}$ enzymes and lipid metabolism.

Flavins also have pro-oxidative and antioxidative functions. They are thought to contribute to oxidative stress by producing superoxide and to catalyze the production of hydrogen peroxide. As an antioxidant, FAD is a coenzyme to glutathione reductase in the regeneration of reduced glutathione from oxidized glutathione, which is necessary for the removal of lipid peroxides. Riboflavin deficiency is associated with increased lipid peroxidation. Flavins also have homocysteine-lowering properties; FAD is a cofactor to methylenetetrahydrofolate reductase in the remethylation of homocysteine.

Requirements and Reference Nutrient Intakes[2]
Assessment of riboflavin requirements is based on the relationship of dietary intake to overt signs of (1) hyporiboflavinosis, (2) urinary excretion of the vitamin, (3) erythrocyte riboflavin content, and (4) erythrocyte glutathione reductase activity. Based on these considerations, the current RDA has been set at 1.3 mg/d for adult men and 1.1 mg/d for adult women . Additional requirements are suggested in pregnancy and lactation.

Deficiency
Deficiency of riboflavin is characterized by (1) sore throat, (2) hyperemia, (3) edema of the pharyngeal and oral mucous membranes, (4) cheilosis, (5) angular stomatitis, (6) glossitis (magenta tongue), (7) seborrheic dermatitis, and (8) normochromic, normocytic anemia. However, some of these symptoms, such as glossitis and dermatitis, when encountered in the field, may have resulted from other complicating deficiencies.

Although riboflavin has a wide distribution in foodstuffs, many people live for long periods on low intakes; consequently, minor signs of deficiency are common in many parts of the world. In addition to poor intake, functional deficiency has been induced by diseases, such as hypothyroidism and adrenal insufficiency, which inhibit the conversion of riboflavin to its coenzyme derivatives. Because flavin coenzymes are widely distributed in intermediary metabolism and are involved in the metabolism of (1) folic acid, (2) pyridoxine, (3) vitamin K, and (4) niacin, deficiency will affect enzyme systems other than those requiring flavin coenzymes.

Toxicity
Probably as a result of its limited solubility and limited gastric absorption, no adverse effects have been associated with ingestion of riboflavin appreciably above RDA concentrations.

Laboratory Assessment of Status[11]
Riboflavin status is assessed by (1) determination of urine riboflavin excretion, (2) a functional assay using the activation coefficient of stimulation of the enzyme glutathione reductase by FAD, or (3) direct measurement of riboflavin or its metabolites in plasma or erythrocytes.

Urinary riboflavin is measured by fluorometric and microbiological procedures, but for specificity, HPLC combined with fluorometric detection is the method of choice. Under conditions of adequate intake, the amount excreted per day is more than 120 μg or 80 μg/g creatinine. Conditions that cause negative nitrogen balance and administration of antibiotics and certain psychotropic drugs (phenothiazine derivatives) increase urinary riboflavin as a consequence of tissue depletion and displacement.

A commonly used functional method for assessing riboflavin status consists of determining erythrocyte glutathione reductase activity and the increase in activity on incubation with exogenous FAD. Most methods measure the rate of change of absorbance at 340 nm caused by oxidation of NADPH and have been automated to produce rapid throughputs and CVs of less than 2% within run, although some have used fluorescence detection. In long-standing riboflavin deficiency, apoenzyme activity may be reduced, leading to a misleading activation coefficient calculation.

The most widely used methods in current clinical practice include direct measurements of riboflavin, FMN, and FAD in plasma or erythrocytes by (1) HPLC, usually with fluorescence detection after protein precipitation or by (2) capillary zone electrophoresis with laser-induced fluorescence detection.

Reference Intervals

The reference intervals when a fluorometric method is used for erythrocyte riboflavin are 10 to 50 μg/dL (266 to 1330 nmol/L), and for plasma concentrations of riboflavin, 4 to 24 μg/dL (106 to 638 nmol/L). Guidance reference intervals for the activation coefficient of erythrocyte glutathione reductase by FAD are 1.20 (adequacy), 1.21 to 1.40 (marginal deficiency), and 1.41 and above (deficiency).

Vitamin B$_6$—Pyridoxine, Pyridoxamine, and Pyridoxal

Pyridoxine (pyridoxol), *pyridoxamine*, and *pyridoxal* are the three natural forms of vitamin B$_6$. They are converted to pyridoxal phosphate, which is required for synthesis, catabolism, and interconversion of amino acids.

Chemistry

The three natural forms—(1) pyridoxine (pyridoxol) (PN), (2) pyridoxamine (PM), and (3) pyridoxal (PL)—are 4-substituted 2-methyl-3-hydroxyl-5-hydroxymethyl pyridines (Figure 27-10). During metabolic conversion, each vitamer becomes phosphorylated at the 5-hydroxymethyl position. Although both pyridoxamine-5′-phosphate (PMP) and pyridoxal-5′-phosphate (PLP, P-5′-P) interconvert as coenzyme forms during aminotransferase (transaminase)-catalyzed reactions, PLP is the coenzyme form that participates in the largest number of B$_6$-dependent enzyme reactions.

Dietary Sources

Vitamin B$_6$ is widely distributed in animal and plant tissue, where phosphorylated forms, particularly PLP, predominate. Meat, poultry, and fish are good sources, as are yeast, certain

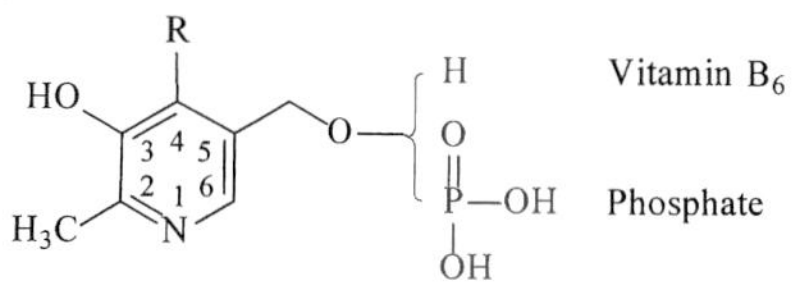

Figure 27-10 Free and phosphorylated forms of vitamin B$_6$. R = CH$_2$OH for pyridoxine, CH$_2$NH$_2$ for pyridoxamine, and CHO for pyridoxal.

seeds, bran, and bananas. Fortified ready-to-eat cereals have become an important dietary source. The common commercial form of the vitamin is pyridoxine hydrochloride, which is a water-soluble, white, crystalline solid.

Absorption, Transport, Metabolism, and Excretion

Food sources of animal origin contain mainly PLP with some PMP, whereas plant sources also contain pyridoxine-5′-glucoside, which is absorbed in a different manner. The phosphorylated sources are hydrolyzed by the intraluminal action of intestinal alkaline phosphatase, but pyridoxine-5′-glucoside is less effectively hydrolyzed by nonspecific glycosidase within cells. The nonphosphorylated vitamers are readily absorbed by the mucosal cells through a process of passive diffusion. Here, as in other cells requiring vitamin B$_6$, the unphosphorylated vitamers may be "metabolically trapped" as the phosphorylated forms by cytoplasmic pyridoxal kinase responsible for catalyzing the ATP-dependent phosphorylation of all three vitamin forms. The vitamers are unphosphorylated before transport to the liver via the portal vein.

Figure 27-11 shows the intracellular metabolism of vitamin B$_6$. Most cells contain a cytosolic FMN-dependent pyridoxine (pyridoxamine)-5′-phosphate oxidase responsible for catalyzing the oxygen-dependent conversion of pyridoxine phosphate and pyridoxamine phosphate to PLP (and hydrogen peroxide). PLP enters directly into subcellular organelles, such as hepatocyte mitochondria, and binds for catalytic function with numerous specific apoenzymes throughout the cell. The erythrocyte, in addition, traps PLP as a conjugate Schiff base with hemoglobin. Vitamin B$_6$ in muscle accounts for 80% of body stores, mostly as PLP bound to glycogen phosphorylase. Total body stores of vitamin B$_6$ are thought to be about 1 mmol.

Release of free vitamin, mainly pyridoxal, occurs when physiological, nonsaturating concentrations of vitamin are absorbed. The phosphates are then hydrolyzed by nonspecific alkaline phosphatase located on the plasma membrane of cells. Some PLP is released into the circulation by the liver. Although PLP is the principal tissue form of vitamin B$_6$ and pyridoxal constitutes much of the circulating vitamin, the main catabolite excreted in urine is 4-pyridoxic acid (4-PA).

Functions

As coenzyme PLP, vitamin B$_6$ functions in more than 100 reactions involved in the metabolism of macronutrients. Especially diverse are PLP-dependent enzymes that are involved in amino acid metabolism, which link amino acid metabolism with ketogenic and glucogenic reactions. Other examples of

Diffusion and/or transport to/from blood

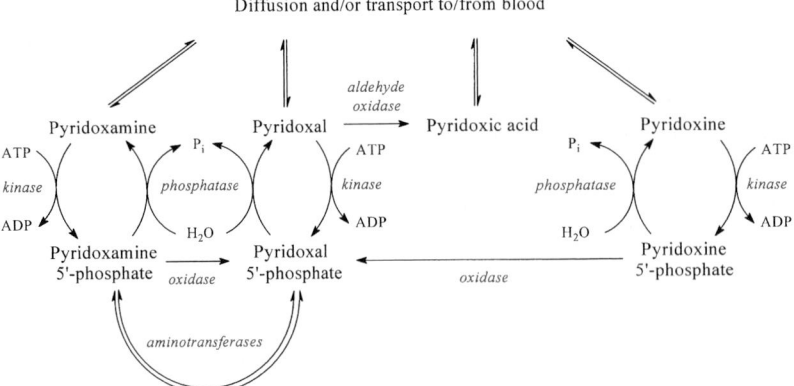

Figure 27-11 Metabolism of vitamin B_6.

PLP-requiring enzymes are (1) the amino acid decarboxylases that lead to formation of amines (e.g., epinephrine, norepinephrine, serotonin, γ-aminobutyrate); (2) cysteine desulfhydrase and serine hydroxymethyltransferase, which use PLP to effect the loss or transfer of amino acid sidechains; (3) phosphorylase, which catalyzes phosphorolysis of the α-1,4-linkages of glycogen; and (4) cystathionine beta-synthase, which is involved in the transsulfuration pathway of homocysteine. Additionally, the biosynthesis of heme depends on the early formation of 5-aminolevulinate from PLP-dependent condensation of glycine and succinyl-CoA, followed by decarboxylation, and an important role in lipid metabolism is the PLP-dependent condensation of L-serine with palmitoyl-CoA to form 3-dehydrosphinganine—a precursor of sphingomyelins.

Requirements and Reference Nutrient Intakes[2]

Requirements for vitamin B_6 are largely dependent upon protein intake. A ratio of 0.016 mg of vitamin B_6/g of protein intake has been suggested for normal adults and may be extrapolated to children and adolescents. Proposed RDAs are 1.3 mg/d for men to age 50 years and 1.7 mg/d for men over 50 years, 1.3 mg/d for women 19 to 50 years and 1.5 mg/d for women over 50 years. Additions of 0.6 and 0.5 mg B_6 per day are suggested in pregnancy and lactation, respectively.

Deficiency

Deficiency of vitamin B_6 alone is uncommon and is more usual in association with deficits in other vitamins of the B-complex. As with other water-soluble vitamins that function as coenzymes, progressive symptoms of deficiency of the vitamin are dependent upon the relative affinity of the coenzyme for a given apoenzyme and the extent to which the **holoenzyme**-catalyzed reaction is essential. Some drug interactions lead to **hypovitaminosis (avitaminosis)** of B_6. These involve the antituberculosis drug isoniazid (isonicotinic acid hydrazide), which forms hydrazones with pyridoxal and PLP; penicillamine; and the antiparkinsonian drugs benserazide, carbidopa, and theophylline.

Vitamin B_6–responsive inborn errors of metabolism include (1) infantile convulsions, in which the apoenzyme for glutamate decarboxylase has poor affinity for the coenzyme;

(2) xanthurenic aciduria, in which affinity of the mutant kynureninase for PLP is decreased; and (3) homocystinuria, which is caused by a similarly defective cystathionine β-synthase . In these cases, increased amounts (200 to 1000 mg/d) of administered vitamin B_6 are required for life. Low vitamin B_6 status (together with low vitamin B_{12} and folate status) in humans has been linked to hyperhomocysteinemia, which is an independent risk factor for cardiovascular disease.

Clinically, electroencephalographic abnormalities appear within 3 weeks and epileptiform convulsions are a common finding in young vitamin B_6–deficient individuals. In addition, skin changes, including dermatitis with cheilosis and glossitis, may occur. Hematological manifestations include a decrease in the number of circulating lymphocytes and possibly a normocytic, microcytic, or sideroblastic anemia.

Toxicity

Although no adverse effects have been observed with high intake of vitamin B_6 from food sources, high oral supplemental doses have been observed to produce neurotoxic and photosensitive effects. Based on the end point of development of sensory neuropathy, current U.S. recommendations have set a tolerable upper intake concentration of 100 mg/d for adults.

Laboratory Assessment of Status[11]

As with other B vitamins that act as coenzymes, biochemical assessment of vitamin B_6 is accomplished by direct chemical analysis of the vitamer or its metabolites or by completion of functional tests. For example, analytical techniques are used to measure (1) PLP in plasma or red cells, (2) its metabolite 4-PA in urine or plasma, (3) the activity and activation coefficient of the red cell aminotransferases (aspartate and alanine), and (4) the tryptophan load metabolite excretion test. As no single analyte adequately reflects status, a combination of these markers is often used.

Plasma PLP and plasma or urine 4-PA are most commonly measured by HPLC. PLP is measured by HPLC with fluorescence detection following precolumn fluorophore formation as a semicarbazone or as a pyridoxic acid phosphate. The natural fluorescence of 4-PA is measured. A homogeneous, nonradioactive recombinant enzymatic method for PLP has been described that uses 5 μL of plasma and has a lower limit of detection of 5 nmol/L.

Functional assessment of vitamin B_6 status is achieved by measuring the activity of red cell aspartate (or alanine) aminotransferase and its activation coefficient on incubation with PLP. These tests are less robust than those for vitamins B_1 and B_2 and are considered less useful. Measurement of urinary tryptophan metabolites, particularly xanthurenic acid, after an oral load (2 to 5 g) of L-tryptophan, is used in studies of vitamin B_6 **nutriture** because changes are recognized early and measurements are relatively easy to obtain.

Reference Intervals

A guidance reference interval for plasma PLP is 5 to 30 ng/mL (20 to 121 nmol/L). Plasma concentrations less than 5 ng/mL (20 nmol/L) are judged deficient. Activation coefficients less than about 1.5 for aspartate aminotransferase and 1.2 for alanine aminotransferase are considered normal but may depend somewhat on the assay method used.

Vitamin B_{12}—Cyanocobalamin

Vitamin B_{12} is also known as cyanocobalamin. It is a water-soluble hematopoietic vitamin that is required for the maturation of erythrocytes.

Chemistry

Vitamin B_{12} is a generic term that refers to a group of physiologically active substances chemically classified as cobalamins or corrinoids. They are composed of tetrapyrrole rings surrounding central cobalt atoms and nucleotide sidechains attached to the cobalt. The cobalamin tetrapyrrole ring, exclusive of cobalt and other sidechains, is called a *corrin*. All compounds that contain this corrin nucleus are corrinoids. The cobalt-corrin complex is termed cobamide (Figure 27-12).

Cobalamins differ in the nature of additional side groups bound to cobalt. Examples include (1) methyl (methylcobalamin), (2) 5′-deoxyadenosine ([deoxyadenosyl or adenosyl] cobalamin), (3) hydroxyl (hydroxocobalamin), (4) H_2O (aquocobalamin), and (4) cyanide (cyanocobalamin). Cyanocobalamin is a stable compound that forms dark red, needle-like crystals. It is the reference compound used to calibrate serum cobalamin methods. The predominant physiological form of cobalamin in serum is methylcobalamin, whereas that in cytosols is adenosylcobalamin. Cyanocobalamin has a molecular weight of 1355 Da and is gradually destroyed on exposure to light.

Dietary Sources

All vitamin B_{12} is ultimately the product of microbial synthesis, and because plants do not use this vitamin, the main dietary sources are (1) meat and meat products, (2) dairy products, (3) fish and shellfish, and (4) fortified ready-to-eat cereals.

Absorption, Transport, Metabolism, and Excretion

Uptake of vitamin B_{12} from the intestine into the circulation is a complex mechanism, involving five separate vitamin B_{12}–binding molecules, receptors, and transporters. Vitamin

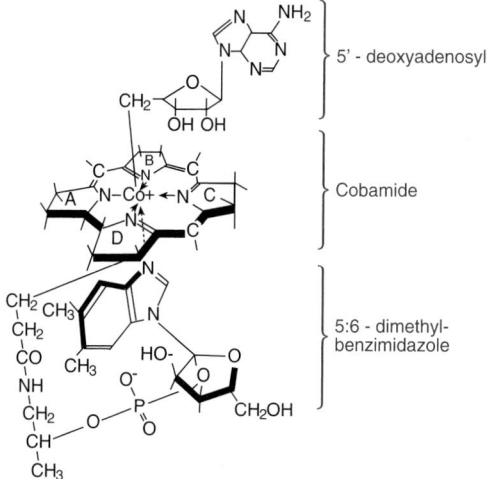

Figure 27-12 The structure of 5′-deoxyadenosyl cobalamin. *(Modified from Chanarin I: The megaloblastic anemias, 2nd edition. Oxford: Blackwell Scientific, 1979.)*

B_{12} released from food in the stomach is bound to haptocorrin (R protein, a salivary protein) and travels with it into the intestine, where haptocorrin is digested by pancreatic enzymes. The liberated vitamin B_{12} then binds to intrinsic factor (IF), a glycoprotein with a molecular weight of approximately 50 kDa, which is produced by the gastric mucosa. When the vitamin B_{12}/IF complex reaches the distal ileum, it is bound by receptors on the surface of mucosal epithelial cells and then enters the cells. Within the mucosal epithelial cells, the vitamin B_{12}/IF complex is dissociated, and the vitamin B_{12} then binds with transcobalamin II (TcII). This complex is transported across the cell membrane bound to a TcII receptor and then is released into the plasma of the mucosal capillaries and subsequently into the blood in the portal vein. Almost all of the vitamin B_{12} is taken up by hepatocytes as the blood in the portal vein passes through the liver. It is stored in the liver and is released to plasma to meet physiological demands. If the quantity of vitamin B_{12} exceeds the capacity of hepatocyte receptors, most of the excess is excreted by the kidneys. Normally, approximately 1 mg of vitamin B_{12} is stored in the liver—a quantity equivalent to the daily metabolic requirement for 2000 days. Thus, when the dietary supply of vitamin B_{12} is interrupted or mechanisms of absorption are impaired, vitamin B_{12} deficiency does not become evident for 5 years or longer.

Vitamin B_{12} is continually secreted in the bile, but most is reabsorbed and available for metabolic functions. If circulating vitamin B_{12} concentrations exceed the binding capacity of the blood, the excess will be excreted in the urine. In most circumstances, however, the greatest losses of vitamin B_{12} occur through the feces.

Functions

Vitamin B_{12} is required in coenzyme form for more than 12 different enzyme systems. In humans it is required for the conversion of (1) L-methylmalonyl CoA to succinyl-CoA and (2) homocysteine to methionine. Congenital defects of mutase synthesis or inability to synthesize adenosyl-cobalamin (adenosyl-Cbl) results in life-threatening methylmalonic aciduria and metabolic ketoacidosis. Congenital defects in methionine synthase or the synthesis of methyl-Cbl results in severe hyperhomocysteinemia.

Requirements and Reference Nutrient Intakes[2]

Total body stores of vitamin B_{12} are estimated to be between 2 and 5 mg in the adult man, of which about 1 mg is found in the liver and a smaller amount in the kidney. A daily obligatory loss of vitamin B_{12} of about 0.1% of body pool, irrespective of size, has been observed,[12] suggesting that the daily requirement to maintain stores would vary from 2 to 5 µg. The daily diet of individuals in Western countries contains between 5 and 30 µg of vitamin B_{12}, with average ingestion of 7 to 8 µg/d by adult men and 4 to 5 µg/d by adult women. Additional small amounts may be available through synthesis of vitamin B_{12} by intestinal microorganisms. Of the amount ingested, between 1 and 5 µg is absorbed.

The RDA for vitamin B_{12} is based on the amount necessary for maintenance of hematological status and normal serum vitamin B_{12} concentrations, and assumes 50% absorbance of ingested vitamin B_{12}. The RDA for adults (19 to 50 years) has been set at 2.4 µg/d, with an increase to 2.6 µg/d during pregnancy and to 2.8 µg/d in lactation.

Deficiency

Deficiency of vitamin B_{12} in humans is associated with megaloblastic anemia and neuropathy. The most common cause of vitamin B_{12} deficiency is **pernicious anemia**, an autoimmune disease in which chronic atrophic gastritis results from antibodies to gastric parietal cells and IF, directed against gastric parietal cell H^+/K^+-ATPase. Pernicious anemia may also occur in children as the result of failure of IF secretion or secretion of biologically inactive IF. Other groups at risk of vitamin B_{12} deficiency include those (1) older than 65 years of age; (2) with malabsorption; (3) who are vegetarians; (4) with autoimmune disorders; or (5) taking prescribed medication known to interfere with vitamin absorption or metabolism, including (1) nitrous oxide, (2) phenytoin, (3) dihydrofolate reductase inhibitors, (4) metformin, (5) proton pump inhibitors, and (6) infants with suspected metabolic disorders.

Intestinal malabsorption of vitamin B_{12} may be caused by gastrectomy or ileal resection, with an inverse relationship between the length of ileum resected and the absorption of vitamin B_{12}. Other causes of malabsorption are (1) tropical sprue, (2) inflammatory disease of the small intestine, (3) intestinal stasis with overgrowth of colonic bacteria, which consume the vitamin B_{12} ingested by the host, and (4) human immunodeficiency virus (HIV) infection. Vegetarians have a lower intake of vitamin B_{12} than omnivores, and although clinical signs of deficiency are uncommon, biochemical markers of status may indicate functional vitamin B_{12} deficiency. A large number of disorders are associated with cobalamin deficiency in infancy or childhood. Of these, the most commonly encountered is the Imerslund-Gräsbeck syndrome, a condition characterized by inability to absorb vitamin B_{12}, with or without IF, and proteinuria. It appears to be due to an inability of intestinal mucosa to absorb the vitamin B_{12}/IF complex. The second most common of these is congenital deficiency of gastric secretion of IF.

The hematological effects of vitamin B_{12} deficiency are indistinguishable from those of folate deficiency. The classic morphological changes in the blood, in approximate order of appearance, are (1) hypersegmentation of neutrophils, (2) macrocytosis, (3) anemia, (4) leukopenia, and (5) thrombocytopenia, with megaloblastic changes in bone marrow accompanying peripheral blood changes. All bone marrow lesions are reversed with vitamin B_{12} therapy.

In addition to hematological changes, vitamin B_{12} deficiency has been known to result in a demyelinating disorder of the central nervous system. This disorder has been known to lead to other serious and often irreversible neurological conditions, such as (1) burning pain or loss of sensation in the extremities, (2) weakness, (3) spasticity and paralysis, (4) confusion, (5) disorientation, and (6) dementia. This disorder has been given the name *subacute combined degeneration of the spinal cord.*

Toxicity

No adverse effects have been associated with excess vitamin B_{12} intake from food or supplements in healthy people.

Laboratory Assessment of Status[11]

Both direct and indirect functional tests are available for assessing vitamin B_{12} status. Indirect tests include (1) assays for urinary and serum concentrations of methylmalonic acid (2) assays for plasma homocysteine, (3) the deoxyuridine suppression test, and (4) the vitamin B_{12} absorption test.

Microbiological competitive protein binding (CPB) and immunoassays have been used for direct quantification of serum vitamin B_{12}. The microbiological assays have been largely replaced by other, more convenient and accurate methods, although they remain reference methods for determination of biologically active vitamin B_{12}. Commercial kits are available for the CPB assays of vitamin B_{12}. In a widely used CPB assay, vitamin B_{12} (cobalamin) competes with ^{57}Co-labeled cobalamin for a limited number of binding sites on IF.

Most immunoassay methods use solid-phase separation by immobilizing the IF binder on beads or magnetic particles. The free vitamin B_{12} then remains in the supernatant, and the bound analytes become part of the solid-phase suspension. For simultaneous folate/vitamin B_{12} measurement, a gamma-scintillation counter that discriminates between the energy concentrations of ^{57}Co (for vitamin B_{12}) and those of ^{125}I (for folate) is required. In addition, multiple automated and semi-automated systems are available for measuring vitamin B_{12} and folate by using, for example, chemiluminescence as a signal.

Indirect tests assess the functional adequacy of vitamin B_{12}. Serum methylmalonic acid concentration is increased when lack of adenyl-Cbl causes a block in the conversion of methylmalonyl-CoA to succinyl-CoA. Plasma total homocysteine concentration is a sensitive indicator of vitamin B_{12} status because methyl-Cbl is required for the remethylation of homocysteine to methionine, but it is not specific because of elevations in deficiency of folate and vitamins B_6 and B_{12}. Measurement of holotranscobalamin II is potentially useful as a specific marker of biologically available vitamin B_{12} because only cobalamin bound to TcII is specifically available for uptake by all cells. Methods have been described for the measurement of holotranscobalamin in serum; one uses an immobilized monoclonal antibody to human transcobalamin, followed by measurement of released cobalamin by CPB. This method is available as a commercial kit.

The Schilling test is primarily a test of vitamin B_{12} absorption, not of status, but it permits differentiation of causes of vitamin B_{12} deficiency (e.g., pernicious anemia, intestinal malabsorption). The usual procedure is to measure radioactivity in a 24-hour urine sample, which is collected after oral administration of 0.5 μg of radioactive Co-labeled vitamin B_{12} after an overnight fast. In healthy individuals, 8% or more of the dose administered is excreted in the urine, whereas in people with pernicious anemia, less than 7% (often 0% to 3%) is excreted. A confirmatory test for lack of IF requires ingestion of vitamin B_{12} and IF.

Reference Intervals

The WHO defined a serum vitamin B_{12} concentration of less than 150 ng/L (110 pmol/L) as deficient, and one of 201 ng/L (147 pmol/L) or higher as acceptable.

Serum methylmalonic acid concentrations less than 376 nmol/L have been considered acceptable in an elderly U.S. population, as have concentrations less than 320 nmol/L in a group of older Dutch subjects.

Vitamin C—Ascorbic Acid

Vitamin C (L-ascorbic acid) serves as a reducing agent in several important hydroxylation reactions in the body.

Chemistry

The term *vitamin C* refers to all molecules that exhibit antiscorbutic properties in humans and includes both ascorbic acid and its oxidized form, dehydroascorbic acid (DHA) (Figure 27-13). Plants and most animals possess the ability to synthesize the vitamin from D-glucose via the lactones of D-glucuronic and L-gulonic acids. Humans and some mammals, however, lack L-gulonolactone oxidase, the enzyme that catalyzes the formation of 2-oxo-L-gulonolactone, which spontaneously tautomerizes to L-ascorbic acid. Hence daily intake for humans and some mammals is essential.

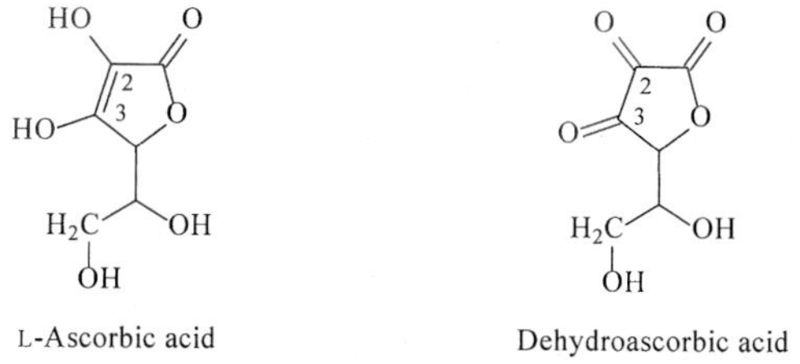

Figure 27-13 L-Ascorbic and dehydroascorbic acids.

Dietary Sources

Excellent sources of the vitamin are (1) citrus fruits, (2) berries, (3) melons, (4) tomatoes, (5) green peppers, (6) broccoli, (7) Brussels sprouts, and (8) leafy green vegetables.

Absorption, Transport, Metabolism, and Excretion

Gastrointestinal absorption of ascorbic acid occurs through a combination of sodium-dependent active transport at low concentrations and simple diffusion at high concentrations. The absorbed ascorbic acid moves rapidly from the intestinal cell into the blood by a process of facilitated diffusion. Ascorbate uptake by cells is mediated by sodium-dependent transporters and DHA via facilitated-diffusion glucose transporters. Vitamin C is found in most tissue, but glandular tissue, such as the (1) pituitary, (2) adrenal cortex, (3) corpus luteum, and (4) thymus, has the highest amounts. The retina has 20 to 30 times the plasma concentration. The body pool of vitamin C is approximately 2 g and the biological half-life about 16 days. Excretion of unchanged ascorbate occurs increasingly with increased dosage, with almost all of an ingested dose greater than 500 mg excreted over 24 hours. DHA that is not recycled may be irreversibly delactonized to 2,3-diketogulonic acid and further degraded to oxalic acid for urine excretion.

Functions

Ascorbic acid acts as a cofactor for a number of mixed function oxidases in processes in which it promotes enzyme activity by maintaining metal ions in their reduced form (particularly iron and copper). These include three different hydroxylating enzymes that take part in the intracellular biosynthesis steps of collagenous proteins. Each has different substrate specificities and two or more isoenzymes (e.g., prolyl 4-hydroxylase [EC 1.14.11.2], has at least 2 isoenzymes; prolyl 3-hydroxylase [EC 1.14.11.7], has at least 2 isoenzymes; and lysyl hydroxylase [EC 1.14.11.4], has at least 3 isoenzymes).[10] Functionally, prolyl 4-hydroxylase is regarded as the most important, as it produces 4-hydroxyproline, the content of which must be above a certain threshold value if the collagen is to be kept in its triple-helical conformation at body temperature. Other processes in which ascorbic acid is involved include (1) carnitine biosynthesis, where it serves as a cofactor to 6-*N*-trimethyl-lysine hydroxylase and butyrobetaine hydroxylase; (2) degradation of tyrosine via 4-OH phenylpyruvate dioxygenase; (3) synthesis of adrenal hormones via dopamine β-hydroxylase; (4) biosynthesis of corticosteroids and aldosterone; (5) hydroxylation of cholesterol in the formation of bile acids; (6) and folate metabolism and leukocyte functions.

Ascorbic acid, one of the most effective water-soluble antioxidants in biological fluids, scavenges physiologically important reactive oxygen species and reactive nitrogen species. The ascorbyl radical is relatively stable because of resonance stabilization of the unpaired electron. Ascorbate will regenerate other small molecule antioxidants, including (1) α-tocopherol, (2) reduced glutathione, (3) urate, and (4) β-carotene, from their respective radical species, and thus may prevent oxidative damage to biological macromolecules, including DNA, lipids, and proteins.

Requirements and Reference Nutrient Intakes[4]

The amount of vitamin C sufficient to alleviate and cure the clinical signs of **scurvy** is only 10 mg/d, which is probably near the minimum requirement in humans. This amount, however, is not adequate to maintain near saturation of tissue in the adult human male or to maintain an optimal nutritional state. Current recommendations of the U.S. Institute of Medicine include an RDA for adult males of 90 mg/d and 75 mg/d for females, with increases for pregnancy and lactation. Some special groups, such as smokers, should take an additional 35 mg/d.

Deficiency

Protracted deficiency of vitamin C leads to the classic disease of scurvy, which still occurs in many countries. Those most at risk of the disease include (1) elderly men, particularly those who live alone, (2) those with alcohol dependence, (3) smokers, (4) those who have unbalanced diets, (5) some mentally ill patients, (6) renal failure patients undergoing peritoneal dialysis or hemodialysis, and (7) some patients with cancer. Lack of vitamin C leads to an inability to form adequate intercellular substance in connective tissue and is reflected in swollen, tender, often bleeding or bruised loci at joints and in other areas where structurally weakened tissue does not withstand stress. Some scorbutic patients may (1) develop anemia, (2) display radiological changes characteristic of osteoporosis, or (3) die suddenly from heart failure. Conditions of vitamin C deficiency that might reflect its role as an antioxidant include (1) increased risk of coronary heart disease, as demonstrated in a cohort of Finnish men, and (2) increased risk of death by stroke in a cohort of elderly British people.

Toxicity

Vitamin C is generally well tolerated by healthy subjects, and ingestion of supplements of 2 to 4 g/d—as taken by some for prevention or amelioration of the common cold—is usually without hazard, although gastrointestinal irritation has been experienced. Other potential but rare adverse effects include (1) increased oxalate excretion and kidney stone formation, (2) increased uric acid excretion, (3) excess iron absorption, (4) lowered vitamin B_{12} concentrations, (5) systemic conditioning, and (6) "rebound" scurvy. Ingestion of amounts of vitamin C greater than 200 mg/d shows little increase in plasma steady-state concentrations, which suggests that overload of vitamin C is unlikely. The tolerable upper limit for vitamin C in adults has been set at 2 g/d.

Laboratory Assessment of Status[11]

At present no useful functional tests of vitamin C adequacy are available, thus laboratory assessment of status is made by direct measurement of (1) plasma, (2) urine, or (3) tissue concentrations of ascorbic acid, total vitamin C, or (rarely) metabolite. Plasma ascorbate concentration is considered to be a reliable indicator of ascorbate intake and has been measured photometrically by oxidation with 2,4-dinitrophenyl-hydrazine to form the red *bis*-hydrazone, or with 2,4-dichlorophenol-indophenol, which is reduced to a colorless form.

A more specific approach is to use the enzyme ascorbate oxidase to convert ascorbate to dehydroascorbate, which is then coupled with o-phenylene diamine to form a product that is measured by fluorimetry or by photometry. HPLC methods are more specific but more time-consuming. Detection may occur by precolumn derivatization to the fluorescent quinoxaline, or by electrochemical or coulometric means. Leukocyte ascorbic acid is considered to be a better indicator of body stores than plasma ascorbate, but it has not been widely adopted because of technical problems. Urinary excretion and red blood cell (RBC) concentrations have not been found to be specific and useful indices of vitamin C status although measurement of urinary concentrations of ascorbic acid, especially after a load test, has been found helpful in the clinical diagnosis of scurvy.

Reference Intervals

With adequate intake of vitamin C, plasma concentrations of total vitamin (ascorbic acid plus dehydroascorbic acid) are between 0.4 and 1.5 mg/dL (23 and 85 μmol/L). A value lower than 0.2 mg/dL (11 μmol/L) is considered deficient. The guidance reference interval for vitamin C concentrations in leukocytes is 20 to 53 μg/10^8 leukocytes (1.14 to 3.01 fmol/leukocyte), with concentrations less than 10 μg/10^8 leukocytes (0.57 fmol/leukocyte) considered deficient.

Biotin

Biotin is also known as vitamin H. It is the prosthetic group for a number of carboxylation reactions.

Chemistry

Biotin is *cis*-tetrahydro-2-oxothieno[3,4-*d*]-imidazoline-4-valeric acid (Figure 27-14). The vitamin in most organisms is found mainly bound to protein. In addition, some biotin is linked noncovalently as a complex with avidin, a protein in egg white.

Dietary Sources

Good sources of biotin include (1) liver, (2) kidney, (3) pancreas, (4) eggs, (5) yeast, and (6) milk. Poor sources of the vitamin include (1) cereal grains, (2) fruits, (3) most vegetables, and (4) meat.

Absorption, Transport, Metabolism, and Excretion

Biotin in the diet is largely protein bound, and digestion by gastrointestinal enzymes produces biotinyl peptides, which may be further hydrolyzed by intestinal biotinidase to release biotin. Avidin, a protein found in raw egg whites, binds biotin tightly and prevents its absorption. The peptide biocytin

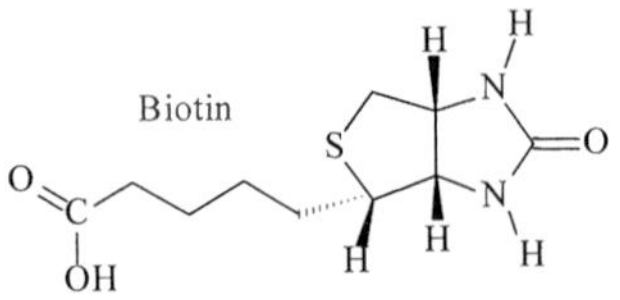

Figure 27-14 Biotin.

(ε-N-biotinyl lysine) is resistant to hydrolysis by proteolytic enzymes in the intestinal tract but together with biotin is readily absorbed. Sodium-dependent multivitamin transporter (SMVT) is a carrier for biotin for which pantothenic acid and lipoate compete. It is located in the intestinal brush border membrane and transports biotin against a sodium ion concentration gradient. The enzyme biocytinase in plasma and erythrocytes catalyzes the hydrolysis of biocytin to yield free biotin. Biotin is cleared from the circulating blood more rapidly in deficient than in normal mammals. It is taken up by such tissues as (1) liver, (2) muscle, and (3) kidney, and (4) is localized in cytosolic and mitochondrial carboxylases.

About half of absorbed biotin is excreted as the metabolites bisnorbiotin and biotin sulfoxide.

Functions

The principal biochemical function of biotin in man is to serve as a cofactor for carboxylation reactions. Five carboxylases are found in human tissue. One of these, an acetyl-CoA carboxylase, is inactive and may act as a storage vehicle for biotin. The others are carboxylases for (1) acetyl-CoA, (2) propionyl-CoA, (3) β-methylcrotonyl-CoA, and (4) pyruvate. These enzymes operate via a common mechanism, which involves phosphorylation of bicarbonate by ATP to form carbonyl phosphate. This is followed by transfer of the carboxyl group to the sterically less hindered nitrogen of the biotin moiety. The resulting N(1)-carboxybiotinyl enzyme then exchanges the carboxylate function with a reactive center in a substrate. With cytosolic acetyl-CoA carboxylase, the product is malonyl-CoA, which is used for fatty acid biosynthesis. In mitochondria, pyruvate carboxylase catalyzes the formation of oxaloacetate, which, together with acetyl-CoA, forms citrate. The other carboxylases are involved in the metabolism of odd-numbered fatty acids and branched chain fatty acids.

Requirements and Reference Nutrient Intakes[2]

Biotin does not have a current RDA. Intestinal microflora makes a significant contribution to the body pool of available biotin, making determination of the dietary requirement difficult. As a consequence, an adequate intake (AI) recommendation for adults 19 years and older is 30 μg/d. An additional 5 μg/d is recommended for the lactating mother.

Deficiency

Biotin deficiency is uncommon but may be seen (1) with prolonged consumption of raw egg whites, (2) in TPN without biotin supplementation, and (3) in patients with a genetic deficiency of biotinidase. Deficiencies 1 and 2 may be complicated by effects on gut flora that produce biotin. Symptoms include (1) anorexia, (2) nausea, (3) vomiting, (4) glossitis, (5) pallor, (6) depression, and (7) a dry scaly dermatitis.

Toxicity

No adverse effects of biotin in doses up to 300 times normal dietary intake have been reported among patients with biotinidase deficiency.

Laboratory Assessment of Status[11]

Traditionally, biotin has been measured in biological samples by microbiological assay, where whole blood is first digested with papain or acid hydrolysis to release free biotin, samples of which are then added to a biotin-deficient medium inoculated with a test organism, such as *Lactobacillus plantarum*. Other methods for unbound biotin include avidin-binding assays, for which a competitive protein-binding radioisotope assay is set up with ³H-labeled biotin or a nonradioactive enzyme-linked sorbent assay using streptavidin as the binding agent. Urinary excretion of biotin and 3-hydroxyisovaleric acid appears to be a better indicator of biotin status than blood concentrations.

Reference Intervals

Typical reference interval values for whole blood biotin by a microbiological method are 0.5 to 2.20 nmol/L.

Folic Acid

Folic acid serves as a carrier of one-carbon groups in many metabolic reactions.

Chemistry

Folate and folic acid are generic terms for a family of compounds that function as coenzymes in the processing of one-carbon units. They are derived from pteroic acid (*Pte*), to which one or more molecules of glutamic acid are attached. Pteroic acid is composed of a pteridine ring joined to a p-aminobenzoic acid residue (Figure 27-15). When pteroic acid is conjugated with one molecule of L-glutamic acid, pteroylglutamic acid (PteGlu) is formed; this is then reduced to dihydrofolic acid ($H_2PteGlu$ or DHF/FH_2) or to tetrahydrofolate ($H_4PteGlu$ or THF/FH_4). Only the reduced forms are biologically active. Other folate derivatives have multiple glutamic acid residues ($H_4PteGlu_n$). Multiple forms of folic acid occur with substitutions of functional groups, such as (1) methyl, (2) formyl, (3) methylene, (4) hydroxymethyl, and (5) others at nitrogen atoms in the pteroic acid residue, usually N^5 or bridging N^5 and N. The principal form is 5-methyltetrahydrofolate.

Dietary Sources

Principal food sources of folate are (1) liver, (2) spinach, (3) other dark green leafy vegetables, (4) legumes, such as kidney and lima beans, and (5) orange juice. In countries where cereal fortification with folate is established, this is often the major source of dietary folate. Since the U.S. Food and Drug Administration (FDA) program of fortification of all enriched grain products with folic acid (140 μg per 100 g) began in 1998, study populations have shown doubling of mean plasma folate concentrations.

Absorption, Transport, Metabolism, and Excretion

Folate is absorbed from dietary sources as reduced methyl- and formyl-tetrahydropteroylpolyglutamates. The bioavailability of folate from food sources, however, is variable. The bioavailability of supplemental folic acid may be as high as 100% for supplements taken on an empty stomach compared with about 50% for food folates. Polyglutamate forms

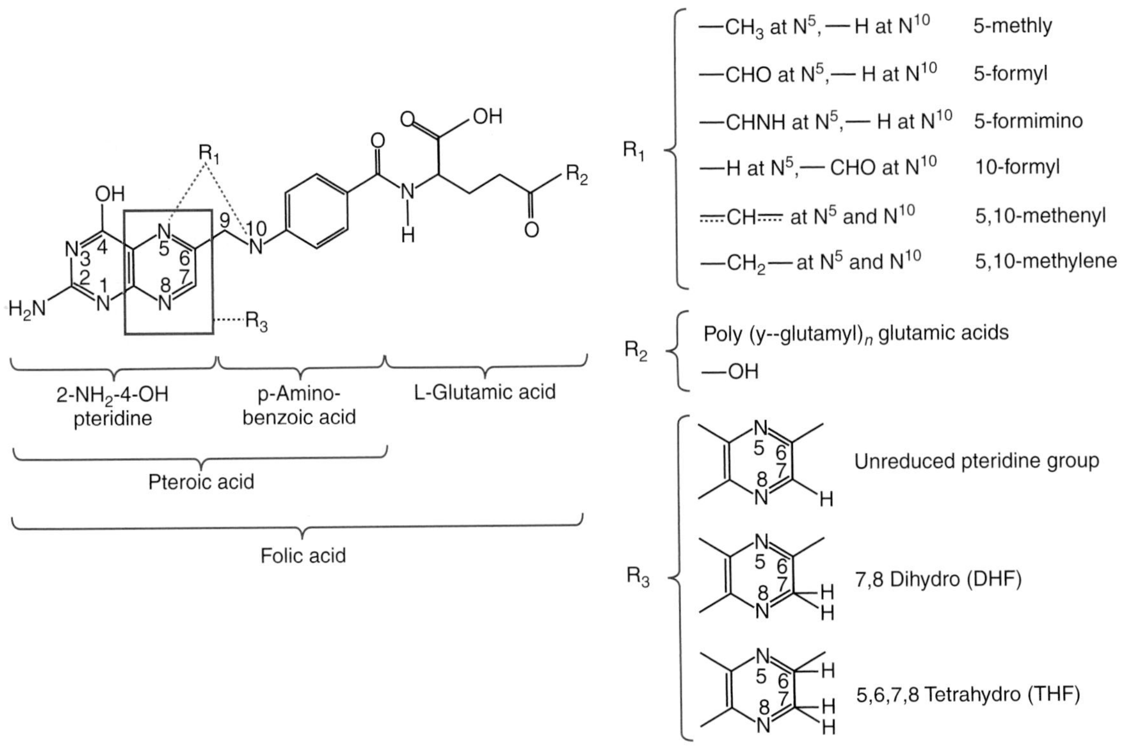

Figure 27-15 Structure of folic acid.

Functions

Folate coenzymes, together with coenzymes derived from vitamins B_{12}, B_6, and B_2, are essential for one-carbon metabolism. Biochemically, a carbon unit from serine or glycine is transferred to THF to form methylene-THF, which is then (1) used in the synthesis of thymidine (and incorporation into DNA), (2) oxidized to formyl-THF for use in the synthesis of purines (precursors of RNA and DNA), or (3) reduced to methyl-THF, which is necessary for the methylation of homocysteine to methionine. Much of this methionine is converted to S-adenosylmethionine, a universal donor of methyl groups to (1) DNA, (2) RNA, (3) hormones, (4) neurotransmitters, (5) membrane lipids, and (6) proteins. Different folates are involved in these reactions, depending on the chemical state of the single-carbon fragments transferred.

Folic acid also is involved in the metabolism of homocysteine. Elevations in plasma homocysteine concentrations have been shown to be independent risk factors for coronary artery disease and probably cerebrovascular disease. The involvement of folate in its coenzyme forms with homocysteine and methionine metabolism is summarized in Figure 27-16. Folate is the principal micronutrient determinant of homocysteine status, and supplementation with folate has been used as a treatment modality to reduce circulating homocysteine concentrations. The extent to which this is associated with clinical benefit remains unclear.

Requirements and Reference Nutrient Intakes[2]

Total body stores of folate are estimated to be between 12 and 28 mg. Studies suggest a minimum daily requirement of between 60 and 280 µg to replace losses. In calculating

of folate present in food are first converted to monoglutamates by pteroylpolyglutamate hydrolase in the intestinal mucosa. Absorption of monoglutamyl folates at low concentration occurs by a saturable transport process with an additional apparently nonsaturable absorption mechanism when intestinal folate concentrations exceed 5 to 10 µmol/L. After cellular uptake, most of the folate is reduced and methylated and enters the circulation as 5-methyltetrahydrofolate (5-MTHF), circulating loosely bound to albumin or to a lesser degree to a high-affinity folate-binding protein. Uptake by (1) kidney, (2) placenta, and (3) choroid plexus cells occurs with membrane-associated folate-binding proteins that act as folate receptors. Once within the cell, 5-MTHF is demethylated and is converted to the polyglutamyl form by folylpolyglutamate synthase, which helps to retain folate within the cell. For release into the circulation, the polyglutamates are reconverted to monoglutamates by polyglutamate hydrolase.

Folic acid and vitamin B_{12} metabolism are linked by the reaction that transfers a methyl group from 5-MTHF to cobalamin. In cases of cobalamin deficiency, folate is "trapped" as 5-MTHF, is "metabolically dead," and is not recycled as tetrahydrofolate (THF).

Protein-free plasma folate is filtered at the glomerulus, and most is reabsorbed by the proximal renal tubules. Folate is predominantly excreted by catabolism after cleavage of the C9-N10 bond to produce p-aminobenzoylpolyglutamates, which then are hydrolyzed to monoglutamates and are N-acetylated before excretion. Biliary excretion of folate has been estimated at about 100 µg/d, but much of this is reabsorbed in an enterohepatic circulation.

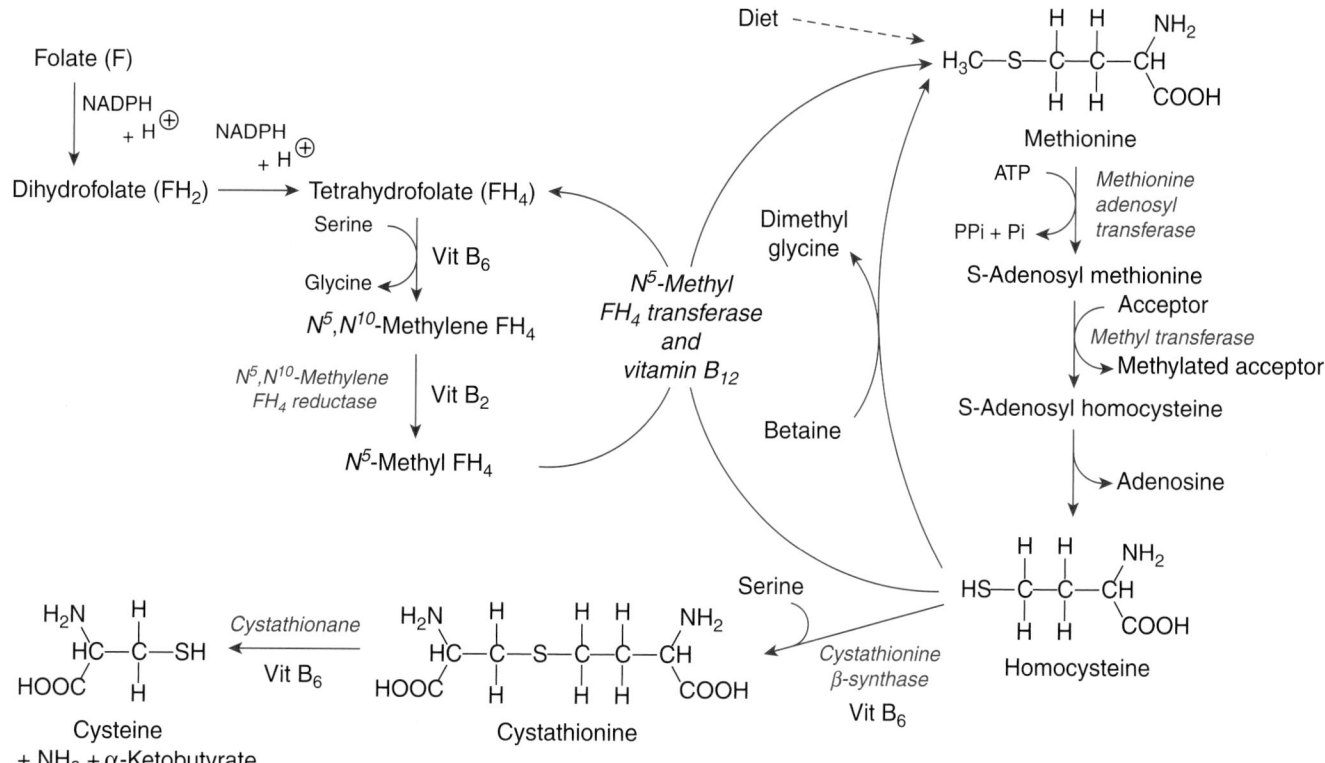

Figure 27-16 Metabolism of homocysteine and methionine.

nutritional requirements, the concept of the dietary folate equivalent (DFE) has been used to adjust for the nearly 50% lower bioavailability of food folate compared with supplemental folic acid. Current RDAs of the U.S. Institute of Medicine are 400 µg/d DFE for adults 19 years and older, 600 µg/d DFE in pregnancy, and 500 µg/d DFE for lactating women.

Deficiency

Deficiency of folate may result from (1) the absence of intestinal microorganisms (gut sterilization), (2) poor intestinal absorption (e.g., after surgical resection, in celiac disease or sprue), (3) insufficient dietary intake (including chronic alcoholism), (4) excessive demands as in pregnancy, liver disease, and malignancies, (5) administration of antifolate drugs (e.g., methotrexate), and (6) anticonvulsant therapy (leading to increased folate requirements, especially during pregnancy). **Megaloblastic anemia** (characterized by large, abnormally nucleated erythrocytes in the bone marrow) is the major clinical manifestation of folate deficiency, although sensory loss and neuropsychiatric changes may also occur.

Pregnancy brings increased demand upon folate stores caused by increased DNA synthesis and one-carbon transfer reactions, and low serum folate concentrations in pregnancy are associated with adverse outcomes. Additionally, many observational studies have confirmed a reduction in risk of neural tube defects (NTDs) with periconceptional folic acid supplementation.

Several enzyme polymorphisms affect folate metabolism. The most extensively studied of these is 5,10-methylenetetrahydrofolate reductase (MTHFR), the enzyme responsible for the irreversible reduction of 5,10-MTHF to 5-methyltetrahydrofolate (5-MTHF), the methyl donor of homocysteine to methionine. The homozygous TT variant has an incidence of around 12% in Asian and Caucasian populations and loss of enzyme activity of about 50%, whereas the heterozygous CT variant has an incidence of up to 50% in some populations. Another enzyme involved in folate metabolism, methionine synthase, has been shown to have at least two relatively prevalent polymorphisms, although these are thought to be benign. Absorption of folate from polyglutamyl folate food sources is thought to be reduced by a variant of glutamate carboxypeptidase II.

Toxicity

No adverse effects have been reported to result from the consumption of folate-fortified foods, thus any signs of toxicity are associated with supplemental folate. Most of the limited evidence suggests that excessive folate supplementation, typically in doses up to 10 mg/d, will precipitate or exacerbate neuropathy in vitamin B_{12}–deficient individuals, and it is this end point that has been used to set a tolerable upper intake concentration of 1 mg/d from fortified food or supplements for adults. One recognized complication of folate supplementation is that it "masks" vitamin B_{12} deficiency because the associated anemia responds to folate alone. This may delay treatment of the deficiency, allowing neurological abnormalities to progress.

Laboratory Assessment of Status[11]

Folate status may be reliably assessed by direct measurement of (1) serum, (2) erythrocyte, or (3) whole blood concentrations, and its metabolic function as coenzyme may be assessed by direct measurement of metabolite concentrations, such as plasma homocysteine. Serum folate concentrations are considered indicative of recent intake, not of tissue stores, but serial measurements have been used to confirm adequate intake. Whole blood or erythrocyte folate concentrations are more indicative of tissue stores and have been shown to have a moderate correlation with liver folate concentrations.

CPB assays have largely replaced microbiological procedures for the measurement of serum, whole blood, or erythrocyte folate.

Reference Intervals

Data collected from the NHANES of 1988 to 1994 in the United States produced reference intervals of 2.6 to 12.2 µg/L (6.0 to 28.0 nmol/L) for serum folate and 103 to 411 µg/L (237 to 945 nmol/L) for erythrocyte folate; however, these data were collected before mandatory flour fortification. Biochemical deficiency has been defined as a concentration <1.4 µg/L (<3.2 nmol/L) for serum folate and <110 µg/L (<253 nmol/L) for erythrocyte folate.

Niacin and Niacinamide

Niacin and niacinamide (nicotinamide and nicotinic acid amide) are converted to the ubiquitous redox coenzymes nicotinamide-adenine dinucleotide (NAD)$^+$ and nicotinamide-adenine dinucleotide phosphate (NADP)$^+$.

Chemistry

The term niacin refers to (1) nicotinic acid (pyridine-3-carboxylic acid), (2) its amide niacinamide (nicotinamide), and (3) derivatives that show the same biological activity as nicotinamide. A distinction between the two primary vitamin forms has to be considered, however, when some aspects of their metabolism are considered, especially their different pharmacological actions at high doses. The structures of both vitamers and of the two coenzyme forms are shown in Figure 27-17.

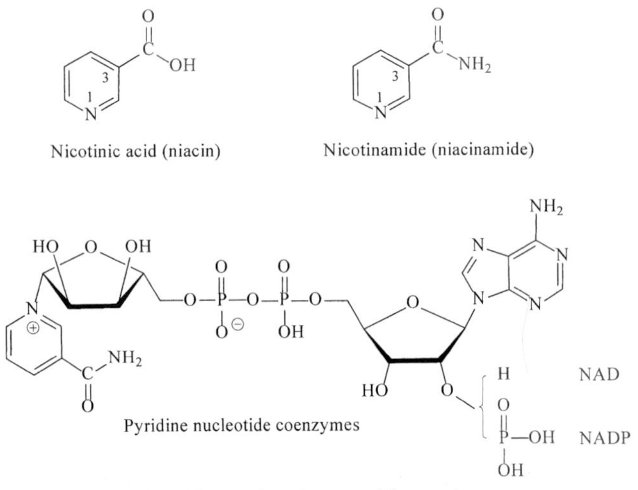

Figure 27-17 Niacin, niacinamide, and coenzyme.

Dietary Sources

Sources of niacin include (1) yeast, (2) lean meats, (3) liver, (4) poultry, (5) milk, (6) canned salmon, and (7) several leafy green vegetables. Additionally, some plant foodstuffs, especially cereals such as corn and wheat, contain niacin bound to various peptides and sugars in forms nutritionally not readily available (niacinogens or niacytin). Because tryptophan is a precursor of niacin, protein provides a considerable portion of niacin equivalent (as much as two-thirds of the niacin requirement). In countries where fortification of processed cereals is practiced, this may provide up to 20% of niacin intake.

Absorption, Transport, Metabolism, and Excretion

Dietary NAD$^+$ and NADP$^+$ are hydrolyzed by enzymes in the intestinal mucosa to release nicotinamide, which, together with any nicotinic acid, is rapidly absorbed in both the stomach and the intestine by Na$^+$-dependent facilitated diffusion at low concentrations and passive diffusion at higher concentrations. Nicotinamide is the main circulating form in the plasma after absorption or release from hydrolyzed liver NAD; it then diffuses into most tissues requiring NAD. Once inside the cells, both nicotinic acid and nicotinamide are converted to coenzyme forms. In the tissue, most of the vitamin is present as nicotinamide in NAD and NADP, although the liver may contain a significant fraction of the free vitamin. Little storage of niacin as such has been noted.

Excess niacin is excreted mainly as *N*-methylnicotinamide (NMN) after methylation in the liver.

Functions

Niacin is essential for the coenzymes NAD and NADP, in which nicotinamide acts as an electron acceptor or a hydrogen donor in a large number of redox reactions. Many of the enzymes function as dehydrogenases and catalyze such diverse reactions as the conversion of (1) alcohols to aldehydes or ketones, (2) hemiacetals to lactones, (3) aldehydes to acids, and (4) certain amino acids to keto acids.

Most dehydrogenases using NAD or NADP function reversibly. Glutamate dehydrogenase, for example, favors the oxidative direction, whereas others, such as glutathione reductase, preferentially catalyze reduction. Nicotinic acid, when used as a pharmaceutical agent, has important antiatherogenic properties. It effectively (1) lowers triglycerides, (2) raises HDL cholesterol, and (3) shifts LDL particles to a less atherogenic phenotype.

Requirements and Reference Nutrient Intakes[2]

Requirements for niacin are expressed as niacin equivalents (NEs), which account for the contribution of tryptophan derived from protein. The median intake of preformed niacin from food in the United States is 28 mg for men and 18 mg for women, and a study of two Canadian populations showed corresponding values of 41 mg and 28 mg/d. Additionally, the average U.S. diet supplies between 0.7 and 1.1 g of tryptophan per day. Based on niacin metabolite excretion data, current RDAs are 16 mg/d of NE for men and 14 mg/d for women. An increase of 4 NE per day during pregnancy is recommended, and an increase of 3 NE is recommended daily for lactation.

Deficiency

Pellagra is the classic deficiency disease of the human that has been found most often among those who subsist chiefly on corn (maize), which is low in both niacin and tryptophan. Although its pathogenesis has been attributed to a deficiency of these two factors, other associated complicating factors include lack of (1) PLP, (2) FAD, and (3) iron, which are functional in the conversion of tryptophan to niacin. Pellagra is an occasional secondary manifestation of carcinoid syndrome, in which up to 60% of tryptophan is catabolized to 5-OH tryptophan and serotonin; **Hartnup disease**, an autosomal recessive disorder in which several amino acids, including tryptophan, are poorly absorbed; and treatment with the antituberculous drug isoniazid, which competes with PLP. The typical presentation of pellagra is that of a chronic wasting disease associated with (1) dermatitis, (2) dementia, and (3) diarrhea.

Toxicity

Although no toxic effects have been associated with niacin intake from naturally occurring food, the use of supplements and pharmacological doses of niacin has produced adverse effects in some individuals. In disorders of reduced tryptophan availability, such as Hartnup disease and carcinoid syndrome, daily niacin doses of 40 to 200 mg may be required, and in the treatment of dyslipidemias, up to 6 g daily may be used. Such doses are commonly associated with vascular dilation or "flushing"—a burning, tingling sensation of the face (that may be reddened), arms, and chest—and are thought to be mediated by prostaglandins. Other side effects of high-dose niacin treatment are (1) pruritus, (2) nausea, (3) vomiting, and (4) diarrhea, although these symptoms often abate with continued therapy. Symptoms of flushing have been taken as an end point sign in the formulation of a tolerable upper intake concentration for niacin, which has been set at 35 mg/d for adults.

Laboratory Assessment of Status[11]

At present, no blood markers are commonly used as indicators of niacin status. Most assessments of niacin nutriture have been based on the urinary measurement of N′-methylnicotinamide and N′-methyl-2-pyridone-5-carboxamide. Normally, adults excrete 20% to 30% of niacin in the form of methylnicotinamide and 40% to 60% as the pyridone. An excretion ratio of pyridone to methylnicotinamide of 1.3 to 4.0 is thus normal, but latent niacin deficiency is indicated by a value below 1.0. HPLC methods are currently the methods of choice, although some capillary electrophoresis methods have been developed.

Reference Intervals

A guidance reference interval for the excretion rate of N′-methylnicotinamide is 2.4 to 6.4 mg/d (17.5 to 46.7 μmol/d) or 1.6 to 4.3 mg/g creatinine (11.7 to 31.4 μmol/g creatinine).

Pantothenic Acid

Pantothenic acid is a component of coenzyme A that is required for the metabolism of fat, protein, and carbohydrate via the citric acid cycle.

Chemistry

Pantothenic acid is of ubiquitous occurrence in nature, where it is synthesized by most microorganisms and plants from pantoic acid (D-2,4-dihydroxy-3,3-dimethylbutyric acid) and β-alanine. Addition of both cysteamine at the C-terminal end and phosphorylation forms 4′-phosphopantetheine, which serves as a covalently attached prosthetic group of acyl carrier proteins and as part of CoA (Figure 27-18). The most common commercial synthetic form is the calcium salt.

Dietary Sources

Pantothenic acid is widely distributed in foods, mostly within CoA-containing compounds, and is particularly abundant in (1) animal sources, (2) legumes, (3) whole grain cereals, (4) egg yolk, (5) kidney, (6) liver, and (7) yeast.

Absorption, Transport, Metabolism, and Excretion

Pantothenic acid is taken in as dietary CoA compounds and 4′-phosphopantetheine and is hydrolyzed by pyrophosphatase and phosphatase in the intestinal lumen to (1) dephospho-CoA, (2) phosphopantetheine, and (3) pantetheine, which are further hydrolyzed to pantothenic acid. The vitamin is primarily absorbed as pantothenic acid through a saturable process at low concentrations and by simple diffusion at higher ones. The saturable process is facilitated by a sodium-dependent multivitamin transporter. After absorption, pantothenic acid enters the circulation and is taken up by cells in a manner similar to its intestinal adsorption. The synthesis of CoA from pantothenate is regulated by pantothenate kinase. Pantothenic acid is excreted in the urine after hydrolysis of CoA compounds by enzymes that cleave phosphate and the cysteamine moieties.

Functions

Pantothenic acid has two major metabolic roles (1) as part of CoA and (2) as the prosthetic group of the acyl-carrier protein (ACP). In the former role, CoA is involved primarily in acetyl

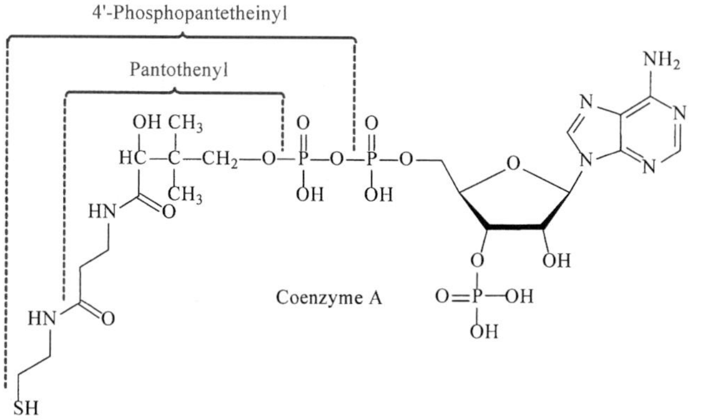

Figure 27-18 Pantothenate and 4′-phosphopantetheine as components of CoA.

and acyl transfer reactions in catabolic processes of carbohydrate, lipid, and protein chemistry. As the 4'-phosphopantetheine moiety of ACP, the phosphodiester-linked prosthetic group uses the sulfhydryl terminus to exchange with malonyl-CoA to form an ACP-S malonyl thioester, which chain-elongates during fatty acid biosynthesis .

Requirements and Reference Nutrient Intakes[2]

The daily intake of pantothenic acid has been set at 5 mg/d for those over 13 years of age. An additional 1 mg/d is suggested in pregnancy, and an additional 2 mg/d is suggested for lactating mothers.

Deficiency

The widespread availability of pantothenic acid in food is commensurate with its many roles and makes an uncomplicated dietary deficiency of pantothenate unlikely in humans. Symptoms produced in volunteers fed pantothenate-antagonist or semisynthetic diets virtually free of pantothenate included (1) irascibility, (2) postural hypotension and rapid heart rate on exertion, (3) epigastric distress with anorexia and constipation, (4) numbness and tingling of the hands and feet, (5) hyperactive deep tendon reflexes, and (6) weakness of finger extensor muscles. Historically, pantothenic acid deficiency has been associated with the syndrome of "burning feet" experienced by prisoners in the Second World War in Asia, which was relieved only by pantothenic acid supplementation, not by other B-group vitamins.

Toxicity

No adverse effects have been reported, with the exception of occasional mild diarrhea, with oral pantothenic acid at doses as high as 20 g/d.

Laboratory Assessment of Status[11]

No convenient or reliable functional tests of pantothenic acid status are available, thus assessment is made by direct measurement of whole blood or urine pantothenic acid concentrations. Urine measurements are perhaps the easiest to conduct and interpret, and concentrations are closely related to dietary intake. Whole blood measurements are preferred to measurements of plasma, which contains only free pantothenic acid and is insensitive to changes in pantothenic acid intake. Concentrations of pantothenic acid in all of the above fluids have been measured by microbiological assay, most commonly with the use of *Lactobacillus plantarum*. Other techniques that have been used include (1) radioimmunoassay, (2) gas chromatography, (3) gas chromatography–mass spectrometry, and (4) a stable isotope dilution assay. CoA and ACP have been measured by enzymatic methods.

Reference Intervals

Urinary excretion of pantothenic acid of less than 1 mg/d is considered abnormally low. Suspicion of inadequate intake is further supported when whole blood concentrations are less than 100 µg/L. A guidance reference interval for pantothenic acid in whole blood or serum is 344 to 583 µg/L (1.57 to 2.66 µmol/L), and for urinary excretion is 1 to 15 mg/d (5 to 68 µmol/d).

Trace Elements[15]

The term trace element was originally used to describe the residual amount of inorganic analyte quantitatively determined in a sample. Sensitive analytical methods now provide accurate determination of most inorganic micronutrients present at very low concentrations in body fluids and tissue.[13,14] Those present in body fluids (µg/dL) and in tissue (mg/kg) are still widely referred to as "trace elements" and those found at ng/dL or µg/kg as "**ultratrace elements.**" The corresponding dietary requirements are quoted in mg/d or µg/d, respectively. An element is considered essential when the signs and symptoms induced by a deficient diet are uniquely reversed by an adequate supply of the particular trace element (Figure 27-19).

Overview of Chemistry

Important factors that need to be considered for the understanding of trace elements and how they function, include (1) ionic forms, (2) relative solubilities, (3) possible organo complex formation, and (4) **chemical speciation**. This approach will serve as a proper basis for understanding physiological function, as well as relevant approaches to measurement.

Analytical Considerations

Analytical factors that have to be considered in the measurement of trace elements include (1) specimen requirements, (2) preanalytical factors, (3) collection equipment, (4) methodology, and (5) quality assurance.

Specimen Requirements

Specimens commonly submitted for direct trace element analysis include (1) whole blood, (2) blood plasma, and (3) serum. Direct determination of trace elements, however, is performed on any body fluid or tissue. For example, tissue samples for analysis may be obtained by needle biopsy (liver or bone) or after autopsy. Hair and nail samples are obtained noninvasively and are used to assess toxic metal exposure, but problems of

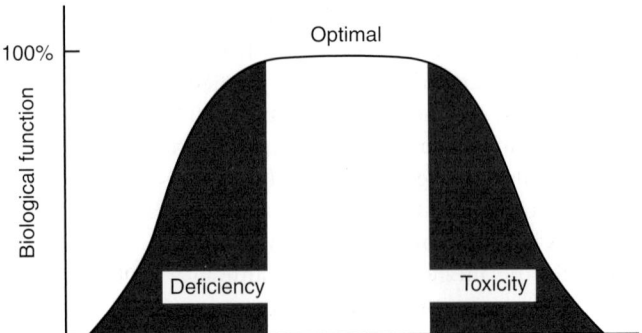

Figure 27-19 Model of the relationship between tissue concentration and intake of an essential nutrient and dependent biological function.

external contamination from (1) environmental pollution, (2) cosmetics, or (3) shampoos, are difficult to control.

The concentration of essential trace elements in nucleated cells has been determined in various types of leukocytes and in platelets. However, separation of white cells and platelets in whole blood before trace element analysis is subject to serious problems of contamination.

Preanalytical Factors

Numerous variables affect trace element determinations before analysis of the sample is undertaken, and these require careful control. For example, (1) age, (2) sex, (3) ethnic origin, (4) time of sampling in relation to food intake, (5) time of day, (6) history of medication, and (7) tobacco usage should be recorded when reference intervals from healthy control populations are established. For interpretation of results, knowledge of the extent of any **acute-phase reaction (APR)** is required.

Note that the APR is a response of the body to inflammation that results in a number of biochemical and physiological changes, including an increase or decrease in the plasma concentrations of a class of proteins known as acute phase reactants. Of particular relevance to this chapter, most trace element and vitamin concentrations in plasma are also markedly affected. In 1992, the Consensus Conference Committee of the American College of Chest Physicians/Society of Critical Care Medicine discussed the topic of sepsis and decided that APR was a part of the more general condition they termed the **systemic inflammatory response syndrome (SIRS)**.[2] As appropriate, SIRS is used instead of APR in the discussions that follow.

Collection Equipment

The choice of container for sample collection is important because contamination from (1) rubber, (2) cork, and (3) colored plastics has been a problem. For blood plasma, plastic tubes with lithium heparin as an anticoagulant are suitable for most analyses. For blood serum, plain glass containers have been used. For the ultratrace metals (Mn, Cr), special arrangements have to be made to collect blood via plastic cannulae or siliconized steel needles, and then the sample is placed into acid-washed containers. Trace metal Vacutainers are available commercially. It is good practice to run dilute acid blanks through all containers and collection systems to ensure that all batches remain as free from contamination as possible.

For 24-hour urine collection, it is important that urine is not collected into disposable fiber or stainless steel containers, and polyethylene bottles with glacial acetic acid should be used as the preservative, although bottles rinsed well with ultrapure deionized water are also appropriate.

Methodology

The detection limits of analytical methods used for determination of trace and ultratrace elements in biological specimens are important because concentrations of trace and ultratrace elements are in the nanogram per gram to microgram per gram range. In practice, the concentration of a trace or ultratrace element should be at least 10 times the detection limit of the method, thus ensuring sufficient accuracy and precision.

The most commonly used analytical methods are summarized in the following sections.

Spectrophotometry

When applied to the analysis of trace elements, spectrophotometric methods are based on the use of a color-forming reagent; however, they lack specificity. Interferences occur in (1) hemolyzed, (2) lipemic, and (3) icteric samples. In practice, this technique is sensitive only for the more abundant trace elements, such as (1) iron, (2) zinc, and (3) copper.

Atomic Absorption Spectrophotometry (AAS)

AAS is widely used for determination of Zn and Cu in serum (see Chapter 9). This technique cannot be used to measure Cu in urine, for which the more sensitive but technically more demanding electrothermal atomization-atomic absorption spectrometry (ETA-AAS) is required. With this technique, sample volumes as small as 10 μL are sequentially volatilized and atomized in a graphite tube. This technique is useful in situations in which the sample volume is limiting, or for which elements with low limits of detection are required, such as selenium or manganese. Optical background correction systems using a deuterium lamp or employing the Zeeman effect are now standard components of ETA-AAS instrumentation (see Chapter 9). Flame and electrothermal types of AAS are single element techniques, and the methods used for different elements have to be run sequentially; this is wasteful in terms of time and sample.

Inductively Coupled Plasma–Optical Emission Spectrometry (ICP-OES)

ICP-OES is replacing AAS, and its use has led to lower limits of detection. It offers a wide dynamic range (e.g., three orders of magnitude for most elements) that allows performance of simultaneous analyses on a single diluted aliquot of sample. The high temperature of the plasma (7500 °C) renders the technique largely free of chemical interferences, but (1) matrix effects, (2) background, and (3) spectral interferences are greater than those in AAS.

Inductively Coupled Plasma–Mass Spectrometry (ICP-MS)

This technique is more sensitive than ETA-AAS or ICP-OES and is now the method of choice for ultratrace elements. Polyatomic interferences are more likely at masses less than 80. ICP-MS has been used to measure stable isotopes and to conduct stable isotope tracer experiments and isotope dilution analysis. The principles of mass spectrometry are discussed in Chapter 13 .

Accelerator Mass Spectrometry

Accelerator mass spectrometry (AMS) differs from other forms of mass spectrometry in that it accelerates ions to extraordinarily high kinetic energies before mass analysis. This makes possible the detection of naturally occurring, long-lived radioisotopes, such as ^{10}Be, ^{36}Cl, ^{26}Al, and ^{14}C. The special property of AMS compared with other mass spectrometric methods is its power to separate a rare isotope from an abundant neighboring mass (e.g., ^{14}C from ^{12}C). For this reason, the technique is particularly useful in drug kinetic studies, where only very small amounts of actual labeled drug are required (i.e., at low µg concentration).

Other Techniques

Other techniques have been applied to elemental analysis, including X-ray–based techniques that have lower limits of detection at the µg/g concentration achievable for most sample materials. For thin sections of tissue, femto gram concentrations have been detected and reported for µ-synchrotron radiation X-ray fluorescence analysis (µ-SRXRF) stations installed at second-generation synchrotrons; with this technique, it is possible to map the three-dimensional (3D) orientation of metal in tissue (e.g., bone).

Speciation Methods of Assessment

Speciation methods involve techniques to separate the chemical complexes of individual elements present in any particular medium; these are now regarded as crucial for an understanding of the (1) absorption, (2) utilization, (3) function of elements and (4) problems of excess and potential toxicity. Recent developments have coupled separative with analytical procedures, in particular with ICP-OES or ICP-MS. This application has enabled analysis of several elements and study of their distribution in plasma in various abnormal clinical states (e.g., uremia). The low limit of detection of ICP-MS has enabled the low sample requirement of capillary electrophoresis to be coupled in this way.

Coupling of analytical procedures such as ICP-MS with ion exchange chromatography specifically configured to measure the elements attached to small molecules (e.g., organic acids) allows chemical speciation not only of the organo complexes but also of chemically ionized states of the elements in solution. It is possible to model such speciation in physiological fluids using established affinity constants and commercial computer programs. Such a model predicts that the major small species of elements will be complexed with citric acid (e.g., iron); obviously this will affect cellular uptake of the elements.

The European Virtual Institute for Speciation Analysis (EVISA) is a service provider in the field of speciation analysis. The EVISA Web portal (www.speciation.net/; accessed October 7, 2013) is a primary source for all those seeking information about chemical species with respect to (1) analysis, (2) biological activity (toxicity, nutritional value, metabolism), (3) legislation (laws, rules, standards), and (4) research in related fields.

Quality Assurance Considerations

An effective quality assurance scheme for trace or ultratrace element analyses requires incorporation of the following into each batch of analyses: (1) reagent blanks, (2) replicate analyses to assess precision, (3) calibrators of trace elements of interest in the expected concentration range of specimens analyzed, and (4) a control or reference solution with known or certified concentrations of trace elements to be determined to assess accuracy and batch-to-batch precision. The reference material should be of the same matrix type and should contain approximately the same quantities of analytes as the specimens. It is essential that trace element laboratories participate in external quality assessment programs.

Individual Trace Elements

Trace elements that are discussed below include (1) chromium, (2) cobalt, (3) copper, (4) fluoride, (5) manganese, (6) molybdenum, (7) selenium, and (8) zinc.

Chromium

Chromium occurs naturally in various crystal materials. It is a transitional element with many industrial uses and is discharged into the environment as industrial waste.

Chemistry

Chromium (atomic number 24, relative atomic mass 51.99) is a transition metal that occurs in biology with valence 3^+ or 6^+, each with markedly different properties. Trivalent Cr^{3+} is considered an essential trace element that enhances the action of insulin. Hexavalent Cr^{6+} is a strong oxidant that causes tissue damage, although it is normally rapidly reduced to Cr^{3+} during contact with foodstuffs and gastric contents.

A biologically active form of Cr^{3+} is known as **glucose tolerance factor** (GTF) and is found in brewer's yeast, but its function remains uncertain. Its structure is thought to be an octahedral chromium complex, with two molecules of nicotinic acid having and four coordination sites linked to glutamic acid, glycine, and cysteine.[13]

Dietary Sources

Estimates of the amount of chromium in foodstuffs vary because of analytical difficulties and contamination associated with contact with stainless steel during food processing, storage, and cooking. Good sources of chromium include (1) processed meats, (2) whole grain products, (3) green beans, (4) broccoli, and (5) some spices. The estimated dietary intake for adults in the United States ranges from 20 to 30 µg/d. Supplements that contain chromium are taken by about 8% of adults in the United States.

Absorption, Transport, Metabolism, and Excretion

Intestinal absorption of Cr^{3+} ranges from 0.4% to 2.5% of the quantity ingested with fecal output being mainly unabsorbed dietary chromium. After absorption, chromium binds to plasma transferrin with an affinity similar to that of iron. It then concentrates in human (1) liver, (2) spleen, (3) other soft tissue, and (4) bone. Urine chromium output is around 0.2 to 0.3 µg/d; the amount excreted is dependent upon intake.

Functions

A low-molecular-weight intracellular octapeptide (LMWCr), also known as chromodulin, is thought to bind Cr^{3+} and enhance the response of insulin receptors. Its proposed mode of action includes the following: (1) Inactive insulin receptors on cell membranes are converted to an active form by binding circulating insulin; (2) this binding stimulates movement into cells of chromium bound to plasma transferrin; (3) chromium then binds to apoLMWCr, converting it to an active form that binds to the insulin receptors and potentiates kinase activity; and (4) as plasma glucose and insulin fall to normoglycemic concentrations, the LMWCr factor is released from the cell to terminate its effects.

Requirements and Reference Nutrient Intakes[6]

Because evidence has been insufficient to set an **estimated average requirement (EAR)**, an average intake based on estimated intakes has been set at 35 µg Cr per day for men and 25 µg Cr per day for women. No tolerable upper limit has been set for dietary Cr^{3+} intake.

Deficiency

Clinical signs of human chromium deficiency were first clearly described in patients receiving parenteral nutrition for a prolonged period. All published case histories have had similar presentations, with previously stable patients developing (1) insulin-resistant glucose intolerance, (2) weight loss, and, in some cases, (3) neurological deficits. Addition of substantial amounts of Cr^{3+} to the intravenous regimen (150 to 200 µg/d) reversed glucose intolerance and reduced insulin requirements with eventual improvement in neurological disorders.

Clinical Significance

Chromium is thought to play a role in (1) impaired glucose tolerance, (2) diabetes, and (3) cardiovascular disease.

Impaired Glucose Tolerance and Diabetes. Poor chromium nutritional status may be a factor in impaired glucose tolerance in some patients. However, the variability of dietary chromium intake and the lack of an easily usable laboratory or clinical marker to identify those patients with poor chromium status have created difficulties. A meta-analysis investigating 15 randomized controlled trials on the effects of chromium on (1) glucose, (2) insulin, and (3) glycated hemoglobin (HbA_{1c})[11] concluded that no effect was caused by chromium on glucose or insulin in nondiabetic participants, and that the data for persons with diabetes were inconclusive.

It has been suggested that a short-term dosage of less than 1000 µg Cr per day may be a useful additional treatment for type 2 diabetes. Monitoring of kidney function and clinical assessment of dermatological changes are required. The dosages used suggest a pharmacological role for chromium, and potential toxicity has to be considered. Chromium therapy in the control and prevention of diabetes is therefore of considerable interest and is the subject of much controversy.

Cardiovascular Disease. Chromium depletion has long been thought to be associated with increased cardiovascular risk. Reports of favorable lipid responses to chromium supplementation have been published.

Toxicity

Hexavalent chromium is a recognized carcinogen, and industrial exposure to fumes and dusts containing this metal is associated with increased incidence of (1) lung cancer, (2) dermatitis, and (3) skin ulcers (see Chapter 32).

Cr^{3+} species are relatively nontoxic, in part because of their poor intestinal absorption and rapid excretion in urine. However, chromium picolinate is a widely used dietary supplement, and this compound has been reported to cause renal and hepatic damage when used at high doses.

In addition, markedly increased concentrations (up to 1000-fold) have been observed in both plasma (12 µg/L [620 nmol/L]) and urine (50 µg/L [2600 nmol/L]) in patients with problem hip prostheses. These may be raised in any patient receiving chrome-cobalt prostheses. No harmful effects of these high concentrations have been observed.

Laboratory Assessment of Status[11]

A beneficial response of glucose-intolerant patients to chromium supplementation is presently the only means of confirming chromium deficiency. No practicable method of assessing intracellular chromium depletion is yet available. Furthermore, it has been known since early animal experiments were conducted that circulating chromium is not in equilibrium with physiologically important reserves.

Direct determination of chromium in blood plasma or serum is possible only if great care is taken to prevent contamination before and during analysis. Sample collection procedures have to avoid any contact with stainless steel, so all-plastic phlebotomy systems or siliconized steel needles should be used, and samples should be stored in acid-washed containers.

Detection of increased amounts of chromium in urine confirms recent occupational or environmental exposure to excess chromium.

Reference Values

Very low values are now considered as normal for serum (0.1 to 0.2 µg/L [2 to 3 nmol/L]) and for urine (<0.2 µg Cr per L (<3 nmol/L).

Cobalt

Cobalt is essential for humans as an integral part of vitamin B_{12} (cobalamin). No other function for cobalt in the human body is known. Details of vitamin B_{12} biochemistry and function were discussed previously. The microflora of the human intestine is not able to use cobalt to synthesize physiologically active cobalamin. The human vitamin B_{12} requirement must be supplied by the diet. Free (nonvitamin B_{12}) cobalt does not interact with the body vitamin B_{12} pool. However, exposure to the kidney of increasing concentrations of cobalt ions may cause release of the hypoxia-inducible factor (HIF), leading to release of erythropoietin and an increase in erythropoiesis.

Reference values in plasma are less than 1 µg/L and in urine are usually less than 2 µg/g creatinine. Increased exposure through industrial uses, particularly with hard metal saw blades, leads to high mean urinary Co concentrations. Increases are also associated with hip prostheses for which concentrations can be markedly raised with no evidence of overt toxicity.

Copper

Copper is an important trace element that is associated with various metalloproteins.

Chemistry

Copper (atomic number 29, relative atomic mass 63.54) has Cu^{1+} and Cu^{2+} oxidation states in biological systems. The simple exchange between these ions gives the element important redox properties. Because of their high electron affinities, these ions are the most strongly bound to organic molecules of all essential trace metals. For example, copper in biological material is complexed with (1) proteins, (2) peptides, and (3) other organic ligands. An elaborate series of binding and transport proteins inside cells protects the genome from copper-generated free-radical attack. This keeps the concentration of free copper in the cytoplasm very low (around 10^{-15} mol/L). The copper metalloenzyme superoxide dismutase (SOD) protects against random free-radical damage both in the cytoplasm and in blood plasma.

Dietary Sources

The copper content of food is variable and is affected by applications to crops of copper-containing fertilizers and fungicidal sprays and the use of copper-containing cooking vessels. The metal is most plentiful in (1) organ meats, such as liver and kidney, with relatively large amounts also found in (2) shellfish, (3) nuts, (4) whole grain cereals, and (5) cocoa-containing products. The median intake of copper in the United States is around 1.0 to 1.6 mg/d.

Absorption, Transport, Metabolism, and Excretion

The extent of small intestinal copper absorption varies with dietary copper content and is around 50% at low copper intakes (less than 1 mg Cu per day) but only 20% at higher intakes (>5 mg Cu per day). Absorption is reduced by other dietary components, such as zinc (via metallothionein), molybdate, and iron, and is increased by amino acids.

Absorbed copper is transported to the liver bound to albumin in portal blood, where it is incorporated by hepatocytes into cuproenzymes and other proteins and then is exported in peripheral blood mainly as ceruloplasmin to tissue and organs. Although two-thirds of the 80 to 100 mg total body copper content is located in skeleton and muscle, the liver is the key organ in copper homeostasis. Ceruloplasmin is a positive acute-phase reactant that is increased during infection and after tissue injury. A smaller amount of copper in plasma (<10%) is bound to albumin. An overview of copper metabolism is illustrated in Figure 27-20.

Between 0.5 and 2.0 mg of copper per day is excreted via bile into feces. Patients with cholestatic jaundice or other forms of liver dysfunction are therefore at risk of copper accumulation caused by failure of excretion. Urine copper output is normally less than 60 µg/d.

Functions

Copper is a catalytic component of numerous enzymes and is a structural component of other important proteins in humans, animals, plants, and microorganisms.

Energy Production. Cytochrome c oxidase is a multisubunit complex that contains copper and iron. Located on the external face of mitochondrial membranes, the enzyme catalyzes a four-electron reduction of molecular oxygen, which is necessary for ATP production.

Connective Tissue Formation. Protein-lysine 6-oxidase (lysyl oxidase) is a cuproenzyme that is essential for stabilization of extracellular matrixes, specifically the enzymatic cross-linking of collagen and elastin. The enzyme is highly associated with connective tissue and is located in (1) aorta, (2) dermal connective tissue, (3) fibroblasts, and (4) cytoskeleton of many other cells.

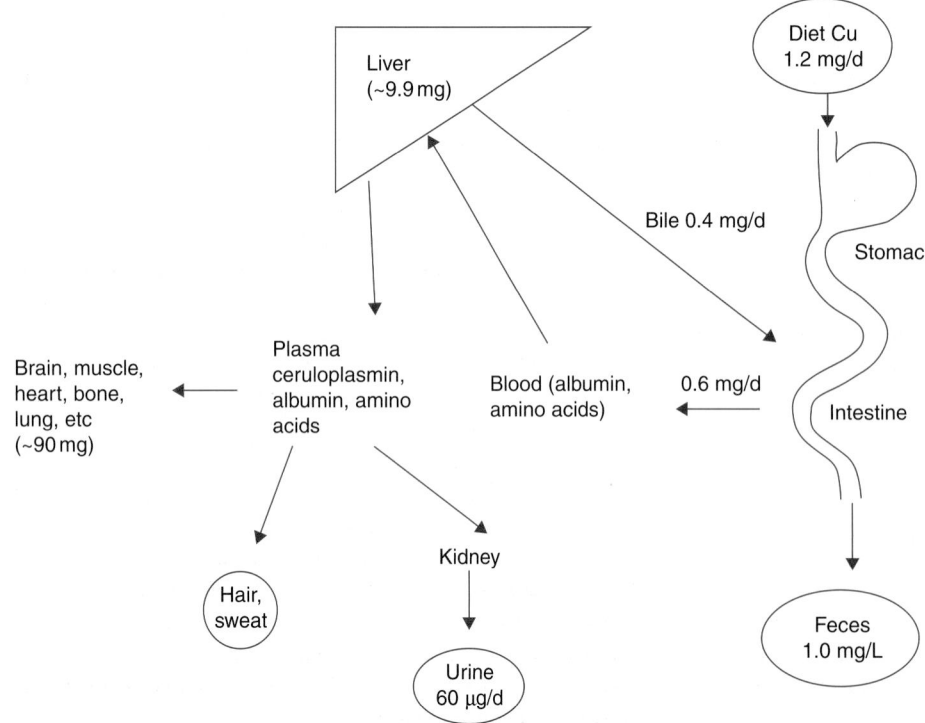

Figure 27-20 Metabolism of copper. *(Modified from Harris ED. Copper. In: O'Dell BL, Sunde RA, editors. Handbook of nutritionally essential mineral elements. New York: Marcel Dekker, 1997:231–73.)*

Iron Metabolism. Copper-containing enzymes—namely, (1) ferroxidase I (ceruloplasmin), (2) ferroxidase II, and (3) hephaestin in the enterocyte—oxidize ferrous iron to ferric iron. This allows incorporation of Fe^{3+} into transferrin and eventually into hemoglobin.

Central Nervous System. Dopamine mono-oxygenase (DMO) is an enzyme that requires copper as a cofactor and uses ascorbate as an electron donor. This enzyme catalyzes the conversion of dopamine to norepinephrine, the important neurotransmitter. Monoamine oxidase is a copper-containing enzyme that catalyzes the degradation of serotonin in the brain.

Melanin Synthesis. Tyrosinase is a copper-containing enzyme that is present in melanocytes and catalyzes the synthesis of melanin.

Antioxidant Functions. Both intracellular and extracellular SODs are copper- and zinc-containing enzymes that are able of converting superoxide radicals to hydrogen peroxide, which is subsequently removed. Ceruloplasmin also binds copper ions, thus preventing oxidative damage from free copper ions, which generate hydroxyl radicals.

Regulation of Gene Expression and Intracellular Copper Handling. Synthesis of metallothionein is controlled by copper-responsive transcription factors, and this protein is important in regulating the intracellular distribution of copper. Additional specialized proteins act as "copper chaperones" to deliver copper to intracellular sites and prevent oxidative damage by free copper ions.

Inborn Errors of Copper Metabolism. Menkes disease is caused by a defective gene that regulates the metabolism of copper in the body. **Wilson disease** is inherited as an autosomal recessive trait that involves a defect in the metabolism of copper, with accumulation of copper in (1) liver, (2) brain, (3) kidney, (4) cornea, and (5) other tissue. Copper-transporting P-type ATPases, known as *ATP7A* and *ATP7B*, are essential factors in maintaining copper balance. Impaired intestinal transport of copper caused by a mutation in the *ATP7A* gene leads to the severe copper deficiency disease seen in Menkes disease. A defect in the *ATP7B* gene affects both incorporation of copper into ceruloplasmin and copper excretion via bile and serves as the basis of Wilson disease.

Requirements and Reference Nutrient Intakes[6]

The recommended dietary intake for adults is 0.9 mg/d. This is near the lower limit of 1.0 mg/d found in dietary surveys and has led to suggestions that marginal copper depletion could be found in the U.S. population. The tolerable upper limit is 10 mg/d.

Deficiency

A deficiency of copper has been noted in a number of conditions.

Malnourished Infants. When malnourished infants with a history of chronic diarrhea were rehabilitated using a formula based upon cow's milk, they developed (1) iron-resistant anemia, (2) neutropenia, (3) other hematological disorders, and (4) bone lesions. Copper supplementation of milk feeds reversed these abnormalities.

Premature Infants. Most of the accumulation of copper in the fetal liver occurs in the last 3 months of pregnancy, and premature infants fed formula lacking sufficient copper are at risk of deficiency disease because they lack adequate liver copper stores. Hematological abnormalities and easily fractured brittle bones have been described.

Nutritional Support. Adults and children fed intravenously without addition of sufficient copper to the nutrient regimen develop symptomatic copper deficiency. Hematological changes of hypochromic anemia and neutropenia are reversed by copper supplementation. Similar effects have been reported during prolonged enteral feeding via jejunostomy. Children may develop the typical bone changes mentioned previously.

Menkes Disease. This disorder typically occurs in male infants at 2 to 3 months who present with (1) loss of previously normal development, (2) hypotonia, (3) seizures, and (4) failure to thrive. Physical changes in the hair (pili torti/corkscrew hair) and in facial appearance, as well as neurological abnormalities, suggest the diagnosis. Local first-line tests would be likely to find plasma copper less than 10 µmol/L, ceruloplasmin less than 220 mg/L, and demonstration of pili torti by microscopic examination of hair.

Malabsorption Syndromes. Patients at risk include those with (1) celiac disease, (2) sprue, (3) cystic fibrosis, and (4) short bowel syndrome. In some cases, excessive intake of oral zinc supplements has caused copper deficiency by zinc induction of metallothionein in the intestinal mucosa, which then sequesters dietary copper, blocking its absorption.

Cardiovascular Disease. Animal studies show that severe copper deficiency causes cardiac damage, but the abnormality differs from that seen in human cardiovascular disease. Epidemiological surveys have shown that increased plasma copper values are a positive cardiovascular risk factor. An increase in plasma ceruloplasmin and hence plasma copper may be a nonspecific response to the inflammation of arteries seen in arteriosclerosis.

Anemia. Copper deficiency is an established cause of hematological abnormalities but is frequently misdiagnosed. Patients with copper deficiency have been known to present with a combination of hematological and neurological abnormalities that may masquerade as a myelodysplastic syndrome. Records between 1970 and 2005 of patients excluding Wilson disease with hypocupremia (mean, 0.23; range, 0 to 0.69 µg/mL; normal plasma zinc) reveal various hematological abnormalities on bone marrow examination, including (1) vacuoles in myeloid precursors, (2) iron-containing plasma cells, and (3) a decrease in granulocyte precursors and ring sideroblasts. Thus copper deficiency is an uncommon but very treatable cause of hematological abnormalities.

Neuropathy. Copper deficiency is an increasingly recognized cause of gait unsteadiness. A case report of copper deficiency due to celiac disease suggested that ataxia associated with celiac disease was likely due to a copper deficiency, myeloneuropathy. Similar findings have resulted from copper deficiency due to excess zinc intake.

Toxicity

Wilson disease is a genetic disorder of copper metabolism that causes an increase in copper to toxic concentrations. The incidence of Wilson disease is estimated to be 1/30,000 live births. Because presentation is highly variable, adolescents or young adults with otherwise unexplained liver disease or neurological symptoms should be screened, especially when there is a family history of suspected Wilson disease. Initial local investigations would include measurements of plasma copper and ceruloplasmin (<50 µg/dL, 8 µmol Cu/L) and ceruloplasmin (<200 mg/L). Although the total plasma copper is decreased, the non–ceruloplasmin-bound fraction is increased, allowing deposition of copper in brain, eyes, and kidneys.

Slit lamp examination of the eye may detect copper deposits in the eye (Kayser-Fleischer rings), and abnormalities may be noted in liver function tests with increased urine copper output (>500 µg Cu/L). Liver biopsy for copper analysis is useful in suspected cases, and results showing more than 250 µg/g Cu dry weight are usually found (normal, 8 to 40 µg Cu/g dry weight). Gene tracking and mutation detection are now possible. Diagnosis often is difficult in Wilson disease cases involving acute liver failure. Greatly increased plasma copper will be found but without an increase in ceruloplasmin.

The chronic form of Wilson disease is treated with oral chelating agents, such as penicillamine and trientine, which remove excess copper from tissue and increase urine copper excretion.

Toxicity has been known to occur as the direct result of copper contamination of diet and water supplies.

Laboratory Assessment of Status[9]

Plasma copper and ceruloplasmin assays are convenient and are widely used to confirm severe copper deficiency. However, they are not sensitive indicators of marginal copper depletion.

Because about 90% of plasma copper is bound to ceruloplasmin, factors that increase the hepatic synthesis of ceruloplasmin, such as APR or the oral contraceptive pill, will increase plasma copper independently of dietary copper intake. In premature infants with liver immaturity and low ceruloplasmin synthesis, plasma copper values less than 30 µg/L (<5 µmol Cu/L) suggest the necessity for increased copper input.

The ratio of immunologically to enzymatically measured ceruloplasmin may be a useful index of marginal copper depletion. Apoceruloplasmin is increased in blood serum during copper depletion, and this contributes to the total ceruloplasmin assay, but enzymatic activity is decreased in even marginal copper depletion.

Reference Intervals

For adults, plasma copper is usually in the interval of 70 to 140 µg/dL (10 to 22 µmol/L). Values in women of child-bearing age, especially in pregnancy, are higher. Plasma copper for adults below 50 µg/dL (8 µmo/L) and for infants below 30 µg/dL (5 µmol/L) indicates probable copper depletion. Adjusting the copper concentration to account for variations in ceruloplasmin is problematic, as it depends on the accuracy of an immunoassay.

The most reliable procedure consists of using plasma ultrafiltration when a reference interval of 0 to 10 µg/dL (0 to 1.6 µmol/L) has been reported in 137 healthy adult (20 to 59 years of age) blood donors. Free copper concentrations for patients diagnosed with Wilson disease were at least sixfold greater than the reference upper limit.

Urine copper output is normally less than 60 µg/24 h (<1.0 µmol/24 h), and values above 200 µg/24 h (3 µmol/L) are found in Wilson disease. A copper concentration in a liver biopsy sample >250 µg Cu/g dry weight (normally 8 to 40 µg/g dry weight) is indicative of Wilson disease, in the absence of other causes of cholestatic disease.

Urine copper output, in response to an oral penicillamine test, greater than 25 µmol/24 h is thought to be diagnostic of Wilson disease. Evidence suggests that this test is valuable in the diagnosis of Wilson disease with active liver disease but is unreliable in excluding the diagnosis in asymptomatic siblings.

Fluoride

Fluoride (Fl) is the most widely used of the "pharmacologically beneficial trace elements" in the area of public health. Dental caries has been described as the last major epidemic of preventable bacterial disease, and dental decay leads to (1) tooth loss, (2) nutritional problems, and (3) systemic infection.

Dietary Sources

Many studies have established that addition of fluoride to drinking water reduces the incidence of tooth decay; more than 60% of the U.S. population now uses fluoridated water. Clinical studies from 1950 to 1980 in 20 different countries found that adding fluoride to community water supplies, within the interval 0.7 to 1.2 mg/L, reduced the incidence of caries by 40% to 50% in primary (infant) teeth and by 50% to 60% in permanent teeth.

Fluoride supplementation of (1) salt, (2) sugar, and (3) milk has been used in areas where fluoride is not added to water supplies.

Function

The fluoride ion is exchanged for hydroxyl in the crystal structure of apatite, a main component of skeletal bone and teeth. This stabilizes the regenerating tooth surface. Fluoride is available from saliva and may be released from dental plaque at low pH. Initially, benefit was considered to involve solely the erupting teeth of children, but topical effects on adult teeth are now thought to reduce decay. Initial evidence from small studies suggests that pharmacological doses of fluoride may reduce the incidence of bone fracture in patients with osteoporosis.

Absorption, Transport, Metabolism, and Excretion

Fluoride ions are absorbed from both the stomach and the small intestine. Soluble salts are efficiently absorbed, and a peak increase in fluoride occurs in blood plasma within 1 hour of ingestion. Ions are rapidly cleared from plasma into tissue in exchange with anions, such as (1) hydroxyl, (2) citrate, and (3) carbonate. At least 95% of the 2.6 g of total body fluoride is located in bones and teeth. Almost 90% of excess fluoride is excreted in urine.

Toxicity

Dental fluorosis—the mottling of enamel in the erupting teeth of children—is now estimated to affect around 20% of the population. This is sometimes a disfiguring condition, and it occurs in a greater proportion of children than was thought at first. This condition is possibly caused by ingestion of fluoride-containing toothpaste by children. It is suggested that "pediatric" toothpastes with lower fluoride content should be made available in areas where the water supply is fluoridated.

Occupational exposure to inhaled fluoride dusts among cryolite workers during aluminum refining has resulted in severe bone abnormalities, but safety equipment now limits such exposure. No cases of skeletal fluorosis have been reported in areas with controlled fluoridation of water supplies. However, skeletal fluorosis may occur in areas of the world where naturally occurring drinking water has high concentrations of fluoride, such as China and the Indian subcontinent.

Laboratory Assessment of Status[3]

Laboratory analysis of drinking water may be required to detect possible fluoride excess in natural well waters and may be necessary during incidents of failure of the equipment used to treat drinking water. Determination of fluoride in urine has been used to assess exposure to different sources of fluoride. For drinking water and urine, direct determination using a fluoride-specific electrode is performed.

Reference Intervals

Concentrations of fluoride in body fluids and tissue vary widely, depending on the fluoride content of drinking water and input from diet, toothpaste, and mouth rinses. For urine, a guideline interval is 0.2 to 3.2 mg/L (10.5 to 168 μmol/L).

Manganese

Manganese is present in biological systems bound to protein in the 2^+ or 3^+ valence state. It is associated mainly with (1) formation of connective and bony tissue, (2) growth and reproductive functions, and (3) carbohydrate and lipid metabolism.

Chemistry

Manganese (atomic number 25, relative atomic mass 54.94) has 11 available oxidation states, but only Mn^{2+} and Mn^{3+} are found in biological systems, most often bound to protein.

Dietary Sources

Manganese-rich sources include (1) whole grain foods, (2) nuts, (3) leafy vegetables, (4) soy products, and (5) teas. Median intake in the United States is about 2 mg/d. Vegetarian diets containing high quantities of whole grains and nuts have been known to supply more than 10 mg/d.

Absorption, Transport, Metabolism, and Excretion

Dietary manganese is absorbed from the small intestine by mechanisms that may have a pathway common to that of iron. Manganese absorption increases at low dietary intakes and decreases at higher intakes, with tracer studies suggesting absorption efficiencies of 2% to 15%. Once absorbed, manganese is transported in portal blood to the liver bound to albumin and then is exported to other tissues bound to transferrin and possibly to α_2-macroglobulin . Excretion of manganese occurs primarily via bile into feces, and urine output is very low.

Functions

Manganese, a constituent of many important metalloenzymes, acts as a nonspecific enzyme activator. Mn^{2+} ions will replace Mg^{2+} during activation of some enzymes.

Superoxide Dismutase. Manganese-dependent **superoxide dismutase** (SOD) is a mitochondrial enzyme that is an important factor in limiting oxygen toxicity. This enzyme catalyzes the breakdown of the superoxide radical O_2^- to H_2O_2, which then is removed by catalase and glutathione peroxidase.

Pyruvate Carboxylase. SOD acts together with phosphoenol pyruvate (PEP) carboxykinase, an enzyme that is activated by manganese ions. These enzymes are required to catalyze the formation of PEP from pyruvate—a key reaction in the hepatic synthesis of glucose.

Arginase. Arginase, the terminal enzyme in the urea cycle, hydrolyzes L-arginine to urea and ornithine. The activity of arginase affects the production of nitric oxide by limiting the availability of L-arginine.

Glycosyl Transferases. These enzymes are responsible for the sequential addition of carbohydrate molecules to proteins to form proteoglycans, and ultimately connective tissue and cartilage. They are therefore important for the structural integrity of bone and skin and for healthy wound healing.

Requirements and Reference Nutrient Intakes[6]

Because of lack of information on manganese dietary requirements, the U.S. Food and Nutrition Board has set an adequate intake for adults at 2.3 mg/d for males and 1.8 mg/d for females. An area of concern is the potential toxicity of manganese for infants, whose immature hepatic development reduces the biliary excretion of excess manganese.

Deficiency

Overt manganese deficiency has not been documented in humans eating natural diets. However, in animal studies, signs of experimentally induced manganese deficiency include (1) impaired growth and reproductive function, (2) skeletal abnormalities, (3) impaired glucose tolerance, and (4) impaired cholesterol synthesis. Young men fed experimental diets low in manganese developed skin lesions and low plasma cholesterol.

Prolidase is a cytosolic dipeptidase that hydrolyzes dipeptides with proline or hydroxyproline at the carboxy terminus. Its deficiency in infants is a rare genetic disorder that is known to be associated with abnormalities of manganese biochemistry.

Toxicity

The occupational health hazard from prolonged exposure to manganese-containing dust or fumes is well recognized (see

Chapter 32). Neurological symptoms resembling Parkinson disease develop slowly over months or years.

Patients with severe liver disease may have neurological and behavioral signs of manganese neurotoxicity due to failure to excrete manganese in bile. Manganese deposition in the globus pallidus during liver failure results in magnetic resonance signal hypersensitivity.

Patients receiving manganese intravenously during TPN have shown evidence of manganese retention and deposition in the midbrain and brainstem. Typical symptoms include a parkinsonian-like tremor and abnormalities of gait.

It is now recommended that only 1 μg Mn per kg (18 nmol/kg) be administered during TPN to infants and no more than 1 μmol/d (55 μg/d) to adults. All patients requiring prolonged intravenous nutrition (IVN), especially those who have cholestasis, should be monitored for evidence of manganese retention.

Laboratory Assessment of Status

Plastic cannulae should be used for phlebotomy, and hemolysis should be prevented during sample separation. Whole blood includes about 10 times as much manganese as plasma or serum and is not as affected by contamination from steel needles during sample collection. Consequently, measurement of whole blood manganese is the most widely used method for monitoring manganese status.

Reference Intervals

The reference interval for serum manganese is 0.5 to 1.3 μg/L (9 to 24 nmol/L). The reference interval for whole blood manganese is 5 to 15 μg/L (90 to 270 nmol/L). Increases in serum manganese to greater than 5.4 μg/L (>30 nmol/L) or blood manganese to greater than 20 μg/L (>360 nmol/L) are indices of manganese retention.

Molybdenum

The essential need for molybdenum by animals and humans is based on its incorporation into metalloenzymes.

Chemistry

Molybdenum (atomic number 42, relative atomic mass 95.94) is a metal that includes several oxidation states, but the most stable in biological systems is Mo^{6+}, as is found in molybdate (MoO_4^{2-}). A close parallel has been noted between the chemistries of (1) molybdenum, (2) tungsten, and (3) vanadium. Molybdenum enzymes facilitate important carbon, nitrogen, and sulfur cycles.

Dietary Sources

Good sources of molybdenum are (1) legumes, such as peas, lentils, and beans; (2) grains; and (3) nuts. In the United States, the average dietary intake for adults is 76 to 109 μg Mo per day.

Absorption, Transport, Metabolism, and Excretion

Molybdenum is efficiently absorbed over a wide range of dietary intakes, mainly as molybdate, although competitive inhibition of absorption by sulfate reduces intestinal uptake. Between 80% and 90% of molybdenum in whole blood is bound to red cell proteins. Transport of the smaller amount in blood plasma may involve α_2-macroglobulin. Urine output directly reflects the dietary intake of molybdenum.

Functions

Several important mammalian enzymes, such as (1) sulfite oxidase, (2) xanthine dehydrogenase, and (3) aldehyde oxidase, require molybdenum as a cofactor. This organic component is a molybdopterin complex. Sulfite oxidase catalyzes the last step in the degradation of sulfur amino acids, oxidizing sulfite to sulfate and transferring electrons to cytochrome c. Xanthine dehydrogenase and aldehyde oxidase hydroxylate various heterocyclic substances, such as purines and pteridines.

Requirements and Reference Nutrient Intakes[6]

The RDA for Mo has been set at 45 μg per day for adults, which is below the estimated average dietary intake.

Deficiency

Molybdenum deficiency has not been observed in healthy people who consume a normal dietIt is now common, especially in Europe, to include a small amount of molybdenum (19 μg/d [0.2 μmol/d]) in trace element additive mixtures.

Very rare recessive inherited diseases result from defects in the biosynthesis of molybdenum cofactor; in most cases, they lead to early childhood death. First symptoms include (1) failure to thrive and seizures; in later stages, (2) lens dislocations are noted, together with (3) cerebral atrophy. Disease-causing mutations have been identified, and the possibility of gene therapy is being investigated.

Biochemical diagnosis has been made by detection of excess sulfite in urine using the a sulfite dipstick test. Note that samples should not be evaluated until at least 10 days after birth and should be tested within 10 minutes of collection. Another type of molybdenum cofactor deficiency is confirmed by finding low plasma uric acid. Specialized centers offer biochemical prenatal diagnosis on chorionic villous samples.

Toxicity

Molybdenum compounds have low toxicity in humans. Excess molybdenum intake induces copper deficiency in ruminants by blocking copper absorption through formation of an insoluble thiomolybdate/copper complex. This discovery has suggested the use of ammonium molybdate in the management of Wilson disease.

Laboratory Assessment of Status

Whole blood and serum or plasma molybdenum concentrations are too low to be used for the detection of deficiency. However, urinary output is responsive to increases or decreases in input. Measuring urate or sulfite in the urine is the most available means of confirming molybdenum cofactor disorders or possible molybdenum deficiency.

Reference Intervals

Approximately 0.5 µg Mo per L (5 nmol/L) is present in plasma or serum and about 1 µg Mo per L (10 nmol/L) in whole blood. Urine molybdenum values determined by ICP-MS are approximately 40 to 60 µg/L.

Selenium

Selenium (Se) is an essential element for humans and is a constituent of the enzyme glutathione peroxidase; it is believed to be closely associated with vitamin E in its functions.

Chemistry

Selenium (atomic number 34, relative atomic mass 78.96) is a nonmetal that has several chemical forms and valences and a bioinorganic chemistry that is related to sulfur. The most important biologically active compounds contain selenocysteine, in which selenium is substituted for sulfur in cysteine. Now considered to be the twenty-first amino acid, selenocysteine is incorporated into proteins by the specific codon UGA, which was previously thought to be solely a stop codon (see Chapter 18).

Ingested selenium compounds include (1) selenate, (2) selenite, (3) selenocysteine, and (4) selenomethionine, which are metabolized largely via selenide that may be associated with a chaperone protein. Selenide is then converted to selenophosphate, which is an important precursor in the synthesis of selenocysteine proteins (Figure 27-21).

Dietary Sources

Selenium enters the food chain mainly as selenomethionine from plants that take the element up from the soil but do not appear to use it. The soil content of selenium is highly variable and is usually low in volcanic soils when soluble salts are leached out by ground water. In the United States and Canada, wheat and other cereal products are a good source of selenium; average intakes in North America vary from 80 to 220 µg Se per day, whereas in the UK, dietary intake is about 30 to 60 µg/d. Intakes in China are as low as 11 µg/d and in New Zealand 28 µg/d.

Absorption, Transport, Metabolism, and Excretion

Intestinal absorption of various dietary forms of selenium is efficient but is not regulated. The inorganic salts selenite and selenate used as dietary supplements and in food fortification are almost completely absorbed, but much of the selenate ion is rapidly excreted in urine. Selenium from inorganic salts is more rapidly incorporated into glutathione peroxidase and other selenoproteins than is selenium from organic sources containing selenomethionine. However, selenium-enriched yeast containing the organic forms is considered less toxic and is widely used as a dietary supplement.

About 50% to 60% of the total plasma selenium is present as the protein selenoprotein P, a highly basic protein that includes multiple histidine residues and about 10 atoms of selenium per molecule. Approximately 30% of plasma selenium is present as glutathione peroxidase (GSHPx-3), and the remainder is incorporated into albumin as selenomethionine.

Urinary output of selenium is the major route of excretion and reflects recent dietary intake. The amounts excreted vary widely, ranging from less than 20 to more than 1000 µg Se/L, depending on the geographic origins of the food.

Functions

Thirty or more biologically active selenocysteine-containing proteins have been identified. Some of the most important ones are listed below.

Glutathione Peroxidase. This enzyme has four isoforms: (1) GSHPx-1 in red cells, (2) GSHPx-2 in gastrointestinal mucosa, (3) blood plasma GSHPx-3, and (4) the cell membrane–located GSHPx-4. These enzymes use the reducing power of glutathione to remove an oxygen atom from hydrogen peroxide and lipid hydroperoxides.

Iodothyronine Deiodinase. Type I, II, and III isoforms of this enzyme are responsible for conversion of the precursor

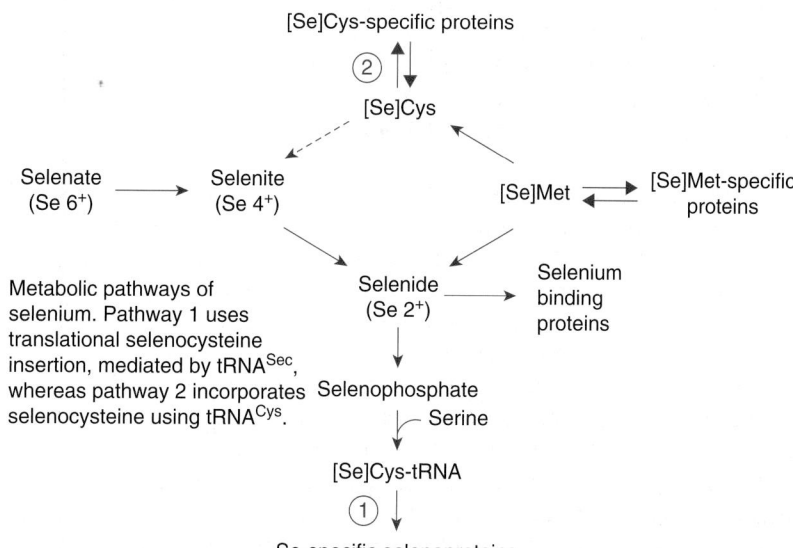

Figure 27-21 Metabolic pathways of selenium. *(Adapted from Sunde.)*

hormone T_4 to the active hormone T_3. Type I, thyroxine-5-deiodinase, is located in the(1) liver, (2) kidney, and (3) muscle and is responsible for more than 90% of plasma T_3 production.

Thioredoxin Reductases. Three isoforms catalyze the NADPH-dependent reduction of thioredoxin and are important in maintaining the intracellular redox state.

Selenoprotein P. This protein, which is the major selenium-containing protein in blood plasma, may be a transport protein for the element and has an antioxidant function.

Requirements and Reference Nutrient Intakes[1]

The RDA for selenium is set at 55 μg/d for adults. In many countries in Europe, intakes are now close to or less than 55 μg/d, and selenium dietary provision may be suboptimal.

Deficiency

Important selenium-dependent diseases have been identified in farm animals, such as white muscle disease in sheep and cattle, and myopathy of cardiac and skeletal muscle in lambs and calves. As is discussed later, a range of deficiency states has been identified in humans.

Severe Deficiency

Keshan Disease. Conclusive evidence of a role for selenium in human nutrition came with publication of the results of large-scale trials in China that showed the protective effects of selenium supplementation on children and young adults suffering from an endemic cardiomyopathy. This was observed in areas of the country (Keshan region (thus, **Keshan disease**)) with low soil selenium concentrations.

Kashin-Beck Disease. **Kashin-Beck disease** is type of severe arthritis is described in parts of China and neighboring areas of Russia where soil selenium is particularly low.

Artificial Nutrition. Inadequate selenium provision in specialized diets used to treat inborn errors and during long-term parenteral nutrition has led to cases of deficiency. Symptoms of severe deficiency include muscle weakness. Cases involving cardiomyopathy, which is usually fatal and resembles Keshan disease, and macrocytosis and pseudoalbinism in children have been described.

Marginal Deficiencies

Thyroid Function. Selenium and other trace elements are necessary for normal thyroid function because the important deiodinase enzymes are selenoproteins. Endemic thyroid disease in Zaire may be related to the combined depletion of iodine and selenium. Care must be taken in giving selenium supplementation under such circumstances because stimulation of thyroid hormone metabolism may induce hypothyroidism.

Immune Function. Deficiency of selenium is accompanied by loss of immunocompetence and this is related to the reduction of selenoproteins in the liver, spleen, and lymph nodes. Both cell-mediated immunity and B-cell function are impaired.

Reproductive Disorders. Adequate selenium supply is necessary for successful reproduction in a variety of farm animals. Male fertility in man may be affected by selenium depletion because selenium is necessary for testosterone synthesis and for maintenance of sperm viability.

Mood Disorders. Marginal selenium depletion has been associated with (1) anxiety, (2) confusion, and (3) hostility, and improvements have been claimed following supplementation.

Inflammatory Conditions. Many conditions associated with inflammation and increased oxidative stress may be influenced by selenium status. Positive effects have been reported following supplementation in arthritis, in pancreatitis, and in intensive care.

Viral Virulence. An unusually virulent strain of the Coxsackie virus is probably part of the cause of cardiomyopathy in selenium-depleted regions of China. This is consistent with seasonal variations in the incidence of disease. In laboratory studies, a nonlethal form of Coxsackie B (CVB 3/0) mutated to a virulent strain when inoculated into selenium-deficient mice, probably as a result of oxidative stress. Further animal studies have demonstrated that a mild strain of influenza virus exhibits increased virulence when given to selenium-deficient mice. The relevance of these study findings for humans needs to be established.

Cancer Chemoprevention. Epidemiological surveys have found a link between cancer incidence and soil selenium content, suggesting a higher incidence of certain cancers in individuals with low selenium intake. Large-scale trials in China on people at high risk for viral hepatitis B and liver cancer demonstrated that selenium-enriched table salt led to a reduced incidence of liver cancer of 35%.

For some years, it was hoped that selenium supplementation above the minimum dietary requirement may have a role in cancer prevention, particularly in relation to prostatic cancer. However, the large selenium and vitamin E cancer prevention study known as the Selenium and Vitamin E Cancer Prevention Trial (SELECT) reported and concluded that selenium or vitamin E, alone or in combination at the doses and formulations used, did not prevent prostate cancer in this population of relatively healthy men.

Toxicity

Soil in areas of China and the United States includes large amounts of selenium, and locally produced food contains excess selenium. Clinical signs of selenosis are (1) garlic odor in the breath, (2) hair loss, and (3) nail damage. The tolerable upper limit has been set at 400 μg/d for adults and less for children.

Laboratory Assessment of Status[1]

Carbon furnace atomic absorption spectroscopy (CFAAS) is widely used to measure plasma and/or serum selenium, although ICP-MS, without the need for dynamic cell reaction to remove polyatomic interference from argon mass 80, is probably the preferred procedure in routine laboratories.

The main components of plasma selenium are extracellular GSHPx-3 and selenoprotein P. Red cell GSHPx-1 and plasma GSHPx-3 are assayed by enzymatic methods, and tertiary-butyl peroxide is a commonly used substrate because it is not as affected by catalase as is hydrogen peroxide.

After 1 year on TPN without selenium supplements, patients have low plasma selenium and red cell GSHPx. With replacement of selenium as selenious acid, a rapid increase in GSHPx-3 is seen within the first 24 hours, and normal concentrations are reached within 1 to 2 weeks. Red cell GSHPx takes 3 to 4 months to recover, consistent with the need for formation of these cells in the presence of selenium.

The major selenium-containing plasma protein selenoprotein P is determined by immunological methods. Selenoprotein P concentration in plasma responds rapidly to supplementation.

Plasma selenoprotein P, plasma GSHPx-3, and total plasma selenium concentrations are all lowered by the SIRS to injury or infection. This effect should be considered when plasma selenium values in postoperative patients or those with infection or inflammatory disease are considered.

Urine selenium output is mainly a reflection of recent dietary input and has not been extensively employed in population surveys. Hair and nail selenium analysis has been used as a measure of long-term dietary selenium intake.

In practice, measurements of plasma selenium and GSHPx provide a good estimate of status, in particular the adequacy of recent intake, provided they are interpreted with knowledge of changes in the SIRS, with red cell GSHPx providing an index of long-term intake.

Reference Intervals

The reference interval for selenium in (1) whole blood, (2) plasma, (3) serum, (4) hair, and (5) nails should be established locally because these indices are affected by dietary selenium intake. Plasma selenium adult values lie in the interval from 63 to 160 µg/L (0.8 to 2.0 µmol/L). Values less than 40 µg Se/L (0.5 µmol/L) indicate probable selenium depletion.

Values in children are lower and in the United Kingdom are as follows: 16 to 71 µg/L (0.2 to 0.9 µmol/L) for those younger than 2 years old; 40 to 103 µg/L (0.5 to 1.3 µmol/L) for 2- to 4-year-olds; and 55 to 134 µg/L (0.7 to 1.7 µmol/L) for 4- to 16-year-olds. Cutoff values less than 8 µg/L (0.1 µmol/L) in neonates are strongly suggestive of selenium depletion. Increased plasma values are found in suspected selenium toxicity, and results greater than 5 µmol/L (400 µg/L) indicate excessive intake.

In cases of toxicity (selenosis), serum concentrations were as high as 1400 µg/L with no obvious effects, and acute fatal poisonings were seen with selenium at up to 30,000 µg/L. However, the nature of the selenium compound is important, as most reports that describe acute selenium poisoning involve ingestion of inorganic compounds such as selenious acid, which is found in gun-bluing agents, and fatalities that occur within the first day are associated with postmortem blood selenium concentrations greater than 1400 µg/L.

Red cell GSHPx-1 activity in adults ranges from 13 to 25 U/g Hb, whereas values in children are slightly lower. Local age-related reference intervals are again required.

Zinc

The discovery of a variety of zinc-related clinical disorders has directly demonstrated the importance of zinc in human nutrition. It is second to iron as the most abundant trace element in the body.

Chemistry

Zinc (atomic number 30, relative atomic mass 65.39) is a particularly stable ion. Zinc is a good electron acceptor (strong Lewis acid) that has no redox reactions. It has been hypothesized that zinc ions, present in the cytoplasm at 10^{-11} mol/L and in equilibrium with numerous zinc metalloenzymes and transcription factors, act as a "master hormone," particularly in relation to cell division and growth.

Dietary Sources

Zinc is widely distributed in food, mainly bound to proteins. The bioavailability of dietary zinc is dependent upon digestion of these proteins to release zinc and allow it to bind to (1) peptides, (2) amino acids, (3) phosphate, and (4) other ligands within the intestinal tract. The most available dietary sources of zinc are red meat and fish. Wheat germ and whole bran are good sources, but their zinc content is reduced by milling and food processing. The median intake for men in the United States is about 14 mg/d and for women 9 mg/d.

Absorption, Transport, Metabolism, and Excretion

The net intestinal uptake of zinc is regulated by control of absorption efficiency and varies from 20% to 50% of the dietary content. At an intake of 12.2 mg Zn per day, the fractional absorption is 26%, but at the very low intake of 0.23 mg Zn per day, this has been shown to increase to 100%. Interaction with other dietary constituents, such as (1) phytate, (2) fiber, (3) calcium, and (4) iron, reduces the net absorption of zinc.

Iron at supplemental dosages (up to 65 mg/d) may decrease zinc absorption, so that pregnant and lactating women taking iron may require zinc supplementation.

New insights into mammalian zinc metabolism have been acquired through the identification and characterization of zinc transporters. All of these proteins have transmembrane domains and are encoded by two solute-linked carrier (SLC) gene families: *ZnT (SLC30)* and *Zip (SLC39)*. At least 9 ZnT and 15 Zip transporters are present in human cells. They appear to have opposite roles in cellular zinc homeostasis. ZnT transporters reduce intracellular zinc availability by promoting zinc efflux from cells or into intracellular vesicles; Zip transporters increase intracellular zinc availability by promoting extracellular zinc uptake and, perhaps, vesicular zinc release into the cytoplasm.

Both ZnT and Zip transporter families exhibit (1) unique tissue-specific expression, (2) differential responsiveness to dietary zinc deficiency and excess, and (3) differential responsiveness to physiological stimuli via hormones and cytokines.

Absorbed zinc is transported to the liver, where active incorporation into metalloenzymes and plasma proteins occurs. About 80% of plasma zinc is associated with albumin, and most of the rest is tightly bound in α_2-macroglobulin. Zinc is present on albumin in equilibrium with plasma amino acids (mostly histidine and cysteine), and this small (<1%) ultrafilterable fraction may be important in cellular uptake mechanisms (Figure 27-22).

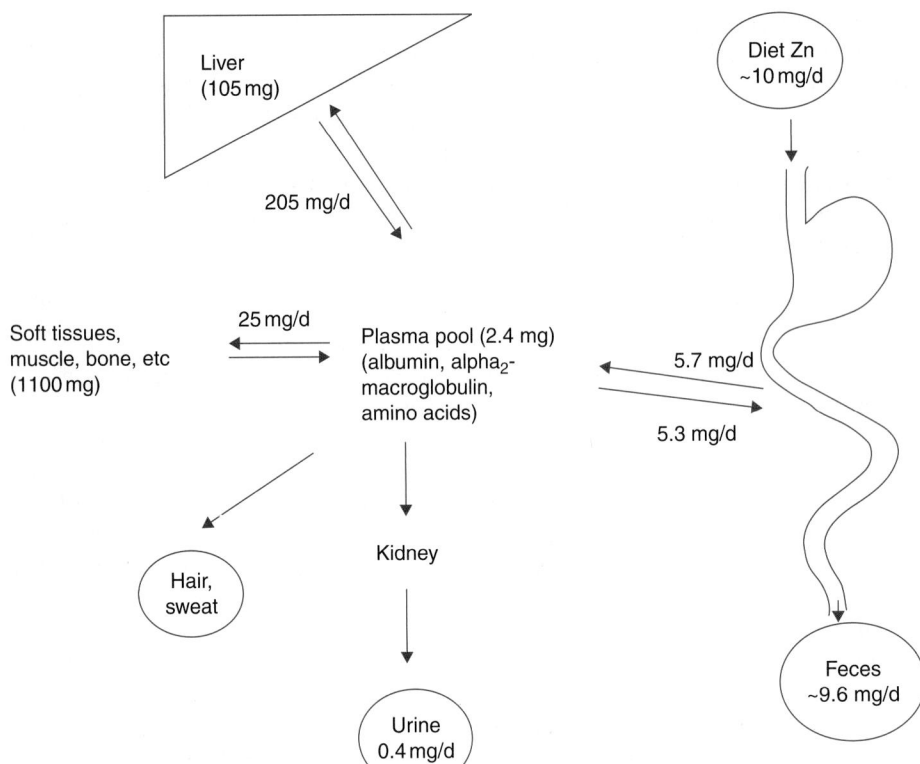

Figure 27-22 Summary of zinc metabolism.

Total adult body content of zinc is about 2 to 2.5 g, and the metal is present in the cells of all metabolically active tissues and organs. About 55% of the total is found in muscle, and approximately 30% in bone. Red cell zinc concentration is about 10 times higher than in plasma because of the large amounts of carbonic anhydrase.

Zinc binding to the metal-regulatory transcription factor 1 (MTF1) activates metallothionein (Mt) expression. This multifunctional, protein (9000 to 10,000 Da) has a high content of cysteine and reversibly binds zinc. Mt is important in intracellular zinc trafficking and helps to maintain intracellular zinc concentrations. Hepatic synthesis of Mt is induced by interleukin-1, interleukin-6, and glucocorticoids in response to (1) infection, (2) trauma, and (3) other stressors.

Fecal excretion includes both unabsorbed dietary zinc and zinc resecreted into the gut. Urine output of zinc is normally only about 0.5 mg/d but increases greatly during catabolic illness and ketosis. Release of intracellular contents from skeletal muscle has been established as the source of excess urinary zinc.

Functions

More than 300 zinc metalloenzymes are present in all six categories of enzyme systems. Important examples in human tissue include (1) carbonic anhydrase, (2) alkaline phosphatase, (3) RNA and DNA polymerases, (4) thymidine kinase carboxypeptidases, and (5) alcohol dehydrogenase. The key role of zinc in protein and nucleic acid synthesis explains the failure of growth and impaired wound healing observed in individuals with zinc deficiency.

Proteins form domains that are able to bind tetrahedral zinc atoms by coordination with histidine and cysteine to form folded structures known as "**zinc fingers**." These have important roles in gene expression by acting as DNA-binding transcription factors and play a key role in developmental biology and in the regulation of (1) steroid, (2) thyroid, and (3) other hormone synthesis.

Prostate Function. Secretion by the prostate of large amounts of zinc (resultant concentration, 1 to 2 mmol/L) is key to the function of sperm, maintaining both vitality and an antibacterial environment. The mechanism of this aspect of zinc function is regulation of motility through interaction of Zn^{2+} ions with semenogelin (Sg1) during semen coagulum formation at ejaculation, as well as during liquefaction of the coagulum in the female reproductive tract. Studies have implicated seminal Zn with parameters of semen quality, in that decreased seminal Zn is considered a risk factor for sperm abnormality and idiopathic male infertility, and smokers in particular are susceptible to Zn deficiency in their seminal fluid. Poor Zn nutrition may therefore be a risk factor for low quality of sperm and idiopathic male infertility. Routine determination of Zn concentrations during infertility investigation is recommended.

Seminal plasma zinc concentrations are normal in chronic prostatitis and adenoma, whereas with prostatic neoplasm, a highly significant decrease (100-fold) in zinc secretion has been noted. Prostate cancer cells do not secrete zinc because they have a reduced capacity for accumulation of intracellular zinc caused by the decrease in ZIP1 protein expression and the intracellular redistribution of intracellular transporter ZIP3.

These neoplastic cells are extremely sensitive to the Zn^{2+} ion; direct tumor injection causes marked cell death and therefore may represent a possible chemoprevention therapy.

Requirements and Reference Nutrient Intakes[6]

In the United States, the dietary reference intake (DRI) for zinc is 11 mg/d for men and 8 mg/d for women. Infants and young children need smaller amounts. Strict vegetarians may need as much as 50% more zinc per day because of the increased phytic acid and fiber in their diet.

Clinical Deficiency

As might be expected from the multiple biochemical functions of zinc, the clinical presentation of deficiency disease is (1) varied, (2) nonspecific, and (3) related to the degree and duration of depletion. Signs and symptoms include (1) depressed growth with stunting; (2) increased incidence of infection, possibly related to alterations in immune function; (3) diarrhea; (4) skin lesions; and (5) alopecia.

Effects on Growth. Dietary zinc deficiency is prevalent in countries worldwide where a cereal-based diet high in phytate and fiber, but low in animal protein, is common. In children, reduced growth and other developmental abnormalities are reversible by zinc supplementation. Zinc in human breast milk is efficiently absorbed because of the presence of factors such as picolinate and citrate.

Acrodermatitis Enteropathica. Acrodermatitis enteropathica (AE) is characterized by (1) periorificial and acral dermatitis, (2) alopecia, and (3) diarrhea; symptoms are reversed by oral zinc supplementation. This formerly fatal condition is an autosomal recessive inborn error that affects zinc absorption from the intestinal mucosa via mutation of the *SLC39a4* gene on chromosome 8 q24.3, which encodes a transporter for zinc uptake.

Parenteral Nutrition. Some patients who require intravenous feeding after surgery are likely to be significantly zinc depleted because of poor oral intake before and after surgery. They may have increased zinc losses from the intestinal tract via diarrhea and in the urine from catabolism of muscle during periods of negative nitrogen balance. Other problems include (1) diarrhea, (2) mental depression, (3) dermatitis, (4) delayed wound healing, and (5) alopecia that may be seen during the anabolic period of weight regain, when zinc in the nutritional regimen is insufficient to support tissue repair. Provision of adequate zinc intravenously to achieve a positive zinc balance is associated with improvement in nitrogen balance.

Infectious Disease. Zinc depletion impairs immunity and has a direct effect on the gastrointestinal tract, which increases the severity of enteric infections. A review of controlled trials of zinc supplementation for children in low-income countries found significant clinical benefit in cases of persistent diarrhea and respiratory disease. Interaction with vitamin A is important because in populations at risk of zinc and vitamin A deficiency, provision of zinc alone increases the incidence of respiratory infection, but when vitamin A is added, respiratory infections are decreased.

Subclinical Effects of Deficiency

When zinc deficiency is not severe enough to cause clinical signs and symptoms, it may still have a subclinical effect on (1) immune function, (2) synthesis and action of hormones, and (3) neurological function.

Immune Function. Patients in the Middle East with zinc deficiency were known to die before the age of 25 because of various infections and parasitic diseases. With zinc deficiency, a reduction is seen in the activity of serum thymulin, the thymus-specific hormone that is involved in T-cell function, and an imbalance develops between Th1 and Th2 helper cells. The lytic activity of natural killer cells also decreases. These complex changes result in impairment of cell-mediated immunity.

Hormones. Zinc has a role in the synthesis and actions of many hormones via zinc transcription factors. Zinc depletion is associated with low circulating concentrations of (1) testosterone, (2) free T_4, (3) insulin-like growth factor (IGF)-1, and (4) thymulin. Both plasma IGF-1 and growth velocity are increased in zinc-supplemented children.

Neurological Effects. Severe zinc deficiency is known to affect mental well-being; varying degrees of confusion and depression are consistent with the important activity of zinc enzymes in brain development and function.

Zinc has been shown to be a neurosecretory product or cofactor and is highly concentrated in the synaptic vesicles of a specific contingent of neurons, called zinc-containing neurons. Zinc in the vesicles probably exceeds 1 mmol/L in concentration and is only weakly coordinated with any endogenous ligand. Zinc-containing neurons are found almost exclusively in the forebrain, where in mammals they have evolved into a complex and elaborate associational network that interconnects most of the cerebral cortices and limbic structures. Alterations in zinc homeostasis may be associated with brain dysfunction, including brain inflammatory status. Zinc ion dyshomeostasis may play a role in the aging neuron through deterioration of synapses.

Toxicity

Clinical effects of ingestion of a zinc-contaminated diet include (1) abdominal pain, (2) diarrhea, (3) nausea, and (4) vomiting. More than 60 mg Zn per day has been known to result in copper depletion by causing blockade of intestinal absorption.

Laboratory Assessment of Status

Although plasma zinc determination is insensitive to dietary zinc intake and subject to a variety of influences, it remains the most widely used laboratory test to confirm severe deficiency. It is also used to monitor adequacy of zinc provision, especially when interpreted together with changes in serum albumin and the SIRS. No laboratory procedures have been established to clearly identify populations with marginal zinc depletion. Clinical and biochemical responses to zinc supplementation are therefore used to postulate a marginally zinc-depleted state.

Plasma Zinc. Plasma samples are preferred to serum samples for zinc analysis because of possible zinc contamination from (1) erythrocytes, (2) platelets, and (3) leukocytes during clotting and centrifugation. Plasma zinc concentrations are most commonly measured by CFAAS.

Care has to be taken in controlling preanalytical factors that will lower plasma zinc independently of dietary intake. These include collection of sample in relation to (1) meals, (2) time of day, and (3) use of steroid-based medications, such as the contraceptive pill. Any cause of hypoalbuminemia will lower plasma zinc. Plasma albumin is a negative acute-phase protein that is redistributed into interstitial spaces from the plasma pool (1) during infection, (2) after trauma, and (3) in chronic disease. Induction of hepatic Mt synthesis during the SIRS and subsequent sequestering of zinc further lower the plasma concentration. It is therefore essential to consider plasma zinc results along with plasma albumin and plasma CRP or another marker of the SIRS.

Blood Cell Zinc. It has been suggested that the zinc content of white cells and platelets better reflects tissue zinc. The zinc content of (1) neutrophils, (2) lymphocytes, and (3) platelets has been shown to decline more rapidly than plasma zinc in experimental studies of zinc depletion in humans. However, the relatively large volume of blood required and problems with contamination make application to patients in the hospital or to population surveys difficult.

Zinc in Hair. Low hair zinc has been associated with poor growth in children. However, variables such as hair growth rate and external contamination from hair dyes and cosmetics have caused inconsistent results.

Zinc-Dependent Enzymes. Despite the large number of zinc metalloenzymes that have been identified, no single enzyme assay has yet found acceptance as an indicator of zinc status.

Urine Zinc. A slight fall in the urinary excretion of zinc has been noted during dietary deficiency. Difficulties of sample contamination during collection limit the practical value of this information.

Zinc Speciation

Relatively few studies have explored the actual chemical species present in physiological fluids. However, studies on wound fluids regarded as an important site of zinc wound healing have revealed complex interactions. Most Zn ions were present as charged species, and the major species was a citrate complex.

Reference Intervals

Serum zinc concentrations are generally 5% to 15% higher than those of plasma because of osmotic fluid shifts from the blood cells when anticoagulants are used. Concentrations are decreased after food and are higher in the morning than in the evening. A guidance reference interval is 80 to 120 µg/dL (12 to 18 µmol/L).

Other Possibly Essential Elements

More than 15 additional trace elements are considered to have a potentially important role in human medicine.

Other trace metals to consider include (1) lead, (2) cadmium, (3) arsenic, (4) aluminum, and (5) nickel, primarily as toxic elements (see Chapter 32). Others, such as (6) lithium and (7) fluoride, are classified as pharmacologically beneficial,

and monitoring of dosage may be required. Some elements are considered "nutritionally beneficial" and are reported to produce "restorative health effects" at lower dosages. Evidence is derived mainly from animal studies, when dietary depletion of the element is combined with other metabolic, hormonal, or physiological "stressors."

For (8) boron, (9) silicon, and (10) vanadium, measurable responses in humans have been observed during variations in the dietary intake of these elements. These and other elements have been promoted by the supplement industry, and the clinical chemist may be asked for advice and possibly for monitoring of dosage in cases of suspected toxicity. AAS, ICP-OES, and ICP-MS methods have been used to measure most of these elements in biological samples.

Contamination of TPN solutions by small quantities of metals, such as Al, Pb, Cd, and Ni, could be a problem, as could the lack of others, such as Si, B, and V, when very long-term nutritional support is required.

Boron

Boron (B) has not been officially designated as essential to human health, although it is considered an essential macronutrient for plants.

Function

Boron normally present in living organisms as the borate ion (BO_3^{3-}) does have essential properties in plants that affect cell wall integrity. However, it still is not known to have any specific physiological function in humans, although various studies have suggested that it may be a beneficial bioactive element.

Dietary Sources

It is thought that the acceptable safe range of boron intake is from 1 to 13 mg/d, and evidence suggests that some people are consuming less than 1 mg/d. Plant foods, especially (1) fruits, (2) leafy vegetables, (3) nuts, and (4) legumes, are good sources, whereas meat, fish, and dairy products are not. Average daily intakes of dietary boron in the United Kingdom are variable (2.8 ± 1.5 mg), and intakes are higher than in the United States (1.5 ± 0.4 mg).

Absorption, Transport, Metabolism, and Excretion

Dietary boron is efficiently absorbed as boric acid—B(OH)$_3$— and is efficiently excreted into urine, with about 85% to 100% of an oral dose of borate appearing in urine over a 5- to 7-day period. The oral toxicity of boron is relatively low; it has been estimated that safe population mean intakes are <13 mg/d, and that individuals are at risk of toxicity when intakes continually exceed 100 mg/d for up to 6 days. The richest food sources of boron are nuts and dried fruits (15 to 30 mg/kg) and wine (8.5 mg/L). The use of boric acid food additives is now prohibited, except for caviar, at 4000 mg/kg.

Laboratory Assessment of Status

Problems with contamination and loss of volatile boron compounds during sample preparation have limited the reliable documentation of boron concentrations in human tissue and body fluids. A complex technique involving a porous graphite column—inductively coupled plasma–atomic emission spectrophotometry (ICP-AES)—and an ICP time-of-flight mass spectrometer (TOF-MS) has been developed for investigation of boron neutron capture in cancer therapy.

Normal concentrations in plasma of less than 30 μg/L were established by ICP-AES—the recommended procedure for assay because of the low atomic mass (10) of boron. Excretion in urine is normally less than 1 mg/d and up to 5 mg/L with boron intake of 0.33 to 3.33 mg/d.

Silicon

Silicon (Si) is a nonmetallic element that has an atomic weight of 28; it is a member of group IV C, Si, Ge, etc. Similar to elements in this group, it forms tetrahedral types of complexes and a multitude of polymer types. Silica is the term used to refer to the naturally occurring materials composed principally of silicon dioxide. The term *silicone* refers to any of a large group of siloxane polymers that do not occur naturally and are based on the structure of alternating oxygen and silicon (…-Si-O-Si-O-Si-O-…), with organic side groups attached to the four-coordinate silicon atoms. In some cases, organic side groups are used to link two or more of these -Si-O- backbones. Through variations in -Si-O- chain lengths, side groups, and cross-linking, silicones with a wide variety of properties and compositions have been synthesized. These compounds have a variety of uses from parchment coatings to sealant and breast implants.

Dietary Sources

Soluble silica (orthosilicic acid) is ubiquitous in the diet (20 to 50 mg Si/d) and in natural waters (0.8 to 44 mg Si/L), and, unlike crystalline silica (quartz), has no associated toxicity. Silicon is widely distributed in plants and is an essential element for structural integrity. Amorphous silica is incorporated as an anticaking agent at concentrations up to 2% in a variety of foods. Beer can also be rich in silicon with content up to 20 mg/L. No values have been suggested for the recommended intake of silicon.

Absorption, Transport, Metabolism, and Excretion

Absorption of silicon seems to be dependent on its polymeric nature; the smaller the molecule (i.e., monomeric orthosilicic acid), the more effective is absorption, whereas the larger polymer forms are poorly absorbed. The efficiency of absorption is up to 60% of an ingested load, with most excreted renally within 24 hours of exposure. As yet, little evidence suggests retention in any tissue-specific site.

Function and Clinical Significance

In veterinary and laboratory animals, silicon has been shown to be important in the synthesis of collagen and bone. The few supplementation studies in humans have reported associated increases in trabecular bone volume and bone mineral density.

Laboratory Assessment of Status

Healthy fasting plasma concentrations of silicon are less than 12 μmol/L. These concentrations are elevated in renal failure, particularly in patients on hemodialysis, to above 150 μmol/L and higher, depending on the content of dialysis water. Urine silicon excretion depends on intake and varies from 100 to 1000 μmol/24 h. Toxicity from silicon has never been reported, although increased concentrations (>3 mmol/L) have resulted in the formation of silica stones.

Vanadium

Vanadium, a group V trace element that belongs to the first transition series of elements, is ubiquitously distributed. It exists in four valency states—2, 3, 4, and 5; thus, its chemistry is complex. Vanadium is found in neutral solutions as meta-vanadate (V_3^-), the predominant species in body fluids, and enters cells through an anion transport system. Exogenously administered vanadyl sulfate and ammonium vanadate have been found to bind serum transferrin tightly, indicating that this protein may serve as a vanadium transporter. Although the vanadium requirement of some organisms has been established, its essential value in humans remains to be proved.

Although most foods contain low concentrations of vanadium (<1 ng/g), food is the major source of exposure to vanadium for the general population; however, absorption of vanadium salts from the gastrointestinal tract is poor. Excretion of vanadium by the kidneys is rapid, with its biological half-life of 20 to 40 hours. Estimated daily intake of the U.S. population ranges from 10 to 60 μg. Vanadyl sulfate is a supplement that is commonly used to enhance weight training in athletes at doses up to 60 mg/d. Most of the toxic effects of vanadium compounds result from local irritation of the eyes and upper respiratory tract, rather than from systemic toxicity.

Functional Aspects

Vanadium plays a limited role in biology. Nevertheless a vanadium-containing nitrogenase is used by some nitrogen-fixing microorganisms. Clinical interest in the vanadate compounds involves their potential role in the treatment of diabetes. Various studies have suggested that these compounds reduce the requirement for insulin by activating the cellular response without the presence of insulin, in effect mimicking its action.

Amounts given in such trials are much greater than suggested normal intake, indicating that vanadium compounds are more likely to work as alternative therapies, rather than revealing the essential function of the element. The possibility of using vanadium compounds is focused on cytotoxicity and cancer treatment.

Assessment of Laboratory Status

Plasma and urine concentrations are usually measured by GF-AAS or ICP-AES. Use of ICP-MS revealed a number of urinary vanadium compounds of 1 to 10 μg/L in healthy volunteers. Detection of the vanadate ion using size exclusion chromatography coupled with ICP-MS with a dynamic reaction cell yielded normal serum concentrations less than 0.05 μg/L. Studies on high-resolution ICP-MS also showed whole blood concentrations close to the detection limit of less than 0.05 μg/L, indicating that careful sampling techniques are required for confident use of analyzed concentrations.

Review Questions

Match the vitamin in column A with its correct function in column B.

A		B	
1.	Ascorbic acid E	a.	red blood cell protection
2.	Folic acid D	b.	antihemorrhagic activity
3.	Phylloquinone B	c.	coenzyme activity
4.	Tocopherol A	d.	nucleic acid synthesis
5.	Niacin C	e.	collagen synthesis

6. Thiamine:
   a. is considered a fat-soluble vitamin.
   b. deficiency is referred to as pellagra.
   c. functions in oxidative decarboxylation reactions.
   d. is also referred to as vitamin B_{12}.

7. A vitamer:
   a. is an essential organic micronutrient that must be supplied exogenously.
   b. is any of a number of compounds that possess a given vitamin activity.
   c. is a natural reactant, usually either a metal ion or a coenzyme, that is required in an enzyme-catalyzed reaction.
   d. is an inorganic molecule that is found in human and animal tissues in milligram per kilogram amounts.

Match the trace element in column A with its correct function listed in column B. Answers may be used once, more than once, or not at all.

A		B	
8.	Molybdenum C	a.	role in glucose tolerance
9.	Cobalt B	b.	structural component of vitamin B_{12}
10.	Zinc D	c.	cofactor in electron transfer reactions
11.	Chromium A	d.	normal growth and development
12.	Manganese D		

13. Ultratrace elements:
    a. are those elements found in ng/dL concentrations in body fluids and in μg/kg concentrations in tissue.
    b. include retinol, iron, and chromium, for example.
    c. are inorganic molecules found in human and animal tissues in mg/kg amounts or less.
    d. are organic micronutrients that must be supplied exogenously.

14. Fat-soluble vitamins include:
    a. B and C vitamins only.
    b. vitamin B_{12} and folic acid.
    c. vitamins D and E only.
    d. vitamins A, D, E, and K.

15. Selenium:
    a. is a constituent of glutathione peroxidase that is associated with vitamin E.
    b. excess will induce copper deficiency by blocking copper absorption.
    c. toxicity results in neurological symptoms resembling Parkinson disease.
    d. stabilizes the regenerating tooth surface by binding the tooth enamel.

References

Note: A detailed reference list to statements in this chapter is found in Reference 12 in the list below.

1. Ashton K, Hooper L, Harvey LJ, Hurst R, Casgrain A, Fairweather-Tait SJ. Methods of assessment of selenium status in humans: a systematic review. Am J Clin Nutr 2009;89:2025S–39S.
2. Bone RC, Balk RA, Cerra FB, Dellinger RP, Fein AM, Knaus WA, et al. Definitions for sepsis and organ failure and guidelines for the use of innovative therapies in sepsis. The ACCP/SCCM Consensus Conference Committee. American College of Chest Physicians/Society of Critical Care Medicine. 1992. Chest 1997; 112:235–43.
3. Food and Nutrition Board IOM. Dietary reference intakes for thiamin, riboflavin, niacin, vitamin B_6, folate, vitamin B_{12}, pantothenic acid, biotin, and choline. Washington, DC: National Academy Press, 1998.
4. Food and Nutrition Board IOM. Dietary reference intakes for calcium, phosphorus, magnesium, vitamin D, and fluoride. Washington, DC: National Academy Press, 1999.
5. Food and Nutrition Board IOM. Dietary reference intakes for vitamin C, vitamin E, selenium, and carotenoids. Washington, DC: National Academy Press, 2000.
6. Food and Nutrition Board IOM. Dietary reference intakes for energy, carbohydrate, fiber, fat, fatty acids, cholesterol, protein, and amino acids. Washington, DC: National Academy Press, 2002.
7. Food and Nutrition Board IOM. Dietary reference intakes for vitamin A, vitamin K, arsenic, boron, chromium, copper, iodine, iron, manganese, molybdenum, nickel, silicon, vanadium, and zinc. Washington, DC: National Academy Press, 2002.
8. Frausto Da Silva JJR, Williams RJP. The biological chemistry of the elements. In: The inorganic chemistry of life, 2nd edition. New York: Oxford University Press, 2001.
9. Harvey LJ, Ashton K, Hopper L, Casgrain A, Fairweather-Tait SJ. Methods of assessment of copper status in humans: a systematic review. Am J Clin Nutr 2009;89:2009S–24S.
10. Myllyharju J, Kivirikko KI: Collagens, modifying enzymes and their mutations in humans, flies and worms. Trends Genet 2004;20:33–43.
11. Sauberlich HE. Laboratory tests for the assessment of nutritional status, 2nd edition. Boca Raton, FL: CRC Press, 1999.
12. Shenkin A, Roberts NB. Vitamins and trace elements. In: Burtis CA, Ashwood ER, Bruns DE, editors. Tietz textbook of clinical chemistry and molecular diagnostics, 5th edition. St Louis, MO: Saunders, 2012:895–983.
13. Tappendam KA, editor. Micronutrients in parenteral nutrition: too little or too much? Gastroenterology 2009;139(Suppl 1):S1–S134.
14. Tonelli M, Wiebe N, Hemmelgarn B, Klarenbach S, Field C, Manns B, et al. Trace elements in hemodialysis patients: a systematic review and meta-analysis. BMC Med 2009;7:25–38.
15. Wiernsperger N, Rapin JR.Trace elements in glucometabolic disorders: an update. Diabetol Metab Syndr 2010;2:70.

Hemoglobin, Iron, and Bilirubin*

Trefor Higgins, F.C.A.C.B., John H. Eckfeldt, M.D., Ph.D., James C. Barton, M.D., and Basil T. Doumas, Ph.D.

Objectives

1. Define the following:

   Bilirubin
   Conjugated (direct)
      bilirubin
   Ferritin
   Hemochromatosis
   Hemoglobin
   Hemoglobinopathy
   Hemosiderin

   Hemosiderosis
   Jaundice
   Kernicterus
   Thalassemia
   Transferrin
   Unconjugated (indirect)
      bilirubin
   Urobilinogen

2. Describe the structure and physiological role of hemoglobin.
3. State the function of hemoglobin and its significance in health and disease.
4. List four different types of hemoglobin and state the makeup of the globin chains in each.
5. State the specific changes in the globin chain in deletional, insertion, deletion/insertion, and elongation hemoglobin variants.
6. List four different types of thalassemia and state the globin deficiency and genetic defect in each.
7. Compare the differences between hemoglobinopathy and thalassemia with regard to causes and laboratory values.
8. List five analytical methods used to assess the presence of a hemoglobinopathy or thalassemia.
9. Describe the principle of the cyanmethemoglobin method of hemoglobin determination.
10. Contrast ferritin with hemosiderin with regard to structure and solubility.
11. State how iron is transported in blood.
12. State how the regulation of body iron is achieved.

13. List three proteins that affect iron homeostasis and the effects of a deficiency of each of these.
14. State the two major disorders of iron metabolism.
15. List two causes of iron deficiency anemia in children and adults; list two causes of increased serum iron.
16. Compare the causes of primary, secondary, and juvenile hemochromatosis.
17. State the principle of chromogenic serum iron determination and the clinical significance of the results.
18. Define total iron-binding capacity (TIBC) and state how TIBC value is determined.
19. State and, given appropriate data, solve the formula used to calculate transferrin saturation (Tsat).
20. List three analytical methods used to assess serum ferritin and state the clinical significance of the results of these.
21. Compare the laboratory results of serum iron, TIBC and Tsat in the following conditions: ingestion of oral contraceptives, hepatitis, inflammation, iron deficiency, and hemochromatosis; describe how serum iron is affected by diurnal variation.
22. Describe the biochemistry of bilirubin including transport in blood, conjugation in the hepatocyte, and hydrolysis in the intestine.
23. List two inherited disorders of bilirubin metabolism and state the bilirubin alteration.
24. List and describe three causes of unconjugated hyperbilirubinemia in the neonate and two causes of conjugated hyperbilirubinemia in the neonate.
25. State the principle of the diazo method of total bilirubin analysis; state what is required in this reaction to measure direct bilirubin.

*The authors gratefully acknowledge the original contributions of Drs. Virgil F. Fairbanks and George G. Klee (hemoglobin and iron) and Drs. Keith G. Tolman and Robert Rej (bilirubin), on which portions of this chapter are based.

Key Words and Definitions

Biliary atresia A condition characterized by failure of a fetus to develop an adequate pathway for bile to drain from the liver to the intestine.

Bilirubin A yellow bile pigment that is a breakdown product of heme mainly formed from the degradation of erythrocyte hemoglobin in reticuloendothelial cells.

Carboxyhemoglobin A form of hemoglobin in which the sites usually bound to oxygen are bound to carbon monoxide.

Complete blood count (CBC) The determination of the quantity of each type of blood cell in a mL of blood, often including the amount of hemoglobin, the hematocrit, and the proportions of various white cells.

Conjugated bilirubin Bilirubin that has been taken up by the liver cells and conjugated to form the water-soluble bilirubin diglucuronide.

Crigler-Najjar syndrome An autosomal recessive form of nonhemolytic jaundice due to the absence of the hepatic enzyme glucuronosyltransferase.

Direct bilirubin The fraction of bilirubin that reacts with the diazo reagent in the absence of alcohol.

Dubin-Johnson syndrome An autosomal recessive disorder that causes an increase of conjugated bilirubin in the serum.

Ferritin The iron/apoferritin complex, which is one of the chief forms in which iron is stored in the body; it occurs in the (1) gastrointestinal mucosa, (2) liver, (3) spleen, (4) bone marrow, and (5) reticuloendothelial cells.

Gilbert syndrome An inborn error of bilirubin metabolism,

Heme Any quadridentate chelate of iron with the four pyrrole groups of a porphyrin, further distinguished as ferroheme or ferriheme, referring to the chelates of Fe(II) and Fe(III), respectively.

Hemin A porphyrin chelate of Fe^{3+} derived from red blood cells.

Hemochromatosis A rare genetic disorder caused by deposition of hemosiderin in the parenchymal cells, resulting in tissue damage and dysfunction of the liver, pancreas, heart, and pituitary. Also called *iron overload disease.*

Hemoglobin The oxygen-carrying pigment of the erythrocytes, formed by the developing erythrocyte in bone marrow. It is a conjugated protein containing four heme groups and globin, with the property of reversible oxygenation.

Hemoglobinopathy Any inherited disorder caused by abnormalities of hemoglobin, resulting in conditions such as sickle cell anemia, hemolytic anemia, or thalassemia.

Hemosiderin An intracellular storage form of iron; the granules consist of an ill-defined complex of ferric hydroxides, polysaccharides, and proteins having an iron content about 33% by weight.

Hemosiderosis A focal or general increase in tissue iron stores without associated tissue damage. Hepatic and pulmonary forms of hemosiderosis are characterized by abnormal quantities of hemosiderin in the liver and lungs, respectively.

Hereditary hemochromatosis A genetically heterogeneous group of inherited disorders of iron metabolism characterized by failure to prevent excessive amounts of iron from entering the circulatory pool and accumulating in the tissues.

Hereditary persistence of fetal hemoglobin A condition characterized by continued production of fetal hemoglobin beyond the point when it is normally replaced by hemoglobin A.

Hyperbilirubinemia Excessive concentrations of bilirubin in the blood, which may lead to jaundice; the hyperbilirubinemias are classified as conjugated or unconjugated, according to the predominant form of bilirubin in the blood.

Icterus A condition characterized by hyperbilirubinemia and deposition of bile pigments in the skin, mucous membranes, and sclera, with resulting yellow appearance of the patient; called also *jaundice.*

Indirect bilirubin Free bilirubin that has not been conjugated with glucuronic acid.

Jaundice A condition characterized by hyperbilirubinemia and deposition of bile pigment in the skin, mucous membranes, and sclera, with resulting yellow appearance of the patient; also called *icterus.*

Kernicterus A clinical syndrome of the neonate resulting from high concentrations of unconjugated bilirubin that passes the immature blood-brain barrier of the newborn and causes degeneration of cells of the basal ganglia and hippocampus.

Ligandin An hepatic transport protein; measurement of it in serum and urine may be a means of estimating the severity of hepatocellular necrosis.

Lucey-Driscoll syndrome A potentially fatal disorder characterized by severe hyperbilirubinemia present at birth, which accumulates in the brain.

Methemoglobin A form of hemoglobin where its iron atom is changed from the ferrous to the ferric state.

Myoglobin A heme-containing protein found in red skeletal muscle.

Rotor syndrome A type of chronic familial nonhemolytic jaundice that differs from Dubin-Johnson syndrome in the lack of liver pigmentation.

Sickle cell anemia An autosomal dominant type of hemolytic anemia that is caused by the presence of hemoglobin S with abnormal sickle-shaped erythrocytes *(sickle cells).*

Thalassemia A heterogeneous group of hereditary hemolytic anemias having a decreased rate of synthesis of one or more hemoglobin polypeptide chains and classified according to the chain involved (α, β, δ); the two major categories are α- and β-thalassemia.

Thalassemia major The homozygous form of β-thalassemia, a severe condition evident from the neonatal period with complete absence of hemoglobin A.

Thalassemia minor The heterozygous form of β-thalassemia; it is usually asymptomatic, although hemoglobin A synthesis may be retarded and there is sometimes moderate anemia and splenomegaly.

Transferrin A beta globulin that carries iron in the blood.

Unconjugated bilirubin Free bilirubin that has not been conjugated with glucuronic acid.

Urobilinogen A colorless compound formed in the intestines by the reduction of bilirubin.

Hemoglobin (Hb), iron, and **bilirubin** are analytes that collectively may be viewed in terms of a manufacturing process in which the raw material (iron) is incorporated with other raw materials in a multistage complex process leading to a finished product (Hb).[16] This finished product has a limited life span, after which degradation into the waste product (bilirubin) occurs. Within this process, many exquisite (1) biochemical control, (2) conservation, and (3) synthesis mechanisms are found. For example, this process may be disrupted by (1) a deficiency in the supply of raw material, (2) lack of control or synthesis mechanisms, (3) excessive loss of finished product, or (4) excessive conversion to or deficiency in the elimination of waste products. These disruptions are manifest in the clinical disorders of (1) **hemoglobinopathies**, (2) **thalassemias**, (3) iron deficiency anemias, (4) liver disease, and (5) various genetic diseases.

Hemoglobin

Hemoglobin is the oxygen-carrying pigment of the erythrocytes that is formed by the developing erythrocyte in bone marrow. It is a conjugated protein containing four **heme** groups and globin (Figure 28-1), having the property of reversible oxygenation.

Chemistry

Hemoglobin is a hemoprotein, globular in shape with a diameter of 6.4 nm and a molecular weight of approximately 64,500 Da. The heme portion is an iron-containing chelate with the globin portion consisting of two pairs of polypeptide globin chains, designated α and non-α. The four globin chains form a thick-walled globular shell surrounding a central cavity, in which the heme portion, attached by interaction of the histidine residues of the globin chains to the iron in heme, is suspended (see Figure 28-1). The heme iron is normally in the ferrous (2^+) oxidation state.

The two pairs of globin chains in normal hemoglobin (HbA) are called α and β. The α-chain contains 141 amino acid residues and the β-chain 146 amino acid residues. In fetal hemoglobin, HbF, the α-chain is the same as that found in HbA, but the non-α chain is the γ-chain that has the same number of amino acid residues and substantial structural homology to the β-chain. HbA₂ has the usual α-chain, but the non-α chain is the δ-chain. By convention, the α-chain is always written first in abbreviations of hemoglobin structure. For example, HbA is written as $\alpha_2\beta_2$, HbF as $\alpha_2\gamma_2$, and HbA₂ as $\alpha_2\delta_2$. In normal adults, HbA forms about 85% to 95% of the total hemoglobin, HbF is less than 1%, and HbA₂ is less than 3.5%. Changes in the amino acid residue sequence of the globin chains (a qualitative change) lead to hemoglobinopathies, whereas decreases in globin chain production (a quantitative change) lead to thalassemias.

Chemically Modified Hemoglobins

Hemoglobin may be modified by attachment of chemicals to form chemically modified hemoglobins. Some of these chemically modified hemoglobins compromise the structural stability and/or functionality of hemoglobin. Carbon monoxide, for example, preferentially replaces oxygen from heme to form **carboxyhemoglobin**, compromising the oxygen-carrying ability of hemoglobin; in extreme cases, death results from the deprivation of oxygen to the tissue. **Methemoglobin** is formed as the result of a change in oxidation state of the iron atom in heme from the normal ferrous oxidation state (2^+) to the ferric (3^+) state, resulting in notably decreased oxygen-carrying ability. The presence of nitrate in well water has been known to cause methemoglobinemia. Sulfhemoglobin, commonly resulting from exposure to certain drugs, is formed when one or more oxygen atoms in the porphyrin rings of heme is replaced by sulfur. Removal of the source of the chemical leads to restoration of normal hemoglobin.

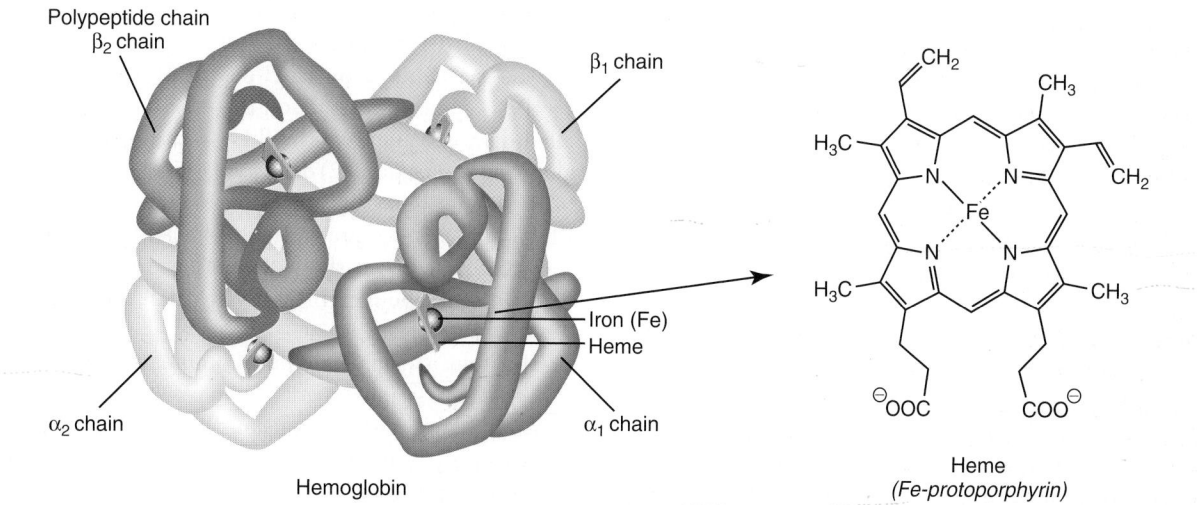

Figure 28-1 Model of the Hb tetramer with the α-chain subunits facing the reader. Each subunit contains a molecule of heme attached to an atom of iron.

Adduct hemoglobins are formed by the attachment of a molecule to the globin chains most commonly at the N-terminal amino acid, although it may occur anywhere along the globin chain. Carbamylated hemoglobin, seen in patients with end-stage renal disease, is formed by the attachment of urea, and glycated hemoglobin is formed by the attachment of glucose to the N terminus of the β-globin chain. The glycated hemoglobin adduct, HbA_{1c}, is important clinically in diagnosis and monitoring of glycemic control in patients with diabetes mellitus (see Chapter 33). Fetal hemoglobin (HbF, $α_2γ_2$) is unique in that it may form an acetylated adduct. Heme, ferrous protoporphyrin IX, consists of four pyrrole rings surrounding an iron atom, with four of the six electron pairs of iron attached to the nitrogen atoms in the pyrrole rings (see Chapter 29).

Hemin results from the relatively easy oxidation of the iron of heme from the ferrous to the ferric state. To remain electrically neutral, a halide molecule, usually chloride, becomes attached to hemin. In alkaline solution, hematin is formed by replacement of the halide atom of hemin by a hydroxyl group.

Biochemistry

Heme is biosynthesized primarily in the bone marrow and the liver (see Chapter 29).

It is an eight-step process, with each step involving a different genetically controlled enzyme. The first and last three steps take place in the mitochondria of the erythroblasts and reticulocytes of the bone marrow. The middle four stages take place in the cytosol.

In common with all genes, the globin genes consist of exons (coding sequences) and introns (intervening noncoding sequences) with codons (triplets of nucleotides) coding for specific amino acids. The globin genes have three exons and two introns, with a promoter region (specific for the globin chain) at the 5′ end of each gene. The transcription and translation processes are the same as in any other synthesis of amino acid chains.

Physiological Role

The iron in heme is normally in the ferrous state (2^+) and is able to act as the major oxygen-carrying entity by combining reversibly with oxygen. *Cooperativity* is the term used to describe the interaction of globin chains in such a way that oxygenation of one heme group enhances the probability of oxygenation of another or all heme groups. The *Bohr effect* refers to the reduction in oxygen affinity to heme with a decrease in pH. This effect is particularly important in exercising muscle, where the products of anaerobic metabolism, CO_2, and carbonic acid lower the pH to 6, and release of the oxygen attached to heme is facilitated.

Clinical Significance

Thalassemias and hemoglobinopathies form two distinct disease groups of genetic origin.[9] Thalassemias originate from insufficient globin chain production. The name is derived from the Greek word for sea, *thalasa,* because all early cases of β-thalassemia were described in children of Mediterranean origin. Hemoglobinopathies, collectively, are structural hemoglobin variants arising from mutations in the globin genes and resulting in disruptions in the normal amino acid sequence in one, or more, of the globin chains of hemoglobin. They are the most common single gene disorder in the world.

Thalassemias

Thalassemias are identified according to the globin chain in which there is a production deficiency. For example, α-thalassemias arise from defective α-globin chain production, β-thalassemias from deficient β-globin chain production, and δβ-thalassemia from deficiencies in production of both δ- and β-globin chains. Thalassemias are further classified by the extent of the reduction in globin chain production and resultant anemia. Four globin genes control the production of α-globin, and deletions or point mutations in any of these genes result in α-thalassemia. The severity of the anemia is a reflection of the number of gene deletions. The diagnosis of α-thalassemia is often one of exclusion, with the presence of thalassemic indices in the **complete blood count** (CBC) and the absence of an elevation in the HbA_2 forming the basis for presumptive diagnosis of α-thalassemia. Confirmation by DNA testing is required for definitive diagnosis.

A single gene deletion written as (αα/α-), sometimes called *silent α-thalassemia,* is usually clinically silent and has no significant hematological feature other than occasionally marginally decreased mean corpuscular volume (MCV).

The two gene deletions, sometimes called *α-thalassemia trait* or *α-thalassemia minor* (written as αα/- or α-/α-), have significant clinical and hematological features. Indices that are all decreased include (1) MCV, (2) mean corpuscular hemoglobin (MCH), and (3) Mentzer index (MCV/red blood count). The peripheral blood smear shows a microcytic, hypochromic anemia. No abnormal peaks are noted on high-performance liquid chromatography (HPLC) or capillary electrophoresis, and no unusual bands on conventional electrophoresis. The deletion is said to be a *cis* deletion when the two deletions are found on the same gene locus (αα/-), and a *trans* deletion when they are on opposite gene loci (α-/α-).

A three α-gene deletion (-/αα-) results in HbH disease. However, a nondeletion HbH disease is seen, which is more severe in clinical presentation than the more typical deletion HbH disease. Patients with HbH disease have (1) low hemoglobin concentration, (2) decreased MCV, (3) decreased MCH, (4) a slightly raised red blood cell count, and (5) increased RDW. Iron studies are normal. The HPLC chromatogram, shown in Figure 28-2, shows the presence of sharp bands close to the injection point. HbH is noted as a distinct peak on capillary electrophoresis.

The four α-gene deletion, commonly called *Hb Bart's hydrops fetalis,* is incompatible with life without massive intrauterine and postnatal transfusion. Typically, mothers carrying a fetus with Hb Bart's present at about weeks 20 to 25 of gestation with manifestation of polyhydramnios. The hemoglobin concentration of the cord blood is greatly decreased for age, and hypoalbuminemia is present. HPLC analysis of cord blood, shown in Figure 28-2, shows a single sharp band at the

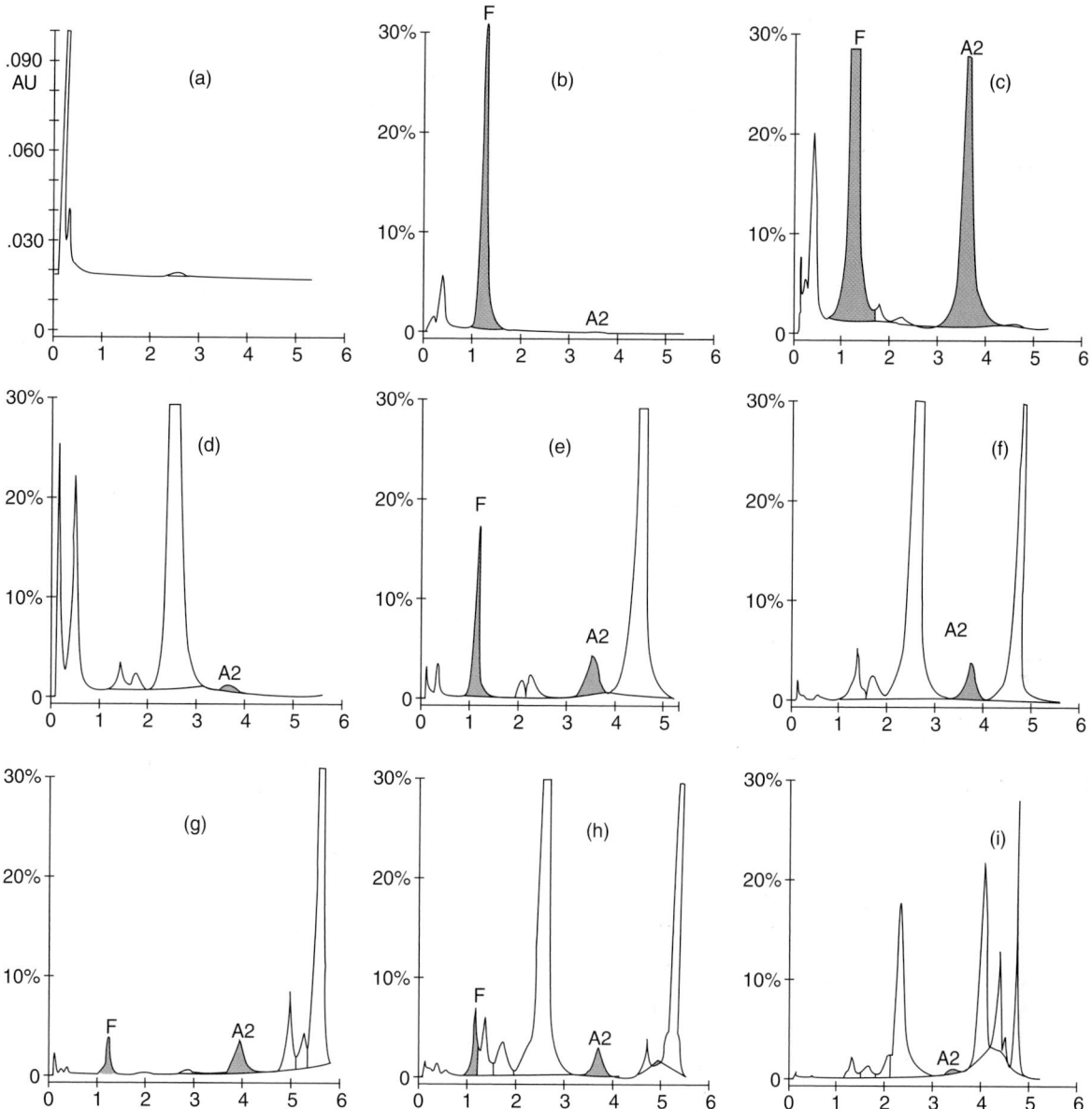

Figure 28-2 HPLC chromatograms obtained from a variety of variants. *a,* Hb Bart's; *b,* β⁰-thalassemia major; *c,* β⁰-thalassemia homozygous E; *d,* HbH; *e,* homozygous S; *f,* S trait; *g,* homozygous C; *h,* C trait; *i,* HbS-HbG Philadelphia. *(From Clarke GM, Trefor N, Higgins TN. Laboratory investigation of hemoglobinopathies and thalassemias: review and update. Clin Chem 2000;46:1284-90.)*

injection point of the chromatogram. Electrophoresis at alkaline pH shows a fast migrating band. In Figure 28-3, HPLC and electrophoresis patterns at alkaline pH of cord blood from a normal 26-week-old fetus and a fetus of similar gestational age with Hb Bart's are shown. The HPLC of the Hb Bart's fetus shows the characteristic single peak at the point of injection, whereas the HPLC from the normal fetus shows HbF (both acetylated and normal) with some HbA. Screening, with appropriate follow-up counseling, is provided for all prospective parents in some parts of the world, where two *cis* α-gene deletions are common.

Beta (β)-thalassemias result from a decrease in synthesis of β-globin chain. These are common in areas surrounding

(1) the Mediterranean, (2) the southern provinces of China, and (3) the Indian subcontinent. Screening programs are in place[2] in several of these locations.

β-Thalassemia is further classified as (1) **thalassemia major**, (2) Thalassemia intermediate, or (3) **thalassemia minor**. δβ-Thalassemia is also a thalassemic condition.

β⁰-Thalassemia (β-Thalassemia Major)

Sometimes called *Cooley's anemia*, β-thalassemia major is evident when individuals (1) have frequent infections, (2) appear pale, (3) are malnourished, and (4) exhibit splenomegaly with facial bone changes. These manifestations primarily reflect the degree of bone expansion associated with ineffective

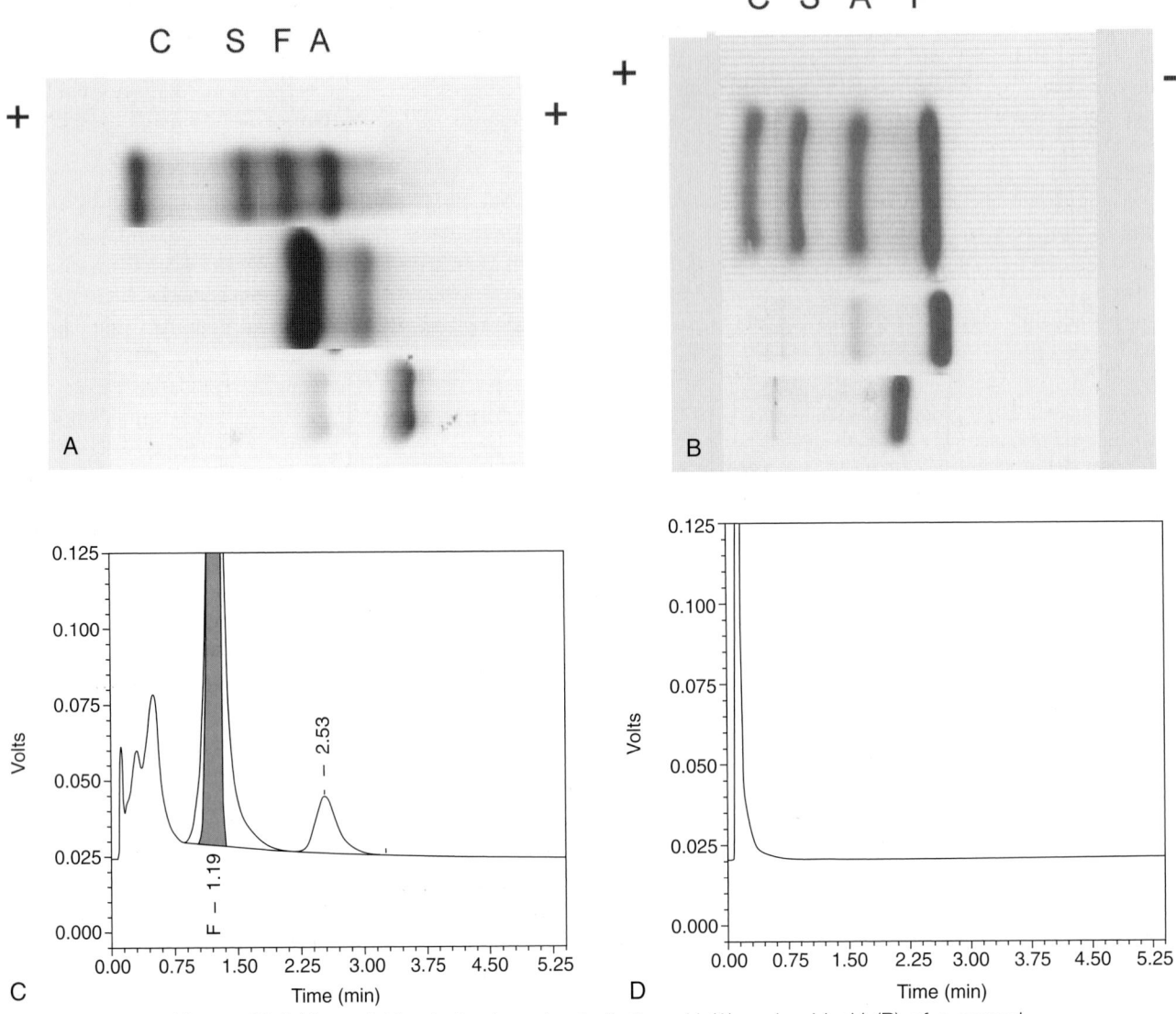

Figure 28-3 Hemoglobin electrophoresis at alkaline pH (A) and acid pH (B) of a normal 26 weeks' gestational age fetus *(lane 2)* and an Hb Bart's fetus of similar gestational age *(lane 3)*. HPLC chromatograms of the same normal fetus (C) and Hb Bart's fetus (D).

erythropoiesis. β^0-Thalassemia results from mutations that interfere with translation or are involved in (1) initiation, (2) elongation, or (3) termination of β-globin chain synthesis.

Clinical presentation usually occurs before 1 year of age with features that include (1) small size for age, (2) abdominal girth expansion, and (3) failure to thrive. Physical examination of the patient may reveal (1) frontal bossing (a rounded eminence on the forehead) caused by thickening of the cranial bones, (2) pallor, and (3) prominence of the cheek bones. In older children, this obscures the base of the nose and exposes the teeth.

Typical CBC results include severe anemia, with the hemoglobin concentration between 30 and 65 g/L, MCV 48 to 72 fL, and mean corpuscular hemoglobin concentration (MCHC) of 230 to 320 g/L. On the peripheral blood smear, a characteristic abnormal red blood cell (RBC) morphology is noted that includes (1) a large number of microcytes,

(2) numerous target cells, which may have a bridge joining the central and peripheral pigment zones, (3) polychromasia, (4) occasional spherocytes, (5) schistocytes, and (6) nucleated red cells. The **ferritin** is within its reference interval. A family study[1] should always be performed on a family with a child with β-thalassemia major. Hemoglobinopathy investigation of blood from children with β-thalassemia major shows a large HbF peak with no HbA peak and a small or absent HbA$_2$ peak (for an HPLC chromatogram, see Figure 28-2). Sometimes a small sharp band at the point of injection is seen that has been called *pseudo Hb Bart's* but is, in fact, bilirubin. Co-inheritance of β^0-thalassemia with a β-chain hemoglobin variant, for example, HbE/β^0-thalassemia, produces a severe anemia.

Lifelong transfusions together with chelation therapy are the primary therapies. Bone marrow transplantation has also been effective.

β⁺-Thalassemia (β-Thalassemia Intermedia)

β⁺-Thalassemia intermedia is attributed to a wide variety of genotypes, but all have in common a significant reduction in production of the β-globin chain, with subsequent reduction in the quantity of HbA present. A reduction in the severity of clinical features is seen with the co-inheritance of α-thalassemia. β⁺-Thalassemia is found in Mediterranean countries, especially in countries in the Eastern Mediterranean.

Clinical presentation varies from symptoms similar to β⁰-thalassemia through to those associated with β-thalassemia trait. Transfusions usually are not necessary, and hydroxyurea therapy is frequently used to increase the production of hemoglobin F and mitigate disease symptoms. The CBC shows decreased hemoglobin, with (1) anisocytosis, (2) hypochromia, (3) basophilic stippling, (4) target cells, and (5) nucleated RBCs observed on the peripheral blood smear.

Co-inheritance of β⁺-thalassemia with a β-chain haemoglobin variant, HbE/β⁺-thalassemia, for example, produces a severe anemia.

β-Thalassemia Minor

Patients with β-thalassemia minor, sometimes called β-*thalassemia trait,* are often asymptomatic, except at times of hematopoietic stress, such as infection or pregnancy, when they may require blood transfusions because of the development of anemia. The CBC on patients with β-thalassemia trait shows low normal or decreased hemoglobin and hematocrit, decreased MCV (<74 fL) and MCH (<27 pg), and a normal or mildly increased RBC distribution width (RDW). However, for patients with liver disease and β-thalassemia, MCV and MCH may be increased to the low end of the reference interval.

The peripheral blood smear shows microcytic RBCs with occasional (1) hypochromia, (2) poikilocytosis, and (3) target cells. The diagnosis of β-thalassemia minor may be made when the HbA_2 is greater than 4% if the patient is iron replete, with appropriate thalassemic indices such as (1) low MCV, (2) high RBC count, and (3) normal or acceptably close to normal RDW in the CBC. Individuals with iron deficiency (Hb <8.0 g/L) should become iron replete before a definitive diagnosis of β-thalassemia is made, as the HbA_2 may be falsely decreased (up to 0.5%) with iron depletion. HPLC is the preferred method for this quantification. In 30% to 40% of all cases of β-thalassemia minor, HbF will also be raised (>1.0%). In β-thalassemia minor, the life span of the RBC may be reduced, and patients with diabetes may show a lower HbA_{1c} compared with normal individuals with equivalent glycemic control. The β-thalassemia mutation may be identified by Southern blot electrophoresis using mutation-specific probes or a sequence-specific polymerase chain reaction (PCR).

δβ-Thalassemia

Deletion of both δ- and β-genes results in δβ-thalassemia, with both heterozygous and homozygous conditions described. The condition is found in a variety of ethnic groups but is most prevalent in countries of the Eastern Mediterranean, especially Greece and Italy. CBC analysis shows reduced hemoglobin (80 to 135 g/L) with low normal or marginally reduced MCV and MCH. HPLC analysis shows an HbA peak with reduced HbA_2 concentration and raised HbF concentration. However, in the Sardinian type of δβ-thalassemia, thalassemic indices are present on the CBC (low MCV and MCH, normal RDW) with a normal HbA_2 concentration and an HbF concentration between 15% and 20%.

Hereditary Persistence of Fetal Hemoglobin

The term **hereditary persistence of fetal hemoglobin** (HPFH) is used to describe a group of genetic conditions in which the concentration of HbF is increased above the reference interval with reduction of β-globin synthesis and a compensatory increase in γ-globin synthesis. Two major classes, of HPFH have been described—heterocellular and deletional. Several deletional variants of HPFH have been described that include (1) Greek, (2) Indian, (3) Italian, (4) Corfu, and (5) Black variants. In these deletional HPFH variants, the HbF concentration may be as high as 36%.

Nondeletional HPFH, sometimes called *heterocellular HPFH,* describes a group of disorders in which the increase in HbF is distributed heterogeneously among the red cells of otherwise hematologically normal individuals. The HbF concentration varies between 1% and 13% of the total hemoglobin in heterozygotes and from 19% to 21% in homozygotes.

Hemoglobinopathies

More than 950 hemoglobinopathies have been described (http://globin.cse.psu.edu/; accessed October 15, 2013); however, only a few have clinical significance. Identification of hemoglobin variants in areas with previously low incidence (Northern Europe, South America, and Canada) has increased in recent years because of immigration from areas of high incidence of hemoglobinopathies (Africa, Southeast Asia). Screening of neonates for hemoglobinopathies is common in the United States and in Northern European countries.

Nomenclature

Hemoglobin variants have been named by using (1) letters (S, C, D, E), (2) the family name of the index case (Hb Lepore), (3) the place of discovery of the variant, or (4) the hometown or river flowing through the town of the propositus (person immediately concerned about or affected by an action). In some cases, both a letter and a secondary name are used, for example, HbG Coushatta, indicating that the variant has electrophoretic mobility similar to other hemoglobin Gs, and that the variant was originally found in the Coushatta Indian tribe in the Southern United States. The term *AS trait* (sometimes abbreviated to *S trait*) is used to describe the heterozygous HbS state, with the term *SS* used to describe the homozygous HbS state. The homozygous HbS state is known as **sickle cell anemia** or sickle cell disease because of the sickle-shaped cells that appear in the blood of afflicted individuals.

A systematic nomenclature system is now used alongside the variant name to describe (1) the affected chain, (2) the chain location, and (3) the amino acid substitution. As an example, Hb Spanish Town ($\alpha 27[B8]^{Glu \rightarrow Val}$) is a hemoglobin variant named after a district in Kingston, Jamaica, and found

TABLE 28-1	Parameters That Constitute a Complete Blood Count (CBC)
Parameter	**Definition**
White blood cell count (WBC)	The number of white blood cells in the blood
WBC differential count (neutrophils, lymphocytes, basophils, eosinophils, and monocytes)	The number (or percentage) of each type of WBC present in the blood
Red blood cell count (RBC)	The number of red blood cells in the blood
Hematocrit (Hct)	The proportion of blood volume that is occupied by red blood cells
Hemoglobin (Hb)	The protein molecule in RBCs that carries oxygen
Mean cell volume (MCV)	The average volume of an RBC
Mean cell hemoglobin (MCH)	The average amount of hemoglobin in the average RBC
Mean cell hemoglobin concentration (MCHC)	The average concentration of hemoglobin in a given volume of blood
Red cell distribution width (RCDW)	A measurement of the variability of red blood cell size
Platelet count	Number of platelets in a volume of blood

in Jamaicans of African descent; it arises from a substitution of valine for glutamic acid in position 27 of the α-globin chain, which is located in position 8 of the B helix of the α-chain.

Classification of Hemoglobin Variants

Hemoglobin variants are classified according to type of mutation. Single-point mutations in a globin chain give rise to a substitution of one amino acid residue [e.g., Hb San Diego (β109[G11]$^{Val \rightarrow Met}$)]. Hemoglobin C Harlem is an example of a hemoglobin variant in which two amino acid residues are substituted, namely, valine replacing glutamic acid at position 6 and asparagine replacing aspartic acid at position 73 of the β-chain.

Types of hemoglobin variants include (1) deletional, (2) insertion, (3) deletion/insertion, (4) elongation, and (5) hybrid/fusion/crossover hemoglobins. *Deletional* hemoglobin variants arise from the deletion of one to five amino acid residues in the globin chain. *Insertion* hemoglobins are seen with insertion of one to three amino acid residues into the globin chain. *Deletion/insertion* hemoglobins are caused by the deletion of a portion of the normal amino acid residue sequence and the insertion of another sequence, with resultant lengthening or shortening of the globin chain. *Elongation* hemoglobins result from a single base pair mutation or frameshift at the 3′ end of exon 3 or at the 5′ end of exon 1 of the α_2- or β-globin chain. *Hybrid/fusion/crossover* hemoglobins result from the fusion of an α- or β-globin chain with a portion of another globin chain.

Analytical Methodology

Hemoglobin and related compounds are measured by several different types of methods. In addition, several technologies provide information leading to the diagnosis of thalassemias and hemoglobinopathies. Methods used for this purpose are divided into (1) those that provide a presumptive identification and (2) those that provide definitive identification. Examples of tests that provide presumptive identification include CBC, HPLC, and electrophoresis. DNA sequencing or mass spectroscopy provides definitive information. The preferred sample for investigation of hemoglobins and thalassemias is a fresh ethylenediaminetetraacetic acid (EDTA) anticoagulated blood sample. Storage for longer than 5 days at 4 °C may compromise sample integrity.

Measurement of Hemoglobin in Whole Blood

Measurement of hemoglobin concentration in venous or capillary blood is typically performed using the cyanmethemoglobin method. The principle of the method is based upon oxidation of the Fe^{2+} of hemoglobin to the Fe^{3+} of methemoglobin by ferricyanide, with methemoglobin then converted into stable cyanmethemoglobin by the addition of potassium cyanide (KCN):

$$HbFe^{2+} + Fe^{3+}(CN)_6^{3-} \rightarrow HbFe^{3+} + Fe^{2+}(CN)_6^{4-}$$

$$HbFe^{3+} + CN^- \rightarrow HbFe^{3+}CN$$

where $HbFe^{2+}$ represents a hemoglobin monomer, $HbFe^{3+}$ a methemoglobin monomer, and $HbFe^{3+}CN$ a monomer of cyanmethemoglobin. The absorbance of cyanmethemoglobin is measured at 540 nm and is used to calculate the concentration of hemoglobin.

Complete Blood Count

A complete blood count is a test (Table 28-1) that evaluates the cells that circulate in blood; it is also known as a full *blood count* (FBC), full *blood* exam (FBE), or *blood* panel. It consists of (1) counts of cells such as RBCs (erythrocytes), white blood cells (leukocytes), and platelets; (2) a measure of Hb; (3) estimates of the volume of red cells; and (4) an estimation of white blood cell subtypes (neutrophils, lymphocytes, basophils, eosinophils, and monocytes).

As a CBC provides the first indication of a thalassemia or hemoglobinopathy, it is essential to perform a CBC as a part of any investigation of hemoglobinopathies and thalassemias. In thalassemias, values for the MCV and MCH are below the reference interval. Hemoglobin may be below or within the reference interval. MCV is sometimes quite notably low, with the RBC count in the upper half of or elevated above the reference interval. The RDW is within the reference interval or is marginally above it. The blood smear should show a microcytic, hypochromic pattern. In hemoglobinopathies, the CBC is very often normal. On the peripheral blood smear, however, changes may be noted that are associated with a particular hemoglobin variant, such as the presence of sickle red cells in sickle cell disease (homozygous HbS) or target cells in homozygous HbE.

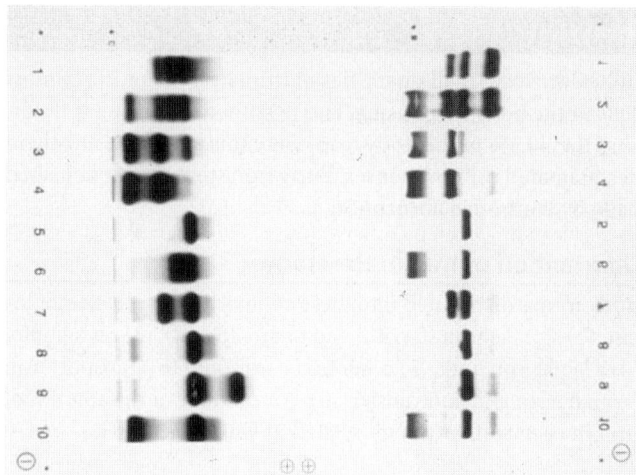

Figure 28-4 Alkaline and acid electrophoresis of various hemoglobinopathies. *Lane 1,* HbS, HbFA control. *Lane 2,* HbS, HbF, HbCA control. *Lane 3,* Transfused SC disease. *Lane 4,* SC disease. *Lane 5,* Hb A (normal). *Lane 6,* Hb Presbyterian. *Lane 7,* HbS. *Lane 8,* Raised HbA2 (β-thalassemia trait). *Lane 9,* HbJ Baltimore. *Lane 10,* HbC.

Several formulas derived from parameters in the CBC have been recommended to determine whether the patient has thalassemia. One study proposes that MCV less than 72 fL (reference interval ≈80 to 100 fL)[20] is suggestive of thalassemia, and that this single parameter is the best discriminator of thalassemia. The Mentzer index (MI) has been proposed as a screening parameter for β-thalassemia,[9] with values less than or equal to 14.69 indicative of thalassemia.

CBC parameters and associated calculations or the peripheral blood smear, however, is unable to provide a definitive diagnosis of thalassemia or hemoglobinopathies. It is also crucial to know the iron status of the patient, as iron deficiency may mimic or blunt the features of an underlying thalassemia. In practice, the measurement of ferritin is the most popular test for determining iron status but has limitations.

Electrophoresis

The most common initial test for hemoglobinopathy or thalassemia screening is electrophoresis using agarose gel and a pH 9.2 barbital buffer. Although this method is commonly used, it has several limitations. First, the HbA2 cannot be accurately quantified, and second, many hemoglobin variants comigrate, making identification difficult. After electrophoresis (Figure 28-4), the hemoglobins are visualized using Ponceau S (reddish staining) or preferably Amido Black (dark blue to black staining).

Variations of electrophoretic techniques that have been used in the identification of hemoglobin variants include isoelectric focusing and capillary isoelectric focusing electrophoresis (see Chapter 11).

HPLC

HPLC using a column packed with cation exchange resin provides in a single analysis quantification of HbA2 and HbF and initial identification of any hemoglobin variant present

(see Figure 28-2). Extensive lists of the retention times of hemoglobin variants on both commercial and laboratory developed methods have been published.[17,23] Advantages of HPLC over electrophoresis include (1) superior resolution of hemoglobin variants, (2) rapid assay time, and (3) accurate quantification of hemoglobin fractions, including HbA2 and HbF.

Capillary Electrophoresis

Capillary electrophoresis systems are now commercially available and used in clinical laboratories to assay for hemoglobin variants. Separation in an alkaline buffer using high voltages is based on (1) charge differences, (2) electrolyte pH, and (3) electro-osmotic flow. Extra manual manipulation is needed to correctly analyze a sample with a homozygous hemoglobin variant. However, several advantages of capillary electrophoresis over HPLC have been noted, including the quantification of HbA2 in the presence of HbE.

Electrospray Mass Spectroscopy

Electrospray mass spectroscopy has become the method of choice for the characterization of hemoglobin variants and hemoglobin adducts. This technique establishes very quickly (1) whether the variant is an α- or β-chain variant, (2) the location and identity of the amino acid residue substitution, and (3) the quantity of variants present. It requires, however, several preparative steps and a mass spectrometer.

DNA Analysis

The primary role of DNA analysis in the investigation of hemoglobinopathies and thalassemias is to identify, in populations with a known high incidence of disease, those specific individuals at risk who may benefit from genetic counseling. The uses of DNA analysis for this purpose are listed in Box 28-1.

Tests for Specific Hemoglobin Variants

HbS Solubility Test

Hemoglobin S, when deoxygenated, is insoluble in concentrated phosphate buffer and produces visible turbidity. Almost all other hemoglobins, including hemoglobins (1) A, (2) F, (3) C, (4) E, and (5) D, are soluble in such solutions. Thus, this test quickly identifies specimens of blood that contain HbS. A reducing substance, sodium hydrosulfite ($Na_2S_2O_4$, sodium dithionite), is used to deoxygenate the hemoglobin, and saponin is used to lyse the RBCs. Increased turbidity in a sample with HbS is noted by viewing a lined card (Figure 28-5) through the treated sample, with decreased clarity of the lined card indicating the presence of HbS. False-positive results are found in samples with (1) Heinz bodies, (2) high concentrations of monoclonal protein, or (3) cold agglutinins. False-negative results are obtained on anemic patients (hemoglobin <80 g/L) or on samples with hematocrit less than 15%. Other hemoglobin variants, including HbC Harlem, Hb Memphis, and HbC Ziguinchor, also yield positive results. Interpretation of the test is highly subjective.

HbH Test

HbH, beta 4 (β_4), is an insoluble tetramer found in patients with α-thalassemia. HbH punctate inclusions, usually described as looking like "golf balls," are found in the RBCs of a peripheral blood smear from a patient with α-thalassemia that has been treated with new methylene blue or brilliant cresyl blue at 37 °C. The method is laborious and is highly subjective. Many such inclusions are present in individuals with HbH disease, whereas cells containing inclusions are rare among individuals with thalassemia trait.

Tests for Unstable Hemoglobins

Treatment of the blood sample with heat at 55 °C to 60 °C or with isopropanol is used to detect the presence of unstable hemoglobins. For example, unstable hemoglobins precipitate under these conditions and are detected by an increase in turbidity or complete precipitation in the sample after treatment. Normal HbA takes about 40 minutes to precipitate, but unstable hemoglobins precipitate in 3 to 4 minutes.

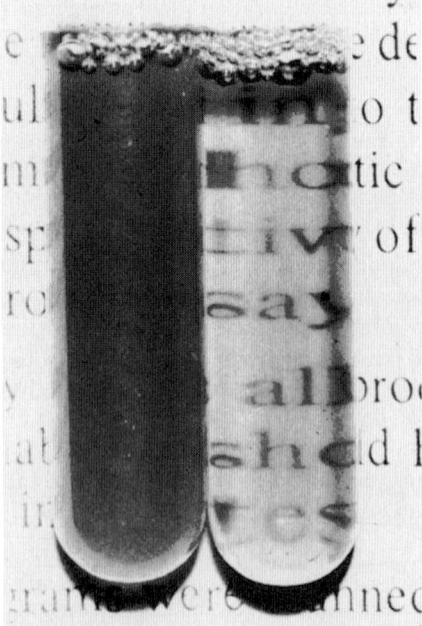

Figure 28-5 Solubility test for HbS. Deoxyhemoglobin S *(left tube)* is insoluble in 2.3 mol/L phosphate buffer. By contrast, normal hemolysate *(right tube)* is sufficiently transparent that print can easily be read through it.

Iron

In health, very small quantities of iron are present in (1) most cells of the body, (2) plasma, and (3) other extracellular fluids. Less than 0.1% of the body iron content is lost daily, mostly in desquamated cells or menses. Body iron stores are replenished daily by controlled absorption.

Distribution of Iron in the Body

Body iron is distributed into these compartments: (1) hemoglobin, (2) storage iron (ferritin and **hemosiderin**), (3) myoglobin, (4) a labile iron pool, (5) other tissue iron, and (6) transport iron (**transferrin** and apotransferrin). An estimate of the amount of iron in each compartment is listed in Table 28-2.

Hemoglobin

The erythrocyte volume in a 70-kg man is about 2 L. Each mL contains approximately 1 mg of iron which is equivalent to the body containing ≈2 g of hemoglobin iron.

Storage Iron

Iron is stored in the form of ferritin and hemosiderin.

Ferritin

Ferritin consists of a protein shell surrounding an iron core. Ferritin consists of an apoferritin shell composed of 24 subunits that are either L (light) or H (heavy) ferritin chains, and an interior ferric oxyhydroxide $(FeOOH)_x$ crystalline core (Figure 28-6).

Ferritin occurs in nearly all body cells and stores iron in a form that is shielded from body fluids and is therefore unable to cause oxidative damage. Ferritin in hepatocytes and macrophages provides a reserve of iron that is available for synthesis of hemoglobin and other heme proteins. In healthy men, ≈800 mg of storage iron is present, mostly as ferritin. In healthy women, storage iron ranges up to ≈200 mg. Minute quantities of ferritin are also present in serum in concentrations roughly proportional to total body iron stores. Relatively large amounts of ferritin, much of it without stored iron, may be released into plasma as the result of liver injury and diverse other pathological conditions.

Hemosiderin

Hemosiderin, a terminus of the intracellular storage iron pathway, is formed when ferritin is aggregated and partially

TABLE 28-2	Average Iron Content of Compartments in an Average 70-kg Male	
Compartment	**Iron Content, mg**	**Total Body Iron, %**
Hemoglobin iron	2000	67
Storage iron (ferritin, hemosiderin)	1000	27
Myoglobin iron	130	3.5
Labile pool	80	2.2
Other tissue iron	8	0.2
Transport iron	3	0.08

deproteinized in secondary lysosomes. Like ferritin, hemosiderin is usually found predominantly in cells of the (1) liver, (2) spleen, and (3) bone marrow. Unlike ferritin, hemosiderin is insoluble in aqueous solutions.

Tissue Iron

Numerous cellular enzymes and coenzymes require iron as an integral part of the molecule or as a cofactor. These include *peroxidases* and *cytochromes,* all of which are heme proteins, like hemoglobin. Other enzymes, such as *aconitase* and *ferredoxin,* contain iron that is coordinated with sulfur in a so-called iron-sulfur cluster. These enzymes and coenzymes occur in all nucleated cells of the body and form the *tissue iron compartment,* normally ≈8 mg of iron.

Myoglobin

Myoglobin very closely resembles a single hemoglobin subunit and contains a single heme per molecule.

The Labile Iron Pool

The labile pool contains ≈80 mg of iron. This compartment has no clear anatomical location and is a concept derived from kinetic measurements with radiolabeled iron.[18]

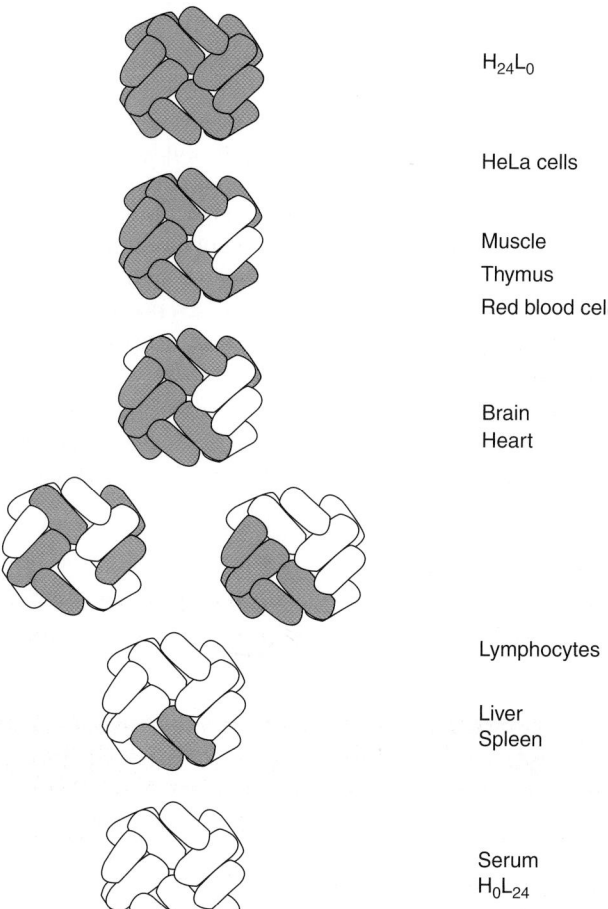

$H_{24}L_0$

HeLa cells

Muscle
Thymus
Red blood cells

Brain
Heart

Lymphocytes

Liver
Spleen

Serum
H_0L_{24}

Figure 28-6 Schematic representation of the subunit structure of ferritins from various tissues. *(From Harrison PM, Arosio P. The ferritins: molecular properties, iron storage function and cellular regulation. Biochim Biophys Acta 1996;1275:161-203.)*

Iron Transport

Iron is transported from one organ to another in the plasma by the transport protein *apotransferrin.* The apotransferrin/Fe^{3+} complex is called transferrin. Normally, ≈2.5 mg of iron is present in plasma. When transferrin binds to the *transferrin receptor* of cells, the transferrin/receptor complex is internalized into an endosome that becomes acidified, releasing the iron from transferrin and reducing it to ferrous iron (Fe^{2+}). This is transported into the cell via the divalent metal transporter, DMT1. The apotransferrin is then transported back to the cell surface, ready to transport another transferrin molecule to the interior of the cell. This series of reactions has been designated the *transferrin cycle.*

Regulation of Iron Homeostasis

Regulation of body iron content in healthy persons is achieved predominantly by controlling the amount of iron absorbed from the upper intestinal tract to that lost.[14] Hepcidin, a peptide hormone produced by the liver, is the central regulator of iron absorption. The amount of unavoidable iron loss in healthy persons depends only minimally upon the iron burden.

Normal Iron Balance

The average daily American diet contains 10 to 15 mg of iron, much of it in the form of (1) heme proteins, (2) hemoglobin, and (3) myoglobin in meat. Normally, ≈1 mg of iron is absorbed each day, mostly by the duodenum. To be absorbed, inorganic iron must be in the ferrous state (Fe^{2+}). Heme is absorbed directly through a specific receptor.[25]

Proteins That Affect Iron Homeostasis

Many proteins influence iron homeostasis. Mutations in genes that encode these proteins may cause iron overload or iron deficiency. Table 28-3 summarizes the effects of some of these proteins on iron homeostasis.

Clinical Significance

Iron deficiency and iron overload are the major disorders of iron metabolism. Abnormal distribution of iron or abnormal production of iron-related proteins may play a primary or secondary role in other heritable or acquired disorders. The latter include (1) *hereditary hyperferritinemia–cataract syndrome,* (2) *aceruloplasminemia,* (3) *GRACILE* (growth retardation, aminoaciduria, cholestasis, iron overload, lactic acidosis, and early death) syndrome, (4) *neuroferritinopathy,* (5) *pantothenate kinase–associated neurodegeneration* (formerly Hallervorden-Spatz disease), (6) *atransferrinemia,* and possibly (7) neurodegenerative disorders such as *Parkinsonism, Alzheimer disease,* and *amyotrophic lateral sclerosis* (Lou Gehrig's disease).

Iron Deficiency

Iron deficiency is a a common disorder of humans and especially affects (1) children, (2) young women, and (3) older persons, but it can occur in people of all ages and social strata. In children, iron deficiency is frequently caused by dietary deficiency because milk has low iron content, and iron

TABLE 28-3   Proteins That Affect Iron Homeostasis

Protein	Putative Function	Effect of Deficiency	Comments
HFE*	May transmit signal that upregulates hepcidin	Increased Fe	Most patients with hereditary hemochromatosis are homozygous for the 845 A→G (C282Y) mutation of this gene
Hemojuvelin	Helps regulate hepcidin	Increased Fe absorption	Mutations cause early age of onset of hemochromatosis
β₂-Microglobulin	Transports HFE to the cell membrane	Increased Fe absorption	Deficiency known to cause iron overload in mice only
Transferrin	Transports iron in the plasma	Increased Fe absorption	
Transferrin receptor-1	Binds and internalizes transferrin at the membrane	Lethal. Increased CNS Fe	
Transferrin receptor-2	May transmit signal that upregulates hepcidin	Increased Fe absorption	Mutations cause rare forms of severe hemochromatosis
Ferroportin (SLC40A1)	Transmembrane iron transport protein that acts as a receptor for hepcidin	Increased Fe absorption	Dominant inheritance of iron overload
Hephaestin	Oxidizes ferrous iron to ferric iron at the intestinal abluminal membrane	Fe deficiency	Encoded by a sex-linked gene. Deletion is cause of sla mouse
DMT1	Transports ferrous iron across membranes	Fe deficiency in rodents; iron overload in humans	The naturally occurring mutations found in the mk mouse and the Belgrade rat are the same
Ceruloplasmin		Fe increased in brain, liver	Brain accumulation and neurological disease
Hepcidin	Central regulator of iron absorption; produced in liver	Increased Fe absorption, hemochromatosis	Rare mutations cause hemochromatosis
Steap3		Fe deficiency	

HFE, Human hemochromatosis protein.

requirements for growth and development are high. In adults, iron deficiency is almost always the result of chronic blood loss or childbearing.[15]

Many different measurements have been advocated for the diagnosis of iron deficiency. Originally, emphasis was placed upon RBC indices. Today, measurements of (1) serum iron, (2) iron-binding capacity, (3) serum ferritin, (4) stainable iron in the bone marrow, and (5) erythrocyte protoporphyrin are used extensively to diagnose iron deficiency. Circulating transferrin receptor and reticulocyte hemoglobin measurements also have diagnostic utility. DNA analyses are necessary to confirm diagnoses in unusual cases. For example, iron-refractory iron deficiency is caused by mutations in the TMPRSS6 gene. Neuroferritinopathy caused by mutations in the ferritin light chain gene (FTL) mimics iron deficiency because affected persons typically have low serum ferritin levels.

Although most methods readily identify severe, uncomplicated iron deficiency, the large number of tests that have been advocated for the diagnosis of iron deficiency reflects the fact that none by itself is sufficient to detect mild iron deficiency or iron deficiency in a clinically complex setting. No one method is superior, and various studies differ in the conclusions that they draw regarding advantages of one method over another.[3]

Iron Overload

Hemochromatosis and types of anemia associated with ineffective erythropoiesis cause increased iron absorption and iron overload that affect the (1) liver, (2) heart, (3) pancreas, and (4) joints. The increased absorption is mediated by subnormal or inappropriately low action of hepcidin. Other heritable disorders such as (1) *aceruloplasminemia*, (2) *neuroferritinopathy*, or (3) *Friedreich's ataxia* cause harmful brain iron overload. **Hemosiderosis** and *siderosis* are terms best used to describe iron overload at the tissue level. Examples include relatively harmless iron deposits at sites of bleeding or inflammation and the life-threatening heart iron overload seen in some persons with hemochromatosis or severe β-thalassemia. Hyperferritinemia without iron overload is usually due to (1) common liver disorders, (2) inflammation, (3) neoplasms, and (4) hereditary hyperferritinemia–cataract syndrome. In general native Africans, African Americans, and Asians have higher mean levels of serum ferritin.

Hereditary Hemochromatosis

Hereditary hemochromatosis is a group of heritable disorders[24] that increase the susceptibility to develop iron overload due to increased iron absorption.[5] Some severely affected persons have (1) bronzing of the skin, (2) cirrhosis, (3) diabetes mellitus, (4) joint disease, (5) hypogonadotrophic hypogonadism, and (6) cardiomyopathy. The term *juvenile hemochromatosis* is used to describe rare severe forms of hemochromatosis and severe iron overload that affect (1) children, (2) adolescents, and (3) young adults. Specific types of hemochromatosis are best designated by the name of the gene in which causative mutations have been detected.

HFE Hemochromatosis. This is the most prevalent type of hemochromatosis worldwide. It occurs predominantly in Caucasians of European descent. Transmitted as an autosomal recessive trait, this disorder is usually caused by inheritance of two copies of the **HFE** mutation designated as *C282Y* (nt.845G→A).[4] Approximately 1 in 200 European Caucasians are *C282Y* homozygotes (two abnormal gene copies). A high proportion of *C282Y* homozygotes diagnosed in nonscreening settings have moderate or severe iron overload. More than 50% of untreated homozygotes have elevated transferrin saturation or serum ferritin concentrations, and ≈10% have elevated levels of serum alanine aminotransferase. In *C282Y* homozygotes discovered in screening programs, severe iron overload (serum ferritin >1000 μg/L) is uncommon. **HFE** H63D and S65C are common mutations that are infrequently associated with severe iron overload.

Hemojuvelin (HJV) Hemochromatosis. This rare disorder is characterized by early age of onset and severe multiorgan iron overload. Most reported patients have European ancestry. Manifestations of iron overload are more prevalent and more severe in *HJV* than in *HFE* hemochromatosis. Heart failure and arrhythmia are the predominant causes of death. Untreated patients have (1) high transferrin saturation, (2) severe hyperferritinemia, and (3) elevated liver transaminase levels. *HJV* hemochromatosis is transmitted as an autosomal recessive disorder. Worldwide, the most common deleterious *HJV* mutation is *G320V* (nt.959G→T). A major attribute of *HJV* hemochromatosis is dysregulation of hepcidin.

Transferrin Receptor-2 *(TFR2)* Hemochromatosis. *TFR2* hemochromatosis is a rare autosomal recessive disorder characterized by (1) elevated serum transferrin saturation, (2) elevated ferritin levels, and (3) liver iron overload. Most patients are of European or Asian ancestry. In some kinships, severe iron overload occurs in children or young adults. Many patients are compound heterozygotes for two different *TFR2* mutations. The *TFR2* gene encodes transferrin receptor-2, a protein that continues to mediate uptake of transferrin-bound iron by the liver after the classical transferrin receptor is downregulated by iron overload. Increased iron absorption in *TFR2* hemochromatosis is due to hepcidin dysregulation.

Ferroportin *(SLC40A1)* Hemochromatosis. Ferroportin, the receptor for hepcidin, occurs on the surfaces of cells responsible for gathering and recycling iron, including macrophages and absorptive cells of the small intestine and placenta. Mutations in the *SLC40A1* gene cause an uncommon, heterogeneous group of iron overload disorders characterized by an autosomal dominant pattern of inheritance. Ferroportin hemochromatosis has been described worldwide in a variety of race/ethnicity groups. In some kinships, (1) serum iron measures are minimally abnormal, (2) mild anemia is often present, and (3) complications of iron overload are uncommon. *In other kinships,* ferroportin mutations cause a serious disorder that resembles *HFE* or *HJV* hemochromatosis.

African Iron Overload and African American Iron Overload. African iron overload occurs in 14% to 18% of Bantu-speaking Natives in many sub-Saharan Africa countries. This disorder is due primarily to the ingestion of large quantities of iron contained in traditional beer, although an African iron overload gene(s) may also exist. Some patients develop harmful iron deposits in the (1) liver, (2) spleen, (3) pancreas, and (4) other organs, predominantly in macrophages. Affected persons have normal or elevated transferrin saturation and elevated serum ferritin levels. A similar disorder occurs in African Americans, but iron overload is typically less severe than in African Natives. Some cases in African Americans are due to (1) *HFE* genotypes typical of Caucasian hemochromatosis, (2) rare mutations of other hemochromatosis-associated genes, or (3) types of hemoglobinopathy or thalassemia.

Iron Overload Due to Anemia With Ineffective Erythropoiesis

Some types of heritable and acquired anemia cause ineffective erythropoiesis and increased GDF15 (growth/differentiation factor-15) production by erythroblasts. This downregulates hepcidin expression and thus increases iron absorption. Transferrin saturation and serum ferritin levels are elevated in untreated patients. These types of anemia include (1) β-thalassemia major, pyruvate kinase deficiency, (2) congenital dyserythropoietic anemia, and (3) refractory anemia with ringed sideroblasts due to myelodysplasia. Increased GDF15 expression probably also occurs in patients with X-linked sideroblastic anemia. Chronic erythrocyte transfusion may exacerbate iron overload due to increased absorption in persons with these types of anemia.

Secondary Iron Overload

Chronic erythrocyte transfusion is the most common cause of this group of disorders.[8] Transfusion iron overload is common in patients with severe β-thalassemia major and sickle cell disease. Transfusion iron overload also occurs in persons with (1) severe aplastic anemia, (2) Blackfan-Diamond syndrome, (3) Fanconi's anemia, (4) acute leukemia, (5) autoimmune hemolytic anemias, and (6) myelodysplasia with refractory anemia.

Daily consumption of traditional beer that contains large amounts of iron is the major cause of African iron overload. Rarely, iron overload develops in persons who ingest large quantities of supplemental iron. Hematite miners and other workers chronically exposed to iron ore dust may develop iron overload of the lungs and adjacent lymph nodes, but serum iron measures are usually normal.

Analytical Methodology

Several methods are used to measure iron and related analytes.[7] These include methods for (1) serum iron, (2) iron-binding capacity, (3) transferrin saturation, and (4) serum ferritin.

Methods for the Determination of Serum Iron, Iron-Binding Capacity, and Transferrin Saturation

Iron is released from transferrin by decreasing the pH of the serum. It is reduced from Fe^{3+} to Fe^{2+} and then is complexed with a chromogen such as bathophenanthroline or ferrozine. Such iron/chromogen complexes have an extremely high absorbance at the applicable wavelength, which is proportional to the iron concentration.

Serum unsaturated iron-binding capacity and total iron-binding capacity (TIBC) are determined by the addition of sufficient Fe^{3+} to saturate iron-binding sites on transferrin. Excess Fe^{3+} is removed (e.g., by adsorption with [1] light magnesium carbonate [$MgCO_3$] powder, [2] a silica column, or

[3] an ion exchange resin], and the assay for iron content is then repeated. From this second measurement, the TIBC is obtained.

$$\text{Transferrin saturation }(\%) = (100 \times \text{serum iron})/\text{TIBC}$$

Many automated chemistry analyzers now measure unsaturated iron-binding capacity (UIBC) and calculate TIBC, rather than measure it directly. UIBC is measured by adding a known excess concentration of iron to serum. By leaving the pH near neutral, only the iron that did not bind to transferrin is measured upon addition of an iron-binding chromogen. TIBC is calculated by adding the UIBC to the serum iron level.

Reference Intervals

Reference intervals for serum iron differ by as much as 35% between commercial methods. Therefore, a generic reference interval is not valid. If an automated commercial method is used, a laboratory should independently define its own reference intervals based on race/ethnicity samples appropriate for the laboratory's clientele.

Clinical Relevance

The serum iron concentration refers to the Fe^{3+} bound to serum transferrin and does not include the iron contained in serum as free hemoglobin. The serum iron concentration is decreased in many, but not all, patients with iron deficiency anemia and with chronic inflammatory disorders, such as (1) acute infection, (2) immunization, and (3) myocardial infarction (Table 28-4). Other conditions that decrease serum iron concentration include (4) blood donation, (5) hemorrhage, and (6) menstruation.

Elevated serum iron levels occur (1) in iron-loading disorders such as hemochromatosis,[22] (2) in patients with aplastic anemia, (3) in children with acute iron poisoning, (4) after oral or parenteral iron use, (5) as the result of acute liver injury, and (6) with the use of hormonal contraceptives.

Because only about one-third of the iron-binding sites of transferrin are occupied by Fe^{3+} in healthy individuals, serum transferrin has much reserve iron-binding capacity (UIBC). TIBC is a measurement of the maximum concentration of iron that transferrin binds. TIBC is increased in many persons with iron deficiency and is decreased in those with chronic inflammatory disorders or malignancies. In many persons with untreated hemochromatosis, TIBC is slightly decreased.

Comments and Precautions

1. Except when atomic absorption spectroscopy is used, hemolysis has very little effect on serum iron assay results because hemoglobin iron is not released from heme by acid treatment. Markedly hemolyzed specimens should be rejected for analysis.
2. Many factors influence serum iron concentration and TIBC. Conditions that affect these measures are listed in Table 28-4. Day-to-day variation is great in many healthy people. Diurnal variation in serum iron concentrations also occurs. Values are lower in the afternoon than in the morning and are very low in the evening (as low as 10 to 20 μg/dL [2 to 4 μmol/L] in healthy individuals). Because many causes of low serum iron levels are known, results must be interpreted with caution. Furthermore, values of serum iron concentration and TIBC are normal in many people with mild iron deficiency.

TABLE 28-4   Conditions Known to Affect Serum Iron Concentration, Total Iron-Binding Capacity, and Transferrin Saturation

Condition	Effect
Diurnal variation	Normal values in morning; low values in midafternoon; very low values near midnight
Menstrual cycle	Premenstrually, elevated values (SI increased by 10%-30%); at menstruation, low values (SI decreased by 10%-30%)
Pregnancy	May elevate SI owing to increased progesterone; may lower SI owing to iron deficiency
Ingestion of iron (including iron-fortified vitamins)	High values; may raise SI by +54 μmol/L (+300 μg/dL) and Tsat to 100%
Oral contraceptives (progesterone-like)	High values; may raise SI to >36 μmol/L (>200 μg/dL) and Tsat to 75%; also elevates TIBC
Iron contamination of syringe, Vacutainer tube, or other glassware (phenomenon may be rare, sporadic, very difficult to prove)	High values; e.g., SI >30 μmol/L (>170 μg/dL); Tsat 75%-100%
Iron dextran injection	Very high values; SI may be >180 μmol/L (>1000 μg/dL), Tsat 100%, probably from circulating iron dextran; effect may persist for several weeks
Hepatitis	Very high values; SI may be >180 μmol/L (>1000 μg/dL) owing to hyperferritinemia from hepatocyte injury
Acute inflammation (respiratory infection), abscess, immunization, myocardial infarction	Low or normal SI; normal or low Tsat
Chronic inflammation or malignancy	Low or normal SI; normal or low Tsat
Iron deficiency	Low or normal SI; low or normal Tsat; increased TIBC
Iron overload (hemochromatosis)	High SI; high Tsat; normal or low TIBC

From Fairbanks VF. Laboratory testing for iron status. Hosp Pract 1991;26:19.
SI, Serum iron concentration; *TIBC,* total iron-binding capacity; *Tsat,* transferrin saturation.

3. Because iron is ubiquitous, scrupulous care is necessary to ensure that glassware, water, and reagents do not become contaminated with extraneous iron.

4. Transferrin saturation (Tsat) may be estimated from the TIBC by the following relationship:

$$\text{Serum transferrin (g/L)} = 0.007 \times \text{TIBC (µg/dL)}$$

Note that the relationship is not entirely linear as a small portion of iron in serum is bound to proteins other than transferrin. Therefore, calculated TIBC values are slightly greater than the amount of transferrin-bound iron. However, these small differences are of no practical consequence. Immunoassays are available for assay of serum transferrin concentration. Results of immunological measurements of transferrin concentration correlate with those of the TIBC assay, but the clinical utility of transferrin measurement is very limited. A slight advantage for the immunoassay of transferrin is that the required volume per specimen is much smaller.

Methods for the Determination of Serum Ferritin

Serum ferritin assay may be performed by any of several methods, including (1) immunoradiometric assay, (2) enzyme-linked immunosorbent assay (ELISA), (3) immunochemiluminescence assays, and (4) immunofluorometric methods. Reagents for these assays are available in kit form and for automated immunoassay instruments from several manufacturers.

Reference Intervals

Reference intervals for serum ferritin concentrations are summarized in Table 28-5. Much variation is seen with different methods for serum ferritin and purposes of testing and test populations. Reference intervals must be determined for each laboratory.

Clinical Significance

Ferritin is present in the blood in very low concentration. Although it is an acute-phase protein, under normal conditions serum ferritin levels are usually proportional to the body iron content. The circulating protein is largely apoferritin. It is iron-poor and largely consists of iron-poor, glycosylated L-chains. The plasma ferritin concentration declines very early in the development of iron deficiency—long before changes are observed in (1) blood hemoglobin concentration, (2) RBC size, or (3) serum iron concentration. Thus measurement of serum ferritin concentration is used as a highly sensitive indicator of iron deficiency that is uncomplicated by other concurrent disease. Alternatively, many chronic diseases cause increased serum ferritin levels (see Table 28-4). Most persons with elevated serum ferritin levels do not have hemochromatosis and other iron overload disorders. In persons with proven hemochromatosis or iron overload, serum ferritin measurements are useful gauges to the progress of phlebotomy therapy in achieving iron depletion.

Method for Red Cell Volume and Hemoglobin Content

MCV and mean corpuscular hemoglobin concentration (MCHC) are indices that are included in the CBC test. One of their uses is to characterize the blood of patients with anemia. Low values of MCV and MCHC are indicators of iron deficiency. The diagnostic utility of MCV and MCHC in detecting iron deficiency is limited in patients with MCV values greater than 100 fL. Values of MCV are elevated in many persons with other chronic medical conditions, including untreated *HFE* hemochromatosis. Common heritable traits may increase or decrease MCV and MCHC.

Method for the Determination of the Serum Transferrin Receptor

The cell membranes of developing erythroid cells in bone marrow are rich in transferrin receptors to which the iron/transferrin complex binds as a normal attribute of the transferrin cycle. The number of transferrin receptors increases in the presence of iron deficiency and decreases in iron excess. These variations in the quantity of transferrin receptors in erythropoietic tissue are reflected in changes in soluble serum transferrin receptor, which are measured by a variety of standard immunoassay techniques. To a large extent, serum transferrin receptor concentrations reflect the rate of erythropoietic activity, regardless of the iron status of the patient.

Bilirubin

Bilirubin is the orange-yellow pigment derived mainly from senescent (*aging*) red blood cells. It is extracted and metabolized mainly in the liver and is excreted in bile and urine. The (1) chemistry, (2) biochemistry, (3) clinical significance, and (4) analytical methods for bilirubin are reviewed in this section.

Chemistry

Bilirubin was discovered in blood in 1849 by Virchow, who called the yellow pigment "hematoidin." The term *bilirubin* was coined by Stadeler in 1864, and in 1874 Tarchanoff demonstrated the direct association of bile pigments with hemoglobin. In 1942, Fisher and Plieninger synthesized bilirubin IXα and proposed the structure shown in the upper portion of Figure 28-7. This linear tetrapyrrolic structure of the bilirubin molecule was accepted for longer than 30 years. However, the insolubility of the bilirubin molecule in water and its solubility in a variety of nonpolar, lipid solvents are not predicted

TABLE 28-5	Reference Intervals for Serum Ferritin	
	ng/mL	**µg/L**
Newborn	25-200	25-200
1 mo	200-600	200-600
2 to 5 mo	50-200	50-200
6 mo to 15 y	7-140	7-140
Adult man	20-250	20-250
Adult woman	20-200	20-200
Iron overload		
• Adult male	>400	>400
• Adult female	>200	>200

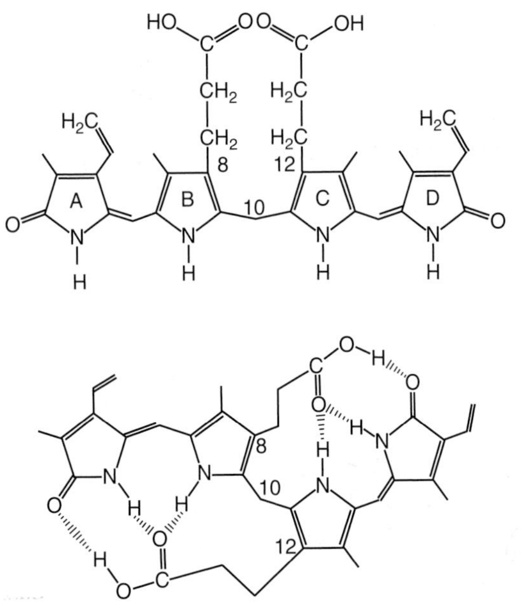

Figure 28-7 Bilirubin IXα structure. *Top,* A linear molecular representation of unconjugated bilirubin. *Bottom,* The preferred structure of unconjugated bilirubin IXα, Z-Z configuration. The folded ridge-tile structure is stabilized by six hydrogen bonds formed between the two carboxyl groups of the sidechains and the two carbonyl- and four imino- groups. The "ridge" involves carbon atoms 8 through 12.

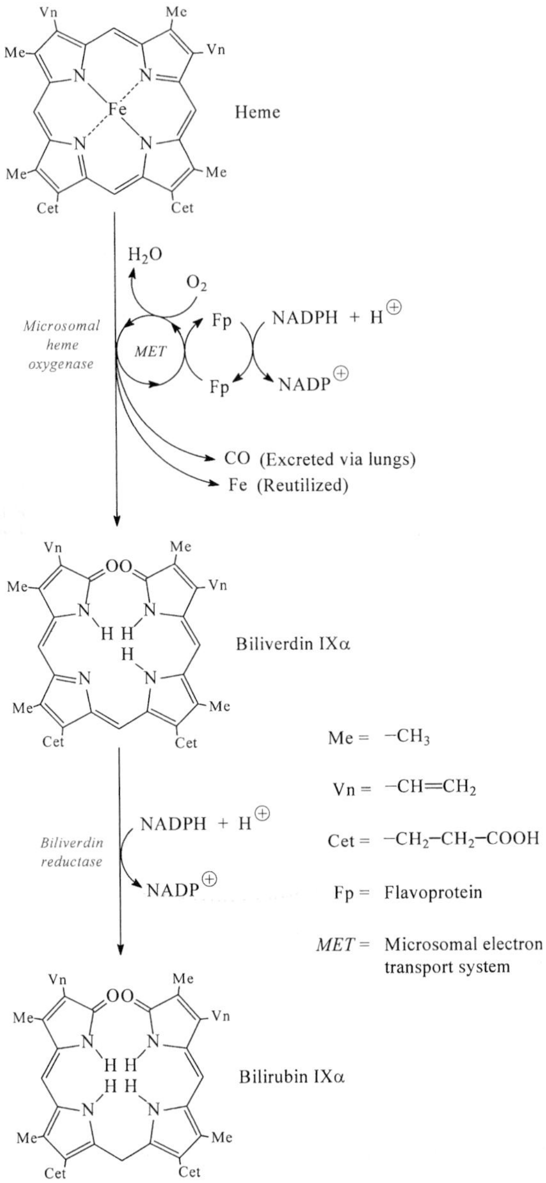

from this linear tetrapyrrole structure; the two propionic acid sidechains would be expected to make the bilirubin molecule highly polar and therefore water soluble.

The overall chemical structure of bilirubin was established by X-ray crystallography. Crystalline bilirubin assumes a ridge-tiled configuration, stabilized by six intramolecular hydrogen bonds. This Z-Z (*trans*) conformation, in which the propionic acid–carboxylic acid groups are hydrogen-bonded to the nitrogen atoms of the pyrrole rings (see Figure 28-7), prevents the interaction of bilirubin with polar groups in aqueous media. When exposed to light, the Z-Z (*trans*) configuration is converted by rupture of the intramolecular double bonds to the E-E (*cis*) conformation, which is more water soluble than the Z-Z conformation. Thus light-exposed forms of bilirubin are more water soluble and are readily excreted in the bile. This is the rationale for irradiating jaundiced newborns with 450 nm light.

Biochemistry

Bilirubin IXα is produced from the catabolism of protoporphyrin IX by a microsomal heme oxygenase (Figure 28-8). The tetrapyrrolic product of the ring opening at the α-methene bridge is the green pigment biliverdin, which is subsequently reduced to bilirubin by the reduced form of nicotinamide adenine dinucleotide phosphate (NADPH)-dependent, cytosolic enzyme biliverdin reductase. For each mole of heme catabolized by this pathway, one mole each of (1) carbon monoxide, (2) bilirubin, and (3) ferric iron is produced. Daily bilirubin production from all sources in humans averages from 250 to 300 mg. Approximately 85% of the total bilirubin produced is

Figure 28-8 Catabolism of heme to bilirubin IXα. *(From Berlin NI, Berk PD. Quantitative aspects of bilirubin metabolism for hematologists. Blood 1981:57:983-99.)*

derived from the heme moiety of hemoglobin released from senescent erythrocytes that are destroyed in the reticuloendothelial cells of the (1) liver, (2) spleen, and (3) bone marrow. The remaining 15% is produced from red blood cell precursors destroyed in the bone marrow (so-called ineffective erythropoiesis) and from the catabolism of other heme-containing proteins, such as (1) myoglobin, (2) cytochromes, and (3) peroxidases.

In blood, bilirubin is bound to albumin and is transported to the liver. It dissociates from albumin at the membrane of the hepatocyte and is transported across the membrane into the liver (Figure 28-9). Inside the liver cells, bilirubin is reversibly bound to soluble proteins known as **ligandins** or *protein Y*. Ligandin also binds a variety of other compounds, such as (1) steroids, (2) bromsulphthalein (BSP), (3) indocyanine green, and (4) some carcinogens. Inside the hepatocytes, bilirubin

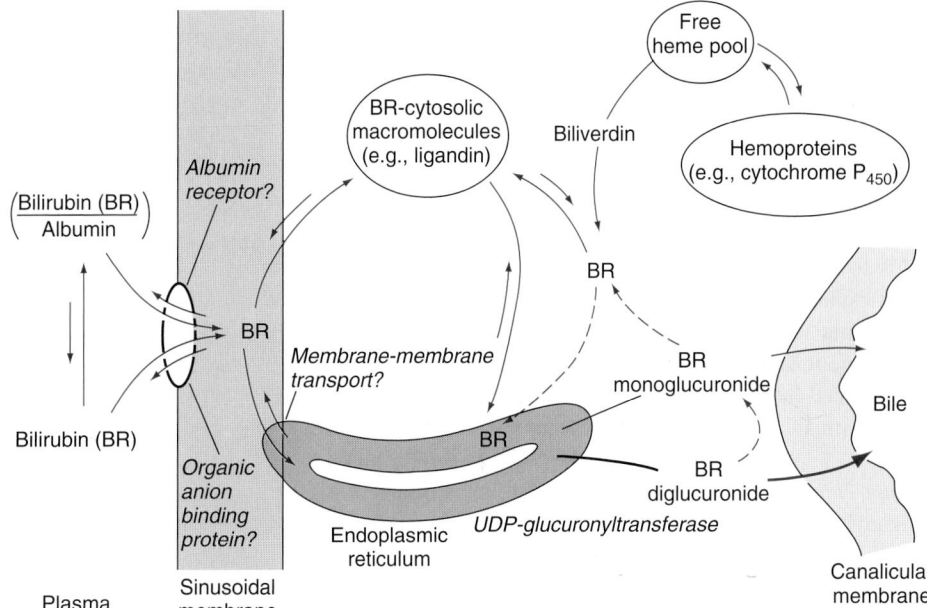

Figure 28-9 Bilirubin uptake, metabolism, and transport in the hepatocyte. *(From Gollan JL, Schmid R. Bilirubin metabolism. In: Popper H, Schaffner F, eds. Progress in liver diseases, vol 7, Chapter 15. Philadelphia: WB Saunders, 1982.)*

is rapidly conjugated with glucuronic acid to produce bilirubin monoglucuronide and diglucuronide, which then are excreted into bile (see Figure 28-9). The microsomal enzyme bilirubin uridine diphosphate (UDP)–glucuronyltransferase (EC 2.4.1.17) catalyzes the formation of bilirubin monoglucuronide. It is not certain whether conversion of the monoglucuronide to the diglucuronide is catalyzed by the same enzyme or by another enzyme located in or near the canaliculus. In adults, virtually all bilirubin excreted in bile is in the form of glycosidic conjugates.

In the intestine, bilirubin glucuronides are hydrolyzed by the catalytic action of β-glucuronidase from the (1) liver, (2) intestinal epithelial cells, and (3) bacteria. The **unconjugated bilirubin** is then reduced by anaerobic intestinal microbial flora to form a group of three colorless tetrapyrroles collectively called **urobilinogens**. The urobilinogens differ from one another in the degree of hydrogenation; they contain 6, 8, or 12 more hydrogen atoms than does bilirubin and are named (1) *stercobilinogen,* (2) *mesobilinogen,* or (3) *urobilinogen,* respectively. In the lower intestinal tract, the three urobilinogens are spontaneously oxidized at the middle methylene bridge to produce the corresponding bile pigments (1) stercobilin, (2) mesobilin, and (3) urobilin, which are orange-brown and the major pigments of stool.

Clinical Significance

Jaundice is a condition characterized by **hyperbilirubinemia** and deposition of bile pigment in the (1) skin, (2) mucous membranes, and (3) sclera, with a resulting yellow appearance of the patient; it is also called **icterus**. Defects in bilirubin metabolism resulting in jaundice occur at each step of the metabolic pathway (see Figure 28-9). The disorders are usually classified as (1) inherited disorders of bilirubin metabolism or (2) jaundice of the newborn. All of these disorders are characterized by elevations in conjugated or unconjugated bilirubin

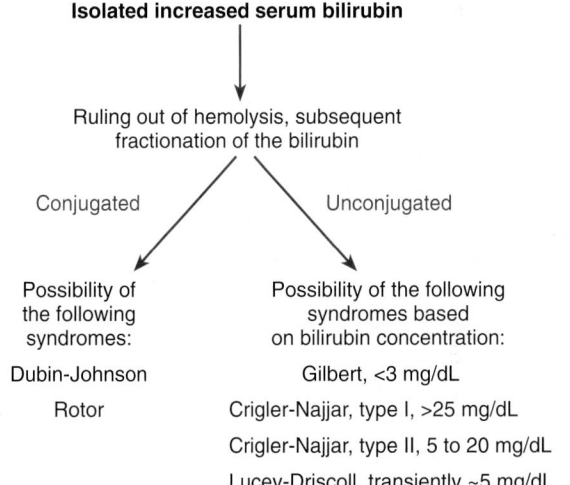

Figure 28-10 Algorithm for differentiating the familial causes of hyperbilirubinemia.

in the absence of other abnormal liver tests. It is only in these disorders that bilirubin fractionation is clinically useful.

Patients are occasionally seen with isolated elevations in bilirubin concentration. In most cases, this is due to (1) inherited disorders of bilirubin metabolism, (2) familial hyperbilirubinemia, or (3) hemolysis. An algorithm for differentiating familial causes of hyperbilirubinemia is presented in Figure 28-10.

Inherited Disorders of Bilirubin Metabolism

Inherited disorders of bilirubin metabolism include (1) **Gilbert, Crigler-Najjar** (Types I and II), (2) **Lucey-Driscoll,** (3) **Dubin-Johnson,** and (4) **Rotor syndromes.**

Gilbert Syndrome

Gilbert syndrome is a benign condition manifested by mild unconjugated hyperbilirubinemia. This abnormality, which affects 3% to 5% of the population, is probably inherited as an autosomal recessive trait; it is clinically important because is often misdiagnosed as chronic hepatitis. (Gilbert syndrome is easily distinguished from chronic hepatitis by the absence of anemia and bilirubin in urine and by normal liver function test results.)

With this syndrome, the serum concentration of bilirubin fluctuates between 1.5 and 3 mg/dL (26 and 51 µmol/L) and tends to increase with fasting. The cause of jaundice is low hepatic glucuronyltransferase activity.

Patients with Gilbert syndrome may be predisposed to acetaminophen toxicity because acetaminophen is primarily metabolized by glucuronidation. No treatment is needed, but patients must be reassured that they do not have liver disease.

Crigler-Najjar Syndrome (Type I)

Crigler-Najjar syndrome type I, a rare disorder caused by complete absence of UDP-glucuronyltransferase, is manifested by very high concentrations of unconjugated bilirubin, often exceeding 25 mg/dL (428 µmol/L). It is inherited as an autosomal recessive trait. Most patients die of severe brain damage caused by kernicterus (encephalopathy related to increased serum bilirubin that leads to permanent brain damage) within the first year of life. Phlebotomy and plasmapheresis reduce the serum bilirubin, but encephalopathy usually develops. Early liver transplantation is the only effective therapy.

Crigler-Najjar Syndrome (Type II)

This rare autosomal dominant disorder is characterized by a partial deficiency of UDP-glucuronyltransferase. Unconjugated bilirubin is usually 5 to 20 mg/dL (85 to 340 µmol/L). Unlike Crigler-Najjar syndrome type I, type II responds dramatically to phenobarbital, and a normal life is expected.

Lucey-Driscoll Syndrome

Lucey-Driscoll syndrome is a familial form of unconjugated hyperbilirubinemia caused by a circulating inhibitor of bilirubin conjugation. The hyperbilirubinemia is mild and lasts for the first 2 to 3 weeks of life.

Dubin-Johnson and Rotor Syndromes

Dubin-Johnson syndrome is due to a rare autosomal recessive disorder and is characterized by jaundice with predominantly elevated **conjugated bilirubin** and a minor elevation of unconjugated bilirubin. Rotor syndrome is similar to Dubin-Johnson syndrome, but without black pigment in the liver. Both conditions are benign.

Jaundice in the Neonate

Disorders that cause jaundice in the neonate are classified as unconjugated or conjugated hyperbilirubinemia (Box 28-2).

Unconjugated Hyperbilirubinemia

Unconjugated hyperbilirubinemia poses a risk for development of **kernicterus** (acute bilirubin encephalopathy), especially in low birth weight infants. Kernicterus refers to a neurological syndrome that results in brain damage owing

BOX 28-2	Physiological Classification of Jaundice

Unconjugated Hyperbilirubinemia
Increased Production of Unconjugated Bilirubin from Heme
Hemolysis
   Hereditary
   Acquired
Ineffective erythropoiesis
Rapid turnover of increased RBC mass (in the neonate)

Decreased Delivery of Unconjugated Bilirubin (in Plasma) to Hepatocyte
Right-sided congestive heart failure
Portacaval shunt

Decreased Uptake of Unconjugated Bilirubin Across Hepatocyte Membrane
Competitive inhibition
   Drugs
   Others
Gilbert syndrome
Sepsis, fasting

Decreased Storage of Unconjugated Bilirubin in Cytosol (Decreased Y and Z Proteins)
Competitive inhibition
Fever

Decreased Biotransformation (Conjugation)
Neonatal jaundice (physiological)
Inhibition (drugs)
Hereditary (Crigler-Najjar)
   Type I (complete enzyme deficiency)
   Type II (partial deficiency)
Hepatocellular dysfunction
Gilbert syndrome

Conjugated Hyperbilirubinemia (Cholestasis)
Decreased Secretion of Conjugated Bilirubin into Canaliculi
Hepatocellular disease
   Hepatitis
   Cholestasis (intrahepatic)
Dubin-Johnson and Rotor syndromes
Drugs (estradiol)

Decreased Drainage
Extrahepatic obstruction
   Stones
   Carcinoma
   Stricture
   Atresia
Sclerosing cholangitis
Intrahepatic obstruction
   Drugs
   Granulomas
   Primary biliary cirrhosis
   Bile duct paucity
   Tumors

to deposition of bilirubin in the basal ganglia and brainstem nuclei. In term infants, early symptoms of kernicterus include (1) poor feeding, (2) lethargy, and (3) vomiting; later, (4) opisthotonos (backward arching of the trunk), (5) seizures, and (6) death may follow. Seventy percent of affected infants die within the first week, and those remaining have severe brain damage. It is possible to prevent this syndrome by phototherapy and exchange transfusion in infants with elevated unconjugated bilirubin concentrations.

Causes of unconjugated hyperbilirubinemia in the neonate are (1) physiological jaundice of the newborn, (2) hemolytic (3) disease owing to Rh or ABO incompatibility, and (4) breast milk hyperbilirubinemia.

Guidelines for Assessing Risk. In 2004, the Subcommittee on Hyperbilirubinemia of the American Academy of Pediatrics issued new guidelines for management of jaundice in the neonate. These guidelines became necessary because newborns are currently discharged between 36 and 72 hours after birth, and severe hyperbilirubinemia may not be present at discharge. The time-honored bilirubin concentration of 20 mg/dL (340 μmol/L), which was considered critical and required action (e.g., phototherapy, exchange transfusion), has now been abandoned and replaced by monitoring the increase in bilirubin concentration from time of birth until time of discharge from the hospital[6]; it is now recommended that a plot of bilirubin concentration (mg/dL) versus time (hours) should be constructed and compared with the similar plot found in Figure 2 of reference 6.

Physiological Jaundice of the Newborn. Babies frequently become jaundiced within a few days of birth; this condition is known as *physiological jaundice of the newborn.* Unconjugated bilirubin concentrations reach a peak within 3 to 5 days of birth and remain elevated for less than 2 weeks. Factors contributing to physiological jaundice include (1) increased bilirubin load in the newborn caused by the shortened life span of red blood cells; (2) decreased conjugation of bilirubin resulting from relative lack of glucuronyltransferase (conjugating enzyme) in the first few days after birth; and (3) exposure of breast-feeding infants to pregnanediol, nonesterified fatty acids, and other inhibitors of bilirubin conjugation present in breast milk.

Physiological jaundice of the newborn is treated with phototherapy; the infant is exposed to light of approximately 450 nm that disrupts intramolecular hydrogen bonds in the bilirubin molecule and yields several photoisomers that are more water soluble than the Z-Z-isomer and thus are excreted in the bile. Exchange transfusions are rarely necessary.

Hemolytic Disease. Hemolytic disease of the newborn results from maternal-fetal incompatibility of Rhesus blood factors, in which the maternal Rh-negative blood becomes sensitized by a previous pregnancy with an Rh-positive fetus or an Rh-positive blood transfusion. The infant becomes jaundiced with unconjugated bilirubin in the first or second day of life and is susceptible to kernicterus. The diagnosis is confirmed by Coombs' test with Rh-positive blood in the infant and Rh-negative blood in the mother.

Breast Milk Hyperbilirubinemia. This type of hyperbilirubinemia affects about 30% of breast-fed newborns. It is due to the presence of α-glucuronidase in breast milk, which hydrolyzes conjugated bilirubin in the intestine. The unconjugated bilirubin, being more lipophilic, is passively absorbed. The condition lasts for a few weeks and is treated by discontinuation of breast-feeding.

Conjugated Hyperbilirubinemias
These syndromes are characterized by hyperbilirubinemia in which conjugated bilirubin exceeds 1.5 mg/dL (26 μmol/L). The most important of these stndromes are idiopathic neonatal hepatitis and biliary atresia. Conjugated hyperbilirubinemia is seen fairly often in the newborn as a complication of parenteral nutrition.

Biliary Atresia
Biliary atresia is a condition in which the bile ducts either fail to develop or develop abnormally. It occurs in one in 10,000 births, and females are more frequently affected.

Having no exit to the intestine, bile accumulates inside the liver and eventually escapes into the blood, causing mixed hyperbilirubinemia. Other possible causes include (1) cytomegalovirus, (2) reovirus III, (3) Epstein-Barr virus, (4) rubella virus, (5) α_1-antitrypsin deficiency, and (6) trisomy 17 or 18.

Extrahepatic biliary atresia, more common than the intrahepatic type, may involve all or part of the extrahepatic biliary tree. If jaundice persists beyond 14 days of age, a direct or conjugated bilirubin measurement must be performed to exclude biliary atresia. If bilirubin is elevated, the urine should be tested for bile. Early identification of this condition is essential if these infants are to benefit from the operation of portoenterostomy, which should be performed no later than 60 days after birth. If portoenterostomy is not successful, liver transplantation is the treatment of choice. Children rarely live beyond 3 years unless the lesion is surgically correctable.

Intrahepatic biliary atresia is characterized by lack of intrahepatic bile ducts. Jaundice usually appears within the first few days of life. Serum bilirubin is elevated, and serum cholesterol may be very high, leading to the formation of xanthomas.

Analytical Methdology
Several analytical techniques are used to measure bilirubin in serum and urine.

Serum Bilirubin
Bilirubin is measured in body fluids by (1) spectrophotometric (diazo—chemical, direct spectrophotometric, enzymatic, and transcutaneous) or (2) chromatographic methods.

Diazo Methods
The reaction of bilirubin with diazotized sulfanilic acid, known as the *diazo reaction,* discovered by Ehrlich in 1883 and applied to the measurement of bilirubin in serum and bile by van den Bergh and Muller in 1916, is the basis of the most widely used methods for measuring bilirubin. The observation that the reaction was slow in sera from jaundiced infants and required an accelerator (ethanol) to proceed and that it was rapid in bile and in adult sera without addition of ethanol led to the terms **indirect bilirubin** and **direct bilirubin**, respectively.

The reaction of the coupling of bilirubin with a diazo compound is shown in Figure 28-11. In this example, diazotized sulfanilic acid (the diazo reagent) reacts with bilirubin to produce two azodipyrroles (azopigments), which are reddish purple at neutral pH and blue at low or high pH values. Numerous

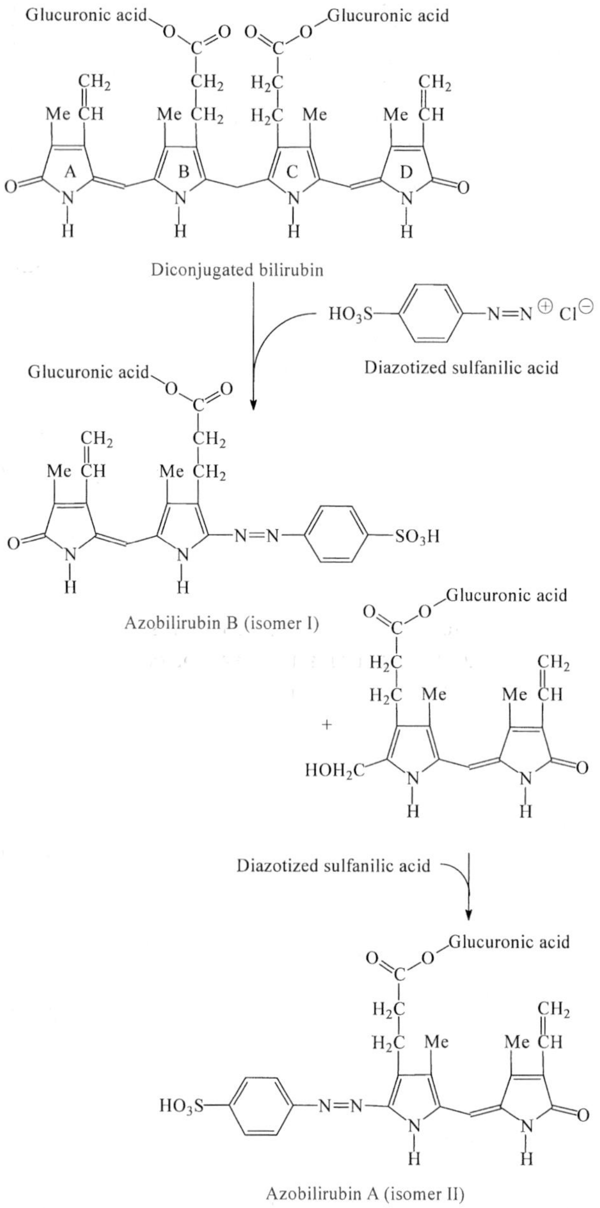

Figure 28-11 The reaction of bilirubin glucuronide with diazotized sulfanilic acid to produce isomers I and II of azobilirubin B. Unconjugated bilirubin reacts in the same way to produce isomers I and II of azobilirubin A.

variations of the van den Bergh method have been developed. All use one of a variety of "accelerators," which facilitate the reaction of unconjugated (indirect) bilirubin with the diazo reagent. The most commonly used accelerators are (1) caffeine,[10] dyphylline, and (3) several surface active agents (surfactans). The diazo method of Malloy and Evelyn, which used methanol as an accelerator and is virtually abandoned today, is mentioned here for historical reasons only.

Total Bilirubin. The diazo method described by Jendrassik and Grof in 1938 and later modified by Doumas and colleagues[11] measures quantitatively the sum of (1) unconjugated, (2) monoconjugated, (3) di-conjugated, and (4) δ-bilirubin fractions in serum, yielding results that are reproducible and reliable.

In this procedure, serum is added to an aqueous solution of caffeine and sodium benzoate (accelerator), which displaces unconjugated bilirubin from its association sites on albumin. Formation of hydrogen bonds with caffeine renders the bilirubin water soluble and facilitates its reaction with diazotized sulfanilic acid. After 10-minute incubation at room temperature, alkaline tartrate is added, and absorbance of the alkaline azobilirubin is measured at 598 nm.

With automated clinical analyzers, addition of alkaline tartrate is omitted and absorbance is measured at 530 nm. The method is calibrated with solutions of known bilirubin concentrations prepared by adding unconjugated bilirubin of known purity to human serum. Such bilirubin, Standard Reference Material (SRM) No. 916, is available from the National Institute of Standards and Technology (NIST), in Gaithersburg, Maryland. This method has acceptable transferability among laboratories and is currently the reference method of choice for measuring total bilirubin in serum.

Direct Bilirubin. Bilirubin monoconjugates and diconjugates (mainly glucuronides) and δ-bilirubin, because they are water soluble, react with the diazo reagents in the absence of accelerators. A reliable method for direct bilirubin should not measure any unconjugated bilirubin. To prevent the unconjugated bilirubin from reacting, it is necessary to keep the pH of the reaction mixture near 1.0.[10] A preferred manual method for direct bilirubin is available.[11] Ditaurobilirubin (bilirubin conjugated with taurine and available as the disodium salt), a water-soluble synthetic material, is used by instrument manufacturers for calibrating direct bilirubin methods; it is also present in materials used for quality control and for proficiency testing.

Direct Spectrophotometry

This method is based on the absorption of light by bilirubin near 460 nm and is restricted primarily to blood specimens from healthy newborns, among whom unconjugated bilirubin is the predominant species. Correction for oxyhemoglobin, invariably present in sera form neonates, is achieved by measuring absorbance at two wavelengths and solving a system of two simultaneous equations with two unknowns. If absorbance (A) is measured at 454 nm and 540 nm—the isosbestic wavelengths for hemoglobin—the concentration of bilirubin is then calculated from a single equation.

Note, this method requires determination of the absorptivity of pure unconjugated bilirubiin in human serum at the chosen wavelengths, and of hemoglobin if the chosen wavelengths are not isosbestic.

Calibrators for Bilirubin Measurements

The primary calibrator for all bilirubin methods should consist of unconjugated bilirubin dissolved in human serum. Several instrument manufacturers are using bovine serum, instead of human serum, as the protein base in preparing fluids for calibrating methods for total and direct bilirubin; the protein base is enriched with unconjugated bilirubin or ditaurobilirubin or both. Unconjugated bilirubin in human serum reacts completely with the reference method and with diazo methods

BOX 28-3 **Bilirubin Fractions**

Unconjugated bilirubin (α-bilirubin)
Monoconjugated bilirubin (β-bilirubin)
Di-conjugated bilirubin (γ-bilirubin)
A fraction irreversibly bound to protein (δ-bilirubin)

available in commonly used clinical analyzers. However, its reaction in bovine serum from commercial sources is incomplete and unpredictable; this makes virtually impossible the assignment of accurate bilirubin values to calibrators, the protein base of which is commercial bovine serum.[21] In human serum, ditaurobilirubin was underestimated by two of seven clinical analyzers tested; the calibrators of these two analyzers were made in bovine serum. Ditaurobilirubin in commercial bovine serum was underestimated by all analyzers and by the reference method. Consequently, it is recommended that the practice of using bilirubin calibrators made in bovine sera be abandoned because it compromises the accuracy of bilirubin measurements in jaundiced neonates.[21]

High-Performance Liquid Chromatography (HPLC)

HPLC methods have been developed for relatively rapid separation and quantification of the four main bilirubin fractions: (1) α-unconjugated bilirubin; (2) β-bilirubin monoglucuronide; (3) γ-bilirubin diglucuronide; and (4) δ-bilirubin (Box 28-3). More complex methods can be used to detect and separate the various bilirubin photoisomers produced in newborns during phototherapy.

δ-Bilirubin is formed in blood and in vitro by a spontaneous reaction between serum albumin and the bilirubin glucuronides; unconjugated bilirubin does not react with albumin to form δ-bilirubin. Because δ-bilirubin is water soluble, it reacts directly (without a promoter) with diazotized sulfanilic acid.

The discovery of δ-bilirubin solved the mystery of persistently high bilirubin concentrations, mostly direct reacting, in patients with intrahepatic or obstructive jaundice long after hepatitis has subsided or obstruction has been relieved. Because δ-bilirubin is the slowest fraction to clear from serum, it follows the catabolism of albumin, which has a half-life of approximately 17 to 19 days.

It should be noted that the various bilirubin fractions have been separated by capillary electrophoresis.

Enzymatic Methods

Enzymatic methods for total and direct bilirubin and for bilirubin conjugates with glucuronic acid are based on the oxidation of bilirubin to biliverdin by bilirubin oxidase and molecular oxygen. At a pH near 8 and in the presence of sodium cholate and sodium dodecylsulfate, all four bilirubin fractions are oxidized to biliverdin, which is further oxidized to purple and finally colorless products. The decrease in absorbance at 425 or 460 nm is proportional to the concentration of total bilirubin. Results obtained by the bilirubin oxidase method have been shown to correlate with those obtained by the Jendrassik-Grof procedure. Direct bilirubin is measured at pH 3.7 to 4.5; at this pH range, the enzyme oxidizes bilirubin conjugates and δ-bilirubin, but not unconjugated bilirubin. At pH 10, the enzyme oxidizes selectively the two glucuronides. δ-Bilirubin is not oxidized, and only 5% of unconjugated bilirubin is measured as conjugates.[12]

Transcutaneous Measurement of Bilirubin

A noninvasive approach for measuring bilirubin was introduced in 1980 by Yamanouchi and colleagues. The first bilirubinometer (icterometer) was a reflectance photometer that used two filters to correct for the color of Hb and required measurements at eight body sites. The accuracy of commercially available devices has improved substantially, and two of them (the BiliChek, http://bilichek.respironics.eu\; accessed October 14, 2013; and the Minolta JM 103 Jaundice Meter, http://www5.konicaminolta.eu/; accessed October 14, 2013) have been cleared by the U.S. Food and Drug Administration for clinical use in the United States[13]; furthermore, the U.S. National Academy of Clinical Biochemistry has approved transcutaneous bilirubin measurement for point-of-care testing.[19] A review of this subject has been published.[13]

Although transcutaneous bilirubin measurements may not substitute for laboratory quantitative determinations, they (1) provide instantaneous information, (2) reduce the necessity for serum bilirubin determinations, (3) spare infants the trauma of heel sticks, and (4) save money. Furthermore, they are useful in determining whether in a jaundiced infant it is necessary to draw blood before initiating treatment, such as phototherapy or exchange transfusion (currently this is extremely rare). Another application involves predicting those babies who require follow-up according to the "hour-specific" serum bilirubin nomogram.[13]

Urine Bilirubin

Because only conjugated bilirubin is excreted in urine, its presence indicates conjugated hyperbilirubinemia. The most commonly used method for detecting bilirubin in urine involves the use of a dipstick impregnated with a diazo reagent. Dipstick methods are capable of detecting bilirubin concentrations as low as 0.5 mg/dL. A number of these methods are available commercially.

Review Questions

1. Heme is a:
   a. chelate of iron with the four pyrrole groups of a porphyrin.
   b. conjugated protein and an oxygen-carrying pigment of the erythrocytes.
   c. protein found in red skeletal muscle that releases oxygen.
   d. colorless compound formed in the intestines by the reduction of bilirubin.

2. The role of hemoglobin is to:
   a. transport iron between organs.
   b. store iron and readily release it when body iron stores are low.

   c. reversibly bind oxygen.

   d. conjugate bilirubin in the liver.

3. What is bilirubin conjugated to in a hepatocyte to form conjugated bilirubin?

   a. Cholic acid

   b. Glycogen

   c. Bile acid

   d. Glucuronic acid

4. In an individual with suspected β-thalassemia, which of the following laboratory results would correctly indicate the presence of this disease?

   a. Increased hemoglobin concentration, MCV and MCHC with the peripheral blood smear showing increased macrocytes and Howell-Jolly bodies

   b. Decreased hemoglobin concentration, MCV and MCHC with the peripheral blood smear indicating microcytosis, target cells and polychromasia

   c. Decreased hemoglobin concentration, increased MCV and MCHC and persistence of hemoglobin F with the peripheral blood smear indicating spherocytosis and nucleated red blood cells

   d. Increased hemoglobin concentration and normal MCV and MCHC with a normal peripheral blood smear

5. Which of the following is associated with low serum iron and high total iron binding capacity (TIBC)?

   a. Hemochromatosis

   b. Iron deficiency anemia

   c. Iron intoxication

   d. Hemosiderosis

6. This readily soluble iron/protein complex is the form in which iron is stored in tissues:

   a. Ferritin

   b. Transferrin

   c. Hemosiderin

   d. Hemoglobin

7. The correct formula for determining the percent of transferrin saturation % is:

   a. MCV < 70 mL = increased transferrin

   b. total iron binding capacity ÷ serum iron

   c. total iron binding capacity × 100

   d. [total iron binding capacity ÷ serum iron] × 100

8. The major difference between thalassemia and hemoglobinopathy is that:

   a. in thalassemia the globin chains of hemoglobin are structurally altered.

   b. in thalassemia the serum level of conjugated bilirubin is dramatically increased.

   c. in a hemoglobinopathy the globin chains of hemoglobin are structurally altered.

   d. in a hemoglobinopathy the globin chains of hemoglobin are insufficiently produced.

9. An inherited disorder caused by an inherited abnormality of proteins that regulate iron hemostasis with excess circulating iron is called:

   a. hemosiderosis.

   b. primary hemochromatosis.

   c. secondary hemochromatosis.

   d. sideroblastic anemia.

10. Hemolytic disease in a newborn results from maternal-fetal Rh incompatibility. This produces physiological jaundice that is characterized by:

   a. unconjugated hyperbilirubinemia.

   b. conjugated bilirubinemia.

   c. hemosiderosis.

   d. hemoglobinopathy.

11. Extrahepatic biliary atresia:

   a. is characterized by lack of bile ducts within the liver.

   b. is less common than intrahepatic biliary atresia.

   c. is characterized by a mixed hyperbilirubinemia.

   d. produces jaundice that can be observed within the first few days of life.

12. Bilirubin:

   a. in the conjugated form is highly toxic to the nervous system when elevated.

   b. in the plasma is bound to albumin before conjugation in hepatocytes.

   c. becomes conjugated to cholic acid in the hepatocyte.

   d. All of the above answers are correct.

References

1. Berendt HL, Blakney GB, Clarke GM, Higgins TN. A case of β thalassemia major detected using HPLC in a child of Chinese ancestry. Clin Biochem 2000;33:311–3.
2. Berenstein LH, Kneifati-Hayek J, Riccioli A. Development and validation of a beta thalassemia screening protocol. Clin Chem 2004;51:A177.
3. Beutler E. Disorders of iron metabolism. In: Lichtman MA, Beutler E, Kipps TJ, Seligsohn U, Kaushansky K, Prchal J, eds. Williams hematology. New York: McGraw-Hill, 2006:511–53.
4. Beutler E, Felitti VJ, Koziol JA, Ho NJ, Gelbart T. Penetrance of the 845G→A (C282Y) HFE hereditary haemochromatosis mutation in the USA. Lancet 2002;359:211–8.
5. Beutler E. The HFE Cys282Tyr mutation as a necessary but not sufficient cause of hereditary hemochromatosis. Blood 2003;101:3347–50.
6. Bhutani VK, Johnson L, Sivieri EM. Predictive ability of predischarge hour-specific serum bilirubin for subsequent significant hyperbilirubinemia in healthy term and near-term newborns. Pediatrics 1999;103:6–14.
7. Canals C, Remacha AF, Sarda MP, et al. Clinical utility of the new Sysmex XE 2100 parameter—reticulocyte hemoglobin equivalent—in the diagnosis of anemia. Haematologica 2005;90:1133–4.
8. Cazzola M, May A, Bergamaschi G, et al. Absent phenotypic expression of X-linked sideroblastic anemia in one of two brothers with a novel ALAS2 mutation. Blood 2002;100:4236–8.
9. Clarke GM, Higgins TN. Laboratory investigation of hemoglobinopathies and thalassemias: review and update. Clin Chem 2000;46:1284–90.
10. Doumas BT, Perry BW, Jendrzejczak B, Katona V. Pitfalls in the American Monitor kit methods for determination of total and "direct" bilirubin. Clin Chem 1982;28:2305–8.
11. Doumas BT, Poon PKC, Perry BW, et al. Candidate reference method for determination of total bilirubin in serum: development and validation. Clin Chem 1985;31:1779–89.
12. Doumas BT, Yein F, Perry B, et al. Determination of the sum of bilirubin sugar conjugates in plasma by bilirubin oxidase. Clin Chem 1999;45:1255–60.
13. El-Beshbishi SN, Shattuck KE, Mohammad AA, Petersen JR. Hyperbilirubinemia and transcutaneous bilirubinometry. Clin Chem 2009;55:1280–7.
14. Fairbanks VF, Beutler E. Iron metabolism. In: Beutler E, Lichtman MA, Coller BS, et al, eds. Williams hematology. New York: McGraw-Hill, 2001:295–304.
15. Fairbanks VF, Brandhagen DJ. Disorders of iron storage and transport. In: Beutler E, Lichtman MA, Coller BS, et al, eds. Williams hematology. New York: McGraw-Hill, 2001:489–502.

16. Higgins T, Eckfeldt JH, Barton JC, Doumas BT. Hemoglobin, iron, and bilirubin. In: Burtis CA, Ashwood ER, Bruns DE, eds. Tietz textbook of clinical chemistry and molecular diagnostics. Philadelphia: Elsevier, 2012:985–1030.

17. Joutovsky A, Hadzi-Nesic J, Nardi MA. HPLC retention time as a diagnostic tool for hemoglobin variants and hemoglobinopathies: a study of 60,000 samples in a clinical diagnostic laboratory. Clin Chem 2004;50:1736–47.

18. Kakhlon O, Cabantchik ZI. The labile iron pool: characterization, measurement, and participation in cellular processes. Free Radic Biol Med 2002;33:1037–46.

19. Kazmierczak S, Bhutani V, Gourley G, et al. Transcutaneous bilirubin testing. In: Laboratory medicine practice guideline: evidence-based practice for point-of-care testing. Washington, DC: AACC Press, 2007:5–12.

20. Lafferty JD, Crowther MA, Ali MA, Levine ML. The evaluation of various mathematical RBC indices and their efficiency in discriminating between thalassemic and non-thalassemic microcytosis. Am J Clin Pathol 1996;106:201–5.

21. Lo SF, Jendrzejczak B, Doumas BT. Bovine serum-based bilirubin calibrators are inappropriate for some diazo methods. Clin Chem 2010;56:869–72.

22. Olynyk JK, Cullen DJ, Aquilia S, et al. A population-based study of the clinical expression of the hemochromatosis gene. N Engl J Med 1999;341:718–24.

23. Ou CN, Rognerud CL. Diagnosis of hemoglobinopathies: electrophoresis vs. HPLC. Clin Chem Acta 2001;313:187–94.

24. Pietrangelo A. Hereditary hemochromatosis—a new look at an old disease. N Engl J Med 2004;350:2383–97.

25. Shayeghi M, Latunde-Dada GO, Oakhill JS, et al. Identification of an intestinal heme transporter. Cell 2005;122:789–801.

Porphyrins and Porphyrias

Michael N. Badminton, M.B.Ch.B., Ph.D., F.R.C.Path., Sharon D. Whatley, Ph.D.,
Allan C. Deacon, Ph.D., F.R.C.Path., and George H. Elder, M.D., F.R.C.P., F.R.C.Path.

Objectives

1. Define the following terms:

    5-Aminolevulinic   Porphyrin

    Amino acid   Porphobilinogen (PBG)

    Ferrochelatase   Porphyria

    Heme   Zinc protoporphyrin

2. Summarize the biosynthetic pathway of heme, including intracellular sites of each synthetic step, rate-limiting step, and enzyme, and incorporation into hemoglobin.

3. List six functions of heme.

4. Compare and contrast the acute and nonacute porphyrias, including causes, symptoms, and laboratory analyses; describe the screening tests that differentiate between the two categories of porphyria.

5. List and categorize seven porphyrias; state the major elevated intermediates involved in each.

6. List the abnormalities of porphyrin metabolism that are unrelated to porphyria.

7. Explain the effects of lead toxicity on the heme biosynthetic pathway and on iron status.

8. List the specimen collection and storage requirements for samples undergoing porphyrin analysis.

9. Describe the laboratory methods of analysis for the following:

    Porphobilinogen   Porphyrins in urine, stool,

    5-Aminolevulinic acid   blood, and plasma

        DNA assessments

10. Analyze and solve case studies related to abnormal porphyrin metabolism and lead toxicity.

Key Words anda Definitions

Acute porphyrias Inherited disorders of heme biosynthesis, characterized by acute attacks of neurovisceral symptoms; potentially life threatening; diagnosed by elevated urine PBG.

Acute intermittent porphyria (AIP) An autosomal dominant hepatic porphyria caused by mutation in the *HMBS* gene (locus: 11q23.3), which encodes hydroxymethylbilane synthase.

5-Aminolevulinic acid (ALA) Immediate precursor of porphobilinogen; two molecules of ALA combine to form one molecule of porphobilinogen.

Congenital erythropoietic porphyria (CEP) An autosomal recessive porphyria due to mutation in the *UROS* gene (locus: 10q25.2-q26.3), which encodes uroporphyrinogen-III synthase.

Coproporphyrin A porphyrin with four methyl and four propionic acid sidechains attached to the tetrapyrrole backbone.

Cutaneous porphyrias Disorders of heme biosynthesis in which accumulations of porphyrins in the skin cause skin damage on exposure to sunlight.

Erythropoietic protoporphyria (EPP) An autosomal dominant disorder due to mutation in the *FECH* gene (locus: 18q21.3), which encodes ferrochelatase, causing a partial deficiency of the enzyme.

Ferrochelatase (FECH) A mitochondrial enzyme of the lyase class that catalyzes the insertion of ferrous iron into protoporphyrin IX to form protoheme IX, the heme of hemoglobin.

Hereditary coproporphyria (HCP) An autosomal dominant hepatic porphyria caused by mutations of the *CPOX* gene (locus: 3q12) that result in partial deficiency of coproporphyrinogen oxidase activity

Porphobilinogen (PBG) Immediate precursor of the porphyrins; a pyrrole ring with acetyl, propionyl, vinyl, and aminomethyl sidechains; four molecules of PBG condense to form one molecule of 1-hydroxymethylbilane, which is then converted successively to uroporphyrinogen-III, coproporphyrinogen-III, protoporphyrinogen-IX, protoporphyrin-IX, and heme.

Porphyrins Any of a group of compounds containing the porphyrin structure; four pyrrole rings connected by methylene bridges in a cyclical configuration, to which a variety of sidechains are attached.

Porphyrias A group of mainly inherited metabolic disorders that result from partial deficiencies of the enzymes of heme biosynthesis, which cause increased formation and excretion of porphyrins, their precursors, or both.

Key Words and Definitions—cont'd

Porphyria cutanea tarda (PCT) The most common form of porphyria, characterized by cutaneous photosensitivity.

Porphyrin precursors ALA and PBG, the biosynthetic intermediates, are metabolized to porphyrinogens and porphyrins.

Protoporphyrin A porphyrin with four methyl, two vinyl, and two propionic acid sidechains attached to the tetrapyrrole backbone; the protoporphyrin-IX//iron complex; heme is the prosthetic group of hemoglobin, cytochromes, and other hemoproteins.

Upregulation A process that results in an increase in the number of receptors on the surface of target cells, making the cells more sensitive to a hormone or another agent. Downregulation is a decrease in the number of receptors on the surface of target cells.

Uroporphyrin A porphyrin with four acetic acid and four propionic acid sidechains attached to the tetrapyrrole backbone.

Variegate porphyria (VP) An autosomal dominant hepatic porphyria due to mutation in the *PPOX* gene (locus: 1q22), which encodes protoporphyrinogen oxidase.

X-linked protoporphyria (XLDPP) A rare genetic disorder characterized by an abnormal sensitivity to the sun (photosensitivity).

Zinc protoporphyrin (ZPP) A normal but minor by-product of heme biosynthesis found in the red blood cell; when insufficient Fe^{2+} is available for heme biosynthesis, increased ZPP is formed.

The **porphyrias** are a group of diseases characterized by either deficiency in one of the enzymes of heme biosynthesis, leading to the overproduction of intermediates of the pathway or, in one rare disorder, an increase in activity of the rate-controlling enzyme of erythroid heme synthesis.[1,17] These intermediates are excreted in excessive amounts in (1) urine, (2) feces, or (3) both. The clinical consequences depend on the nature of the heme precursors that accumulate. In the **acute porphyrias**, excess **porphyrin precursors (5-aminolevulinic acid [ALA]** and **porphobilinogen [PBG])** are associated with potentially fatal acute neurovisceral attacks, which are often provoked by (1) a number of commonly prescribed or illicit drugs, (2) hormonal factors, (3) alcohol, (4) starvation, (5) stress, or (6) infection. In the nonacute porphyrias, and in those acute porphyrias in which the skin may be affected, accumulation of porphyrins results in photosensitization and skin lesions. Diagnosis depends on laboratory investigation to demonstrate the pattern of heme precursor accumulation specific for each type of porphyria. This requires examination of appropriate specimens for key metabolites using adequately sensitive and specific methods.

Technical advances in the field of molecular genetics have made it possible to investigate all porphyrias at the molecular level. Although not essential for diagnosis of symptomatic cases, these techniques are important for the investigation of families with porphyria.

1 through 8. Variation in the distribution of the same substituents around the peripheral positions of the tetrapyrrole ring gives rise to porphyrin isomers, which are usually depicted by Roman numerals (I, II, III, etc.). The reduced form of a porphyrin, known as a porphyrinogen (see Figure 29-1), differs by the presence of six additional hydrogens (four on the methylene bridges and two on the ring nitrogens). Porphyrinogens are unstable in vitro and are spontaneously oxidized to the corresponding porphyrins. Under the lower oxygen tension of the cell, porphyrinogens are stable and form intermediates of the heme biosynthetic pathway; aromatization to **protoporphyrin** at the penultimate step requires an enzyme.

Chelation of Metals

The arrangement of four nitrogen atoms at the center of the porphyrin ring enables porphyrins to chelate various metal ions. Protoporphyrin that contains iron is known as heme; ferroheme refers specifically to the Fe^{2+} complex and ferriheme to Fe^{3+}. Ferriheme associated with a chloride counter ion is known as *hemin*, or hematin when the counter ion is hydroxide.

Spectral Properties

Porphyrins were named from the Greek root for "purple" (*porphyra*) and owe their color to the conjugated double-bond structure of the tetrapyrrole ring. The porphyrinogens

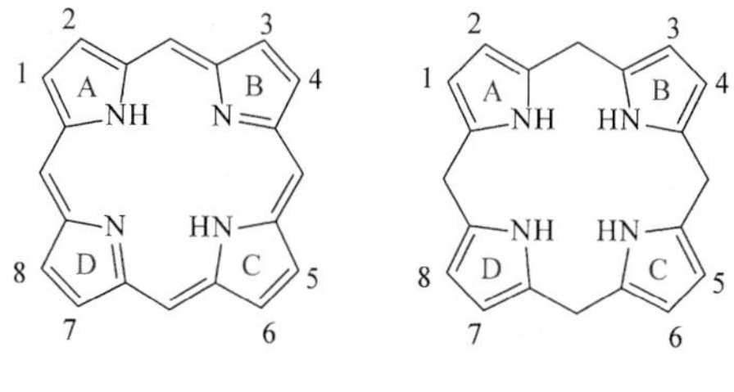

Porphyrin and Heme Chemistry

In this section, porphyrin (1) structure, (2) nomenclature, and (3) chemical characteristics are reviewed.

Porphyrin Structure and Nomenclature

The basic **porphyrin** structure consists of four monopyrrole rings connected by methene bridges to form a tetrapyrrole ring (Figure 29-1). Many porphyrin compounds are known, but only a limited number are of clinical interest. The porphyrin compounds of relevance to the porphyrias (Table 29-1) differ in the substituents occupying peripheral positions

Figure 29-1 Representations of porphyrin and porphyrinogen. Numbering system and ring designations are based on the Fischer system.

TABLE 29-1   Substituents Around the Macrocycle in Porphyrins of Clinical Importance

Porphyrin	Position							
	1	2	3	4	5	6	7	8
Uroporphyrin-I	C_m	C_{et}	C_m	C_{et}	C_m	C_{et}	C_m	C_{et}
Uroporphyrin-III	C_m	C_{et}	C_m	C_{et}	C_m	C_{et}	C_{et}	C_m
Heptacarboxylate porphyrin-III	C_m	C_{et}	C_m	C_{et}	C_m	C_{et}	C_{et}	Me
Hexacarboxylate porphyrin-III	Me	C_{et}	C_m	C_{et}	C_m	C_{et}	C_{et}	Me
Pentacarboxylate porphyrin-III	Me	C_{et}	Me	C_{et}	C_m	C_{et}	C_{et}	Me
Coproporphyrin-III	Me	C_{et}	Me	C_{et}	Me	C_{et}	C_{et}	Me
Coproporphyrin-I	Me	C_{et}	Me	C_{et}	Me	C_{et}	Me	C_{et}
Isocoproporphyrin	Me	Et	Me	C_{et}	C_m	C_{et}	C_{et}	Me
Dehydroisocoproporphyrin	Me	Vn	Me	C_{et}	C_m	C_{et}	C_{et}	Me
Deethylisocoproporphyrin	Me	H	Me	C_{et}	C_m	C_{et}	C_{et}	Me
Protoporphyrin	Me	Vn	Me	Vn	Me	C_{et}	C_{et}	Me
Pemptoporphyrin	Me	H	Me	Vn	Me	C_{et}	C_{et}	Me
Deuteroporphyrin	Me	H	Me	H	Me	C_{et}	C_{et}	Me
Mesoporphyrin	Me	Et	Me	Et	Me	C_{et}	C_{et}	Me

C_m, carboxymethyl (—CH_2COOH); C_{et}, C_{et}, carboxyethyl (—CH_2CH_2COOH); Me, methyl (—CH_3); Et, ethyl (—CH_2CH_3); Vn, vinyl (—$CH_2 = CH_3$).

have no conjugated double bonds and are colorless. Porphyrins show a particularly strong absorbance near 400 nm, often called the *Soret band*. When exposed to light in the 400-nm region, porphyrins display a characteristic orange-red fluorescence in the range of 550 to 650 nm. Absorbance and fluorescence are altered by substituents around the porphyrin ring and by metal binding. Zinc chelation shifts the fluorescence peak of protoporphyrin to shorter wavelengths and reduces the fluorescence intensity. The strong binding of iron alters the character of protoporphyrin to the extent that heme lacks significant fluorescence.

Solubility

Porphyrins are only marginally soluble in water. The differing solubilities of individual porphyrins are of importance not only in the design of analytical methods for their extraction and fractionation but in determination of the route of excretion from the body. At pH 7, the carboxyl groups are ionized, and the molecule has a net negative charge. Below pH 2, the pyrrole nitrogens and the carboxyl groups become protonated so that the molecule has a net positive charge.

At physiological pH, the solubility of a given porphyrin is determined by the number of substituent carboxyl groups. For example, **uroporphyrin** has eight carboxylate groups and is the most soluble porphyrin in aqueous media. As protoporphyrin has only two carboxylate groups, it is essentially insoluble in water but dissolves readily in lipid environments and binds readily to the hydrophobic regions of proteins, such as albumin. **Coproporphyrin**, with four carboxylate groups, has intermediate solubility.

Porphyrin Precursors

ALA and PBG are known as porphyrin precursors (Figure 29-2). ALA is sometimes referred to as aminolevulinate (to emphasize its ionic nature at physiological pH). PBG contains a single pyrrole ring (unlike porphyrins, which contain four)

and is often referred to as a *monopyrrole*. PBG polymerizes readily, particularly at high concentrations in acid solution to form primarily the I-isomer of uroporphyrin. Both ALA and PBG are highly water soluble.

Heme Biosynthesis

The complex tetrapyrrole ring structure of heme is built up in a stepwise fashion from the very simple precursors succinyl-coenzyme A (CoA) and glycine (see Figure 29-2).[1] The pathway is present in all nucleated cells, and it has been estimated that daily synthesis of heme in humans consists of 5 to 8 mmol/kg body weight. The pathway is compartmentalized, with some steps occurring in the mitochondrion and others in the cytoplasm. No transport defect has yet been reported in the porphyrias.

5-Aminolevulinate Synthase (EC 2.3.1.37), ALAS

ALAS is the initial enzyme of the pathway with a housekeeping (ALAS1) and an erythroid (ALAS2) isozyme; it catalyzes the formation of ALA from succinyl-CoA and glycine. The enzyme is mitochondrial and requires pyridoxal phosphate as a cofactor, which forms a Schiff base with the amino group of glycine at the enzyme surface. The carbanion of the Schiff base displaces CoA from succinyl-CoA with the formation of α-amino-β-ketoadipic acid, which is then decarboxylated to ALA. The activity of ALAS is rate limiting as long as the catalytic capacities of other enzymes in the pathway are normal.

5-Aminolevulinic Acid Dehydratase (EC 4.2.1.24), ALAD

ALAD (also known as *porphobilinogen synthase*) is a cytoplasmic enzyme that catalyzes the formation of the monopyrrole PBG from two molecules of ALA with elimination of two molecules of water. The enzyme requires zinc ions as a cofactor and reduced sulfhydryl groups at the active site and is therefore susceptible to inhibition by lead.

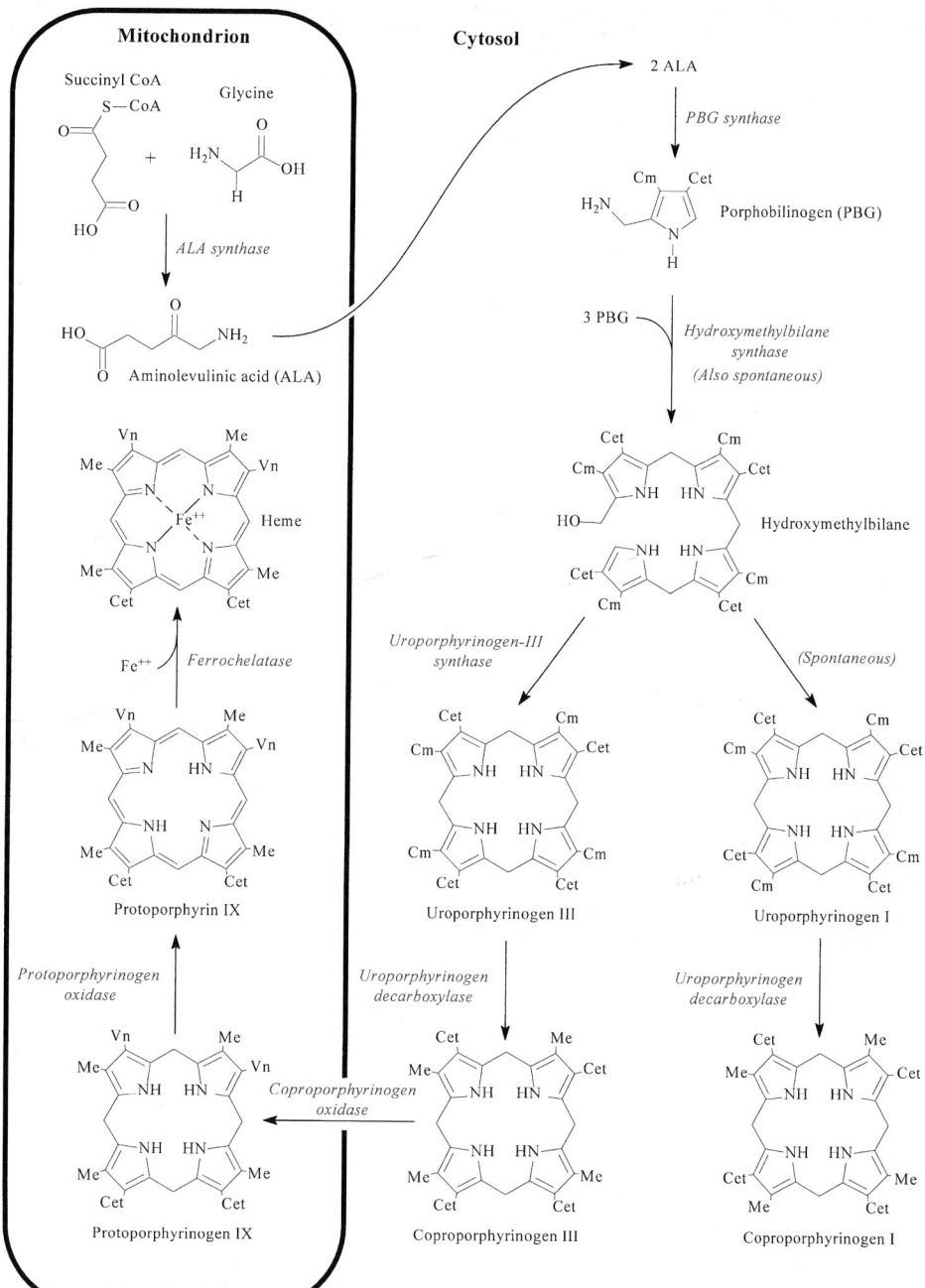

Figure 29-2 Biosynthetic pathway of porphyrins and heme. C_{et}, $-CH_2CH_2COOH$; C_m, $-CH_2COOH$; Me, $-CH_3$; Vn, $-CH=CH_2$.

Hydroxymethylbilane Synthase (EC 2.5.1.61), HMBS

HMBS (also known as *PBG deaminase*) is a cytoplasmic enzyme that catalyzes the formation of one molecule of the linear tetrapyrrole 1-hydroxymethylbilane (HMB; also known as *pre-uroporphyrinogen*) from four molecules of PBG with the release of four molecules of ammonia. The enzyme is susceptible to allosteric inhibition by intermediates farther down the heme biosynthetic pathway, notably coproporphyrinogen-III and protoporphyrinogen-IX.[16]

Uroporphyrinogen-III Synthase (EC 4.2.1.75), UROS

UROS is a cytoplasmic enzyme that rearranges and cyclizes HMB to form uroporphyrinogen-III. Each pyrrole ring of

HMB contains methylcarboxylate and ethylcarboxylate substituents, which are in the same orientation. By the rotation of (1) no, (2) one, or (3) two alternate pyrrole rings or (4) two adjacent pyrrole rings, it is possible to arrive at four different isomers (I to IV). Apart from closing the ring structure, the enzyme rotates the D-ring via a spirane intermediate, producing the type III isomer—this rotation is vital because only the type III isomer contributes to heme biosynthesis. HMB is unstable, and in those porphyrias in which excess HMB accumulates, cyclization occurs non-enzymatically with formation of the type I isomer. Normally, only minimal amounts of uroporphyrinogen-I are formed.

Uroporphyrinogen Decarboxylase (EC 4.1.1.37), UROD

This last cytoplasmic enzyme in the pathway catalyzes the decarboxylation of all four carboxymethyl groups to form the tetracarboxylic coproporphyrinogen. The enzyme uses both I and III isomers of uroporphyrinogen as substrate. Decarboxylation commences on ring D and proceeds stepwise through rings A, B, and C with formation of heptacarboxylate, hexacarboxylate, and pentacarboxylate intermediates at a single active site. A UROD deficiency causes accumulation of these intermediates in addition to its substrate, uroporphyrinogen. At high substrate concentrations, decarboxylation occurs by a random mechanism.

Coproporphyrinogen Oxidase (EC 1.3.3.3), CPOX

CPOX is situated in the intermembrane space of mitochondria and catalyzes the sequential oxidative decarboxylation of the 2- and 4-carboxyethyl groups to vinyl groups to produce the more lipophilic protoporphyrinogen-IX, with formation of a tricarboxylic intermediate, harderoporphyrinogen. Oxygen is required as the oxidant. The enzyme requires sulfhydryl groups for activity, making it a target for inhibition by metals. The enzyme is specific for the type III isomer, so that metabolism of the I-series of porphyrins does not occur beyond coproporphyrinogen-I. The product of the enzyme differs from the substrate in that replacement of two of the carboxyethyl groups by vinyl groups has introduced a third substituent into the molecule. Therefore the number of possible isomeric forms increases, and conventionally the numbering system changes, so that the III isomer becomes the IX isomer. In UROD-deficient states, one of the ethylcarboxylate groups of accumulated pentacarboxylate porphyrinogen is decarboxylated by an unknown mechanism to form the isocoproporphyrin series of porphyrins.

Protoporphyrinogen Oxidase (EC 1.3.3.4), PPOX

PPOX is a flavoprotein located in the inner mitochondrial membrane that catalyzes the removal of six hydrogens (four from methylene bridges and two from ring nitrogens) to form protoporphyrin IX. Nonenzymatic oxidation also occurs in vitro. However, under the oxygen tension in the cell, PPOX is essential for the oxidation to occur. The protoporphyrin produced is the only porphyrin that functions in the heme pathway. Other porphyrins are produced by nonenzymatic oxidation and represent porphyrinogens that have irreversibly escaped from the pathway.

Ferrochelatase (EC 4.99.1.1)

Ferrochelatase (FECH/also known as *heme synthase*) is an iron-sulfur protein located in the inner mitochondrial membrane. This enzyme inserts ferrous iron into protoporphyrin to form heme. During this process, two hydrogens are displaced from the ring nitrogens. Other metals in the divalent state will also act as substrate, yielding the corresponding chelate (e.g., incorporation of Zn^{2+} into protoporphyrin to yield **zinc protoporphyrin [ZPP]**). In iron-deficient states Zn^{2+} successfully competes with Fe^{2+} in developing red cells, so that the concentration of zinc protoporphyrin in erythrocytes

is increased. Furthermore, other dicarboxylic porphyrins will also serve as substrates (e.g., mesoporphyrin).

Function of Heme

Heme functions as a prosthetic group in various proteins in which, depending on the function of the protein, the iron shifts freely between different valence states. Seventy percent to 80% of heme synthesis occurs in the bone marrow, and approximately an additional 15% in the liver. Heme-containing proteins participate in a variety of redox reactions, including:

1. Oxygen transport (by hemoglobin in the blood) and storage (by myoglobin in muscle)
2. Mitochondrial respiration (by cytochromes b_1, c_1, and a_3)
3. Enzymatic destruction of peroxides (by catalase and peroxidase)
4. Drug metabolism (by microsomal cytochrome P-450 mixed function oxidases)
5. Desaturation of fatty acids (by microsomal cytochrome b_5)
6. Tryptophan metabolism (by tryptophan oxygenase)

Reactions of nitric oxide (NO) are often mediated by the reaction of heme with NO in control enzymes such as guanylate cyclase.

Other naturally occurring tetrapyrrole derivatives include vitamin B_{12} and chlorophyll, each of which contains an atom of chelated cobalt and magnesium, respectively.

Excretion of Heme Precursors

Normally, only minute amounts of heme precursors accumulate in the body. The route of excretion largely depends on solubility. The porphyrin precursors ALA and PBG are water soluble and are excreted almost exclusively in urine. Uroporphyrinogen, with eight carboxylate groups, is readily water soluble and is also excreted via the kidney. The last intermediate of the pathway, protoporphyrin and protoporphyrinogen, is excreted in the feces via the biliary tract. The other porphyrins are of intermediate solubility and appear in both urine and feces. Coproporphyrinogen-I is taken up and excreted by the liver in preference to the III isomer so that coproporphyrinogen-I predominates in feces and coproporphyrinogen-III in urine. All porphyrinogens in the urine or feces are slowly oxidized to the corresponding porphyrins.

Once in the gut, porphyrins are susceptible to modification by gut flora. The two vinyl groups of protoporphyrins are (1) reduced to ethyl groups, (2) hydrated to hydroxyethyl groups, or (3) removed, giving rise to a variety of secondary porphyrins. Gut flora also metabolizes heme to produce a variety of dicarboxylic porphyrins. Furthermore, some bacteria are capable of de novo synthesis of porphyrins.

Regulation of Heme Biosynthesis

Heme supply in all tissues is controlled by the activity of mitochondrial ALAS, the first enzyme of the pathway. Two isoforms of ALAS are known. The ubiquitous isoform, ALAS1, is encoded by a gene on chromosome 3p21 and is expressed in all tissue. Because it has a half-life of approximately an hour, changes in its rate of synthesis produce short-term alterations in enzyme concentration and cellular ALAS activity.

Synthesis of ALAS1 is under negative feedback control by heme. In the liver, ALAS1 is induced by a wide range of drugs and chemicals that induce microsomal cytochrome P-450–dependent oxidases (CYPs). This effect is thought to be mediated primarily by direct transcriptional activation by drug-responsive nuclear receptors rather than being secondary to depletion of an intracellular regulatory heme pool. Induction of ALAS1 is prevented by heme, which acts by destabilizing messenger ribonucleic acid (mRNA) for ALAS1, by blocking mitochondrial import of pre-ALAS1, and possibly by inhibiting transcription.

The erythroid isoform, ALAS2, is encoded by a gene on chromosome Xq21-22 and is expressed only in erythroid cells. Its activity is regulated by two main mechanisms. One: Transcription is enhanced during erythroid differentiation by the action of erythroid-specific transcription factors. Two: mRNA concentrations are regulated by iron. Iron deficiency in erythroid cells promotes specific binding of iron regulatory proteins to an iron-responsive element in the 5′ untranslated region (UTR) of ALAS2 mRNA with consequent inhibition of translation.

Primary Porphyrin Disorders

The porphyrias are a group of metabolic disorders that result from partial deficiencies of the enzymes of heme biosynthesis, or in one disorder, a gain of function mutation[18] (Table 29-2). All are inherited in monogenic patterns, except some forms of **porphyria cutanea tarda (PCT)** and rare types of erythropoietic porphyria. Large numbers of disease-specific mutations have now been identified in each of the genes encoding the defective enzymes (www.hgmd.cf.ac.uk/; accessed October 29, 2013). Each type of porphyria is defined by the association of characteristic clinical features with a specific pattern of accumulation of heme precursors. These patterns reflect increased formation of substrates for the enzyme that is deficient in that type of porphyria (Table 29-3).

The porphyrias are characterized clinically by two main features: skin lesions on sun-exposed areas and acute neurovisceral attacks, typically comprising (1) abdominal pain,

(2) peripheral neuropathy, and (3) mental disturbance. The skin lesions are caused by porphyrin-catalyzed photo damage, of which singlet oxygen is the main mediator. Acute attacks are associated with increased formation of ALA from induced activity of hepatic ALAS1 and partial hepatic heme deficiency, often in response to induction of hepatic CYPs by drugs and other factors. The relationship of these biochemical changes to the neuronal dysfunction that underlies all clinical features of the acute attack is uncertain.

As listed in Table 29-2, the porphyrias are categorized as (1) acute porphyrias, in which acute neurovisceral attacks occur, and (2) nonacute porphyrias.

Acute Porphyrias

Acute porphyrias include (1) acute intermittent porphyria (AIP), (2) **variegate porphyria (VP)**, and (3) **hereditary coproporphyria (HCP)**. The inherited defect in autosomal dominant acute porphyrias is a mutation leading to complete or near complete inactivation of one of the pairs of allelic genes that encode the enzyme whose partial deficiency causes the disorder. Enzyme activities are therefore half normal in all tissue in which they are expressed, reflecting the activity of the normal gene *trans* to the mutant allele. Heme supply is maintained at healthy or near healthy amounts by **upregulation** of ALAS with a consequent increase in the substrate concentration of the defective enzyme. These compensatory changes vary between tissues and are most prominent in the liver and undetectable in most other organs. These changes also vary between individuals with (1) some showing no evidence of overproduction of heme precursors and (2) some biochemically manifesting disease. Low clinical penetrance is a prominent feature of all the autosomal dominant acute porphyrias. Family studies indicate that about 80% of affected individuals are asymptomatic throughout life. Long-term complications of acute porphyria include chronic renal failure, hypertension, and hepatocellular carcinoma.[1,17]

In AIP the primary defect is a deficiency of HMBS, which results in accumulation of its substrate PBG (and to a lesser

Disorder	Defective Enzyme	Prevalence*	Neurovisceral Crises	Skin Lesions	Inheritance
Acute Porphyrias					
ALA dehydratase deficiency porphyria (ALADP)	ALAD	Very rare	+	—	AR
Acute intermittent porphyria (AIP)	HMBS	1-2:100,000	+	—	AD
Hereditary coproporphyria (HCP)	CPO	1-2:1,000,000	+	+†,‡	AD
Variegate porphyria (VP)	PPOX	1:250,000	+	+†,‡	AD
Nonacute Porphyrias					
Congenital erythropoietic porphyria (CEP)	UROS	1:3,000,000	—	+‡	AR
Porphyria cutanea tarda (PCT)	UROD	1:25,000	—	+‡	Complex (20% AD)
Erythropoietic protoporphyria (EPP)	FECH	1:140,000	—	+§	AR
X-linked dominant protoporphyria	ALAS2	1:3,000,000	—	+§	X linked

TABLE 29-2 The Main Types of Human Porphyria

AD, Autosomal dominant; *AR*, autosomal recessive.
*Estimated prevalence of clinically overt disease in the United Kingdom.
†Skin lesions and neurovisceral crises may occur alone or together.
‡Fragile skin, bullae.
§Acute photosensitivity without fragile skin, bullae.

TABLE 29-3   The Porphyrias: Patterns of Overproduction of Heme Precursors During Clinically Overt Phase of Disease

Porphyria	Urine PBG/ALA	Urine Porphyrins	Fecal Porphyrins	Erythrocyte Porphyrins	Plasma Fluorescence Emission Peak
ALADP	ALA	Copro-III	Not increased	Zn-proto	—
AIP	PBG > ALA	Mainly uroporphyrin from PBG	Normal, or slight increase in Copro, ProtoProto[*]	Not increased	615-620 nm[†]
CEP	Not increased	Uro-I, Copro-I	Copro-I	Zn-proto, Proto, Copro-I, Uro-I	615-620 nm
PCT	Not increased	Uro, Hepta[‡]	Isocopro, Hepta[‡]	Not increased	615-620 nm
HCP	PBG > ALA[§]	Copro-III, uroporphyrin from PBG	Copro-III	Not increased	615-620 nm[†]
VP	PBG > ALA[§]	Copro-III, uroporphyrin from PBG	Proto-IX > Copro-III, X-porphyrin	Not increased	624-628 nm
EPP	Not increased	Not increased	±Proto±Proto[∥]	Proto	626-634 nm[¶]
XLDPP	Not increased	Not increased	±Proto	Zn-proto, Proto,	626-634 nm[¶]

[*]Total porphyrin may be increased because of the presence of excess uroporphyrin.
[†]Not always increased during acute attack.
[‡]Other methylcarboxylate substituted porphyrins are increased to a smaller extent; uroporphyrin is a mixture of type I and III isomers; heptacarboxylate porphyrin is mainly type III.
[§]PBG and ALA may be normal when only skin lesions are present.
[∥]Not increased in about 40% of patients.
[¶]Protoporphyrin[¶] bound to globin (if hemolysis is in the sample) has a peak at 626 to 628 nm.

extent ALA). In VP and HCP inherited deficiencies of enzymes further down the pathway lead to the accumulation of porphyrinogens, which are potent allosteric inhibitors of HMBS,[16] and lead to secondary accumulation of PBG (and ALA). In the very rare recessive disorder ALADP (ALA dehydratase deficiency porphyria), an inherited deficiency of ALAD leads to accumulation of ALA and coproporphyrin-III but not PBG.

The life-threatening, acute neurovisceral attacks that occur in AIP, VP, and HCP are clinically identical.[17] Acute attacks are more common in women, usually occurring first between the ages of 15 and 40 years. They are very rare before puberty.

Acute attacks of porphyrias almost always start with abdominal pain that rapidly becomes very severe. However, they are not accompanied by *peritonism* or other signs of an acute surgical condition. Pain may also be present in the back and thighs and may occasionally be most severe in these regions. Signs of autonomic neuropathy, such as (1) vomiting, (2) constipation, (3) tachycardia, and (4) hypertension, are frequent. When convulsions occur, they are often caused by hyponatremia. Pain may resolve within a few days, but in severe cases a predominant motor neuropathy develops that may progress to flaccid quadriparesis (weakness of both arms and both legs). Persistent pain and vomiting may lead to weight loss and malnutrition. The acute phase may be accompanied by mental confusion with abrupt changes in (1) mood, (2) hallucinations, and (3) other psychotic features. However, these mental disturbances disappear with remission. Persistent psychiatric illness is not a feature of the acute porphyrias, although mild anxiety or depression may be present in some patients. Abdominal pain usually resolves within 2 weeks, but recovery from neuropathy may take many months and is not always complete. In fact, most patients have one or a few attacks followed by complete recovery and prolonged remission. About 5% have repeated acute attacks that in women may be premenstrual.

Precipitating factors have been identified in about two-thirds of patients who have acute attacks. The most important are (1) drugs, (2) alcohol, especially binge drinking, (3) the menstrual cycle, (4) calorie restriction, (5) infection, and (6) stress. Although pregnancy is typically uncomplicated in acute porphyria patients, acute attacks can occasionally occur. Drugs known to provoke acute attacks include (1) barbiturates, (2) sulfonamides, (3) progestogens, and (4) many anticonvulsants, but many others have been implicated in the precipitation of acute attacks[1] (www.porphyria-europe.org/; accessed October 29, 2013). Many of these precipitating factors induce hepatic CYPs.

Skin lesions similar to those of PCT and other bullous porphyrias are present in about 80% of patients with clinically manifest VP (see Table 29-2). About 60% of patients with this condition have skin lesions alone. The skin is less commonly affected in HCP; skin lesions without an acute attack are uncommon and are usually provoked by intercurrent cholestasis.

Nonacute Porphyrias

These fall into two categories, depending upon whether patients have (1) bullous skin lesions or (2) acute photosensitivity.

Nonacute Porphyrias with Bullous Skin Lesions

These include PCT and **congenital erythropoietic porphyria (CEP)**. In addition the acute porphyrias, VP and HCP, may have identical skin lesions. Lesions on sun-exposed skin, particularly the (1) backs of the hands, (2) forearm, and (3) face, are present in all patients. Increased mechanical fragility of the skin, with trivial trauma leading to erosions, and subepidermal bullae are present in virtually all patients. Hypertrichosis (excess growth of hair) of the face and patchy pigmentation are also common. Erosions and bullae heal slowly to leave

(1) atrophic scars, (2) milia (small, white or yellowish cyst-like masses just below the surface of the skin), and (3) depigmentated areas.

CEP is a rare condition that usually occurs in early childhood and is transmitted in an autosomal recessive manner. The skin lesions resemble those of PCT, VP, and HCP but are more severe and persistent throughout life. With advancing age, progressive scarring, particularly if erosions become infected, and atrophic changes lead to photomutilation with erosions of the terminal phalanges; destruction of ears, nose, and eyelids; and alopecia. Accumulation of porphyrin in bone is visible as erythrodontia—brownish-red teeth that fluoresce red in ultraviolet A (UVA) light. Hemolytic anemia with splenomegaly is common in CEP. Hemolysis may be fully compensated or mild, but in some patients, anemia is severe enough to require repeated transfusion.

PCT is the most common of all the porphyrias, usually occurring during the fifth and sixth decades, with most patients having evidence of liver cell damage, usually minor, and some degree of hepatic siderosis (deposition of iron in tissue). PCT results from a decrease in activity of UROD in the liver, which leads to overproduction of uroporphyrinogen and other carboxymethyl-substituted porphyrinogens. Two main types of PCT are identified by measurement of UROD activity in liver and extrahepatic tissue, or by analysis of the UROD gene. About 80% of patients have the sporadic (type I) form of PCT in which the enzyme defect is restricted to the liver and the UROD gene appears to be normal. The rest have familial (type II) PCT. In this form, mutation of one UROD gene leads to half-normal UROD activity in all tissue, which is inherited in an autosomal dominant manner. In both types, clinically overt PCT is strongly associated with (1) alcohol abuse, (2) estrogens, (3) infection with hepatotropic viruses, particularly hepatitis C (HCV) and human immunodeficiency virus (HIV), (4) increased hepatic iron stores, and (5) mutations in the hemochromatosis (HFE) gene.[4] PCT may also be caused by exposure to certain polyhalogenated aromatic hydrocarbons, such as hexachlorobenzene and 2,3,7,8-tetrachlorodibenzo-p-dioxin.

Nonacute Porphyria with Acute Photosensitivity

Erythropoietic protoporphyria (EPP) and **X-linked dominant protoporphyria** (XLDPP) are characterized by lifelong acute photosensitivity caused by accumulation of protoporphyrin-IX in the skin.[12,18] The absence of (1) fragile skin, (2) subepidermal bullae, and (3) hypertrichosis distinguishes protoporphyria clinically from all other **cutaneous porphyrias.** Onset of acute photosensitivity typically occurs between the ages of 1 and 6 years, and both sexes are equally affected. Once a child within an EPP or XLDPP family reaches the age of 14, the risk of developing acute photosensitivity becomes very low. Onset during adult life is very rare; most cases have been associated with myelodysplasia and are caused by acquired somatic mutations of the FECH or ALAS2 gene in hematopoietic cells.

Exposure to sun is followed, usually within 5 to 30 minutes, by an intensely painful, burning, prickling, itching sensation in the skin, most frequently on the face and backs of the hands. Symptoms persist for several hours or occasionally for days and are not relieved by shielding the skin from light. Patients characteristically seek relief by plunging their hands into water or covering their skin with wet towels. Young children may become very distressed by the pain. The skin may appear normal throughout, although there is often erythema (redness of the skin), which may be followed by edematous swelling with crusting. These changes usually subside within a few hours, so that by the time the child reaches the doctor, there is nothing to be seen, and the episode may be dismissed as severe sunburn. Recurrent episodes lead to chronic skin changes that are often minor and hard to detect. Typical lesions are shallow linear scars over the bridge of the nose and elsewhere on the face; the skin may become thickened and waxy, especially over the knuckles. Symptoms tend to be more severe during spring and summer and may improve during pregnancy.

The most severe complication of EPP and XLDPP is progressive hepatic failure, which is caused by accumulation of protoporphyrin in the liver.[17,18] About 15% of patients have abnormal biochemical tests of liver function, particularly increased aspartate aminotransferase, but only about 2% develop liver failure. EPP may also increase the risk of cholelithiasis—the formation of gallstones being promoted by high concentrations of protoporphyrin in the bile.

In EPP, overproduction of protoporphyrin-IX results from decreased activity of FECH, whereas in XLDPP, gain-of-function mutations in *ALAS2*, usually deletions within the C-terminal region, lead to formation and accumulation of protoporphyrin in excess of the amount required for hemoglobinization. Although FECH activity is decreased in all tissue in EPP, as in XLDPP, the excess protoporphyrin is formed mainly in erythroid cells. XLDPP is inherited in an X-linked pattern with expression of disease in males and in most females. EPP is an autosomal recessive disease; most individuals are compound heterozygotes for an *FECH* mutation that abolishes or severely decreases FECH activity and a hypomorphic *FECH* IVS3-48C allele.[9] In about 4% of EPP families, clinically affected individuals are heteroallelic or homoallelic for rare *FECH* mutations. Patients in these families, as in XLDPP, are at greater risk of severe liver disease than those with a hypomorphic *FECH* allele. Most *FECH* mutations are restricted to one or a few families; more than 130 have been identified (www.hgmd.cf.ac.uk/; accessed October 29, 2013).

Abnormalities of Porphyrin Metabolism not Caused by Porphyria

Abnormalities of porphyrin metabolism or excretion or both may occur in the absence of porphyria. A number of other diseases need to be considered when data from patients in whom porphyria is suspected are interpreted. These include: (1) exposure to various toxins, (2) *hereditary tyrosinemia* type I (3) renal disorders, (4) hepatobiliary disorders, (5) hematological disorders, (6) dietary, bacterial, and gastrointestinal bleeding factors, and (7) pseudoporphyria.

Exposure to Lead and Other Toxins

Lead exposure increases urinary ALA and coproporphyrin-III excretion and causes accumulation of ZPP in erythrocytes. The definitive test for lead toxicity is measurement of blood lead, but occasionally lead exposure is responsible for porphyria-like symptoms and sometimes is an unexpected finding when patients are investigated for suspected porphyria.

Increased ALA excretion is secondary to inhibition of ALAD caused by lead displacing zinc at its catalytic center. Lead also leads to increased excretion of coproporphyrin-III in urine. CPO requires sulfhydryl groups for activity and so is potentially a target for inhibition by lead. However, if lead-induced coproporphyrinuria is caused by inhibition of this enzyme, then it is not clear why fecal excretion of coproporphyrin is not increased. Increased concentrations of red cell ZPP associated with lead exposure probably are not caused by inhibition of FECH because inhibition of this enzyme requires higher lead concentrations than are usually encountered after lead exposure. The current view is that lead exposure creates an intracellular iron deficiency (perhaps by affecting iron transport into the cell or inhibition of iron reductase) so that zinc replaces iron as a substrate for FECH. Once formed, erythrocyte ZPP remains elevated for the life of the red cell. Because the half-life of an erythrocyte is longer than that of blood lead, monitoring of lead workers requires both whole-blood lead and ZPP testing. ZPP measurement also offers the advantage that there is no interference from lead contamination via the skin when the blood sample is collected, especially if a finger-prick sample is used.

Secondary coproporphyrinuria also is caused by the toxic effects of (1) alcohol, (2) arsenic, (3) other heavy metals, and (4) various drugs.

Hereditary Tyrosinemia Type I

Succinylacetone, which accumulates in this disease, has a structural resemblance to ALA and is therefore a competitive inhibitor of ALAD. Consequently ALA accumulates, and excess amounts are excreted in urine. Patients with hereditary tyrosinemia suffer neurological crises very similar to attacks of acute porphyria.

Renal Disorders

Impaired glomerular function reduces the clearance of water-soluble porphyrins normally excreted in the urine. Furthermore, these porphyrins are poorly cleared by dialysis, and, as a consequence, concentrations of plasma porphyrins are raised in end-stage renal failure. Even in the absence of biochemical evidence of porphyria, dermatological problems commonly affect dialysis patients and often share common features with PCT such as (1) melanosis, (2) actinic elastosis, (3) fragility, and (4) bullae. The concentrations of plasma porphyrin found in dialysis patients are often much higher than normal but rarely approach those found in patients with the active skin lesions caused by PCT. The term "dialysis porphyria" has been coined for these patients, even though it is unlikely that raised porphyrins are responsible for the skin lesions. Genuine PCT may occur in dialysis patients, and some cases of dialysis porphyria in the literature have not been adequately investigated

to exclude PCT. Patients are often anuric, and without the benefit of urinary analysis, careful evaluation of plasma and fecal porphyrins is necessary to distinguish pseudoporphyria from PCT and acute porphyrias in which skin lesions may occur.

Hepatobiliary Disorders

In diseases such as (1) obstructive jaundice, (2) cholestatic jaundice, (3) hepatitis, and (4) cirrhosis, urinary excretion of predominantly coproporphyrin-I is increased because liver disease causes a diversion of the secretion of coproporphyrin-I from the biliary to the renal route.

In the Dubin-Johnson syndrome, urinary excretion of coproporphyrin-I is increased and excretion of coproporphyrin-III is reduced. In the Rotor syndrome, urinary excretion of coproporphyrin-I is increased with normal coproporphyrin-III excretion, and in Gilbert disease urinary excretion of both isomers is increased.

Hematological Disorders

In iron deficiency anemia, zinc acts as an alternative substrate for FECH, leading to increased ZPP. Increased red cell protoporphyrin (mostly ZPP) may also occur in (1) sideroblastic, (2) megaloblastic, and (3) hemolytic anemias.

Dietary, Bacterial, and Gastrointestinal Bleeding Factors

The dicarboxylic porphyrin fraction of feces contains protoporphyrin and other dicarboxylic porphyrins derived from it by bacterial reduction or removal of vinyl side groups. Additional protoporphyrin and other dicarboxylic porphyrins may be formed by the action of gut flora on heme-containing proteins derived from the diet or by gastrointestinal hemorrhage. Even minor gastrointestinal hemorrhage, particularly if it occurs high in the gut, which may not give rise to a positive occult blood test, greatly increases the concentration of dicarboxylic porphyrins in feces. Confusion with EPP may occur when associated iron deficiency increases erythrocyte total porphyrin, and skin lesions from some other causes are present, or with VP when coexisting liver disease causes coproporphyrinuria. Porphyria is excluded when no porphyrin fluorescence is detectable on fluorescence emission spectroscopy of plasma. Porphyrins may also come directly from the diet.

Pseudoporphyria

The term "pseudoporphyria" was originally applied to patients with PCT-like skin lesions in whom no abnormality of accumulation or excretion of porphyrins could be demonstrated.[10] Many drugs are potent photosensitizers and may produce porphyria-like lesions.

Laboratory Diagnosis of Porphyria

A number of clinical situations are known to benefit from laboratory testing for porphyrins and precursors. These include patients with symptoms of (1) acute porphyria or (2) typical cutaneous lesions, and (3) relatives of patients known to have porphyria.

Patients with Symptoms of Porphyria

The clinical features of the porphyrias are not specific enough to enable their diagnosis without laboratory investigation. In patients with current symptoms caused by porphyria, it is always possible to demonstrate excessive production of porphyrins and/or porphyrin precursors. Diagnosis depends on demonstrating specific patterns of overproduction of heme precursors (see Table 29-3) and is usually straightforward, provided appropriate specimens are examined for the relevant intermediates using adequately sensitive techniques.[3,6] DNA and enzyme studies (1) give no information about disease activity, (2) are rarely necessary to confirm the diagnosis in clinically overt porphyria, and (3) are mainly useful for family studies.

Patients with Acute Neurovisceral Symptoms

The single essential investigation in patients with suspected acute porphyria is an adequately sensitive test for excess urinary PBG.[3,6] Failure to correctly diagnose an attack of acute porphyria not only delays appropriate life-saving treatment, but may lead to unnecessary surgery or the administration of porphyrinogenic drugs. Either of these risky medical interventions may further aggravate the attack with potentially fatal consequences. A false diagnosis of porphyria may be just as serious by delaying vital surgery or other treatment and may lead to analgesic (e.g., opiates) misuse and dependency.

During an attack, PBG excretion is grossly elevated, and the increase is usually in excess of 10 times the upper reference limit. Normal PBG, at a time when symptoms are present, excludes all acute porphyrias, except the very rare ALADP, as its cause. In AIP, PBG usually remains elevated for years after an attack.[14] However, in VP or HCP, PBG may rapidly return to normal (sometimes within days) once the attack starts to resolve, although urine porphyrin excretion will still be increased. Therefore, if a suspected attack is entering remission, or clinical suspicion of acute porphyria persists, analysis of fecal and plasma porphyrins, with measurement of ALA if these are normal, is advisable even if PBG excretion is normal. Increased urinary PBG requires careful evaluation; although the patient clearly has an acute porphyria, the disease may not be the cause of current symptoms. Some patients with AIP have very high rates of PBG excretion in the absence of symptoms, and there is poor correlation between urinary PBG and symptoms, with no "threshold" above which symptoms appear. PBG excretion increases during an acute attack, but detection of this change requires information about the patient's baseline excretion. The higher the urinary PBG excretion, the greater the likelihood that porphyria is responsible for symptoms; however, the final diagnosis must always be made on clinical grounds.

If elevated urinary PBG was found by a qualitative/semi-quantitative screening test, then this finding must be confirmed by a specific, quantitative method[12] to eliminate the possibility of a false-positive test. This is best done on the original urine specimen (ideally stored frozen) because by the time a new specimen is obtained, PBG may have returned to normal.

Management of the attack is the same regardless of the type of porphyria, so further investigation is not a matter of urgency. Differentiation between the acute porphyrias is essential for the selection of appropriate tests for family studies; the absence of skin lesions does not exclude VP or HCP (see Table 29-2). If total fecal porphyrin is normal, then VP and HCP are excluded, and the patient must have AIP. Assay of red cell HMBS activity is not essential and may mislead. If total fecal porphyrin is elevated, porphyrins should be fractionated by a high-performance liquid chromatography (HPLC) technique capable of resolving coproporphyrin isomers.[13] In HCP, coproporphyrin-III is grossly elevated and protoporphyrin-IX minimally raised or normal. In VP, protoporphyrin-IX and other dicarboxylate porphyrins are elevated, and a smaller increase in coproporphyrin is seen (with the type III isomer predominating) (see Table 29-3). It is important to remember that protoporphyrin-IX and other dicarboxylate porphyrins may arise by the action of gut flora on heme (whether the heme is of dietary origin or is the result of gastrointestinal bleeding). Therefore, if the fecal porphyrin pattern resembles VP, plasma should be examined by fluorescence emission spectroscopy for the characteristic fluorescence maximum at 624 to 628 nm (see Table 29-3).[11]

Sometimes the laboratory is asked to make a retrospective diagnosis of porphyria after the patient has fully recovered from an attack or as the cause of a chronic neuropsychiatric disorder sometime after the onset of illness. The first step is to quantify urinary PBG, but it should be noted that screening tests are too insensitive for this purpose. Fecal porphyrin is measured (to exclude HCP) and plasma fluorescence emission spectroscopy performed (to exclude VP). If all of these tests are negative, it is very unlikely that symptoms are or were caused by porphyria. However, it is difficult to exclude porphyria after periods as long as several years of clinical remission. Depending on the degree of clinical suspicion, enzyme and DNA studies may be pursued but are often unrewarding.

Patients with Cutaneous Symptoms

Skin lesions of the **cutaneous porphyrias** are always accompanied by overproduction of porphyrins. The route of investigation should be dictated by the clinical presentation (see Table 29-2).

Patients with Bullae, Fragility, and Scarring

Four main porphyrias have been identified in which clinically indistinguishable skin lesions of fragile skin and bullae occur (see Table 29-2). Total urinary and fecal porphyrin should be measured by a spectrophotometric[3,6] or fluorometric[3] method with adequate sensitivity. Plasma porphyrins are then determined by fluorescence emission spectroscopy.[11] In practice, fecal analysis is often unnecessary because the two most common bullous porphyrias—PCT and VP—are identified by analysis of urine and plasma (see Table 29-3). If these tests are normal, then porphyria is excluded as the cause of any active skin lesions. Any increase in total urinary or fecal porphyrin should be further investigated by determination of individual porphyrins using a technique capable of resolving all porphyrins of clinical interest, including isomers.[13] The pattern observed in each of these porphyrias is unique.

Patients with Acute Photosensitivity

For suspected EPP or XLDPP, the essential investigation consists of measurement of whole blood (or erythrocyte) porphyrin using a sensitive fluorometric method. Screening tests using solvent extraction of blood or fluorescence microscopy of erythrocytes are unreliable and should not be used. If the erythrocyte/whole-blood porphyrin concentration is within reference limits, EPP is excluded. If the erythrocyte/whole-blood porphyrin concentration is high, it is important to determine whether the increase could be caused by (1) free protoporphyrin (as in EPP); (2) free protoporphyrin and/or ZPP (as in XLDPP); or (3) ZPP in iron deficiency, or lead toxicity.). Distinguishing between the protoporphyrins requires first extraction with a neutral solvent such as ethanol[8] to avoid the removal of metal caused by strong acids. Extraction is followed by fluorescence spectroscopy or HPLC to distinguish free protoporphyrin from ZPP (fluorescence emission maxima 630 nm and 587 nm, respectively) (Figure 29-3). Of note, the measurement of fecal protoporphyrin is not of use in the diagnosis of EPP or XLDPP because increases may be caused by the action of gut flora on heme from the diet or from gastrointestinal bleeding.

Relatives of Patients with Porphyria

Screening family members to identify asymptomatic individuals who have inherited AIP, VP, or HCP and therefore are at risk for acute attacks is an essential part of management of

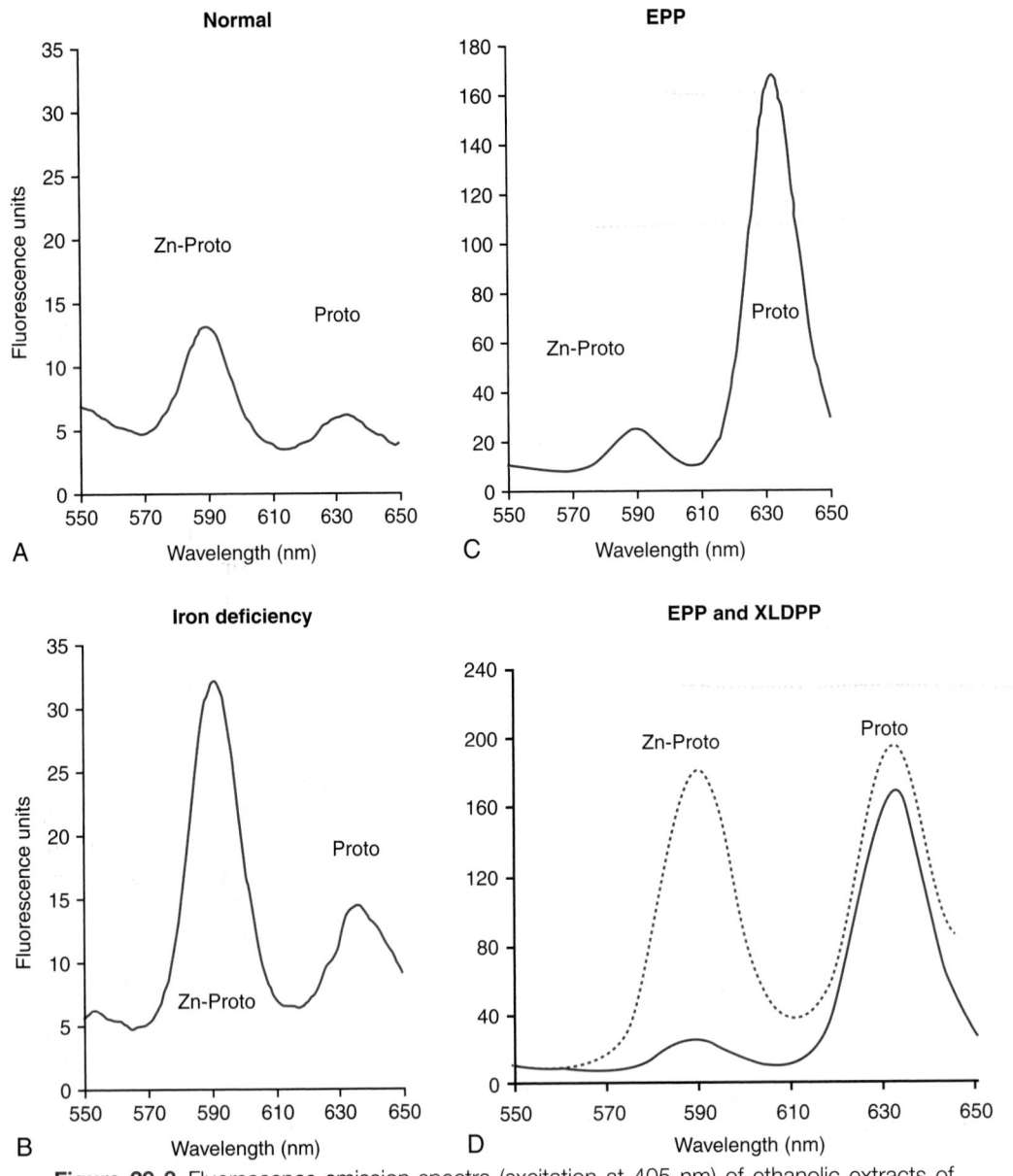

Figure 29-3 Fluorescence emission spectra (excitation at 405 nm) of ethanolic extracts of erythrocytes from individuals who are healthy *(Panel A)*, who have iron deficiency *(Panel B)*, who have been diagnosed with erythropoietic protoporphyria—EPP *(Panel C)*, and who have been diagnosed with X-linked dominant protoporphyria—XLDPP *(Panel D)*. Note that different scales are used.

families with these disorders. Screening may be carried out by (1) metabolite measurement, (2) enzyme assay, (3) DNA analysis, or (4) a combination of these approaches. Metabolite measurement is simple but has low sensitivity; furthermore these tests are almost always normal before puberty and therefore are not suitable for the investigation of children. Measurement of defective enzyme activity is clinically more sensitive, but both clinical sensitivity and specificity are limited by the overlap between activities in disease and in a healthy population. Mutation detection by DNA analysis is more specific and sensitive than biochemical methods. In practice, it is quickly replacing other methods, particularly because it offers the additional advantage of enabling asymptomatic disease to be excluded with certainty. However, its use depends on prior identification of a disease-specific mutation in the family under investigation.

Family investigation has a more limited role in the clinical management of other porphyrias. In PCT, the autosomal dominant familial form is identified by erythrocyte UROD assay or mutational analysis, but as yet no evidence suggests that family studies are necessary unless requested by anxious relatives. However, patients of Northern European ancestry should be tested for the C282Y mutation in the hemochromatosis (HFE) gene. Hemochromatosis should be considered in families shown to have a C282Y homozygous member.

In EPP testing, the unaffected parent for the presence of the IVS3-48C low-expression FECH allele is helpful for assessing the risk that a future child will have clinically overt disease. Mutational analysis of the FECH gene may be required for genetic counseling of some families.[9] Mutational analysis of the ALAS2 gene is essential for confirming the diagnosis of XLDPP.

Analytical Methods

The analytical methods used to diagnosis and monitor porphyria are described here briefly. These are described in greater detail in an expanded version of this chapter.[2]

Specimen Collection and Stability

It is important that all samples for porphyrin assay be protected from light. For example, urinary porphyrin concentrations have been observed to decrease by up to 50% if kept in the light for 24 hours. Urinary porphyrins and PBG are best analyzed in fresh, early morning (10 to 20 mL) specimens collected without preservative. Dilute urine (creatinine <2 mmol/L [23 mg/dL]) is unsuitable for analysis.

Twenty-four-hour collections (1) offer little advantage, (2) delay diagnosis, and (3) increase the risks of incomplete collection and light exposure during the collection period. PBG and porphyrins are stable in urine in the dark at 4 °C for up to 48 hours and for at least a month at –20 °C. Specimens for ALA estimation should be promptly refrigerated. Urine specimens can be stored at 4 °C in the dark for at least 2 weeks without significant loss of ALA, and frozen specimens are stable for weeks. Whereas PBG is more stable around pH 8 to 9,

ALA is more stable around pH 3 to 4, although more acidic environments greatly reduce ALA stability.

About 5 to 10 g wet weight of feces is adequate for porphyrin measurements. Diagnostically important changes in concentration are unlikely to occur within 36 hours at room temperature, and samples are stable for many months at –20 °C.

Whole blood, anticoagulated with ethylenediamine tetraacetic acid (EDTA), shows no loss of protoporphyrin for up to 8 days at room temperature and for at least 8 weeks at 4 °C in the dark.

It is good practice to treat all samples received from patients with suspected bullous porphyria as "high risk" because the frequency of infection with hepatotropic viruses, particularly HCV, is increased in PCT.

Methods for Metabolites

Porphobilinogen

Most methods for PBG are based on the reaction of Ehrlich's reagent (4-dimethylaminobenzaldehyde in acidic solution) with the α-methene carbon of the pyrrole ring to form a colored product variously described as "rose-red" or "magenta." It has a characteristic absorption spectrum with a peak at 553 nm and a shoulder at 540 nm. Porphyrins do not contain any α-methene hydrogens and so do not react. Some other substances in urine may react with the reagent to give red products, notably urobilinogen, may inhibit the reaction, or are pigmented themselves and so mask the red chromogen. All interferences need to be removed. This is best achieved by ion exchange chromatography, as in methods for the accurate quantification of PBG based on the procedure first described by Mauzerall and Granick[15]. Methods based on HPLC and tandem-mass spectrometry (MS) that are sufficiently sensitive to measure PBG in plasma have recently been described.[7]

Qualitative screening tests in which urine is reacted directly with Ehrlich's reagent and is assessed visually for the formation of the red chromogen (e.g., the Watson-Schwartz- and Hoesch tests) are convenient but have been criticized for low analytical sensitivity and specificity, even when solvent extraction has been used to separate the PBG-Ehrlich compound from the urobilinogen/Ehrlich complex. The Mauzerall and Granick method has been modified in attempts to produce an alternative that is acceptable for screening purposes. Buttery and Stuart[5] avoided the use of columns by employing batchwise treatment with resin, and visually compared the final color with that of a surrogate reference solution. Blake et al[3] eliminated the centrifugation steps by using resin-filled syringes with detachable filters and compared the final color with a range of artificial reference solutions. These modifications reduced the time taken to perform the test to 10 minutes and produced a semi-quantitative result. A commercial kit based on Blake's method is available (PBG Kit, Thermo Scientific, Pittsburgh, PAPA; http://www.thermoscientific.com/; accessed October 29, 2013) and is advertised to be more sensitive and specific for initial screening than qualitative, solvent extraction procedures. If a qualitative screening test is used, it is essential to include appropriate reference solutions and controls and to confirm all positive tests using a specific quantitative method.

5-Aminolevulinic Acid

ALA is measured directly but is more usually converted into an Ehrlich-reacting pyrrole by condensation with a reagent, such as acetylacetone, after separation from PBG by two-stage anion exchange chromatography. A method for the measurement of PBG and ALA, based on that of Mauzerall and Granick,[15] is available commercially (Bio-Rad Laboratories, Hercules, CA; http://www.bio-rad.com/; accessed October 29, 2013).

Analysis of Porphyrin in Urine and Feces

Methods of porphyrin fractionation are complex and time-consuming and are not available in every laboratory. For this reason, simple qualitative screening tests are often used to exclude most specimens that do not require further investigation from the few that justify fractionation of the individual porphyrins. Screening tests in which extracts of urine or feces are examined visually for typical red-pink fluorescence of porphyrins lack sensitivity and should not be used. Methods based on spectrophotometric scanning of acidified urine or fecal extracts for the presence of the Soret band are recommended and yield semi-quantitative information.[6] Quantitative fluorometric methods are also available.[3]

All methods used for the fractionation of porphyrins are based on the different solubilities of individual porphyrins because of their different β-substituents, and to a lesser extent on their order around the macrocycle. These methods include (1) differential extraction with solvents, (2) paper and thin-layer chromatography, and (3) HPLC. Solvent extraction methods yield only limited and sometimes misleading information and should not be used. Reversed-phase HPLC,[13] the current method of choice, separates all porphyrins of clinical interest, including isomers and metal chelates, without the need for prior methylation.

Analysis of Blood Porphyrins

All of the methods described next require a spectrofluorometer fitted with a red sensitive photomultiplier. If such equipment is not available locally, samples should be referred to a reference laboratory.

The simplest method for whole-blood or erythrocyte protoporphyrin is that described by Piomelli and modified by Blake et al.[3] Porphyrins are extracted, and hemoglobin and other proteins are precipitated by mixing diluted blood with a diethyl ether–acetic acid mixture. Porphyrins are then back-extracted into hydrochloric acid and are measured fluorometrically (see Figure 29-3). This method has the disadvantage that the acidic conditions result in the release of zinc from ZPP, and it therefore provides a measure of total protoporphyrin. To preserve the zinc chelate, neutral or basic extraction conditions are required. Diluted cells are mixed with ethanol, which precipitates hemoglobin and other proteins and extracts porphyrins without dissociating heme from hemoglobin.[8] The extract is scanned in a spectrofluorometer to distinguish the emission maxima of protoporphyrin from its zinc chelate.

Analysis of Plasma Porphyrins

Plasma porphyrins have been determined by fluorescence emission spectroscopy of saline-diluted plasma[9] or deproteinized extracts, or by HPLC. The first of these methods provides the advantages of simplicity and inclusion of porphyrins that are bound covalently to plasma proteins. Porphyrins at neutral pH fluoresce in the 610 to 640 nm region; the wavelength of maximum emission depends primarily on the porphyrin structure but is also influenced by the nature of the porphyrin/protein complex. This method is useful in front-line investigation for suspected cutaneous porphyria.

Enzyme Measurements

Assay of individual enzymes of the heme biosynthetic pathway is rarely required for the investigation of patients with symptoms of porphyria. However, measurement of enzyme activities is useful for family studies (1) when the individual mutation cannot be identified, (2) when DNA analysis is not available, and (3) for the identification of subtypes, such as nonerythroid AIP and "homozygous" forms of autosomal dominant porphyrias. Erythrocytes are a convenient source of cytoplasmic enzymes (ALAD, HMBS, UROS, and UROD), but assay of the mitochondrial enzymes (CPO, PPOX, and FECH) requires nucleated cells, such as lymphocytes or cultured fibroblasts. Assays for enzymes that use porphyrinogens as substrates are technically difficult because the substrate (1) is unstable, (2) has to be prepared in situ, and, particularly with protoporphyrinogen, (3) undergoes nonenzymatic oxidation during the assay.

DNA Analysis

Screening families for porphyria by DNA analysis is a two-stage process. First, the mutation that causes porphyria in the family under investigation needs to be identified by analysis of DNA from a family member in whom the diagnosis of a specific type of porphyria has been established unequivocally. Second, that patient's relatives are screened for the mutation. The first part of this process is the more complex task. Because most mutations are restricted to one family or a few families, identification of a mutation in a new family almost always requires at least analysis of all exons with their flanking intronic sequences and the promoter region. Only in those countries where founder mutations predominate, as with VP in South Africa and AIP in Sweden, is initial testing for a single mutation worthwhile. Standard techniques of mutation analysis are employed.

Review Questions

1. The precursors of the tetrapyrrole ring structure of porphyrin are:
   a. 5-aminolevulinic acid and iron.
   b. acetyl CoA and porphyrin.
   c. succinyl CoA and glycine.
   d. zinc and porphyrinogen.

2. The important initial screening test that allows for differentiation between the two categories of porphyria is:
   a. serum coproporphyrin.
   b. urine aminolevulinic acid (ALA) and porphobilinogen (PBG).
   c. serum zinc protophyrin.
   d. red blood cell zinc protoporphyrin.

3. Another name for protoporphyrin that contains iron is:
   a. heme.
   b. PBG.
   c. coproporphyrin.
   d. ferrochelatase.

4. The skin lesions and photosensitivity observed in patients with nonacute cutaneous porphyrias are the result of:
   a. autonomic neuropathy.
   b. excessive production of ALA.
   c. accumulation of porphyrins in the liver.
   d. excess presence of porphyrins in skin that generate oxygen radicals.

5. In lead toxicity, what replaces iron as a substrate for ferrochelatase to be incorporated into protoporphyrin?
   a. Carbon dioxide
   b. Zinc
   c. Copper
   d. Lead

6. The most common of all the porphyria disorders is:
   a. variegate porphyria.
   b. acute intermittent porphyria.
   c. porphyria cutanea tarda.
   d. congenital erythropoietic porphyria.

7. The initial steps of heme synthesis occur in the:
   a. mitochondrion.
   b. cytosol.
   c. endoplasmic reticulum.
   d. cell nucleus.

8. The best specimen type for analyzing porphobilinogen is:
   a. heparinized plasma separated and frozen immediately after collection.
   b. a 24-hour urine collection collected in a dark brown container and preserved with 0.1% HCl.
   c. a fresh early morning urine specimen collected without preservative and protected from light.
   d. blood anticoagulated with EDTA and protected from light.

9. Erythropoietic protoporphyria is characterized by which of the following symptoms?
   a. Flaccid quadriparesis caused by accumulation of porphobilinogen in muscle
   b. Lifelong acute photosensitivity caused by protoporphyrin-IX accumulation in skin
   c. Liver damage and hepatic siderosis caused by iron accumulation in cells
   d. Severe abdominal pain and peripheral neuropathy caused by induction of hepatic cytochromes

10. The reduced form of a porphyrin is known as a:
    a. protoporphyrin.
    b. heme molecule.
    c. pyrrole ring.
    d. porphyrinogen.

References

1. Anderson KE, Sassa S, Bishop D, Desnick RJ. Disorders of heme biosynthesis: X-linked sideroblastic anemia and the porphyrias. In: Scriver CR, Beaudet AL, Sly WS, Valle D, eds. The metabolic and molecular basis of inherited disease, 8th edition. New York: McGraw-Hill, 2000: 2961–3062.

2. Badminton MN, Whatley SD, Deacon AC, Elder GH. The porphyrias and other disorders of porphyrin metabolism. In: Burtis CA, Ashwood ER, Bruns DE, eds. Tietz textbook of clinical chemistry and molecular diagnostics. St Louis: Elsevier, 2012:1031–55.

3. Blake D, Poulos V, Rossi R. Diagnosis of porphyria—recommended methods for peripheral laboratories. Clin Biochem Rev 1992;13(Suppl 1): S1–24.

4. Bulaj ZJ, Phillips JD, Ajioka RS, et al. Hemochromatosis genes and other factors contributing to the pathogenesis of porphyria cutanea tarda. Blood 2000;95:1565–71.

5. Buttery JE, Stuart S. Measurement of porphobilinogen in urine by a simple resin method with use of a surrogate standard. Clin Chem 1991;37:2133–6.

6. Deacon AC, Elder GH. ACP Best Practice No. 165. Front line tests for the investigation of suspected porphyria. J Clin Pathol 2001;54:500–7.

7. Floderus Y, Sardh E, Möller C, et al. Variations in porphobilinogen and 5-aminolevulinic acid concentrations in plasma and urine from asymptomatic carriers of the acute intermittent porphyria gene with increased porphyrin precursor excretion. Clin Chem. 2006; 52:701–7.

8. Garden JS, Mitchell DG, Jackson KW. Improved ethanol extraction procedure for determining zinc protoporphyrin in whole blood. Clin Chem 1977;23:264–9.

9. Gouya L, Martin-Schmitt C, Robreau AM, et al. Contribution of a single nucleotide polymorphism to the genetic predisposition for erythropoietic protoporphyria. Am J Hum Genet 2006;78:2–14.

10. Green JJ, Manders SM. Pseudoporphyria. J Am Acad Dermatol 2001;44:100–8.

11. Hift R, Davidson BP, van der Hooft C, et al. Plasma fluorescence scanning and fecal porphyrin analysis for the diagnosis of variegate porphyria: precise determination of sensitivity and specificity with determination of protoporphyrinogen oxidase mutations as a reference standard. Clin Chem 2004;50:915–23.

12. Holme SA, Anstey AV, Finlay AY, et al. Erythropoietic protoporphyria in the United Kingdom: clinical features and effect on quality of life. Br J Dermatol 2006;155:574–81.

13. Lim CK, Peters TJ. Urine and faecal porphyrin profiles by reversed-phase HPLC in the porphyrias. Clin Chim Acta 1984;139:55–63.

14. Marsden JT, Rees DC. Urinary excretion of porphyrins, porphobilinogen and δ-aminolaevulinic acid following an attack of acute intermittent porphyria. J Clin Pathol. 2013 Aug 1. doi: 10.1136/jclinpath-2012-201367.

15. Mauzerall D, Granick S. The occurrence and determination of δ-amino-levulinic acid and porphobilinogen in urine. J Biol Chem 1956;219:435–46.

16. Meissner P, Adams P, Kirsch R. Allosteric inhibition of human lymphoblast and purified PBG-deaminase by protoporphyrinogen and coproporphyrinogen. J Clin Invest 1991;91:1436–44.

17. Puy H, Gouya L, Deybach J-C. Porphyrias. Lancet 2010;375:924–37.

18. Whatley SD, Ducamp S, Gouya L, et al. C-Terminal deletions in the ALAS2 gene lead to gain of function and cause a previously undefined type of human porphyria, X-linked dominant protoporphyria, without anemia or iron overload. Am J Hum Genet 2008; 83: 408–14.

CHAPTER

30

Therapeutic Drugs and Their Management[*]

Christine L.H. Snozek, Ph.D., D.A.B.C.C., and Gwendolyn A. McMillin, Ph.D., D.A.B.C.C.

Objectives

1. Define the following terms:
   Bioavailability
   First-order metabolism
   Half-life
   Mechanism of action
   Peak and trough (pre-dose) drug concentration
   Pharmacodynamics
   Pharmacokinetics
   Prodrug
   Steady state
   Therapeutic range

2. List and describe the four processes of drug disposition and the physiological or pathological factors that affect these.

3. State the need for therapeutic drug management; state the criteria that make a drug a candidate for therapeutic drug monitoring.

4. Explain the difference between protein-bound and free drug concentration; state the physiological effect of free drug concentration and the physiological systems that affect equilibrium between bound and free components.

5. List three prodrugs and their active metabolites.

6. Describe the phases of drug metabolism in relation to pharmacokinetics, including the metabolic phases and processes, the enzymes involved, and what can affect each of these.

7. State six categories of therapeutic drugs and give examples of drugs in each category; describe each drug's mechanism of action and major active metabolite; state which specimen type is best suited for specific drugs.

8. Discuss the importance of timing of specimen collection when managing drug dosing, including time of draw and rationale, result interpretation, and possible problems if the protocol is not followed.

9. Describe sources of drug interactions and how these affect laboratory analysis.

10. List common laboratory methods available for measuring drug concentration; discuss the advantages and disadvantages of using immunoassays for therapeutic drug monitoring.

11. Analyze and solve case studies related to the use and management of therapeutic drugs.

Key Words and Definitions

Bioavailability The degree to which a drug or other substance becomes available to the target tissue after administration.

Cytochrome P$_{450}$ A generic term for mixed-function, oxidative enzymes important in animal, plant, and bacterial physiology. Note: Often abbreviated as CYP usually followed by an arabic numeral, a letter, and another arabic numeral (e.g., CYP 2D6).

Drug half-life Time required for one-half of an administered drug to be lost through metabolism and elimination.

Drug interactions The effects of a drug on absorption, metabolism, or action of another drug.

Drug monitoring The process of studying the effects of a chemical substance administered to an individual.

Enzyme induction Increased synthesis of an enzyme in response to an inducer or other stimulus.

Enzyme inhibition Decreased enzymatic activity due to substrate competition or the presence of a compound that reduces enzyme function.

First-pass metabolism Extensive hepatic metabolism of a drug before it reaches the systemic circulation.

Generic form A drug not protected by a trademark. Also, the scientific name as opposed to the proprietary, brand name.

[*]The authors gratefully acknowledge the original contributions of Thomas P. Moyer, Charles E. Pippenger, and Leslie M. Shaw, on which portions of this chapter are based.

Key Words and Definitions—cont'd

Immunosuppression The prevention or diminution of the immune response by irradiation or by administration of antimetabolites, antilymphocyte serum, or specific antibody.

Mechanism of action The mechanism by which a pharmacologically active substance produces an effect on a living organism or in a biochemical system.

Peak concentration The highest concentration achieved within the dosing cycle.

Pharmacodynamics (PD) The study of the physiological response to drugs (what the drug does to the body); encompasses the interaction of drugs with target sites, and the biochemical and physiological consequences that lead to therapeutic or adverse effects.

Pharmacogenomics The study of the inherited variations in genes that dictate drug response and the way these can be used to predict individual responses to a drug, using a genome-wide approach.

Pharmacokinetics (PK) The activity or fate of drugs in the body over a period of time, including the processes of absorption, distribution, metabolism, and elimination (what the body does to the drug).

Prodrug A drug that is administered in a form that is pharmacologically inactive or only weakly active. Once absorbed, the prodrug is biotransformed (enzymatic or nonenzymatic) into a pharmacologically active compound(s).

Therapeutic drug monitoring/management (TDM) A process used to measure blood drug levels so that the most effective dosage is maintained and toxicity prevented.

Therapeutic range The interval between the minimum and maximum doses of a drug.

Trough concentration The lowest concentration achieved just before the next dose.

Xenobiotic A chemical foreign to a given biologic system.

It has long been recognized that individuals respond very differently to the same dose of the same drug. Physicians have traditionally used clinical judgment and factors such as weight and comorbidities to individualize each patient's drug dosage. Over time, individualization of drug dosage has evolved into a multidisciplinary science, known as **therapeutic drug monitoring** and **therapeutic drug management (TDM)**. Ideally, this activity synthesizes clinical information and laboratory testing results to facilitate selection of the optimal drug and dose for each patient; it also allows assessment of therapeutic compliance and efficacy, and detection of **drug interactions** and drug-induced toxicity. TDM traditionally involves quantitation of drugs and active metabolites in biological fluids, but it is evolving to include assessment of biomarkers indicative of response, and of genetic variants that may affect drug response (i.e., **pharmacogenomics,** see Chapter 46).

TDM essentially provides a photograph of the disposition of a drug at the moment the specimen is drawn, indicating how much has been (1) absorbed, (2) distributed, (3) metabolized, and (4) eliminated. These processes constitute the **pharmacokinetics (PK)** of a drug. PK is often described as "what the body does to a drug," in contrast to **pharmacodynamics (PD)**, "what the drug does to the body"), which consists of the physiological responses to a compound. Individual deviations in PK will indicate (1) genetic variants, (2) drug-drug or drug-food interactions, (3) organ failure, or (4) patient noncompliance. Note that *pharmacology* refers to broad knowledge of the systemic effects of a drug, encompassing both PD and PK; PD relates to the interaction of a drug at its site of action and at off-target sites, whereas PK is a mathematical description of drug disposition. These terms are quite different and should not be used interchangeably.

Toxicology is the subdiscipline of pharmacology concerned with adverse effects of chemicals on living systems (see Chapter 31). The toxic effects and metabolism may be different from the therapeutic effects and metabolism for the same drug. Similarly, at the high dose of drugs at which toxic effects may be produced, the rates of processes such as metabolism are frequently altered compared with those at therapeutic doses. For these reasons, the terms *toxicodynamics* and *toxicokinetics* are applied to these special situations.

More detailed discussion of the concepts and specific drugs outlined in this chapter, as well as a more extensive reference list, is found in Chapter 34 of *Tietz Textbook of Clinical Chemistry and Molecular Diagnostics.*[12]

Basic Concepts

The pharmacological effects of a drug arise by interaction of the drug with receptors or other target molecules involved in physiological processes. This interaction and its downstream consequences are referred to as the drug's **mechanism of action**. The location (organ or specific cell type) of the target molecules upon which a drug acts is called the *site of action* of the drug. Most drugs exert their effects by binding to a protein target such as an enzyme or a transporter. For example, most antidepressants act upon the transporters that regulate synaptic concentrations of monoamine neurotransmitters such as serotonin. Drugs also may target nonprotein molecules such as lipids or nucleic acids; one example is topoisomerase, a chemotherapeutic agent that binds DNA to prevent tumor cell replication.

The utility of monitoring drug concentration is based on the premise that physiological response correlates with the concentration of drug. This is true for many drugs, which demonstrate increasing clinical effects with increasing dose (Figure 30-1). Often, a maximum effect or plateau is reached, for example, as the result of saturation at the receptor or overload of a drug transporter. Ideally, one would monitor drug concentrations at the site of action (receptor), but this generally

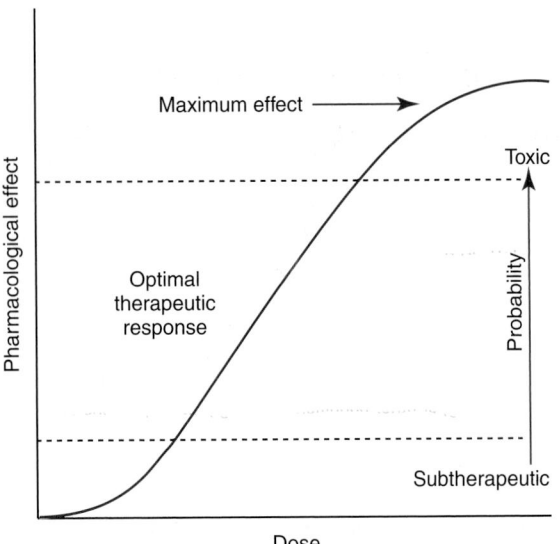

Figure 30-1 The dose-effect relationship. The probability of increasing pharmacological response and risk of toxicity parallels concentration for most drugs. The plateau (maximum effect) is likely due to saturation at the receptor.

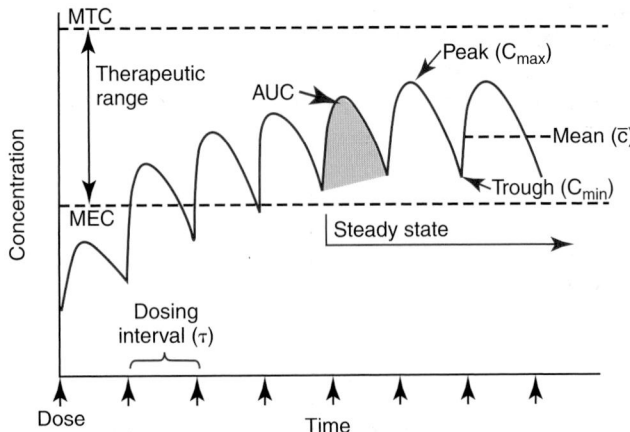

Figure 30-2 Peak, mean, and trough drug concentrations increase with multiple identical doses administered once each half-life until they reach steady state. For most drugs, it takes five to seven half-lives to reach steady state. At steady state, optimal peak and trough concentrations are less than the MTC and greater than the MEC. The range of values between MEC and MTC is referred to as the *therapeutic range. AUC,* Area under the concentration-time curve; *MEC,* minimum effective concentration; *MTC,* minimum toxic concentration. *(Modified from Gilman AG, Goodman L, Gilman A, eds. The pharmacological basis of therapeutics, 6th edition. New York: Macmillan, 1980. Reproduced with permission of The McGraw-Hill Companies.)*

is not feasible, so a surrogate such as serum concentration must be used. Differences in physiological responses between individuals have been known to occur despite similar serum drug concentrations; thus measurement of biomarkers—if available—will complement TDM and improve prediction of individual responses to drug therapy.

The use of a surrogate for drug concentration at the receptor is important in TDM because it is the basis upon which all therapeutic and toxic concentration reference values are established. Drug concentrations in a surrogate matrix such as serum are measured to define a **therapeutic range** (Figure 30-2) that represents the relationship between *minimum effective concentration* (MEC) and *minimum toxic concentration* (MTC). In an optimal dosing cycle, the **trough concentration** (the lowest concentration achieved just before the next dose) should not fall below the MEC, and the **peak concentration** (the highest concentration achieved within the dosing cycle) should not rise higher than the MTC. Dosing regimens should achieve *steady-state* serum drug concentrations consistently within the therapeutic range defined by the MEC and the MTC. *Steady state* requires equilibrium between the rate of drug administration (dosing) and elimination; this occurs roughly 5 half-lives after initiation of therapy if the dose interval (τ) is the same as the **drug half-life**.

MTC and MEC are useful guidelines in therapy because concentrations greater than the MTC put patients at risk for toxicity, whereas concentrations less than the MEC put them at risk for the disorder that the drug is supposed to treat. The therapeutic range, therefore, represents the range of drug concentrations within which the probability of the desired clinical response is relatively high, and the probability of unacceptable toxicity or failure to achieve further clinical benefit is relatively low. The smaller the difference between MEC and MTC, the narrower the therapeutic index and the more likely TDM will be necessary.

Pharmacokinetics

Pharmacokinetics is the mathematical description of the physiological disposition of **xenobiotics** (a chemical compound that is foreign to a living organism) or endogenous chemicals. The key processes of drug disposition include (1) **absorption**, (2) **distribution**, (3) **metabolism**, and (4) **excretion**, commonly referred to by the acronym ADME. These processes are affected by factors specific to the individual receiving the drug, including (1) disease state, (2) co-medication, (3) age, and (4) sex (Box 30-1). Such factors contribute to interindividual and intraindividual variability in both drug concentration and pharmacological response, as summarized in Figure 30-3.

Absorption

Generally, the most direct route of administering a drug is intravenous delivery, which places the entire dose into immediate circulation. However, drugs are frequently delivered by alternate means, most commonly via oral administration. Oral dosing requires the drug to pass from the gastrointestinal tract into the vascular system through a process known as *absorption*. To be absorbed, a compound must dissociate from its dosing formulation into digestive fluids (called *liberation*), then must cross through cell membranes by passive diffusion or, less commonly, by active transport. The ability to negotiate these steps determines the rate and extent of drug absorption and is affected greatly by the nature of the drug itself (e.g., solubility, pK_a), the formulation matrix (e.g., immediate-release, sustained-release), and the physiological environment (e.g., pH, gastrointestinal motility).

Most drugs are weak acids or bases that assume ionized or nonionized forms depending on the surrounding pH.

BOX 30-1   Factors That Influence Drug Disposition in Humans

Demographic Factors

Age category (premature infant, neonate, infant, child, adolescent adult, elderly adult)

Weight (obesity, malnourishment)

Sex

Race

Genetic constitution (metabolic enzyme polymorphisms)

Disease-Related Factors

Liver disease (cirrhosis, hepatitis, cholestasis)

Kidney disease

Thyroid disorders (hypothyroidism or hyperthyroidism)

Cardiovascular disease (arrhythmias, congestive heart failure)

Gastrointestinal disease or disorder (sprue or other malabsorption syndromes, peptic ulcer, colitis)

Cancer

Surgery

Burns

Volume status (e.g., dehydration)

Nutritional status (cachectic or anorexic state)

Extracorporeal Factors

Hemodialysis

Peritoneal dialysis

Cardiopulmonary bypass

Hypothermia or hyperthermia

Chemical and Environmental Factors Influencing

Absorption of Drug

Food or coadministered drug affecting extent and rate of absorption

Immediate- or extended-release formulation

Gastric pH and motility

Activity of transporters (e.g., P-glycoprotein) and GI metabolic enzymes (e.g., CYP3A4)

Distribution of Drug

Coadministered drug affecting binding to plasma proteins or tissue receptors

Changes in physiological composition (e.g., rapid weight loss)

Pregnancy, aging, or other condition affecting plasma proteins and body composition

Metabolism of Drug

Food, herbs, or drugs competing for metabolism

Coadministration of drug that induces metabolic enzymes (e.g., phenobarbital)

Coadministration of drug that inhibits metabolic enzymes (e.g., cimetidine)

Excretion of Drug

Coadministration of drug that competes for renal tubular secretory paths (e.g., probenecid, penicillin)

Changes in urinary flow rate

Coadministration of compounds that enhance tubular reabsorption (e.g., sodium bicarbonate, phenobarbital)

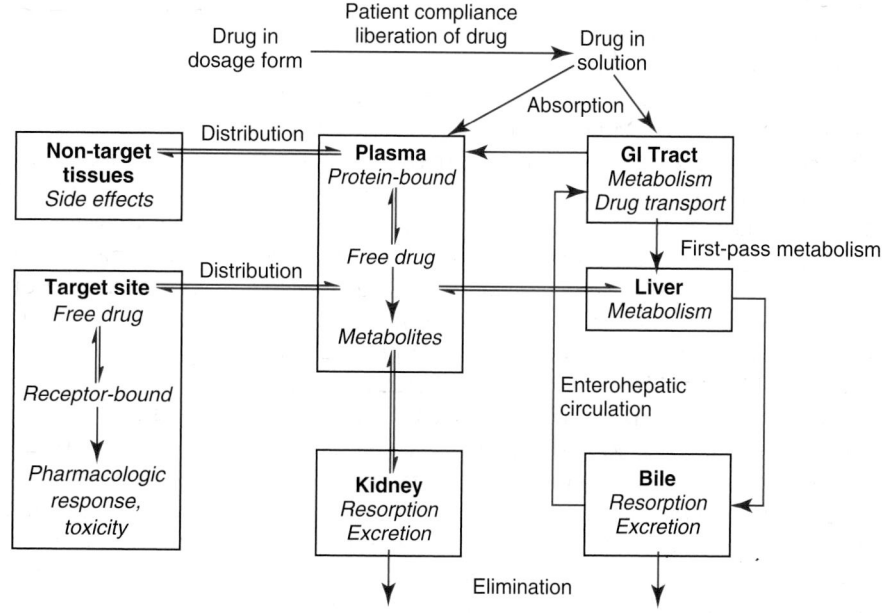

Figure 30-3 Factors affecting plasma drug concentration. **Absorption:** Patients must comply with administration, and the formulation must ensure bioavailability from the GI tract or other site of absorption. First-pass metabolism occurs for many drugs absorbed via the GI. **Distribution:** The drug may be found in both target and nontarget tissues. Interaction with a receptor or other target molecule can induce intended (therapeutic), unintended (side), or toxic effects. **Metabolism:** Conversion of the drug to pharmacologically active or inactive compounds may occur in tissue other than the liver. **Elimination:** Excretion in urine or feces is most common, but it can also occur via saliva, expired air, breast milk, or other means.

Passive diffusion across lipid membranes requires the drug to be nonionized; thus absorption will occur most readily at a pH at which the nonionized form is favored. For this reason, alterations in gastrointestinal pH (e.g., antacid use) affect the ability of a compound to enter the circulation. Likewise, ingestion of absorptive resins or medications and diseases that influence gastrointestinal motility change the extent or rate of drug absorption. Absorption generally occurs more rapidly than elimination; however, sustained-release formulations prolong the rate of drug absorption, allowing less frequent dosing and lessening the variability in drug concentrations between doses.

The amount of drug absorbed relative to the quantity given is referred to as its **bioavailability** (f). This is calculated as the ratio of drug exposure after equivalent doses of oral and intravenous forms, where exposure is measured as the area under the curve (AUC) of plasma drug concentration over time:

$$f = \frac{AUC_{oral}}{AUC_{iv}} \qquad (1)$$

Thus, the more efficiently a drug is absorbed, the more its exposure (AUC) after oral dosing resembles exposure after intravenous administration, up to a maximum of 100% bioavailability or identical exposure for the two formulations. To be useful as an oral agent, a compound must be absorbed rapidly and extensively enough to provide therapeutically effective concentrations.

Bioavailability is affected by **first-pass metabolism**, which reflects the activity of metabolic enzymes in the intestine and liver. After absorption from the gastrointestinal lumen, drugs are metabolized in intestinal cells before reaching the bloodstream. In addition, drugs absorbed from the small intestine are transported via the portal vein directly to the liver, where they are exposed to hepatic metabolic enzymes. Thus, first-pass metabolism after absorption will reduce the quantity of drug to reach the systemic circulation. Drug transporters in the gastrointestinal tract or liver also are able to expel an absorbed drug, further reducing the apparent bioavailability.

Distribution

Once in the bloodstream, drugs undergo *distribution and* spreads throughout the systemic circulation and into various tissues. Some drugs remain primarily in the blood plasma (e.g., ibuprofen, warfarin); others localize extensively to tissue (e.g., amiodarone, chloroquine). The distribution of a drug to a particular site in the body depends on numerous factors, including (1) molecular size, (2) degree of ionization, (3) lipid solubility, (4) extent of protein binding, and (5) body composition. In general, drugs that distribute extensively into tissues tend to be lipophilic, as this facilitates passage through cell membranes. Widely distributed compounds often show relatively slow clearance because of the need to remove drug stored in tissue.

Many drugs bind to one or more plasma proteins, most notably, (1) albumin, (2) globulins such as α_1-acid glycoprotein (AAG), and (3) lipoproteins. In general, acidic drugs associate primarily with albumin, whereas basic drugs preferentially bind globulins and lipoproteins. An equilibrium exists between the amount of drug that is *protein-bound* and the amount of *free* or *unbound* drug. As free drug is more accessible to drug receptors, the free fraction is considered the active component. Serum-free drug concentrations have been estimated with the use of ultrafiltration or ultracentrifugation techniques. In addition, measurement in oral fluid (saliva) has been proposed as an estimate of free concentrations but is unacceptable for many compounds.

Changes in equilibrium between free and bound drug will greatly affect the physiological response to that compound. Drugs that bind the same plasma macromolecules are capable of displacing one another, increasing the free fraction. Physiological (e.g., pregnancy, aging) or pathological conditions affect the concentrations of drug-binding molecules, or the rate of elimination of free drug. Patients may experience adverse effects, even severe toxicity, as a direct consequence of increased free drug concentrations.

For highly protein-bound drugs, clinically significant changes in the free fraction often go unnoticed if only the total (bound plus free drug) concentration is monitored; the total serum drug concentration may not change or may even decrease in situations that significantly elevate the free fraction. Management of these situations requires careful attention to clinical presentation and, if available, free drug measurements.

Metabolism

Metabolism is the biotransformation of a compound, whether endogenous or exogenous. In the context of drug therapy, metabolism is typically thought to enhance excretion by increasing water solubility. Note that this does not necessarily inactivate or detoxify the drug; for example, acetaminophen hepatotoxicity is the result of a minor metabolite (N-acetyl-p-benzoquinone imine) rather than the parent compound. Many drug metabolites are active, and this must be considered when the clinical effect of a medication is assessed. Some therapeutics (e.g., acetylsalicylate [aspirin], codeine) are delivered as inactive or low-activity compounds, called **prodrugs**, which require metabolism by the body to exert the desired physiological effect.

Drug metabolism in humans is typically the result of enzymatic activity. Metabolic enzymes are expressed throughout the body, with largest concentrations in (1) liver, (2) gastrointestinal tract, and (3) kidneys. Mathematically, it is possible to describe metabolism by using similar models as those applied to other enzymatic processes (see Chapter 14). Most drugs exhibit *first-order* metabolism, in which excess metabolic capacity is available and the rate of metabolism depends primarily on the drug concentration. First-order metabolism leads to a log-linear association of drug concentration versus time, meaning that a given *fraction* of drug is metabolized per unit time. This is frequently expressed as the *half-life* ($t_{1/2}$), the time required to metabolize 50% of the drug present.

Some agents (e.g., ethanol, salicylate) instead follow *zero-order* or nonlinear kinetics; many other drugs will convert to zero-order in overdoses. Nonlinear kinetics occurs when drug concentrations exceed the available metabolic capacity. In this situation, the amount of enzyme is the rate-limiting factor and the rate of metabolism is independent of drug concentration. A familiar example is the "one drink per hour" clearance estimate used for alcoholic beverages: The same quantity of ethanol is eliminated per hour, regardless of the number of drinks consumed. Compounds with zero-order kinetics do not have a true half-life because a constant amount of drug, rather than a constant percentage, is eliminated per unit time. However, for a given quantity of a drug, an *apparent half-life* is defined, reflecting the time required to eliminate 50% of the initial concentration. Apparent half-life changes as the amount of drug changes increasing with higher concentrations and decreasing with lower concentrations. For this reason, in nonlinear kinetics, small dose increases create disproportionately large elevations in drug concentrations (Figure 30-4).

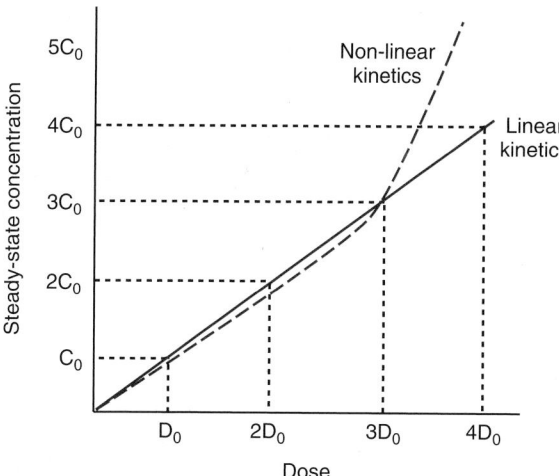

Figure 30-4 Nonlinear and linear responses to dose changes. Drugs with linear kinetics *(solid line)* display serum steady-state concentrations (C) that vary proportionately with dose (D). In contrast, for drugs with nonlinear kinetics *(dotted line),* an increase in dose may result in a disproportionate elevation in serum steady-state concentrations.

Metabolic processes are typically classified as *phase I* or *phase II.* Phase I metabolism is chemical modification (e.g., reduction/oxidation, hydrolysis). Phase II involves conjugation to another moiety such as glucuronic acid. The names do not indicate the order in which metabolic processes occur. The most important phase I enzymes are the **cytochromes P$_{450}$** (CYPs), with just a few CYP isoenzymes accounting for biotransformation of the vast majority of current pharmaceuticals. Several families of phase II enzymes are known (e.g., glucuronyltransferases, methyltransferases).

Genes that encode for the P$_{450}$ enzymes, and the enzymes themselves, are designated with the abbreviation CYP, followed by an Arabic numeral for the subfamily and another numeral for the individual gene. The convention is to italicize when referring to the gene. For example, *CYP2E1* is the gene that encodes for the enzyme CYP2E1—one of the enzymes involved in paracetamol (acetaminophen) metabolism. Cytochromes CYP 1 to 3 are the ones involved with drug metabolism, and most human drug oxidation is due to CYP isoenzymes (1) CPY1A2, (2) CPY2B6, (3) CPY2C9, (4) CPY2C19, (5) CPY2D6, (6) CPY2E1, and (7) CPY3A4. Drug metabolism displays a great deal of interindividual variability, both genetic and environmental. Genetic variability is covered extensively in later chapters and will not be discussed here. Environmental variability often occurs by **enzyme induction** or **enzyme inhibition.** *Induction* refers to enhanced metabolic activity, typically due to increased expression of genes encoding drug-metabolizing enzymes. An example of this is upregulation of *CYP3A4* by the herbal product St. John's Wort, which accelerates metabolism of other CYP3A4 substrates, including oral contraceptives and immunosuppressive drugs, leading to unintended pregnancies and transplant rejection. Enzyme inhibition is more common than induction and frequently occurs via substrate competition, wherein more than one compound must compete for a limited number of enzyme binding sites. This slows the metabolism of all substrates of that enzyme, although the difference may be more apparent for one of the involved drugs.

Many therapeutic drugs, herbal products, and foods have been reported to inhibit metabolic enzymes. In practice, the site of inhibition is important, for example, grapefruit juice inhibits CYP3A4 in intestinal cells, reducing first-pass metabolism and increasing bioavailability of CYP3A4 substrates. Several algorithms are available to predict potential drug-drug interactions by using current information on metabolic enzyme (mainly CYP) inhibitors, inducers, and substrates.

Elimination

Elimination is the final removal of drugs from the body. The most common routes of elimination are excretion into (1) urine or (2) stool, although drugs are also eliminated into (3) breast milk, (4) sweat, and (5) hair. Clearance can be measured directly, and renal elimination can be estimated by using the glomerular filtration rate. Direct measurement of drug clearance requires multiple samples from the patient. However, it is infrequently done, except to monitor certain therapeutic agents or to more accurately define the glomerular filtration rate.

Although urine is used extensively in toxicology testing, the correlation between urine drug concentrations and serum concentrations is poor at best. This is the result of wide variability in several factors that affect renal drug elimination, including (1) patient hydration status, (2) urine pH, and (3) circadian fluctuations in renal function. It is theoretically possible to normalize urine drug concentrations with the use of 24-hour urine samples and correction to a marker of renal function such as creatinine. In practice, however, urine is rarely used for TDM purposes.

Pharmacokinetic Models

The ADME processes are not completely independent steps, but rather occur in an overlapping fashion, often simultaneously, within the body. This is especially true if a subsequent dose is given before the first dose has been completely eliminated. Thus, pharmacokinetic models have been developed to estimate factors such as (1) the amount of drug present at a given time, (2) the rate of clearance of a drug from the system, and (3) overall exposure to a drug for a given dose.

The concept of physiological compartments is used to envision the systemic distribution of a drug. A compartment is not a true corollary to a particular organ or fluid; rather, a compartment is a representation of the regions of the body to which a compound displays similar affinity. For example, some drugs remain preferentially in blood, while others distribute extensively into tissues. For the former, only a single pool of drug (in the blood) needs to be considered, whereas the latter drug has a pool in blood and a second pool in tissues. The first compound could be described by a one-compartment model, but the second may be more accurately represented by a two-compartment model (Figure 30-5). A drug that

One-compartment model

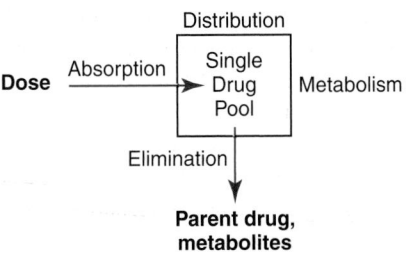

Two-compartment model

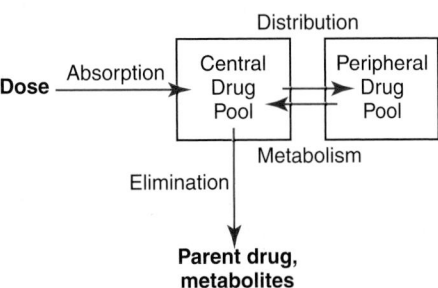

Figure 30-5 One- and two-compartment pharmacokinetic models. For a one-compartment model *(top)*, an administered dose is considered as being contained within a single pool of drug in the body. All pharmacokinetic processes affect that single pool. For a two-compartment model *(bottom)*, pharmacokinetic estimates must consider the equilibrium of drug between the central and peripheral compartments. Final elimination from the body generally occurs from the pool of drug contained in the central compartment, thus peripherally distributed drug must re-enter the central compartment to be removed.

distributes to tissue is modeled reasonably accurately with one compartment, so long as the drug exhibits similar kinetics in the tissues and fluids involved; the compartments are not regions of the body, merely representations of distinct aspects of drug kinetics.

In a one-compartment model, the rate of elimination is governed by metabolism or clearance from a single pool of distributed drug. First-order elimination from a single compartment is shown graphically in Figure 30-6. The slope of the line describing the decline is the *elimination constant, k,* which is a measure of overall elimination that includes loss of drug into urine or feces, metabolism, and so on. The elimination constant is related to half-life according to the following formula:

$$t_{1/2} = \frac{0.693}{k} \quad (2)$$

In this model, the concentration of drug at any time (C_t) after a single dose is calculated from the original concentration (C_0), the elimination constant, and the time *(t)*:

$$c_t = C_0 e^{-Kt} \quad (3)$$

In a two-compartment model, the kinetics of distribution and elimination are distinct from one another (Figure 30-7). The initial plasma concentration of drug declines rapidly as

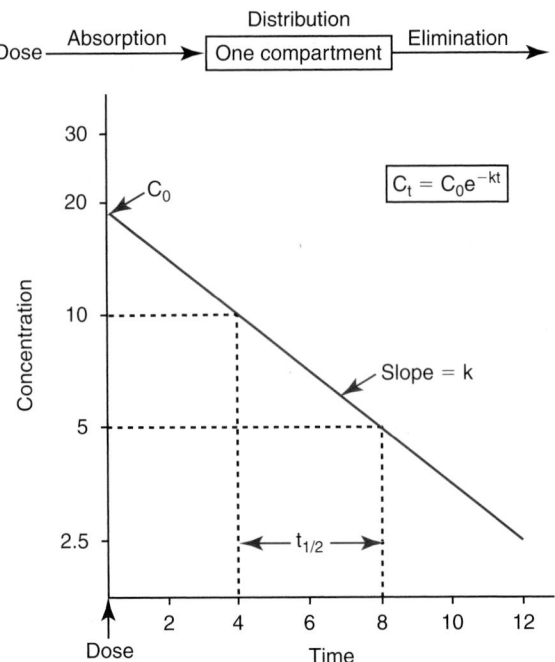

Figure 30-6 Drug concentration in plasma after administration of a dose for a one-compartment model. Monoexponential decline from the original concentration (C_0) is described by the elimination constant *(k)*, which is related to the drug half-life $(t_{1/2})$. Drug concentration at any time (C_t) can be estimated with knowledge of C_0, k, and the time *(t)*.

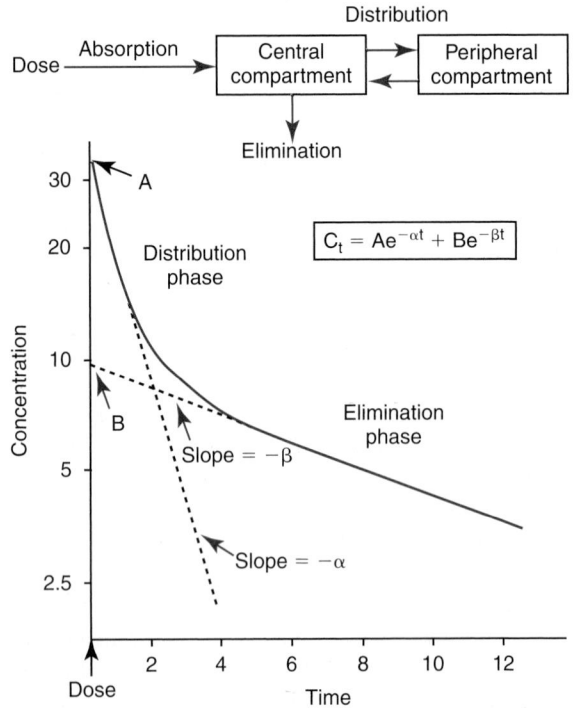

Figure 30-7 Drug concentration in plasma after administration of a dose for a two-compartment model. Decline from the original concentration (C_0) is affected by both the distribution phase (characterized by the constant α) and the elimination phase (characterized by the constant β).

the compound equilibrates between the two compartments *(distribution phase)*. After distribution, the dominant kinetic mechanism becomes the elimination of drug from the central pool *(elimination phase)*. The slopes of each phase are the distribution (α) and elimination (β) constants, respectively, which are related to the distribution or *alpha half-life*, and the elimination or *beta half-life*. Calculation of concentration incorporates both phases, as is evident in the following equation:

$$C_t = Ae^{-\alpha t} + Be^{-\beta t} \qquad (4)$$

As was discussed earlier, the extent of distribution into tissue varies between drugs. This difference is reflected in the *volume of distribution (V_d)* of each drug. The V_d is defined by the relationship between a single dose *(D_0)* corrected for bioavailability *(f)* and the plasma concentration *(C_0)* observed after dosing:

$$V_d = \frac{D_0 X f}{C_0} \qquad (5)$$

The V_d is not an actual physiological volume; rather, it is a calculated parameter that can be much larger than the volume of a human body. A helpful description is that the V_d is the volume of blood theoretically required to dilute a given dose to the measured drug concentration in blood. If most of a compound enters tissue, its measured concentration will be low, resulting in a higher calculated V_d. Thus a large V_d reflects extensive distribution, and a small V_d suggests that the drug is preferentially retained in the vasculature. V_d is expressed as a volume (e.g., in liters) or as a volume per unit body weight (e.g., L/kg).

The V_d is useful for estimating drug concentrations after dosing and for predicting the clearance rate of a drug. Total body *clearance* (Cl_T), the amount of blood or plasma completely cleared of drug per unit time, depends on both the V_d and the elimination constant *k*:

$$Cl_T = V_d k \qquad (6)$$

Steady State

Although the example of a single dose is helpful for understanding basic pharmacokinetic principles, in practice TDM is performed for drugs administered multiple times. Almost invariably, doses are administered before the preceding dose has been completely eliminated; thus TDM models must account for both residual and newly introduced drug. As seen in Figure 30-2, at *steady state* the amount of drug administered is in balance with the amount being eliminated. Each dose produces a peak *(C_{max})* and a trough *(C_{min})*, but at steady state each dose provides a similar profile of drug concentration versus time. For this discussion, the dosing interval (τ) will be assumed to equal the half-life, although this is not universally true in practice.

If doses are given at each half-life, a drug requires approximately five doses to approach steady-state concentrations (>95% of C_{ss}). Similarly, at the end of therapy, five to seven half-lives after the last dose must pass for >95% of the steady-state

concentration to be eliminated. Reaching steady state typically takes many days to weeks for drugs with long half-lives; such agents are often given in a larger, initial bolus known as a *loading dose* to rapidly elevate plasma concentrations closer to steady-state concentrations.

Once steady state is achieved, TDM measurements are generally made at trough, that is, immediately before a scheduled dose. Trough sampling minimizes interpatient variability in ADME and improves the reliability of comparison of a single plasma concentration versus population therapeutic ranges.

Calculation of trough C_{ss} is possible if several parameters (D_0, f, V_d, k, τ, and t [time since last dose]) are known:

$$C_{ss} = \frac{(D_0 \times f)\, e^{-kt}}{V_d \left(1 - e^{-kt}\right)} \qquad (7)$$

It is also possible to estimate a median steady-state concentration *(C)* using D_0, f, Cl_T, and τ:

$$C = \frac{D_{0 \times f}}{Cl_T \times \tau} \qquad (8)$$

Clinical and Analytical Considerations

A robust TDM program offers clinicians the means to better manage patients and has the potential to improve patient quality of life by (1) optimizing dose, (2) supporting compliance, and (3) minimizing toxicity. The practice of TDM has been expanded and enhanced by advancements in rapid, sensitive, and specific analytical techniques for a wide variety of therapeutic agents.

Clinical Utility

The best candidate drugs for TDM are those that meet one or more of the following criteria: (1) a narrow therapeutic index; (2) used for long-term therapy; (3) correlation between serum concentration and clinical response; (4) wide interindividual or intraindividual variability in pharmacokinetics; (5) absence of a biomarker associated with therapeutic outcome; and (6) administered with other, potentially interacting compounds. Ideally, TDM allows determination of a baseline drug concentration at a time when the patient is responding well clinically and is known to be compliant; this baseline therapeutic concentration is then used over time to (1) assess compliance, (2) address physiological or pathological changes, and (3) maintain optimal dosing for each individual patient. Single measurements of serum drug concentrations should always be interpreted in the context of (1) clinical presentation, (2) length of therapy, (3) comedications, and (4) other factors capable of affecting serum concentrations.

Long-term pharmacological therapy is a necessary component in the management of many conditions. Some therapeutic agents have convenient biomarkers or clinical indicators of their efficacy, for example, statin treatment is assessed by quantifying cholesterol, and antihypertensive therapy is evaluated by following blood pressure. However, for many drugs, biomarkers and clinical indicators are absent or are not visible until after the onset of therapeutic failure (e.g., transplant rejection resulting from inadequate immunosuppression). Such drugs are frequently managed using TDM, particularly when the condition for which they are prescribed involves the potential for serious risk to the patient, as with antiseizure therapy or post-transplant immunosuppression. Even for agents with available biomarkers, use of TDM often assists clinical decision making. For example, if a patient receiving antiarrhythmic therapy fails to improve cardiac rhythm, TDM may be used to clarify whether (1) the patient requires a different dose, (2) is refractory to that particular drug, or (3) is simply noncompliant.

The potential to detect noncompliance is a major asset of consistent use of TDM. The World Health Organization estimates that only half of patients receiving long-term drug therapy comply with the prescribed regimen. It should be noted that noncompliance may be a result of taking the medication (1) erratically, (2) too often, (3) too infrequently, or (4) not at all. Noncompliance is often very costly to the patient and to society. Patients at particular risk include (1) the elderly, who frequently must manage several drug regimens for comorbidities; (2) those with conditions prone to reducing ability or will to comply (e.g., severe depression); and (3) individuals whose conditions include asymptomatic periods, wherein patients feel better and forget or do not feel the need to continue treatment. Without routine TDM, noncompliance with therapy may remain unnoticed until symptoms resume (e.g., renewed seizure activity in an epileptic individual) or the treatment fails (e.g., rejection of a transplanted organ).

Serum drug concentrations are useful at many stages of treatment. Initial selection and dosing of a drug may be guided by TDM, particularly if wide interpatient variability in (1) absorption, (2) metabolism, or (3) other parameters of drug disposition is noted. Without measuring drug concentrations, it is difficult to discern which patients respond poorly to therapeutic concentrations of a particular drug and which patients simply are not within the therapeutic range. Similarly, the presence of comorbidities (e.g., hepatic failure, renal dysfunction) or the use of comedications will complicate the process of establishing an effective dose; population pharmacokinetics often does not adequately address comorbidities or drug interactions, necessitating TDM for such patients.

Routine TDM is also helpful for detecting and managing alterations in drug disposition within an individual. Such changes occur with physiological processes such as (1) puberty, (2) pregnancy, and (3) aging. However, they may also reflect development or progression of a pathological state. Conditions that seem as simple as weight loss or as complex as severe illness radically affect the disposition of a drug within a single patient; these changes occur rapidly and may be very difficult to manage clinically. Both acute and chronic shifts in pharmacokinetic behavior are addressed more effectively with TDM because dose adjustments are guided by each individual patient's serum drug concentrations.

Analytical Concerns

A wide variety of analytical techniques, including numerous permutations of immunoassay methods, are available to facilitate TDM. Chromatographic techniques, such as (1) gas chromatography–mass spectrometry (GC-MS), (2) liquid chromatography–mass spectrometry/mass spectrometry (LC-MS/MS), and (3) high performance liquid chromatography–ultraviolet (HPLC-UV), are often used. These techniques are discussed in Chapters 12 through 15. Immunoassays provide rapid results and ready automation; chromatographic techniques improve specificity and limits of detection, although at a lower throughput. Unfortunately, commercial immunoassays are not available for many of the newer-generation drugs. LC-MS/MS is progressively replacing other HPLC-based methods; it displays greater selectivity and permits less analytical interference, allowing development of multianalyte assays with higher throughput and less influence from metabolites or other potentially coeluting compounds. The choice of analytical method typically depends on the availability of resources (e.g., technologist expertise, laboratory funding) and the clinical demand for turnaround.

TDM analysis embodies many of the same concerns as other areas of clinical chemistry, including (1) the need for accurate, reproducible methods; (2) the requirement for quality assurance and proficiency testing programs; and (3) the necessity of establishing target ranges (therapeutic indices) and critical values (e.g., toxic concentrations). Certain preanalytical and analytical issues are of particular importance for drug assays, for example, some pharmaceuticals adsorb to the gel matrix in serum or plasma separator tubes, causing falsely low apparent drug concentrations and making these collection devices unacceptable for many tests. Similarly, the time of blood draw relative to administration of the drug is often a key factor in the interpretation of TDM results. Most TDM protocols require sampling at trough immediately before the next scheduled dose, particularly for compounds with short half-lives or variable pharmacokinetics.

Other considerations for TDM include the determination of which metabolites and which drug fractions (e.g., free, protein-bound) are clinically relevant. Active metabolites should be quantified, and if the parent compound is also active (i.e., not a prodrug), the concentrations of parent and metabolite should be considered together when the results are interpreted. Inactive metabolites are often of interest as well. They may be associated with toxicity that is independent of the drug's intended activity (e.g., the acetaminophen metabolite N-acetyl-p-benzoquinone imine) or may serve as a reservoir for conversion to active drug (e.g., the glucuronide conjugate of the immunosuppressant mycophenolic acid). Metabolites often accumulate at a different rate than the parent drug; thus inactive metabolites may provide longer detection windows or in vivo assessment of an individual's metabolic capacity.

TDM of drugs with extensive protein binding may benefit from monitoring of free drug concentrations. In reasonably healthy individuals free of conditions affecting protein concentrations (e.g., pregnancy, malnutrition) or of comedications capable of altering the free versus bound equilibrium, analysis of free drug concentrations typically is not necessary. However, illness, physiological alterations, or changes in comedications may shift the balance of free drug concentrations; similarly, free drug measurements are helpful in the management of digoxin overdose treated with a drug-binding agent that nullifies but does not remove the excess digoxin. Equilibrium dialysis is the reference method for most free drug assays but is extremely time-consuming. In practice, ultrafiltration is used to remove larger molecules, including protein-bound drug; removal is followed by analysis of the remaining unbound fraction.

Finally, one further issue of clinical and analytical relevance to TDM is the format in which concentration units are expressed. Measured therapeutic drug concentrations are often expressed in units of micrograms per milliliter (μg/mL) or milligrams per liter (mg/L). However, it is recognized that use of the abbreviation μ could adversely affect patient safety. For example, in prescribing medication, a handwritten "μg" can be mistaken for mg (milligram), resulting in a thousand-fold overdose of drug, which clearly has the potential to harm a patient. Institutions accredited by The Joint Commission now use "mcg" rather than μg when prescribing medication. Drug concentrations in this chapter are provided as mg/L (equivalent to μg/mL) or as μg/L (equivalent to ng/mL) unless conventionally reported in molar units.

Specific Drug Groups

Drugs that are routinely monitored are conveniently classified by the type of therapy they support, such as (1) control of epilepsy or infection, (2) management of respiratory or cardiac function, and (3) suppression of immune response. The following discussion is organized in accordance with classifications commonly recognized. Proprietary (brand) names are provided in parentheses after the compound name where pertinent. Note that some drugs such as salicylate are discussed in Chapter 31.

Antiepileptics

Many drugs are available for treating seizures (Table 30-1). In general, antiepileptic drugs prevent or minimize seizures by augmenting inhibitory processes, for example, by enhancing γ-aminobutyric acid (GABA)-mediated neurotransmission or inhibiting excitatory processes (e.g., voltage- or ligand-gated ion channels, glutamate-mediated neurotransmission) in the brain. Therefore, some of these drugs are also used as sedatives and are used to treat (1) neuropathic pain, (2) migraine headache, and (3) psychiatric conditions, as well as (4) to manage addictions. The discussion presented here is limited to application of antiepileptic TDM to support management of seizures.

Antiepileptic drugs were among the first class of drugs monitored to establish appropriate dosing, in part because both underdosing and overdosing are manifested by seizure activity, making it difficult to titrate and optimize dose clinically. In addition, therapeutic and toxic effects of early drugs such as phenobarbital and phenytoin were shown to be related to serum concentrations. Antiepileptic drugs are frequently described as first-generation or classical (introduced clinically before 1990) versus newer or second-generation drugs (introduced clinically after 1990).

TABLE 30-1	Pharmacokinetic Parameters of Antiepileptic Drugs						
Drug	Recommended[9,14] Therapeutic Range, mg/L	Mean Time to Steady State, d	Observed Range of Half-life in Adults, h[†]	Mean Volume of Distribution, L/kg	Mean Oral Bioavailability, %	Protein Binding, %	Important Metabolizing Enzymes
Carbamazepine	4-12	2-4	8-12	1.4	70	75	CYP3A4
Clonazepam	0.02-0.07	3-10	17-56	3.2	>90	85	CYP3A4
Ethosuximide	40-100	7-10	30-60	0.7	>90	0	CYP3A4
Gabapentin	2-20	1-2	5-9	0.9	Variable	0	NA
Lamotrigine	2.5-15	3-6	20-30	1.2	>90	55	NA
Levetiracetam	12-46	1-2	6-8	0.6	>90	0	NA
Monohydroxy oxcarbazepine (MHD)*	3-35	2-3	8-15	0.8	>90	40	NA
Phenobarbital	10-40	12-24	70-140	0.7	>90	50	CYP2C19
Phenytoin	10-20 (free: 1.0-2.0)	5-17	30-100	0.6	80	90	CYP2C9, 2C19
Primidone	5-10	2-4	3-22	0.7	>90	20	CYP2C9, 2C19
Topiramate	5-20	4-5	20-30	0.7	80	15	NA
Valproic acid	50-100	2-4	11-20	0.2	>90	90	CYP2C9, 2C19, 2B6, 2E1, 2A6
Zonisamide	10-40	9-12	50-70	1.4	65	50	CYP2C19, 3A4

*Active metabolite not available as a unique drug.
†Based on average half-life and no interfering medications.
NA, Not applicable.

Although therapeutic ranges and toxic thresholds are proposed for all antiepileptic drugs, the overwhelming caution is to "treat the patient, not the level." Consequently, most antiepileptic therapy is administered over the long term, possibly on a lifelong basis, meaning that dosing requirements will change with (1) age, (2) stage of development, and (3) clinical status. In addition to comparing steady-state concentrations of antiepileptic drugs, TDM for antiepileptics is used early in therapy to ensure that steady-state concentrations have been achieved before efficacy is evaluated, particularly for drugs that exhibit nonlinear and/or variable pharmacokinetics. With maintenance therapy, TDM is useful for (1) identifying and managing drug-drug interactions, (2) managing changes in dose or drug formulation, and (3) evaluating compliance, particularly when signs of therapeutic failure or toxicity are evident. In general, older antiepileptic drugs are monitored more frequently than the newer drugs, in part because of the wide availability of automated immunoassays. In general, immunoassay procedures target a single analyte (usually the parent drug) and are (1) fast, (2) inexpensive, and (3) available for a wide variety of analyzers. When immunoassays are not available, or in certain clinical situations for which higher sensitivity and specificity are needed, chromatographic methods are applied to support antiepileptic TDM.

Some antiepileptics (e.g., phenytoin) are extensively bound to circulating plasma proteins. As with most drugs, only the unbound (free) fraction of drug passes through membranes to exert pharmacological activity, and many drug-drug interactions occur as a result of competition for protein-binding sites. For patients with unpredictable protein concentrations, or for whom drug-drug interactions are a significant concern, it may be appropriate to provide TDM for the free fraction of drug. For example, if the proportion of drug bound to proteins changes from 95% to 80%, the amount of active (free) drug in circulation will increase dramatically, while the total drug concentration for that patient may not change. As such, risk of toxicity could be missed and TDM results could be misinterpreted, particularly for pregnant women and elderly persons with poor nutritional status who are managed with multiple medications. Most analytical techniques are designed to measure total drug concentrations and do not distinguish between free and bound drug concentrations. To accommodate TDM of free drug concentrations, protein-bound drug is separated and removed from plasma using physical or chemical techniques. Resulting free drug concentrations are determined by immunoassays or chromatographic techniques, with the method's calibration and lower limit of detection designed to accommodate lower concentrations than those observed when total drug concentrations are measured.

A brief discussion of TDM support for specific antiepileptic drugs is provided here. They have been organized as: (1) Traditional and still widely used, (2) contemporary, and (3) historical and no longer widely used.

Traditional Antiepileptics, Still Widely Used

Antiepileptic drugs introduced before 1990 and currently in use include (1) benzodiazepines (diazepam and clonazepam), (2) carbamazepine, (3) ethosuximide, (4) phenobarbital and primidone, (5) phenytoin and fosphenytoin, and (6) valproic acid.

Benzodiazepines (e.g., Diazepam, Clonazepam)

Benzodiazepines are a diverse class of drugs that reduce neuronal excitation through agonist activity at the $GABA_A$ receptor. Although many benzodiazepines have antiseizure activity, those used most often in management of seizures include diazepam (Valium) and clonazepam (Klonopin). Both drugs are available in a wide variety of formulations and are sold under other names. Diazepam is frequently administered by the rectal or intravenous route in emergency situations, such as to gain control of status epilepticus (a life-threatening condition in which the brain is in a state of persistent seizure). Diazepam is not used for long-term control of seizure disorders and is not monitored routinely for this purpose because tolerance at the $GABA_A$ receptor develops rapidly, and the drug becomes ineffective within 2 to 3 days. Also, because tolerance to clonazepam does not develop rapidly, it is used to manage seizures and may be monitored through TDM.

Clonazepam is rapidly and completely absorbed after oral dosing, and peak plasma concentrations occur after 1 to 4 hours. Clonazepam is extensively metabolized by CYP3A4, as well as by glucuronidation and sulfation reactions. As such, modulators of CYP3A4 will affect plasma concentrations of clonazepam. The 7-amino-clonazepam metabolite has some pharmacological activity and is present in approximately equal concentrations to parent drug at steady state.

Serum concentrations of clonazepam increase in a linear fashion with doses for both children and adults; however, serum concentrations are not well correlated with efficacy or toxicity because of the development of tolerance that occurs to some extent with long-term administration. The proposed therapeutic range is 20 to 70 µg/L. At concentrations higher than 80 µg/L, no additional seizure protection is observed, and toxicity (drowsiness and ataxia) ensues.

Carbamazepine

Carbamazepine (Tegretol) is available under other names and in **generic form**. Similar to phenytoin, carbamazepine modulates the synaptic sodium channel, which acts to reduce central synaptic transmission, aiding in control of abnormal neuronal excitability. Carbamazepine also has an antidiuretic effect, reducing concentrations of antidiuretic hormone, although it is unlikely that this contributes to antiepileptic activity.

After oral administration, carbamazepine is slowly but erratically absorbed with wide individual formulation–based variability. The active metabolite of carbamazepine is carbamazepine-10,11-epoxide, formed by the action of CYP3A4. This metabolite has been found to accumulate in children and exists in concentrations equivalent to carbamazepine. Monitoring of ratios may be useful for evaluating compliance and drug-drug interactions. Cross-reactivity of this metabolite in commercial immunoassays is variable and should be considered when carbamazepine TDM is provided. The therapeutic concentration range for optimal pharmacological effects of carbamazepine is 4 to 12 mg/L. Toxicity associated with excessive carbamazepine may occur at plasma concentrations in excess of 15 mg/L (or free carbamazepine >3 mg/L) and is characterized by symptoms of (1) blurred vision, (2) paresthesia, (3) nystagmus, (4) ataxia, (5) drowsiness, and (6) diplopia. Side effects unrelated to plasma concentration include development of an urticarial rash, which usually disappears on discontinuation of the drug, and hematological depression (leukopenia, thrombocytopenia, and aplastic anemia).

Ethosuximide

Ethosuximide (Zarontin) is used for the treatment of absence seizures characterized by brief loss of consciousness. Ethosuximide reduces the flow of calcium through T-type calcium channels in the synapse and slows the rate of these seizure-inducing pulses. Ethosuximide is a chiral molecule that is used clinically as a racemic mixture.

Ethosuximide is readily absorbed from the gastrointestinal tract with near complete bioavailability. The drug is cleared primarily by metabolism mediated by CYP3A4 (hydroxyethyl metabolite) and the glucuronide. Drug-drug interactions occur primarily as a result of enzyme induction or through CYP3A4.

The established therapeutic range of ethosuximide is 40 to 100 mg/L, although it is not uncommon that higher concentrations are required. Toxicity related to an excessive blood concentration of ethosuximide is rare. Symptoms of gastrointestinal distress, lethargy, dizziness, and euphoria may be encountered early in therapy, but patients usually become tolerant to these symptoms.

Phenobarbital and Primidone

Phenobarbital is a broad-spectrum antiepileptic drug that was introduced clinically in 1912 under the name Luminal. It is now (1) known by a wide variety of proprietary names, (2) given alone or in combination with many other drugs, and (3) used to manage all but absence seizure types. It is also the active component of the prodrug primidone (Mysoline) and is known to reduce synaptic transmission through action on the $GABA_A$ receptor, resulting in decreased neuronal excitability.

Serum concentrations of phenobarbital are well correlated with dose; however, pharmacokinetics is widely variable. Absorption of oral phenobarbital is near complete, but the rate of absorption is age dependent—rapid in adults, slow in children. Thus, the time at which peak plasma concentrations are reached ranges from 4 to 10 hours after the dose. Primidone is rapidly and nearly completely absorbed after oral administration. Phenobarbital is metabolized by CYP2C19 to p-hydroxyphenobarbital, which is largely excreted as the glucuronide. Phenobarbital is also recognized to induce hepatic enzymes, which will affect the concentrations of other coadministered medications.

The widely recognized therapeutic range of phenobarbital for adults is between 15 and 40 mg/L. The predominant side effect observed in adults at blood concentrations greater than 40 mg/L is sedation, although tolerance to this effect develops with long-term therapy. Actual optimal concentrations vary and may not be realized until tolerance to the sedative effects has occurred. Because of the long elimination half-life of phenobarbital, the blood concentration does not change rapidly. Therefore, it is possible to collect blood for TDM at any time of day, once steady state has been achieved.

The optimal therapeutic concentration of primidone has been established as 5 to 10 mg/L. Because phenobarbital is an active metabolite of primidone, concurrent analysis of phenobarbital is required for complete interpretation of results. In addition to revealing drug-drug interactions, evaluating the ratio of phenobarbital to primidone may assist with detection of noncompliance.

Phenytoin and Fosphenytoin

Phenytoin (diphenylhydantoin), most commonly available as Dilantin but also available under other names and in generic form, is used in the treatment of all but absence seizures. Phenytoin interferes with sodium channel activity by prolonging inactivation, which reduces synaptic transmission and assists in control of abnormal neuronal excitability.

The pharmacokinetics of phenytoin is complex and unpredictable as the result of variable absorption, high (>90%) protein binding, saturable metabolism, and drug-drug interactions. Phenytoin is not readily soluble in aqueous solutions. When administered by intramuscular injection, most of the dose precipitates at the site of injection and then is slowly absorbed. A prodrug called fosphenytoin (Cerebyx) allows intramuscular injection and rapid conversion to and liberation of phenytoin. Monitoring of fosphenytoin is accomplished through the use of routine phenytoin assays. However, specimens collected shortly after administration of fosphenytoin may not accurately reflect active drug concentrations; interpretation of TDM for fosphenytoin should be performed after phenytoin concentrations reach steady state.

Phenytoin is metabolized by CYP2C19 and CYP2C9. The principal metabolite is 5-(p-hydroxyphenyl)-5-phenylhydantoin, which is excreted principally as a glucuronide. Hepatic metabolism of phenytoin may become saturated within the therapeutic range. Once metabolism is saturated, small dose increments result in large changes in blood concentration. This phenomenon partially explains the wide variation in dose among patients that is required to achieve a therapeutic effect. Because of this saturation phenomenon, the half-life of phenytoin varies tremendously.

The optimal therapeutic concentration for seizure control without side effects is 10 to 20 mg/L. Free phenytoin concentrations of 1 to 2 mg/L are optimal. Total phenytoin concentrations greater than 20 mg/L usually do not enhance seizure control and often are associated with nystagmus and ataxia. Total phenytoin plasma concentrations greater than 35 mg/L have been shown to precipitate seizure activity. A side effect of phenytoin not related to plasma concentration is development of gingival hyperplasia.

Valproic Acid

Valproic acid (Depakote) is most commonly used for the treatment of absence seizures. The drug inhibits the enzyme GABA transaminase, resulting in increased concentrations of GABA and overall inhibition of neuronal activity in the brain.

Valproic acid is rapidly and almost completely absorbed after oral administration. Peak concentrations occur 1 to 4 hours after an oral dose of conventional tablets or solutions is given, but they are extended for enteric-coated and sustained-release formulations, as well as when taken with food. The metabolism of valproic acid is extensive, involving β-oxidation and production of several glucuronide conjugates. The half-life is shortened from approximately 20 hours with the initial dose to approximately 12 hours as steady state is achieved. The half-life is shorter in children than in adults, with the exception of neonates with hepatic disease, in whom the half-life becomes prolonged. Relatively poor correlation has been noted between dose and serum concentrations. Valproic acid modulates the pharmacokinetics of many other antiepileptic drugs.

The minimum effective therapeutic concentration of valproic acid is 50 mg/L. Concentrations greater than 100 mg/L have been associated with hepatic toxicity and acute toxic encephalopathy. Free concentrations are sometimes clinically useful.

Contemporary Antiepileptics

Examples of antiepileptic drugs introduced after 1990 and currently in use include (1) gabapentin, (2) levetiracetam, (3) lamotrigine, (4) oxcarbazepine, (5) topiramate, and (6) zonisamide

Gabapentin

Gabapentin (Neurontin) is a chemical analog of GABA that promotes the release of GABA. It does not interact directly with the GABA receptor, and its mechanism of action is somewhat unclear.

Absorption of oral gabapentin is mediated by the L-amino transport system in the small intestines through a saturable process. Thus, bioavailability is dose dependent. Peak concentrations are observed 2 to 3 hours after a dose. Absorption is reduced by concomitant use of antacids. The minimum effective concentration of gabapentin is 2 mg/L, and the optimally effective therapeutic serum concentration of gabapentin is reported as between 2 and 20 mg/L. Side effects observed in adults at serum concentrations greater than 12 mg/L include somnolence, ataxia, dizziness, and fatigue.

Lamotrigine

Lamotrigine (Lamictal) is a broad-spectrum antiepileptic drug that is thought to act through multiple mechanisms, including blocking sodium and calcium channels and reducing glutamate release.

Lamotrigine is completely absorbed from the gastrointestinal tract after oral administration, with peak concentrations occurring at 1 to 3 hours. A linear relationship between dose and serum concentrations is observed. Lamotrigine is extensively metabolized and is eliminated primarily as the glucuronide ester. Autoinduction reduces serum concentrations by ≈20% with approximately 2 weeks of therapy.

Enzyme-inducing drugs such as (1) phenobarbital, (2) phenytoin, or (3) carbamazepine lead to reduced lamotrigine concentrations. Clearance is greater in children and increases up to 300% in pregnancy.

The proposed therapeutic range for lamotrigine is between 2.5 and 15 mg/L. Signs of toxicity that have been reported include (1) dizziness, (2) ataxia, (3) diplopia, (4) blurred vision, (5) nausea, and (6) vomiting. However, these effects are rare when plasma concentrations are less than 15 mg/L. Lamotrigine is a potent inhibitor of dihydrofolate reductase. Folate concentrations are decreased when this drug is administered. If folate replacement is not implemented, rash and anemia may be experienced when lamotrigine is within the therapeutic range. Lamotrigine has been associated with the development of severe rash that is not dose-related (Stevens-Johnson syndrome) in approximately 1% of patients.

Levetiracetam

Levetiracetam (Keppra) is a broad-spectrum antiepileptic that acts through synaptic vesicle protein SV2A, which is involved in the release of neurotransmitters from presynaptic terminals. This drug is chiral, and its antiepileptic activity is highly enantioselective.

Levetiracetam is 100% bioavailable after an oral dose and reaches maximum concentration in approximately 1 hour. Levetiracetam is not extensively metabolized. Renal function and age are the major determinants of elimination kinetics. The possibility of in vitro metabolism by blood esterases (after the specimen is collected) has been proposed, so plasma should be separated from cells promptly. The half-life ranges from 16 to 18 hours for newborns and from 6 to 8 hours in healthy adults.

The minimal effective serum concentration of levetiracetam for seizure control is 3 mg/L, but the effective concentration is not well defined. A proposed therapeutic range is 12 to 46 mg/L. Toxicity known to be associated with levetiracetam, sometimes at therapeutic concentrations, includes (1) decreased RBC count, (2) decreased hematocrit, (3) decreased neutrophil count, (4) somnolence, (5) asthenia, and (6) dizziness.

Oxcarbazepine

Oxcarbazepine (Trileptal), a 10-keto analogue of carbamazepine, is a chiral prodrug that is metabolized to 10-hydroxy-10,11-dihydrocarbamazepine, known commonly as monohydroxycarbamazepine (MHD), the metabolite responsible for the therapeutic effect. MHD, similar to carbamazepine, blocks sodium channels; MHD also exhibits inhibitory activity at calcium channels.

Oxcarbazepine is rapidly and completely absorbed, with peak concentrations observed at 1 to 2 hours; food has no effect on rate or extent of absorption. Concentrations of MHD peak at 3 to 5 hours. Concentrations of the S-enantiomer of MHD are much higher than those of the R-enantiomer because conversion is stereoselective. The metabolism of MHD is extensive; about 96% of the dose is excreted in the urine as metabolites. Most of the dose is eliminated and recovered as the glucuronide ester of oxcarbazepine or MHD. Metabolism does not involve inducible enzymes; however, drug-drug interactions are minimal.

Optimal response is reported in the range of 3 to 35 mg/L. Toxicities that may be observed at therapeutic concentrations include (1) hyponatremia, (2) dizziness, (3) somnolence, (4) diplopia, (5) fatigue, (6) nausea, (7) vomiting, (8) ataxia, (9) abnormal vision, (10) abdominal pain, (11) tremor, (12) dyspepsia, and (13) abnormal gait. Serum sodium concentration less than 125 mmol/L and decreased thyroxine (T_4) have also been seen in patients treated with MHD.

Topiramate

Topiramate (Topamax) is a broad-spectrum antiepileptic drug that exerts activity through several mechanisms. It has sodium and calcium channel blocking activity, potentiates the activity of GABA, and inhibits glutamate release.

Topiramate is absorbed rapidly and peaks at 2 to 4 hours. Approximately 50% of topiramate is metabolized. Most studies have reported a therapeutic range for topiramate of 5.0 to 20 mg/L, yet considerable overlap is seen in serum concentrations between responders and nonresponders.

Zonisamide

Zonisamide (Zonegran) is a sodium and calcium channel blocker. Therefore it is considered a broad-spectrum antiepileptic.

Peak concentrations of zonisamide are observed 2 to 6 hours after dose administration. Pharmacokinetics becomes nonlinear at high concentrations. Zonisamide is extensively metabolized, with a primary pathway mediated by CYP2C19 and CYP3A4. The proposed therapeutic range of zonisamide is 10 to 40 mg/L, but overlap in plasma concentrations between responders and nonresponders occurs. Adverse effects on cognition are reported at concentrations that exceed 30 mg/L. Toxicity is likely at concentrations that exceed 70 mg/L.

Historical and No Longer Widely Used

Antiepileptics of historical interest include (1) bromides, (2) methsuximide, (3) ethotoin, and (4) mephobarbital. As they are no longer widely used they are not discussed here.

Antimicrobial Agents

Antimicrobial agents include a wide range of compounds with very different (1) target organisms, (2) mechanisms of activity, and (3) pharmacokinetics. Efficacy of therapy is dependent on both the drug and the infectious agent, thus TDM for these compounds requires knowledge not only of the pharmacological and toxicological characteristics of the drug itself, but also of the nature of the infection it is intended to treat. Pharmacokinetic details of select antibacterial and antifungal agents are summarized in Table 30-2.

Antibacterials

Bacterial susceptibility to antibiotics is commonly measured in terms of the minimum inhibitory concentration (MIC), that is, the concentration of drug sufficient to inhibit growth of an organism. The MIC varies widely for different strains of the same species; TDM for antibiotics often involves relating the serum drug concentration to the MIC of the specific infectious agent being treated.

Aminoglycosides

Aminoglycoside antibiotics such as (1) amikacin, (2) gentamicin, and (3) tobramycin (available as generics) inhibit protein synthesis to kill aerobic, gram-negative bacteria. Because oral absorption is poor, aminoglycosides are administered intravenously or by intramuscular injection. Elimination is largely renal with minimal metabolism; kidney dysfunction is therefore a concern with use of these agents and may necessitate adjustment of dose or dosing intervals. Aminoglycosides are associated with risk of serious toxicity, particularly nephrotoxicity (renal tubular necrosis) and potentially irreversible ototoxicity (auditory nerve degeneration) leading to hearing loss.

For optimal efficacy, the peak (C_{max}) aminoglycoside concentration must rise to significantly above the minimum inhibitory concentration (MIC) of the organism being treated. This characteristic is termed *concentration-dependent killing*. However, to avoid toxicity, trough concentrations must be allowed to decline substantially before the next dose; thus these drugs do not reach steady state. Allowing the drug to clear does not adversely affect therapy because aminoglycosides show a

TABLE 30-2 Pharmacokinetic Parameters of Antibiotics and Antifungals

Drug	Therapeutic Targets*	Mean Half-life, h	Mean Volume of Distribution, L/kg	Mean Oral Bioavailability, %	Protein Binding, %	Enzymes Inhibited or Induced
Aminoglycoside Antibiotics[5]						
Amikacin	C_{max}: 25-35; C_{min}: 1-8	2.3	0.3	NA	5	
Gentamicin	C_{max}: 5-12; C_{min}: <1	2.5	0.3	NA	5	
Tobramycin	C_{max}: 5-12; C_{min}: <1	2	0.3	NA	<10	
Glycopeptide Antibiotics[10]						
Vancomycin	C_{min} > 10-15 mg/L	4-12	0.4-1.0	Low	50-55	
Triazole Antifungals[1,4]						
Posaconazole	C_{min}: >1.25 mg/L	24	>100	High, varies	98	3A4
Voriconazole	C_{min}: 1-6 mg/L Toxic: >6 mg/L	6	4.6	96	60	2C9, 3A4, 2C19

*C_{max}, Peak concentration; C_{min}, trough concentration; *NA*, data not available.

considerable *postantibiotic effect,* that is, they enhance bactericidal activity that lasts after the drug has been cleared from the body. For these reasons, aminoglycoside TDM samples are drawn at peak (1 hour postdose) and at trough (immediately predose, or at minimum 10 to 12 hours postinfusion) to monitor efficacy and risk of toxicity, respectively.

Vancomycin

Vancomycin (Vancocin) is a glycopeptide antibiotic with activity against antibiotic-resistant bacteria, including methicillin-resistant *Staphylococcus aureus* (MRSA). In earlier years, vancomycin was suspected to cause nephrotoxicity and ototoxicity (damage to the ear); however, these concerns were likely due to impurities in early formulations of the drug. More recent studies show lower (although not absent) risk for adverse effects unless administered with other agents capable of damaging hearing or renal function, such as aminoglycosides.

TDM of vancomycin has been associated with improved therapy and reduced risk of toxicity. Current guidelines suggest that the preferred means of monitoring vancomycin is the trough serum concentration, obtained immediately before the fourth dose. For most infections, trough vancomycin concentrations should be maintained above 10 mg/L, depending on the MIC of the pathogen; for more severe infection, trough concentrations should be sustained in the range of 15 to 20 mg/L. Peak vancomycin concentrations do not appear to be helpful in monitoring risk of toxicity.

Other Antibiotics

Analytical methods to detect many other types of antibiotics have been described, but TDM is uncommon, and testing remains limited to methods developed in-house or at reference laboratories. TDM for other antibacterial drugs is potentially useful in the management of patients with (1) renal dysfunction, (2) severe hepatic disease, or (3) suspicion of atypical pharmacokinetics (e.g., poor absorption, altered distribution).

Antifungal Agents

The incidence of fungal infection is increasing with the growth in prevalence of immunocompromised individuals (e.g., transplant recipients). The most common pathogens are species of *Candida* yeasts or *Aspergillus* molds. Advances have expanded the number of fungicidal drugs available to combat such infections; however, data regarding optimal use of TDM for patient management are insufficient. The triazole group of antifungal drugs is discussed below.

Triazoles

This group includes two newer agents: voriconazole (Vfend) and posaconazole (Noxafil). These broad-spectrum compounds kill by inhibiting synthesis of the major fungal sterol, ergosterol. Bioavailability varies greatly, thus it is recommended to administer these agents while fasting (voriconazole) or with a high-fat meal (posaconazole). All triazoles inhibit one or more of the CYP enzymes, thus their administration can greatly affect concentrations of commonly coadministered drugs such as immunosuppressants. Triazoles are also CYP substrates and subject to induction or inhibition of metabolism. Drug interactions and bioavailability concerns are common rationales for performing triazole TDM.

Voriconazole and posaconazole have broad-spectrum activity and are effective against fungi that are resistant to older triazoles. Voriconazole displays nonlinear kinetics at therapeutic doses. Posaconazole generally follows linear kinetics but converts to nonlinear behavior (saturation) at high doses. Both agents show progressively greater risk of toxicity as serum concentrations increase, but there does not appear to be a single cutoff that clearly delineates toxic concentrations from nontoxic. Target concentrations vary depending on whether the drug is used for active infection or for prophylaxis. Recommended steady-state trough concentrations for voriconazole are 1 to 6 mg/L; targets for posaconazole are as yet poorly defined, although concentrations greater than 1.5 mg/L appear to be effective against invasive fungal infection.

Antineoplastics (Anticancer Drugs)

Treatment of cancer is based on clinical protocols that often utilize a series of drugs or combinations of drugs. TDM is not common for most of the drugs utilized. Two drugs that are sometimes monitored in cancer therapy are busulfan and methotrexate.

Busulfan

Busulfan is a chemotherapeutic drug that inhibits the growth of malignant cells by alkylating DNA. An orally administered formulation was introduced in 1953 as a possible treatment for chronic myelogenous leukemia and was largely replaced by the introduction of an IV formulation (Busulfex). Studies have shown that high-dose oral busulfan combined with 2 or 4 days of cyclophosphamide or fludarabine, before bone marrow transplant, is an effective alternative to cyclophosphamide and total body irradiation. In addition to being an effective antitumor agent, the regimen has been reported to minimize the risk of secondary tumor development and growth retardation in children when compared with irradiation. As such, busulfan is also used to treat malignant and nonmalignant bone marrow disorders, such as (1) acute and chronic leukemias, (2) myelodysplastic syndromes, (3) β-thalassemia major, (4) polycythemia vera, (5) sickle cell anemia, (6) inborn errors of metabolism, and (7) severe immune deficiencies.

A well-accepted dosing paradigm for IV busulfan to replace the historical 1-mg/kg PO dosing consists of 0.8 mg/kg IV (adult) and 1.0 mg/kg IV (children), administered as a 2-hour infusion every 6 hours for 16 doses (4 days). Busulfan pharmacokinetics is affected by (1) age, (2) weight, (3) disease status, (4) hepatic function, and (5) drug interactions. The optimal range of therapeutic area under the plasma concentration versus time curve (AUC) for standard dose busulfan is 900 to 1350 μmol•min/L. Patients with busulfan concentrations below the therapeutic range are thought to have increased risk of relapse as well as of rejection, even though the immunosuppressive capability of busulfan is controversial. Conversely, patients with plasma concentrations greater than 1500 μmol•min/L are at increased risk of severe treatment-related toxicity, such as sinusoidal obstruction syndrome (SOS; previously called *veno-occlusive disease of the liver*) and oral mucositis.

Methotrexate

Methotrexate has proved useful in the management of (1) acute lymphoblastic leukemia, (2) choriocarcinoma, (3) elated trophoblastic tumors, and (4) various carcinomas, and in (5) maintenance of remission in leukemia and (6) treatment of severe psoriasis.

Methotrexate inhibits DNA synthesis and competitively inhibits the enzyme dihydrofolate reductase. This decreases the concentrations of tetrahydrofolate essential for the methylation of the pyrimidine nucleotides and consequently the rate of pyrimidine nucleotide synthesis. Leucovorin, a folate analog, is used to rescue host cells from methotrexate inhibition and as a synthetic substrate for dihydrofolate reductase. Methotrexate is a nonspecific cytotoxin, and prolongation of blood concentrations appropriate to killing tumor cells may lead to severe, unwanted cytotoxic effects such as (1) myelosuppression, (2) gastrointestinal mucositis, and (3) hepatic cirrhosis.

Serum concentrations of methotrexate are commonly monitored during high-dose therapy (>50 mg/m^2) to identify the time at which active intervention by leucovorin rescue should be initiated. Criteria for serum concentrations indicative of potential for toxicity after single-bolus, high-dose therapy are as follows:

1. Methotrexate concentration greater than 10 μmol/L 24 hours after dose.
2. Methotrexate concentration greater than 1 μmol/L 48 hours after dose.
3. Methotrexate concentration greater than 0.1 μmol/L 72 hours after dose.

Characteristically, serum concentrations are monitored at 24, 48, and 72 hours after the single dose, and leucovorin is administered when methotrexate concentrations are inappropriately high for a postdose phase. The route of elimination for methotrexate is primarily renal excretion. During the period of high serum concentrations, particular attention must be paid to maintaining output of a large volume of alkaline urine.

The pK_a of methotrexate is 5.5; thus small decreases in urine pH result in significant reduction in its solubility. Keeping urinary pH alkaline diminishes risks of intratubular precipitation of the drug and obstructive nephropathy during the treatment period. Monitoring serum concentrations therefore serves as the basis for decisions related to timing of initiation and continuance of leucovorin treatment and for management of urinary pH.

Cardioactive Drugs

The major cardioactive drugs requiring TDM are the antiarrhythmic agents and the glycoside digoxin. For over a decade, use of these compounds has benefited from well-established monitoring guidelines that are still valid. However, prescription trends have shifted over time, resulting in less use of older, relatively difficult-to-manage drugs. Pharmacokinetic parameters of select cardioactive drugs are listed in Table 30-3.

Antiarrhythmic Agents

Arrhythmias are disturbances in normal cardiac sinus rhythm and are sometimes associated with substantial morbidity and mortality. Atrial fibrillation is the most common serious arrhythmia. Many antiarrhythmic drugs regulate cation channels (Na$^+$, K$^+$, or Ca^{2+}) and are associated with drug interactions and serious toxicity arising at concentrations only slightly above the upper limit of the therapeutic range.

Class I antiarrhythmics primarily affect sodium channel function. Class IA agents are moderate Na$^+$ channel blockers and include (1) quinidine (generic), (2) disopyramide (Norpace), and (3) procainamide (Pronestyl; monitored with its active metabolite, N-acetylprocainamide). Class IB agents are weak Na$^+$ channel blockers such as lidocaine (Xylocaine) and mexiletine (Mexitil); these agents are used in acute management of cardiac arrhythmia but are less frequently used as long-term therapy. Immunoassays are available for several class IA and IB agents, making TDM convenient for most providers. Serum concentrations are typically measured to ensure adequate therapy and to minimize toxicity.

Use of strong Na$^+$ channel blockers (class IC agents) has increased slowly over time, possibly in part because of their

TABLE 30-3 Pharmacokinetic Parameters of Cardioactive Drugs

Drug	Therapeutic Range,[13] mg/L*	Minimum Toxic Concentration, mg/L	Mean Half-life, h	Mean Volume of Distribution, L/kg	Mean Oral Bioavailability, %	Protein Binding, %	Enzymes Involved in Metabolism
Amiodarone	0.5-2	>2.5	45 days	60	45	99	CYP3A4, 2C8
Digoxin	0.5-2 μg/L	>3 μg/L	40	5	70	25	CYP3A4
Disopyramide	2-5	>7	8	0.6	83	65	CYP2D6, 3A4
Flecainide	0.2-1	>1	14	5	70	45	CYP2D6
Lidocaine	1.5-5	6	1.8	1.1	35	70	CYP2D6, 3A4, Pg
Mexiletine	0.5-2	>2	10	5	90	60	CYP2D6, 1A2
Procainamide	4-8	>10	6	1.9	83	20	NAT
N-acetylprocainamide	10-20	>40	8	NA	NA	NA	NA
Quinidine	2-5	>6	6	3	80	85	CYP3A4

NA, Data not available; *NAT*, N-acetyl transferase.
*Except where noted.

comparatively lower association with serious toxicity. Class IC agents include flecainide (Tambocor) and propafenone (Rythmol). Monitoring is typically performed with the use of chromatographic assays. TDM is recommended to prevent concentration-dependent toxicity (flecainide) and to ensure adequate concentrations after first-pass metabolism (propafenone).

Class III antiarrhythmics such as amiodarone (Cordarone) act primarily via K⁺ channel blockade. Amiodarone is used to manage atrial fibrillation; it is less prone to inducing arrhythmia than many of the class I agents but is nonetheless associated with adverse events such as (1) pulmonary fibrosis, (2) hepatic failure (both uncommon, but serious), and (3) disruption of thyroid function (relatively common, but generally manageable). TDM for amiodarone should include measurement of its active metabolite, desethylamiodarone, although recommended therapeutic ranges tend to address only the parent drug.

Acceptance of TDM for antiarrhythmic agents is not universal, although the benefits of a robust program have been shown. Common situations that call strongly for the use of TDM include drug interactions and comorbidities such as renal failure.

Digoxin

Obtained from *Digitalis* plants such as foxglove, digoxin (Lanoxin) is a cardiac glycoside used in treatment of arrhythmias and heart failure. Cardiac glycosides are a group of related compounds found in a variety of plants, many of which are poisonous (e.g., oleandrin, the toxic component of oleander). Thus, digoxin use is accompanied by the risk of serious toxicity, necessitating TDM. Digoxin is thought to act through several mechanisms to (1) slow heart rate, (2) increase the strength and velocity of cardiac contraction, and (3) regulate the nervous (sympathetic) and endocrine (renin-angiotensin) systems. Digoxin use has declined but the drug is still prescribed, particularly in cases of congestive heart failure, for which it is successful in relieving symptoms, although without substantial improvement in mortality.

Serum digoxin concentrations are an unreliable predictor of efficacy. Digoxin distributes extensively into tissue over several hours after an administered dose. For this reason, TDM samples should be drawn at least 8 hours after the last dose; serum drawn earlier will provide elevated results that are not representative of the true serum concentration after distribution. Similarly, because of its long half-life, digoxin requires 8 to 10 days after a dose adjustment to reach steady state.

However, TDM is essential in assessing risk of digoxin toxicity, particularly in patients with suspicious symptoms. Certain populations (e.g., women, the elderly) are at increased risk for elevated digoxin concentrations and thus toxicity, which begins with nonspecific effects (nausea, vomiting, anorexia) but can progress to severe, potentially lethal cardiac manifestations. Patients with electrolyte imbalances (high calcium, low magnesium, or low potassium) or with renal dysfunction are predisposed to developing toxicity, even at digoxin concentrations within the therapeutic window. Digoxin-binding antibodies are available to treat toxicity by sequestering the drug and preventing its physiological effects. The antidote-bound drug remains in serum for some time after treatment and is detectable in assays measuring total digoxin concentrations. The active fraction (i.e., that which is not bound to antibody) is determined by measuring free digoxin concentrations.

Immunosuppressants

Immunosuppressants (drugs capable of suppressing immune responses) are used to treat (1) autoimmune disease, (2) allergies, (3) multiple myeloma, (4) other cancers, and (5) chronic nephritis, and (most important) (6) to prevent rejection in organ or bone marrow transplantation. Therapeutic ranges and toxic thresholds are proposed and are widely used to optimize dosing of these drugs. TDM is important for optimizing immunosuppressant therapy because serious consequences of underdosing (e.g., graft rejection) and overdosing (e.g., risk of opportunistic infection) are known. TDM also prevents drug-related toxicity (e.g., kidney damage) and is used to evaluate compliance.

Drug regimens used today vary widely according to the transplanted organ type and the specific clinical scenario. All immunosuppressant drugs have narrow therapeutic indices, and their pharmacokinetics is highly variable in transplant patients, particularly in the early post-transplant period. Frequent (sometimes daily) monitoring during the early post-transplant stage of therapy requires rapid response from the laboratory until a stable therapeutic dosing strategy is established. TDM support during the maintenance stage of therapy, often a few weeks post-transplant and potentially lifelong afterward, remains important but is often provided only periodically to verify compliance, to respond to anticipated changes in pharmacokinetics, or as otherwise indicated clinically. Consensus guidelines and position papers regarding immunosuppression and TDM methods and application are available.

Interest in application of LC-MS/MS methods to immunosuppressive TDM is prominent because of increased analytical sensitivity and specificity compared with common immunoassay methods, and as a result of multianalyte capabilities. Note that, because of metabolite cross-reactivity of the detection antibodies on which commercially available immunoassays are based, therapeutic ranges for immunosuppressant drugs may vary with the analytical technique. Values obtained by immunoassay may be 20% to 60% higher than those obtained by chromatographic techniques such as HPLC or LC-MS/MS. The therapeutic ranges and toxic thresholds provided within this chapter are intended to serve as general guidelines but should not be applied to clinical practice without consideration of the analytical technique used and the circumstances surrounding the patient, such as (1) clinical indication, (2) clinical status of the patient, (3) time post-transplant (for tissue or organ transplant recipients), (4) time of specimen collection relative to drug administration, and (5) comedications. In general, therapeutic ranges are higher in the immediate post-transplant period (0 to 3 months) and are lower during maintenance therapy. They may also be lower for combination therapies and specialized protocols, such as those designed to minimize calcineurin inhibitors.

Discussion here will focus on the common immunosuppressants currently monitored clinically to support initiation and maintenance of immunosuppression in solid organ and bone marrow transplant patients. These include (1) two calcineurin inhibitors (cyclosporine, tacrolimus), (2) an inosine-5′-monophosphate dehydrogenase (IMPDH) inhibitor (mycophenolate mofetil), and (3) two mammalian target of rapamycin (mTOR) inhibitors (sirolimus and everolimus). Pharmacokinetic parameters for immunosuppressants are summarized in Table 30-4.

Calcineurin Inhibitors

Calcineurin inhibitors discussed next include cyclosporine and tacrolimus.

Cyclosporine

Cyclosporine is a fat-soluble cyclical peptide composed of 11 amino acids, some of novel structure, isolated from the fungus *Trichoderma polysporum*. It is available in many formulations and brand names (e.g., Sandimmune, Neoral). Cyclosporine is considered a calcineurin inhibitor, but it provides **immunosuppression** by blocking the activation of T lymphocytes via a multifaceted mechanism. Cyclosporine formulations are not bioequivalent and cannot be used interchangeably. All formulations are considered to have erratic and incomplete absorption after oral administration, ranging from 5% to 60%, and averaging 30%. Peak concentrations are 1 to 6 hours after oral administration. Cyclosporine undergoes extensive metabolism mediated by CYP3A4. The combination of variable expression of CYP3A4 and the associated multidrug efflux pump known as P-glycoprotein in the small intestine is thought to form a natural barrier to the absorption of cyclosporine after oral administration, and it is thought to explain much of the extensive interpatient range of bioavailability. Because many other drugs are substrates for these two systems, the gastrointestinal tract is an important site for drug-drug interactions. Elimination of cyclosporine is biphasic and is primarily biliary.

Terminal half-life is variable with formulation and patient, ranging from 5 to 27 hours.

TDM for cyclosporine is best performed with whole blood. The degree of concentration in erythrocytes is temperature dependent in vitro. Consequently, measurement of plasma concentration is not recommended. Conventional therapeutic concentrations of cyclosporine for renal transplants are 150 to 300 µg/L immediately post-transplant, and 100 to 200 µg/L thereafter. Efforts to minimize toxicity have led to evaluation of lower cyclosporine target ranges, such as 50 to 100 µg/L. Rates of acute rejection have not been different with low-dose versus conventional dosing. Higher target concentrations are commonly used for (1) cardiac, (2) hepatic, and (3) pancreatic transplants.

Tacrolimus

Tacrolimus (Prograf, formerly known as FK506) is a macrolide lactone isolated from *Streptomyces tsukubaensis*. It is is considered a calcineurin inhibitor that acts by blocking T-lymphocyte function. Tacrolimus is administered in much lower doses than cyclosporine because of its substantially higher potency.

Absorption from the small intestine is generally low, averaging 25%, but is highly variable from patient to patient and with time post-transplant. Low tacrolimus bioavailability, as with cyclosporine, is thought to be due to the presence of CYP3A4 and P-glycoprotein in the small intestinal enterocytes. Peak concentrations are observed 0.5 to 4 hours after administration. The elimination half-life of tacrolimus is variable, averaging 8 to 12 hours, but has been known to range from 4 to 41 hours. As with cyclosporine, CYP3A4 (coupled to P-glycoprotein) is primarily responsible for tacrolimus metabolism; nine metabolites have been identified, including one active metabolite—31-O-desmethyl tacrolimus. This metabolite is generally present at very low concentrations and therefore is negligible in most patients. Most TDM for tacrolimus occurs with single predose blood samples, and, as with cyclosporine, whole blood is the preferred specimen. The originally proposed therapeutic range for tacrolimus was 5 to 20 µg/L, although efficacy has been demonstrated at lower

TABLE 30-4	Pharmacokinetic Parameters of Immunosuppressant Drugs						
Drug[2,3,7,8,11]	Minimum Effective Concentration, MEC, µg/L	Minimum Toxic Concentration, MTC*, µg/L	Average Half-life, h	Average Volume of Distribution, L/kg	Average Oral Bioavailability, %	Average Protein Binding, %	Important Metabolizing Enzymes
Cyclosporin A†	50	350*	8.4	3-5	30	90	CYP 3A4, Pg
Everolimus	3	15*	24	NA	16	74	CYP 3A4, Pg
Mycophenolic acid	1.3 mg/L	12 mg/L	18	4	94	97	UGT
Sirolimus	4	20*	62	12	10	90	CYP 3A4, Pg
Tacrolimus	3	20*	21	0.85	15	85	CYP 3A4, Pg

*Trough (predose) concentrations. The minimum effective and toxic concentrations are intended to provide general guidelines but should not be applied to clinical practice without consideration of the analytical technique used, the clinical indication, the clinical status of the patient, time post-transplant (for tissue or organ transplant recipients), time of specimen collection relative to drug administration, and comedications. In general, therapeutic ranges are higher in the immediate post-transplant period (0-3 months) and lower during maintenance therapy. They may also be lower for combination therapies and specialized protocols.
†Refers to data for Neoral.
NA, Data not available; *Pg*, P-glycoprotein; *UGT*, uridine diphosphate glucuronosyltransferase.

concentrations, particularly for protocols designed to minimize renal toxicity by lowering concentrations of calcineurin inhibitors. The European Consensus Conference of 2007 recommended that laboratories seek methods with lower limits of quantification of 1 µg/L or less to support sparing protocols that lower and narrow the therapeutic range to 3 to 7 µg/L.

IMPDH Inhibitor: Mycophenolate Mofetil

Mycophenolate mofetil (MMF) (CellCept, Myfortic) is the ester prodrug form of the active immunosuppressant mycophenolic acid (MPA). It is derived from a fermentation product of several *Penicillium* species. MPA is a reversible and uncompetitive inhibitor of IMPDH. T-cell proliferation is arrested by the suppression of guanine nucleotide production when IMPDH is inhibited by MPA

MMF has near complete bioavailability after oral administration and is rapidly hydrolyzed by widely distributed esterases in blood and tissues to produce MPA. MPA usually reaches maximal concentrations within an hour of oral administration of MMF. Clearance of MPA is affected by glucuronidation and enterohepatic circulation. The appearance of a secondary MPA concentration peak anywhere from 4 to 12 hours after the morning dose of MMF is believed to result from enterohepatic circulation, which is inhibited by coadministration of cyclosporine. MPA forms mycophenolic acid glucuronide (MPAG) and is cleared by the kidney. MPAG accumulates to several hundred–fold higher plasma concentrations than MPA in uremic patients.

The specimen of choice for TDM of MPA is plasma or serum. A well-accepted therapeutic range for predose MPA is 1.0 to 3.5 mg/L when combined with cyclosporine, and 1.9 to 4.0 mg/L when combined with tacrolimus. It has been shown that MMF becomes hydrolyzed in vitro, which may lead to determinations that overestimate the proportion of active MPA if specimen is collected too soon after administration of MMF. Of note, a functional method that uses IMPDH, the natural target receptor of MPA, is available. Inhibition of IMPDH activity by MPA in an aliquot of patient serum or plasma is the basis for this method.

mTOR Inhibitors

Examples of mTOR inhibitors include sirolimus and Everolimus.

Sirolimus

Sirolimus (Rapamune, formerly known as rapamycin) is a lipophilic macrocyclic lactone composed of a 31-member macrolide ring. Sirolimus inhibits T-lymphocyte activation and proliferation by inhibiting the mTOR through a mechanism of action unique from calcineurin or IMPDH inhibitors. Briefly, the complex of sirolimus and the intracellular immunophilin FK-BP12 inhibits the specific cell cycle regulatory protein mTOR, preventing cell cycle progression from the G_1 to the S phase.

Formulations of sirolimus are not bioequivalent. Sirolimus is rapidly absorbed from the gastrointestinal tract but has average bioavailability of 15%. As with calcineurin inhibitors, the low bioavailability is attributable to extensive intestinal and hepatic metabolism by CYP3A4 and to countertransport by the multidrug efflux pump P-glycoprotein in the gastrointestinal tract. Metabolism of sirolimus by the human body is driven by CYP3A4, and at least seven metabolites are characterized, which are pharmacologically inactive.

The specimen of choice for sirolimus TDM is whole blood. In practice, an accepted range is 4 to 12 µg/L when sirolimus is used in conjunction with cyclosporine and corticosteroids. Alternative ranges proposed include 5 to 10 µg/L when sirolimus is combined with MMF and corticosteroids, and 12 to 20 µg/L when used with just corticosteroids.

Everolimus

Everolimus (Zortress) is a structural analog of sirolimus with potent immunosuppressive and antitumor activity; it has the same mechanism of action as sirolimus. Everolimus for immunosuppression is typically used in conjunction with cyclosporine. The primary difference between everolimus and sirolimus is the half-life (approximately 32 hours), which is approximately half that of sirolimus (approximately 62 hours), theoretically leading to more rapid attainment of steady-state concentrations.

Everolimus is rapidly absorbed from the gastrointestinal tract, with average time to reach maximal concentration in whole blood of about 3 hours. Low bioavailability (≈30%) is explained by CYP3A4 and P-glycoprotein in the gastrointestinal tract. Cyclosporine inhibits the metabolism of everolimus, requiring everolimus dose reduction when coadministered. Everolimus does not affect cyclosporine metabolism. The primary side effects of concern with everolimus therapy are hyperlipidemia and thrombocytopenia at concentrations >8 µg/L.

The current specimen of choice for supporting TDM of everolimus is predose whole blood, and for kidney transplant patients comedicated with cyclosporine, the target therapeutic range is 3 to 8 µg/L.

Pain Management

Chronic noncancer pain affects approximately one in three Americans during their lifetime and is the leading cause of health-related absenteeism. Escalating medical costs and lost productivity, as well as increased risk of depressive and anxiety disorders associated with chronic pain, have created a tremendous social burden. Pharmacological management of pain involves mechanistically diverse drugs, including (1) antiepileptics, (2) tricyclic antidepressants, (3) muscle relaxants, (4) benzodiazepines, (5) anesthetics, and (6) opioids. Therapeutic ranges for these drugs in the management of pain have not been established, but compliance with prescribed therapy is often evaluated by random urine drug testing. Of particular interest is detection of compliance with opioid therapy because (1) safety concerns, (2) risk of drug diversion, (3) risk of drug abuse, and (4) tolerance to the analgesic properties of these drugs sometimes require dramatic escalation in dosing for continued efficacy. Detection of nonprescribed opioids and classical drugs of abuse (e.g., marijuana, cocaine, amphetamines) is another objective of **drug monitoring** in this population. However, conventional drugs of abuse tests designed for occupational or forensic purposes may not meet the needs of medical testing because conventional tests have relatively high cutoff concentrations and may not detect drugs of interest such as oxycodone and methadone.

Opioids

Drugs that produce analgesia through interaction with opioid receptors found in the central nervous system are referred to as *opioids*. Opioids include (1) opiates—those drugs derived naturally from the opium poppy plant (e.g., codeine, morphine), (2) semi-synthetic opiates (e.g., hydromorphone, hydrocodone, oxycodone, oxymorphone, heroin), and (3) fully synthetic opioids (e.g., fentanyl, methadone, tramadol, propoxyphene, buprenorphine, meperidine). These drugs are widely used to manage chronic pain and are commonly monitored in urine to detect (1) compliance, (2) diversion, and (3) use of nonprescribed opioids.

Laboratories that provide testing for opioids to verify compliance must recognize that common immunoassays for opiates do not detect all opioids and may have inadequate sensitivity for testing with random urine specimens. Other factors to be evaluated include (1) concentrations of various opioids relative to prescribed doses, (2) individual drug pharmacokinetics, (3) dosing intervals, and (4) consideration of complex metabolism. Figure 30-8 depicts the complexity of opioid metabolism.

Psychiatric Therapies

Psychiatry is one area of clinical practice that has welcomed the use of TDM. Therapy in psychiatric illness fits many of the criteria for monitoring. For example, (1) treatment is usually long term; (2) efficacy is difficult to assess from clinical indicators alone; and (3) the toxicity of many psychoactive drugs is concentration dependent and preventable. Compliance rates are often lower in mental disorders than in nonpsychological illnesses, supporting the rationale for measuring psychotropic drug concentrations.

Antidepressants

Antidepressants are commonly used to treat a variety of psychological and mood-related conditions, such as (1) depression, (2) anxiety disorders, (3) obsessive-compulsive behavior, (4) eating disorders, (5) substance abuse, (6) insomnia, and (7) chronic pain. Their primary mechanism for activity is thought to be modulation of catecholamine neurotransmitters such as (1) serotonin, (2) norepinephrine, and (3) dopamine in the central nervous system. Published guidelines strongly recommend TDM for several tricyclic antidepressants (TCAs) because of the correlation between serum concentration and response, especially toxicity. TDM of other antidepressants is also useful in (1) evaluating individual pharmacokinetics, (2) assessing compliance, (3) managing comedication, and (4) caring for patients with renal or hepatic disease. Pharmacological parameters of antidepressants are shown in Table 30-5.

Tricyclic Antidepressants

TCAs represent one of the first drug classes available to treat depression. Strong evidence supports the utility of monitoring

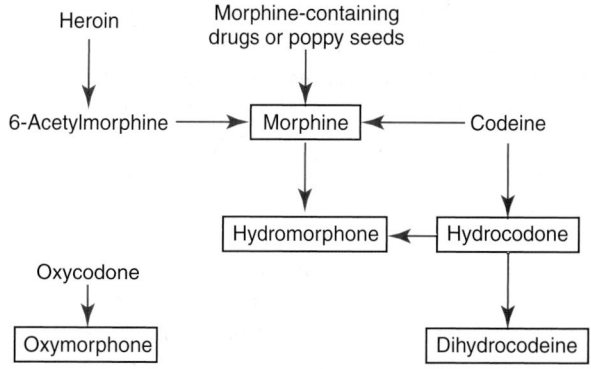

Note: *Drugs shown in boxes could be parent drug or metabolite of another drug.*

Figure 30-8 Opiate metabolism. Metabolic relationships between several of the major natural and semisynthetic opiates are shown. Drugs that appear in boxes could be present in patient specimens as a result of administration of that compound (i.e., parent drug) or as a metabolic product resulting from administration of a related agent.

serum TCA concentrations to improve patient management and reduce toxicity. Common TCAs include (1) amitriptyline (many proprietary names, e.g., Elavil), (2) clomipramine (Anafranil), (3) desipramine (Norpramin), (4) imipramine (Tofranil), and (5) nortriptyline (Aventyl, Pamelor).

Of note, several TCAs, including (1) amitriptyline (active metabolite/nortriptyline), (2) clomipramine (active metabolite/norclomipramine), and (3) imipramine (active metabolite/desipramine), are metabolized into compounds with comparable pharmacological activity that must be included in TDM measurements. TCAs generally show an initial positive correlation between increasing serum concentration and clinical improvement; however, they exhibit a threshold concentration past which clinical progress may decline because of return of symptoms (e.g., mood worsening) or development of toxicity. Adverse responses to TCA excess include (1) dry mouth, (2) fever, (3) urinary retention, (4) agitation, (5) confusion, and (6) seizures. Additional cardiovascular complications include hypotension and electrocardiographic changes (QRS widening) that are characteristic of TCA overdose. Serum concentrations correlate with the risk of toxicity but are poor predictors of cardiovascular change or seizures.

Combination of TCAs with other regulators of monoamine neurotransmitters creates the potential for serotonin toxicity, characterized by increased synaptic serotonin, which leads to (1) neuromuscular hyperactivity, (2) fever, (3) tachycardia, (4) tachypnea, and (5) agitation. Severe toxicity is capable of producing (1) dangerously high fever (>38.5 °C), (2) confusion, (3) seizures, and (4) death. Numerous compounds regulate serotonin concentrations, including (1) antidepressants, (2) antipsychotics, (3) anti-Parkinson agents, (4) migraine therapies, and (5) several drugs of abuse such as MDMA (3,4-methylenedioxymethamphetamine; Ecstasy), amphetamine, and cocaine. Overdose of a single agent or use of more than one of these drugs increases the risk of serotonin toxicity.

TABLE 30-5	Pharmacokinetic Parameters of Antidepressants and Antipsychotics						
Drug	Recommended[6] Therapeutic Range, μg/L*	Minimum Toxic Concentration, μg/L	Mean Half-life, h	Volume of Distribution, L/kg	Oral Bioavailability, %	Protein Binding, %	CYP Enzymes Involved in Metabolism
Tricyclic Antidepressants							
Amitriptyline + nortriptyline	80-200	>300 (sum)	21	15	50	95	2D6, 2C19, 2C9, 1A2, 3A4
Clomipramine + norclomipramine	230-450	>450 (sum)	21	12	36-62	96	2C19, 3A4, 2D6
Desipramine	100-300	>300	22	24-60	35-51	90	2D6
Imipramine + desipramine	175-300	>300 (sum)	12	18	40	90	2D6, 2C19, 1A2, 3A4
Nortriptyline	70-170	>300	30	18	50	92	2D6, 3A4
Newer Antidepressants							
Citalopram	50-110	>220	33	12	80	80	2C19, 2D6, 3A4
Duloxetine	30-120	>240	12	23	NA	>90	1A2, 2D6
Escitalopram	15-80	>160	22	15	80	56	2C19, 3A4
Fluoxetine + norfluoxetine	120-500	>1000	55	35	60	95	2D6, 2C9
Fluvoxamine	60-230	>500	17	5	53	77	1A2, 2D6
Paroxetine	30-120	>240	21	13	90	95	2D6
Sertraline	10-150	>300	26	25-50	>44	98	2D6, 2C9, 2C19, 3A4
Trazodone	700-1000	>1200	7	1	75	93	3A4, 2D6
Venlafaxine + desmethylvenlafaxine	100-400	>800 (sum)	5	6.5	92	27	2D6, 3A4
Antipsychotic Agents							
Amisulpride	100-320	>640	12	5.8	50	17	none
Clozapine	350-600	>1000	13	5	40	95	1A2, 2C19, 3A4, 2D6
Fluphenazine	1-10	>15	13	11	3	99	2D6
Haloperidol	1-10	>15	18	18	60	92	3A4, 2D6
Olanzapine	20-80	>150	33	16	80	93	1A2, 2D6
Perazine	100-230	>460	8-16	NA	NA	NA	2C19, 1A2, 3A4
Perphenazine	0.6-2.4	>5	10	20	20	92	2D6
Thioridazine	100-200	>400	6.5	18	NA	98	2D6
Lithium	0.5-1.2 mmol/L	>1.2	24	1	99	0	none

*Except where noted.
NA, Not available.

Selective Serotonin Reuptake Inhibitors

Selective serotonin reuptake inhibitors (SSRIs) are second-generation antidepressants whose primary activity is modulation of synaptic serotonin concentrations. In general, they are less toxic than older antidepressants, although serotonin toxicity is a greater potential risk for SSRIs than for most other drugs. SSRIs include (1) citalopram (Celexa), (2) escitalopram (S-citalopram; Lexapro), (3) fluoxetine (Prozac, Sarafem), (4) fluvoxamine (Luvox), (5) paroxetine (Paxil), and (6) sertraline (Zoloft). Many other compounds are nonselective regulators of serotonin but are not strictly considered SSRIs.

Most SSRIs are substrates for multiple CYP enzymes, and several such as fluoxetine and citalopram are CYP inhibitors,

resulting in (1) complex metabolism, (2) significant risk for drug-drug interactions, and (3) wide interindividual variability in serum concentrations at a given dose of drug. The usefulness of TDM is less well established for SSRIs than for TCAs because the correlation among serum concentrations, response, and toxicity is weaker. TDM is largely used to assess compliance; this saves costs by preventing hospitalizations and time away from work due to relapse, or by guiding dose adjustment in select populations such as the elderly.

Other Antidepressants

Several other classes of antidepressants are available, including serotonin-norepinephrine reuptake inhibitors (SNRIs) such as (1) venlafaxine (Effexor) and (2) duloxetine (Cymbalta) and (3) catecholamine receptor antagonists (e.g., trazodone [Desyrel]). Older antidepressants include monoamine oxidase (MAO) inhibitors and tetracyclic antidepressants, which have fallen in popularity with the availability of better tolerated alternatives. TDM for these drugs is less common; when it occurs, primary clinical uses include (1) assessing nonresponders, (2) confirming compliance, and (3) managing comorbidities (e.g., renal or hepatic dysfunction).

Neuroleptic Agents

Neuroleptics are used to treat patients with mental illness involving a psychotic component such as schizophrenia and bipolar disorder, as well as other neurological conditions such as Tourette's syndrome. Most antipsychotics are antagonists or partial agonists of D_2-like dopamine receptors. Several have numerous metabolites, but with one exception (risperidone), current guidelines do not include active metabolites in TDM interpretation.

Classical Antipsychotics

Older antipsychotic agents (called *classical* or *atypical antipsychotics*) successfully treat the "positive" aspects of psychotic disorders, including hallucinations and delusions, but are less effective in managing "negative" aspects such as social withdrawal. Many of these agents induce (1) severe cardiac toxicity, (2) prolactin elevation, and (3) involuntary motor activity such as tardive dyskinesia (uncontrollable repetition of purposeless facial motions). They are associated with a rare but potentially fatal condition, neuroleptic malignant syndrome, which is characterized by (1) muscle rigidity, (2) fever, (3) unstable blood pressure, and (4) poor mental status. Risk of this syndrome may be increased with concomitant SSRI use.

Consensus guidelines recommend TDM of haloperidol (Haldol) and several phenothiazines such as (1) fluphenazine (Permitil, Prolixin), (2) perazine (not available in the United States), (3) perphenazine (Trilafon), and (4) thioridazine (Mellaril). Evidence suggests that TDM is best used for optimizing quality of life when concentration-dependent effects such as seizures and tardive dyskinesia are reduced by maintaining patients at the minimum effective concentration for clinical response. Life-threatening adverse responses (e.g., neuroleptic malignant syndrome) are generally unrelated to serum concentration.

Atypical Antipsychotics

Newer antipsychotics are often called *atypical antipsychotics,* although this nomenclature is somewhat deceiving, given that the mechanism of both classes of drugs is modulation of dopamine receptors. However, atypical antipsychotics have less effect on areas of the brain involved in motor control, leading to reduced incidence of extrapyramidal effects such as tardive dyskinesia. Atypical antipsychotics that are strongly recommended for routine TDM include (1) clozapine (Clozaril), (2) olanzapine (Zyprexa), and (3) amisulpride (not available in the United States), although some studies show promise for monitoring other drugs in the class.

Clozapine is one of the oldest and most toxic atypical antipsychotics. Its adverse effects include several potentially fatal conditions such as severe myocarditis (particularly at the start of therapy), seizures, and agranulocytosis; this last necessitates monitoring of white blood cell counts throughout treatment. Most newer atypical antipsychotics show better safety profiles, although several atypical agents are metabolized by CYP isoforms, and this creates the potential for drug interactions.

Lithium

The monovalent cation lithium (Eskalith, Lithobid) has long been used as a mood-stabilizing agent in the treatment of bipolar disorder and other conditions with a manic component. Lithium exhibits a narrow therapeutic window, with toxic concentrations (>1.5 mmol/L) very near the upper threshold for effective therapy (up to 1.2 mmol/L). The severity of toxicity is concentration related. Early signs include (1) lethargy, (2) muscle weakness, (3) tremors, and (4) speech difficulties. Concentrations greater than 2.5 mmol/L produce signs of severe intoxication, including muscle rigidity and life-threatening seizures.

Bronchodilators

Drugs used as bronchodilators include the β-adrenergic agonists, theophylline and caffeine. These two agents, although not used extensively, may be monitored to benefit management of neonatal apnea.

Theophylline

Theophylline is used primarily to treat persistent asthma and neonatal apnea. The therapeutic effect is likely due to antagonism of adenosine receptors in smooth muscle, whereas the toxic effects are due to inhibition of cyclical nucleotide phosphodiesterase.

Theophylline is readily absorbed, and the blood concentration peaks within 2 hours. If it is administered with food or as the slow-release formula, peak concentrations occur 3 to 5 hours after the dose is given. Once absorbed, it is 50% protein bound. Theophylline is metabolized by CYP1A2. Nonsmoking adults in good health have an elimination half-life averaging 9 hours, and it is 3 to 4 hours in smokers. The half-life in neonates is 20 to 30 hours, depending on the degree of liver immaturity or loss of liver function.

At serum concentrations greater than 20 mg/mL, small dose increases lead to disproportionately large increases in serum concentration and intoxication. Symptoms of theophylline toxicity include (1) nausea, (2) vomiting, (3) headache, (4) diarrhea, (5) irritability, and (6) insomnia. Serious toxicity characterized by cardiac arrhythmias and seizures is usually associated with serum concentrations in excess of 30 mg/mL. TDM for theophylline in neonates should also include caffeine.

Caffeine

A minor metabolite of theophylline in adults, caffeine has been shown to accumulate to significant concentrations in neonates. Therapy with caffeine alone has been demonstrated to be as effective in the treatment of neonatal apnea as theophylline; caffeine is gaining popularity because of its long half-life in neonates (>30 hours). Caffeine is metabolized by CYP1A2. The optimal therapeutic concentration of caffeine ranges from 8 to 14 mg/mL.

Review Questions

1. The interaction between a drug and its receptors or other target molecules involved in physiological processes, in addition to the consequences of this interaction, is referred to as a drug's:
   a. therapeutic index.
   b. peak and trough concentrations.
   c. mechanism of action.
   d. volume of distribution.

2. A category of therapeutic drug that must be closely monitored because of the serious consequences of underdosing, which might lead to graft rejection, is:
   a. antiarrhythmics.
   b. bronchodilators.
   c. antineoplastics.
   d. immunosuppressants.

3. A glycopeptide antibiotic antimicrobial agent that has activity against methicillin-resistant *Staphylococcus aureus* is:
   a. vancomycin.
   b. gentamicin.
   c. triazole.
   d. busulfan.

4. The type of therapeutic drug that is inactive when taken and that requires metabolism by the body before it exerts its physiological effect is referred to as a(n):
   a. toxic drug.
   b. immunosuppressant.
   c. prodrug.
   d. free drug.

5. Disorders that affect the synthesis of drug transport proteins alter which component of drug disposition?
   a. Absorption
   b. Distribution
   c. Metabolism
   d. Elimination

6. The amount of body fluid in liters required to dissolve the total amount of drug required to achieve a specific concentration in blood is referred to as:
   a. bioavailability.
   b. pharmacokinetics.
   c. steady-state level.
   d. volume of distribution.

7. The drug group that functions to inhibit DNA synthesis and stop cell division is the:
   a. immunosuppressant group.
   b. antimetabolite group.
   c. antiarrhythmic group.
   d. anticonvulsive group.

8. Pharmacokinetics describes the:
   a. half-life curve.
   b. concentration of drug at its sites of action.
   c. blood concentration of a drug over time.
   d. relationship between blood and tissue drug levels.

9. When would a blood sample be collected to determine the trough level of a drug?
   a. Immediately before the next scheduled dose
   b. Immediately after the dose is given
   c. Two hours after the dose is given
   d. Trough levels cannot be determined.

10. When the amount of a drug in the body is in balance between administration and elimination, it is said to be at:
    a. its bioavailability phase.
    b. normal distribution.
    c. phase 1 metabolism.
    d. steady state.

References

1. Andes D, Pascual A, Marchetti O. Antifungal therapeutic drug monitoring: established and emerging indications. Antimicrob Agents Chemother 2009;53:24–34.
2. de Jonge H, Naesens M, Kuypers DR. New insights into the pharmacokinetics and pharmacodynamics of the calcineurin inhibitors and mycophenolic acid: possible consequences for therapeutic drug monitoring in solid organ transplantation. Ther Drug Monit 2009;31:416–35.
3. Ekberg H, Tedesco-Silva H, Demirbas A, Vitko S, Nashan B, Gurkan A, et al. Reduced exposure to calcineurin inhibitors in renal transplantation. N Engl J Med 2007;357:2562–75.
4. Goodwin ML, Drew RH. Antifungal serum concentration monitoring: an update. J Antimicrob Chemother 2008;61:17–25.
5. Hammett-Stabler CA, Johns T. Laboratory guidelines for monitoring of antimicrobial drugs. National Academy of Clinical Biochemistry. Clin Chem 1998;44:1129–40.
6. Hiemke C, Baumann P, Bergemann N, et al. AGNP consensus guidelines for therapeutic drug monitoring in psychiatry: update 2011. Pharmacopsychiatry 2011;44:195–235.
7. Moore J, Middleton L, Cockwell P, et al. Calcineurin inhibitor sparing with mycophenolate in kidney transplantation: a systematic review and meta-analysis. Transplantation 2009;87:591-605.
8. Oellerich M, Armstrong VW. The role of therapeutic drug monitoring in individualizing immunosuppressive drug therapy: recent developments. Ther Drug Monit 2006;28:720–5.
9. Patsalos PN, Berry DJ, Bourgeois BF, et al. Antiepileptic drugs—best practice guidelines for therapeutic drug monitoring: a position paper by the Subcommission on Therapeutic Drug Monitoring, ILAE Commission on Therapeutic Strategies. Epilepsia 2008;49:1239–76.
10. Rybak M, Lomaestro B, Rotschafer JC, et al. Therapeutic monitoring of vancomycin in adult patients: a consensus review of the American Society of Health-System Pharmacists, the Infectious Diseases Society of America, and the Society of Infectious Diseases Pharmacists. Am J Health Syst Pharm 2009;66:82-98.
11. Sanchez-Fructuoso AI. Everolimus: an update on the mechanism of action, pharmacokinetics and recent clinical trials. Expert Opin Drug Metab Toxicol 2008;4:807–19.
12. Snozek CLH, McMillin GA, Moyer TP. Therapeutic drugs and their management. In: Burtis C, Ashwood E, Bruns D, eds. Tietz textbook of clinical chemistry and molecular diagnostics. 5th edition. St Louis: Elsevier, 2011:1057–108.
13. Valdes R Jr, Jortani SA, Gheorghiade M. Standards of laboratory practice: cardiac drug monitoring. National Academy of Clinical Biochemistry. Clin Chem 1998;44:1096–109.
14. Warner A, Privitera M, Bates D. Standards of laboratory practice: antiepileptic drug monitoring. National Academy of Clinical Biochemistry. Clin Chem 1998;44:1085–95.

Clinical Toxicology*†

Loralie Langman, Ph.D., Laura K. Bechtel, Ph.D., and Chris Holstege, M.D.

Objectives

1. Define the following terms:

   Anion gap   Spot test

   Confirmatory test   Sympathomimetic

   Osmol gap   Toxicology

   Screening test   Toxidrome

2. State and explain the formulas for calculating anion gap and osmol gap; given appropriate information, calculate and interpret the results of these formulas and list possible interferences with these calculated measurements.

3. For each of the following cellular hypoxia causative agents, describe the agent, the toxic effects, the treatment, and the method(s) of analysis, including specimen requirements and laboratory results, for each:

   Carbon monoxide

   Cyanide

   Methemoglobin-forming agents

4. For each of the following alcohols, describe the pharmacological action, the metabolites, the antidote, and the method(s) of analysis, including specimen requirements and laboratory results, for each:

   Ethanol   Isopropanol

   Ethylene glycol   Methanol

5. For each of the following analgesics, describe the toxic effects of overdose, the dose and time of symptom onset, the metabolizing enzyme and metabolite, the antidote, and the method(s) of analysis, including specimen requirements and laboratory results, for each:

   Acetaminophen

   Salicylate

6. For the following cholinergic/anticholinergic toxidrome agents, describe the clinical uses if any, the mechanism of action, the metabolites, the methods of analysis, and the laboratory results for each:

   Antihistamines   Organophosphates/carbamates

   Antimuscarinics   Tricyclic antidepressants

   Antipsychotics

7. For the following drugs, describe the manifestations of intoxication, the metabolizing enzyme and metabolite, the pharmacological response, clinical uses if any, the antidote, and the screening tests and confirmatory methods for each:

   Amphetamines/   Marijuana

      methamphetamines   Opioids

   Barbiturates   Phencyclidine

   Benzodiazepines   Synthetic opioids

   Cannabinoid

   Cocaine

8. List and describe five drugs used in drug-facilitated sexual assault, including drug classification, pharmacological effects, and methods of analysis.

9. For the following specimen types, state the advantages and disadvantages of each when used for drug analysis, and list a method of analysis for each:

   Hair   Saliva (oral fluid)

   Meconium   Sweat

10. Evaluate and analyze case studies related to clinical toxicology and toxic drug analysis.

Key Words and Definitions

Amphetamine A sympathomimetic amine that has a stimulating effect on the central and peripheral nervous systems.

Analgesics Agents that relieve pain without causing loss of consciousness.

Anticholinergic agent An agent that opposes the effects of impulses conveyed by adrenergic postganglionic fibers.

Antihistamines Antagonists of the H_1 or H_2 histamine receptors that are used to treat allergic reactions or gastric hyperacidity.

*The authors gratefully acknowledge the original contributions of William H. Porter, on which portions of this chapter are based.

†A more extensive review of the subject and additional references are found in: Langman LJ, Bechtel L, Holstege CP. Clinical toxicology (Chapter 35). In: Burtis CA, Ashwood ER, Bruns DE, eds. Tietz textbook of clinical chemistry and molecular diagnostics. St Louis: Elsevier, 2012:1109-88.

Key Words and Definitions—cont'd

Barbiturate Any of a class of sedative-hypnotic agents derived from barbituric acid or thiobarbituric acid and classified into long-, intermediate-, short-, and ultrashort-acting classes.

Benzodiazepines Any of a group of minor tranquilizers that have a common molecular structure and similar pharmacological activity, including antianxiety, sedative, hypnotic, amnestic, anticonvulsant, and muscle-relaxing effects.

Bezoar A concretion of foreign material found in the gastrointestinal tract or urinary tract.

Cholinergic toxidrome A toxidrome that represents the acute phase of cholinesterase inhibitor poisoning.

Clinical toxicology A subdivision of toxicology that involves the analysis of drugs, heavy metals, and other chemical agents in body fluids and tissues for the purpose of patient care.

Cocaine A crystalline alkaloid, obtained from leaves of *Erythroxylon coca* (coca leaves) and other *Erythroxylon* species, or by synthesis from ecgonine or its derivatives.

Confirmatory testing As used in programs that test for drugs of abuse, confirmatory tests are used to confirm a positive or sometimes negative result that had been presumptively classified as positive for a specific drug.

Crack cocaine The freebase form of cocaine that can be smoked.

Diuresis Increased excretion of urine.

Drug-facilitated sexual assault (DFSA) The use of (1) alcohol, (2) drugs, and/or (3) chemical agents to incapacitate an individual and facilitate sexual assault.

Drugs of abuse Drugs that are repeatedly and deliberately used in a way other than prescribed or socially sanctioned (i.e., a drug that is taken for nonmedicinal reasons).

Drug half-life ($t_{1/2}$) The length of time it takes for one-half of an administered drug to decrease due to a biological processes.

Enantiomer A molecule that exhibits stereoisomerism through the presence of one or more chiral centers (i.e., stereoisomers that are nonsuperimposable mirror images).

Ethylene glycol An ethylene compound with two hydroxy groups located on adjacent carbons. It is a common ingredient in antifreeze and is highly toxic if ingested.

Gamma-hydroxybutyric acid (GHB) A potent sedative, hypnotic, euphorigenic agent that is illicitly ingested for its pleasurable effects.

Intoxication A state of impaired mental or physical functioning resulting from ingestion of alcohol or drug.

Lysergic acid diethylamide (LSD) A derivative of an alkaloid found in certain fungi that has hallucinogenic properties.

Marijuana A crude preparation of the leaves and flowering tops of (male or female plants) *Cannabis sativa,* usually used in cigarettes and inhaled as smoke for its euphoric properties.

MDA (3,4-methylenedioxyamphetamine) A psychedelic drug of the phenethylamine and amphetamine classes of drugs.

MDMA (3,4-methylenedioxy-N-methylamphetamine) A drug of the phenethylamine and amphetamine classes of drugs. Known as "ecstasy."

Methadone A synthetic opioid analgesic, possessing pharmacologic actions similar to those of morphine and heroin and similar potential for addiction; used as an analgesic and as a narcotic abstinence syndrome suppressant in the treatment of heroin addiction.

Methamphetamine (Ritalin) A sympathomimetic amine closely related chemically to both amphetamine and ephedrine, having actions similar to those of amphetamine.

Methylphenidate (MPH) A central stimulant used in the treatment of attention-deficit/hyperactivity disorder, narcolepsy, and certain forms of depression.

Miosis Constriction of the pupil of the eye, resulting from a normal response to an increase in light or caused by certain drugs or pathological conditions.

Mnemonics A mnemonic or mnemonic device is any learning technique that aids information retention.

Opiate/Opioid *Opiate* refers to any of a group of naturally occurring (poppy plant) or semi-synthetic narcotic alkaloids with pharmacological actions and chemical structure similar to morphine. *Opioid* is a general term that is applied to all substances with morphine-like properties, regardless of origin or chemical structure.

Phencyclidine A potent veterinary analgesic and anesthetic, sometimes used as a drug of abuse by humans but capable of causing serious psychological disturbances.

Poison Any substance that, when relatively small amounts are ingested, inhaled, or absorbed, or when it is applied to, injected into, or developed within the body, has chemical action that may cause damage to structure or disturbance of function, producing symptoms, illness, or death.

Screening test An initial test, such as an immunoassay or a TLC, that is used to "screen" urine specimens to eliminate "negative" ones from further consideration and to identify presumptively positive specimens that then require confirmatory testing.

Sedative A drug that depresses activity of the central nervous system and reduces anxiety and induces sleep.

Toxidrome A syndrome caused by a dangerous concentration of toxins in the body.

Toxins Poisonous substances that are produced by living cells or organisms and is capable of causing disease when introduced into the body tissues and is often capable of inducing neutralizing antibodies or antitoxins.

Toxicology is a broad, multidisciplinary science whose goal is to determine the effects of chemical agents on living systems. Innumerable potential **toxins** inflict harm, including (1) pharmaceuticals, (2) herbals, (3) household products, (4) environmental agents, (5) occupational chemicals, (6) **drugs of abuse,** (7) drugs used in sexual attacks, and (8) drugs used by athletes for their performance-enhancing effects. Each year, millions of human exposure cases are reported to the American Association of **Poison** Control Centers. The Centers for Disease Control and Prevention has reported that poisoning (both intentional and unintentional) is one of the top 10 causes of injury-related death in the United States in all adult age groups.

This chapter provides a general overview of **clinical toxicology** and the laboratory services necessary to support the care of poisoned patients. Because a comprehensive discussion of all aspects of toxicology is beyond the scope of this chapter, the clinical significance and toxicity of only a select number of (1) common drugs, (2) drugs of abuse, and (3) other chemicals are discussed.

Basic Information

In practice, it is neither possible nor necessary to test for all of the hundreds or thousands of clinical toxins that may be encountered. In reality, up to 24 drugs or agents account for 80% or more of cases of **intoxication** treated in most emergency departments. The scope of clinical toxicology testing provided by the laboratory depends on the pattern of local drug use and on the available resources of the institution.

The value of drug and/or substance testing is well established (1) in the workplace, (2) for some athletic competitions, (3) to monitor drug use during pregnancy, (4) to evaluate drug exposure and/or withdrawal in newborns, (5) to monitor patients in pain management and drug abuse treatment programs, and (6) to aid in the prompt diagnosis of toxicity for a number of commonly encountered drugs or agents for which a specific antidote or treatment modality is required (Table 31-1). In many other instances of drug toxicity, the value of drug testing, especially on an emergency basis, is controversial.[13]

Clinical Considerations

To operate effectively, the laboratory should be closely associated with the healthcare team that is directly managing the patient. Through close and collaborative work, clinical information provided will help to guide appropriate ordering of tests and to ensure that interpretation of results is complete and accurate. For example, the team caring for the patient should provide the following information with the laboratory request:

1. The time and date of the suspected exposure along with the time and date of sample collection.
2. History obtained from the patient or from witnesses that might aid in identification of the toxin.
3. Assessment of the physical state of the patient at the time of presentation. Such information is useful for guiding test selection and interpretation of results.

Analytical Considerations

Because of the wide variety of drugs, no single analytical technique is adequate for broad-spectrum drug detection. Therefore, several analytical approaches in combination are generally required. Other critical issues include (1) speed of analysis, (2) turnaround time, and (3) availability of services. A drug analysis that requires several hours to complete or that is not available at all hours of the day may be of little value in a clinical emergency. Alternatively, a rapid test that may provide false information could result in erroneous diagnostic and therapeutic decisions.

TABLE 31-1	Antidote or Specific Treatment for Intoxication
Toxin	**Antidote/Treatment**
Acetaminophen	N-Acetylcysteine
Aluminum, iron	Deferoxamine
Anticholinergic agents	Physostigmine
Arsenic	Dimercaprol; 2,3-dimercaptosuccinic acid; D-penicillamine
Barbiturates	Multiple-dose oral activated charcoal; alkaline diuresis (phenobarbital only)
Benzodiazepines	Flumazenil
β-Blockers	Glucagon
Calcium channel blockers	Calcium; glucagon; high-dose insulin infusion
Carbamazepine	Multiple-dose oral activated charcoal; charcoal hemoperfusion
Carbon monoxide	Oxygen
Cyanide	Amyl nitrite, sodium nitrite, sodium thiosulfate; hydroxocobalamin
Digoxin	Anti-digoxin Fab fragments
Ethylene glycol, methanol	Fomepizole (4-methylpyrazol) or ethanol; hemodialysis
Isoniazid	Pyridoxine
Lead	Calcium disodium edetate; dimercaprol; 2,3-dimercaptosuccinic acid
Lithium	Hemodialysis
Mercury	Dimercaprol; 2,3-dimercaptosuccinic acid; D-penicillamine
Methanol	Fomepizole (4-methylpyrazol) or ethanol; hemodialysis; folate
Nitrites, nitrates	Methylene blue
Opioids	Naloxone
Organophosphate or carbamate	Atropine; pralidoxime (controversial for carbamates)
Salicylates	Bicarbonate; hemodialysis, activated charcoal, alkaline diuresis
Theophylline	Multiple-dose oral activated charcoal; hemodialysis
Tricyclic antidepressants	Bicarbonate; benzodiazepines

Clinical Evaluation

When a healthcare team initially evaluates a patient who presents with a potentially toxicologically induced problem, the final diagnosis is often determined by (1) reviewing the history, (2) performing a directed physical examination, (3) using ancillary tests (e.g., electrocardiogram, radiology), and (4) laboratory testing.

Toxic Syndromes

Toxic syndromes ("**toxidromes**") are clinical syndromes that are essential for the successful recognition of poisoning patterns. A toxidrome is a constellation of clinical signs and symptoms that suggests a specific class of poisoning. An important purpose of the secondary survey is to determine whether a specific toxic syndrome is present. The most commonly encountered toxidromes include (1) anticholinergic, (2) cholinergic, (3) opioid, (4) sedative-hypnotic, and

(5) sympathomimetic toxidromes (Table 31-2). Many toxidromes have several overlapping features. For example, anticholinergic findings are highly similar to sympathomimetic findings, with one exception being their effect on sweat glands. In this exception, **anticholinergic agents** produce warm, flushed dry skin, but sympathomimetic agents produce diaphoresis (purfuse perspiration). Toxidrome findings may also be affected by (1) individual variability, (1) comorbid conditions, and (3) co-ingestants. For example, tachycardia associated with sympathomimetic or anticholinergic toxidromes may be absent in a patient who is concurrently taking beta-antagonist medications. Additionally, although toxidromes may be applied to classes of drugs, one or more toxidrome findings may be absent for some individual agents within these classes. For instance, meperidine is an opioid **analgesic**, but it does not induce **miosis** (constriction of the pupil), which helps to define the "classic" opioid toxidrome. When accurately identified, the toxidrome may provide invaluable information for diagnosis and subsequent treatment, although the many limitations that impede acute toxidrome diagnosis must be carefully considered.

Screening Procedures for Detection of Drugs

Screening procedures are designed for the relatively rapid and generally qualitative detection of drugs or other toxic substances. Screening procedures may be designed to detect a particular drug or drug class. In general, **screening tests** have adequate clinical sensitivity but lack specificity. Thus a negative result may rule out with reasonable certainty the presence of clinically significant concentrations of a particular analyte. Because of possible interferences, a positive result should be considered "presumptive positive" and should be confirmed by an alternate procedure of greater specificity. Screening tests include simple visual color tests (spot tests) and immunoassays.

Spot Tests

Spot tests are qualitative procedures that are (1) rapid, (2) easily performed, and (3) non–instrument based. They are potentially valuable to rule out the presence of drugs or to suggest (but not prove) the presence of a drug of a particular group. In practice, spot tests have been largely replaced by rapid immunoassays that may be performed at the point of care or in the central laboratory. Two examples of such tests are the ferric chloride and Trinder tests for rapid identification of the patient with salicylate toxicity. Both involve simply applying a few drops of a prepared reagent to a small sample of a patient's urine and watching for a characteristic color change.[13] Both have been used for rapid point-of-care testing and should be followed by determination of serum salicylate concentrations to confirm toxicity and quantitate the salicylate concentration.

Determination of Anion Gap

A basic metabolic panel is recommended and is an important initial screening test for all poisoned patients. When

TABLE 31-2	Symptoms of the Important Toxidromes
Toxidrome	**Symptom**
Anticholinergic	Agitation
	Blurred vision
	Decreased bowel sounds
	Dry skin
	Fever
	Flushing
	Hallucinations
	Ileus
	Lethargy/coma
	Mydriasis
	Myoclonus
	Psychosis
	Seizures
	Tachycardia
	Urinary retention
Cholinergic	Diarrhea
	Miosis
	Bradycardia
	Bronchorrhea
	Emesis
	Lacrimation
	Salivation
	Urination
Opioid	Bradycardia
	Decreased bowel sounds
	Hypotension
	Hypothermia
	Lethargy/coma
	Miosis
	Shallow respirations
	Slow respiratory rate
Sedative-hypnotic	Ataxia
	Blurred vision
	Confusion
	Diplopia
	Dysesthesias
	Hypotension
	Lethargy/coma
	Nystagmus
	Respiratory depression
	Sedation
	Slurred speech
Sympathomimetic	Agitation
	Diaphoresis
	Excessive motor activity
	Excessive speech
	Hallucinations
	Hypertension
	Hyperthermia
	Insomnia
	Restlessness
	Tachycardia
	Tremor

low concentration of serum bicarbonate is discovered on a metabolic panel, the clinician should determine whether an elevated anion gap exists. The formula most commonly used for the anion gap (AG) calculation is as follows:

$$AG = \left[Na^+\right] - \left[Cl^- + HCO_3^-\right]$$

The reference interval for this anion gap is accepted to be 8 to 16 mmol/L.[13] An increase in the anion gap, accompanied by a metabolic acidosis, represents an increase in unmeasured endogenous (e.g., lactate) or exogenous (e.g., salicylates) anions. A list of the more common causes is described using the classic MUDPILES **mnemonic** (Box 31-1). It is imperative that clinicians who admit poisoned patients initially presenting with an increased anion gap metabolic acidosis investigate the cause of that acidosis. Many symptomatic poisoned patients may have an initial mild metabolic acidosis upon presentation, caused by processes resulting in elevated serum lactate. However, with adequate supportive care, including hydration and oxygenation, the anion gap acidosis should improve. If, despite adequate supportive care, an anion gap metabolic acidosis worsens in a poisoned patient, the clinician should consider as potential causes (1) continued absorption of exogenous acids (e.g., salicylate, **ethylene glycol**, methanol), (2) formation of acidic metabolites (e.g., glycolic acid, toluene metabolites), and (3) cellular ischemia with worsening lactic acidosis (e.g., cyanide).

Electrocardiogram

Because numerous drugs cause changes in the electrocardiogram (ECG), interpretation of the ECG in the poisoned patient has been known to significantly facilitate appropriate (1) laboratory testing, (2) diagnosis, and (3) management of care.

Determination of Osmol Gap

The main osmotically active constituents of serum are (1) Na^+, (2) Cl^-, (3) HCO_3^-, (4) glucose, and (5) urea. Several empirical formulas based on measurement of these substances have been used to estimate serum osmolality.[13] In practice, one has not shown itself to be superior to the others, yet each equation demonstrates significant differences in the

osmol gap reference interval. Therefore, reference intervals must be validated on appropriate patient populations. Two commonly used formulas (in conventional and SI units) are presented here:

$$\begin{aligned} OSMc\ (mOsm/kg) =\ &2\ Na\ (mmol/L) \\ &+ glucose\ (mg/dL)/18 \\ &+ urea\ (mg/dL)/2.8 \end{aligned}$$

$$\begin{aligned} OSMc\ (mOsm/kg) =\ &2\ Na\ (mmol/L) + glucose\ (mmol/L) \\ &+ urea\ (mmol/L) \end{aligned}$$

or

$$\begin{aligned} OSMc\ (mOsm/kg) =\ &1.86\ Na\ (mmol/L) \\ &+ glucose\ (mg/dL)/18 \\ &+ urea\ (mg/dL)/2.8 + 9 \end{aligned}$$

$$\begin{aligned} OSMc\ (mOsm/kg) =\ &1.86\ Na\ (mmol/L) \\ &+ glucose\ (mmol/L) \\ &+ urea\ (mmol/L) + 9 \end{aligned}$$

The difference between the actual osmolality (OSMm), measured by freezing-point depression, and the calculated osmolality (OSMc) is referred to as delta-osmolality, or the osmol gap (OSMg).

$$OSMg = OSMm - OSMc$$

Elevated OSMg implies the presence of unmeasured osmotically active substances. Compounds that increase serum osmolality when present in significant concentrations include volatile alcohols such as (1) ethanol, (2) methanol, (3) isopropanol, (4) acetone, and (5) ethylene glycol. The calculation of OSMg is commonly used as a screen. However, it is important to remember that volatile alcohols are not detected when osmolality is measured with a vapor pressure osmometer. Therefore, for the purpose of determining the OSMg, only osmolality measurements based on freezing-point depression are acceptable.

What constitutes a normal osmol gap is widely debated. Large variability is seen in the normal population.[13] It would be expected that each 100 mg/dL (21.7 mmol/L) of ethanol (molecular weight = 46.068 g/mol) in serum results in an approximate increase of 21.7 mOsm/kg. However, this is not found to be the case. Applying a correction factor of 0.83 to the ethanol value will more closely approximate the contribution of ethanol to the OSMg. However, it has been observed that ethanol does not follow a completely predictable relationship with OSMg. In severe ethanol intoxication, OSMg is increased with increasing concentration, implying that something is present besides the alcohol.

A significant residual osmol gap (>10 mOsm/kg) after correction for ethanol suggests the possible presence of (1) isopropanol, (2) methanol, (3) acetone, or (4) ethylene glycol. This information, in conjunction with the presence or

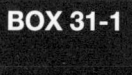

BOX 31-1 Use of the MUDPILES Mnemonic to Remember the Common Causes of Increased Anion Gap

Methanol
Uremia
Diabetic ketoacidosis
Paraldehyde
Iron, inhalants (i.e., carbon monoxide, cyanide, toluene), isoniazid, ibuprofen
Lactic acidosis
Ethylene glycol, ethanol ketoacidosis
Salicylates, starvation ketoacidosis, sympathomimetics

TABLE 31-3 Laboratory Findings Characteristic of Ingestion of Alcohols

Alcohol	Serum Osmol Gap	Metabolic Acidosis with Anion Gap	Serum Acetone	Urine Oxalate
Ethanol	+	−	−	−
Methanol	+	+	−	−
Isopropanol	+	−	+	−
Ethylene glycol	+	+	−	+

absence of metabolic acidosis or serum acetone, is helpful to the clinician when specific measurements of alcohols other than ethanol are not available on an emergency basis (Table 31-3). Unfortunately, OSMg as a screening method is insensitive to low, but clinically significant, concentrations of ethylene glycol (<50 mg/dL) and methanol (<30 mg/dL). It must be realized that ketones (for example, in patients with diabetes) and substances administered to patients such as polyethylene glycol, mannitol (osmotic diuretic), and propylene glycol (solvents in some drug formulations) may increase serum osmolality.[13]

Use of Immunoassay

Different types of immunoassays are useful in screening specimens for drugs (see Chapter 15). Some immunoassays are relatively specific for a single drug, but in others, several drugs of a similar class are detected (e.g., **opiates**). The detection limit for various members of a class of drugs or the degree of cross-reactivity for similar drugs varies, and each manufacturer of immunoassay reagents should be consulted for specific information. These assays (1) are easy to perform, (2) are available for use on automated instrumentation, and (3) often are capable of providing "semiquantitative" results. Several portable noninstrumental immunoassay-based drug detection devices are available for use in point-of-care testing (POCT). For the vast majority of drugs of abuse, immunoassays are the methods of choice for initial screening. However, for more comprehensive drug screening, chromatographic procedures complement immunoassays.

Use of Planar Chromatography

Planar chromatography, commonly known as *thin-layer chromatography (TLC)*, is a versatile procedure that requires no instrumentation and thus is operationally relatively simple and inexpensive (see Chapter 12). With this technique, a large number of drugs may be detected and it has been applied to the analysis of (1) serum, (2) gastric contents, or (3) urine. However, urine is the specimen of choice because most drugs and drug metabolites are present in urine in relatively high concentrations. However, application of TLC to drug screening requires considerable experience and skill on the part of the laboratorian to recognize drug and metabolite patterns and various color hues

for detection; it has largely been replaced by other chromatographic techniques[3]

Use of Gas Chromatography

Gas liquid chromatography (GC) is (1) relatively rapid, (2) capable of resolving a broad spectrum of drugs, and is (3) widely used for qualitative and quantitative drug analysis.[11] Capillary columns are analytical columns that are commonly used for drug detection by GC (see Chapter 12). In many instances, nonderivatized drugs have good GC properties when capillary columns are used. However, derivatization to a less polar or a more volatile compound is often necessary. Common detectors for drug detection by GC are flame ionization and alkali flame ionization (nitrogen phosphorus) detectors. A GC coupled to a mass spectrometer (GC-MS) provides an analytical system with the greatest accuracy of identification. Numerous methods for general drug screening by GC-MS spectrometry have been published

Use of High-Performance Liquid Chromatography

High-performance liquid chromatography (HPLC) (see Chapter 12) has been applied to the complex challenge of comprehensive drug screening in biological fluids. Advantages of HPLC over GC include its usefulness in analyzing (1) polar compounds without derivatization (e.g., morphine, benzoylecgonine) and (2) thermally labile drugs (e.g., chlordiazepoxide). The advent of diode array detectors that provide a spectral scan of compounds as they elute from the column has greatly increased the discriminatory power of this technique. Analytical systems based on coupling of liquid chromatography (LC) with mass spectrometry (MS) (LC-MS or LC-MS/MS) are rapidly gaining in popularity.[13]

Use of Point-of-Care Devices

Numerous point-of-care (POC) drug test devices for urine (and oral fluid) are designed for easy, rugged, and portable use by nontechnical personnel. Although these devices are relatively simple to use, proper training of nonlaboratory users is important for optimal results (see Chapter 17). These noninstrumental immunoassay test devices are designed for use at the site of collection; results are available within minutes and are variously configured to detect only one drug or many drugs simultaneously. The assay principles of POC test devices are found in the package insert for each specific test kit.

Pharmacology and Analysis of Specific Drugs and Toxic Agents

The toxic consequences of several drugs and toxins are individually discussed in this section. They include (1) agents that cause cellular hypoxia, (2) alcohols, (3) analgesics (nonprescription), (4) agents related to anticholinergic toxidrome, (5) agents related to cholinergic toxidrome, (6) drugs of abuse, and (7) drugs used in sexual assault.

Agents That Cause Cellular Hypoxia

Carbon monoxide (CO) and methemoglobin-forming agents interfere with oxygen transport, resulting in cellular hypoxia. Cyanide interferes with oxygen use and therefore causes an apparent cellular hypoxia.

Carbon Monoxide

CO is a colorless, odorless, tasteless gas that is a product of incomplete combustion of carbonaceous material. Small amounts of CO are produced endogenously in the metabolic conversion of heme to biliverdin.

Toxic Effects

When inhaled, CO combines tightly with the heme Fe^{2+} of hemoglobin to form *carboxyhemoglobin*. The binding affinity of hemoglobin for carbon monoxide is about 250 times greater than that for oxygen. Moreover, the binding of carbon monoxide to a hemoglobin subunit increases the oxygen affinity for the remaining subunits in the hemoglobin tetramer. Thus at a given tissue PO_2 value, less oxygen dissociates from hemoglobin when carbon monoxide is also bound, shifting the hemoglobin-oxygen dissociation curve to the left. Consequently, carbon monoxide not only decreases the oxygen content of blood, it also decreases oxygen availability to tissue. This produces a greater degree of tissue hypoxia than would result from an equivalent reduction in oxyhemoglobin due to hypoxia alone. Carbon monoxide may also bind to other heme proteins, such as myoglobin and mitochondrial cytochrome oxidase a_3; this may limit oxygen use when tissue PO_2 is very low.[13]

Treatment for carbon monoxide poisoning involves removal of the individual from the contaminated area and administration of oxygen. The **drug half-life ($t_{1/2}$)** of carboxyhemoglobin in the body is variable. Low carboxyhemoglobin concentrations relative to the severity of poisoning may be observed if the patient was removed from the CO-contaminated environment several hours before blood sampling. Hyperbaric oxygen therapy for CO is highly debated, and current position papers have reported no evidence to support its use.

Analytical Methods

Carbon monoxide may be released from hemoglobin and then measured by GC, or it may be determined indirectly as carboxyhemoglobin by spectrophotometry. Gas chromatographic methods are accurate and precise even for very low concentrations of carbon monoxide. Spectrophotometric methods are (1) rapid, (2) convenient, (3) accurate, and (4) precise, except at very low concentrations of carboxyhemoglobin (<3%).

Gas chromatographic methods measure the carbon monoxide content of blood and are considered to be reference procedures. When blood is treated with potassium ferricyanide, carboxyhemoglobin is converted to methemoglobin, and carbon monoxide is released into the gas phase. Measurement of the released carbon monoxide may be performed by GC using various methods and detectors.[13] In clinical practice,

CO binding capacity is determined after an aliquot of the blood specimen is treated with carbon monoxide to saturate the hemoglobin. The results are then expressed as percentage of carboxyhemoglobin:

$$\% \, HbCO = \frac{CO_{content}}{CO_{capacity}} \times 100$$

Spectrophotometric methods rely on the characteristic spectral absorption properties of carboxyhemoglobin. The most common are based on automated, multi-wavelength measurements of several hemoglobin species, and they are rapid and convenient. Spectrophotometric methods generally compare favorably with gas chromatographic procedures at carboxyhemoglobin concentrations greater than 2% to 3%, but their precision is poor below these concentrations. Therefore, they are sufficiently accurate and precise for measurement of carbon monoxide after exogenous exposure, but they are too insensitive to detect the increased endogenous production of carbon monoxide that occurs in hemolytic anemia.

Fetal hemoglobin and adult hemoglobin differ slightly in their spectral properties. Consequently, falsely high carboxyhemoglobin values of 4% to 7% may occur when blood from neonates is measured by some spectrophotometric methods by using fewer wavelengths. Moreover, erroneous results may occur with lipemic and icteric specimens and in the presence of methylene blue (see later section, "Methemoglobin-Forming Agents").

Cyanide

Cyanide consists of one atom of carbon triple-bonded to one atom of nitrogen (C≡N). Inorganic cyanides (also known as *cyanide salts*) contain cyanide in anion form (CN^-) and are used in numerous industries. Organic compounds that have a cyano group bonded to an alkyl residue are called *nitriles*. Iatrogenic cyanide poisoning may occur during use of nitroprusside.

Toxic Effects

Cyanide in serum readily crosses all biological membranes and avidly binds to heme iron (Fe^{3+}) in the cytochrome a-a_3 complex within mitochondria. When bound to cytochrome a-a_3, cyanide is a competitive inhibitor that causes decoupling of oxidative phosphorylation. Patients exposed to toxic concentrations of cyanide exhibit rapid onset of symptoms typical of cellular hypoxia, such as (1) flushing, (2) headache, (3) tachypnea, (4) dizziness, and (5) respiratory depression. Subsequently, cellular hypoxia progresses rapidly to (1) coma, (2) seizures, (3) complete heart block, and (4) death if the cyanide dose is sufficiently large. Hydroxycobalamin or the cyanide antidote kit should be administered as soon as cyanide poisoning is suspected.

Analytical Methods

After microdiffusion, whole blood CN^- is measured by spectrophotometry or by headspace gas chromatography.[13]

Methemoglobin-Forming Agents

The heme iron in hemoglobin is typically present in the ferrous state (Fe^{2+}). When oxidized to the ferric state (Fe^{3+}), methemoglobin is formed, and this form of hemoglobin does not bind oxygen. The principal physiological system that maintains hemoglobin iron in the reduced state is nicotinamide adenine dinucleotide (NADH)-methemoglobin reductase. A minor pathway for methemoglobin reduction involves nicotinamide adenine dinucleotide phosphate (NADPH)-methemoglobin reductase. Congenital methemoglobinemia may result from a deficiency of NADH-methemoglobin reductase or, more rarely, from hemoglobin variants (hemoglobin M) in which heme iron is both more susceptible to oxidation and more resistant to reduction by the methemoglobin reductase system.

Toxic Effects

An acquired (toxic) methemoglobinemia may be caused by various drugs and chemicals (Table 31-4). The normal percentage of methemoglobin is <1.5% of total hemoglobin. All symptoms associated with methemoglobinemia are consequences of hypoxia associated both with diminished O_2 content of blood and with decreased O_2 dissociation from hemoglobin species. The PO_2 is normal in these patients, and therefore so is the calculated hemoglobin oxygen saturation. Thus, a normal PO_2 in a cyanotic patient is a significant indication of the possible presence of *methemoglobinemia*. Direct measurement of methemoglobin is important in these cases. Specific therapy for toxic methemoglobinemia involves the administration of methylene blue. Methylene blue and sulfhemoglobin cause spectral interference in the measurement of methemoglobin with some co-oximeters but not with the Evelyn-Malloy method.

Analytical Methods

Methemoglobin is measured in blood manually or by taking automated multi-wavelength measurements with a co-oximeter. Methemoglobin interferes with the noninvasive pulse oximetry method, measuring the absorbance of light at 660 nm (oxyhemoglobin) and 940 nm (deoxyhemoglobin). Because methemoglobin is not stable at room temperature, specimens should be kept on ice or refrigerated but not frozen. The stability of methemoglobin at 4 °C has not been well studied. Some sources report significant decreases in methemoglobin concentration after 4 to 8 hours, whereas others describe little or no change after 24 hours. Freezing results in an increase in methemoglobin concentration.

Alcohols

Several alcohols are toxic and medically important. They include (1) ethanol, (2) methanol, (3) isopropanol and acetone, and (4) ethylene glycol.

Ethanol

Ethanol is the most widely used and often abused chemical substance. Consequently, measurement of ethanol is one of the more frequently performed tests in the toxicology laboratory. The principal pharmacological action of ethanol involves central nervous system (CNS) depression, and effects vary depending on the blood ethanol concentration (Table 31-5) and an individual's tolerance. A blood alcohol concentration of 80 mg/dL (0.08%) has been established as the per se limit for operation of a motor vehicle in North America.[13]

Ethanol is metabolized principally by liver alcohol dehydrogenase to acetaldehyde, which is subsequently oxidized to acetic acid by aldehyde dehydrogenase (Figure 31-1). The rate of elimination of ethanol from blood approximates a zero-order process. This rate varies among individuals, averaging about 15 mg/dL/h for males and 18 mg/dL/h for females. At both low (<20 mg/dL) and high (>300 mg/dL) ethanol concentrations, elimination becomes more nearly first-order; it is accelerated at high concentrations. The elimination rate is also influenced by drinking practices (e.g., alcoholics have increased elimination rates caused by enzyme induction).

When consumed with other CNS depressant drugs, ethanol exerts a potentiation or synergistic depressant effect. This occurs at relatively low alcohol concentrations, and numerous deaths have resulted from combined ethanol and drug ingestion.[13] Ethanol is a teratogen, and alcohol consumption during pregnancy can result in the birth of a baby with fetal alcohol spectrum disorder (FASD). FASD is an umbrella term that describes the variety of effects that occur in an individual whose mother drank alcohol during pregnancy. These effects may include (1) physical, (2) mental, (3) behavioral, and (4) learning disabilities with lifelong implications. They are, however, 100% preventable when a woman completely **abstains** from alcohol during her pregnancy.

Methanol

Methanol is used as a solvent in several commercial products and is sold in numerous consumer products such as de-icers and windshield washer fluids. Methanol poisoning can be lethal if not recognized early. Unfortunately, in some instances, the latent period is as long as 24 hours before toxicity is recognized, making laboratory identification of this poisoning critical.[13]

Methanol is oxidized by liver alcohol dehydrogenase (at about one-tenth the rate of ethanol) to formaldehyde. Formaldehyde in turn is rapidly oxidized by aldehyde dehydrogenase to formic

TABLE 31-4	Examples of Acquired Causes of Methemoglobinemia
Drugs	**Chemical Agents**
Amyl nitrite	Aniline
Benzocaine	Amyl nitrite
Chloroquine	Butyl nitrite
Dapsone	Chlorobenzene
Nitroglycerin	Naphthalene
Phenacetin	Nitrates
Phenazopyridine	Nitrites
Primaquine	Nitrophenol
Sulfonamides	Nitrous oxide

acid, which may cause serious acidosis and optic neuropathy, resulting in blindness or death. The mainstay of therapy for methanol toxicity includes (1) administration of ethanol or fomepizole as a competitive alcohol dehydrogenase inhibitor, (2) administration of either folate or folinic acid, and (3) dialysis.

Isopropanol and Acetone

Isopropanol is readily available to the general population, commonly as a 70% aqueous solution, for use as rubbing alcohol. It has about twice the CNS depressant action as ethanol. Isopropanol is rapidly metabolized by alcohol dehydrogenase to acetone, which is eliminated much more slowly. Therefore, concentrations of acetone in serum often exceed those of isopropanol during the elimination phase after isopropanol ingestion. Acetone has CNS depressant activity similar to that of ethanol, and because of its longer half-life, it may prolong the apparent CNS effects of isopropanol. Supportive care is the mainstay of treatment, with rare reports of dialysis in severe intoxication.

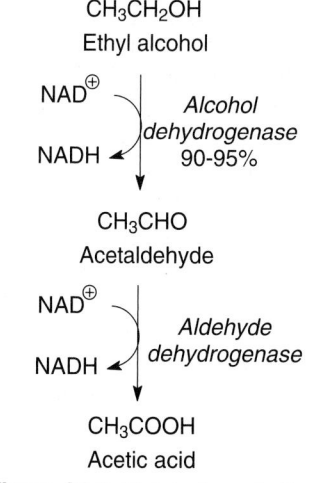

Figure 31-1 Metabolism of ethanol.

Blood Alcohol Concentration, g/100 mL or mg/dL	Influence	Clinical Signs/Symptoms
0.01-0.05	Subclinical	Influence/effects not apparent or obvious
		Behavior nearly normal by ordinary observation
		Impairment detectable by special tests
0.03-0.12	Euphoria	Mild euphoria, sociability, talkativeness
		Increased self-confidence; decreased inhibitions
		Diminution of attention, judgment, and control
		Some sensorimotor impairment
		Slowed information processing
		Loss of efficiency in finer performance tests
		Impairment of perception, memory
0.09-0.25	Excitement	Emotional instability; loss of critical judgment comprehension
		Decreased sensory response; increased reaction time
		Reduced visual acuity, peripheral vision, and glare recovery
		Sensorimotor incoordination; impaired balance
		Drowsiness
0.18-0.30	Confusion	Disorientation, mental confusion; dizziness
		Exaggerated emotional states (fear, rage, grief, etc.)
		Disturbances of vision (diplopia, etc.) and of perception of color, form, motion, dimensions
		Increased pain threshold
		Increased muscular incoordination; staggering gait; slurred speech
		Apathy, lethargy
0.25-0.40	Stupor	General inertia; approaching loss of motor functions
		Markedly decreased response to stimuli
		Marked muscular incoordination; inability to stand or walk
		Vomiting; incontinence of urine and feces
		Impaired consciousness; sleep or stupor
0.35-0.50	Coma	Complete unconsciousness; coma; anesthesia
		Depressed or abolished reflexes
		Subnormal temperature
		Impairment of circulation and respiration
		Possible death
0.45 +	Death	Death from respiratory arrest

TABLE 31-5 Stages of Acute Alcoholic Influence/Intoxication

Ethylene Glycol

Ethylene glycol, present in products such as antifreeze, may be ingested accidentally or for the purpose of inebriation or suicide. Ethylene glycol itself is relatively nontoxic, and its initial CNS effects resemble those of ethanol. However, metabolism of ethylene glycol by alcohol dehydrogenase (ADH) results in the formation of numerous acid metabolites, including oxalic acid and glycolic acid, which are responsible for much of the toxicity of ethylene glycol. Serum ethylene glycol concentrations associated with death from ethylene glycol ingestion have no correlation with severity of toxicity. It is thus impossible to define a serum ethylene glycol concentration associated with a high probability of death. However, the serum concentration of the metabolite glycolic acid correlates more closely with clinical symptoms and mortality. Because of the rapid elimination of ethylene glycol, its serum concentration may be low or undetectable at a time when glycolic acid remains elevated. Thus the determination of ethylene glycol and glycolic acid provides useful clinical and confirmatory analytical information in cases of ethylene glycol ingestion. The mainstay of therapy for ethylene glycol toxicity includes administration of ethanol or fomepizole as a competitive alcohol dehydrogenase inhibitor and dialysis.

Analysis of Ethanol

Serum, plasma, and whole blood are suitable blood-related specimens for the determination of ethanol. The venipuncture site should be cleansed with an alcohol-free disinfectant, such as aqueous benzalkonium chloride.

Serum/Plasma and Blood Ethanol

Alcohol distributes into the aqueous compartments of blood; because the water content of serum is greater than that of whole blood. Higher alcohol concentrations are obtained with serum as compared with whole blood. Experimentally, the serum-to-whole blood ethanol ratio is 1.18 and varies slightly with hematocrit. Therefore, laboratories that perform alcohol determinations should make clear the choice of specimen.

Because of the volatile nature of alcohols, specimens should be kept capped to avoid evaporative loss. Blood may be stored, when properly sealed, for 14 days at room temperature or at 4 °C, with or without preservative. For longer storage or for nonsterile postmortem specimens, sodium fluoride should be used as a preservative to prevent a decrease or occasionally an increase (via fermentation) in ethanol concentration.

To measure ethanol in serum/plasma, the enzymatic assay is the method of choice in many clinical laboratories. With this method, ethanol is measured by oxidation to acetaldehyde with NAD, a reaction catalyzed by ADH. With this reaction, the formation of NADH, measured at 340 nm, is proportional to the amount of ethanol in the specimen.

$$\text{Ethanol} + \text{NAD} \xrightarrow{\text{ADH}} \text{Acetaldehyde} + \text{NADH}$$

Under most assay conditions, ADH is reasonably specific for ethanol, with interferences by (1) isopropanol, (2) acetone, (3) methanol, and (4) ethylene glycol of typically <1%. Results obtained with these methods generally compare closely with gas chromatographic methods. However, spuriously increased results for ethanol have been described in the presence of high concentrations of lactate dehydrogenase (LD) and lactate, resulting from the production of NADH by LD.

Breath Ethanol

Statutory laws for driving under the influence of alcohol were originally based on the concentration of ethanol in venous whole blood. Because collection of blood is invasive and requires the participation of medical personnel, determination of alcohol in expired air (breath) has long been the mainstay of evidential alcohol measurements. Clinical interest in determination of breath alcohol at the point of care is growing. The fundamental principle for the use of breath analysis is that alcohol in capillary alveolar blood rapidly equilibrates with alveolar air in a ratio of approximately 2100:1 (blood/breath). This blood/breath ratio may actually be closer to 2300:1 but in any case is variable. Nevertheless, in the United States, evidential breath alcohol measurements are based on the ratio of 2100:1. To alleviate confusion and uncertainty surrounding conversion from breath to blood alcohol concentration, the traffic laws in many countries specify per se limits for blood and/or breath.

Before breath alcohol analysis, a deprivation period of at least 15 minutes is recommended to allow for clearance of any residual alcohol that may have been present in the mouth from (1) very recent drinking, (2) use of alcohol-containing mouthwash, or (3) vomiting of alcohol-rich gastric fluid. Duplicate tests, performed 3 to 10 minutes apart, typically must agree within 20 mg/dL (0.02%) as an additional safeguard against mouth alcohol contamination.

Determination of ethanol in expired air requires specialized breath alcohol analyzers. Several commercial evidential breath alcohol measurement devices are available. Breath alcohol devices also may be used for the medical evaluation of patients at the point of care (e.g., emergency department).

Urine Ethanol

Urine has been used as an alternative, less invasive specimen for determination of alcohol use. During the postabsorptive phase that follows alcohol ingestion, the concentration of alcohol in urine is roughly 1.3 times that in blood.[2] However, the use of urine alcohol measurements to estimate blood concentrations is discouraged because the ratio is highly variable, and, perhaps more important, because the urine alcohol concentration reflects an average of the blood alcohol concentration during the period in which urine is collected in the bladder. The detection of alcohol in urine represents ingestion of alcohol within the previous 8 to 12 hours.

Effects of Minor Metabolites

Ethyl glucuronide (EtG) and ethyl sulfate (EtS) are minor metabolites of alcohol. EtG is a phase II metabolite formed through UDP-glucuronosyltransferase, and EtS is formed directly by conjugation of the ethanol with sulfate group. In practice, it is possible to detect EtG in urine 80 hours post alcohol consumption, and it is found even when small amounts of alcohol are consumed. Because of its long urinary elimination time and its specificity for ethanol exposure, its use as a marker of recent ethanol intake has been proposed. However, challenges associated with factors such as (1) establishing appropriate cutoff concentrations capable of distinguishing between drinking and nonbeverage sources of ethanol exposure, (2) sample stability, and (3) microbial activity substantially complicate accurate interpretation of results.

Analysis of Volatile Alcohols

Flame ionization GC remains the most common method used to detect and quantify volatile alcohols in biological samples.[2] Not only does it distinguish between (1) ethanol, (2) methanol, (3) isopropanol, and (4) acetone, it has the capability to measure concentrations as low as 10 mg/dL (0.01%). Specimens are prepared by a variety of methods; the two most common are direct injection and headspace analysis. Direct injection involves injection of a sample prepared by dilution with an aqueous solution of internal standard. However, repeated injection of this matrix into the GC may cause buildup on the injector and on the front of the analytical column, requiring frequent maintenance and column replacement. In practice, this problem is mitigated by the use of headspace injection. The volatility of the alcohols is used to separate them from the matrix. Specifically, the "Gas Law" states that at a given temperature, the amount of volatile substance in the air space above the liquid—headspace—is proportional to the concentration of the volatile alcohol in the solution. Therefore, the sample in the headspace allows calculation of the concentration in the specimen. Conversely, direct injection GC is the method of choice for ethylene glycol because it has a higher boiling point and is not as amenable to headspace analysis.[13]

Analgesics (Nonprescription)

Analgesics are substances that relieve pain without causing loss of consciousness.

Acetaminophen

Acetaminophen has analgesic and antipyretic actions. In normal doses, acetaminophen is safe and effective, but it may cause severe hepatic and renal toxicity when consumed in overdose quantities. Initial clinical findings in acetaminophen toxicity are relatively mild and nonspecific and include (1) nausea, (2) vomiting, and (3) abdominal discomfort. However, these conditions are not predictive of impending hepatic necrosis. Antidotal therapy with *N*-acetylcysteine (NAC) is most effective when administered before hepatic injury occurs, as signified by elevation of activities of aspartate aminotransaminase (AST) and alanine aminotransaminase (ALT). Thus the measurement of serum acetaminophen concentration becomes paramount for proper assessment of the severity of overdose and for appropriate decision making for antidotal therapy. The Rumack-Matthew nomogram relates serum acetaminophen concentration and time after acute ingestion to the probability of hepatic necrosis (Figure 31-2).

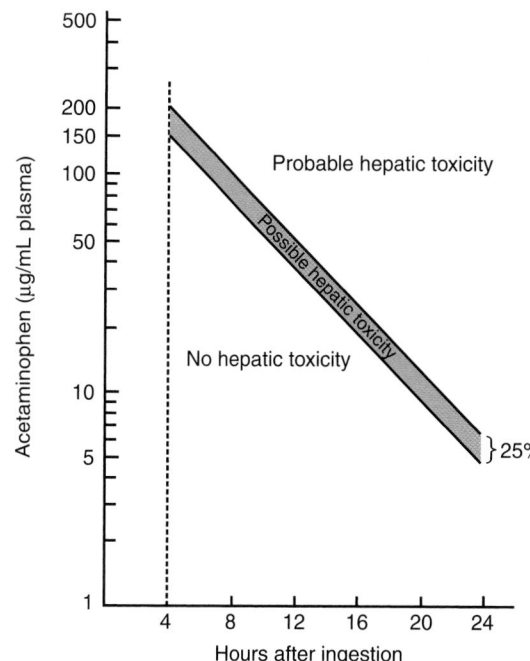

Figure 31-2 Rumack-Matthew nomogram. *(From Rumack BH, Matthew H. Acetaminophen poisoning and toxicity. Pediatrics 1975;55:871-6. Reproduced by permission of Pediatrics.)*

Acetaminophen is normally metabolized in the liver to glucuronide (50% to 60%) and sulfate (≈30%) conjugates. A smaller amount (≈10%) is metabolized by a cytochrome P450 mixed-function oxidase pathway that is thought to involve formation of a highly reactive intermediate (Figure 31-3), *N*-acetyl-*p*-benzoquinoneimine (NAPQI). This intermediate normally undergoes electrophilic conjugation with glutathione and then subsequent transformation to cysteine and mercapturic acid conjugates of acetaminophen. With acetaminophen overdose, the sulfation pathway becomes saturated; consequently, a greater portion is metabolized by the P450 mixed-function oxidase pathway. When the tissue stores of glutathione become depleted, arylation of cellular molecules by the benzoquinoneimine intermediate leads to hepatic necrosis. Specific therapy for acetaminophen overdose is administration of NAC, which acts as a glutathione substitute.

Many spectrophotometric methods are available for determination of acetaminophen.[13] In general, these methods are simple and relatively easy to perform but are subject to various interferences such as bilirubin or bilirubin byproducts absorbing at similar wavelengths. Some methods measure the nontoxic metabolites and the potentially toxic parent acetaminophen, and thus may produce especially misleading results. Therefore, only methods specific for parent acetaminophen should be used. Immunoassays are widely used for this purpose, as they are (1) rapid, (2) easily performed, and (3) accurate. A different spectrophotometric approach uses arylacrylamide amidohydrolase to hydrolyze acetaminophen (but not conjugates) to *p*-aminophenol and acetate. Subsequent formation of the absorbing species depends on the reaction of generated *p*-aminophenol with 8-hydroxyquinoline or *o*-cresol. Arylacrylamide amidohydrolase methods are susceptible

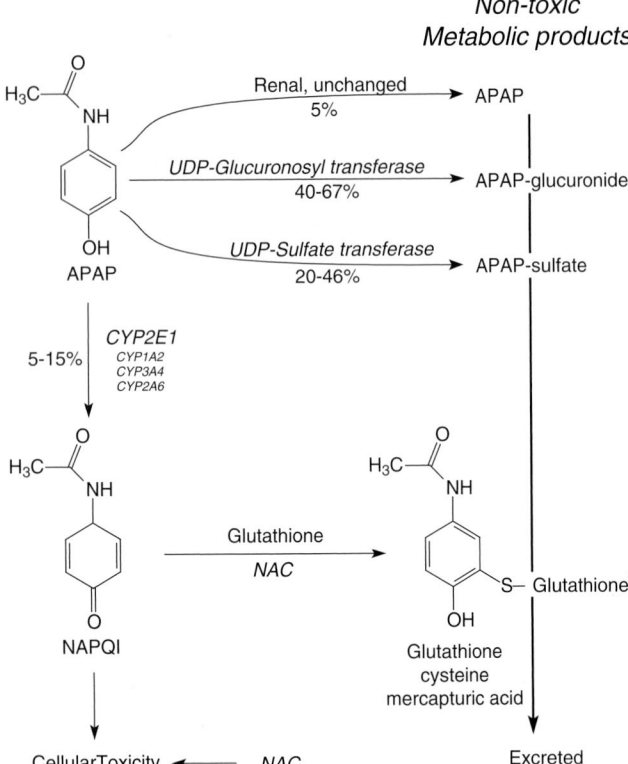

Figure 31-3 Pathways of acetaminophen metabolism. APAP (*N*-acetyl-*p*-aminophenol/acetaminophen), NAPQI (*N*-acetyl-*p*-benzoquinoneimine), and NAC (*N*-acetylcysteine).

to interference by (1) NAC, (2) bilirubin, and (3) immunoglobulin (Ig)M monoclonal immunoglobulins. A qualitative, one-step lateral flow immunoassay (cutoff of 25 µg/mL) may be suitable for point-of-care application, yet it has a low positive predictive value. Most chromatographic methods are very accurate and are considered reference procedures.

Salicylates

Acetylsalicylic acid (aspirin) is a salicylate that has (1) analgesic, (2) antipyretic, and (3) anti-inflammatory properties. Salicylates directly stimulate the central respiratory center, thereby causing hyperventilation and respiratory alkalosis. Moreover, salicylates cause uncoupling of oxidative phosphorylation. As a result, (1) heat production (hyperthermia), (2) oxygen consumption, and (3) metabolic rate may be increased. In addition, salicylates enhance anaerobic glycolysis but inhibit the Krebs cycle and transaminase enzymes, all of which lead to accumulation of organic acids and thus to metabolic acidosis.

After acute salicylate overdose, patients initially may be asymptomatic, especially if that product is enteric coated. Salicylate toxic patients may develop (1) nausea, (2) vomiting, (3) abdominal pain, (4) tinnitus (ringing of the ear), (5) tachypnea (rapid breathing), (6) oliguria (decreased urine output), and (7) altered mental status ranging from lethargy to coma. Individuals with chronic intoxication present in a similar fashion as those with acute exposures, yet such exposures typically are more insidious and therefore are often misdiagnosed.

Use of salicylate concentrations to guide management must be done cautiously and only in conjunction with careful evaluation of a patient's clinical status. Although toxic concentrations alone are of poor prognostic value, certain clinical findings predict a poor prognosis, including (1) pulmonary edema, (2) fever, (3) coma, and (4) acidosis. The absorptive phase of salicylates is often unpredictable (delayed or erratic) as a result of (1) **bezoar** formation, (2) enteric-coated product, (3) gastric outlet obstruction, or (4) pylorospasm. Therefore, a specimen drawn soon after the original ingestion may not be reflective of the potential peak concentration. Initial serial concentrations should be obtained every 2 hours while the patient is monitored clinically. When the concentrations begin to decline and the patient's clinical status is improved, concentrations are measured less frequently.

Treatment for salicylate intoxication is directed toward (1) decreasing further absorption, (2) increasing elimination, and (3) correcting acid-base and electrolyte disturbances. Activated charcoal binds aspirin and prevents its absorption. Elimination of salicylate may be enhanced by alkaline **diuresis** and in severe cases by hemodialysis. Sodium bicarbonate may be given to alleviate metabolic acidosis. Indications for hemodialysis include (1) serum salicylate >1000 mg/L, (2) severe CNS depression, (3) intractable metabolic acidosis, (4) hepatic failure with coagulopathy, and (5) renal failure.

Classic methods for measurement of salicylate in serum are based on the method of Trinder (see the section, "Spot Tests"). These procedures rely on the reaction between salicylate and Fe^{3+} to form a colored complex that is measured at 540 nm. To lessen endogenous background interference, a protein precipitation step or a serum blank is necessary. Nevertheless, blank readings equivalent to about 20 to 25 mg/L are generally observed. Moreover, interference by (1) salicylate metabolites, (2) endogenous compounds, and (3) some drugs, especially structurally related drugs such as diflunisal (difluorophenyl salicylate), may occur. Azide, which is present as a preservative in some commercial control sera, also interferes. Despite these limitations, photometric methods continue to be successfully used to assess salicylate overdose. The Trinder method results agreed very closely with those of a reference HPLC procedure.[10] Other methods for salicylate quantitation include fluorescent polarization immunoassay and a salicylate hydroxylase–mediated photometric procedure. These procedures are subject to some of the same interferences as the Trinder method, but the salicylate hydroxylase method is considered more specific and has been adapted to automated analyzers. Gas and liquid chromatographic methods are the most specific methods for salicylate, but their general availability, especially for emergency use, is limited and probably is not necessary. A qualitative, one-step lateral flow immunoassay (cutoff of 100 µg/mL) is commercially available for point-of-care application but has a low positive predictive value (0.47).

Agents Related to Anticholinergic Toxidrome

Agents related to anticholinergic toxidrome include (1) tricyclic antidepressants, (2) antipsychotics, and (3) **antihistamines**.

These agents have divergent therapeutic applications. However, in overdose, they often share similar anticholinergic and antihistaminic toxidromes as principal components of their overall toxic effects.

Tricyclic Antidepressants and Related Drugs

Tricyclic antidepressants (TCAs) are so named because of their three-ring structure (Figure 31-4). They represent a class of drugs frequently prescribed for the treatment of depression. The *N*-demethylated metabolites of several tricyclic antidepressants are pharmacologically active and contribute variably to overall pharmacodynamic activity (see Chapter 30). Because TCAs have had a history of problems with toxicity, they have been largely supplanted by newer, less toxic agents. However, because of (1) their continued use as an inexpensive alternative to new-generation antidepressants, (2) their narrow therapeutic range, and (3) the nature of the illness for which they are typically prescribed, TCAs are frequently associated with severe or fatal toxicity.

The therapeutic mechanism of tricyclic antidepressants is the blockade of neuronal reuptake of serotonin and/or norepinephrine. However, TCAs have many other pharmacological actions, including (1) anticholinergic; (2) antihistaminic; (3) α_1-receptor blocker actions; (4) inhibition of the GABA channel; and (5) of cardiac potassium efflux and fast sodium channels. They apparently do not contribute to therapeutic effects, but they do contribute to adverse effects, both at therapeutic dosing and in overdose.

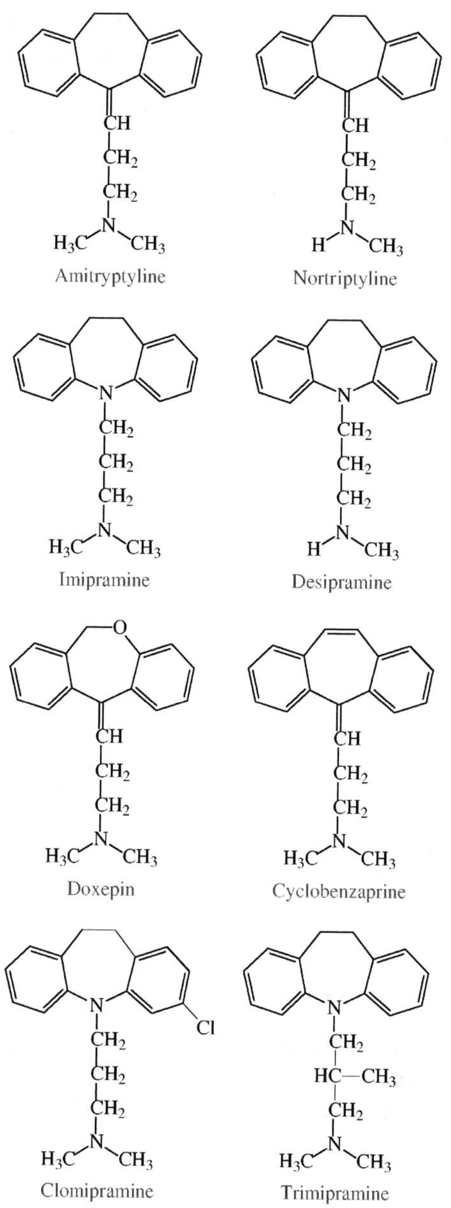

Analytical Methods

Tricyclic antidepressants are measured by chromatographic methods or by immunoassay. Immunoassays are rapid and relatively easy to perform but may be subject to interference by other drugs,[13] and they cannot necessarily be used to identify which TCA is being quantitated. In cases of overdose, qualitative identification (serum or urine) is sufficient because the severity of intoxication is more reliably indicated by an increase in the QRS interval than by the serum concentration.

Cyclobenzaprine, a tricyclic amine that is structurally very similar to amitriptyline (see Figure 31-4), is used as a centrally acting skeletal muscle relaxant. Similar to amitriptyline, cyclobenzaprine (1) causes sedation, (2) produces central and peripheral muscarinic blockade, and (3) potentiates adrenergic actions. In overdose, cyclobenzaprine may cause (1) a typical anticholinergic toxidrome, (2) cardiac arrhythmias, (3) hypotension, and (4) coma. The analytical distinction between amitriptyline and cyclobenzaprine is often difficult. Cyclobenzaprine cross-reacts with immunoassays for tricyclic antidepressants; however, it is possible to distinguish between them by using chromatographic methods.[13]

Antipsychotic Drugs

Antipsychotic drugs are generally used for numerous psychiatric disorders. In addition to their psychotherapeutic effects, certain members of this group are used for other indications.[13]

Figure 31-4 Structure of tricyclic antidepressants and related drugs.

Antipsychotic compounds are traditionally divided and subdivided according to their chemical structure (Table 31-6 and Figure 31-5).

The principal manifestations of phenothiazine toxicity involve the CNS and the cardiovascular system. The presentation for most of these drugs is related to their mechanisms of action, which include (1) dopamine blockade (CNS depression), (2) α_1-blockade (hypotension and miosis), (3) anticholinergic blockade (tachycardia), and (4) K-efflux blockade (QT prolongation). Toxicity is strongly correlated with peak serum concentrations.

Neuroleptics are measured by chromatographic methods and by immunoassay. Chromatographically, GC methods with (1) nitrogen phosphorus (NP), (2) electron capture (EC), and (3) MS detectors are used, along with HPLC, LC-MS, and LC-MS/MS methods.[13]

TABLE 31-6 Examples of Classical and Atypical Antipsychotics

Antipsychotics	Examples
Classical Antipsychotics	
Phenothiazines	Chlorpromazine
	Promethazine
	Trichlorperazine
	Perphenazine
	Fluphenazine
	Thioridazine
	Mesoridazine
	Trifluoperazine
Thioxanthenes	Flupenthixol
	Zuclopenthixol
Dibenzoxazepine	Loxapine
Dihydroindole	Molindone
Butyrophenones	Droperidol
	Haloperidol
Diphenylbutylpiperidines	Pimozide
Benzamides	Sulpiride
Atypical Antipsychotics	
Dibenzodiazepine derivatives	Clozapine
	Olanzapine
Benzothiapine derivatives	Quetiapine
	Zotepine
Benzisoxazole derivatives	Risperidone
Benzothiazole piperazine	Ziprasidone
Imidazolindone derivatives	Setindole

Antihistamines

Antihistamines are medications that are popular among the general public for treatment of allergic reactions and as common sleep aids. Antihistamines are widely available, and many do not require a prescription. Histamine is released from mast cells and plays an important physiological role in immediate hypersensitivity and allergic responses. Histamine functions as a neurotransmitter in the CNS and stimulates gastric acid secretion. Currently available antihistamine drugs clinically antagonize H_1 and H_2 histamine receptors. First-generation liphophilic antihistamines, such as diphenhydramine (Benadryl), bind H_1 receptors, exhibit peripheral and central nervous system effects, and bind to muscarinic and adrenergic receptors, resulting in anticholinergic activity. The principal H_2 receptor response is stimulation of gastric acid secretion, whereas other actions of histamine such as (1) smooth muscle contraction, (2) vasodilation, (3) increased capillary permeability, (4) pain, and (5) itching are primarily mediated by H_1 receptors. Second-generation antihistamines, such as fexofenadine (Allegra), are highly specific for peripheral H_1 receptors and do not penetrate the CNS. Therefore, second-generation H_1 receptor antagonists display minimal **sedative** and anticholinergic effects. Individuals overdosed with first-generation H_1 antihistamines present clinically with CNS depression or stimulation and peripheral anticholinergic effects.

Commonly available antihistamines are detected qualitatively and quantitatively in blood and urine specimens.

Methods of choice for their measurement include GC-MS/MS, and LC-MS/MS. However, the clinical necessity of quantitative serum antihistamine concentrations is questionable, as poor correlation has been noted among patient's (1) age, (2) dose, (3) blood concentration, (4) clinical effects, and (5) death. Antihistamines are detected by forensic laboratories as agents potentially used in facilitating sexual assault.

Although detection of antihistamines is not typically clinically relevant for the acutely toxic patient, it is important to note that very high concentrations of first-generation antihistamines, such as promethazine and diphenhydramine, have been documented to cross-react with urine drug immunomethods used for screening purposes. Therefore, physicians and medical review officers (MROs) should be aware of potential false-positive results from on-site drug testing devices, as well as immuno-screening methods for (1) **amphetamine**, (2) propoxyphene, and (3) tricyclic antidepressants.

Antimuscarinic Agents

Besides numerous pharmaceutical agents, several plant and mushroom species contain antimuscarinic compounds that mimic anticholinergic symptoms when ingested. Plants are commonly ingested or brewed as tea. Patients are clinically managed on the basis of clinical presentation, rather than by identification of ingested plants or drug-specific testing. Testing for atropine and scopolamine is performed by LC-MS methods.

Agents Related to Cholinergic Toxidrome

Agents inducing cholinergic toxidrome are diverse and act by producing uncontrolled acetylcholine transmission through inactivation of cholinesterase enzymes or direct stimulation of acetylcholine receptors. Acetylcholine is an essential neurotransmitter that affects (1) parasympathetic synapses (autonomic and central nervous systems), (2) sympathetic preganglionic synapses, and (3) the neuromuscular junction (see also prior section, "Toxic Syndromes"). Clinical manifestations in cholinergic toxidrome include (1) muscarinic, (2) nicotinic, and (3) central effects (see Table 31-2). The duration of acetylcholine action is controlled by acetylcholinesterase and butyrylcholinesterase/pseudocholinesterase (see Chapter 19). Acetylcholinesterase is found in (1) red blood cells, (2) nervous tissue, and (3) skeletal muscle. Butyrylcholinesterase is found in (1) plasma, (2) liver, (3) heart, (4) pancreas, and (5) brain.

Organophosphate and Carbamate Compounds

Organophosphate insecticides are toxic because they inactivate acetylcholinesterases that are required for hydrolyzing acetylcholine at nerve junctions. This inhibition is a consequence of phosphorylation of the serine hydroxyl group at the active site of the cholinesterase enzyme catalytic triad (Ser-Glu-His). Subsequent hydrolysis results in irreversible dealkylation of AChE. Although carbamates are structurally different from organophosphates, carbamates exert their toxicity at the active site of AChE but inhibit enzyme activity through carbamylation rather than phosphorylation of the serine hydroxyl group. Regeneration of

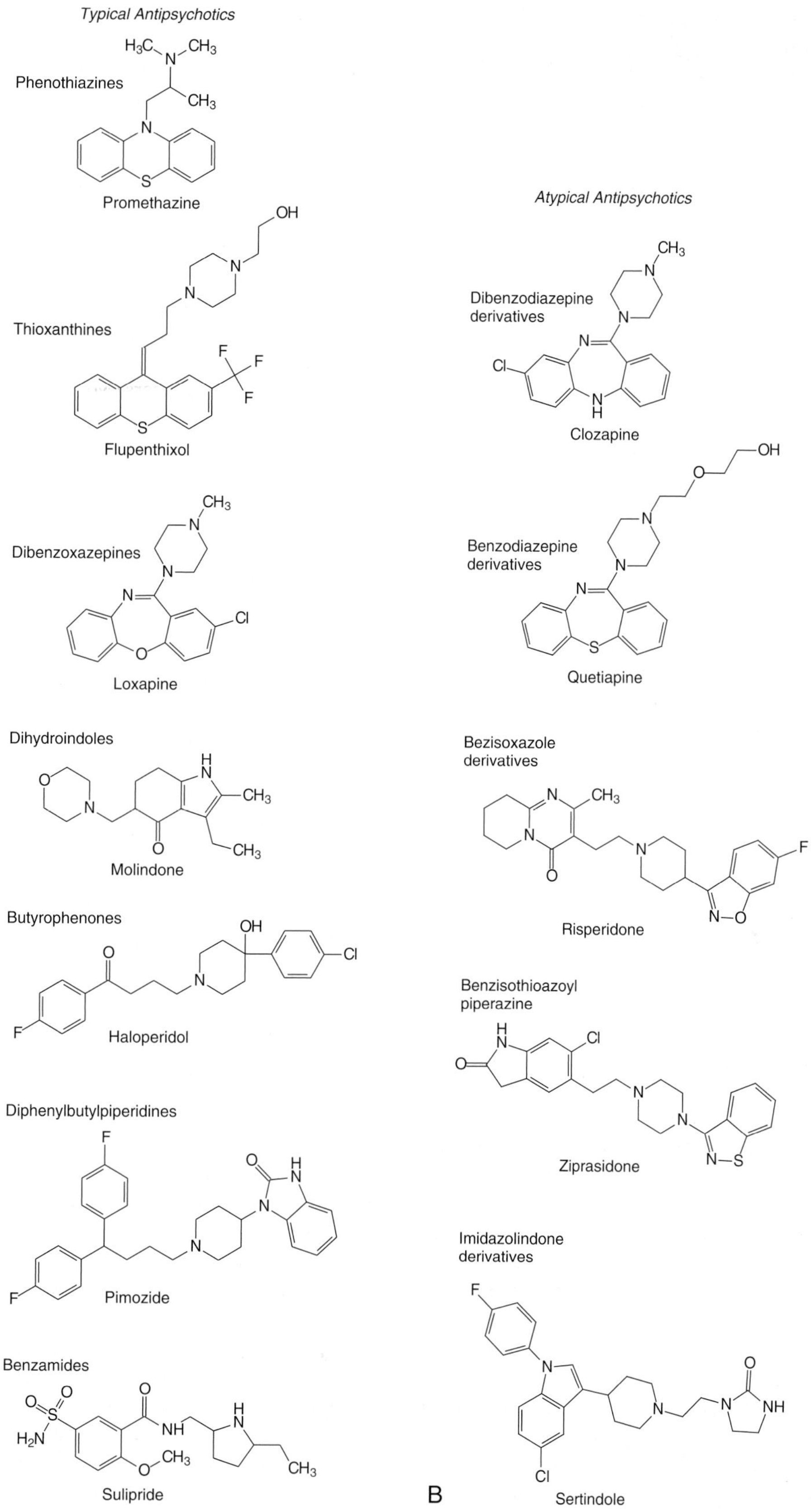

Figure 31-5 Classification and structure of select antipsychotic drugs. **A,** Typical antipsychotics. **B,** Atypical antipsychotics.

enzyme activity occurs in hours rather than days. Carbamates exhibit poor CNS penetration and have a shorter duration of action. In addition, their neurotoxicity is usually less severe.

Excess synaptic acetylcholine stimulates muscarinic receptors (peripheral and central nervous systems) and stimulates but then depresses or paralyzes nicotinic receptors. Activation of peripheral muscarinic receptors causes signs and symptoms described by the mnemonics SLUDGE (Salivation, Lacrimation, Urination, Defecation, GI distress, Emesi) or DUMBBELS (Diarrhea, Urination, Miosis, Bradycardia, and Bronchorrhea-bronchoconstriction, Emesis, Lacrimation, Sweating-salivation). Stimulation or paralysis of nicotinic receptors at the neuromuscular junction causes (1) muscle twitching, (2) cramping, (3) weakness, and (4) respiratory muscle paralysis. Stimulation of nicotinic receptors at sympathetic ganglia results in (1) hypertension, (2) tachycardia, (3) pallor, and (4) mydriasis. Thus, the actual signs and symptoms observed with these toxins depend on the balance of muscarinic and nicotinic receptor activation.

Diagnosis of organophosphate and carbamate toxicity depends mainly on (1) exposure history, (2) physical presentation, (3) clinical suspicion, and (4) laboratory support. Specific therapy for organophosphate and carbamate insecticide poisoning includes administration of atropine to block the muscarinic (but not the nicotinic) actions of acetylcholine. In addition, pralidoxime is given to reactivate cholinesterase in organophosphate poisoning. Treatment requires immediate attention and should not rely on **confirmatory testing** by the laboratory. Yet cholinesterase activity is often monitored by clinicians in occupational exposure, acute intentional and accidental exposure, and response to therapy.

Cholinesterase activity is measured to assess exposure and to monitor reactivation during treatment. Acetylcholinesterase and butyrylcholinesterase enzyme activities are typically monitored using spectrophotometric analyses (see Chapter 19). Acetylcholinesterase activity present at nerve junctions is similar to that present in red blood cells and is an appropriate index of neurotoxicity. This assay is more sensitive than serum cholinesterase activity and often is used to confirm exposure and to predict enzyme reactivation during treatment. Butyrylcholinesterase (pseudocholinesterase), also present in serum, is inhibited by these insecticides. The activity of butyrylcholinesterase declines then returns to normal more rapidly than is observed for the red cell enzyme. Serum butyrylcholinesterase is readily measured on hemolyzed samples and in clinical laboratories without isolation of red blood cells. However, interindividual variability is high; therefore pre-exposure activities are optimal when butyrylcholinesterase activities are interpreted. Because butyrylcholinesterases are synthesized in the liver, this assay is particularly sensitive to interferences associated with pregnancy and liver disease such as (1) acute and chronic hepatitis, (2) cirrhosis, and (3) malignancy. Thus, red cell cholinesterase activity theoretically should correlate more closely with the degree of neurotoxicity. In acute poisoning, symptoms generally begin when cholinesterase activity is inhibited by about 50% of the lower limits of the reference interval, and this degree of inhibition is of diagnostic value.

However, the degree of cholinesterase inhibition generally does not correlate well with the clinical severity of poisoning. Interpretation of test results is made more difficult by considerable individual variability of reference activities. The presence of urinary organophosphate and carbamate metabolites is generally assessed by GC-MS and GC-MS/MS. These methods are labor-intensive and typically are reserved for monitoring chronic occupational exposure to specific agents rather than for emergency management of acute toxicity.

Drugs of Abuse

Many definitions exist for the term "drugs of abuse." For this chapter, this term is defined as "a drug that is repeatedly and deliberately used in a way other than prescribed or socially sanctioned (i.e., a drug that is taken for nonmedicinal reasons)." The spectrum of drugs tested includes (1) tricyclic antidepressants, (2) **barbiturates**, (3) **benzodiazepines**, (4) **methadone**, (5) **methylenedioxymethamphetamine (MDMA)**, (6) **methylenedioxyethylamphetamine (MDEA)**, (7) oxycodone, (8) amphetamine, (9) **cocaine**, (10) **marijuana**, (11) opiates, and (12) **phencyclidine**. Note: these last 5 drugs are known collectively as the SAMHSA (Substance Abuse and Mental Health Services Administration) or NIDA (National Institute on Drug Abuse).[5] They are the drugs for which tests are required under the Department of Transportation's (DOT) rule, 49 CFR Part 40, regulations.

Testing for drugs of abuse usually involves analyzing a single urine specimen for various drugs. It should be noted, however, that a single urine drug test detects only fairly recent drug use and does not differentiate casual use from chronic drug abuse. The latter requires sequential drug testing and clinical evaluation. Moreover, urine drug testing alone cannot determine (1) the degree of impairment, (2) the dose of drug taken, or (3) the exact time of use. Because of these and other limitations of testing for drugs in urine, integrating the use of alternate biological specimens for drug testing is a matter of growing interest (see later section on alternate specimens).

Several techniques have been used to mask or adulterate samples to avoid detection. These include (1) exchange of urine from a drug-free individual, (2) dilution of the urine specimen by excessive consumption of water, (3) dilution by addition of water to the specimen, and (4) use of a diuretic. Also, readily available adulterants, such as (1) detergent, (2) bleach, (3) salt, (4) alkali, (5) ammonia, (6) tetrahydrozoline, or (7) acid, may be added to the specimen after collection in an attempt to interfere with immunoassay screening procedures. Other adulterants specifically marketed to avoid drug detection include those that contain (1) glutaraldehyde, (2) nitrite, (3) chromate, and (4) a combination of peroxide and peroxidase.[13] These adulterants also interfere with immunoassays to a variable degree, and the oxidizing agents may result in destruction of morphine, codeine, and the principal metabolite resulting from marijuana use, thus interfering with their GC-MS or LC-MS confirmatory testing.

Direct observation of urine collection is the most stringent means to guard against specimen exchange or adulteration.

However, an individual's right to privacy and dignity must be weighed against the need for the highest degree of certainty of specimen integrity. Alternative measures to prevent specimen adulteration include (1) limitations on clothing or other personal belongings allowed in the specimen collection area, (2) addition of coloring agent to toilet water, and (3) inactivation of the hot water tap. In addition, several validity checks for specimen integrity may be made at the collection site and at the testing site. Validity testing criteria have been established by the U.S. Department of Health and Human Services (DHHS) for the drug testing program mandated for U.S. federal employees.[8] Numerous commercial reagents for validity testing are available in both test strip and liquid forms. Detailed information on the collection and processing analytes to be tested and on storage of specimens for drug testing has been presented in the federal rules for employee drug testing[8] and in the federal regulations promulgated by the Department of Transportation and the Nuclear Regulatory Commission. Testing programs for participants engaged in athletic competition typically are much more extensive.

Initial screening tests for the previously listed drugs are typically immunoassays (see Chapter 15). These assays are calibrated at established cutoff concentrations. Specimens yielding responses greater than the cutoff (threshold) value are considered "*presumptively positive*," whereas values below the cutoff are considered negative. Immunoassays may demonstrate limited and variable specificity within certain drug classes. Similar drugs may result in a positive test, for example, pseudoephedrine, present in cold medications, may produce a positive response in immunoassays designed to detect amphetamine and **methamphetamine**. Therefore, it is important that positive screening tests be confirmed by an alternate, more definitive test. The most widely accepted method for confirmatory testing is GC-MS; however, LC-MS/MS is also used and accepted.

In the following sections, the pharmacological and analytical aspects of commonly measured drugs will be discussed.

Barbiturates

The success of barbital in 1903 and phenobarbital (Figure 31-6) in 1912 led to the synthesis and testing of more than 2500 barbiturate derivatives, of which approximately 50 were distributed commercially. However, because of their low therapeutic index and high potential for abuse, they have been largely replaced by the much safer benzodiazepines. Nevertheless, barbiturates continue to be available.[13] The classification of barbiturates as (1) ultra-short-acting, (2) short-acting, (3) intermediate-acting, and (4) long-acting refers to the duration of effect, not to the elimination half-life (Table 31-7). The barbiturates produce all degrees of depression of the CNS, ranging from mild sedation to general anesthesia.

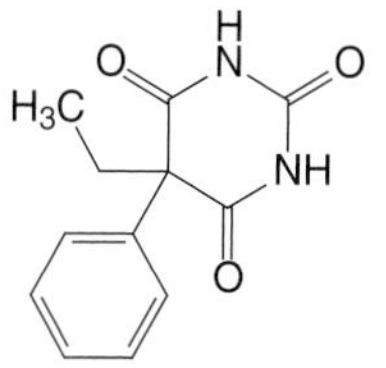

Analytical Methods
Screening
Numerous commercial immunoassays for barbiturates are available, and although the degree of cross-reactivity of other barbiturates varies with each assay, most have sufficient

Figure 31-6 Structure of phenobarbital.

TABLE 31-7	Half-life and Significant Active Metabolites of Select Barbiturates	
Drug	**Half-life**	**Active Metabolite**
Ultrashort-Acting		
Thiopental	6-46 hours	Pentobarbital
Methohexital	1.2-2.1 hours	
Thiamylal	0.6-0.8 hours initial	
	12-34 hours terminal	
Short-Acting and Intermediate-Acting		
Pentobarbital	15-48 hours	
Secobarbital	22-29 hours	
Butalbital	35-88 hours	
Aprobarbital	14-34 hours	
Amobarbital	15-40 hours (dose dependent)	
Butabarbital	34-42 hours	
Long-Acting		
Phenobarbital	2-6 days	
Mephobarbital	48-52 hours	Phenobarbital

cross-reactivity to detect the major therapeutically used barbiturates.

Confirmatory Testing
Numerous confirmatory methods for barbiturates have been described. These include (1) GC with flame ionization detection, nitrogen phosphorous detection, and MS detection; (2) capillary electrophoresis-ultraviolet (UV) detection; (3) liquid chromatography using ultraviolet (LC-UV) detection; and (4) LC-MS.[13]

Benzodiazepines

Benzodiazepines include any of a group of compounds that have a common molecular structure and act similarly as depressants of the CNS. The prototype benzodiazepines are diazepam and nordiazepam (*N*-desmethyldiazepam) (Figure 31-7). Over 30 members of this group are presently used worldwide. Commonly used ones are listed in Table 31-8. As a class of drugs, benzodiazepines are among the most commonly prescribed drugs in the Western hemisphere because of their (1) efficacy, (2) safety, (3) low addiction potential, and (4) minimal side effects, and (5) because of the high public demand for sedative and anxiolytic agents. They have largely replaced barbiturates for sedative-hypnotic use because they (1) have fewer side effects, (2) cause fewer problems with liver enzyme induction, and (3) are safer in occurrences of overdose. New-generation sedative-hypnotics such as (1) zolpidem (Ambien), (2) eszopiclone (Lunesta), and (3) zaleplon (Sonata) modulate the $GABA_A$

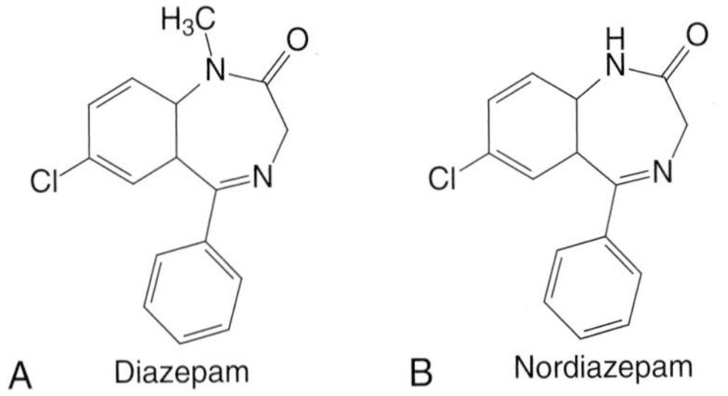

Figure 31-7 Structure of **(A)** diazepam and **(B)** nordiazepam.

receptor, as do benzodiazepines, yet they are structurally different, permitting unique physiological properties that will be discussed in a subsequent section (see "Drugs Used in Sexual Assault"). The benzodiazepines given by themselves or in combination with other drugs, particularly narcotic analgesics (opioids), are among the most widely abused drugs.

Benzodiazepines may be divided into three categories based on their onset time and elimination half-lives: (1) short-acting agents, (2) intermediate-acting agents, and (3) long-acting agents (see Table 31-8). These pharmacokinetic properties in part determine the primary clinical applications for some benzodiazepines.

Treatment of benzodiazepine toxicity is primarily supportive. Flumazenil may be used in select cases and is a competitive inhibitor of the benzodiazepine site on the GABA complex. It finds its greatest utility in the reversal of benzodiazepine-induced sedation from minor surgical procedures. However, flumazenil should not be administered as a nonspecific coma-reversal drug and should be used with extreme caution after intentional benzodiazepine overdose because it has the potential to precipitate withdrawal in benzodiazepine-dependent individuals and/or to induce seizures in those at risk.

Analytical Methods

Benzodiazepines are measured through a variety of techniques. However, their structural diversity and wide variation in potency provide a challenge for laboratories seeking to detect all relevant members in one analytical scheme. Reviews of analysis of benzodiazepines have been published.[6,7,14] These cover the range of techniques used to screen for the presence of the class of drugs and to confirm the presence of one or more members.

Screening

Several commercial immunoassay systems are available for detection and screening for a wide variety of benzodiazepines and metabolites, but they differ in their ability to detect (1) the various benzodiazepines, (2) their metabolites, and (3) glucuronide conjugates.[6] Cross-reactivity in screening immunoassays of the various benzodiazepines and their metabolites varies considerably from manufacturer to manufacturer, and screening assays cannot be used to distinguish between the individual benzodiazepines. Most assays are calibrated to a common metabolite such as (1) oxazepam, (2) temazepam, or (3) nordiazepam. However, the large number of different

TABLE 31-8 Half-life of Select Benzodiazepines

Drug	Half-life, hours	Significant Phase I Metabolites
Short-Acting		
Midazolam	1-4	α-Hydroxy-midazolam
Estazolam	10-24	3-Hydroxy-estazolam
Flurazepam	1-3	Hydroxy-ethyl-flurazepam
	47-100 (N-desalkyl-flurazepam)	N-desalkyl-flurazepam*
Temazepam	3-13	
Triazolam	1.8-3.9	α-Hydroxy-triazolam
Intermediate-Acting		
Flunitrazepam†	9-25	7-Amino-flunitrazepam
Long-Acting Agents		
Diazepam	21-37	Nordiazepam*
		Oxazepam*
		Temazepam*
Quazepam	39-53	3-Hydroxy-quazepam
		N-desalkyl-2-oxo-quazepam
		2-Oxo-3-hydroxy-quazepam
Alprazolam	6-27	α-Hydroxy-alprazolam
Chlordiazepoxide	6-27	Nordiazepam*
		Oxazepam*
Clonazepam	19-60	7-Amino-clonazepam
Clorazepate‡	2	Nordiazepam*
	31-97 (nordiazepam)	Oxazepam*
Lorazepam	9-16	
Oxazepam	4-11	

*Active metabolite.
†Not available in the United States.
‡Converted to nordiazepam by gastric HCl.

functional groups that may be present on the benzodiazepine nucleus makes it difficult to detect all drugs in this class, and some compounds such as (1) midazolam, (2) chlordiazepoxide, and (3) flunitrazepam may not be detected by many assays. Other factors, such as low doses and short half-lives, make the detection of some benzodiazepines especially challenging. In the absence of sufficiently sensitive or specific immunoassays, direct analysis by a confirmatory method is warranted in suspected cases.

It should be noted that benzodiazepines may be identified and quantified in serum, but such quantitative information is not warranted in cases of benzodiazepine overdose because serum concentrations are not predictive of the severity of intoxication. However, a urine or serum immunoassay screening test for benzodiazepines is valuable in the evaluation of patients with an unknown cause of CNS depression.

Confirmatory Testing

Analysts need to be aware that the specimen type will dictate the target substance. Blood analyses invariably will target the parent benzodiazepine and perhaps the major active metabolite (e.g., nordiazepam for diazepam and other analogues metabolized to nordiazepam). This applies similarly to analyses targeted for saliva. In urine, a metabolite is often the required target species.

Benzodiazepines and their metabolites have been extracted from biological specimens by liquid-liquid extraction (LLE) or solid-phase extraction (SPE). When urine specimens are analyzed by GC-MS, a hydrolysis step is necessary to cleave the glucuronide conjugates. Enzymatic hydrolysis is preferred over acid hydrolysis because some benzodiazepines are unstable and rearrange to form benzophenones.

Many benzodiazepines are analyzed without derivatization by GC; these include (1) diazepam, (2) nordiazepam, (3) flurazepam, and (4) alprazolam. Drugs that are more polar, including those with hydroxyl groups such as (1) oxazepam, (2) temazepam, and (3) lorazepam or a nitro group (clonazepam, nitrazepam), display poor chromatographic characteristics and require derivatization. Chlordiazepoxide is thermally unstable and may degrade at high temperatures in the GC. Some consider GC-MS as the definitive confirmatory method; however, LC with UV detection (240 nm) has been used to detect benzodiazepines and metabolites without derivatization. LC-MS and LC-MS/MS are becoming increasingly useful and popular methods for benzodiazepine parent drugs and their metabolites.

Cannabinoids

Cannabinoids are a group of compounds found in the marijuana plant *Cannabis sativa*. Cannabis is the most extensively abused illicit drug in the world. Cannabis has been used for centuries as a medicinal and a psychotropic agent. The main psychotropic effects are (1) euphoria, (2) distorted perceptions, (3) relaxation, and (4) a feeling of well-being.

Delta-9-tetrahydrocannabinol (THC) is the primary psychoactive component of the *C. sativa* plant (Figure 31-8). It binds to the endogenous cannabinoid receptors, CB1 (neuronal) and CB2 (immune cells). These transmembrane receptors are G-protein–coupled receptors that mediate signal transduction through inhibition of adenylate cyclase and calcium ions, and through activation of potassium ion channels. The distribution pattern of CB1 receptors in the CNS accounts for most of the clinical effects of THC such as those affecting (1) mood, (2) memory, (3) cognition, (4) pain, and (5) appetite. CB2 may regulate immune and inflammatory processes.

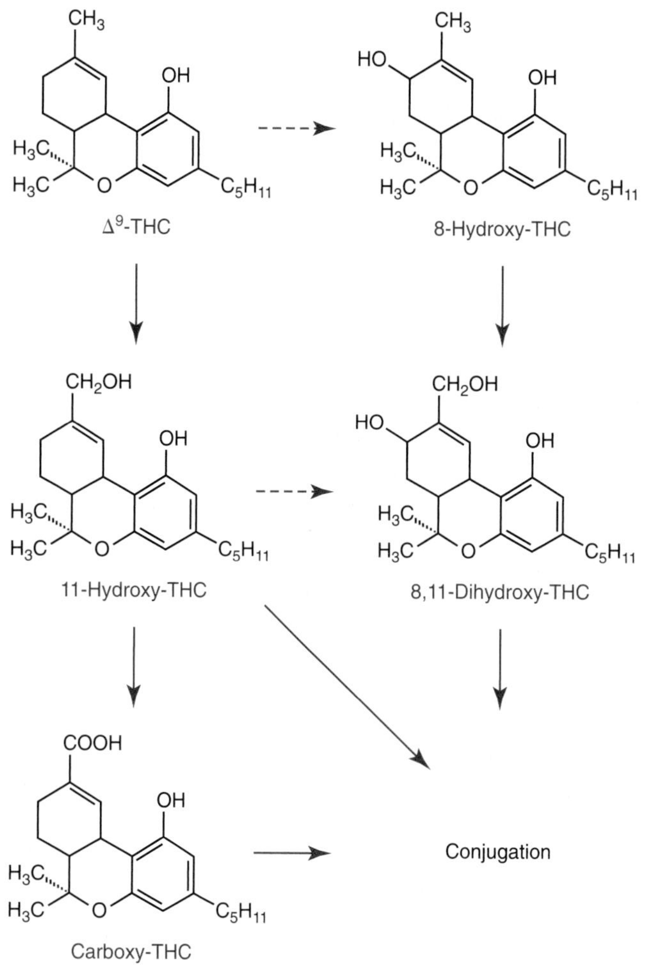

Pharmacological Response

When marijuana is smoked, THC diffuses into the plasma in seconds and is distributed into multiple phases. First, it distributes to highly vascularized tissues in minutes because of its lipophilic nature. THC then (1) is redistributed back into the bloodstream, (2) undergoes hepatic metabolism, and (3) slowly accumulates into less vascularized and fatty tissues. After cessation of marijuana smoking, THC and its metabolites are slowly released from fat stores.

The main psychotropic effects after inhalation of marijuana occur within minutes and persist for several hours. The peak plasma concentration of THC is dependent on the dose and occurs during the early acute phase (6 to 10 minutes). Numerous factors contribute to the variability in dose, such as

Figure 31-8 Principal metabolic route for delta-9-tetrahydrocannabinol (THC) in humans.

(1) method of consumption, (2) depth of inhalation, (3) exposure frequency, and (4) cannabis potency. Onset of clinical symptoms and peak plasma concentrations after oral ingestion of THC is slower (2 to 6 hours) than after inhalation, primarily as the result of first-pass hepatic clearance. The intensity of clinical effects described for smoked cannabis occurs during multiple phases. These phases are categorized as (1) acute (0 to 60 minutes), (2) postacute (60 to 150 minutes), and (3) residual (>150 minutes). The ratio of THC to 11-nor-delta-9-tetrahydrocannabinol-9-carboxylic acid (THC-COOH) metabolite has been used to estimate the time of exposure to marijuana. This approach may be useful in naive users but is unreliable in chronic abusers of marijuana.

Although marijuana is the most frequently used illicit drug, it does have some limited legitimate medicinal use. For example, dronabinol (Marinol) contains synthetic THC and is used to treat anorexia and nausea in patients with (1) acquired immunodeficiency syndrome (AIDS), (2) nausea and vomiting associated with chemotherapy, or (3) asthma and glaucoma. Measurement in urine of the principal THC metabolite, THC-COOH, present in cannabis but not in dronabinol has been proposed as a means to distinguish ingestion of marijuana from ingestion of Marinol.

Analytical Methods

An immunoassay method is typically used to screen for potential cannabinoid use in (1) workplace drug testing, (2) athlete drug testing, and (3) clinical specimens. A presumptive positive sample should be confirmed by quantitative GC-MS for at least THC-COOH. Confirmatory testing of quantitative concentrations of the parent compound, THC, is typically reserved for forensic samples.

Screening

Legitimate concern has been raised concerning the potential for false-positive results with "passive inhalation" from nearby users, or for use or consumption of hemp products causing positive results in cannabinoid screens and confirmatory analyses. Since 1998, the U.S. Federal Government has prohibited the importation of *Cannabis sativa* seeds and oil containing greater than 0.3% THC to reduce human exposure to THC. The concentration of THC consumed in drug use is 2% to 20%. Subsequent studies have suggested that these measures were successful in reducing potential positive cannabinoid drug screen results from dietary sources.

TCH is metabolized by cytochrome liver enzymes to greater than 100 metabolites. The main active metabolite, 11-hydroxy-delta-9-THC, is further oxidized to the most abundant inactive THC-COOH (see Figure 31-8). Immunoassay screens have been designed to detect cannabis use in urine samples using antibody reagents developed against the inactive THC-COOH metabolite; these reagents cross-react with numerous other THC metabolites. Therefore the presence of multiple cannabinoid metabolites in a patient specimen will have an additive effect in immune-screen analyses, leading to screening results that estimate concentrations 1.5 to 8 times greater than the actual concentration of THC-COOH as determined by GC-MS.

A positive result from a urine cannabinoid screen or a positive result found by confirmatory testing does not indicate intoxication or degree of exposure. The window of detection for the urine concentration of THC-COOH varies among casual (2 to 7 days) and chronic abusers (up to 73 days) of marijuana and is dose dependent. Variables affecting the duration of detection include (1) dose, (2) frequency of exposure, (3) route of exposure, (4) body composition, (5) fluid excretion, and (6) method of detection. In practice, monitoring of abstinence is particularly challenging, as dilution of urine due to normal biological fluctuations (hydration) or ingested adulterants has caused a negative result one day and a positive on the next. To correct for hydration fluctuations, urine concentrations of THC-COOH are normalized per milligram creatinine in monitoring individuals who are resuming cannabis use. With the use of these normalized THC-COOH/creatinine concentrations, a ratio is calculated by comparing any normalized urine specimen (U2) with a previously collected normalized urine specimen (U1). "New use" is defined as a U2/U1 ratio ≥0.5 to 1.5 in urine specimens taken more than 24 hours apart and containing THC-COOH concentrations >15 ng/mL. Using the 1.5 cutoff rate results in decreased false-positive but increased false-negative decisions.

Confirmatory Testing

A positive screening result for THC obtained by immunoassay is confirmed by detection of THC-COOH by GC-MS/MS or LC-MS/MS analysis of the urine specimens.

Opiates and Opioids

The term *opioid* describes compounds that encompass the natural and semi-synthetic opiates that include variations on the structure of morphine and fully synthetic opioids with minimal structural homology to the natural alkaloids (Figure 31-9). The defining characteristic of this class of drugs is their morphine-like activity stemming from interaction with opioid receptors. Other compounds that are referred to as "*opioids*" include receptor antagonists and mixed agonist/antagonists, as well as other opium-derived alkaloids such as papaverine.

Pharmacological Response

Opioids interact with the family of opioid receptors that are variably distributed throughout the body. Opioid receptor agonists typically produce analgesia, and antagonists block this response. Most opioids have both substantial addictive capacity and potentially life-threatening side effects. Thus the benefits of their use in non–end-stage patients must be carefully weighed against the chance of rather serious consequences. The development of tolerance and the risk of prescription diversion complicate even further the process of monitoring long-term opioid therapy for compliance and efficacy.[15]

The metabolism of opioids is varied, but numerous biotransformations are common to these drugs. Several of the most commonly used opiates are formed in vivo by metabolism of other compounds, as seen with codeine demethylation resulting in conversion to morphine. This interconversion is a frequent source of confusion and must be considered when results of opiate screens are interpreted; specific details are provided below for key opioids with active metabolites.

One of the more important CYP cytochrome enzymes, CYP2D6, is particularly notable for its role in variable clinical response to opioids; it will be discussed in greater detail in a later section. Many additional CYP enzymes, including CYP3A and CYP2C and others, are involved in opioid metabolism. It is important to note that several of these enzymes are subject to substrate inhibition and/or induction. Substrate-dependent changes in metabolic activity are affected by (1) other drugs, (2) herbal supplements, and (3) endogenous compounds that are substrates of the same enzyme. For example, methadone concentrations may be lower than expected in a patient taking St. John's Wort—a noted CYP3A4 inducer—but higher in a patient ingesting a CYP3A4 inhibitor such as grapefruit juice.

Types of Opiates

Types of opiates include (1) natural opium alkaloids, (2) semi-synthetic opiates, (3) fully synthetic opioids, and (4) opioid antagonists and mixed agonists/antagonists.

Natural Opium Alkaloids

Opiates are classified as phenanthrenes or benzylisoquinolines. The principal phenanthrenes are (1) morphine (10%

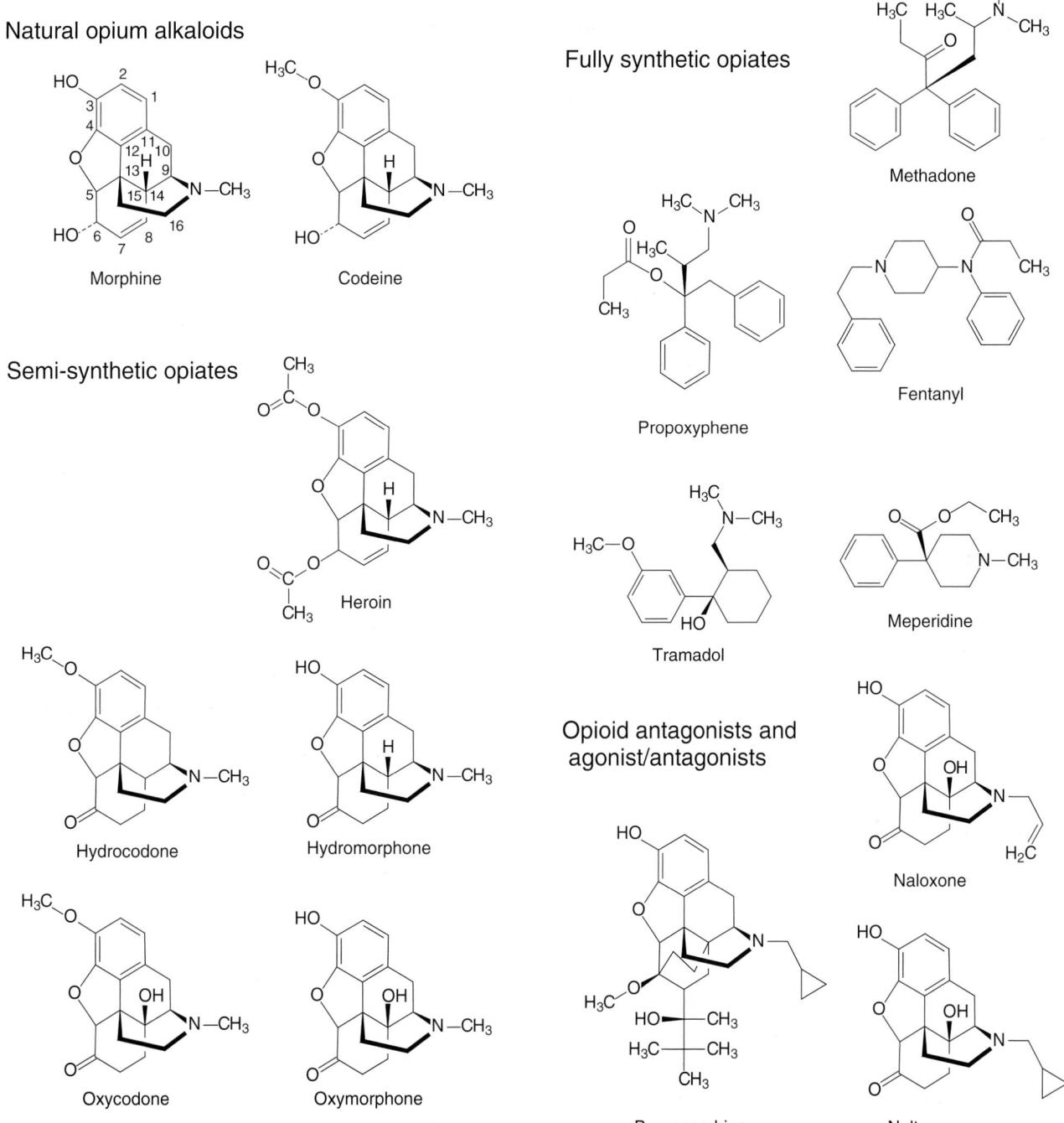

Figure 31-9 Structure and half-life of common opioids.

of opium), (2) codeine (0.5%), and (3) thebaine (0.2%). The principal benzylisoquinoline is papaverine (1%), which is a smooth muscle relaxant, and noscapine (6%).

Poppy seeds from the poppy plant *Papaver somniferum* contain morphine and to a lesser extent codeine. Because of first-pass metabolism, no pharmacological effect is experienced from poppy seed ingestion. Ingestion of bakery products containing poppy seeds leads to excretion of morphine (and codeine) in urine. In practice, caution is required when the results of a positive urine test for morphine and codeine are interpreted.

Morphine. Morphine is used as the basis of comparison for relative characterizations of the opioid class. Its major metabolites are glucuronide conjugates, including (1) inactive morphine-3-glucuronide (M3G; ≈60%), (2) active morphine-6-glucuronide (M6G; ≈10%), and (3) a small amount of morphine-3,6-diglucuronide mediated primarily by UGT2B7 (UDP-Glucuronosyltransferase-2B7), but also to a lesser extent by UGT1A3 (UDP-glucuronosyltransferase 1-3).[1,12] Note: The UGTs serve a major role in the conjugation and subsequent elimination of potentially toxic xenobiotics and endogenous compounds.

With long-term administration, and when morphine concentrations are high, a minor fraction is converted to hydromorphone (up to 2.5% of the urine morphine concentration). Therefore, glucuronides accumulate in serum to greater concentrations than morphine, and in patients with renal insufficiency, morphine glucuronides are thought to significantly contribute to opioid toxicity, as patients are unable to excrete the water-soluble metabolites. The detection time for morphine in urine is usually 48 to 72 hours, but this varies with individual differences in metabolism excretion and route and frequency of use.

Codeine. Because of its antitussive and analgesic properties, codeine is one of the most frequently prescribed opiates in the world; it is frequently combined with nonopiate analgesic agents such as aspirin and acetaminophen. Codeine has only about one-tenth the analgesic potency of morphine and is generally considered a prodrug.[3] The small fraction of codeine converted to morphine by CYP2D6 via O-demethylation is considered to be responsible for the analgesic effect. During the early phase of excretion, codeine and conjugates predominate, but after this time, morphine conjugates are the major product. Approximately three days after codeine use, morphine and its conjugates are the only metabolites detected.[3]

Genetic variation may play a significant role in the metabolism of codeine and several other opioids. More than 60 alleles have been described for CYP2D6, with resultant enzymatic activity ranging from essentially zero, in the case of null alleles, to many times higher than normal, in the case of amplified alleles (http://www.cypalleles.ki.se/cyp2d6.htm/; accessed on October 31, 2013). Thus, at the same codeine dose, patients with minimal CYP2D6 activity (poor metabolizers) would likely receive inadequate analgesia because of lack of conversion to morphine; however, patients with very high CYP2D6 activity would be at risk for adverse responses to excessive morphine. Without knowledge of the CYP2D6 genotype, these clinical presentations are confusing. Therefore, the possibility of pharmacogenetic effects is important to consider when (1) appropriate dosing, (2) patient compliance, and (3) potential diversion or illicit uses are assessed.

Semi-synthetic Opiates

Examples of semisynthetic opiates include (1) heroin, (2) hydrocodone, (3) hydromorphone, (4) oxycodone, and (5) oxymorphone.

Heroin. Heroin is a synthetic opiate that is made from morphine and is also called *diacetylmorphine* or *diamorphine.* It has an analgesic potency two to three times that of morphine because of its better penetration across the blood-brain barrier. This penetration is the result of the two acetyl groups that enhance CNS distribution. Heroin is no longer legally produced in the United States, but it is still used elsewhere for fast-acting analgesia. Heroin itself is rarely found in body fluids because of its extremely short half-life (2 to 6 minutes). Given that acetylcodeine is a common contaminant of heroin, both morphine and low concentrations of codeine are frequently detected in urine after heroin use.[3]

A metabolite of heroin is 6-monoacetylmorphine (6-MAM). It is hydrolyzed to morphine, and although it has a longer half-life (6 to 25 minutes), it is detectable in urine only for about 8 hours after administration. Both 6-MAM and morphine are pharmacologically active, and 6-MAM is four to six times more potent than morphine. Because 6-MAM is a unique metabolite to heroin, its presence in the urine confirms that heroin was the opioid used.

Hydrocodone. Hydrocodone has about six times the potency and greater oral bioavailability than codeine[3] but it is thought to be more toxic than codeine. Similar to codeine, hydrocodone is metabolized by CYP2D6 to an active metabolite (hydromorphone) and therefore may be subject to pharmacogenetic variability in patients with abnormal CYP2D6 activity.

Hydromorphone. Oral hydromorphone is five to seven times more potent than morphine. Although it is used as an analgesic in its own right, hydromorphone is also an active metabolite of hydrocodone.[4] Similar to morphine, hydromorphone is metabolized in large part to a 3-glucuronide by UGT2B7, but also to a lesser extent by UGT1A3.[1,12] Hydromorphone lacks a free hydroxyl group at the 6-position. Two minor metabolites of hydromorphone—dihydromorphine and dihydroisomorphine—have demonstrated pharmacological activity, but their contribution may be minimal because of the small amount formed.[3]

Oxycodone. Oxycodone is a potent analgesic with high oral bioavailability that is frequently formulated in combination with aspirin or acetaminophen. Noncombination oxycodone is also available in immediate- and extended-release dosage forms. During illicit use, the pills may be (1) chewed, (2) crushed, (3) snorted, or (4) solubilized for IV injection to permit immediate availability of the entire dose, which is intended for extended release over a 12-hour period.[3]

Although its own strong analgesic activity precludes consideration of oxycodone as a prodrug, it is converted to the active metabolite, oxymorphone, through the activity of CYP2D6. This conversion appears to be less of a concern for CYP2D6 poor metabolizers, in whom oxycodone itself still provides analgesia, than for ultra-rapid metabolizers.[3]

Oxymorphone. Oxymorphone provides potent analgesia with minimal interaction with CYP enzymes. Most oxymorphone is metabolized by UGT2B7 to the 3-glucuronide, which is a minor metabolite. 6-Hydroxyoxymorphone is an active analgesic with a steady-state area under the curve (AUC) similar to the parent compound. Oxymorphone is a metabolite of oxycodone that is formed via CYP2D6.

Fully Synthetic Opioids

Examples of fully synthetic opioids include (1) fentanyl, (2) meperidine, (3) methadone, (4) propoxyphene, and (5) tramadol.

Fentanyl. Fentanyl is a lipophilic drug with numerous routes of administration that is used in applications ranging from anesthesia to rapid management of breakthrough pain. It provides the structural backbone for a number of opioids, including remifentanil and sufentanil. Norfentanyl, the primary metabolite, is generated by CYP3A and is inactive; the high potency of fentanyl and the clinical insignificance of its metabolites make it a preferred analgesic for patients with major organ failure. Transdermal fentanyl patches are used for longer-term administration among drug abusers, unfortunately, nonstandard application of the patch (e.g., chewing, extraction) carries substantial risk for overdose.

Meperidine. Originally synthesized as an anticholinergic, meperidine has analgesic potency comparable with or somewhat less than that of morphine. One major metabolite, normeperidine, also has analgesic activity. (1) It is thought to be responsible for the serotonergic toxicity of meperidine, (2) it is eliminated renally, and (3) its use results in seizure activity in patients with renal failure.

Methadone. A relatively long-acting opiate, methadone is used both for analgesia and in the treatment of opioid addiction. It is thought to provide (1) milder withdrawal, (2) somewhat lower potential for abuse, and (3) reduced exposure to the risks of illicit intravenous drug use. Substantial interindividual and intraindividual variability in metabolism and elimination has been noted. Both urine pH and seemingly self-inducible metabolism substantially influence the pharmacokinetics of this compound, as do commonly coadministered drugs such as benzodiazepines and antiretrovirals. Although a large fraction of methadone is excreted unchanged, measurement of a metabolite such as EDDP (2-ethylidene-1,5-dimethyl-3,3-diphenylpyrrolidine) in the setting of addiction treatment provides evidence of patient compliance rather than an exogenously spiked sample. EDDP excretion is less pH dependent than is clearance of the parent drug.[3] Use of the methadone/EDDP ratio to assess compliance has been suggested but is complicated by the pharmacokinetic variability already described.

Propoxyphene. A relatively weak analgesic, propoxyphene is less potent than codeine but carries significant risk of atypical adverse effects such as cardiac arrhythmia and seizure. The incidence of such negative responses is particularly high in the elderly. In November 2010, the FDA announced that medications containing propoxyphene were being withdrawn from the U.S. market.

Tramadol. Unlike most opioid agonists, tramadol has low abuse potential and therefore is unscheduled. It has low affinity for opioid receptors and mediates analgesia through opioid-independent regulation of neurotransmitter uptake; however, its main active metabolite (O-desmethyltramadol) is formed via CYP2D6 and is a potent opioid receptor agonist. These mechanisms are thought to work synergistically to provide greater total pain relief than the sum of each individual component. However, because of its effects on neurotransmission, tramadol has the potential to cause serotonergic toxicity. In fact, several synthetic phenylpiperidine opioids such as (1) tramadol, (2) methadone, (3) dextromethorphan, and (4) propoxyphene have been associated with increased risk of serotonin toxicity caused by weak reuptake inhibition of monoamines when used in combination with serotonin reuptake inhibitors, monoamine oxidase inhibitors, and amphetamine-type stimulants.

Opioid Antagonists and Mixed Agonists/Antagonists

These clinically useful compounds produce very different physiological responses, depending on the situation. For example, in opioid-naive patients, mixed agonists/antagonists (MAAs) provide μ-opioid receptor (MOR)-mediated analgesia with less risk of an adverse reaction, but the same dose in an opioid-tolerant patient may precipitate immediate withdrawal. In medical usage, coadministration of low-dose antagonists or MAAs alleviates minor opioid-induced side effects and appears useful in preventing opioid tolerance. In opioid addiction treatment, the addition of a low-dose antagonist to maintenance therapy seems to minimize subjective "feel-good" effects without substantially worsening withdrawal symptoms. Examples of opioid antagonists and mixed agonists/antagonists include (1) buprenorphine, (2) naloxone, and (3) naltrexone.

Buprenorphine. A semisynthetic derivative of thebaine, buprenorphine is an MOR partial analgesia. Low doses provide analgesia through MOR activation, but unlike full agonists, pain relief has a maximal threshold or "ceiling effect." Buprenorphine is available as sublingual tablets (with or without naloxone) for the treatment of opioid dependence. Buprenorphine is metabolized via N-dealkylation by CYP3A4 to the active compound, norbuprenorphine, both of which are further conjugated to inactive glucuronides by UGT1A1. CYP3A4 and UGT1A1 are subject to environmental and genetic variability, although the effects of these factors on buprenorphine are not well characterized. Only a small amount is found in urine, and it is usually detectable for 1 to 3 days.

Naloxone. Naloxone binds nonspecifically to all three opioid receptor types, with the greatest effect at MOR. Naloxone is commonly used in comatose patients as a therapeutic and diagnostic agent to (1) restore respiratory function, (2) protect the airway, and (3) improve level of consciousness, and (4) as an antidote for opioid intoxication. Its clinical efficacy lasts for as little as 45 minutes. Therefore, patients are at risk for recurrence of narcotic effect. This is particularly true for patients exposed to opioids with long elimination half-lives, such as methadone and sustained-release opioid products. Patients should be observed for re-sedation for at least 4 hours after reversal with naloxone. Because naloxone is renally eliminated, patients with renal dysfunction may have delayed re-sedation past 4 hours and therefore should be observed for a longer time.

Naloxone has been known to precipitate profound withdrawal symptoms in opioid-dependent patients. Its efficacy is much greater by intravenous administration as compared with oral and sublingual routes.

Naltrexone. Commonly used for the treatment of alcoholism, naltrexone is a potent antagonist of all three opioid receptors. Its combined formulation with opioid agonists is less common than are naloxone/opioid combinations; however, the greater oral bioavailability of naltrexone suggests that it may be useful in applications where poor oral delivery limits the utility of naloxone.

Analytical Methods

Many different immunoassay methods are used to screen for opiates. Gas chromatography (GC) with mass spectroscopic detection (GC-MS) is the technique of choice for confirmatory testing after a positive screening result.

Screening Assay

Given their ability to detect several opiates, immunoassays are the methods of choice to screen urine samples for their opiate content. Antibodies in opiate abuse screens commonly target morphine, and variability in cross-reactivity; thus some opiates or opioids (see Figure 31-9) with high abuse potential such as oxycodone are often poorly detected. For clinical application, a cutoff of 300 ng/mL morphine (or morphine equivalents) is commonly used to distinguish negative from positive urine specimens. Other general opiate screening methods are available, including thin-layer chromatography, but these techniques are more labor-intensive and may not provide adequate turnaround time for stat or emergency testing. In this setting, point-of-care devices are being used more frequently.

The cutoff concentrations used for drugs in federally regulated tests, in particular, opioids (2000 ng/mL), are too high to be of value in monitoring compliance of pain management patients or other clinical settings. Nonregulated testing of opioid cutoff concentrations (300 ng/mL) allows for a considerably more sensitive screening assay.[15] It is important for drug testing laboratories to communicate relevant aspects of the metabolic interconversion of opiates to physicians responsible for these programs. Monitoring compliance for oxycodone in pain management programs is problematic because of the low cross-reactivity of oxycodone in most opiate immunoassays. In this instance, a false-negative opiate immunoassay test may lead to an accusation of oxycodone diversion. Direct determination of oxycodone by a confirmatory method such as (1) GC-MS, (2) LC-MS, or (3) LC-MS/MS is more appropriate in monitoring compliance for this drug.[13]

Confirmatory Testing

For compound-specific confirmatory assays, GC-MS has historically been considered the method of choice. In addition, it is considered the reference method for determination of most natural and semi-synthetic opiates, particularly in forensic settings, although other detectors are available and have been used for GC applications. Despite the long-standing role of GC in opiate analysis, LC methods are common and are often analytically advantageous. One notable example is that LC provides the ability to analyze glucuronide-conjugated metabolites, as well as parent compounds. In addition, in practice, LC methods are used to measure polar metabolites without prior derivatization, and on-column extraction is possible with some LC systems. One trend in method development is the ability to quantitate/identify combinations of (1) morphine, (2) other opiates, and (3) opioids and their metabolites.[13]

Drugs of Abuse Related to the Sympathomimetic Syndrome

Several stimulants and hallucinogens chemically related to *phenylethylamine* are referred to collectively as amphetamine-type stimulants (ATSs). They are considered to be sympathomimetic drugs, as they mimic endogenous transmitters in the sympathetic nervous system. Amphetamine and methamphetamine (Figure 31-10) are CNS stimulant drugs that have limited legitimate pharmacological uses such as treatment for (1) narcolepsy, (2) obesity, and (3) attention-deficit hyperactivity disorders. They produce an initial euphoria and have a high abuse potential. Other sympathomimetic amines that have high potential for abuse include (1) ephedrine, (2) pseudoephedrine, and (3) phenylpropanolamine.

Amphetamine and Methamphetamine

These drugs have a stimulating effect on both the central and peripheral nervous systems. In the brain, a primary action is to elevate the concentrations of extracellular monoamine neurotransmitters such as (1) dopamine, (2) serotonin, and (3) norepinephrine. These drugs promote presynaptic release from the nerve endings rather than blockade of reuptake.[13] Amphetamine and methamphetamine are substrates for the dopamine, serotonin, and norepinephrine transporters.

Amphetamine and methamphetamine increase (1) blood pressure, (2) heart rate, (3) body temperature, and (4) motor activity, (5) relax bronchial muscle, and (6) depress the appetite. Abuse of these drugs may lead to (1) strong psychological dependence, (2) marked tolerance, (3) mild physical dependence associated with tachycardia, (4) increased blood pressure, (5) restlessness, (6) irritability, (7) insomnia, (8) personality changes, and (9) a severe form of chronic intoxication psychosis similar to schizophrenia. These unpleasant responses reinforce repetitive use of the drugs to maintain the "high." Tolerance and psychological dependence develop with repeated use of amphetamines. Long-term effects may include depression and impaired memory and motor skills, probably caused by a decrease in dopamine transporters and by damage to dopaminergic and serotonergic neurons.

The optical isomers of amphetamine and methamphetamine exhibit stereoselective pharmacological properties. The CNS activity of S(+) amphetamine (D-amphetamine) is three to four times greater than that of R(−) amphetamine (L-amphetamine), but the latter drug has more potent cardiovascular

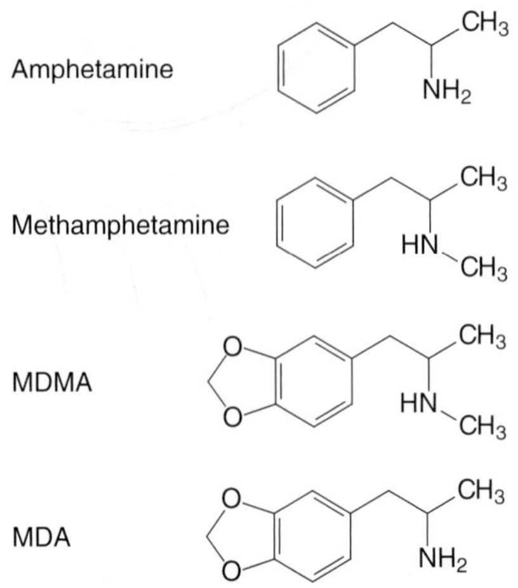

Figure 31-10 Select amphetamine-type stimulants.

effects than the former.[3] The CNS effects of S(+) methamphetamine (D-methamphetamine) are about 10 times greater than those of R(−) methamphetamine (L-methamphetamine), but the latter drug has greater vasoconstrictive properties than the former. Because of minimal CNS activity, low abuse potential, and vasoconstrictive properties, R(−) methamphetamine had been included in some nonprescription nasal inhalants (e.g., Vick's).

The main metabolic pathways of amphetamine and methamphetamine include (1) aromatic hydroxylation, (2) aliphatic hydroxylation, (3) *N*-demethylation, (4) oxidative deamination, (5) *N*-oxidation, and (6) conjugation of nitrogen. In addition to hepatic metabolism, amphetamine is eliminated as unchanged drug in urine. Elimination is dependent on urine pH.[3] Therefore, elimination half-life (renal excretion and hepatic metabolism) varies with urine pH from 7 to 14 hours at acid pH to 18 to 34 hours at alkaline pH.[13] These effects of urine pH on the elimination of unchanged amphetamines are a consequence of tubular reabsorption of nonionized amphetamine (pK_a, 9.9). Similarly methamphetamine is eliminated in urine in a pH-dependent manner, similar to that used for amphetamine.

Pharmacogenetics is thought to play a role in differences seen in the metabolism/elimination of these drugs. CYP2D6 is responsible for 4-hydroxylation of amphetamine and methamphetamine and *N*-demethylation of methamphetamine. However, the effects of methamphetamine are not reliably predicted from serum concentrations.

Ephedrine and Pseudoephedrine

These amines are diastereoisomers that possess two asymmetrical carbon atoms and exist as isomers designated as 1R,2S- and 1S,2R-ephedrine and 1R,2R- and 1S,2S-pseudoephedrine. The 1R,2S-ephedrine (ephedrine) and 1S,2S-pseudoephedrine (pseudoephedrine) isomers occur naturally in various plants of the *Ephedra* genus.

Ephedrine is both an α-adrenergic and a β-adrenergic receptor agonist. In addition, it enhances the release of norepinephrine from sympathetic neurons and is considered a mixed-acting sympathomimetic drug. Adverse effects such as (1) hypertension, (2) tremors, (3) myocardial infarction, (4) seizures, and (5) stroke have resulted in fatalities. Because of this, the FDA banned the sale of dietary supplements containing ephedra in 2004.

Pseudoephedrine is used primarily as a decongestant because of its vasoconstrictive properties (α-adrenergic action).[3] Pseudoephedrine is also used as a precursor for the illicit synthesis of methamphetamine. Because of this, the quantity per purchase of products containing these drugs is now restricted in many places.

PPA (Phenylpropanolamine)

PPA is a metabolite of ephedrine and pseudoephedrine and was once widely available in a number of nonprescription cold medications and diet control products. Adverse effects are similar to those described for ephedrine. In response to an FDA warning of increased risk of hemorrhagic

stroke, PPA has been withdrawn from the market by most manufacturers.[3]

Designer Amphetamines

The terms "designer drugs" and "club drugs" originated in the 1980 and include derivatives of amphetamine-type stimulants such as (1) benzylpiperazine, (2) phenylpiperazine, and (3) pyrolidinophenone.[13] The moniker "club drug" does not imply that recreational use is restricted to this social environment. Most designer drugs (1) produce feelings of euphoria and energy and (2) a desire to socialize, (3) promote social and physical interactions, and (4) distort or enhance visual and auditory sensations. Designer drugs mistakenly have the reputation of being safe and several studies have revealed the increased risk of (1) serotonin syndrome, (2) hepatotoxicity, (3) neurotoxicity, and (4) psychopathology, and (5) the abuse potential of such drugs. Some of the more common designer amphetamines are listed in Box 31-2.

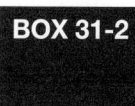

BOX 31-2   Designer Drugs Related to Phenylethylamine, Benzylpiperazine, Phenylpiperazine, and Pyrrolidinophenone[13]

Phenylethylamines
- 3,4-Methylenedioxymethamphetamine (MDMA; Ecstasy)
- 3,4-Methylenedioxyethylamphetamine (MDEA; "Eve")
- 3,4-Methylenedioxyamphetamine (MDA), which is also a metabolite of MDMA
- Paramethoxyamphetamine (PMA)
- Paramethoxymethamphetamine (PMMA)
- 2,5-Dimethoxy-4-methylamphetamine (DOM)
- 2,5-Dimethoxy-4-methylthioamphetamine (DOT)
- 4-Iodo-2,5-dimethoxyamphetamine (DOI)
- 2,5-Dimethoxy-4-bromo-amphetamine (DOB)
- 2,5-Dimethoxy-4-bromo-methamphetamine (MDOB)
- 3,4-(Methylenedioxyphenyl)-2-butanamine (BDB)
- *N*-Methyl-1-(3,4-methylenedioxy-phenyl)-2-butanamine (MBDB)
- 6-Chloro-3,4-methylenedioxymethamphetamine (Cl-MDMA)
- 3,4-Methylenedioxymethcathinone
- 4-Bromo-2,5-diemthoxy-phenylethylamine (2C-B)
- 2,5-Dimethoxy-4ethylthio-phenylethylamine (2C-T-2)
- 2,5-Dimethoxy-4 propylthio-phenylethylamine (2C-T-7)

Benzylpiperazines
- 1-Benzylpiperazine (BZP)
- 1-(3,4-Methylenedioxybenzyl)-piperazine (MDBP)

Phenylpiperazines
- 1-(3-Trifluoromethylphenyl)piperazine (TFMPP)
- 1-(3-Chlorophenyl)piperazine (mCPP)
- 1-(4-Methoxyphenyl)piperazine (MeOPP)

Pyrrolidinophenone
- α-Pyrrolidinopropiophenone (PPP)
- 4-Methoxy-α-pyrrolidinopropiophenone (MOPPP)
- 3,4-Methylenedioxy-α-pyrrolidinopropiophenone (MDPPP)
- 4-Methyl-α-pyrrolidinopropiophenone (MPPP)
- 4-Methyl-α-pyrrolidinohexanophenone (MPHP)

Methylphenidate (Ritalin)

Methylphenidate (MPH) is a phenethylamine derivative with psychostimulant properties similar to those of S(+) amphetamine. It is commonly used to treat attention-deficit hyperactivity disorder (ADHD) and narcolepsy.[3] Like many of its related amphetamine-type stimulants, it exists as an isomer, as (R,R)-methylphenidate (D-MPH) and as (S,S)-methylphenidate (L-MPH). The pharmacological actions of MPH are almost solely performed by the D-isomer. Diversion and abuse of methylphenidate have been increasing among children and adults because of its stimulant and purported aphrodisiac properties. In overdose, the clinical effects of methylphenidate are similar to those of amphetamines.

Analytical Methods

The initial screening test for amphetamines and related drugs is typically immunoassay. For confirmatory testing of a presumptive positive test, a quantitative drug measurement is performed using GC-MS.

Immunoassay. Most "amphetamine" immunoassays have been designed to detect amphetamine/methamphetamine; others have been designed to detect MDMA and MDA; and others to more broadly capture the ATS group—all with varying cross-reactivity. Not all amphetamine immunoassays were suitable for detection of the amphetamine-derived designer drugs PMA, PMMA, and MDEA, and especially not for the tryptamine, cathinones, and piperazine-derived substances. Alternatively, other chemically related compounds such as pseudoephedrine have been shown to produce positive results. Additionally, many psychotropic medications have been reported to interfere with immunoassays. Regarding methylphenidate, it should be noted that its detection by urine drug immunoassay is problematic, as it does not cross-react well with amphetamine immunoassays, and because of its low concentration.[3]

Confirmatory Methods. All positive immunoassay results should be confirmed by a second independent method. However, if the other designer amphetamines (see Box 31-2) are suspected, a negative amphetamine immunoassay screen cannot rule out the presence of these drugs. Fortunately, numerous GC- and LC-based methods for identification and quantitation of these drugs in biological samples have been described.[13]

Most published methods for analysis of members of the amphetamine class in (1) urine, (2) plasma, and (3) blood employ liquid-liquid extraction (LLE) or solid-phase extraction (SPE). Amphetamine-type stimulants are considered volatile and are lost during a dry-down or evaporation step during extraction. Also, because of their extreme volatility at the high temperatures encountered in GC-MS, derivatization before analysis lowers the limit of detection. Additionally, (1) the molecular weight of amphetamine-type stimulants, (2) the low intensity of their mass fragments in electron impact mode, and (3) the structural similarity of many endogenous and exogenous compounds result in a mass spectrum that is not highly characteristic. The issue of lack of specificity of the mass spectrum is resolved by derivatization. Although many derivatives are available for GC-MS use, the 4-CB derivative in the presence of ephedrine/pseudoephedrine may generate methamphetamine, which leads to the DHHS rule that amphetamine must also be detected before a positive methamphetamine result can be reported. The poor UV absorption properties of this class of drugs make it an unsuitable candidate for HPLC with UV detection, and it has no native fluorescence and no significant oxidative electrochemical properties at low voltages. However, LC-MS and LC-MS/MS have been gained in popularity.[13] Other prescription drugs that are metabolized to amphetamine or methamphetamine are listed in Table 31-9. Care must be taken in interpreting the results of drug screens.

Cocaine

Cocaine is an alkaloid found in *Erythroxylon coca,* which grows principally in (1) the northern South American Andes and to a lesser extent in (2) India, (3) Africa, and (4) Java. In clinical medicine, it is used for local anesthesia and vasoconstriction in nasal surgery, and to dilate pupils in ophthalmology. Cocaine abuse has a long history, and it iss still one of the most common illicit drugs of abuse.

Cocaine is sold on the street in two forms: (1) a hydrochloride salt (powder) and (2) a free-base product known as **crack cocaine.** The hydrochloride salt form of cocaine is administered by nasal insufflation ("snorting") or, less frequently, intravenously. Crack is a free-base form and comes as a rock crystal that is heated and its vapors inhaled. The term refers to the crackling sound heard when it is heated.

It should be noted that "crack" cocaine is not to be confused with "free-basing," which is a process in which the user purifies cocaine HCl by mixing an aqueous solution of cocaine with baking soda or ammonia and adding diethyl ether, thereby extracting the free form of the drug into the organic solvent. However, because of the extremely flammable nature of diethyl ether, and therefore the risk of igniting any remaining ether, free-basing is no longer a common practice.

Chemically, cocaine is methylbenzoylecgnine (COC). Its metabolism is complex (Figure 31-11) and occurs via both nonenzymatic hydrolysis and enzymatic transformation in the plasma and liver, producing both active and inactive metabolites. COC is rapidly metabolized to benzoylecgonine (BE) and ecgonine methyl ester, both of which are inactive. It should be noted that cocaethylene, produced when cocaine and ethyl alcohol are used simultaneously, possesses the same CNS

TABLE 31-9	Prescription Drugs That Are Metabolized to Amphetamine or Methamphetamine	
Drug	**Chemical Name**	**Drugs Detected**
Adderall	Amphetamine	Amphetamine
Dexedrine	D-Amphetamine	D-Amphetamine
Deprenyl	Selegiline	L-Methamphetamine
		L-Amphetamine
Didrex	Benzphetamine	Methamphetamine
		Amphetamine

stimulatory activity as cocaine in experimental animals. Nor-cocaine (NC) is of clinical interest because of its conversion to potentially hepatotoxic metabolites: hydroxyl-norcocaine and then norcocaine-nitroxide.

BE has a half-life longer than that of COC. It is the most commonly monitored analyte in urine for determination of COC use. BE is further metabolized to minor metabolites such as m-hydroxybenzoylecgonine (m-HOBE), which has been shown to be an important metabolite in the meconium of cocaine-exposed babies. Anhydroecgonine methyl ester (AEME; methyl ecgonidine) has been identified as a unique COC metabolite after smoked COC ("crack") administration. Anhydroecgonine ethyl ester (AEEE; ethyl ecgonidine) has been identified in COC smokers who also use ethyl alcohol.

Pharmacological Response

Cocaine has cardiovascular effects and is a potent CNS stimulant that elicits a state of increased alertness and euphoria with actions similar to those of amphetamine but of shorter duration. These CNS effects are thought to be largely associated with the ability of cocaine to block dopamine reuptake at nerve synapses, thereby prolonging the action of dopamine in the CNS. It is this response that leads to recreational abuse of cocaine. Cocaine also blocks the reuptake of norepinephrine at presynaptic nerve terminals; this produces a sympathomimetic response. Sudden death due to cardiotoxicity may occur after cocaine use.[13] Death may also occur after the sequential development of hyperthermia, agitated delirium, and respiratory arrest. Excited delirium and extreme physical activity may lead to (1) rhabdomyolysis, (2) acute renal failure, and (3) disseminated intravascular coagulopathy.

The CNS and cardiovascular effects of cocaine exhibit acute tolerance; its effects are more pronounced when the concentration of cocaine in blood is increasing than when it is at a decreasing concentration (*clockwise hysteresis*). Thus, it is difficult to correlate isolated blood concentration values with psychomotor effects.[13]

COC is frequently used with other drugs, most commonly ethanol. This combination produces greater euphoria and an enhanced perception of well-being relative to COC. CE appears to be equipotent to COC with regard to dopamine transporter affinity but is less potent than cocaine pharmacologically. As a consequence, large amounts of COC and ethanol may be ingested, placing users at greater risk for toxicity than if either drug is used alone. The longer elimination half-life of CE may contribute to its toxicity. Additionally, with simultaneous administration of COC and ethanol, the production of NC may be increased, along with the potential for toxicity. It has been suggested that simultaneous COC and ethanol use carries an 18- to 25-fold increase in risk for immediate death over that associated with COC alone.

Analytical Methods

The half-life of COC is 0.5 to 1.5 hours, whereas the half-life of BE is 4 to 7 hours. Thus, BE is the analyte of choice in screening for cocaine use. The initial screening test for cocaine use is the immunoassay detection directed against the primary metabolite BE.[13]

Most confirmatory assays offer quantification of both parent drug and metabolite. Numerous methods have been described for measurement of COC and various metabolites. GC techniques for analysis of COC and its metabolites require derivatization, especially of polar metabolites.

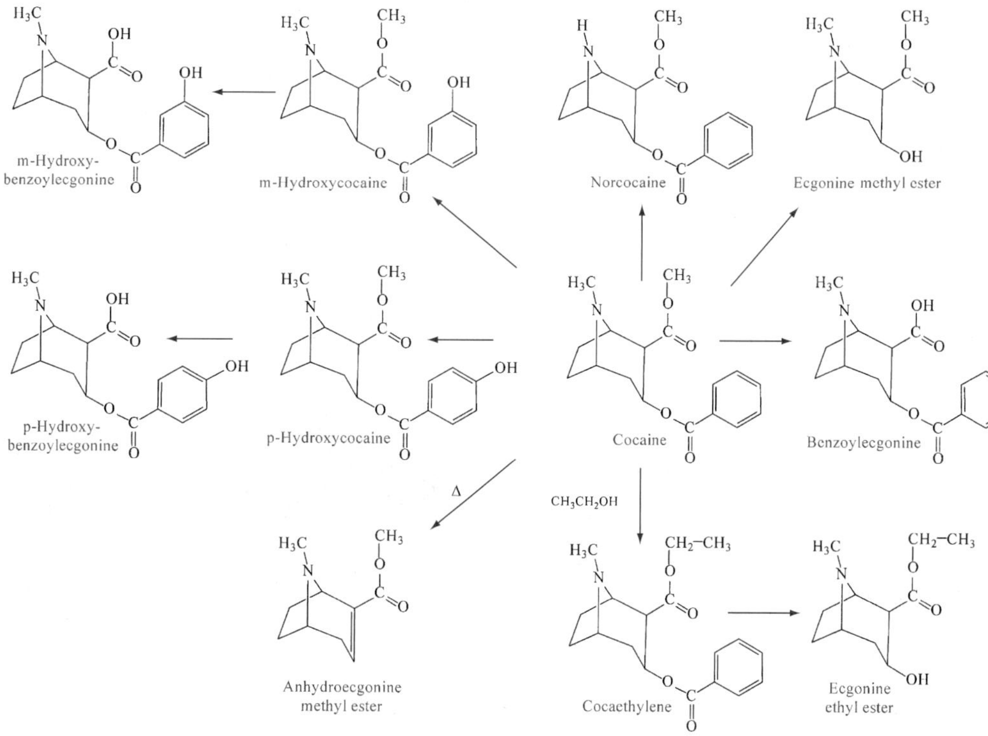

Figure 31-11 Metabolism of cocaine.

GC-MS is the method of choice for many laboratories.[13] However, some reports have suggested that AEME is not a truly unique indicator of smoked cocaine use because it has been reported to be produced in the injector port of a GC at high temperatures. With an LC method, high temperatures are not present in the injector or in any other part of the LC; therefore, AEME is not generated, and its presence identifies a smoked route of COC use. Additionally, LC methods measure simultaneously many of the more polar potentially significant secondary metabolites such as (1) CE, (2) NC, (3) AEME, and (4) AEEE. For these reasons, LC-MS/MS methods are gaining in popularity.[13]

Lysergic Acid Diethylamide (LSD)

Lysergic acid diethylamide (LSD) is an extremely potent psychedelic ergot alkaloid derived from the fungus *Claviceps purpurea*, which grows on wheat and other grains.

Pharmacological Response

LSD shares structural features with serotonin (5-hydroxytryptamine), a major CNS neurotransmitter and neuromodulator. The drug LSD binds to serotonin receptors in the CNS and acts as a serotonin agonist. The principal psychological effects of LSD are (1) perceptual distortions of color, sound, distance, and shape; (2) depersonalization and loss of body image; and (3) rapidly changing emotions from ecstasy to depression or paranoia.

Popular dosage forms include (1) powder, (2) gelatin capsule, (3) tablet, (4) LSD-impregnated sugar cubes, (5) filter paper, and (6) postage stamps. The drug is rapidly absorbed from the GI tract, and its effects (1) begin within 40 to 60 minutes, (2) peak at about 2 to 4 hours, and (3) subside by 6 to 8 hours. The elimination half-life is about 3 hours. The metabolism of LSD in humans is incompletely understood, but 2-oxo-3-hydroxy-LSD is present in urine at concentrations 10- to 43-fold greater than those of LSD. *N*-demethyl-LSD and other metabolites are present in urine specimens but at concentrations less than or equal to those of LSD. Iso-LSD is not a metabolite but is formed by nonenzymatic epimerization of LSD during synthesis or storage of urine at alkaline pH and elevated temperature.

Analytical Methods

Because of the very high potency of LSD and its subsequent rapid and extensive metabolism, only about 1% to 2% of the drug is excreted unchanged in urine. Thus, detection of LSD presents an especially difficult analytical challenge. Even with sensitive assays, the detection window for LSD is generally only 12 to 24 hours. The detection window may be extended, perhaps twofold to threefold, by including 2-oxo-3-hydroxy-LSD in the confirmatory test, while using sensitive techniques such as (1) GC-MS-MS, (2) LC-MS-MS, or (3) LC-MS. To avoid degradation of LSD and 2-oxo-3-hydroxy-LSD or epimerization of LSD to iso-LSD, urine specimens should be protected from (1) sunlight, (2) bright fluorescent light, and (3) elevated temperature at alkaline pH.

Drugs Used in Sexual Assault

Drug-facilitated sexual assault (DFSA) is defined as the use of (1) alcohol, (2) drugs, and/or (3) chemical agents to incapacitate an individual and facilitate sexual assault. In addition to alcohol, the drugs most often implicated in drug-facilitated sexual assault include (1) benzodiazepines, (2) choral hydrate, (3) nonbenzodiazepine sedative-hypnotics, (4) **gamma-hydroxybutyric acid (GHB)**, (5) 1,4-butanediol, (6) γ-butyrolactone, (7) dextromethorphan, (8) ketamine, and (9) nonprescription medications such as antihistamines and anticholinergics. These drugs share similar characteristics that are desired by an assailant such as (1) fast onset, (2) colorlessness, (3) tastelessness, and (4) easy access. Similar clinical effects permit the victim to be easily incapacitated. They include (1) impaired judgment, (2) confusion, (3) reduced inhibitions, (4) sedation, (5) hypnosis, (6) loss of muscle coordination, and (7) sometimes anterograde amnesia. These effects are intensified when these agents are coadministered willingly or involuntarily with other psychotropic medications that produce CNS depression, most notably ethanol. This or involuntarily administration is a commonly reported occurrence. Because of the amnesic properties of these drugs, victims often may not report their sexual assault for several days. Therefore, sensitive analytical techniques are necessary to detect these drugs and their metabolites in urine or hair samples after a single dose.

Benzodiazepines

It is estimated that 8% of sexual assault cases are positive for benzodiazepines. Benzodiazepines that have been reported in sexual assault victims are (1) diazepam, (2) triazolam, (3) temazepam, and (4) clonazepam (see benzodiazepine section above for more details). Flunitrazepam (Rohypnol) has achieved significant public awareness. It is a fast-acting sedative-hypnotic categorized as a Schedule I drug in the United States. Because it is still licensed for use in Europe, Asia, and Latin America, sexual predators are able to acquire this drug through illegal trafficking. Sexual assault predators use flunitrazepam because (1) it is easily dissolved into a beverage, (2) it is relatively tasteless and odorless, (3) it quickly incapacitates their victims, and (4) routine drug screens do not detect its presence.

Pharmacological Effects

Flunitrazepam is more potent than diazepam because of its slower dissociation from the GABA receptor. It is rapidly absorbed and distributed into tissues upon oral administration. Onset of its (1) sedative, (2) amnesic, (3) hypnotic, and (4) disinhibitory effects occurs within 20 to 30 minutes. Flunitrazepam has a long half-life (up to 25 hours), permitting an extended window of detection in blood and urine.[3] Although the effects of flunitrazepam occur rapidly when it is used alone, it is often co-ingested with alcohol, which amplifies its effects.

Analytical Methods

Detection of flunitrazepam (Rohypnol) is especially challenging because of the low doses and the low degree of cross-reactivity of most immunoassays with the principal urinary metabolite, 7-aminoflunitrazepam, although specific immunoassays have been developed. As with other benzodiazepines, prior glucuronidase hydrolysis may improve immunoassay detection. Direct analysis or confirmatory testing of 7-aminoflunitrazepam by GC-MS or LC-MS/MS is indicated in suspected cases.

Choral Hydrate

Chloral hydrate is classified as a sedative and as a hypnotic. The CNS depressant effects of chloral hydrate are believed to be due to its active metabolite trichloroethanol.

Pharmacological Effects

The clinical diagnosis of chloral hydrate intoxication is difficult to differentiate from (1) alcohol, (2) benzodiazepine, and (3) barbiturate intoxication, as all share similar clinical effects. The exact mechanism of action of chloral hydrate has not been determined. The elimination half-life of choral hydrate is very short (4 minutes), but the half-life of its metabolite trichloroethanol is 6 to 10 hours.[3] If co-ingested with alcohol, the metabolism of chloral hydrate may be seriously impaired. Because both ethanol and chloral hydrate are metabolized by CYP2E1 and alcohol dehydrogenase, co-ingestion not only may exacerbate their clinical effects but also may prolong their duration of action.

Analytical Methods

Chloral hydrate is not detected on routine drug screens. Chloral hydrate and its metabolite trichloroethanol (TCE) are detected with the use of LC-MS and capillary gas chromatography with electron-capture detection (GC-ECD), or GC-flame ion detection (GC-FID).

Nonbenzodiazepine Sedative-Hypnotics

A new generation of sedative-hypnotics are available that are structurally different from benzodiazepines (Figure 31-12). They include (1) zopiclone, (2) eszopiclone (Lunesta), (3) zolpidem (Ambien), and (4) zaleplon (Sonata). As a group, they are prescribed as sleep aids through a prescription for a Schedule IV drug. However, they are also used in DFSAs as they are (1) readily prescribed, (2) easily shared, and (3) sold illegally. The rapid onset and amnesic properties of this class of drugs result in (1) disinhibition, (2) passivity, and (3) retrograde amnesia, making it a favored DFSA drug. These drugs require only a low dosage to cause an effect and are rapidly metabolized. CNS-depressant effects are additive when they are co-administered with other psychotropic medications such as (1) anticonvulsants, (2) antihistamines, (3) ethanol, and (4) other drugs that produce CNS depression.[13]

Pharmacological Effects

The pharmacological effects of these agents result from their interaction with a specific subtype of $GABA_A$ receptor complex. These drugs modulate the $GABA_A$ receptor chloride channel by binding to the benzodiazepine (BZ) receptors in the brain without binding to peripheral BZ receptors. Therefore, these drugs have fewer muscle relaxant properties.

Analytical Methods

Although these drugs do not cross-react with most benzodiazepine immunoassays, specific reagent systems (ELISA) directed against the nonbenzodiazepine hypnotics are available. Screening and confirmatory testing are performed by GC-MS or LC-MS/MS.

Four Carbon (C4) Compounds

Gamma-Hydroxybutyric acid (GHB) and its synthetic precursor compounds, 1,4-butanediol (1,4-BD) and γ-butyrolactone (GBL), are Schedule I agents in the United States, and availability is restricted in numerous other countries. GHB is an odorless and colorless liquid, or it can be obtained as an off-white powder that easily dissolves in liquids. When ingested, it has CNS depressant effects, resulting in sedation and hypnosis.

Pharmacological Effects

GHB is a naturally occurring substance that is produced in the brain. It is metabolized to GABA by multiple endogenous enzymes. Consumption of GHB, or the synthetic GHB precursor compound 1,4-BD or GBL, will promote GABA activity. In addition to increased metabolism to GABA, GHB has direct effects on the CNS by binding GHB-specific receptors and $GABA_B$ receptors.

GHB is rapidly metabolized ($t_{1/2} \approx 30$ minutes).[3] Onset of its effects occurs in approximately 15 to 30 minutes and the duration of response is short, typically 1 to 3 hours for a normal dose (1 to 5 g) and 2 to 4 hours with excessive doses.[13]

Analytical Methods

GHB is not detected on immunoassay-screens but can be identified with the use of GC-FID or GC-MS. Because GBH is metabolized rapidly, timely sample collection is an important

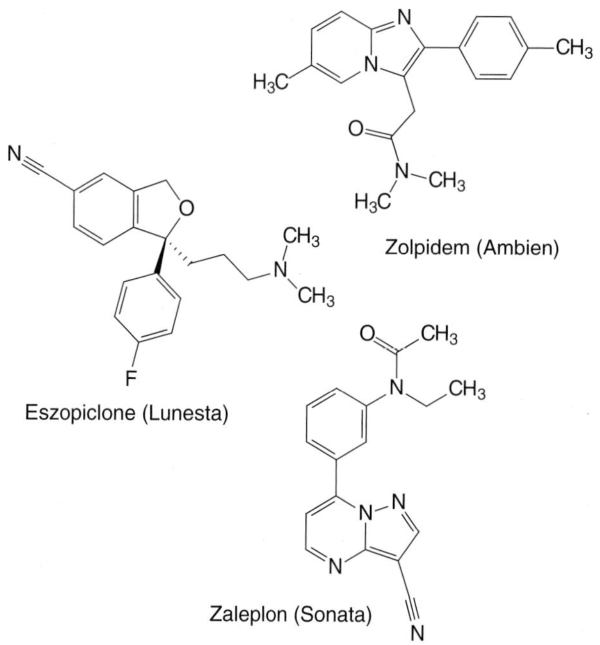

Figure 31-12 Chemical structures of the nonbenzodiazepine sedative-hypnotics (zolpidem, eszopiclone, zaleplon).

facet of GBH assay. Plasma samples should be collected within 6 to 8 hours after ingestion, and urine samples within 10 to 12 hours. Endogenous concentrations of GHB are typically 1.0 mg/L[3] and after exogenous exposure may return to normal levels within 8 to 12 hours after ingestion.

Dextromethorphan

Dextromethorphan (DXM) is structurally related to the opioids, but it does not bind to opioid receptors at normal dose. The (L−) isomer of dextromethorphan, levorphan (not available in the United States), is a potent opioid analgesic and is an example of the stereoselective nature of opioid receptor binding. DXM lacks analgesic activity but does have antitussive activity comparable with that of codeine. DXM is present in (1) numerous over-the-counter (OTC) cough medications, often in combination with (2) antihistamines, (3) nasal decongestants, (4) guaifenesin, (5) aspirin, and (6) acetaminophen. At high doses, DXM binds opioid receptors to produce (1) miosis, (2) respiratory depression, and (3) CNS depression. High doses may also cause (1) lethargy, (2) agitation, (3) ataxia, (4) nystagmus, (5) diaphoresis, and (6) hypertension.[3]

Pharmacological Effects

Dextromethorphan is metabolized to dextrophan by CYP2D6. Dextrophan may be responsible for the more pleasant psychotropic effects of high-dose dextromethorphan, whereas the parent drug may cause (1) dysphoria, (2) sedation, and (3) ataxia. Thus, poor metabolizers (deficient in CYP2D6 activity) may be less prone and extensive metabolizers more prone to continue the abuse of dextromethorphan.[13] Dextrophan and to a lesser degree DXM bind to PCP- and ketamine-binding sites on the NMDA receptor; this may account for their similar psychotropic actions (see phencyclidine and ketamine sections).

Analytical Methods

Clinically approved doses of DXM are not detected by most clinical opiate immunoassays, but larger doses may cross-react. ELISA assays are available to detect DXM and its major metabolite, dextrorphan. Because most preparations contain dextromethorphan as the bromide salt, excessive ingestion of dextromethorphan may result in bromide poisoning and in a negative serum aniongap. The presence of DXM or dextrophan in a sample is confirmed by GC-MS or LC-MS/MS.[13] Dextrophan is the **enantiomer** of levorphanol, a potent opioid agonist available in the United States (Levo-Dromoran). Unless chiral analytical techniques are used, these enantiomers are not resolved.

Ketamine and Phencyclidine

Ketamine and phencyclidine (PCP) are potent analgesics and general anesthetics. PCP is listed as a Schedule II drug in the U.S. Federal Controlled Substance Act and is not approved for human use. Ketamine is a Schedule III drug that is commonly used as an anesthetic in pediatric medicine for short surgical procedures. Both drugs have been used illicitly in human cases of drug abuse, as well as in cases of drug-facilitated sexual assault. They are sold under a variety of names and are available as a colorless, odorless liquid or as a white powder.

Pharmacological Effects

Ketamine and PCP share similar structural features and pharmacological actions. They are classified as dissociative anesthetics because they produce rapid-acting (1) dissociation of perception, (2) consciousness, (3) movement, and (4) memory.[13] The effects are dose dependent and vary between individuals. An anesthetic dose produces profound analgesia, but the individual is awake yet incapacitated, with limited voluntary limb movement. The mechanism of action for these compounds consists of complex integration of neurological pathways. They bind and antagonize the excitatory glutaminergic system by binding to NMDA receptors. They also (1) decrease GABA transmission, (2) disrupt cortical activity, and (3) increase dopamine and norepinephrine synaptic reuptake.[13]

Analytical Methods

Initial screening is typically done by immunoassay. Immunoassays for PCP are generally reliable; however, false positives have been reported because of high concentrations of (1) dextromethorphan, (2) diphenhydramine, and (3) thioridazine. Immunoassay-positive specimens should be confirmed using GC-MS or LC-MS techniques. Note, these techniques will also detect norketamine and dehydronorketamine, the active metabolites of ketamine.[13]

Athletes and Drug Testing

"Doping" in athletic competitions has a history of abuse in a variety of sports for centuries. Regulation of performance-enhancing substances was initiated in 1967 in response to the death of Danish cyclist, Knud Jensen, at the 1960 Olympic Games in Rome. After decades of global reform between governments and sporting agencies,[16] the World Anti-Doping Agency (WDA) was established in 1999. Approximately 30 facilities around the world are accredited for detecting drug use among competitive athletes. Prohibited drugs are substances or methods that conform to two of three criteria: (1) performance enhancing, (2) may endanger the athlete's health, (3) go against the spirit of the sport. "In-competition" testing was established to detect drugs such as (1) stimulants, (2) narcotics, (3) cannabinoids, and (4) glucocorticosteroids in specimens taken at the time of a competition to temporarily enhance performance.

"Out-of-competition" testing is performed to detect substances and methods such as (1) anabolic-androgenic steroids, (2) hormones, (3) hormone modulators, (4) oxygen transfer enhancement, and (5) genetic manipulations. These compounds and methods are used by an athletic for their performance-enhancing effects. In practice, they have a gradual onset to allow for more intense and efficient training, and their use is then abruptly discontinued before competition begins.[16]

Detection of Drugs of Abuse Using Other Types of Specimens

Blood, serum, and urine samples are typically collected for the purpose of determining exposure to various agents. However, sampling of blood is considered invasive, and collection of urine may require some invasion of privacy and loss of dignity. In addition, urine specimens are subject to adulteration or manipulation to evade detection. For these reasons, alternate biological specimens have been investigated as alternative types of samples for drug analysis. They include (1) meconium, (2) oral fluid, (3) hair, and (4) sweat.

Meconium

The first intestinal discharge from newborns is meconium, which is a viscous, dark green substance contains (1) intestinal secretions, (2) desquamated squamous cells, (3) lanugo hair, (4) bile pigments, (5) blood, (6) pancreatic enzymes, (7) free fatty acids, (8) porphyrins, (9) interleukins, (10) phospholipase A_2, and (11) bile acids. Meconium begins to form during the second trimester and continues to accumulate until birth; drugs taken by the mother can be detected in the meconium of the newborn.

Illicit drug use during pregnancy is a major social and medical issue. Drug abuse during pregnancy is associated with significant perinatal complications, including a high incidence of (1) stillbirth, (2) meconium-stained fluid, (3) premature rupture of the membranes, (4) maternal hemorrhage (abruptio placentae or placenta previa), and (5) fetal distress. In the neonate, conditions that contribute to increases in the rates of mortality and morbidity include (1) asphyxia, (2) prematurity, (3) low birth weight, (4) hyaline membrane disease, (5) infection, (6) aspiration pneumonia, (7) cerebral infarction, (8) abnormal heart rate and breathing patterns, and (9) drug withdrawal.

In practice, identification of the drug-exposed mother or her neonate is not easy. Maternal admission of the use of drugs is often inaccurate principally because of denial about addiction or fear of the consequences stemming from such admission. Likewise, many infants who have been exposed to drugs in utero may appear normal at birth and show no overt manifestations of drug effects. Drug testing, on the other hand, is an objective means of determining drug exposure in both mother and infant. Thus, drug testing is necessary in infants to document proof of the infant's exposure to illicit drugs. Urine testing of the mother or newborn will detect only recent drug use (within a few days before birth), and urine collection from newborns may be problematic.

Meconium testing has some limitations. For example, meconium is usually passed by full-term newborns within 1 to 2 days; however, low-birth-weight infants may have delayed passage (median age of 3 days). Thus, meconium collection is missed completely, or significant delay is seen in detection of intrauterine drug exposure.

In the clinical laboratory, meconium is an unfamiliar matrix; it is a sticky material that is difficult to process. Meconium drug screening has been adapted to various analytical

TABLE 31-10	Drugs and Metabolites of Significance in Meconium
Drug Class	**Confirmation Compound**
Cocaine	Cocaine
	Benzoylecgonine
	Cocaethylene
	m-Hydroxybenzoylecgonine
Opiates	Morphine
	Codeine
	6-Monoacetylmorphine (6-MAM)
	Hydromorphone
	Hydrocodone
	Oxycodone
Cannabinoids	9-Carboxy-11-nor-delta-9-THC
	11-Hydroxy-delta-9-tetrahydrocannabinol
	8,11-Dihydroxy-delta-9-tetrahydrocannabinol
Amphetamines	Amphetamine
	p-Hydroxyamphetamine
	Methamphetamine
	MDMA
	MDA
	MDEA
Ethanol	Fatty acid ethyl esters
PCP	PCP

techniques, including (1) radioimmunoassay, (2) enzyme immunoassay, and (3) fluorescence polarization immunoassay. As with any immunoassay-based drug screen, confirmatory testing by MS is necessary.

A variety of (1) GC-MS, (2) LC-MS, and (3) LC-MS/MS methods and their advantages and disadvantages have been described. Confirmatory assays for meconium are more difficult than those for urine. Recovery of drugs from meconium is low (10% to 50%). Some debate continues as to which are the most appropriate drug analytes that should be measured in meconium; Table 31-10 attempts to summarize current knowledge.[9,13] Meconium drug testing is far less standardized than urine drug testing. Assay cutoff limits and units (ng/g meconium or ng/mL extract) may vary; suitable reference or control materials are not yet available.

A word of caution, interpretation of meconium data should be approached carefully. For example, some investigators believe that tremendous, and potentially inappropriate, value has been placed on meconium results. On occasion, decisions about treatment or custody of the infant have been based solely on meconium drug screen results. It is critical to remember that a positive test could indicate drug exposure. However, a negative result does not rule it out. It is clear that additional work is necessary to address these important issues and to improve our understanding of the disposition of drugs in meconium.

Oral Fluid (Saliva)

Reports concerning the appearance of organic solutes in oral fluid have been included in the scientific literature for longer than 70 years. Analysis of saliva for drugs was first done almost 30 years ago for the purpose of therapeutic drug monitoring. It has since been evaluated for use in forensic toxicology, with recognition of its advantages over other biological matrices. Most studies on saliva in humans use whole saliva. It should be noted that the term "oral fluid" is now preferred for the specimen collected from the mouth.

Several advantages are associated with monitoring oral fluid as contrasted with monitoring plasma or serum concentrations. For example, collection of oral fluid is considered to be a noninvasive procedure, direct observation is possible minimizing risk of adulteration, and some of the risks associated with drawing of blood are avoided. Furthermore, for the patient, the (1) fear, (2) anxiety, and (3) discomfort that may accompany the drawing of blood are diminished. One significant disadvantage of oral fluid is that the window of detection is about equivalent to that of blood or serum and is short compared with that of urine. Another disadvantage is the small volume of sample collected. The problem of small sample size is usually overcome by using methods that simultaneously extract multiple drug groups.

In principle, oral fluid drug concentration is related to plasma free drug concentration; therefore oral fluid has the potential to show a relation between behavior/impairment and drug concentration, making it a possible medium for monitoring drug intoxication or for conducting therapeutic drug management. Since disposition of drugs in oral fluid is dependent upon chemical and metabolic processes appropriate interpretation is required.[5] In recent years, great interest has been expressed in the use of oral fluid testing for (1) roadside drug screening, (2) monitoring the compliance of individuals on drug maintenance programs, and (3) workplace drug testing. Low concentrations of drugs and metabolites necessitate sensitive screening methods, which typically are immunoassays. Again, low concentrations of drugs have necessitated that confirmatory methods be equally sensitive. Many confirmatory methods have been developed for oral fluid testing of abused drugs, including (1) GC-MS, (2) LC-MS, and (3) LC-MS/MS.[13]

Hair

For longer than 30 years, hair has been analyzed for trace metals, including (1) lead, (2) arsenic, and (3) mercury (see Chapter 32). This was achieved with the use of atomic absorption spectroscopy (see Chapter 9). Subsequently, interest in analysis of hair for the purpose of detecting drug use has increased.[13]

Hair is advantageous as a biological specimen for drug analysis because (1) it is easily obtained, (2) it is obtained with less embarrassment, and (3) it is not easily altered or manipulated to avoid drug detection. Hair also differs from other human materials used for toxicological analysis in that it has a substantially longer detection window (months to years) depending on the length. The rate of hair growth depends on (1) anatomical location, (2) race, (3) sex, and (4) age. Once deposited in hair, drugs are very stable, and analysis can be performed even after centuries.

The exact mechanism by which chemicals are incorporated into hair is still being studied. It has been suggested, however, that passive diffusion may be augmented by binding of the drug to intracellular components of hair cells such as the hair pigment melanin. Factors that may affect how efficiently drugs are incorporated into hair are not well established but may include (1) rate of hair growth, (2) anatomical location of hair, (3) hair color (melanin content), and (4) hair texture (thick or fine, porous or not). These factors are determined by genetic factors and by the effects of various hair treatments. For example, in vitro studies suggest that melanin pigment plays an important role in drug binding. Studies have demonstrated that after the same dosage is given, dark hair incorporates much more of the drug than is incorporated by light hair. This may lead to biases in hair testing for drugs of abuse.[13]

Drugs, when deposited in hair, are generally present in relatively low concentrations; thus sensitive analytical techniques are required for detection. Immunoassay procedures have been modified for use with hair. For confirmatory testing, GC-MS is generally the method of choice; however, various GC-MS/MS or LC-MS/MS methods have been used.[13] External exposure to drugs causes them to be detected in hair; one of most crucial issues facing hair analysts today is technical and false positives. The need to distinguish between passive exposure (environmental contamination) and active consumption is fundamental; consequently, decontamination procedures for hair are compulsory. These usually involve a washing step.

Sweat

Drugs may be excreted in sweat, and sweat analysis may provide an alternative detection technique. Sweat patch collection devices that resemble an adhesive bandage may be worn for several days to several weeks. During this time, a drug, if present, accumulates in the absorbent pad in the patch, while water vapor escapes through the semi-permeable covering. Thus sweat drug testing offers the possibility of monitoring drug use over extended periods without the need for frequent collection of urine.[13] Sweat drug excretion may also be an important mechanism by which drugs enter hair.

Review Questions

1. The best specimen type used to determine whether a neonate has been exposed to drugs drug during the second or third trimester of her pregnancy is:
   a. fetal oral fluid.
   b. meconium.
   c. fetal hair.
   d. newborn infant urine.
2. The antidotal therapy for acetaminophen overdose is:
   a. forced alkaline diuresis.
   b. inhibition of the GABA channel.
   c. pralidoxime.
   d. N-acetylcysteine.

3. The best advantage of using high-performance liquid chromatography (HPLC) over gas chromatography (GC) for comprehensive drug screening for a broad range of chemicals is that:
   a. HPLC does not require a derivatization step.
   b. HPLC can be performed at the individual's bedside.
   c. GC gives diverse color hues and requires considerable technical skill.
   d. GC drug testing methods are subject to many types of interference.

4. The *principal* pharmacological action of ethanol is:
   a. binding to heme iron in the cytochrome complex within mitochondria.
   b. respiratory acidosis.
   c. central nervous system depression.
   d. increased metabolism of GABA.

5. A phenethylamine derivative that has properties similar to amphetamine and is used to treat attention-deficit hyperactivity disorder and narcolepsy is:
   a. methylphenidate.
   b. methamphetamine.
   c. pyridoxime.
   d. ephedrine.

6. To confirm heroin use, testing of which of the following urinary metabolites is considered unique and specific for this drug?
   a. morphine
   b. codeine
   c. meperidine
   d. 6-Monoacetylmorphine

7. For assessment of drugs of abuse, the most widely accepted laboratory method for drug *confirmation* is:
   a. immunoassay.
   b. gas chromatography-mass spectrometry.
   c. HPLC.
   d. reflectance photometry.

8. An example of an agent that induces the cholinergic syndrome when present in overdose amounts would be a(n):
   a. tricyclic antidepressant.
   b. antihistamine.
   c. organophosphate compound.
   d. barbiturate.

9. The correct formula for determining osmol gap is:
   a. measured cations – measured anions
   b. calculated osmolality – measured osmolality
   c. measured osmolality – calculated osmolality
   d. measured anions – measured cations

10. An increased anion gap value associated with acidosis likely indicates:
    a. methanol overdose.
    b. overuse of antihistamines.
    c. carbon monoxide inhalation.
    d. treatment of opioid overdose with naloxone.

References

1. Armstrong SC, Cozza KL. Pharmacokinetic drug interactions of morphine, codeine, and their derivatives: theory and clinical reality, Part I. Psychosomatics 2003;44:167–71.
2. Baselt RC. Dispositition of toxic drugs and chemicals in man, 9th edition. Foster City, Ca: Biomedical Publications, 2011.
3. Blanke R, Decker W. Analysis of toxic substances. In: Tietz N, ed. Textbook of clinical chemistry, 1st edition. Philadelphia, Pa: WB Saunders, 1986:1670–744.
4. Cone EJ, Heit HA, Caplan YH, Gourlay D. Evidence of morphine metabolism to hydromorphone in pain patients chronically treated with morphine. J Anal Toxicol 2006;30:1–5.
5. Cone EJ, Huestis M A. Interpretation of oral fluid tests for drugs of abuse. Ann N Y Acad Sci U S A 2007;1098:51–103.
6. Drummer OH. Methods for the measurement of benzodiazepines in biological samples. J Chromatogr 1998;713:201–25.
7. Drummer OH. Chromatographic screening techniques in systematic toxicological analysis. J Chromatogr 1999;733:27–45.
8. Federal Register 49 CFR Part 40—Procedures for transportation workplace drug and alcohol testing programs. Updated as of August 31, 2009.
9. Gray TR, Kelly T, LaGasse LL, et al. New meconium biomarkers of prenatal methamphetamine exposure increase identification of affected neonates. Clin Chem 2010;56:856–60.
10. Jarvie DR, Heyworth R, Simpson D. Plasma salicylate analysis: a comparison of colorimetric, HPLC and enzymatic techniques. Ann Clin Biochem 1987;24(Pt 4):364–73.
11. Jones G. Post-mortem toxicology. In: Moffat A, ed. Clarke's analysis of drugs and poisons, 3rd edition. London, UK: Pharmaceutical Press, 2004:95–108.
12. Kadiev E, Patel V, Rad P, et al. Role of pharmacogenetics in variable response to drugs: focus on opioids. Exp Opin Drug Metab Toxicol 2008;4:77–91.
13. Langman LJ, Bechtel L, Holstege CP. Clinical toxicology (Chapter 35). In: Burtis CA, Ashwood ER, Bruns DE, eds. Tietz textbook of clinical chemistry and molecular diagnostics, 5th edition. St Louis: Elsevier, 2012:1109–88.
14. Maurer HH. Systematic toxicological analysis of drugs and their metabolites by gas chromatography-mass spectrometry. J Chromatogr 1992;580:3–41.
15. Trescot AM, Datta S, Lee M, Hansen H. Opioid pharmacology. Pain Physician 2008;11:S133–53.
16. World Anti-Doping Code. The 2013 prohibited list; international standard. Montreal, Canada: World Anti-Doping Agency, 2013.

Toxic Metals*

Thomas P. Moyer, Ph.D.

Objectives

1. Define the following terms:

Adverse Reaction to Metal Debris	Chelation therapy
Argyria	Dimercaprol
Berylliosis	Mees' lines
British anti-Lewisite	Penicillamine
Cardiomyopathy	

2. List three factors that must be demonstrated before a diagnosis of metal toxicity is made.
3. Describe the location and classification of essential and nonessential metals in the periodic table, including row, column, and characteristics of these metals.
4. For the following metals, list common uses, physiological significance (if any), metabolism, therapeutic uses (if any), physiological effects of overexposure, therapy (if any), and methods of analysis:

Aluminum	Manganese
Antimony	Mercury
Arsenic	Nickel

Beryllium	Platinum
Cadmium	Selenium
Chromium	Silicon
Cobalt	Silver
Copper	Thallium
Gadolinium	Titanium
Lead	Vanadium

5. Describe the specimen requirements for quantification of metal, including special collection procedures, how results are reported, and possible inferences.
6. Evaluate and analyze case studies involving metal overexposure and analysis.

Key Words and Definitions

Adverse Reaction to Metal Debris (ARMD) A condition characterized by severe hip pain that results from metal release when the ball and joint of the prosthesis used in a hip replacement are both metal.

Argyria A permanent ash gray discoloration of the skin, conjunctiva, and internal organs that results from long-continued use of silver salts.

ATSDR Agency for Toxic Substances and Disease Registry

Berylliosis A hypersensitivity response to beryllium, usually involving the lungs and less often the skin, subcutaneous tissues, lymph nodes, liver, or other structures. Two varieties are distinguished: *acute b.* and *chronic b.* Called also *beryllium poisoning.*

Cardiomyopathy A general diagnostic term designating primary noninflammatory disease of the heart muscle.

CERCLA Comprehensive Environmental Response, Compensation, and Liability Act. (see **SARA** and **Superfund**).

Chelation therapy Administration of chelating agents to remove metals from the body.

Mees' lines Lines of discoloration across the nails of the fingers and toes.

Minamata disease A condition characterized by symptoms of alkyl mercury poisoning that were seen between 1953 and 1958 among individuals who ate seafood from a bay in Japan that was polluted with alkyl mercury compound.

NIOSH U.S. National Institute for Occupational Safety and Health

OSHA U.S. Occupational Safety and Health Administration

Pneumoconiosis Deposition of large amounts of dust or other particulate matter in the lungs.

SARA Superfund Amendments and Reauthorization Act. The Superfund Amendments and Reauthorization Act (SARA) amended the Comprehensive Environmental Response, Compensation, and Liability Act (CERCLA) on October 17, 1986.

---

*A more extensive review of this subject and additional references are found in Moyer TP. Toxic metals. In: Burtis C, Ashwood E, Bruns D, eds. Tietz textbook of clinical chemistry and molecular diagnostics, 7th edition. St Louis: Saunders Elsevier, 2012:1189–205.

Key Words and Definitions—cont'd

Superfund A program of the U.S. Government to clean up the nation's uncontrolled hazardous waste sites. Under the Superfund program, abandoned, accidentally spilled, or illegally dumped hazardous waste that poses a current or future threat to human health or the environment is cleaned up.

Toxic metals Metals that are elements with high molecular weight and generally toxic in low concentrations to plant and animal life. *Note:* The International Union of Pure and Applied

Chemistry (IUPAC) considers the term "heavy metal" to be both meaningless and misleading and recommends that it no longer be used.

Threshold limit value (TLV) The maximum concentration of a chemical allowable for repeated exposure without producing adverse health effects.

WHO World Health Organization.

Metals have been recognized as toxins for centuries. For example, arsenic (As) poisoning was a favored way to dethrone royalty in the Renaissance era, and mercury (Hg) poisoning was common in eighteenth century Europe, where it was used in the generation of felt from beaver pelts to make the popular top hat. This resulted in behavioral changes and common use of the phrase "mad as a hatter."

This chapter explores these and other **toxic metals** and the role of the clinical laboratory in diagnosing and monitoring toxicity associated with exposure to them.

Assessment of Metal Poisoning

Important questions to address when metal toxicity is considered are listed in Box 32-1. These questions are addressed generally in the first section of this chapter. In the second section, the unique characteristics of the more common metals known to be associated with toxicity are discussed.

Prevalence of Metal-Based Toxicity

As the twenty-first century begins, one would might assume that metal toxicities would be thoroughly known and avoidable. However, humans still encounter elemental toxins, and chronic, low-concentration exposure occurs more frequently in individuals than in large population groups. Concern continues regarding low-concentration exposure to lead and the effect that such exposure has on mental development in the young. As is common in our environment, individuals are occasionally exposed because of lack of knowledge of the household products they are using. Many insecticides contain As as an active ingredient, the most common source of exposure causing peripheral neuropathy among patients who

have been unwittingly exposed. Another problematic metal is cadmium (Cd), which is used to manufacture brightly colored paint pigments. Painters who fail to use adequate respiratory protection have been known to experience significant exposure. It is also significantly present in tobacco products. Studies indicate that apoptotic pathways are initiated by metals such as As, Cd, chromium (Cr), nickel (Ni), and beryllium (Be), and possibly lead (Pb), antimony (Sb), and cobalt (Co).

Although rare, manufacturing errors have caused the production of products that contain toxic metals. For example, in the early 1960s, a Canadian beer brewery accidentally contaminated a large lot of its product with Co. The product was sold to and consumed by the public, resulting in an outbreak of renal disease and **cardiomyopathy**. In this type of situation, the Public Health Service is often called in to identify the cause of an outbreak of unusual symptoms. The clinical laboratory should be prepared to support these types of investigations.

Diagnosing Toxicity

Confirming the diagnosis of metal toxicity is difficult because signs and symptoms are similar to those of a number of non–element-dependent diseases. Consequently, diagnosis of metal toxicity requires demonstration of *all* of the following factors: (1) A source of metal exposure must be evident, (2) the patient must demonstrate signs and symptoms typical of the metal, and (3) abnormal metal concentration in the appropriate tissue or body fluid must be evident.

In clinical practice, analysis of toxic elements should always be considered in the clinical work-up of the patient with (1) renal disease of unexplained origin, (2) bilateral peripheral neuropathy, (3) acute change in mental function, (4) acute inflammation of the nasal or laryngeal epithelium, or (5) a history of exposure. Certain elements should be considered as the (1) active, (2) causative, or (3) deficient agents in specific circumstances (Table 32-1).

Classification of Metals

Some metals are essential for life (see Chapter 27), but if their concentration in one's body exceeds a certain threshold, toxicity may develop. Also, some nonessential metals are toxic even at low concentrations. Review of the periodic table provides some insight into the determination of a metal's potential toxicity (Figure 32-1).

BOX 32-1   Pertinent Questions Relative to Metal Toxicity

1. Is the metal of concern toxic?
2. What is the prevalence associated with the metal of concern?
3. What are the signs and symptoms of exposure to that metal?
4. Is the degree of exposure known?
5. Are adequate analytical techniques available to analyze the metal?
6. Are appropriate body fluids and tissues and analytical techniques available to identify and quantify the metal?

TABLE 32-1	Conditions That Result from Various Metal Toxicities
Metal	**Condition**
Aluminum	Dialysis, encephalopathy, or dementia
Arsenic	Bilateral pain radiating from feet to legs or peripheral neuropathy, or unexplained impaired renal function
Cadmium	Impaired renal function in aerosol painters
Cobalt	Pulmonary edema, allergy, hemorrhage, renal failure, or neurologic impairment
Copper-zinc deficiency	Impaired wound healing
Gadolinium	Nephrogenic systemic fibrosis
Lead	Children younger than 2 years living in older homes, or unexplained gastric upset, anemia, or impaired renal function at any age
Mercury	Acute changes in behavior, impaired speech, visual field constriction, hearing loss, and somatosensory disorders
Manganese	Onset of parkinsonism in individuals younger than age 50
Selenium (deficiency)	Patients undergoing total parenteral nutrition
Thallium	Acute hair loss
Zinc (deficiency)	Burn patients exhibiting erythema

Elements in rows 3 and 4 of groups 1 and 2 of the periodic table are essential elements. The gastrointestinal tract and the dermis are very effective in regulating the body burden of these compounds. Consequently, patients rarely experience toxicity from one of these elements unless the element is injected directly into the vascular system. Elements in groups 6 through 12 in row 4 are essential for life but are required at low concentrations; many are protein cofactors required for enzymatic activity. The gastrointestinal tract and the dermis regulate intake to some degree, but overload will induce passive diffusion that leads to excessive concentrations and toxicity. Elements in rows 5 and below are classified as nonessential (or if essential, are required at picomolar concentrations or less). As one moves from right to left across the periodic table, the elements become more prevalent and therefore have greater potential to induce toxicity. Elements in groups 13 through 16 in rows 4 through 6 are of particular interest as toxins because they have electron configuration that allows them to bond covalently with sulfur. This characteristic has been identified as a significant factor in the mechanism of action of this group of metals. These metals include (1) As, (2) Cd, (3) Pb, (4) Hg, and (5) thallium (Tl), which are toxins of considerable concern. Elements in group 17 (halides) are essential for life but are toxic when present in excess. The inert elements that constitute group 18 are toxic in the gas phase because they can cause anoxia; their inert characteristic is the very cause of their toxicity.

Occupational Monitoring

Employees are frequently monitored when working in an environment where exposure to toxic metals is a possibility. The most common form of monitoring involves quantification of airborne concentrations of metals in the production

process. **Threshold limit values (TLV)** for airborne concentrations and time interval exposure concentrations are specified by the U.S. National Institute for Occupational Safety and Health (**NIOSH**). TLVs are air quality standards developed by the American Conference of Governmental Industrial Hygienists (ACGIH). They are the model for many other air quality limits such as the permissible exposure limits (PELs) of the Occupational Safety and Health Administration (**OSHA**). They are defined generally as the maximum concentration of a chemical allowable for repeated exposure to ensure worker safety without producing adverse health effects.

Workers may also be monitored by quantification of biological samples. The most common sample used is a random urine sample, and results are expressed in concentration units for the metal of interest per gram of creatinine to normalize for excretion volume variances. Cd, Cr, and Pb have defined urine excretion concentrations set by a U.S. federal agency to ensure worker safety.[15-17] Additional technical and regulatory information about toxic metals is available at the OSHA website at http://www.osha.gov/SLTC/metalsheavy/index. html/; (accessed November 5, 2013).

The World Health Organization (**WHO**) and OSHA have defined blood concentrations for Pb that are designed to warn employers when workers are overexposed. Safety limits for other metals have been set by professional organizations, such as the American Conference of Governmental Hygienists.[7]

Analytical Methods

Analytical techniques used to measure metals in biological fluid include (1) atomic absorption spectrometry with flame (AA-F) or electrothermal atomization furnace (AA-ETA), (2) inductively coupled plasma emission spectroscopy (ICP-ES), (3) inductively coupled plasma mass spectrometry (ICP-MS), and (4) high-performance liquid chromatography–inductively coupled plasma mass spectrometry (LC-ICP/MS). These techniques are specific and sensitive and provide the clinical laboratory with the capability to measure a broad array of metals at clinically significant concentrations. For example, ICP-MS and ICP-ES are used to measure several metals simultaneously.[2] Photometric assays are available but require large volumes of sample and have limited specificity. Spot tests are also available but should be considered obsolete because they are error prone, often yielding false-positive results.

Specific Metals

Certain metals are known to be toxic when humans are exposed to elevated concentrations; five metals are listed in the top 20 of the 2007 **CERCLA** (Comprehensive Environmental Response, Compensation, and Liability Act) Priority List of Hazardous Substances (http://www.atsdr.cdc.gov/SPL/index.html/; accessed November 5, 2013).[12] They include As (No. 1), Pb (No. 2), Hg (No. 3), Cd (No. 7), and Cr (No. 18). Other metals of concern include (1) aluminum (Al), (2) Be, (3) Co, (4) copper (Cu), (5) gadolinium (Gd), (6) iron (Fe), (7) manganese (Mn), (8) Ni, (9) platinum (Pt), (10) selenium (Se), (11) silicon (Si), (12) silver (Ag), and (13) Ti. The Agency

IUPAC Periodic Table of the Elements

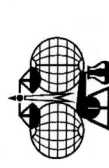

Group																		
1																		18
1 **H** hydrogen [1.007, 1.009]	2											13	14	15	16	17		**2** **He** helium 4.003
3 **Li** lithium [6.938, 6.997]	**4** **Be** beryllium 9.012											**5** **B** boron [10.80, 10.83]	**6** **C** carbon [12.00, 12.02]	**7** **N** nitrogen [14.00, 14.01]	**8** **O** oxygen [15.99, 16.00]	**9** **F** fluorine 19.00		**10** **Ne** neon 20.18
11 **Na** sodium 22.99	**12** **Mg** magnesium [24.30, 24.31]	3	4	5	6	7	8	9	10	11	12	**13** **Al** aluminium 26.98	**14** **Si** silicon [28.08, 28.09]	**15** **P** phosphorus 30.97	**16** **S** sulfur [32.05, 32.08]	**17** **Cl** chlorine [35.44, 35.46]		**18** **Ar** argon 39.95
19 **K** potassium 39.10	**20** **Ca** calcium 40.08	**21** **Sc** scandium 44.96	**22** **Ti** titanium 47.87	**23** **V** vanadium 50.94	**24** **Cr** chromium 52.00	**25** **Mn** manganese 54.94	**26** **Fe** iron 55.85	**27** **Co** cobalt 58.93	**28** **Ni** nickel 58.69	**29** **Cu** copper 63.55	**30** **Zn** zinc 65.38(2)	**31** **Ga** gallium 69.72	**32** **Ge** germanium 72.63	**33** **As** arsenic 74.92	**34** **Se** selenium 78.96(3)	**35** **Br** bromine [79.90, 79.91]		**36** **Kr** krypton 83.80
37 **Rb** rubidium 85.47	**38** **Sr** strontium 87.62	**39** **Y** yttrium 88.91	**40** **Zr** zirconium 91.22	**41** **Nb** niobium 92.91	**42** **Mo** molybdenum 95.96(2)	**43** **Tc** technetium	**44** **Ru** ruthenium 101.1	**45** **Rh** rhodium 102.9	**46** **Pd** palladium 106.4	**47** **Ag** silver 107.9	**48** **Cd** cadmium 112.4	**49** **In** indium 114.8	**50** **Sn** tin 118.7	**51** **Sb** antimony 121.8	**52** **Te** tellurium 127.6	**53** **I** iodine 126.9		**54** **Xe** xenon 131.3
55 **Cs** caesium 132.9	**56** **Ba** barium 137.3	57-71 lanthanoids	**72** **Hf** hafnium 178.5	**73** **Ta** tantalum 180.9	**74** **W** tungsten 183.8	**75** **Re** rhenium 186.2	**76** **Os** osmium 190.2	**77** **Ir** iridium 192.2	**78** **Pt** platinum 195.1	**79** **Au** gold 197.0	**80** **Hg** mercury 200.6	**81** **Tl** thallium [204.3, 204.4]	**82** **Pb** lead 207.2	**83** **Bi** bismuth 209.0	**84** **Po** polonium	**85** **At** astatine		**86** **Rn** radon
87 **Fr** francium	**88** **Ra** radium	89-103 actinoids	**104** **Rf** rutherfordium	**105** **Db** dubnium	**106** **Sg** seaborgium	**107** **Bh** bohrium	**108** **Hs** hassium	**109** **Mt** meitnerium	**110** **Ds** darmstadtium	**111** **Rg** roentgenium	**112** **Cn** copernicium		**114** **Fl** flerovium		**116** **Lv** livermorium			

Key:

atomic number
Symbol
name
standard atomic weight

57 **La** lanthanum 138.9	**58** **Ce** cerium 140.1	**59** **Pr** praseodymium 140.9	**60** **Nd** neodymium 144.2	**61** **Pm** promethium	**62** **Sm** samarium 150.4	**63** **Eu** europium 152.0	**64** **Gd** gadolinium 157.3	**65** **Tb** terbium 158.9	**66** **Dy** dysprosium 162.5	**67** **Ho** holmium 164.9	**68** **Er** erbium 167.3	**69** **Tm** thulium 168.9	**70** **Yb** ytterbium 173.1	**71** **Lu** lutetium 175.0
89 **Ac** actinium	**90** **Th** thorium 232.0	**91** **Pa** protactinium 231.0	**92** **U** uranium 238.0	**93** **Np** neptunium	**94** **Pu** plutonium	**95** **Am** americium	**96** **Cm** curium	**97** **Bk** berkelium	**98** **Cf** californium	**99** **Es** einsteinium	**100** **Fm** fermium	**101** **Md** mendelevium	**102** **No** nobelium	**103** **Lr** lawrencium

Notes

- IUPAC 2011 Standard atomic weights abridged to four significant digits [Table 4 published in *Pure Appl. Chem.* 85, 1047-1078 (2013); http://dx.doi.org/10.1351/PAC-REP-13-03-02. The uncertainty in the last digit of the standard atomic weight value is listed in parentheses following the value. In the absence of parentheses, the uncertainty is one in that last digit. An interval in square brackets provides the lower and upper bounds of the standard atomic weight for that element. No values are listed for elements which lack isotopes with a characteristic isotopic abundance in natural terrestrial samples. See PAC for more details.

- "Aluminum" and "cesium" are commonly used alternative spellings for "aluminium" and "caesium."

- Claims for the discovery of all the remaining elements in the last row of the Table, namely elements with atomic numbers 113, 115, 117 and 118, and for which no assignments have yet been made, are being considered by a IUPAC and IUPAP Joint Working Party.

For updates to this table, see iupac.org/reports/periodic_table/. This version is dated 1 May 2013.
Copyright © 2013 IUPAC, the International Union of Pure and Applied Chemistry.

INTERNATIONAL UNION OF
PURE AND APPLIED CHEMISTRY

Figure 32-1 2011 IUPAC Periodic Table of the Elements. *(From Pure Appl Chem 2013;85:1047–78.)*

for Toxic Substances and Disease Registry (**ATSDR**) provides toxicological profiles for many of these.

Several of these metals are also considered essential trace elements and are discussed in Chapter 27. Risk assessments for essentiality versus toxicity for Cr, Cu, iodine (I), Fe, Mn, molybdenum (Mo), Se, and zinc (Zn) have been performed by several U.S. governmental and private organizations.

Aluminum

Under normal physiological conditions, the usual daily dietary intake of Aluminum (Al) is 5 to 10 mg, which is completely excreted. This excretion is accomplished by filtration of Al from the blood by the glomerulus of the kidney. Patients in renal failure lose this ability and are candidates for Al toxicity. The dialysis process is not highly effective in eliminating Al and can be a significant source of exposure. Furthermore, it is common practice to administer Al-based gels orally to patients in renal failure to reduce the amount of phosphate absorbed from their diet to avoid excessive phosphate accumulation. A small fraction of this Al may be absorbed, and patients in renal failure accumulate this Al. After dialysis, albumin is sometimes administered to replace that which is removed during dialysis. A note of caution, some albumin products have high Al content resulting from the pharmaceutical purification process of passing the product through Al silicate filters.

As a consequence of Al intake, it (1) accumulates in blood if not filtered by the kidney; (2) binds firmly to proteins, such as transferrin; and (3) is rapidly distributed throughout the body. Deposition of Al in bone interrupts physiological calcium exchange; the calcium in bone becomes unavailable for resorption into blood—a process under the physiological control of parathyroid hormone (PTH) and 1,25-dihydroxy vitamin D (see Chapter 39). The normal physiological action of PTH on bone is blunted in patients with renal failure because their renal cells are not synthesizing the 1,25-dihydroxy vitamin D required for normal PTH action. It is typical for patients in renal failure to have high serum PTH values and low serum calcium; this represents secondary hyperparathyroidism—the normal physiological response to vitamin D deficit. Deposition of Al at the bone mineralization front and its binding to parathyroid calcium receptors interfere with this physiological process. Clinical guidelines suggest that patients with no signs or symptoms of osteomalacia or encephalopathy are likely to have serum Al concentrations <20 µg/L and PTH whole molecule concentrations 150 to 300 ng/L—typical for secondary hyperparathyroidism associated with renal failure. Patients with osteomalacia or encephalopathy typically have serum Al concentrations >60 µg/L, and PTH concentrations <65 ng/L indicating Al-related bone disease. Patients with serum Al concentrations >20 and <60 µg/L were identified as candidates for likely onset of Al-related bone disease; these patients required aggressive efforts to reduce their daily Al exposure. Efforts to reduce Al intake include (1) switching from Al-containing phosphate binders to calcium-containing phosphate binders, (2) ensuring that dialysis water contains less than 10 µg/L of Al, and (3) ensuring that albumin used during postdialysis therapy is Al-free.

Al has been implicated as a factor in Alzheimer's disease (AD) because Al accumulates in the neurofibrillary tangle of patients with AD. Although a cause-and-effect relationship between accumulation of Al in brain and AD has not been conclusively demonstrated,[1] studies have clearly shown an increased concentration of Al in the brain. It is probable that accumulation of Al in the neurofibrillary tangle of AD patients is a secondary finding associated with the disease but not directly related to the cause. The neurofibrillary tangle has a higher than normal affinity for Al that may explain increased accumulation of Al in brain tissue of Alzheimer's patients.

Antimony

Compounds containing antimony (Sb) have been known since ancient Egyptian times and were used as cosmetics by the women of that era. In the sixteenth century, Sb preparations were thought to be wonder drugs that in the nineteenth century were prescribed for a number of conditions. Today antimony compounds are used to treat parasitic diseases such as (1) leishmaniasis, (2) schistosomiasis, and (3) bilharziasis.

Workplace exposure to Sb dust over a period of years leads to **pneumoconiosis**. The size of the dust particles of Sb trioxide significantly increases the occurrence of pneumoconiosis, with smaller particles being more dangerous. The workers at greatest danger are those in underground facilities and in metal production. Smoking may also contribute to respiratory problems. Other conditions of damage to the liver and spleen resulting from antimony exposure are (1) lymphocytosis, (2) eosinophilia, and (3) reduction in leukocyte and platelet counts. It is important to remember that when intoxication occurs with metallic Sb, the effect is caused not only by Sb, but also by the lead, arsenic, and other metals that may accompany it.

Arsenic

Arsenic (As) is one of the most widely known toxic metals, having gained notoriety from its extensive use by Renaissance nobility as an antisyphilitic agent and an antidote against acute arsenic poisoning. This agent was memorably used in the well-known tale "Arsenic and Old Lace" as a means of terminating undesirable acquaintances. Currently, As is still a dangerous toxicant, as evidenced by the Bangladesh incident wherein several hundred persons were poisoned by drinking ground water contaminated with As leaching from bedrock. As mentioned earlier, As is listed as the No. 1 toxicant on the 2011 U.S. CERCLA Priority List of Hazardous Substances (http://www.atsdr.cdc.gov/SPL/index.html/; accessed November 5, 2013), and it is still used extensively in insecticides.

Arsenic exists in numerous toxic and nontoxic forms. Toxic forms include (1) the inorganic species As^{3+}, also denoted as As(III); (2) the more toxic As^{5+}, also known as As(V), and their partially detoxified metabolites; (3) monomethylarsine (MMA); and (4) dimethylarsine (DMA). Detoxification occurs in the liver as As^{5+} is reduced to As^{3+} and then is methylated to MMA and DMA. (The structures of these and related As species are shown in Figure 32-2.)

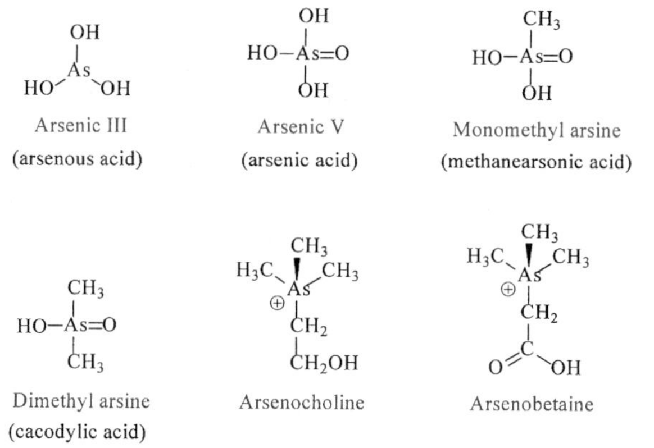

Figure 32-2 Structures of arsenic species.

As a result of detoxification, As^{3+} and As^{5+} are found in the urine shortly after ingestion, whereas MMA and DMA are the species that predominate longer than 24 hours after ingestion. Urinary As^{3+} and As^{5+} concentrations peak in urine at approximately 10 hours and return to normal 20 to 30 hours after ingestion. Urinary MMA and DMA concentrations normally peak at about 40 to 60 hours and return to baseline 6 to 20 days after ingestion. In a large U.S. population study, for all participants aged >6 years, dimethylarsinic acid and arsenobetaine made the greatest contribution to the quantity of total urinary arsenic. Arsenobetaine was the primary contributor to high total urinary arsenic concentrations (see further discussion on this later).[3]

The half-life of inorganic As in blood is 4 to 6 hours, and the half-life of the methylated metabolites is 20 to 30 hours. Blood concentrations of As are elevated for only a short time after administration, after which As rapidly disappears into the large body phosphate pool. Abnormal blood As concentrations in the 5 to 50 ng/mL range can be detected shortly after exposure. Nontoxic forms of As are present in many foods. Arsenobetaine and arsenocholine are the two most common forms of organic As that are found in food. The foods that most commonly contain significant concentrations of organic As are shellfish and other predators in the seafood chain (e.g., cod, haddock). In a large U.S. population study, for all participants aged >6 years, dimethylarsinic acid and arsenobetaine made the greatest contribution to the total urinary arsenic. Arsenobetaine was the primary contributor to high total urinary arsenic concentrations.[3] Arsenic excretion in healthy individuals who have ingested arsenobetaine-containing foods is >120 µg per 24-hour specimen. After ingestion, arsenobetaine and arsenocholine undergo rapid renal clearance to become concentrated in the urine. Arsenobetaine and arsenocholine are completely excreted within 1 to 2 days after ingestion, and no residual toxic metabolites are present. The apparent half-life of organic As is 4 to 6 hours. Consumption of seafood before collection of a urine sample for As testing is likely to result in an elevated concentration of As in the urine.

The toxicity of As is due to three different mechanisms, two of which are related to energy transfer. Firstly, As avidly binds to dihydrolipoic acid, a necessary cofactor for pyruvate dehydrogenase. Absence of the cofactor inhibits the conversion of pyruvate to acetyl coenzyme A—the first step in gluconeogenesis. Secondly, As competes with phosphate for reaction with adenosine diphosphate (ADP), resulting in formation of the lower-energy adipic acids (ADPAs) rather than adenosine triphosphate (ATP). Thirdly, As also binds with any hydrated sulfhydryl group on protein, distorting the three-dimensional configuration of the protein, thus causing it to lose activity.

British antilewisite (BAL) is an effective antidote for treating As intoxication; the active agent in BAL is dimercaprol, a sulfhydryl-reducing agent. This suggests that the primary mechanism of action of the toxicity of As is related to sulfhydryl binding. Arsenic also interferes with the activity of several enzymes of the heme biosynthetic pathway. Arsenic is also a known carcinogen, as evidence suggests increased risk of bladder, skin, and lung cancers, as well as lung cancer associated with smoking, following consumption of water with high As contamination.

Of note is the fact that As compounds are also used for therapeutic reasons. For example, arsenic compounds have been used for decades in the management of protozoal infections such as trypanosomiasis. A preparation of arsenic trioxide called Fowler's agent was used in the nineteenth century as a health tonic and for a variety of ailments ranging from skin disease to leukemia. Arsphenamine was used intravenously to treat (1) syphilis, (2) yaws (a tropical infection of the skin, bones, and joints), and some (3) protozoal infections. Arsenic is still a key ingredient of certain herbal remedies, and arsenic trioxide is currently used in the management of refractory promyelocytic leukemia.

To distinguish among toxic inorganic species and nontoxic organic species of As of seafood origin, high-performance liquid chromatography (HPLC) techniques have been developed.[3] A typical finding in a urine specimen with total 24-hour excretion of As of 350 µg/24 h is that more than 95% is present as the organic nontoxic seafood species, and less than 5% is present as the inorganic toxic species. Such a finding indicates that the elevated total As concentration was likely due to ingestion of seafood.

Hair analysis is frequently used to document time of As exposure. Arsenic circulating in the blood will bind to protein by formation of a covalent complex with sulfhydryl groups of the amino acid cysteine. Because As has a high affinity for keratin, which has high cysteine content, the As concentration in hair or nails is greater than in other tissue. Several weeks after exposure, transverse white striae, called **Mees' lines**, may appear in the fingernails; this event is caused by denaturation of keratin by metals such as (1) As, (2) Cd, (3) Pb, and (4) Hg. Because hair grows at a rate of approximately 0.5 cm/mo, hair collected from the nape of the neck can be used to document recent exposure. Axillary or pubic hair is used to document long-term (6 months to 1 year) exposure. Hair As >1 µg/g dry weight indicates excessive exposure. Blood is the least useful specimen for identifying As exposure because blood As concentrations are elevated for only a short time after administration and rapidly disappear into the large body phosphate pool. This occurs because the body treats As like phosphate, incorporating it wherever phosphate would be incorporated.

Absorbed As is rapidly circulated and distributed into tissue storage sites. Abnormal blood As concentrations are detected for only a few hours (<4 hours) after ingestion. This test is useful only to document an acute exposure when the As is likely to be >20 ng/mL for a short time. Typically, serum As is <4.0 ng/mL.

Arsenic has been accurately analyzed by ICP-MS. The specimen is prepared in dilute acid containing gallium as an internal standard and is aspirated directly into the argon plasma. Mass response from the argon plasma is monitored for As (75 m/z), gallium (70 m/z), and $^{16}O^{35}Cl$ (51 m/z) to allow for correction for $^{40}Ar^{35}Cl$ (75 m/z) interference. The operator must be aware of the potential for interference from argon chloride. A correction is made by accounting for chloride by measuring 51 m/z and subtracting that residual from 75 m/z. Urine is the sample of choice for As analysis because As is excreted predominantly by the kidney, where it becomes concentrated.

Beryllium

Beryllium (Be) metal and alloys and Be ceramics are used in a wide range of applications, including (1) dental appliances, (2) golf clubs, (3) nonsparking tools, (4) wheelchairs, (5) satellite and spacecraft manufacture, (6) circuit board production, and (7) the nuclear power industry, as well as in (8) weapons as a neutron modulator.

The general population is exposed to low concentrations of Be through food and drinking water; these exposures are of no clinical consequence. The major route by which Be enters the body is via the respiratory tract, and industrial exposure usually occurs from inhalation and ingestion of Be dust. Inhaled Be compounds are cleared very slowly from the lungs. Soluble compounds are absorbed to a much greater degree than others, such as Be oxide, which is much less soluble. Beryllium salts are strongly acidic when dissolved in water, and this is thought to have a major toxic effect on human tissue. Absorbed Be accumulates in the skeleton. Renal clearance is very slow.

Acute exposure to Be (1) is rare, (2) is usually caused by an industrial accident or explosion, and (3) typically results in chemical pneumonitis. Chronic Be exposure in the workplace has led to occupational health concerns because of its potential to cause a progressive and potentially fatal respiratory condition called *chronic Be disease (CBD)*. This disease, also known as **berylliosis**, is characterized by the formation of granulomas resulting from an immune reaction to Be particles in the lung. To reduce the number of workers currently exposed to beryllium in the course of their work at the U.S. Department of Energy (DOE) facilities or among its contractors, the DOE has established a chronic beryllium disease prevention program (CBDPP) to minimize the concentrations of, and the potential for, exposure to beryllium, and has put forth medical surveillance requirements to ensure early detection of the disease.

Studies have suggested that the size of the Be particles affects not only the site of deposition but also the amount deposited. This in turn may influence the clearance rate and thus the time of contact between immune cells and Be. Several years ago, researchers noted that blood and lung cells from CBD patients proliferated when exposed to Be in culture. This assay has been refined and is offered as the Be lymphocyte proliferation test (BeLPT) (http://www.hss.doe.gov/nuclearsafety/techstds/docs/specification/SPEC11422001.pdf/; accessed on November 4, 2013). Unfortunately, because of the nature of the test and variability from laboratory to laboratory, the BeLPT has been known to produce false-negative and problematic results. Efforts are under way by several groups to standardize the assay. Despite these issues, the BeLPT in bronchoalveolar cells is part of the current "gold standard" diagnosis for CBD. Quantification of Be in serum or urine is not useful in making this diagnosis. Air analysis (TLV) is the preferred method of exposure evaluation.

Cadmium

Cd is a byproduct of zinc and lead smelting. It is used (1) in industrial electroplating, (2) in the production of rechargeable batteries, (3) as a common pigment in organicbased paints, and (4) in tobacco products. Breathing the fumes of Cd vapors leads to nasal epithelial deterioration and pulmonary congestion resembling chronic emphysema. Spray painting of organic-based paints without the use of protective breathing apparatus is a common source of chronic exposure. Auto repair mechanics represent a work group that has significant opportunity for exposure to Cd.

The toxicity of Cd resembles that of As, Hg, and Pb in that it attacks the kidney. Patients suffering from Cd toxicity typically present with renal dysfunction with proteinuria of slow onset (over a period of years). Chronic exposure to Cd causes accumulated renal damage.[15] Breathing the fumes of Cd vapors leads to nasal epithelial deterioration and pulmonary congestion resembling chronic emphysema. Cadmium toxicity is expressed via formation of protein-Cd adducts that change the conformational structure of the protein, causing it to denature. This protein denaturation occurs at the site of highest concentration—in the alveoli if exposure is due to dust inhalation—and in the proximal tubule of the kidney because this is a major route of excretion.

NIOSH regulations mandate that employees exposed to Cd in the workplace must be monitored with the use of quantification of the urinary concentrations of Cd and creatinine, with results in µg of Cd expressed per gram of creatinine. This is based on the finding that renal damage caused by Cd exposure is detected by increased Cd excretion relative to creatinine. Cadmium excretion >3 µg Cd/g of creatinine indicates significant exposure to Cd. Results >15 µg Cd/g of creatinine are considered indicative of severe exposure. The urinary concentration of Cd is a more specific measure of Cd exposure than are other markers of renal function, such as (1) β_2-microglobulin, (2) retinol-binding protein, and (3) N-acetyl glucosaminidase. Normal blood Cd concentration is less than 5 ng/mL, and most concentrations are in the interval of 0.5 to 2 ng/mL. Moderately increased blood Cd (3 to 7 ng/mL) may be associated with tobacco use. Acute toxicity is observed when the blood concentration exceeds 50 ng/mL. Usual daily excretion of Cd is less than 3 µg/d. Collection of urine samples using a rubber catheter has been known to result in elevated results because latex rubber contains trace amounts of Cd that are extracted as urine passes through it. Brightly colored plastic urine collection containers should be avoided because the pigment in the plastic may be Cd-based. Cadmium concentrations also increase with age and may be involved with senescence. Cadmium is usually quantified by atomic absorption spectrometry, but it also has been accurately quantified by ICP-MS.

Chromium

Occupational exposure to Cr represents a significant health hazard.[16] Chromium is used extensively (1) in the manufacture of stainless steel, (2) in chrome plating, (3) in the tanning of leather, (4) as a dye for printing and textile manufacture, (5) as a cleaning solution, (6) as an anticorrosive in cooling systems, and (7) in metallic orthopedic implants.[9]

The toxic form of Cr is Cr^{6+} [Cr(VI)], which is rare; a strong oxidizing environment is required to convert the common form Cr^{3+} [Cr(III)] to Cr^{6+}, as might be found when Cr^{3+} is exposed to high temperatures in the presence of oxygen or during high-voltage electroplating. Inhalation of the vapors of Cr^{6+} causes erosion of the epithelium of the nasal passages and produces squamous cell carcinomas of the lung. Cr^{6+} is highly lipid soluble and readily crosses cell membranes, whereas Cr^{3+} is rather insoluble and does not readily cross membranes. Clinically, monitoring biological specimens for Cr^{6+} is neither practical nor clinically useful to detect Cr toxicity because the instant it enters a cell, it is reduced to nontoxic Cr^{3+}. Instead, monitoring the air at the manufacturing site for Cr^{6+} is the usual way to test for Cr^{6+} exposure.

Quantification of total Cr in urine can be used to assess exposure to total Cr. NIOSH has proposed <30 µg chromium/g creatinine as the concentration of concern when employees are monitored, but this concentration does not indicate that the specific exposure was to Cr^{6+}. The presence of chromium in erythrocytes is suggestive of exposure to Cr^{6+} within the past 120 days, because Cr^{6+} crosses biological membranes but Cr^{3+} does not.[13] Increased serum chromium concentrations are observed in association with orthopedic implants made from chromium alloys. ICP-MS is the preferred technology for quantification of Cr in body fluids.

Total hip replacement is a successful treatment for advanced joint disease; more than 1 million total hip replacements are surgically inserted worldwide each year.[9] Bearing surfaces such as ceramic on ceramic and metal on metal (MoM) have become the dominant forms in the prosthesis market, with the expectation that these forms could be used in younger, more active individuals, and wear would no longer be an issue. Although these patients benefit from joint replacement with improved mobility and quality of life, implant-specific local and systemic adverse effects due to hypersensitivity to the metal or hyperreactivity due to the wear of MoM surfaces affect a small number of implant recipients.[9] Metal implants made up of various combinations of (1) Al, (2) Cr, (3) Co, (4) Fe, (5) Mg, (6) Mo, (7) Ni, and/or (8) V, wear as the result of continuous motion at the MoM surfaces, resulting in release of

microparticles into the surrounding tissues. These microparticles can corrode, resulting in the release of metal ions into the systemic circulation.

DeSmet and coworkers have provided data relating serum and joint synovial fluid concentrations to orthopedic implant status.[6] Joint fluid concentrations of metal ions were at least an order of magnitude higher than those measured in the serum. The median serum Cr concentration in the patients with documented MoM wear were approximately ten times higher than those in patients without MoM wear. Joint fluid Cr concentration correlates with serum Cr concentrations; significantly elevated serum Cr in the context of severe joint pain associated with hip implant is known as **Adverse Reaction to Metal Debris (ARMD)**.

Serum Cr analysis is useful for evaluation of implant wear. All patients with an orthopedic implant will have Cr concentrations higher than individuals without implants. Patients experiencing implant joint pain with serum Cr >15 ng/mL or Co >10 ng/mL are likely to have significant implant deterioration.

Preanalytical handling of the specimen for Cr analysis is critically important. Many specimen collection products contain Cr in the rubber stopper or O-rings to add plasticity to the rubber. Special rubber was created to manufacture evacuated blood collection tubes suitable for use in trace metal testing. Attention to detail during specimen collection is essential for achieving successful and clinically valid testing. Blood for Cr testing should be collected in tubes that are approved by the U.S. Food and Drug Administration (FDA) for trace metal testing.

Cobalt

Co is widely distributed in the environment and is the essential cofactor in vitamin B_{12}. Quantification of active vitamin B_{12} (see Chapter 27) is the usual way to assess nutritional status. Cobalt deficiency has not been reported in humans. Exposure to Co is of growing concern among patients with metallic orthopedic implants.[6,9]

Cobalt is found in metal alloys that (1) are very hard, (2) have high melting points, and (3) are resistant to oxidation. Cobalt is not highly toxic, but large exposures will produce (1) pulmonary edema, (2) allergy, (3) nausea, (4) vomiting, (5) hemorrhage, (6) renal failure, and (7) neurologic impairment. Occupational exposure occurs during production and machining of these metal alloys and has been known to result in interstitial lung disease. Cardiomyopathy and renal failure are symptomatic of acute Co exposure. These symptoms were discovered in an incidence of mass population exposure to Co when beer contaminated with the metal was consumed. Chronic exposure may cause (1) pulmonary syndrome, (2) skin irritation, (3) allergy, (4) gastrointestinal irritation, (5) nausea, (6) cardiomyopathy, (7) hematological disorders, and (8) thyroid abnormalities. Cobalt exposure alone may not lead to toxicity and must be considered within the context of exposure to multiple metals.

Quantification of urinary Co is an effective means of identifying individuals with excessive exposure. For example, the National Health and Nutrition Examination Survey

(NHANES/; http://www.cdc.gov/nchs/nhanes.html/; accessed November 5, 2013) reported that the geometric mean of cobalt excretions in a large population was 0.54 µg/g creatinine in children and 0.34 µg/g creatinine in adults. Serum cobalt concentrations are increased above normal (>1 µg/L) in patients with orthopedic implants made from cobalt alloys. Cobalt is quantified in biological tissues by atomic absorption spectrometry or by ICP-MS.

DeSmet and coworkers have provided data relating serum and joint synovial fluid concentrations to orthopedic implant status.[6] Joint fluid concentrations of metal ions were at least an order of magnitude higher than those measured in the serum. The median serum Co concentration in the patients with documented MoM wear were 5 to 20 times higher than those in patients without MoM wear. As with Cr, joint fluid concentration of Co correlates with serum Co concentration, and significantly elevated serum Co in the context of severe joint pain associated with hip implant is known as Adverse Reaction to Metal Debris (ARMD).

Copper

The homeostasis and analysis of Cu are discussed in Chapter 27. Copper ingestion has been known to cause serious toxicity, and exposure may be caused by common pesticides. Copper arsenate is one of the active agents in marine antifouling paints and in the wood preservative used with green "treated" wood. Copper arsenate wood products have been taken off the market in the United States because of this concern. Ingestion of copper produces (1) severe gastrointestinal pain with erosion of the epithelial layer of the gastrointestinal tract, (2) hemolytic anemia, (3) centrilobular hepatitis with jaundice, and (4) renal damage. The classical presentation of Cu toxicosis is represented by the genetic disease of Cu accumulation known as *Wilson's disease*. This disease is typified by hepatocellular damage (increased transferases) and/or changes in mood and behavior caused by accumulation of Cu in central neurons.

Evaluation of serum and urine copper concentration is useful in diagnosing Wilson's disease (see Chapter 18). Because most Cu circulating in blood is bound to ceruloplasmin, and ceruloplasmin formation is decreased in Wilson's disease, serum copper concentration is less than the reference interval for serum (Cu, 0.7 to 1.4 µg/mL), and urinary Cu concentrations are increased to 15 to 60 µg/L. Increased hepatic Cu >2.0 (adjusted for age and reported as the hepatic iron index) is diagnostic for Wilson's disease. Increased serum Cu is observed in patients prescribed estrogen. Excess Zn ingestion interferes with absorption of copper and leads to copper deficiency, which is characterized by myeloneuropathy.

Gadolinium

Gd is a chemical element found in image contrast agents that are used during magnetic resonance imaging (MRI) and magnetic resonance angiography (MRA) procedures. These agents have come under scrutiny by the FDA (http://www.fda.gov/; accessed November 5, 2013) because gadolinium-based contrast agent (GBCA) is thought to be involved in nephrogenic systemic fibrosis (NSF), a debilitating disorder characterized by (1) edema, (2) plaques, (3) discoloration, and (4) severe thickening of the skin, resulting in contractures and immobility. In addition to GBCA exposure, proposed contributing factors and associations with NSF include (1) renal insufficiency, (2) pharmaceutical erythropoietin usage, (3) hypocalcemia acidosis, (4) low serum albumin concentrations, and (5) high serum ferritin concentrations. Exposure to GBCA during a condition of low glomerular filtration rate (GFR) appears to be the most consistent risk factor. Because GBCA is excreted by the kidney, exposure is prolonged in patients with renal insufficiency. It is thought that extended exposure permits transmetallation to occur; this allows free gadolinium to come in contact with proteins and other cellular components. Although several different attempted therapies have been administered, some leading to moderate disease regression, no known cure is uniformly effective.

Iron

The homeostasis and analysis of iron (Fe) are reviewed in Chapter 28. Iron supplements are used frequently to maintain an adequate body burden of Fe. Occasionally, ingestion exceeds the needed daily requirement, resulting in Fe toxicity. For example, ingestion of more than 0.5 g of Fe has been known to produce severe irritation of the epithelial lining of the gastrointestinal tract, resulting in hemosiderosis, which may develop into hepatic cirrhosis. The presence of Fe >350 µg/dL or transferrin >125 micromole/L in serum corroborates this diagnosis.

Lead

Lead (Pb) is a metal commonly found in the environment that is an acute and a chronic toxin. It is present at high concentration (up to 35% w/w) in many paints manufactured before 1972. The Pb content of paints intended for household use was limited to <0.5% in 1978, but Pb is still found in paint products intended for nondomestic use and in artists' pigments. Ceramic products for use in homes available from noncommercial suppliers such as local artists have been known to contain significant amounts of Pb. Also, lead is leached from the ceramic products by weak acids such as vinegar and fruit juices. Leaded crystal contains up to 10% Pb, which is leached during long-term storage of acidic fluids such as fruit juice. Lead is also found (1) in dirt from areas adjacent to homes painted with Pb-based paints and (2) on highways, where it has accumulated from the use of leaded gasoline in automobiles. Use of leaded gasoline has diminished significantly since the introduction of unleaded gasoline, which has been required in personal automobiles in the United States since 1978. Lead is also found in soil near abandoned industrial sites where Pb may have been used. Water transported through Pb or Pb-soldered pipe contains some Pb, with higher concentrations found in water that is weakly acidic. Some foods such as moonshine distilled in Pb pipes and some traditional home medicines also contain Pb. Exposure to Pb from any of these sources by (1) ingestion, (2) inhalation, or (3) dermal contact has been known to cause significant toxicity.

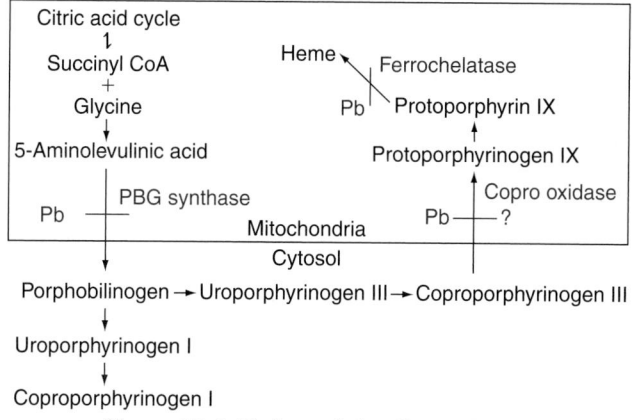

Figure 32-3 Erythropoietic effects of lead.

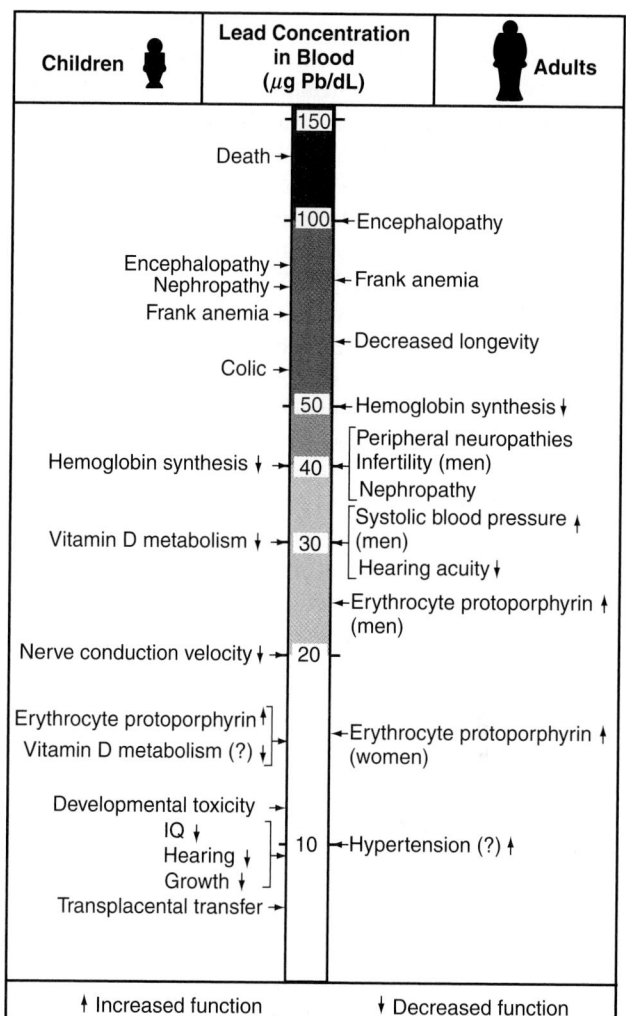

Figure 32-4 Effects of inorganic lead on children and adults (lowest observable adverse effect concentrations). *(From Royce SE, Needleman HL, eds. Case studies in environmental medicine: lead toxicity. Washington, DC: U.S. Public Health Service, ATSDR, 1990.)*

A typical diet in the United States contributes approximately 3 μg of Pb per day, of which 1% to 10% is absorbed. Children may absorb as much as 50% of the dietary intake. The fraction of Pb absorbed is enhanced by nutritional deficiency. Most of the daily intake is excreted in the stool after direct passage through the gastrointestinal tract. Although a significant fraction of the absorbed Pb is rapidly incorporated into bone and erythrocytes, Pb is ultimately distributed among all tissues. Lipid-dense tissues, such as the central nervous system, are particularly sensitive to organic forms of Pb. Erythrocyte turnover of Pb occurs within approximately 120 days. Lead is ultimately excreted in bile or urine.

Lead expresses its toxicity by several mechanisms that are described graphically in Figure 32-3. It avidly inhibits amino levulinic acid dehydratase (ALAD), which is an enzyme that catalyzes the synthesis of heme from porphyrin. Inhibition of ALAD causes accumulation of protoporphyrin in erythrocytes (see Chapter 29), which is a significant marker for Pb exposure. Anemia caused by lack of heme is frequently observed in Pb toxicity. Lead also is an electrophile that avidly forms covalent bonds with the sulfhydryl group of cysteines in proteins. Thus proteins in all tissues exposed to Pb will have Pb bound to them. Keratin in hair contains a high fraction of cysteine relative to other amino acids and actively binds Pb. Consequently, hair analysis for Pb is a good marker for exposure. Some proteins become labile as Pb binds with them because Pb causes the tertiary structure of the protein to change. Cells of the nervous system are particularly susceptible to this effect. Some Pb-bound proteins change their tertiary configuration sufficiently that they become antigenic. Renal tubular cells are particularly susceptible to this effect because they are exposed to relatively high Pb concentrations during clearance.

The development of Pb toxicity follows a progressive pattern. Figure 32-4 describes this progression through a series of symptoms.[4] The finding that Pb contributes significantly to decreased intellectual capability in the very young is of particular concern. Young children are particularly prone to the effects of Pb because they have greater opportunity for exposure. For example, in older homes that have been previously treated with Pb-based paints, Pb-laden paint chips and dust accumulate on the floor where they are likely to be ingested by children.

The definitive test for Pb toxicity is measurement of blood Pb. Over the past 3 decades, studies have shown an inverse relationship between blood Pb concentrations and children's IQ at increasingly lower Pb concentrations. In response, the Centers for Disease Control and Prevention (CDC) has continued to lower the upper limit of normal for children, which is now stated at less than 10 μg/dL, with 5 per μg/dL the reference concentration at which the CDC recommends that public health actions be initiated. (http://www.cdc.gov/nceh/lead/; accessed November 5, 2013). It is important to note that the median blood Pb concentration in children fell from 15 μg/dL in 1978 to 2 μg/dL in 1999. Consequently, renewed interest in determining safe blood Pb concentrations resulted in additional studies. Preliminary data have revealed an inverse relationship between Pb concentrations and children's IQ even at blood Pb concentrations <10 μg/dL. On the basis of these findings, New York State has recommended that blood lead concentrations for children be lowered to <5 μg/dL (www.health.state.ny.us/environmental/lead/; accessed November 5, 2013).[14]

The WHO has defined blood Pb concentrations >30 µg/dL in adults as indicative of significant exposure. Lead concentrations >60 µg/dL require **chelation therapy** (administration of chelating agents to remove metals from the body). In 2000, CDC recommended that, as a preventive health measure, blood Pb concentrations in exposed workers be reduced to <25 µg/dL by the year 2010. Similar to the situation seen in children, adult blood Pb concentrations have dropped to a mean value of 1.4 µg/dL for ages 20 to 49 and a mean value of 1.9 µg/dL for ages 50 to 69. Studies have shown a number of adverse health effects in adults exposed to Pb at concentrations below existing regulatory exposure limits. These include hypertension, adverse reproductive outcomes, and subtle central nervous system problems.

Although erythrocyte protoporphyrin concentrations are not a sensitive indicator of low-concentration Pb exposure, they are definitive markers for significant Pb exposure. For example, an erythrocyte protoporphyrin concentration greater than 60 µg/dL is a significant indicator of Pb exposure[17] (see Chapter 29). Serum activities of ALAD are also a useful indicator of medium to high concentrations of Pb exposure; however, they do not correlate with low concentrations of Pb exposure. Serum Pb analysis is of very limited utility because Pb concentrations are abnormal only for a short time after exposure. The National Health and Nutrition Examination Survey (NHANES) reported a median urine excretion of 3 µg/L lead or 2.4 µg lead per g creatinine in a large population (http://www.cdc.gov/; accessed November 5, 2013). Quantification of urine excretion rates before or after chelation therapy has been used as an indicator of Pb exposure. Normally, the hair Pb content is lower than 5 µg/g; hair Pb concentration >5 µg/g indicates significant Pb exposure. Blood Pb concentrations have the strongest correlation with toxicity.

Avoidance of continued exposure to Pb is paramount when blood Pb concentrations exceed acceptable limits. Oral dimercaprol has become a standard therapy and is being used in the outpatient setting for all except those with the most severe Pb poisoning. Although chelation therapy is effective in reducing blood Pb concentrations, a 2003 study indicated that chelation therapy given to preschool children with Pb concentrations in the range of 20 to 44 µg/dL showed no beneficial effect on tests of cognition or behavior.[12] Thus, prevention is the best therapeutic option.

Analysis of Pb is routinely performed by (1) ICP-MS,[2] (2) electrothermal atomic absorption spectrometry, or (3) anodic stripping voltammetry. Because Pb is concentrated in the erythrocytes, blood containing ethylenediaminetetraacetic acid (EDTA) as an anticoagulant is the specimen of choice for Pb analysis. Sodium heparin is also used; however, samples that are not analyzed within 48 hours are frequently clotted and must be rejected. Care must be taken when obtaining capillary blood. For example, samples having (1) surface contamination, (2) insufficient collection volume, or (3) inadequate mixing with EDTA should be rejected. Urinalysis is also used, as urine quantification correlates with exposure.

If ICP-MS is used to measure Pb concentrations, care must be taken to sum the masses of 206, 207, and 208 m/z to account for the natural isotopic variation of Pb in the environment. Failure to sum masses will skew results above or below the actual concentration, as the isotopic abundance of a particular mass in the calibrator might not match the sample. However, this isotopic variation has been exploited to determine the source of Pb exposure. By determining the relative abundances of Pb in blood and of potential sources of exposure (e.g., paint chips, soil), it is possible to identify a matching pattern. The exposure source with the same ratio of major Pb isotopes as the blood should then be avoided or removed from the patient's environment.

Manganese

Mn is ubiquitous in the environment and is used as (1) a binding agent in red brick, (2) an anticorrosive in most steel alloys, (3) a cleaning agent for glassware, and (4) a common pigment in paints and glazes. Humans exhibit toxicity to Mn when exposed to large quantities of dust containing the metal, which occurs in (1) mining, (2) ore crushing, (3) machining of Mn alloys, and (4) construction and destruction of brick.

After chronic exposure, Mn accumulates in the substantia nigra of the brain, causing a Parkinson-like neurodegenerative disorder known as *manganism*. Manganese toxicity is also a concern in newborns and children receiving long-term parenteral nutrition.

Blood or urine Mn concentrations are good indicators of exposure. Adult reference +intervals for blood Mn are 0.4 to 1.1 ng/mL (7.0 to 20.0 nmol/L) for serum or plasma and 7.7 to 12.1 ng/mL (140 to 220 nmol/L) for whole blood. Typical daily excretion of Mn in urine varies from 0.2 to 0.5 µg/d. However, approximately 5% of healthy individuals excrete up to 2 µg of the metal per day, probably because of greater than average exposure.

Most of the Mn in daily diets is not absorbed. Because Mn-containing dust is common, contamination of urine with the metal occurs easily. Trace contamination of acid preservatives used for stabilizing the urine has also been observed. Manganese is quantified by electrothermal atomization atomic absorption spectrometry and ICP-MS.

Mercury

Metallic mercury is a liquid at room temperature; its elemental symbol, Hg, is derived from the Greek word *hydrargyrias*, meaning "water silver" (http://emedicine.medscape.com/article/819872-overview/; accessed November 5, 2013). As mentioned earlier, mercury is listed as No. 3 on the 2007 CERCLA Priority List of Hazardous Substances.[19]

Hg is widely found in the environment and occurs both naturally and as the result of industrial processes, with the single largest source of Hg being its natural out-gassing from granite rock. Hg is also found in deposits throughout the world, mostly as cinnabar (mercuric sulfide), which is the source of the red pigment vermilion.

In the past, Hg was extensively used in the manufacture of devices such as (1) thermometers, (2) barometers, (3) manometers, and (4) sphygmomanometers. However, concerns about its toxicity have resulted in the phasing out of Hg-based instruments, which have been replaced by (1) alcohol-filled, (2) digital, or (3) thermistor-based ones. It is still used as a dental amalgam and in lighting as mercury vapor lamps, although these are being replaced by sodium vapor bulbs. Hg also is used (1) in the pulp and paper industry as a whitener, (2) as a catalyst in the synthesis of plastics, and (3) as a potent fungicide in antifouling and latex paints.

Mercury is essentially nontoxic in its elemental form (Hg^0). In the absence of any chemical or biological system that chemically alters Hg^0, it is possible to consume it orally with no significant side effects. However, once Hg^0 is chemically modified to the ionized, inorganic species, Hg^{2+}, it becomes toxic. Further bioconversion to an alkyl Hg, such as methyl Hg (CH_3Hg^+), yields a very toxic species of Hg that is highly selective for lipid-rich tissue, such as the neuron. The relative order of toxicity is as follows:

$$Hg^0 <<<<<<< Hg^+ << Monomethyl - Hg \ (CH_3Hg) \ or$$
$$Dimethyl - Hg \ [(CH_3)_2 - Hg]$$

Chemically, it is possible to convert Hg from its elemental state to its ionized state; in industry, this is frequently accomplished by exposing Hg^0 to a strong oxidant, such as chlorine. Elemental Hg is also bioconverted to both Hg^{2+} and alkyl Hg by microorganisms that exist both in the normal human gut and in the bottom sediment of lakes and rivers. When Hg^0 enters bottom sediment, it is absorbed by (1) bacteria, (2) fungi, and (3) related microorganisms that metabolically convert it to Hg^{2+}, CH_3Hg^+, $(CH_3)_2Hg$, and similar species. Consequently, the methyl mercurials are accumulated in the aquatic food chain and reach their highest concentrations in predatory fish.

As a consequence of accumulation of methylmercury in the aquatic food chain, most human exposure to mercury happens through the eating of contaminated (1) fish, (2) shellfish, and (3) sea mammals. In adults, cases of methylmercury poisoning are characterized by the focal degeneration of neurons in regions of the brain such as the cerebral cortex and the cerebellum. Depending on the degree of in utero exposure, methylmercury may result in effects ranging from fetal death to subtle neurodevelopmental delays. Consequently, because pregnant women, women of childbearing age, and young children are particularly at risk, the FDA recommends that they avoid eating (1) shark, (2) swordfish, (3) mackerel, and (4) tilefish (http://www.fda.gov/; accessed November 5, 2013).

Mercury toxicity is expressed in three ways. First, Hg^{2+} avidly reacts with sulfhydryl groups of protein, causing a change in the tertiary structure of the protein with subsequent loss of the biological activity associated with that protein. As Hg^{2+} becomes concentrated in the kidney during regular clearance processes, this is the target organ that experiences the greatest toxicity. Second, with the tertiary change noted previously, some proteins become immunogenic, eliciting a proliferation of β-lymphocytes that generate immunoglobulins to bind the new antigen (collagen tissues are particularly sensitive to this). Third, alkyl Hg species, such as methylmercury, are particularly lipophilic and actively bind to proteins

in lipid-rich tissue, such as neurons; myelin is particularly susceptible to disruption by this mechanism.[12] Mercury has also been found to alter porphyrin excretion patterns.

Experience with Hg poisoning has been gained from the investigation of the 1951 to 1963 industrial dumping of Hg-laden waste sludge into Minamata Bay, Japan. Fish in Minamata Bay became heavily laden with Hg through the food chain. The local human population, whose diet was dependent on fish from the bay, exhibited symptoms of methylmercury poisoning, which include (1) ataxia, (2) impaired speech, (3) visual field constriction, (4) hearing loss, and (5) somatosensory change, characterized histologically by cerebral cortex necrosis. Collectively, these symptoms have become known as **Minamata disease**.

In the late 1980s, the public became concerned about exposure to Hg from dental amalgams.[21] However, later studies failed to confirm a causal relationship.[18] Basic to the initial concerns was the fact that restorative dentistry used an Hg-silver amalgam for approximately 90 years as a filling material. In 2010, the FDA issued rules that classify dental amalgam, reclassify dental mercury, and specify special controls for dental amalgam, mercury, and amalgam alloy (21 CFR Part 872 /http://www.accessdata.fda.gov/; accessed November 5, 2013).

Concerns have been raised about the possible relationship between Hg exposure from vaccines and autistic disorders. In the United States, the prevalence of autism has risen from 1 in approximately 2500 in the mid-1980s to 1 in approximately 300 children in the mid-1990s.[20] Some investigators believe that this rise has occurred because of the Hg that is present in vaccines as the preservative thimerosal (sodium ethyl mercury thiosulfate). However, this causality has been questioned by numerous other studies, which have not been able to confirm the relationship.[22] In 2001, the Committee on Immunization Safety Review of the Board on Health Promotion and Disease Prevention of the Institute of Medicine initiated a study to review the connection between Hg-containing vaccines and neurodevelopmental disorders, including autism. The Committee has issued several reports; in its eighth and final report, put forth in 2004, the Committee reported that the hypothesis was biologically plausible, but that evidence was insufficient to accept or reject a causal connection. At that time, the Committee recommended a comprehensive research program. The findings of this report have been challenged, and thimerosal has been removed from most vaccines in the United States.

The reader should note that the issue of linking Hg exposure from vaccines with autistic disorders became highly controversial and resulted in the journal *Lancet* retracting the article linking autism to MMR (measles, mumps, and rubella) vaccines. However, the senior author involved with this publication has challenged this retraction and has initiated a lawsuit.[8]

Dietary sources also contribute to Hg body burden, as many foods contain Hg. For example, commercially distributed fish considered safe for consumption contain less than 0.3 µg/g, but some game fish contain more than 2 µg/g and, if consumed on a regular basis, contribute to significant body burdens of Hg.

Of note is the fact that Hg compounds have been used for therapeutic reasons. For example, Hg has been used (1) in medications that were touted as cures for syphilis and dysentery, (2) to treat constipation, and (3) as diuretics.

Analysis of blood, urine, and hair for Hg concentrations is used to determine exposure. The quantity of Hg found in blood and urine correlates with the degree of toxicity, and hair analysis has been used historically to document the time of peak exposure. However, it should be noted that hair analysis for metals in general is difficult because of contamination. Reference whole blood Hg concentration is usually lower than 10 μg/L. Individuals who have mild occupational exposure (e.g., dentists) may routinely have whole blood Hg concentrations up to 15 μg/L. Significant exposure is indicated when the whole blood Hg concentration is greater than 50 μg/L (if exposure is to methylmercury) or greater than 200 μg/L (if exposure is to Hg^{2+}). The WHO safety standard for daily exposure of Hg is 45 μg/d; daily urine excretion exceeding 50 μg/d indicates significant exposure. Normally, hair contains less than 1 μg/g of Hg; greater amounts indicate increased exposure. Treatment with BAL or penicillamine will mobilize Hg, allowing for its excretion in the urine. Therapy is usually monitored by following urinary excretion of Hg; therapy may be terminated after the daily urine excretion rate falls below 50 μg/L.

Nickel

Ni is frequently used (1) in the production of metal alloys, (2) in Ni-based rechargeable batteries, and (3) as a catalyst in the hydrogenation of oils. Nickel alloyed with transition metals is considered nontoxic, except that it will induce inflammation at the point of contact. Nickel oxides and sulfides and aqueous solution of Ni in the oxidation state of 1^+, 2^+, or 3^+ are considered group I carcinogens. If Ni is essential for life, it is so only at very low concentrations, below the detection limit of most analytical techniques. Nickel carbonyl $[Ni(CO)_4]$, used in petroleum refining, is one of the most toxic chemicals known to humans, as it is absorbed after inhalation, readily crosses all biological membranes, and noncompetitively inhibits ATPase and RNA polymerase. Patients exposed to Ni carbonyl exhibit rapid onset of pulmonary congestion and inability to oxygenate hemoglobin, followed by development of lesions of the (1) lung, (2) liver, (3) kidney, (4) adrenal glands, and (5) spleen.

Patients undergoing dialysis are exposed to Ni and accumulate Ni in blood and other organs. No adverse health effects have been associated with this exposure. Nickel is quantified by AA-ETA or ICP-MS.

Platinum

A variety of Pt-containing antineoplastic agents are used in chemotherapy, typified by cisplatin (cis-diamminedichloroplatinum)[10] and carboplatin (cyclobutanedicarboxylatoplatinum).[11] These compounds have nephrotoxicity that is related to the concentration of Pt circulating in the blood. Patients responding to carboplatin therapy had serum platinum concentration in the range of 0.6 to 1.8 μg/mL. Trough concentrations varied from 0.1 to 0.4 μg/mL. Platinum concentrations maintained at >1.8 μg/mL can induce neutropenia and renal failure if coadministered with nephrotoxic antibiotics. Both AA-ETA and ICP-MS are used to measure Pt.

Selenium

Se is an essential element (see Chapters 18 and 27) that may play a role in mitigating biological damage caused by oxidative damage. It is a cofactor required to maintain activity of glutathione peroxidase, an enzyme that catalyzes the degradation of organic hydroperoxides. Absence of Se correlates with loss of glutathione peroxidase activity and is associated with damage to cell membranes caused by the accumulation of free radicals. In a situation of Se deficiency associated with loss of glutathione peroxidase activity, the serum concentration is less than 40 ng/mL.

In humans, cardiac muscle is the tissue most susceptible to Se deficiency; with cell membrane damage, normal cells are replaced by fibroblasts.[5] This condition, known as cardiomyopathy, is characterized by an enlarged heart consisting of predominantly nonfunctioning fibrotic tissue.

The geographic source of plant and animal foodstuffs determines the amount of dietary intake. In the United States and Canada, wheat and other cereal products are a good source of selenium; average intakes in North America range from 80 to 220 μg Se/d, whereas in the United Kingdom, dietary intake is about 30 to 60 μg/d. Intakes in China are as low as 11 μg/d, and in New Zealand 28 μg/d (see Chapter 27). Symptoms of selenium toxicity vary among individuals and are dependent on a number of factors such as (1) dose, (2) type, and (3) form of selenium ingested, and length of time the product was used. Symptoms of selenium poisoning include (1) hair loss, (2) muscle cramps, (3) nausea, (4) vomiting, (5) diarrhea, (6) joint pain, (7) fatigue, (8) fingernail changes, and (9) blistering skin. The tolerable upper limit has been set at 400 μg/d for adults and less for children.

Selenium deficiency among people who consume food only from a particular region has been related to the low soil content of the metal in that region. For example, the soil of the Keshan region of China is noted for this characteristic. Children living in the Keshan region who receive no Se supplement develop cardiomyopathy. Deficiency is also related to use of total parenteral nutrition, which is administered to patients who have no functional bowel (e.g., those who have undergone surgical removal of the small and large intestines because of cancer) or who have acute inflammatory bowel disease, such as Crohn's disease (see Chapter 38). Selenium supplementation to raise serum concentration to above 90 ng/mL is the usual practice in these patients, and serum monitoring is performed on a semi-annual basis to ensure the adequacy of supplementation.

Selenium toxicity has been observed in animals when daily intake exceeds 400 μg/d. Teratogenic effects are frequently noted in the offspring of animals living in regions where Se soil content is high, such as in south central South Dakota and the northern coastal regions of California. Selenium toxicity in humans is not known to be a significant problem except in acute overdose cases, and Se is not classified as a human teratogen. Selenium is found in many over-the-counter vitamin preparations because its antioxidant activity is thought to be anticarcinogenic.

Selenium is quantified by ICP-MS or by atomic absorption spectrometry after the specimen has been mixed with a matrix modifier.

Silicon

Si is the most abundant element in the earth's environment; it constitutes 26% of the earth's crust. From the toxicological viewpoint, several forms of Si are of interest, including asbestos (amorphous oxides of Si) and methylated polymers of Si (e.g., silicone).

Inhalation of asbestos-containing dust leads to deposition of asbestos fibers in the pulmonary alveoli. These fibers are needle-shaped spicules approximately 150 micrometers in length and up to 15 micrometers in diameter. When these fibers are inhaled, they deposit in the alveoli, where they are surrounded by macrophages and become coated with protein and mucopolysaccharide to form "asbestos bodies." The diagnosis of asbestosis is made by (1) interpretation of a chest X-ray by a qualified radiologist, (2) demonstration of asbestos in sputum, and (3) documentation of asbestos bodies in a lung biopsy by electron microscopy. Direct analysis of lung tissue for Si is not useful because all lung tissue is infiltrated with Si, most of which is not asbestos. Thus, direct analysis for Si cannot distinguish asbestosis from normal background Si.

Silver

Clinical interest in Ag analysis is limited to two applications: (1) monitoring burn patients treated with Ag sulfadiazine, and (2) monitoring patients treated with Ag-containing nasal decongestants. In both cases, Ag is deposited in many organs, including the subepithelium of the skin and mucous membranes, producing a syndrome called **argyria** (graying of the skin). Argyria is associated with (1) growth retardation, (2) hemopoiesis, (3) cardiac enlargement, (4) degeneration of the liver, and (5) destruction of renal tubules. The customary concentration of serum Ag is less than 2 ng/mL. Typical Ag concentrations observed in serum of unaffected patients during treatment range up to 300 ng/mL, and their urine output has been found to be as high as 550 μg/d.

Thallium

Tl is a byproduct of lead smelting. Interest in Tl derives primarily from its former use as a rodenticide, and accidental contact represents the most likely source of exposure. Additionally, environmental concerns are growing because thallium is a waste product of coal combustion and the manufacturing of cement. Thallium is rapidly absorbed via (1) ingestion, (2) inhalation, and (3) skin contact. It is considered to be as toxic as lead and mercury and has similar sites of action. The mechanism of Tl toxicity consists of (1) competition with potassium at cell receptors to affect ion pumps, (2) inhibition of DNA synthesis, (3) binding to sulfhydryl groups on proteins in neural axons, and (4) concentration in renal tubular cells to cause necrosis. Patients exposed to high doses of Tl (>1 g) demonstrate alopecia (hair loss), peripheral neuropathy and seizures, and renal failure. Typical serum concentrations are less than 10 ng/mL, and daily urine excretion is less than 10 μg/d. Exposed patients have been observed to have serum concentrations as high as 50 μg/mL, with urine output in excess of 500 μg/d.

Titanium

Ti is the ninth most abundant element in the earth's crust. No evidence indicates that titanium is an essential element. In part because of the formation propensity of titanium oxide, the element is considered to be nontoxic. Average daily oral intake through food consumption is 0.1 to 1 mg/d, which accounts for more than 99% of exposure. Gastrointestinal absorption of titanium is low (≈3%), and most ingested titanium is rapidly excreted in the urine and stool. The total body burden of titanium is typically in the range of 9 to 15 mg, a significant portion of which is contained in the lung. Titanium dust entering the respiratory tract is nonirritating and is almost completely nonfibrogenic in humans.

Titanium-containing alloys are used in (1) artificial joints, (2) prosthetic devices, and (3) implants. Titanium dioxide allows osseointegration between an artificial medical implant and bone. Despite their wide use, exposure to these materials has not been linked to toxicity. However, as implant wear occurs, a significant increase in detectable serum titanium becomes evident. Although titanium concentrations are not a measure of toxicity, they are useful in determining whether implant breakdown is occurring. Serum titanium <1.0 ng/mL suggests that a prosthetic device is in good condition. Serum concentrations >3 ng/mL in a patient with a titanium-based implant suggest prosthesis wear. An increased serum titanium concentration in the absence of corroborating clinical information does not independently predict prosthesis wear or failure.

Vanadium

V is naturally found in minerals and rocks and is considered an essential element for mammals (see Chapter 27), although conclusive evidence for humans is lacking. V is recovered from minerals or is derived as a byproduct of (1) iron, (2) titanium, and (3) uranium refining. Vanadium compounds are used in (1) dyes, (2) photography, and (3) ceramics, and (4) in the production of special glasses. V is also a component of many fiber mesh prosthetic devices.

The main source of V intake for the general population is food, with an estimated daily intake of 20 μg, of which most is not absorbed and excreted in the feces. Absorption through the inhalation route results in more effective uptake. The clearance half-life is not well documented, but it appears to be on the order of several days. V has been recognized as an occupational hazard for many years. Elevated atmospheric V concentration results from burning fossil fuels with a high V content. Inhalation and ingestion are the primary exposure routes. V exposure results in a metallic taste and so-called "green tongue." Sensitization has been known to result in asthma or eczema.

Because the kidney is primarily responsible for V elimination, increased serum concentrations are observed in dialysis patients and those with compromised renal function. Serum V values <1.0 ng/mL are typical; values >5.0 ng/mL indicate probable exposure. Elevated serum V concentrations have been observed in patients with joint replacement; concentrations are likely to be increased above the reference interval in patients with metallic joint prosthesis. A modest increase (1 to 2 ng/mL) in serum V concentration is likely to be associated with a prosthetic device in good condition. Serum concentrations >5 ng/mL in a patient with a vanadium-based implant suggest significant prosthesis wear. Increased serum trace element concentrations in the absence of corroborating clinical information do not independently predict prosthesis wear.

Review Questions

1. A modest increase in this metal occurs in the blood of an individual who has a prosthetic device in good condition, and greater increases occur when a prosthetic device is becoming worn out; however, blood analysis of this metal is not considered to be a good indicator of prosthetic damage. Increased exposure to this same metal can result in a "green tongue."
   a. Cadmium
   b. Copper
   c. Vanadium
   d. Aluminum

2. An individual has eaten a large meal of seafood including shellfish and haddock before submitting a urine specimen for metal analysis. He had also been recently treated for trypanosomiasis. What metal would be present in a high concentration in his urine specimen?
   a. Arsenic
   b. Copper
   c. Mercury
   d. Cadmium

3. Lead inhibits _____, an enzyme that catalyzes synthesis of heme from porphyrin.
   a. ATPase
   b. RNA polymerase
   c. glutathione peroxidase
   d. aminolevulinic acid dehydratase

4. Occupational overexposure via inhalation of this metal can produce squamous cell carcinoma in lungs, and blood analysis of this metal can provide useful information regarding orthopedic implant wear.
   a. Cadmium
   b. Copper
   c. Vanadium
   d. Aluminum

5. A serum level >60 µg/L of which of the following metals interrupts normal calcium exchange in bone and leads to osteomalacia?
   a. Aluminum
   b. Arsenic
   c. Copper
   d. Antimony

6. Which of the following metals is considered to be an essential trace element in humans?
   a. Vanadium
   b. Manganese
   c. Arsenic
   d. Aluminum

7. Amorphous oxides of silicon are also known as:
   a. silicone.
   b. thimerosal.
   c. asbestos.
   d. keratin.

8. A chemical element found in image contrast agents used during magnetic resonance imaging and angiography procedures that is thought to be involved in nephrogenic systemic fibrosis is:
   a. mercury.
   b. gadolinium.
   c. cobalt.
   d. lead.

9. Certain metals that express toxicity have in common an ability to react with sulfhydryl groups of protein to denature these proteins. These metals include:
   a. arsenic.
   b. lead.
   c. mercury.
   d. All of the above metals react with sulfhydryl groups.

10. In the periodic table, elements with a particular electron configuration that allows them to bind covalently with sulfur are located in which group(s) and row(s)?
    a. Groups 6 through 12, row 4
    b. Groups 1 and 2, rows 3 and 4
    c. Group 1, row 5
    d. Groups 13 through 16, rows 4 through 6

References

1. Bondy SC. The neurotoxicity of environmental aluminum is still an issue. Neurotoxicology 2010;31:575–81.
2. Burritt M, Butz J. Modified from Forrer R, Guatschi K, Lutz H. Simultaneous measurement of trace element Al, As, B, Be, Cd, Co, Cu, Fe, Li, Mn, Mo, Ni, Rb, Se, Sr. and Zn in human serum and their reference ranges by ICP-MS. Biol Trace Elem Res 2001;80:77–93.
3. Caldwell K, LJones RL, Verdon CP, et al. Levels of urinary total and speciated arsenic in the US population: National Health and Nutrition Examination Survey 2003–2004. J Exp Sci Environ Epidemiol 2009;19:59–68.
4. Case studies in environmental medicine: lead toxicity. Washington, DC: U.S. Public Health Service, ATSDR. 2010. http://www.atsdr.cdc.gov/csem/lead/; (accessed on March 10, 2013).
5. Chariot P, Bignani O. Skeletal muscle disorders associated with selenium deficiency in humans. Muscle Nerve 2003;27:662–8.
6. De Smet K, De Hann R, Calistri A, Campbell KV. Metal ion measurement as a diagnostic tool to identify problems with metal-on-metal hip resurfacing. J Bone Joint Surg Am 2008;90:202–8.
7. Documentation of the 2011 threshold limit values and biological exposure indices. www.acgih.org/store/ (accessed on November 5, 2013).
8. Dyer C. Wakefield sues BMJ over MMR articles. BMJ 2012 Jan 10;344.
9. Estey MP, Diamandis EP, Van Der Straeten C, et al. Cobalt and chromium measurement in patients with metal hip prostheses. Clin Chemi 2013;59:880–86.
10. Katano K, Tsujitani S, Oka S, et al. Pharmacokinetics of hypotonic cisplatin chemotherapy administered into the peritoneal and pleural cavities in experimental model. Anticancer Res 2000;20:1603–8.
11. Kaufmann SJ, Karp JE, Letendre L, et al. Phase I and pharmacologic study of infusional topotecan and carboplatin in relapsed and refractory acute leukemia. Clin Cancer Res 2005;11:6641–9.
12. Moyer T. Toxic metals. In: Burtis C, Ashwood E, Bruns D, eds. Tietz textbook of clinical chemistry and molecular diagnostics. St Louis: Elsevier, 2012:1189–205.

13. National Institute for Occupational Safety and Health. Chromium-NIOSH. http://www.cdc.gov/niosh/review/public/144/default.html/ (accessed on November 5, 2013).

14. New York State Department of Health. Lead poisoning prevention. www.health.state.ny.us/environmental/lead/ (accessed on November 05, 2013).

15. Occupational Safety and Health Administration. Cadmium-OSHA. http://www.osha.gov/SLTC/cadmium/evaluation.html/ (accessed on November 5, 2013).

16. Occupational Safety and Health Administration. Chromium-OSHA. http://www/cdc.gov.nisoh/review/public/144/default.html/ (accessed on November 5, 2013).

17. Occupational Safety and Health Administration. Lead-OSHA. http://www.osha.gov/ (accessed on November 5, 2013).

18. Park JD, Zheng W. Human exposure and health effects of inorganic and elemental mercury. J Prev Med Public Health 2012;45:344–52.

19. Priority List of Hazardous Substances. http://www.atsdr.cdc.gov/SPL/index.html / (accessed on November 5, 2013).

20. Ratajczak HV. Theoretical aspects of autism: causes—a review. J Immunotoxicol 2011;8:68–79.

21. Roberts HW, Charlton DG. The release of mercury from amalgam restorations and its health effects: a review. Oper Dent 2009;34:605–14.

22. Schultz ST. Does thimerosal or other mercury exposure increase the risk for autism? A review of current literature. Acta Neurobiol Exp (Wars) 2010;70:187–95.

CHAPTER

33 Diabetes

David B. Sacks, M.B., Ch.B., F.R.C.Path.

Objectives

1. Define the following:

    Advanced glycation end product
    Albuminuria
    C-peptide
    Diabetes mellitus
    Epinephrine
    Fatty acid
    Fructosamine
    Gestational diabetes mellitus
    Glucagon
    Glucose tolerance
    Glycated hemoglobin
    Hemoglobin A_{1c}
    Hyperglycemia
    Insulin
    Insulin-like growth factor 1
    Insulin resistance syndrome
    Ketoacidosis
    Ketone bodies
    Proinsulin
    Type 1 and 2 diabetes

2. Compare and contrast type 1 and type 2 diabetes mellitus including the following:

    Causes
    Symptoms
    Insulin concentration in blood
    Appearance of symptoms versus clinical diagnosis
    Development of chronic complications
    Genetic factors

3. Compare impaired glucose tolerance with impaired fasting glucose including the fasting blood glucose concentration in each and the usefulness of these classifications as risk factors for diabetes and cardiovascular disease.

4. List the three important functions of insulin.

5. Summarize how the following hormones specifically affect blood glucose concentration: insulin, glucagon, epinephrine, cortisol, somatostatin, and growth hormone.

6. Briefly describe the function of the facilitative glucose transporters, including the importance of GLUT4 in glucose uptake by skeletal muscle.

7. List five antibodies that are involved in the pathogenesis of type 1 diabetes mellitus.

8. Describe insulin resistance and the role it plays in the pathogenesis of type 2 diabetes mellitus; explain how loss of β-cell function results in development of type 2 diabetes mellitus.

9. State how diet and exercise are related to development of type 2 diabetes mellitus.

10. State the basic criteria for the diagnosis of diabetes mellitus including fasting plasma glucose concentration, casual* plasma glucose concentration, oral glucose tolerance test results, and inclusion of glycated hemoglobin results.

11. Outline the procedure for administration and collection of an oral glucose tolerance test; analyze and interpret the results of this test in the diagnosis of type 2 diabetes mellitus, impaired glucose tolerance, and gestational diabetes mellitus.

12. Summarize the role of the clinical laboratory in the diagnosis and short- and long-term management of diabetes mellitus.

13. Describe the assay of whole blood glucose used in a blood glucose meter; calculate the difference between whole blood and plasma glucose concentrations.

14. List five variables that affect the accuracy and reproducibility of blood glucose meters; state how dehydration affects the reliability of a blood glucose meter.

15. Describe a typical implanted sensor for monitoring blood glucose including assay method, calibration, and usefulness in a person with type 1 diabetes.

16. Discuss the metabolic relationships between glucose, ketones, fatty acids, and metabolic acids including how they are altered, the effects of increased counter-regulatory hormones, and the clinical significance of ketonemia and ketonuria in uncontrolled diabetes mellitus.

17. Describe the glycation of hemoglobin A_{1c}; state the percentage of hemoglobin A_1 constituted by A_{1c}.

18. Explain how measurement of glycated hemoglobin is useful in diagnosis of diabetes and in monitoring control of blood glucose concentration; state the cutoff value of hemoglobin A_{1c} used to diagnose diabetes.

19. Specify the effects that young and old erythrocytes have on hemoglobin A_{1c} values.

---

*Casual is defined as any time of day without regard to time since last meal.

Objectives—cont'd

20. List and discuss three techniques used to determine glycated hemoglobin values including principles of analysis, possible interference by hemoglobin variants, and specimen requirements.
21. Describe the effects of hyperglycemia on advanced glycation end products and in turn how advanced glycation end products contribute to certain complications of diabetes.

22. State how urinary albumin excretion is useful in determining diabetic nephropathy; list the specimen collection requirements for this urine test.
23. Describe three semi-quantitative analyses of urinary albumin.
24. State the healthy reference intervals used for fasting plasma glucose, oral glucose tolerance, and glycated hemoglobin analyses.
25. Analyze and solve case studies related to the different types of diabetes and impaired glucose tolerance using descriptions of symptoms and results of laboratory analyses.

Key Words and Definitions

Advanced glycation end products (AGEs) Proteins that have been irreversibly modified by nonenzymatic attachment of glucose; may contribute to the chronic complications of diabetes.

C-peptide A 31-amino-acid protein that connects insulin's A-chain to its B-chain in the proinsulin molecule.

Diabetes mellitus A group of metabolic disorders of carbohydrate metabolism in which glucose is underutilized, producing hyperglycemia.

Diabetic nephropathy The nephropathy that commonly accompanies later stages of diabetes mellitus.

Diabetic retinopathy The retinal changes associated with diabetes mellitus.

Diabetogenes Genes that contribute to the development of diabetes; a genetic basis is identified in less than 5% of individuals with type 2 diabetes.

Facilitative glucose transporters A group of membrane proteins that facilitate the transport of glucose over a plasma membrane.

Fasting Abstinence from all food and drink except water for a prescribed period.

Gestational diabetes mellitus (GDM) Carbohydrate intolerance with onset during pregnancy.

Glucagon A polypeptide hormone secreted by the alpha cells of the islets of Langerhans in response to hypoglycemia or the presence of acetylcholine, certain amino acids, or growth hormone.

Glucose A six-carbon simple sugar that is the premier fuel for most organisms and an important precursor of other body constituents.

Glycated hemoglobin Hemoglobin that has a sugar residue attached; HbA_{1c} is the major fraction of glycated hemoglobin; also known as *glycohemoglobin.*

Glycogen A polysaccharide with a formula of $(C_6H_{10}O_5)$ used by muscle and liver for carbohydrate storage.

Glycogen storage disease A group of rare inborn errors of metabolism caused by defects in specific enzymes or transporters involved in the metabolism of glycogen (also known as *Von Gierke disease*).

Hyperglycemia Increased glucose concentrations in the blood.

Hypoglycemia Decreased glucose concentrations in the blood.

Impaired glucose tolerance (IGT) A term denoting values of fasting plasma glucose or results of an oral glucose tolerance test that are abnormal but not high enough to be diagnostic of diabetes mellitus.

Insulin A protein hormone produced by β-cells of the pancreas that decreases blood glucose concentrations.

Insulin-like growth factors (IGF) Serum peptides with insulin-like actions, formerly called somatomedins.

Insulin resistance Impairment of normal biologic responses to insulin.

Ketones Compounds that arise from free fatty acid breakdown; insulin deficiency leads to increased serum ketones, which are the major contributors to the metabolic acidosis that occurs in individuals with diabetic ketoacidosis.

Oral Glucose tolerance test (OGTT) A test whereby glucose is ingested into a fasting stomach and measurements of plasma glucose are taken over time; if glucose levels do not return to normal within 2 to 2.5 hours the patient may have impaired glucose tolerance or diabetes mellitus.

Proinsulin A precursor of insulin, with a molecular weight of 8,000 to 10,000; it has minimal hormonal activity and is converted to insulin by removal of the connecting C peptide, leaving the two (A and B)-chain, active insulin molecule.

Self-monitoring of blood glucose (SMBG) A procedure for collecting concentrations of blood glucose at several time points to enable maintenance of a constant glucose concentration.

Type 1 diabetes mellitus (T1DM) One of the two major types of diabetes mellitus. It is an autoimmune disease that results in the destruction beta cells of the pancreas, leading to loss of the ability to secrete insulin. Also called insulin-dependent diabetes, type 1A diabetes.

Type 2 diabetes mellitus (T2DM) One of the two major types of diabetes mellitus, characterized by peak age of onset between 50 and 60 years.

Diabetes mellitus is a group of metabolic disorders of carbohydrate metabolism in which **glucose** is underused, producing **hyperglycemia**. Some patients may experience acute life-threatening hyperglycemic episodes, such as ketoacidosis or hyperosmolar coma. As the disease progresses, patients are at increased risk for the development of specific complications, including **diabetic retinopathy** leading to blindness, **diabetic nephropathy** leading to renal failure, and nerve damage, collectively known as microvascular complications, as well as *atherosclerosis*, which is considered a *macrovascular complication*. The last may result in stroke, gangrene, or coronary artery disease.

Diabetes is a common disease, although the exact prevalence is unknown. Current estimates range from ≈285 to 366 million people with diabetes, and by 2030, this number is predicted to reach 552 million, 80% of whom will live in developing countries. In the United States, the number of people with diabetes has increased dramatically. The prevalence in 1999-2002 was 9.3%, 30% of whom were undiagnosed. Recent analysis, using both fasting glucose and hemoglobin A_{1c} (but not **oral glucose tolerance testing [OGTT]**) indicates a 2010 prevalence of diabetes in the United States in persons 20 years of age and older of 11.3% (equivalent to ≈26 million people). Of these, ≈27% are undiagnosed. Similarly, the prevalence of diabetes in Asian populations has increased rapidly in recent decades, reaching more than 110 million in 2007. These statistics led to a description of diabetes as "one of the main threats to human health in the twenty-first century." The prevalence of diabetes increases with age, and approximately half of all cases occur in people older than 55 years. In the United States, more than 25% of the population older than 65 years has diabetes. A racial predilection has been noted, and by the age of 65, 33%, 25%, and 17% of Hispanics, blacks, and whites, respectively, in the United States have diabetes. In 2007, diabetes was estimated to be responsible for $174 billion in healthcare expenditures in the United States. Direct costs were $116 billion, with 56% of that total incurred by those 65 years of age and older. An estimated 3.8 million people worldwide died from diabetes-related causes in 2007. Diabetes is the fourth most common cause of death in the developed world.

Classification

Diabetes was initially diagnosed by OGTT. In 1979 a workgroup of the National Diabetes Data Group proposed modified criteria for diagnosis. This classification scheme recognized two major forms of diabetes: type I (**insulin**-dependent) diabetes mellitus (IDDM) and type II (non–insulin-dependent) diabetes mellitus (NIDDM). The terms *juvenile-onset* and *adult-onset diabetes* were abolished. To base the classification on cause rather than on treatment, the American Diabetes Association (ADA) revised the classification, in 1997, eliminating the terms *insulin-dependent diabetes mellitus* and *non-insulin-dependent diabetes mellitus,* which now are termed **Type 1 diabetes mellitus (T1DM)** and **Type 2 diabetes mellitus (T2DM)** respectively (Box 33-1). The previous categories of abnormality of glucose tolerance and potential abnormality of glucose tolerance have been abolished.

BOX 33-1　Classification of Diabetes Mellitus

I　Type 1 diabetes
II　Type 2 diabetes
III　Other specific types of diabetes
IV　Gestational diabetes mellitus (GDM)

From the American Diabetes Association, Diabetes Care 2013;36(Suppl 1):S11-66.

Type 1 Diabetes Mellitus

Approximately 5% to 10% of all cases of diabetes are included in this category. Patients usually have abrupt onset of symptoms such as (1) polyuria, (2) polydipsia, and (3) rapid weight loss. They have insulinopenia (a deficiency of insulin) caused by loss of pancreatic islet β-cells and are dependent on insulin to sustain life and prevent ketosis. Most patients have antibodies that identify an autoimmune process (see later discussion) and some have no evidence of autoimmunity and are classified as type 1 idiopathic. The peak incidence occurs in childhood and adolescence. Approximately 75% acquire this disease before the age of 18, but onset in the remainder may occur at any age. Age at presentation is not a criterion for classification.

Type 2 Diabetes Mellitus

This group accounts for approximately 90% of all cases of diabetes. Patients have minimal symptoms, are not prone to ketosis, and *are not dependent on insulin* to prevent ketonuria. Insulin concentrations may be *(1) normal, (2) decreased, or (3) increased,* and most individuals with this form of diabetes have impaired insulin action. *Obesity* is commonly associated, and weight loss alone usually improves hyperglycemia in these persons. However, many individuals with type 2 diabetes may require (1) dietary manipulation, (2) oral hypoglycemic agents, or (3) insulin to control hyperglycemia. Most patients acquire the disease after age 40, but it may occur in younger people. Type 2 diabetes in children and adolescents is an emerging, significant problem. Among children in Japan, type 2 diabetes is now more common than type 1.

Other Specific Types of Diabetes Mellitus

This subclass includes uncommon patients in whom hyperglycemia is due to a specific underlying disorder, such as (1) genetic defects of β-cell function; (2) genetic defects in insulin action; (3) disease of the exocrine pancreas; (4) endocrinopathies (e.g., Cushing syndrome, acromegaly, glucagonoma); (5) administration of hormones or drugs known to induce β-cell dysfunction (e.g., dilantin, pentamidine) or to impair insulin action (e.g., glucocorticoids, thiazides, β-adrenergics); (6) infection; (7) uncommon forms of immune-mediated diabetes; or (8) other genetic conditions (e.g., Down syndrome, Klinefelter syndrome, porphyria; see Reference 2 for a detailed list). This was formerly termed *secondary diabetes.*

Gestational Diabetes Mellitus

This is defined as carbohydrate intolerance of variable severity *with onset or first recognition during pregnancy.* (Note that women with diabetes who become pregnant are not included in this category.) Estimates of the frequency of abnormal glucose tolerance during pregnancy vary from 1% to 14%, depending on the population studied and the diagnostic tests employed. In the United States, **gestational diabetes mellitus (GDM)** occurs in 6% to 8% of pregnancies (≈200,000 cases annually). Women with GDM are at significantly increased risk for the subsequent development of type 2 diabetes. The risk is particularly high in women (1) who have marked hyperglycemia during or soon after pregnancy, (2) who are obese, and (3) whose GDM was diagnosed before 24 weeks' gestation. At 6 to 12 weeks postpartum, all patients who had GDM should be evaluated for diabetes according to nonpregnant OGTT criteria. If diabetes is not present, patients should be re-evaluated for diabetes at least every 3 years.

Impaired Glucose Tolerance

Impaired glucose tolerance (IGT) is diagnosed in people who have fasting blood glucose concentrations less than those required for a diagnosis of diabetes but have a plasma glucose response during the OGTT between normal and diabetic states. The 2-hour postload plasma glucose following an OGTT is 140 to 199 (7.8-11.1 mmol/L) for this classification. An OGTT is required to assign a patient to this class. Development of overt diabetes occurs at a rate of 1% to 5% per year, but a large proportion of cases spontaneously revert to normal glucose tolerance. Microvascular disease is rare in this group, and patients usually do not experience the renal or retinal complications of diabetes. Patients have an increased prevalence of atherosclerosis and mortality from cardiovascular disease.

Impaired Fasting Glucose

This category is analogous to IGT, but it is diagnosed by a *fasting* glucose concentration between the reference interval for a healthy individual and that diagnostic of diabetes. For example, a fasting plasma glucose (FPG) between 100 and 125 mg/dL (5.6-6.9 mmol/L). It is a metabolic stage between healthy glucose homeostasis and diabetes. As with IGT, persons with impaired fasting glucose (IFG) are at increased risk for the development of diabetes and cardiovascular disease. IFG and IGT are not clinical entities but rather are risk factors for diabetes and cardiovascular disease.

Hormones that Regulate Blood Glucose Concentration

During a brief fast, a precipitous decline in the concentration of blood glucose is prevented by breakdown of **glycogen** stored in the liver and synthesis of glucose in the liver. Some glucose is derived from gluconeogenesis in the kidneys. These organs contain glucose-6-phosphatase, which is necessary to convert glucose-6-phosphate (derived from gluconeogenesis or glycogenolysis) to glucose. Skeletal muscle lacks this enzyme; muscle glycogen therefore cannot contribute directly to blood glucose. With more prolonged fasting (>42 hours), gluconeogenesis accounts for essentially all glucose production. In contrast, after a meal, the absorbed glucose is converted to glycogen (for storage in the liver and skeletal muscle) or fat (for storage in adipose tissue). Despite large fluctuations in the supply and demand of carbohydrates, the concentration of glucose in the blood is typically maintained within a fairly narrow interval by hormones that modulate the movement of glucose into and out of the circulation. These include (1) insulin, which decreases blood glucose, and the counter-regulatory hormones (2) glucagon, (3) epinephrine, (4) cortisol, and (5) growth hormone, which increase blood glucose concentrations (Figure 33-1). Normal glucose disposal depends on (1) the ability of the pancreas to secrete

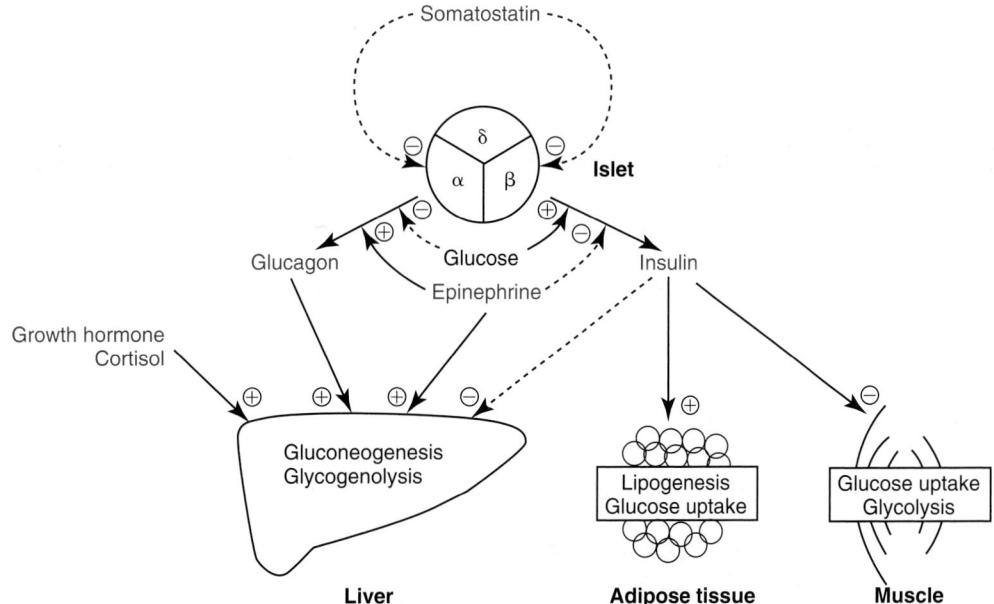

Figure 33-1 Hormonal regulation of blood glucose. Key: +, stimulation; –, inhibition. Cortisol, growth hormone, and epinephrine antagonize the effects of insulin.

insulin, (2) the ability of insulin to promote uptake of glucose into peripheral tissue, and (3) the ability of insulin to suppress hepatic glucose production. The major insulin target organs are (1) liver, (2) skeletal muscle, and (3) adipose tissue. These organs exhibit some differences in their responses to insulin. For example, the hormone stimulates glucose uptake through a specific glucose transporter—GLUT4—into muscle and fat cells but not into liver cells.

Insulin

Insulin is a protein hormone produced by the β-cells of the islets of Langerhans in the pancreas. Insulin was the first protein hormone to be sequenced, the first substance to be measured by radioimmunoassay (RIA), and the first compound produced by recombinant DNA technology for clinical use. It is an anabolic hormone that stimulates the uptake of glucose into fat and muscle, promotes the conversion of glucose to glycogen or fat for storage, inhibits glucose production by the liver, stimulates protein synthesis, and inhibits protein breakdown. The release and mechanisms of action of insulin are discussed in greater detail on pages 1417 to 1422 in an expanded version of this chapter in the 5th edition of *Tietz Textbook of Clinical Chemistry and Molecular Diagnostics*.[12]

Human insulin (molecular mass 5808 Da) consists of 51 amino acids in two chains (A and B) joined by two disulfide bridges, with a third disulfide bridge within the A chain. Insulin from most animals is immunologically and biologically similar to human insulin, and in the past, patients were treated with insulin purified from beef or pig pancreas. Virtually all patients are now treated with recombinant human insulin.

Preproinsulin, a protein of about 100 amino acids, is not detectable in the circulation under normal conditions because it is rapidly converted by cleaving enzymes to proinsulin. **Proinsulin** is stored in secretory granules in the Golgi complex of the β-cells, where proteolytic cleavage to insulin and connecting peptide (**C-peptide**) occurs. This post-translational processing is catalyzed by two Ca^{2+}-regulated endopeptidases: prohormone convertases 1 and 2 (PC1 and PC2). The split proinsulin intermediates,

split-32,33-proinsulin and split-65,66-proinsulin, are further hydrolyzed to insulin and C-peptide. At the cell membrane, insulin and C-peptide are released into the portal circulation in equimolar amounts. In addition, small amounts of proinsulin and intermediate cleavage forms enter the circulation.

Proinsulin which has relatively low biological activity (approximately 10% of insulin potency), is the major storage form of insulin. Normally, only small amounts (about 3% of the amount of insulin, on a molar basis) of proinsulin enter the circulation. However, the hepatic clearance rate for proinsulin is only 25% of insulin clearance, the half-life of proinsulin is twofold to threefold longer, and concentrations in the fasting state are ≈10% to 15% of insulin concentrations.

C-peptide is devoid of biological activity but appears necessary to ensure the correct structure of insulin. Fasting C-peptide concentrations are fivefold to 10-fold higher than those of insulin owing to the longer half-life of C-peptide (≈35 minutes). The liver does not extract C-peptide, which is removed from the circulation by the kidneys and is degraded, with a fraction excreted unchanged in the urine.

Glucose Transport

One of the fundamental effects of insulin is to increase glucose uptake into cells. The molecular mechanism of this action of insulin is extremely complex. The transport of glucose into cells is modulated by two families of proteins. The sodium-dependent glucose transporter promotes the uptake of glucose and galactose from the lumen of the small bowel and their reabsorption from urine in the kidney. The second family of glucose carriers, termed **facilitative glucose transporters** (GLUTs), is located on the surface of all cells (Table 33-1). These transporters are designated GLUT1 to GLUT14, according to the order in which they were identified. Eleven have been shown to mediate glucose transport. On the basis of sequence similarities, they have been divided into three subfamilies, namely, class I (GLUT 1 to 4), class II (GLUT 5, 7, 9, and 11), and class III (GLUT 6, 8, 10, 12, and 14). GLUT1 is widely expressed and provides many cells with their basal glucose requirement. GLUT1 in the blood-brain barrier and GLUT3 in neuronal cells

TABLE 33-1	Facilitative Human Glucose Transporters		
Name	**Class**	**Tissue**	**Function**
GLUT1	I	Wide distribution, especially brain, kidney, colon, and fetal tissues	Basal glucose transport
GLUT2	I	Liver, β-cells of pancreas, small intestine, and kidney	Non–rate-limiting glucose transport
GLUT3	I	Wide distribution, especially neurons, placenta, and testis	Glucose transport in neurons
GLUT4	I	Skeletal muscle, cardiac muscle, adipose tissue	Insulin-stimulated glucose transport
GLUT5	II	Small intestine, kidney, skeletal muscle, brain, and adipose tissue	Transports fructose (not glucose)
GLUT6	III	Brain, spleen, leukocytes	
GLUT7	II	Intestine, testis, prostate	
GLUT8	III	Testis, heart, brain	
GLUT9	II	Kidney, liver	
GLUT10	III	Liver, pancreas	
GLUT11	II	Pancreas, kidney, placenta, skeletal muscle	
GLUT12	III	Heart, prostate	
HMIT		Brain	Transports *myo*-inositol (not glucose)
GLUT14	III	Testis	

provide the constant high concentrations of glucose required by the brain. GLUT2 is expressed in hepatocytes, β-cells of the pancreas, and basolateral membranes of intestinal and renal epithelial cells. It is a low-affinity, high-capacity transport system that allows non–rate-limiting movement of glucose into and from these cells. GLUT4 catalyzes the rate-limiting step for glucose uptake and metabolism in skeletal muscle, the major organ of glucose consumption.

When circulating insulin concentrations are low, most of the GLUT4 is localized in intracellular compartments and is inactive. After a meal, the pancreas releases insulin, which stimulates the translocation of GLUT4 to the plasma membrane, thereby promoting glucose uptake into skeletal muscle and fat. Insulin-stimulated glucose transport into skeletal muscle is impaired in individuals with type 2 diabetes, but the mechanism of the defect has not been established. GLUT5 is responsible for fructose uptake in the intestine. Less is known about the other GLUTs. Glucose transport has been reported for GLUT 6, 8, 11, and 12.

Insulin-Like Growth Factors

Insulin-like growth factors (IGF) 1 and 2 (IGF-1 and IGF-2) are polypeptides structurally related to insulin (see Chapter 40). These hormones (previously referred to as *nonsuppressible insulin-like activity* or *somatomedin*) exhibit metabolic and growth-promoting effects similar to those of insulin. Accumulating evidence implicates the IGF axis in the development of several common cancers. IGF-1 (previously known as *somatomedin C*) is an important mediator of growth hormone action and is one of the major regulators of cell growth and differentiation. The physiological role of IGF-2 is not known. Synthesis of IGF-1 depends on growth hormone and occurs predominantly in the liver. In addition, many other cells produce IGF-1 that does not enter the circulation but acts locally. Circulating IGF concentrations are approximately 1000-fold higher than insulin concentrations, and the hormone is kept inactive by binding to a family of at least six specific binding proteins. These proteins regulate IGF by protecting the ligands in the circulation and delivering them to their target tissue. In contrast to insulin, which is unbound in the circulation, less than 10% of total serum IGF-1 is free. The biological actions of IGF are exerted through specific IGF receptors or the insulin receptor. The IGF-1 receptor is closely related to the insulin receptor in structure and biochemical properties. In contrast, the IGF-2 receptor is quite different; it lacks tyrosine kinase activity, and its physiological relevance is not understood. The IGF-1 receptor has a high affinity for both IGF-1 and IGF-2 but a low affinity for insulin. The IGF-2 receptor has (1) high, (2) low, and (3) no affinity for IGF-2, IGF-1, and insulin, respectively. The insulin receptor binds insulin with high affinity and IGF-1 and IGF-2 with low affinity.

The significance of IGFs in normal carbohydrate metabolism is not known. Exogenous administration produces **hypoglycemia**, whereas a deficiency of IGF-1 results in dwarfism (pygmies and Laron dwarfs). IGFs, particularly IGF-2, may be produced in excess by extrapancreatic neoplasms, and patients may have fasting hypoglycemia. High concentrations of both IGF-2 protein in the blood and IGF-2 messenger RNA (mRNA) in tumor extracts led to the proposal that IGF-2 is the humoral mediator of non–islet cell tumor–induced hypoglycemia. Hypoglycemia resolves after removal of the tumors. Clinically, measurements of plasma IGF-1 concentrations are used primarily to evaluate growth hormone deficiency and to detect and monitor treatment of growth hormone excess (acromegaly).

Counter-Regulatory Hormones

Several hormones have actions opposite to those of insulin. These counter-regulatory hormones are catabolic and increase hepatic glucose production initially by enhancing the breakdown of glycogen to glucose (glycogenolysis), and later by stimulating the synthesis of glucose (gluconeogenesis). The initial response (within minutes) to low blood glucose is an increase in glucose production, stimulated by glucagon and epinephrine. Over time (3 to 4 hours), growth hormone and cortisol increase glucose mobilization and decrease glucose use (see Figure 33-1). Evidence suggests that glucose production by the liver is an inverse function of ambient glucose concentration, independent of hormonal factors (*glucose autoregulation*). The role of other hormones or neurotransmitters is not clear but appears relatively unimportant. Multiple counter-regulatory hormones exhibit both redundancy and hierarchy. Glucagon is the most important, and epinephrine becomes critical when glucagon is deficient. The other factors have lesser roles. Note: These hormones, briefly described here, are discussed further in Chapters 25, 26, 40, and 42.

Glucagon

Glucagon is a 29-amino-acid polypeptide secreted by α-cells of the pancreas. The major target organ for glucagon is the liver, where it binds to specific receptors and increases both intracellular adenosine-5′-monophosphate and calcium. Glucagon stimulates the production of glucose in the liver by glycogenolysis and gluconeogenesis and enhances ketogenesis in the liver. A minor target organ for glucagon is adipose tissue, where the hormone increases lipolysis. Glucagon secretion is regulated primarily by plasma glucose concentrations, with low and high concentrations of plasma glucose being stimulatory and inhibitory, respectively. Long-standing diabetes impairs the glucagon response to hypoglycemia, resulting in an increased incidence of hypoglycemic episodes. Stress, exercise, and amino acids induce glucagon release. Insulin inhibits glucagon release from the pancreas and decreases glucagon gene expression, thereby attenuating its biosynthesis. Increased glucagon concentrations, secondary to insulin deficiency, are believed to contribute to the hyperglycemia and ketosis of diabetes.

Proglucagon is also produced in the distal gut by L-cells, which process it into glucagon, glucagon-like peptide-1 (GLP-1), and GLP-2. Food ingestion stimulates release of GLP-1, which acts on β-cells of the pancreas to stimulate insulin gene transcription and potentiate glucose-induced insulin secretion. GLP-1 and glucose-dependent insulinotropic polypeptide (GIP) are incretin hormones that are responsible for 70% of postprandial insulin secretion. GLP-1 reduces hyperglycemia by regulating insulin and glucagon secretion. It also inhibits acid secretion and emptying in the stomach and decreases food intake by increasing satiety. For these reasons, GLP-1 analogues are now used in the treatment of type 2 diabetes,

Epinephrine

Epinephrine (see Chapter 26), a catecholamine secreted by the adrenal medulla, stimulates glucose production (via gluconeogenesis and glycogenolysis) and decreases glucose use, thereby increasing blood glucose concentrations. It also stimulates glucagon secretion and inhibits insulin secretion by the pancreas (see Figure 33-1). Epinephrine appears to have a key role in glucose counter-regulation when glucagon secretion is impaired (e.g., in type 1 diabetes). Physical or emotional stress increases epinephrine production, releasing glucose for energy. Tumors of the adrenal medulla, known as *pheochromocytomas,* secrete excess epinephrine or norepinephrine and produce moderate hyperglycemia as long as glycogen stores are available in the liver.

Growth Hormone

Growth hormone (see Chapter 40) is a polypeptide secreted by the anterior pituitary gland. It stimulates gluconeogenesis, enhances lipolysis, and antagonizes insulin-stimulated glucose uptake.

Cortisol

Cortisol (see Chapter 41), secreted by the adrenal cortex in response to adrenocorticotropic hormone (ACTH), stimulates gluconeogenesis and increases the breakdown of protein and fat. Patients with Cushing syndrome have *increased cortisol* owing to tumor or hyperplasia of the adrenal cortex and may become hyperglycemic. In contrast, people with Addison's disease have *adrenocortical insufficiency* caused by destruction or atrophy of the adrenal cortex and may exhibit hypoglycemia.

Other Hormones Influencing Glucose Metabolism

Thyroxine

Thyroxine (see Chapter 42), secreted by the thyroid gland, is not directly involved in glucose homeostasis, but it stimulates glycogenolysis and increases the rates of gastric emptying and intestinal glucose absorption. These factors may produce glucose intolerance in thyrotoxic individuals, but patients usually have a fasting plasma glucose concentration in the reference interval.

Somatostatin

Somatostatin, also called *growth hormone–inhibiting hormone,* is a 14-amino-acid peptide found in the (1) gastrointestinal tract, (2) hypothalamus, and (3) δ-cells of the pancreatic islets. Although somatostatin does not appear to have a direct effect on carbohydrate metabolism, it inhibits the release of growth hormone from the pituitary. In addition, *somatostatin inhibits secretion of glucagon and insulin by the pancreas,* thus modulating the reciprocal relationship between these two hormones.

Measurement of Insulin, Proinsulin, C-Peptide, and Glucagon

Although interest in the possible clinical value of measuring the concentrations of insulin and its precursors continues, the assays are useful primarily for research purposes. No role is known for routine testing for insulin, proinsulin, or C-peptide in most patients with diabetes. Measurement of C-peptide is sometimes necessary in the United States for patients to obtain insurance coverage for continuous subcutaneous insulin infusion pumps. It must be emphasized that the diagnostic criteria for diabetes do not include measurements of hormones.

Various methods are used to measure (1) insulin, (2) proinsulin, (3) C-peptide, and (4) glucagon. A brief overview is provided here. For additional details, readers are referred to the expanded version of this chapter in the 5th edition of *Tietz Textbook of Clinical Chemistry and Molecular Diagnostics.*[12]

Insulin

The primary clinical application of insulin measurement is for the evaluation of patients with fasting hypoglycemia (see Chapter 22). Measurement of circulating insulin, however, could be helpful in evaluating **insulin resistance** and insulin secretion. Insulin determination has also been proposed to be of value in selecting the optimal initial therapy for patients with type 2 diabetes. In theory, the lower the pretreatment insulin concentration, the more appropriate might be insulin or an insulin secretagogue (a substance that causes another substance to be secreted) as the treatment of choice. Although intellectually appealing, no evidence suggests that knowledge of the insulin concentration leads to more efficacious treatment. Moreover, lack of harmonization of insulin assays hampers use of the assays.

In the past, measurement of insulin was advocated in the evaluation and management of patients with polycystic ovary syndrome. Women with this condition have insulin resistance and abnormal carbohydrate metabolism that may respond to oral hypoglycemic agents. However, it is not clear whether assessing insulin resistance by measuring insulin concentrations affords any advantage over clinical signs of insulin resistance (body mass index, acanthosis nigricans), and the American College of Obstetrics and Gynecology does not recommend routine measurements of insulin.

A few investigators have recommended measuring insulin along with glucose during an OGTT as an aid to early diagnosis of diabetes, but this approach also is not recommended.

Although insulin has been assayed for more than 50 years, there is still no (1) highly accurate, (2) precise, and (3) reliable procedure available to measure insulin. Many insulin assays, however, are commercially available. The most widely used techniques are immunoassays and, isotope dilution mass spectrometry (IDMS) assay. The term *immunoreactive insulin* is used in reference to assays that may recognize, in addition to insulin, substrates that share antigenic epitopes with insulin. Examples include (1) proinsulin, (2) proinsulin conversion intermediates, and (3) insulin derivatives, produced by glycation or dimerization. Antisera raised against insulin show some cross-reactivity with proinsulin but not with C-peptide. Specificity is not a problem in healthy individuals because the low proinsulin concentrations do not appreciably affect the absolute values of insulin. In certain situations (e.g., patients with diabetes or islet cell tumors), proinsulin is present at higher concentrations, and direct assay of plasma may falsely overestimate the true insulin concentration. Because proinsulin has very low activity, incorrect conclusions regarding the availability of biologically active insulin may be reached in patients with diabetes. The magnitude of the error depends on the concentration of proinsulin and the extent of cross-reactivity of the antiserum with proinsulin. The various immunoassays also show different cross-reactivities with pharmacological insulins.

An IDMS assay has been developed to measure the concentrations of (1) insulin, (2) proinsulin, and (3) C-peptide. Comparison of patient samples revealed that most, but not all, results were higher by immunoassay than by mass spectrometry. Thus immunoassays may overestimate insulin, particularly at low concentrations. The high protein concentration in the serum requires extraction of proteins (e.g., by immunoaffinity) and purification by high-performance liquid chromatography (HPLC) before quantification by mass spectrometry. This method is not suitable for routine laboratory analysis, but it is the best higher-order measurement procedure available and is used as a candidate reference procedure.

In 2004 the ADA convened an international workgroup to standardize insulin assays. Evaluation of 10 commercial insulin methods from nine manufacturers revealed within-assay CVs ranging from 3.7% to 39% and among-assay CVs of 12% to 66%. A common insulin reference preparation failed to improve harmonization of results. The report concluded that not all commercial insulin assays have acceptable performance characteristics.

Reference intervals vary among assays. After an overnight fast, insulin concentrations in healthy, normal, non-obese people vary from 12 to 150 pmol/L (2 to 25 µIU/mL). More specific assays that have minimal cross-reactivity with proinsulin reveal a fasting plasma insulin concentration less than 60 pmol/L (10 µIU/mL). Concentrations up to 1200 pmol/L (200 µIU/mL) have been reached during a glucose tolerance test.[12] **Fasting** insulin values are higher in obesity and lower in trained athletes.

Proinsulin

High proinsulin concentrations are usually noted in patients with benign or malignant β-cell tumors of the pancreas. Most patients with β-cell tumors have increased (1) insulin, (2) C-peptide, and (3) proinsulin concentrations, but occasionally only proinsulin is increased. Despite its low biological activity, proinsulin production may be adequate to produce hypoglycemia. In addition, a rare form of familial hyperproinsulinemia, produced by impaired conversion to insulin, has been described.[12] Measurement of proinsulin can be useful to determine the amount of proinsulin-like material that cross-reacts in an insulin assay. Patients with type 2 diabetes have increased proportions of proinsulin and proinsulin conversion

intermediates, high concentrations of which are associated with cardiovascular risk factors. Even relatively mild hyperglycemia produces hyperproinsulinemia, with values greater than 40% of insulin concentration in type 2 diabetes. Increased proinsulin concentrations may also be detected in patients with chronic renal failure, cirrhosis, or hyperthyroidism.

Accurate measurement of proinsulin has been difficult because (1) normal blood concentrations are low; (2) antibody production is difficult; (3) most antisera cross-react with insulin and C-peptide, which are present in much higher concentrations; (4) the assays measure intermediate cleavage forms of proinsulin; and (5) reference preparations of pure proinsulin are not readily available. Biosynthetic proinsulins have more recently allowed the production of monoclonal antibodies to proinsulin and have been used in the manufacture of proinsulin calibrators and reference preparations.

Reference intervals for proinsulin are highly dependent on the method of analysis, the degree of cross-reactivity of the antisera, and the purity of proinsulin calibrators. Each laboratory should establish its own reference intervals. Reference intervals in healthy, fasting individuals reported in the literature vary from 1.1 to 6.9 pmol/L to 2.1 to 12.6 pmol/L.

C-Peptide

Measurement of C-peptide has several advantages over insulin measurement. Because hepatic metabolism is negligible, C-peptide concentrations are better indicators of β-cell function than are insulin concentrations. Furthermore, C-peptide assays do not measure exogenous insulin and are not affected by insulin antibodies, which interfere with insulin immunoassays.

The primary reason for measuring C-peptide is to evaluate fasting hypoglycemia. Some patients with insulin-producing β-cell tumors, particularly if hyperinsulinism is intermittent, may exhibit increased C-peptide concentrations with normal insulin concentrations. When hypoglycemia is due to surreptitious insulin injection, *insulin* concentrations will be high but C-peptide values will be low; this occurs because C-peptide is not found in commercial insulin preparations and exogenous insulin suppresses β-cell function.

Basal or stimulated (by glucagon or glucose) C-peptide concentrations provide estimates of a patient's insulin secretory capacity and rate. Although valuable in clinical research, C-peptide measurement has a negligible role in the routine management of patients with diabetes. A relatively new indication for C-peptide analysis is the requirement that Medicare patients in the United States must have low C-peptide concentrations to be eligible for coverage of insulin pumps.

Measurement of C-peptide also is used to monitor patients' response to pancreatic surgery. C-peptide should be undetectable after a radical pancreatectomy and should increase after a successful pancreas or islet cell transplant. In addition, a stable C-peptide concentration is used as an end point in immunomodulatory trials for the prevention of type 1 diabetes.

Measurements of urine C-peptide are useful when continuous assessment of β-cell function is desired, or when frequent blood sampling is not practical. The 24-hour urine C-peptide content (in the absence of renal failure, which produces increased concentrations) correlates well with fasting serum C-peptide concentration or with the sum of C-peptide concentrations in sequential specimens after a glucose load. However, the fraction of secreted C-peptide that is excreted in the urine exhibits high intersubject and intrasubject variability, limiting the value of urine C-peptide as a measure of insulin secretion.

Assays are not affected by anti-insulin antibodies, but methodological problems produce large between-method variation. These difficulties include variable specificity among different antisera, variable cross-reactivity with proinsulin, and various types of C-peptide preparations used as a calibrator. Fasting serum concentrations of C-peptide in healthy people vary from 0.78 to 1.89 ng/mL (0.25 to 0.6 nmol/L). After stimulation with glucose or glucagon, values vary from 2.73 to 5.64 ng/mL (0.9 to 1.87 nmol/L), or three to five times the prestimulation value. Urinary C-peptide is usually in the interval of 74 ± 26 µg/L (25 ± 8.8 µmol/L).

Glucagon

Very high concentrations of glucagon are seen in patients with α-cell tumors of the pancreas called *glucagonomas*. Patients with this tumor frequently have (1) weight loss, (2) necrolytic migratory erythema, (3) diabetes, (4) stomatitis, and (5) diarrhea. Skin lesions often occur first and are frequently overlooked. Most tumors have metastasized when finally diagnosed. Low glucagon concentrations are associated with chronic pancreatitis and long-term sulfonylurea therapy.

Immunoassays are commercially available for measuring glucagon. The WHO glucagon international standard (69/194) has been used to calibrate some of these assays.

Fasting plasma concentrations of glucagon vary from 70 to 180 ng/L (20 to 52 pmol/L). Values up to 500 times the upper reference limit may be found in patients with autonomously secreting α-cell neoplasms.

Pathogenesis of Type 1 Diabetes Mellitus

Type 1 diabetes results from cell-mediated autoimmune destruction of the insulin-secreting cells of pancreatic β-cells.[3] In the vast majority of patients, destruction is mediated by T cells. This is termed type 1A or immune-mediated diabetes (see Box 3-1). The α-, δ-, and other islet cells are preserved. The islet cells have a chronic mononuclear cell infiltrate, called *insulitis*. The autoimmune process leading to type 1 diabetes begins months or years before the clinical presentation, and an 80% to 90% reduction in the volume of β-cells is required to induce symptomatic type 1 diabetes. The rate of islet cell destruction is variable and is usually more rapid in children than in adults.

The other subtype of type 1 diabetes is called *idiopathic*, or type 1B diabetes. Individuals who have idiopathic type 1 diabetes also experience beta cell destruction, but it is due to a chromosomal abnormality or an unknown cause rather than any autoimmune process.

Antibodies

The most practical markers of β-cell autoimmunity are circulating antibodies, which have been detected in the serum years before the onset of hyperglycemia. The best characterized antibodies are as follows:

Islet cell cytoplasmic antibodies (ICAs) react with a sialoglycoconjugate antigen present in the cytoplasm of all endocrine cells of the pancreatic islets. These antibodies are detected in the serum of 0.5% of normal individuals and in 75% to 85% of patients with newly diagnosed type 1 diabetes.

Insulin autoantibodies (IAAs) are present in more than 90% of children who develop type 1 diabetes before age 5, but in less than 40% of individuals who develop diabetes after age 12. Their frequency in healthy people is similar to that of ICA.

Antibodies to the 65 kDa isoform of glutamic acid decarboxylase (GAD_{65}) have been found up to 10 years before the onset of clinical type 1 diabetes and are present in ≈60% of patients with newly diagnosed diabetes.

Insulinoma-associated antigens (IA-2A and IA-2βA), directed against two tyrosine phosphatases, have been detected in more than 50% of newly diagnosed type 1 diabetes patients.

Zinc transporter ZnT8 was identified recently as a major autoantigen in type 1 diabetes. Initial analysis identified ZnT8 in 60% to 80% of patients with new-onset type 1 diabetes compared with less than 2% of controls.

The American Diabetes Association's "Standards of Medical Care in Diabetes—2013" indicates that antibody tests may be used, in the context of clinical research studies,[1] in relatives of individuals with type 1 diabetes to assess their risk of developing diabetes.

Genetics

Susceptibility to type 1 diabetes is inherited, but the mode of inheritance is complex and has not been defined. It is a multigenic trait, and the major locus is the major histocompatibility complex on chromosome 6. At least 11 other loci on 9 chromosomes also contribute, with the regulatory region of the insulin gene *INS* on chromosome 11p15 serving as an important locus. The human leukocyte antigen (HLA)-DQ and -DR genetic factors are by far the most important determinants for risk of type 1 diabetes. The concordance rate between identical twins is approximately 30%, and approximately 95% of whites with type 1 diabetes express HLA-DR3 or HLA-DR4 histocompatibility antigens. However, up to 40% of the nondiabetic population also expresses these alleles. In contrast, the *HLA-DQB1*0602* allele significantly decreases the risk of type 1 diabetes. HLA typing can indicate absolute risk of diabetes. The risk of a sibling developing diabetes is 1%, 5%, and 10% to 20% if the number of haplotypes shared is none, one, and two, respectively. Nevertheless, only 10% of patients with type 1 diabetes have an affected first-degree relative. Genome-wide association studies have also identified non-HLA genetic factors that increase risk, including the insulin gene variable number tandem repeat (*INS* VNTR, *CTLA4,* and *PTPN22*). The multiplicity of independent chromosomal regions associated with a predisposition to type 1 diabetes suggests that other susceptibility genes will be identified. Routine measurement of genetic markers is not of value at this time for the diagnosis or management of patients with type 1 diabetes.

Environment

Environmental factors are reported to contribute to the onset of diabetes. Viruses, such as (1) rubella, (2) mumps, and (3) coxsackie virus B, have been implicated. It seems likely that autoimmunity to β-cells is initiated by a viral protein (that shares amino acid sequence with a β-cell protein) or some other environmental insult. Genetic susceptibility and other host factors (e.g., HLA type) determine the progression of the β-cell destruction.

Pathogenesis of Type 2 Diabetes Mellitus

At least two major identifiable pathological defects have been reported in patients with type 2 diabetes. One is a decreased ability of insulin to act on peripheral tissue. This is called **insulin resistance** and is thought by many to be the primary underlying pathological process. The other is β-*cell dysfunction,* which is an inability of the pancreas to produce sufficient insulin to compensate for the insulin resistance. Thus a relative deficiency of insulin occurs early in the disease, and absolute insulin deficiency occurs late in the disease. The debate over whether type 2 diabetes is due primarily to a defect in β-cell secretion or to peripheral resistance to insulin, or to both, has been raging for decades. However, data are available to support the concept that insulin resistance is the primary defect, preceding the derangement in insulin secretion and clinical diabetes by as much as 20 years. Despite the lack of consensus, it is clear that type 2 diabetes is an extremely heterogeneous disease, and no single cause is adequate to explain the progression from normal glucose tolerance to diabetes. The fundamental molecular defects in insulin resistance and insulin secretion result from a combination of environmental and genetic factors.

Insulin Resistance

Insulin resistance is defined as "a decreased biological response to normal concentrations of circulating insulin"; it is found in obese individuals without diabetes and in patients with type 2 diabetes. The underlying pathophysiological defects have not been identified, but insulin resistance is usually attributed to a defect in insulin action. Measurement of insulin resistance in a routine clinical setting is difficult, and surrogate measures, namely, fasting insulin concentration and the euglycemic insulin clamp, are used to provide an indirect assessment of insulin function. The euglycemic clamp is performed in hospital under close supervision. The patient receives a constant intravenous infusion of insulin in one arm with concurrent intravenous infusion of variable amounts of glucose in the other arm to maintain blood glucose at a normal fasting concentration. A broad clinical spectrum of insulin resistance varies from euglycemia (with marked increase in endogenous insulin) to hyperglycemia (despite large doses of exogenous insulin). Several rare clinical syndromes are also associated with insulin resistance. The prototype is the type A insulin resistance syndrome, which is characterized by hyperinsulinemia, acanthosis nigricans, and ovarian hyperandrogenism.

The *insulin resistance syndrome* (also known as *syndrome X,* or *the metabolic syndrome*) is a constellation of associated clinical and laboratory findings, consisting of (1) insulin resistance, (2) hyperinsulinemia, (3) obesity, (4) dyslipidemia (high triglyceride and low high-density lipoprotein [HDL] cholesterol), and (5) hypertension.[11] Individuals with this syndrome are at increased risk for cardiovascular disease. The metabolic syndrome is diagnosed if an individual meets three or more of the following criteria:

- Abdominal obesity: waist circumference greater than 35 inches (women) or 40 inches (men)
- Triglycerides greater than 150 mg/dL (1.70 mmol/L)
- HDL cholesterol less than 50 mg/dL/(1.30 mmol/L) (women) or less than 40 mg/dL/1.1 mmol/L (men)
- Blood pressure greater than or equal to 130/85 mm Hg
- Fasting plasma glucose greater than or equal to 110 mg/dL (6.1 mmol/L)

The diagnostic criteria proposed by the WHO differ from those listed here. The concept of the "metabolic syndrome" has been questioned by several experts, including the person who first described it, and by major clinical diabetes organizations.

Loss of β-cell Function

Increased β-cell demand induced by insulin resistance is ultimately associated with progressive loss of β-cell function that is necessary for the development of fasting hyperglycemia. The major defect is a *loss of glucose-induced insulin release,* which is termed *selective glucose unresponsiveness.* Hyperglycemia appears to render the β-cells increasingly unresponsive to glucose (called *glucotoxicity*), and the degree of dysfunction correlates with both glucose concentration and duration of hyperglycemia. Restoration of euglycemia rapidly resolves the defect. Increased free fatty acids in serum have also been implicated in β-cell failure. Other insulin secretory abnormalities in type 2 diabetes include disruption of the normal pulsatile release of insulin and an increased ratio of plasma proinsulin to insulin. Evidence obtained from knockout mice reveals that insulin resistance in the β-cells may contribute to alterations in insulin secretion, as occur in type 2 diabetes.

Environment

Environmental factors, such as diet and exercise, are important determinants of the pathogenesis of type 2 diabetes. Convincing evidence links obesity to the development of type 2 diabetes, but the association is complex. Although 60% to 80% of patients with type 2 diabetes are obese, diabetes develops in less than 15% of obese individuals. In contrast, virtually all obese individuals, even those with normal carbohydrate tolerance, have hyperinsulinemia and are insulin resistant. Other factors that are important include (1) family history of type 2 diabetes (genetic predisposition), (2) the duration of obesity, and (3) the distribution of fat. Nevertheless, the rising prevalence of diabetes is believed to be a consequence of the increase in obesity (defined as a body mass index ≥ 30 kg/m^2), which was reported to be 35.7% in U.S. adults in 2009 to 2010.

An inverse relationship has been noted between the degree of physical activity and the prevalence of type 2 diabetes. For every 500-kcal increase in daily energy expenditure, a 6% decrease in age-adjusted risk of type 2 diabetes occurs. This effect is independent of both body weight and a parental history of diabetes. The mechanism of the protective effect of exercise is thought to be increased sensitivity to insulin in skeletal muscle and adipose tissue.

Diabetogenes

Genetic factors contribute to the development of type 2 diabetes. For example, the concordance rate for type 2 diabetes in identical twins approaches 100%. Type 2 diabetes is 10 times more likely to occur in an obese person with a parent who has diabetes than in an equally obese person without a diabetic family history. However, the mode of inheritance is unknown, and type 2 diabetes has been described as a "geneticist's nightmare." It is genetically more complex than mendelian disorders and is not inherited according to simple mendelian rules. Multiple genetic factors interact with exogenous influences (such as environmental factors) to produce the phenotype.

Numerous factors complicate the search for **diabetogenes** in type 2 diabetes. A variety of approaches have produced several genes that are associated with type 2 diabetes. Recent genome-wide association studies (GWAS) have substantially contributed to our understanding of the genetic architecture of type 2 diabetes, with >30 genetic loci identified. Most of these genetic loci are associated with the insulin secretion pathway, rather than with insulin resistance. Despite considerable effort to identify the genetic basis of type 2 diabetes, *genetic defects identified to date account for only $\approx$5% of patients with type 2 diabetes.* Therefore, the gene or genes causing common forms of type 2 diabetes remain unknown. Moreover, all of the risk alleles in these loci have small effects (odds ratios, 1.1 to 1.3). Incorporation of 18 different risk loci to construct a genotype score did not significantly improve clinical prediction based on current phenotype risk factors.

Diagnosis of Diabetes

For many years, the diagnosis of diabetes was dependent solely on the demonstration of *hyperglycemia* (Box 33-2).[2] Several influential clinical organizations now include hemoglobin A_{1c} (HbA$_{1c}$), which reflects long-term blood glucose concentrations, as a diagnostic criterion for diabetes (for additional information, see the "**Glycated Hemoglobins**" section, later in this chapter). For type 1 diabetes, the diagnosis is usually easy because hyperglycemia (1) appears abruptly, (2) is severe, and (3) is accompanied by serious metabolic derangements. Diagnosis of type 2 diabetes may be difficult because hyperglycemia often is not severe enough for the patient to notice

---

BOX 33-2 Criteria for the Diagnosis of Diabetes Mellitus

Any of the following is diagnostic:
Hemoglobin A_{1c} (HbA1c)* $\geq$6.5%
OR
Fasting plasma glucose (FPG) $\geq$ 126 mg/dL (7.0 mmol/L) †
OR
2-hour plasma glucose $\geq$200 mg/dL (11.1 mmol/L) during an oral glucose tolerance test (OGTT)

*The test should be performed in a laboratory that is NGSP-certified and standardized to the DCCT assay. Point-of-care assays should not be used for diagnosis.
†In the absence of unequivocal hyperglycemia, these criteria should be confirmed by repeating the same test on a different day. Mixing different methods to diagnose diabetes should be avoided.
From the American Diabetes Association. Diagnosis and classification of diabetes mellitus. Diabetes Care 2013;36(Suppl 1):S67-74.

---

symptoms of diabetes. Nevertheless, the risk of complications makes it important to identify people with the disease.

Fasting Plasma Glucose Concentrations

FPG concentrations of *126 mg/dL (7.0 mmol/L) or greater on more than one occasion* are diagnostic of diabetes mellitus (see Box 33-2). The diagnosis of most cases of diabetes is often established with this criterion. However, some investigators believe that fasting hyperglycemia may be a relatively late development in the course of type 2 diabetes, delaying the diagnosis and leading to underestimation of the prevalence of diabetes in the population. Complications of diabetes, such as (1) retinopathy, (2) proteinuria, and (3) neuromuscular disease, are present in approximately 30% of patients at clinical diagnosis of type 2 diabetes, and onset of type 2 diabetes probably occurs at least 4 to 7 years before clinical diagnosis. Screening of high-risk individuals for diabetes is now recommended. Fasting glucose (or HbA$_{1c}$) should be measured in all asymptomatic persons at age 45 (or younger in patients at increased risk), with follow-up testing every 3 years. However, no published evidence indicates that treatment based on screening is efficacious.

Oral Glucose Tolerance Test

Serial measurement of plasma glucose before and after a specific amount of glucose given orally should provide a standard method by which to evaluate individuals and establish values for healthy and diseased individuals. Although more sensitive than FPG determinations, glucose tolerance testing is affected by multiple factors that result in *poor reproducibility* (Box 33-3). Moreover, approximately 20% of OGTTs fall into the nondiagnostic category (e.g., only one blood sample exhibits increased glucose concentration). Unless results are grossly abnormal initially, *the OGTT should be performed on two separate occasions* to establish the diagnosis of diabetes.

The following conditions should be met before an OGTT is performed: (1) discontinue, when possible, medications known to affect glucose tolerance; (2) perform test in the morning after 3 days of unrestricted diet (containing at least 150 g of carbohydrate per day) and activity; and (3) perform

BOX 33-3	Factors Other Than Diabetes That Influence the Oral Glucose Tolerance Test

Patient Preparation
Duration of fast
Prior carbohydrate intake
Medications (e.g., thiazides, oral contraceptives, corticosteroids)
Trauma
Intercurrent illness
Age
Activity
Weight

Administration of Glucose
Form of glucose (anhydrous or monohydrate)
Quantity of glucose ingested
Volume in which administered
Rate of ingestion

During the Test
Posture
Anxiety
Caffeine
Smoking
Activity
Time of day
Sample preservation

TABLE 33-2	Screening and Diagnosis of Gestational Diabetes Mellitus

Screening

1. Perform at between 24 and 28 weeks' gestation on all average and very high-risk pregnant women not identified as having glucose intolerance.
2. Give 50 g oral glucose load without regard to time of day or time of last meal.
3. Measure venous plasma glucose at 1 hour.
4. If glucose is ≥140 mg/dL (7.8 mmol/L),* perform glucose tolerance test.

Diagnosis

1. Perform in the morning after an overnight fast of at least 8 hours.
2. Measure fasting venous plasma glucose.
3. Give 75 or 100 g of glucose orally.
4. Measure plasma glucose hourly for 3 hours (or for 2 hours if 75 g of glucose is given).
5. At least two values must meet or exceed the following:

	100 g Load	**75 g Load**
Fasting	95 mg/dL (5.3 mmol/L)	95 mg/dL (5.3 mmol/L)
1 hour	180 mg/dL (10 mmol/L)	180 mg/dL (10 mmol/L)
2 hour	155 mg/dL (8.6 mmol/L)	155 mg/dL (8.6 mmol/L)
3 hour	140 mg/dL (7.8mol/L)	—

6. If results are normal in a clinically suspect situation, repeat during the third trimester.

*Some experts recommend a cutoff of 130 mg/dL (7.2 mmol/L).

the test after a 10- to 16-hour fast only in ambulatory outpatients (bed rest impairs glucose tolerance), who should remain seated during the test without smoking cigarettes. Glucose tolerance testing should not be performed on hospitalized, acutely ill, or inactive patients. The test should begin between 7 AM and 9 AM. Concentrations of venous plasma glucose should be measured fasting, and then 2 hours after the oral glucose load. For nonpregnant adults, the recommended load is 75 g, which may not be a maximum stimulus; for children, 1.75 g/kg, up to 75 g maximum, is given. The glucose should be dissolved in 300 mL of water and ingested over 5 minutes. A commercial, more palatable form of glucose may be ingested, but whether the anhydrous or monohydrate form of glucose should be used is still in question.

Diagnosis of Gestational Diabetes

Normal pregnancy is associated with increased insulin resistance, especially in the late second and third trimesters. Euglycemia (glucose concentrations within healthy reference interval) is maintained by increased insulin secretion, with GDM developing in those women who fail to augment insulin sufficiently. Risk factors for GDM include (1) a family history of diabetes in a first-degree relative, (2) obesity, (3) advanced maternal age, (4) glycosuria, and (5) selected adverse outcomes in a previous pregnancy (e.g., stillbirth, macrosomia). ADA recommendations for laboratory diagnosis of GDM have been modified extensively since the publication in 2008 of the Hyperglycemia in Pregnancy and Adverse Outcome (HAPO) study (http://www.ncbi.nlm.nih.gov/; accessed November 11, 2013).[8] This large prospective, multinational study of ≈25,000

pregnant women revealed strong, graded, linear associations between maternal glycemia and adverse outcomes. All pregnant women not previously known to have diabetes should be evaluated for GDM by a 75-g OGTT at 24 to 28 weeks' gestation. Diagnostic cutpoints for fasting, 1-hour and 2-hour plasma glucose concentrations have been established.

These new criteria, which increase the incidence of GDM by ~2.5-fold, have not been accepted by all clinical organizations. For example, the American College of Obstetrics and Gynecology in the United States continues to advocate prior diagnostic criteria (Table 33-2). These state that all pregnant women should be evaluated by a two-step method:

1. Screen by history, clinical risk factors, or a 50-gram oral glucose load (the patient does not need to be fasting). A plasma glucose value greater than or equal to 140 mg/dL (7.7 mmol/L) at 1 hour after glucose ingestion indicates the necessity for definitive testing. Approximately 15% of pregnant women meet this criterion and require a full OGTT. This subgroup includes ≈80% of all women with GDM. Some experts recommend a cutoff of 130 mg/dL (7.1 mmol/L), which increases sensitivity for GDM to 90% but includes ≈25% of all pregnant women.
2. The diagnosis of GDM can be made on the basis of the result of the 100-gram, 3-hour OGTT. This should be performed on a different day from the 50-gram OGTT.

Although usually asymptomatic and not life-threatening to the mother, GDM is associated with increased neonatal mortality and morbidity, including (1) hypocalcemia, (2) hypoglycemia, and (3) macrosomia. Maternal hyperglycemia causes the fetus to secrete more insulin, resulting in stimulation of fetal growth and macrosomia. Recognition is important because therapy can reduce perinatal morbidity and mortality. Maternal complications include a high rate of cesarean delivery and hypertension. In addition, mothers with GDM are at significantly increased risk of subsequent type 2 diabetes.

Distinct from GDM is pregnancy in a patient with preexisting diabetes ($\approx$19,000 per annum in the United States). This is associated with an increased incidence of congenital malformation, but meticulous glycemic control during the first 8 weeks of pregnancy can significantly decrease the risk of congenital malformation. Tight control results in an increased incidence of maternal hypoglycemia, which is teratogenic in animals but does not cause malformation in humans.

Chronic Complications of Diabetes Mellitus

Patients with type 1 or type 2 diabetes are at high risk for the development of chronic complications. Diabetes-specific microvascular pathology in the (1) retina, (2) renal glomeruli, and (3) peripheral nerves produces (1) retinopathy, (2) nephropathy, and (3) neuropathy, respectively. As a result, diabetes is the most frequent cause of new cases of blindness in the industrialized world in persons between 25 and 74 years of age and is the leading cause of end-stage renal disease. Diabetes is also associated with a marked increase in atherosclerotic macrovascular disease involving (1) cardiac, (2) cerebral, and (3) peripheral large vessels. Therefore, patients with diabetes have a high rate of (1) myocardial infarction (the major cause of mortality in diabetes), (2) stroke, and (3) limb amputation.

Type 1 Diabetes

Although it was theorized for many years that better glycemic control would decrease rates of long-term complications of diabetes, it was not until the publication of the Diabetes Control and Complications Trial (DCCT) in 1993 that this hypothesis was verified (http://www.diabetes.niddk.nih.gov/; accessed November 11, 2013). The DCCT was a multicenter, randomized trial that compared the effects of intensive and conventional therapy on the development and progression of complications in 1441 patients with type 1 diabetes, all of whom required insulin. During the study period, which averaged 6.5 years, intensively managed patients maintained significantly lower mean blood glucose concentrations. Compared with conventional therapy, intensive therapy reduced the risks of (1) retinopathy, (2) nephropathy, and (3) neuropathy by 40% to 75%. Intensive therapy delayed the onset and slowed the progression of these complications, regardless of age, sex, or duration of diabetes. Absolute risks of retinopathy and nephropathy were proportional to the mean HbA_{1c} values (discussed later in the chapter). Although intensive therapy also reduced the development of hypercholesterolemia, macrovascular complications were not significantly decreased in the initial assessment. However, analysis after 17 years of follow-up documented a 42% lower incidence of cardiovascular disease in the intensively treated group. This landmark study has had a considerable impact on therapeutic goals and comprehension of the pathogenesis of complications of diabetes.

At the conclusion of the DCCT, 95% of participants enrolled in the long-term follow-up study, termed the Epidemiology of Diabetes Interventions and Complications (EDIC)/ http://www.ncbi.nlm.nih.gov/; accessed November 11, 2013). Five years after the end of the DCCT, no difference in metabolic control (as assessed by HbA_{1c} measurements) was noted between the former conventional and intensively treated groups. Nevertheless, further progression of retinopathy and neuropathy was significantly lower in the former intensive group, demonstrating that the beneficial effects of intensive treatment persisted for at least several years beyond the period of strictest intervention.[5]

Type 2 Diabetes

The role of hyperglycemia in the development of complications in individuals with type 2 diabetes was established in the United Kingdom Prospective Diabetes Study (UKPDS/ http://www.dtu.ox.ac.uk/; accessed November 11, 2013). The UKPDS was a major randomized, multicenter clinical study that included 5102 patients with newly diagnosed type 2 diabetes who were followed for an average of 10 years. Analogous to the findings of the DCCT, the UKPDS demonstrated in patients with type 2 diabetes that intensive treatment diminishes by approximately 10% to 40% the development of microvascular complications. Intensive treatment also decreased the rate of occurrence of macrovascular complications. Although the reduction was not statistically significant initially, follow-up 10 years after the study ended showed a significant reduction in myocardial infarction among patients who had received intensive therapy. Analogous to the EDIC findings, long-term benefits for microvascular complications were observed with follow-up of patients in the UKPDS despite loss of glycemic separation between intensive and standard cohorts after the study ended. An important caveat of both the DCCT and the UKPDS was that intensive therapy produced a threefold increase in the incidence of severe hypoglycemia.

Role of the Clinical Laboratory in Diabetes Mellitus

The clinical laboratory has a vital role in both the diagnosis and management of diabetes.[13] Some of the important variables assayed are outlined in Table 33-3. In 2002 the National Academy of Clinical Biochemistry (NACB) published evidence-based guidelines for laboratory analysis in diabetes. These guidelines were reviewed by the Professional Practice Committee of the ADA and were consistent in those areas where the ADA also published recommendations. Specific recommendations for laboratory testing based on published data or derived from expert consensus are presented. An updated version of these guidelines was published in 2011 (http://www.aacc.org/; accessed November 11, 2013). The revised guidelines were also published as a Position Statement by the ADA.

TABLE 33-3	Role of the Laboratory in Diabetes Mellitus
Diagnosis	
Preclinical (screening)	Immunological markers
	ICA
	IAA
	GAD antibodies
	Protein tyrosine phosphatase antibodies (IA-2)
	Zinc transporter ZnT8 antibodies
	Genetic markers (e.g., human leukocyte antigen [HLA])
	Insulin secretion
	Fasting
	Pulses
	In response to a glucose challenge
	Blood glucose
	Hemoglobin A1c (HbA$_{1c}$)
Clinical	Blood glucose
	Oral glucose tolerance test (OGTT)
	HbA$_{1c}$
	Ketones (urine and blood)
	Other (e.g., insulin, C-peptide, stimulation tests)
Management	
Acute	Glucose
	Blood
	Urine
	Ketones
	Blood
	Urine
	Acid-base status (pH, bicarbonate)
	Lactate
	Other abnormalities related to cellular dehydration or therapy (e.g., potassium, sodium, phosphate, osmolality)
Chronic	Glucose
	Blood (fasting-random)
	Urine
	Glycated proteins
	Glycated hemoglobin (GHb) (HbA$_{1c}$)
	Fructosamine
	Glycated serum albumin
	Urinary protein
	Urinary albumin excretion (UAE) (high albuminuria)
	Proteinuria
	Evaluation of complications (e.g., creatinine, cholesterol, triglycerides)
	Evaluation of pancreas transplant (C-peptide, insulin)
	Eligibility for insulin pump (C-peptide)

Diagnosis

Preclinical (Screening)

Evidence from animal studies suggests that immune intervention therapy provided before the appearance of clinical symptoms is capable of delaying or preventing type 1 diabetes. Results from human studies, however, have been disappointing. Nevertheless, several large clinical trials are under way to assess a variety of therapeutic strategies designed to delay or prevent the onset of type 1 diabetes. Until effective intervention therapy becomes available and cost-effective screening strategies are developed for young children, screening for antibodies outside of clinical studies is not recommended. Also, screening by determining HLA type is not currently warranted, except in research studies. A decrease in glucose-stimulated insulin secretion is the first functional abnormality in both type 1 and type 2 diabetes. Nevertheless, tests of insulin secretion are not currently recommended for routine clinical use.

Screening asymptomatic individuals for type 2 diabetes has been the subject of much controversy. The ADA, which previously did not support screening, now advocates screening in all asymptomatic individuals over the age of 45 years. If the HbA$_{1c}$ is less than 5.7% or the FPG is less than 100 mg/dL (5.5 mmol/L), testing should be repeated at 3-year intervals.

Clinical

The laboratory diagnosis of diabetes is made exclusively by the demonstration of hyperglycemia, as evidenced by measurements of venous plasma glucose or HbA$_{1c}$. Although other tests (e.g., C-peptide, insulin analysis) have been proposed to assist in the diagnosis and classification of the disease, they do not at present have a role outside of research studies.

Management

Acute

In disorders such as (1) diabetic ketoacidosis, (2) hyperosmolar nonketotic coma, and (3) hypoglycemia, the clinical laboratory has an essential role in both diagnosis and monitoring of therapy. Several analytes are frequently measured to guide clinicians in treatment regimens to restore euglycemia and correct other metabolic disturbances. The metabolic abnormalities of these conditions are beyond the scope of this book, and interested readers are referred to a standard textbook of medicine. The NACB guidelines (http://www.aacc.org/accessed November 11, 2013) also provide information on the tests that are used.

Chronic

The DCCT and UKPDS studies documented a correlation between blood glucose concentrations and the development of long-term complications of diabetes.[15] Measurement of glucose and glycated proteins provides an index of short- and long-term glycemic control. Detection of and monitoring for complications are achieved by assaying (1) creatinine, (2) urine albumin, and (3) serum lipids. In practice, the success of newer therapies, such as islet cell or pancreas transplantation, is monitored by measuring serum C-peptide or insulin concentrations.

Self-Monitoring of Blood Glucose

Patients with diabetes, especially those who need insulin, require careful monitoring to maintain control of blood glucose. This has become particularly important with the results of the DCCT and the recommendation that patients use intensive therapy to achieve nearly normal glycemia. These regimens include (1) multiple daily insulin injections, (2) insulin pumps, and (3) continuous subcutaneous insulin injections. However, testing urine for glucose is not adequate for monitoring patients on insulin therapy. Although some evidence suggests that it may be effective for monitoring type 2 diabetes, the ADA states that limitations of urine testing make blood glucose measurements the preferred method for assessing glycemic control.

Portable meters for measurement of blood glucose concentrations are used in three major settings: (1) in acute and chronic care facilities (at the patient's bedside and in clinics or hospitals); (2) in physicians' offices; and (3) by patients at home, work, and school. The last, **self-monitoring of blood glucose (SMBG),** used by approximately 1 million people with diabetes, is performed in the United States at least once a day by 40% and 26% of individuals with type 1 and 2 diabetes, respectively.

Using SMBG, patients measure their own blood glucose concentrations and modify their insulin doses on the basis of the result. It is impractical for patients themselves to perform glucose determinations by the methods described earlier, but a large number of simple test strips that are available permit rapid measurements on a drop of whole blood. These use the same enzyme-catalyzed reactions as described earlier for glucose analysis—predominantly glucose oxidase or glucose dehydrogenase. The reagents are combined in dry form on a small surface area of a test strip. More than 80 different blood glucose meters are commercially available. To perform the measurement, a sample of blood, usually from a fingerstick, but anticoagulated whole blood collected in ethylenediaminetetraacetic acid (EDTA) or heparin, is placed on the test pad, which is attached to a plastic support. The test strip is then inserted into the meter. (In some devices, the strip is inserted into the meter before the sample is applied.) After a fixed time, the result appears on a digital display screen. These meters use reflectance photometry or electrochemistry to measure the rate of the reaction or the final concentration of the products. Large variability has been noted among meters as to the test time (5 to 45 seconds) and the claimed reading range of 30 to 500 mg/dL (1.65-27.5 mmol/L) to 0 to 600 mg/dL (0-33.0 mmol/L). Calibration is automatic on some devices, whereas others use lot-specific code chips or strips. All manufacturers supply control solutions. Strict adherence to the instructions is necessary for accurate results to be obtained. Some meters have a porous membrane that separates erythrocytes, and analysis is performed on the resultant plasma. Of note, whole blood glucose concentrations are approximately 10% to 15% lower than plasma or serum concentrations, but meters can be calibrated and adjusted to report plasma glucose values, even when the sample is whole blood. For example a study group of the International Federation of Clinical Chemistry and Laboratory Medicine (IFCC) recommended a factor of 1.11× to convert concentrations of glucose measured per volume of whole blood to the concentration of glucose in plasma.[12]

Analytical Goals for Glucose Meters

Multiple analytical goals have been proposed for the performance of glucose meters. The recommendations promulgated by the Clinical and Laboratory Standards Institute (CLSI) and the International Organization for Standardization (ISO) are that 95% of results should fall within 20% of laboratory-measured glucose concentrations when >75 mg/dL (4.2 mmol/L), and within 15 mg/dL (0.83 mmol/L) of laboratory glucose when the glucose concentration is ≤75 mg/dL (4.2 mmol/L). Many experts consider these acceptance criteria to be too wide. In 2013, a new guideline from CLSI on Point-of-Care Blood Glucose Testing in Acute and Chronic Care Facilities (POCY12-A3/WWW.CLSI.org/; accessed November 11, 2013) concluded that "meter performance is acceptable for use in hospitals when 95% of the individual results from the POC glucose meter system agree within ±12 mg/dL (0.67 mmol/L) of the laboratory analyzer values at glucose concentrations below 100 mg/dL (5.55 mmol/L) and within ±12.5% of the laboratory analyzer values at glucose concentrations at or above 100 mg/dL (5.55 mmol/L). In addition, the sum of the number of individual results with (1) errors that exceed 15 mg/dL (0.83 mmol/L) at glucose concentrations below 75 mg/dL (4.2 mmol/L) and (2) errors that exceed 20% at glucose concentrations at or above 75 mg/dL (4.2 mmol/L) should not exceed 2% of all results." It also indicated that samples used to validate meter performance should be taken from the patient care area where the meter is intended to be used. Shortly after publication of the CLSI guideline, this higher standard was shown to be achievable, with at least one glucose meter validated with the challenging samples that come from patients in ICUs where patients receive multiple drugs and have extremes of hematocrit and sodium that may adversely affect meter performance.[12]

A different method uses an error grid to try to define clinically important errors by identifying fairly broad target ranges. An approach using simulation modeling concluded that meters that achieve both a CV and a bias less than 5% rarely lead to major errors in insulin dose. It should be noted, however, that lack of consensus on quality goals for glucose meters reflects the absence of agreed-upon objective criteria. When biological variation criteria are used, a goal for total error (including both bias and imprecision) of ≤6.9% has been proposed.

Glucose meters are also used to calculate insulin dose in patients without diabetes on tight glucose control protocols in intensive care units (ICUs). Evidence in 2001 showed that intensive insulin therapy significantly reduced mortality and morbidity of critically ill patients in the surgical ICU. Although some subsequent studies were unable to replicate these findings, aggressive glucose control with intravenous infusion of insulin still is used extensively in hospital ICUs. Many factors, such as (1) hypoxia, (2) shock, and (3) low hematocrit, are common in these patients and can compromise glucose analysis in capillary blood samples.[6] The use of glucose meters in these settings has been questioned by some experts. Some meters may have adequate analytical performance (as noted earlier), but the use of skin puncture (fingerstick) samples introduces serious error in patients who have conditions such as shock.

Performance of Glucose Meters

The most common errors in SMBG, such as (1) proper application, (2) timing, and (3) removal of excess blood, have been reduced by advances in technology but still can occur. Additional innovations that reduce operator error include (1) systems that abort testing if the sample volume is inadequate, (2) built-in programs that simplify quality control, and (3) increased memory that allows the instrument to store up to several hundred glucose readings that can be downloaded into a computer.

Several factors affect the accuracy and reproducibility of SMBG. These include (1) user variability—up to 50% of values may vary by more than 20% from reference values; (2) hematocrit—the presence of anemia (false increase) or polycythemia (false depression) may result in up to 30% variability; and (3) defective reagent strips or instrument malfunction (rare). Other variables include changes in (1) altitude, (2) environmental temperature, (3) humidity; (4) hypotension; (5) hypoxia; and (6) high triglyceride concentrations. In addition, these assays are unreliable at very high and very low glucose concentrations, for example, <60 mg/dL (3.3 mmol/L) and >500 mg/dL (27.5 mmol/L). Because dehydration, a common feature of diabetic ketoacidosis, greatly increases blood viscosity, inaccurately low blood glucose results may be obtained. Several drugs interfere, but not with all meters. Another important factor is the lack of correlation among meters, even from a single manufacturer, caused by different assay methods and architecture. Moreover, results from two meters of the same brand have been observed to differ substantially. Patient factors are also important, particularly adequate training when the meter is used for SMBG. Recurrent education at clinic visits and comparison of SMBG with concurrent laboratory glucose analysis improved the accuracy of patients' blood glucose readings. It is important to evaluate the patient's technique at regular intervals.

Meter performance varies widely. Under carefully controlled conditions in which all assays were performed by a single medical technologist, ≈50% of analyses met the ADA criterion of less than 5% deviation from reference values. Performance of older meters was substantially worse. Note that medical technologists perform better than patients. Comparison with laboratory values of almost 22,000 measurements of capillary glucose by patients using meters revealed no significant improvement in meter performance between 1989 and 1999. The imprecision of most meters precludes their use in the diagnosis of diabetes.

Alternatives to Meters for Monitoring of Blood Glucose

A major limitation to performing SMBG is that it is painful and inconvenient. Since the 1960s, attempts have been made to develop a painless method for monitoring blood glucose concentrations. Three general approaches have been used, namely, (1) implanted sensors, (2) minimally invasive monitoring, and (3) noninvasive monitoring.

Implanted Sensors

Several implanted biosensors have been developed and evaluated in both animals and humans. Detection systems are based on (1) enzymes, (2) electrodes, or (3) fluorescence. The most widely studied method is an electrochemical sensor that is usually implanted subcutaneously. All monitoring devices use glucose oxidase to measure glucose every 1 to 5 minutes. The values are sent to a monitor. Results are recorded and may be downloaded later in the physician's office and usually are available to the patient in real time. These devices are subject to some limitations. Implantation of a needle type of sensor into the subcutaneous tissue induces inflammatory responses in the host that alter the sensitivity of the device, limiting to 3 to 7 days the time the devices can be worn. The sensors require calibration by the user initially and at least twice a day with a glucose meter and are subject to the imprecision of the meter. In addition, changes in glucose concentration in the interstitial fluid occur 4 to 20 minutes later than changes in the blood. Nevertheless, real-time continuous glucose monitoring improves long-term glycemic control in a subset of patients with type 1 diabetes.[14]

Minimally Invasive Glucose Monitoring

The concept underlying these methods is that the concentration of glucose in the interstitial fluid correlates with the blood glucose concentration. The principle of the GlucoWatch Biographer involved the application of a low-level electrical current to the skin. This induced movement by electro-osmosis of glucose across the skin, where it is measured by a glucose oxidase detector. Glucose concentrations in transdermal fluid and plasma are highly correlated. The clearest application of the GlucoWatch, which is designed to measure glucose three times per hour for up to 12 hours, appears to be in the detection of unsuspected hypoglycemia. Initial clinical studies reveal reasonable correlation of the GlucoWatch with SMBG. Of note, this device has been withdrawn from the market.

Nonivasive Glucose Monitoring

Noninvasive in vivo monitoring of glucose has been an area of active investigation for many years. Near-infrared spectroscopic devices measure absorption or reflection of light from subcutaneous tissue. Although glucose has a specific absorption at 1035 nm, many substances interfere. A computer, individually calibrated, screens out interfering information to obtain the glucose result. Alternative approaches include Raman scattering spectroscopy and photoacoustic spectroscopy. Notwithstanding the investment of considerable resources, no noninvasive sensing technology has been approved by the FDA for glucose measurement in patients.

Ketone Bodies

The development of ketosis requires changes in both adipose tissue and the liver. The primary substrates for ketone body formation are free fatty acids from adipose stores. Normally, long-chain fatty acids are (1) taken up by the liver, (2) re-esterified to triglycerides, (3) stored in the liver or incorporated in very low-density lipoproteins and (4) returned to the plasma. In contrast to other tissues, the brain cannot use free fatty acids for energy. When glucose is unavailable, ketone bodies supply the vast majority of the brain's energy. After a 3-day fast, ketone bodies provide 30% to 40% of the body's energy requirements. In uncontrolled diabetes, the low insulin concentrations result in increased lipolysis and decreased re-esterification, thereby increasing plasma free fatty acids. In addition, the increased glucagon/insulin ratio enhances fatty acid oxidation in the liver. Increased counter-regulatory hormones also augment lipolysis and ketogenesis in fat and liver, respectively. Thus increased hepatic ketone production and decreased peripheral tissue metabolism lead to acetoacetate accumulation in the blood. A small fraction undergoes spontaneous decarboxylation to form acetone, but most of it is converted to β-hydroxybutyrate.

The relative proportions in which the three ketone bodies are present in blood vary, depending on the redox state of the cell. In healthy people, β-hydroxybutyrate and acetoacetate—which are present at approximately equimolar concentrations—constitute virtually all the serum **ketones**. Acetone is a minor component. In severe diabetes, the ratio of β-hydroxybutyrate to acetoacetate may increase to 6:1 owing to the presence of a high concentration of nicotinamide adenine dinucleotide (NADH), which favors β-hydroxybutyrate production.

Clinical Significance of Ketones

Excessive formation of ketone bodies results in increased blood concentrations of ketones *(ketonemia)* and increased excretion of ketones in the urine *(ketonuria)*. This process is observed in conditions associated with decreased availability of carbohydrates (such as starvation or frequent vomiting) or decreased use of carbohydrates such as (1) diabetes mellitus, (2) **glycogen storage disease** (von Gierke disease), and (3) alkalosis. The popular high-fat, low-carbohydrate diets are ketogenic and increase ketone bodies in the circulation. Diabetes and alcohol consumption are the most common causes of ketoacidosis. Urine ketone test results are positive in ≈30% of first-morning-void specimens from pregnant women. Semiquantitative determination of ketone bodies in blood is more accurate than determination of these compounds in urine in the treatment of diabetic ketoacidosis. Although not always excreted in proportion to blood ketone concentrations, urine ketones are widely used for monitoring control in patients with type 1 diabetes because of convenience. Patients with type 1 diabetes should test for ketones during acute illness or stress, with consistent increases in blood glucose (greater than 300 mg/dL/16.5 mmol/L), during pregnancy, or when symptoms of ketoacidosis are present.[7] Measurement of ketones in urine and blood is widely performed in patients with diabetes for both diagnosis and monitoring of diabetic ketoacidosis.

None of the commonly used methods for the detection and determination of ketone bodies in serum or urine reacts with all three ketone bodies. Gerhardt's ferric chloride test reacts with acetoacetate only. Tests using nitroprusside are at least 10 times more sensitive to acetoacetate than to acetone and give no reaction at all with β-hydroxybutyrate. Thus, most of the tests used for this purpose essentially detect or measure acetoacetate only.

Measurement of Ketones in Body Fluids

In general, the tests described above are not used as routine tests. The semi-quantitative (1) Acetest, (2) Ketostix, and (3) DiaScreen 1K are frequently used but are insensitive to β-hydroxybutyrate. It is important to bear in mind, therefore, that a negative nitroprusside test result does not rule out ketoacidosis.

Acetest

Acetest tablets contain a mixture of glycine, sodium nitroprusside, disodium phosphate, and lactose. Acetoacetate or acetone (to a lesser extent) in the presence of glycine forms a lavender-purple complex with nitroprusside. β-Hydroxybutyrate does not react with nitroprusside. Disodium phosphate provides an optimum pH for the reaction, and lactose enhances the color.

Ketostix

Ketostix is a modification of the nitroprusside test, in which a reagent strip is used instead of a tablet. The Ketostix test gives a positive reaction within 15 seconds with a specimen containing at least 50 mg of acetoacetate per liter. The color chart from the manufacturer gives readings for ketone concentrations of 50, 150, 400, 800, and 1600 mg/L. Acetone also reacts, but the test is less sensitive to it.

Determination of β-Hydroxybutyrate

In this test, β-hydroxybutyrate in the presence of nicotinamide adenine dinucleotide (NAD⁺) is converted by β-hydroxybutyrate dehydrogenase to acetoacetate, producing reduced nicotinamide adenine dinucleotide (NADH). Diaphorase catalyzes the reduction of nitroblue tetrazolium (NBT) by NADH to produce a purple compound, and its absorbance is read in a special meter that provides a digital readout.

β-Hydroxybutyrate concentrations range from 0.02 to 0.27 mmol/L (0.21 to 2.81 mg/dL) in healthy people after an overnight fast. Ketone bodies in the blood can reach 2 mmol/L (20 mg/dL) with prolonged exercise.[9] Patients with diabetic ketoacidosis usually have β-hydroxybutyrate concentrations greater than 2 mmol/L (20 mg/dL).

Determination of Ketone Bodies in Urine

Acetest and Ketostix are also suitable for detecting ketone bodies in urine. The sensitivity and specificity of these tests are the same as outlined for serum.

Glycated Proteins

Measurement of glycated proteins, primarily GHb, is effective in monitoring long-term glucose control in people with diabetes. It provides a retrospective index of integrated plasma glucose concentrations over an extended time and is not subject to the wide fluctuations observed when blood glucose concentrations are assayed. GHb concentrations therefore are a valuable and widely used adjunct to blood glucose determinations for monitoring long-term glycemic control. In addition, HbA_{1c} has recently been recommended for the diagnosis of diabetes and is a measure of risk for the development of microvascular complications of diabetes.

Glycated Hemoglobins

Glycation is the nonenzymatic addition of a sugar residue to amino groups of proteins. Human adult hemoglobin (Hb) usually consists of HbA (≈97% of the total), HbA_2 (2.5%), and HbF (0.5%). HbA is made up of four polypeptide chains, two α-chains and two β-chains. Chromatographic analysis of HbA identifies several minor hemoglobins, namely, HbA_{1a}, HbA_{1b}, and HbA_{1c}, which are collectively referred to as HbA_1, *fast hemoglobins* (because they migrate more rapidly than HbA in an electrical field), *glycohemoglobins*, or *glycated hemoglobins*. The Joint Commission on Biochemical Nomenclature of the International Union of Pure and Applied Chemistry recommends the term *neoglycoprotein* for such derivatives and the term *glycation* to describe this process. Therefore, although *glycosylated* and *glucosylated* have been widely used in the literature, the term *glycated* now is preferred. HbA_{1c} is formed by the condensation of glucose with the *N*-terminal valine residue of each β-chain of HbA to form an unstable Schiff base (aldimine, pre-HbA_{1c}; see Figure 33-2). The Schiff base may dissociate or may undergo an Amadori rearrangement to form a stable ketoamine, HbA_{1c}.

Also HbA_{1a1} and HbA_{1a2}, which make up HbA_{1a}, have fructose-1,6-diphosphate and glucose-6-phosphate, respectively, attached to the amino terminal of the β-chain. HbA_{1b} contains pyruvic acid linked to the amino terminal valine of the β-chain, probably by a ketamine bond. *HbA1c is the major fraction*, constituting approximately 80% of HbA_1.

Glycation may also occur at sites other than the end of the β-chain, such as lysine residues, or the α-chain. The sum of all GHbs, referred to as total glycated hemoglobin, cannot be separated from nonglycated hemoglobin by methods based on charge but are measured by boronate affinity chromatography.

Formation of GHb is essentially irreversible, and the concentration in the blood depends on both the life span of the red blood cell (RBC; average 120 days) and the blood glucose concentration. Because the rate of formation of GHb is directly proportional to the concentration of glucose in the blood, *the GHb concentration represents integrated values for glucose over the preceding 8 to 12 weeks.* This provides an additional criterion for assessing glucose control because GHb values are free of day-to-day and hour-to-hour glucose fluctuations and are unaffected by exercise or food ingestion immediately before collection of the blood sample. The contribution of the plasma glucose concentration to GHb depends on the time interval, with more recent values (such as during the preceding month) providing a larger contribution than earlier values (such as 3 months earlier). The plasma glucose in the preceding 1 month determines 50% of the HbA_{1c}, whereas days 60 to 120 determine only 25%. After a sudden alteration in blood glucose concentrations, the rate of change in HbA_{1c} is rapid during the initial 2 months, followed by a more gradual change approaching steady state 3 months later.

Interpretation of GHb depends on RBCs having a normal life span. Patients with hemolytic disease or other conditions with shortened RBC survival exhibit a substantial reduction in HbA_{1c}.[4] HbA_{1c} can still be used to monitor these patients, but values must be compared with previous values from the same patient—not with published reference intervals. Similarly, individuals with recent significant blood loss have falsely low values owing to a higher fraction of young erythrocytes. High HbA_{1c} concentrations have been reported in iron deficiency anemia, probably because of the high proportion of old erythrocytes. The effects of hemoglobin variants such as (1) HbF, (2) HbS, and (3) HbC depend on the specific method of analysis used. Depending on the particular hemoglobinopathy and assay, results may be spuriously increased or decreased. Most manufacturers of HbA_{1c} assays have modified their assays to

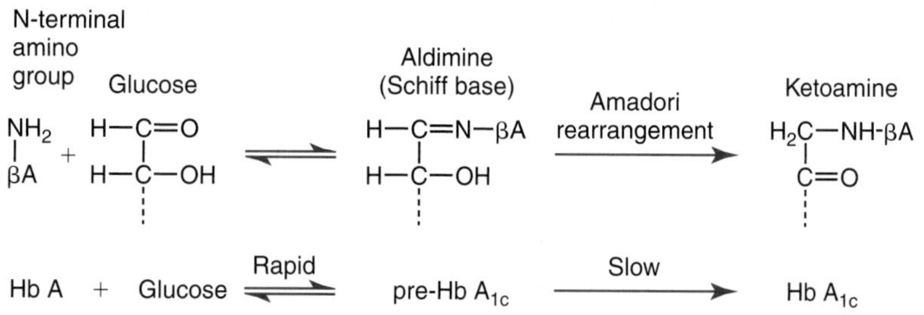

Figure 33-2 Formation of hemoglobin A_{1c}.

eliminate interference from many of the common hemoglobin variants. Therefore, HbA_{1c} can be accurately measured by selecting an appropriate instrument, and is useful provided the RBC life span is not altered by the hemoglobinopathy (see www.NGSP.org/accessed November 11, 2013 for additional information). Another source of error in selected methods is *carbamylated hemoglobin*, formed by attachment of urea. It is present in large amounts in renal failure, which is more common in people with diabetes. Most interferents produce small effects, and HbA_{1c} is measured accurately in the vast majority of patients with diabetes.

Hemoglobin A_{1c} in Diagnosis of Diabetes

A major change in the diagnosis of diabetes was recommended in 2009. An International Expert Committee advised that HbA_{1c} could be used for the diagnosis of diabetes (see Box 33-2). An HbA_{1c} value ≥6.5% was selected as the decision point, based on the prevalence of retinopathy. This recommendation has been endorsed by both the ADA and the WHO. HbA_{1c} values from 5.7% to 6.4% indicate individuals at high risk of developing diabetes. HbA_{1c} was also recommended as an alternative to glucose for screening for diabetes. This last recommendation has been accepted by the ADA.

Hemoglobin A_{1c} in Monitoring of Diabetes

HbA_{1c} is firmly established as an index of long-term blood glucose concentrations and a measure of the risk for developing microvascular complications in patients with diabetes. Absolute risks of retinopathy and nephropathy are directly proportional to the mean HbA_{1c} concentration. In persons without diabetes, HbA_{1c} is directly related to risk of cardiovascular disease.

Methods for Determination of Glycated Hemoglobins

More than 130 different methods may be used to determine GHb. These methods separate glycated from nonglycated hemoglobin using techniques based on (1) *charge differences* (ion exchange chromatography, HPLC, electrophoresis, and isoelectric focusing), (2) *structural differences* (affinity chromatography and immunoassay), or (3) *chemical analysis* (photometry and spectrophotometry). The result is expressed as a percentage of total hemoglobin. Most laboratories in the United States use immunoassay or HPLC and report % HbA_{1c}. The selection of method by a laboratory is influenced by several factors, including (1) sample volume, (2) patient population, and (3) cost. It is advisable to consult clinicians in this process. The ADA recommends that laboratories use only HbA_{1c} assays that are certified by the National Glycohemoglobin Standardization Program (NGSP) as traceable to the DCCT reference. The list of these assays on the NGSP website (www.NGSP.org/accessed November 12 2013) is updated at least annually.

High-Performance Liquid Chromatography

HbA_{1c} and other hemoglobin fractions are separated by HPLC, with cation exchange chromatography. Several fully automated systems are commercially available. Assays require only 5 µL of whole blood, and fingerstick samples are collected in a capillary tube for analysis. Anticoagulated blood is diluted with a hemolysis reagent containing borate. Samples are incubated at 37 °C for 30 minutes to remove the Schiff base and are inserted into the autosampler. (Some instruments have a shorter preincubation step, and others separate labile GHb chromatographically, eliminating the step to remove the Schiff base.) A step gradient using three phosphate buffers of increasing ionic strength is passed through the column. Detection is performed at both 415 and 690 nm, and results are quantified by integrating the areas under the peaks. Analysis time is as short as 3 minutes. HbA_{1c} by HPLC was used for analysis of all patient samples in the DCCT.

Immunoassay

Assays for HbA_{1c} have been developed using antibodies raised against the Amadori product (acid or base catalyzed isomerization or rearrangement reaction of the N-glycoside of the glycosylamine) of glucose (ketoamine linkage) plus the first few (four to eight) amino acids at the N-terminal end of the β-chain of hemoglobin. A widely used assay measures HbA_{1c} in whole blood by inhibition of latex agglutination. The agglutinator, a synthetic polymer containing multiple copies of the immunoreactive portion of HbA_{1c}, binds the anti-HbA_{1c} monoclonal antibody that is attached to latex beads. This agglutination produces light scattering, measured as an increase in absorbance. HbA_{1c} in the patient's sample competes for the antibody on the latex, inhibiting agglutination, thereby decreasing light scattering. Immunoassays are generally calibrated to give values that match HPLC values. The antibodies do not recognize labile intermediates or other GHbs (such as HbA_{1a} or HbA_{1b}) because both the ketoamine with glucose and specific amino acid sequences are required for binding. Similarly, several hemoglobin variants, such as HbF, HbA_2, HbS, and carbamylated hemoglobin, are not detected. The procedure has been adapted for capillary blood samples using a bench-top analyzer with reagent cartridges designed for use in physicians' office laboratories.

Affinity Chromatography

Affinity gel columns are used to separate GHb, which binds to *m*-aminophenylboronic acid on the column, from the nonglycated fraction. The boronic acid reacts with the *cis*-diol groups of glucose bound to hemoglobin to form a reversible five-member ring complex, thus selectively holding the GHb on the column. Nonglycated hemoglobin does not bind. Sorbitol is added to elute the GHb. Absorbance of bound and nonbound fractions, measured at 415 nm, is used to calculate the percentage of GHb.

The major advantages of affinity chromatography are no interference from nonglycated hemoglobins and negligible interference from the labile intermediate form of HbA_{1c}. It is unaffected by variations in temperature and has reasonably good precision. Hemoglobin variants such as HbS, HbC, HbD, or HbE produce little effect.

Affinity methods measure total GHb. This includes components other than HbA_{1c} because the assay detects ketoamine structures on lysine and valine residues on both α- and β-chains of hemoglobin.

Although the method detects all GHbs, most commercial systems are calibrated to report a standardized HbA_{1c} value. The value is derived from an equation obtained from linear regression between total GHb and HbA_{1c} analysis by HPLC. A linear relationship has been demonstrated, and standardized HbA_{1c} values are thus comparable with values obtained by methods specific for HbA_{1c}. Columns and reagents are commercially available.

Removal of Labile Glycated Hemoglobin from Red Blood Cells

The concentration of the labile form of HbA_{1c} (Schiff base) fluctuates rapidly in response to acute changes in plasma glucose concentrations, and it should be removed before analysis by charge-based assays. This may be accomplished by any of several methods including incubation of RBCs in saline or in buffer at pH 5 to 6. Most reagent sets for column assays contain reagents to remove this labile component.

Assay Standardization

Clinical laboratories measure GHb with diverse assays that use multiple methods and quantify different components. The DCCT results accentuated the need for accurate GHb measurement and provided a strong impetus for harmonization. At the end of the DCCT, it was noted that absence of both a reference method and a single GHb standard had generated confusion. Interlaboratory comparisons were not possible, and a single quality control sample analyzed by a single method exhibited interlaboratory CVs of 16.5%. Committees were established under the auspices of the American Association for Clinical Chemistry (AACC) in 1993 and the IFCC in 1995 to standardize GHb assays.

The NGSP was established in 1996 to implement the protocol developed by the AACC to calibrate GHb results to DCCT-equivalent values. Employing a network of reference laboratories, the NGSP interacts with manufacturers of GHb methods to help them calibrate their methods and trace values to the DCCT. Manufacturers apply for certification by performing precision testing and reporting results in DCCT-equivalent HbA_{1c} values. This calibration effort has markedly improved harmonization of results and reduced imprecision. Results obtained using NGSP-certified assays can be compared with results of the DCCT and the UKPDS, allowing alignment with clinical outcomes data. The ADA recommends that clinical laboratories use only assays certified by the NGSP and participate in proficiency testing offered by the College of American Pathologists (CAP). The CAP-GH2 survey uses pooled whole blood specimens at three HbA_{1c} concentrations. Target values are assigned by the NGSP network. Thus individual laboratories can directly compare their HbA_{1c} results with those of the DCCT and the UKPDS. Note: Beginning January 2014, 37 of 40 results (38 of 40 for Level I laboratories) will need to be within ±6% (relative) of the NGSP Secondary Reference Laboratory (SRL) in order to pass certification (current limits are ±7%).

A different approach was adopted by the IFCC. The IFCC Working Group isolated standards of pure HbA_{1c} and HbA_0 as primary reference materials and developed two reference methods, namely, HPLC electrospray ionization mass spectrometry (ESI-MS) and HPLC-capillary electrophoresis. These specifically measure the glycated N-terminal valine of the β-chain of hemoglobin. Analysis is performed by digesting the hemoglobin molecule with endoproteinase Glu-C, which cleaves the β-chain between Glu-6 and Glu-7, releasing the N-terminal hexapeptide. Glycated and nonglycated hexapeptides are separated and quantified by HPLC-ESI-MS or by HPLC-capillary electrophoresis. HbA_{1c} is measured as the ratio between glycated and nonglycated N-terminal hexapeptides. The IFCC method is (1) time-consuming, (2) technically complex, and (3) not designed to be used for routine analysis of patient samples. The IFCC Working Group has established a network of laboratories to implement and maintain the reference system. Comparisons between IFCC and NGSP reference methods (and reference systems from Japan and Sweden) indicate a close and stable relationship and allow manufacturers to calibrate their instruments to a higher-level reference method. However, HbA_{1c} results obtained using IFCC reference methods are 1.5% to 2% absolute HbA_{1c} units lower than those of the NGSP (and lower than other reference systems).

Units for Reporting of HbA_{1c}

HbA_{1c} is reported in the NGSP system as a percentage of total hemoglobin. These values, which are equivalent to those reported in the DCCT and the UKPDS, represent the most widely used reporting system in patient care and in the published literature. The IFCC method reports HbA_{1c} in System International (SI) units, namely, mmol HbA_{1c}/mol total Hb. Comparison between the IFCC and NGSP networks produced a master equation that permits conversion between the two reference systems. For example, an HbA_{1c} result of 7% (in NGSP/DCCT/UKPDS units) is equivalent to 53 mmol/mol (in IFCC units). A calculator to convert between units is available at http://www.ngsp.org/convert1.asp/; accessed November 11, 2013. Some countries have elected to report HbA_{1c} exclusively in SI units.

In some countries, an estimated average glucose (eAG) is reported together with HbA_{1c}. A conversion table is available at http://www.ngsp.org/A1ceAG.asp/; accessed November 11, 2013. A large, prospective clinical study revealed a significant correlation between HbA_{1c} and mean plasma glucose concentrations. The concept of reporting eAG with HbA_{1c} is not accepted by all and is controversial.[10]

Specimen Collection and Storage

Patients need not be fasting to submit a specimen for HbA_{1c} analysis. Venous blood should be collected in tubes containing EDTA, oxalate, or fluoride. Sample stability depends on the assay method used. Whole blood may be stored at 4 °C for up to 1 week. Above 4 °C, HbA_{1a+b} increases in a time- and temperature-dependent manner, but HbA$_{1c}$ is only slightly affected. Samples are not stable at −20 °C. For most methods, whole blood samples stored at −70 °C or colder are stable for at least 18 months.

Reference Intervals

Values for GHbs are expressed as a proportion of total blood hemoglobin. HbA$_{1c}$ should be reported. The reference interval (using an NGSP-certified method) is 4% to 5.6% (20 to 38 mmol/mol).

Results are not affected by acute illness. Intraindividual variability is minimal (CV ≈1%). HbA$_{1c}$ increases slightly with age and differs among racial groups and is higher in African Americans and Hispanics than Caucasians. It is not known whether this has clinical significance. In patients with poorly controlled diabetes, values rarely exceed 15%. HbA$_{1c}$ greater than 15% or below 4% should prompt additional studies to determine the possible presence of variant hemoglobin. Note that ADA target values derived from DCCT and UKPDS, not the reference values, are used to evaluate metabolic control in patients with diabetes.

There is no specific value of HbA$_{1c}$ below which the risk of diabetic complications is eliminated completely. The ADA states that for most patients the goal of treatment should be to maintain HbA$_{1c}$ at less than 7%. (Some organizations recommend an HbA$_{1c}$ target of less than 6.5%.) These goals are applicable only if the assay method is certified as traceable to the DCCT reference. Each laboratory should establish its own reference interval. Assay precision is important because each 1% change in HbA$_{1c}$ represents an approximate 30-mg/dL (1.7 mmol/L) change in average blood glucose.

No consensus has been reached on optimum frequency of testing. The ADA recommends that *HbA1c should be routinely monitored at least every 6 months in patients meeting treatment goals (and who have stable glycemic control).* These recommendations are for patients with type 1 or type 2 diabetes.

Fructosamine

In selected patients with diabetes (e.g., GDM), assays may be needed that are more sensitive than HbA$_{1c}$ to shorter-term alterations in average blood glucose concentrations. Nonenzymatic attachment of glucose to amino groups of proteins other than hemoglobin (e.g., serum proteins, membrane proteins, lens crystallins) to form ketoamines also occurs. Because serum proteins turn over more rapidly than erythrocytes (the circulating half-life for albumin is about 20 days), *the concentration of glycated serum albumin reflects glucose control over a period of 2 to 3 weeks.* Therefore, deterioration of control and improvement with therapy are evident earlier than with HbA$_{1c}$.

Fructosamine is the generic name for plasma protein ketoamines. The name refers to the structure of the ketoamine rearrangement product formed by the interaction of glucose with the ε-amino group on lysine residues of albumin. Analogous to HbA$_{1c}$, fructosamine may be used as an index of the average concentration of blood glucose over an extended time.

Because all glycated serum proteins are fructosamines and albumin is the most abundant serum protein, measurement of fructosamine is thought to be largely a measure of glycated albumin, but this has been questioned by some investigators. Although the fructosamine assay has been automated and is less expensive and faster than HbA$_{1c}$ assay, *there is a lack of consensus on its clinical utility.* The clinical value of fructosamine has not been firmly established, and no convincing evidence relates its concentration to the chronic complications of diabetes.

Fructosamine may be useful in circumstances where HbA$_{1c}$ is of little value, such as in patients with hemoglobin variants that are associated with decreased erythrocyte life span. Gross changes in protein concentration and half-life may have large effects on the proportion of protein that is glycated. Thus fructosamine results may be invalid in patients with (1) nephrotic syndrome, (2) cirrhosis of the liver, or (3) dysproteinemias, or (4) after rapid changes in acute-phase reactants. However, in current practice, there is no role for fructosamine in the diagnosis of diabetes.

Determination of Fructosamine

Methods for measuring glycated proteins such as fructosamine include (1) affinity chromatography using immobilized phenylboronic acid (similar to the GHb assay); (2) HPLC of glycated lysine residues after hydrolysis; (3) a photometric procedure in which mild acid hydrolysis releases 5-hydroxymethylfurfural—proteins are precipitated with trichloroacetic acid and the supernatant is reacted with 2-thiobarbituric acid; and (4) other procedures using phenylhydrazine and ε-N-(2-furoylmethyl)-L-lysine (furosine). None of these assays is popular because they are not suitable for routine clinical laboratories. The development of monoclonal antibodies to glycated albumin, although theoretically advantageous, has not yet resulted in the widespread availability of commercial glycated albumin assays. Prolonged storage at ultra-low temperatures (−96 °C) prevents in vitro glycation of serum proteins.

An alternative method used to measure fructosamine is based on the principle that under alkaline conditions, fructosamine undergoes an Amadori rearrangement. The resultant compounds have reducing activity that is different from other reducing substances. In the presence of carbonate buffer, fructosamine rearranges to the eneaminol form, which reduces NBT to a formazan. Absorbance at 530 nm is measured at two time points, and the absorbance change is proportional to the fructosamine concentration. A 10-minute preincubation period is necessary to allow fast-reacting interfering reducing substances to react. The assay is easily automated and has excellent between-batch analytical precision. Hemoglobin (>100 mg/dL) and bilirubin (>4 mg/dL/27.7 μmol/L) may interfere; therefore moderate to grossly hemolyzed and icteric samples should not be used. Ascorbic acid concentrations greater than 5 mg/dL may cause negative interference.

In one method to measure glycated albumin the molecule is first hydrolyzed by proteinases to glycated amino acids, which are oxidized by ketoamine oxidase, producing H_2O_2. The H_2O_2 is then quantified and glycated albumin is expressed as a percentage of total albumin. This assay is not available in the United States at the time of this writing.

Reference Intervals for Fructosamine

Values in a nondiabetic population vary from 205 to 285 μmol/L. The reference interval for results that are adjusted to account for high or low concentrations of (total) albumin is slightly different (e.g., 191 to 265 μmol/L).

Advanced Glycation End Products

The molecular mechanism by which hyperglycemia produces toxic effects is unknown, but glycation of tissue proteins may be important. Nonenzymatic attachment of glucose to long-lived proteins, lipids, or nucleic acids produces stable Amadori early-glycated products. These undergo a series of additional (1) rearrangements, (2) dehydration, and (3) fragmentation reactions, resulting in stable **advanced glycation end products (AGEs)**. The amounts of these products do not return to normal when hyperglycemia is corrected, and they accumulate continuously over the life span of the protein. Hyperglycemia accelerates the formation of protein-bound AGE, and patients with diabetes thus have more AGE than healthy subjects. Through effects on the functional properties of protein and the extracellular matrix, AGEs may contribute to the microvascular and macrovascular complications of diabetes. AGEs are also able to activate the receptor for AGE (RAGE) to induce intracellular signaling that leads to enhanced oxidative stress and the production of proinflammatory cytokines. Moreover, inhibitors of AGE formation, such as aminoguanidine, prevent some of the complications of diabetes in animal models. The clinical role of AGE is yet to be elucidated and defined.

Urinary Albumin Excretion

Patients with diabetes are at high risk of suffering renal damage. End-stage renal disease requiring dialysis or transplantation develops in approximately one-third of patients with type 1 diabetes, and diabetes is the most common cause of end-stage renal disease in the United States and Europe. Although nephropathy is less common in patients with type 2 diabetes, approximately 60% of all cases of diabetic nephropathy occur in these patients because of the considerably higher incidence of this form of diabetes. Persistent proteinuria detectable by routine screening tests (equivalent to a urinary albumin excretion [UAE] rate ≥200 μg/min) indicates overt diabetic nephropathy. This condition is usually associated with long-standing disease and is unusual less than 5 years after the onset of type 1 diabetes. Once diabetic nephropathy occurs, renal function deteriorates rapidly and renal insufficiency evolves. Treatment at this stage can retard the rate of progression without stopping or reversing the renal damage. Preceding this stage is a period of increased UAE not detected by routine dipstick methods. This range of 20 to 200 μg/min (or 30 to 300 mg/24 h) of increased UAE is termed high albuminuria, formerly called *microalbuminuria*. The term *microalbuminuria*, although widely used, is misleading. It implies a small version of the albumin molecule rather than an excretion rate of albumin greater than normal but less than that detectable by routine methods. Use of the term is discouraged.

The presence of increased UAE denotes an increase in the transcapillary escape rate of albumin and therefore is a marker of microvascular disease. Persistent UAE greater than 20 μg/min represents a 20-fold greater risk for the development of clinically overt renal disease in patients with type 1 and type 2 diabetes. Prospective studies have demonstrated that increased UAE precedes and is highly predictive of (1) diabetic nephropathy, (2) end-stage renal disease, (3) cardiovascular mortality, and (4) total mortality in patients with diabetes. Intensive glucose-lowering therapy can significantly reduce the risk of development of increased UAE and overt nephropathy in individuals with diabetes.[12] In addition, increased UAE identifies a group of people without diabetes who are at increased risk for coronary artery disease. Interventions such as control of blood glucose concentrations and blood pressure, particularly with angiotensin-converting enzyme (ACE) inhibitors, slow the rate of decline in renal function.

Specimen Collection and Storage

Variations in urine flow rate may be corrected by expressing albumin as a ratio to creatinine (i.e., albumin/creatinine). UAE is increased by physiological factors (e.g., exercise, posture, diuresis), and the method of urine collection must be standardized. Samples should not be collected (1) after exertion, (2) in the presence of urinary tract infection, (3) during acute illness, (4) immediately after surgery, or (5) after an acute fluid load. All the following urine samples are currently acceptable: (1) 24-hour collection; (2) overnight (8 to 12 hours, timed) collection; (3) 1- to 2-hour timed collection (in laboratory or clinic); and (4) first-morning sample for simultaneous albumin and creatinine measurement. Timed specimens are most sensitive, but the albumin/creatinine ratio is more practical and convenient for the patient and is the recommended method. A first-morning-void sample is best because it has lower within-person variation than a random urine sample. At least three separate specimens, collected on different days, should be assayed because of high intraindividual variation (CV of 30% to 50%) and diurnal variation (50% to 100% higher during the day). Urine should be stored at 4 °C after collection. Alternatively, 2 mL of 50 g/L sodium azide can be added per 500 mL of urine, but preservatives are not recommended for some assays. Bacterial contamination and glucose have no effect. Specimens are stable for 1 week at 4 °C and for at least 5 months at −80 °C. Albumin concentration decreases by 0.27%/d at −20 °C.

Semi-quantitative Assays

Several semi-quantitative assays are available for screening for increased UAE.[12] These test strips, most of which are optimized to read "positive" at a predetermined albumin concentration, have been recommended for screening programs. In view of the wide variability in UAE, a "normal" value does not rule out renal disease. *Because these assays measure albumin concentration, dilute urine may yield a false-negative test result.* Refrigerated urine samples should be allowed to reach at least 10 °C before analysis.

Quantitative Assays

All quantitative sensitive, specific assays for urine albumin use immunochemistry with antibodies to human albumin. Methods available include (1) RIA, (2) ELISA, (3) radial immunodiffusion, and (4) immunoturbidimetry. Each method has advantages and disadvantages, and the choice depends on local experience and technical support. In general, these methods have similar (1) imprecisions, (2) detection limits, and (3) reference intervals. Details of these methods are found in an expanded version of this chapter.[12]

Reference Intervals

Albuminuria

	μg/min	mg/24 h	Albumin/Creatinine Ratio (μg/mg Urine Creatinine)
Normal	<20	<30	<30
High albuminuria (formerly microalbuminuria)	20-200	30-300	30-300
Very high albuminuria*	>200	>300	>300

*Also termed *overt nephropathy.*

The ADA recommends initial albuminuria measurement in patients with type 1 diabetes who have had diabetes for 5 years or longer, and at the time of diagnosis of type 2 diabetes. Analysis should be performed annually in all patients who have a negative screening result. Screening may be performed with a semi-quantitative assay. If the screening result is positive, albuminuria should be evaluated by a quantitative assay. Diagnosis requires the demonstration of increased UAE in at least two of three tests measured within a 3- to 6-month period.

If the confirmatory test result is positive, treatment with an ACE inhibitor or an angiotensin-receptor blocker should be initiated. ACE inhibitors delay progression to overt nephropathy, and the National Kidney Foundation recommends their use in both normotensive and hypertensive patients with type 1 or type 2 diabetes. Untreated, the UAE would increase by 10% to 30% per year, whereas the albumin/creatinine ratio in patients taking ACE inhibitors should stabilize or decrease by up to 50%.

Review Questions

1. Glycated hemoglobin indicates compliance of a patient with diabetes with his or her insulin-taking regimen by monitoring glucose control. GHb concentration represents the integrated glucose value in the blood over what period?
   a. 8 to 12 days
   b. 8 to 12 weeks
   c. 8 to 12 months
   d. One day

2. Which of the following values obtained during an oral glucose tolerance test (OGTT) is above the appropriate cutpoint for diagnosis of diabetes mellitus?
   a. 2-Hour specimen = 125 mg/dL (6.9 mmol/L)
   b. Fasting glucose = 138 mg/dL (7.7 mmol/L)
   c. Fasting glucose = 110 mg/dL (6.1 mmol/L)
   d. 2-Hour specimen = 80 mg/dL (4.4 mmol/L)

3. Type 2 diabetes:
   a. is associated with resistance to the action of insulin.
   b. is caused by destruction of pancreatic β-cells.
   c. is also known as insulin-dependent diabetes mellitus.
   d. occurs less frequently than type 1 diabetes.

4. All of the following results are confirmatory and diagnostic laboratory values for diabetes mellitus *except*:
   a. nonfasting blood glucose >200 mg/dL (11.1 mmol/L).
   b. 2-hour oral glucose tolerance values >200 mg/dL. (11.1 mmol/L)
   c. urine glucose >250 mg/dL. (13.9 mmol/L)
   d. fasting plasma glucose >126 mg/dL (7.0 mmol/L)

5. Release of glucose from its storage form is referred to as:
   a. glycogenesis.
   b. glycogenolysis.
   c. glycolysis.
   d. glyconeogenesis.

6. Which of the following hormones produces *hyperglycemia*?
   a. Epinephrine
   b. Glucagon
   c. Thyroid hormone
   d. All of the above hormones produce hyperglycemia.

7. Whole blood glucose values are approximately what percent different from plasma glucose values?
   a. 20% higher
   b. 15% lower
   c. 50% higher
   d. There is no difference between whole blood glucose and plasma glucose values.

8. The development of ketosis in uncontrolled diabetes is a result of:
   a. increased lipolysis of fatty acids from adipose stores and decreased re-esterification of these fatty acids to triglycerides.
   b. increased nonenzymatic addition of glucose to proteins, lipids, and nucleic acids that form ketoamines.
   c. increased formation of advanced glycation end products that do not return to normal levels when diabetes is controlled.
   d. formation of circulating antibodies that are formed against the excess adipose tissue present in a person with diabetes.

9. Which of the following hormones promotes *decreased* blood glucose?
   a. Epinephrine
   b. Glucagon
   c. Cortisol
   d. Insulin

10. The purpose of examining urinary albumin excretion in an individual with type 1 or type 2 diabetes is to:

a. assess the ability of the pancreas to synthesize sufficient insulin.

b. determine the rate of formation of advanced glycation end products.

c. assess the possibility of overt diabetic nephropathy.

d. examine the health of the liver in its ability to synthesize albumin.

References

1. American Diabetes Association. Standards of medical care in diabetes—2012. Diabetes Care 2013;36(Suppl 1):S11–63.

2. American Diabetes Association. Diagnosis and classification of diabetes mellitus. Diabetes Care 2012;35(Suppl 1):S67–74.

3. Atkinson MA, Eisenbarth GS. Type 1 diabetes: new perspectives on disease pathogenesis and treatment. Lancet 2001;358:221–9

4. Bry L, Chen PC, Sacks DB. Effects of hemoglobin variants and chemically modified derivatives on assays for glycohemoglobin [Review]. Clin Chem 2001;47:153–63.

5. DCCT. The effect of intensive treatment of diabetes on the development and progression of long-term complications in insulin-dependent diabetes mellitus. N Engl J Med 1993;329:977–86.

6. Dungan K, Chapman J, Braithwaite SS, Buse J. Glucose measurement: confounding issues in setting targets for inpatient management. Diabetes Care 2007;30:403–9.

7. Goldstein DE, Little RR, Lorenz RA, et al. Tests of glycemia in diabetes. Diabetes Care 2004;27:1761–73.

8. HAPO Study Cooperative Research Group, Metzger BE, Lowe LP, Dyer AR, Trimble ER, Chaovarindr U, Coustan DR, et al. Hyperglycemia and adverse pregnancy outcomes. N Engl J Med 2008;358:1991–2002.

9. Laffel L. Ketone bodies: a review of physiology, pathophysiology and application of monitoring to diabetes. Diabetes Metab Res Rev 1999;15:412–26.

10. Little RR, Sacks DB. HbA1c: how do we measure it and what does it mean? Curr Opin Endocrinol Diabetes Obes 2009;16:113–8.

11. Reaven GM. Banting Lecture 1988. Role of insulin resistance in human disease. Diabetes 1988;37:1595–607.

12. Sacks DB. Diabetes mellitus. In: Burtis C, Ashwood E, Bruns D, eds. Tietz textbook of clinical chemistry and molecular diagnostics, 5th edition. St Louis: Saunders, 2012:1415–56.

13. Sacks DB, Arnold M, Bakris GL, Bruns DE, Horvath AR, Kirkman MS, et al. Guidelines and recommendations for laboratory analysis in the diagnosis and management of diabetes mellitus. Clin Chem 2011;57:e1–47.

14. Tamborlane WV, Beck RW, Bode BW, Buckingham B, Chase HP, Clemons R. Continuous glucose monitoring and intensive treatment of type 1 diabetes. N Engl J Med 2008;359:1464–76.

15. U.K.Prospective Diabetes Study (UKPDS) Group. Intensive blood-glucose control with sulphonylureas or insulin compared with conventional treatment and risk of complications in patients with type 2 diabetes (UKPDS 33). Lancet 1998;352:837–53.

Cardiovascular Disease

Fred S. Apple, Ph.D., Jens Peter Goetze, M.D., D.M.Sc., and Allan S. Jaffe, M.D.

Objectives

1. Define the following terms:

   Acute coronary syndrome (ACS)

   Acute myocardial infarction (AMI)

   Angina

   Atherosclerosis

   Cardiac biomarker

   Congestive heart failure (CHF)

   Coronary artery disease (CAD)

   Creatine kinase (CK)

   Electrocardiogram (ECG)

   Ischemia

   Myocardium

   Myocardial infarction

   Myoglobin

   Natriuretic peptide (NP)

   Plaque

   Troponin

2. Describe the anatomy of the heart, including layers, chambers, and protein makeup of muscle.
3. List the events in the process of atherosclerotic plaque formation.
4. Describe an ideal cardiac biomarker, including necessary characteristics, analytical considerations, and persistence in blood following an acute myocardial infarction (AMI).
5. Compare troponin I and T, including structural differences, physiological function, localization, and usefulness in diagnosing an AMI.
6. List six proposed elements of the guidelines of the National Academy of Clinical Biochemistry for point-of-care testing (POCT) of cardiac biomarkers.
7. For the following cardiac biomarkers, list and describe location with heart tissue, physiological function if known, clinical utility as a cardiac biomarker, specificity, and other conditions that cause increased values, laboratory analysis of choice and specimen requirements:

   Creatine kinase (CK)

   CK isoforms

   Myoglobin

   Natriuretic peptides (NPs)

   NT-proBNP

   Troponins

8. List four preanalytical considerations that must be assessed by a clinical laboratory that uses NP assays; state what units must be used to report these analytes.
9. Evaluate and analyze case studies related to cardiovascular disease and the use of cardiac biomarkers in the diagnosis of cardiovascular disease.

Key Words and Definitions

Acute coronary syndrome (ACS) A sudden cardiac disorder that varies from angina (chest pain on exertion with reversible tissue injury), to unstable angina (with minor myocardial injury), and to myocardial infarction (with extensive tissue necrosis, which is irreversible).

Acute myocardial infarction (AMI) An acute infarction (obstruction of circulation) of the heart muscle occurring during the period when circulation to a region of the heart is obstructed and necrosis is occurring.

Angina A condition marked by severe pain in the chest, often also spreading to the shoulders, arms, and neck, caused by an inadequate blood supply to the heart.

Arrhythmia Any variation from the normal rhythm of the heartbeat; alternative (and broader) term: *dysrhythmia*, especially to indicate an abnormally slow or fast heartbeat which may have rhythmic beating.

Atherosclerosis Any of a group of diseases characterized by thickening and loss of elasticity of arterial walls.

Atherosclerotic plaque A pearly white area within the wall of an artery that causes the intimal (interior) surface to bulge into the lumen; composed of lipid, cell debris, smooth muscle cells, collagen, and sometimes calcium; also known as an *atheroma*; vulnerable to rupture that causes the formation of a platelet- and fibrin-rich thrombus leading to myocardial infarction and ischemic stroke.

Cardiac biomarker A biological compound whose measurement is useful in the diagnosis of cardiac disease; used to (1) detect cardiac disorders, (2) detect risk of developing cardiac disorders, (3) monitor the disorder, or (4) predict the response of a disorder to a treatment.

Congestive heart failure (CHF) A clinical syndrome due to heart disease, characterized by breathlessness and abnormal sodium and water retention, often resulting in edema; also called *heart failure*.

Key Words and Definitions—cont'd

Coronary arteries The two main arteries that provide blood to the heart, surrounding the heart like a crown, coming out of the aorta, arching down over the top of the heart, and dividing into two branches.

Electrocardiogram (ECG) A graphic recording of the electrical activity produced by the heart.

Myocardial ischemia Deficiency of blood supply to the heart muscle due to obstruction or constriction of the coronary arteries

Myocardium The middle and thickest layer of the heart wall, composed of cardiac muscle.

Necrosis The sum of the morphological changes indicative of cell death and caused by the progressive degradative action of enzymes.

Non–ST segment elevation myocardial infarction (NSTEMI) A myocardial infarction in which the ST segment is not elevated in one lead or several leads of the ECG.

Percutaneous coronary intervention (PCI) The management of coronary artery occlusion by any of various catheter-based techniques.

Risk stratification A statistical process used to determine detectable characteristics associated with an increased chance of experiencing unwanted outcomes.

ST segment elevation myocardial infarction (STEMI) Any type of myocardial infarction in which the ST segment is elevated in one lead or several leads of the ECG.

Thrombolysis Lysis of a thrombus or thrombi.

Unstable angina An angina that occurs unpredictably or suddenly increases in severity or frequency.

Ventricles (right and left) The two lower chambers of the heart, responsible, respectively, for pumping blood into the lungs via the pulmonary artery and into the systemic circulation via the aorta.

Acute ischemic disease and heart failure are the two most common cardiovascular diseases that rely on a biochemical diagnosis. They, and the **cardiac biomarkers** used in their diagnosis, are the major focus of this chapter.

The most serious form of ischemic heart disease is **acute myocardial infarction (AMI)**. AMI occurs when there is an imbalance between supply and demand for oxygen in the **myocardium** (heart muscle) resulting in injury to and the eventual death of muscle cells (myocytes). When the blood supply to the muscle in a region of the heart is blocked for more than a few minutes, many or most of the muscle cells in the affected region die. This is called **necrosis** (cell death) of the myocardium. Other events of lesser severity may be missed entirely or be called **angina**, which ranges from stable to **unstable angina**. The ischemic events in the heart, ranging from angina (no cell death) to AMI (cell death), are known as **acute coronary syndromes (ACSs)**.

In the United States, approximately 700,000 patients every year suffer a first AMI, and another 500,000 people who had suffered an AMI in the past suffer another one (called *recurrent AMI*). About 1.7 million patients are hospitalized each year in the United States with ACS. The yearly economic burden of coronary artery disease (CAD) is in excess of $133.2 billion, more than a third of the total of $368.4 billion due to cardiovascular disease overall. Today the management of AMI suggested by most guidelines is aggressive and invasively oriented in the hope of reducing the extent of the myocardial damage and thus improving prognosis.

In acute ischemic heart disease, the clinical laboratory plays an important role in detection of myocardial injury. For example, the measurement of the cardiac troponins (cTns) is an important test for this purpose. These proteins are found exclusively in heart muscle cells and released into the circulation when cells die. Increased concentrations of cTns in the blood are sensitive signs of damage to heart muscle.

Conversely, reference concentrations provide powerful evidence for the healthcare provider that a patient's symptoms are not related to cardiac injury.

Heart failure is often termed **congestive heart failure (CHF)**. The National Heart, Lung, Blood Institute estimates that the current prevalence of CHF in America is 4.9 million individuals with an annual incidence of approximately 400,000 new cases each year. It is the leading cause of hospitalization in individuals 65 years and older. Prognosis is dependent on disease severity, but overall it is poor. Five-year mortality is (1) approximately 10% in mild CHF, (2) 20% to 30% in moderate CHF, and (3) up to 80% in end-stage disease. The cost of these poor outcomes is estimated at $18.8 billion per year in the United States.

Clinical chemistry testing has become important in detection of CHF. The key tests are B-type natriuretic peptide (BNP) and the N-terminal [portion of] proBNP (NT-proBNP) molecules, which are breakdown products of proBNP. BNP and NT-proBNP are released by the stressed heart and are found in the circulation. As the name "natriuretic" implies, BNP increases the renal excretion of sodium. Unlike cTns, which are intracellular proteins that escape from heart muscle cells only because the cells are dead or seriously injured, BNP is a hormone that is secreted into the blood. The secretion of BNP is stimulated by the stretch of the heart wall that occurs in heart failure. Measurement of BNP in plasma has proven to be clinically valuable as will be explored in this chapter. (Note that the general use of the term *BNP* in this chapter refers to either BNP or NT-proBNP unless specifically indicated.)

Anatomy and Physiology of the Heart

The average human adult heart weighs approximately 325 g in men and 275 g in women. It is enclosed in a sac called the *pericardium*. The cardiac wall is composed of three layers: the *epicardium* (the outer most layer), a middle layer, and an inner layer called the *endocardium.* The heart has four chambers. The two upper chambers are termed the *right* and *left atria,* and the two lower chambers are termed the *right* and *left* **ventricles** (Figure 34-1). The endocardium is the layer most susceptible to **myocardial ischemia,** a condition where the heart tissue is slowly or suddenly starved of oxygen and other nutrients. Note that the **coronary arteries,** which supply the blood to the

wall of the heart, are on the epicardium. The myocardium contains bundles of striated muscle fibers. The work of the heart is generated by the alternating contraction and relaxation of these fibers. The fibers contain the contractile proteins actin and myosin. The fibers also contain the troponins that regulate contraction. Two of the troponins, the cardiac forms of troponins I and T, have become the definitive biomarkers of cardiac injury.

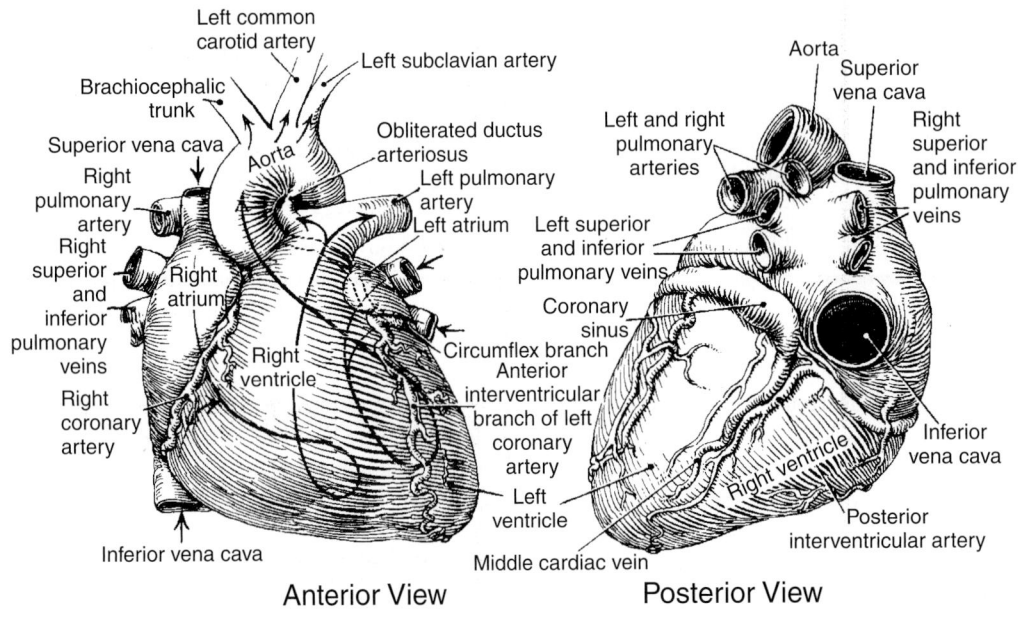

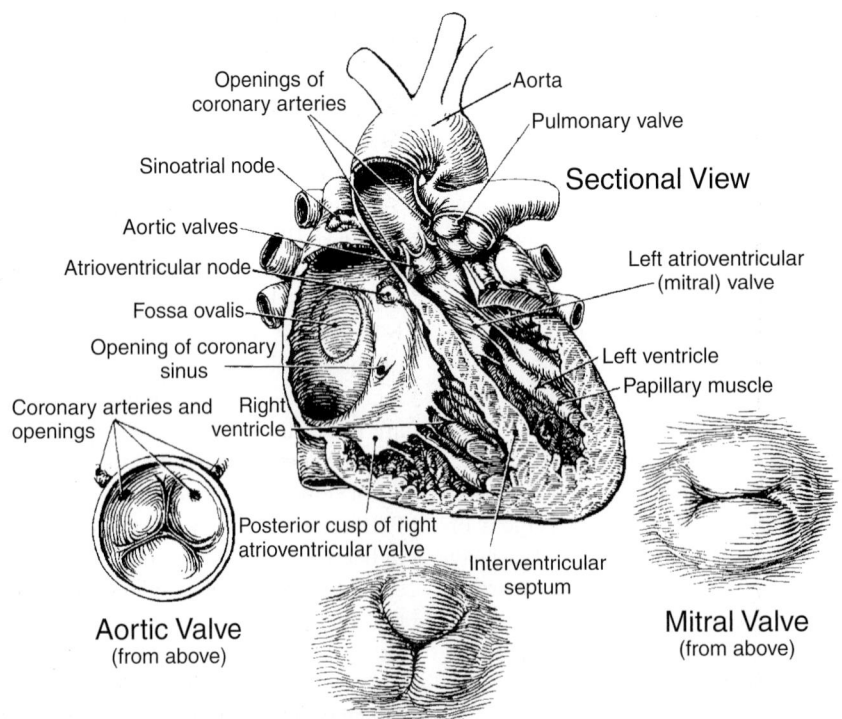

Figure 34-1 Anatomy of the heart. *(From Dorland's illustrated medical dictionary, 30th edition. Philadelphia: WB Saunders, 2003: Panel 20.)*

A typical cardiac cycle consists of two intervals known as *systole* and *diastole* (Figure 34-2). During systole, the blood pressure (BP) in the aorta is typically about 120 mm Hg. During diastole, the BP falls to about 70 mm Hg. At rest, the heart pumps between 60 and 80 times per minute. The cardiac cycle is tightly controlled by the cardiac conducting system, which initiates electrical impulses and carries them, via a specialized conducting system, to the myocardium. The **electrocardiogram (ECG)** records changes in electrical potential and is a graphic tracing of the variations in electrical potential caused by the excitation of the heart muscle. The surface ECG is a recording of the electrical potential as detected at the body surface. Clinically, the ECG is used to identify (1) anatomic, (2) metabolic, (3) ionic, and (4) hemodynamic changes. The clinical sensitivity and specificity of ECG abnormalities for detecting ACSs are influenced by a wide spectrum of physiological and anatomical changes and the clinical situation.

Under normal circumstances, each cardiac cycle's electrical potential changes, with each being similar to that of every other cycle, and includes three major components (Figure 34-3): the atrial depolarization (the P wave), ventricular depolarization (the QRS complex), and repolarization (the ST segment and T wave). A routine ECG is composed of twelve leads. Six are called *limb leads*, because they are recorded between arm and leg electrodes, and six are called *precordial* or *chest leads* and are recorded across the sternum and left precordium. Each lead records the same electrical impulse but in a different position relative to the heart. Areas of pathology shown on the ECG are localized by analyzing differences between the tracing in question and what is considered normal in the twelve different leads.

Cardiac Disease

In this section, ACS and heart failure are discussed in more detail.

Acute Coronary Syndromes

The term, acute coronary syndrome (ACS), includes patients who have a variety of forms of unstable ischemic heart disease. In the severe form of AMI, the ECG typically shows elevation of a portion called the *ST segment*. The associated clinical picture is known as **ST segment elevation myocardial infarction (STEMI)**. Partial loss of coronary perfusion, if severe, also leads to necrosis, but the magnitude of cell death is generally less and the ECG does not show elevation of the ST segment. The condition is known as **non–ST segment elevation myocardial infarction (NSTEMI)**, or non-STEMI. Patients with STEMI usually will develop Q waves on their ECGs (see Figure 34-3) hence the term *Q-wave MI*. If they

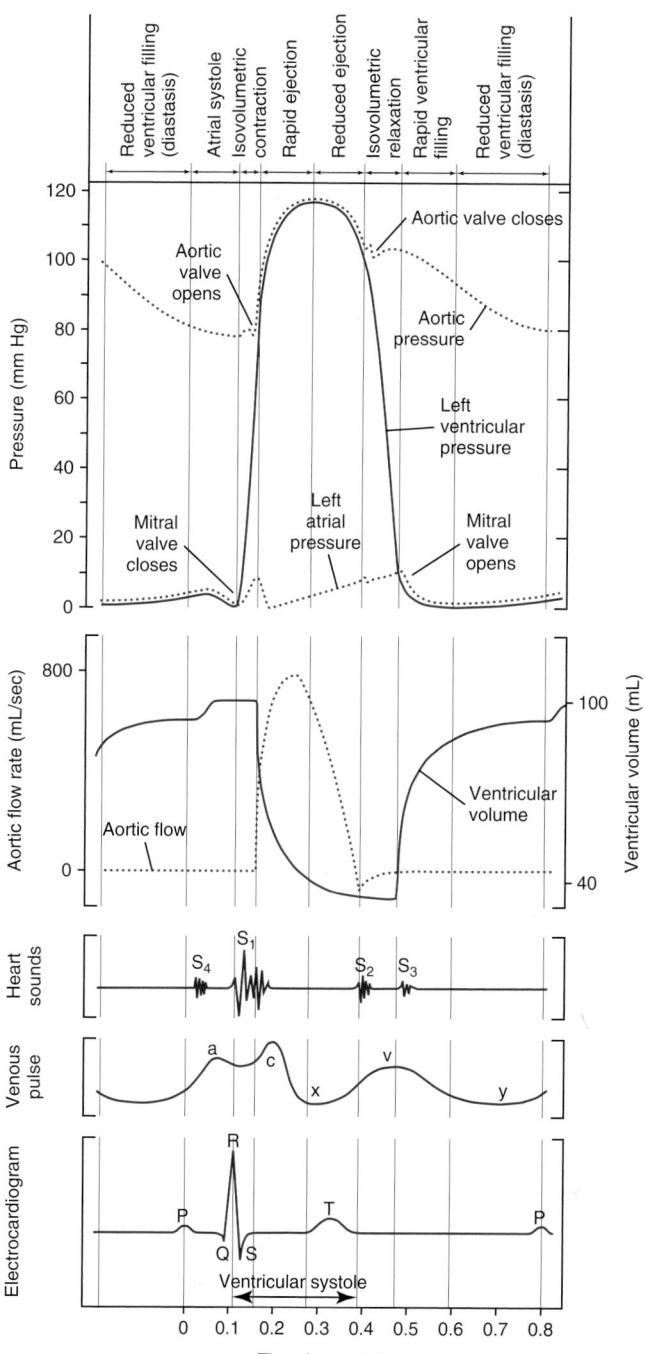

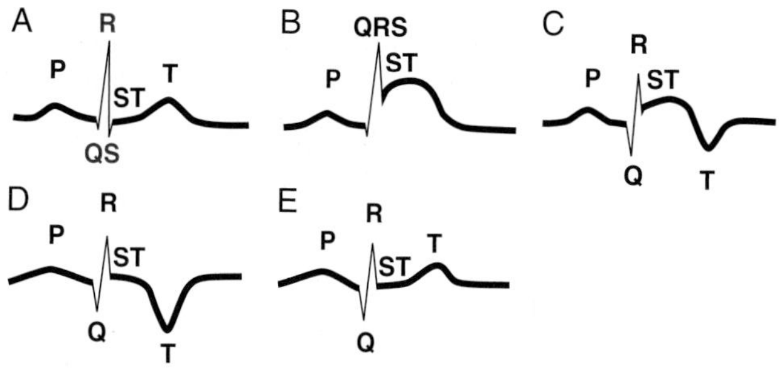

Figure 34-2 The cardiac cycle. *(From Dorland's illustrated medical dictionary, 30th edition. Philadelphia: WB Saunders, 2003, with permission from the National Kidney Foundation.)*

Figure 34-3 Electrocardiograms (ECGs) from a patient with an acute myocardial infarction (AMI). The sequence is **(A)** normal, **(B)** hours after infarction, the ST segment becomes elevated, **(C)** hours to days later, the T wave inverts and the Q wave becomes larger, **(D)** days to weeks later, the ST segment returns to near normal, and **(E)** weeks to months later, the T wave becomes upright again, but the large Q wave may remain.

do not have STE but have biochemical evidence of cardiac injury (e.g., an increasing cTnI or cTnT in blood), they are called *NSTEMI*. Those who have unstable ischemia and do not show evidence of cardiac necrosis (cell death) as indicated by increased blood concentrations of a cTn are classified as having unstable angina. Most of these syndromes occur in response to an acute event in the coronary artery that obstructs circulation to a region of the heart. If the obstruction blocks much of the passageway for blood in the vessel and persists, then necrosis usually results. Since necrosis is known to take some time to develop, it is apparent that opening the blocked coronary artery in a timely fashion often will prevent some of the death of myocardial tissue.

The major cause of ACS is **atherosclerosis**. This is a disease caused by plaque (a deposit of fatty material) being formed on the inner lining of the coronary arteries that feed the surface of the heart, which contributes to significant narrowing of the artery's lumen. Such plaques are vulnerable to rupture that results in the formation of a platelet- and fibrin-rich thrombus leading to myocardial infarction and ischemic stroke.

Atherosclerosis is also considered a chronic inflammatory disease that results after some event damages the internal lining cells (endothelium) of blood vessels, which facilitates the passage of lipid into the subendothelial space. The process of atherosclerosis progresses slowly with the involvement of (1) lymphocytes, (2) monocytes, (3) macrophages, and (4) smooth muscle cells. This process also involves adherence of white blood cells to the damaged endothelial surface with subsequent degranulation of the white cells and release of myeloperoxidase (MPO). There also is a procoagulant component attributable predominantly to the presence of tissue factor, which is localized immediately under the cap of the plaque. There also is intermittent instability because of inflammatory products within the plaque that release chemicals that degrade ground substances. These processes, in addition to a reduction in flow, lead to necrosis or at least recurrent myocardial ischemia. It is also thought that the process that eventually leads to acute events involves a systemic tendency to platelet aggregation and inflammation. Finally, necrosis when present also stimulates an acute phase reaction, including an inflammatory component. Given this pathophysiology, many therapies are now oriented toward inhibition of (1) thrombosis, (2) fibrinolysis, (3) platelet aggregation, and (4) inflammation.

In addition, **atherosclerotic plaque** has a tendency to break open (plaque disruption) and form blood clots (thrombi) within the vessel, further blocking or completely stopping blood flow. Myocardial ischemia and subsequent infarction usually begin in the endocardium and spread toward the epicardium. The extent of myocardial injury reflects: (1) extent of the occlusion, (2) the metabolic needs of the area deprived of perfusion, and (3) the duration of the imbalance between coronary supply, substrate availability, and the metabolic needs of the tissue. Irreversible cardiac injury consistently occurs when the occlusion is complete for at least 15 to 20 minutes. Most of the damage occurs within the first 2 to 3 hours.

Restoration of coronary blood flow within the first 60 to 90 minutes results in the maximal salvage of tissue, but treatment even up to 4 to 6 hours is associated with increased survival. For patients with STEMI, earlier opening the vessel can be achieved with clot dissolving agents (**thrombolysis**) and/or **percutaneous coronary intervention (PCI)**, which is a non-surgical method used to open narrowed arteries that supply the heart muscle with blood. With PCI, a catheter typically is inserted into a femoral artery, and its tip is maneuvered through the aorta and into the coronary artery. There the blockage is opened, often by inflating a balloon that is on the catheter, near its tip. The cardiologist may then insert a stent, a wire mesh tube placed inside the vessel to keep it open. This approach yields the highest acute opening rate and fewer bleeding problems than do other interventions, such as use of agents to dissolve clots. However, many hospitals cannot or do not offer urgent PCI 24 hours a day, 365 days per year. Thus administration of clot-dissolving medications without the use of PCI still plays a major role in treatment. In addition, it is now apparent that urgent invasive revascularization also benefits those with NSTEMI. It is now known that many treatments, such as newer (1) anticoagulant, (2) antiplatelet, and (3) antiinflammatory agents, when used in conjunction with PCI and other approaches to coronary revascularization, save lives in this group.

Precipitating Factors

In medical terminology, a *precipitating factor* is defined as an element that causes or contributes to the occurrence of a disorder. In many patients with AMI, the following precipitating factors have been observed for patient activities at the onset of AMI: (1) heavy physical exertion, 13%; (2) modest or usual exertion, 18%; (3) surgical procedure, 6%; (4) rest, 51%; and (5) sleep, 8%.

Role of Clinical History in Diagnosis of Acute Coronary Syndrome

The clinical history remains of substantial value in establishing a diagnosis. A prodromal history of angina is elicited in 40% to 50% of patients with AMI. Approximately one-third have had symptoms from 1 to 4 weeks before hospitalization. In the remaining two-thirds, symptoms predate admission by a week or less, with one-third of these patients having had symptoms for 24 hours or less.

In most patients, the pain of an ACS is severe but rarely intolerable. Such pain is described as (1) constricting, (2) crushing, (3) oppressing, or (4) compressing. In addition, the patient often complains of something sitting on or squeezing the chest. The pain is usually felt behind the sternum (retrosternal), spreading frequently to both sides of the chest, favoring the left side. Often the pain radiates down the left arm. In some instances, the pain of AMI may begin in the upper abdomen (epigastrium) and simulate a variety of abdominal disorders, which may lead to a misdiagnosis of indigestion. In other patients, the discomfort of AMI radiates to the (1) shoulders, (2) upper extremities, (3) neck, and (4) jaw, again usually favoring the left side. In patients with preexisting angina, the pain of infarction usually resembles that of angina with respect to features and location, but it is generally (1) much more severe, (2) lasts longer (more than 30 minutes), and/or (3) is not relieved by rest and nitroglycerin. Older individuals, diabetics, and women are more likely to present atypically, without pain or with nonspecific symptoms. Sometimes, the pain of AMI may have disappeared by the time a physician first encounters the patient, or it may persist for a few hours.

Role of Cardiac Biomarkers in Acute Coronary Syndrome

A cardiac biomarker is a biochemical compound whose measurement is useful in detecting cardiac disease, most commonly for detecting AMI or myocardial injury. In the latter setting, they are most useful when patients have nondiagnostic ECGs. For a biomarker to be clinically useful in detecting AMI, it must be released rapidly from the heart into the circulation and provide sensitive and specific diagnostic information. Furthermore, the analytical assays must be rapid and able to measure low concentrations of the biomarker in serum, plasma or whole blood samples. Also, the ideal biomarker of myocardial injury would persist in the circulation for several days to provide a late diagnostic time window for patients who arrive late after the event (for example, those with minimal pain).

Diagnosis of Acute Myocardial Infarction

Historically, the use of cardiac biomarkers in the diagnosis of AMI began in the 1950s. Initially, measurement of serum biomarkers for this purpose included (1) aspartate amino-transferase (AST), (2) lactate dehydrogenase (LD), (3) total creatine kinase (CK) and (4) α-hydroxybutyrate. In 1986 the World Health Organization (WHO) produced criteria for the diagnosis of AMI. These criteria required that at least two of the following be met for diagnosing AMI: (1) a history of chest pain, (2) evolutionary changes on the ECG, and/or (3) elevations of serial cardiac biomarkers to a level two times the normal value. (http://www.who.int/classifications/; accessed April 1, 2013).[26] These criteria are have been superseded by newer guidelines.

A 2000 European Society of Cardiology/American College of Cardiology (ESC/ACC) consensus conference updated in 2007 and 2012 (Global Task Force)[24,25] codified the role of cardiac biomarkers by advocating that the diagnosis should be based on biomarkers of cardiac damage in the appropriate clinical situation (Box 34-1).[24,25] The recommendations of the Biochemistry Panel of the ESC/ACC Committee for the use of biomarkers in the diagnosis of an established AMI are listed in Box 34-2.

Congestive Heart Failure

CHF is defined as a condition in which the heart has lost the ability to pump enough blood to the body's tissues. With too little blood being delivered, the organs and other tissues do not receive enough oxygen and nutrients to function properly. Encompassed in the definition of heart failure is a wide spectrum of clinical conditions, ranging from (1) a primary impairment in pump function, such as might occur after a large AMI; (2) increased cardiac stiffness, which causes increases in pressure in the heart, restricts filling, and increases hydrostatic pressures behind the area of reduced compliance; and (3) situations in which peripheral demand

---

BOX 34-1   Criteria for the Definition of Acute Myocardial Infarction

1. Detection of rise and/or fall of cardiac biomarkers (preferably troponin) above the 99th percentile of the upper reference limit, together with evidence of ischemia with at least one of the following:
   a. Ischemic symptoms
   b. Electrocardiogram (ECG) changes of new ischemia (new ST-T changes or new left bundle branch block [LBBB])
   c. Development of pathologic Q waves on the ECG
   d. Imaging evidence of new loss of viable myocardium or new regional wall motion abnormality
   e. Identification of an intracoronary thrombus by angiography or autopsy

From Thygesen K, Alpert JS, Jaffe AS, et al. Third universal definition of myocardial infarction. ESC/ACCF/AHA/WHF expert consensus document. Circulation 2012;126:2020-35.

BOX 34-2   European Society of Cardiology/ American College of Cardiology Recommendations for Use of Cardiac Biomarkers for Detection of Myocardial Injury and Myocardial Infarction

- Increases in biomarkers of cardiac injury are indicative of injury to the myocardium, but not an ischemic mechanism of injury.
- cTns (I or T) are preferred biomarkers for diagnosis of myocardial injury.
- Increases in cardiac biomarker proteins reflect irreversible injury.
- Improved quality control of troponin assays is essential.
- Myocardial infarction is present when there is cardiac damage, as detected by biomarker proteins (an increase above the 99th percentile of the reference interval) in a clinical setting consistent with myocardial ischemia.
- For patients with an ischemic mechanism of injury, prognosis is related to the extent of troponin increases.
- If an ischemic mechanism is unlikely, other causes for cardiac injury should be pursued.
- Samples must be obtained at least 6 to 9 hours after the symptoms begin.
- After PCI and CABG, the significance of biomarker elevations and patient care should be individualized.

CABG, Coronary artery bypass grafting; cTn, cardiac troponin; PCI, percutaneous coronary intervention.

---

is excessive. The latter results in what is known as *high output heart failure*, which is defined as the inability of the heart to increase its output sufficiently to meet the peripheral demands for blood.

To functionally stage CHF patients, the New York Heart Association (NYHA) classification system is often used (Table 34-1). In this system, Class I patients are generally considered asymptomatic with no restrictions on physical activity. In the highest class (Class IV), patients are often symptomatic at rest with severe limitations on physical activity. The clinical manifestations of heart failure vary considerably and many are non-specific. The findings depend on many factors, including (1) the clinical characteristics of the patient, (2) the extent and rate at which the heart's performance becomes abnormal, (3) the cause of the heart disease, (4) concomitant co-morbidities, and (5) the part of the heart that is affected by abnormal functioning. The severity of impairment ranges from mild—manifested

<table>
<tr><td colspan="2">TABLE 34-1 New York Heart Association Functional Classification Used to Classify the Extent of Heart Failure*</td></tr>
</table>

NYHA Class	Symptoms
I	Cardiac disease, but no symptoms and no limitation in ordinary physical activity (e.g., shortness of breath when walking, climbing stairs, etc.)
II	Mild symptoms (mild shortness of breath and/or angina) and slight limitation during ordinary activity
III	Marked limitation in activity due to symptoms, even during less-than-ordinary activity (e.g., walking short distances [20-100m]). Comfortable only at rest.
IV	Severe limitations; experiences symptoms even while *at rest* (mostly bedbound patients)

*As of April 1, 2013.
NYHA, New York Heart Association.

clinically only during stress—to advanced, in which cardiac pump function is unable to sustain life without external support.

Because the symptoms and signs of heart failure are nonspecific, an objective test for heart failure would be extremely useful. Ideally, the biomarker would increase progressively with increasing severity of disease and not be increased (or decreased) in conditions that mimic CHF. Furthermore, as for biomarkers of cardiac injury, rapid assays are desirable.

Cardiac Biomarkers

Numerous biomarkers have been monitored to assess myocardial injury and dysfunction (Table 34-2 and Table 34-3). Most are myocardial proteins and differ in their (1) location within the myocyte, (2) release kinetics after damage, and (3) clearance from the circulation. In this section, cTns (used as biomarkers of myocardial injury and in diagnosis of AMI) and natriuretic peptides (used in CHF) are described first and followed by brief discussions of three other biomarkers of myocardial injury (CK and CKMB, high-sensitivity C-reactive protein [hsCRP], and myoglobin) that are available but are not used as widely.[21] The section ends with a discussion of other cardiac biomarkers that may find utility in the next few years for various purposes.

Cardiac Troponins I and T

cTns are specific proteins found in cardiac muscle (Figure 34-4) and are measured in the diagnosis of myocardial infarction. Cardiac troponins I and T are the two main types of troponin and are referred to as *cTnT* and *cTnI*, respectively.

Biochemistry

Three troponin subunits form a complex that regulates the interaction of actin and myosin and thus regulates cardiac contraction (see Figure 34-4). The three troponins are (1) troponin T (the tropomyosin-binding component), (2) troponin I (the inhibitory component), and (3) troponin C (the calcium-binding component).

<table>
<tr><td colspan="2">TABLE 34-2 Biomarkers in Heart Failure</td></tr>
</table>

Inflammation*,†,‡	CRP
	Tumor necrosis factor-α
	Fas (APO-1)
	IL-1, IL-6, and IL-18
Oxidative stress*,†,§	Oxidized LDLs
	MPO
	Urinary biopyrrins
	Urinary and plasma isoprostanes
	Plasma malondialdehyde
Myocyte injury*,†,§	Cardiac-specific troponins I and T
	Myosin light-chain kinase I
	Heart-type fatty acid protein
	Creatine kinase MB fraction
Myocyte stress†,§,¶	BNP
	NT-proBNP
	Midregional proANP (MR-proANP)
	ST2
Extracellular matrix remodeling*,†,§	MMPs
	Tissue inhibitors of metalloproteinases
	Collagen propeptides
New biomarkers†	Chromogranin
	Galectin-3
	Osteoprotegerin
	Adiponectin
	Growth differentiation factor 15
Neurohormones*,†,§	Norepinephrine
	Renin
	Angiotensin II
	Arginine vasopressin
	Endothelin

Fas (APO-1), FAS receptor (FasR), also known as apoptosis antigen 1 (APO-1); *BNP*, B-type natriuretic peptide; *CRP*, C-reactive protein; *IL*, interleukin; *LDL*, low-density lipoproteins; *MMP*, matrix metalloproteinase; *MPO*, myeloperoxidase; *NT-proBNP*, N-terminal proBNP.
*Biomarkers in this category aid in elucidating the pathogenesis of heart failure.
†Biomarkers in this category provide prognostic information and enhance risk stratification.
‡Biomarkers in this category can be used to identify subjects at risk for heart failure.
§Biomarkers in this category are potential targets of therapy.
¶Biomarkers in this category are useful in the diagnosis of heart failure and in monitoring of therapy.
Adapted from Braunwald E. Biomarkers in heart failure. N Engl J Med 2008;358:2148-59.

component). Troponins are localized primarily in the myofibrils (94% to 97%) with a smaller cytoplasmic fraction (3% to 6%). cTnI and cTnT have different amino acid sequences encoded by different genes, and are different from the predominant troponins found in other muscle such as skeletal muscle. Human cTnI has an additional post translational 31–amino acid residue on the amino terminal end compared with skeletal muscle TnI, giving it cardiac specificity. Only one isoform of cTnI has been identified. cTnI is not expressed in normal, regenerating, or diseased human or animal skeletal muscle. cTnT is also encoded by a different gene than the one that encodes skeletal muscle isoforms. An 11–amino acid amino terminal residue gives this biomarker cardiac specificity. However, during human fetal development, in regenerating rat skeletal muscle, and in diseased human skeletal muscle, small amounts of

TABLE 34-3	Biomarkers in Acute Coronary Syndrome
Type	**Markers**
Serologic biomarkers of arterial vulnerability	Lipid profile
	Apolipoprotein B
	Lp(a)
	LDL particle number
	CETP
	Lp-PLA$_2$
	Inflammation
	hsCRP
	sICAM-1
	IL-6
	IL-18
	SAA
	MPO
	sCD40
	Oxidized LDL
	Glutathione peroxidase activity
	Nitrotyrosine
	Homocysteine
	Cystatin-C
	NPs
	ADMA
	MMP-9
	TIMP-1
Structural markers of arterial vulnerability	Carotid IMT
	Coronary artery calcium
Functional markers of arterial vulnerability	BP
	Endothelial dysfunction
	Arterial stiffness
	Ankle-brachial index
	Urine albumin excretion
Serologic markers of blood vulnerability	Fibrinogen
	D-Dimer
Decreased fibrinolysis	TPA/PAI-1
Increased coagulation	von Willebrand factor
Structural markers of myocardial vulnerability	Exercise stress echo
	PET
Serologic markers of myocardial injury	cTns

ADMA, Asymmetric dimethylarginine; *Apo,* apolipoprotein; *BP,* blood pressure; *CETP,* cholesterol ester transfer protein; *cTn,* cardiac troponin; *hsCRP,* high-sensitivity C-reactive protein; *IL,* interleukin; *IMT,* intimal-medial thickness; *LDL,* low-density lipoprotein; *Lp(a),* lipoprotein a; *Lp-PLA$_2$,* lipoprotein-associated phospholipase A$_2$; *MMP,* matrix metalloproteinase; *MPO,* myeloperoxidase; *NP,* natriuretic peptide; *PET,* positron emission tomography; *SAA,* ribonucleoprotein; *sCD40,* soluble CD40 ligand; *sICAM,* soluble intracellular adhesion molecule; *TIMP,* tissue inhibitor of metalloproteinase; *TPA/PAI-1,* tissue plasminogen activator, plasminogen activator inhibitor 1.
Adapted from Vasan RS. Biomarkers of cardiovascular disease: molecular basis and practical considerations. Circulation 2006;113:2335-62.

cTnT are expressed as one of four identified isoforms in skeletal muscle. In humans, cTnT isoform expression has been reported in skeletal muscle specimens obtained from patients with (1) muscular dystrophy, (2) polymyositis, (3) dermatomyositis, and (4) end-stage renal disease; there is some evidence that diseased skeletal muscle increases circulating cTnT immunoreactivity measured by the current cTnT immunoassay. The other

troponin, troponin C, is not useful as a cardiac biomarker as the troponin C expressed in the heart is not specific for the heart.

Following myocardial injury or because of genetic disposition, multiple forms of troponin appear both in tissue and in blood. These include (1) the complexes of cardiac troponins T, I, and C (T-I-C, or ternary complex); (2) complexes of I and C (I-C binary complex); and (3) free I. Multiple modifications of these three forms exist resulting from biochemical processes involving (1) oxidation, (2) reduction, (3) phosphorylation, (4) dephosphorylation, and (5) removal of the amino acids at the ends (C or N) of the molecules. Clinically useful immunoassays ideally recognize epitopes in the stable region of the measured molecule and measure equally the various forms (have an "equimolar response" to the various forms) that circulate in the blood.

Analytical Considerations

Many assays have been developed to measure cTns. However, these assays have been difficult to standardize, resulting in unique reference intervals for each assay.

Types of Assays

In general, immunoassay is the technique of choice for measuring cTns. Cummins and coworkers were the first to develop a cTn immunoassay. They measured cTnI by use of a radioimmunoassay (RIA) and (polyclonal) anti-cTnI antisera.[3] This RIA was followed by an enzyme-linked immunosorbent cTnI assay that eliminated the need for radioactivity and achieved high specificity by use of monoclonal antibodies.[3]

Numerous manufacturers have since developed monoclonal antibody-based diagnostic immunoassays for the measurement of cTnI in serum. Typically, these assays have lower limits of detection in the range of 0.01 to 0.10 µg/ L.[1,2,5] Many of these assays have been approved by the US Food and Drug Administration (FDA) for patient testing within the United States on central laboratory and point-of-care testing (POCT) platforms. In addition to these quantitative assays, several assays have been approved by the FDA for the qualitative determination of cTnI. Further development has led to the design of high-sensitivity cTnI (hs-cTnI) assays and a hs-cTnT assay that have lower limits of detection of 0.1-3.0 ng/L.[2,11,16,18] In practice, two obstacles limit the ease of switching from one cTnI assay to another in clinical practice or research. First, no primary reference cTnI material is currently available for manufacturers to use in standardizing cTnI assays. Second, assay concentrations are not consistent between assays because cTnI circulates in its various forms and the different antibodies used in the available assays recognize different epitopes of cTnI.

In addition to the immunoassays developed for use in clinical laboratories, assays and devices have been developed for POCT. To guide their use, the National Academy of Clinical Biochemistry (NACB) has developed Laboratory Medicine Practice Guidelines for POCT for the use of cardiac biomarkers in ACS. (American Association for Clinical Chemistry. NACB: laboratory medicine practice guidelines [LMPG]. http://www.aacc.org/members/nacb/LMPG/; accessed September 9, 2013).

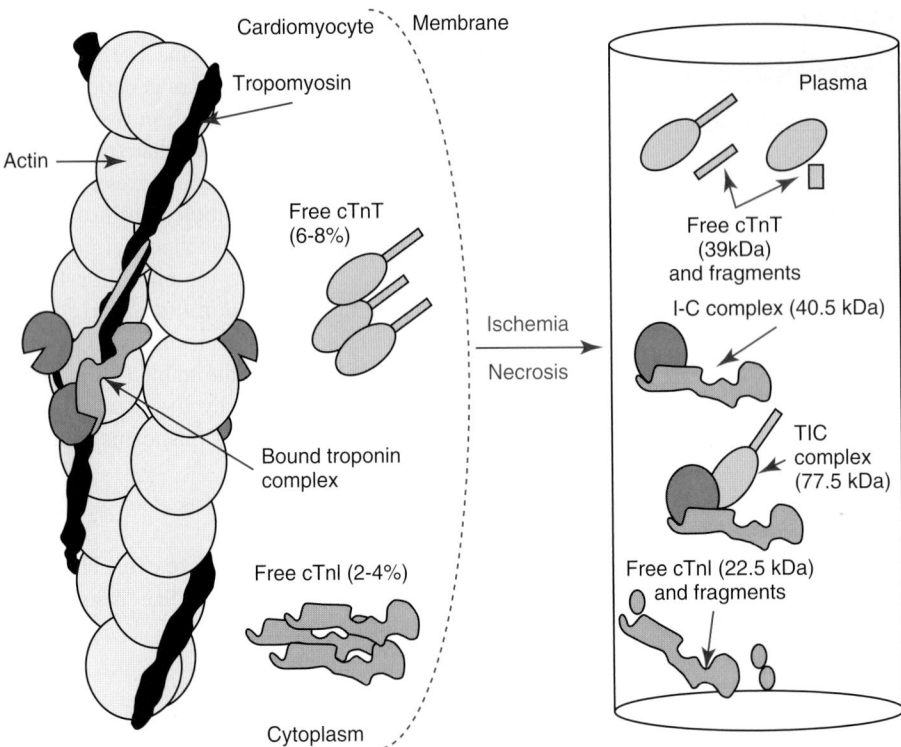

Figure 34-4 Structure of cardiac troponin (cTn) complex and troponin forms released following myofibril necrosis. *(From Gaze DC, Collinson PO. Multiple molecular forms of circulating cardiac troponin: analytical and clinical significance. Ann Clin Biochem 2008;45:349-59. Figure courtesy of Paul Collinson.)*

These guidelines address (1) administrative issues, (2) cost-effective utilization, and (3) clinical and technical performance of cardiac biomarkers in the emergency medicine department. Proposed elements of the guidelines include:

1. Members of emergency medicine departments, primary care physicians, cardiologists, hospital administrators, and clinical laboratory staff should work collectively to develop an accelerated protocol for the use of biomarkers in the evaluation of patients with possible ACS.
2. Quality assurance measures should be used with monitoring to reduce medical errors and improve patient treatment.
3. The laboratory should perform biomarker testing with a maximum turnaround time (TAT) of 1 hour, optimally 30 minutes. The TAT is defined as the time from blood collection to reporting of results to the provider. Institutions that cannot consistently provide a 1 hour TAT should implement POCT assays. Performance specifications and characteristics for central laboratory and POCT assays should not differ. POCT assays should provide quantitative results.

Specimen Requirements
For both laboratory and POCT, and for practical considerations, anticoagulated whole blood or plasma appears to be the optimal specimen for rapid processing and testing. This eliminates the extra time needed for clotting and additional sample handling. However, differences have been described between plasma, whole blood, and serum specimens for cTnI concentration measurement by an individual assay. Both ethylenediaminetetraacetic acid (EDTA) and heparin are known to interfere with cTnI and cTnT antibody-binding affinity, as well as produce matrix effects. In addition, it is

recommended that different sample types should not be used during an individual's workup when serial, timed samples are being drawn to rule in or out a myocardial infarction. It should be noted that at present, results obtained from POCT assays are substantially less sensitive than laboratory-based assays and that should be acknowledged by both laboratorians and clinicians when such assays are used. The higher limits of quantification mean that small increases of cTn at early time points after AMI will not be detected with these assays. This fact works against the goal of early detection of AMI.

Standardization/Harmonization
Standardization of cTn assays remains elusive. The cTnI Standardization Subcommittee of the American Association for Clinical Chemistry (AACC) in collaboration with the National Institute of Standards and Technology (NIST) have produced a cTnI standard reference material (SRM #2921) that is a TnC-cTnI-cTnT complex purified from human heart under nondenaturing conditions. Since this material was found to be commutable with only 50% of current cTnI assays, it is of limited value for assay harmonization of current assays and is not useful as a common calibrator. It does, however, allow for traceability to a common reference material. Currently an International Federation of Clinical Chemistry and Laboratory Medicine (IFCC) Working Group is working toward developing a secondary serum-based reference material.

In 2001, the IFCC Committee on Standardization of Markers of Cardiac Damage (C-SMCD) updated quality specifications for cTn assays that were intended for use by the manufacturers of commercial assays and by clinical laboratories utilizing cTn assays.[20] The overall goal was to attempt to establish uniform criteria so that all assays could be

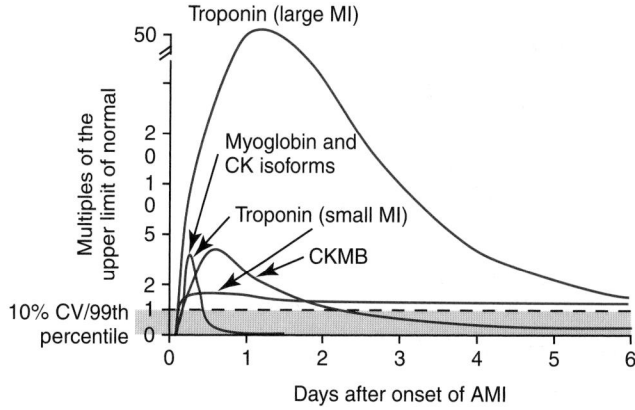

Figure 34-5 Kinetics of myoglobin, troponin, and CK-MB. With contemporary assays, cardiac troponin (cTn) rises more rapidly than do other markers. With small myocardial infarctions, two types of time courses are possible, as indicated by the two sets of arrows.

BOX 34-3   Quality Specifications—Cardiac Troponin Assays

Analytical Factors
1. Antibody specificity—recognize epitopes as part of molecule and equimolar for all forms
2. Influence of anticoagulants
3. Calibration against natural form of molecule
4. Defined type of material useful for dilutions
5. Demonstrated recovery and linearity of method
6. Described detection limit and imprecision (10% CV)
7. Addressing interferants (e.g., RF, heterophile antibodies)

Preanalytical Factors
1. Storage time and temperature conditions
2. Centrifugation effects—gel separators
3. Serum-plasma—WB correlations

CV, Coefficient of variation; RF, rheumatoid factor; WB, whole blood.
Adapted from Panteghini M, Gerhardt W, Apple FS, et al. Quality specifications for cardiac troponin assays. Clin Chem Lab Med 2001;39:174-8.

---

evaluated objectively for their analytical qualities and clinical performance. A description of the (1) analytical principles, (2) method design, and (3) assay components developed by this group is found in Box 34-3.

Reference Intervals

There are many ways to obtain reference intervals for biomarkers of AMI, including those described in Chapter 5 and those published in the literature and in manufacturer's package inserts. However, different methods for the same analyte may yield different values, depending on calibration and other technical considerations.[20] Consequently, different reference intervals and results are often obtained in different laboratories. Variability among methods is particularly characteristic of methods that use antibodies to detect the analyte of interest. Values from apparently "healthy" and diseased people may overlap significantly. Therefore reference intervals, although useful as a guide for clinicians, should not be used as absolute indicators of health and disease (see Chapter 5). The reference intervals presented in this chapter and in Chapter 50 are for *general informational purposes only*. Guidelines for defining and determining reference intervals have been discussed in Chapter 5 and published in the 2010 Clinical Laboratory Standards Institute (CLSI) EP28-A3C guideline (Defining, Establishing, and Verifying Reference Intervals in the Clinical Laboratory; Approved Guideline—Third Edition, which is available at http://www.clsi.org/ (accessed September 9, 2013). As stated in several chapters in this textbook, each individual laboratory should generate its own set of reference intervals.

Guidelines

In addition to the "how to" guidelines mentioned earlier, guidelines have also been generated to define AMI. For example, consensus guidelines have been developed by the (1) Global Task Force for the Third Universal Definition of Myocardial Infarction,[24,25] (2) NACB/IFCC,[4,19] (3) ESC/ACC,[8] (4) American Heart Association (AHA)/ACC[23] and (5) Acute Decompensated Heart Failure National Registry (ADHERE)

Scientific Advisory Committee.[13] Additional guidelines have been published in 2012[12] and 2013.[10]

To quote the NACB/IFCC recommendations "The 99th percentile of a reference decision-limit (medical decision cutoff) for cTn assays should be determined in each local laboratory by internal studies using the specific assay that is used in clinical practice or validating a reference interval that is based on findings in the literature".[7] Desirable imprecision (expressed as % coefficient of variation [CV]) of each cTn assay (and CK-MB mass assay) has been defined as less than 10% CV at the 99th percentile reference limit. Unfortunately, some laboratories do not have (1) the resources to perform adequately powered 99th percentile reference studies, nor (2) the ability to carry out CLSI protocols to establish total imprecision criteria. Therefore, these clinical laboratories must rely on the peer-reviewed published literature to assist in establishing both local reference limits and imprecision characteristics. Caution must be taken when comparing the findings reported in the manufacturers' package inserts, which have been cleared by the FDA with the findings reported in journals because of differences in (1) total sample size, (2) distributions by sex and ethnicity, (3) age ranges, and (4) statistical methods used to calculate the 99th percentile.

Clinical Utility

As discussed earlier, cardiac biomarkers have been used since the 1950s in the diagnosis of AMI. Because of their high clinical sensitivity and specificity, the assays for the measurement of troponins have become the cornerstone of the diagnosis of myocardial infarction (Figure 34-5 and Figure 34-6). Therefore, in practice, an increased value of cardiac cTn is required in the appropriate clinical setting with values that manifest a rising pattern for the diagnosis of AMI. It should be noted, however, that other conditions (Box 34-4) also cause the death of cardiomyocytes and lead to increases of cTn in the blood, thus indicating myocyte damage.

Guidelines have been developed for their use in a clinical setting. Individuals with spontaneous AMI typically

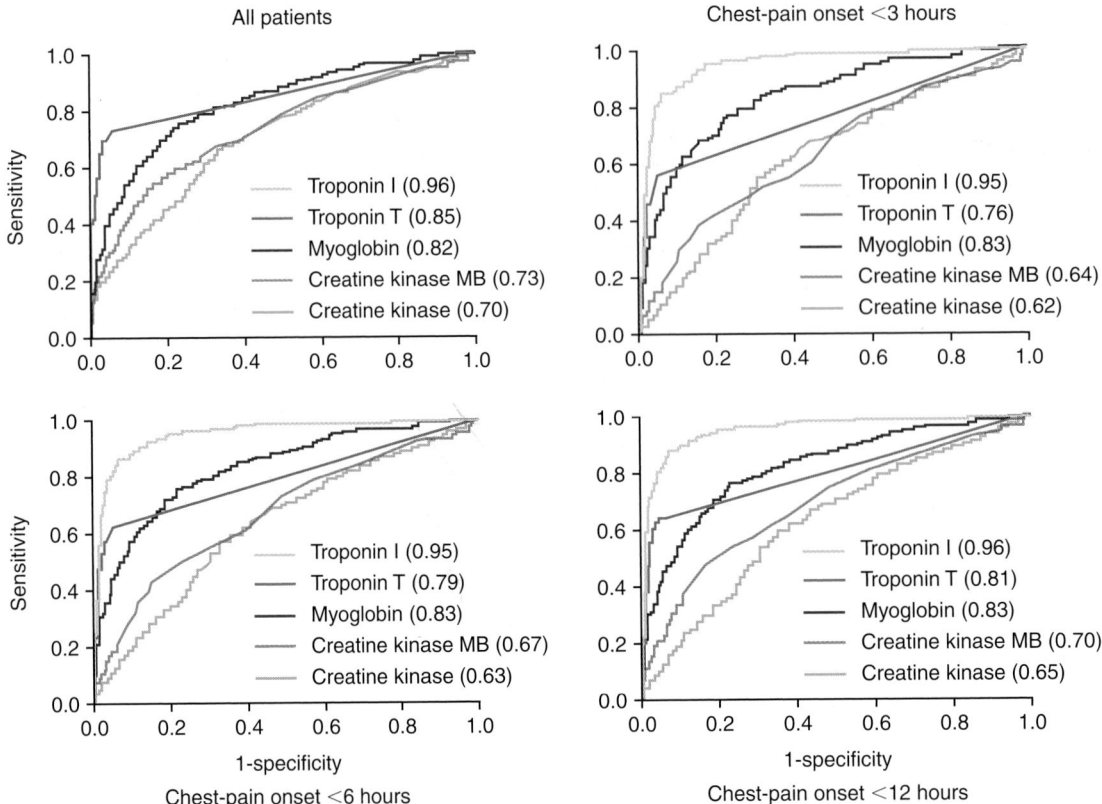

Figure 34-6 Receiver operating characteristic (ROC) curve analysis of troponin, myoglobin, and CK-MB by time from onset of symptoms to presentation.

BOX 34-4 Conditions That Increase Blood Concentrations of Troponins without Overt Ischemic Heart Disease

Trauma (including contusion, ablation, pacing, and cardioversion)
CHF—acute and chronic*
Aortic valve disease and HOCM with significant LVH*
Hypertension
Hypotension, often with **arrhythmias**
Postoperative noncardiac surgery patients who seem to do well*
Renal failure*
Critically ill patients, especially with diabetes; respiratory failure*
Drug toxicity (e.g., Adriamycin, 5-FU, Herceptin, snake venoms)*
Hypothyroidism
Coronary vasospasm, including apical ballooning syndrome
Inflammatory diseases (e.g., myocarditis, with parvovirus B19, Kawasaki disease, sarcoidosis, smallpox vaccination, or myocardial extension of PE)
Post-PCI patients who appear to be uncomplicated*
Pulmonary embolism, severe pulmonary hypertension*
Sepsis*
Burns, especially if TBSA >30%*
Infiltrative diseases, including amyloidosis, hemochromatosis, sarcoidosis, and scleroderma*
Acute neurologic disease, including CVA, subarachnoid hemorrhage*
Rhabdomyolysis with cardiac injury
Transplant vasculopathy
Vital exhaustion

*Troponin concentrations have been reported to carry prognostic information in these conditions.
5-FU, Fluorouracil cream 5%; *CHF,* congestive heart failure; *CVA,* cardiovascular accident; *HOCM,* hypertrophic obstructive cardiomyopathy; *LVH,* left ventricular hypertrophy; *PCI,* percutaneous coronary intervention; *PE,* pulmonary embolus; *TBSA,* total body surface area.

---

have either STEMI or NSTEMI as indicated by their ECG pattern. For patients with STEMI, immediate treatment aimed at opening the occluded artery is mandatory and is initiated based on the ECG pattern alone. (Note: This is even before the cTn values become available to assist with diagnosis.) Primary PCI and/or prescription of thrombolytic agents currently are the treatments of choice for opening the artery. Primary PCI is preferred whenever the two treatments are available in similar timeframes. With prompt coronary recanalization, the amount of myocardium that is lost is minimized, and mortality is reduced. (Note: Coronary recanalization increases the rapidity of cTn release; thus the rate of rise of the time-concentration curve is increased, and the time to peak values is shortened.)

An NSTEMI is typically not associated with total coronary occlusion and is identified by ECG changes. Such changes show ST segment depression or T wave changes. Given the sensitivity of cTn for this diagnosis, the ECG is sometimes totally normal. Patients who have symptoms of chest pain due to CAD should have (1) risk factors, (2) an appropriate presentation, or (3) imaging evidence of this syndrome. Patients with an increased concentration of cTn are known to have more severe coronary heart disease than individuals without increased cTns. Thus, they also have more procoagulant activity and multiple intervention studies have shown that these patients benefit from aggressive anticoagulation. This therapy includes (1) treatment with heparin, (2) administration of glycoprotein IIb/IIIa antiplatelet agents, and (3) an early invasive strategy consisting of PCI or coronary artery bypass grafting

(CABG). Use of these strategies in patients without increased cTn values has been shown to be of no benefit and, in some trials, has actually proved detrimental.[3]

Brain Natriuretic Peptide

In 1981, the Canadian physiologist Adolfo de Bold and his colleagues reported that infusion of atrial tissue extracts produced (1) an increase in the renal excretion of sodium and water, (2) a rapid decrease in BP, and (3) an increase in blood hematocrit. The responsible substance was named the *atrial natriuretic factor*. This factor was subsequently purified and identified as a peptide comprising 28–amino acid residues and renamed *atrial natriuretic peptide (ANP)*. Later, brain natriuretic peptide (BNP) and C-type natriuretic peptide (CNP), two structurally related peptides, were isolated and identified in the porcine brain. However, as BNP is mainly expressed in the heart, it was later renamed *B-type natriuretic peptide* (Figure 34-7).

Biochemistry[14]

B-type natriuretic peptide (BNP) is a hormone that is mainly released from the myocardial ventricles.[22] Figure 34-8 illustrates the synthesis of the preprohormone and subsequent secretion of BNP from the cardiac myocytes. It is not known whether proBNP is split in the myocyte or later in the plasma. It is known, however, that there are circulating

proteases that are capable of cleaving the N-terminal and the active BNP moiety. The major circulating forms are the N-terminal portion (or fragment) of proBNP (NT-proBNP), which has unknown function; proBNP, function unknown; and BNP (the physiologically active hormone, which is the C-terminal part of pro-BNP). BNP is cleared via degradation by (neutral) endopeptidases, by receptor-mediated clearance, and perhaps via the kidneys, which also secretes BNP. The NT-proBNP fragment is not cleared via receptor-mediated mechanisms, but is thought

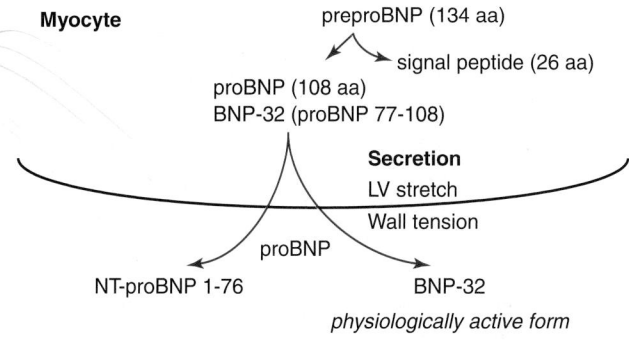

Figure 34-8 The biotransformation and release of BNP and NT-proBNP from the myocyte into the circulation (*aa, amino acid*).

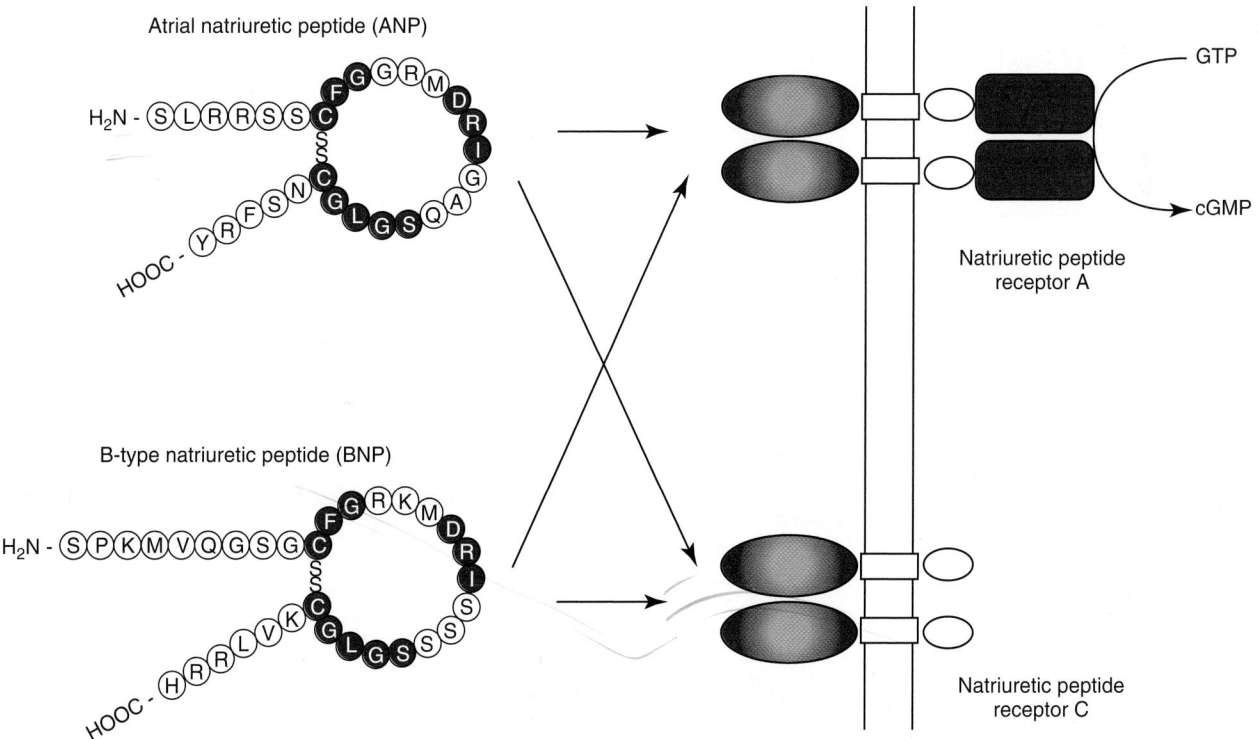

Figure 34-7 Schematic presentation of human atrial and B-type natriuretic peptides (BNPs) with their principal receptors. Homolog amino acid residues between the natriuretic peptides (NPs) are marked in *bold circles*. The natriuretic peptide receptor (NPR)-A mediates atrial natriuretic peptide (ANP) and brain natriuretic peptide (BNP) signal transduction through induction of cyclic guanosine monophosphate (cGMP); NPR-C lacks the intracellular domain and has been classed primarily as a clearance receptor.

to be cleared predominantly by the kidneys. Therefore, it is more sensitive to changes in renal function. The majority of research on NPs in CHF has focused on BNP and NT-proBNP. However, investigations have now described substantial amounts of circulating proBNP, which cross-reacts in BNP and NT-proBNP assays.

Analytical Considerations

Generally, the concentrations of BNP and NT-proBNP are measured by immunoassay. A number of immunoassays are available that use antibodies directed to different epitopes located on the antigen molecules.[4] Degradation of BNP is known to occur by cleavage at serine and proline residues in vivo and in vitro (Figure 34-9); cleavage is mediated by proteases, which make the concentration of BNP unstable in collected blood.[7] For monitoring of patients by measurements of NT-proBNP (amino acids 1-76), an improved understanding of potential cross-reactivity with split products of the N-terminal portion of NT-proBNP and proBNP itself is needed.[17] For both assays—BNP and NT-proBNP—minimizing interference from heterophilic antibodies and rheumatoid factor, for example, needs to be optimized. For BNP, EDTA-anticoagulated whole blood or plasma appears to be the only acceptable specimen choice. For NT-proBNP, serum, heparin plasma, and EDTA plasma appear acceptable, although results are 10% lower with the latter. Plastic blood collection tubes are necessary for BNP; for NT-proBNP, either glass or plastic is acceptable.

Guidelines

In 2005, the IFCC C-SMCD established recommended analytical and preanalytical quality specifications for NP assays.[6]

These specifications were intended for use by the manufacturers of commercial assays and by clinical laboratories utilizing NP assays. The overall goal of this committee was to establish uniform analytical and clinical criteria for their measurement and clinical use. Subsequently, the NACB and the IFCC committee developed guidelines pertaining to analytical issues for biomarkers of heart failure.[4]

Recommendations from these guidelines include:

1. Reference limits (95th or 97.5th percentile) should be established independently for both BNP and NT-proBNP based on age (by decade) and by sex. Each commercial assay should be validated separately. The effects of ethnicity and renal function need to be evaluated as possible independent variables.

2. Receiver operating characteristic (ROC) curves (Figure 34-10) should be established to evaluate clinical effectiveness and to establish optimal medical decision cutoffs for BNP and NT-proBNP assays for diagnostic usefulness.

3. Assays for BNP and NT-proBNP should have total imprecision (%CV) ≤15% at their age- and sex-defined upper reference limits, as well as at the NYHA-defined medical decision concentrations.

Before introduction into clinical practice, BNP and NT-proBNP assays must be characterized with respect to the following preanalytical and analytical issues:

1. Preanalytical:
   a. Effects of storage time and temperature
   b. Influence of different anticoagulants
   c. Influence of gel separator tubes
   d. Need for plastic blood collection tubes for BNP; for NT-proBNP, either glass or plastic is acceptable

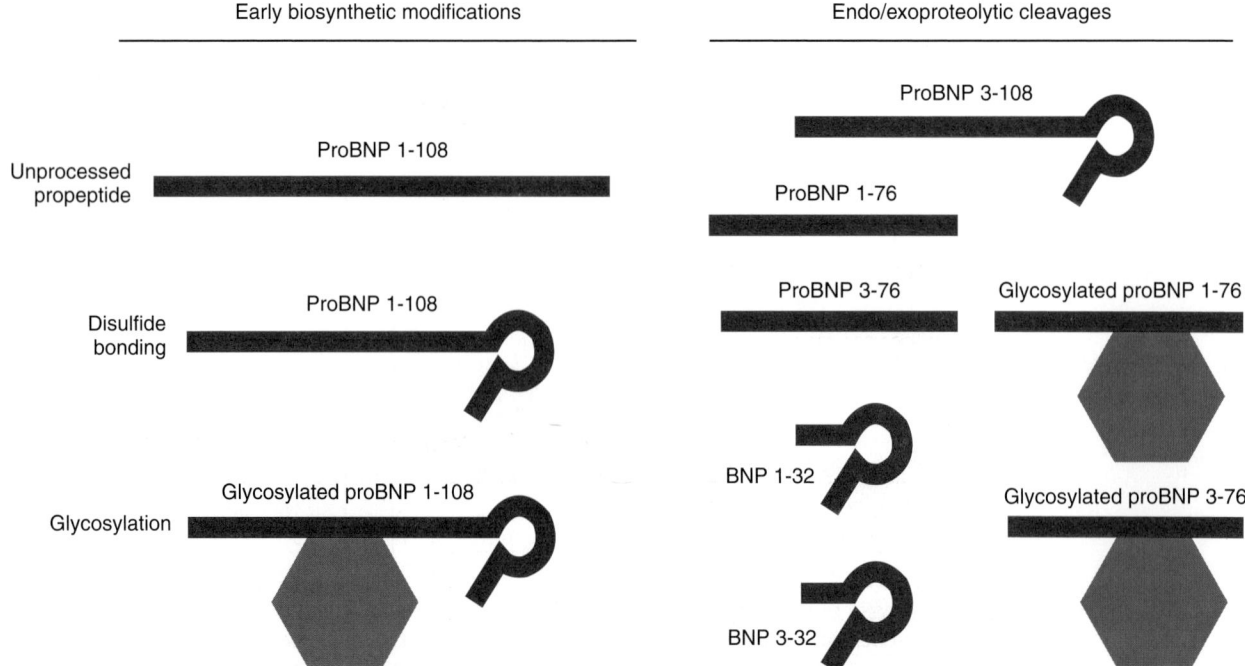

| Early biosynthetic modifications | Endo/exoproteolytic cleavages |

Figure 34-9 Schematic presentation of possible proBNP-derived peptide products. Note that most peptides are not chemically identified but rather are suggested by biochemical methods that rely on antibody recognition. Carbohydrate is indicated by the shaded hexagons.

PRIDE

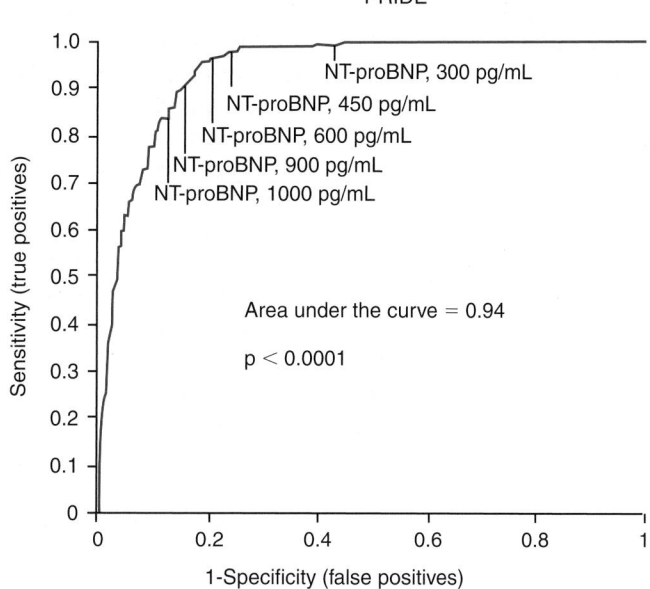

Cut point	Sensitivity	Specificity	Positive predictive value	Negative predictive value	Accuracy
300 pg/mL	99%	68%	62%	99%	79%
450 pg/mL	98%	76%	68%	99%	83%
600 pg/mL	96%	81%	73%	97%	86%
900 pg/mL	90%	85%	76%	94%	87%
1000 pg/mL	87%	86%	78%	91%	87%

Breathing Not Properly

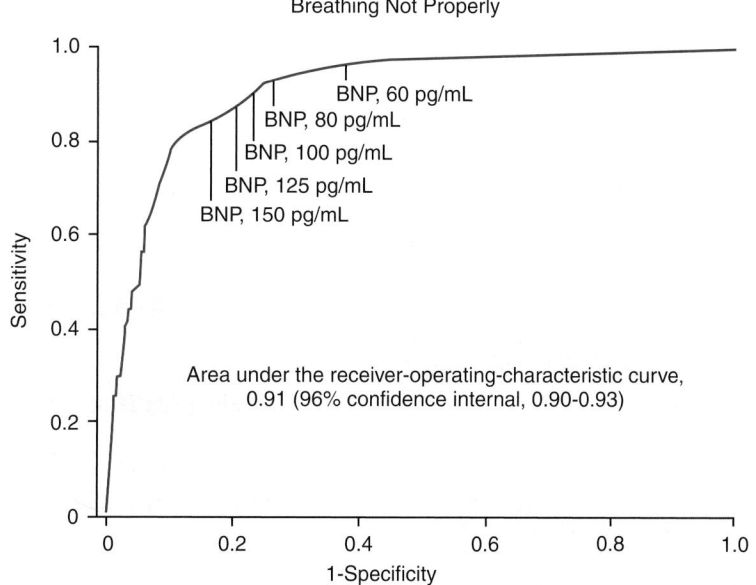

BNP pg//mL	Sensitivity	Specificity	Positive predictive value	Negative predictive value	Accuracy
50	97 (98-98)	62 (60-66)	71 (68-74)	96 (94-97)	79
80	98 (91-96)	74 (70-77)	77 (76-80)	92 (89-94)	83
100	90 (88-92)	76 (73-78)	79 (78-81)	92 (87-91)	83
125	87 (86-90)	79 (78-82)	80 (78-83)	87 (84-89)	83
150	86 (82-88)	83 (80-86)	83 (80-86)	85 (83-88)	84

Figure 34-10 Receiver operating characteristic (ROC) analysis for brain natriuretic peptide (BNP) and N-terminal pro B-type natriuretic peptide (NT-proBNP) for the diagnosis of acute heart failure.

2. Analytical:
   a. Identification of the epitopes in the NP that are recognized by the reagent antibodies
   b. Cross-reactivity characteristics with related NPs, including NT-proANP, ANP, CNP, BNP, and glycosylated and nonglycosylated NT-proBNP and proBNP
   c. Identification of interference from heterophile antibodies, rheumatoid factors, human antimouse antibodies
   d. Description of calibration material used, how the material was defined, and the concentration value assigned
   e. Clarification of dilution response
3. For both BNP and NT-proBNP, in the interim until a primary reference material is defined for either assay for appropriate calibration of assays, measurements should be reported in ng/L, not in pmol/L; and patient specimen comparisons and regression analysis should be performed, in accordance with CLSI guidelines, to establish the degree or lack of harmonization across the dynamic range of each assay. Specifically, harmonization around the current presumed optimal diagnostic medical decision cutoff of 100 ng/L for BNP should be validated.
4. For both BNP and NT-proBNP, biological variability has been determined to be at least 50%,. Therefore, caution should be exercised in interpreting concentration changes of less than 50% to 80% as reflective of medical therapy. However, consistent trends should be followed as clinically important.

Reference Intervals

As recommended (Chapters 5 and 50), each laboratory should determine a reference interval based on a reference group for with the specific assay used in clinical practice or validate the reference interval in the literature. In the case of BNP and NT-proBNP, there are several practical issues regarding the use of serum/plasma/whole blood monitoring of them. First, reference intervals vary depending on which assay is used and the nature of the reference population used. Second, a number of clinical factors affect the BNP and NT-proBNP concentrations, most importantly (1) age, (2) sex, (3) obesity, and (4) renal function. Significant differences are observed between men and women (higher), and concentrations increase with age, as shown in Figure 34-11 for NT-proBNP. For both BNP and NT-proBNP, there is an inverse relationship between concentrations and body mass index. For NT-proBNP, establishing reference intervals has been challenging. For example, review of both the FDA-approved U.S. package insert and the European assay package insert reveals substantial differences in the concentrations that are considered as reference intervals by age and sex.

For BNP, a single cutoff has been designated at 100 pg/mL. However, as shown in Figure 34-11, many subjects older than 75 years have concentrations above the 100 pg/mL cutoff. For NT-proBNP, the FDA-cleared cutoff concentrations are based on age. For example, for patients younger than 75 years the cutoff concentration is 125 pg/mL. For patients older than 75 years, the cutoff concentration is 450 pg/mL.

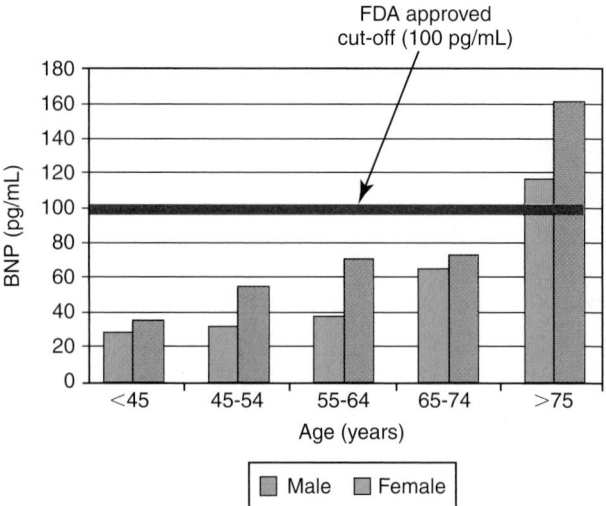

Figure 34-11 Representative brain natriuretic peptide (BNP) concentration distributions in normal males and females by decade (years) with indication of the U.S. Food and Drug Administration (FDA)-cleared 100 pg/mL cutoff value.

Clinical Utility[15]

BNP has a multiplicity of cardiac functions and is released as a counter-regulatory hormone in response to a variety of cardiac stresses but most particularly cardiac stretch. It is significantly affected by changes in volume and in cardiac performance, and among its effects are fluid-volume reduction and vasodilation. Thus, this hormone is a sensitive biomarker for changes in ventricular physiology.[15] Circulating concentrations of BNP and NT-proBNP depend on age and sex (see Figure 34-11). In addition, they are increased in chronic heart failure and are correlated with its severity. Early studies have demonstrated that BNP secretion reflects regional wall stress in the ventricles and is thus associated with adverse ventricular remodeling and poor prognosis after AMI. It is now apparent that BNP measurements are useful (1) in identifying patients with moderate to severe CHF and (2) **risk stratification**[13] of CHF patients and of patients who present with ACS. The data suggest that both BNP and NT-proBNP assays provide information that is synergistic with the measurement of troponin in these settings and is especially useful for risk stratification when cTn concentrations are within the reference intervals.

Creatine Kinase Isoenzymes and Isoforms

CK is an enzyme present in (1) heart muscle, (2) skeletal muscle, and (3) the brain (see Chapter 19 for details of its measurement). Three cytosolic isoenzymes (CK-3, CK-2, CK-1) and one mitochondrial isoenzyme (CK-Mt) of CK (approximately 80,000 Da for all 4 isoenzymes) have been identified. The cytosolic enzymes are dimers of two subunits called M and B. Distinct genes encode the M and B subunits, and a third encodes mitochondrial CK. CK-3 (CK-MM) is predominant in both heart and skeletal muscle, and CK-1 (CK-BB) is the dominant form in brain and smooth muscle. CK-2 (CK-MB) is sometimes called the *cardiac isoenzyme* because 10% to 20% of the total CK activity in myocardium is from CK-MB, whereas in skeletal muscle this percentage ranges from less than 2% to 5%. Electrophoresis of CK isoenzymes, using extended electrophoresis times or electrophoresis at high voltages, reveals at least three CK-MM isoforms and at least 4 CK-MB isoforms (subtypes of the individual isoenzymes).

The proportion of CK-MB is much lower in the surrounding normal areas of tissue than in infarcted myocardium in humans. When studied more completely in humans, CK-MB concentrations ranged from 15% to 24% of total CK in myocardial tissue obtained from patients with either (1) left ventricular hypertrophy (LVH) caused by aortic stenosis, (2) CAD without LVH, or (3) CAD and LVH due to aortic stenosis. In contrast, patients with normal left ventricular tissue had a low percentage of CK-MB (less than 2%). Diseased cells also have less total CK per cell. Normal skeletal muscle, depending on its location, contains very little CK-MB. Percentages as high as 5% to 7% have been reported, but less than 2% is most common. Severe skeletal muscle injury following trauma or surgery is known to lead to elevations of CK-MB above the upper reference limit of CK-MB in serum. However, the percent CK-MB in serum is less than 5%. Increases in serum total CK and CK-MB often present a diagnostic challenge to the clinician as they are also increased in other conditions. For example, elevations of serum CK-MB resulting from chronic muscle disease occur in (1) muscular dystrophy, (2) end-stage renal disease, (3) polymyositis, and (4) healthy subjects who undergo extreme exercise or physical activities (for example, the increase in serum CK-MB in runners). In all these pathologies, cTn has been shown to be normal when the myocardium is not injured.

C-Reactive Protein

C-reactive protein (CRP) is an acute-phase reactant that was initially developed to evaluate patients with infection. It now appears that concentrations below those seen in infection but above healthy values (as measured by so-called high-sensitivity CRP, or hsCRP, assays) are biomarkers of the atherosclerotic process (see Chapter 23 for further information on the use of hsCRP for this purpose).[16]

Myoglobin

Myoglobin is an oxygen-binding protein of cardiac and skeletal muscle with a molecular mass of 17,800 Da. Measurement of serum myoglobin was advocated because it appeared to increase sooner than CK-2 after AMI. Increases in serum myoglobin occur after trauma to either skeletal or cardiac muscle, as in crush injuries or AMI. Increases of the serum concentrations of myoglobin are cleared rapidly, leading to false-negative results after a few hours. Even minor injury to skeletal muscle may result in increased serum concentrations of myoglobin, creating a potential for misinterpretation as myocardial injury (false-positive results for AMI). Myoglobin is cleared by the kidneys so that abnormalities in renal function can cause elevations.

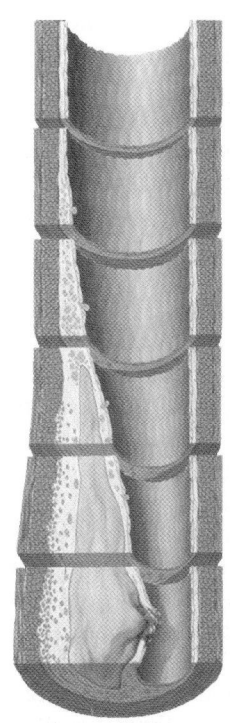

- Proinflammatory Cytokines
  - IL-6, TNFa
- Plaque Destabilization
  - MPO, MMPs, CAMs
- Plaque Rupture
  - sCD40L, PlGF, PAPP-A
- Acute Phase Reactants
  - hs-CRP, serum amyloid
- Ischemia
  - Choline, FFAu, copeptin, GPBB
- Necrosis
  - cTnT, cTnI, CKMB, myoglobin, FABP
- Myocardial Dysfunction/CHF
  - BNP, NT-proBNP, MR-proANP, proBNP, ST2, GDF-15, galactin

Figure 34-12 Spectrum of acute coronary pathophysiological process from initiation of atherosclerosis to cell death with potential biomarkers listed for each. *(From personal communication, Robert Jesse, MD.)*

Other Potential Biomarkers

Figure 34-12 portrays a biochemical profile in coronary vascular disease that correlates staging of biomarker release into the circulation with various pathophysiologic mechanisms of ACS and heart failure. As shown in Tables 34-2 and 34-3, numerous biomarkers have been studied and used for different clinical reasons, and other promising novel biomarkers are trying to establish themselves alongside cTn and NPs as routine clinical tools.[9] In this section, selected characteristics of several of these are briefly discussed (in alphabetical order). It should also be noted that, in general, these potential biomarkers do not have (1) standardized assays, (2) reference interval studies, and (3) consistent assay validations.

Adhesion Molecules

Adhesion molecules are a wide variety of molecules that can potentially be measured as a way of assessing the adherence of leukocytes and/or platelets or other adhesive proteins to the endothelial matrix. Some are receptors. Examples include platelet-endothelial adhesion molecule 1 (PECAM-1), P-selectin, e-selectin, and vascular cell adhesion molecule 1 (VCAM-1).

sCD40 Ligand

sCD40 Ligand is a transmembrane protein related to tissue necrosis factor (TNF) alpha. It has multiple prothrombotic and proatherogenic effects. Assays are usually designed to measure the circulating soluble form of the receptor, which has been shown to be a predictor of events after acute ACS presentations.

Choline

Choline is released after stimulation of phospholipase D and has been touted as a test of prognosis in patients with chest discomfort.

Copeptin

Copeptin is a 30-amino-acid glycoprotein that constitutes the C-terminal portion of arginine vasopressin. Measurement of copeptin serves as a rapid and early rule-out biomarker for AMI at presentation in patients with symptoms suggestive of ACS with a normal cTn value.

Cytokines

A variety of stimulatory and inhibitory interleukins (ILs) (TNF, IL-1, IL-6, IL-8, IL-12, and IL-18) are thought to help mediate the elaboration of CRP and the development of atherosclerosis and acute events. These cytokines may stimulate or inhibit leukocytes, often through T cell–mediated processes and effects on monocytes. In some studies, IL-6 has been found to be more prognostic than hsCRP.[3] These cytokines often have inhibitors and/or binding proteins that modulate their effects.

Galectin-3

Galectin-3 is protein that is a member of the lectin family that contains a carbohydrate-recognition-binding domain (CRD) of about 130 amino acids that enable the specific binding of β-galactosides. It has been shown to be involved in several biological processes including (1) cell adhesion, (2) cell activation, (2) chemoattraction, (3) cell growth and differentiation, (4) cell cycle, and (5) apoptosis. Clinically, galectin-3 has been found to be involved in (1) cancer, (2) inflammation, (3) fibrosis, (4) stroke, and (5) heart disease. It has also been shown that the expression of galectin-3 is implicated in a variety of processes associated with (1) heart failure, (2) myofibroblast proliferation, (3) fibrogenesis, (4) tissue repair, (5) inflammation, and (6) remodeling of ventricles.

Isoprostanes

Isoprostanes are the end breakdown products of lipid per-oxidation; urinary levels have been used to assess the level of oxidative stress. It is thought that oxidation of low-density lipoprotein (LDL) is essential for the development of atherosclerosis, and that high-density lipoprotein (HDL) and other antioxidants work by antagonizing this oxidative stress. Urinary isoprostanes give some assessment of this critical process. The most commonly measured are F_2-iso-prostanes, but a large number of others are available for measurement.

Lipoprotein-Associated Phospholipase A$_2$

Lipoprotein-associated phospholipase A$_2$ (Lp-PLA$_2$) is a phospholipase enzyme associated with LDL that is thought to be an inflammatory biomarker. It was previously known as *platelet-activating factor (PAF) acetyl hydrolase*. It is synthesized by monocytes and lymphocytes and is thought to cleave oxidized lipids to produce lipid fragments that are more atherogenic and that increase endothelial adhesion.

Matrix Metalloproteinases

Matrix metalloproteinases (MMPs) degrade the collagen matrix in the coronary artery or myocardium. They are integral to remodeling of the coronary artery and/or the heart after acute events. Elaboration of MMP-9, a gelatinase, is thought to be important in plaque destabilization; thus some have tried to measure it as a prognostic index. Other MMPs participate in the elaboration of extracellular matrix in the heart. Many MMPs also have inhibitors (such as, tissue inhibitors of metalloproteinase [TIMPs]) that modulate their effects.

Monocyte Chemotactic Protein

Monocyte chemotactic protein (MCP-1) is a chemokine that is thought to be responsible for the recruitment of monocytes into atherosclerotic plaque. It has been reported to be elevated in patients with ACS and to have long-term predictive value.[3]

Myeloperoxidase

MPO is released when neutrophils aggregate. This release may indicate an active inflammatory response in blood vessels. It is elevated chronically when chronic CAD is present. Also, it is increased when patients present with ACS. A multi-biomarker study has shown that MPO as a prognostic tool was dependent on the outcomes studied (cardiac death) and the demographics of the patient population enrolled.

Nourin

Nourin I is a small protein released rapidly by "stressed myocytes." It induces changes in a variety of inflammatory cytokines and attracts neutrophils. Preliminary studies have been done to attempt to validate its use.

Oxidized Low-Density Lipoprotein

Oxidized LDL has been attributed a key role in the development of atherosclerosis (see Chapter 23). Several methods have been used to measure it, but they yield potentially different data. Some have correlated malondialdehyde LDL with the development of atherosclerosis and short-term events. Direct identification with antibodies suggests that oxidized LDL may be released from vessels and may colocalize with lipoprotein a (Lp[a]) after acute events.

Placental Growth Factor

Placental growth factor is an angiogenic factor related to vascular endothelial growth factor (VEGF), which stimulates smooth muscle cells and macrophages. It also increases TNF and MCP-1. A novel assay for this analyte is thought to provide additional prognostic information on patients who present with ACS.[3]

Pregnancy-Associated Plasma Protein A

Pregnancy-associated plasma protein A (PAPP-A) is a metalloproteinase that is thought to be expressed in plaques that may be prone to rupture. Although the literature in this regard is mixed concerning its use, data suggest that heparin administration in myocardial infarction patients is associated with increased PAPP-A concentrations.

Secreted Platelet Granular Substances

Both platelet factor 4 (PF4) and beta thromboglobulin (BTG) are secreted when platelets aggregate. PF4 has a short half-life and is released by heparin. BTG is not released by heparin and has a longer half-life. Both biomarkers have been used to assess platelet aggregation.

Serum Amyloid Protein A

Serum amyloid protein A is an acute-phase protein and an apolipoprotein. It has been used with hsCRP in cross-sectional studies. It thought to be synergistic with hsCRP but is much less commonly used than the assay for hsCRP.

ST2

ST2 is a receptor protein that is a member of the IL-1 receptor family and a marker of cardiac stress. It signals the presence and severity of adverse cardiac remodeling and tissue fibrosis, which occurs in response to (1) myocardial infarction, (2) ACS, or (3) heart failure. The ST2 protein has two isoforms and is directly implicated in the progression of cardiac disease: a soluble form (referred to as soluble ST2 or sST2) and a membrane-bound receptor form (referred to as the ST2 receptor or ST2L). The ligand for ST2 is the cytokine IL-33.

Tissue Plasminogen Activator Antigen and Plasminogen Activator Inhibitor 1

Tissue plasminogen activator (t-PA) is the body's physiologic fibrinolytic activator. Plasminogen activator inhibitor 1 (PAI-1) is the endogenous inhibitor of t-PA and binds to it. Inhibition of fibrinolysis has been suggested to cause recurrent infarction. As maximal inhibition usually occurs in the early morning hours, this may explain the circadian variability of AMI. It may also be the reason that persons with diabetes have such an unstable disease, because the growth factor properties of insulin stimulate increases in PAI-1.

Unbound Free Fatty Acid

Unbound free fatty acid (uFFA) has also been touted as a marker of ischemia. Most fatty acid in plasma is bound (to proteins), and ischemia is thought to increase the small unbound fraction.

Urinary Thromboxane

Urinary thromboxane is the end metabolite of thromboxane A2, which is a measure of platelet aggregation. Urinary concentrations are elevated in patients with unstable coronary disease.

Review Questions

1. The technique of choice for measuring cTns is a(n):
   a. Photometric assay
   b. Immunoassay
   c. Potentiometric assay
   d. Amperometric assay
2. What are the names of the contractile proteins that are located in the striated muscle fibers of the heart?
   a. Natriuretic peptides
   b. Modified albumins
   c. Troponins
   d. Actin and myosin
3. Which one of the following cardiac biomarkers is important in detecting moderate to severe CHF?
   a. B-type natriuretic peptide
   b. Troponin
   c. Nourin
   d. Myoglobin
4. An oxygen-binding protein of cardiac and skeletal muscle that is thought to increase sooner than the isoform CK-2 after an AMI is:
   a. Troponin
   b. Myoglobin
   c. B-type natriuretic peptide
   d. CK
5. A protein that is involved in a number of disease processes including cancer, inflammation, and heart disease and that is expressed in the process of cardiac ventricular remodeling is:
   a. Isoprostane
   b. Phospholipase A_2
   c. Galectin-3
   d. MPO
6. The most common cause of ACS is:
   a. Myocardial ischemia due to incomplete occlusion of a coronary artery
   b. Atherosclerosis in coronary arteries
   c. Reduced outflow of blood from left side of heart
   d. Decreased output of the right side of the heart due to cardiac valve destruction
7. Which one of the following is not a requirement for an ideal cardiac biomarker?
   a. Specificity
   b. Rapid release from heart into circulation
   c. Rapid removal from circulation
   d. Sensitivity
8. Which one of the following CK isoenzymes is referred to as the "cardiac isoenzyme" because it makes up at least 10% of total CK activity in the myocardium?
   a. CK-1
   b. CK-2
   c. CK-3
   d. Total CK
9. Loss of oxygen in the form of arterial blood supply to an area of cardiac tissue is referred to as:
   a. Ischemia
   b. Infarct

   c. Necrosis

   d. Atherosclerosis

10. The condition resulting from ineffective pumping of blood to the body's tissues is referred to as:

   a. Coronary artery syndrome

   b. AMI

   c. Atable angina

   d. CHF

References

1. Apple FS. A new season for cardiac troponin assays: it's time to keep a scorecard. Clin Chem 2009;55:1303–6.

2. Apple FS, Collinson PO, IFCC Task Force on Clinical Applications of Cardiac Biomarkers. Analytical characteristics of high-sensitivity cardiac troponin assays, Clin Chem 2012;58:54–61.

3. Apple FS, Goetz JP, Jaffe AS. Cardiac function. In: Burtis CA, Ashwood ER, Bruns DE, eds. Tietz textbook of clinical chemistry and molecular diagnostics, 5th edition. St Louis: Saunders/Elsevier, 2012:1457–522.

4. Apple FS, Jesse RL, Newby LK, et al. National Academy of Clinical Biochemistry and IFCC Committee for Standardization of Markers of Cardiac Damage Laboratory Medicine Practice guidelines: analytical issues for biochemical markers of acute coronary syndromes. Clin Chem 2007;53:547–51.

5. Apple FS, Ler R, Murakami MM. Determination of 19 cardiac troponin I and T assay 99th percentile values from a common presumably healthy population. Clin Chem 2012;58:1574–81.

6. Apple FS, Panteghini M, Ravkilde J, et al. Quality specifications for B-type natriuretic peptide assays. Clin Chem 2005;51:486–93.

7. Apple FS, Quist HE, Doyle PJ, et al. Plasma 99th percentile reference limits for cardiac troponin and creatine kinase MB mass for use with European Society of Cardiology/American College of Cardiology consensus recommendations. Clin Chem 2003;49:1331–6.

8. Apple FS, Wu AHB, Jaffe AS. European Society of Cardiology and American College of Cardiology guidelines for redefinition of myocardial infarction: how to use existing assays clinically and for clinical trials. Am Heart J 2002;144:981–6.

9. Apple FS, Wu AHB, Mair J, et al. Future biomarkers for detection of ischemia and risk stratification in acute coronary syndrome. Clin Chem 2005;51:810–24.

10. Cannon CP, Brindis RG, Chaitman BR, et al. 2013 ACCF/AHA key data elements and definitions for measuring the clinical management and outcomes of patients with acute coronary syndromes and coronary artery disease. Circulation 2013;127:1052–89.

11. de Lemos JA, Drazner MH, Omland T, et al. Association of troponin T detected with a highly sensitive assay and cardiac structure and mortality risk in general population. JAMA 2010;304:2503–12.

12. Fihn SD, Gardin JM, Abrams J, et al. 2012 ACCF/AHA/ACP/AATS/PCNA/SCAI/STS Guideline for the diagnosis and management of patients with stable ischemic heart disease: a report of the American College of Cardiology Foundation/American Heart Association Task Force on Practice Guidelines, and the American College of Physicians, American Association for Thoracic Surgery, Preventive Cardiovascular Nurses Association, Society for Cardiovascular Angiography and Interventions, and Society of Thoracic Surgeons. J Am Coll Cardiol 2012;60:e44-e164; Circulation 2012;126:e354–471.

13. Fonarow GC, Adam KF, Abraham WT, et al. Risk Stratification for in-hospital mortality in acutely decompensated heart failure classification and regression tree analysis. JAMA 2005;293:581–88.

14. Goetze JP. Biochemistry of pro-B-type natriuretic peptide-derived peptides: the endocrine heart revisited. Clin Chem 2004;50:1503–10.

15. Januzzi JL, van Kimmenade R, Lainchbury J, et al. NT-proBNP testing for diagnosis and short-term prognosis in acute destabilized heart failure: an international pooled analysis of 1256 patients: the International Collaborative of NT-proBNP Study. Eur Heart J 2006;27:330–7.

16. Korley FK, Jaffe AS. Preparing the United States for high sensitivity cardiac troponin assays. J Am Coll Cardiol 2013; 61:1753–8.

17. Luckenbill KN, Christenson RH, Jaffe AS, et al. Cross reactivity of BNP, NT-proBNP, and proBNP in commercial BNP and NT-proBNP assays: preliminary observations from the IFCC Committee for Standardization of Markers of Cardiac Damage. Clin Chem 2008;54:619–21.

18. Mills NL, Churchhouse AMD, Lee KK, et al. Implementation of a sensitive troponin I assay and risk of recurrent myocardial infarction and death in patients with suspected acute coronary syndrome. JAMA 2011;305:1210–6.

19. Morrow DA, Cannon CP, Jesse RL, et al. National Academy of Clinical Biochemistry Laboratory Medicine practice guidelines: clinical characteristics and utilization of biochemical markers in acute coronary syndromes. Clin Chem 2007;53:552–74.

20. Panteghini M, Gerhardt W, Apple FS, et al. Quality specifications for cardiac troponin assays. Clin Chem Lab Med 2001;39:175–9.

21. Saenger AK, Jaffe AS. Requiem for a heavyweight: the demise of creatine kinase-MB. Circulation 2008;118:2200–6.

22. Schellenberger U, O'Rear J, Guzzetta A, et al. The precursor to B-type natriuretic peptide is an O-linked glycoprotein. Arch Biochem Biophys 2006;451:160–6.

23. Smith SC Jr, Allen J, Blair SN, et al. AHA/ACC guidelines for secondary prevention for patients with coronary and other atherosclerotic vascular disease: 2006 update: endorsed by the National Heart, Lung, and Blood Institute. Circulation 2006;113:2363–72.

24. Thygesen K, Alpert JS, Jaffe AS, et al. Third universal definition of myocardial infarction. J Am Coll Cardiol 2012;60:1581–98.

25. Thygesen K, Alpert JS, White HD. Universal definition of myocardial infarction. Eur Heart J 2007;28:2525–38.

26. World Health Organization: Classifications: the WHO family of international classifications. http://www.who.int/classifications/en/. Accessed on September 9, 2013.

Kidney Disease[*]

Michael P. Delaney, B.Sc., M.D., F.R.C.P., Christopher P. Price, Ph.D., F.R.C.Path., and Edmund J. Lamb, Ph.D., F.R.C.Path.

Objectives

1. Define the following:

Bence-Jones protein	Juxtaglomerular apparatus
Clearance	Micturition
Cystatin-C	Nephrolithiasis
Diabetes insipidus (DI)	Nephron
Diabetic nephropathy	Pyelonephritis
Dialysis	Renal pelvis
Diuretic	Renal replacement therapy
Glomerulus	(RRT)
Glomerular filtration rate	Ureter
(GFR)	Urine

2. Describe the following components of the renal system, including structure, function, contribution to urine formation and clinical significance:

Bladder	Juxtaglomerular apparatus
Bowman capsule	Kidneys
Collecting tubules	Loop of Henle
Distal convoluted tubule	Nephron
Glomerulus	Proximal convoluted tubule

3. State the significance of kidney blood supply in the formation of urine within the structure of the glomerulus; list the arteries that form the glomerular capillary bed.

4. List and describe the three major functions of the kidneys, including processes involved, laboratory analytes affected in each process, and how each function is controlled.

5. Describe glomerular filtration rate (GFR) and clearance in terms of clinical usefulness and effects of renal disease and age on each process; list the markers used to assess clearance; state and calculate the formula used to determine GFR.

6. Describe the renal handling of electrolytes and water, including normal physiology, hormones involved, and effect of disease on each function.

7. List and describe the proteins found in urine including their characteristics, how they are affected in disease and laboratory methods of protein measurement.

8. Discuss the following conditions including the causes (such as, drugs and toxins), symptoms, acid-base disturbances (if any), laboratory methods used to assess, and pertinent laboratory results obtained:

Acute kidney injury (AKI)	Glomerular disease
Acute nephritic syndrome	Interstitial nephritis
Acute tubular necrosis (ATN)	Nephrotic syndrome
Chronic kidney disease (CKD)	Pyelonephritis
Diabetes insipidus (DI)	Renal tubular acidoses
End-stage renal disease	(RTAs)
(ESRD) (including uremic	Uremic syndrome
syndrome)	Urinary tract obstruction

9. Describe two options for renal replacement therapy (RRT), including the clinical need for the therapy and laboratory assessment of each therapy.

10. Evaluate and analyze case studies related to renal disease and laboratory analysis of renal disease.

[*]We are grateful for data supplied by the US Renal Data System (USRDS). Interpretation and reporting of these data are the responsibility of the authors and in no way should be seen as an official policy or interpretation of the US government. We are also grateful for data supplied by the UK Renal Registry. Interpretation and reporting of these data are the responsibility of the authors and in no way should be seen as an official policy or interpretation of the UK Renal Registry.

Key Words and Definitions

Acidosis Accumulation of acid and hydrogen ions or depletion of the alkaline reserve (bicarbonate content) in the blood and body tissues.

Acute kidney injury (AKI) A rapid decline in kidney function that occurs over hours and days.

Acute nephritic syndrome The sudden onset of hematuria, proteinuria, diminished urine production, azotemia, hypertension, and edema.

Acute tubular necrosis (ATN) Acute renal failure with mild to severe damage or necrosis of tubule cells.

Antidiuretic hormone (ADH; vasopressin) An octapeptide hormone formed by the neuronal cells of the hypothalamic nuclei and stored in the posterior lobe of the pituitary gland (neurohypophysis). It has both antidiuretic and vasopressor actions.

Azotemia An excess of urea or other nitrogenous compounds in the blood.

Bartter syndrome Hypertrophy and hyperplasia of the juxtaglomerular cells, producing hypokalemic alkalosis and hyperaldosteronism.

Bence-Jones protein An abnormal plasma or urinary protein, consisting of monoclonal immunoglobulin light chains, excreted in some neoplastic diseases. It is a characteristic protein found in the urine of most patients with multiple myeloma.

Bowman capsule The double-walled globular kidney structure that forms the beginning of a renal tubule and surrounds the glomerulus.

Chronic kidney disease (CKD) Abnormalities of kidney structure or function, present for greater than 3 months, with implications for health.

Continuous ambulatory peritoneal dialysis (CAPD) A common method of peritoneal dialysis, involving the continuous presence of dialysis solution in the peritoneal cavity.

Dent disease Tubulopathy of the proximal renal tubules with low molecular weight proteinuria, hypercalciuria, hypokalemia, nephrocalcinosis, rickets, and progressive renal failure.

Diabetes insipidus (DI) A diabetic (defined as the excessive production of urine) disorder due either to insufficient synthesis of antidiuretic hormone (ADH) or defective ADH receptors or endorgan resistance to its action. This results in failure of tubular reabsorption of water in the kidney.

Diabetic nephropathy The nephropathy that commonly accompanies later stages of diabetes mellitus; it begins with hyperfiltration, renal hypertrophy, albuminuria, and hypertension.

Dialysis The removal of certain elements from the blood by virtue of the difference in the rates of their diffusion through a semipermeable membrane, for example, by means of a hemodialysis (HD) machine or filter.

End-stage renal disease (ESRD) A condition where renal function is inadequate to support life.

Erythropoietin A glycoprotein hormone secreted chiefly by the kidney in the adult; it increases production of red blood cells.

Fanconi syndrome A rare recessive disorder with a poor prognosis, characterized by pancytopenia, bone marrow hypoplasia, and patchy brown skin and multiple congenital anomalies of the musculoskeletal and genitourinary systems.

Gitelman syndrome A syndrome of hypertrophy of juxtaglomerular cells similar to Bartter syndrome but with hypocalciuria and hypomagnesemia.

Glomerular filtration rate (GFR) The rate in milliliters per minute at which small molecules are filtered through the kidney's glomeruli. It is a measure of the number of functioning nephrons.

Glomerulonephritis Nephritis accompanied by inflammation of the capillary loops of the glomeruli of the kidney. It occurs in acute, subacute, and chronic forms.

Glomerulus A tuft of blood vessels found in each nephron of the kidney that are involved in the filtration of the blood.

Hematuria Blood in the urine.

Hemodiafiltration A type of hemofiltration with a dialytic component added. With it, blood flow is accelerated to twice that of conventional dialysis.

Hypertension A medical condition characterized by high arterial blood pressure.

IgA nephropathy A common, chronic form of glomerulonephritis marked by hematuria and proteinuria and by deposits of immunoglobulin A in the mesangial areas of the renal glomeruli.

Interstitial nephritis Primary or secondary disease of the renal interstitial tissue.

Juxtaglomerular apparatus (JGA) A complex in the kidney whose function is the autoregulation of the glomerular filtration rate.

Liddle syndrome A rare autosomal dominant syndrome resulting from epithelial sodium channel mutations that lead to abnormally increased channel function.

Lithotripsy The crushing of a calculus within the urinary system or gallbladder, followed at once by the washing out of the fragments; it is done either surgically or by several different noninvasive methods.

Loop of Henle The U-shaped part of the renal tubule, extending through the medulla from the end of the proximal convoluted tubule to the beginning of the distal convoluted tubule.

Metabolic acidosis Any of the various kinds of acidosis in which the acid-base status of the body shifts toward the acid side because of loss of base or retention of acids other than carbonic acid.

Nephritis Inflammation of the kidney with focal or diffuse proliferation or destructive processes that may involve the glomerulus, tubule, or interstitial renal tissue.

Nephrolithiasis A condition marked by the presence of renal calculi (stones).

Nephron The anatomical and functional unit of the kidney, consisting of the (1) renal corpuscle, (2) proximal convoluted tubule, (3) descending and ascending limbs of loop of Henle, (4) distal convoluted tubule, and (5) collecting tubule.

Nephrotic syndrome General name for a group of diseases involving defective kidney glomeruli, characterized by massive proteinuria and lipiduria with varying degrees of edema, hypoalbuminemia, and hyperlipidemia.

Obstructive uropathy Uropathy resulting from an obstruction in the tract.

Oliguria Diminished urine production and excretion.

Key Words and Definitions—cont'd

Peritoneal dialysis (PD) Diffusion of solutes and convection of fluid through the peritoneal membrane. The dialyzing solution is introduced into and removed from the peritoneal cavity as either a continuous or an intermittent procedure.

Polycystic kidney disease The most common renal cystic condition, with deterioration of renal function.

Polyuria The passage of a large volume of urine in a given period

Proteinuria Excessive serum proteins in the urine, such as in renal disease, after strenuous exercise, and with dehydration.

Pseudohypoaldosteronism type 1 A hereditary disorder of infancy characterized by severe salt wasting, failure to thrive, and other signs of aldosterone deficiency.

Pyelonephritis An inflammation of the kidney and its pelvis as a result of infection.

Rapidly progressive glomerulonephritis (RPGN) Acute glomerulonephritis marked by a rapid progression to end-stage renal disease.

Renal clearance The volume of plasma from which a given substance is completely cleared by the kidneys per unit of time.

Renal replacement therapy (RRT) Any treatment that replaces kidney function, including dialysis and transplantation.

Renal tubular acidosis (RTA) A variety of metabolic acidosis resulting from impairment of renal function.

Renin An enzyme of the hydrolase class that catalyzes cleavage of the leucine-leucine bond in angiotensinogen to generate angiotensin I

Toxic nephropathy Kidney damage caused by the effects of a nephrotoxin.

Uremia An excess in the blood of urea, creatinine, and other nitrogenous end products of protein and amino acid metabolism; also referred to as *azotemia*.

Uremic syndrome The spectrum of symptoms accompanying uremia.

X-linked hypophosphatemia A form of familial hypophosphatemic rickets, with X-linked dominant inheritance.

The kidneys play a central role in the homeostatic mechanisms of the human body. Reduced renal function strongly correlates with increasing morbidity and mortality. The basic anatomy and physiology of the kidneys are described as a foundation to understanding the pathophysiology of disease and the rationale for diagnostic and management strategies in kidney disease. The key analytical methods employed during the investigation of kidney disease are discussed in Chapter 21.

Anatomy

The kidneys are a paired organ system located in the lumbar region. Their function is to (1) filter the blood and excrete the end-products of body metabolism in the form of urine; (2) regulate the concentrations of (a) hydrogen, (b) sodium, (c) potassium, (d) phosphate, and (e) other ions in the extracellular fluid; and (3) produce hormones in an adult, each kidney is about 12 cm long and weighs about 150 g in men and 135 g in women. A kidney is of a characteristic bean shape through which pass the (1) vessels, (2) nerves, and (3) ureter (Figure 35-1).

Nephron

The functional unit of the kidney is the **nephron**. Each kidney may contain up to 1 million nephrons. The nephron consists of a (1) glomerulus, (2) proximal tubule, (3) **loop of Henle**, (4) distal tubule, and (5) collecting duct (Figure 35-2). The collecting ducts ultimately combine to develop into the renal calyces, where the urine collects before passing along the ureter and into the bladder. The kidney is divided into several lobes. The cortex is the outer, darker region of each lobe and consists of most of the glomeruli and the proximal and distal tubules. It surrounds a paler inner region, the medulla, which is further divided into a number of conical areas known as the renal pyramids, the apex of which extends toward the renal

pelvis, forming papillae. Medullary rays are visible striations in the renal pyramids, which connect the kidney cortex with the medulla. They are composed of (1) descending (straight proximal) and (2) ascending (straight distal) thick limbs of Henle, and (3) collecting ducts and associated blood vessels

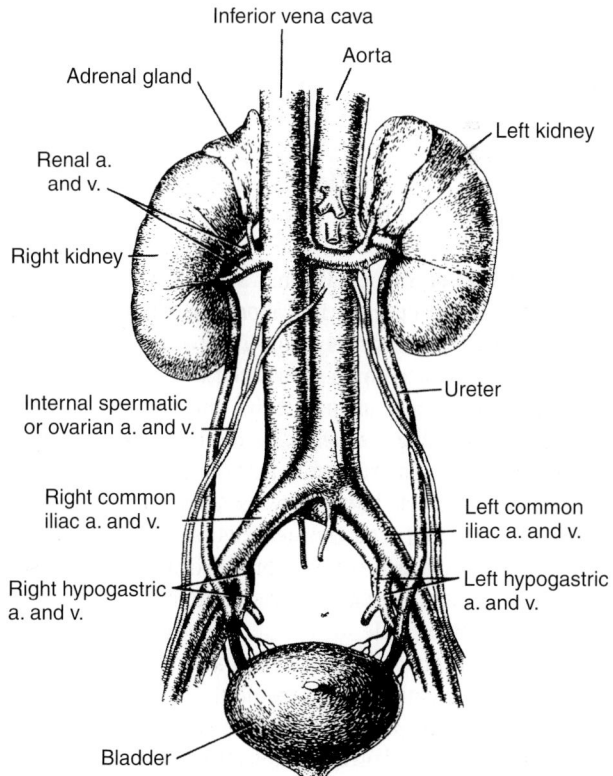

Figure 35-1 The vascular and anatomical relationships of the kidneys in humans. *(From Leaf A, Cotran RS. Renal pathophysiology, 3rd edition. Oxford: Oxford University Press, 1985. By permission of Oxford University Press, Inc.)*

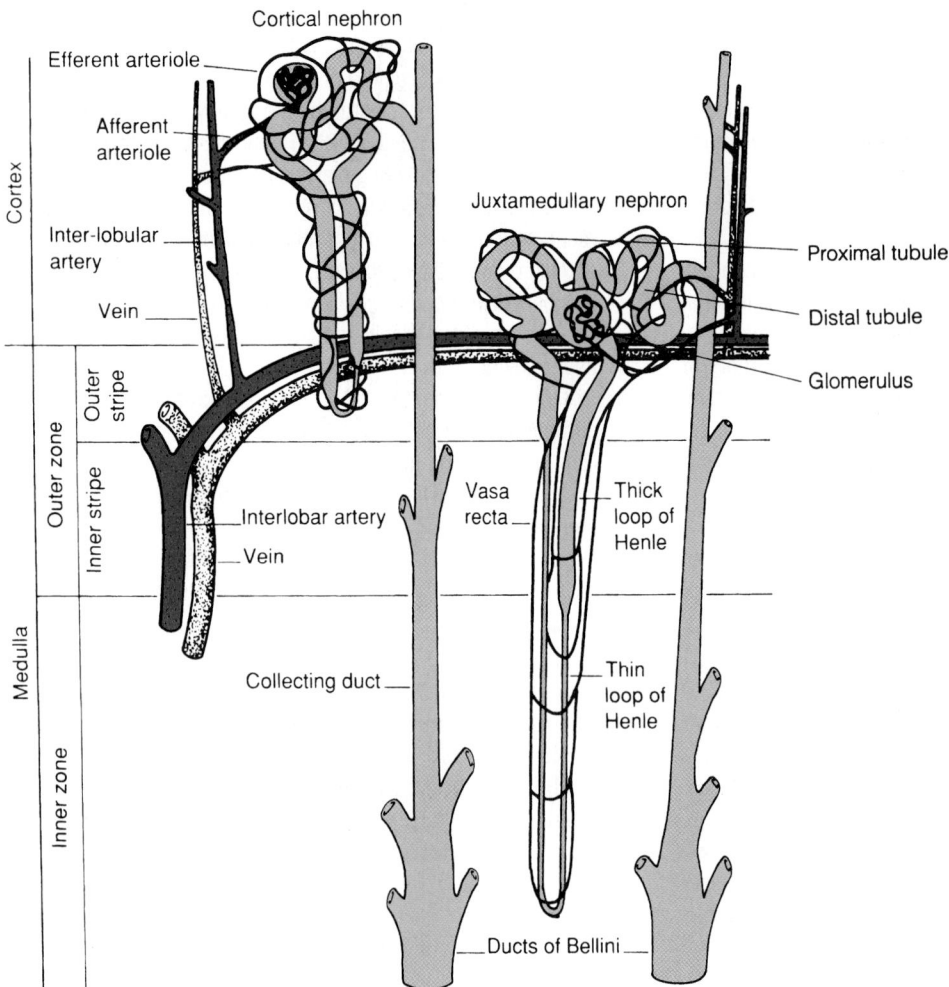

Figure 35-2 Diagrammatic representation of the nephron, the functional unit of the kidney, illustrating the anatomical and vascular arrangements. *(From Pitts RF. Physiology of the kidney and body fluids, 3rd edition. Chicago: Year Book Medical Publishers, 1974.)*

(the vasa recta). The central hilus is where blood vessels, lymphatics, and the renal pelvis (containing the ureter) join the kidney.

The **glomerulus** is formed from a specialized capillary network. Each capillary develops into approximately 40 glomerular loops around 200 μm in size and consisting of a variety of different cell types supported on a specialized basement membrane (see Figure 35-2). There are endothelial and epithelial cells that act in concert with the specialized glomerular basement membrane to form the glomerular filtration barrier. The glomerular capillaries are supported by a network of mesangial cells and mesangial matrix that act as connective tissue for the glomerular apparatus. The basement membrane forms the main size-discriminant barrier to protein passage into the tubular lumen.

The **Bowman capsule** forms the beginning of the tightly coiled, proximal convoluted tubule (pars convoluta), which on its progress toward the renal medulla becomes straightened and is then called the pars recta. The human proximal tubule is about 15 mm long. The proximal tubule is the most metabolically active part of the nephron, facilitating the reabsorption of 60% to 80% of the glomerular filtrate volume—including 70% of the filtered load of (1) sodium and (2) chloride, most of the (3) potassium, (4) glucose, (5) bicarbonate, (6) phosphate,

and (7) sulfate—and secreting 90% of the (8) hydrogen ion excreted by the kidney.

The pars recta drains into the descending thin limb of the loop of Henle, which after passing through a hairpin loop becomes first the ascending thin limb and then the thick ascending limb. At the end of the thick ascending limb, there is a cluster of cells known as the *macula densa* (Figure 35-3). The main role of the loop of Henle is to provide the ability to generate a concentrated urine, hypertonic with respect to plasma.

The cells forming the distal tubule of the nephron start at the macula densa and extend to the first fusion with other tubules to form the collecting ducts. Sodium chloride reabsorption and some potassium and hydrogen ion excretion occur at this site.

The collecting ducts are formed from approximately six distal tubules. These are successively joined by other tubules to form ducts of Bellini, which ultimately drain into a renal calyx.

Juxtaglomerular Apparatus

Where the ascending loop of Henle passes very close to the Bowman capsule of its own nephron, the cells of the tubule and the afferent arteriole show regional specialization (see Figure 35-3). The tubule forms the macula densa and the

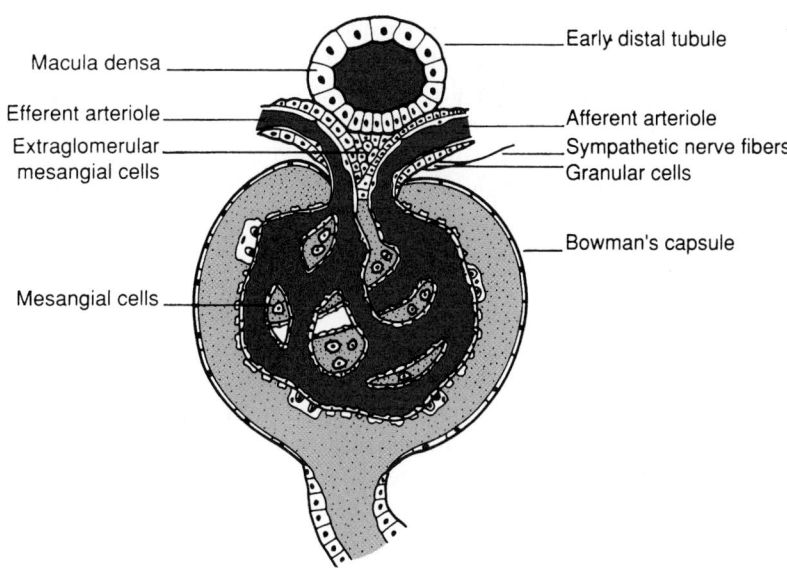

Figure 35-3 The juxtaglomerular apparatus. The beginning of the distal tubule (i.e., where the loop of Henle reenters the cortex) lies very close to the afferent and efferent arterioles, and the cells of both the afferent arteriole and the tubule show specialization. The cells of the afferent arteriole are thickened granular (juxtaglomerular) cells and are innervated by sympathetic nerve fibers. The mesangial cells are irregularly shaped and contain filaments of contractile proteins. Identical cells are found just outside the glomerulus and are termed extraglomerular mesangial cells or Goormaghtigh cells. *(From Lote CJ. Principles of renal physiology, 4th edition. London: Kluwer Academic Publishers, 2000. With kind permission of Springer Science and Business Media.)*

arteriolar cells are filled with granules (containing **renin**) and are innervated with sympathetic nerve fibers. This area is called the **juxtaglomerular apparatus (JGA)**. The JGA plays an important part in maintaining systemic blood pressure through regulation of the circulating intravascular blood volume and sodium concentration. The proteolytic enzyme renin is released primarily in response to decreased afferent arteriolar pressure and decreased intraluminal sodium delivery to the macula densa. Renin release from the macula densa is also influenced by renal cortical prostaglandins (predominantly PGI_2) and the sympathetic nervous system. The released renin then acts on the plasma protein angiotensinogen to generate angiotensin I. This is converted in the lungs by angiotensin converting enzyme (ACE) to the potent vasoconstrictor and stimulator of aldosterone release, angiotensin II (AII). The vasoconstriction and aldosterone release (with increased distal tubular sodium retention) act in concert with the other action of AII, to increase the release of **antidiuretic hormone (ADH, vasopressin)** and to increase proximal tubular sodium reabsorption, intravascular volume, and pressure. AII also has an inhibitory effect on renin release as part of a negative feedback loop.

Blood Supply

The renal artery divides into posterior and anterior elements, which then divide into interlobar, arcuate, interlobular, and ultimately into the afferent arterioles, which expand into the capillary bed that forms the glomerulus (see Figure 35-2). These capillaries then rejoin to form the efferent arteriole, which then forms the capillary plexuses and the elongated vessels (the vasa recta). These pass around the remaining parts of the (1) nephron, (2) proximal and distal tubules, (3) loop of Henle, and (4) collecting duct, providing oxygen and nutrients and removing ions, molecules, and water, which are reabsorbed by the nephron. The efferent arteriole then merges with renal venules to form the renal veins, which emerge into the inferior vena cava. The complex architecture of the intrarenal

vascular tree is ordered in three dimensions in a characteristic arrangement that probably serves to distribute the blood pressure and flow appropriately to the glomeruli.

In the adult, the kidneys receive approximately 25% of the cardiac output. In the newborn infant, however, it is 5%, only reaching adult proportions by the end of the first year of life. About 90% of this blood flow supplies the renal cortex, maintaining the highly active tubular cells. The maintenance of renal blood flow is essential to renal function, and there is a complex array of intrarenal regulatory mechanisms that ensure that it is maintained across a wide range of systemic blood pressures. The renal glomerular perfusion pressure is independent of the systemic pressure between 90 and 200 mm Hg, being maintained at a constant 45 mm Hg.

Kidney Function

The main biological functions of the kidneys are (1) excretion, (2) homeostatic regulation, and (3) endocrine. The kidneys integrate these functions to maintain homeostasis and regulate the internal milieu.

Excretory Function

Urine is (1) excreted by the kidneys, (2) passed through the ureters, (3) stored in the bladder, and (4) discharged through the urethra. In health, it (1) is sterile and clear, (2) has an amber color, (3) has a slightly acidic pH (5.0 to 6.0), and (4) has a characteristic odor, and specific gravity of about 1.024. In addition to dissolved compounds, it contains a number of (1) cellular fragments, (2) complete cells, (3) proteinaceous casts, and (4) crystals (formed elements). Changes in these formed elements are studied using urine microscopy.

Urination, also termed *micturition,* is the discharge of urine. In normal adults, adequate homeostasis is maintained with a urine output of about 500 mL/day. Alterations in urinary output are described as *anuria* (<100 mL/day), **oliguria** (<400 mL/day), or **polyuria** (>3 L/day or 50 mL/kg body weight/day). The most common disorder of urination is altered frequency, which may be associated with increased urinary volume or with partial urinary tract obstruction (e.g., in prostatic hypertrophy).

The first step in urine formation is filtration of plasma water at the glomeruli. A net filtration pressure of about 17 mm Hg in the capillary bed of the tuft drives the ultrafiltrate through the glomerular membrane. Each nephron produces about 100 μL of ultrafiltrate per day. Overall, approximately 170 to 200 L of ultrafiltrate pass through the glomeruli in 24 hours. In the passage of ultrafiltrate through the tubules, reabsorption of solutes and water in various regions of the tubules reduces the total urine volume, which typically varies from 0.4 to 2 L/day.

Transport of solutes and water occurs both across and between the epithelial cells that line the renal tubules. Transport is both active (energy requiring) and passive. Direct coupling of adenosine triphosphate (ATP) hydrolysis is an example of an active transport process. The most important of these in the nephron is Na^+,K^+-ATPase, which is located on the basolateral membranes of the tubuloepithelial cells. This enzymatic transporter accounts for much of renal oxygen consumption and drives more than 99% of renal sodium reabsorption.

Renal epithelial cell membranes also contain proteins that act as ion channels. For example, there is one for sodium that is closed by amiloride and modulated by hormones such as atrial natriuretic peptide (ANP). Ion channels enable much faster rates of transport than ATPases, but are relatively fewer in number—approximately 100 sodium and chloride channels as against 10^7 Na^+,K^+-ATPase molecules per cell.

In the tubules, the solute composition of the ultrafiltrate is altered by the processes of reabsorption and secretion, so the urine excreted may have a very different composition from that of the original filtrate. Different regions of the tubule have been shown to specialize in certain functions. For example, in the proximal tubule, 60% to 80% of the ultrafiltrate is reabsorbed in an obligatory fashion, along with (1) sodium, (2) chloride, (3) bicarbonate, (4) calcium, (5) phosphate, (6) sulfate, and (7) other ions. Glucose is virtually completely reabsorbed, predominantly in the proximal tubule by a passive process. Uric acid is also reabsorbed in the proximal tubule by a passive sodium-dependent mechanism, but there is also an active secretory mechanism.

In the loop of Henle, chloride and more sodium without water are reabsorbed, generating dilute urine. Water reabsorption in the more distal tubules and collecting ducts is then regulated by hypothalamic ADH. In the distal tubule, secretion is the prominent activity with (1) organic, (2) potassium, and (3) hydrogen ions being transported from the blood in the efferent arteriole into the tubular fluid. It is also this region that secretes hydrogen ions and reabsorbs sodium and bicarbonate to aid in acid-base regulation. Paracellular (between cell) movement is driven predominantly by concentration, osmotic, or electrical gradients.

Regulatory Function

The regulatory function of the kidneys has a major role in homeostasis. The mechanisms of differential reabsorption and

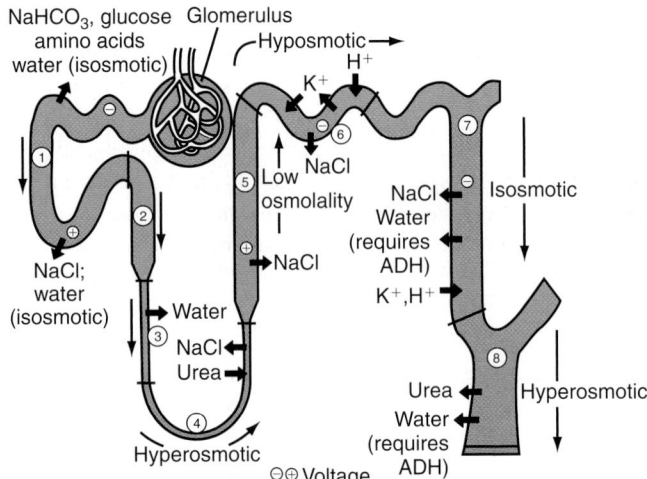

Figure 35-4 Countercurrent multiplication mechanism: schematic representation of the principal processes of transport in the nephron. In the convoluted portion of the proximal tubule *(1)*, salts and water are reabsorbed at high rates in isotonic proportions. Bulk reabsorption of most of the filtrate (65% to 70%) and virtually complete reabsorption of glucose, amino acids, and bicarbonate take place in this segment. In the pars recta *(2)*, organic acids are secreted and continuous reabsorption of sodium chloride takes place. The loop of Henle comprises three segments: the thin descending *(3)* and ascending *(4)* limbs and the thick ascending limb *(5)*. The fluid becomes hyperosmotic, because of water abstraction, as it flows toward the bend of the loop, and hyposmotic, because of sodium chloride reabsorption, as it flows toward the distal convoluted tubule *(6)*. Active sodium reabsorption occurs in the distal convoluted tubule and in the cortical collecting tubule *(7)*. This latter segment is water-impermeable in the absence of ADH, and the reabsorption of sodium in this segment is increased by aldosterone. The collecting duct *(8)* allows equilibration of water with the hyperosmotic interstitium when ADH is present. *(From Burg MB. The nephron in transport of sodium, amino acids, and glucose. Hosp Pract 1978;13:100. Adapted from a drawing by A. Iselin.)*

secretion, located in the tubule of a nephron, are the effectors of regulation. The mechanisms operate under a complex system of control in which both extrarenal and intrarenal humoral factors participate.

Electrolyte Homeostasis

The proximal convoluted tubule is predominantly concerned with reabsorption (Figure 35-4). Water reabsorption in the proximal convoluted tubule is termed "obligatory" because its volume is related to the heavy load of solutes being returned to the blood in the efferent arteriole. The amount of bicarbonate reabsorption is related to the **glomerular filtration rate (GFR)** and the hydrogen ion secretory rate. The amount of phosphate reabsorption is controlled in part by (1) plasma calcium concentration and (2) the effect of parathyroid hormone (PTH) on the tubular cells. Normally, the high-threshold substances such as glucose and, to a great extent, amino acids are reabsorbed here by means of specific intracellular active transport systems. Uric acid may be either reabsorbed or secreted in the proximal convoluted tubule by a two-way carrier-mediated process.

In the ascending limb of the loop of Henle, 20% to 25% of filtered sodium is reabsorbed without concomitant reabsorption of water. This process generates dilute urine with an osmolality of 100 to 150 mOsm/kg of water and helps establish the corticomedullary osmotic gradient. The resulting hypertonicity of the interstitium is important in the pathogenesis of renal infections because the hypertonic environment interferes with leukocyte function. Subsequent water reabsorption is regulated by ADH. The distal tubule is functionally the most active region of the nephron for the homeostatic regulation of plasma electrolytes and plasma acid-base concentrations. Here a combination of secretion and reabsorption takes place among Na^+, K^+, and H^+. Although excess plasma hydrogen ions are secreted all along the tubule, it is in the distal tubule that exchange of H^+ for Na^+ (which is reabsorbed) fine tunes the balance between H^+ loss and retention (see Chapter 36). Potassium ions are also secreted in the distal tubule. The aldosterone produced by the adrenal gland is a potent modulator of Na^+ reabsorption in the distal tubule, particularly when the need arises to conserve Na^+. Production of aldosterone in the adrenal cortex is stimulated by the renin-angiotensin system and by high plasma potassium concentration. Renal secretion of renin is complex, but is at least partly regulated by renal perfusion and plasma sodium concentration. Both inadequate perfusion and a low concentration of plasma sodium stimulate renin secretion. Organic anions, such as acetoacetate and β-hydroxybutyrate, also consume H^+ as they are eliminated in part in their nondissociated acid form. When H^+ must be conserved to maintain blood pH, distal tubule cells (1) reduce the secretion of H^+, (2) reduce NH_4^+ generation, (3) reduce Na^+-H^+ exchange, and (4) increase bicarbonate excretion. The net effect is a reduction in plasma bicarbonate and restoration of normal blood pH.

Water Homeostasis

The production of glomerular filtrate normally amounts to about 180 L/day. The unique physiology of the kidney enables approximately 99% of this to be reabsorbed in the production of urine with variable osmolality: between 50 and 1400 mOsmol/kg H_2O at extremes of water intake. Different segments of the nephron show differing permeability to water, enabling the body to both retain water and produce urine of variable concentration. Approximately (1) 70% of the water content of the tubular fluid is reabsorbed in the proximal tubule, (2) 5% in the loop of Henle, (3) 10% in the distal tubule, and (4) the remainder in the collecting ducts.

Water reabsorption occurs both isosmotically, in association with electrolyte reabsorption in the proximal tubule, and differentially, in the (1) loop of Henle, (2) distal tubule, and (3) collecting duct in response to the action of the nonapeptide ADH. Absorption of water depends on the driving force for water reabsorption (predominantly active sodium transport) and the osmotic equilibration of water across the tubular epithelium. The generation of concentrated urine depends upon medullary hyperosmolality, which in turn requires low water permeability in some kidney segments (ascending limb of the loop of Henle). In other kidney segments there is a requirement for high water permeability. This difference in permeability and the need for hormonal control is largely caused by the differential expression along the nephron of a family of proteins known as the aquaporins (AQP), which act as water channels.

Urinary concentration is predominantly achieved by countercurrent multiplication in the loop of Henle (see Figure 35-4). Although the descending thin limb is very permeable to water, the ascending limb and the collecting duct are not (the collecting ducts are also poorly permeable to urea). The fluid entering the loop of Henle is isotonic to plasma but is hypotonic on leaving it. The ascending limb has active sodium reabsorption driven by Na^+, K^+-ATPase with electroneutralizing transport of chloride, a combined process that is inhibited by the so-called loop diuretics (e.g., furosemide). In this section of the nephron, sodium reabsorption is not accompanied by water, creating a hypertonic medullary interstitium and facilitating water reabsorption from the anatomically adjacent descending limb. The descending limb cells are permeable to sodium chloride, which is cycled from the descending limb back to the ascending limb. The continuous flow along the loop generates an osmotic gradient at the tip of the loop that can reach 1400 mOsmol/kg/H_2O. The regulation of ADH excretion is of vital importance to fluid homeostasis. The normal plasma osmolality is maintained very tightly between 280 and 290 mOsmol/kg H_2O and is regulated by means of specific osmoreceptors found in the anterior hypothalamus. These receptors modulate the release of ADH and also affect thirst. ADH release may also be stimulated by (1) hypotension, (2) hypovolemia, and (3) vomiting independently of osmoregulation.

Endocrine Function

The endocrine functions of the kidneys may be regarded either as (1) primary, because the kidneys are endocrine organs producing hormones, or (2) secondary, because the kidneys are a site of action for hormones produced or activated elsewhere. In addition, the kidneys are a site of degradation for hormones, such as insulin and aldosterone. In their primary endocrine function, the kidneys produce (1) **erythropoietin** (EPO), (2) prostaglandins and thromboxanes, (3) renin, and (4) 1,25(OH)$_2$ vitamin D$_3$.

Erythropoietin

EPO is a glycoprotein hormone secreted chiefly by the kidney in the adult and by the liver in the fetus that acts on the bone marrow cells to stimulate erythropoiesis. It is an α-globulin having a molecular weight of 38 kDa. Physiologically, the kidneys sense a reduction in O_2 delivery to tissue by blood and release EPO, thereby stimulating the bone marrow to produce more red blood cells (RBCs). Conversely, with a surplus of O_2 in blood traversing the kidneys, as in some forms of polycythemia, the release of EPO into blood is diminished. The use of recombinant human erythropoietin (rhEPO, Epoetin) in the management of anemia of kidney disease is discussed later.

Prostaglandins and Thromboxanes

Prostaglandins and thromboxanes are synthesized from arachidonic acid by the cyclooxygenase enzyme system (see Chapter 23). This system is present in many parts of the kidneys. The predominant metabolite of its vascular endothelial activity is prostacyclin (PGI_2). Prostaglandin E_2 (PGE_2) appears to be the major metabolite of mesangial and tubular cells. The production and activity of these biologically active compounds have an important role in regulating the physiological action of other hormones on (1) renal vascular tone, (2) mesangial contractility, and (3) tubular processing of salt and water.

Renin

Renin is produced within the juxtaglomerular cells after processing and cleavage of prorenin, which is produced in the liver. Increased production of renin results in formation of angiotensin II in the liver, which is a powerful intrarenal vasoconstrictor and also a key stimulus of aldosterone release from zona glomerulosa cells in the adrenal glands. The net effect is (1) systemic vasoconstriction, (2) intrarenal vasoconstriction, and (3) increased aldosterone release. Aldosterone controls salt and water balance in the kidney. Its effect is predominantly on the distal tubular network, effecting an increase in sodium reabsorption in exchange for potassium.

1,25(OH$_2$) Vitamin D$_3$

The kidneys are primarily responsible for producing 1,25(OH$_2$) vitamin D_3 from 25-hydroxycholecalciferol as a result of the action of the enzyme 25-hydroxycholecalciferol 1α-hydroxylase found in proximal tubular epithelial cells. The regulation of this system is discussed in Chapter 39.

Kidney Physiology

The (1) GFR, (2) renal blood flow, and (3) glomerular permeability are important physiological components of renal function.

Glomerular Filtration Rate

The GFR is considered to be a reliable measure of the functional capacity of the kidneys and is often thought of as indicative of the number of functioning nephrons. As a physiological measurement, it has proved to be a useful marker of changes in overall renal function. The rate of formation of the glomerular filtrate depends upon the balance between hydrostatic and oncotic forces along the afferent arteriole and across the glomerular filter. The net pressure difference must be sufficient not only to drive filtration across the glomerular filtration barrier but also to drive the ultrafiltrate along the tubules against their inherent resistance to flow. In the absence of sufficient pressure, the lumina of the tubules will collapse.

A decrease in GFR precedes kidney failure in all forms of progressive disease. Different pathological kidney conditions have been known to progress to (1) **end-stage renal disease (ESRD)** and (2) **dialysis** dependency at rates varying from weeks to several decades. The symptoms accompanying progressive kidney disease and their correlation with falling GFR are influenced by this rate of progression. Measuring GFR in established disease is useful in (1) targeting treatment, (2) monitoring progression, and (3) predicting when **renal replacement therapy (RRT)** will be required and (4) as a guide to dosage of drugs excreted by the kidneys to prevent potential drug toxicity. A number of methods are used to measure the GFR; most involve the kidneys' ability to clear either an exogenous or endogenous marker.

The Concept of Renal Clearance

GFR measurements may be based on either the urinary or plasma clearance of a marker. The **renal clearance** of a substance is defined as "the volume of plasma from which the substance is completely cleared by the kidneys per unit of time." For a substance (S) to be used to measure renal clearance, it must be (1) in stable concentration in the plasma; (2) physiologically inert; (3) freely filtered at the glomerulus; (4) neither secreted; (5) neither reabsorbed; (6) neither synthesized; and (7) not metabolized by the kidney. If a substance possesses these qualities, then the amount of that substance filtered at the glomerulus is equal to the amount excreted in the urine. The amount of S filtered at the glomerulus is equal to the GFR multiplied by plasma S concentration: GFR × [P_S]. The amount of S excreted equals the urine S concentration (U_S) multiplied by the urinary flow rate (V, volume excreted per unit of time).

Since filtered S = excreted S, then

$$GFR \times [P_S] = [U_S] \times V \qquad (1)$$
$$GFR = ([U_S] \times V) / [P_S] \qquad (2)$$

where GFR = clearance in units of milliliters of plasma cleared of a substance per minute

[U_S] = urinary concentration of the substance
V = volumetric flow rate of urine in milliliters per minute
[P_S] = plasma concentration of the substance

The term ($[U_S] \times V)/[P_S]$ is defined as the clearance of substance S and is an accurate estimate of GFR providing the aforementioned criteria are satisfied. Inulin satisfies these criteria and has long been regarded as the most accurate estimate of GFR (see later). Kidney size and GFR are roughly proportional to body size. It is conventional therefore to adjust clearance estimates to a standard body surface area (BSA) of 1.73 m^2.

Markers Used

A variety of exogenous and endogenous markers have been used to estimate clearance (Table 35-1). Measurement of clearance may require accurate measurements of both plasma and urinary concentrations of the marker used plus a reliable urine collection. For a reliable plasma measurement, the substance must have reached a steady-state concentration and not be rapidly changing. For a reliable urine collection (1) the urine flow must be adequate (several mL/min), (2) the collection

TABLE 35-1 Markers Used to Measure Glomerular Filtration Rate

Hierarchy	Marker	Advantages	Disadvantages
Gold standard	Inulin (sinistrin) continuous infusion urinary clearance method	Gold standard	Exogenous
Silver standard	Inulin (sinistrin) single bolus plasma clearance method		Time-consuming Requires a timed urine collection Poor specificity of analysis Extrarenal clearance = 0.083 mL/min/kg Exogenous
	^{51}Cr-EDTA	Radioisotopic (simple measurement) Close correlation with inulin clearance	Time-consuming Poor specificity of analysis Extrarenal clearance = 0.083 mL/min/kg Exogenous Radioisotopic (risks of ionizing radiation) Time-consuming Extrarenal clearance = 0.079 mL/min/kg ^{51}Cr less readily available than ^{99m}Tc
	^{99m}Tc-DTPA	Radioisotopic (simple measurement) Has been used for gamma camera imaging	Exogenous Radioisotopic (risks of ionizing radiation) Time-consuming Protein binding
	^{125}I-iothalamate	Radioisotopic (simple measurement)	Exogenous Radioisotopic (risks of ionizing radiation) Not available in all countries Reports of allergic reactions
	Iohexol	Nonradioisotopic	Exogenous Extrarenal clearance = 0.087 mL/min/kg Reports of allergic reactions
Bronze standard	Creatinine	Endogenous Inexpensive Is used to generate GFR from formula (e.g., MDRD Study)	Poor sensitivity and specificity
	Cystatin C	Not secreted/reabsorbed Constitutively expressed More sensitive and specific than creatinine	Influence of thyroid function
Of uncertain clinical use	Creatinine clearance	Endogenous Inexpensive	Requires a timed urine collection Inaccurate
	Urea	Endogenous Inexpensive	Poor sensitivity and specificity
	RBP	Endogenous Not secreted/reabsorbed	Nonrenal influences on production rate
	α_1-microglobulin	Endogenous Not secreted/reabsorbed	Nonrenal influences on production rate Less freely filtered than RBP

EDTA, Ethylenediaminetetraacetic acid; *DTPA*, diethylenetriaminepentaacetic acid; *GFR*, glomerular filtration rate; *MDRD*, Modification of Diet in Renal Disease; *RBP*, retinol-binding protein; *Tc*, technetium.

period of long enough duration (typically more than 4 hours), and (3) complete bladder emptying achieved. In addition, to ensure accuracy when measuring GFR using urinary clearance methods, it is essential that (1) renal tubular secretion or reabsorption does not contribute to the elimination of the compound and (2) plasma protein binding of the pharmaceutical is negligible.

Exogenous Markers of Glomerular Filtration Rate

Both nonradioisotopic and radioisotopic markers are used as exogenous markers. Nonradioactive compounds used to measure GFR include inulin and iohexol. Radiopharmaceuticals that have been used include (1) ^{51}Cr-ethylenediaminetetraacetic acid (EDTA), (2) ^{99m}Tc-diethylenetriaminepentaacetic acid (DTPA), and (3) ^{125}I-iothalamate. Using these markers, the biological variability of GFR in patients with kidney disease has been reported to be between 6% and 12%.

Inulin Clearance. The fructose polymer inulin (molecular mass approximately 5 kDa) satisfies the criteria as an ideal marker of GFR. Inulin clearance using a constant infusion urinary clearance approach has long been regarded as the "gold standard" measure of GFR. Acceptable single bolus plasma clearance approaches have also been evaluated. However, lack of availability of simple laboratory methods of measurement of inulin remains an impediment to universal usage.

Iohexol Clearance. The clearance of the nonradioactive x-ray contrast agent iohexol has been proposed as a simpler alternative to inulin clearance. In one method, plasma iohexol is measured by high-performance liquid chromatography (HPLC) with reversed-phase separation and ultraviolet (UV) detection, following prior deproteinization with perchloric acid. Analytical imprecision (CV) is less than 3% intraassay and 5% interassay. Isotope-dilution mass spectrometry (ID-MS) methods have also been used. Single-bolus plasma clearance of iohexol demonstrates excellent agreement with constant-infusion urinary inulin clearance.

Single-bolus plasma clearance methods have obvious practical advantages compared with the complex continuous-infusion methods. A single dose of the marker such as (1) inulin, (2) iohexol or (3) Cr-EDTA, 50 to 100 μCi is injected and venous blood samples are then collected at timed intervals (e.g., typically 120, 180, and 240 minutes after the start of the injection of the marker). The GFR is calculated using the amount of marker injected and the decrease in marker concentration (or radioactivity) as a function of time. The elimination of the marker is described by a two-compartment model (see Chapter 31). This comprises an initial equilibration or distribution phase while the marker mixes between the vascular and extravascular space while also being cleared from the plasma by the kidney. The distribution phase lasts between 2 and 8 hours, depending on the (1) size of the subject, (2) distribution volume of the molecule (e.g., longer in patients with an excessive accumulation of serous fluid), and (3) GFR of the subject (the lower the GFR, the longer the distribution phase). This gives rise to a biexponential clearance curve. However, GFR is normally calculated using single-exponential analysis by plotting log marker concentration against time. The half-life is calculated from the slope (k) and the volume of distribution (C_0) of the marker just after injection.

$$GFR = k \times C_0 \tag{3}$$

Because this model ignores the distribution phase, GFR is overestimated. Various corrections are used to adjust for this.

Endogenous Markers of Glomerular Filtration Rate
Although the clearance of infused exogenous markers is generally considered an accurate assessment of GFR, to date these procedures have been considered too costly and cumbersome for routine use, particularly in cases where the GFR is assessed on a regular basis. Creatinine and certain low molecular weight proteins (such as cystatin C) have been used as endogenous markers of GFR. These markers obviate the necessity for injection and require only a single blood sample thereby simplifying the procedure and increasing its utility.

Creatinine Concentration. The most widely used endogenous marker of GFR is creatinine,[10] expressed as its (1) plasma concentration, (2) serum concentration plasma and serum concentrations of creatinine are equivalent, or (3) renal clearance (see Chapter 21) and efforts continue to standardize the measurement of creatinine.[6,14,18] Creatinine (molecular mass 113 Da) is freely filtered at the glomerulus and its concentration is inversely related to GFR. As a GFR marker, it is convenient and inexpensive to measure but its measured concentration is affected by (1) age, (2) sex, (3) exercise, (4) certain drugs (e.g., cimetidine and trimethoprim), (5) muscle mass, (6) nutritional status, and (7) meat intake. Further, a small (but significant) and variable proportion of the creatinine appearing in the urine is derived from tubular secretion. Typically, 7% to 10% is due to tubular secretion, but this percentage is increased in the presence of renal insufficiency. Significant analytical interferences continue to be a problem. Perhaps most importantly, plasma creatinine remains within the reference interval until significant renal function has been lost. Since plasma creatinine is derived from creatine and phosphocreatine breakdown in muscle, the reference interval encompasses the variety of muscle mass observed in the population. This contributes to the insensitivity of creatinine as a marker of diminished GFR. Additionally, in patients with **chronic kidney disease (CKD)**, extrarenal clearance of creatinine further blunts the anticipated increase in plasma creatinine in response to falling GFR. Consequently, plasma creatinine measurement does not detect mild CKD (GFR 60 to 89 mL/min/1.73 m^2) and also fails to identify many patients with moderate CKD (GFR 30 to 59 mL/min/1.73 m^2). Thus, although an increased plasma creatinine concentration does generally equate with impaired kidney function, a healthy plasma creatinine does not necessarily equate with normal kidney function. Because of all these limitations, it is recommended that plasma creatinine measurement alone not be used to assess kidney function.

Creatinine Clearance. Because creatinine is endogenously produced and released into body fluids at a constant rate, its clearance has been measured as an indicator of GFR. Historically, creatinine clearance has been seen as more sensitive for detection of renal dysfunction than measuring plasma creatinine. However, it requires a timed urine collection, which (1) introduces its own inaccuracies, (2) is inconvenient, and (3) is unpleasant. In addition, it is imprecise as the intraindividual day-to-day coefficient of variation (CV) for repeated measures of creatinine clearance can exceed 25%. Hence, at best creatinine clearance only provides a crude index of GFR.

Estimated Glomerular Filtration Rate. The mathematical relationship between plasma creatinine and GFR is improved by correcting for the confounding variables that make that relationship nonlinear. Many equations have been derived that estimate GFR using plasma creatinine corrected for some or all of (1) sex, (2) body size, (3) race, and (4) age. Their use is thought to produce a better estimate of GFR than plasma creatinine alone. The Modification of Diet in Renal Disease (MDRD) study equation was developed in 1999 by Levey and co-workers among 1628 predominantly middle-aged patients enrolled in the MDRD Study. An abbreviated version of this equation was subsequently published and later aligned for use with creatinine assays with standardization traceable to the international reference system[10,11]:

$$
\begin{aligned}
\text{GFR (mL/min/1.73 m}^2) = {} & 175 \\
& \times [\text{plasma creatinine (mg/dL)}]^{-1.154} \\
& \times [\text{age}]^{-0.203} \\
& \times [1.210 \text{ if black}] \\
& \times [0.742 \text{ if female}]
\end{aligned}
$$

or,

$$
\begin{aligned}
\text{GFR (mL/min/1.73 m}^2) = {} & 175 \\
& \times [\text{plasma creatinine }(\mu\text{mol/L}) \times 0.011]^{-1.154} \\
& \times [\text{age}]^{-0.203} \\
& \times [1.210 \text{ if black}] \\
& \times [0.742 \text{ if female}]
\end{aligned}
$$

The MDRD Study equation has been widely adopted internationally; although it is acknowledged that at GFR levels greater than 60 mL/min/1.73 m², it suffers from negative bias. An alternative equation, the Chronic Kidney Disease Epidemiology Collaboration (CKD-EPI) equation has been proposed.[12] This is favored by some workers on the basis that, at least in people with less advanced kidney disease, it is less biased than the MDRD Study equation and enables GFR values in excess of 90 mL/min/1.73 m² to be reported. It also has a smaller coefficient for black ethnicity than the MDRD Study equation, and there are some indications that it is possible to use it without adjustment for race in some other ethnic groups.

$$
\begin{aligned}
\text{GFR (mL/min/1.73 m}^2) = {} & 141 \\
& \times \min(\text{Scr}/\kappa, 1)^{\alpha} \\
& \times \max(\text{Scr}/\kappa, 1)^{-1.209} \\
& \times 0.993^{\text{Age}} \\
& \times 1.018 \text{ [if female]} \\
& \times 1.159 \text{ [if black]},
\end{aligned}
$$

where Scr is serum creatinine in mg/dL, κ is 0.7 for females and 0.9 for males, α is -0.329 for females and -0.411 for males, min indicates the minimum of Scr/κ or 1, and max indicates the maximum of Scr/κ or 1.

Alternative equations are available for use in children (e.g., the Schwartz equation). The equations are clearly complex: software is available for such calculations (e.g., see http://www.nkdep.nih.gov/; accessed September 16, 2013).

It must be remembered, however, that plasma creatinine is an imperfect marker of GFR and therefore equations based upon it are imperfect. Use of the equation does not circumvent the very significant optical interferences affecting plasma creatinine measurement, such as (1) hemolysis, (2) icterus, and (3) lipemia, and (4) it does not address the inter-individual variability in concentrations of non-creatinine chromogens.

Low-Molecular-Weight Proteins. A number of proteins with molecular weights of less than 30 kDa are mostly cleared from the circulation by renal filtration and are considered to be relatively freely filtered at the glomerular filtration barrier. These include (1) α_2-microglobulin, (2) retinol-binding protein (RBP), (3) α_1-microglobulin, (4) β-trace protein, and (5) cystatin C.[2] These proteins are (1) filtered at the glomerulus, (2) reabsorbed and metabolized in the proximal tubule or excreted into the urine, and (3) entirely eliminated from the circulation. Therefore they have the potential to meet the criteria for use as a marker of GFR. However, all these proteins have been shown to have plasma concentrations that are influenced by other, nonrenal factors, such as (1) inflammation (α_2-microglobulin), (2) liver disease (RBP, α_1-microglobulin) and (3) thyroid disease (cystatin C). The relationship between the circulating concentrations of these proteins shows the same curvilinear form as plasma creatinine, but several groups have demonstrated that cystatin C measurement may offer a more sensitive and specific means of monitoring changes in GFR than plasma creatinine.

Cystatin C is a low molecular weight (12.8 kDa) protein synthesized by all nucleated cells whose physiological role is that of a cysteine protease inhibitor. With regard to renal function, its most important attributes are its small size and high isoelectric point (pI = 9.2), which enable it to be more freely filtered than the above-mentioned proteins at the glomerulus. Plasma concentrations of cystatin C appear to be unaffected by (1) muscle mass, (2) diet, or (3) sex. Also, there are no known extrarenal routes of elimination, and clearance from the circulation is only by glomerular filtration. Further, cystatin C measurement appears unaffected by the optical interferences affecting creatinine assays. Because of its multiple advantages, cystatin C is considered by some to be a superior marker for determining GFR. It appears to be especially useful when trying to detect mild to moderate impairment of kidney function. A GFR estimating equation based upon cystatin C has recently been proposed by the CKD-EPI collaboration[2,3,4]:

$$
\begin{aligned}
\text{GFR (mL/min/1.73 m}^2) = {} & 133 \\
& \times \min(\text{Scys}/0.8, 1)^{-0.499} \\
& \times \max(\text{Scys}/0.8, 1)^{-1.328} \\
& \times 0.996^{\text{Age}} \\
& \times 0.932 \text{ [if female]}
\end{aligned}
$$

where Scys is serum cystatin C in mg/L, min indicates the minimum of Scr/κ or 1, and max indicates the maximum of Scr/κ or 1.

Glomerular Filtration Rate and Age

GFR is not constant throughout life. For example, in utero, urine is produced by the developing fetus from about the ninth week of gestation. The GFR at birth is approximately 30 mL/min/1.73 m². It increases rapidly during the first weeks of life to reach approximately 70 mL/min/1.73 m² by age 16 days with adult values of BSA-corrected GFR being achieved by 2 years of age. On average, GFR declines with age by approximately 1 mL/min/1.73 m²/yr over the age of 40 and the rate of decline in GFR accelerates after age 65 years.

Recommendations and Reference Intervals

The measurement of the urinary clearance of inulin, after continuous infusion, is considered the reference method for the determination of GFR. However, because the necessary plasma and urine assays for inulin often are not practical in clinical laboratories, plasma creatinine or creatinine clearance has almost universally been used for assessment of GFR. With increasing recognition of the importance of early detection and management of CKD, the requirement for more accurate assessment of GFR is being emphasized. Consequently, creatinine clearance is no longer considered acceptable as a measure of GFR and plasma creatinine measurements should not be reported in isolation but should be used to generate estimations of GFR. However, the susceptibility of these equations to creatinine assay calibration variations must be recognized. The success of alternative markers (such as cystatin C) will depend on understanding the benefit of the superior diagnostic accuracy and improved clinical and economic outcomes in relation to the greater cost of the assay when compared with the Jaffe creatinine methods.

As indicated earlier, reference data for GFR are dependent on the age of the population studied. A reference value in young adult men and women of approximately 125 mL/min/1.73 m is used by many.

Glomerular Permeability, Filtration, and Protein Loss

The glomerular permeability and filtration capabilities of the kidney control the amount of protein lost in the urine.

Glomerular Permeability and Filtration

The glomerulus acts as a selective filter of the blood passing through its capillaries. The combination of a (1) fenestrated (porous) endothelial layer, (2) basement membrane rich in negatively charged proteoglycans, and (3) highly specialized terminally differentiated epithelial cell barrier produces a filter that restricts the passage of macromolecules in a (1) size-, (2) charge-, and (3) shape-dependent manner. The epithelial cells (podocytes) have foot processes that are connected to the glomerular basement membrane and form the final barrier to filtration via interdigitating with neighboring cell foot processes connected by a slit diaphragm. Examples of the relationships between (1) size, (2) charge, and (3) mass of the major urinary proteins and their glomerular processing are listed in Table 35-2. In general, proteins of molecular weights greater than albumin (66 kDa, diameter 3.5 nm) are retained by the healthy glomerulus and are termed high molecular weight proteins. However, lower molecular weight proteins are also retained to a significant extent.

Urinary Protein Loss

Increased urinary protein loss (**proteinuria**) results from (1) any increase in the filtered load, (2) increased circulating concentration of low molecular weight proteins, or (3) decrease in reabsorptive capacity. Historically, the pattern of urinary protein loss has been used to identify the cause and to classify the proteinuria, of which there are three main types: (1) glomerular, (2) overflow, and (3) tubular proteinuria.

The normal urinary total protein loss is less than 150 mg/24 hr. The proteins lost are made up of mostly albumin (50% to 60%) and some smaller proteins, together with proteins secreted by the tubules, of which Tamm-Horsfall glycoprotein (THG) is one. The normal concentrations of proteins found in urine are listed in Table 35-2. Investigation for increased urinary protein loss is required for the examination of any patient with suspected kidney disease. Clinical or overt proteinuria is often detected using reagent strip methods, the detection limit of which is 200 to 300 mg/L. Proteinuria above 300 mg/day is generally pathological. However, there are exceptions to this. For example, proteinuria has been observed to occur as a result of fever

---

TABLE 35-2	**Characteristics of the Major Urinary Proteins**						
Protein	M_r (kDa)	Free Plasma Concentration (g/L)	Diameter (nm)	Glomerular Sieving Coefficient*	Filtered Load (mg/L)†	Urinary Concentration (mg/L)	% Reabsorbed
IgG	150	10	5.5	0.0001	1	0.1	99
Albumin	66	40	3.5	0.0002	8	5	99
α_1-microglobulin	31	0.025	2.9	~0.3	7.5	5	99
RBP	22	0.025	2.1	~0.7	17.5	0.1	99
Cystatin C	12.8	0.01	—	~0.7	0.7	0.1	99
β_2-microglobulin	11.8	0.015	1.6	0.7	1.1	0.1	99
Total Protein	—	70	—	NA‡	700	< 150	NA‡

*The glomerular sieving coefficient of a molecule that is freely filtered is 1.0.
†Concentration in the glomular filtrate.
‡Not applicable because of tubular secretion of proteins (e.g., Tamm-Horsfall glycoprotein (THG), which forms ~50% of urinary total proteins in health).
IgG, Immunoglobulin G; *M_r*, molecular mass; *RBP*, retinol-binding protein.

and exercise (functional) or related to posture (orthostatic). These sporadic changes cause interpretative difficulties when pathology is suspected. Upright posture increases protein loss in both normal subjects and those with kidney disease. Proteinuria above 1000 mg/day implies glomerular proteinuria. Glomerular proteinuria may be heavy and a mixed proteinuria with the elevation of both high and low molecular weight proteins may be observed.

There is a growing consensus that urinary total protein measurement should be replaced by urinary albumin measurement when assessing patients for proteinuria in most clinical situations. Albumin is the predominant protein in urine in the majority of kidney diseases and is accurately and specifically measured using immunoassay techniques.[8]

Consequences of Proteinuria
Many physicians believe that proteinuria is not just a consequence of, but contributes directly to, progression of kidney disease. The accumulation of proteins in abnormal amounts in the tubular lumen may trigger an inflammatory reaction, which contributes to interstitial structural damage and expansion, and progression of kidney disease. Evidence gathered from in vitro studies suggests that glomerular filtration of an abnormal amount or types of protein induces mesangial cell injury, leading to glomerulosclerosis, and that these same proteins also have adverse effects on proximal tubular cell function. Numerous studies have demonstrated that proteinuria is a potent risk marker for progression of renal disease in both nondiabetic and diabetic kidney disease. Furthermore, reducing protein excretion slows the rate of progression of proteinuric kidney disease. This has been observed in clinical trials in patients treated with (1) angiotensin-converting enzyme (ACE) inhibitors and (2) angiotensin II receptor blockers (ARBs), either alone or in combination. These drugs reduce protein loss by reducing intraglomerular filtration pressure and possibly by stabilizing the glomerular epithelial cell slit diaphragm proteins. Consequently, reduction of proteinuria is an important therapeutic target.

Sample Collection Considerations
Extensive discussion has occurred in the literature about the appropriate urine sample to use for the investigation of protein loss. It is generally recognized that a 24-hour sample is the definitive means of demonstrating the presence of proteinuria. However, in practice, (1) overnight, (2) first void in the morning (early morning urine [EMU]), (3) second void in the morning, or (4) random sample collections have also been used. Since creatinine excretion in the urine is fairly constant throughout the 24-hour period, measurement of protein/creatinine (or albumin/creatinine) ratios allows correction for variations in urinary concentration. It is now a generally accepted practice to substitute the protein/creatinine ratio for 24-hour total protein excretion measured from a 24-hour collection. An EMU sample is preferred since it correlates well with 24-hour protein excretion and is required to exclude the diagnosis of orthostatic (postural) proteinuria. However, a random urine sample is acceptable if no early morning sample is available. If required, daily protein excretion (in mg/24 hours) is roughly estimated as numerically equal to the protein/creatinine ratio (measured as mg/g) as creatinine excretion is about 1g/day. In SI units, multiply the protein/creatinine ratio (measured in mg/mmol) by a factor of ten since an average figure of 10 mmol creatinine per day is assumed. A suitable protocol for the further investigation of patients found to have proteinuria at screening is given in Figure 35-5.

Measurement of Urinary Protein
There are numerous methods used for the measurement of total protein in urine. Discussion of several of these methods is found in Chapter 18. Detection of protein using reagent strips is discussed later.

Pathophysiology of Kidney Disease
Despite the diverse initial causes of injury to the kidney, progression of kidney disease leading to loss of function and ultimately to kidney failure is a process characterized by (1) early inflammation, (2) accumulation and deposition of extracellular matrix, (3) tubulointerstitial fibrosis, (4) tubular atrophy, and (5) glomerulosclerosis (scarring). Upregulation of angiotensin II within the kidney directly (causing increasing glomerular permeability to protein) and indirectly (stimulating pro-inflammatory cytokines) contributes to these changes. Proteinuria is one of the most important risk factors for progression of kidney disease. Angiotensin II is an important therapeutic target in kidney disease.

The kidneys have considerable ability to increase their functional capacity in response to injury. Thus, a significant reduction in functioning renal mass (50% to 60%) may occur before any major biochemical alterations appear and symptoms appear. The most sensitive and specific measure of functional change, the GFR, is reduced to less than 60 mL/min/1.73 m² before signs and symptoms of kidney failure are observed. An increase in workload per nephron is thought to be an important cause of progressive renal injury.

Diagnosis and Screening for Kidney Disease
The patient with kidney disease generally presented with (1) an abnormality detected on a routine biochemical blood screen or urinalysis, (2) a symptom or physical sign, or (3) with a systemic disease with a known renal involvement, such as diabetes mellitus. Unfortunately, as many as 30% of individuals see a clinician very late in their disease and may require urgent dialysis with no previous experience with the specialist nephrology service. These patients have a poor prognosis. Therefore, early recognition of kidney disease is thought to be of vital importance to outcome.

Effective management of the patient with kidney disease is dependent upon establishing a definitive diagnosis. Initial management includes a (1) detailed clinical history, (2) clinical examination, and (3) urinalysis and assessment of the urinary sediment.

Urinalysis
Examination of the urine is an important step in the assessment of a patient suspected of having, or confirmed to have

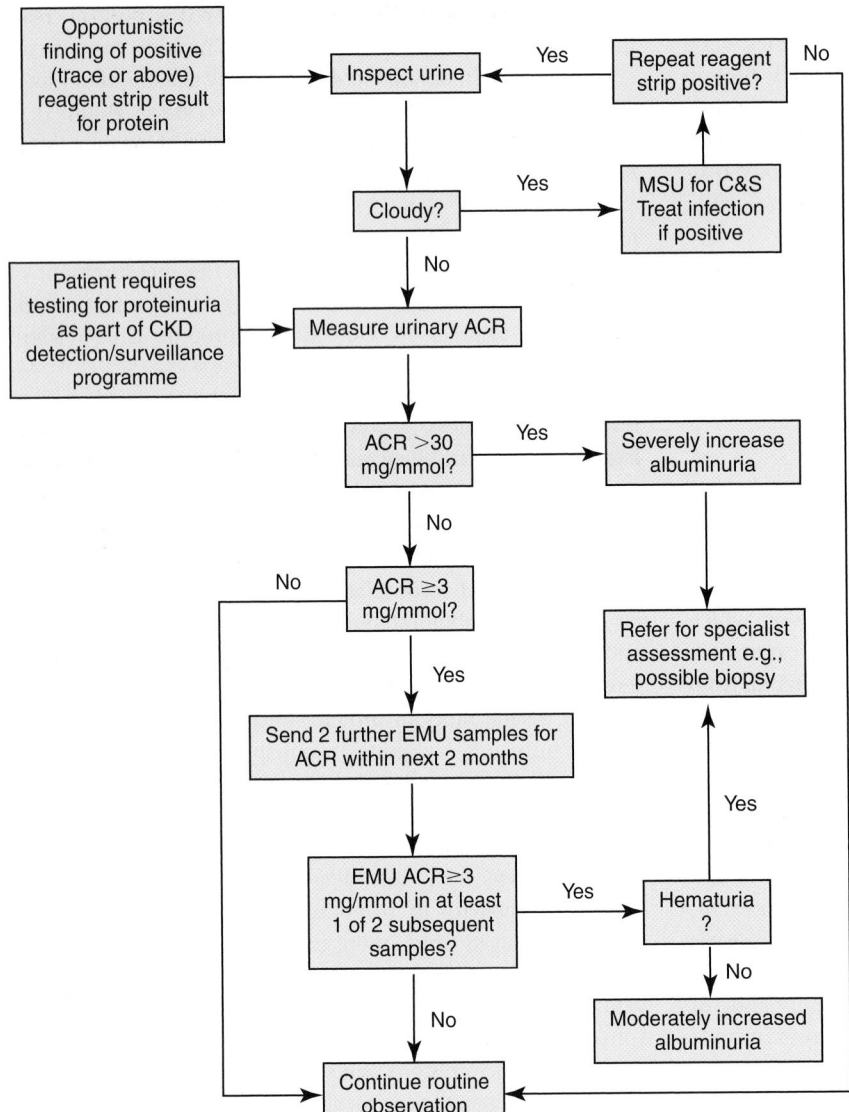

Figure 35-5 Suggested protocol for the further investigation of an individual demonstrating a positive reagent strip test for albuminuria/proteinuria or quantitative albuminuria/proteinuria test. Reagent strip device results should be confirmed using laboratory testing of the albumin-to-creatinine ratio (ACR) on at least two further occasions. Patients with two or more positive (≥ 3 mg albumin/mmol creatinine) tests on early morning samples 1 to 2 weeks apart should be diagnosed as having persistent albuminuria. The possibility of postural proteinuria should be excluded by the examination of an early morning urine *(EMU)* specimen. Protein-to-creatinine ratio (PCR) measurement can be substituted for the ACR but is insensitive in the detection of moderately increased albuminuria/proteinuria: approximate PCR equivalent to an ACR of 30 mg/mmol is 50 mg/mmol. Consider other causes of increased ACR, such as (1) menstrual contamination, (2) uncontrolled hypertension, (3) symptomatic urinary tract infection, (4) heart failure, (5) other transitory illnesses, and (6) strenuous exercise, especially in the case of type 1 diabetes present for less than 5 years. The presence of hematuria may indicate non-diabetic renal disease. *C&S,* Culture and sensitivity; *CKD,* chronic kidney disease; *MSU,* mid-stream urine.

deterioration in kidney function. In the laboratory, urine is examined (1) visually, (2) chemically, and (3) microscopically. The appearance (color and odor) of urine itself is often helpful with a darkening from the pale normal straw color indicating more concentrated urine or the presence of another pigment. Hemoglobin and myoglobin give a pink-red-brown coloration, depending on the concentration. Turbidity in a fresh sample may indicate infection, but may also be due to fat particles in a patient with **nephrotic syndrome.** Excessive foaming of urine when shaken suggests proteinuria. Urine is often chemically evaluated with the help of reagent strip ("dipstick") tests. Regarding dipstick technology, many tests of renal significance have been adapted for use on strips of cellulose or pads of cellulose on strips of plastic that have been coated or impregnated with reagents for the analyte in question. A reagent strip may contain reagents for just one test per stick or reagents for multiple tests on a single stick. For example, up to 10 constituents are now measured on a single strip allowing for detection of multiple abnormalities simultaneously.

Clinically, proteinuria and **hematuria** are the most important of these in suspected kidney disease. Urine samples for testing should be collected in sterile containers and testing performed on the fresh urine. Reagent strips should be used only if they have been stored properly desiccated, because some deteriorate in a matter of hours.

Proteinuria is a common finding in patients with kidney disease, and the use of a reagent strip is a common screening test in any individual suspected of having renal disease. Annual urinalysis for proteinuria is accepted as a useful way of identifying patients at risk of progressive kidney disease but is inadequate for the detection of CKD among patients with diabetes, who should undergo annual testing for albuminuria using sensitive immunoassay techniques. Increasingly, it is argued that quantitative measurement of albumin or total protein should *replace* reagent strip approaches in all patients with, or at risk of, CKD. The reagent strip for total protein includes a cellulose test pad impregnated with tetrabromophenol blue and a citrate buffer having a pH of 3. The reaction is based on the "protein error of indicators" phenomenon in which certain chemical indicators demonstrate one color in the presence of protein and another in its absence. Thus tetrabromophenol blue is green in the presence of protein at pH 3 but yellow in its absence. The color is read after exactly 60 s and the test has a lower limit of detection of 150 to 300 mg/L, depending on the type and proportions of proteins present. The reagent is most sensitive to albumin and less sensitive to (1) globulins, (2) **Bence-Jones protein**, (3) mucoproteins, and (4) hemoglobin.

The presence of hemoglobin in the urine may be due to (1) glomerular, (2) tubulointerstitial, or (3) postrenal disease, although the latter two causes are the more common. The presence of blood in urine is detected by the use of a phase contrast microscope to determine the presence of red cells in urine sediment or by use of a reagent strip test. The chemical detection of hemoglobin in urine depends on the peroxidase activity of the protein, employing a peroxide substrate and an oxygen acceptor. For this test, the reagent pad is impregnated with buffered tetramethyl benzidine (TMB) and an organic peroxide, cumene hydroperoxide. The color change varies from orange through pale to dark green, and red cells or free hemoglobin are detected together with myoglobin. Again the color of the reagent pad should be compared with a color chart after exactly 60 s. Two reagent pads are employed for the low hemoglobin concentration. If intact red cells are present, the low-concentration pad will have a speckled appearance; a solid color indicates hemolyzed red cells. The test is equally sensitive to hemoglobin and to myoglobin. The presence of free hemoglobin or red cells in the urine indicates the presence of renal or bladder disease. Hematuria is often present in a number of kidney diseases, including (1) **glomerulonephritis**, (2) polycystic kidney disease, (3) sickle cell disease, (4) vasculitis, and (5) several infections. A spectrum of urological diseases may also give rise to hematuria, including (1) bladder malignancy, (2) prostate malignancy, (3) pelvic malignancy, (4) ureteral malignancy, (5) kidney stones, (6) trauma, (7) bladder damage, and (8) ureteral stricture.

Microscopic examination of the sediment obtained from the centrifugation of a fresh urine sample will show the presence of (1) a few cells (erythrocytes, leukocytes, and cells derived from the kidney and urinary tract), (2) casts (composed predominantly of THG), and (3) possibly fat or pigmented particles. An increase in red cells or casts implies hematuria, possibly caused by glomerular disease. White cells or casts imply the presence of white cells in the tubules. Inflammation of the upper urinary tract may result in polymorphonuclear leukocytes and various types of casts, and in lower urinary tract inflammation the casts will not be present. In acute glomerulonephritis, hematuria may lead to coloration of urine and the presence of large numbers of red cells and white cells; as the duration of the disease increases, the amount of sediment diminishes.

Biochemical measurements, particularly of plasma creatinine concentration (see earlier and Chapter 21) and estimated GFR, play an important role in the discovery that kidney damage has occurred and in monitoring progress and treatment.

Noninvasive imaging using ultrasonography is invaluable for identifying the size and shape of the kidneys along with any evidence of obstruction. However, percutaneous kidney biopsy is routinely performed to (1) confirm the diagnosis, (2) guide treatment, and (3) gain information regarding prognosis.

Classification of Kidney Failure

The terminology associated with kidney diseases has been revised. Previously, renal failure was divided into either acute renal failure (ARF) or chronic renal failure (CRF). These terms indicate the rate at which damage occurs rather than the mechanism by which it occurs. Seminal guidelines published in 2002 by the United States National Kidney Foundation-Kidney Disease Outcomes Quality Initiative (NKF KDOQI) classified CKD by categories of GFR, characterized by differing levels of metabolic decompensation (Table 35-3).[15] The term "renal" has largely been replaced by "kidney" when referring to *chronic* disease since it is more easily understood by patients and nonspecialists. In addition, "acute renal failure" has been replaced by **acute kidney injury (AKI)**.

Acute Kidney Injury

The definition of AKI, endorsed by the Kidney Disease Improving Global Outcomes (KDIGO) during 2012, is the occurrence of any one of the following[4,7]:

(1) Increase of plasma creatinine by $\geq$ 0.3 mg/dL ($\geq$ 26 umol/L) within 48 hours

(2) Increase in plasma creatinine to $\geq$ 1.5 times baseline, which is known or presumed to have occurred within the prior 7 days

(3) Reduction in urine output (documented oliguria < 0.5 mL/kg/h for > 6 hours)

In addition, AKI is staged 1 to 3, depending on severity. In the UK, the National Confidential Enquiry into Patient Outcome and Death reported that failure (1) to identify intravascular volume depletion, (2) to withhold nephrotoxic drugs, and (3) of early diagnosis of causative conditions (such as, sepsis) directly contributed to in-hospital mortality associated with AKI (http://www.ncepod.org.uk/ 2009report1/Downloads/AKI_summary.pdf/accessed September 16, 2013).

Patients at risk for AKI include (1) older persons; those with (2) pre-existing CKD, (3) sepsis, (4) diabetes, and (5) heart disease; and (6) patients receiving nephrotoxic drugs, particularly in the setting of hypovolemia. Clinical assessment of AKI should consider whether the precipitant is (1) prerenal, (2) intrarenal (intrinsic), or (3) postrenal. The most common causes are listed in Box 35-1. As intrinsic AKI is caused by primary (1) vascular, (2) glomerular, or (3) interstitial disorders, it is important that all patients presenting with AKI undergo urinalysis to test for (1) infection, (2) hematuria, and (3) proteinuria. In most cases, the kidney lesion seen on histology is referred to as **acute tubular necrosis (ATN)**. ATN is caused by ischemic or nephrotoxic

TABLE 35-3 Kidney Disease Improving Global Outcomes 2012 Classification of Chronic Kidney Disease by Glomerular Filtration Rate and Albumin Excretion Rate*

Glomerular Filtration Rate (GFR)

Category	GFR (mL/min/1.73 m²)	Terms	Metabolic consequences	Management
G1†	≥ 90	Normal or high		• Diagnosis and treatment • Treatment of comorbid conditions • Slowing progression • CVD risk reduction
G2†	60-89	Mildly decreased‡	• Concentration of PTH starts to rise (GFR 60-80)	• Estimating progression
G3a	45-59	Mildly to moderately decreased	• Decrease in calcium absorption (GFR < 50) • Lipoprotein lipase activity falls	• Evaluating and treating complications
G3b	30-44	Moderately to severely decreased	• Malnutrition • Onset of LVH • Onset of anemia (EPO deficiency)	
G4	15-29	Severely decreased	• Triglyceride concentrations start to rise • Hyperphosphatemia • Metabolic acidosis • Tendency to hyperkalemia	• Preparation for RRT if appropriate
G5	< 15	Kidney failure (add D if treated by dialysis)	• Uremic syndrome	• RRT if appropriate

Albumin Excretion Rate (AER)

Category	AER	Approximately Equivalent ACR		Terms
	(mg/d)	(mg/mmol)	(mg/g)	
A1	< 30	< 3	< 30	Normal to mildly increased
A2	30-300	3-30	30-300	Moderately increased†
A3	> 300	> 30	> 300	Severely increased§

*Broad metabolic consequences and management are indicated.
†Neither GFR category G1 nor G2 without markers of kidney damage fulfil the criteria for chronic kidney disease (CKD).
‡Relative to young adult level.
§Including nephrotic syndrome (albumin excretion usually >2200 mg/d).
AER, Albumin exretion rate; ACR, albumin-to-creatinine ratio; CVD, cardiovascular disease; EPO, erythropoietin; GFR, glomerular filtration rate; LVH, left ventricular hypertrophy; PTH, parathyroid hormone; RRT, renal replacement therapy.
Adapted from Improving Global Outcomes (KDIGO) CKD Work Group. KDIGO 2012 clinical practice guideline for the evaluation and management of chronic kidney disease. Kidney Inter. 2013(Suppl);3:1-150.

BOX 35-1 Causes of Acute Kidney Injury

Prerenal AKI
  Hemorrhage
  Diarrhea
  Postoperative fluid and blood losses
  Sepsis
  Acute cardiac failure
Intrinsic renal disease
  Tubular
  Glomerular
  Vascular
Any of the prerenal causes that are severe or that are not corrected promptly leading to ATN
Other causes of ATN
  Drug nephrotoxicity
  NSAIDs, ACE inhibitors
  Aminoglycoside antibiotics
  Amphotericin
TIN
  Allergic TIN associated with antibiotics and NSAIDs
  Sarcoidosis
  Pyelonephritis
Renal parenchymal disease

RPGN: (1) ANCA-associated vasculitides, (2) Goodpasture disease, (3) SLE, (4) other crescentic glomerulonephritides
  Thrombotic microangiopathies
  Cryoglobulinemia
Myeloma
Miscellaneous
  Contrast nephropathy
  Poisoning
  Rhabdomyolysis
  Atheroembolism
  Urate nephropathy
  Hepatorenal syndrome
Vascular causes
  Aortic dissection
  Renal vein thrombosis
Postrenal AKI
Bladder outflow obstruction
  Benign and malignant prostate disease
  Invasive bladder carcinoma
Bilateral renal calculi or calculi within a single kidney
Retroperitoneal fibrosis

ACE, Angiotensin-converting enzyme; AKI, acute kidney injury; ANCA, antineutrophil cytoplasmic antibody; ATN, acute tubular necrosis; NSAIDs, nonsteroidal antiinflammatory drugs; RPGN, rapidly progressive glomerulonephritis; SLE, systemic lupus erythematosus; TIN, tubulointerstitial nephritis.

TABLE 35-4 Investigation of Acute Kidney Injury

Test	Indication/Comments
Urine Testing	
Urine reagent strip ("dipstick")	Hematuria and proteinuria may indicate glomerular origin
Red cell casts on microscopy	Not available universally; may need bedside microscope
Urine microscopy and culture	Identify urinary tract infection
Urine protein electrophoresis and immunofixation	
Blood Tests	
Baseline Studies	
Urea, electrolytes, creatinine, and calcium, phosphate, albumin	Check previous laboratory reports: AKI or AKI with preexisting CKD
Liver function tests	Suspected multiorgan involvement or abnormal coagulation
Acid-base studies	Arterial blood gas or venous plasma bicarbonate concentration
Full blood count	Anemia, hemolysis, thrombocytopenia
Coagulation studies	Evidence of intravascular coagulation; need to normalize if considering kidney biopsy and central line insertion
Selected Additional Investigations	
Blood culture	Any infection but especially endocarditis, severe pneumonia, or urinary tract sepsis
CK	Very high in cases of muscle inflammation and necrosis (rhabdomyolysis)
LD	If high, suspect renal infarction and consider hemolysis
Antineutrophil cytoplasmic antibodies	Vasculitides
Anti–glomerular basement membrane antibody	Anti–glomerular basement membrane disease
Antinuclear antibodies	SLE
Anti-dsDNA antibodies, ENAs	SLE
Low C4 complement	SLE, atheroembolism, cryoglobulinemia
Cryoglobulin	Cryoglobulinemia
Urate	Urate nephropathy
Serum protein electrophoresis	Myeloma
Virology studies	Hepatitis serology, antistreptolysin O titer, HIV
Imaging	
Chest x-ray	Pulmonary edema, pneumonia, effusions, malignancy, granulomas
Abdominal x-ray (kidney, ureter, and bladder)	Renal stones
Renal tract ultrasound scan	Identify size and symmetry of kidneys
	Evidence of an obstructed system
	Small shrunken kidneys in advanced CKD
CT scan	Anatomy and perfusion
Magnetic resonance imaging	Angiography to identify renovascular lesions
Formal angiography	Critical renal artery stenosis
Kidney biopsy	Reserved for patients with unexplained AKI in whom ATN is not suspected; it is anticipated that additional therapy (such as, steroids, cytotoxic drugs, and plasma exchange) may be required

AKI, acute kidney injury; *ATN,* acute tubular necrosis; *CK,* creatine kinase; *CKD,* chronic kidney disease; *CT,* computed tomography; *dsDNA,* double-stranded DNA; *ENA,* extractable nuclear antigen; *HIV,* human immunodeficiency virus; *LD,* lactate dehydrogenase; *SLE,* systemic lupus erythematosus.

injury to the kidney. In 50% of cases of hospital-acquired AKI, the cause is multifactorial.[17]

Laboratory testing of blood is crucial in the management of AKI. Blood tests also assist in establishing the underlying diagnosis, and specific investigations are requested if kidney function has not improved following volume correction. An acute renal screen should clearly focus on most likely diagnoses and include the tests shown in Table 35-4.

In addition to biochemical testing, there is a role for ultrasound and radiological imaging in kidney disease and in particular exclusion of obstruction is important. Kidney biopsy is generally reserved for cases of AKI wherein an ultrasound scan has excluded obstructed kidneys, kidney sizes are maintained and the cause of AKI is otherwise unexplained, and an intrinsic pathology is suspected.

Metabolic acidosis is the most common acid-base disorder in patients with AKI. Reduced renal excretion of potassium and the effects of **acidosis** on the generation of extracellular potassium may lead to a very high concentration of potassium in the plasma. Severe hyperkalemia (plasma potassium concentration more than 6.5 mmol/L) is associated with life-threatening cardiac arrhythmias. Emergency treatment of hyperkalemia should be instituted as necessary. When hyperkalemia persists despite appropriate medical measures, then dialysis should be considered. Recovery from AKI usually occurs within days or weeks following removal of the initiating event. However, uncomplicated AKI has a mortality rate of 5% to 10% although AKI complicating nonrenal organ system failure in the intensive care unit setting is associated with mortality rates approaching 50% to 70%.

Chronic Kidney Disease

Studies established to identify the (1) incidence, (2) causes, and (3) complications of CKD have focused on advanced disease and kidney failure. Markers used to to identify CKD include (1) plasma creatinine, (2) estimated GFR, and (3) measured creatinine. Guidelines introduced over the past 10 years have attempted to evaluate, classify, and stratify CKD (see Table 35-3).[5,9,15] In these Guidelines, CKD is defined as abnormalities of kidney structure or function, present for more than 3 months with implications for health. A GFR of less than 60 mL/min/1.73 m^2 is considered decreased, and a GFR of less than 15 mL/min/1.73 m is considered kidney failure. Kidney damage is defined by structural abnormalities or functional abnormalities other than decreased GFR and may include (1) albuminuria, (2) urine sediment abnormalities, (3) electrolyte and other abnormalities due to tubular disorders, (4) abnormalities detected by histology, (5) structural abnormalities detected by imaging, or (6) a history of kidney transplantation.[5]

The 2002 NKF KDOQI guideline[15] stratified CKD by GFR from stage 1 at the mild end of the spectrum to stage 5, kidney failure, or a GFR of less than 15 mL/min/1.73 m^2, which encompasses those patients that require RRT to sustain life. Although the cutoff values between these stages are arbitrary, the scheme allows for consistency in prevalence reporting for epidemiological studies and also focused treatment schedules for individual patients (see Table 35-3). Guidelines published in 2013 by KDIGO[5] built upon and refined this classification. The GFR categories have been retained, with the exception that GFR category 3 has been split into 3a (mildly to moderately decreased, 45 to 59 mL/min/1.73 m^2) and 3b (moderately to severely decreased, 30 to 44 mL/min/1.73 m^{2}s), reflecting the different (1) metabolic, (2) prognostic, and (3) management features of these two situations. In addition, a second dimension has been added to the classification scheme based on the degree of albuminuria (see Table 35-3). Albuminuria categories are assigned based on daily urinary albumin loss, generally measured as an albumin-to-creatinine ratio (ACR): A1 (< 30 mg/day, ACR < 30 mg/g, < 3 mg/mmol), A2 (30 to 300 mg/day, ACR 30 to 300 mg/g, 3 to 30 mg/mmol) and A3 (> 300 mg/day, ACR > 300 mg/g, > 30 mg/mmol). Risk of death and kidney disease progression increases incrementally with declining GFR and increasing albuminuria. As an example of how the system is applied, a patient with a GFR of 50 mL/min/1.73 m^2 and no albuminuria would be assigned CKD stage G3a, A1, whereas a patient with a GFR of 20 mL/min/1.73 m^2 and ACR 50 mg/mmol would be assigned CKD stage G4, A3.

The main causes of CKD leading to kidney failure from 1990 to 2009 in the United States are indicated in Figure 35-6. As indicated, diabetes mellitus is the largest single cause of advanced CKD and accounts for 44% of new dialysis patients in the United States. **Hypertension** is the underlying diagnosis in around 28% of new dialysis patients and is particularly prevalent among African-Americans. In addition the rate of new ESRD in African-Americans is 3.5 times higher than whites. The myriad of kidney diseases, including

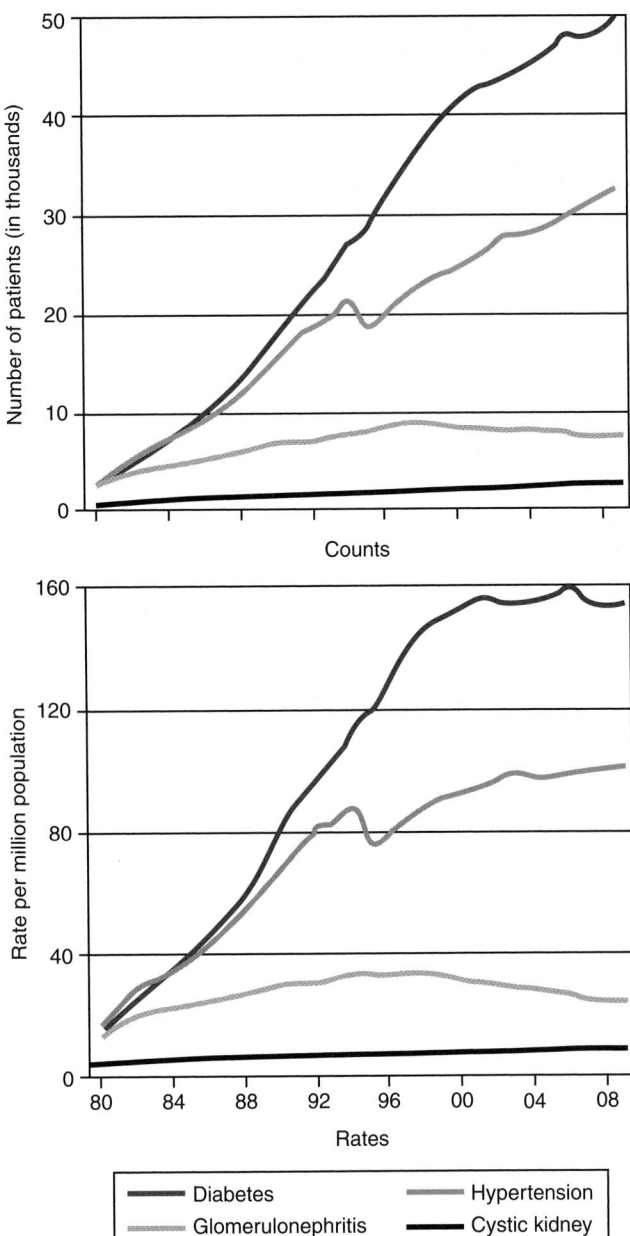

Figure 35-6 Trends in incident rates of end-stage renal disease (ESRD) by primary diagnosis. Diabetes is the primary cause of ESRD in 44% of adult dialysis patients in the United States in 2009. The overall incidence of ESRD has increased since the 1980s, and diabetes and hypertension account for this increase. The incidence of ESRD as a consequence of glomerulonephritis and cystic kidney diseases has not increased. (http://www.usrds.org/2011/pdf/v2_ch01_11.pdf, accessed online April 09, 2013.) *(US Renal Data System, USRDS 2011 Annual Data Report: Atlas of End-Stage Renal Disease in the United States, National Institutes of Health, National Institute of Diabetes and Digestive and Kidney Diseases, Bethesda, MD, 2011. The data reported here have been supplied by the United States Renal Data System (USRDS). The interpretation and reporting of these data are the responsibility of the author(s) and in no way should be seen as an official policy or interpretation of the US government. http://www.usrds.org/2011/pdf/v2_ch01_11.pdf; accessed online September 16, 2013.)*

(1) glomerulonephritis, (2) infection, (3) hereditary conditions, (4) systemic conditions, (5) interstitial conditions, (6) obstructive conditions, and (7) those of unknown origin.

Management of Chronic Kidney Disease

Rate of progression of CKD is dependent on both non-modifiable and modifiable factors. Non-modifiable factors include (1) age, (2) sex, (3) race, and (4) level of kidney function at diagnosis. Modifiable factors include (1) proteinuria, (2) blood pressure, and (3) smoking.

Lowering blood pressure and reduction of proteinuria have been shown to decrease the progression of CKD. The MDRD Study compared the rates of decline in GFR in patients with various causes of CKD assigned to either a "usual" or "low" blood pressure goal. Outcome data suggest that the low blood pressure goal had some beneficial effect in those patients with higher concentrations of proteins in their urine. In practice, medications that inhibit parts of the renin-angiotensin-aldosterone system (RAAS) blockade are typically preferred, because these drugs have been demonstrated to reduce proteinuria and rate of progression of CKD.

Protein intake is restricted spontaneously to approximately 0.6 to 0.8 g/kg/day in uremic patients not receiving dietary advice. To prevent malnutrition, patients receive professional dietary advice with diets containing an increased proportion of high quality protein and increased calorie content of up to 35 kcal/kg/day. General health measures, including cessation of cigarette smoking, are encouraged. Complications of CKD that develop before the need for RRT are numerous and include (1) cardiovascular disease, (2) bone disease, and (3) anemia. Albuminuria and proteinuria have been shown to be associated with increased risk of cardiovascular disease, cardiovascular mortality, and all-cause mortality.

Cardiovascular Complications of Chronic Kidney Disease

The incidence of cardiovascular disease is sevenfold to tenfold greater in patients with CKD than in non-CKD age- and sex-matched controls and by the time patients develop the need for RRT the risk increases to approximately seventeen times greater.

The spectrum of cardiovascular disease studied in CKD includes (1) angina, (2) congestive heart failure, (3) myocardial infarction, (4) peripheral vascular disease, (5) stroke, and (6) transient ischemic attack. Structural heart disease, such as left ventricular hypertrophy (LVH) and valvular heart disease, is very common. The risk factors for cardiovascular disease in CKD are a mixture of the traditional and CKD-specific (Table 35-5). Vascular calcification is highly prevalent in dialysis patients and is associated with reduced survival.

Dyslipidemia in Chronic Kidney Disease

The pattern of dyslipidemia (abnormal amount of lipids in the blood) in CKD differs from that seen in non-CKD. Although total cholesterol concentration may be within reference intervals for a healthy population, there is often a highly abnormal

TABLE 35-5	Traditional and Chronic Kidney Disease–Related Risk Factors for Cardiovascular Disease
Traditional Risk Factors for Cardiovascular Disease	**CKD-Related Risk Factors for Cardiovascular Disease**
Older age	Extracellular fluid overload
Male sex	LVH
White race	Proteinuria
Hypertension	Anemia
Elevated LDL cholesterol	Abnormal calcium phosphorus metabolism
Decreased HDL cholesterol	Dyslipidemia
Diabetes mellitus	MIA syndrome
	Infection
Smoking	Thrombogenic factors
Sedentary life-style	Oxidative stress
Menopause	Elevated homocysteine
Family history	Uremic toxins

CKD, Chronic kidney disease; *HDL,* high-density lipoprotein; *LDL,* Low-density lipoprotein; *LVH,* left ventricular hypertrophy; *MIA,* malnutrition inflammation atherosclerosis.

lipid subfraction profile with a predominance of atherogenic, small, dense LDL particles. In addition triglyceride concentrations are high. Low cholesterol is associated with increased mortality in dialysis patients, likely reflecting coincident inflammation and malnutrition ("reverse causality").

Although there are no data to suggest that statins are of benefit in patients receiving dialysis the Study of Heart and Renal Protection (SHARP) evaluated the use of cholesterol lowering with simvastatin and ezetimibe in 9,000 patients (including 3,000 dialysis patients) and demonstrated significant reductions in stroke and arterial revascularization in the treated patients followed for a median of 4.9 years.[1]

Disturbances in Calcium and Phosphate Metabolism and Bone Disease in Chronic Kidney Disease

Bone disease as a consequence of CKD has long been recognized.[13] As GFR declines, both renal excretion of phosphorus and renal activation of vitamin D decrease reducing ionized calcium. Consequently, the parathyroid glands increase the production of PTH. This increased secretion of PTH stimulates resorption of calcium and phosphate from the bone, the body's major calcium reservoir. Problems develop early, typically once GFR has fallen to approximately 45 mL/min/1.73 m². Secondary hyperparathyroidism classically causes (1) bone changes, (2) so-called high turnover bone disease, and (3) increased risk of fracture. In addition, up regulation of the phosphaturic, fibroblast growth factor 23 (FGF23) occurs early in CKD and this contributes to maintaining plasma phosphate concentrations within the reference interval despite GFR falling below 30 mL/min/1.73 m² (and often much lower).

"Adynamic" bone disease is also highly prevalent in patients with CKD and is characterized by poor bone formation. It is more common in the elderly and those with diabetes and malnutrition. Adynamic bone is associated with (1) a low PTH concentration, (2) abnormal calcium balance,

(3) hyperphosphatemia, (4) acidosis and (5) the use of high doses of vitamin D analogs. Vascular calcification is commonly associated with adynamic bone disease.

High concentrations of plasma phosphate are associated with increased mortality in hemodialysis (HD) patients. Tactics to reduce phosphate concentrations are employed routinely in the treatment of patients on dialysis. Phosphate is present in many foods and is linearly associated with protein ingestion. The recommended allowance of phosphate is reduced for patients on dialysis to around 800 mg/d. Treatment with vitamin D analogs increases gut absorption of phosphate from approximately 65% to almost 85%. The use of phosphate binders, taken with meals, is almost universal in dialysis patients and reduces phosphate absorption to 30% to 40%. It has been possible to regulate phosphate balance in patients treated by daily HD.

Anemia

The World Health Organization (WHO) defines anemia as a hemoglobin concentration of less than 13 g/dL in men and less than 12 g/dL in women. It is clearly established that anemia is inevitable as CKD progresses. Therapies are available to correct anemia, and therefore it is mandatory to assess a patient with CKD for anemia. The NKF KDOQI guideline recommends that an estimated GFR of less than 60 mL/min/1.73 m² should be the cutoff value for determining presence or absence of anemia.[16] Detection is important since treatment may alleviate many of the symptoms of CKD and hopefully reduce risk of LVH. The pathology of anemia in CKD is multifactorial but the predominant cause is loss of peritubular fibroblasts (specialized cells that produce collagen and other materials) within the renal cortex that synthesize EPO. Failure to produce EPO leads to decreased numbers of red cells and concomitant decreased concentrations of hemoglobin. Other causes of anemia include (1) absolute or functional iron deficiency, (2) folic acid and vitamin B_{12} deficiencies, and (3) chronic inflammation. Red cell survival may also be reduced. Treatment with recombinant erythropoiesis stimulating agents is recommended to correct anemia. The gene for human EPO was cloned in 1985 and (1) recombinant forms of EPO (rhEPO), (2) epoetin, or (3) erythropoietin stimulating agents [ESA]) were introduced into clinical practice shortly afterwards. The most common side effect is hypertension, and therefore blood pressure should be controlled before the introduction of treatment. The majority of patients respond to treatment. However, failure to respond requires thorough investigation for many potential causes, such as (1) occult blood loss, (2) hyperparathyroidism, (3) iron deficiency, (4) vitamin B_{12} deficiency (5) folate deficiency, and (6) inadequate dialysis. Many clinical benefits are derived from correcting anemia with ESAs, including (1) improved exercise capacity, (2) improved cognitive function, (3) better quality of life, and (4) increased libido. Later studies have, however, highlighted risks of high doses of ESA in non-dialysis CKD patients with associated increases mortality and cardiovascular morbidity. These studies have been instructive in setting the current

hemoglobin target of 10.0 to 12.0 g/dL and in recommending ESA dose adjustments when hemoglobin is less than 10.5 or greater than 11.5 g/dL, to balance benefit versus safety to patients.

Assessment of Iron

Treatment of anemia in CKD requires adequate iron stores. For example, in patients with CKD, a concentration of plasma ferritin of less than 100 µg/L suggests iron deficiency, and a plasma ferritin of 100 to 200 µg/L in association with a transferrin saturation (TSAT) of less than 20% represents "functional" iron deficiency. Parenteral iron is the treatment of choice for absolute and functional iron deficiency since oral iron has low efficacy in CKD.

The Uremic Syndrome

The **uremic syndrome** is the group of (1) symptoms, (2) physical signs, and (3) abnormal findings on diagnostic studies that result from the failure of the kidneys to maintain adequate (1) excretory, (2) regulatory, and (3) endocrine function. It is considered the terminal clinical manifestation of kidney failure. At least 90 organic compounds have been shown to be retained in **uremia** (Box 35-2).

The classic signs of uremia (**azotemia**) include (1) progressive weakness and easy fatigue, (2) loss of appetite followed by (3) nausea and vomiting, (4) muscle wasting, (5) tremors, (6) abnormal mental function, (7) frequent but shallow respirations, and (8) metabolic acidosis. The syndrome evolves to produce (1) stupor, (2) coma, and (3) ultimately death unless support is provided by dialysis or successful kidney transplantation. The composition of plasma is abnormally labile in response to such factors as (1) diet, (2) state of hydration, (3) gastrointestinal bleeding, (4) vomiting, (5) diarrhea, and (6) intake of therapeutic drugs. Patients with stage 5 CKD (GFR of less than or equal to 15 mL/min/m²) will generally exhibit signs and symptoms of uremia, or a need for RRT.

The most characteristic laboratory findings are increased concentrations of nitrogenous compounds in plasma, such as urea and creatinine, as a result of reduced GFR and decreased tubular function. Retention of these compounds and of metabolic acids is followed by progressive (1) hyperphosphatemia, (2) hypocalcemia, and potentially dangerous (3) hyperkalemia. Although most patients eventually exhibit acidemia, respiratory compensation by elimination of carbon dioxide is extremely important. In addition, reduced endocrine function is manifested by inadequate synthesis of EPO and calcitriol with resulting anemia and osteomalacia. Disordered regulation of blood pressure generally leads to hypertension. Biochemical characteristics of the uremic syndrome are summarized in Box 35-2.

In addition to the consequences of reduced (1) excretory, (2) regulatory, and (3) endocrine function of the kidneys, the uremic syndrome has several systemic manifestations—among them (1) pericarditis, (2) pleuritis, (3) disordered platelet and granulocyte function, and (4) encephalopathy.

Many retained metabolites have been implicated in the systemic toxicity of the uremic syndrome. Although urea was the

BOX 35-2 Biochemical Characteristics of the Uremic Syndrome

Retained Nitrogenous Metabolites
Urea
Cyanate
Creatinine
Guanidine compounds
"Middle molecules"
Uric acid

Fluid, Acid-Base, and Electrolyte Disturbances
Fixed urine osmolality
Metabolic acidosis (decreased blood pH, bicarbonate)
Hyponatremia or hypernatremia or hyperkalemia
Hyperchloremia
Hypocalcemia
Hyperphosphatemia
Hypermagnesemia

Carbohydrate Intolerance
Insulin resistance (hypoglycemia may also occur)
Plasma insulin within reference interval or increased
Delayed response to carbohydrate loading
Hyperglucagonemia

Abnormal Lipid Metabolism
Hypertriglyceridemia
Decreased high-density lipoprotein cholesterol
Hyperlipoproteinemia

Altered Endocrine Function
Secondary hyperparathyroidism
Osteomalacia (secondary to abnormal vitamin D metabolism)
Hyperreninemia and hyperaldosteronism
Hyporeninemia
Hypoaldosteronism
Decreased erythropoietin production
Altered thyroxine metabolism
Gonadal dysfunction (increased prolactin and luteinizing hormone, decreased testosterone)

first of these metabolites to be identified as being increased in uremia, it does not appear to be responsible for the systemic manifestations of uremia. Urea is a 60 Da water-soluble compound (see Chapter 21) that has the highest concentration of presently known uremic retention solutes in uremic plasma. Although its removal by dialysis is directly related to patient survival, the effects of urea on biological systems are not clear. Urea removal by dialysis is not necessarily representative of other molecules retained in the uremic syndrome, particularly protein bound solutes or middle molecules, such as PTH and cystatin C.

Other Diseases of the Kidney

Other kidney diseases discussed in this section include (1) diabetic nephropathy, (2) hypertensive nephropathy, (3) glomerular diseases, (4) interstitial **nephritis**, (5) polycystic kidney disease, (6) toxic nephropathy, (7) obstructive uropathy, (8) tubular diseases, (9) renal calculi, and (10) cystinuria. In addition, this section also includes discussions on prostaglandins

and NSAIDs in kidney disease, and monoclonal light chains and kidney disease.

Diabetic Nephropathy

Diabetic nephropathy is a clinical diagnosis based on the finding of proteinuria in a patient with diabetes. Overt nephropathy is characterized by protein loss greater than 0.5 g/day. This is equivalent to albumin loss of around 300 mg/day. It is preferable to assess proteinuria as albuminuria, because it is a more sensitive marker for CKD due to diabetes. Consequently, there has been a uniform adoption of albumin as the "criterion standard" in evaluating diabetes-related kidney damage. Patients with a urinary albumin "excretion" rate exceeding 30 mg/day have pathologically increased albuminuria. Diabetic nephropathy is the most common cause of ESRD in the United States and accounts for approximately 40% of incident patients[*] in RRT programs. More than 100,000 people receiving HD in the United States have diabetes as the cause of their ESRD. Among patients who require dialysis, those with diabetes have a 22% higher mortality at 1 year and a 15% higher mortality at 5 years than patients without diabetes. Patients with type 1 diabetes and kidney failure with limited secondary complications of diabetes may be considered for simultaneous pancreas and kidney (SPK) transplantation. Tactics to reduce progression of CKD in patients with diabetes include (1) RAAS blockade, (2) attention to complications of CKD, and (3) reduction of cardiovascular risk. In addition, reaching optimal targets for glycemic control reduces the risk of progression.

Hypertension

Hypertension is second only to diabetes as a primary diagnosis of ESRD for incident patients commencing dialysis in the United States. From 2000-2009, there was an increase of approximately 9% in hypertension as the primary cause of ESRD accounting for around 33% of new ESRD patients. The incidence is higher in the elderly and especially among the black population in the United States. In addition, hypertension often develops as a *consequence* of CKD because of alterations in salt and water metabolism and activation of the sympathetic nervous and renin-angiotensin systems. Hypertension has been known to act as an accelerating force in the development of ESRD. Treatment of hypertension to predefined target blood pressure values is critical to preventing the progression to ESRD.

Glomerular Diseases

Clinically, there are a number of distinctive clinical syndromes that result from glomerular injury. Some of the more important are discussed below.

Individuals with primary glomerular disease present clinically with (1) abnormalities of the urine, including

---

[*]An incident patient is one who is receiving regular in-center hemodialysis or any type of peritoneal dialysis treatments for chronic renal failure at least once weekly for the first time. (http://www.usrds.org/download/1997/ch04.pdf/accessed September 16, 2013)

proteinuria and hematuria, (2) hypertension, (3) edema and, often, (4) reduced renal excretory function. Urinalysis should be ordered for patients presenting with hypertension or renal impairment or suspected of having kidney disease. Urinary casts are identified by microscopy, and red cell casts are indicative of glomerular bleeding and glomerular pathology. Laboratory tests performed to investigate glomerular disease and systemic disorders include (1) urinary protein, (2) plasma creatinine concentration and estimated GFR, (3) liver function tests, (4) plasma glucose concentration, (5) urinary examination for Bence Jones protein and, if myeloma is suspected, (6) serum protein electrophoresis. Serological testing for the presence of autoantibodies to (1) antinuclear antigens (ANAs), (2) double-stranded DNA (dsDNA), (3) extractable nuclear antigens (ENAs), and (4) antineutrophil cytoplasmic antibody (ANCA). The latter is measured if either SLE or systemic vasculitis is suspected. Antiglomerular basement membrane (anti-GBM) antibodies may be detected in rare cases of renal-limited anti-GBM disease (Goodpasture disease) and pulmonary-renal syndromes (Goodpasture syndrome). Components of the complement system sometimes are affected (e.g., reduced concentrations of complement C3 and C4) in several conditions, including (1) SLE, (2) infection, (3) cryoglobulinemia, and (4) mesangiocapillary (also referred to as *membranoproliferative*) glomerulonephritis. Blood cultures are taken for bacteriological examination in a case of suspected infection.

Immunoglobulin A Nephropathy

IgA nephropathy is the most common type of glomerulonephritis worldwide. The disease tends to be slowly progressive. For example, in 20 years 30% to 40% of affected patients will develop ESRD depending on the degree of (1) proteinuria and (2) GFR at the time of diagnosis and (3) interstitial fibrosis on biopsy. Biopsy findings are pathognomonic with deposition of polymeric IgA. Up to 50% of patients exhibit elevated concentrations of plasma IgA, although diagnosis depends on kidney biopsy findings. Current treatment strategies are unsatisfactory, but involve general measures to reduce proteinuria, and prednisolone therapy in selected cases.

Rapidly Progressive Glomerulonephritis

Rapidly progressive glomerulonephritis (RPGN) is a heterogeneous group of disorders characterized by a fulminating clinical course that leads to kidney failure in only weeks or a few months. These syndromes are often characterized by focal necrotizing glomerulonephritis and extracapillary crescent formation within the parietal layer of Bowman capsules. Proliferating epithelial cells and macrophages eventually compress the glomeruli and obstruct the proximal convoluted tubules, thus severely compromising nephron function.

Acute Nephritic Syndrome

The **acute nephritic syndrome** is characterized by the rapid onset of (1) hematuria, (2) proteinuria, (3) reduced GFR, and (4) sodium and water retention with resulting hypertension and localized peripheral edema. This is generally caused by a proliferative process causing marked glomerular inflammation. In contrast, nephrotic syndrome is characterized by heavy proteinuria but not typically hematuria.

Nephrotic Syndrome

Gross changes in glomerular permeability characterize the nephrotic syndrome. The diagnostic criteria for establishing nephrotic syndrome are the presence of (1) proteinuria (total protein >3 g/day or albumin >1.5 g/day), (2) hypoalbuminemia, (3) hypercholesterolemia, and finally (4) edema. Nephrotic syndrome results from a variety of causes, including (1) minimal change nephropathy (most common in children); (2) focal segmental glomerulosclerosis (FSGS); (3) membranous nephropathy, which may be idiopathic or associated with carcinoma, drugs, or infection; (4) SLE; and (5) diabetic nephropathy.

Interstitial Nephritis

A variety of chemical, bacterial, and immunological injuries to the kidney cause either generalized or localized changes that primarily affect the tubulointerstitium rather than the glomerulus. This group of disorders is characterized by alterations in tubular function that, in advanced cases, may cause secondary vascular and glomerular damage. **Interstitial nephritis**, including chronic pyelonephritis, is the primary diagnosis, accounting for 3.8% of patients admitted into dialysis programs in the United States. **Pyelonephritis** is the term associated with a bacterial infection that causes this kind of damage and is the most common of the interstitial nephritides. Acute allergic interstitial nephritis presents with AKI and marked inflammation of the interstitium. Blood cells that are prominent upon inspection include (1) lymphocytes, (2) polymorphonuclear cells, and (3) eosinophils. A drug hypersensitivity reaction is the most common form of acute interstitial nephritis. Urinary findings may be typical, or there may be blood and proteinuria. More than 100 different drugs have been implicated, but NSAIDs and β-lactam antibiotics are the drugs most commonly identified.

Polycystic Kidney Disease

Autosomal dominant **polycystic kidney disease** (ADPKD) is the second most common inherited monogenic disease (after familial hypercholesterolemia), and is the most common inherited kidney disease. Approximately 12.5 million people worldwide are affected. In the United Kingdom, ADPKD is responsible for 10% of new ESRD in patients younger than 65 years with approximately 50% of ADPKD patients developing kidney failure by age 55 years. An important clinical observation is the highly variable phenotype within families. The disease causes the development of multiple kidney cysts and extrarenal cysts occurring in the liver and pancreas. About 10% of ADPKD families have a strong family history of intracranial arterial aneurysm rupture. Hypertension is an early and frequent manifestation, and gross hematuria is a common presenting symptom. On the basis of its (1) effectiveness,

(2) cost, and (3) safety, ultrasound is the imaging modality most commonly used to make the diagnosis.

ADPKD is caused by mutations in the genes (*PKD1* and *PKD2*) that encode polycystin 1 and 2, which are located in primary cilia. A definite diagnosis of ADPKD relies on imaging or molecular genetic testing. Genetic testing is not used routinely as a screening tool because current techniques identify only 70% of the hundreds of different *PKD1* and *PKD2* mutations. Specific treatments for ADPKD in clinical practice are currently lacking although generic therapy of CKD is used including treatment of hypertension with ACE inhibitors and/ or ARBs and maintaining a fluid intake of 2 to 3 L/d to reduce risk of kidney stone disease. Specific therapies in development include vasopressin receptor antagonists and antiproliferative drugs that may reduce cyst progression.

Toxic Nephropathy

A wide variety of nephrotoxins exist in the environment that result in a condition known as **toxic nephropathy**. For example, a variety of metals (such as cadmium and lead) have long been known to be associated with kidney disease, often causing proximal tubular dysfunction and glomerular damage. A summary of the drugs and environmental toxins known to cause kidney damage is given in Table 35-6. Both glomerular and tubulointerstitial damage result from exposure to these toxins. Detection of both requires biochemical monitoring of GFR and tubular and glomerular proteinuria.

Obstructive Uropathy

Benign prostatic hypertrophy (BPH) is one of the most common types of **obstructive uropathy** and an almost universal finding in aging men. Among the most common symptoms are disorders of micturition, in particular increased frequency; and in many cases, this progresses to bladder outflow obstruction. There is a tendency to slower progression to ESRD in obstructive uropathy compared with other kidney diseases.

Tubular Diseases

Renal tubular acidoses (RTAs) and inherited tubulopathies are types of renal tubular disease.

Renal Tubular Acidoses

The **renal tubular acidoses (RTAs)** comprise a diverse group of both inherited and acquired disorders. They affect either the proximal or distal tubule. They are characterized by a (1) hyperchloremic, (2) normal-anion-gap, (3) metabolic acidosis, with (3) urinary bicarbonate or (4) hydrogen ion excretion inappropriate for the plasma pH. They are the result of either failure to retain bicarbonate or inability of the renal tubules to secrete hydrogen ion. Typically the GFR in RTA is normal, or slightly reduced, and there is no retention of anions, such as phosphate and sulfate (as occurs with the acidosis of renal failure).

The three categories of RTA are (1) distal (dRTA, type I); (2) proximal (pRTA, type II); and (3) type IV, which is secondary to aldosterone deficiency or resistance. Note: The term "type III RTA" (mixed proximal/distal defect) has been abandoned, because it is no longer considered a separate entity.

TABLE 35-6	Drugs and Environmental Toxins Associated with the Development of Nephropathy
Drug	**Toxic Action**
ACE inhibitors	Drastic drop in GFR in patients with bilateral renal artery stenosis
	High-dose captopril known to cause proteinuria
NSAIDs/COX-2 inhibitors	Drastic drop in GFR in patients with circulatory insufficiency (e.g., cardiac failure)
	Hypovolemia; known to cause acute and chronic interstitial nephritis
Antirheumatoid Drugs	
Calcineurin inhibitors	Vasoconstriction, glomerular vasculopathy, and interstitial fibrosis (cyclosporine and tacrolimus)
Gold salts	Membranous-type picture with nephrotic syndrome (mechanism unknown)
Mercury compounds	Membranous-type picture with nephrotic syndrome (mechanism unknown)
D-penicillamine	Membranous-type picture with nephrotic syndrome (mechanism unknown)
Antitumor Drugs	
Mitomycin	Hemolytic-uremic syndrome
Cisplatin	ATN
Methotrexate	Intraluminal precipitation and ATN
Antibiotics/Antifungals	
Aminoglycosides	ATN and interstitial nephritis
Cephalosporins	Interstitial nephritis
Penicillin G	Interstitial nephritis
Ampicillin	Interstitial nephritis
Amoxicillin	Interstitial nephritis
Amphotericin	Nephrotoxicity
Lithium	Distal tubular damage with nephrogenic DI
Allopurinol	Interstitial nephritis
Environmental Toxins	
Mercury	Glomerulonephritis
Cadmium	Chronic interstitial nephritis
Lead	Hypertension and tubulointerstitial nephritis
Chromium	Increased tubular proteins and enzymuria
Vanadium	Increased tubular proteins and enzymuria
Nickel	Increased tubular proteins and enzymuria
Paraquat	Free radical generator; acute tubular damage
Solvents	
Dry cleaning/paints	Glomerulonephritis

ACE, Angiotensin converting enzyme; *ATN*, acute tubular necrosis; *COX*, cyclooxygenase; *DI*, diabetes insipidus; *GFR*, glomerular filtration rate; *NSAID*, nonsteroidal anti-inflammatory drug.

The finding of a hyperchloremic metabolic acidosis in a patient without evidence of gastrointestinal bicarbonate losses and with no obvious pharmacological cause should prompt suspicion of an RTA. In addition to plasma electrolyte (including potassium) measurements, preliminary investigation should include measurement of urinary pH in a fresh, EMU sample. The finding of a urine pH greater than 5.5 in the presence of a systemic acidosis supports the diagnosis of dRTA.[19]

Inherited Tubulopathies

The inherited tubulopathies comprise a heterogeneous set of rare disorders, including (1) **Bartter syndrome**, (2) **Gitelman syndrome**, (3) **Liddle syndrome**, (4) **pseudohypoaldosteronism type I**, (5) **Dent disease**, and (6) **X-linked dominant hypophosphatemic** rickets (previously known as vitamin D–resistant rickets). Most are characterized by electrolyte disturbances. In addition to these, general reasons to suspect a tubulopathy include (1) a familial disease pattern, (2) renal impairment, (3) nephrocalcinosis, and (4) stone formation, especially if these should present at an early age. In cases in which a diuretic-sensitive channel is affected, these disorders will clearly mimic the effects of diuretic use, and exclusion of covert use of diuretics is important. Although they are individually uncommon or rare, an awareness of these disorders is critical for the clinical laboratorian when considering the potential differential diagnoses in patients having electrolyte imbalances.[20]

Diuretics

Diuretics are predominantly prescribed to treat hypertension and/or disorders associated with fluid overload. All diuretics act by interfering with tubular reabsorption of sodium and/or chloride and therefore have accompanying effects on water retention. Different classes of diuretics act at different sites along the nephron. Classes include (1) loop, (2) thiazide, and (3) "potassium-sparing" diuretics. Many diuretics will cause hypokalemia to some degree, depending on the (1) potency, (2) dose, (3) duration of treatment, and (4) patient's underlying potassium balance.[21]

Diabetes Insipidus

Diabetes insipidus (DI) is a disorder in which there is an abnormal increase in urine output, fluid intake, and often thirst. DI is due to the absence of an ADH effect, either because of impaired or failed secretion (cranial or central DI) or lack of end-organ response to ADH (nephrogenic DI). A further disorder, psychogenic polydipsia, or compulsive water drinking, has been known to present as DI. The investigation of DI involves firstly demonstrating that the patient is unable to form a concentrated urine by undertaking a water deprivation test (see Chapter 40). The patient is then given synthetic ADH to establish whether the defect in concentrating ability is at the renal or pituitary level.

Renal Calculi

Nephrolithiasis is a condition marked by the presence of renal calculi. Such calculi ("kidney stones") occur in the (1) renal pelvis, (2) ureter, and (3) bladder. Kidney stone formation is often considered to be a nutritional or environmental disease, linked to affluence, but genetic or anatomical abnormalities also play a role. Approximately 5% to 10% of the population of the western world are thought to have formed at least one kidney stone by the age of 70 years and the prevalence of kidney stones may be increasing. In both males and females, the average age of first stone formation is decreasing. For most stone types, there is a male preponderance. The passage of a stone is associated with severe pain called "renal colic", which may last for 15 minutes to several hours and is commonly associated with nausea and vomiting.

The majority of kidney stones found in the western world are composed of one or more of the following substances: (1) calcium oxalate with or without phosphate (frequency 67%); (2) magnesium ammonium phosphate (12%); (3) calcium phosphate (8%); (4) urate (8%); (5) cystine (1% to 2%); and (6) complex mixtures of the above (2% to 3%). These poorly soluble substances crystallize within an organic matrix, the nature of which is not well understood. Most kidney stones are treated by **lithotripsy** that entails crushing a calculus within the urinary system or gallbladder, followed at once by the washing out of the fragments.

Prostaglandins and Nonsteroidal Antiinflammatory Drugs in Kidney Disease

The prostaglandins are a series of twenty-carbon unsaturated fatty acid derivatives arachidonic acid synthesized by the cyclooxygenase (cox) enzyme system (see Chapter 23). The major renal vasodilatory prostaglandin is PGE_2, which is synthesized predominantly in the medulla of the kidney. The major vasoconstrictor prostaglandin is thromboxane A_2, which is produced primarily within the renal cortex. PGE_2 (1) increases renal blood flow rate, (2) inhibits sodium reabsorption in the distal nephron and collecting duct, and (3) stimulates renin release. These actions promote natriuresis (process of excretion of sodium in the urine) and diuresis. In patients with CKD, renal PGE_2 excretion rates are three to five times higher than those in healthy subjects, and therefore PGE_2 production represents a compensatory response to loss of nephron mass. Vasodilatory prostaglandins are synthesized following stimulation with renal sympathetic adrenergic and AII-dependent mechanisms to offset or modulate vasoconstriction. In the tubule, prostaglandins act as autocoids, exerting their effects locally, near the site of synthesis.

NSAIDs have (1) analgesic, (2) antipyretic, and (3) antiinflammatory effects. They block the synthesis of COX products of arachidonic acid, which have a critical role in (1) renal hemodynamics, (2) control of tubular function, and (3) renin release. Analgesic nephropathy is a common cause of ESRD in a number of countries, reaching 10% in Switzerland and Australia, but is essentially a preventable condition for which biochemical monitoring has proved useful. Older people demonstrate significant reduction of GFR within 1 week of ingestion of NSAIDs. Acute interstitial nephritis and nephrotic syndrome have been reported to occur with NSAIDs.

Monoclonal Light Chains and Kidney Disease

Immunoglobulin (Ig) molecules are formed in secretory B cells from polypeptide heavy (H) and light (L) chains. The molecular weight of light chains is around 22.5 kDa. In healthy individuals, the small quantity of circulating polyclonal light chains is filtered by the glomerulus with approximately 90%

reabsorbed in the proximal tubule. When the concentration of filtered light chains is increased, this leads to pathological alteration in the proximal tubule cells. For example, light chains have been known to deposit in the kidney as (1) casts, (2) fibrils, (3) precipitates and (4) crystals, giving rise to a spectrum of disease, including (1) cast nephropathy, (2) amyloid, (3) light chain deposition disease (LCDD), and (4) **Fanconi syndrome**. However, not all patients with a large excess production of monoclonal light chains develop disease. Other promoters include (1) dehydration, (2) hypercalcemia, and (3) contrast medium. NSAIDs also have been implicated.

Myeloma or multiple myeloma is a neoplastic proliferation of secretory B cells (plasma cells) that produce excess amounts of a monoclonal Ig (paraprotein), so-called M protein, because of the characteristic peaks obtained from serum protein electrophoresis on agarose gel. This clonal production is associated with an excess of pure light chain production. In multiple myeloma complete monoclonal Igs (usually IgG or IgA) are accompanied in the plasma by variable concentrations of free light chains that appear in the urine as Bence Jones proteins. M proteins and light chains are identified in the blood and/or the urine in 98% of patients with myeloma using protein electrophoresis and immunofixation. Impairment of kidney function at presentation occurs in almost 50% of patients.

Light chains may cause tubular dysfunction, especially of the proximal tubular cells. Characteristically the light chain variable domain is resistant to degradation by proteases in lysosomes in the tubular cells. The variable domain fragments accumulate in proximal tubular cells, and clinical features include RTA and phosphate wasting.

Treatment of cast nephropathy in myeloma includes (1) fluid resuscitation and (2) treatment of hypercalcemia and (3) infection as supportive measures. In addition chemotherapy is commenced to reduce the light chain load from the proliferating plasma cells.

Renal Replacement Therapy

ESRD is an administrative term in the United States that is related to (1) the conditions for payment for healthcare by the Medicare ESRD Program and specifically the level of GFR and (2) the occurrence of signs and symptoms of kidney failure necessitating initiation of treatment by RRT. No absolute recommendation of commencement of dialysis based on GFR alone is to be made, although commencement of dialysis is typically considered as GFR falls below 15 mL/min/1.73 m^2. The USRDS reports the mean GFR on initiation of dialysis is 10 mL/min/1.73 m^2. RRT includes dialysis procedures and transplantation. Extensive laboratory support is required by an RRT program (Table 35-7).

Dialysis

Dialysis is the process of separating macromolecules from ions and low molecular weight compounds in solution by the difference in their rates of diffusion through a semipermeable

TABLE 35-7	Clinical Laboratory Support for Dialysis Programs
Clinical Condition	**Laboratory Tests**
Acute Dialysis	
Dialysis disequilibrium	Urea and electrolyes, bicarbonate, calcium
Pyrexia	C-reactive protein, white cell count, blood cultures
Bleeding	Clotting screen, platelets
Chronic Dialysis Programs	
Anemia	Ferritin, TSAT, vitamin B12, folate Blood film, PTH, C-reactive protein
Sepsis	C-reactive protein, blood, urine specimens for microscopy, culture and sensitivity
Nutrition	Albumin, phosphate
Cardiovascular disease risk	Lipid profile
Dialysis-related amyloid	β2-Microglobulin (not routinely measured)
CKD-MBD	Predialysis plasma calcium, phosphate (monthly in HD patients; 3X monthly in PD patients)
	ALP
	PTH (at least every 3 months)
	Aluminum in patients receiving aluminum-based phosphate binders (3X-monthly)
Adequacy of HD as assessed by urea clearance	Predialysis and postdialysis urea
Sepsis, abdominal pain in PD	Microscopy and culture of peritoneal dialysate
Adequacy of PD as assessed by weekly small solute clearance	Dialysate creatinine, urea
Peritoneal membrane characteristics assessed by PET	Plasma and dialysate glucose and creatinine

ALP, alkaline phosphatase; *CKD*, chronic kidney disease; *HD*, hemodialysis; *MBD*, mineral and bone disorder; *PD*, peritoneal dialysis; *PET*, peritoneal equilibration test; *PTH*, parathyroid hormone; *TSAT*, transferrin saturation .

membrane. Crystalloids (aqueous solutions of mineral salt) pass readily through this membrane, but larger substances (colloids) pass very slowly or not at all. Two distinct physical processes are involved: diffusion and convection.

Dialysis procedures include (1) hemodialysis (HD), (2) **hemodiafiltration** (HDF), and (3) **peritoneal dialysis (PD)**.

Hemodialysis

HD is the most common method used to treat advanced and permanent kidney failure. Operationally, it involves connecting the patient to a hemodialyzer into which their blood flows.

A concentration gradient is established between the blood side and the dialysate side of a semi-permanent membrane ("artificial kidney") to allow rapid diffusion of waste products from the blood. In addition, a hydrostatic pressure gradient is established across the membrane to facilitate fluid removal and further metabolite clearances by filtration. The cleaned blood is returned to the patient. It

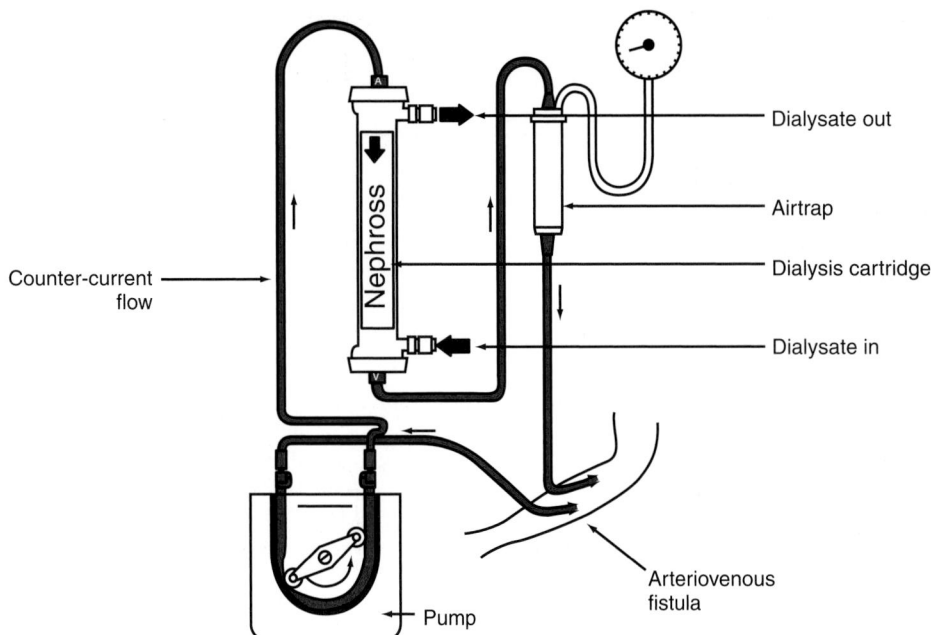

Figure 35-7 A hemodialyzer setup with inset flow diagram.

is a complicated and inconvenient therapy and requires a coordinated effort from a healthcare team and patient and care givers.

An example of a hemodialyzer is shown in Figure 35-7. The most important functional part is the dialyzer membrane. A variety of membranes are available with different surface areas and filtration characteristics. The oldest type of membrane was made from cuprophane and cellulose acetate; however, these have been replaced by more biocompatible synthetic membranes made from polysulfone and polyacrylonitrile. Patients are dialyzed in home-based or hospital-based units with dialysis usually performed three times a week for sessions lasting between 3 and 5 hours.

Hemodiafiltration

HDF is a method of treatment that combines HD and hemofiltration. It offers the advantages of HD (predominantly diffusion based) and high filtration volumes in a single therapy. The result is that HDF provides a 10% to 15% increase in urea clearance compared with HD as well as increased middle molecule clearances from convection.

Peritoneal Dialysis

Peritoneal dialysis (PD) is a type of dialysis in which dialysate is introduced into the patient's peritoneal cavity and is the peritoneum employed as the dialysis membrane (Figure 35-8). **Continuous ambulatory peritoneal dialysis (CAPD)** is performed in ambulatory patients during normal activities.

Operationally, CAPD uses the patient's own peritoneal membrane (surface area approximately 2 m²) across which fluid and solutes are exchanged between the peritoneal capillary blood and the dialysis solution placed in the peritoneal

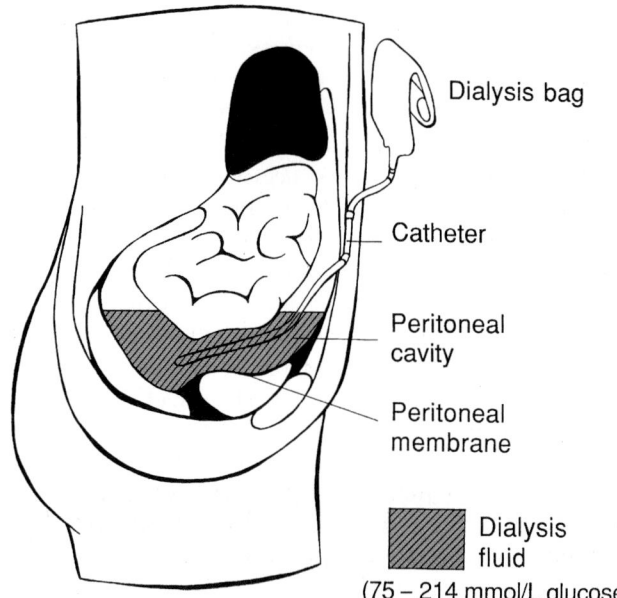

Figure 35-8 Diagrammatic sketch of peritoneal dialysis (PD). To convert glucose concentration in mmol/L to mg/dL, multiply by 18. *(Redrawn from Nolph KD. Peritoneal anatomy and transport physiology. In: Maher JF, ed. Replacement of renal function by dialysis, 3rd edition. Dordrecht, The Netherlands: Kluwer Academic Publishers/Springer, 1989, Chapter 23. With kind permission of Springer Science and Business Media.)*

cavity. Fluid removal or ultrafiltration is achieved by using dialysis fluids containing high concentrations of dextrose acting as an osmotic agent; as the dextrose passes across the peritoneal membrane, the rate of fluid removal decreases. Conventional therapies use four daily exchanges of approximately

2 L of fluid with approximately 10 L of spent dialysate generated, including UF.

Kidney Transplantation

Kidney transplantation is the most effective form of RRT, in terms of long-term survival and quality of life. Approximately 30% of patients on dialysis are selected to be placed on the waiting list for a transplant. Successful transplantation requires (1) preoperative assessment, (2) postoperative assessment, and (3) therapeutic drug management. In addition to cadaveric donation there has been increased utilization of live donors in many countries with excellent outcomes. All these advancements have led to increases in graft and patient survival with 1-year graft survival of approximately 90% being the norm. By contrast, long-term graft survival remains a major problem, with half of transplants failing within 14 years, usually as a result of chronic allograft injury or death with a functioning graft.

Preoperative Assessment

The criteria for acceptance into a transplant program differ slightly from center to center, and it is easier to consider reasons for exclusion. Candidates should not be obese (body mass index [BMI] less than 40 kg/m^2) and should not have (1) severe chronic lung disease, (2) inoperable ischemic heart disease, (3) active infective liver or immunological disease, (4) chronic infection (e.g., tuberculosis), (5) pre-existing malignancy, or (6) lower urinary tract dysfunction. There are also two important psychological issues to be considered: (1) the concept of organ receipt and (2) the potential difficulty in complying with immunosuppressive therapies. Age is no longer a primary issue in an otherwise healthy individual.

Laboratory assessment includes indicators of general operative health, such as (1) electrolytes, (2) acid-base status, (3) clotting profile, (4) full blood cell count, and (5) tissue crossmatching. Full human leukocyte antigen (HLA) tissue typing is also undertaken, in addition to a full screen for infectious diseases, particularly (1) cytomegalovirus (CMV), (2) hepatitis, (3) herpes, and (4) HIV, as these infections are sometimes activated by immunosuppressive therapy.

Postoperative Assessment

During the initial postoperative phase of 1 to 2 weeks, careful monitoring of plasma creatinine (Figure 35-9) and urine output is required to monitor graft function. Most grafts produce measurable amounts of urine within a matter of hours, and this is a clear sign of a functioning graft; however, in perhaps 5% to 10% of cases, there is apparently primary non-function. In this subgroup, continuing dialysis support is necessary. Since in nearly all cases the transplant has different tissue

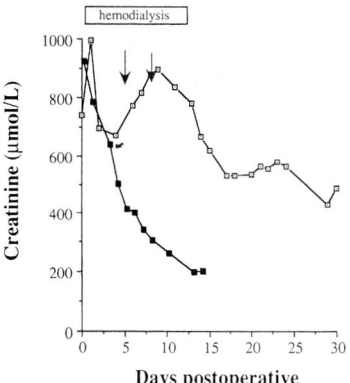

Figure 35-9 Posttransplantation biochemical profile. *Open squares* represent the course of a patient who experienced an early rejection episode (confirmed by biopsy, ↓) and requiring initial hemodialysis (HD) support. *Solid squares* represent the typical profile of an uncomplicated transplant recipient. To convert creatinine concentration in μmol/L to mg/dL, multiply by 0.011.

antigens to the recipient, it will be recognized as foreign by the recipient's immune system, which could result in rejection of the transplant.

Immunosuppression and Therapeutic Drug Management

The introduction of immunosuppressive drugs in the 1970s led to a vast improvement in the success rate of kidney transplantations. Despite their obvious benefits, immunosuppressive drugs have numerous and potentially serious side effects. Therefore, therapeutic drug management and monitoring are required, details of which are given in Chapter 30. In the very early postoperative phase, in addition to rejection, graft dysfunction may be a consequence of (1) delayed graft function, (2) immunosuppressive drug toxicity, and (3) acute tubular damage. Relative hypotension and dehydration may also contribute. Renal artery and vein thromboses are rare complications, and ureteric obstruction is readily diagnosed using ultrasonography. Histologic examination of a transplant biopsy is necessary to aid diagnosis and treatment adjustment. Regular monitoring of (1) kidney function, (2) drug concentrations, and (3) viral assay—particularly for CMV viremia and polyoma viruses, such as BK virus—is mandated following kidney transplantation in many centers. In addition vigilance for post-transplant lymphoproliferative disorders (PTLD), particularly driven by Epstein-Barr virus, is necessary. In the long-term, consideration is given to increased cardiovascular risk and regular assessment of bone mineral mass since osteoporosis is more prevalent in the transplanted population than in age- and sex-matched normal population. Non-infectious complications of immunosuppressive drugs are outlined in Table 35-8.

TABLE 35-8   Non-Infectious Complications of Immunosuppressant Drugs

Drug	Drug Dose	Target Therapeutic Range*	Selected Toxicity Profile
Corticosteroids (e.g., prednisone)	Dose depends on weight of patient and time since transplant.	Not appropriate	Increased risk of developing diabetes mellitus Osteoporosis Psychosis Hypertension Weight gain
Calcineurin Inhibitors			
Cyclosporine	Variable Depends on weight, time since transplant, and achieved drug concentration. Given in two divided doses and predose trough concentration measured in morning blood sample.	200-300 µg/L for first 3 to 12 months. Thereafter aim for 100 µg/L	Nephrotoxicity Hypertension Tubular electrolyte abnormalities (hypophosphatemia, hypomagnesemia, hyperkalemia) Hirsutism Gingival hyperplasia
Tacrolimus			As for cyclosporine, except no hirsutism or gingival hyperplasia Increased risk of diabetes mellitus Cardiomyopathy (children) Alopecia
Mycophenolate mofetil	Aim for 2 g daily in divided doses.	Not routinely measured although active compound, mycophenolic acid (MPA), measured in some institutions	Abdominal pain Diarrhea Myelosuppression
Sirolimus	Dose depends on weight and achieved drug concentration. The drug is administered once daily.	Concentration depends on time since transplant. Typical early (< 3 months) targets are 8-12 µg/L and thereafter 4-8 µg/L	Lymphocele (a fluid-filled collection near to transplanted kidney) Low platelets Hyperlipidemia
Azathioprine	Usual starting dose of 2 mg/kg body weight in a single daily dose.	Concentrations not measured. Because the enzyme TPMT metabolizes azathioprine, the risk of myelosuppression is increased in patients with low activity of the enzyme.	Myelosuppression Severe interaction if used with allopurinol (treatment for gout)
Biological Agents			
Anti-CD25 monoclonal antibodies Basiliximab and daclizumab	Given at time of transplant and once thereafter.		Very well tolerated
Polyclonal ATG and ALG, and monoclonal	Given in response to refractory rejection episodes in selected patients.		Increased risk of malignancy, post-transplant lymphoproliferative disease, hypersensitivity reactions

*These are not recommendations but are illustrative and will vary between centers.
ALG, Antilymphocyte globulin; *ATG*, antithymocyte globulin; *TPMT*, thiopurine methyltransferase.

Review Questions

1. It is difficult to directly measure the GFR of a kidney; therefore, which one of the following is assessed to determine GFR?
   a. Renal blood flow
   b. Renal threshold
   c. Serum creatinine
   d. Urine albumin
2. Which one of the following tests evaluates renal tubular (including loop of Henle) function?
   a. Urine osmolality
   b. Inulin clearance
   c. Urine albumin
   d. Urine protein
3. The structural and functional unit of the kidney is the nephron. What structures make up a nephron?
   a. Only the structures located in the kidney cortex
   b. The glomeruli, tubules, and associated blood vessels
   c. The ureters, bladder, and urethra
   d. Only the structures located in the kidney medulla
4. Pyelonephritis is:
   a. Caused by a lack of intrinsic factor
   b. The destruction of kidney glomeruli by immune complexes
   c. A tumor of the stomach
   d. A kidney tubule disease involving the renal pelvis

5. Which one of the following hormones synthesized in cells of the JGA is involved in control of blood pressure through its action on angiotensinogen?
   a. Erythropoietin
   b. Anti-diuretic hormone
   c. Renin
   d. Aldosterone

6. Regarding laboratory findings, uremia/azotemia specifically refers to:
   a. Reduced renal function
   b. Elevated nitrogenous compounds in blood
   c. Elevated serum proteins in blood
   d. Decreased urine albumin

7. The most common glomerular disease caused by damage to the glomerular membrane from deposition of immune complexes is:
   a. IgA nephropathy
   b. Chronic glomerulonephritis
   c. Uremic syndrome
   d. Pyelonephritis

8. A disorder in which there is an abnormal increase in urine output, fluid intake, and often thirst and that is caused by the absence of anti-diuretic hormone is:
   a. Diabetes mellitus
   b. IgA nephropathy
   c. Diabetes insipidus
   d. Nephrolithiasis

9. Which one of the following hormones affects water reabsorption in the proximal tubule, the loop of Henle, the distal tubule, and the collecting duct of the kidney?
   a. Aldosterone
   b. Renin
   c. $1,25(OH_2)$ vitamin D_3
   d. Anti-diuretic hormone

10. A drug prescribed to an individual to treat hypertension and/or disorders associated with fluid overload is referred to as a(n):
    a. ACE inhibitor
    b. Diuretic
    c. Cystatin C
    d. Exogenous marker

References

1. Baigent C, Landray MJ, Reith C, et al. The effects of lowering LDL cholesterol with simvastatin plus ezetimibe in patients with chronic kidney disease (Study of Heart and Renal Protection): a randomised placebo-controlled trial. Lancet 2011;377(9784):2181–92.

2. Delanaye P, Cavalier E, Moranne O, et al. Creatinine-or cystatin C-based equations to estimate glomerular filtration in the general population: impact on the epidemiology of chronic kidney disease. BMC Nephrol. 2013;14(1):57.

3. Inker LA, Schmid CH, Tighiouart H, et al. A new equation to estimate glomerular filtration rate from standardized creatinine and cystatin C. N Engl J Med. 2012;367(1):20–9.

4. Kidney Disease Improving Global Outcomes Acute Kidney Injury Working Party. KDIGO clinical practice guideline for acute kidney injury. Kidney Int 2012; 2(Supplement 1):1–138.

5. Kidney Disease Improving Global Outcomes. KDIGO 2012 clinical practice guideline for the evaluation and management of chronic kidney disease. Kidney Int 2013;3(Supplement 1):1–150.

6. Killeen AA, Ashwood ER, Ventura CB, et al. Recent trends in performance and current state of creatinine assays. Arch Pathol Lab Med. 2013;137(4):496–502.

7. Lamb EJ, Levey AS, Stevens PE. The Kidney Disease Improving Global Outcomes (KDIGO) guideline update for chronic kidney disease: evolution not revolution. Clin Chem 2013;59:462–5.

8. Lamb EJ, Mackenzie F, Stevens PE. How should proteinuria be detected and measured? Ann Clin Biochem. 2009;46:205–17.

9. Levey AS, Eckardt KU, Tsukamoto Y, et al. Definition and classification of chronic kidney disease: a position statement from Kidney Disease: Improving Global Outcomes (KDIGO). Kidney Int 2005;67(6):2089–100.

10. Levey AS, Coresh J, Greene T, et al. Using standardized serum creatinine values in the modification of diet in renal disease study equation for estimating glomerular filtration rate. Ann Intern Med. 2006;145(4):247–54.

11. Levey AS, Coresh J, Greene T, et al. Expressing the modification of diet in renal disease study equation for estimating glomerular filtration rate with standardized serum creatinine values. Clin Chem 2007;53(4):766–72.

12. Levey AS, Stevens LA, Schmid CH, et al. A new equation to estimate glomerular filtration rate. Ann Intern Med. 2009;150(9):604–12.

13. Lewis R. Mineral and bone disorders in chronic kidney disease: new insights into mechanism and management. Ann Clin Biochem. 2012;49:432–40.

14. Myers GL, Miller WG, Coresh J, et al. Recommendations for improving serum creatinine measurement: a report from the Laboratory Working Group of the National Kidney Disease Education Program. Clin Chem 2006;52(1):5–18.

15. National Kidney Foundation. K/DOQI clinical practice guidelines for chronic kidney disease: evaluation, classification, and stratification. Am J Kidney Dis 2002;39(2 Suppl 1):S1–266.

16. National Kidney Foundation. KDOQI clinical practice guideline and clinical practice recommendations for anemia in chronic kidney disease: 2007 update of hemoglobin target. Am J Kidney Dis. 2007;50(3):471–530.

17. Nisula S, Kaukonen KM, Vaara ST,, et al. Incidence, risk factors and 90-day mortality of patients with acute kidney injury in Finnish intensive care units: the FINNAKI study. Intensive Care Med 2013;39(3):420–8.

18. Panteghini M, Myers GL, Miller WG, et al. The importance of metrological traceability on the validity of creatinine measurement as an index of renal function. International Federation of Clinical Chemistry and Laboratory Medicine; Working Group on Standardization of Glomerular Filtration Rate Assessment (WG-GFRA), Clin Chem Lab Med 2006;44(10):1287–92.

19. Penney MD, Oleesky DA. Renal tubular acidosis. Ann Clin Biochem 1999;36:408–22.

20. Sayer JA, Pearce SH. Diagnosis and clinical biochemistry of inherited tubulopathies. Ann Clin Biochem 2001;38(Pt 5):459–70.

21. Wile D. Diuretics: a review. Ann Clin Biochem 2012;49:419–31.

Physiology and Disorders of Water, Electrolyte, and Acid-Base Metabolism

Emily I. Schindler, M.D., Ph.D., and Mitchell G. Scott, Ph.D.

Objectives

1. Define the following:

Acid-base balance	Depletional hyponatremia
Aldosterone	Dilutional hyponatremia
Anion gap	Hyper- and hypovolemia
Anti-diuretic hormone	Interstitial fluid
Compensation	Respiration, internal and external

2. State the significance of and describe the total body water (TBW) distribution between compartments, including approximate volume and composition of each compartment, electrolyte distribution and active/passive transport for ion exchange; list the hormonal regulators of water and sodium.

3. For each of the following electrolytes, state and describe regulatory mechanisms, disorders and causes/effects of these disorders:

   Chloride
   Potassium
   Sodium

4. State the Henderson-Hasselbalch equation, and explain each of its components; explain its relation to compensatory mechanisms in acid-base disturbances.

5. Categorize the physiological buffer systems relative to their specific roles in the regulation of blood pH.

6. Explain the specific respiratory and renal mechanisms important in the regulation of acid-base balance.

7. For each of the acid-base imbalances listed below, list the causes, state the primary deficit, compensatory mechanisms and laboratory values obtained with each:

Metabolic acidosis	Respiratory acidosis
Metabolic alkalosis	Respiratory alkalosis

8. State the formula for and calculate anion gap; discuss the clinical usefulness of anion gap, including eight causes of an increased anion gap and four causes of normal anion gap acidosis.

9. Compare chloride responsive, chloride resistant, and exogenous base metabolic alkalosis, including causes and lab values.

10. Assess and solve case studies related to electrolyte disturbances and acid-base balance disorders.

Key Words and Definitions

Acid-base balance The homeostatic maintenance of acids and bases within the body to achieve a physiological pH (approximately 7.40).

Acidemia An arterial blood pH <7.35.

Alkalemia An arterial blood pH >7.45.

Anion gap (AG) The difference between the serum sodium concentration and the sum of the serum chloride and bicarbonate concentrations; the anion gap is high in some forms of metabolic acidosis.

Antiporter A membrane transport protein that mediates the cotransport of substances in opposite directions.

Chronic obstructive pulmonary disease (COPD) Any disorder characterized by persistent or recurring obstruction of bronchial air flow, such as chronic bronchitis, asthma, or pulmonary emphysema.

Compensated metabolic acidosis A state of acidosis in which the pH of the blood has been returned toward normal by respiratory compensation.

Depletional hyponatremia A condition characterized by low plasma concentration of sodium associated with low total body sodium and normal blood volume; called also euvolemic hyponatremia.

Diabetes insipidus Any of several types of polyuria in which the volume of urine exceeds 3 liters per day, causing dehydration and great thirst, as well as sometimes emaciation and great hunger.

Dilutional hyponatremia A condition characterized by low plasma concentration of sodium resulting from loss of sodium from the body with nonosmotic retention of water.

Extracellular fluid (ECF) A general term for all the body fluids outside the cells, including the interstitial fluid, plasma, lymph, and cerebrospinal fluid (CSF); this fluid provides a constant external environment for the cells.

Henderson-Hasselbalch equation An equation that defines the relationship between pH, bicarbonate, and the partial pressure of dissolved carbon dioxide gas.

Key Words and Definitions—cont'd

Hyperkalemia A concentration of serum potassium above the reference interval limit of 5.0 mmol/L.

Hypernatremia A concentration of serum sodium above the reference interval limit of 150 mmol/L.

Hypervolemia Abnormal increase in the volume of circulating fluid (plasma) in the body.

Hypokalemia A concentration of serum potassium below the reference interval limit of 3.5 mmol/L.

Hyponatremia A concentration of serum sodium below the reference interval limit of 136 mmol/L.

Hypovolemia Abnormally decreased volume of circulating fluid (plasma) in the body.

Intracellular fluid (ICF) The portion of the total body water (TBW) with its dissolved solutes that is within the cell membranes.

Ketoacidosis A condition characterized as acidosis accompanied by the accumulation of ketone bodies (ketosis) in the body tissues and fluids.

Metabolic acidosis A pathological process that leads to the accumulation of acid that lowers the bicarbonate concentration and decreases the pH; also known as primary bicarbonate deficit.

Metabolic alkalosis A pathological process that leads to the accumulation of base that raises the bicarbonate concentration and increases the pH; also known as *primary bicarbonate excess.*

Mixed acid-base disturbance The occurrence of more than one acid-base disorder simultaneously; the blood pH may be low, high, or within the reference interval.

Respiratory acidosis A pathological process that leads to the accumulation of carbon dioxide that raises the PCO_2 and decreases the pH; usually caused by emphysema or hypoventilation.

Respiratory alkalosis A pathological process that leads to the excessive elimination of carbon dioxide which lowers the PCO_2 and increases the pH; caused by hyperventilation.

Sodium–hydrogen exchanger (NHE) A membrane protein that is primarily responsible for maintaining the balance of sodium; also called the sodium–hydrogen antiporter.

Total body water (TBW) Any of various estimates of the water content of the human body, taking into consideration the person's height, weight, and age.

Adaptation to terrestrial life led to the evolution of physiological systems to maintain the composition of the internal milieu of animals, including humans. These systems include a variety of chemical buffers and highly specialized mechanisms of the lungs and kidneys that work in concert to regulate (1) water, (2) electrolytes, and (3) pH between intracellular and extracellular compartments. Small changes (perturbations) in the dynamic equilibria that exist for (1) water, (2) electrolytes, and (3) pH may arise from external sources, such as (1) trauma, (2) changes in altitude, (3) ingestion of toxic substances, or (4) internal sources, such as healthy metabolism and disease state. Endogenous correction of these imbalances may not always be adequate; at these times, the clinical laboratory provides valuable information for guiding therapy.

Total Body Water—Volume and Distribution

Approximately two thirds of **total body water (TBW)** is distributed into the **intracellular fluid (ICF)** compartment, and one third exists in the **extracellular fluid (ECF)** compartment. These compartments are physically separated by the cellular plasma membrane. The ECF may be subdivided into interstitial ($\approx$75% of ECF) and intravascular ($\approx$25% of ECF) fluid compartments, which are separated by the capillary endothelium. The average adult has $\approx$5 L blood volume (intravascular compartment) and a plasma volume of $\approx$3.0 L when the hematocrit is $\approx$40%.

Factors that influence daily water and electrolyte requirements include (1) activity of the individual, (2) environmental conditions, and (3) disease. However, on average, an adult must take in $\approx$1.5 to 2.0 L of water daily to maintain fluid balance.

Because primary regulatory mechanisms are designed to first maintain intracellular hydration status, imbalances in TBW are initially reflected in the ECF compartment. Table 36-1 lists common causes and clinical manifestations of expansion and contraction of the ECF compartment.

Water and Electrolytes—Composition of Body Fluids

The primary cationic (positively charged) electrolytes are (1) sodium (Na^+), (2) potassium (K^+), (3) calcium (Ca^{2+}), and (4) magnesium (Mg^{2+}). The primary anionic (negatively

TABLE 36-1	Causes and Clinical Manifestations of Changes in Extracellular Fluid Volume
	Clinical Manifestations	**Causes**
ECF Loss	Thirst, anorexia, nausea, lightheadedness, orthostatic hypotension, syncope, tachycardia, oliguria, decreased skin turgor and "sunken eyes," shock, coma, death	Trauma (and other causes of acute blood loss), "third-spacing" of fluid (e.g., burns, pancreatitis, peritonitis), vomiting, diarrhea, diuretics, renal or adrenal (sodium wasting) disease
ECF Gain	Weight gain, edema, dyspnea (due to pulmonary edema), tachycardia, jugular venous distention, portal hypertension (ascites), esophageal varices	Heart failure, cirrhosis, nephrotic syndrome, iatrogenic (intravenous fluid overload)

ECF, Extracellular fluid.

charged) electrolytes include (1) chloride (Cl^-), (2) bicarbonate (HCO_3^-), (3) phosphate (HPO_4^{2-}, HPO_4^-), (4) sulfate (SO_4^{2-}), (5) organic ions (such as, lactate), and (6) negatively charged proteins. Electrolyte concentrations of the body fluid compartments are shown in Table 36-2. Na^+, K^+, and Cl^- in the plasma or serum are commonly analyzed in an *electrolyte profile,* because their concentrations provide the most relevant information about the (1) osmotic, (2) hydration, and (3) acid-base status of the body.[3] Although hydrogen ion (H^+) is a cation, its concentration is approximately 1 million–fold lower in plasma than the major electrolytes listed in Table 36-2 (10^{-9} mol/L vs. 10^{-3} mol/L) and thus is negligible in terms of osmotic activity.

Extracellular and Intracellular Compartments

The compartments of fluid found in the human body are (1) plasma, (2) interstitial fluid, and (3) ICF.

Plasma

Plasma generally has a volume of 1300 to 1800 mL/m[2] of body surface and constitutes approximately 5% of the body volume ($\approx$3.5 L for a 66 kg subject). Table 36-2 describes the electrolyte composition of plasma. The mass concentration of water in normal plasma is about 0.933 kg/L, depending on the protein and lipid content (see "Electrolyte Exclusion Effect" in Chapter 24). Thus a concentration of sodium in the plasma of 140 mmol/L would correspond to a molality of sodium in plasma water of 150 mmol/kg H_2O (140 mmol/L divided by 0.933 kg/L). The concentration of net protein ions in plasma is $\approx$12 mmol/L with the charge mainly caused by albumin.

Interstitial Fluid

Interstitial fluid is essentially an ultrafiltrate of blood plasma. When all extracellular spaces except plasma are included, the volume accounts for about 26% (10.5 L) of the total body volume. Plasma is separated from the interstitial fluid by the endothelial lining of the capillaries, which acts as a semipermeable membrane and allows passage of water and diffusible solutes but not compounds of high molecular mass, such as proteins.

Intracellular Fluid

The exact composition of ICF is extremely difficult to measure because of the relative unavailability of cells free of contamination. Data for ICF (see Table 36-2), therefore, are considered only approximations. As indicated in the table, the ICF constitutes $\approx$66% of the total body volume. The composition of ICF differs markedly from that of ECF because of separation of these compartments by the cell membrane. The composition differences are primarily a consequence of active and passive transport of ions.

Distribution of Ions by Active and Passive Transport

Examination of Table 36-2 reveals that the electrolyte compositions of blood plasma and interstitial fluid (both ECFs) are similar, but their compositions differ markedly from that of ICF. The major ECF ions are Na^+, Cl^-, and HCO_3^-, but in ICF, the main ions are (1) K^+, (2) Mg^{2+}, (3) organic phosphates, and (4) protein. This unequal distribution of ions is due to active transport of Na^+ from inside to outside the cell against an electrochemical gradient. This process requires energy supplied by metabolic processes in the cell such as glycolysis. An active sodium pump deriving its energy from adenosine triphosphate (ATP) is present in most cell membranes and frequently is coupled with transport of K^+ into the cell.

In addition to the Na^+/K^+-ATPase, a ubiquitous Na^+-H^+ exchanger (often referred to as an **antiporter**) actively pumps H^+ out of the ICF in exchange for Na^+. This exchanger is critical for maintaining intracellular pH homeostasis.

Electrolytes

Individual electrolytes having a strong influence on electrolyte disorders and maintenance of water homeostasis include (1) Na^+, (2) K^+, (3) Cl^-, and (4) HCO_3^-

Sodium

Disorders of Na^+ homeostasis occur because of (1) excessive loss, (2) excessive gain, (3) and/or retention of Na^+ or H_2O. As described in detail in Chapter 35, the kidney is the primary organ for regulating body water and extracellular Na^+.

Kidney Function

In the proximal tubules, 70% to 80% of filtered Na^+ is actively reabsorbed, with H_2O and Cl^- following passively to maintain electrical neutrality and osmotic equivalence. In the descending loop of Henle, H_2O, but not electrolytes, is passively reabsorbed because of the high osmotic strength of interstitial fluid

TABLE 36-2	**Electrolyte and Water Composition of Body Fluid Compartments***		
Component	Plasma	Interstitial Fluid	Intracellular Fluid[†]
Volume, H_2O (TBW = 42 L)	3.5 L	10.5 L	28 L
Na^+	142	145	12
K^+	4	4	156
Ca^{2+}	2.4	2-3	0.3
Mg^{2+}	2	1-2	26
Trace elements	1	—	—
Total cations	155	—	—
Cl^-	103	114	4
HCO_3^-	27	31	12
Protein$^-$	16	—	55
Organic acids$^-$	5	—	—
HPO_4^{2-}	2	—	—
SO_4^{2-}	1	—	—
Total anions	154	—	—

TBW, Total body water.
*All electrolyte values are expressed in mEq/L of *fluid.* Because the H_2O content of plasma is $\approx$93% by volume, the corresponding electrolyte concentrations in plasma water are $\approx$10% higher. Note that the *molar concentration* of divalent ions is one half the depicted value.
[†]These values are derived from skeletal muscle.

in the renal medulla. In the ascending loop of Henle, Cl^- is reabsorbed actively with Na^+ following. At the distal tubule, the first of the two primary Na^+/H_2O regulating processes occurs. Here, aldosterone stimulates the cortical collecting ducts to reabsorb Na^+ (with water following passively) and secrete K^+ (and to a lesser extent, H^+) to maintain electrical neutrality. Aldosterone is produced by the adrenal cortex in response to angiotensin II derived via the action of renin. The secretion of renin by renal juxtaglomerular cells is stimulated by low chloride, by β-adrenergic activity, and by low arteriolar pressure.[12] Thus, when the kidneys are hypoperfused (as occurs when blood volume decreases, or when the renal arteries are obstructed), the distal tubules, under the influence of aldosterone, reclaim Na^+.

Further water regulation in the kidney occurs from the distal tubule through the collecting duct, where tubular permeability to H_2O is under the influence of antidiuretic hormone (ADH) (see Chapters 35 and 40). ADH (also called *vasopressin*) is released by the posterior pituitary under the influence of baroreceptors in the aortic arch and of hypothalamic chemoreceptors responsive to circulating osmolality. When blood volume is decreased, or when plasma osmolality is increased, (1) ADH is secreted, (2) tubular permeability to H_2O increases, and (3) H_2O is reabsorbed in an attempt to restore blood volume or to decrease osmolality. In contrast, when blood volume is increased or osmolality decreased, ADH secretion is inhibited, and more H_2O is excreted in the urine (diuresis).

Besides the kidney, the body's other mechanism for restoring Na^+/H_2O homeostasis is ingestion of H_2O. Thirst is stimulated by decreased blood volume or by a hyperosmotic condition. It is important to remember that receptors that influence renal handling of Na^+ and H_2O, and thirst, sense changes only in the intravascular blood volume and not the total ECF. Furthermore, laboratory assessment of water and electrolyte disorders is made primarily from the blood volume (plasma). As discussed in subsequent sections, the clinician must assess the status of TBW and blood volume before interpreting laboratory values in the diagnosis of water and electrolyte disorders (see Table 36-1).

Hyponatremia

Hyponatremia is defined as a decreased plasma Na^+ concentration (<130 to 135 mmol/L). Hyponatremia typically manifests clinically as (1) nausea, (2) generalized weakness, and (3) mental confusion. For example, Na^+ values are typically (1) <120 mmol/L for mental confusion, (2) <110 mmol/L for ocular palsy, and (3) between 90 and 105 mmol/L for severe mental impairment.[11]

It is important to note, however, that symptoms are due to changes in osmolality rather than to the Na^+ concentration per se. For example, hyponatremia is categorized as (1) hypo-osmotic, (2) hyperosmotic, or (3) isosmotic. Thus, measurement of plasma osmolality is an important initial step in the assessment of hyponatremia. Of these, the most common form is hypo-osmotic hyponatremia. Figure 36-1 describes an algorithm for laboratory measurements and physical examination findings in the differential diagnosis of plasma Na^+ <135mmol/L.

Hypo-Osmotic Hyponatremia

Typically, when plasma Na^+ concentration is low, calculated or measured osmolality will also be low. This type of hyponatremia is due to excess loss of Na^+ (**depletional hyponatremia**) or increased ECF volume (**dilutional hyponatremia**). Differentiating these initially requires clinical assessment of TBW and ECF volume by history and physical examination.

Depletional hyponatremia (excess loss of Na^+) is almost always accompanied by loss of ECF water, but to a lesser extent than Na^+ loss. This occurs because thirst leads to ingestion of water, which obviously is more hypotonic than the lost fluids. **Hypovolemia** is apparent in the physical examination with the observation of (1) orthostatic hypotension, (2) tachycardia, and (3) decreased skin turgor. If urine Na^+ is low (generally <10 mmol/L), the loss is extrarenal (see Figure 36-1), because the kidneys are retaining filtered Na^+ in response to aldosterone, which is stimulated by hypovolemia. Causes of extrarenal loss of Na^+ in excess of H_2O include losses from the gastrointestinal tract or skin (see Figure 36-1).

Alternatively, if urine Na^+ is elevated in this setting (generally >20 mmol/L), renal loss of Na^+ is likely. Renal loss of Na^+ occurs with (1) osmotic diuresis, (2) use of diuretics that inhibit reabsorption of Cl^- and Na^+ in the ascending loop, (3) adrenal insufficiency (no aldosterone or cortisone prevents distal tubule reabsorption of Na^+), and (4) salt wasting nephropathies that occurs after acute tubular necrosis or obstructive nephropathy. Renal loss of Na^+ in excess of H_2O has been known to occur in **metabolic alkalosis** from prolonged vomiting, because increased renal HCO_3^- excretion is accompanied by Na^+ ions.

Dilutional hyponatremia is a result of excess H_2O retention and often is detected during the physical examination as edema. In advanced renal failure, water is retained because of decreased filtration and H_2O excretion. When ECF is increased but the blood volume is decreased, as occurs in (1) congestive heart failure (CHF), (2) hepatic cirrhosis, or (3) nephrotic syndrome, a vicious cycle is established. For example, the decreased blood volume is sensed by baroreceptors and results in increased aldosterone and ADH, even though ECF volume is excessive. The kidneys reabsorb Na^+ and H_2O in response to increased aldosterone and ADH in an attempt to restore the blood volume, but this simply results in further increases in ECF and further dilution of Na^+.

In hypo-osmotic hyponatremia with a normal volume status, the most common causes are the (1) syndrome of inappropriate ADH (SIADH), (2) primary polydipsia, and (3) hypothyroidism (see Figure 36-1). SIADH is usually a result of ectopic or otherwise "inappropriate" ADH production arising from a variety of conditions[6] (see Chapters 35 and 40) and results in excessive H_2O retention.

Hyperosmotic Hyponatremia

Hyponatremia that occurs in the presence of increased quantities of other solutes in the ECF is the result of an extracellular shift of water or an intracellular shift of Na^+ to maintain osmotic balance between ECF and ICF compartments. The

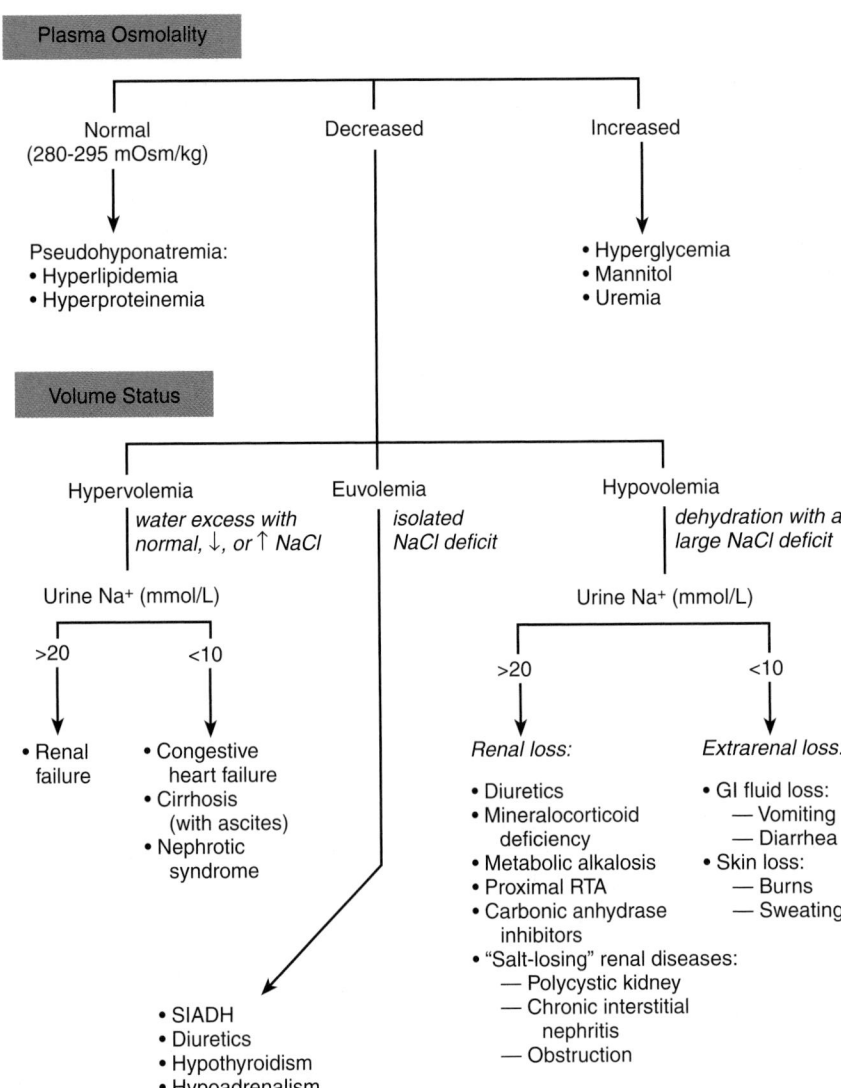

Figure 36-1 Algorithm for the differential diagnosis of hyponatremia. *(Modified from Kirkpatrick W, Kreisberg R. Acid-base and electrolyte disorders. In: Liu P, ed. Blue book of diagnostic tests. Philadelphia: WB Saunders, 1986:239-54.)*

most common cause of this type of hyponatremia is severe hyperglycemia (see Figure 36-1). As a general rule, Na^+ is decreased by ≈ 1.6 to 2.4 mmol/L for every 100 mg/dL increase in glucose above 100 mg/dL.[13]

Isosmotic Hyponatremia

If the measured Na^+ concentration in plasma is decreased, but measured (1) plasma osmolality, (2) glucose, and (3) urea are within their reference interval, the most likely explanation is pseudohyponatremia caused by the *electrolyte exclusion effect* (see Chapter 24).

Hypernatremia[1]

Hypernatremia (plasma Na^+ >150 mmol/L) is always hyperosmolar. Symptoms of hypernatremia are primarily neurologic (because of neuronal cell loss of H_2O to the ECF) and include (1) tremors, (2) irritability, (3) ataxia, (4) confusion, and (5) coma. Most cases of hypernatremia occur in patients with altered mental status or in infants, both of whom may have difficulty in rehydrating themselves despite a normal thirst reflex.

Hypernatremia arises in the setting of (1) hypovolemia (excessive water loss or failure to replace normal water losses), (2) **hypervolemia** (a net Na^+ gain in excess of water gain), or (3) normovolemia. Again, assessment of TBW status by physical examination and measurement of urine Na^+ and osmolality are important steps in establishing a diagnosis (Figure 36-2).

Hypovolemic Hypernatremia

Hypernatremia in the setting of decreased ECF is caused by renal or extrarenal loss of hypo-osmotic fluid, leading to dehydration. Thus, once hypovolemia is established by physical examination, measurement of urine Na^+ and osmolality is used to determine the source of fluid loss. Patients who have large extrarenal losses will have concentrated urine (often >800 mOsmol/L) with low urine Na^+ (<20 mmol/L), reflecting a proper renal response to conserve Na^+ and water to restore ECF volume.

Hypervolemic Hypernatremia

The presence of excess TBW and hypernatremia indicates a net gain of water and Na^+ with Na^+ gain in excess of water

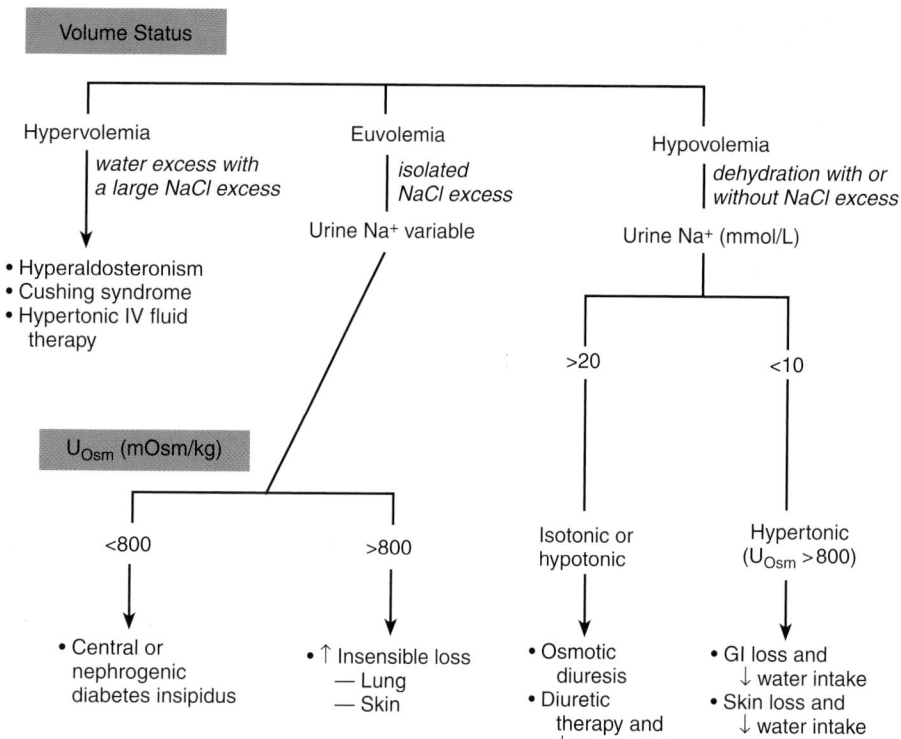

Figure 36-2 Algorithm for the differential diagnosis of hypernatremia. *(Modified from Kirkpatrick W, Kreisberg R. Acid-base and electrolyte disorders. In: Liu P, ed. Blue book of diagnostic tests. Philadelphia: WB Saunders, 1986:239-54.)*

(see Figure 36-2). This rare condition is observed most commonly in hospital patients receiving hypertonic saline or sodium bicarbonate.

Normovolemic Hypernatremia

Hypernatremia in the presence of normal ECF volume is often a prelude to hypovolemic hypernatremia. Insensible losses through the lung or skin again must be suspected and are characterized by concentrated urine as the kidneys conserve water. Another cause of normovolemic hypernatremia is water diuresis, which is manifested by polyuria (see Figure 36-2). The differential for polyuria (generally defined as >3 L urine output/d) is a water or solute diuresis. Solute diuresis is exemplified by the osmotic diuresis of diabetes mellitus and generally is characterized by urine osmolality >300 mOsmol/L and hyponatremia. Water diuresis, a manifestation of **diabetes insipidus** (DI), is characterized by dilute urine (osmolality <250 mOsmol/L) and slight hypernatremia. DI is either central or nephrogenic. Central DI is due to decreased or absent ADH secretion resulting from (1) head trauma, (2) hypophysectomy, (3) pituitary tumor, or (4) granulomatous disease. Nephrogenic DI is due to renal resistance to ADH as a result of drugs, such as (1) lithium, (2) demeclocycline, (3) amphotericin, or (4) propoxyphene. Nephrogenic DI also results from sickle cell anemia and Sjögren syndrome as they affect collecting duct responsiveness to ADH; or, more rarely, mutant ADH receptors.[2]

Potassium

The total body potassium of a 70 kg subject is ≈3.5 mol (40 to 59 mmol/kg) of which only 1.5% to 2% is present in the ECF.

Nevertheless, plasma K[+] is often a good indicator of total K[+] stores, unless abnormal K[+] is due to abnormal cellular shifts. Disturbance of K[+] homeostasis has serious consequences. For example, a decrease in extracellular K[+] (**hypokalemia**) is characterized by (1) muscle weakness, (2) irritability, and (3) paralysis. Plasma K[+] concentrations less than 3.0 mmol/L are often associated with marked neuromuscular symptoms. At lower concentrations, tachycardia and cardiac conduction defects are apparent by electrocardiogram (flattened T waves) and has been known to lead to cardiac arrest.[11]

High extracellular K[+] (**hyperkalemia**) concentrations may produce symptoms of (1) mental confusion, (2) weakness, (3) tingling, (4) flaccid paralysis of the extremities, and (5) weakness of the respiratory muscles.[11] Cardiac effects of hyperkalemia include bradycardia and conduction defects. Prolonged severe hyperkalemia >7.0 mmol/L can lead to peripheral vascular collapse and cardiac arrest. Symptoms are almost always present at K[+] concentrations >6.5 mmol/L. Concentrations >10.0 mmol/L in most cases are fatal.

Hypokalemia

Causes of hypokalemia (plasma K[+] <3.5 mmol/L) are classified as redistribution of extracellular K[+] into ICF, or true K[+] deficits, caused by decreased intake or loss of potassium-rich body fluids (Figure 36-3).

Redistribution

Intracellular redistribution of K[+] is illustrated by the fall in plasma K[+] that occurs following insulin therapy for diabetic hyperglycemia when cells take up K[+] as a consequence of glucose transport. Redistribution hypokalemia is also a feature of

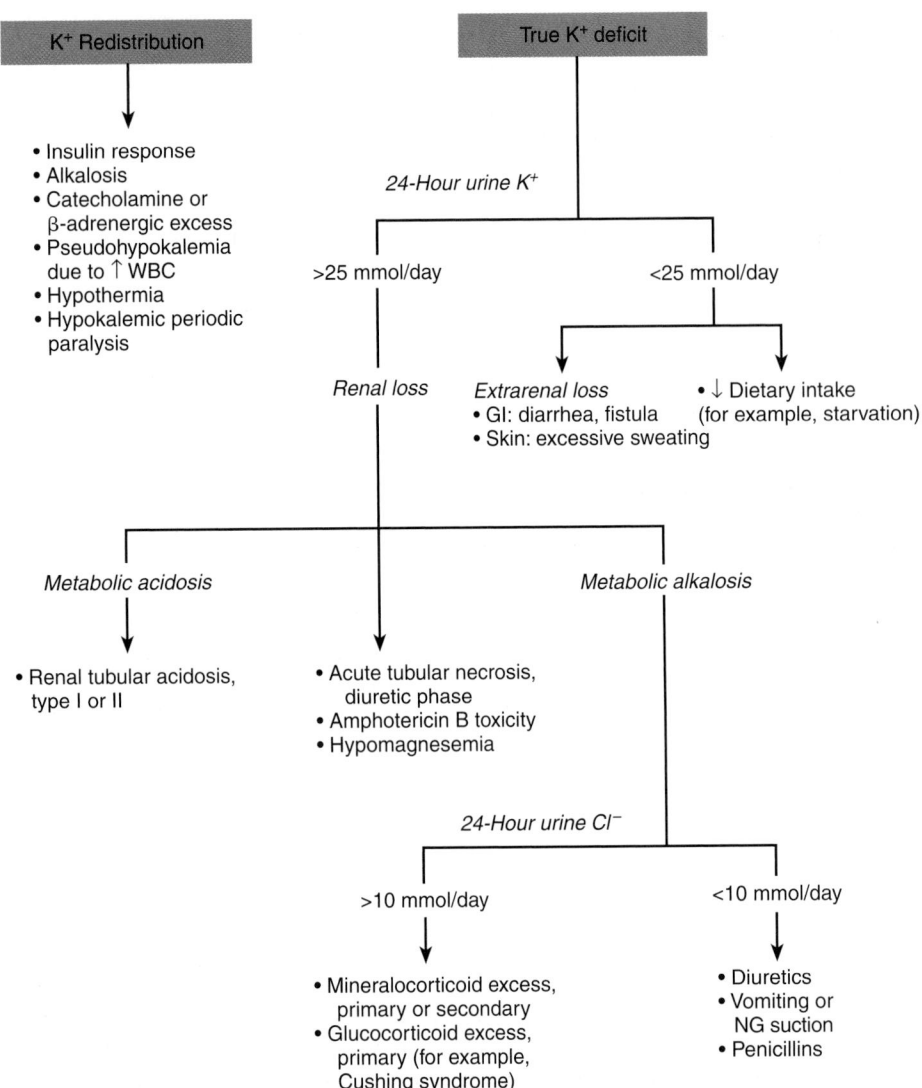

Figure 36-3 Algorithm for the differential diagnosis of hypokalemia. *(Modified from Kirkpatrick W, Kreisberg R. Acid-base and electrolyte disorders. In: Liu P, ed. Blue book of diagnostic tests. Philadelphia: WB Saunders, 1986:239-54.)*

alkalosis, in which K^+ moves from ECF into cells as increased H^+ alters activity of the Na^+/K^+-ATPase. In addition, renal conservation of H^+ in the distal tubule occurs at the expense of K^+. Causes of intracellular redistribution are listed in Figure 36-3.

True Potassium Deficit
Hypokalemia reflecting true total body deficits of K^+ is classified into renal and nonrenal losses, based on daily excretion of K^+ in the urine (see Figure 36-3). If urine excretion of K^+ is <30 mmol/d, it is judged that the kidneys are properly functioning and are attempting to reabsorb K^+ as appropriate in a hypokalemic setting. The cause may be decreased K^+ intake or extrarenal loss of K^+-rich fluid. Situations of decreased intake include chronic starvation and postoperative intravenous fluid therapy with K^+-poor solutions. Gastrointestinal loss of K^+ occurs most commonly with diarrhea.

Urine excretion exceeding 25 to 30 mmol/d in a hypokalemic setting indicates that the kidneys are the primary source of lost amounts of K^+. Renal losses of K^+ may occur during the diuretic (recovery) phase of acute tubular necrosis and

during states of excess mineralocorticoid (primary or secondary aldosteronism) or glucocorticoid (Cushing syndrome) production. When this occurs the distal tubules increase Na^+ reabsorption and K^+ excretion. Renal loss of K^+ is also caused by thiazide and loop diuretics.[9] In addition to redistribution of K^+ into cells in an alkalotic setting, K^+ is lost from the kidneys in exchange for reclaimed H^+ ions.

Hyperkalemia

Hyperkalemia (plasma K^+ >5.0 mmol/L) is a result of singly or in combination: (1) redistribution, (2) increased intake, or (3) increased retention. In addition, preanalytical conditions—such as, (1) hemolysis, (2) thrombocytosis (>10^6/μL), and (3) leukocytosis (>10^5/μL)—have been known to cause marked pseudohyperkalemia (Figure 36-4), as described in detail in Chapter 24.

Redistribution
The transfer of intracellular K^+ into ECF invariably occurs in acidosis as K^+ shifts outward as the result of pH-induced

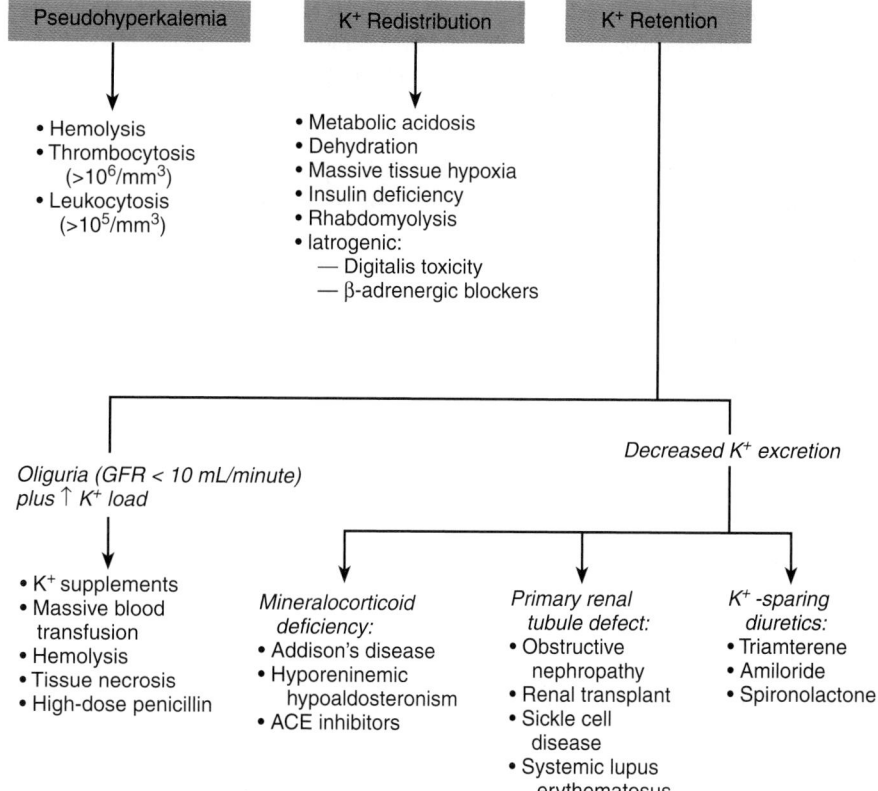

Figure 36-4 Algorithm for the differential diagnosis of hyperkalemia. *(Modified from Kirkpatrick W, Kreisberg R. Acid-base and electrolyte disorders. In: Liu P, ed. Blue book of diagnostic tests. Philadelphia: WB Saunders, 1986:239-54.)*

changes in Na^+/K^+-ATPase activity. When acidosis is corrected, normokalemia will be restored rapidly. Extracellular redistribution of K^+ may also occur in (1) tissue hypoxia; (2) insulin deficiency (e.g., diabetic ketoacidosis); (3) massive intravascular hemolysis; (4) severe burns; (5) violent muscular activity, as in status epilepticus; (6) rhabdomyolysis; and (7) tumor lysis syndrome. Finally, important iatrogenic causes of redistribution hyperkalemia include digoxin toxicity and β-adrenergic blockade, especially in patients with diabetes or on dialysis.[11]

Potassium Retention

When glomerular filtration or renal tubular function is decreased, hyperkalemia may be precipitated by intravenous infusion of K^+. When renal function is natural , overtreatment with K^+ solutions is unlikely to produce hyperkalemia, because renal capacity is more than adequate to excrete the excess K^+. Decreased excretion of K^+ in moderate and acute renal disease and end-stage renal failure (with oliguria or anuria) are the most common causes of prolonged hyperkalemia (see Figure 36-4). Hyperkalemia occurs along with Na^+ depletion in adrenocortical insufficiency (e.g., Addison disease) because diminished Na^+ reabsorption results in decreased tubular K^+ secretion. Drugs that block the production of aldosterone, such as (1) inhibitors of angiotensin-converting enzyme (ACE inhibitors; e.g., lisinopril), (2) nonsteroidal antiinflammatory drugs, and (3) angiotensin II receptor blockers, may also cause hyperkalemia.

Chloride

In the absence of acid-base disturbances, Cl^- concentrations in plasma generally will follow those of Na^+. However, determination of plasma Cl^- concentration is useful in the differential diagnosis of acid-base disturbances and is essential for calculating the **anion gap (AG)**. Fluctuations in serum or plasma Cl^- have little clinical consequence.

Hypochloremia

In general, causes of hypochloremia will parallel causes of hyponatremia. **Respiratory acidosis**, which is accompanied by increased HCO_3^-, is another common cause of decreased Cl^- with normal Na^+.

Hyperchloremia

Increased plasma Cl^- concentration, similar to increased Na^+ concentration, occurs with (1) dehydration, (2) prolonged diarrhea with loss of sodium bicarbonate, (3) DI, and (4) overtreatment with normal saline solutions, which have a Cl^- content of 154 mmol/L. A rise in Cl^- concentration may also be seen in **respiratory alkalosis** because of renal compensation for excreting HCO_3^-.

Bicarbonate

The total carbon dioxide (CO_2) content of plasma consists of carbon dioxide dissolved in an aqueous solution (dCO_2), CO_3 loosely bound to amine groups in proteins (carbamino compounds), HCO_3^-, and very small quantities of CO_3^{2-} ions and carbonic acid (H_2CO_3). Bicarbonate ions make up all but ≈2 mmol/L of the total carbon dioxide of plasma. Alterations in HCO_3^- and CO_2 dissolved in plasma are characteristic of acid-base imbalances.

Acid-Base Physiology

Normal metabolic processes result in the production of large amounts of (1) carbonic acid and lesser amounts of (2) sulfuric, (3) phosphoric, and (4) other acids. For example, during a 24-hour period, a person weighing 70 kg respires approximately 20 mol of carbon dioxide (the volatile form of carbonic acid) through the lungs, and about 70 to 100 mmol (or ≈1 mmol/kg) of nonvolatile acids (mainly sulfuric and phosphoric acids) through the kidneys. These products of metabolism are transported to the lungs and kidneys via the ECF and blood with no appreciable change in the ECF pH, and with only a minimal difference between arterial (pH 7.35 to 7.45) and venous (pH 7.32 to 7.38) blood. This is accomplished by the buffering capacity of blood and by respiratory and renal regulatory mechanisms.

Acid-Base Balance and Acid-Base Status

The bicarbonate/carbonic acid system is the most important mammalian buffering system. The acid-base status of body fluids is typically assessed by measurements of (1) total CO_2, (2) plasma pH, and (3) PCO_2.

The following clinical terms are used to describe acid-base status. **Acidemia** is defined as an arterial blood pH <7.35, and **alkalemia** indicates an arterial blood pH >7.45. Acidosis and alkalosis refer to pathological states that often lead to acidemia or alkalemia. It should be noted that more than one type of pathological process can occur simultaneously, giving rise to a **mixed acid-base disturbance**, in which the blood pH may be (1) low, (2) high, or (3) within the reference interval. To understand how these and other perturbations of acid-base metabolism affect human physiology, it will be necessary to examine briefly the concepts of (1) acids, (2) bases, (3) pH, and (4) buffers in relation to the relevant systems that function to maintain normal **acid-base balance** in the human body.

Acid-Base Parameters—Definitions and Abbreviations

Acids are chemical substances that donate protons (H^+ ions) in solution, and *bases* are substances that accept protons. Strong acids readily give up H^+, whereas strong bases readily accept H^+. Thus the conjugate base of a strong acid is a weak base and vice versa.

pH and pK

The pH of a solution is defined as the negative logarithm of the hydrogen ion activity (pH = $-\log aH^+$). Thus *pH is a dimensionless quantity*, and a decrease in one pH unit represents a tenfold increase in H^+ activity (see Chapter 8 for a more detailed discussion of this topic). Potentiometric determinations of blood pH measure H^+ activity and not H^+ concentration, although

the activity is assumed to equal the concentration. The average pH of blood (7.40) corresponds to a hydrogen ion concentration of 40 nmol/L, but this assumes an activity coefficient of 1 (see Figure 36-5). This relationship is inverse and is obviously nonlinear.

The pK is the pH at which an acid is half dissociated, existing as equal proportions of acid and conjugate base. Thus acids have pK values <7.0, whereas bases have pK values >7.0. The lower the pK, the stronger the acid is, and the higher the pK, the stronger the conjugate base is. For example, the pK of lactic acid is 3.86, and that of ammonium ion NH_4^+ is 9.5.

The pH of plasma may be considered to be a function of two independent variables: (1) the PCO_2, which is regulated by the lungs and represents the acid component of the carbonic acid/bicarbonate buffer system, and (2) the concentration of titratable base (base excess or deficit, which is defined later), which is regulated by the kidneys. The plasma total CO_2 (bicarbonate) concentration generally is taken as a measure of the base excess or deficit in plasma and ECF, although conditions exist in which it may not accurately reflect the true base excess or deficit.

Bicarbonate and Dissolved CO$_2$

Bicarbonate is the second largest fraction (behind Cl^-) of plasma anions (≈26 mmol/L). Conventionally, it is defined to include (1) plasma bicarbonate ion (HCO_3^-), (2) carbonate ion (CO_3^{2-}), and (3) CO_2 bound in plasma carbamino compounds. At the pH of blood, the plasma carbonate concentration is ≈26 μmol/L, which is $\approx1/700$ to $1/1000$ of the total bicarbonate fraction. CO_2-bound carbamino compounds (RCNHCOOH) are 0.2 mmol/L in plasma and 1.5 mmol/L in erythrocytes. Actual bicarbonate ion concentration is not measured, but rather is calculated from the **Henderson-Hasselbalch equation** as described later (and discussed in detail in

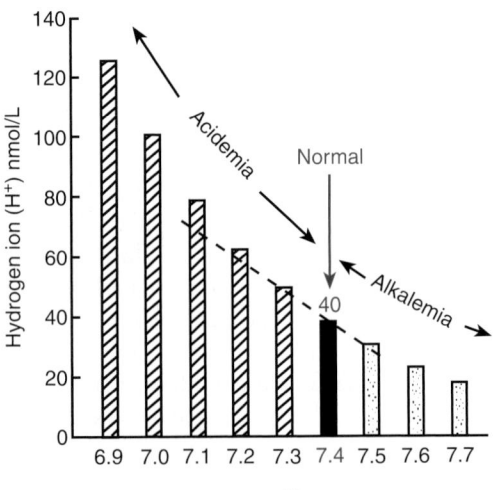

Figure 36-5 Relationship of pH to hydrogen ion concentration. A *broken line* is drawn to emphasize the (approximate) linear relationship between hydrogen ion concentration and pH over the pH range of 7.2 to 7.5. *(From Narins RG, Emmett M. Simple and mixed acid-base disorders: a practical approach. Medicine 1980;59:161-87.)*

Chapter 24). Also as described in Chapter 24, the analyte usually measured in plasma is total CO_2, which includes bicarbonate and dissolved CO_2 (dCO_2). At the pH of the blood, the amount of dissolved CO_2 is 700 to 1000 times greater than the amount of carbonic acid (H_2CO_3); therefore $cdCO_2$ is the term used to express their combined concentration. It is calculated from the solubility coefficient of CO_2 in blood at 37 °C ($\alpha = 0.031$ mmol/L per mm Hg) multiplied by the measured PCO_2 in mm Hg. Thus at a PCO_2 of 40 mm Hg, $cdCO_2$ is 1.224 mmol/L (0.031 mmol/L × 40 mm Hg). This $cdCO_2$ value is then used, in the Henderson-Hasselbalch equation, to calculate the total bicarbonate concentration.

Henderson-Hasselbalch Equation

The Henderson-Hasselbalch equation is described in detail in Chapter 24. However, it is important to review this equation here, because it enhances understanding of pH regulation of body fluids as it relates to compensatory mechanisms of the body in acid-base disturbances. The equation derived in Chapter 24 is also written as follows:

$$pH = 6.1 + \frac{cHCO_3^-}{cdCO_2}$$

where $cdCO_2$ is equal to α (0.031 mmol/L per mm Hg) PCO_2, and 6.1 is the pK for the carbonic acid/bicarbonate system.

The average typical ratio of the concentrations of bicarbonate and dissolved carbon dioxide in plasma is 26 (mmol/L)/1.25 (mmol/L) ≈ 20/1. Thus, any change in the concentration of bicarbonate or dissolved CO_2 relative to each other is accompanied by a change in pH. Such changes in this important ratio also occurs through a change in $cHCO_3^-$ (the renal component) or in PCO_2 (the respiratory component). Clinical conditions characterized as *metabolic* disturbances of acid-base balance are classified as primary disturbances in $cHCO_3^-$. Those characterized as *respiratory* disturbances are classified as primary disturbances in $cdCO_2$ (PCO_2). Various compensatory mechanisms attempting to re-establish the normal ratio of $cHCO_3^-/cdCO_2$ may result in changes in bicarbonate concentration, dissolved CO_2 concentration, or both. Application of the Henderson-Hasselbalch equation to human acid-base physiology is illustrated with the use of a lever-fulcrum (teeter-totter) diagram (Figure 36-6).

Buffer Systems and Their Role in Regulating the pH of Body Fluids

A buffer is a mixture of a weak acid and a salt of its conjugate base that resists changes in pH when a strong acid or base is added to the solution (see Chapter 8). If concentrations of the acid and base components of a buffer are equal, the pH will equal the pK. Generally, buffers work best at resisting pH changes in the interval ±1 pH unit of its pK, (buffers work best when the ratio of acid/base is within the range of 10:1 to 1:10). Buffers are also more effective at higher concentrations, so that a 10 mmol/L buffer solution is more effective than a 1.0 mmol/L solution.

The action of buffers in the regulation of body pH is explained by using the bicarbonate buffer system as an example. If a strong acid is added to a solution containing HCO_3^- and H_2CO_3, the H^+ will react with HCO_3^- to form more H_2CO_3, and subsequently CO_2 and H_2O. The hydrogen ions are thereby bound, and the increase in the H^+ concentration will be minimal.

$$H^+ + HCO_3^- \rightleftharpoons H_2CO_3 \rightleftharpoons CO_2 + H_2O$$

Bicarbonate/Carbonic Acid Buffer System

The most important buffer of plasma is the bicarbonate/carbonic acid pair. Upon inspection, it is not initially apparent

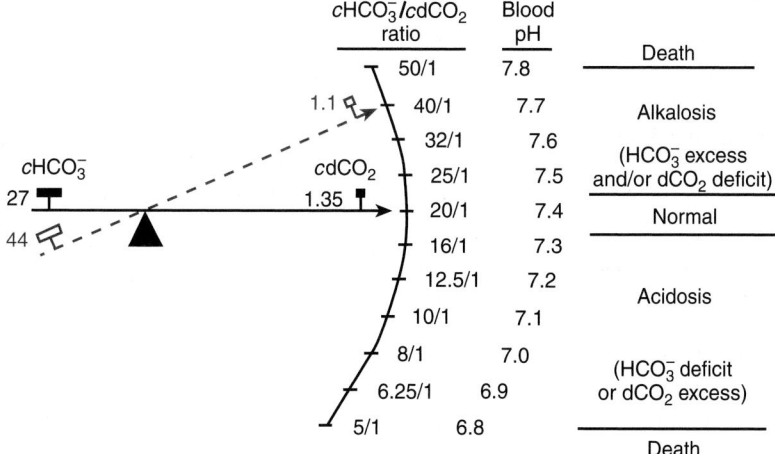

Figure 36-6 Scheme demonstrating the relation between pH and the ratio of bicarbonate concentration to the concentration of dissolved CO_2. If the ratio in blood is 20:1 ($cHCO_3^-$ = 27 mmol/ $cdCO_2$ = 1.35 mmol/L), the resultant pH will be 7.4, as demonstrated by the solid beam. The *dotted line* shows a case of uncompensated alkalosis (bicarbonate excess) with a bicarbonate concentration of 44 mmol/L and a $cdCO_2$ of 1.1 mmol/L. The ratio therefore is 40:1, and the resultant pH is 7.7. In a case of uncompensated acidosis, the pointer of the balance would point to a pH between 6.8 and 7.35, depending on the $cHCO_3^-/cdCO_2$ ratio. *(From Weisberg HF. A better understanding of anion-cation ("acid-base") balance. Surg Clin North Am 1959;39:93-120.)*

that this buffer would be very effective because its pK is 6.1, whereas normal plasma pH is 7.4. Also note that the normal bicarbonate/dCO$_2$ ratio is 20:1, which is outside the 10:1 or 1:10 ratio at which buffers are most effective. However, the effectiveness of the bicarbonate buffer is based on the fact that the lungs are able to readily dispose of or retain CO$_2$. In addition, the renal tubules are able to increase or decrease the rate of reclamation of bicarbonate from the glomerular filtrate (see Chapter 35).

Phosphate Buffer System

At a plasma pH of 7.4, the ratio $\left(cHPO_4^{2-}/cH_2PO_4^{-}\right)$ is 4:1 (pK = 6.8). The total concentration of this buffer in both erythrocytes and plasma accounts for about 5% of the nonbicarbonate buffer value of plasma. Organic phosphate, however, in the form of 2,3-diphosphoglycerate (present in erythrocytes in a concentration of about 4.5 mmol/L), accounts for about 16% of the nonbicarbonate buffer value of erythrocytes.

Plasma Protein and Hemoglobin Buffer System

Proteins, especially albumin, account for the greatest portion (>90%) of the nonbicarbonate buffer value of plasma. The most important buffer groups of proteins in the physiological pH range are the imidazole groups of histidines (pK ≈7.3). Each albumin molecule contains 16 histidines. In addition, hemoglobin accounts for the major part of nonbicarbonate buffers of erythrocyte fluid.

Respiratory Mechanism in the Regulation of Acid-Base Balance

In addition to supplying O$_2$ to tissue cells for normal metabolism, the respiratory mechanism contributes to maintenance of typical body pH through elimination or retention of CO$_2$ in **metabolic acidosis** and alkalosis, respectively.

Respiration

Exchange of O$_2$ and CO$_2$ in the lungs between alveolar air and blood is called *external respiration,* in contrast to internal respiration, which occurs at the cellular level. At inspiration, muscular contraction expands intrathoracic volume and creates a fall in intrapulmonary pressure. Atmospheric air is drawn into the bronchial tree, which terminates at the alveoli, where the exchange of gases between alveolar air and pulmonary blood occurs. Expiration takes place passively as the elastic tissues of the lungs and chest wall rebound and the intrathoracic volume is decreased.

Peripheral venous blood reaches the pulmonary circulation from the right ventricle of the heart and is *arterialized* in the capillaries of the lungs by uptake of O$_2$ and loss of CO$_2$. Pulmonary venous blood then returns to the left ventricle by way of the left atrium and is pumped through the aorta to the peripheral tissues. In the capillaries of peripheral tissues, the arterial blood releases O$_2$ to the tissue cells and takes up CO$_2$.

In a resting state, the respiration rate is normally 12 to 15 breaths/min. Involuntary increases in rate and depth of respiration are regulated by the medullary respiratory center in the brainstem, which is (1) stimulated by central chemoreceptors located on the anterior surface of the medulla oblongata and (2) by peripheral chemoreceptors located in the carotid arteries and aorta. Peripheral chemoreceptors are stimulated by a fall in pH caused by accumulation of CO$_2$ or by a decrease in PO$_2$. Central chemoreceptors are stimulated only by a decrease in pH of the cerebrospinal fluid (CSF). Pathologically, the response of these receptors is perturbed by adverse conditions in the circulatory or respiratory system. When this occurs, the patient may require assisted ventilation that uses a mechanical device to provide gas mixtures via an endotracheal tube. Adjustments of gas mixtures and rates of mechanical ventilation depend greatly on the results of laboratory blood gas and pH determinations.

Exchange of Gases in the Lungs and Peripheral Tissues

Diffusion of O$_2$ and CO$_2$ across alveolar and cell membranes is governed by gradients in the partial pressure of each gas (Figure 36-7). Dry air inspired at a pressure of 1 atm (760 mm Hg) consists of 21% O$_2$ (PO$_2$ ≈160 mm Hg), 0.03% CO$_2$ (PCO$_2$ ≈0.25 mm Hg), 78% nitrogen, and ≈0.1% other inert gases. As inspired air passes over the moist mucous membranes of the upper respiratory tract, it is (1) warmed to 37 °C, (2) becomes saturated with water vapor, and (3) mixes with air in the respiratory tree. This results in partial pressures of ≈150 mm Hg for O$_2$, ≈0.3 mm Hg for CO$_2$, ≈47 mm Hg for H$_2$O, and ≈563 mm Hg for nitrogen. Further mixing with alveolar air results leads to partial pressures at the alveolar membrane of ≈105 mm Hg for O$_2$, ≈40 mm Hg for CO$_2$, and ≈47 mm Hg for H$_2$O. Venous blood on the opposite side of the alveolar membrane has PO$_2$ ≈40 mm Hg and PCO$_2$ ≈46 mm Hg. Thus the gradient for O$_2$ is inward, toward the blood; and for CO$_2$, it is outward, toward the alveoli. CO$_2$ removal is so efficient that the PCO$_2$ in expired air is more than 100 times the PCO$_2$ in inspired air (see Figure 36-7). In arterial blood, the PO$_2$ is slightly lower than in alveolar air (90 to 100 vs. 105 mm Hg).

At the arterial end of capillaries of peripheral tissues, the PO$_2$ at 95 mm Hg is substantially higher than the average PO$_2$ at the surface of tissue cells (20 mm Hg). The PCO$_2$ at 40 mm Hg is substantially lower than that in the cells (50 to 70 mm Hg). Thus, in the tissue capillary, the gradient for O$_2$ is inward to the cell; for CO$_2$, it is outward to the capillary blood. The arteriovenous difference in partial pressures is approximately 60 mm Hg for O$_2$ and 6 mm Hg or less for CO$_2$. This difference in arteriovenous (affecting an artery and a vein) PO$_2$ is one indicator of the efficiency of O$_2$ extraction in the passage of blood through the capillaries.

Respiratory Response to Acid-Base Perturbations

The respiratory system responds immediately to a change in acid-base status. However, several hours may be required for the response to become maximal and is not attained until both central and peripheral chemoreceptors are fully stimulated. For example, in the early stages of metabolic acidosis, plasma pH decreases, but because H$^+$ ions equilibrate rather slowly across the blood-brain barrier, the pH in CSF remains nearly normal. However, because peripheral chemoreceptors are stimulated by decreased plasma pH, hyperventilation occurs, and plasma PCO_2 is decreased. Consequently, the PCO_2 of the CSF decreases immediately because CO_2 equilibrates rapidly across the blood-brain barrier, leading to a rise in pH of the CSF that inhibits the central chemoreceptors. As plasma bicarbonate gradually falls because of acidosis, bicarbonate concentration and pH in the CSF will also eventually fall. At this point, stimulation of respiration becomes maximal from both central and peripheral chemoreceptors.

The reverse is true when a patient with metabolic acidosis is treated with HCO_3^-. When the pH in plasma increases as the result of HCO_3^- administration, stimulation of the peripheral chemoreceptors returns to normal. However, because of slow equilibration of HCO_3^- between plasma and CSF, the central chemoreceptors continue to be stimulated and the patient continues to hyperventilate. Respiration does not return to normal until normal acid-base balance in the CSF is restored.

Renal Mechanisms in the Regulation of Acid-Base Balance

The average pH of plasma and of the glomerular filtrate is ≈ 7.4, whereas the average urinary pH is ≈ 6.0, reflecting the renal excretion of nonvolatile acids. Various functions of the kidneys respond to different alterations in acid-base status. In the case of acidosis, excretion of acids is increased and that of base is conserved. In alkalosis, the opposite occurs. The pH of the urine changes correspondingly and may vary in *random* specimens from pH 4.5 to 8.0. Renal excretion of acid and conservation of HCO_3^- occur through several mechanisms, including (1) Na^+-H^+ exchange, (2) production of ammonia and excretion of NH_4, and (3) reclamation of HCO_3^-.

Na⁺-H⁺ Exchange

Nearly all mammalian cells contain a plasma membrane ATP-hydrolyzing protein capable of exchanging sodium ions for protons—the so-called **sodium hydrogen exchanger (NHE)**. In the renal tubules, Na^+-H^+ exchangers extrude H^+ ions into the tubular fluid in exchange for Na^+ ions. Na^+-H^+ exchange is enhanced in states of acidosis and is inhibited in alkalosis.

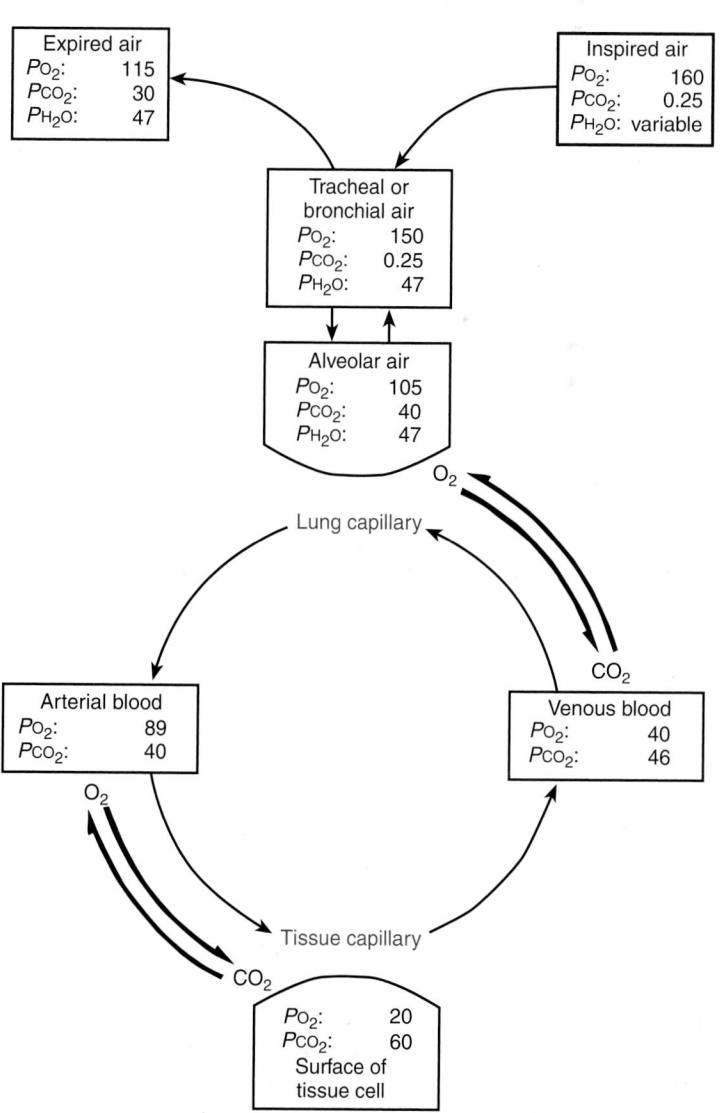

Figure 36-7 Partial pressures of oxygen and carbon dioxide in air, blood, and tissue. Values shown are approximations in mm Hg and are calculated assuming a 5% shunt. *Red arrows* show directions of gradients. *(Modified from Tietz NW. Fundamentals of clinical chemistry, 3rd edition. Philadelphia: WB Saunders, 1987.)*

The proximal tubules cannot maintain an H^+ gradient of more than ≈ 1 pH unit, whereas the distal tubules cannot maintain one of more than ≈ 3 pH units. Thus maximum urine acidity is reached at $\approx$pH 4.4. In type I and type IV renal tubular acidosis (RTA), this exchange process is defective and may lead to a decrease in blood pH.

Potassium ions compete with H^+ in the renal tubular Na^+-H^+ exchanger. If the concentration of intracellular K^+ in renal tubular cells is high, more K^+ and less H^+ are exchanged for Na^+. As a result, the urine becomes less acidic, thereby increasing the acidity of body fluids. If K^+ is depleted, more H^+ ions are exchanged for Na^+; the urine becomes more acidic and the body fluids more alkaline. Thus hyperkalemia contributes to acidosis and hypokalemia to alkalosis.

Renal Production of Ammonia and Excretion of Ammonium Ions

Renal tubular cells are able to generate ammonia from glutamine and other amino acids derived from muscle and liver cells according to the following reaction:

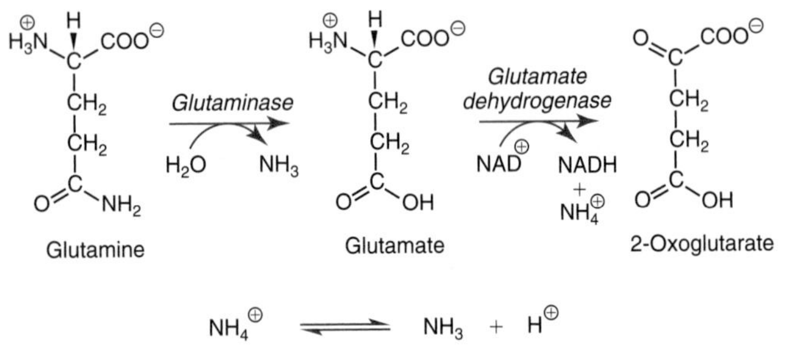

The ammonium ion produced dissociates into ammonia and hydrogen ions to a degree dependent on the pH. At physiological blood pH, the ratio of NH_4 to NH_3 is about 100 to 1. Ammonia is a gas that diffuses readily across the cell membrane into the tubular lumen, where it combines with hydrogen ions to form ammonium ions. At the acid pH of urine, the equilibrium between NH_4 and NH_3 shifts markedly to the left ($\approx 10,000$ to 1), strongly favoring formation of NH_4. The NH_4 formed in the tubular lumen will not easily cross cell membranes and thus is trapped in the tubular urine and excreted with anions, such as (1) phosphate, (2) chloride, and (3) sulfate. In healthy individuals, NH_4 production in the tubular lumen accounts for the excretion of $\approx 60\%$ (30 to 60 mmol) of the hydrogen ions.

Excretion of H^+ as $H_2PO_4^-$

H^+ secreted into the tubular lumen by the Na^+-H^+ exchanger may also react with HPO_4^{2-} to form $H_2PO_4^-$. This process depends on the amount of phosphate filtered by the glomeruli and the pH of urine. Under normal physiological conditions, ≈ 30 mmol of H^+ is excreted per day as $H_2PO_4^-$. Acidemia increases phosphate excretion and thus provides additional buffer for reaction with H^+. A decrease in the glomerular filtration rate (GFR), as observed in renal disease, results in a decrease in $H_2PO_4^-$ excretion.

Reclamation of Filtered Bicarbonate

The unmodified glomerular filtrate has the same concentration of HCO_3^- as does plasma; however, with increasing acidification of proximal tubular urine, the HCO_3^- concentration is decreased. Excreted H^+ reacts with HCO_3^- catalyzed by carbonic anhydrase in the proximal tubular cells) to form H_2CO_3 and subsequently CO_2 and H_2O.

This increase in urinary CO_2 causes carbon dioxide to diffuse across the tubular cell membrane into the tubular cell, where it reacts with H_2O in the presence of *cytoplasmic* carbonic anhydrase to form H_2CO_3 and subsequently H^+ and HCO_3^-. Thus reclamation of bicarbonate consists of diffusion of CO_2 into tubular cells and its subsequent conversion to HCO_3^-. The increase in HCO_3^- helps to maintain or restore a normal pH in the circulation. Typically in a healthy individual, $\approx 90\%$ of filtered HCO_3^- (or about 4500 mmol/d) is reclaimed in the proximal tubule, which parallels Na^+ reabsorption. Thus for each mmol H^+ secreted into the tubular fluid, 1 mmol Na^+ and 1 mmol HCO_3^- enter the tubular cell and return to the general circulation. When plasma HCO_3^- concentration is above ≈ 28 mmol/L, the capacity of the proximal and distal tubules to reclaim HCO_3^- is exceeded, and HCO_3^- is excreted in the urine.

Conditions Associated with Abnormal Acid-Base Status and Abnormal Electrolyte Composition of the Blood[5,10,11]

Many pathological conditions are accompanied by acid-base and electrolyte disturbances in the blood. Abnormalities in acid-base status of the blood are always accompanied by characteristic changes in electrolyte concentrations in the plasma. Hydrogen ions cannot accumulate without concomitant accumulation of anions (such as, Cl^- or lactate), or without exchange for cations (such as, K^+ or Na^+). Consequently, the electrolyte composition of blood serum or plasma is often determined along with measurements of blood gases and pH to assess acid-base disturbances.

Acid-base disturbances are traditionally classified as (1) metabolic acidosis, (2) metabolic alkalosis, (3) respiratory acidosis, or (4) respiratory alkalosis. For simple acid-base disorders, the laboratory parameters observed for these groups are shown in Table 36-2. However, interpretation of laboratory values to classify these disorders is rarely straightforward because of compensatory responses by the respiratory and renal systems in attempting to correct the imbalance.

Causes of acid-base disorders, resultant laboratory values, and compensatory responses are discussed here in the traditional categorization of these disorders. However, it is often difficult to remember which disorders fall into which categories, and so it is common for mnemonic devices or tables to be used to facilitate description of these disorders. A useful and more logical approach is to realize that an acidosis only occurs as the result of one (or a combination) of three mechanisms: (1) increased addition of acid, (2) decreased elimination of acid, and (3) increased loss of base. Similarly, alkalosis occurs only by (1) increased addition of base, (2) decreased

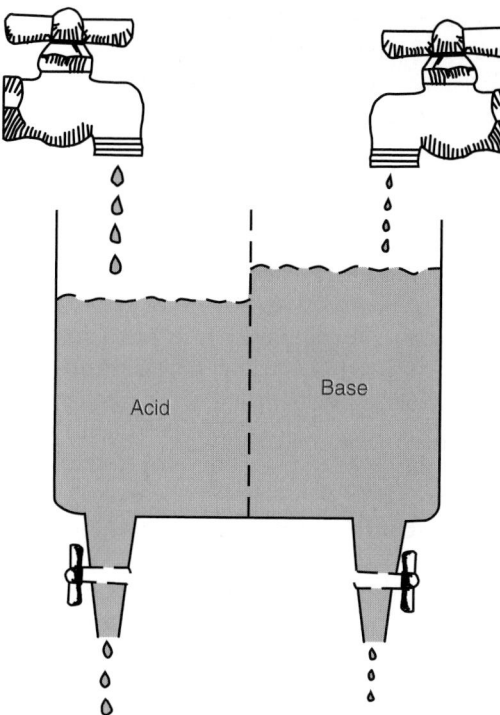

Figure 36-8 Simple depiction of the body as a two-vat system of acid and base. At equilibrium, input and output from each "vat" are equal. *(From Dufour DR. Acid-base disorders. In: Dufour DR, Christenson RH, eds: Professional practice in clinical chemistry: a review. Washington, DC: AACC Press, 1995:604-35.)*

elimination of base, and (3) increased loss of acid. Dufour has illustrated this simple concept by depicting the body as a two-tank vat, one of acid and one of base with inputs and outputs for each vat (Figure 36-8).[5] In the normal setting, these inputs and outputs are balanced. An acid-base disorder then involves a perturbation in the input or output of these body reservoirs, as is discussed in the next section.

Metabolic Acidosis (Primary Bicarbonate Deficit)

Metabolic acidosis is readily detected by decreased plasma bicarbonate (or a negative base excess). Causes include the following:

1. Production of organic acids that exceeds the rate of elimination (e.g., production of acetoacetic acid and β-hydroxybutyric acid in diabetic **ketoacidosis** and of lactic acid in lactic acidosis). Bicarbonate is "lost" in the buffering of excess acid.

2. Reduced excretion of acids (H^+) as occurs in renal failure and some RTAs, resulting in an accumulation of acid that consumes bicarbonate.

3. Excessive loss of bicarbonate due to increased renal excretion (decreased tubular reclamation) or excessive loss of duodenal fluid (as in diarrhea). Plasma $cHCO_3^-$ decreases with the fall associated with a rise in the concentration of inorganic anions (mostly chloride) or, rarely, a concomitant fall in the sodium concentration.

When any of these conditions exists, the ratio of $cHCO_3^-/cCO_2$ is decreased because of the primary decrease

in bicarbonate. The resulting drop in pH stimulates respiratory compensation via hyperventilation, which lowers PCO2 and thereby raises the pH.

Increased Anion Gap Acidosis (Organic Acidosis)

Metabolic acidoses are classified as those associated with an increased anion gap or a normal anion gap (Table 36-3). The concept of the anion gap was originally devised as a quality control rule when it was noted that if the sum of Cl^- and HCO_3^- values was subtracted from the Na^+ value [$Na^+ - (Cl^- + HCO_3^-)$], the difference, or "gap," averaged 12 mmol/L in healthy subjects.[7] This *apparent* gap is due to unmeasured anions (e.g., proteins, SO_4^{2-}, $H_2PO_4^{2-}$) that are present in plasma. It is important to note that infrequently, low serum anion gaps (<2 mEq/L) occur. Laboratory error is the most common cause, but (1) bromide, (2) lithium, or (3) iodide intoxication also leads to a low anion gap, as does (4) low albumin/increased immunoglobulin in cirrhosis and (5) monoclonal gammopathies.[7] The anion gap is increased in many patients with a metabolic acidosis, and the presence of an elevated anion gap is often the first indication of a metabolic acidosis and should be assessed in the electrolyte profiles of all patients (Figure 36-9).[7]

All anion gap metabolic acidoses, besides inborn errors of metabolism, are able to be explained by one (or a combination) of eight underlying mechanisms listed here according to the common mnemonic device, MUDPILES. The physiologic basis for the anion gap in these conditions is the consumption of bicarbonate in buffering excess acid. Cl^- values remain normal when the excess acid is any other than HCl, because lost bicarbonate is replaced by the unmeasured anions.

Methanol

Although nontoxic itself, methanol is metabolized by the liver to formaldehyde and formic acid (see Chapter 31). Accumulation of this acid leads to metabolic acidosis with a high anion gap and to clinical symptoms of optic papillitis ("snowfield" blindness), and ultimately blindness as well as neurologic defects that may lead to coma. Methanol and other ingested alcohols, such as (1) ethylene glycol, (2) ethanol, and (3) isopropanol will increase the osmolality of plasma. Thus in the presence of a high anion gap acidosis, determination of the osmolal gap (see Chapter 24) will help determine the source of the unmeasured anion and will suggest specific toxicologic analyses.[4]

Uremia of Renal Failure

Loss of functional renal tubular mass results in (1) decreased ammonia formation, (2) decreased Na^+-H^+ exchange, and (3) decreased GFR. All result in decreased acid excretion (see Chapter 35). Acidosis usually develops if GFR falls below 20 mL/min.

Diabetes or Ketoacidosis

The pathogenesis of ketoacidosis is discussed in detail in Chapter 22. Ketoacids (such as, β-hydroxybutyrate and 2-oxoglutarate accumulate) represent the unmeasured anions. Accumulation

TABLE 36-3	Conditions of Metabolic Acidoses with High and Normal Anion Gaps		
Etiology		**Retained Acids**	**Other Laboratory Findings**
High Anion Gap*			
Methanol toxicity		Formate	↑Osmolal gap (>15 mOsmol/kg)
Uremia of renal failure		Sulfuric, phosphoric, organic	↑BUN† and serum creatinine
Ketoacidoses			
Diabetes mellitus		Acetoacetate and β-hydroxybutyrate	↑Plasma and urine glucose
Ethyl alcohol toxicity			↑Osmolal gap (>15 mOsmol/kg)
Starvation			
Paraldehyde toxicity			
Isoniazid or iron toxicity, also ischemia		Organic, mainly lactate	Isoniazid and iron act as mitochondrial poisons
Lactic acidosis		Lactate	
Ethylene glycol toxicity		Hippurate, glycolate, oxalate	↑Osmolal gap (>15 mOsmol/kg), urine oxalate crystals
Salicylate toxicity		Salicylate, organic	Respiratory alkalosis
Normal Anion Gap			
Gastrointestinal fluid loss		Primary loss of bicarbonate	
Severe diarrhea			Hypokalemia
Pancreatitis			K+ variable
Intestinal fistula			
Renal tubular acidoses			
Proximal (type II) RTA			Urine pH <5.5, with K+ normal or low
Distal (type I) RTA			Urine pH >5.5 with hypokalemia (usually)
Type IV RTA			Urine pH <5.5 with hyperkalemia

*Although there is considerable variability, the anion gap is often >25 mmol/L in these conditions with the exception of uremic renal failure.
†Blood urea nitrogen (reference interval: 8 to 25 mg/dL, or ≈3.0 to 9.0 mmol/L).
RTA, Renal tubular acidosis.

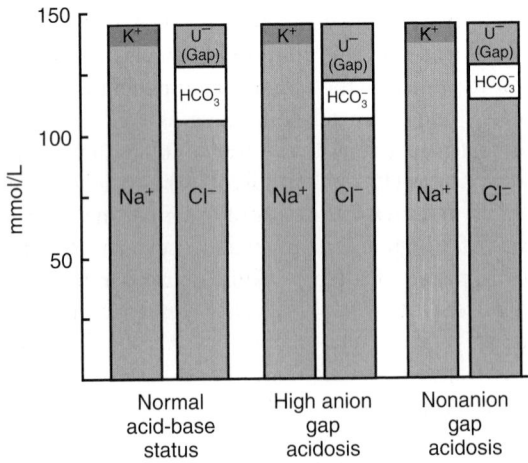

Figure 36-9 Simple "Gambelgram" depiction of normal gap, anion gap acidosis, and nonanion gap acidosis. Cations, Na+ and K+, are in left bar for each condition, whereas measured (Cl− and HCO₃⁻) and unmeasured (U−) anions are in right bar for each condition.

of these "ketone bodies" causes a decrease in HCO_3^- and a high anion gap. Ketoacids also accumulate in states of starvation and alcoholic malnutrition.

Paraldehyde Toxicity

Paraldehyde toxicity may develop after chronic paraldehyde ingestion. The pathogenesis is poorly defined, but the acidosis includes β-hydroxybutyric acid. Patients with paraldehyde toxicity have a pungent, apple-like odor to their breath.

Isoniazid, Iron, or Ischemia ("Three I's")

These causes of high anion gap acidosis share the common feature of accumulating organic acids with a predominance of lactic acid. Thus the "three I's" actually represent special cases in the general category of lactic acidosis, which is described later. Both isoniazid, an antimycobacterial agent commonly used in the treatment of tuberculosis, and iron toxicity involve the production of toxic peroxides that act as mitochondrial poisons and interfere with normal cellular respiration.

Tissue ischemia results from many causes; one of which is hypoperfusion that leads to hypoxia of cells. This results in anaerobic metabolism with accumulation of organic (mainly lactic) acids.

Lactic Acid Acidosis

Lactic acid, present in blood entirely as the lactate ion ($pK = 3.86$), is an intermediate of carbohydrate metabolism that is derived mainly from muscle cells and erythrocytes (see Chapter 22). It represents the end product of anaerobic metabolism and is normally metabolized by the liver. Therefore, the blood lactate concentration is affected by its rate of production and rate of metabolism, both of which are dependent on adequate tissue perfusion. An increase in the concentration of lactate to >3 mmol/L with the associated increase in H^+ is considered lactic acidosis.

Lactic acidosis caused by severe tissue hypoxia is seen in (1) severe anemia, (2) shock, (3) cardiac arrest, and (4) pulmonary insufficiency. If the origin of lactate (e.g., seizure, hypoxic tissue) is rectified, it is rapidly metabolized to CO_2, which then is eliminated by an intact respiratory system.

Lactic acidosis is also caused by (1) drugs and toxins, (2) acquired and hereditary defects in enzymes involved in gluconeogenesis, (3) uremia, (4) liver failure, (5) tumors, (6) seizures, (7) anesthesia, and (8) abnormal intestinal bacteria producing D-lactate.

Ethylene Glycol

Ingested ethylene glycol is metabolized primarily to glycolic and oxalic acids. Its metabolism leads to an acidosis with high anion and osmolal gaps. Accumulation of toxic metabolites may also contribute to lactic acid production that further contributes to the acidosis. Precipitation of calcium oxalate and hippurate crystals in the urinary tract may lead to acute renal failure. Clinically, patients develop a variety of neurologic symptoms that may lead to coma. The minimal lethal dose of ethylene glycol is ≈ 100 mL for an average 70 kg adult.

Salicylate Intoxication

Acidosis generally occurs with blood salicylate concentrations above 30 mg/dL. Salicylate, itself an unmeasured anion, alters peripheral metabolism, leading to the production of various organic acids without dominance of any specific acid. These processes eventually result in a metabolic acidosis with a high anion gap. Salicylate also stimulates the respiratory center to increase the rate and depth of respiration, resulting in a low PCO_2 and thus a mixed respiratory alkalosis and metabolic acidosis.

Normal Anion Gap Acidosis (Inorganic Acidosis)

In contrast to high anion gap acidoses, in which bicarbonate is consumed from buffering excess H^+, the cause of acidosis in the presence of a normal anion gap is the loss of bicarbonate-rich fluid from the kidney or the gastrointestinal tract. As bicarbonate is lost, more Cl^- ions are reabsorbed with Na^+ or K^+ to maintain electrical neutrality so that hyperchloremia ensues (see Figure 36-9). Normal anion gap acidosis is divided into (1) hypokalemic, (2) normokalemic, and (3) hyperkalemic acidoses, which is helpful in the differential diagnosis of this type of disorder (see Table 36-3).

Gastrointestinal Losses

Diarrhea may cause acidosis as a result of loss of (1) Na^+, (2) K^+, and (3) HCO_3^-. One of the primary exocrine functions of the pancreas is production of HCO_3^- to neutralize gastric contents on entry into the duodenum. If the water, K^+, and HCO_3^- in the intestine are not reabsorbed, a hypokalemic, normal anion gap metabolic acidosis develops. The resulting hyperchloremia is due to replacement of lost bicarbonate with Cl^- to maintain electrical balance.

Renal Tubular Acidoses, Types I and II

These syndromes are characterized predominantly by loss of bicarbonate due to decreased tubular secretion of H^+ (distal or type I RTA) or decreased reabsorption of HCO_3^- (proximal or type II RTA).[8] Because the major urine-acidifying power of the kidneys rests in the distal tubules, proximal and distal RTAs may be differentiated by measurement of urine pH after administration of acid. In proximal RTA, urine pH becomes <5.5, whereas in distal RTA, the distal tubules are compromised and urine pH is >5.5.[8]

Carbonic Anhydrase Inhibitors

Acetazolamide is the most commonly used drug in this class of therapeutic agents. It is rarely used as a mild diuretic. More often, it is used for urine alkalinization and in patients suffering from open-angle glaucoma or acute mountain (altitude) sickness. Inhibition of carbonic anhydrase causes wasting of (1) Na^+, (2) K^+, and (3) HCO_3^- in the proximal tubules and represents a pharmacologically-induced proximal RTA.

Hyperkalemic Normal Anion Gap Acidosis (RTA Type IV)

Common causes of hyperkalemic normal anion gap acidosis—often called *RTA type IV*—include (1) failure of the kidneys to synthesize renin, (2) failure of the adrenal cortex to secrete aldosterone, and (3) renal tubular resistance to aldosterone. This type of acidosis inhibits Na^+ reabsorption, and both K^+ and H^+ are thus abnormally retained. The result is decreased renal ammonia formation and therefore decreased elimination of H^+. Hyperkalemia is also usually present.

Compensatory Mechanisms in Metabolic Acidosis

The buffer systems of the blood (mainly the bicarbonate/carbonic acid buffer) minimize changes in pH. In acidoses, the bicarbonate concentration decreases to yield a ratio of $cHCO_3^-/cdCO_2$ of less than 20:1. The respiratory compensatory mechanism responds to correct the ratio with increased rate and depth of respiration to eliminate CO_2. Table 36-4 depicts expected compensation in acidoses and alkaloses and corresponding laboratory values.

Respiratory Compensatory Mechanism

The decrease in pH in metabolic acidosis stimulates hyperventilation (Kussmaul respiration), which results in (1) the elimination of carbonic acid as CO_2, (2) a decrease in PCO_2 (hypocapnia), and (3) ultimately a decrease in $cdCO_2$. There is also a decrease in $cHCO_3^-$ that is smaller than that in $cdCO_2$. For example, the ratio of $cHCO_3^-/cdCO_2$ might be 16:1.28 (12.5:1) for a pH of 7.2 before compensation, and 14.5:0.9 (16:1) for a pH of 7.30 after compensation (see Figure 36-6).

TABLE 36-4	Classification and Characteristics of Simple Acid-Base Disorders		
	Primary Change	**Compensatory Response**	**Expected Compensation**
Metabolic			
Acidosis	$\downarrow cHCO_3^-$	$\downarrow PCO_2$	$PCO_2 = 1.5\ (cHCO_3^- + 8 \pm 2 PCO_2$ falls by 1 to 1.3 mm Hg for each mmol/L fall in $cHCO_3^-$ Last 2 digits of pH $= PCO_2$ (e.g., if $PCO_2 = 28$, pH $= 7.28$)$cHCO_3^- + 15 =$ last two digits of pH ($cHCO_3^- = 15$, pH $= 7.30$)
Alkalosis	$\uparrow cHCO_3^-$	$\uparrow PCO_2$	PCO_2 increases 6 mm Hg for each 10 mmol/L rise in HCO_3^- $cHCO_3^- + 15 =$ last two digits of pH $cHCO_3^- = 35$, pH $= 7.50$)
Respiratory			
Acidosis			
Acute	$\uparrow PCO_2$	$\uparrow cHCO_3^-$	$cHCO_3^-$ increases by 1 mmol/L for each 10 mm Hg rise in PCO_2
Chronic	$\uparrow PCO_2$	$\uparrow cHCO_3^-$	$cHCO_3^-$ increases by 3.5 mmol/L for each 10 mm Hg rise in PCO_2
Alkalosis			
Acute	$\downarrow PCO_2$	$\downarrow cHCO_3^-$	$cHCO_3^-$ falls by 2 mmol/L for each 10 mm Hg fall in PCO_2
Chronic	$\downarrow PCO_2$	$\downarrow cHCO_3^-$	$cHCO_3^-$ falls by 5 mmol/L for each 10 mm Hg fall in PCO_2

Modified from Narins RG, Gardner LB. Simple acid-base disturbances. Med Clin North Am 1981;65:321-46.

Renal Compensatory Mechanism

Functional kidneys respond to restore the normal pH through increased excretion of acid and preservation of base by an increased (1) rate of Na^+-H^+ exchange, (2) ammonia formation, and (3) reabsorption of bicarbonate. When the renal compensating mechanisms are functioning, urine acidity and ammonia are increased.

Metabolic Alkalosis (Primary Bicarbonate Excess)

Alkalosis occurs when (1) excess base is added to the system, (2) base elimination is decreased, or (3) acid-rich fluids are lost (Box 36-1). All lead to a primary bicarbonate excess, such that the ratio of $cHCO_3^-/cdCO_2$ becomes greater than 20:1. For instance, a primary increase in bicarbonate to 48 mmol/L will alter the $cHCO_3^-/cdCO_2$ to 48:1.5 (32:1) for a pH of 7.6 (see Figure 36-9). The patient will hypoventilate to raise PCO_2, thereby lowering the pH toward normal. However, hypoxia usually prevents the patient from achieving a PCO_2 greater than 55 mm Hg. Above pH 7.55, tetany may develop, even in the presence of a normal serum total calcium concentration. The cause of the tetany is a decreased concentration of ionized calcium due to increased binding of calcium ions by albumin as H^+ ions decrease. Measurement of urine Cl^- is often helpful, as causes of metabolic alkalosis fall into (1) Cl^- responsive, (2) Cl^- resistant, and (3) exogenous base categories (see Box 36-1 and Figure 36-3).

Cl⁻ Responsive Metabolic Alkalosis

Most causes of Cl^- responsive metabolic alkalosis occur as a result of *hypovolemia* (see Box 36-1). When the ECF is severely depleted, the resulting acid-base disorder is often referred to as *contraction alkalosis*. Hypovolemia will result in (1) increased reabsorption of Na^+, (2) increased HCO_3^- absorption and (3) excretion of K^+ and H^+. Urine Cl^- will be less than 10 mmol/L, as both the available Cl^- and HCO_3^- are reabsorbed with Na^+. Urine Na^+ is not useful for classifying metabolic alkalosis because an obligatory loss of Na^+ will

BOX 36-1	**Conditions Leading to Metabolic Alkalosis**

Chloride-Responsive (Urine Cl⁻ <10 mmol/L)
Contraction alkaloses
    Prolonged vomiting or nasogastric suction
    Pyloric or upper duodenal obstruction
    Prolonged or abusive diuretic therapy (loop diuretics)
    Dehydration
Posthypercapnic state
Cystic fibrosis (systemic ineffective reabsorption of Cl⁻)

Chloride-Resistant (Urine Cl⁻ >20 mmol/L)
Mineralocorticoid excess
    Primary hyperaldosteronism (adrenal adenoma or, rarely, carcinoma)
    Bilateral adrenal hyperplasia
    Secondary hyperaldosteronism
    Congenital adrenal hyperplasia (due to adrenal enzyme deficiencies in cortisol production [11β- or 17α-hydroxylase])
Glucocorticoid excess
    Primary adrenal adenoma (Cushing syndrome)
    Pituitary adenoma secreting ACTH (Cushing disease)
    Exogenous cortisol therapy
    Excessive licorice ingestion
Bartter syndrome (defective renal Cl⁻ reabsorption)

Exogenous Base
Iatrogenic
    Bicarbonate-containing intravenous fluid therapy
    Massive blood transfusion (sodium citrate overload)
    Antacids and cation-exchange resins in dialysis patients
    High-dose carbenicillin or penicillin (associated with hypokalemia)
Milk-alkali syndrome

ACTH, Adrenocorticotropic hormone.

occur when filtered HCO_3^- exceeds reclamation. Common causes of contraction alkalosis include prolonged vomiting or nasogastric suction and the use of certain diuretics. Treatment consists of replacing TBW with (1) water, (2) NaCl tablets, or (3) saline infusion.

Cl⁻ Resistant Metabolic Alkalosis

This condition is far less common than Cl⁻ responsive metabolic alkalosis and is almost always associated with an underlying disease, such as (1) primary hyperaldosteronism, (2) Cushing syndrome, or (3) Bartter syndrome, or with excess addition of exogenous base. In these conditions, urine Cl⁻ will usually be greater than 20 mmol/L.

In states of adrenocortical excess (endogenous or pharmacologic, primary or secondary), K^+ and H^+ are "wasted" by the kidneys as a consequence of increased Na^+ reabsorption stimulated by elevated aldosterone or cortisol. The attendant hypokalemia often further contributes to the alkalosis and should be treated with K^+ replacement therapy. The decreased tubular K^+ concentration stimulates NH_3 production and thus renal H^+ excretion as NH_4^+. Diseases in which endogenous mineralocorticoids, glucocorticoids, or both are elevated include (1) primary and secondary hyperaldosteronism, (2) bilateral adrenal hyperplasia, (3) pituitary adrenocorticotropic hormone (ACTH)-producing adenoma (Cushing disease), and (4) primary adrenal adenomas producing glucocorticoids (Cushing syndrome) or aldosterone.

Exogenous Base

Examples in this category include (1) citrate toxicity following massive blood transfusion, (2) aggressive intravenous therapy with bicarbonate solutions, and (3) ingestion of large quantities of antacids in the treatment of gastritis or peptic ulcer (*milk-alkali syndrome*). The latter is far less commonly seen since the introduction and now widespread use of H_2-receptor antagonists (drugs used to block the action of histamine on parietal cells) and proton pump inhibitors (drugs that reduce gastric acid production).

Compensatory Mechanisms in Metabolic Alkalosis

The compensatory mechanisms for metabolic alkalosis include both respiratory compensation and, if physiologically possible, renal compensation. The increase in pH depresses the respiratory center, causing retention of carbon dioxide (hypercapnia), which in turn causes an increase in cH_2CO_3 and $cdCO_2$. Thus the ratio of $cHCO_3^-/cdCO_2$, which was originally increased, approaches its normal value, although the actual concentrations of both $cHCO_3^-$ and $cdCO_2$ remain increased. The kidneys respond to the state of alkalosis by decreased (1) Na^+-H^+ exchange, (2) formation of ammonia, and (3) reclamation of bicarbonate. This response is blunted, however, in conditions of hypokalemia and hypovolemia.

Respiratory Acidosis

Any condition that decreases elimination of carbon dioxide through the lungs results in an increase in PCO_2 (hypercapnia) and dCO_2 (respiratory acidosis). Thus respiratory acidosis occurs only through decreased elimination of CO_2. Causes of decreased CO_2 elimination (Box 36-2) are classified as acute or chronic. Alternatively, these conditions may be separated into those caused by factors that directly depress the respiratory center, such as (1) centrally acting drugs, (2) CNS trauma, or (3) infection, and (4) those that affect the respiratory apparatus or cause mechanical obstruction of the airways. **Chronic**

BOX 36-2   Conditions Leading to Respiratory Acidosis

Factors That Directly Depress the Respiratory Center
Drugs, such as narcotics and barbiturates
CNS trauma, tumors, and degenerative disorders
Infections of the CNS, such as encephalitis and meningitis
Comatose states, such as cerebrovascular accident due to intracranial hemorrhage
Primary central hypoventilation

Conditions That Affect the Respiratory Apparatus
COPD (most common cause)
Severe pulmonary fibrosis
Status asthmaticus (severe)
Disease of the upper airways, such as laryngospasm or tumor
Pulmonary infection (severe)
Impaired lung motion due to pleural effusion or pneumothorax
Adult respiratory distress syndrome
Chest wall disease and chest wall deformity
Neurologic disorders affecting the muscles of respiration

Others
Abdominal distention, as in peritonitis and ascites
Extreme obesity (pickwickian syndrome)
Sleep disorders, such as sleep apnea

CNS, Central nervous system; COPD, chronic obstructive pulmonary disease.

---

obstructive pulmonary disease (COPD) is the most common cause. Rebreathing, or breathing air high in CO_2 content, may also cause a high PCO_2. An increase in PCO_2 results in an increase in $cdCO_2$ (and thus H_2CO_3, which dissociates to H^+ and HCO_3^-), which in turn causes a decrease in the $cHCO_3^-/cdCO_2$ ratio (e.g., the ratio may be 28:1.7 [16:1] for a pH of ≈7.30; see Figure 36-6). Doubling of PCO_2 will cause a fall in pH of about 0.23 when other factors remain constant.

Compensatory Mechanisms in Respiratory Acidosis

Compensation for respiratory acidosis occurs immediately via buffers, and over time via the kidneys and, if possible, the lungs. Excess carbonic acid present in blood is buffered to a great extent by the hemoglobin and protein buffer systems. Buffering of CO_2 causes a slight rise in $cHCO_3^-$. Thus in the immediate posthypercapnic state, this compensation may appear as a metabolic alkalosis (see Box 36-2). The kidneys respond to respiratory acidosis similarly to the way that they respond to metabolic acidosis, namely, with increased (1) Na^+-H^+ exchange, (2) ammonia formation, and (3) reclamation of bicarbonate. In a partially chronic compensated respiratory acidosis at steady state, the plasma pH is returned about halfway toward normal as compared with the acute (uncompensated) situation. Renal compensation is not effective before 6 to 12 hours and is not optimal until 2 to 3 days. In chronic respiratory acidosis, such as occurs in patients with COPD, full renal compensation may be seen even in those patients with very high PCO_2 (>50 mm Hg). However, patients with severe COPD often present with a superimposed metabolic alkalosis arising from a variety of causes, such as prolonged administration of diuretics.

The increase in PCO_2 stimulates the respiratory center, resulting in an increased pulmonary rate and depth of respiration, provided that the primary defect is not in the respiratory center. Elimination of carbon dioxide through the lungs results in a decrease in $cdCO_2$; thus the ratio of $cHCO_3^-/cdCO_2$ and pH approach normal.

Respiratory Alkalosis

A decrease in PCO_2 (hypocapnia) and the resulting primary deficit in $cdCO_2$ (respiratory alkalosis) are caused by an increased rate and/or depth of respiration. Therefore, the basic cause of respiratory alkalosis is excess elimination of acid via the respiratory route. Excessive elimination of carbon dioxide reduces the PCO_2 and causes an increase in the $cHCO_3^-/cdCO_2$ ratio. The latter shifts the normal equilibrium of the bicarbonate/carbonic acid buffer system, reducing the hydrogen ion concentration and increasing the pH. This shift also results in a decrease in $cHCO_3^-$, which somewhat improves the change in pH. Analogous to causes of respiratory acidosis, causes of respiratory alkalosis have been classified as those with a direct stimulatory effect on the respiratory center and those due to effects on the pulmonary system. These and some additional conditions underlying respiratory alkaloses are listed in Box 36-3.

Compensatory mechanisms for respiratory alkalosis respond in two stages. In the first stage, erythrocyte and tissue buffers provide H^+ ions that consume a small amount of HCO_3^-. The second stage becomes operational in prolonged respiratory alkalosis and depends on renal compensation as described for metabolic alkalosis (decreased reclamation of bicarbonate).

BOX 36-3 **Factors Causing Respiratory Alkalosis**

Nonpulmonary Stimulation of Respiratory Center
Anxiety, hysteria
Febrile state
Gram-negative septicemia
Metabolic encephalopathy (e.g., from liver disease)
CNS infection, such as meningitis, encephalitis
Cerebrovascular accident
Intracranial surgery
Hypoxia (e.g., severe anemia, high altitudes [acute condition])
Drugs and agents, such as salicylates, catecholamines, and progesterone
Pregnancy, mainly third trimester (↑ progesterone?)
Hyperthyroidism

Pulmonary Disorders*
Pneumonia
Pulmonary emboli
Interstitial lung disease
Large right-to-left shunt (PCO_2 <50 mm Hg)
CHF
Respiratory compensation after correction of metabolic acidosis

Others
Ventilator-induced hyperventilation

*The severe stages of some of these disorders may be associated with respiratory acidosis if elimination of CO_2 is severely impaired.
CHF, Congestive heart failure; *CNS*, central nervous system.

Review Questions

1. External respiration is defined as:
   a. the exchange of oxygen (O_2) and carbon dioxide (CO_2) at the tissue level.
   b. decreased O_2 due to the decreased availability of O_2 as in suffocation.
   c. the exchange of O_2 and CO_2 in the lungs between alveoli and blood.
   d. the number of breaths an individual takes in one minute.

2. Total body water (TBW) makes up approximately 60% of body weight. The majority of TBW is located in which one of the following compartments?
   a. Extracellular fluid (ECF)
   b. Intracellular fluid (ICF)
   c. Interstitial fluid
   d. Plasma

3. The anion gap, an estimate of anions not directly measured in serum, is correctly calculated by which one of the following formulae?
   a. $(Na) + (Cl + HCO_3)$
   b. $(Na) - (Cl + HCO_3)$
   c. $(Cl) + (HCO_3 + Na)$
   d. $(HCO_3 - Na) - (Cl)$

4. Hypernatremia commonly occurs in:
   a. decreased production of antidiuretic hormone (ADH).
   b. decreased aldosterone.
   c. the syndrome of inappropriate ADH (SIADH) secretion.
   d. all of the above.

5. A decrease in PCO_2 and a resulting primary deficit in $cdCO_2$ is referred to as:
   a. metabolic acidosis.
   b. metabolic alkalosis.
   c. respiratory acidosis.
   d. respiratory alkalosis.

6. Low blood volume will cause synthesis of this hormone by the kidneys, which in turn causes production of aldosterone, which will increase kidney reabsorption of sodium and retention of water.
   a. Insulin
   b. Renin
   c. Antidiuretic hormone (ADH)
   d. Erythropoietin

7. Because of *increased* dietary intake of this particular electrolyte, an individual with this disorder will demonstrate mental confusion, bradycardia, and possible eventual cardiac arrest.
   a. Sodium; hypernatremia
   b. Sodium; hyponatremia
   c. Potassium; hyperkalemia
   d. Potassium; hypokalemia

8. Which one of the following is the primary cause of *respiratory* acidosis?
   a. Hyperventilation
   b. Overdose of antacids
   c. Chronic obstructive pulmonary disease (COPD)
   d. Uncontrolled diabetes mellitus

9. The *metabolic* component of acid-base balance is the:
   a. hepatic system.
   b. respiratory system.
   c. gastrointestinal tract.
   d. renal system.

10. In whole blood, the normal ratio of bicarbonate to dissolved carbon dioxide is approximately:
    a. 10:1
    b. 1:20
    c. 20:1
    d. 1:10

References

1. Adrogué HJ, Madias NE. Hypernatremia. N Engl J Med 2002;342:1493–9.
2. Birnbaumer M. The V2 vasopressin receptor mutations and fluid homeostasis. Cardiovasc Res 2001;51:409–15.
3. Brown D, Bouley R, Păunescu TG, Breton S, Lu HA. New insights into the dynamic regulation of water and acid-base balance by renal epithelial cells. Am J Physiol Cell Physiol 2012;302(10):C1421–33.
4. Dorwart WV, Chalmers L. Comparison of methods for calculating serum osmolality form chemical concentrations, and the prognostic value of such calculations. Clin Chem 1975;21:190.
5. Dufour DR. Acid-base disorders. In: Dufour R, Christenson RH, eds. Professional practice in clinical chemistry: a review. Washington, DC: AACC Press, 1995:604–35.
6. Ellison DH, Berl T. The syndrome of inappropriate antidiuresis. N Engl J Med 2007;356:2064–72.
7. Kraut JA, Madias NE. Serum anion gap: its uses and limitations in clinical medicine. Clin J Am Soc Nephrol 2007;2:162–74.
8. Lash JP, Arruda JA. Laboratory evaluation of renal tubular acidosis. Clin Lab Med 1993;13:117–29.
9. Petri WA. Antimicrobial agents. In: Hardman JG, Linbird LE, eds. Goodman and Gilman's the pharmacological basis of therapeutics, 10th edition. New York: McGraw-Hill, 2001:1111–26.
10. Preuss HG. Fundamentals of clinical acid-base evaluation. Clin Lab Med 1993;13:103–16.
11. Singer G. Fluid and electrode management. In: Ahya SL, Flood K, Paranjothi S, Schaiff R, eds. The Washington manual of medical therapeutics, 30th edition. Philadelphia: Lippincott, Williams and Wilkins, 2001:3–75.
12. Skott O. Renin. Am J Physiol Regul Integr Comp Physiol 2002;282:R937–9.
13. Verbalis JG. Hyponatremia and hypoosmolar disorders. In: Greenberg A, Cheung AK, eds. Primer on kidney diseases, Philadelphia: Elsevier Saunders, 2005:55–65.

Liver Disease*

D. Robert Dufour, M.D.

Objectives

1. Define the following:

Acinus	Hepatitis
Ascites	Hepcidin
Bilirubin	Jaundice
Cholestasis	Model for end-stage liver
Cirrhosis	disease (MELD) score
Gallbladder	Portal hypertension
Hepatic lobule	Portal triad
	Xenobiotics

2. Describe the microscopic and macroscopic anatomy of the hepatic system, including functional units, lobules, hepatobiliary ducts, blood supply, intrinsic cell types, and functional organization.

3. Detail the major functions of the liver, including the mechanisms of bilirubin excretion, substances synthesized and their functions, and substances metabolized and their sources.

4. List the causes and consequences of each of the following clinical manifestations of liver disease:

Disordered hemostasis	Liver enzyme release
Jaundice	Portal hypertension

5. List the enzymes synthesized in the liver, their subcellular location, tissue specificity, and mechanisms of enzyme release and clearance.

6. Compare and contrast acute liver injury with chronic liver injury, including manifestations of injury, target cells involved, specific means of cell death, and laboratory analyses used to distinguish between them.

7. List and describe five types of viral hepatitis, including type of virus, mode of transmission, involvement in liver cancer, methods of prevention, and laboratory tests used to diagnose the presence of the virus.

8. Describe the following types of liver disease, including causes, clinical presentation, and laboratory findings:

Acute alcoholic hepatitis	Drug-induced liver injury
Alcoholic liver disease	(DILI)
Autoimmune hepatitis	Ischemic hepatitis
Cholestatic hepatitis	Primary biliary cirrhosis
Cholestatic liver diseases	(PBC)
Cirrhosis	Primary sclerosing
	cholangitis (PSC)
	Toxic hepatitis

9. State the formula for calculating a MELD score; calculate a MELD score given appropriate values and determine prognosis in cirrhosis.

10. Describe hepatocellular carcinoma (HCC) including prevalence, risk factors, screening tests, and laboratory findings.

11. Assess and solve case studies related to liver disease.

Key Words and Definitions

Alcoholic hepatitis An acute or chronic degenerative and inflammatory lesion of the liver in the alcoholic that is potentially progressive though sometimes reversible.

Alcoholic liver disease Liver injury caused by excessive ethanol (alcohol) ingestion.

Apoptosis Programmed cell death as signaled by the nuclei in normally functioning human and animal cells when age or state of cell health and condition dictates

Ascites Serous fluid that accumulates in the abdominal cavity.

Autoimmune hepatitis (AIH) A form of hepatitis, usually with hypergammaglobulinemia and serum autoantibodies.

Bile A greenish-yellow fluid secreted by the liver and stored in the gallbladder.

Biliprotein The conjugated bilirubin-protein complex (also known as *delta-bilirubin*).

Biotransformation The series of chemical alterations of a compound (for example, a drug) that occurs within the body, as by enzymatic activity.

Cholestasis Suppression of the normal flow of bile.

---

*The author gratefully acknowledges the original contributions by Drs. Keith G. Tolman and Robert Rej, on which portions of this chapter are based.

Key Words and Definitions—cont'd

Chronic hepatitis A collective term for a clinical and pathological syndrome that has several causes and is characterized by varying degrees of hepatocellular necrosis and inflammation for at least 6 months.

Cirrhosis Liver disease characterized pathologically by loss of the normal microscopic lobular architecture with fibrosis and nodular regeneration.

Drug-induced liver injury (DILI) A diseases of the liver that is caused by prescribed medications, over-the-counter medications, vitamins, hormones, herbs, illicit ("recreational") drugs, and environmental toxins.

Fulminant hepatitis A rare and frequently fatal form of acute hepatitis B in which the patient's condition rapidly deteriorates with hepatic encephalopathy, necrosis of the hepatic parenchyma, coagulopathy, renal failure, and coma.

Fulminant hepatic failure A condition characterized by the development of severe liver injury with impaired synthetic capacity and encephalopathy in patients with previous normal liver or at least well-compensated liver disease.

Gallstone A solid formation in the gallbladder, most commonly composed of cholesterol and bile salts.

Hemochromatosis A rare genetic disorder, due to abnormalities in genes that regulate iron metabolism.

Hepatic encephalopathy A condition used to describe the deleterious effects of liver failure on the central nervous system. Features include confusion ranging to unresponsiveness (coma).

Hepatic failure A condition of severe liver dysfunction that is accompanied by a loss of normal liver functions.

Hepatitis Inflammation of the liver. Typically divided into acute (duration of weeks to months) and chronic (lasting for more than 6 months).

Hepatocellular carcinoma (HCC) A cancer arising from hepatocytes.

Hepatocyte An epithelial liver cell that performs most of the synthetic and metabolic functions of the liver.

Hepcidin A hormone produced by liver cells, in response to signals from a complex pathway, that decreases iron mobilization across intestinal and macrophage membranes, preventing excess iron in the blood.

Jaundice A clinical finding characterized by hyperbilirubinemia and deposition of pigment in the skin, mucous membranes, and sclera with resulting yellow appearance; also called *icterus*.

Model for End-Stage Liver Disease (MELD) Score A scoring system for assessing the severity of chronic liver disease.

Necrosis The sum of the morphological changes indicative of cell death and caused by the progressive degradative action of enzymes; it may affect groups of cells or part of a structure or an organ.

Non alcoholic fatty liver disease (NAFLD) A condition characterized by the buildup of extra fat in liver cells that is not caused by alcohol.

Non alcoholic steatohepatitis (NASH) An inflammatory disease of the liver of uncertain pathogenesis.

Portal hypertension Any increase in the pressure in the portal vein (which carries venous blood from the intestines and spleen to the liver) due to anatomical or functional obstruction (for example, cirrhosis) to blood flow in the portal venous system.

Primary biliary cirrhosis (PBC) A rare form of liver disease that results in the irreversible destruction of the small bile ducts within the liver.

Primary sclerosing cholangitis (PSC) A chronic, nonbacterial inflammatory narrowing of the bile ducts (usually the larger ducts outside of the liver.

Reye syndrome A sudden, sometimes fatal, disease of the brain (encephalopathy) caused by specific forms of acute injury to the liver.

Seroconversion Development of antibodies in blood serum as a result of infection or immunization.

Sjögren syndrome A systemic autoimmune disease in which immune cells attack and destroy the glands that produce tears and saliva.

Varices Enlarged and tortuous veins, most commonly found in the esophagus (termed *esophageal varices*).

Viral hepatitis Liver inflammation caused by viruses. Specific hepatitis viruses have been labeled A, B, C, D, and E.

Viral load The measurement of the amount of virus in the blood. It is expressed as the copies of virus per milliliter of body fluid and used to guide treatment decisions and monitor response to treatment.

Wilson disease An autosomal recessive disorder associated with excessive quantities of copper in the tissue, particularly the liver and central nervous system.

Xenobiotics Chemical substances foreign to the biological system. They include naturally occurring compounds, drugs, environmental agents, carcinogens, insecticides, etc.

The liver has a central and critical biochemical role in (1) metabolism, (2) digestion, (3) detoxification, and (4) the elimination of substances from the body. All blood from the intestinal tract initially passes through the portal vein to the liver, where products derived from digestion of food are (1) processed, (2) transformed, and (3) stored. The liver also has a central role in (1) protein, (2) carbohydrate, (3) lipid metabolism, (4) synthesizing bile acids from cholesterol to facilitate dietary fat, and (5) vitamin absorption. The liver metabolizes both endogenous and exogenous compounds (such as, drugs and toxins) by **biotransformation**, allowing their elimination.[15] The liver performs endocrine functions as it catabolizes (1) thyroid hormone, (2) cortisol, and (3) vitamin D, and synthesizes (4) insulin-like growth factor I, (5) angiotensinogen, (6) **hepcidin**, (7) thrombopoietin, and (8) small amounts of erythropoietin. Many of these hepatic functions may be assessed by laboratory procedures to gain insight into the integrity of the liver.[4]

As a large organ, the liver performs its functions with extensive reserve capacity. In many cases, individuals with liver disease maintain normal function despite extensive liver damage. In such cases, liver disease may only be recognized by using tests that detect liver injury. Most commonly, this is accomplished by measurement of plasma activities of enzymes found within liver cells released in somewhat specific patterns with different forms of injury. Chronic liver injury often involves fibrosis in the liver. Consequently, detection of markers of the fibrotic process might be indicators of degree of liver injury.

The chapter begins with a discussion of the anatomy and biochemical functions of the liver. The various disease states that involve the liver are then discussed. The chapter concludes with a discussion of use of laboratory test results in recognizing and characterizing patterns of liver injury.

Anatomy of the Liver

The adult liver weighs approximately 1.2 to 1.5 kg. It is located beneath the diaphragm in the right upper quadrant of the abdomen and is protected by the ribs and held in place by ligamentous attachments (Figure 37-1).

Blood Supply

The liver has a dual blood supply. The first is the portal vein, which carries blood from the spleen and nutrient-enriched blood from the gastrointestinal (GI) tract. It supplies approximately 70% of the blood flow to the liver. The second blood supply is the hepatic artery, which is a branch of the celiac axis. It carries oxygen-enriched arterial blood from the central circulation to the liver. Ultimately, these two blood supplies

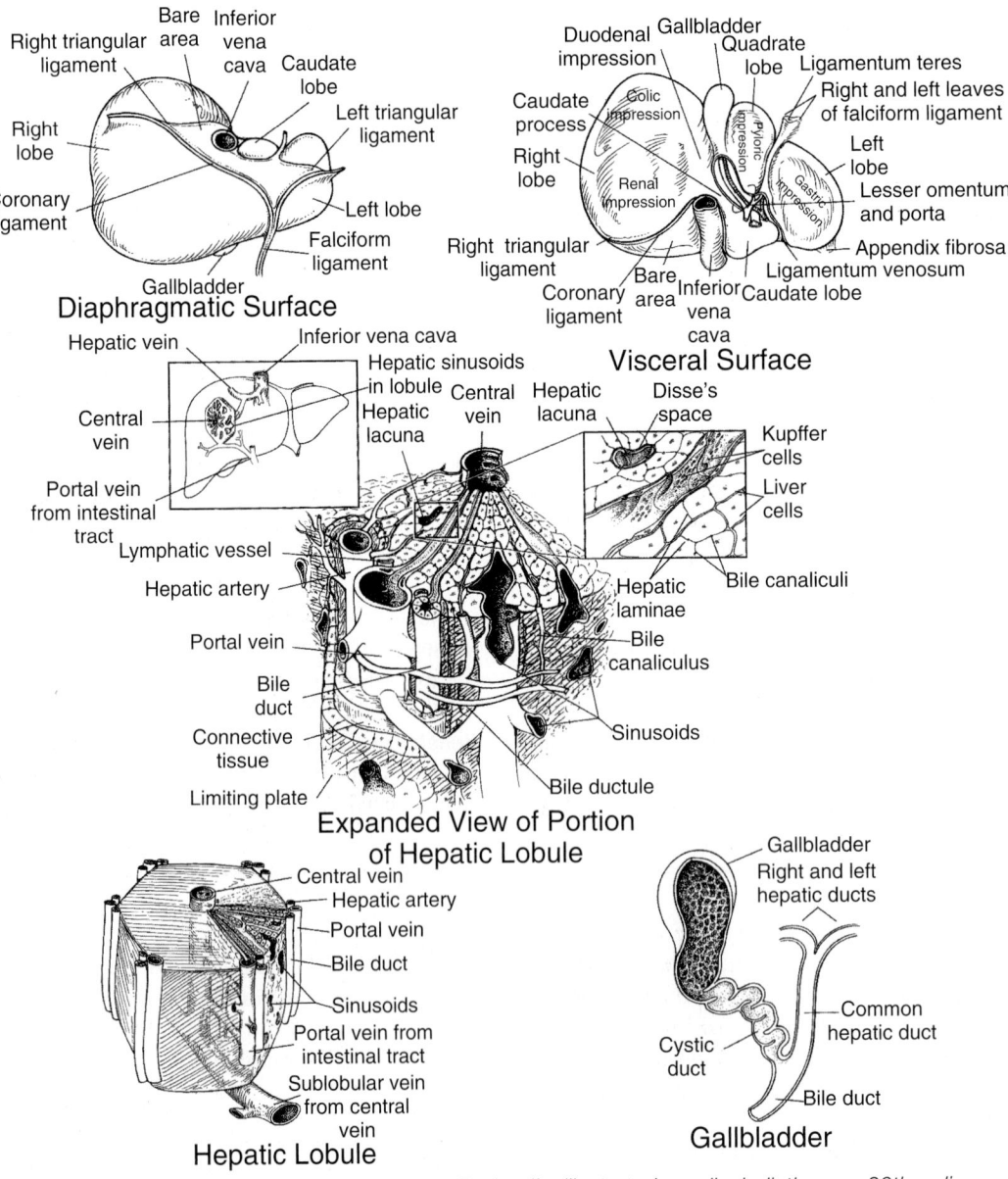

Figure 37-1 Structure of the liver. *(From Dorland's illustrated medical dictionary, 30th edition. Philadelphia: WB Saunders, 2003, plate 26.)*

merge and flow into the sinusoids that course between individual hepatocytes. The venous drainage from the liver converges into the hepatic veins, which join the inferior vena cava near its entry into the right atrium.

Biliary Drainage

Biliary drainage originates at the bile canaliculi, grooves between adjacent hepatocytes, which form ductules that merge to form the intrahepatic bile ducts. These ultimately join to form the right and left hepatic ducts, which exit from the liver at the porta hepatis and unite to form the common hepatic duct. The hepatic duct is joined by the cystic duct from the gallbladder, creating the common bile duct (see Figure 37-1), which enters the duodenum (usually with the pancreatic duct) at the ampulla of Vater. The gallbladder, located on the undersurface of the right lobe of the liver, stores and concentrates **bile**, which is a mixture of bile salts and waste products. Hormonal stimuli initiated by food ingestion cause contraction of the muscular wall of the gallbladder, releasing bile salts into the intestine to facilitate digestion of fat.

Microscopic Anatomy

The functional anatomical unit of the liver is the *acinus*, adjacent to the portal triad, which consists of a branch of the (1) portal vein, (2) hepatic artery, and (3) bile duct. Each acinus is a diamond-shaped mass of liver parenchyma that is supplied by a terminal branch of the portal vein and of the hepatic artery and drained by a terminal branch of the bile duct. At the periphery of the portal triad, the hepatic artery and portal vein branches fuse to form sinusoids, which perfuse the liver and ultimately drain into the central (terminal) hepatic vein (see Figure 37-1). The sinusoids are lined by fenestrated endothelial cells that contain pores that allow free filtration of blood and phagocytic Kupffer cells (see Figure 37-1). The fenestrations (pores) allow passage of (1) nutrients into hepatocytes, (2) larger blood proteins into the space surrounding the hepatocyts, and (3) the liver's synthetic products into the systemic circulation. The Kupffer cells, derived from monocytes, contain lysosomes that break down phagocytized bacteria, and are the main site for clearance of antigen-antibody complexes from blood.

The major functioning cells in the liver are the hepatocytes, responsible for most of its metabolic and synthetic functions. Stellate cells (formerly referred to as *Ito cells*) are located between the endothelial lining of sinusoids and the hepatocytes. In their normal, quiescent state, stellate cells store vitamin A, and synthesize nitric oxide (among other bioactive substances), which helps to regulate intrahepatic blood flow. When stimulated, stellate cells are transformed to collagen producing cells, and are responsible for fibrosis and, eventually, **cirrhosis**. Oval cells are located within periportal bile ductules; these are believed to be liver progenitor cells, which proliferate following liver injury and regenerate both bile ducts and hepatocytes.

The blood supply to each acinus passes hepatocytes loosely arranged in three zones (Figure 37-2). Zone 1 is the area immediately adjacent to the portal tract, and these hepatocytes are

enriched with lysosomes and mitochondria. The periphery of the acinus, zone 3, has (1) hepatocytes enriched with endoplasmic reticulum, (2) is very active metabolically, and (3) has relatively low oxygen tension. This area is most susceptible to injury, although zone 1 appears to be involved with protecting the liver from external injury and providing a base for hepatic regeneration.

Ultrastructure of the Hepatocyte

Hepatocytes contain a well-developed organelle substructure (Figure 37-3). Mitochondria are the site of oxidative phosphorylation and energy production. The rough endoplasmic reticulum is the site of protein synthesis, while the smooth endoplasmic reticulum contains microsomes involved in drug and toxin metabolism and cholesterol and bile acid synthesis. Peroxisomes catalyze the β-oxidation of medium-chain fatty acids with chain lengths from 7 to 18 carbons and enzymes that participate in ethanol metabolism. Lysosomes contain hydrolytic enzymes that act as scavengers. Deposition of (1) iron, (2) lipofuscin (an iron-negative lipid pigment), (3) bile pigments, and (4) copper occurs in the lysosomes. The Golgi

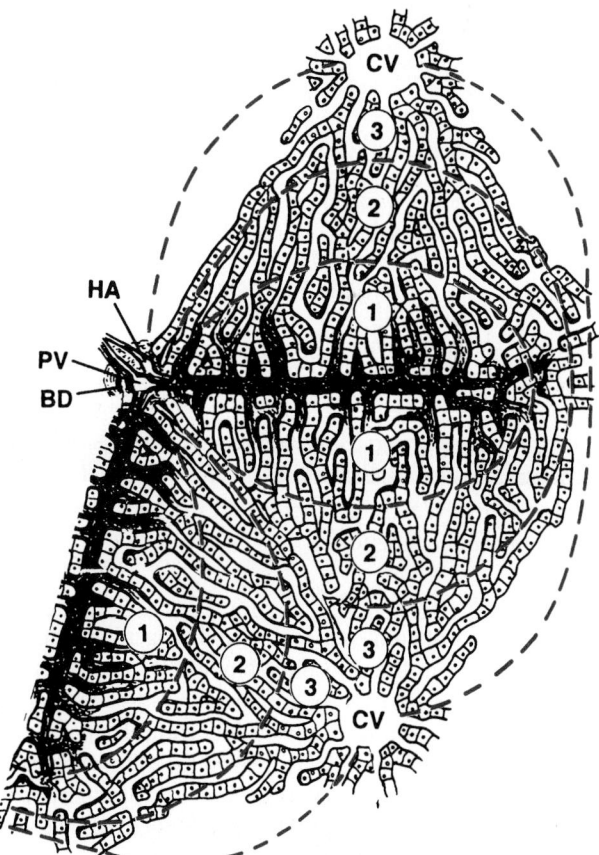

Figure 37-2 Blood supply of the simple liver acinus. *Zones 1, 2,* and *3* indicate corresponding volumes in a portion of an adjacent acinar unit. Oxygen tension and the nutrient concentration in the blood in sinusoids decrease from zone 1 through zone 3. *BD,* Bile duct; *CV,* central vein; *HA,* hepatic artery; *PV,* portal vein. *(From Zakim O, Boyer TD. Hepatology: A textbook of liver disease, 3rd edition. Philadelphia: WB Saunders, 1996:10.)*

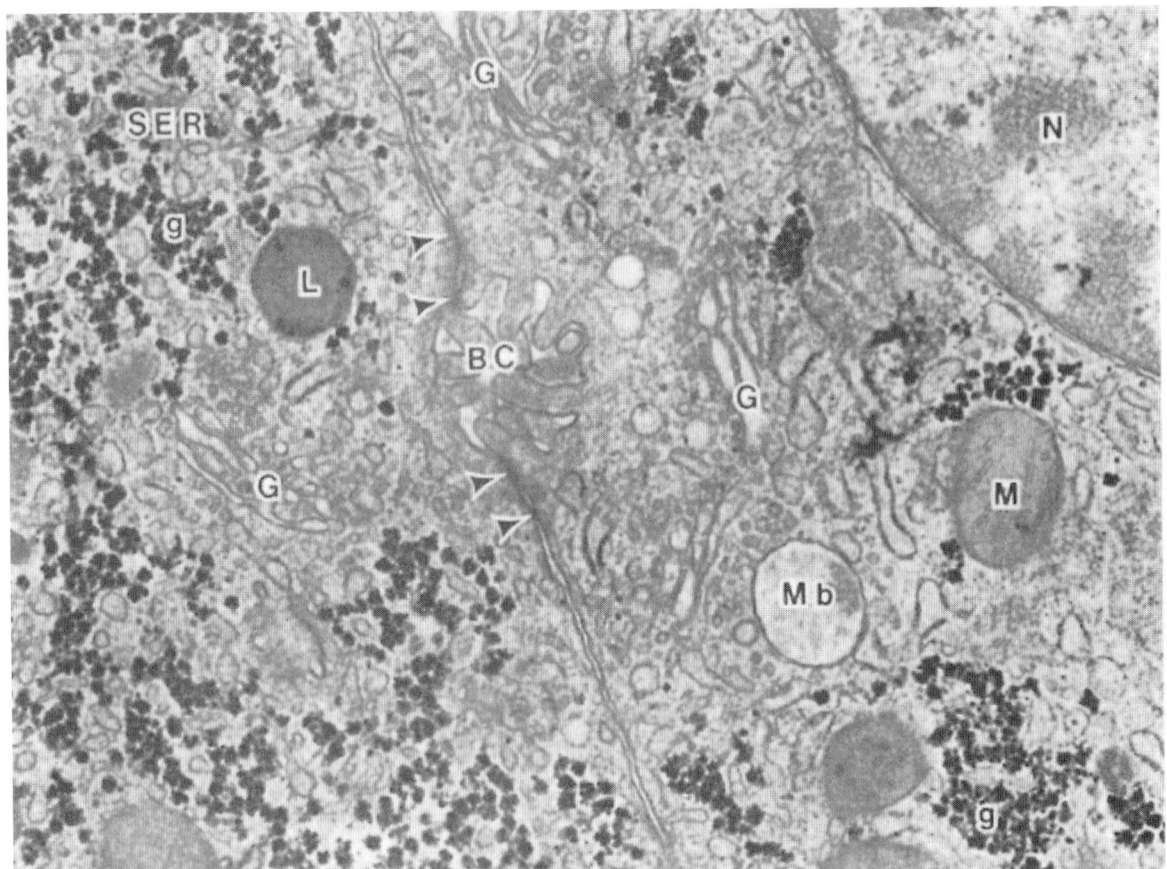

Figure 37-3 Portions of two human liver cells showing the relationship of the organelles and a typical bile canaliculus (BC). *Arrowheads* indicate light junctions. *g,* Glycogen; *G,* golgi; *L,* lysosome; *M,* mitochondria; *Mb,* microbody; *N,* nucleus; *SER,* smooth endoplasmic reticulum. *(From Zakim O, Boyer TD. Hepatology: A textbook of liver disease, 3rd edition. Philadelphia: WB Saunders, 1996:20.)*

apparatus is involved with secretion of various substances, including bile acids and albumin.

Biochemical Functions of the Liver

The liver is involved in a number of (1) excretory, (2) synthetic, and (3) metabolic functions.

Hepatic Excretory Function

Organic anions of both endogenous and exogenous origin are (1) extracted from the sinusoidal blood, (2) biotransformed, and (3) excreted into the bile or urine. Assessment of this excretory function provides valuable clinical information. The most frequently used tests involve the (1) measurement of plasma concentrations of endogenously produced compounds, such as bilirubin and (less commonly used) bile acids, and (2) determination of the rate of clearance of exogenous compounds, such as aminopyrine, lidocaine, and caffeine. Drug metabolic tests also are used as markers of function in liver transplants and in advanced liver disease.

Bilirubin is a pigment derived from heme turnover. It is extracted and biotransformed in the liver and excreted in bile and urine. The (1) chemistry, (2) biochemistry, and (3) analytical methodology for bilirubin and related compounds are discussed in Chapter 28. Only a brief overview of factors relevant to understanding of liver disease is included here.

Bilirubin is carried to the liver, loosely bound to albumin, in its native, unconjugated form. Bilirubin is transported across the hepatocyte membrane and rapidly conjugated to produce bilirubin glucuronides, which are then excreted into bile by an energy-dependent process. This process is highly efficient, and bilirubin conjugates are detectable in normal plasma only using highly sensitive techniques. In the presence of bilirubin monoglucuronide, albumin (and other proteins) is modified by covalent attachment of bilirubin to lysine residues, producing **biliprotein** or δ-bilirubin. Increases in conjugated bilirubin or δ-bilirubin are highly specific markers of hepatic dysfunction (except in rare inherited disorders, such as Dubin-Johnson syndrome). In the intestinal tract, bilirubin glucuronides are hydrolyzed and reduced by bacteria to *urobilinogens,* which undergo an enterohepatic circulation, and then to stool pigments stercobilin, mesobilin, and urobilin.

Increased plasma bilirubin is typically classified as unconjugated (indirect: an approximation of unconjugated bilirubin) or conjugated (direct: an approximation of the sum of conjugated bilirubin and biliprotein). Increased unconjugated bilirubin indicates either overproduction of bilirubin, usually caused by (1) hemolysis, (2) decreased delivery of bilirubin to the liver (in **portal hypertension**), or (3) decreased metabolism by the liver (primarily because of congenital defects involving uridine 5'-phosphate [UDP]-glucuronyl transferase). With severe liver injury, liver disease may cause primarily unconjugated hyperbilirubinemia. Increased conjugated bilirubin generally results from *acute hepatitis* or **cholestasis** (stoppage or suppression of the flow of bile); the percentage of conjugated bilirubin is similar in both types of liver disease. Conjugated bilirubin is often mildly elevated in advanced forms of *chronic* **hepatitis** or chronic cholestasis, and it is often the only evidence of dysfunction of the liver. Urine bilirubin is typically elevated in the presence of increased conjugated bilirubin. With resolution of liver disease, conjugated bilirubin is rapidly cleared, and biliprotein may become the only form present. Urine bilirubin is typically absent in such circumstances. Increased conjugated bilirubin is also rarely seen with congenital defects in bilirubin excretion (such as, Dubin-Johnson syndrome) and with impaired bilirubin excretion (as occurs in sepsis or other acute illness).

Hepatic Synthetic Function

The liver has extensive synthetic capacity and plays a major role in the regulation of protein, carbohydrate, and lipid metabolism. For example, (1) protein, (2) glucose, (3) glycogen, (4) triglyceride, (5) fatty acid, (6) cholesterol, and (7) bile acid synthesis all occur within the liver. Because details of these are discussed in other chapters (see Chapters 18, 22, and 23), discussion in this section is limited to tests useful for evaluation of liver function.

Protein Synthesis

The liver has a significant reserve capacity, preventing protein concentrations from decreasing unless there is extensive liver damage. In addition, many liver proteins have relatively long half-lives, such as albumin at approximately 3 weeks. The clinical sensitivity and specificity of protein concentrations for diagnosis of liver disease are far from ideal. The patterns of plasma protein alterations seen in liver disease depend on the (1) type, (2) severity, and (3) duration of liver injury. For example, in *acute hepatic dysfunction,* there is usually little change in the plasma protein profile or the total plasma protein concentration. With **fulminant hepatic failure** or severe liver injury, concentrations of short-lived hepatic proteins (such as, transthyretin and prothrombin) will decrease quickly and become abnormal. Proteins with longer half-lives may not be affected. In advanced cirrhosis, concentrations of all liver-synthesized plasma proteins decrease, whereas immunoglobulins increase (probably related to impaired Kupffer cell function). Serial determination of plasma proteins provides prognostic information; for example, a worsening of prothrombin time (PT) during *acute hepatitis* suggests a poor prognosis, while PT has been used as part of the **Model for End-Stage Liver Disease (MELD)** score for predicting prognosis in patients with cirrhosis.

Plasma Proteins

The plasma proteins discussed below are discussed in more detail in Chapter 18.

Albumin. Albumin is the most commonly measured serum protein and is synthesized exclusively by the liver. With liver disease, hypoalbuminemia is noted primarily in (1) cirrhosis, (2) autoimmune hepatitis, and (3) **alcoholic hepatitis**. One important consideration in measurement of albumin is the inaccuracy of dye-binding methods in patients with liver disease. Although bromcresol green measurements tend to overestimate albumin concentration at low concentrations, bromcresol purple methods give falsely low values in patients with **jaundice** because of interference of bilirubin at the site of binding.

Transthyretin. This protein has a short half-life of 24 to 48 hours, making it a sensitive indicator of current synthetic ability. Failure of transthyretin to increase is an indicator of fulminant hepatic failure in acute hepatitis and is associated with a poor prognosis. It is more commonly used as a measurement of nutritional status.

Immunoglobulins. Immunoglobulins are commonly increased in (1) cirrhosis, (2) autoimmune hepatitis, and (3) **primary biliary cirrhosis (PBC)** but are normal in most other types of liver disease. Immunoglobulin G (IgG) is increased in **autoimmune hepatitis (AIH)** and cirrhosis; Immunoglobulin M (IgM) is increased in PBC. Immunoglobulin A (IgA) tends to be increased in all types of cirrhosis. None of these findings is specific, and they are seldom used in the diagnosis of liver disease.

Ceruloplasmin. This protein is decreased in (1) **Wilson disease**, (2) cirrhosis, and (3) many causes of chronic hepatitis. It may also be increased by (1) inflammation, (2) cholestasis, (3) **hemochromatosis**, (4) pregnancy, and (5) estrogen therapy, masking the decrease expected in Wilson disease. It is discussed in more detail later in the section on Wilson disease.

α₁-Antitrypsin. This protein is the major serine protease inhibitor (serpin) in plasma, and is decreased in homozygous deficiency and cirrhosis and increased by acute inflammation. It is discussed in more detail later in the section on α₁-antitrypsin deficiency.

α-Fetoprotein. This protein, a normal, major component of fetal blood, falls to adult concentrations by 1 year of age. Mild increases are seen in patients with acute and chronic hepatitis and indicate hepatocellular regeneration. High levels in the setting of acute liver failure indicate **hepatocyte** regeneration and indicate a good prognosis. It is present at higher concentrations in **hepatocellular carcinoma (HCC)** and is discussed in more detail later and in Chapters 20 and 44.

Coagulation Proteins

Because of the large functional reserve of the liver, failure of hemostasis usually does not occur except in severe or long-standing liver disease. The PT measures activity of (1) fibrinogen (factor I), (2) prothrombin (factor II), and (3) factors V, VII, and X. Since all of these factors are synthesized in the liver, a prolonged PT often indicates the presence of significant liver disease. In cholestasis, vitamin K deficiency may also cause an increase in PT. In this case, the coagulation abnormality is corrected within a few days by parenteral injection of 10 mg of vitamin K. In contrast, if PT is prolonged because of hepatocellular disease, factor synthesis is decreased and administration of vitamin K does not

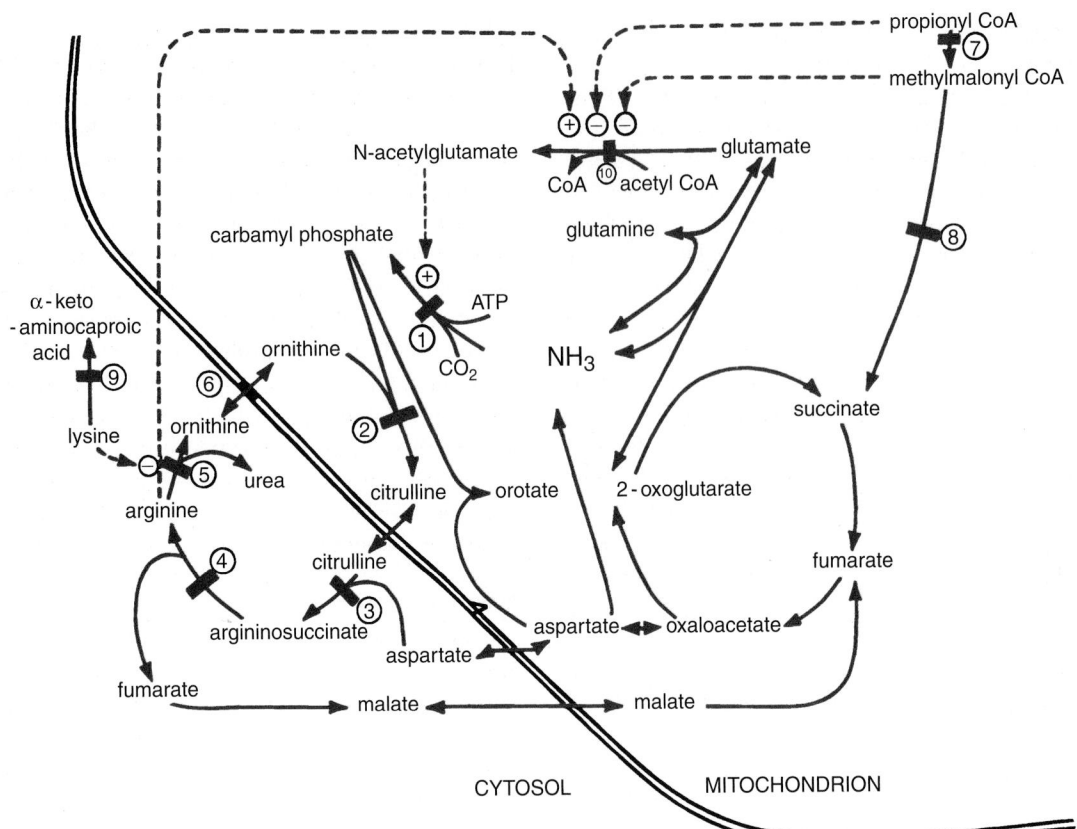

Figure 37-4 The major metabolic pathways for the use of ammonia by the hepatocyte. *Solid bars* indicate the sites of primary enzyme defects in various metabolic disorders associated with hyperammonemia: *(1)* carbamyl phosphate synthetase 1, *(2)* ornithine transcarbamylase, *(3)* argininosuccinate synthetase, *(4)* argininosuccinate lyase, *(5)* arginase, *(6)* mitochondrial ornithine transport, *(7)* propionyl CoA carboxylase, *(8)* methylmalonyl CoA mutase, *(9)* L-lysine dehydrogenase, and *(10)* N-acetyl glutamine synthetase. *Dotted lines* indicate the site of pathway activation (+) or inhibition (–). *(From Flannery OB, Hsia YE, Wolf B. Current status of hyperammonemia syndromes. Hepatology 1982;2:495-506. Copyright 1996 American Association for the Study of Liver Diseases. Reprinted with permission of Wiley-Liss, Inc., a subsidiary of John Wiley & Sons, Inc.)*

typically correct the problem. The method for reporting PT in liver disease remains controversial, but the International Normalized Ratio (INR)*does not standardize PT measurement in liver disease as it does in warfarin therapy.

Urea Synthesis

Patients with end-stage liver disease may have low concentrations of urea in plasma. The rate of urea excretion in urine is lower than in healthy individuals. In addition, plasma concentrations of urea precursors ammonia (see later) and amino acids are increased in end-stage liver disease.

Hepatic Metabolic Function

The liver has a central and important role in several metabolic and regulatory pathways. For example, the functional expression of the complex, integrated organelle structure includes the

metabolism of drugs (activation and detoxification) and the disposal of exogenous and endogenous substances, such as ammonia. A classic example, for example, is galactosemia. In this condition, the congenital absence of the galactose-1-phosphate uridyltransferase enzyme allows accumulation of the toxic metabolite galactose 1-phosphate, which causes injury to the (1) liver, (2) brain, and (3) kidneys.

Ammonia Metabolism

The major source of circulating ammonia is the action of (1) bacterial proteases, (2) ureases, and (3) amine oxidases acting on GI tract contents. The ammonia concentration in the portal vein is typically fivefold to tenfold higher than that in the systemic circulation. Under normal circumstances, most ammonia is metabolized to urea in hepatocytes in the Krebs-Henseleit urea cycle (Figure 37-4).

Animal and human studies have shown that an elevated concentration of ammonia in the brain that results from high plasma ammonia concentration (hyperammonemia) exerts toxic effects on the central nervous system. There are several causes, both inherited and acquired, of hyperammonemia.

*The INR is a system established by the World Health Organization (WHO) and the International Committee on Thrombosis and Hemostasis for reporting the results of blood *coagulation* (clotting) tests. All results are standardized using the international sensitivity index for the particular thromboplastin reagent and instrument combination utilized to perform the test.

The inherited deficiencies of urea cycle enzymes are the major cause of hyperammonemia in infants.

The common acquired causes of hyperammonemia are advanced liver disease and renal failure. Severe or chronic liver failure (as occurs in **fulminant hepatitis** and cirrhosis, respectively) leads to a significant impairment of normal ammonia metabolism. **Reye syndrome**, which is primarily a central nervous system disorder with minor hepatic dysfunction, is also associated with hyperammonemia.

Hepatic encephalopathy, in the cirrhotic patient, is often precipitated by GI bleeding that enhances ammonia production. Other precipitating causes of encephalopathy include (1) excess dietary protein, (2) constipation, (3) infections, (4) drugs, or (5) electrolyte and acid-base imbalance. Because these conditions also increase ammonia concentrations, there is a small correlation between the degree of elevation in ammonia and the degree of impairment of liver function. There is, however, little correlation in an individual patient between plasma ammonia concentrations and degree of encephalopathy. The fasting venous plasma ammonia concentration is useful in the differential diagnosis of encephalopathy when it is unclear if encephalopathy is of hepatic origin. It is especially helpful in diagnosing Reye syndrome and the inherited disorders of urea metabolism. However, it is not useful in patients with known liver disease.

Should ammonia values in healthy subjects be much higher than expected, consideration should be given to the existence and correction of sources of preanalytical error. These include errors resulting from (1) contamination (from cigarette smoke, use of ammonium heparin anticoagulation), (2) the collection process (prolonged tourniquet use, fist clenching during collection), or (3) sample handling (delayed analysis, failure to put sample in ice water).

Xenobiotic Metabolism and Excretion

Xenobiotics are foreign substances that are cleared and metabolized by the liver and some have been used as tests of liver function. For example, certain lipophilic substances, such as (1) bromsulfophthalein (BSP), (2) indocyanine green (ICG), (3) aminopyrine, (4) caffeine, (5) lidocaine, and (6) the stain rose bengal are excreted into bile as the intact parent compound, its conjugates, or both. The clearance of these xenobiotics by the liver is normally very rapid, and it is believed that uptake by hepatocytes is a carrier-mediated, active-transport process. Little, if any, is cleared by other tissue. Excretion into bile is slow. The elimination of these compounds from the bloodstream therefore depends on (1) hepatic blood flow, (2) patency—the quality or state of being open or unobstructed—of the biliary tree, and (3) hepatic parenchymal function.

Clinical Manifestations of Liver Disease

A number of conditions are indicative of liver disease, including (1) jaundice, (2) portal hypertension, (3) disordered hemostasis, and (4) the release of enzymes into various body fluids.

Jaundice

Jaundice (also known as *icterus*) is characterized by a yellow appearance of the skin, mucous membranes, and sclera caused by bilirubin deposition. It is the most specific clinical manifestation of hepatic dysfunction. It is, however, not present in many individuals with liver disease (especially chronic liver disease), and also may occur with bilirubin overproduction (hemolysis) or congenital disorders of bilirubin metabolism. Jaundice is usually apparent clinically in older children and adults when the plasma bilirubin concentration reaches 2 to 3 mg/dL (34 to 51 μmol/L). When bilirubin clearance from the liver to the intestinal tract is impaired (as in acute hepatitis and bile duct obstruction), it may be accompanied by acholic (gray-colored) stools. Increases in water-soluble conjugated bilirubin lead to tea-colored urine. Bilirubin metabolism is discussed in Chapter 28. A classification of jaundice, based on the site of altered bilirubin metabolism, is shown in Box 28-3 in Chapter 28.

Portal Hypertension

The venous outflow of the GI tract, spleen, and pancreas passes through the portal circulation (Figure 37-5). Portal hypertension occurs when there is obstruction to portal flow anywhere along its course. The causes of obstruction leading to portal hypertension are classified by site as (1) presinusoidal, (2) sinusoidal, and (3) postsinusoidal. Presinusoidal portal hypertension is most commonly caused by portal vein thrombosis or schistosomiasis. Important causes of postsinusoidal hypertension include hepatic vein occlusion (Budd-Chiari syndrome) and congestive heart failure. The vast majority of cases of portal hypertension represent sinusoidal hypertension, most commonly caused by cirrhosis.

When portal pressure increases, the portal venous system becomes dilated and forms collateral connections to the systemic venous flow (Figure 37-6), leading to portosystemic shunting. Initially, this is clinically silent, but as portal hypertension worsens, it compromises many of the metabolic functions of the liver. One such abnormality is altered estrogen metabolism, leading to skin findings, such as spider telangiectasias and palmar erythema, gynecomastia in men, and abnormal vaginal bleeding and irregular menstrual periods in women. Impaired metabolic functions lead to the accumulation of ammonia and abnormal neurotransmitters and ultimately to hepatic encephalopathy. Because most nutrients arrive through the portal vein, synthetic functions are also impaired, resulting in decreased concentrations of most plasma proteins. This includes clotting factors and clotting factor inhibitors, such as antithrombin and proteins C and S. Patients with portal hypertension are thus predisposed to both excessive bleeding and to venous thrombosis.

Bleeding Esophageal Varices

The most life-threatening consequence of portosystemic shunting is the development of **varices** (enlarged and tortuous veins), which occur throughout the GI tract but are most common in the esophagus and stomach. Bleeding from varices is one of the leading causes of morbidity and mortality in patients with cirrhosis. Varices are present at the time of

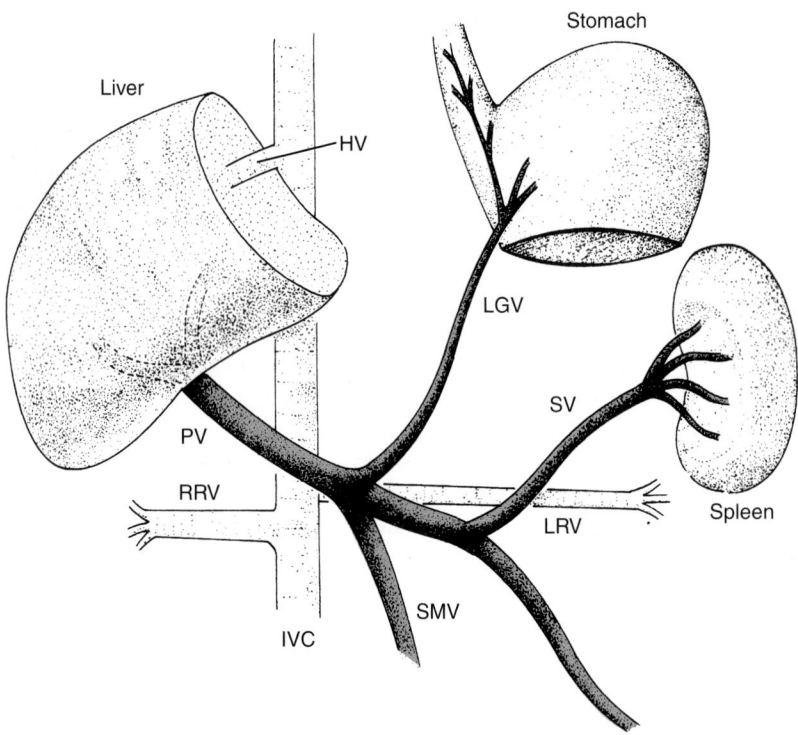

Figure 37-5 The portal-venous system. *HV,* Hepatic vein; *IVC,* inferior vena cava; *IMV,* inferior mesenteric vein; *LGV,* left gastric vein; *LRV,* left renal vein; *PV,* portal vein; *RRV,* right renal vein; *SV,* splenic vein; *SMV,* superior mesenteric vein. *(From Zakim O, Boyer TD. Hepatology: A textbook of liver disease, 3rd edition. Philadelphia: WB Saunders, 1996:721.)*

diagnosis of cirrhosis in about 40% of patients and develop in an additional 6% per year.

Ascites

Ascites is the accumulation of fluid in the abdominal cavity. Ascites is the most common clinical finding in patients with portal hypertension. Ascites itself is usually not life threatening, but is uncomfortable and may compromise respiration. It also predisposes individuals to spontaneous bacterial peritonitis, which is life threatening. Since there are many causes of ascites, the feature that most distinguishes portal hypertension is an increase in the difference in albumin concentrations between plasma and ascitic fluid. This is sometimes called the *serum-ascites albumin gradient (SAAG).* A gradient >1.1 g/dL is diagnostic of ascites caused by portal hypertension.

Spontaneous Bacterial Peritonitis

Ascites predisposes to spontaneous bacterial peritonitis, defined as bacteremia (typically gram negative) in the absence of mechanical disruption of the bowel. It usually presents in an individual with known cirrhosis who develops (1) abdominal pain, (2) fever, or (3) leukocytosis. The diagnosis is established by examination of the ascitic fluid. Values of >250 neutrophils per microliter, or >500 in the absence of a positive blood culture, is considered diagnostic. In contrast, secondary peritonitis is usually associated with (1) higher neutrophil counts, (2) low glucose in ascitic fluid, and (3) high concentration of protein.

Hepatic (Portosystemic) Encephalopathy

Hepatic encephalopathy is a metabolic disorder characterized by a wide spectrum of neuropsychiatric dysfunction. It may occur (1) as an acute syndrome in patients with acute **hepatic failure** from viral or drug-induced hepatitis, or (2) as a chronic syndrome associated with liver failure and cirrhosis. A variety of neurotransmitter systems are dysfunctional in hepatic encephalopathy, but the exact cause for the changes is not known. Plasma ammonia concentrations are rarely helpful, either for diagnosis or for monitoring the patient's disorder. Normal ammonia concentrations, however, are helpful in excluding hepatic encephalopathy as a cause of cerebral dysfunction.

Hepatorenal Syndrome

Hepatorenal syndrome (HRS) refers to decreased renal function secondary to hepatic disease. Portal hypertension is a common factor in all cases of HRS developing in chronic liver disease.[1] HRS, however, also may develop in acute liver failure. Although formerly thought to be a rapidly progressing, terminal event in a person with end-stage liver disease, it is now recognized that HRS falls into two major groups. Type 2 HRS, a slowly progressive or stable decline in renal function that is due to peripheral vasodilation and renal vasoconstriction, is the most common form. Type 1, or classic, HRS represents rapidly declining renal function, usually developing in a person with preexisting type 2 HRS. Type 1 HRS usually develops in the setting of an acute decrease in blood pressure, often due to (1) spontaneous bacterial peritonitis, (2) variceal bleeding, or (3) excessive use of diuretics to treat ascites.

A common feature in both forms of HRS is activation of the renin-angiotensin-aldosterone axis caused by intravascular volume depletion, leading to salt and water retention. This leads to development of (1) hyponatremia, (2) hypokalemia, (3) metabolic alkalosis, (4) low urine sodium and high urine potassium excretion, and (5) high urine osmolality.

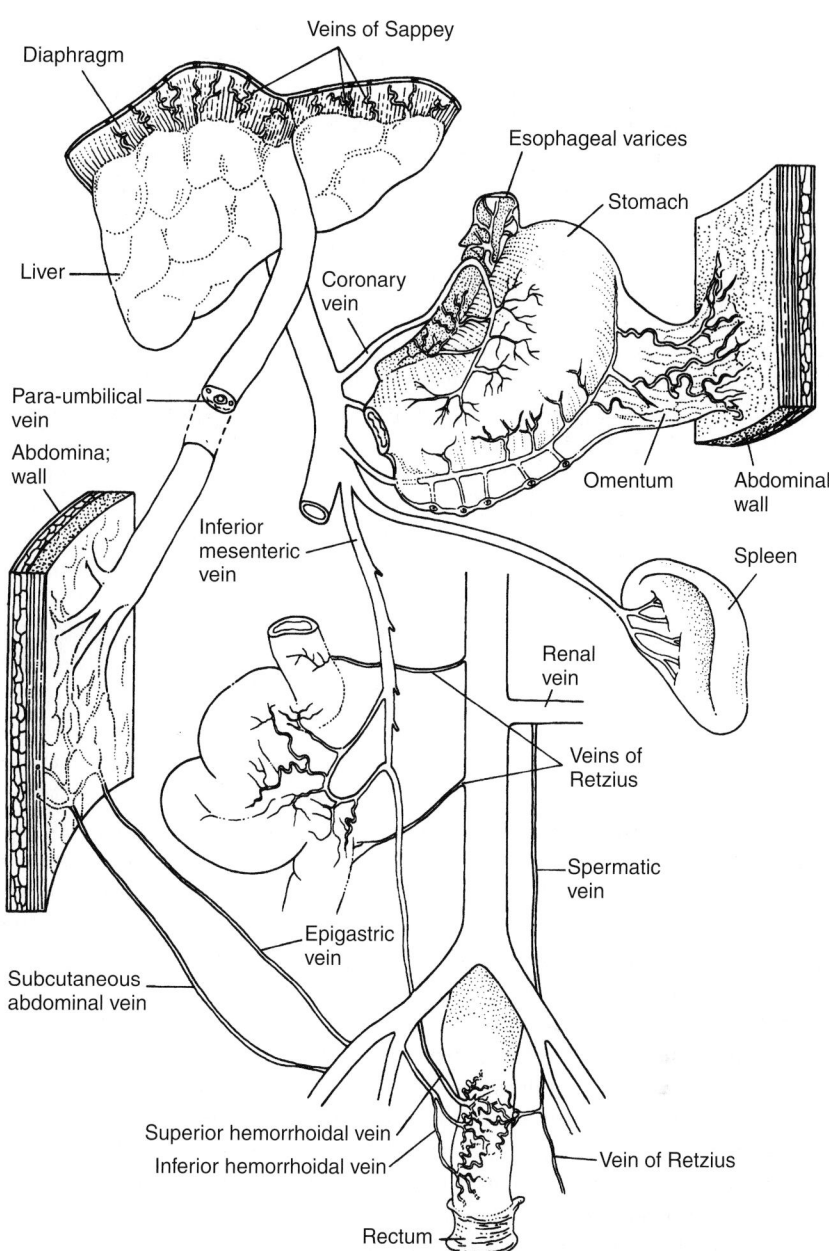

Figure 37-6 The sites of the portosystemic collateral circulation in cirrhosis of the liver. *(From Sherlock S, Dooley J, eds. Diseases of the liver and biliary system, 9th edition. London: Blackwell Scientific Publications, 1993:134.)*

Disordered Hemostasis in Liver Disease

Numerous coagulation factors are manufactured by the liver. Thus, abnormal hemostasis is common in liver disease, particularly cirrhosis and acute liver failure. Disorders of fibrinogen (such as, dysfibrinogenemia) may also be seen in both acute and chronic liver disease, leading to prolongation of the partial thromboplastin time. Disseminated intravascular coagulation occurs with acute hepatic **necrosis**, presumably as a result of the release of tissue thromboplastin and defective clearance of inhibitors, such as antithrombin and protein C. Thrombocytopenia (common in persons with cirrhosis) may contribute to ineffective intravascular coagulation. Although commonly attributed to splenic sequestration (hypersplenism), there is evidence of antibody-mediated platelet destruction, and decreased production of thrombopoietin

by the liver contributes to thrombocytopenia. Patients with AIH may have anticardiolipin antibodies and antibodies to platelets.

Enzymes Released from Diseased Liver Tissue

Because hepatic function is often normal in many patients with liver disease, the plasma activities of numerous enzymes are more reliable indicators of liver disease. For example, the pattern and degree of elevation of enzyme activity vary with the type of liver disease, their measurement is extremely helpful in the recognition and differential diagnosis of liver damage (see Chapter 19). A number of factors govern the ability of liver enzymes to assist in diagnosis, including their (1) tissue specificity, (2) subcellular distribution, (3) relative degree of enzyme activity in liver and plasma, (4) patterns of release, and (5) clearance from plasma

Tissue Specificity

The five enzymes that are commonly measured and used in the diagnosis of liver disease include (1) aspartate aminotransferase (AST; EC 2.6.1.1); (2) alanine aminotransferase (ALT; EC 2.6.1.2); (3) alkaline phosphatase (ALP; 3.1.3.1); (4) γ-glutamyltransferase (GGT; EC 2.3.2.2), all of which are commonly used to detect liver injury; and (5) lactate dehydrogenase (LD; EC 1.1.1.27), which is occasionally used. ALT and GGT are present in several tissues, but plasma activities primarily reflect liver injury. AST is found in (1) liver, (2) muscle (cardiac and skeletal), and to a limited extent in (3) red cells. LD has wide tissue distribution, and is thus relatively nonspecific. ALP is found in a number of tissues, but in normal individuals primarily reflects bone and liver sources. Thus, based on tissue distribution, ALT and GGT are considered the most specific markers for liver injury.

Subcellular Distribution

Enzymes are found at different locations within cells. AST, ALT, and LD are cytosolic enzymes. As such, they are released with cell injury, and appear in plasma relatively rapidly. In the case of AST and ALT, there are both mitochondrial and cytosolic isoenzymes in hepatocytes and other cells containing these enzymes. With ALT, the relative amount of mitochondrial isoenzyme is small, and its plasma half-life is extremely short, making it of no diagnostic significance. With AST, the mitochondrial isoenzyme represents a significant fraction of total AST within hepatocytes, although little is released in most forms of liver disease. In contrast, ALP and GGT are membrane-bound glycoprotein enzymes. The most important location of both enzymes is on the canalicular membrane of hepatocytes.

Relative Activity in Liver and Plasma

For cytoplasmic enzymes, the relative amount of enzyme in the liver relative to plasma is an important determinant of clinical utility. The activity of AST within hepatocytes is about twice that of ALT, although plasma activities are similar. In contrast, hepatocyte activities of LD are much lower (relative to plasma) than those of the other two enzymes, and plasma activities of LD are several times higher than those of AST and ALT. This causes less of an increase in LD with liver injury than occurs with AST and ALT. The relative amount of enzyme in tissue is not necessarily the same in disease. In (1) cirrhosis, (2) alcohol abuse, and (3) malnutrition, there are greater decreases in cytoplasmic ALT than in cytoplasmic AST.

Mechanisms of Release

Several mechanisms appear to be involved in release of enzymes from hepatocytes. Cell injury is the simplest mechanism and appears to allow leakage of cytoplasmic enzymes, but minimal release of other types of enzymes. Alcohol appears to induce expression of mitochondrial AST on the surface of hepatocytes. Not surprisingly, alcoholic hepatitis is associated with increased plasma activities of this isoenzyme. The mechanism of release of membrane-bound enzymes such as GGT and ALP into the circulation is less well understood, but there appears to be (1) increased synthesis, (2) membrane fragmentation by bile acids, and (3) solubilization of membrane-bound enzymes by the action of bile acids.

Rate of Clearance of Enzyme from Plasma

Clearance of liver enzymes from plasma occurs at variable rates. The half-life of ALT is about 48 hours, whereas that of cytosolic AST (the main form found in plasma) is about 16-18 hours; thus although more AST is released from liver, the much longer half-life of ALT leads to higher activities of ALT than AST in most forms of hepatocellular injury. The half-life of the liver isoenzyme of ALP has been variously reported as from 1 to 10 days; the former figure appears to correspond better to the changes seen with removal of **gallstones**. The half-life of GGT has been reported as 4.1 days. The mechanism by which enzymes are removed from circulation is not completely known, although receptor-mediated endocytosis by liver macrophages is likely involved.

Diseases of the Liver

The liver has a limited number of ways of responding to injury. Acute injury to the liver may be asymptomatic, but it often presents as jaundice. The two major acute liver diseases are acute hepatitis and cholestasis. Chronic liver injury generally takes the clinical form of chronic hepatitis; its long-term complications include cirrhosis and HCC. The discussion of liver disease will focus mainly on these patterns, and a few diseases that differ from this general pattern.

Mechanisms and Patterns of Injury

The target cell determines the pattern of injury with hepatocyte injury leading to hepatocellular disease and biliary cell injury leading to cholestasis. All cellular injury may induce fibrosis as an adaptive or healing response with the duration of injury and genetic factors determining whether cirrhosis and ultimately carcinoma occur (Figure 37-7).

Cell death occurs by necrosis or **apoptosis**, or both. Cellular necrosis occurs as the result of an injurious environment and has been referred to as "cell murder." Ischemic injury and toxic injury from compounds, such as (1) carbon tetrachloride, (2) aspirin, and (3) acetaminophen[9] occur for the most

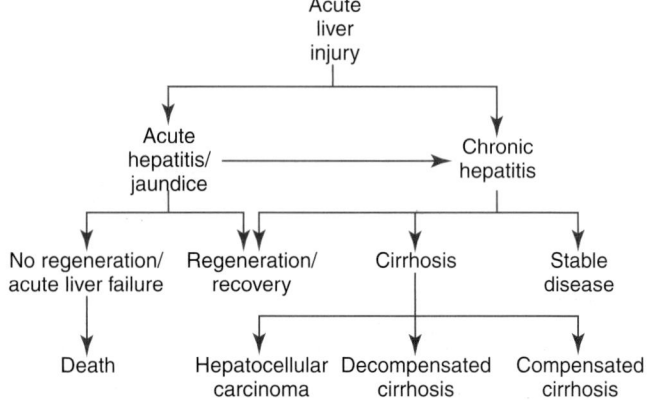

Figure 37-7 Natural history of liver disease.

part by necrosis. Apoptosis occurs as the result of accelerated programmed death in which the cell participates in its own demise and thus commits "cell suicide." Most forms of acute and chronic hepatitis are associated with apoptosis. Regardless of the cause, cell death typically results in leakage of cytoplasmic enzymes. Laboratory tests are helpful in distinguishing the (1) pattern of injury (hepatocellular versus cholestatic), (2) chronicity of injury (acute versus chronic), and (3) severity of injury (mild versus severe). In general, the aminotransferase enzymes and ALP are used to distinguish the pattern. With acute liver injury, the PT or factor V concentration are used to determine the severity. In chronic liver injury (detected by persistently elevated enzymes for over 6 months), prognosis is related to the degree of impairment in liver function, such as (1) increased bilirubin, (2) decreased albumin and platelets, and 3) prolonged PT. At the present time, the only way to accurately detect fibrosis is by a liver biopsy.

Disorders of Bilirubin Metabolism

Defects in bilirubin metabolism resulting in jaundice are known to occur at each step in the metabolic pathway. The pathway and the disorders related to these defects are discussed in Chapter 28.

Hepatic Viral Infection

Five viruses have been identified (A, B, C, D, E) as causes of infection that primarily targets the liver. In addition, certain other viruses may infect the liver as part of a more generalized infection, among them (1) cytomegalovirus (CMV), (2) Epstein-Barr virus (EBV), and (3) herpes simplex virus (HSV). The various hepatitis viruses are outlined in Table 37-1. Only hepatitis A, B, and C will be discussed in this section.

Hepatitis A Virus

Hepatitis A virus (HAV) is the most common cause of acute **viral hepatitis** in North America, although its incidence has markedly declined with the use of vaccination. Epidemics have been associated with waterborne and food-borne contamination. While most adults with acute HAV infection become jaundiced, most children remain asymptomatic. There is no chronic form of hepatitis A, but cholestasis (manifested by several weeks of jaundice and pruritus) may occur in some adults.

Tests commonly used to evaluate a patient for exposure to HAV include the measurement of total antibody to HAV and IgM anti-HAV. Total antibody to HAV develops after natural exposure or following immunization, and appears to persist for life with natural infection and for at least 20 years following vaccination. IgM anti-HAV develops rapidly with acute exposure, and generally remains detectable for 3 to 6 months. With the falling incidence of acute HAV infection, most positive IgM anti-HAV results represent false positives; the Centers for Disease Control and Prevention (CDC) recommends the test be used only in the setting of acute hepatitis.

Hepatitis B Virus

Hepatitis B virus (HBV) is the most common chronic viral infection. An estimated 350 million individuals are chronically infected with HBV, and approximately one third of the world population has been exposed to HBV. The frequency of chronic HBV is high in most of (1) Asia, (2) central Africa, and (3) southern Europe, but much less common among those born in North America (except Alaska) and northern Europe. HBV is transmitted through body fluids, primarily by parenteral or sexual contact. It has been found to be transmitted

---

TABLE 37-1 Types of Viral Hepatitis

	A	B	C	D	E
Type	RNA	DNA	RNA	Partial	RNA
Incubation period (d)	45-50	30-150	15-160	30-150	20-40
Transmission					
Fecal-oral	Yes	No	Min	No	Yes
Household	Yes	Min	Min	Yes	Yes
Vertical	No	Yes	Min	Yes	No
Blood	Rare	Yes	Yes	Yes	Unknown
Sexual	No	Yes	Min	Yes	Unknown
Diagnosis	Anti-HAV IgM	HBsAg, HBV DNA, anti-HBc IgM	Anti-HCV, HCV RNA	Anti-HDV, HDV RNA	Anti-HEV
Carrier state	No	Yes	Yes	Yes	Yes
Chronic hepatitis	No	Depends on age and immune system	50%-80%	Yes	Yes (in immunocompromised)
Liver cancer	No	Yes	Yes	Yes	No
Prevention					
Vaccine	Yes	Yes	No	Yes*	Yes
Immunoglobulin	Yes	Yes	No	Yes*	No
Response to interferon	Not used	50%	20%-45%	Yes	Not used

*Vaccination and passive immunization against HBV protects against HDV infection.

anti-HBc, Antibody to the hepatitis B core antigen; *DNA,* deoxyribonucleic acid; *HAV,* hepatitis A virus; *HBsAg,* hepatitis B surface antigen; *HBV,* hepatitis B virus; *HCV,* hepatitis C virus; *HDV,* hepatitis D virus; *HEV,* hepatitis E virus; *HGV,* hepatitis G virus; *IgM,* immunoglobulin M; *Min,* minimal; *PCR,* polymerase chain reaction; *RNA,* ribonucleic acid.

from mother to child, usually at or after delivery (termed *vertical transmission*). In parts of the world with high rates of chronic infection, much of the transmission is vertical. As discussed later, chronic HBV infection may take several forms, not all of which have the same significance.

Hepatitis B is caused by a 42-nm DNA virus that is a member of the hepadna virus family. Hepadna viruses are unusual in that they reproduce from an RNA template using reverse transcriptase and are prone to developing mutant strains. Several mutants have clinical importance. Mutants that prevent production of the hepatitis B e antigen (HBeAg), but allow production of antibody to the e antigen (anti-HBe) are common in much of the world, and represent up to 25% of chronic infections in North America. This limits the utility of HBeAg as a marker of viral replication. Mutants resistant to reverse transcriptase inhibitors, commonly used to treat chronic HBV, develop in many individuals treated long-term (although they are uncommon in those treated with entecavir and tenofovir). Rare mutants involve the portion of the surface antigen (HBsAg) recognized both by HBsAg kits and by antibodies developed in response to the HBV vaccine, and may cause infection that is not detected by routine laboratory tests.

Immunization

Hepatitis B may be prevented by either passive (hepatitis B immune globulin [HBIG]) or active (hepatitis B recombinant vaccine) immunization. Many countries require routine vaccination of children, which has markedly reduced the incidence of hepatitis B infection.

Diagnostic Tests for Hepatitis B

HBsAg is produced in excess by the virus, and its measurement is used as a laboratory test to detect current HBV infection. It is typically present with both acute and chronic infection. Antibody to the hepatitis B core antigen (anti-HBc) is the most commonly detected antibody against HBV. Two assays are usually employed: IgM and total anti-HBc. The total antibody assay measures both IgM and IgG antibodies and is usually positive for life after exposure. IgM anti-HBc is usually positive for 3 to 6 months after acute infection, but is occasionally present with chronic HBV infection as well. Antibody to the hepatitis B surface antigen (anti-HBs) is considered evidence of immunity to hepatitis B and is the only marker found in those receiving the hepatitis B vaccine; with "recovery" from natural infection, most individuals develop both anti-HBs and anti-HBc.

HBeAg and anti-HBe are typically used only in the setting of chronic HBV infection. HBeAg is produced along with, but is not part of the HBV viral particle. It is used as a marker of persistence of infectious virus; its clearance and the appearance of anti-HBe have been used as indicators of conversion to the nonreplicating state and as goals of antiviral treatment. Presence of HBeAg in untreated individuals always indicates persistent viremia; its absence is not reliable in indicating loss of circulating virus, as will be discussed later.

Hepatitis B viral DNA is a direct measure of circulating virus; it is most commonly measured by amplification assays.

It is unclear how many copies of HBV DNA represents clinically important viremia. Clinical practice guidelines, however, have adopted 100,000 copies/mL (20,000 IU/mL) as a "clinically significant" level of viremia. Studies have shown that risk of complication begins to increase with **viral loads** between 1000 and 10,000 copies/mL.[11] With treatment, the first evidence of response is a fall in HBV DNA.

Hepatitis C Virus

The hepatitis C virus (HCV)[5] is the most common cause of chronic hepatitis in (1) North America, (2) Europe, and (3) Japan. It is estimated to infect approximately 170 million individuals worldwide. HCV infection primarily occurs through plasma. The major risk factors are injection drug use and transfusion before testing the blood supply, which began in 1990. HCV is an RNA flavivirus with a high rate of spontaneous mutation. There are six major genotypes (<70% nucleotide homology), along with a number of subtypes (77% to 80% homology).[5]

Prevention

Prevention of HCV has proved to be more difficult than with HAV and HBV. However, there has been an 80% decrease in incidence of acute HCV over the past decade, which is thought to be due to testing blood donors for HCV and to safe injection practices instituted to reduce risk of human immunodeficiency virus (HIV) infection. No successful vaccine has been developed against HCV.

Diagnostic Tests for Hepatitis C

Measurement of the antibody to HCV (anti-HCV) is the principal screening test for HCV exposure. Second generation assays become positive an average of 12 weeks after exposure, whereas third generation assays become positive an average of 9 weeks after exposure. The CDC have identified signal to cutoff ratios for most commercial anti-HCV assays that are associated with high likelihood of true positive results.

HCV RNA is used to detect active infection. Rapid separation of serum from clot is critical for accurate measurement of HCV RNA. Of note, EDTA plasma is more stable and is often preferred for testing. Assays for HCV RNA have generally used qualitative and quantitative reporting, although many laboratories no longer perform qualitative testing because newer quantitative tests (particularly those using real-time PCR) have limits of detection similar to or lower than the original qualitative assays. Also, quantitative testing is preferred over qualitative testing because treatment decisions require knowledge of the actual viral load. HCV genotype is an important pretreatment parameter. Genotype is determined by direct sequencing or line probe assay.

Acute Hepatitis

Acute hepatitis refers to an acute injury directed against the hepatocytes. The injury may be mediated either directly or indirectly. Direct injury occurs with certain drugs, such as acetaminophen, or with ischemia. Indirect injury is immunologically mediated injury that occurs with hepatitis viruses and most drugs, including ethanol. In direct injury, there is typically a rapid rise in cytosolic enzymes, such as (1) AST, (2) ALT, and (3) LD, followed by a rapid fall with rates of decline similar to known half-lives of the enzymes. With indirect injury, there is a (1) gradual rise in cytosolic enzymes, (2) plateau phase, and (3) gradual resolution of enzyme elevation. Although jaundice is a key clinical finding leading to recognition of acute hepatitis, it is often absent. An increase of AST activity to greater than 200 IU/L, or of ALT activity to greater than 300 IU/L, has clinical sensitivity and specificity of greater than 90% for acute hepatitis. ALP is usually mildly elevated and is less than three times the upper reference limit in 90% of cases of acute hepatitis. Bilirubin elevation, when present, typically is predominantly direct-reacting bilirubin, in a percentage of total similar to that in bile duct obstruction. Liver synthetic function is usually well-preserved in most forms of acute hepatitis. However, impaired synthetic function is an important predictor of acute liver failure. These and other features that are helpful in the differential diagnosis of acute hepatitis are summarized in Table 37-2.

The outcome of acute hepatitis is variable. In most cases, complete recovery occurs and liver regeneration leads to normal structure and function. With some viruses, failure to clear infection results in the development of chronic hepatitis. In a small percentage of cases, massive destruction of the liver leads to acute (fulminant) hepatic failure, which is associated with high mortality unless liver transplantation occurs.

Acute Viral Hepatitis

All forms of acute viral hepatitis have a similar clinical course, with marked elevations in aminotransferases, usually between 8 and 50 times the upper reference limits. ALT is typically higher than AST because of slower clearance. Enzyme elevations typically peak before peak bilirubin occurs and remain increased for an average of 4 to 5 weeks (longer for ALT than AST because of its longer half-life). The incidence of acute viral hepatitis has declined to less than 10% of rates in the late 1980s, likely due to immunization for HAV and HBV and use of safer injection and sex practices.

Acute Hepatitis A

In adults, about 70% of those with acute HAV infection develop jaundice. In children, acute HAV infection typically goes unrecognized, and only 10% exhibit jaundice. IgM antibody (anti-HAV IgM) appears early in the course of illness and persists for an average of 2 to 6 months, and is the best test to diagnosis acute HAV infection.

Acute Hepatitis B

As with HAV, most infections in children are clinically silent. An estimated 30% to 50% of adolescents and adults with acute HBV infection develop jaundice. The outcome in acute HBV infection is strongly influenced by age and immune status. The serological course of acute hepatitis B infection is illustrated in Figure 37-8. HBsAg is the first serological marker to appear (1 to 2 months after infection, before evidence of hepatitis), and is the last protein marker to disappear. The first antibody to appear, usually coinciding with the onset of clinical evidence of hepatitis 3 to 6 months after infection, is anti-HBc, which usually persists for 3 to 6 months. It is usually considered diagnostic of acute hepatitis B infection. In practice, it is extremely rare to have individuals have negative HBsAg and anti-HBs at the time of initial presentation, leaving IgM anti-HBc as the only commonly measured

TABLE 37-2   Laboratory Features of Different Forms of Acute Hepatitis

Type	AST/ALT	ALP	Bilirubin	PT	Serology	Other
Viral HAV HBV HCV	8-50 × URL	<3 URL	5-15 mg/dL	<15 s	Positive IgM anti-HAV HBsAg, IgM anti-HBc HCV RNA, ±anti-HCV	
Alcoholic	<8 × URL	>3 × URL in 25%	5-15 mg/dL	<15 s	Negative	AST > ALT
Toxic	>50 × URL	Normal	<5 mg/dL	>15 s	Negative	Toxin usually detectable; acute renal failure common
Ischemic	>50 × URL	Normal	<5 mg/dL	>15 s	Negative	Acute renal failure common
Drug induced	8-50 × URL	>3 × URL in 50%	5-15 mg/dL	<15 s	Negative	Eosinophilia, skin rash common
Autoimmune	8-50 × URL	<3 × URL	5-15 mg/dL	<15 s	Positive ANA or ASMA	Low albumin, high globulins
Wilson disease	3-10 × URL	Low normal or decreased	5-15 mg/dL	<15 s	Negative	Hemolytic anemia, renal failure common; low ceruloplasmin often absent

ALP, Alkaline phosphatase; *ALT,* alanine transaminase; *ANA,* antinuclear antibody; *ASMA,* anti-smooth muscle antibody; *AST,* aspartate transaminase; *HAV,* hepatitis A virus; *HBsAg,* hepatitis B surface antigen; *HBV,* hepatitis B virus; *HCV,* hepatitis C virus; *IgM,* immunoglobulin M; *PT,* prothrombin time; *URL,* upper reference limit.

marker to be positive. This finding has been termed the "core window." "Recovery" is associated with loss of HBsAg and appearance of anti-HBs; more than 95% of healthy adults and adolescents have such an outcome, whereas the figure is lower in younger children or those who are immunosuppressed. Accumulating evidence indicates that HBV remains dormant in the body and HBV DNA circulates in low concentrations in "recovery." This has been termed "occult" HBV infection. "Reactivation" of infection may occur with chemotherapy or severe immunosuppression.

Acute Hepatitis C

Acute HCV infection[5] is responsible for 10% to 15% of cases of acute hepatitis in the United States, but only 10% to 30% develop jaundice. HCV RNA is detectable in plasma 2 to 4 weeks after initial exposure with aminotransferases activities increasing about 6 to 8 weeks after infection. Anti-HCV is present in a little more than half of cases at the time of presentation. Diagnosis of acute HCV is likely if (1) anti-HCV is absent but HCV RNA is present, (2) HCV RNA viral load is high and anti-HCV titer is low, (3) anti-HCV titer increases with time, or (4) an initially positive HCV RNA becomes negative without treatment. Viral load falls with development of antibody to one or more HCV proteins, and may become transiently negative even in those who progress to chronic infection. An estimated 30% to 50% of those infected clear the virus spontaneously (more commonly in younger individuals); those who clear virus may fail to develop anti-HCV, or may lose antibody years after exposure.

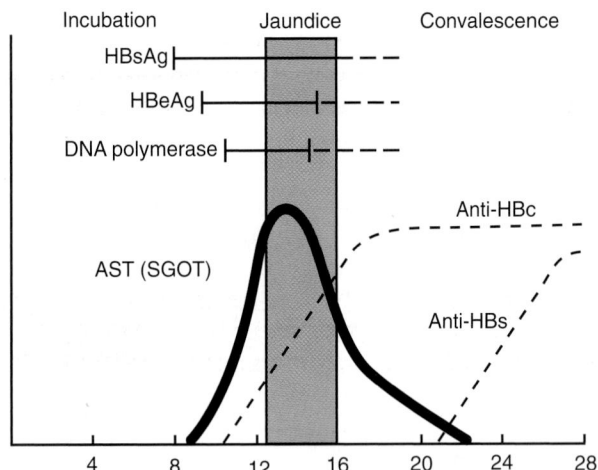

Figure 37-8 Course of acute type B hepatitis with recovery.
1, Onset of hepatitis with jaundice 3 months after exposure; *2,* detection of hepatitis B surface antigen (HBsAg) 2 to 8 weeks after exposure, followed by appearance of its antibody (anti-HBs) 2 to 4 weeks after HBsAg is no longer detectable; *3,* detection of hepatitis Be antigen (HBeAg) shortly after appearance of HBsAg disappears (this is usually followed by the appearance of antibody to HBeAg [anti-HBe], which persists); *4,* detection of hepatitis B core antibody (anti-HBc) at the time of onset of disease 2 to 3 months after exposure. Anti-HBc IgM will be detectable at high levels for 5 months. *(From Balistreri WF. Viral hepatitis: Unique aspects of infection during childhood. Consultant 1984;24:131-53.)*

Acute Alcoholic Hepatitis

Alcoholic liver disease is discussed more fully below under chronic hepatitis. Acute alcoholic hepatitis clinically is an acute febrile illness, characteristically associated with leukocytosis and increased concentrations of acute phase response proteins.[13-14] It also causes mild increases in cytosolic enzymes. For example, AST activity is typically more than two times that of ALT, and it is rare for AST activity to be more than eight times the upper reference limit. A cholestatic form of the disease, with increases in ALP activity to greater than three times the upper reference limit, is seen in up to 20% of cases, and is associated with higher mortality. Increases in bilirubin concentration are common, and reduced liver-synthesized protein concentrations are also commonly present. Increased bilirubin, decreased albumin, and prolonged PT are poor prognostic markers in alcoholic hepatitis. A discriminant function [4.6 × (PT-control PT) + plasma bilirubin (mg/dL)] value >32 indicates individuals with a high mortality rate.

Toxic Hepatitis

Toxic hepatitis refers to direct damage of hepatocytes by a toxin or toxic metabolite. Toxic reactions are usually predictable, and are directly related to the dose of the agent ingested. In North America and Europe, the most common cause of toxic hepatitis is acetaminophen (Figure 37-9)[9]. The first laboratory abnormality to appear is an increase in PT, followed by increased activities of cytosolic enzymes. Initially, LD activity is often increased to higher absolute amounts than AST, and AST tends to be higher than ALT. Peak activities (typically >100 times the upper reference limits) usually occur by 24 to 48 hours, followed by rapid clearance at rates approximating the known half-lives of the enzymes. PT elevations are typical and are >4 seconds above the control value in most cases. Prognosis is related most closely to the prolonged increase in PT. Persistent elevation of PT 4 days after ingestion is associated with a poor prognosis. Other markers of risk include development of acute renal failure or lactic acidosis with pH <7.30.

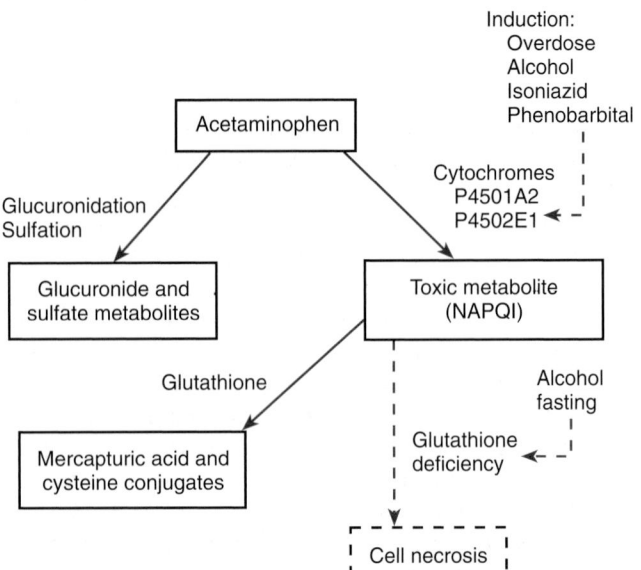

Figure 37-9 Metabolism of acetaminophen by the liver.

Ischemic Hepatitis ("Shock Liver")

Hepatic hypoperfusion (ischemic hepatitis) is one of the most common causes of elevated cytosolic enzymes in hospital patients. It is the cause of the majority of cases of acute liver injury identified clinically. Elevations of bilirubin concentration typically are minimal and usually peak several days after enzyme activities are highest. Laboratory findings are similar to those in toxic hepatitis (including having high LDH), and acute renal failure is a common complicating factor.

Other Causes of Acute Hepatitis

Drug-induced liver injury (DILI) occurs by a number of mechanisms, but the most common is idiosyncratic, immune-mediated injury to hepatocytes, characterized by elevations in the activities of ALT or AST. Cholestatic hepatitis, with increased aminotransferases and ALP, is more common in drug-induced hepatitis than with other causes of acute hepatitis. DILI is becoming more commonly recognized as a cause of acute liver injury. Approximately 60% of cases cause severe acute hepatitis with jaundice, and fatalities occur. Serious reactions are more common in individuals who are continued on the medication. In about one third of cases, liver injury becomes chronic following cessation of the drug.

Some disorders that eventually produce chronic hepatitis may occasionally present in an acute fashion. AIH (see later discussion) has an acute component in up to 40% of cases; it differs from other forms in having (1) decreased albumin, (2) increased globulins, and (3) a more protracted increase in aminotransferases. Wilson disease may also present as an acute hepatitis, often associated with fulminant hepatic failure. The classic biochemical findings of Wilson disease are often absent, and high urine copper is common to all forms of acute hepatitis. A number of additional features that may suggest the diagnosis include (1) hemolytic anemia, (2) acute tubular necrosis, (3) minimally elevated (usually <10×) AST activity, which typically remains higher than ALT activity, and (4) very low ALP activity with a ratio of ALP (in IU/L) to bilirubin (in mg/dL) of <2.

Follow-Up of Acute Hepatitis

The most important tests in determining extent of injury are tests of liver function, especially prolonged PT. In acute viral or alcoholic hepatitis, PT more than 15 seconds is associated with a poor prognosis, whereas persistent elevation more than 4 days after acetaminophen ingestion indicates high risk for liver failure. Other markers of synthetic function, such as transthyretin, or markers of hepatocyte regeneration, such as alpha-fetoprotein, have also been found to predict prognosis. With both hepatitis B and C, serological tests (loss of HBsAg or HCV RNA) are the most reliable way to determine resolution of infection.

Chronic Hepatitis

Chronic hepatitis is characterized by continuing inflammatory damage to hepatocytes (lasting more than 6 months), often accompanied by hepatocyte regeneration and scarring.[5]

The common causes of chronic hepatitis and the tests used to make a specific etiological diagnosis are listed in Table 37-3. Most patients are asymptomatic, but nonspecific features, such as (1) fatigue, (2) lack of concentration, and (3) weakness may be present. Despite this relatively mild clinical picture, gradual scarring of the liver may occur, leading to cirrhosis. After 20 years of chronic viral hepatitis, 20% to 30% of individuals have developed cirrhosis, and ultimately this number increases to 50% developing cirrhosis. Most cases of chronic hepatitis are diagnosed because of increased activities of the aminotransferases (typically 1 to 5 times upper reference limits) or detection of positive tests for a cause of chronic hepatitis. Aminotransferases may sometimes be normal either intermittently or for a prolonged period in chronic hepatitis, especially with HCV and **nonalcoholic steatohepatitis (NASH)**. Characteristically, ALT activity is elevated to a greater degree than AST. Reversal of the AST:ALT ratio to >1 suggests coexisting alcohol abuse or development of cirrhosis. Results of most other tests are normal. The most common causes of chronic hepatitis are (1) chronic HBV, (2) chronic HCV, and (3) NASH, but a variety of other disease processes also cause chronic hepatitis.

Significance of Chronic Hepatitis

Fibrosis and necroinflammatory activity are the two major components of chronic hepatitis. The extent of fibrosis (stage) is strongly related to risk of progression to cirrhosis, whereas necroinflammatory activity (grade) is correlated with progression in some, but not all, studies. ALT activity is strongly correlated with necroinflammatory activity, but not with fibrosis. Fibrosis in the liver involves collagen. Proteoglycans, especially hyaluronate, are also part of scar formation.

Various combinations of (1) markers of cell injury (such as, AST, ALT, and GGT), (2) substances deposited in scar tissue (such as procollagen and hyaluronate), (3) inflammatory markers (such as, α_2-macroglobulin and haptoglobin), and (4) tests that are related to liver function (such, as bilirubin and platelet count) have been proposed to predict the degree

TABLE 37-3	Causes of Chronic Hepatitis and Diagnostic Strategies
Cause	**Diagnosis**
Hepatitis B	History, HBsAg, anti-HBs, anti-HBc, HBV DNA
Hepatitis C	Anti-HCV, HCV RNA by PCR
Autoimmune type 1	ANA, ASMA
Autoimmune type 2	SLA, anti-LKM$_1$
Wilson disease	Ceruloplasmin
Drugs	History
α_1-Antitrypsin deficiency	α_1-AT phenotype
Idiopathic	Liver biopsy, absence of markers

ANA, Antinuclear antibodies; *anti-HBs,* hepatitis B surface antigen; *anti-HBc,* hepatitis B core antigen antibody; *anti-HCV,* hepatitis C virus antibody; *anti-LKM$_1$,* liver kidney microsomal type 1 antibody; *ASMA,* anti-smooth muscle antibody; *AT,* antitrypsin; *DNA,* deoxyribonucleic acid; *HBsAg,* hepatitis B surface antigen; *HBV,* hepatitis B virus; *HCV,* hepatitis C virus; *PCR,* polymerase chain reaction; *RNA,* ribonucleic acid; *SLA;* smooth muscle antibody.

of fibrosis in the liver. There is, however, significant overlap in concentrations of markers in those with varying stages of fibrosis. Marker concentrations change with necroinflammatory activity and may reflect disease activity at the time of sampling, rather than cumulative fibrosis. Consequently, interest has focused more on identifying individuals with minimal fibrosis, who have little risk of progression to cirrhosis, or those likely to already have severe fibrosis or cirrhosis. The most commonly used predictive indices include the FIB4 (involving age, platelet count, and AST/ALT ratio), APRI (the ratio of AST activity to platelet count), and Fibrotest (a combination α_2-macroglobulin, apolipoprotein A_1, total bilirubin, GGT, and haptoglobin, along with age and sex).

Chronic Hepatitis B

Chronic HBV infection (identified by the persistence of HBsAg) exists in multiple forms, largely determined by the interaction between the virus and host immune response.[11] In persons infected early in life or with severe immune suppression, viral replication and circulating viral loads are high, but liver damage is minimal. This has been referred to as the *immune tolerant phase of infection*. In others, the immune response to the high amounts of circulating virus causes damage to the liver, but is inadequate to clear the infection. This is termed the *immune active or chronic hepatitis phase*. In some patients, the immune response is adequate to clear circulating virus and prevent further liver damage, but not to clear the virus completely. In this immune control phase, individuals have no circulating HBV DNA but remain HBsAg positive. As mentioned earlier, those whose immune system "clears" HBsAg often continue to have low levels of circulating and hepatocyte viral DNA, and in this "occult" phase of infection no further liver damage occurs unless the immune system becomes suppressed.

Historically, the measurement of plasma HBeAg has been used as a test to clarify stages of viremia (presence of viruses in the blood). Subsequently, it was recognized that persons who are HBeAg negative may have any of the four phases of HBV infection (while those who are HBeAg positive typically are only in the immune tolerant or immune active phases). In HBeAg positive persons, about 3% to 5% will convert to HBeAg negative status each year; this **seroconversion** is often associated with a worsening of liver injury, sometimes accompanied by jaundice that clinically mimics acute hepatitis. After the conversion, patients are typically in the immune control phase. A small percentage of patients (about 0.5% to 1% per year) will convert from one of the first three phases to the "occult" phase, again often associated with a flare up of liver injury before conversion to occult infection.

A variety of agents are used to treat chronic HBV, and are used in persons with positive HBV DNA, particularly if they also have elevated activities of ALT or significant liver injury on biopsy. The primary goals of treatment is (1) suppression of viral replication, detected first by a decrease in HBV DNA (preferably to undetectable), and (2) improvement in degree of liver injury, detected by normalization of ALT activity.

These two goals are achieved in a high percentage of those treated with the most active agents available currently. Treatment is continued indefinitely except in the minority (about 30% in the first year, fewer in subsequent years) of those who were HBeAg positive before treatment and who clear HBeAg and develop anti-HBe. HBsAg rarely becomes undetectable. With the most active agents (entecavir, tenofovir), resistance rarely occurs as long as the patient continues to take the drug regularly.

Chronic Hepatitis C

Chronic HCV is defined by the persistent presence of HCV RNA for more than 6 months, accompanied in most patients by chronically or intermittently elevated ALT activity and chronic liver injury. The genotype of the patient is typically determined before patients are treated, as there are differences in treatment duration and agents, as well as likelihood of response, based on the genotype of the HCV infecting the person. The genotypes and subgenotypes used to categorize patients with chronic Hepatitis C are listed in Box 37-1. Genotype 1 is the most common type of Hepatitis C genotype in the United States and responds the least well to two drug treatment and requires 48 weeks of therapy. Individuals with genotypes 2 and 3 are almost three times more likely than individuals with genotype 1 to respond to therapy with alpha interferon or the combination of alpha interferon and ribavirin. They require only 24 weeks of therapy. Genotpye 4 responds well to two drug treatment given for 48 weeks. Genotype 1, the most commonly encountered form, responds the least well to two drug treatment and requires 48 weeks of therapy.

Treatment of patients with chronic HCV typically uses a combination of pegylated (polyethylene glycol [PEG]) interferon plus ribavirin. In patients infected with genotype 1, addition of a protease inhibitor produces rates of response similar to those in the other genotypes.[6] Currently, protease inhibitors cannot be used by themselves because of the very high likelihood of resistance developing. Combinations of protease inhibitors with other direct acting anti-viral agents has shown promise in early clinical trials, and future treatments may not require the use of interferon (which causes many of the complications of therapy). Treatment of HCV is often successful in permanently eradicating circulating virus.

Table 37-4 summarizes terms used for interpreting response to treatment of HCV with different agents. They include (1) rapid virologic response (RVR), (2) early virological response

BOX 37-1   Genotypes of Chronic Hepatitis C
Genotype 1a
Genotype 1b
Genotype 2a, 2b, 2c, 2d
Genotype 3a, 3b, 3c, 3d, 3e, 3f
Genotype 4a, 4b, 4c, 4d, 4e, 4f, 4g, 4h, 4i, 4j
Genotype 5a
Genotype 6a

(EVR), and (3) sustained virological response (SVR). An important consideration in monitoring treatment with HCV RNA is the detection limit used; because of the frequency of resistance, any residual virus (with detection limits of 10 to 15 IU/mL) indicates the need for longer treatment duration. In those achieving SVR, long-term control of HCV RNA replication occurs in 99% of patients, and histologic and clinical resolution of chronic hepatitis occurs in most. A number of factors influence response to treatment. The most important is genotype, as mentioned earlier. Persons who (1) are obese, (2) have excess iron in their liver, or (3) have significant scarring (especially those with cirrhosis) have lower rates of response to treatment. Response rates are lower in those of African or Hispanic ancestry. Genome-wide association studies have found a marker near the gene for IL-28b (which codes for a form of interferon) that is associated with response to interferon treatment. Those having the favourable CC genotype have approximately two times the response rate to interferon as those having CT or TT genotype, and at least half of the

racial difference in response is related to frequency of the favourable genotype in those of different ancestry.[8]

Nonalcoholic Fatty Liver Disease and Nonalcoholic Steatohepatitis

Nonalcoholic fatty liver disease (NAFLD) and NASH refers to a disease entity associated with fat and inflammation in the liver in persons with minimal to no alcohol intake. It is most commonly observed in association with (1) diabetes, (2) obesity, and/or (3) dyslipidemia (high triglycerides, low high-density lipoprotein [HDL]-cholesterol). There is increasing recognition that fat accumulation in the liver without inflammation is also commonly found in individuals with obesity and diabetes, and those with other components of the metabolic syndrome. The more encompassing term, nonalcoholic fatty liver disease, has been introduced to include this latter form and NASH. The frequency of NAFLD is high in North America and Europe; it has been estimated that NAFLD occurs in 30% of the population and NASH in 2% to 3%.[3] Thus, NASH is as

TABLE 37-4 Tests for Evaluating Chronic Hepatitis C Infection and Its Treatment

Time of Testing	Test	Condition	Use/Interpretation
Pretreatment	HCV viral load	Detectable	To confirm current infection; as a baseline (to compare to 4-week and 12-week value)
	Genotype	2 or 3 vs. other	Length of treatment (24-week genotype 2 or 3, 48-week if other genotype), use of additional protease inhibitor (genotype 1)
4 weeks on treatment	HCV viral load*	a) Undetectable b) <1 log drop c) >1000 IU/mL	a) RVR—with PR or TPR, high likelihood of response to shorter duration treatment b) With BPR, longer treatment c) With TPR, discontinue treatment
8 weeks on treatment (used only for BPR)		a) Undetectable b) >100 IU/mL	a) Possible shorter treatment depending on patient characteristics b) Nonresponder, discontinue therapy
12 weeks on treatment	HCV viral load*	a) Undetectable b) <2 log drop c) >1000 IU/mL d) >100 IU/mL >2 log drop	a) With TPR or BPR, may use shorter treatment depending on patient characteristics (for TPR, termed extended RVR; with PR, termed EVR) b) Stop treatment (nonresponder)† c) With TPR, discontinue treatment d) With BPR, discontinue treatment Continue treatment (on treatment responder)
24 weeks on treatment‡	Sensitive HCV RNA§	a) Detectable b) Not detectable	a) Stop treatment (nonresponder) b) Continue treatment (if genotype 2/3, treatment completed; with TPR or BPR, may discontinue treatment if eRVR depending on patient characteristics)
End of treatment	Sensitive HCV RNA§	a) Detectable b) Not detectable	a) Nonresponder b) Treatment responder
24 weeks after completion	Sensitive HCV RNA¶¶	a) Detectable b) Not detectable	a) Relapser b) SVR

*With PR, detection limit <50 IU/mL; with TPR or BPR, detection limit <10 to 15 IU/mL.
†Less than 3% chance of SVR; some continue treatment to 24 weeks and reevaluate.
‡With genotype 2/3, considered end of treatment.
§With PR, qualitative or quantitative assay with lower detection limit <50 IU/mL; with BPR or TPR, quantitative assay with detection limit <10 to 15 IU/mL.
¶¶Either qualitative or quantitative HCV RNA with detection limit <50 IU/mL.
BPR, Boceprevir/pegylated interferon/ribavirin (times are from start of PR, boceprevir introduced after week 4); *EVR,* early virologic response; *HCV,* hepatitis C; *PR,* pegylated interferon/ribavirin; *RNA,* ribonucleic acid; *RVR,* rapid virologic response; *SVR,* sustained virologic response; *TPR,* telaprevir/pegylated interferon/ribavirin.

common as chronic HCV. NASH has progressed to cirrhosis in 15% of cases in the small number of published prospective studies, although likelihood of progression seems much lower in those with only NAFLD. Laboratory diagnosis of NASH and NAFLD is not currently possible. The clinical features are similar to those of other causes of chronic hepatitis. To date, the major treatment has been weight loss, which is often associated with decreased ALT values.

Autoimmune Hepatitis

Autoimmune hepatitis (AIH) represents a rapidly progressing form of chronic hepatitis (up to 40% 6-month mortality in untreated individuals) associated with the presence of autoimmune markers and substantial hypergammaglobulinemia.[12] It most commonly occurs in young to middle-aged women. The most important antibodies for diagnosis include (1) antinuclear antibody (ANA), (2) antismooth muscle antibody (ASMA, now often tested for as anti-actin), and (3) anti-liver-kidney microsomal antigen type 1 (LKM_1). A summary of (1) the most common autoantibodies, (2) their associations, and (3) their molecular targets (when known) is given in Table 37-5. Immunosuppressive treatment using prednisone, alone or in combination with azathioprine, is effective in inducing a clinical remission of disease in about 80% of cases.

Drug-Induced Liver Diseases

As discussed earlier, most cases of drug-induced liver disease present as acute hepatitis. Less commonly, drugs have produced a chronic liver injury, in a pattern mimicking chronic hepatitis or other chronic liver injury (chronic cholestasis and hepatic granulomas). The most common drugs linked to chronic hepatitis are (1) nitrofurantoin, (2) methyldopa, and (3) HMG-CoA reductase inhibitors. Herbal medications also have been linked to chronic hepatitis. Establishing drugs as the cause of chronic hepatitis is often difficult as temporal relationships to drug ingestion are not as definitive as with acute hepatitis. Reactions are first seen in those who have been taking the medication for many months. Most chronic drug reactions resolve when the drug is discontinued.

Inherited Liver Diseases Presenting as Chronic Hepatitis

Inherited liver diseases that present as chronic hepatitis include (1) hemochromatosis (discussed in Chapter 28), (2) alpha$_1$-antitrypsin (AAT) deficiency (discussed in Chapter 18), and (3) Wilson disease (discussed in Chapters 18 and 32).

Alcoholic Liver Disease

Alcoholic liver disease[13] differs clinically and biochemically from other forms of hepatitis and liver disease. It is a common cause of liver disease in the developed world. The incidence of acute alcoholic hepatitis, however, seems to be declining in North America and Europe. Risk factors for developing alcoholic liver disease include (1) duration and magnitude of alcohol abuse (rare if intake <40 g/day in men and 10 g/day in women), (2) sex (women may be more likely to develop cirrhosis), (3) presence of co-infection with HBV or HCV (both of which increase risk of cirrhosis), and (4) nutritional state (poor nutrition increases risk of cirrhosis). In addition, there is evidence for an immunological component in alcoholic liver disease, and there is evidence that modification of liver proteins by ethanol metabolites is involved in the pathogenesis. Compared with other causes of chronic hepatitis, alcoholic hepatitis is less likely to have increased activities of AST or ALT, and more likely to have activities of AST higher than those of ALT. The prognosis of chronic alcoholic liver disease

TABLE 37-5   Serological Markers of Autoimmune Liver Disease

Antibody Name	Antigen Target	Associations
Antiactin	Actin	AIH type 1; more specific than ASMA, poor response to corticosteroids, early age onset
Antiasialoglycoprotein receptor (ASGPR)	Transmembrane antigen binding protein	AIH, correlate with activity, disappear with successful treatment
Anti-LKM$_1$	Cytochrome P450 IID6	AIH type 2; seen in only 4% of US cases; usually in children
Antiliver specific cytosol (LC$_1$)	Enzyme (possibly formimino-transferase cyclodeaminase or argininosuccinate lyase)	AIH in younger patients, often with anti-LKM$_1$, PSC; vary with activity of disease
Antimitochondrial antibody (AMA M2 type)	Dihydrolipoamide acyltransferase	PBC
Antineutrophil cytoplasmic antibodies (ANCA)	Bactericidal/permeability protein, cathepsin G, lactoferrin	PSC (50%-70%), ulcerative colitis (50%-70%), AIH; nonspecific
Antinuclear antibody (ANA)	Multiple targets (centromere, ribonucleoproteins); may not be detected by ELISA	AIH type 1, some PSC cases
ASMA	Actin, tubulin, vimentin, desmin, Skelitin	AIH type 1, seen in other autoimmune diseases in lower titers
Antisoluble liver antigen/liver pancreas (SLA)	Selenocysteine pathway protein serine hydroxymethyltransferase)	AIH type 3; very specific for AIH, correlate with relapse after corticosteroid withdrawal

AIH, Autoimmune hepatitis; *anti-LKM$_1$*, anti-liver kidney microsome; *ASMA*, antismooth muscle antibody; *ELISA*, enzyme-linked immunosorbent assay; *PBC*, primary biliary cirrhosis; *PSC*, primary sclerosing cholangitis.

is thought to be similar to that of other causes of chronic hepatitis. The primary treatment is abstinence from alcohol.

Cirrhosis

Cirrhosis, defined anatomically as diffuse fibrosis with nodular regeneration, represents the end stage of scar formation and regeneration in chronic liver injury. The common causes of chronic hepatitis that lead to cirrhosis and their therapies (which may prevent or, in some cases, reverse cirrhosis) are listed in Table 37-3. Virtually all chronic liver diseases are known to lead to cirrhosis, but most cases of cirrhosis occur as a result of chronic hepatitis.

In the early stages of transition from chronic hepatitis to cirrhosis, termed compensated cirrhosis, there may be no signs or symptoms of liver damage. Laboratory abnormalities usually appear before clinical findings begin to develop. The latter include (1) ascites, (2) gynecomastia, (3) palmar erythema, and (4) portal hypertension. The earliest laboratory abnormalities are (1) fall in platelet count, (2) increase in PT, (3) decrease in the albumin to globulin concentration ratio to <1, and (4) increase in the AST/ALT activity ratio to >1. Survival in those with compensated cirrhosis is good; in one large study, 10-year survival rate was 90%. As cirrhosis progresses, decompensation (loss of functionality) occurs with clinical evidence of portal hypertension. Once decompensation occurs, 10-year survival is only about 20%. Currently, prognosis in cirrhosis is usually based on the Model for End-Stage Liver Disease (MELD) score,[7] which is calculated as:

$$
\begin{aligned}
\text{MELD score} = \\
3.8 + \ln \text{bilirubin (mg/dL)} \\
+ 11.2 \ln \text{INR} \\
+ 9.6 \ln \text{creatinine (mg/dL)} \\
+ 6.4 \times \text{etiology score (0 if alcohol or obstruction 1,} \\
\text{for all other causes)}
\end{aligned}
$$

Risk of death over 3 months is low in those with MELD scores below 10, intermediate in those with scores of 10 to 20, and high in those with scores above 20.[7] MELD scores are the primary means used to assign priority for liver transplantation.

Laboratory findings in cirrhosis reflect ongoing liver injury and decreased hepatic function. Activities of aminotransferases are variable in cirrhosis, and reflect underlying necroinflammatory activity. If the cause of cirrhosis has been eliminated (as by abstinence from ethanol or successful treatment of viral hepatitis), aminotransferase activity is often within the reference interval. Persistence of elevation is a risk factor for development of HCC. Increases in alpha fetoprotein (AFP) are common in cirrhotic patients, even in the absence of HCC.

Cholestatic Liver Diseases

Cholestasis (stoppage or suppression of the flow of bile) is associated with retention of bile within the excretory system. The term *obstruction* is often used inappropriately, since cholestasis also occurs without mechanical obstruction to the biliary tract. Although intrahepatic cholestasis may be due to either functional or mechanical problems, extrahepatic cholestasis is always due to physical obstruction of the bile ducts by processes, such as (1) gallstones in the bile ducts (choledocholithiasis), (2) narrowing (strictures), and (3) tumors, both primary in the bile ducts (cholangiocarcinoma) or head of the pancreas, or involving the lymph nodes adjacent to the bile ducts. The major cholestatic diseases are (1) physical obstruction of the bile ducts, (2) primary biliary cirrhosis PBC[10], and (3) **primary sclerosing cholangitis (PSC)**.[4] Cholestatic hepatitis, which has been discussed previously, may also cause cholestasis, but generally presents in a manner closer to hepatitis.

Prolonged cholestasis may lead to bile acid deficiency, causing malabsorption of fat and the fat-soluble vitamins A, D, E, and K (see Chapter 27). Accumulation of normal bile contents leads to jaundice and development of an abnormal lipoprotein-X, containing (1) phospholipids, (2) cholesterol, (3) fragments of cell membrane (along with ALP), and (4) albumin. Lipoprotein-X will be included in low-density lipoprotein (LDL) cholesterol in the Friedewald formula (see Chapter 23) and in most direct LDL cholesterol methods.

Laboratory indicators of cholestasis include an increase in plasma activities of canalicular enzymes, such as ALP and GGT. In general, there is a short lag period between the onset of cholestasis and the increase in plasma activities. In the early stages of mechanical obstruction (especially from gallstones), there may be transient increases in plasma activities of liver cytosolic enzymes, such as AST and ALT, which may exceed 400 IU/L and, in 1% to 2% of cases, may be over 2000 IU/L. Even with continued obstruction, AST and ALT activity gradually decrease, and AST is typically within the reference interval within 8 to 10 days. Increases in total bilirubin, with predominance of conjugated bilirubin, reflect extent of obstruction, and are seen with both extrahepatic or intrahepatic cholestasis. Prolonged PT is the most commonly detected coagulation abnormality. It usually is corrected by administration of parenteral vitamin K. Transient increases in the quantity of Cancer Antigen 19-9 (CA 19-9) occur with bile duct obstruction. This is an important consideration, as CA 19-9 is often used as a diagnostic test for pancreatic and bile duct carcinomas. A key feature of extrahepatic obstruction is dilation of more proximal and intrahepatic bile ducts, which are visualized by imaging studies.

Primary Biliary Cirrhosis

Primary biliary cirrhosis (PBC), or nonsuppurative destructive cholangitis, is an uncommon autoimmune disorder targeting intrahepatic bile ducts primarily in middle-aged women (6:1 female to male ratio, median age at onset 50 years). There is an association with human leukocyte antigen (HLA) class II antigen DR8, and up to 80% of cases are associated with other autoimmune processes, most commonly **Sjögren syndrome** and hypothyroidism (which often develop before onset of PBC). At least 95% of patients have antimitochondrial antibodies that react against the dihydrolipoamide acyltransferase component of the pyruvate decarboxylase complex. Part of this complex is found on the apical surface of biliary epithelial cells, suggesting a role for this antigen as an immune target.

PBC typically presents as an asymptomatic elevation of ALP, but may occur with cholestasis or fatigue. Aminotransferase activities are increased in 50% of cases, but are more than twice the upper reference limit in only 20% of cases. An increased concentration of bilirubin is a late finding and is important in predicting decompensation. PBC progresses slowly in most patients and ultimately leads to portal hypertension, and increases risk of development of HCC.

Primary Sclerosing Cholangitis

PSC is a chronic inflammatory disease of the biliary tree, most commonly affecting extrahepatic bile ducts. Involvement of intrahepatic ducts, either with extrahepatic involvement or as an isolated finding, is also possible. In contrast to PBC, PSC has a male predominance and a younger median age at onset of 30 years. In 80% of patients, PSC is associated with ulcerative colitis, which usually (but not always) precedes onset of PSC. An autoimmune component is likely, as 97% of patients with PSC have one or more plasma autoantibodies present in their plasma. *Antineutrophil cytoplasmic antibodies* (ANCA), usually with an atypical perinuclear pattern, are present in approximately 50% to 80% of patients, but are not specific for PSC; they are also present in PBC and autoimmune hepatitis. Antigens include (1) lactoferrin, (2) bactericidal/permeability increasing protein, and (3) cathepsin G.

The clinical presentation of PSC, like that of PBC, is typically an asymptomatic patient with elevated activities of ALP found during routine laboratory screening. Symptoms are ultimately present in most patients with PSC; the most common are (1) pruritus, (2) intermittent abdominal pain, but (3) fever may also occur. The major cause of death in individuals with PSC is cholangiocarcinoma, which ultimately develops in up to one third of patients.

Drug-Induced Cholestasis

Drugs are a common cause of cholestasis, causing about 15% of cases. Drug reactions are especially common in older individuals, where up to 50% of individuals have increased enzyme activities because of medications. Drugs cause a cholestatic picture by two major mechanisms. In some cases, only conjugated bilirubin is increased, whereas the activities of canalicular enzymes are not elevated.[11] This condition is often seen with estrogen and anabolic steroids. More commonly, drugs induce a cholestatic hepatitis.

Gallstones

Gallstones are solid formations in the gallbladder that are composed of cholesterol and bile salts. Although they vary in chemical composition, they generally contain a mixture of (1) cholesterol, (2) bilirubin, (3) calcium, and (4) mucoproteins. In the United States, 70% to 85% of all gallstones are predominantly cholesterol and more than 10% of the adult population is affected.

Hepatic Tumors

The liver is host to a wide variety of both benign and malignant primary tumors. It is also the second most common site of metastases, which account for 90% to 95% of all hepatic malignancies. While primary tumors may arise from many cell lines in the liver, the most important primary liver tumor is HCC.

HCC is the fifth most common cancer worldwide and a leading cause of cancer death. Historically, approximately 75% of HCC cases occurred in Asia, but the falling prevalence of cases due to HBV in Asia and the increase in cases in Europe and North America due to HCV and NASH cirrhosis are changing this percentage. The incidence is twofold to threefold higher among men than it is among women. Although cirrhosis is present in most patients with HCC, it is absent in about 25% to 30% of cases, often in association with HBV. The major risk factor for development of HCC is infection with HBV or HCV, but any cause of chronic hepatitis and cirrhosis appears equally likely to cause HCC.

Clinical features of HCC usually do not occur until late in the course of disease, when the tumor is large and resection is impossible. Nonspecific signs and symptoms, such as (1) fever, (2) malaise, (3) anorexia, and (4) anemia are common, and (5) jaundice may occur with central tumors that obstruct biliary drainage. In a small number of cases, paraneoplastic features, such as (1) hypoglycemia, (2) hypercalcemia (due to parathyroid hormone–related peptide [PTHrP] production), or (3) erythrocytosis (due to erythropoietin production), may be the initial presenting findings. Laboratory findings include those of cirrhosis and cholestasis, and (except for tumor markers discussed later) are nonspecific.

Because treatment is usually not possible with advanced HCC, there has been much interest in screening high-risk individuals.[2] Smaller tumors detected by screening may be treatable by (1) resection of part of the liver, (2) local/regional treatment (most frequently radiofrequency ablation [RFA] and/or transarterial chemoembolization [TACE]), or (3) liver transplantation in some cases. The most common screening programs use plasma tumor markers and/or imaging studies. The most widely used tumor marker is AFP; recently, the more specific L3 isoform has also been used. *Des-gammacarboxy prothrombin* (DCP, also called *PIVKA-II*) appears a more sensitive and specific marker of HCC than AFP but is not widely used. Elevation of AFP (and less frequently DCP) is also common in individuals with cirrhosis, the group at highest risk for HCC. In the author's experience, AFP above the upper reference limit has a positive predictive value of only 16% for HCC. Use of higher cutoff values than the upper reference limit improves clinical specificity of total AFP at the expense of clinical sensitivity.

Diagnostic Strategy

Liver function and integrity tests are useful in (1) detecting, (2) diagnosing, (3) evaluating severity, (4) monitoring therapy, and (5) assessing the prognosis of liver disease and dysfunction (Table 37-6).

By using a combination of the tests listed in Table 37-6, it is possible to categorize broad types of liver disease, which then are more accurately diagnosed through disease-specific tests. An algorithm for that process is presented in Figure 37-10.

TABLE 37-6	Tests of Hepatic Function
Test	**Utility**
Bilirubin	Diagnosing jaundice, modest correlation with severity
ALP	Diagnosing cholestasis and space-occupying lesions
Bilirubin fractionation	Diagnosing disorders of metabolism and disorders of the newborn
AST	Sensitive test of hepatocellular disease; AST > ALT in alcoholic disease, cirrhosis
ALT	Sensitive and more specific test of hepatocellular disease
Albumin	Indicator of chronicity and severity
PT	Indicator of severity, early indicator of cirrhosis in chronic hepatitis

ALP, Alkaline phosphatase; *ALT,* alanine aminotransferase; *AST,* aspartate aminotransferase; *PT,* prothrombin time.

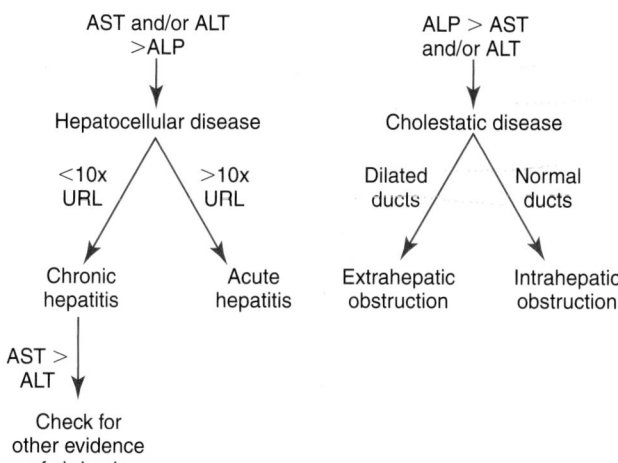

Figure 37-10 Algorithm for using abnormal liver function tests to classify and diagnose various types of liver disease. *ALP,* Alkaline phosphatase; *AST,* aspartate aminotransferase; *URL,* upper reference limit.

Plasma Enzymes

In practice, serum activities of AST, ALT, and ALP are the most useful tests because they allow differentiation of hepatocellular disease from cholestatic disease. Timely differentiation is important because failure to recognize cholestatic disease caused by extrahepatic biliary obstruction will result in liver failure if the obstruction is not quickly corrected. It also is important to recognize that there may be a gray zone of mixed hepatocellular and cholestatic disease where the tests do not distinguish one disease from the other. In this case, it is wise to assume that the problem is cholestatic and to rule out biliary obstruction.

Patients are occasionally seen with isolated elevations in ALP or aminotransferase enzyme activities. In practice, an isolated increase in ALP activity is difficult to interpret. In children, *benign transient hyperphosphatasemia* should always be considered, and it is important to use age-appropriate reference intervals because bone growth causes ALP values to be as much as several times the upper reference limit for adults. In adults, it is necessary to first confirm that the ALP is of hepatobiliary origin. This has been done by isoenzyme fractionation or by measuring another canalicular enzyme (such as, GGT), which should be normal if ALP increases are not of liver origin. The most important aspect of the work-up is to rule out space-occupying lesions by visualizing the liver and biliary tract with various imaging techniques.

Elevated plasma activities of AST and ALT are common in many disorders. The liver is the likely source of elevation if ALT activity is greater than that of AST. If AST activity is greater than that of ALT, other evidence to suggest liver as the origin would include abnormalities in liver function (albumin, PT, bilirubin) and increased ALP activity. If the values for all of these related tests are within their reference intervals in an individual with an AST activity greater than that of ALT, it is reasonable to measure creatine kinase (CK) activity to assure that muscle injury is not the cause. If liver is determined to be the source, administration of all potentially hepatotoxic drugs and alcohol intake (especially if AST is higher than ALT) should be discontinued. If the elevation persists, ultrasound (looking for nonalcoholic fatty liver) and hepatitis B and C serology should be performed. More than 90% of isolated enzyme elevations of liver origin will be caused by these disorders. A liver biopsy is often needed to make a more specific diagnosis, as well as to determine extent of damage. There is no reliable test other than a liver biopsy to detect fibrosis, although there is promise that laboratory tests may at least help to exclude serious fibrosis.

Serum Albumin

Serum albumin measurements are useful in assessing the chronicity and severity of liver disease. For example, the serum albumin concentration is decreased in chronic liver disease. However, its utility for this purpose is somewhat limited, as the serum albumin concentration is also decreased in (1) severe acute liver disease, as well as in (2) inflammatory disorders and (3) malnutrition, and with (4) nephrotic syndrome. Serial measurements of serum albumin also are used to assess the severity of liver disease.

Prothrombin Time

Serial PT measurements are used to determine synthetic liver function. They are thought to be more reliable than the measurement of the concentration of albumin because fewer conditions (other than warfarin administration) affect PT than affect albumin. PT is the most important prognostic marker in acute liver disease and is usually the first function test to become abnormal as chronic hepatitis evolves into cirrhosis. PT is also one of the parameters used in calculating the MELD score, which is used to predict need for transplantation in cirrhosis.

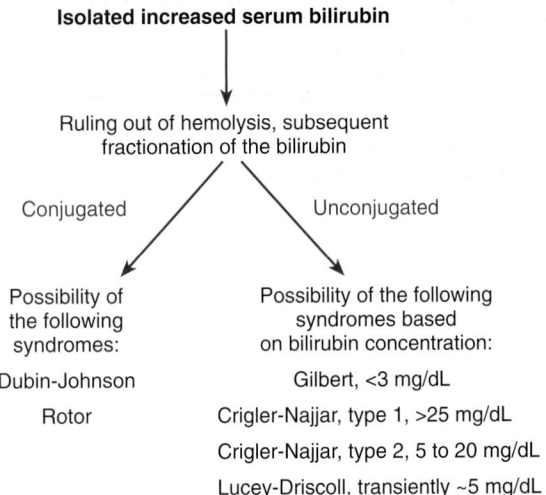

Isolated increased serum bilirubin

Ruling out of hemolysis, subsequent
fractionation of the bilirubin

Conjugated   Unconjugated

Possibility of   Possibility of the following
the following   syndromes based
syndromes: on bilirubin concentration:

Dubin-Johnson   Gilbert, <3 mg/dL

Rotor   Crigler-Najjar, type 1, >25 mg/dL

Crigler-Najjar, type 2, 5 to 20 mg/dL

Lucey-Driscoll, transiently ~5 mg/dL

Figure 37-11 Algorithm for differentiating the familial causes of
hyperbilirubinemia.

Plasma Bilirubin

Serial measurement of bilirubin is helpful in measuring the
severity of acute and chronic liver disease.

Patients are occasionally seen with isolated elevations in
their bilirubin concentration. In most cases, this is due to
inherited disorders of bilirubin metabolism, or hemolysis. It
is not difficult to distinguish hemolysis severe enough to cause
hyperbilirubinemia, because the patient with hemolysis will
have anemia and may have other disease manifestations. An
algorithm for differentiating the familial causes of hyperbilirubinemia is presented in Figure 37-11.

Review Questions

1. In the liver, bilirubin is conjugated to:
   a. vinyl groups.
   b. methyl groups.
   c. hydroxyl groups.
   d. glucuronide.
2. Functions of the liver include the synthesis of all of the
   following *except*:
   a. albumin.
   b. immunoglobulins.
   c. glycogen.
   d. coagulation factors.
3. In the liver, the small grooves between adjacent hepatocytes that carry bile to the gall bladder are the:
   a. cords.
   b. canaliculi.
   c. lobules.
   d. sinusoids.
4. Hepatocellular carcinoma (HCC) can be directly related to:
   a. an acute viral hepatitis infection.
   b. cholestasis.
   c. a chronic hepatitis B infection.
   d. the synthetic function of the liver.

5. Which type of viral hepatitis is usually spread parenterally by transfusion, shared needles, or dialysis and is
   considered the most common chronic viral infection in
   North America?
   a. Hepatitis B
   b. Hepatitis C
   c. Hepatitis A
   d. Cirrhosis
6. Laboratory tests that are initially run to determine the
   presence of any liver disease include:
   a. liver enzymes only.
   b. viral antigens and antibodies, serum cholesterol.
   c. hepatitis antigens and antibodies, coagulation times,
      and serum proteins.
   d. bilirubin, liver enzymes, prothrombin time (PT), and
      albumin.
7. Blockage of the bile ducts or blockage of bile flow from
   within the liver due to inflammation will stop normal bile
   flow. This is referred to as:
   a. hepatitis.
   b. hepatocellular carcinoma (HCC).
   c. cholestasis.
   d. cirrhosis.
8. A genetic disorder that is associated with elevated
   amounts of copper in the liver and other tissues and leads
   to decreased ceruloplasmin concentration in blood is:
   a. Wilson disease.
   b. Reye syndrome.
   c. cholestasis.
   d. autoimmune hepatitis.
9. A woman visits her physician with symptoms of jaundice,
   hepatic pain, and chalky-appearing stools. Lab values
   indicate elevated conjugated bilirubin, alkaline phosphatase (ALP) and γ–glutamyltransferase (GGT). These
   findings are most likely due to:
   a. hemolytic anemia.
   b. ineffective erythropoiesis.
   c. cholestasis due to gallstones.
   d. Reye syndrome.
10. The type of portal hypertension seen in the majority of
    cases is sinusoidal hypertension, which is most com-
    monly caused by:
    a. blockage of the portal veins.
    b. hepatic vein occlusion.
    c. congestive heart failure.
    d. cirrhosis.

References

1. Arroyo V, Fernandez J, Ginès P. Pathogenesis and treatment of hepatorenal syndrome. Semin Liver Dis 2008;28:81–95.
2. Bruix J, Sherman M. Management of hepatocellular carcinoma: an
   update. Hepatology 2011;53:1020–2.
3. Chalasani N, Younossi Z, Lavine JE, et al. The diagnosis and management
   of non-alcoholic fatty liver disease: practice guideline by the American Association for the Study of Liver Diseases, American College of
   Gastroenterology, and the American Gastroenterological Association.
   Hepatology 2012;55:2005–23.

4. Chapman R, Fevery J, Kalloo A, et al. Diagnosis and management of primary sclerosing cholangitis. Hepatology 2010;51:660–78.

5. Ghany M, Strader D, Thomas D, Seeff L. Diagnosis, management, and treatment of hepatitis C: an update. Hepatology 2009;49:1335–74.

6. Ghany MG, Nelson DR, Strader DB, Thomas DL, Seeff LB. An update on treatment of genotype 1 chronic hepatitis C virus infection: 2011 practice guideline by the American Association for the Study of Liver Diseases. Hepatology 2011;54:1433–44.

7. Kamath P, Wiesner R, Malinchoc M, et al. A model to predict survival in patients with end-stage liver disease. Hepatology 2001;33:464–70.

8. Lai M, Afdhal NH. Clinical utility of interleukin-28B testing in patients with genotype 1. Hepatology 2012;56:367–72.

9. Lee W. Acetaminophen-related acute liver failure in the United States. Hepatology Research 2008;38:S3–S8.

10. Lindor KD, Gershwin ME, Poupon R, Kaplan M, Bergasa NV, Heathcote EJ. Primary biliary cirrhosis. Hepatology 2009;50:291–308.

11. Lok A, McMahon B. Chronic hepatitis B. Hepatology 2007;45:507–39.

12. Manns M, Czaja A, Gorham J, et al. Diagnosis and management of auto-immune hepatitis. Hepatology 2010;51:2193–213.

13. McCullough AJ, O'Shea RS, Dasarathy S. Diagnosis and management of alcoholic liver disease. J Dig Dis 2011;12(4):257–62.

14. O'Shea RS, Dasarathy S, McCullough AJ, et al. Alcoholic liver disease. Hepatology 2010;51:307–28.

15. Zimmerman H. Hepatotoxicology: The adverse effects of drugs and other chemicals on the liver. 2nd edition. Philadelphia: JB Lippincott; 1999.

38   Gastrointestinal and Pancreatic Diseases

Peter G. Hill, Ph.D., F.R.C.Path.

Objectives

1. Define the following:

   Diarrhea
   Digestive process
   Disaccharidase
   Gastritis
   Inflammatory bowel
   disease (IBD)
   Lactose intolerance

   Malabsorption
   Maldigestion
   Pancreatitis
   Protein-losing enteropathy
   Steatorrhea
   Zollinger-Ellison syndrome

2. List the components of the gastrointestinal (GI) tract and state the function of each component.
3. Outline the three phases of the digestive process including the specific events and peptide hormones involved during each phase.
4. List five hormones/regulatory peptides synthesized by the intestinal tract.
5. State the function of cholecystokinin (CCK), gastrin, secretin, vasoactive intestinal polypeptide, and glucose-dependent insulinotropic peptide (GIP).
6. List and describe three diseases of the stomach; list possible causes of each disease.
7. State the involvement of *Helicobacter pylori* in peptic ulcer disease and gastric cancer.
8. List four invasive tests and four noninvasive tests used to diagnose the presence of *H. pylori*.
9. Describe urea breath testing and its use in analysis of peptic ulcer disease.
10. State the cause of Zollinger-Ellison syndrome; list and describe two laboratory tests used to diagnose this syndrome, including special specimen requirements and handling.
11. Describe celiac disease, including possible causes; define a laboratory test used to diagnose this disease.
12. Compare congenital and acquired lactase deficiency.
13. Describe the oral lactose tolerance test.
14. Outline the protocol for noninvasive breath-hydrogen testing for lactase deficiency; state how results are interpreted.
15. State how bacterial overgrowth in the intestine leads to fat malabsorption.
16. Describe inflammatory bowel disease (IBD); compare IBD to irritable bowel syndrome (IBS).
17. List two hormones, three enzymes, and one regulatory peptide synthesized in the pancreas.
18. State the functions of amylase, lipase, insulin, and somatostatin.
19. Define *pancreatic insufficiency.*
20. List the most common autosomal recessive disease involving the pancreas, and state one diagnostic test for this disorder in children over the age of 2 weeks.
21. List three adult disorders of the exocrine pancreas; list causes of acute and chronic pancreatitis.
22. List three invasive and two noninvasive tests of pancreatic exocrine function; discuss the issues involved with the two types of testing.
23. Describe a GI neuroendocrine tumor, and list five of them.
24. State the use of the fecal osmolal gap in testing for diarrhea; calculate the formula used to determine fecal osmotic gap (FOG).

Key Words and Definitions

Acute pancreatitis An acute episode of enzymatic destruction of the pancreatic substance due to the escape of active pancreatic enzymes into the pancreatic tissue.

Breath tests Tests that detect products of bacterial metabolism in the gut or products of human metabolism by measuring, most commonly, CO_2 and H_2 in the breath.

Celiac disease A disease caused by the destructive interaction of gluten with the intestinal mucosa causing malabsorption. In most cases, the mucosal damage is reversed by withdrawing all gluten-containing foods from the diet. Also called *gluten-sensitive enteropathy.*

Cholecystokinin (CCK) A 33–amino-acid peptide secreted by the upper intestinal mucosa and also found in the central nervous system. It causes gallbladder contraction and release of pancreatic exocrine (or digestive) enzymes, and affects other gastrointestinal (GI) functions.

Chronic pancreatitis An inflammatory disease characterized by persistent and progressive destruction of the pancreas.

Key Words and Definitions—cont'd

Chyme Food that has been acted upon by the churning action of the stomach and by stomach juices and expelled by the stomach into the duodenum.

Crohn disease A chronic inflammatory disease that may affect any part of the intestine from the mouth to the anus.

Cystic fibrosis (CF) An inherited disease caused by genetic alteration of a cystic fibrosis transmembrane conductance regulator (CFTR) protein that leads to chronic pancreatic and obstructive pulmonary disease.

Diarrhea The passage of loose or liquid stools more than three times daily and/or a stool weight greater than 200 g/day.

Digestion The conversion of food, in the stomach and intestines, into soluble and diffusible products, capable of being absorbed.

Digestive process A three-phase process—neurogenic, gastric, and intestinal. The neurogenic (vagal) phase is initiated by the sight, smell, and taste of food. The gastric phase is initiated by the distention of the stomach by the entry of food. The intestinal phase begins when the partly digested food enters the duodenum from the stomach.

Dumping syndrome Following gastric surgery, hyperosmolar chyme is "dumped" into the small intestine causing rapid hypovolemia and hemoconcentration.

Gastrin A group of peptide hormones secreted by gastrointestinal (GI) mucosa cells in response to mechanical stress or high pH, both of which are produced by the presence of food in the stomach. Gastrin stimulates the stomach parietal cells to produce hydrochloric acid (HCl).

Gastrinoma A tumor of the pancreatic islet cells that results in an overproduction of gastric acid, leading to fulminant ulceration of the esophagus, stomach, duodenum, and jejunum. Gastrinomas may also occur in the stomach, duodenum, spleen, and regional lymph nodes.

Gastritis Mucosal inflammation of the stomach.

Glucose-dependent insulinotropic peptide (GIP, gastric inhibitory polypeptide) A peptide hormone (42 amino acids) that stimulates insulin release and at supraphysiological concentrations inhibits the release of gastric acid and pepsin.

Helicobacter pylori A bacterium found in the mucous layer of the stomach. All strains secrete (1) proteins that cause inflammation of the mucosa and (2) the enzyme urease that produces ammonia from urea; some strains produce toxins that injure the gastric cells.

Lactose intolerance A condition due to lactase deficiency leading to malabsorption of lactose and causing symptoms of flatulence, abdominal discomfort, bloating, or diarrhea after ingesting milk or foods containing lactose.

Malabsorption An abnormality in the absorption of nutrients.

Maldigestion An abnormality of the digestive process due to dysfunction of the pancreas or small intestine.

Peptic ulcer disease The collective name given to duodenal and gastric ulceration.

Postgastrectomy syndrome A syndrome following surgery for peptic ulcer disease that includes the dumping syndrome, diarrhea, maldigestion, weight loss, anemia, bone disease, and gastric cancer.

Secretin A peptide hormone of the gastrointestinal (GI) tract (27 amino acids) found in the mucosal cells of the duodenum. Among its multiple functions, secretin increases water and bicarbonate secretion to buffer the incoming protons of the acidic chyme. It has considerable homology with GIP, vasoactive intestinal polypeptide (VIP), and glucagon.

Sprue A chronic form of malabsorption syndrome occurring in tropical and nontropical forms.

Steatorrhea A condition of excessive fat in feces (more than 5 g/day).

Ulcerative colitis Recurrent inflammatory disease of the large bowel that involves the rectum and spreads to involve a variable amount of colon. Ulcerative colitis, like Crohn disease, is a form of inflammatory bowel disease (IBD).

Vasoactive intestinal polypeptide (VIP) A peptide of 28 amino acids found in the central and peripheral nervous systems where it acts as a neurotransmitter. It is located in the enteric nerves in the gut. It relaxes smooth muscle in the gut and increases water and electrolyte secretion from the gut.

Zollinger-Ellison (Z-E) syndrome A condition resulting from a gastrin-producing tumor (gastrinoma) that results in an overproduction of gastric acid, leading to ulceration of the esophagus, stomach, duodenum, and jejunum, and causing hypergastrinemia, diarrhea, and steatorrhea.

Efficient **digestion** of food and absorption of nutrients are the result of coordinated functions that occur in the gastrointestinal (GI) tract. Coordination and regulation of these functions depend on hormones that stimulate or inhibit secretion of fluids containing hydrochloric acid (HCl), bile acids, bicarbonate, and digestive enzymes.

Anatomy

The GI tract is an 8-meter-long tube beginning with the mouth and ending with the anus. The esophagus, which is about 25 cm in length, is a muscular tube connecting the pharynx to the stomach. The major organs of the GI tract include the (1) stomach, (2) small and large intestines, (3) pancreas, and (4) gallbladder, all of which are involved in the digestive processes that commence with the ingestion of food and water and culminate in the excretion of feces.

Stomach

The stomach consists of three major zones: the cardiac zone, the body, and the pyloric zone (Figure 38-1). The upper cardiac zone, which includes the fundus, contains mucus-secreting

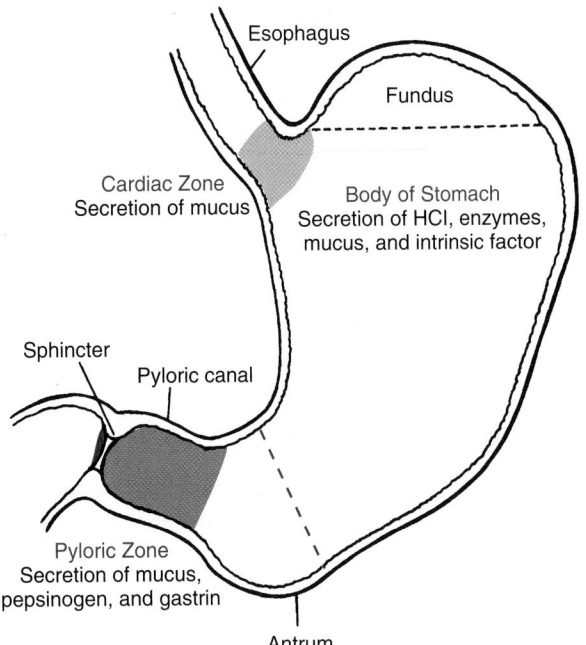

Figure 38-1 Schematic drawing of the stomach with major zones.

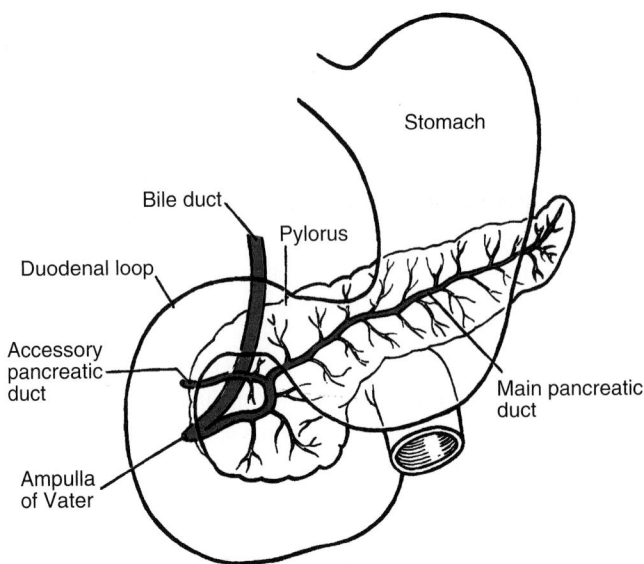

Figure 38-2 Cross-section through the pancreas.

surface epithelial cells and several types of endocrine secreting cells. The body of the stomach contains cells of many different types, including mucus-secreting cells and parietal (oxyntic) cells, which secrete HCl and intrinsic factor. Cells in all three zones of the stomach produce pepsinogens, the precursors of the enzyme pepsin that degrades proteins in the food. The pyloric zone is subdivided into the antrum (the distal third of the stomach), the pyloric canal, and the sphincter. The cells of the pyloric zone secrete mucus, pepsinogens, serotonin, **gastrin**, and several other hormones but no HCl.

Small Intestine

Food is converted in the stomach into a homogeneous, gruel-like material (**chyme**) that passes through the pyloric sphincter into the small intestine, which consists of three parts: the duodenum, jejunum, and ileum. In the adult human, the small intestine is approximately 6 m long and decreases in cross-section as it proceeds distally. The duodenum (about 25 cm long) is the shortest and widest part of the small intestine. The jejunum and ileum make up the remainder of the small intestine.

The internal surface of the upper small intestine contains valvelike circular folds projecting 3 to 10 mm into the lumen of the intestine. Very small (1 mm) fingerlike projections (villi) cover the entire internal surface of the small intestine, giving it a "velvety" appearance. The absorptive surface area of the small intestine is about 250 m², comparable to the area of a doubles tennis court.

Large Intestine

The large intestine is approximately 1.5 m long and includes the cecum, appendix, colon, rectum, and anal canal.

Pancreas

The pancreas is 12 to 15 cm in length and lies across the posterior wall of the abdominal cavity. The head is located in the

duodenal curve; the body and tail are directed toward the left (Figure 38-2).

The Digestive Process

The neurogenic, gastric, and intestinal phases constitute the **digestive process**. The neurogenic (vagal) phase is initiated by the (1) sight, (2) smell, and (3) taste of food. These all stimulate the cerebral cortex and subsequently the vagal nuclei and result in secretion of pepsinogen, HCl, and gastrin. The process is chemically mediated by acetylcholine from postganglionic parasympathetic nerve endings, which act on gastric parietal cells. The vagus also stimulates gastric chief and parietal cells to secrete pepsinogen and HCl. Hydrogen ion secretion takes place against a 1 million-fold concentration gradient, an energy-dependent process catalyzed by H⁺, K⁺-ATPase; it is mediated by acetylcholine, histamine, and gastrin acting through their respective neurocrine, paracrine, and endocrine pathways to stimulate the parietal cells.

The parietal cell is transformed morphologically when acid secretion is stimulated. Cimetidine (Tagamet) and other H₂-receptor antagonists (such as ranitidine [Zantac] and famotidine [Pepcid]) block both the morphological transformation of the parietal cell and H⁺ secretion. Proton pump inhibitors (PPIs) have a different mechanism of action. Omeprazole (a PPI) is taken up by the parietal cell and converted to an active metabolite that inactivates the parietal H⁺, K⁺-ATPase, inhibiting hydrogen ion secretion until new ATPase is synthesized—a process that requires at least 24 hours.

The distention caused by food entry into the stomach initiates the gastric phase of digestion. HCl release is caused by (1) direct stimulation of the parietal cells by the vagus nerve; (2) local distention of the antrum and stimulation of antral cells by the vagus nerve to secrete gastrin, which in turn causes HCl release from parietal cells; and (3) release of gastrin, stimulated by the near neutralization (pH 5 to 7) of gastric

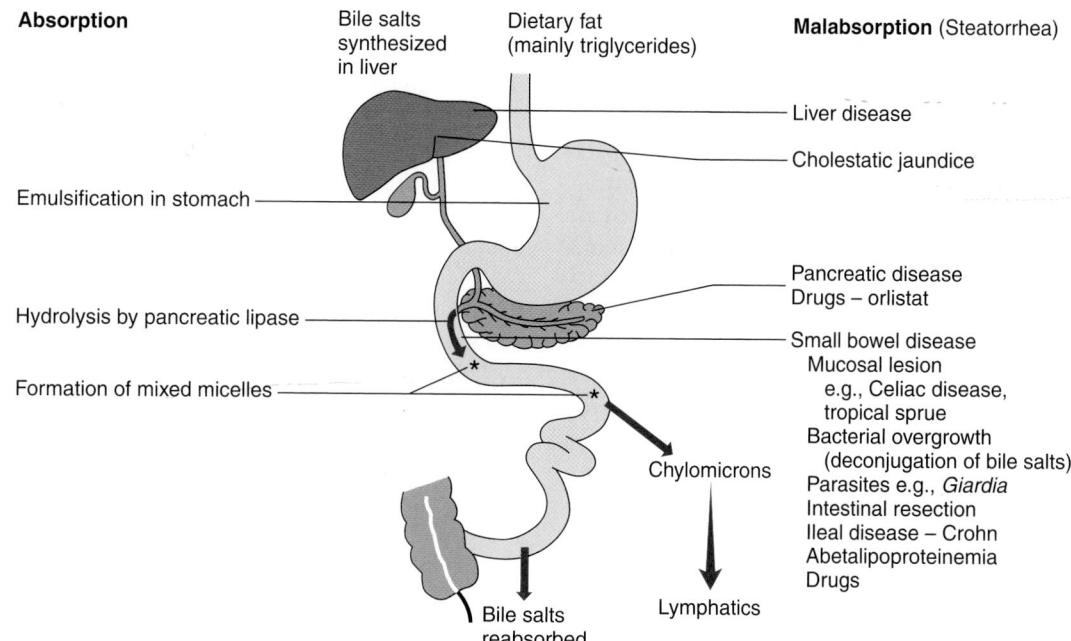

Figure 38-3 Summary of the processes involved in fat absorption and malabsorption. *(From Clark ML, Silk DB. Gastrointestinal disease. In: Kumar P, Clark M, eds. Clinical medicine, 6th edition. Edinburgh: WB Saunders, 2005:265-345.)*

HCl by ingested food entering the pyloric zone. Gastrin also stimulates (1) antral motility, (2) the secretion of pepsinogens and pancreatic fluid rich in enzymes, and (3) the release of GI hormones, such as **secretin**, insulin, acetylcholine, somatostatin, and pancreatic polypeptide (PP). As a result of the acidic environment, pepsinogens are converted rapidly to the active proteolytic enzyme, pepsin. As food enters the stomach, it is mixed by the contractions of the stomach. Chemical secretions of the stomach then partially degrade the food into a mucus-containing mixture called *chyme,* which then is moved through the pylorus into the duodenum. The pylorus plays a role in emptying food into the duodenum by virtue of its strong musculature.

The intestinal phase of digestion begins when the weakly acidic digestive products of proteins and lipids (Figure 38-3) enter the duodenum. Several GI hormones, including gastrin, are released by both neural and local stimulation and act on various regions of the GI tract to regulate digestion and absorption. In addition, the action of gastrin is potentiated by the secretion of **cholecystokinin (CCK).** Additional gastrin is released as the upper duodenal mucosa comes in contact with partially digested proteins and lipids and gastric HCl. CCK is released in the duodenum in response to the presence of fat, protein, and HCl. Its principal actions are stimulation of gallbladder contraction; secretion of enzymes, bicarbonate, insulin, and glucagon from the pancreas; and stimulation of intestinal motility and stomach contraction.

Secretin is released by gastric acid in the duodenum and (1) augments the effect of CCK on gallbladder contraction and pancreatic secretions, (2) stimulates pepsinogen secretion by the stomach, (3) inhibits gastrin and gastric

acid secretion, and (4) reduces gastric and duodenal motility. Gastric inhibitory polypeptide (GIP) is secreted by the duodenum and jejunum. It reduces intestinal motility and increases insulin secretion in the presence of hyperglycemia. **Vasoactive intestinal polypeptide (VIP),** present throughout the gut and in nerve fibers, is a potent vasodilator and aids in the relaxation of smooth muscle. It has a large number of physiological actions, some of which are shared with secretin and GIP. Somatostatin is secreted to inhibit most GI secretory and motor functions, thus preventing excessive reactions.

Pancreatic digestive enzymes, in a bicarbonate-rich juice, enter the duodenum through the ampulla of Vater and sphincter of Oddi (see Figure 38-2) and mix with the food bolus in the duodenum. During passage through the small intestine, carbohydrates are broken down by amylase and saccharidases into monosaccharides, which then are absorbed actively into the bloodstream. Protein is degraded further in the duodenum by trypsin, chymotrypsin, and carboxypeptidase from the pancreas and aminopeptidases from the small intestine. The resulting dipeptides and amino acids are absorbed in the jejunum and ileum by specialized absorptive mechanisms in the mucosal surface. Dietary fats are emulsified in the duodenum by the action of bile. They are hydrolyzed by lipase (aided by colipase) to individual fatty acids, monoacylglycerols (monoglycerides), and glycerol and then are absorbed in the remainder of the small intestine. Most nutrients, including vitamins and minerals, have been absorbed by the time the food passes into the large intestine, where water is absorbed actively, electrolyte balance is regulated, and bacterial actions take place. These processes end ultimately in the formation of feces.

Gut largest endocrine organ

Gastrointestinal Regulatory Peptides[13]

The gut is the largest endocrine organ in the body and also a major target for many hormones, released locally and from other sites. GI regulatory peptides are released from the pancreatic islets (e.g., somatostatin) or from endocrine cells within the gut mucosa (e.g., CCK). Many of these peptides (such as, VIP and somatostatin) are present in the enteric nerves and are also found in the central nervous system and have important roles in the neuroendocrine control of the gut. Although many of them (such as, secretin and gastrin) fulfill the classic criteria for a hormone by acting on distant cells (see Chapter 25), others function as neurotransmitters or have local (paracrine) effects on adjacent cells. Collectively, they influence motility, secretion, digestion, and absorption in the gut. They regulate bile flow and secretion of pancreatic hormones and affect tonicity of vascular walls, blood pressure, and cardiac output.

There is a growing understanding of the role of the neuroendocrine system and gut peptides, and of the importance of the gut-hypothalamic pathway, in the normal control of food intake, and of the possibility of disorders in these mechanisms as causes of obesity. The gastric peptide ghrelin and CCK act as short-term regulators of appetite and satiety. The neuropeptide $PYY_{(3-36)}$ is secreted by endocrine cells in the distal small intestine and colon in response to the ingestion of food. Infusion of $PYY_{(3-36)}$ to physiological plasma concentrations in humans significantly decreases appetite with a 33% reduction in food intake over 24 hours. $PYY_{(3-36)}$ is therefore a further addition to a growing list of hormones with a role in the regulation of energy balance.

Table 38-1 summarizes basic chemical characteristics of five of the major GI regulatory peptides and indicates their site of origin and major functions.

Cholecystokinin   *regulate appetite*

Cholecystokinin (CCK) is a linear polypeptide that exists in multiple molecular forms. In all of them, the five C-terminal amino acids are identical to those of gastrin and are necessary, together with a sulfated tyrosyl residue, for physiological activity. All of the forms of CCK are produced by enzymatic cleavage of a single 115–amino acid precursor, preprocholecystokinin.

CCK is found in the cells of the upper small intestinal mucosa. Circulating concentrations of CCK are increased following ingestion of a mixed meal. CCK secretion is stimulated by mixtures of polypeptides and amino acids (especially tryptophan and phenylalanine), but not by undigested protein. Secretion is also stimulated by gastric acid entering the duodenum and by fatty acids with chains of nine or more carbons, especially in the form of micelles. CCK is rapidly cleared from plasma (half-life of less than 3 min), predominantly by the kidneys. Secretion of CCK is completely inhibited after somatostatin infusion.

CCK regulates gallbladder contraction and increases small intestinal motility. Because it has the same terminal pentapeptide as gastrin, it has a mild stimulatory effect on (1) gastric HCl and pepsinogen secretion, (2) antral motility, and (3) pancreatic bicarbonate secretion. Gastrin and CCK are additive in their stimulation of the pancreas, and both increase the effect of secretin on pancreatic function. CCK also (1) stimulates pancreatic growth, (2) relaxes the sphincter of Oddi, and (3) stimulates secretions from Brunner (duodenal) glands.

TABLE 38-1	Characteristics of Prominent Forms of Principal Gut Regulatory Peptides			
Hormone/Peptide	Molecular Weight (Da)	Number of Amino Acids	Main Gut Localization	Principal Physiological Actions
Gastrin Family				
CCK	3918	33 (also 385, 59)	Duodenum and jejunum Enteric nerves	Stimulates gallbladder contraction and intestinal motility; stimulates secretion of pancreatic enzymes, insulin, glucagon, and PPs; has a role in indicating satiety; the C-terminal 8–amino acid peptide CCK-8 retains full activity
Little gastrin	2098	17	Both forms of gastrin are found in the gastric antrum and duodenum	Gastrins stimulate the secretion of gastric acid, pepsinogen, intrinsic factor, and secretin; stimulate intestinal mucosal growth; increase gastric and intestinal motility
Big gastrin	3839	34		
Secretin-Glucagon Family				
Secretin	3056	27	Duodenum and jejunum	Stimulates pancreatic secretion of HCO_3, enzymes, and insulin; reduces gastric and duodenal motility, inhibits gastrin release and gastric acid secretion
VIP	3326	28	Enteric nerves	Relaxes smooth muscle of gut, blood, and genitourinary system; increases water and electrolyte secretion from pancreas and gut; releases hormones from pancreas, gut, and hypothalamus
GIP	4976	42	Duodenum and jejunum	Stimulates insulin release; reduces gastric and intestinal motility; increases fluid and electrolyte secretion from small intestine

CCK, Cholecystokinin; *GIP,* glucose-dependent insulinotropic peptide; *PP,* pancreatic polypeptide; *VIP,* vasoactive intestinal polypeptide.

CCK is widely distributed throughout both the central and peripheral nervous systems, with highest concentrations in the cerebral cortex; its function in the central nervous system is unclear. When released from the GI tract, it acts as a short-term, meal-related satiety signal, thus regulating appetite.

Gastrin

Gastrin also occurs in multiple molecular forms in blood and tissue; the most important of these are big gastrin (G-34), a linear polypeptide of 34 amino acids and little gastrin (G-17). The principal circulating form of gastrin is G-34 in healthy individuals and in patients with hypergastrinemia. All forms of gastrin originate from a single precursor, preprogastrin, a peptide consisting of 101 amino acids. The smallest peptide sequence of gastrin possessing biological activity is the carboxy-terminal tetrapeptide (G-4, tetrin). A synthetic penta-peptide (pentagastrin) has been used for stimulation of HCl secretion in gastric function testing.

Gastrin is produced and stored mainly by endocrine cells of the antral mucosa and to a lesser extent in the proximal duodenum and in cells of the pancreatic islets. After secretion, gastrin is transported by the blood through the liver to the parietal cells of the fundus of the stomach. There it stimulates the secretion of gastric acid. It also stimulates (1) secretion of gastric pepsinogens and intrinsic factor by the gastric mucosa, (2) release of secretin by the small intestinal mucosa, (3) secretion of pancreatic bicarbonate and enzymes and hepatic bile. It increases (1) gastric and intestinal motility, (2) mucosal growth, and (3) blood flow to the stomach. It is secreted in response to antral distension by meals, and by amino acids, peptides, and polypeptides from partially digested proteins in the stomach. Other stimuli of gastrin include alcohol, caffeine, insulin-induced hypoglycemia, ingestion or intravenous infusion of calcium, and vagal stimulation initiated by smelling, tasting, chewing, and swallowing food.

Maximal secretion of gastrin occurs at an antral pH of 5 to 7. At pH 2.5, secretion is reduced by about 80%; maximal suppression occurs at pH 1.0. Secretion is inhibited by the direct action of acid on the endocrine cells producing gastrin. This negative feedback safeguards against overacidification by any and all stimulants.

Secretin

Secretin is a linear polypeptide containing 27 amino acids and has structural similarities to several hormones, including glucagon, VIP, and GIP. The intact secretin molecule is required for biological activity, and in contrast to gastrin there is no minimum active fragment.

It is secreted by the mucosal granular S cells located in greatest concentration in the duodenum but present throughout the small intestine. It is released primarily on contact of the S cells with gastric HCl; however, as pancreatic juice flows into the duodenum, it neutralizes gastric acid and thereby removes one stimulus for its own secretion. Secretin is not released until the pH is lowered to at least 4.5. However a pH less than 4.5 normally occurs only in the first few centimeters of the duodenum, causing little increase in plasma secretin after a normal meal. Thus secretin release after exposure of S cells to HCl may not be an important physiological stimulus. However, plasma secretin concentrations that are too low to measure may stimulate the pancreas in the presence of physiological concentrations of CCK, which strongly potentiates the action of secretin. Undigested fat does not stimulate secretin release, but fatty acids with chains of ten or more carbons are weak stimulants. Alcohol increases secretin release by stimulation of gastric acid secretion with subsequent lowering of duodenal pH rather than by a direct stimulatory effect. The half-life of secretin is about 4 minutes. The kidney is the major site of its degradation. The only known physiological inhibitor of secretin release is somatostatin.

The primary physiological role of secretin is the stimulation of the pancreas to secrete an increased volume of juice with high bicarbonate content. Other actions include (1) stimulation of bicarbonate and water secretion from the liver and from Brunner glands, (2) augmentation of gallbladder contraction and increased hepatic bile flow, (3) stimulation of parathyroid hormone (PTH) secretion, (4) release of pancreatic enzymes and of pepsinogen by the chief cells of the stomach, (5) reduction of gastric and duodenal motility, (6) reduction of the lower esophageal sphincter pressure, and (7) promotion of pancreatic growth. Secretin inhibits normal gastrin secretion (but does not decrease serum gastrin in the Zollinger-Ellison syndrome) and therefore gastric acid secretion.

Vasoactive Intestinal Polypeptide

Vasoactive intestinal polypeptide (VIP) is a linear polypeptide of 28 amino acids and has structural similarities to secretin, GIP, and glucagon. VIP is present throughout the body and is found in highest concentrations in the nervous system and gut. Unlike secretin and other GI hormones, VIP is not found in the mucosal endocrine cells of the GI tract. It is believed to be a neurotransmitter limited to peripheral and central nervous tissue. VIP-containing nerve fibers are found throughout the GI tract from the esophagus to the colon.

Little is known about the conditions that cause VIP to be released into the circulation. There is no evidence that VIP is released during digestion, but its secretion is increased by vagal stimulation. It has a plasma half-life of about 1 minute, and most of the hormone is inactivated by a single passage through the liver. It has a large number of physiological actions, which are summarized in Table 38-1. Most of the actions of VIP tend to be of short duration because of its rapid degradation.

Glucose-Dependent Insulinotropic Peptide (GIP, Gastric Inhibitory Polypeptide)

Glucose-dependent insulinotropic peptide (GIP) is a linear peptide consisting of 42 amino acids. Its N-terminal end has a close resemblance to glucagon and secretin, but the C-terminal amino acid sequence of 17 residues is not common to any other known intestinal hormone.

GIP is synthesized and released by cells located in the duodenal and jejunal mucosa. Plasma GIP is increased by oral administration of glucose or triacylglycerols or by intraduodenal infusions of solutions containing a mixture of amino acids.

Protein ingestion does not significantly increase GIP. For food components to stimulate GIP release, they must be absorbed by the intestinal mucosa.

The biological actions of GIP are summarized in Table 38-1. The insulinotropic action of GIP appears to be the most important of its biological actions, and as a result, this hormone has more recently been called "glucose-dependent insulinotropic peptide" as a more accurate description of its physiological action.

Other Regulatory Peptides

A large number of other GI regulatory peptides, hormones, and growth factors have now been shown to be localized within the gut although the function of some of these is still unclear. Growth factors belonging to several families of peptides have important roles in the control of a wide range of cell functions in the intestine. The current clinical use of GI hormones/regulatory peptide measurements is in the diagnosis of neuroendocrine tumors of the pancreas and GI tract. It is likely that they will have wider applications as understanding of their functions grow (e.g., in the fields of obesity and appetite modulation).

Stomach, Intestinal, and Pancreatic Diseases and Disorders

Diseases of the GI tract include those for the stomach, intestines, and pancreas.

Diseases of the Stomach

The growth in endoscopic procedures, with direct visualization of the interior of the stomach, has largely removed the need for the clinical laboratory to carry out the analysis of gastric contents. Situations remain, however, in which the laboratory continues to play a significant role in the diagnosis of gastric diseases and in monitoring the effectiveness of treatment. For example, the laboratory provides such services for peptic ulcer disease, the Zollinger-Ellison (Z-E) syndrome, and **gastritis**.

Peptic Ulcer Disease and *Helicobacter pylori*[12]
Description

Spiral-shaped organisms have been observed in the stomach for many years but it was only in 1985 that the association was made between *Helicobacter pylori* (known then as *Campylobacter pylori*) and **peptic ulcer disease**. Most estimates suggest that the bacterium is present in the mucous layer of the stomach in half of the population of the world. In Europe 30% to 50% of adults, and in the United States at least 20% of the adult population, are infected with the organism. Colonization with *H. pylori* causes a chronic inflammatory reaction in the gastric mucosa even when direct endoscopic observation appears normal. Carriers of the organism are at increased risk of gastric cancer (twofold to tenfold) and peptic ulcer (threefold to tenfold). About 90% of gastric cancer patients are infected with *H. pylori*, compared with 40% to 60% of age-matched controls and there is a significant correlation between infection rates and gastric cancer incidence and mortality. However, although a large proportion of gastric cancer can be attributed to infection with *H. pylori*, only in a minority of infected subjects will the inflammatory reaction progress to gastric cancer. Gastric cancer rates have declined in Western countries in recent decades but the incidence remains high in less developed countries.

At least 95% of patients with duodenal ulcer disease are infected with *H. pylori*, and eradication of *H. pylori* is the recommended treatment for patients with duodenal or gastric ulcer who are *H. pylori*–positive. Effective combined antibiotic and acid suppression regimens (using PPIs) are available with eradication rates of about 90%.

The reason for a gastric mucosal infection causing duodenal ulceration is complex but involves a number of pathways leading to increased acid production. Before the role of *H. pylori* in the development of peptic ulcer disease was understood, vagotomy (surgical sectioning, or cutting, of the vagus nerve) was the main form of treatment used to reduce gastric acid output, thereby leading to an environment more conducive to healing of the ulcer.

H. pylori produces urease, and hydrolysis of endogenous urea to bicarbonate and ammonia may create a more hospitable microenvironment for its survival in the stomach. The ability of the organism to rapidly hydrolyze urea is the basis of the urea **breath tests** and of the direct urease tests on gastric biopsy samples. Mammalian cells do not produce urease.

Diagnostic Tests for Helicobacter pylori
Tests for *H. pylori* (Box 38-1) are required for diagnosis of the infection and to ascertain, when symptoms continue, that eradication therapy has been successful. High clinical sensitivity is required to ensure that positives are not missed; similarly, high clinical specificity is essential to prevent inappropriate use of eradication therapy. The Maastricht III Consensus guidelines[12] recommend a "test and treat" strategy in adults with appropriate dyspeptic symptoms under the age of 45 years using either the breath test or stool antigen test. The age limit may vary depending on local prevalence and the age

---

BOX 38-1   **Diagnostic Tests for *Helicobacter pylori***

Invasive Tests—Using Gastric Mucosal Biopsy Samples
Histology: Microscopy after Giemsa or silver staining
Histology: Microscopy after immunohistochemical staining
Direct urease test: A biopsy incubated in urea/indicator solution; visual endpoint
Culture: Incubation on suitable media for 4 to 10 days
Polymerase chain reaction: Amplification of specific DNA sequences

Noninvasive Tests—Using Breath, Blood, Saliva, or Feces
Breath tests: Rise in breath $^{14}CO_2$ or $^{13}CO_2$ after ingestion of ^{14}C- or ^{13}C-labeled urea
Serum tests: Laboratory measurement of specific IgG antibody
Whole blood tests: Point-of-care tests for specific IgG antibody
Saliva tests: Detection of specific IgG antibody
Fecal tests: Detection of specific antigen

IgG, Immunoglobulin G.

distribution of gastric cancer. Successful eradication should be confirmed with the urea breath test or by a direct urease test when endoscopy is clinically indicated; a monoclonal antibody-based stool antigen test may be used if urea breath tests are not available. Currently the urea breath test is the preferred procedure, both for initial diagnosis and for confirmation of eradication. Testing to confirm eradication should be done at least 4 weeks after completion of the course of treatment. PPIs can lead to falsely negative urea breath test results. If PPIs cannot be withheld for at least 2 weeks before a breath test, a negative result must be interpreted with caution.

Urea breath tests are simple to perform, with sensitivity and specificity both greater than 95%. Urea labeled with either ^{14}C or ^{13}C is given orally as a drink or a capsule to swallow with water; urease from gastric *H. pylori* rapidly hydrolyzes the ingested urea to produce labeled bicarbonate, which is absorbed into the blood and exhaled as $^{14}CO_2$ or $^{13}CO_2$. The principal advantages of the stable isotope ^{13}C-urea breath test over the radioactive ^{14}C-urea breath test are the simplicity of breath collection and the avoidance of the regulations related to the use and disposal of radioisotopes. In the ^{13}C-urea breath test, the patient blows through a straw into an empty 15 mL tube, which is then capped. $^{13}CO_2/^{12}CO_2$ ratios are compared for basal and postdose samples using isotope ratio mass spectrometry or alternative infrared measurement methods.

In the stool test, specific *H. pylori* antigens are detected in microtiter plates coated with monoclonal antibodies. The test is currently recommended for posteradication testing if the urea breath test is not available.[12] Serological tests are recommended only in specific situations, e.g. when PPI therapy cannot be withheld or when a patient with a bleeding ulcer is investigated. Their diagnostic accuracy in subjects more than 50 years of age is unsatisfactory although laboratory-based tests generally perform well in younger people. Office-based serology has inadequate sensitivity and specificity and is not recommended.

Zollinger-Ellison Syndrome[1,2]

Description

The Zollinger-Ellison (Z-E) syndrome results from a tumor (**gastrinoma**) of the pancreatic islet cells. Its characteristics include (1) fulminant peptic ulcers, (2) massive gastric hypersecretion, (3) hypergastrinemia, (4) **diarrhea**, and (5) **steatorrhea**. The primary tumors classicaly occur in the pancreas, duodenum or intestinal lymph nodes, but also occur in other organs. About half of all gastrinomas are multiple, and about two thirds are malignant. One fourth of all gastrinomas occur in people with multiple endocrine neoplasia syndrome, type 1 (MEN 1), with associated tumors, or hyperplasia, in pancreatic islets and parathyroid and pituitary glands. In individuals with Z-E syndrome, fasting gastrin concentrations usually are increased substantially, ranging from 2 to 2000 times normal. Fasting plasma gastrin is usually greatly increased, also ranging from 2 to 2000 times normal. Concentrations more than 10 times the upper limit of normal, in the presence of gastric acid hypersecretion, are virtually diagnostic of gastrinoma. The fasting plasma gastrin concentration at presentation in

sporadic Z-E syndrome correlates with the size and site of the tumor and the presence of hepatic metastases and therefore has prognostic value.

Because management of the patient with Z-E syndrome usually requires surgical intervention, it is important to distinguish hypergastrinemia caused by gastrinoma from other conditions that may lead to similar increases in plasma gastrin. For example, increased concentration of plasma gastrin occurs in (1) hypochlorhydria or achlorhydria, (2) patients being treated with acid-suppressing drugs (e.g., histamine H_2-receptor antagonists or PPIs), (3) *H. pylori* infection, (4) pernicious anemia, and (5) patients with chronic atrophic gastritis associated with parietal cell antibodies. Surgical resection or diseases of the kidneys or small intestine also can cause hypergastrinemia, possibly because these are important sites of gastrin degradation or excretion.

Increased basal gastrin concentrations may be classified as "appropriate" or "inappropriate" according to their association with decreased or increased gastric acid secretion. For example, in patients with very low or absent acid secretion and a functionally intact gastric antrum, an increase in plasma gastrin is physiologically appropriate and is expected.

Measurement of Plasma Gastrin

In serum from healthy subjects, the predominant forms of gastrin are amidated G-34 and G-17. In subjects with gastrinomas, the circulating gastrins display unpredictable heterogeneity with a shift toward larger peptides. For the detection of gastrinomas, immunoassays are designed to detect all secreted forms of gastrin to prevent false negatives

Gastrin is unstable in serum or plasma, with up to 50% loss of immunoreactivity during 48 hours at 2 °C to 8 °C, due to the action of proteolytic enzymes. Blood samples should be collected into tubes containing heparin as anticoagulant and aprotinin (e.g., Trasylol, 0.2 mL, 2000 KIU, in a 10-mL tube) to prevent proteolysis. Samples should be mixed by inversion, transported rapidly on ice to the laboratory, and the plasma separated in a refrigerated centrifuge. The plasma should be frozen at - 20 °C within 15 minutes of venipuncture. Samples collected in this way are suitable for the analysis of gastrin, VIP, PP, somatostatin, neurotensin, and chromogranins A and B.

Determination of Basal Acid Output

The documentation of an increased basal acid output (BAO) in gastric juice provides strong evidence that a high serum gastrin concentration is caused by Z-E syndrome. The test is therefore used in patients with duodenal ulceration and a raised serum gastrin concentration. The test is not appropriate in patients with atrophic gastritis. Pernicious anemia, which also causes hypergastrinemia, should be excluded before assessing BAO. PPIs must be stopped for at least 14 days, and H_2-receptor antagonists for at least 3 days, before the test. *H. pylori* as a cause of increased serum gastrin should also be excluded before BAO estimation.

Typically, a 12-hour overnight collection of gastric juice is used to measure BAO. A satisfactory alternative is the collection of gastric juice for 60 minutes after the patient has had a satisfactory night's sleep in a quiet separate room. After waking, the patient must remain fasting; smoking and exercise must be avoided before and during the test. To collect a specimen, a gastric tube is inserted orally, or nasal intubation may be used if the patient has a hyperactive gag reflex. X-ray or fluoroscopic confirmation that the tip of the radiopaque tube is in the lowest portion of the stomach is necessary. Ten or 15 minutes after the patient has become calm and adjusted to the presence of the tube, the patient is positioned with the trunk upright and inclined slightly to the left. Gastric juice is then aspirated and discarded. The total volume of the collected juice is recorded and free acid determined by titration with sodium hydroxide to a pH end-point of 3.5.

BAO reference intervals are 0 to 10.5 mmol/hr for males and 0 to 5.6 mmol/hr for females. Patients with the Z-E syndrome have BAO values of 15 to 100 mmol/hr, or more than 5 mmol/hr if there was previous acid-reducing surgery. A free acid output more than 15 mmol/hr should prompt a suspicion of gastrinoma but is not diagnostic; a value more than 25 mmol/hr with high serum gastrin is virtually diagnostic of Z-E syndrome.

Gastritis

Gastritis is the term used to denote mucosal inflammation of the stomach. Different types of gastritis are classified as (1) erosive, (2) nonerosive, and (3) specific (very rare).

Erosive Gastritis

Erosive gastritis (acute gastritis) occurs in individuals after severe trauma or severe burns (Curling ulcer) and craniotomy or traumatic head injuries. It also is found in individuals with intracranial disease (Cushing ulcer) and in those who chronically ingest drugs, such as corticosteroids, ethanol, or aspirin or other nonsteroidal antiinflammatory drugs (NSAIDs). Endoscopy is usually the definitive technique to establish the diagnosis.

Nonerosive Gastritis

Nonerosive gastritis (chronic gastritis) is associated with peptic ulcer disease or gastric carcinoma, the period after partial gastrectomy, pernicious anemia, *H. pylori* infection, and healthy elderly individuals. Serum gastrin is increased in achlorhydric individuals because of the absence of negative feedback by HCl.

Diseases of the Intestine

Diseases of the intestine include (1) **celiac disease**, (2) disaccharidase deficiency, (3) bacterial overgrowth, (4) bile salt **malabsorption**, (5) inflammatory bowel disease (IBD), and (6) protein-losing enteropathy. The main laboratory tests associated with these diagnoses are described here.

Celiac Disease (Celiac Sprue, Gluten-Sensitive Enteropathy)[5,15]

Celiac disease is sometimes called *nontropical sprue, celiac sprue,* or *gluten-sensitive enteropathy.*

Description

Celiac disease is a lifelong autoimmune intestinal disorder that is found in individuals who are genetically susceptible.[6] The external trigger to its development in these individuals is found in gluten, which is a complex group of proteins present in wheat. All of the proteins (and peptides) that are toxic to the small bowel mucosa in subjects with celiac disease contain large amounts of glutamine. The major toxic proteins of wheat are the gliadins with homologous proteins (the hordeins and secalins) occurring in barley and rye, respectively. The gliadins account for about 50% of the wheat protein. The development of celiac disease is believed to be initiated by these toxic cereal proteins causing intestinal epithelial damage, which releases tissue transglutaminase (tTG).[3] Cross linking by the enzyme produces gliadin-gliadin or gliadin-enzyme complexes, which in genetically susceptible individuals produces an immune response by gut-derived T cells. The characteristic enteropathy is then induced by the release of interferon-γ and other proinflammatory cytokines.

A 33–amino acid peptide of gluten is probably the primary initiator of the inflammatory response. It is resistant to breakdown by all gastric, pancreatic, and intestinal brush-border membrane proteases, thus allowing it to reach the small intestine intact. After deamidation by tTG, it is a potent inducer of gut-derived human T-cell lines from patients with celiac disease.

There is a wide spectrum in the clinical presentation of celiac disease, with the majority of diagnoses made in adult life. Most adults have nonspecific symptoms, such as (1) abdominal pain, (2) fatigue, (3) weight loss, (4) osteoporosis, (5) short stature, and often (6) mild iron deficiency. In addition, there is a strong association with other autoimmune disease, especially with type 1 diabetes mellitus and autoimmune thyroid disease.

Tests for Celiac Disease

Serological tests played a significant role in raising awareness of the high prevalence of the disorder (1% in Caucasian populations). Appropriately standardized tests have high clinical sensitivity and specificity for diagnosis and for monitoring treatment compliance with a gluten-free diet.

Immunoglobulin A (IgA) antibodies are used to diagnose celiac disease. The measurement of tTG antibodies has several advantages over the older tests for endomesial antibodies (EMA), antireticulin antibodies (ARA) and antigliadin antiboides. A laboratory strategy based on tTG antibody testing as a first-line test has been described.[10] The tTG antibody test is now preferred for serological testing and for assessing dietary compliance of subjects on a gluten-free diet. The tTG test is a quantitative procedure; several reagent sets are now commercially available to measure IgA-class anti-tTG antibodies using human recombinant tTG or purified human enzyme as antigen ("second generation methods"). In patients with IgA deficiency, tests for IgG antibodies may be useful. Tests for antibodies against gliadin are rarely if ever indicated, but measurements of antibodies against *deamidated gliadin* have recently been shown to be useful for diagnosis.

For a definitive diagnosis, current guidelines require a jejunal biopsy with (1) the characteristic changes of villous atrophy, (2) increased intraepithelial lymphocytes, and (3) hyperplasia of the crypts. Wider use of serology has led to the recognition of more cases and to the development of the concept of the "celiac iceberg" to highlight the fact that many cases remain hidden if serology is restricted to those having classic signs of the disorder.

Subjects with selective IgA deficiency (IgA less than 0.05 g/L, incidence about 1:600) are at greater risk of celiac disease and small bowel biopsy should be considered in all IgA-deficient subjects with symptoms of celiac disease.

With the availability now of serological tests with high diagnostic accuracy, older tests used to investigate celiac disease should be abandoned. These include the xylose absorption test and tests of fat malabsorption. Tests of pancreatic function (e.g., fecal elastase) may be indicated in patients diagnosed with celiac disease who fail to respond to a gluten-free diet.

Disaccharidase Deficiencies

Brush-border disaccharidases are essential for carbohydrate absorption and a reduction in their activity has been known to result in carbohydrate malabsorption and intolerance. Carbohydrate malabsorption, however, does not always lead to clinical symptoms, but when symptoms occur such as (1) abdominal pain, (2) flatulence, and (3) diarrhea as a consequence of the malabsorption, the patient is described as having carbohydrate intolerance. **Lactose intolerance** is the single most common absorptive defect in adults with an incidence of 5% to 90% depending on the racial group.

Description

Lactase deficiency may be congenital or acquired. Sucrase-isomaltase and trehalase deficiencies also are disaccharidase deficiencies and affect carbohydrate absorption.

Congenital Lactase Deficiency. Intestinal lactase is essential in infancy, and congenital lactase deficiency is a very rare disorder in which lactase activities in the mucosa are low or undetectable at birth. Symptoms occur as soon as milk is taken; stools have a low pH and contain glucose produced by bacterial action on undigested lactose. A definitive diagnosis must be deferred until maturation of the lactase synthesis system has occurred.

Acquired Lactase Deficiency. Expression of the enzyme diminishes with age and by adulthood the concentrations of lactase activity are 10% or less of those seen in infancy. If symptoms of (1) flatulence, (2) abdominal discomfort, (3) bloating, or (4) diarrhea occur after consumption of one or two glasses of milk or of a large portion of ice cream or yogurt, lactose intolerance should be suspected.

Secondary lactose intolerance may occur as a result of reduced enzyme activity following diffuse intestinal damage from (1) infections (giardiasis, bacterial overgrowth, or viral gastroenteritis), (2) **ulcerative colitis**, (3) celiac disease, and (4) tropical **sprue**. This deficiency is usually reversible following recovery from the disorder.

Sucrase-Isomaltase and Trehalase Deficiencies. Sucrase-isomaltase deficiency usually presents clinically in infancy when sucrose and fruit are introduced in the diet, but also may present in adults. Deficiencies of both lactase and sucrase-isomaltase may occur secondary to other small bowel diseases (e.g., celiac disease, **Crohn disease**, or acute gastroenteritis). Trehalase deficiency is a rare disorder, except in Greenland, where it occurs in 8% of the population. It is manifested by diarrhea following the ingestion of mushrooms.

Malabsorption of Monosaccharides. Malabsorption of monosaccharides may cause intestinal symptoms similar to those attributed to **maldigestion** of disaccharides. For example, glucose-galactose malabsorption is inherited as an autosomal recessive trait. Symptoms occur in the affected neonate as soon as milk (lactose) is taken, but also follow ingestion of glucose- or galactose-containing foods. Symptoms caused by fructose malabsorption occur on ingestion of fruit. This dietary intolerance is a different disorder from hereditary fructose intolerance in which the hepatic enzyme aldolase is defective.

Diagnostic Tests for Lactase Deficiency

Many methods have been proposed for detecting lactase deficiency (Box 38-2).

Oral Lactose Tolerance Tests. Oral tolerance tests measure the increase in plasma glucose or galactose following the ingestion of lactose and are used to diagnose lactase deficiency. The usual dose of lactose is 50 g in 200 mL water, although lower doses should be used in children (2 g/kg, up to a maximum of 50 g). Multiple blood samples are collected over a 2-hour period, and the peak increment in glucose (or galactose) is noted.

Because of problems with the oral tolerance test, noninvasive breath-hydrogen testing (Box 38-3) is now the technique of choice for diagnosing lactase deficiency. This technique is based on hydrogen not being an end-product of mammalian metabolism and consequently breath hydrogen is derived from bacterial

---

BOX 38-2 Methods for Detecting Lactase Deficiency

Lactase in mucosal biopsy
Oral lactose tolerance
    Measure increase in plasma glucose
    Measure increase in plasma galactose
    Measure increase in breath H_2
    Measure increase in breath $^{13}CO_2$

BOX 38-3 Protocol for Lactose Tolerance Test with Measurement of Breath Hydrogen

Meal before 1900 hours (restriction on wheat and fiber), then fasting until test completed.
Brush teeth (night and morning) or use mouthwash.
Measure end-expiratory fasting breath H_2.
Give lactose solution (50 g in 180 mL water).
Rinse mouth with further 20 mL water and swallow.
Measure breath H_2 at 15, 30, 60, 90, and 120 min.
Test can be stopped early if H_2 increases more than 20 ppm above fasting concentration.

metabolism in the intestine. Following an oral dose of lactose, the disaccharide will normally be split into its constituent monosaccharides and absorbed. With lactase deficiency, unabsorbed disaccharide will pass into the large bowel and bacterial metabolism will produce hydrogen that is absorbed into the systemic circulation and exhaled in the breath. Breath hydrogen is then measured in end-expiratory breath using laboratory or hand-held direct-reading electrochemical hydrogen monitors.

In most patients with normal lactose absorption, breath hydrogen concentrations will remain at 2 to 5 µL/L (2 to 5 ppm) throughout the test. In lactose malabsorption, breath hydrogen is typically increased (30 to 100 µL/L, 30 to 100 ppm) at 60 to 120 minutes after lactose ingestion. In a few subjects, the large bowel bacteria do not produce hydrogen; in such patients a normal result does not exclude lactase deficiency. Very low hydrogen concentrations (fasting and throughout the test) may therefore indicate a false-negative result. Such false negatives can be confirmed by the failure to produce hydrogen at 45 to 180 minutes after ingestion of lactulose (10 g), which is a nonabsorbable disaccharide and therefore available for bacterial metabolism in the large bowel.

A positive breath hydrogen result following ingestion of lactose may also occur in glucose-galactose malabsorption, which also causes intestinal symptoms. When necessary, glucose-galactose malabsorption can be confirmed or excluded by a breath test in which 25 g each of glucose and galactose are substituted for 50 g lactose. An increase in breath hydrogen confirms the diagnosis.

Sucrose and Trehalose Tolerance Tests. Sucrase deficiency is investigated by using 50 g sucrose instead of lactose. An increase in breath hydrogen of more than 20 µL/L (>20 ppm) within 2 hours is diagnostic. It is rarely necessary to test for trehalase deficiency.

Bacterial Overgrowth

The duodenum and jejunum normally contain few bacteria. Most ingested bacteria do not survive the acidic environment of the stomach and therefore few live organisms normally enter the small bowel. The motility of the jejunum prevents fecal-type organisms from progressing up into the jejunum from the cecum. The ileum normally contains some fecal type of bacteria. Colonization of the upper small bowel is described as bacterial overgrowth and usually occurs as a consequence of other abnormalities (structural or motility disorders) of the small intestine (Box 38-4). Use of PPIs is associated with an increased risk of bacterial colonization.

The bacteria colonizing the small bowel (such as, *Escherichia coli* and *Bacteroides* species) deconjugate and dehydroxylate

---

BOX 38-4   Abnormalities of the Small Intestine Associated with Bacterial Overgrowth

Jejunal diverticuli
Crohn disease
Autonomic neuropathy
Scleroderma (systemic sclerosis)
Pseudo-obstruction
Postgastrectomy

---

bile salts, leading to conjugated bile salt deficiency, which causes fat malabsorption. Bacterial metabolism of vitamin B_{12} may also occur, leading to vitamin B_{12} deficiency. The clinical symptoms of bacterial overgrowth are (1) abdominal pain, (2) diarrhea, and (3) steatorrhea.

The diagnostic "gold standard" requires intubation with aspiration of jejunal contents and the demonstration of a bacterial count of >10^7 organisms/mL and >10^4 anaerobes/mL. In practice, hydrogen breath tests that have glucose or lactulose as substrates are used more frequently.

Bile Salt Malabsorption

Bile acids are synthesized in the liver and pass into the lumen of the small bowel via the gallbladder. They are present in bile as taurine or glycine conjugates. As the pH of bile is slightly alkaline and contains significant amounts of sodium and potassium, most of the bile acids and their conjugates exist as salts (i.e., bile salts). The terms *bile acids* and *bile salts* are frequently used as synonyms. Their major function is to act as surface-active agents, forming micelles and facilitating the digestion of triglycerides and the absorption of cholesterol and fat-soluble vitamins. Little reabsorption of bile acids occurs in the proximal small bowel, but normally more than 90% is reabsorbed in the terminal ileum. They return to the liver in the portal circulation and are resecreted into the bile. This is known as the *enterohepatic circulation*. Less than 10% of secreted bile acids are lost in the feces, or about 0.2 to 0.6 g/day.

Bile acid malabsorption leading to chronic diarrhea occurs when there is ileal disease (e.g., Crohn disease), or after resection of the terminal ileum; it may also occur following cholecystectomy and in some patients with irritable bowel syndrome (IBS). Malabsorption of bile salts produces diarrhea by two different mechanisms. In one, significant deficiency of intraluminal bile salts leads to fat malabsorption and steatorrhea. In the second, which is typically more common, malabsorption of bile salts in the ileum leads to higher concentrations in the colon where they alter water and electrolyte absorption leading to net secretion of water into the lumen and diarrhea. Bile salt malabsorption is probably underdiagnosed and should be suspected in patients with unexplained chronic diarrhea.

Procedures used in the diagnosis of bile salt malabsorption include (1) the [75]selenohomocholyltaurine ([75]SeHCAT) test, (2) measurement of serum 7α-hydroxy-4-cholesten-3-one in serum, and (3) a therapeutic trial of bile acid sequestrants, such as cholestyramine. The first is the most widely used and involves the oral administration of the synthetic radioactive bile acid [75]SeHCAT. Whole body gamma counting is carried out to estimate the basal activity 1 hour after the dose. The gamma count is measured again after 7 days, when normally more than 15% of the administered dose is retained. Retention of l10% indicates bile salt malabsorption.

Inflammatory Bowel Disease[11]

IBD includes Crohn disease, ulcerative colitis, and a number of microscopic inflammatory bowel disorders. IBD has a high prevalence in the United States and Europe and a much lower, although increasing, prevalence in most Asian countries.

Significant overlap in the clinical presentation has been noted, as well as in radiologic and histologic findings, in Crohn disease (which may affect any part of the GI tract) and ulcerative colitis (which is confined to the large bowel). Both conditions present with diarrhea and abdominal pain or discomfort, often associated with fatigue and anemia, and less commonly with inflammation of the joints, skin, and eyes.

Intestinal symptoms are common to both IBD and IBS, although the latter is not an inflammatory disorder and is not associated with organic disease of the bowel. Fecal lactoferrin or calprotectin can be used to differentiate between IBD and IBS when required and to monitor disease activity or response to anti-inflammatory treatment in patients with IBD. The two tests have similar diagnostic accuracies and are markers of the infiltration of neutrophils into the mucosa. Negative tests for these proteins therefore exclude significant neutrophilic intestinal inflammation but may not exclude other organic bowel diseases, such as celiac disease. Lactoferrin and calprotectin can also be used as predictors of relapse in IBD and as markers of mucosal healing following treatment.

Protein-Losing Enteropathy

Loss of significant amounts of serum proteins into the bowel lumen and their passage in the feces occurs in a wide range of GI disorders associated with (1) inflammation or ulceration of a segment of the small or large bowel (as in Crohn disease and ulcerative colitis) or stomach, (2) diseases in which the intestinal lymphatics are obstructed, (3) conditions where there is increased lymphatic pressure (e.g., lymphoma and Whipple disease), or (4) disorders with altered immune status, such as systemic lupus erythematosus and some food allergies.

The diagnosis of protein-losing enteropathy is considered in patients with hypoalbuminemia in whom renal loss, liver disease, and malnutrition have been excluded. The diagnosis can be made by measuring the fecal clearance of alpha$_1$-antitrypsin (AT) as a marker of GI protein loss. AT in feces and serum is measured most conveniently by radial immunodiffusion. Feces should be collected quantitatively, preferably for 3 days, in preweighed containers and kept refrigerated. The AT is extracted into saline before analysis. AT clearance (mL/d) is calculated as [(fecal weight × fecal AT concentration)/serum AT] where fecal weight is expressed in g/day, fecal AT in mg/kg feces, and serum AT in mg/L.

Diseases of the Pancreas and Assessment of Exocrine Pancreatic Function[8]

Pancreatic insufficiency is the inability of the pancreas to produce and/or transport enough digestive enzymes to metabolize food in the intestine and allow its absorption. It typically occurs as a result of chronic pancreatic damage. It is most frequently associated with **cystic fibrosis** (**CF**) in children and with **chronic pancreatitis** in adults. It is less frequently but sometimes associated with pancreatic cancer. In addition, disorders of the exocrine pancreas are frequently associated with GI symptoms of malabsorption or diarrhea because of its central role in the absorption of carbohydrates, fats, and proteins. In this section, pediatric and adult exocrine pancreatic

disorders are briefly discussed and tests for assessing exocrine pancreatic function are described.

Pediatric Disorders of the Exocrine Pancreas

Pancreatic disorders in childhood are summarized in Box 38-5.

Cystic fibrosis (**CF**) is the most common severe autosomal recessive disease with an estimated gene frequency in Western Europe and the United States of between 1:25 and 1:35 and a disease incidence of about 1 in 2500 to 1 in 3200. The pathogenesis and diagnosis of CF are described in Chapter 24. Pancreatic insufficiency is present at birth in 65% of infants with CF, and a further 15% develop it during infancy and early childhood. The 20% who do not develop pancreatic insufficiency have a better prognosis and develop fewer complications.

The measurement of pancreatic elastase-1 in feces is a reliable test for pancreatic insufficiency in infants over the age of 2 weeks with CF and in older children at diagnosis of the disorder. The test also is used to detect the onset of pancreatic insufficiency in those previously pancreatic sufficient.

Adult Disorders of the Exocrine Pancreas

The major exocrine pancreatic disorders presenting in adult life are (1) **acute pancreatitis,** (2) chronic pancreatitis, and (3) carcinoma of the pancreas.[8] The use of enzyme tests in the diagnosis of acute pancreatitis is discussed in Chapter 19. The causes of pancreatitis are given in Box 38-6.

Chronic pancreatitis is an inflammatory disease characterized by persistent and progressive destruction of the pancreas leading to destruction of both endocrine and exocrine function. In Western countries, the most common cause is alcohol (60% to 90% of all cases); however there are clearly other predisposing factors (e.g., smoking and diets high in fat and protein), because only 5% to 15% of heavy drinkers develop the disease.

BOX 38-5	**The Spectrum of Pancreatic Disease in Childhood**

Disorders of Morphogenesis
Annular pancreas, pancreas divisum, pancreatic hypoplasia and agenesis, heterotopic pancreas

Inherited Syndromes Affecting the Pancreas
Cystic fibrosis (CF)
Shwachman-Diamond syndrome, Johanson-Blizzard syndrome, Pearson bone marrow pancreas syndrome

Gene Mutations Leading to Pancreatic Disease
Hereditary pancreatitis; cationic trypsinogen gene mutations, trypsin inhibitor gene mutations

Pancreatic Insufficiency Syndrome
Isolated enzyme deficiencies, lipase, colipase, enterokinase

Pancreatic Insufficiency Secondary to Other Disorders
Celiac disease

Acquired Pancreatitis in Childhood
Idiopathic, traumatic, drugs, viral, metabolic, collagen vascular diseases, autoimmune, fibrosing, nutritional (tropical)

BOX 38-6 Causes of Pancreatitis in Adults

Acute
Gallstones
Alcohol
Infections (e.g., mumps, Coxsackie B)
Pancreatic tumors
Drugs (e.g., azathioprine, estrogens, corticosteroids, didanosine)
Iatrogenic (e.g., postsurgical, ERCP)
Hyperlipidemias
Miscellaneous—trauma, scorpion bite, cardiac surgery
Idiopathic

Chronic
Alcohol
Tropical (nutritional)
Hereditary (trypsinogen and inhibitory protein defects, CF)
Idiopathic
Trauma
Hypercalcemia

CF, Cystic fibrosis; *ERCP,* endoscopic retrograde cholangiopancreatography.
From Burroughs AK, Westaby D. Liver, biliary tract disease and pancreatic disease. In: Kumar P, Clark M, eds. Clinical medicine, 7th edition. Edinburgh: WB Saunders, 2009:319-85.

TABLE 38-2 Summary of Invasive Tests of Pancreatic Exocrine Function

Procedure	Pancreatic Stimulant	Analysis of Duodenal Contents
Lundh test	Standardized meal	Enzyme output
Secretin stimulation test	Purified or synthetic porcine secretin	Bicarbonate output
Secretin-CCK test	Secretin as above plus CCK analogue (CCK-8 or ceruletide)	Bicarbonate and enzymes

CCK, Cholecystokinin.

Tests of Exocrine Function of the Pancreas

The predominant exocrine functions of the pancreas are the production and secretion of pancreatic juice, which is rich in enzymes and bicarbonate. Normal pancreatic juice (1) is colorless and odorless, (2) has a pH of 8.0 to 8.3, and (3) has a specific gravity of 1.007 to 1.042. The total 24-hour secretion volume may be as high as 3000 mL.

A number of invasive (Table 38-2) and noninvasive laboratory tests are available to measure exocrine function in the investigation of pancreatic insufficiency. Invasive tests require GI intubation to collect pancreatic samples. Noninvasive tests (or "tubeless tests") were developed to avoid intubation, which is (1) uncomfortable for the patient, (2) time-consuming, and (3) expensive. Noninvasive tests are simpler and less expensive to perform, but in general they lack the clinical sensitivity and specificity of the invasive tests, particularly for the diagnosis of mild pancreatic insufficiency.

Invasive Tests of Exocrine Pancreatic Function

Invasive tests include measuring the (1) total volume of pancreatic juice, (2) amount or concentration of bicarbonate, and

---

BOX 38-7 Noninvasive Tests Used to Assess Pancreatic Exocrine Function

Fecal chymotrypsin
Fecal elastase-1
N-benzoyl-L-tyrosyl-p-aminobenzoic acid (NBT-PABA)
Pancreolauryl
^{13}C-Mixed chain triglyceride absorption

---

(3) activities of pancreatic enzymes in duodenal contents. The enzyme most commonly measured is (1) trypsin, but (2) amylase, (3) lipase, (4) chymotrypsin, and (5) elastase are also measured. The *Lundh test* consists of giving a standardized meal as a physiological stimulus to the pancreas. Administration of the meal, however, prevents determination of the total enzyme and bicarbonate output or secretory volume. Moreover, it provides inadequate stimulation in the presence of mucosal diseases (e.g., celiac disease), in which hormone release from the duodenal mucosa is impaired. In view of these limitations, the Lundh test is largely of historical interest.

The *secretin test* is based on the principle that secretion of pancreatic juice and bicarbonate output are related to the functional mass of pancreatic tissue. After an overnight fast, basal samples of fluid are collected from the stomach and duodenum. Secretin is then administered intravenously, and duodenal fluid is collected at 15-minute intervals for at least 1 hour. Secretin stimulates the secretion of pancreatic juice and bicarbonate, but stimulation of the secretion of pancreatic enzymes is inconsistent. Addition of CCK (or a synthetic equivalent) stimulates the secretion of pancreatic enzymes, giving a more complete assessment of pancreatic function than with secretin alone.

Noninvasive Tests of Exocrine Pancreatic Function

A variety of noninvasive tests have been used (Box 38-7), but none has adequate clinical sensitivity for reliably detecting early pancreatic disease. When malabsorption is present, such tests are of value in confirming or excluding pancreatic disease. Considerable overlap often occurs between results observed in normal individuals and those found in patients with pancreatic disorders, which is mainly due to the large functional reserve of the pancreas. An estimate has been made that pancreatic insufficiency cannot clearly be demonstrated until at least 50% of the acinar cells have been destroyed. Clinical signs of pancreatic insufficiency often do not appear until the destruction of 90% of acinar tissue. In general, these tests may be used when investigating causes of malabsorption but have inadequate sensitivity for diagnosing chronic pancreatitis. Fecal elastase (measured by the monoclonal antibody method) is currently the noninvasive test of choice for assessing pancreatic insufficiency. Further information on noninvasive tests is found in an expanded version of this chapter. [9]

Neuroendocrine Tumors

The watery diarrhea hypokalemia achlorhydria (WDHA) syndrome also is known as the *Werner-Morrison syndrome* and as a *VIPoma.* This syndrome may be suspected in a patient producing large volumes of secretory diarrhea (more than 1 L per 24 hours) with dehydration and hypokalemia. The diagnosis is confirmed by finding a high plasma VIP concentration and demonstration of the tumor by somatostatin-receptor imaging.

GI neuroendocrine tumors are either endocrine pancreatic tumors or carcinoid tumors arising from enterochromaffin cells, which occur throughout the GI tract. Carcinoid tumors are discussed in Chapter 26.

Approximately two thirds of patients with tumors arising from pancreatic islet cells have clinical syndromes associated with excessive hormone production. This group of tumors includes (1) insulinomas, (2) gastrinomas, (3) VIPomas, (4) glucagonomas, and (5) somatostatinomas. Insulinomas and glucagonomas are not usually associated with GI symptoms. The somatostatinoma syndrome is associated with steatorrhea, gallstones, and diabetes. The remaining one third of patients with endocrine pancreatic tumors have no specific clinical symptoms associated with the tumors, which are described as nonfunctional.

The pattern of hormone and precursor production by neuroendocrine tumors is complex. Most secrete several tumor markers. Measurement of the circulating concentration of chromogranin A provides the highest diagnostic sensitivity (94%) for endocrine pancreatic tumors, followed by measurements of PP (74%). Measurement of chromogranin A is an alternative to more specific markers in monitoring the effectiveness of surgery or drug therapy. However, as with other protein and peptide tumor markers, the epitope specificity of the antiserum has a profound effect on the diagnostic sensitivity of the assay. Although chromogranin A has high sensitivity, false positives have been observed in a number of nonendocrine tumors including prostatic cancer.

Disorders of Maldigestion/Malabsorption

Box 38-8 summarizes the main causes of malabsorption. Clinical presentation of the patient suffering from malabsorption or maldigestion classically includes the following features:

- *Evidence of general ill health,* including (1) anorexia, (2) weight loss, (3) fatigue following minor effort, and (4) dyspnea. In addition, edema (due to hypoalbuminemia), or weakness, tetany, and dehydration due to electrolyte imbalance and water loss may be present. In pancreatic exocrine insufficiency, however, hyperphagia is the rule; patients often report a very high (5000 kcal/day) food intake.
- *Isolated nutritional deficiencies.* Iron, folate, or vitamin B_{12} deficiency may manifest as anemia, which may be mild; vitamin K deficiency as a bleeding tendency; and vitamin D deficiency as bone disease. They are reflected by a variety of signs and symptoms including (1) glossitis, (2) pallor, (3) dermatitis, (4) petechiae, (5) bruising, (6) hematuria, (7) muscle or bone pain, or (8) neurological abnormalities.

BOX 38-8	**Summary of Disorders Leading to Malabsorption**
Disorders of Intraluminal Digestion	
a. Altered gastric function	Postgastrectomy syndrome
	Zollinger-Ellison syndrome
b. Pancreatic insufficiency	Chronic pancreatitis
	Cystic fibrosis (CF)
	Pancreatic cancer
c. Bile acid deficiency	Disease/resection of terminal ileum
	Small bowel bacterial overgrowth
Disorders of Transport into the Mucosal Cell	
a. Generalized disorders due to reduction in absorptive surface area	Celiac disease, tropical sprue
b. Specific disorders	Hypolactasia
	Vitamin B_{12} in pernicious anemia
	Zn in acrodermatitis enteropathica
Disorders of Transport Out of the Mucosal Cell	
a. Blockage of the lymphatics	Abdominal lymphoma, primary lymphangiectasia
b. Inherited disorders	a-β-lipoproteinemia

- *Abdominal symptoms,* such as discomfort, distension, flatulence, and borborygmi (rumbling and gurgling sounds due to movement of gas in the intestine). Such symptoms may also occur after gastric surgery leading to the **postgastrectomy** and **dumping syndromes**.
- *Watery diarrhea and possibly steatorrhea.* In severe cases of steatorrhea (excess fat in feces), the stool is typically loose, bulky, offensive, greasy, light-colored, and difficult to flush away. Alternatively the stools may appear normal, but be more bulky or be passed with greater frequency.

Early presentation of malabsorption is often subtle. For example, there may be only a slight alteration in volume or consistency of the stool and only mild symptoms attributable to the GI tract. The patient may complain only of anorexia, fatigue, and lack of interest in daily activities. It is in such cases that the physician who suspects malabsorption on clinical grounds will rely on the laboratory to assist in the diagnosis. The initial laboratory investigations are (1) routine tests; (2) tests where abnormalities may point to the possibility of malabsorption (e.g., blood hemoglobin concentration; mean red cell volume; serum concentrations of folate, ferritin, calcium, albumin, and alkaline phosphatase); and (3) tests for antibodies in celiac disease (celiac serology).

Chronic Diarrhea[7,14]

Although diarrhea is a common problem, no clear definition has existed to distinguish it from the range of stool weight, frequency, consistency, or volume that occurs in the normal population. In 2003, for a Western diet, diarrhea was defined as "the abnormal passage of loose or liquid stools more than three times daily and/or a volume of stool [with a weight]

BOX 38-9   Causes of Chronic Diarrhea

Colonic	Pancreatic
Colonic neoplasia	Chronic pancreatitis
Ulcerative and Crohn colitis	Pancreatic carcinoma
Microscopic colitis	Cystic fibrosis (CF)
Small bowel	**Endocrine**
Celiac disease	Hyperthyroidism
Crohn disease	Diabetes
Other small bowel enteropathies (e.g., Whipple disease, tropical sprue,	Hypoparathyroidism
amyloid, intestinal lymphangiectasia)	Addison disease
Bile salt malabsorption	Hormone secreting tumors (VIPoma, gastrinoma, carcinoid)
Disaccharidase deficiency	**Other**
Small bowel bacterial overgrowth	Factitious diarrhea
Mesenteric ischemia	"Surgical" causes (e.g., small bowel resection, internal fistulae)
Radiation enteritis	Drugs
Lymphoma	Alcohol
Giardiasis (and other chronic infection)	Autonomic neuropathy

From Thomas PD, Forbes A, Green J, et al. Guidelines for the investigation of chronic diarrhoea, 2nd edition. Gut 2003;52(Suppl V):Vol. 1-Vol. 15; reproduced by permission from the BMJ Publishing Group.

greater than 200 g/day."[14] It may be defined as chronic when it has continued for 4 weeks; such persistence indicates the likelihood of a noninfectious cause requiring further investigation.

Several quite different mechanisms lead to diarrhea. In carbohydrate malabsorption, the presence of unabsorbed solutes in the bowel causes an osmotic diarrhea as water enters the bowel from the tissue. By contrast, the diarrhea of most laxative abuse and in VIPomas is due to active secretion of water and electrolytes into the bowel, which is described as secretory diarrhea. IBDs (ulcerative colitis and Crohn disease) cause diarrhea as a consequence of the inflammatory process with loss of fluid into the bowel.

Many diseases commonly thought to cause "diarrhea" in fact lead to more frequent passage of stools but not usually to an increased stool weight (or volume). Such disorders (e.g., IBS) generally fall outside the scope of the definition of "chronic diarrhea." Box 38-9 describes the many causes of chronic diarrhea; most is due to disease of the colon in which laboratory diagnostic tests are currently of little value. An algorithm for the investigation of chronic diarrhea is given in Figure 38-4.

Surreptitious laxative abuse is an important, often overlooked, cause of chronic diarrhea and is a diagnosis in which laboratory investigations have a significant role (Table 38-3).[4] The main initial prerequisite for making a diagnosis of surreptitious laxative abuse is a high index of clinical suspicion, followed by a request for appropriate analyses in urine and fecal samples at a time when the patient has diarrhea.

Measurement of the fecal osmotic (osmolal) gap (FOG) may be helpful in investigating diarrhea. It is based in the fact that the osmolality of stool "water" will normally be that of serum (290 mOsm/kg), but the contribution of electrolytes and of nonelectrolytes to the total osmolality will vary depending on the cause of the diarrhea. FOG expresses the difference between the theoretical normal osmolality (290 mOsm/kg) and the contribution of Na^+ and K^+ as follows:

$$FOG = 290 - [2 \, (fecal \, Na^+ + K^+)]$$

Fecal sodium and potassium are measured in the fluid obtained by rapid centrifugation of a fecal sample. Total fecal osmolality increases significantly in unrefrigerated samples and use of the serum osmolality or 290 mOsm/kg is recommended rather than a measurement of total fecal osmolality.

Measurement of FOG enables an estimate to be made of the contribution of electrolytes or nonelectrolytes to the retention of water in the bowel and therefore assists in distinguishing between secretory and osmotic diarrhea. In osmotic diarrhea, unabsorbed solutes lead to water retention and thus make a larger contribution than normal to fecal osmolality; fecal sodium and potassium will therefore be present at lower concentrations than normal, leading to a larger "osmotic gap." Conversely, in secretory diarrhea, it is electrolytes that lead to water retention, and the FOG will therefore be small. FOG >50 mOsm/kg is consistent with an osmotic diarrhea from carbohydrate malabsorption or magnesium-induced diarrhea. By contrast FOG <50 mOsm/kg suggests a secretory diarrhea, and further investigations might include a laxative screen for colonic stimulants or rarely tests for a neuroendocrine tumor.[7] A low FOG will be found in factitious diarrhea because of the addition of water to the stool; if this is suspected and if other causes are excluded, then measurement of total stool osmolality may be helpful.

Measurement of creatinine has been used as an indication of contamination of the fecal sample with urine.

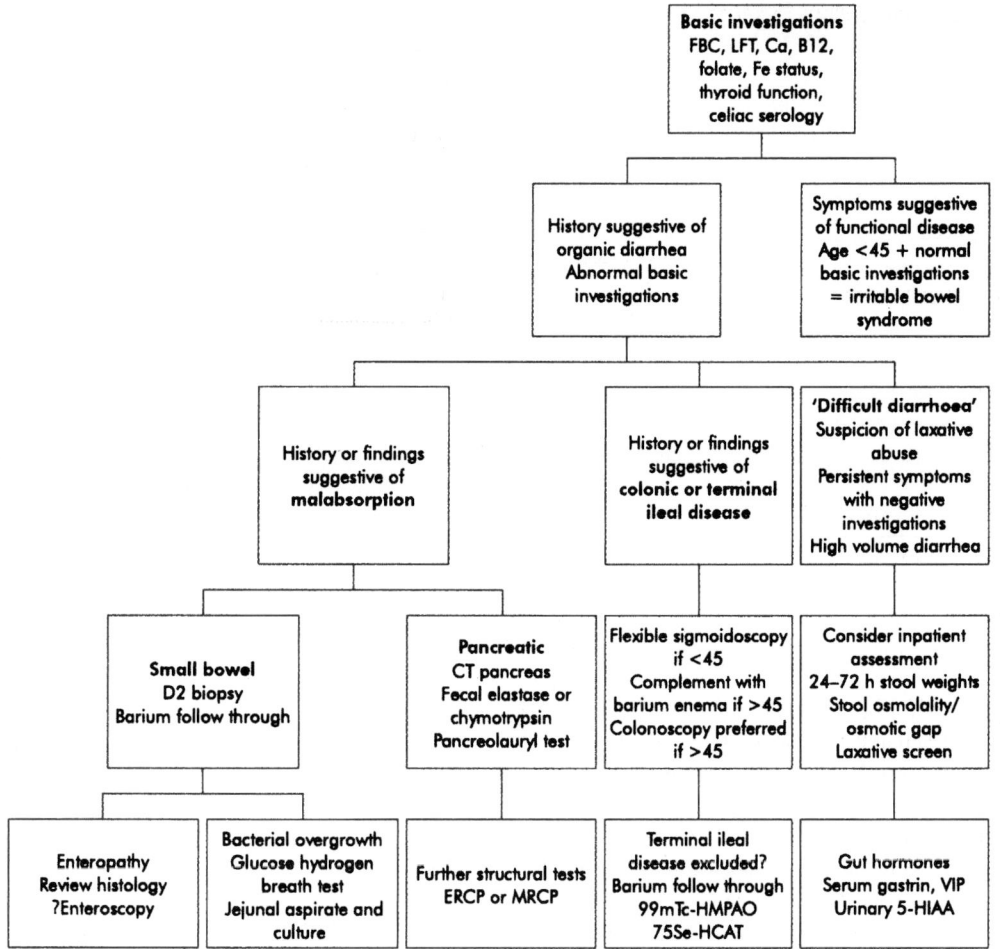

Figure 38-4 An algorithm for the investigation of chronic diarrhea. *5-HIAA,* 5-hydroxyindoleacetic acid; *75Se-HCAT,* 75Se homotaurocholate; *CT,* computed tomography; *ERCP,* endoscopic retrograde cholangiopancreatography; *FBC,* full blood count; *LFT,* liver function tests; *MRCP,* magnetic resonance cholangiopancreatography; *Tc-HMPAO,* technetium hexa-methyl-propyleneamine oxime. *(From Thomas PD, Forbes A, Green J, et al. Guidelines for the investigation of chronic diarrhoea, 2nd edition. Gut 2003;52(Suppl V):v1-v15. Used with permission from the BMJ Publishing Group.)*

TABLE 38-3	Laboratory Tests to Assess Gastrointestinal Function
Clinical Application	**Appropriate Laboratory Investigations**
Investigating diarrhea	Possible lactase deficiency: breath hydrogen after oral lactose
	Possible bacterial overgrowth: breath hydrogen after oral glucose or lactulose
	Possible laxative abuse: urine laxative screen
	Possibly induced by bile acid: ^{75}selenohomocholyltaurine (^{75}SeHCAT) whole body retention or serum 7α-hydroxy-4-cholesten-3-one
	Fecal osmotic gap (FOG); fecal Na, K
Assessing pancreatic function	Pancreolauryl test, fecal elastase
Screening for celiac disease	Tissue transglutaminase (tTG) antibodies
Assessing fat absorption	^{14}C-triolein absorption (breath ^{14}CO$_2$) or fecal microscopy
Other tests	Fecal α-1-antitrypsin for protein-losing enteropathy; gut hormones (gastrin)

From Hill PG. Faecal fat: time to give it up. Ann Clin Biochem 2001;38:164-7.

Review Questions

1. Gastrin
   a. is secreted by the liver and stomach.
   b. is secreted when stomach pH is low.
   c. stimulates gastric acid secretion.
   d. inhibits secretion of intrinsic factor.
2. The hydrogen breath test using glucose or lactulose as substrates is assessing
   a. intestinal bacterial overgrowth.
   b. celiac disease.
   c. the presence of *H. pylori*.
   d. bile acid malabsorption.
3. A peptide neurotransmitter that relaxes smooth muscle in the gut and increases water and electrolyte secretion is
   a. cholecystokinin (CCK).
   b. secretin.
   c. vasoactive intestinal polypeptide (VIP).
   d. gastric inhibitory polypeptide.
4. The three phases of the digestive process include the neurogenic, gastric and the intestinal phases. The intestinal phase is initiated
   a. by distention of the stomach.
   b. by the sight, smell and taste of food.
   c. upon stimulation of the cerebral cortex in the brain.
   d. when weakly acidic digestive products of proteins and lipids enter the duodenum.
5. An example of an invasive test for detection of *H. pylori* in peptic ulcer disease would be
   a. breath testing following ingestion of ^{14}C-labeled urea.
   b. microbiological culture of a gastric biopsy sample.
   c. lab measurement of a specific IgG antibody.
   d. detection of a specific fecal antigen.
6. Which one of the following is considered to be a disease of the intestine?
   a. Zollinger-Ellison syndrome.
   b. peptic ulcer disease.
   c. celiac disease.
   d. cystic fibrosis (CF).
7. The correct formula for determining the fecal osmotic gap (FOG) of a fecal specimen is
   a. $290 - [2(fecal\ Na^+ + K^+)]$.
   b. fecal Na^+ + fecal K^+.
   c. $[fecal\ Na^+ - fecal\ K^+] + 290$.
   d. $2 - [fecal\ Na^+ + fecal\ K^+]$.
8. In Western countries, the most common cause of chronic pancreatitis in adults is
   a. gallstones.
   b. infections.
   c. pancreatic tumors.
   d. alcohol consumption.
9. Which one of the following peptides stimulates increased pancreatic secretion of bicarbonate?
   a. Glucose-dependent insulinotropic peptide (GIP)
   b. Gluten
   c. Secretin
   d. Vasoactive intestinal polypeptide (VIP)
10. A tumor of the pancreatic islet cells that produces in part massive gastric hypersecretion, diarrhea, and steatorrhea causes
    a. the Zollinger-Ellison syndrome.
    b. celiac disease.
    c. lactose intolerance.
    d. cystic fibrosis (CF).

References

1. Barakat MT, Meeran K, Bloom SR. Neuroendocrine tumours. Endocrine-Related Cancer 2004;11:1–18.
2. Del Valle J. Zollinger-Ellison syndrome. In: Yamada T, ed. Textbook of gastroenterology, 5th edition. Oxford, United Kingdom: Wiley-Blackwell, 2009;982–1004.
3. Dieterich W, Ehnis T, Bauer M, et al. Identification of tissue transglutaminase as the autoantigen of celiac disease. Nat Med 1997;3:797–801.
4. Duncan A, Phillips IJ. Evaluation of thin-layer chromatography methods for laxative detection. Ann Clin Biochem 2001;38:64–6.
5. Farrell JJ. Digestion and absorption of nutrients and vitamins. In: Feldman M, Friedman LS, Brandt LJ, eds. Sleisenger and Fordtran's gastrointestinal and liver disease, 8th edition. Philadelphia: WB Saunders, 2006:2147–97.
6. Fasano A, Berti I, Gerarduzzi T, et al. Prevalence of celiac disease in at-risk and not-at-risk groups in the United States: a large multicenter study. Arch Intern Med 2003;163:286–92.
7. Fine KD, Schiller LR. AGA technical review on the evaluation and management of chronic diarrhea. Gastroenterology 1999;116:1464–86.
8. Forsmark CE. Chronic pancreatitis. In: Feldman M, Friedman LS, Brandt LJ, eds. Sleisenger and Fordtran's gastrointestinal and liver isease, 8th edition. Philadelphia: WB Saunders, 2006:1271–308.
9. Hill PG. Gastric, pancreatic, and intestinal function. In: Burtis CA, Ashwood ER, Bruns DE, eds. Tietz textbook of clinical chemistry and molecular diagnostics, 5th edition. St Louis: Saunders, 2012:1695–732.
10. Hill PG, McMillan SA. Anti-tissue transglutaminase antibodies and their role in the investigation of coeliac disease. Ann Clin Biochem 2006;43:105–17.
11. Lewis JD. The utility of biomarkers in the diagnosis and therapy of inflammatory bowel disease. Gastroenterol 2011;140:1817–20.
12. Malfertheiner P, Megraud F, O'Morain C, et al. Current concepts in the management of *Helicobacter pylori* infection—the Maastricht IIIConsensus Report. Gut 2007;56:772–81.
13. Miller LJ. Gastrointestinal hormones and receptors. In: Yamada T, ed. Textbook of gastroenterology, 5th edition. Oxford, United Kingdom: Wiley-Blackwell, 2009:56–85.
14. Thomas PD, Forbes A, Green J, et al. Guidelines for the investigation of chronic diarrhoea, 2nd edition. Gut 2003;52(Suppl V):v1–v15.
15. van Heel DA, West J. Recent advances in coeliac disease. Gut 2006;55:1037–46.

Disorders of Bone and Mineral Metabolism*

*Juha Risteli, M.D, Ph.D., F.E.B.M.B., William E. Winter, M.D.,
Michael Kleerekoper, M.D., F.A.C.B., M.A.C.E., and
Leila Risteli, M.D., Ph.D., M.A., F.E.B.M.B.*

Objectives

1. Define the following:
   Bone marker
   Matrix
   Osteoblast
   Osteoclast
   Osteomalacia
   Osteopenia
   Osteoporosis
   Rickets
   Type I collagen
2. Describe the structure and function of bone, including organic matrix, cellular components, mineral makeup and remodeling units.
3. Detail the physiology and regulation of calcium and phosphate, including biochemical states, factors that alter the distribution of calcium between these states, and the roles of parathyroid hormone (PTH), calcitonin, and vitamin D.
4. List causes, symptoms, and laboratory analyses used in the differential diagnosis of the following:
   Hypercalcemia
   Hypermagnesemia
   Hyperphosphatemia
   Hypocalcemia
   Hypomagnesemia
   Hypophosphatemia
5. List and describe commonly used methods in the measurement of the following analytes, including principles of reactions, specimen requirements, potential preanalytical errors in the measurement of total/free calcium, and how these analytes are affected in bone or mineral disorders:
   Bone alkaline
     phosphatase (BALP)
   Magnesium
   Parathyroid hormone
     (PTH)

Parathyroid-related protein
Phosphate
Total/free calcium
Vitamin D and
   metabolites

6. State the effect each of the following disorders has on total and free calcium, phosphate, albumin, and parathyroid hormone (PTH):
   Primary and secondary hyperparathyroidism
   Primary and secondary hypoparathyroidism
   Pseudohypoparathyroidism
7. Discuss 1,25-dihydroxyvitamin D, including its metabolism, physiology, and roles in bone health, mineral metabolism, and disease.
8. List and describe five markers of bone formation and resorption, including what they are products of, how they reflect specific bone diseases, specimen requirements, and controllable pre-analytical variables.
9. For the following disorders, state the cause(s), symptoms, laboratory analyses, and lab results used to diagnose:
   Adynamic bone disease
   Osteitis fibrosa
   Osteomalacia
   Osteoporosis
   Paget disease
   Rickets
10. Analyze and solve case studies related to bone disorders, biochemical bone markers, and laboratory analysis of these.

Key Words and Definitions

Adynamic bone disease (ABD) A type of renal osteodystrophy characterized by reduced osteoblasts and osteoclasts, and low bone turnover of bone.

Bone alkaline phosphatase (BALP) An isoenzyme of alkaline phosphatase and a biochemical marker of bone formation.

Calcitonin A 32-amino-acid polypeptide hormone elaborated by the parafollicular cells of the thyroid gland in response to hypercalcemia.

CTx An antigen produced when type I collagen is digested by the proteinase cathepsin K yielding cross-linked carboxy-terminal telopeptide of type I collagen; a serum marker for bone resorption and action of cathepsin K.

Deoxypyridinoline (DPD) A deoxypyridinoline crosslink of type I collagen present in bone that is excreted, free or protein-bound, in urine and serves as a marker of bone resorption.

*The authors gratefully acknowledge the original contributions by David B. Endres and Robert K. Rude, on which portions of this chapter are based.

Key Words and Definitions—cont'd

Familial hypophosphatemic rickets Any of several inherited disorders of proximal renal tubular function causing phosphate loss, hypophosphatemia, and skeletal deformities, including rickets and osteomalacia.

Humoral hypercalcemia of malignancy (HHM) A malignancy caused by bone resorption mediated by circulating factors released from distant tumor cells.

Hypercalcemia Increased concentration of calcium in plasma; manifestations include fatigability, muscle weakness, depression, anorexia, nausea, and constipation; most commonly caused by primary hyperparathyroidism or malignancy.

Hypercalcemia-associated malignancy (HAM) A malignancy characterized by hypercalcemia.

Hypermagnesemia A condition characterized by abnormally high concentrations of magnesium in blood plasma.

Hyperphosphatemia A condition characterized by abnormally high concentrations of phosphates in blood plasma.

Hypocalcemia A condition characterized by a low concentration of calcium in plasma.

Hypomagnesemia A condition characterized by a low concentration of magnesium in blood.

Hypoparathyroidism The condition produced by greatly reduced function of the parathyroid glands.

Hypophosphatemia A condition characterized by a low concentration of phosphate in blood.

ICTP An antigen produced when type I collagen is digested by matrix metalloproteinases, yielding cross-linked carboxy-terminal telopeptide of type I collagen; a serum marker for bone resorption.

Mineralization The process by which the body uses minerals to build bone structure.

N-telopeptide (NTx) A biochemical marker of bone resorption.

Osteitis fibrosa A complication of hyperparathyroidism in which the bones are soft and often deformed; also called osteitis *fibrosa cystica*.

Osteoblasts Cells responsible for formation of bone, including synthesis of type I collagen and noncollagenous proteins and mineralization of osteoid.

Osteocalcin (OC) A protein found in the extracellular matrix of bone and dentin and involved in regulating mineralization in the bones and teeth.

Osteoclasts Large, multinuclear cells responsible for resorption of bone.

Osteomalacia Inadequate or delayed mineralization of osteoid; the adult equivalent of rickets (interruption in the development and mineralization of the growth plate in children).

Osteopenia A condition characterized by decreased bone density occurs that is often predecessor to osteoporosis. It is diagnosed with a bone density test.

Osteoporosis A condition characterized by reduction in bone mass, leading to fractures with minimal trauma; postmenopausal osteoporosis occurs in women after menopause; senile osteoporosis occurs in both men and women later in life.

Paget disease A localized, not metabolic bone disease characterized by osteoclastic bone resorption followed by replacement of bone in a chaotic fashion. Prevalance varies strongly between different countries.

Parathyroid hormone (PTH) A peptide hormone secreted by parathyroid glands in response to hypocalcemia that increases calcium in blood by increasing bone resorption, increasing renal reabsorption of calcium, and increasing the synthesis of 1,25-hydroxyvitamin D; the latter increases intestinal absorption of calcium and phosphate.

Parathyroid hormone–related protein (PTHrP) A protein that mimics many actions of PTH, but is a product of a different gene that is expressed in many normal tissues and overexpressed by tumors in most cases of humoral hypercalcemia of malignancy (HHM).

Procollagen type I carboxy-terminal propeptide (PICP) A biochemical marker of bone formation.

Procollagen type I N-terminal propeptide (PINP) A biochemical marker of bone formation.

Pyridium crosslinks A family of molecules that links collagen molecules to each other; the breakdown products are excreted in the urine with attached crosslinks including pyridinoline (PYD) and deoxypyridinoline (DPD).

Renal osteodystrophy Bone diseases associated with chronic renal failure, including high turnover (osteitis fibrosa or secondary hyperparathyroidism) and low turnover (osteomalacia and adynamic bone) diseases.

Rickets A disorder in children caused by a lack of vitamin D, calcium, or phosphate that leads to softening and weakening of the bones. In adults it is known as osteomalacia.

Secondary hyperparathyroidism Excessive secretion of parathyroid hormone (PTH) in response to low plasma calcium that, in turn, is caused by another condition; seen in patients with chronic renal failure and in people with inadequate vitamin D.

Tartrate-resistant acid phosphatase 5b (TRACP5b) An enzyme derived from osteoclasts; it is a marker of bone resorption.

Vitamin D Fat-soluble vitamin produced by skin upon exposure to sunlight (vitamin D_3, also called cholecalciferol) or adsorbed from foods that contain it (vitamin D_2 or ergocalciferol); deficiency causes rickets in children and osteomalacia in adults. Related tests with clinical utility include assays for 25-hydroxyvitamin D [25(OH)D] and 1,25 dihydroxyvitamin D (calcitriol).

The skeletal system is one of the largest organs in the body and the storehouse for 99% of the body's calcium. Bones are mineralized connective tissue in which type I collagen forms a network of flexible fibers. **Mineralization** of this network, or matrix, with calcium salts is required to produce the rigid skeleton. Bones are a living tissue that is constantly being remodeled by degradation of old tissue and its replacement with new bone matrix. Two bone cell types, **osteoclasts** and **osteoblasts**, are mainly responsible for remodeling. It is now possible to analyze both bone formation and resorption by clinical laboratory methods.

The metabolism of calcium is a tightly controlled processes in the body. Calcium has critical roles in intracellular signaling, at the plasma membrane of cells, and in control of function of extracellular proteins, such as those in the coagulation cascade. The body's handling of extracellular (1) calcium is closely intertwined with that of (2) phosphate and to a somewhat lesser extent of (3) magnesium. It is also intricately connected with the active cellular processes in bone, a metabolically and functionally important system in its own right.

After an overview of bone and mineral metabolism, this chapter presents the clinical chemistry of (1) calcium, (2) phosphate, (3) magnesium, (4) hormones regulating these minerals, (5) markers of bone formation and degradation, and (6) major disorders of bone.

Overview of Bone and Mineral Metabolism

The main functions of bone are (1) mechanical, (2) protective, and (3) metabolic. Bones are composed of cortical (about 80 % of mineral) and trabecular (about 20 % of mineral) bone.

The function of cortical bone is primarily mechanical and protective, whereas trabecular bone is more metabolically active. Bone is composed primarily of an extracellular mineralized matrix with a smaller cellular fraction. The organic matrix is primarily type I collagen (about 90%) with lesser amounts of other proteins. The organic matrix is mineralized primarily by the deposition of inorganic calcium and phosphate. Osteoclasts and osteoblasts are the two main types of bone cells. Osteoclasts *resorb bone*, whereas osteoblasts *synthesize new bone*.

Turnover or *remodeling* of bone occurs continuously, enabling the bone to repair damage and adjust strength. Bone remodeling does not occur at random, but instead in discrete packets known as *bone remodeling units* (Figure 39-1). The remodeling cycle includes (1) activation, (2) resorption, (3) reversal, (4) formation, and (5) resting phases. Circulating osteoclast precursors are recruited, proliferate, and fuse to form osteoclasts. These giant multinucleated cells resorb bone by producing hydrogen ions to mobilize minerals and lysosomal enzymes to digest the organic matrix. After resorption ceases, a cement line is deposited in the resorption cavity, probably by mononucleated cells. Stromal lining cells differentiate to osteoblasts. Osteoblasts form bone by synthesizing the organic matrix, including type I collagen, and participating in the mineralization of the newly synthesized matrix. An estimated 10% to 30% of the skeleton is remodeled each year. Bone growth and turnover are influenced by the metabolism of calcium, phosphate, magnesium and by many hormones, especially **parathyroid hormone (PTH)**, 1,25-dihydroxyvitamin D (1,25[OH]$_2$D), and several cytokines.

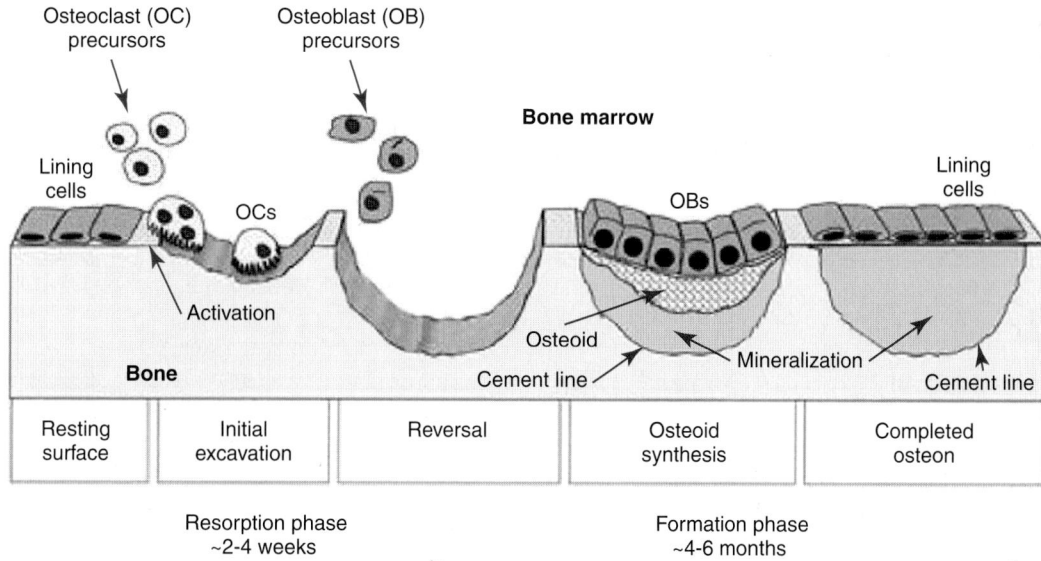

Figure 39-1 Bone remodeling sequence. A depiction of the sequential action of osteoclasts and osteoblasts in removing old bone and replacing it with new bone. For simplicity of illustration, the figure shows remodeling in only two dimensions, whereas in vivo, it occurs in three dimensions with osteoclasts continuing to enlarge the cavity at one end and osteoblasts beginning to fill it in at the other end. *(From Riggs BL, Parfitt AM. Drugs used to treat osteoporosis: the critical need for a uniform nomenclature based on their action on bone remodeling. J Bone Miner Res 2005;20:177-84.)*

Two products of the osteoblast appear to coordinate osteoblast and osteoclast activity. The first, receptor activator of nuclear factor-κB (RANK) ligand, binds to a receptor on osteoclast progenitor cells and increases osteoclast differentiation and activity. The second, osteoprotegerin (OPG), serves as a decoy receptor for RANK ligand. When OPG binds to RANK ligand, the osteoclast-stimulation activity is prevented. The relative ratios of these two molecules determine bone turnover.

Bone contains (1) nearly all of the calcium (99%), (2) most of the phosphate (85%), and (3) much of the magnesium (55%) of the body. Their concentrations in plasma depend on the net effect of (1) bone mineral deposition and resorption, (2) intestinal absorption, and (3) renal excretion. PTH and $1,25(OH)_2D$ are the principal hormones regulating these three processes.

Calcium

Calcium is the fifth most common element in the body and the most prevalent cation. The skeleton contains 99% of the body's calcium (Table 39-1), predominantly as extracellular crystals of unknown structure with a composition approaching that of hydroxyapatite, $Ca_{10}(PO_4)_6(OH)_2$.

TABLE 39-1	Distribution of Calcium, Phosphate, and Magnesium in the Body		
Tissue	**Calcium**	**Phosphate**	**Magnesium**
Skeleton	99%	85%	55%
Soft tissue	1%	15%	45%
Extracellular fluid	<0.2%	<0.1%	1%
Total	1000 g (25 mol)	600 g (19.4 mol)	25 g (1.0 mol)

Modified from Aurbach GD, Marx SJ, Speigel AM. Parathyroid hormone, calcitonin, and the calciferols. In: Wilson JD, Foster DW, eds. Williams textbook of endocrinology, 8th edition. Philadelphia: WB Saunders, 1992:1397-476.

Biochemistry and Physiology

In blood, virtually all of the calcium is in the plasma, which has a mean calcium concentration of approximately 9.5 mg/dL (2.38 mmol/L). Calcium exists in three physicochemical states in plasma (Figure 39-2) with approximately (1) 50% free (ionized), (2) 40% bound to plasma proteins, primarily albumin, and (3) 10% complexed with small anions (see Table 39-1). Calcium is redistributed among these three plasma pools, acutely or chronically, by (1) alterations in the concentration of protein and small anions, (2) changes in pH, or (3) changes in the quantities of free calcium and total calcium in the serum.

The free calcium fraction is the biologically active form. Its concentration in plasma is tightly regulated by the calcium-regulating hormones PTH and $1,25(OH)_2D$. Intracellular calcium has key roles in many important physiological functions, including (1) muscle contraction, (2) hormone secretion, (3) glycogen metabolism, and (4) cell division. The intracellular concentration of calcium in the cytosol of unstimulated cells is $<10^{-6}$ to 10^{-7} mol/L (1 to 0.1 μmol/L), which is less than one one-thousandth of that in the extracellular fluid (10^{-3} mol/L).

Extracellular calcium is needed for (1) bone mineralization, (2) blood coagulation, and (3) other functions. Calcium stabilizes the plasma membranes and influences permeability and excitability. A decrease in the serum free calcium concentration causes increased neuromuscular excitability and tetany. An increased concentration reduces neuromuscular excitability.

Clinical Significance

Disorders of calcium metabolism are separated into those causing **hypocalcemia** and **hypercalcemia**.[3,6,9,10]

Hypocalcemia

Low total serum calcium (hypocalcemia) may be due to a reduction in either the albumin-bound calcium or the free fraction of calcium, or both (Box 39-1). Hypoalbuminemia is the most common cause of decreased total calcium with

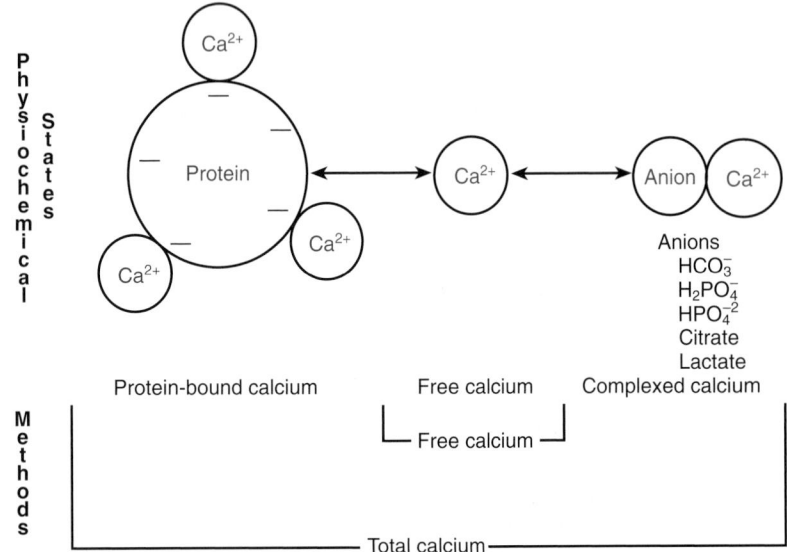

Physiochemical States

Methods

Ca²⁺

Protein

Ca²⁺

Ca²⁺

Ca²⁺

Anion Ca²⁺

Anions
HCO_3^-
$H_2PO_4^-$
HPO_4^{-2}
Citrate
Lactate

Protein-bound calcium

Free calcium

Complexed calcium

Free calcium

Total calcium

Figure 39-2 Equilibria and determinations of calcium in serum. Calcium moves among three physiochemical pools: (1) free calcium, (2) protein-bound calcium, and (3) calcium complexed with inorganic and organic anions. Methods for determining total calcium measure the calcium in all three pools, whereas methods for determining free calcium measure only that pool.

normal free calcium (sometimes called *pseudohypocalcemia*); serum calcium concentration is lower when serum albumin is low because 1 g/dL of albumin binds approximately 0.8 mg/dL of calcium. Common clinical conditions associated with low serum albumin include (1) chronic liver disease, (2) nephrotic syndrome, (3) congestive heart failure, and (4) malnutrition. In such states it is preferable to measure free calcium with a specific assay or, if such is not available, to use an adjustment calculation for the total calcium concentration (discussed later).

In chronic renal failure, (1) hypoproteinemia, (2) hyperphosphatemia, and (3) low serum $1,25(OH)_2D$ (caused by reduced renal synthesis) contribute to hypocalcemia. Magnesium deficiency, as discussed in a later section of this chapter, impairs PTH secretion and causes PTH end-organ resistance.

Hypoparathyroidism is caused most commonly by parathyroid gland destruction during neck surgery (90%). Pseudohypoparathyroidism is characterized by resistance to PTH and increased concentrations of PTH.

Rapid remineralization of bone after (1) surgery for primary hyperparathyroidism (hungry bone syndrome), (2) treatment for hyperthyroidism, or (3) treatment for hematological malignancy may result in hypocalcemia. Acute pancreatitis is frequently complicated by hypocalcemia. **Vitamin D** deficiency may also be associated with hypocalcemia because of impaired intestinal absorption of calcium.

Hypocalcemia most commonly presents with signs and symptoms of neuromuscular hyperexcitability, such as (1) tetany, (2) paresthesias, and (3) seizures. A rapid fall in the serum calcium may also be associated with hypotension and electrocardiographic abnormalities.

The initial laboratory evaluation includes assessment of renal function and measurement of serum albumin and magnesium concentrations. Serum intact PTH concentrations are low or inappropriately normal in hypoparathyroidism and elevated in pseudohypoparathyroidism. Vitamin D deficiency is characterized by low serum 25(OH)D, high PTH (**secondary hyperparathyroidism**), and high serum alkaline phosphatase (ALP).

For symptomatic hypocalcemia, calcium may be administered intravenously.

Hypercalcemia

Hypercalcemia is commonly encountered in clinical practice and results when the flux of calcium into the extracellular fluid compartment from the (1) skeleton, (2) intestine, or (3) kidney is greater than its efflux. Hypercalcemia is caused by (1) increased intestinal absorption, (2) increased renal retention, (3) increased skeletal resorption, or (4) a combination of mechanisms.

Common and many of the uncommon causes of hypercalcemia are listed in Box 39-2. Primary hyperparathyroidism is the most common cause in outpatients, whereas malignancy is the most common cause in hospitalized patients. Together, these two disorders account for 90% to 95% of all cases of hypercalcemia.

Primary hyperparathyroidism is most often caused by an adenoma, but may be caused by hyperplasia involving multiple parathyroid glands, or, rarely, by parathyroid carcinoma.

Greater than 80% of hyperparathyroid patients are relatively free of symptoms on presentation because of the early detection of this disorder by the widespread use of chemistry testing panels that include calcium. The most common signs and symptoms of hypercalcemia are nonspecific and related to the neuromuscular system. With mild hypercalcemia (calcium <12 mg/dL or <3 mmol/L) symptoms include (1) fatigue,

---

BOX 39-1   Causes of Hypocalcemia

Hypoalbuminemia
Chronic renal failure
Magnesium deficiency
Hypoparathyroidism
Pseudohypoparathyroidism
Osteomalacia and rickets due to vitamin D deficiency or resistance
Acute hemorrhagic and edematous pancreatitis
Healing phase of bone disease of treated hyperparathyroidism, hyperthyroidism, and hematological malignancies (hungry bone syndrome)

BOX 39-2   Causes of Hypercalcemia

Primary hyperparathyroidism
   Parathyroid adenoma, hyperplasia, carcinoma
   Familial
      Multiple endocrine neoplasia type I
      Multiple endocrine neoplasia type II
Malignancy
   Skeletal metastases
   Humoral hypercalcemia
      Parathyroid hormone—related protein (PTHrP)
      Growth factor(s) (e.g., epidermal and platelet-derived)
   Hematological malignancy
      Cytokines (interleukin-1, tumor necrosis factor, etc.)
      1,25-Dihydroxyvitamin D (lymphoma)
   Coexistent primary hyperparathyroidism
Other endocrine disorders
   Hyperthyroidism
   Hypothyroidism
   Acromegaly
   Acute adrenal insufficiency
   Pheochromocytoma
Familial hypocalciuric hypercalcemia
Idiopathic hypercalcemia of infancy
Vitamin overdose, vitamin D or A
Granulomatous diseases (e.g., sarcoidosis, tuberculosis)
Renal failure
   Chronic, acute (diuretic phase) or after transplant
Chlorothiazide diuretics
Lithium therapy
Milk-alkali syndrome
Hyperalimentation regimens
Immobilization
Increased serum proteins
   Hemoconcentration
   Paraprotein

(2) malaise, and (3) weakness; at higher concentrations, (4) depression, (5) apathy, and (6) inability to concentrate may be present. Hypercalcemia may induce mild nephrogenic *diabetes insipidus* with increased thirst and increased urination. Chronic hypercalcemia with hypercalciuria has been known to lead to formation of calcium-containing kidney stones, which, in some cases, leads to slowly developing renal failure. The majority of patients with primary hyperparathyroidism (>60%) are postmenopausal women.

Primary hyperparathyroidism is diagnosed by laboratory investigations. Hypercalcemia should be documented by measuring total calcium and serum albumin, or ideally free calcium, on more than one occasion before initiating further testing. Measurement of intact PTH (with concomitant measurement of calcium) is the most sensitive and specific test for parathyroid function and is central to the differential diagnosis of hypercalcemia. In parathyroid-related hypercalcemia, plasma PTH is not suppressed (below its reference interval). In other causes of hypercalcemia, the high circulating calcium concentration suppresses PTH production by the parathyroid glands. Serum $1,25(OH)_2D$ concentration is usually above the middle of the reference interval in primary hyperparathyroidism, as PTH stimulates its production. By contrast, $1,25(OH)_2D$ (like PTH) is low-normal or suppressed in (1) nonparathyroid hypercalcemia, except in sarcoidosis, (2) other granulomatous diseases, and (3) certain lymphomas in which the pathological tissues contain the 25-hydroxyvitamin D-1α-hydroxylase required to produce $1,25(OH)_2D$.

PTH increases the renal clearance of bicarbonate and phosphate. In hyperparathyroidism, a mild hyperchloremic metabolic acidosis is often present, whereas in nonparathyroid hypercalcemia a mild hypochloremic metabolic alkalosis is likely. Although **hypophosphatemia** is often seen in hyperparathyroidism, the measurement of serum phosphate is of limited value, because hypophosphatemia is also found in hypercalcemic cancer patients.

Patients with primary hyperparathyroidism who have signs of adverse effects of the disorder, such as nephrolithiasis and **osteitis fibrosa**, should undergo parathyroid surgery. If the patient is asymptomatic, guidelines have been established recommending surgery over monitoring depending on the (1) serum calcium concentration, (2) creatinine clearance, (3) concentration of urine calcium, and (4) bone density (http://jcem.endojournals.org/content/87/12/5353.long/accessed November 14, 2013).

Hypercalcemia occurs in 5% to 30% of individuals with cancer. Tumors most commonly cause hypercalcemia by (1) producing **parathyroid hormone–related protein** (PTHrP), which is secreted into the circulation and stimulates bone resorption and/or (2) invasion of the bone by metastatic tumor, which produces local factors that stimulate bone resorption. PTHrP binds to the PTH receptor and is the principal mediator of **humoral hypercalcemia of malignancy** (HHM). Cytokines and PTHrP appear to mediate hypercalcemia in multiple myeloma and other hematological malignancies. Some lymphomas associated with acquired immunodeficiency syndrome or human T-lymphotrophic

virus—1 (HTLV-1) infections cause hypercalcemia by producing $1,25(OH)_2D$. Some patients with cancer have coexisting primary hyperparathyroidism.

Signs and symptoms of hypercalcemia in patients with hypercalcemia due to malignancy include (1) rapid increase in serum calcium concentration, (2) lethargy, (3) obtundation, (4) nausea, and (6) vomiting.

Laboratory test selection is similar to that in suspected hyperparathyroidism. Measurement of PTHrP is rarely needed. In specific instances (e.g., sarcoidosis, lymphoma), measurement of $1,25(OH)_2D$ may be useful.

Therapies are directed toward (1) treating the malignancy, (2) decreasing the serum calcium concentration by saline diuresis, and (3) decreasing osteoclastic resorption (by treatment with bisphosphonate drugs). Glucocorticoids are effective in reducing intestinal adsorption of calcium.

Measurement of Calcium

The methods most widely used for quantifying calcium measure either free (ionized) calcium or total calcium. The term *ionized calcium* is a misnomer, because all plasma or serum calcium is ionized, whether or not it is associated with protein or small anions by ionic binding. Throughout this chapter, the term *free calcium* is used.

Free calcium is considered the best indicator of calcium status because it is biologically active and tightly regulated by PTH and $1,25(OH)_2D$.

Measurement of Total Calcium

Methods used to measure the total serum concentrationos calcium include (1) spectrophotometric methods, (2) ion-specific electrode (ISE) methods , and (3) atomic absorption methods.

Spectrophotometric Methods

These methods use metallochromic indicators that change color when they bind calcium. Although less accurate than atomic absorption spectrometry, they have been easier to automate.

o-Cresolphthalein Complexone Method. In alkaline solution, o-cresolphthalein complexone (CPC) forms a red chromophore with calcium, which is measured at a wavelength between 570 and 580 nm. The sample is diluted with acid to release protein-bound and complexed calcium. Interference by magnesium ions is reduced by (1) the addition of 8-hydroxyquinoline, (2) buffering the reaction mixture to near pH 12, and (3) measurement of the absorbance near 580 nm. Additives reduce the turbidity of lipemic specimens and enhance complex formation. Ethanol or other organic solvents may be included to reduce blank absorbance. Multipoint calibration is recommended, and linearity may be improved by adding sodium acetate. Temperature is controlled because the reaction is temperature-sensitive. The CPC and alkaline reagents are stable separately but have limited stability when combined.

Arsenazo III Method. Arsenazo III, at mildly acidic pH (approximately 6), has much higher affinity for calcium than for magnesium. The solution must be thoroughly buffered, because the spectral properties of arsenazo III are dependent on pH. Binding of calcium to arsenazo III is influenced by buffer and sodium concentration. Interference from most biological pigments is reduced by measuring the calcium-dye complex near 650 nm. With the dry-slide technique, clinically significant interference may be noted in patients receiving citrated blood or blood products. Unlike CPC, arsenazo III is stable as a single reagent.

Ion-Specific Electrode Methods

With ISEs, the specimen is acidified to convert protein-bound and complexed calcium to free calcium before measurement of total calcium. Calcium ISEs are discussed later in this chapter.

Atomic Absorption Methods

Atomic absorption is described in detail in Chapter 9.

Specimen Requirements

Serum and heparinized plasma are the preferred specimens for the measurement of total calcium. Citrate, oxalate, and ethylenediaminetetraacetic acid (EDTA) anticoagulants should not be used because they interfere by forming complexes with calcium. Co-precipitation of calcium with fibrin in heparinized plasma or lipids has been reported with storage or freezing.

Urine specimens should be preserved by adding 20 to 30 mL of 6 mol/L HCl per 24-hour specimen (1 to 2 mL for a random specimen) to prevent calcium salt precipitation. Addition of acid after the collection may not completely dissolve precipitated calcium salts.

Interferences

Hemolysis, icterus, lipemia, paraproteins, magnesium, and gadolinium chelates in contrast agents have been reported to interfere with photometric methods. Many methods use (1) bichromatic analysis, (2) multiwavelength corrections, or (3) blanking to reduce interference. Although hemolysis causes a negative error because red blood cells contain lower concentrations of calcium than does serum, more significant errors may be caused by the spectral interference of hemoglobin. Depending on the method, hemoglobin has been reported to produce either negative or positive interference. In photometric methods, if hemolyzed specimens must be analyzed, blanking with ethylene glycol tetraacetic acid (EGTA) is suggested. Individual instruments and methods should be evaluated for their susceptibility to interferants. Gadolinium magnetic resonance contrast agents (gadodiamide [Omniscan] and gadoversetamide [OptiMARK]) cause a significant error (usually underestimation) in spectrophotometric methods.

How the patient is prepared and the specimen obtained affect both free and total calcium measurements as discussed later in this chapter.

Adjusted or Corrected Total Calcium

Various calculations have been used to adjust or correct total calcium for variations in protein concentration. The following

BOX 39-3	Factors Altering the Distribution of Calcium among the Protein-Bound, Complexed, and Free Pools

Factors Altering Protein Binding of Calcium	Factors Altering Complex Formation
Altered concentration of albumin or globulins	Citrate
Abnormal proteins	Bicarbonate
Heparin	Lactate
pH	Phosphate
Free fatty acids	Pyruvate and β-hydroxybutyrate
Bilirubin	Sulfate
Drugs	Anion gap
Temperature	

equation is often seen in textbooks, but fails to consider the lack of harmonization of albumin and calcium methods, and differences in patient populations:

$$\text{Adjusted Total Calcium (mg/dL)} = \text{Total Calcium (mg/dL)} + 0.8\,[4 - \text{Albumin (g/dL)}]$$

$$\text{Adjusted Total Calcium (mmol/L)} = \text{Total Calcium (mmol/L)} + 0.02\,[40 - \text{Albumin (g/L)}]$$

Some factors limiting the ability of total and adjusted calcium to predict free calcium are listed in Box 39-3. When possible, mathematical adjustments or corrections should be replaced by direct determination of free calcium.

Measurement of Free Calcium

ISEs are widely used for the rapid measurement of free calcium, electrolytes, and blood gases (see Chapters 10 and 24). Calcium ISEs contain a calcium-selective membrane and an internal reference electrode.

Modern calcium ISEs use liquid membranes containing the ion-selective calcium sensor dissolved in an organic liquid trapped in a polymeric matrix. Neutral carriers (e.g., ETH 1001) are the most commonly used calcium sensors, followed by ion exchangers, such as organophosphate.

Temperature affects electrode response and the extent of calcium binding by protein and small anions. Most free calcium analyzers adjust and maintain samples at 37 °C, thereby ensuring that results are physiologically relevant for the majority of patients and allowing samples to be chilled before analysis (see discussion below).

Interferences

Because ISEs measure ion activity, they are affected by the ionic strength of a specimen. Free calcium analyzers and calibrators are optimized for specimens of (1) serum, (2) plasma, or (3) whole blood. Because the ionic strength of these fluids is primarily a result of Na^+ and Cl^- in the plasma or serum, calibrators are usually prepared in buffer and NaCl with a final ionic strength of 160 mmol/kg. Errors occur with specimens other than serum, plasma, or whole blood unless the matrices and ionic strength of the calibrators and samples are matched closely.

Modern electrodes have a high selectivity for calcium over (1) Na^+, (2) K^+, (3) Mg^{2+}, (4) H^+, and (5) Li^+. At physiological concentrations, these cations have little effect on the measurement of free calcium. Wide variations, however, in the concentration of Na^+ and high concentrations of Mg^{2+} and Li^+ may influence the apparent concentration of free calcium.

Newer electrodes use a dialysis membrane or neutral carrier to reduce or eliminate the protein effect observed with earlier electrodes. With current electrodes, the effect is less than 0.02 mmol/L for 1 g/dL (10 g/L) of protein. Protein deposits on the electrode may also act as a divalent cation exchanger, resulting in positive interference with high concentrations of Mg^{2+} Regular instrument maintenance and protein removal are reported to minimize this interference.

A number of chemicals may interfere with calcium ISEs or alter free calcium concentrations. Anionic surfactants and ethanol affect the calcium-selective membrane. Physiological anions, including (1) protein, (2) phosphate, (3) citrate, (4) lactate, (5) sulfate, and (6) oxalate, and chemicals, such as (7) EDTA and (8) EGTA, form complexes with calcium and reduce free calcium.

Effect of pH

The binding of calcium by protein and small anions is influenced by pH in vitro and in vivo. Albumin, with up to 30 binding sites for calcium, accounts for approximately 80% of the protein-bound calcium. Increasing the pH of a specimen in vitro increases the ionization and negative charge on albumin and other proteins, leading to an increase in protein-bound calcium and a decrease in free calcium. Decreasing pH in vitro decreases ionization and negative charge, decreasing protein-bound calcium and increasing free calcium. Free calcium changes by about 5% for each 0.1 unit change in pH.

Because of this inverse relationship between free calcium and pH, specimens should be analyzed at the patient's in vivo blood pH.

Specimen Requirements

Specimens for free calcium measurement must be collected and handled anaerobically and promptly to minimize alterations in pH and free calcium due to the loss of CO_2 and the metabolism of blood cells. Syringes and evacuated tubes should be filled completely and sealed to prevent the loss of CO_2 (increase in pH). Specimens should also be handled to prevent the production of lactic acid (decrease in pH) by erythrocytes or white blood cells during anaerobic metabolism or glycolysis. Unless the specimens can be analyzed or processed promptly, specimens should be (1) collected, (2) transported, and (3) maintained on ice to prevent anaerobic metabolism.

Free calcium is measured in (1) heparinized whole blood, (2) heparinized plasma, or (3) serum. For the majority of laboratories in which specimens are analyzed within 30 minutes, heparinized whole blood may be preferable because it reduces processing time and specimen volume requirements and avoids the alteration in pH associated with centrifugation

at temperatures other than 37 °C. Free calcium is reported to be stable in whole blood specimens for 1 hour at room temperature and for 4 hours at 4 °C. If specimens are not promptly analyzed, they should be collected in an ice water slurry to minimize metabolism, but plasma K^+ concentrations may be significantly increased because of the inhibition of Na^+,K^+-ATPase. If analysis is not completed within 1 hour, serum collected in evacuated gel tubes may be the optimal specimen. The tubes should be filled completely. Once centrifuged, specimens are stable for hours at 25 °C and for days at 4 °C, provided the tube remains sealed. Free calcium has been reported to be less stable in specimens from both acidotic and nonacidotic patients with uremia.

The free calcium concentration and the actual pH of the specimen should be reported on each specimen. The pH is useful in verifying that the specimen has been properly handled. Aerobic handling of specimens and correction of the free calcium to pH 7.4 may be misleading in patients with alkalosis or acidosis and should be avoided.

Effects of Anticoagulants

Heparin is the only acceptable anticoagulant for free calcium determinations, but it lowers free calcium at the concentrations (30 to 100 U/mL or more) found in many conventional blood gas syringes. The use of liquid heparin should be avoided; it may result in falsely low free calcium because of (1) dilution of the blood specimen with liquid heparin, and (2) binding of free calcium by high concentrations of heparin. Citrate, oxalate, and EDTA bind calcium and unacceptably decrease free calcium concentrations.

Several commercially-available syringes are suitable for free calcium determinations: (1) electrolyte-balanced or calcium-titrated heparin syringes (final concentration of 40 to 50 U/mL); (2) very low heparin syringes with heparin in an inert filler, providing a final heparin concentration of 2 to 3 U/mL; and (3) lithium-zinc heparin (50 U/mL) syringes. With electrolyte-balanced or calcium-titrated heparin syringes, the heparin is titrated with calcium so that the plasma free calcium concentration is not appreciably altered at most observed concentrations (3.6 to 6.4 mg/dL, or 0.9 to 1.6 mmol/L); however, some bias may be apparent at very low and high free calcium concentrations. Unlike electrolyte-balanced or calcium-titrated heparin, lithium-zinc heparin does not alter total calcium concentration; magnesium, however, was increased by 0.19 mg/dL or 0.08 mmol/L.

Most evacuated collection tubes, when filled completely, contain concentrations of heparin (15 U/mL) that only slightly decrease free calcium. Specific brands or even batches of syringes, evacuated tubes, and heparin should be carefully evaluated.

Patient Preparation and Sources of Preanalytical Error for Total and Free Calcium Measurements

Patient preparation and specimen collection affect the results of total and free calcium measurements (Box 39-4).

A common and important source of preanalytical error is the increase in total, but not free, calcium associated with tourniquet use and venous occlusion during sampling. Errors of 0.5 to 1.0 mg/dL or 0.12 to 0.25 mmol/L in total calcium may result because of the increase in protein-bound calcium caused by the efflux of water from the vascular compartment during stasis. If a tourniquet is required, it should be applied just before sampling and released within 1 minute.

Fist clenching or other forearm exercise should be avoided before phlebotomy because forearm exercise causes a decrease in pH (lactic acid production) and an increase in free calcium.

Changes in posture cause fluid shifts and alter the concentration of cells and large molecules, including albumin and total calcium (as part of it is protein-bound) in the vascular compartment. Postural changes of about 10% in the concentrations of albumin and other proteins are common, but usually not noticed. By contrast, the changes in calcium are noticed, because the reference interval for calcium is narrow and small differences in measured calcium concentrations move the results from within the reference interval outside it or vice versa. Standing decreases intravascular water and increases the total calcium concentration by 0.2 to 0.8 mg/dL or 0.05 to 0.20 mmol/L. The hemodilution caused by recumbency (along with hypoalbuminemia) contributes to the increased prevalence of hypocalcemia (total, but not free calcium) often observed in hospital patients.

Most other preanalytical factors are less likely to lead to confusion. In a few patients, prolonged immobilization and bed rest lead to bone resorption and increase total and free calcium in blood. Hyperventilation and exercise decrease and increase the concentration of free calcium, respectively, because of changes in serum pH. Both serum free calcium and calcium excretion are lower during the night. Food ingestion has been reported to have various effects, but usually causes a slight increase in serum calcium. Ingestion of calcium salts may increase serum calcium. Hemolysis can alter free calcium because of dilution and alterations in pH and its binding (see previous discussion under Interferences).

Reference Intervals

The reference interval for total calcium in adults is approximately 8.6 to 10.3 mg/dL or 2.15 to 2.57 mmol/L. The reference interval for free calcium in adults is about 4.6 to 5.3 mg/dL or 1.15 to 1.33 mmol/L.

Total calcium declines in parallel with serum albumin during pregnancy, whereas free calcium remains unchanged.

Healthy men and women excrete up to 300 mg or 7.5 mmol of calcium per day on a diet with unrestricted calcium content, and up to 200 mg/day or 5 mmol/day on a calcium-restricted diet (500 mg or 12.5 mmol dietary calcium per day or less for several days).

Because of the dependence of free calcium on pH, it is recommended that pH be measured and reported with all free calcium determinations. This will assist the laboratory and physician in identifying specimens in which inappropriate preanalytical handling has led to an in vitro change in pH.

Whole blood specimens develop a liquid-junction potential different from that of serum or plasma because of the presence of cells. A positive bias in free calcium that is directly proportional to the hematocrit has been reported. In addition, free calcium values have been reported to differ among capillary blood, venous blood, and serum samples because of differences in pH.

The desirable analytical coefficients of variation, based on within-person biological variation, are 0.9% and 1.0% or less, respectively, for free and total calcium.

Phosphate

Phosphorus in the form of inorganic and organic phosphate is an important and widely distributed element in the human body (see Table 39-1 and Table 39-2). Inorganic phosphate is the fraction measured in serum and plasma by clinical laboratories.

Biochemistry and Physiology

Phosphate in plasma exists as both monovalent ($H_2PO_4^-$) and divalent (HPO_4^{2-}) phosphate anions. In blood, organic phosphate esters are located primarily within cells. Inorganic phosphate is a major component of hydroxyapatite in bone.

In the soft tissue, most phosphate is cellular. Most of the phosphate in cells is organic and incorporated into nucleic acids, phospholipids, phosphoproteins, and high-energy compounds, such as adenosine triphosphate (ATP). Phosphate is also an essential element of cyclic nucleotides (such as, cyclic adenosine monophosphate [cAMP]) and

---

BOX 39-4   Preanalytical Factors in Measurement of Serum Total or Free Calcium

In Vivo	In Vitro
Tourniquet use and venous occlusion	Inappropriate anticoagulants
Changes in posture: 10% to 12% increase of total calcium and 5% to 6% increase of free calcium on standing	Dilution with liquid heparin
	Interfering concentrations of heparin
	Contamination with calcium
	Corks, glassware, tubes
Exercise	Specimen handling
Hyperventilation	Alterations in pH (free calcium)
Fist clenching	Adsorption or precipitation of calcium
Alimentary status	
Alterations in protein binding	Spectrophotometric interference
Alterations in complex formation	Hemolysis, icterus, lipemia

TABLE 39-2   Physiochemical States of Calcium, Phosphate, and Magnesium in Normal Plasma

State	Approximate Percent of Total		
	Calcium	Phosphate	Magnesium
Free (ionized)	50	55	55
Protein-bound	40	10	30
Complexed	10	35	15
Total (mg/dL)	8.6-10.3	2.5-4.5	1.7-2.4
(mmol/L)	2.15-2.57	0.81-1.45	0.70-0.99

Modified from Marshall RW. Plasma fractions. In: Nordin BEC, ed. Calcium, phosphate, and magnesium metabolism. London: Churchill Livingstone, 1976:162-85.

nicotinamide-adenine dinucleotide phosphate (NADP). It is important for the activity of several enzymes.

Hypophosphatemia

Hypophosphatemia, defined as the concentration of inorganic phosphate in the serum below the reference interval, usually <2.5 mg/dL or <0.81 mmol/L, is relatively common in hospitalized patients (approximately 2%).

Hypophosphatemia may be present when cellular concentrations are within physiological reference intervals, and cellular phosphate depletion may exist when serum concentrations are within serum reference intervals or even elevated. Hypophosphatemia or phosphate depletion may be caused by (1) a shift of phosphate from extracellular to intracellular spaces, (2) renal phosphate wasting, (3) decreased intestinal absorption, and (4) loss from intracellular phosphate. Box 39-5 lists the commonly encountered causes of hypophosphatemia and phosphate depletion.

Injected insulin and carbohydrate-induced stimulation of insulin secretion increase the transport of phosphate and glucose into cells and thus are common causes of hypophosphatemia. Refeeding of malnourished individuals causes an intracellular shift of phosphate. Respiratory alkalosis leads to an increase in intracellular pH, which activates phosphofructokinase and accelerates glycolysis, causing a shift of phosphate into the cell.

In some instances, (1) excessive PTH secretion, (2) Fanconi syndrome, (3) X-linked hypophosphatemic **rickets**, and (4) tumor-induced **osteomalacia** will result in loss of phosphate in urine and may also cause hypophosphatemia or phosphate depletion.

Hypophosphatemia or phosphate depletion due to inadequate phosphate absorption is less common, given the abundance of phosphate in the diet, but may occur in individuals taking aluminum- or magnesium-containing antacids and in patients with malabsorption. The antacids bind phosphate, thus hindering its absorption. The hypophosphatemia and phosphate depletion in patients with malabsorption may be more closely related to their secondary hyperparathyroidism (and resulting loss of phosphorus in urine) than to malabsorption of phosphate.

Intracellular phosphate may be lost in acidosis as a result of the catabolism of organic compounds within the cell. Diabetic ketoacidosis is associated initially with high-normal to increased serum phosphate. Treatment of the ketosis and acidosis with insulin and intravenous fluids, however, results in a rapid decrease in the serum phosphate concentration. Consequently, patients being treated for diabetic ketoacidosis may have both intracellular phosphate depletion and hyperphosphatemia.

The clinical manifestations of serum phosphate depletion depend on the length and degree of the deficiency. Plasma concentrations <1.5 mg/dL or <0.48 mmol/L may produce clinical manifestations. Because phosphate is necessary for the formation of ATP, both glycolysis and cellular function are impaired by low intracellular phosphate concentrations. Other conditions that may occur in phosphate depletion include (1) muscle

BOX 39-5	Causes of Hypophosphatemia and Phosphate Depletion

Intracellular shift	Decreased net intestinal
Glucose	phosphate absorption
Oral or intravenous	Increased loss
Hyperalimentation	Vomiting
Insulin	Diarrhea
Respiratory alkalosis	Phosphate-binding
Lowered renal phosphate	antacids
threshold	Decreased absorption
Primary or secondary	Malabsorption syndrome
hyperparathyroidism	Vitamin D deficiency
Renal tubular defects	Intracellular phosphate loss
Familial	Acidosis
hypophosphatemia	Ketoacidosis
Fanconi syndrome	Lactic acidosis

weakness, (2) acute respiratory failure, and (3) decreased cardiac output. At very low serum phosphate (<1 mg/dL or <0.32 mmol/L), rhabdomyolysis may occur. Phosphate depletion in erythrocytes decreases erythrocyte 2,3-diphosphoglycerate, which causes tissue hypoxia because of increased affinity of hemoglobin for oxygen. Severe hypophosphatemia (serum phosphate concentration <0.5 mg/dL or <0.16 mmol/L) may result in hemolysis of red blood cells. Mental confusion and frank coma also may be secondary to the low ATP and tissue hypoxia. If hypophosphatemia is chronic, rickets (in children) and osteomalacia (in adults) may develop.

Treatment of hypophosphatemia depends on the degree of hypophosphatemia and the presence of symptoms. Patients with moderate hypophosphatemia may require only treatment of the underlying disorder or oral phosphate supplementation. In patients with severe symptoms of hypophosphatemia, particularly if respiratory muscle weakness is present, parenteral administration of phosphate may be indicated.

Hyperphosphatemia

Hyperphosphatemia is usually secondary to the inability of the kidneys to excrete phosphate, as in renal failure. Moderate increases of serum phosphate occur in individuals with (1) low PTH (hypoparathyroidism), (2) PTH resistance (pseudohypoparathyroidism), or (3) acromegaly (increased growth hormone), caused by an elevated renal phosphate threshold. Other common causes of hyperphosphatemia are listed in Box 39-6.

A rapid increase in serum phosphate may be associated with hypocalcemia. Therefore symptoms may include (1) tetany, (2) seizures, and (3) hypotension. Long-term hyperphosphatemia may be associated with (1) secondary hyperparathyroidism, (2) osteitis fibrosa, and (3) soft tissue calcification of the kidneys, blood vessels, cornea, skin, and periarticular tissue.

Therapy for hyperphosphatemia is directed toward correcting the cause of the high serum phosphate. In renal failure and in hypoparathyroidism, dietary restriction of phosphate and agents that bind phosphate in the intestine (calcium carbonate and others) are useful in lowering the serum phosphate concentrations.

BOX 39-6	Causes of Hyperphosphatemia
Decreased renal phosphate excretion	Increased extracellular phosphate load
Decreased glomerular filtration rate	Transcellular shift
Renal failure, chronic and acute	Lactic acidosis
Increased tubular reabsorption	Respiratory acidosis
Hypoparathyroidism	Untreated diabetic ketoacidosis
Pseudohypoparathyroidism	Cell lysis
Acromegaly	Rhabdomyolysis
Disodium etidronate ingestion	Intravascular hemolysis
Increased phosphate intake	Cytotoxic therapy
Oral or intravenous administration	Leukemia
Phosphate-containing laxatives or enemas	Lymphoma

Measurement of Phosphate

All widely used methods for serum inorganic phosphate are based on the reaction of phosphate ions with ammonium molybdate to form a phosphomolybdate complex that is then measured spectrophotometrically. The colorless phosphomolybdate complex is measured directly by ultraviolet (UV) absorption (340 nm), or it is reduced to colored molybdenum blue (600 to 700 nm) by one of several reducing agents, such as aminonaphtholsulfonic acid (ANS). An acid pH is necessary for the formation of the complexes but must be controlled because both complex formation and reduction of molybdate are dependent on pH. Measurement of unreduced complexes has several advantages, including (1) simplicity, (2) speed, and (3) stability. One disadvantage is the greater interference of hemolysis, icterus, and lipemia at 340 nm.

Specimen Requirements

Serum and heparinized plasma are the preferred specimens for the measurement of phosphate. Concentrations of inorganic phosphate are about 0.2 to 0.3 mg/dL or 0.06 to 0.10 mmol/L lower in heparinized plasma than in serum. Anticoagulants (such as, citrate, oxalate, and EDTA) should not be used because they interfere with the formation of the phosphomolybdate complex.

Phosphate concentrations in plasma or serum are increased by prolonged storage with cells at room temperature or 37 °C. Hemolyzed specimens are unacceptable because erythrocytes contain high concentrations of organic phosphate esters, which hydrolyze to inorganic phosphate. Inorganic phosphate increases by 4 to 5 mg/dL or 1.29 to 1.61 mmol/L per day in hemolyzed specimens stored at 4 °C, more rapidly at room temperature or 37 °C.

Phosphate is stable in separated serum for days at 4 °C and for months when frozen, provided evaporation is prevented.

Interferences

Depending on the method used, positive or negative interference has been noted with (1) hemolyzed, (2) icteric, and (3) lipemic specimens. Mannitol, fluoride, and monoclonal immunoglobulins have also been reported to interfere. Phosphate is a common component of detergents.

Reference Intervals

In adults, the reference interval for serum phosphate is 2.5 to 4.5 milligram of phosphorus per deciliter or 0.81 to 1.45 mmol/L. In children it is higher, 4.0 to 7.0 milligram of phosphorus per deciliter or 1.29 to 2.26 mmol/L, because growth hormone increases the renal phosphate threshold. Serum phosphate is lower during pregnancy. Serum phosphate increases after meals and exercise and exhibits a diurnal variation with higher concentrations in the afternoon and evening.

Urinary phosphate varies with (1) age, (2) muscle mass, (3) renal function, (4) PTH activity, (5) time of day, and (6) other factors. Urinary excretion of phosphate varies widely with diet and is essentially equivalent to dietary intake. On a nonrestricted diet, the reference interval for urinary phosphate is 0.4 to 1.3 g/day or 12.9 to 42.0 mmol/day.

Urine should be collected in 6 mol/L HCl, 20 to 30 mL for a 24-hour specimen, to prevent precipitation of phosphate.

Magnesium

Magnesium is the fourth most abundant cation in the body. Approximately 55% of the total body magnesium is in the skeleton and 45% is intracellular; in cells it is the most prevalent cation (see Table 39-1).

Biochemistry and Physiology

The concentration of magnesium in cells is approximately 2.4 to 7.3 mg/dL or 1 to 3 mmol/L. Within the cell, most of the magnesium is bound to proteins and negatively charged molecules, notably ATP. Extracellular magnesium accounts for about 1% of the total body magnesium content. About 55% of plasma magnesium is free (see Table 39-2).

Magnesium is (1) a cofactor for more than 300 enzymes, (2) required for enzyme substrate complex formation (e.g., MgATP), and (3) an allosteric activator of many enzyme systems. Reducing the serum magnesium concentration results in increased neuromuscular excitability, because magnesium competitively inhibits the entry of calcium into neurons.

Hypomagnesemia/Magnesium Deficiency

Hypomagnesemia is common in hospitals. Ten percent of the patients admitted to city hospitals and as many as 65% of patients in intensive care units may be hypomagnesemic. In many cases, the hypomagnesemia appears to reflect a shift into cells because it resolves without magnesium replacement. The causes of magnesium deficiency are shown in Box 39-7. Moderate or severe magnesium deficiency is usually due to losses of magnesium from the gastrointestinal (GI) tract or kidneys.

Magnesium deficiency is commonly associated with losses from the lower intestine in diarrhea. Because magnesium is

BOX 39-7   Causes of Magnesium Deficiency

Gastrointestinal disorders
   Prolonged nasogastric
      suction
   Malabsorption syndromes
   Extensive bowel resection
   Acute and chronic diarrhea
   Intestinal and biliary fistulas
   Protein-calorie malnutrition
   Acute hemorrhagic
      pancreatitis
   Primary hypomagnesemia
      (neonatal)
Renal loss
   Chronic parenteral fluid
      therapy
   Osmotic diuresis
      Glucose (diabetes
         mellitus)
      Mannitol
      Urea
   Hypercalcemia
   Alcohol
   Drugs
      Diuretics (furosemide,
         ethacrynic acid)

Aminoglycosides
Cisplatin
Cyclosporine
Amphotericin B
Cardiac glycosides
Pentamidine
Tacrolimus
Metabolic acidosis (star-
   vation, ketoacidosis,
   alcoholism)
Renal diseases
   Chronic pyelonephritis,
      interstitial nephritis,
      and glomerulonephritis
   Diuretic phase of acute
      tubular necrosis
   Postobstructive
      nephropathy
   Renal tubular acidosis
   Postrenal transplantation
Primary hypomagnesemia
Phosphate depletion

BOX 39-8   Causes of Hypermagnesemia

Excessive intake
   Orally (usually in the presence of chronic renal failure)
      Antacids
      Cathartic
   Rectally
      Purgation
   Parenterally
      Treatment of pregnancy-induced hypertension
      Treatment of magnesium deficiency
Renal failure
   Chronic, usually with administration of magnesium:
      Antacid
      Cathartic
      Enema
      Infusion
      Dialysis fluid
   Acute
      Rhabdomyolysis
Familial hypocalciuric hypercalcemia
Lithium ingestion

most efficiently absorbed from the distal small bowel, malabsorption and bypass surgery for obesity are also associated with magnesium malabsorption. Nasogastric suction or vomiting may deplete body stores of magnesium as upper GI fluids contain approximately 0.5 mmol/L of magnesium.

Excessive urinary losses of magnesium from the kidneys are important causes of magnesium deficiency in (1) in alcoholism, (2) in diabetes mellitus (osmotic diuresis), (3) with loop diuretics (furosemide) and (4) with aminoglycoside antibiotics. Increased sodium excretion (parenteral fluid therapy) and increased calcium excretion (hypercalcemia) also result in renal magnesium wasting.

Neuromuscular hyperexcitability with tetany and seizures may be present. Magnesium deficiency impairs PTH secretion and causes end-organ resistance to PTH, which may result in hypocalcemia. Cardiac arrhythmias have been associated with magnesium deficiency and are partly caused by the hypokalemia and intracellular potassium depletion that occur in magnesium deficiency.

Hypomagnesemia is not necessarily an indication of magnesium deficiency. Conversely, intracellular magnesium depletion and magnesium deficiency may exist despite a normal serum magnesium concentration.

Acute symptomatic magnesium deficiency is usually treated with parenteral magnesium; mild depletion may be treated with oral magnesium.

Hypermagnesemia

Magnesium intoxication is not common, although serum magnesium concentrations may be mildly or moderately increased in as many as 12% of hospital patients. Symptomatic **hypermagnesemia** is usually caused by excessive intake, resulting from the administration of (1) antacids, (2) enemas, and (3) parenteral fluids containing magnesium (Box 39-8). Most symptomatic patients have concomitant renal failure, which limits the ability of the kidneys to excrete excess magnesium. Magnesium is a standard therapy for pregnancy-induced hypertension (preeclampsia and eclampsia); magnesium intoxication may be seen in mothers and their neonates.

Depression of the neuromuscular system is the most common manifestation of magnesium intoxication. Deep tendon reflexes disappear at a serum magnesium concentration above 5 to 9 mg/dL or 2.06 to 3.70 mmol/L, whereas depressed respiration and apnea, caused by paralysis of voluntary muscles, may occur at serum magnesium concentrations >10 to 12 mg/dL (or >4.11 to 4.94 mmol/L) with cardiac arrest at even higher concentrations.

Because calcium acutely antagonizes the toxic effects of magnesium, patients with severe magnesium intoxication may be treated with intravenous calcium. If necessary, peritoneal dialysis or hemodialysis against a low-magnesium dialysis bath effectively lowers the serum magnesium concentration.

Measurement of Total Magnesium

Serum and plasma total magnesium are commonly measured by spectrophotometric methods and occasionally by atomic absorption methods.

Spectrophotometric Methods

Spectrophotometric methods are commonly used to measure magnesium. These methods are defined by the key reagents which include (1) calmagite and methylthymol blue, (2) formazan dye, (2), magon (xylidyl blue), (3) chlorophosphonazo III, and (4) arsenazol. These metallochromic indicators generally form a colored complex (red or blue) with magnesium in alkaline solution, which is measured at around 600 nm. Specific calcium chelating agents (such as EGTA) are added to reduce interference by calcium.

Measurement of Free (Ionized) Magnesium

Free magnesium is determined in (1) whole blood, (2) plasma, or (3) serum by use of commercially-available instruments using ISEs with neutral carrier ionophores. Current ionophores and electrodes, however, have insufficient selectivity for magnesium over calcium. Free calcium is simultaneously determined and used with the signal from the magnesium electrode to calculate free magnesium concentrations.

Specimen Requirements

Serum and heparinized plasma are the preferred specimens for measuring magnesium. Anticoagulants such as (1) zinc heparin, (2) lithium-zinc heparin, and (3) some of the newer heparins developed for free calcium determinations should be avoided because they increase magnesium. Other anticoagulants such as (1) citrate, (2) oxalate, and (3) EDTA also should not be used as they form complexes with magnesium. Storage of serum for days at 4 °C and for months frozen does not affect measured concentrations of total magnesium, provided evaporation of the specimen is prevented.

Serum or plasma must be separated from the clot or red blood cells as soon as possible to prevent an increase in serum magnesium because of cell leakage. Because erythrocytes contain higher concentrations of magnesium than serum or plasma, hemolyzed specimens are unacceptable. Interference by icterus or lipemia depends on the method and can be decreased by use of bichromatic analysis or blanking with EDTA. Lipemic specimens should be ultracentrifuged.

Urine specimens should be collected in acid (e.g., HCl, 20 to 30 mL of 6 mol/L for a 24-hour specimen) to prevent precipitation of magnesium complexes.

Reference Intervals for Total Magnesium

For adults, the reference interval for serum magnesium is approximately 1.7 to 2.4 mg/dL (0.66 to 1.07 mmol/L). Erythrocytes have magnesium concentrations approximately three times those of serum. Care should be taken when interpreting magnesium concentrations, because results in mg/dL and mEq/L are not readily distinguishable unless the units are attached.

Hormones Regulating Mineral Metabolism

PTH and 1,25(OH)$_2$D are the primary hormones regulating bone and mineral metabolism.[1,3,9,10] Calcitonin has pharmacological actions, but a physiological role has not been established in adults. PTHrP is the principal mediator of HHM.

Parathyroid Hormone

Parathyroid hormone (PTH) is synthesized and secreted by the four parathyroid glands located bilaterally in the neck (two on the left and two on the right), on or near the thyroid gland capsule. The glands are composed of chief and oxyphil cells. These cells (1) synthesize, (2) store, and (3) secrete PTH. Ectopic parathyroid glands in the thorax are not uncommon.

Biochemistry and Physiology

The concentration of PTH in plasma is determined by its synthesis and secretion by the parathyroids and by its metabolism and clearance by the liver and kidneys. PTH acts directly on bone and kidney.

Synthesis and Secretion

PTH is synthesized as a precursor, pre-pro-PTH (Figure 39-3). Both the "pre" and "pro" sequences are cleaved off enzymatically within the cell. Intact PTH (84 amino acids, molecular mass of 9425 Da) is either secreted, stored, or degraded intracellularly.

The concentration of free calcium in blood or extracellular fluid is the primary physiological regulator of PTH synthesis and secretion. Free calcium is sensed by a calcium-sensing receptor in the plasma membrane of parathyroid cells. This receptor activates intracellular events that lead to (1) inhibition of PTH synthesis and secretion and (2) enhancement of PTH metabolism. A decrease of plasma calcium has the opposite effect.

Magnesium and 1,25(OH)$_2$D also influence the synthesis and secretion of PTH. The 1,25(OH)$_2$D interacts with vitamin D receptors in the parathyroid glands to chronically suppress PTH synthesis. Chronic severe hypomagnesemia, such as that occurring in alcoholism, has been associated with impaired PTH secretion, whereas acute hypomagnesemia may stimulate secretion. Hypomagnesemia has also been reported to impair the action of PTH on target cells.

Biological Actions

PTH influences both calcium and phosphate homeostasis, directly through its own actions on both bone and kidney and indirectly on the intestine through 1,25(OH)$_2$D. Biological activity resides in the first third or N-terminal region of PTH. Synthetic PTH(1-34) is at least as potent as PTH(1-84) at stimulating (1) calcemic, (2) phosphaturic, and (3) other biological responses in kidney and bone. PTH exerts its actions by interacting with PTH/PTHrP receptors located in the plasma membrane of target cells; it increases cyclic AMP and initiates a cascade of intracellular events.

In the kidneys, PTH (1) increases calcium reabsorption in the distal convoluted tubule of the nephron, (2) decreases reabsorption of phosphate by the proximal tubule, and (3) inhibits Na$^+$-H$^+$ antiporter activity, which favors a mild hyperchloremic metabolic acidosis in hyperparathyroid states, and (4) induces 25-hydroxyvitamin D-1α-hydroxylase, increasing the production of 1,25(OH)$_2$D, which stimulates intestinal absorption of both calcium and phosphate.

The effects of PTH on bone are complex, as evidenced by its stimulation of either bone resorption or bone formation, depending on the concentration of PTH and on the duration

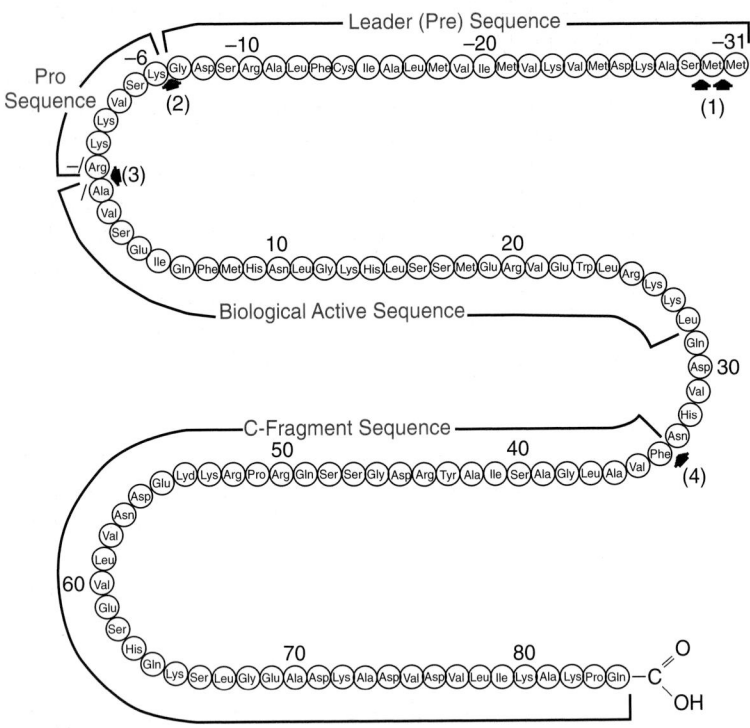

Figure 39-3 Amino acid sequence of pre-proparathyroid hormone. Arrows indicate the sites of cleavage by proteases to remove the N-terminal methionines *(1)*, the leader (pre) sequence *(2)*, and the pro sequence *(3)*, producing intact parathyroid hormone (PTH) (1-84). Cleavage at position *(4)* produces inactive carboxyl (C)-terminal fragments. *(From Habener JF, Rosenblatt M, Potts JT Jr. Parathyroid hormone: biochemical aspects of biosynthesis, secretion, action, and metabolism. Physiol Rev 1984;64:985-1053.)*

of exposure. Bone resorption, a prompt effect, is important for the maintenance of calcium homeostasis, whereas delayed effects are important for extreme systemic needs and skeletal homeostasis.

PTH (1) increases total and free plasma calcium, (2) decreases plasma phosphate, and (3) increases urinary excretion of inorganic phosphate. Urinary calcium is usually increased, because the larger filtered load of calcium (deriving from bone resorption and intestinal calcium absorption) overrides the increased tubular reabsorption of calcium.

Metabolism and Circulating Heterogeneity

PTH circulates as intact hormone and inactive carboxyl (C)-terminal fragments. Its heterogeneity is a consequence of (1) the secretion of both intact and inactive hormone by the parathyroids, (2) peripheral metabolism of intact hormone by liver and kidney, and (3) renal clearance of intact hormone and inactive fragments. In the parathyroids, secretion of intact PTH is increased by hypocalcemia and greatly reduced or absent in hypercalcemia, whereas secretion of inactive fragments persists in hypercalcemia.

Biologically active intact PTH has a half-life in plasma of less than 5 minutes. It is metabolized to inactive fragments in the liver and kidneys. C-terminal fragments are cleared by glomerular filtration and normally have a half-life of less than 1 hour. Their half-life and circulating concentration are increased in individuals with impaired renal function. Generally, 5% to 25% of the total immunoreactive PTH in blood is intact hormone, and 75% to 95% is C-terminal fragments. The relative concentrations of intact hormone and fragments vary with physiology and pathology. More recently, evidence has been presented for circulating forms of PTH missing the first few N-terminal amino acids.[11]

Clinical Significance

Determination of PTH is useful (1) in the differential diagnosis of both hypercalcemia and hypocalcemia, (2) for assessing parathyroid function in renal failure, and (3) for evaluating parathyroid function in bone and mineral disorders. Free or total calcium is usually measured in the same specimen as the PTH because the measured PTH concentration should be interpreted in light of the concomitant calcium result.

PTH is the most important test for differential diagnosis of hypercalcemia. PTH is increased in most patients with primary hyperparathyroidism and below the reference interval in most patients with nonparathyroid hypercalcemia, including those with **hypercalcemia-associated malignancy (HAM)**, the most common cause of nonparathyroid hypercalcemia (Figure 39-4). Primary hyperparathyroidism is (1) most often caused by excessive secretion of PTH by a solitary adenoma, (2) less commonly by multiple hyperplastic glands and (3) uncommonly (<1%) by parathyroid carcinoma. Primary hyperparathyroidism is treated by surgical removal of the adenoma. Intraoperative determination of PTH is helpful in assessing the completeness of parathyroid surgery. A decline of 50% or more from the preoperative concentration is usually considered indicative of successful removal of hyperfunctioning tissue. HAM is usually associated with bone metastases and/or production of PTHrP. Of note, PTHrP does not cross-react in any intact PTH immunoassays that have been evaluated.

PTH is also useful in the differential diagnosis of hypocalcemia. In secondary hyperparathyroidism, PTH is increased before total or free calcium becomes abnormally low. Chronic renal failure is a common cause of hypocalcemia. Magnesium deficiency may impair PTH secretion resulting in unexpectedly low or normal concentrations of PTH. Patients with

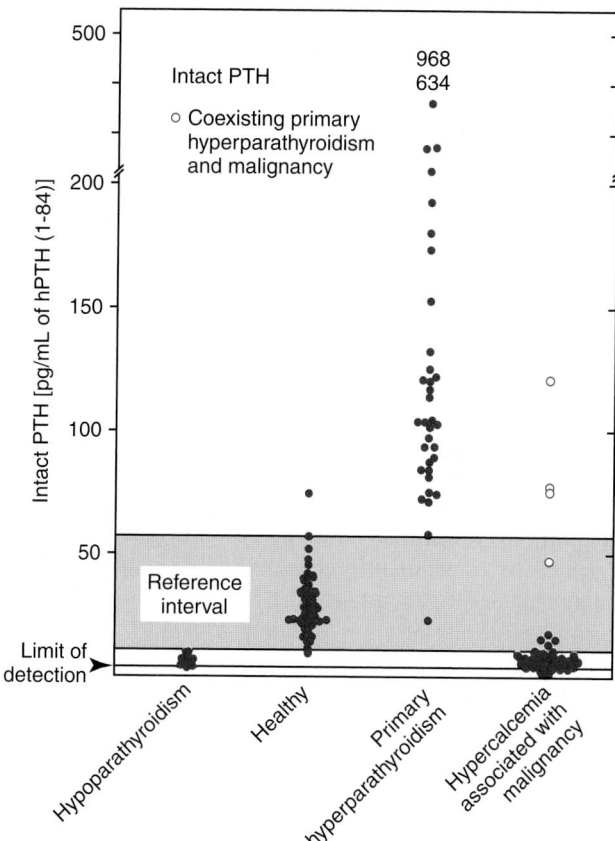

Figure 39-4 Intact parathyroid hormone (PTH) in healthy subjects and patients with primary hyperparathyroidism, hypercalcemia associated with malignancy, and hypoparathyroidism. *(From Endres DB, Villanueva R, Sharp CF Jr, et al. Measurement of parathyroid hormone. Endocrinol Metab Clin North Am 1989;18:611-29.)*

hypoparathyroidism have low concentrations of PTH, whereas PTH is increased in patients with pseudohypoparathyroidism.

In patients with end-stage renal disease, measurement of PTH is helpful in (1) assessing parathyroid function, (2) estimating bone turnover, and (3) improving management (see later section on Metabolic Bone Diseases). Patients with high-turnover bone disease (advanced osteitis fibrosa) have the highest concentration of PTH whereas patients with low-turnover **adynamic bone disease (ABD)**, including osteomalacia, have the lowest concentrations of PTH. A therapeutic goal for intact PTH (as measured with first generation assays) of two to four times the upper limit of the reference interval has been proposed to prevent bone diseases in these patients.

Measurement of Parathyroid Hormone

Two-site or sandwich immunoassays are used to measure intact PTH. These methods require two antibodies capable of simultaneously binding PTH: (1) a solid-phase capture antibody, often directed against the C-terminal region (e.g., amino acid sequences 39-84) and (2) a signal or labeled antibody, often directed against the N-terminal region (e.g., amino acid sequences 1-34). Both antibodies are added in excess to ensure that all PTH is measured. Excess labeled antibody is removed by washing prior to quantification of the labeled antibody

attached to the PTH that is captured by the immobilized capture antibody.

A problem in most first-generation methods for intact PTH is that N-terminal—truncated fragment(s) cross-react. The degree of overestimation of intact PTH by first-generation intact PTH assays is method-dependent. Overestimation of intact PTH by 50% in patients with chronic renal failure or primary hyperparathyroidism and by 20% in healthy individuals is not unusual. Radioimmunoassays and other competitive immunoassays should not be used because they primarily measure inactive C-terminal fragments or are not sensitive enough to adequately measure intact PTH.

Specimen Requirements

Serum or EDTA plasma is generally preferred. After separation, the serum or plasma should be frozen if the analysis is delayed. Lower concentrations of PTH are observed in serum incubated at room temperature for more than a few hours or held a day or more at 4 °C. PTH has been reported to be more stable in EDTA plasma.

Reference Intervals

Reference intervals for PTH are method dependent. Typical reference intervals are 10 to 65 pg/mL or 1.1 to 6.8 pmol/L for first-generation intact PTH and 6 to 40 pg/mL or 0.6 to 4.2 pmol/L for second-generation intact PTH assays. The reported upper limits of the reference intervals may be inappropriately high because of the high prevalence of vitamin D insufficiency, with mild secondary hyperparathyroidism, in the population. Intact PTH concentration is low or normal during pregnancy, but higher during the first few days of life. PTH increases with aging, a possible consequence of mild secondary hyperparathyroidism due to vitamin D insufficiency.

Vitamin D and Its Metabolites

Vitamin D is both produced endogenously by exposure of skin to sunlight and absorbed from foods. Vitamin D is first metabolized to its main circulating form, 25-hydroxyvitamin D [25(OH)D], and then to its biologically more active form, 1,25-dihydroxyvitamin D [1,25(OH)$_2$D], a hormone regulating calcium and phosphate metabolism. The circulating concentration of 25(OH)D reflects vitamin D nutritional status.[3,5,9,10] Deficiency of vitamin D results in impaired formation of bone, producing rickets in children and osteomalacia in adults.

Biochemistry and Physiology

Vitamin D and its metabolites may be categorized as either cholecalciferols or ergocalciferols (Figure 39-5). Cholecalciferol (vitamin D$_3$) is the parent compound of the naturally occurring family and is produced in the skin from 7-dehydrocholesterol on exposure to the UV B portion of sunlight. Factors that influence production of vitamin D$_3$ by the skin include (1) latitude, (2) season of the year, (3) aging, (4) sunscreen use, and (5) skin pigmentation. Vitamin D$_2$ (ergocalciferol), the parent compound of the other vitamin D family, is manufactured by irradiation of ergosterol produced by yeasts. Vitamin D$_2$ differs from vitamin D$_3$ by the presence of

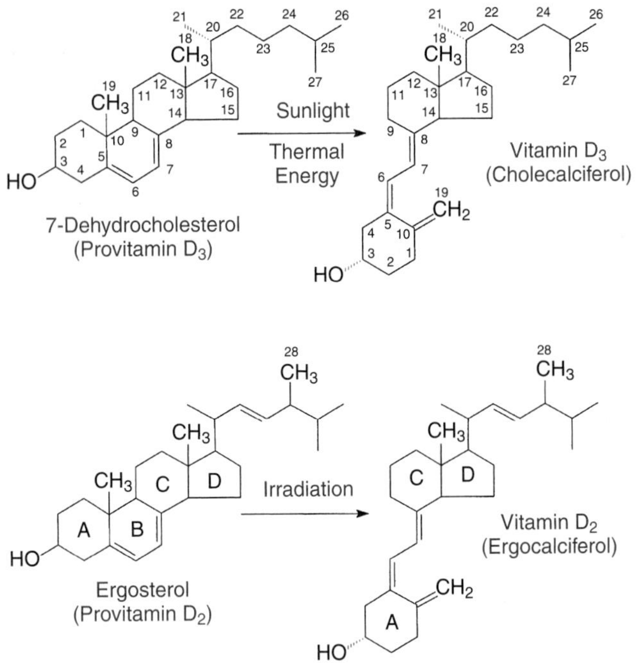

Figure 39-5 Structure of vitamin D$_3$ (cholecalciferol) and vitamin D$_2$ (ergocalciferol) and their precursors. 7-Cholecalciferol is produced in the skin from exposure of 7-dehydrocholesterol to sunlight. Ergocalciferol is produced commercially by irradiation of ergosterol. *(Modified from Holick MF, Adams JS. Vitamin D metabolism and biological function. In: Avioli LV, Krane SM, eds. Metabolic bone disease, 2nd edition. Philadelphia: WB Saunders, 1990:155-95.)*

a double bond between carbon 22 and carbon 23 and a methyl group on carbon 24. When vitamin D or its metabolites are written without a subscript, both families are included.

Vitamin D may be acquired by exposure of skin to sunlight or ingestion of foods containing vitamin D or its metabolites. Only a few foods, primarily (1) fish liver oils, (2) fatty fish, (3) egg yolks, and (4) liver, naturally contain significant amounts of vitamin D. Consequently, before foods were supplemented with vitamin D$_2$ or vitamin D$_3$, most vitamin D in the body was produced by synthesis in skin. In North America, a considerable fraction of vitamin D is acquired by ingestion of fortified foods such as (1) cereals, (2) bread products, (3) milk and (4) vitamin D supplements. The recommended daily allowance is 400 IU (10 µg), although higher requirements (800 to 1000 IU) may be needed in the elderly.

Metabolism, Regulation, and Transport

Vitamin D$_2$ and vitamin D$_3$ are metabolized to 25(OH)D$_2$ and 25(OH)D$_3$, respectively, in the liver by vitamin D-25-hydroxylase. These metabolites are then further metabolized to 1,25(OH)$_2$D$_2$ and 1,25(OH)$_2$D$_3$, respectively, in the kidneys (and also in the placenta in pregnant women) by 25(OH)D-1α-hydroxylase (Figure 39-6). The biologically most-active form of vitamin D is 1,25(OH)$_2$D, whereas 25(OH)D is the main circulating form of vitamin D (Table 39-3). Circulating concentrations of 1,25(OH)$_2$D are approximately 15 to 60 pg/mL (36 to 144 pmol/L), and those of 25(OH)D are 10 to 65 ng/mL (25 to 162 nmol/L) . The half-life of 1,25(OH)$_2$D in

plasma is 4 to 6 hours, whereas the half-life of 25(OH)D is 2 to 3 weeks.

Circulating concentrations of 1,25(OH)$_2$D are tightly regulated, primarily by circulating concentrations of (1) PTH, (2) phosphate, (3) calcium, and (4) 1,25(OH)$_2$D itself. PTH and hypophosphatemia increase the synthesis of 1,25(OH)$_2$D by increasing 25(OH)D-1α-hydroxylase activity, whereas hypocalcemia acts indirectly by stimulating the secretion of PTH. Hypercalcemia, hyperphosphatemia, and 1,25(OH)$_2$D reduce 25(OH)D-1α-hydroxylase activity and production of 1,25(OH)$_2$D. 1,25[OH]$_2$D also induces 25(OH)D-24-hydroxylase, an enzyme producing 24,25-dihydroxyvitamin D (24,25[OH]$_2$D), which is the most prevalent dihydroxylated vitamin D form in serum. The activity of this enzyme may reduce the formation of biologically active 1,25(OH)$_2$D.

In the circulation, vitamin D, 25(OH)D, and 1,25(OH)$_2$D are bound to vitamin D—binding protein (DBP), a specific, high-affinity transport protein also known as *group-specific component*. DBP is synthesized by the liver and circulates in concentrations of approximately 400 mg/L, with fewer than 5% of its binding sites normally occupied. Vitamin D and its metabolites are bound with the following preference: 25(OH)D > 1,25(OH)$_2$D >> vitamin D. Only 0.03% of 25(OH)D and 0.4% of 1,25(OH)$_2$D are normally free in plasma (see Table 39-3). DBP concentrations are increased in pregnancy and with estrogen therapy and decreased in nephrotic syndrome.

Biological Actions of 1,25-Dihydroxyvitamin D

Calcium and phosphate concentrations in serum are maintained by the actions of 1,25(OH)$_2$D on (1) intestine, (2) bone, (3) kidney, and the (4) parathyroids. In the small intestine, 1,25(OH)$_2$D stimulates calcium absorption, primarily in the duodenum, and phosphate absorption in the jejunum and ileum. At high concentrations, it increases bone resorption by inducing monocytic stem cells in bone marrow to differentiate into osteoclasts and by stimulating osteoblasts to produce cytokines and other factors that influence osteoclast activity. By stimulating osteoblasts, 1,25(OH)$_2$D also increases the circulating concentration of **bone alkaline phosphatase (BALP)** and the noncollagenous bone protein **osteocalcin (OC)** (see section on Biochemical Markers of Bone Turnover). In the kidneys, 1,25(OH)$_2$D inhibits its own synthesis and stimulates its metabolism. It also acts directly on the parathyroids to inhibit the synthesis and secretion of PTH. 1,25(OH)$_2$D exerts its actions by associating with a specific nuclear vitamin D receptor.

Clinical Significance

The preferred method for determining vitamin D nutritional status is the measurement of 25(OH)D (Box 39-9), because (1) 25(OH)D is the main circulating form of vitamin D, (2) it has a long half-life, (3) its concentration varies less day-to-day with exposure to sunlight and with dietary intake, and (4) the measurement of 25(OH)D is relatively easy compared with the more technically complicated methods for vitamin D. Groups at higher risk for developing nutritional vitamin D

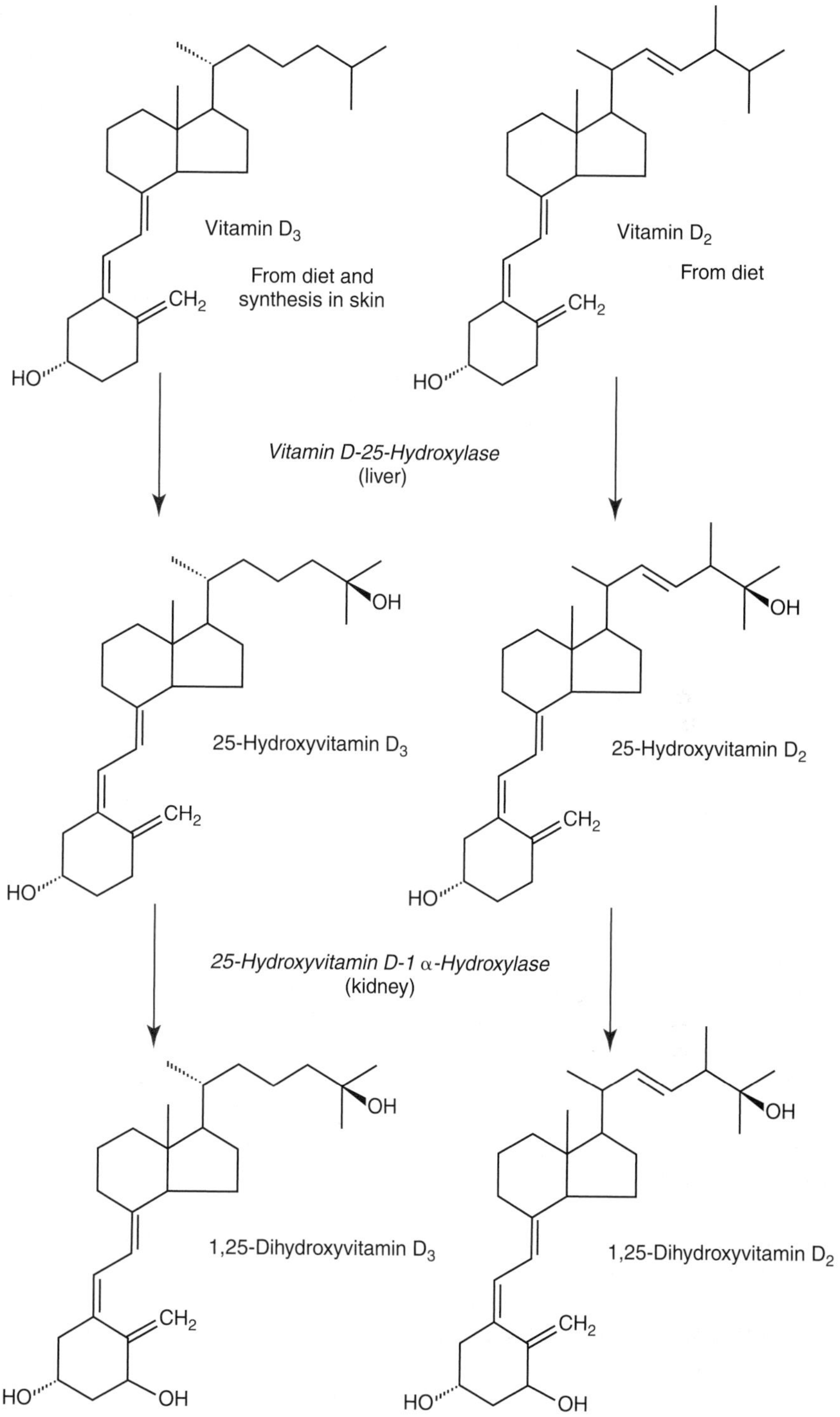

Figure 39-6 Metabolism of vitamin D. Vitamin D_2 and vitamin D_3 are enzymatically hydroxylated to 25-hydroxyvitamin D_2 and D_3 in the liver which are converted to the corresponding two forms of 1,25-dihydroxyvitamin D by the kidneys. 1,25-Dihydroxyvitamin D_2 and 1,25-dihydroxyvitamin D_3 are the most-biologically active forms of vitamin D.

TABLE 39-3 Vitamin D and Its Metabolites in Plasma

Compound	Concentration	Free (%)	Half-Life
Vitamin D	<0.2-20 ng/mL (μg/L) <0.5-52 nmol/L	—	1 to 2 days
25(OH)D	10-65 ng/mL (μg/L) 25-162 nmol/L	0.03	2 to 3 weeks
1,25(OH)₂D	15-60 pg/mL (ng/L) 36-144 pmol/L	0.4	4 to 6 hours

25(OH)D, 25-Hydroxyvitamin D; 1,25(OH)₂D, 1,25-dihydroxyvitamin D.

BOX 39-9 Abnormal Circulating Concentrations of Total 25(OH)D

Decreased 25(OH)D
   Inadequate exposure to sunlight combined with inadaquate dietary
   Inadequate dietary vitamin D combined with inadequate sunlight
   Vitamin D malabsorption combined with inadequate sunlight
   Severe hepatocellular disease
   Increased catabolism (e.g., drugs, such as anticonvulsants)
   Increased loss (nephrotic syndrome)
Increased 25(OH)D
   Vitamin D or 25(OH)D intoxication

deficiency include (1) breast-fed infants, (2) strict vegetarians who abstain from eggs and milk, (3) individuals of color, and (4) the elderly.

Knowing the concentration of 25(OH)D is useful in evaluating (1) hypocalcemia, (2) vitamin D status, (3) bone disease, and (4) other disorders of mineral metabolism. Circulating concentrations of 25(OH)D may be decreased by (1) reduced availability of vitamin D, (2) inadequate conversion of vitamin D to 25(OH)D, (3) accelerated metabolism of 25(OH)D, and (4) urinary loss of 25(OH)D with its transport protein. Reduced availability of vitamin D occurs with (1) inadequate exposure to sunlight, (2) dietary deficiency, (3) malabsorption syndromes, or (4) gastric or small bowel resection. Severe hepatocellular disease has been associated with inadequate conversion of vitamin D to 25(OH)D. Drugs such as (1) phenytoin, (2) phenobarbital, and (3) rifampin induce drug-metabolizing enzymes that accelerate the metabolism of vitamin D and its metabolites. Serum 25(OH)D concentrations may be reduced in patients with nephrotic syndrome because of the urinary loss of DBP and 25(OH)D.

Measurement of 25(OH)D has limited value in hypercalcemia. Its most common use in hypercalcemia is in confirming intoxication after ingestion of large amounts of vitamin D or 25(OH)D. The concentration of the latter is typically greater than 100 ng/mL or 250 nmol/L in such patients.

Measurement of 1,25(OH)$_2$D is useful in detecting inadequate or excessive hormone production in the evaluation of (1) hypercalcemia, (2) hypercalciuria, (3) hypocalcemia, and (4) bone and mineral disorders (Box 39-10). Because activated macrophages convert 25(OH)D to 1,25(OH)$_2$D, serum concentrations of 1,25(OH)$_2$D are often increased in (1) sarcoidosis, (2) tuberculosis, and (3) other granulomatous diseases. Lymphoma may also be associated with increased concentrations of 1,25(OH)$_2$D. Concentrations of 1,25(OH)$_2$D are elevated in vitamin D—dependent rickets type II and in 1,25(OH)$_2$D intoxication, and may be elevated in primary hyperparathyroidism. Those patients with primary hyperparathyroidism who have high concentrations of 1,25(OH)$_2$D appear to be more prone to developing

hypercalciuria and renal stones. Reduced concentrations of 1,25(OH)$_2$D are observed in patients with (1) renal failure, (2) hypercalcemia of malignancy, (3) hyperphosphatemia, (4) hypoparathyroidism, (5) pseudohypoparathyroidism, (6) type I vitamin D—dependent rickets, (7) hypomagnesemia, (8) nephrotic syndrome, and (9) severe hepatocellular disease. Measurement of 1,25(OH)$_2$D, however, is not useful in confirming intoxication with vitamin D or 25(OH)D, because 1,25(OH)$_2$D concentrations may be (1) low, (2) within physiological limits, or (3) elevated.

Measurement of Vitamin D Metabolites

Specific and sensitive assays have been developed for 25(OH)D and 1,25(OH)$_2$D. The assays for 25(OH)D and 1,25(OH)$_2$D should measure D$_2$ and D$_3$ metabolites equally (with equimolar reactivity), since both D$_2$ and D$_3$ are metabolized to produce biologically active 1,25(OH)$_2$D. Separate measurement of the D$_2$ and D$_3$ forms does not necessarily distinguish between dietary and endogenous sources of vitamin D, as food is supplemented with D$_2$ and D$_3$.

Most assays for 25(OH)D and 1,25(OH)$_2$D require the following steps: (1) deproteinization or extraction, (2) purification, and (3) quantification. Deproteinization or extraction, usually with acetonitrile, frees the metabolites from DBP. The differences in their polarities because of the numbers of hydroxyl groups have been used to separate vitamin D and its metabolites. With three hydroxyl groups, 1,25(OH)$_2$D is more polar than 25(OH)D with two hydroxyls, which is more polar than vitamin D with only one hydroxyl group. Solid-phase extraction using octadecyl (C$_{18}$)-silica was widely used for partially purifying 1,25(OH)$_2$D. The most popular method used both a reversed-phase C$_{18}$-silica minicolumn and a normal-phase silica minicolumn to separate vitamin D metabolites. This method was modified by eliminating the silica cartridge and using "phase switching" with a single C$_{18}$OH cartridge. The method of quantification depends on the metabolite being measured.

Serum 25(OH)D has been measured by (1) competitive protein binding assay (CPBA), (2) immunoassay, (3) UV absorbance after separation by high-performance liquid chromatography (HPLC), and (4) liquid chromatography-tandem mass spectrometry (LC-MS/MS). CPBAs based on DBP measure both 25(OH)D$_2$ and 25(OH)D$_3$. CPBAs that do not chromatographically separate 25(OH)D from other metabolites overestimate 25(OH)D concentrations by about 10% in healthy individuals. With immunoassays, samples and calibrators are deproteinized with acetonitrile and analyzed after chromatography or directly without chromatography. Although antisera also recognize 24,25(OH)$_2$D, 25,26(OH)$_2$D, and 25(OH)D-26,23-lactone, results are comparable with HPLC because of the much lower concentration of these other metabolites. In practice, HPLC and LC-MS/MS methods are being more used because of evidence that some immunoassays underestimate the vitamin D$_2$ form of 25(OH)D. HPLC and LC-MS/MS methods measure 25(OH)D$_2$ and 25(OH)D$_3$ separately. The sum of the two concentrations is used to determine whether a patient is deficient in vitamin D (or, also, whether a patient

---

BOX 39-10   Abnormal Concentrations of 1,25-Dihydroxyvitamin D

Decreased 1,25(OH)$_2$D
   Renal failure
   Hyperphosphatemia
   Hypomagnesemia
   Hypoparathyroidism
   Pseudohypoparathyroidism
   Vitamin D—dependent rickets, type I
   Hypercalcemia of malignancy
Increased 1,25(OH)$_2$D
   Granulomatous diseases such as sarcoidosis, tuberculosis
   Primary hyperparathyroidism
   Lymphoma
   1,25(OH)$_2$D intoxication
   Vitamin D—dependent rickets, type II

has a vitamin D overdose). It is not appropriate to "treat" an increased or decreased concentration of 25(OH)D$_2$ or 25(OH)D$_3$ when the sum of the two concentrations is normal.

1,25(OH)$_2$D circulates at concentrations 1 X 10^{-3} lower than that of 25(OH)D and at significantly lower concentrations than other dihydroxylated metabolites, greatly complicating its specific determination in serum. The most widely used method requires (1) deproteinization with acetonitrile, (2) oxidation with sodium metaperiodate to eliminate interference from more abundant dihydroxylated metabolites, and (3) purification using a single C$_{18}$-OH cartridge followed by quantification by radioimmunoassay using a radioiodinated analogue of 1,25(OH)$_2$D. In a newer method, purification of 1,25(OH)$_2$D is carried out with immunocapsules containing a gel with immobilized monoclonal anti-1,25OH)$_2$D antibody, followed then by quantification with an automated chemiluminescent immunoassay.[11]

Specimen Requirements

Serum is typically used in the measurement of vitamin D metabolites. Once separated from the clot, metabolites are relatively stable at both room temperature and 4 °C; however, specimens should be frozen if the analysis is delayed. Vitamin D metabolites in serum do not appear to be sensitive to light and do not require special handling in the laboratory.

Reference Intervals

Reference intervals for vitamin D metabolites are method dependent, and the lower limit of 25(OH)D that is optimal for health is controversial. Representative reference intervals are:

25(OH)D: 20 to 65 ng/mL (50 to 162 nmol/L)
1,25(OH)$_2$D: 15 to 60 pg/mL (36 to 144 pmol/L)

Concentrations of <20 to 30 ng/mL (<50 to 75 nmol/L) are associated with increased circulating PTH and reduced calcium absorption. The National Health and Nutrition Examination Survey (NHANES) III study published in 2002 and 2003 reported an unexpectedly high prevalence of low 25(OH)D concentrations; during the winter in the southern United States, 25(OH)D was <20 ng/mL(<50 nmol/L) in 15% of adult Caucasian men and 30% of women with especially high rates in Blacks and intermediate rates in Hispanics.

Circulating concentrations of 25(OH)D are increased by exposure to sunlight and show seasonal variation with the highest concentrations in summer or fall and the lowest concentrations in winter or spring. Concentrations are influenced by latitude, sunscreen use, and skin pigmentation. Serum 25(OH)D concentrations of 100 ng/mL (250 nmol/)L are not uncommon in individuals highly exposed to sunlight, such as lifeguards.

Concentrations of vitamin D metabolites vary with age and are increased in pregnancy. Concentrations of 1,25(OH)$_2$D are higher in pregnancy and in children than adults with the highest concentrations occurring during periods of greatest growth. Although 25(OH)D and 1,25(OH)$_2$D concentrations have been reported to decrease with age, this decline may be a consequence of (1) poor nutrition, (2) reduced exposure to sunlight, and (3) declining health. Concentrations of these metabolites have been unchanged with age in studies limited to healthy and active subjects.

Calcitonin

Calcitonin is secreted by the parafollicular or C cells, which arise from the neural crest and are distributed throughout the thyroid gland. These cells are included in the APUD (*a*mine *p*recursor *u*ptake and *d*ecarboxylation) family, which explains the association of medullary thyroid carcinoma (a tumor of the C cells) and other tumors of the APUD family in multiple endocrine neoplasia types 2A and 2B (MEN-2A and MEN-2B). Calcitonin as a tumor marker is discussed in Chapter 20. It is unclear whether calcitonin has any physiological role in mineral homeostasis in adult humans.

Parathyroid Hormone–Related Protein

Parathyroid hormone–related protein (PTHrP) was discovered by investigators studying the mechanism by which certain cancers produce HHM.

Biochemistry and Physiology

PTHrP is derived from a gene on chromosome 12 that is distinct from the PTH gene on chromosome 11. Three isoforms of (1) 139, (2) 141, and (3) 173 amino acids are predicted by alternative messenger RNA (mRNA) splicing. The PTH-like activity of PTHrP is contained within the 36 N-terminal amino acids. At the N-terminal end of the molecule, 8 of the first 13 amino acids are identical with those of PTH. PTHrP interacts with the PTH type 1 receptor, mimicking the biological actions of PTH in classic target tissues, including bone and kidney. Like PTH, PTHrP causes (1) hypercalcemia, (2) hypophosphatemia and (3) increased urinary cyclic AMP. When compared with patients with primary hyperparathyroidism, patients with PTHrP-induced hypercalcemia have lower concentrations of 1,25(OH)$_2$D and more typically have (1) metabolic alkalosis (instead of hyperchloremic metabolic acidosis), (2) less distal tubular calcium reabsorption, and (3) less (and uncoupled) bone formation.

Besides its endocrine role in the pathophysiology of HHM, PTHrP appears to participate in healthy physiology by acting locally on cells or tissue as an autocrine or paracrine factor. PTHrP is widely expressed in most healthy tissues of fetuses and adults. Although it is unlikely that the low circulating concentrations of PTHrP have a significant effect on calcium homeostasis in healthy adults, PTHrP may exert endocrine effects on calcium homeostasis during fetal life and lactation. Body fluids that contain high concentrations of PTHrP include breast milk and amniotic fluid.

Clinical Significance

Hypercalcemia-associated malignancy (HAM) is the second most common cause of hypercalcemia. This frequent paraneoplastic syndrome occurs primarily through HHM and/or local osteolysis with the former accounting for the majority of cases of HAM. HHM is common in patients with (1) squamous (lung, head and neck, esophagus, cervix, vulva, skin, and other sites), (2) renal, (3) bladder, and (4) ovarian carcinomas.

Hypercalcemia due to skeletal metastases and local osteolysis is common in (1) breast cancer, (2) multiple myeloma, (3) lymphomas, and (4) other hematological malignancies. The hypercalcemia of a subset of lymphomas appears to be caused by HHM. Breast carcinomas may cause hypercalcemia by HHM and/or skeletal metastases with local osteolysis.

PTHrP is the principal mediator of HHM. After being secreted by tumors, PTHrP circulates and acts on its target tissues (skeleton and kidney) as an endocrine hormone causing hypercalcemia. PTHrP is increased in 50% to 90% of patients with HAM. PTHrP concentrations have been less frequently elevated in patients with hypercalcemia associated with hematological malignancies (e.g., multiple myeloma). PTHrP is undetectable or within the reference interval for healthy individuals in most, but not all, patients with malignancy not associated with hypercalcemia. Increased concentrations of PTHrP have been reported to precede hypercalcemia in some patients with malignancy.

PTHrP determinations are usually considered investigational, because HHM nearly always occurs in advanced disease when the diagnosis is obvious. The need for PTHrP determinations may increase if it becomes important in prognosis, selection of therapy, or monitoring.

Measurement of Parathyroid Hormone–Related Protein

A number of competitive and noncompetitive immunoassays have been used for measuring PTHrP in plasma from patients with HHM.

Specimen Requirements

PTHrP is unstable in serum and plasma at 4 °C and at room temperature unless collected in the presence of protease inhibitors. A combined mixture of (1) aprotinin, (2) leupeptin, (3) pepstatin, and (4) EDTA provides the greatest protection. In general, specimens should be collected with protease inhibitors and kept on ice. Serum or plasma should be promptly separated from the clot or cells and should be frozen.

Reference Intervals

Reference intervals for PTHrP are method dependent. One of the most widely used commercially-available noncompetitive immunoassays has a reference interval of 1.3 pmol/L or less. PTHrP is reported to be detectable in approximately 50% to 80% of healthy individuals with the most sensitive methods.

Integrated Control of Mineral Metabolism

The metabolism of calcium is linked intimately with that of phosphate (Figure 39-7). The homeostatic mechanisms are directed principally toward the maintenance of normal extracellular calcium and phosphate concentrations, which sustain extracellular and intracellular processes and provide substrates for skeletal mineralization. The parathyroid glands respond to a decrease in free calcium concentration within seconds. During a time of calcium deprivation, the increase in serum PTH rapidly alters both renal and skeletal metabolism.

Of the approximately 10 g (250 mmol) of calcium filtered by the kidneys each day, 65% is reabsorbed in the proximal tubule. Calcium reabsorption here is closely linked to sodium and is independent of PTH. Approximately 10% to 20% of calcium is reclaimed in the thick ascending loop of Henle and 5% to 10% in the distal convoluted tubule. PTH enhances calcium reabsorption at the distal tubule, presumably through a cyclic AMP-dependent mechanism. A small portion of filtered calcium, about 5%, is reabsorbed in the collecting duct via a PTH-independent mechanism.

In contrast to the calcium-conserving effect of PTH on the kidneys, PTH increases renal phosphate excretion at the proximal tubule by directly lowering the renal phosphate threshold. Approximately 6.5 g (210 mmol) of phosphate is filtered by the kidneys each day. Typically, 85% to 90% is reabsorbed by the renal tubules (proximal and distal convoluted tubule). PTH is one of the most important factors regulating the renal phosphate threshold and therefore the serum phosphate concentration.

PTH also increases intestinal calcium absorption by increasing $1,25(OH)_2D$. PTH is a major trophic factor for

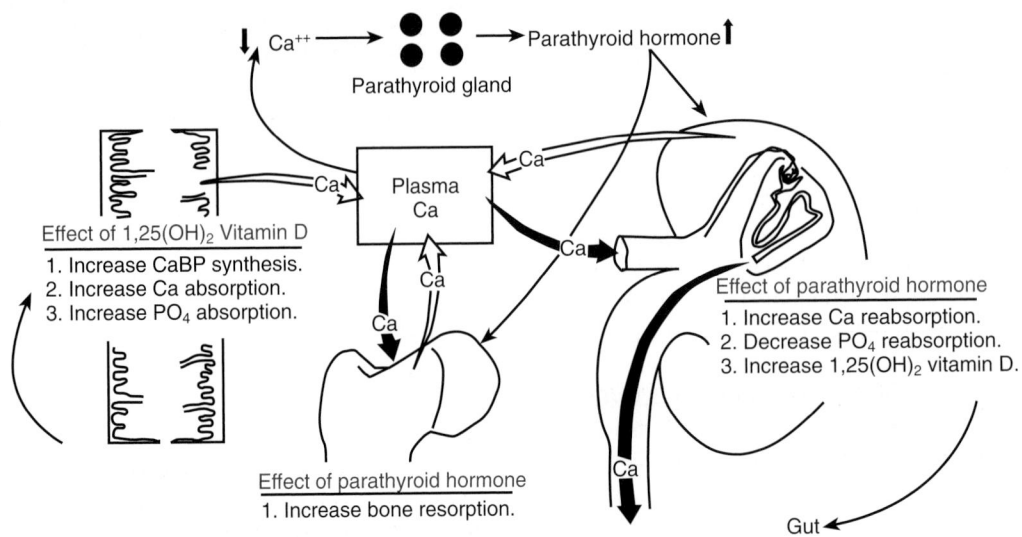

Figure 39-7 Integrated control of mineral metabolism. *CaBP,* Calcium-binding protein.

renal 25(OH)D-1α-hydroxylase. It thus increases the conversion of 25(OH)D to the active vitamin D metabolite, 1,25(OH)₂D. Calcium is absorbed principally in the duodenum, although it also is absorbed by the distal small bowel and colon. About 30% of a daily calcium intake of 1 g (25 mmol) is absorbed. Approximately 100 mg (2.5 mmol) of calcium is secreted into gut lumen by intestinal secretion. Consequently, the net calcium absorption is 200 mg (5.0 mmol)/day. Calcium is absorbed by passive diffusion and by an active transport system. It is estimated that passive diffusion accounts for absorption of about 10% of ingested calcium per day. Active calcium absorption in the duodenum is increased by 1,25(OH)₂D.

Dietary phosphate intake is usually 1.2 to 1.4 g (39 to 45 mmol) per day, nearly twice the recommended intake, of which approximately 60% to 70% is absorbed, principally in the jejunum. As with calcium, both passive and active transport systems exist, with 1,25(OH)₂D being the principal regulator of the active transport of phosphate. PTH-stimulated synthesis of 1,25(OH)₂D thus offsets the phosphaturic effect of PTH. The prevailing serum phosphate concentration also modulates renal 25(OH)D-1α-hydroxylase. Phosphate depletion or hypophosphatemia stimulates formation of 1,25(OH)₂D by the kidneys. In general, at pharmacological concentrations, calcitonin has an effect that is opposite to that of PTH.

PTH also has an acute effect on the skeleton. PTH decreases osteoblastic collagen synthesis, but osteoclastic bone resorption increases with a net increase of mineral (calcium and phosphate) release from bone into the extracellular fluid. PTH is able to act directly on osteoblasts by interacting with their PTH receptors. The effect of PTH on osteoclasts appears to be indirect, through local mediators produced by the osteoblast (e.g., RANK ligand and OPG) or released from the bone matrix (e.g., tissue growth factor beta [TGF-β]). Prolonged calcium deprivation results in enhanced recruitment of osteoclasts and an increased number of mature osteoclasts, which continue to resorb bone, releasing calcium and phosphate and degradation products of the organic bone matrix. Prolonged exposure to PTH eventually also increases osteoblast activity and bone formation.

Despite the critical importance of magnesium in physiology, no hormone or factor has been described as regulating magnesium homeostasis. Magnesium is absorbed efficiently in the intestinal tract (most efficiently in the distal small bowel). In the kidneys, about 25% to 35% of filtered magnesium is passively reabsorbed in the proximal convoluted tubule. The major site of active absorption is the ascending loop of Henle, where 60% to 70% is reabsorbed. During times of magnesium deprivation, urinary magnesium excretion is less than 0.5 mmol/day. When magnesium intake is excessive, any amount greater than the renal threshold is excreted.

Biochemical Markers of Bone Turnover

Biochemical markers of bone turnover are classified as markers of bone formation or bone resorption.

These markers listed in (Table 39-4) have been used for (1) monitoring the effectiveness of therapy, (2) selection of patients for therapy, (3) prediction of bone loss, and (4) prediction of fracture risk. Of these indications, they are mostly used for monitoring the effectiveness of therapy.

Osteoporosis is often characterized by modest alterations in bone turnover, and thus only small changes may occur during therapy. Measurements of bone mass (for example, dual energy x-ray absorptiometry) will identify statistically significant changes in bone mass after 1 to 3 years of treatment. Measurements of bone markers provide earlier assessments than do measurements of bone mass.

In addition to their use in metabolic bone disease, markers of bone turnover are potentially useful tools in diagnosing and monitoring metastatic bone disease.

Preanalytical and Analytical Variables of Bone Turnover Markers

Controllable sources of preanalytical variability include (1) sampling time, (2) sample preservation procedures, and (3) food intake. Bone marker concentrations in urine and serum vary with the time of day because of the diurnal variation of bone resorption and formation. Because of the nocturnal peak in bone turnover, the concentrations of most bone markers peak in the early morning hours (0400 to 0800) and reach their lowest concentrations in the afternoon (1300 to 2300). The amplitude of this variation is greatest for resorption markers with the afternoon values averaging 70% of peak values. Consequently, specimens should be collected at a standardized time of day to minimize the impact of diurnal variability. For urinary markers, collection of the second morning void is often recommended.

Concentrations of urinary resorption markers are usually standardized by dividing by the urinary creatinine concentration. Factors that contribute to the overall variability of urinary resorption markers include (1) the within- and between-method variation in creatinine measurements, (2) the within-subject biological variation in urinary creatinine excretion rates, and (3) the dependence of creatinine excretion rates on muscle mass.

TABLE 39-4	Biochemical Markers of Bone Formation and Resorption
Name	**Abbreviation**
Formation	
Propeptides of Type I Procollagen	PINP and PICP
Bone alkaline phosphatase	BALP
Osteocalcin	OC
Resorption	
Type I Collagen Telopeptides	
N-telopeptide	NTx
C-telopeptide (formed by cathepsin K)	CTx
C-telopeptide (formed by MMPs)	ICTP
Pyridinium Crosslinks	
Free deoxypyridinoline	fDPD
Free deoxypyridinoline and free pyridinoline	fDPD and fPYD
Total deoxypyridinoline and free pyridinoline	tDPD and tPYD
Tartrate-resistant acid phosphatase 5b	TRACP5b

Long-term, within-individual variability of urine markers is generally higher (15% to 60%) than that of serum markers (5% to 10%). Compared with other bone markers, BALP and TRACP5b do not demonstrate significant diurnal variation because of their long half-lives in serum. Food intake has a marked effect only on serum CTx concentration. The variation of serum CTx during the day has a magnitude of about ±±40% around the 24 hour mean mainly due to fasting. With other bone markers, the clinical impact of feeding versus fasting is small. Collection of samples in the fasting state is advantageous for many other tests that are likely to be performed on samples collected for bone-marker testing.

Markers of Bone Formation

Markers of bone formation (Table 39-4) include (1) the amino- or carboxy-terminal propeptides of type I procollagen, (2) **procollagen type I N-terminal propeptide (PINP)**, (3) **procollagen type I carboxy-terminal propeptide (PICP)**, (4) BALP, and (5) OC.

Propeptides of Type I Procollagen (PINP and PICP)

Type I collagen accounts for about 90% of the organic matrix of bone, and is synthesized as a precursor, type I procollagen. Each end (the carboxy-terminal end and the amino-terminal end) of procollagen contains a large domain known as a *propeptide*. The amino- or N-terminal propeptide and the carboxyl- (or C-) terminal propeptide are called PINP and PICP, respectively. To form collagen from procollagen, these propeptides are enzymatically cleaved from the procollagen molecule (in the extracellular space, by two different enzymes), leaving the rod-like collagen molecule in bone. The propeptides are taken up from the circulation via two specific receptor-mediated pathways and degraded by the endothelial cells of the liver.

Clinical Significance

Serum PINP is recommended for use as a reference marker for osteoporosis studies. For example, during the first 2 days of teriparatide (a recombinant form of parathyroid hormone) treatment that induces bone formation, PINP and PICP increase rapidly and continue to increase until the end of 1 month of treatment to a net increase of 110%, whereas resorption markers initially decrease (Figure 39-8). By contrast, during effective *antiresorptive* therapy, markers of bone formation respond more slowly than resorption markers.

Measurement of N-Terminal Propeptide of Type I Procollagen

Assays for PINP are divided into two families (1) intact PINP and (2) total PINP. Intact PINP assays measure only the trimeric form of the propeptide, whereas total PINP measures, in addition, smaller forms, most likely degradation products of the propeptide.

Specimen Requirements

The preferred sample for measuring PINP or PICP is serum where they are very stable. Storage of a serum sample at room temperature for 1 week does not change measurable concentrations.

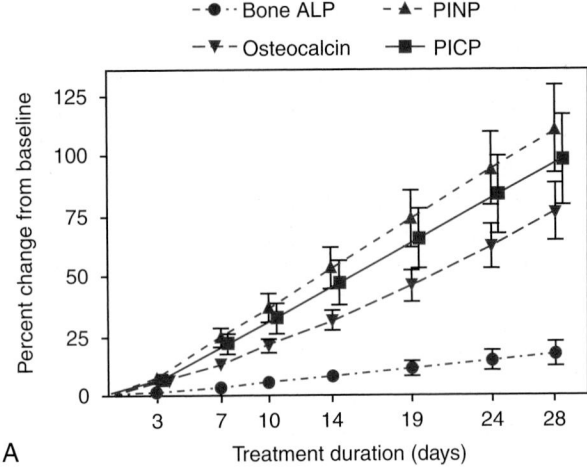

A

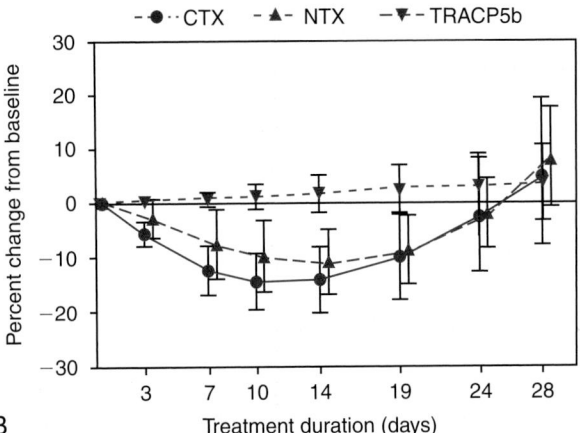

B

Figure 39-8 Changes in biochemical markers of bone metabolism during 28 days of teriparatide [PTH(1-34)] treatment of osteoporosis. *Line plots* show estimated mean and 90% confidence intervals for percentage change from baseline in **(A)** markers of bone formation and **(B)** markers of bone resorption. *Bullet points* at some time points have been slightly shifted horizontally to increase readability. For bone alkaline phosphatase (ALP), osteocalcin (OC), **procollagen type I N-terminal propeptide** (PINP), and procollagen type I carboxy-terminal propeptide (PICP), all changes from baseline are statistically significant (P < 0.0001). For CTx, all changes from baseline until day 19 are statistically significant (P < 0.0004). For N-telopeptide (NTx), all changes from baseline to days 7 to 10 are statistically significant (P < 0.03). For tartrate-resistant acid phosphatase 5b (TRACP5b), no changes are statistically significant. *(From Glover SJ, Eastell R, McCloskey EV, Rogers A, Garnero P, Lowery J, et al. Rapid and robust response of biochemical markers of bone formation to teriparatide therapy. Bone 2009;45:1053-8.)*

Reference Intervals

The reference intervals for PICP are 38 to 202 μg/L in men and 50 to 170 μg/L in women. For intact PINP, the reference intervals in men are 20 to 78 μg/L and in women 19 to 84 μg/L. The reference interval for total PINPI in young healthy premenopausal women (n = 637; age 30 to 39 years) is 16 to 72 μg/L and in men is 14 to 86 μg/L. Conentrations are higher in children, reflecting the child's growth rate. Concentrations increase during growth spurts.

Bone Alkaline Phosphatase

BALPs are membrane-bound ectoenzymes that are found in many tissues, including (1) bone, (2) liver, (3) kidney, (4) intestine, and (5) placenta. The ALP from the first three are isoforms of the same gene product. During mineralization of bone, the main function of BALP is to hydrolyze inorganic pyrophosphate (PPi) to generate phosphate (Pi). BALP is produced by the osteoblast during the matrix maturation phase, when the newly formed collagenous matrix is prepared for the deposition of mineral. Since BALP is firmly bound to the cell membrane, its release to plasma can be delayed. Because of its long half-life ($\approx\approx$40 hours), it is less sensitive than other markers of bone formation to acute changes and is relatively unaffected by diurnal variation.

Clinical Significance

BALP and total alkaline phosphatase (ALP) provide the highest clinical sensitivity and specificity in the diagnosis and monitoring of **Paget disease** of bone. Although total ALP is used most often, BALP is more sensitive than total ALP in mild disease. In severe osteomalacia, BALP may be markedly increased without an increase in bone mineralization because of a mineralizing defect. During teriparatide treatment, BALP is not increased as early or as much as PINP or OC (see Figure 39-8).

Measurement of Bone Alkaline Phosphatase

The activity assays of BALP tend to be technically complicated. A method using wheat germ agglutinin to precipitate BALP does not precipitate all forms from serum from Paget disease patients and fails to completely separate bone and liver activity. Several immunoassays have been reported for BALP, but none of the monoclonal antibodies are completely specific.[11] BALP is stable in serum and does not require special specimen handling.

Reference Intervals

Serum concentrations of BALP are influenced by age and sex. The reference interval of BALP with the IRMA is 5 to 20 µg/L. Children have much higher concentrations, especially during growth spurts.

Osteocalcin

Osteocalcin (OC) is a small protein of 49 amino acids which is the most abundant noncollagenous protein in bone. OC contains three glutamyl residues at amino acid positions 17, 21, and 24, which are formed by vitamin K—dependent enzymatic carboxylation. These carboxylated amino acids bind calcium ions and hydroxyapatite. The exact role of OC in bone formation is unknown. OC knockout mice have increased bone formation, but they also show decreased insulin and higher glucose concentrations in serum. Undercarboxylated OC (about 20% of total) is regarded as an osteoblast-secreted hormone regulating insulin secretion and sensitivity.

Serum OC is cleared by the kidneys and has a half-life of approximately 5 minutes. OC exhibits a diurnal variation with a nocturnal peak, dropping by as much as 50% to a morning nadir. Blood contains both the intact molecule and several proteolytic fragments.

Clinical Significance

The concentration of OC changes rapidly in situations that affect bone turnover. OC is not a pure marker of bone formation since freshly synthesized OC is either secreted into the bloodstream or incorporated into the bone matrix. OC is also released from the bone matrix during bone resorption. During teriparatide treatment, OC increases rapidly but less pronouncedly than PINP and continues to increase until the end of the first month of treatment (see Figure 39-8).

Measurement of Osteocalcin

Many immunoassay methods have been developed for OC. For most assays, specificities with respect to carboxylated and undercarboxylated forms of OC are not known. An immunoassay for the undercarboxylated form of OC uses recombinant human undercarboxylated OC for calibration and two monoclonal antibodies.

Specimen Requirements

OC is rapidly degraded in blood samples at room temperature or at 4 °C. Measured serum OC concentrations are more stable when assessed with methods measuring both intact OC and the N-terminal/midregion fragment (1-43).

Reference Intervals

OC concentrations are influenced by age and sex. In a commercially-available OC enzyme-linked immunosorbent assay (ELISA),[11] the reference interval is 9.6 to 40.0 µg/L in men, 8.4 to 33.9 µg/L in premenopausal women, and 12.8 to 55.0 µg/L in postmenopausal women. Concentrations are higher in children and the highest concentrations are observed during periods of rapid growth.

Markers of Bone Resorption

Except for **tartrate-resistant acid phosphatase 5b (TRACP5b)**, markers of bone resorption (see Table 39-4) are breakdown products of type I collagen.[2,4,9,12] These markers were initially measured in urine, but more recently serum-based methods have been developed.

Collagen Crosslinks

During synthesis, type I collagen molecules are modified extracellularly by formation of intramolecular and intermolecular covalent bonds or crosslinks. Intermolecular cross-linking sites have been located in short non—triple-helical domains at each end of the type I collagen molecule, called *telopeptides*. There are a series of divalent and later trivalent crosslinks (e.g., PYD and DPD). Trivalent crosslinks are also found in soft tissues and in collagen types other than type I (type II, III, etc.).

Degradation of Bone Collagen

Cathepsin K is the main enzyme that degrades bone collagen within the lacuna of the osteoclast. Osteoclasts also produce other proteases, including several *matrix metalloproteinase*

(MMP) enzymes. Cross-linked telopeptides are released from type I collagen during bone resorption. This generates neo-epitopes (such as, **N-telopeptide [NTx]**) that are measured by immunoassays. For C-terminal telopeptides, two distinct immunoassays, **ICTP** and CTx, reflect different enzymatic pathways of bone breakdown. Cathepsin K releases CTx antigen but destroys reactivity in the ICTP assay. ICTP antigen is stable after MMP digestion.

Excretion of hydroxyproline has been used to assess bone turnover or bone resorption because of the relatively high hydroxyproline content of bone proteins, but it is a poor test and is rarely used today.

Comparison of Urine and Serum Analyses

Urine has been used for measuring bone collagen degradation, but urine measurements needs to be corrected for creatinine excretion to adjust for effects of urine concentration or dilution. This includes a second analyte, which has its own analytical variation that adds to the uncertainty of the result. During antiresorptive treatment, urinary telopeptide assessment may overestimate the decrease in bone resorption because the renal metabolism of these peptides can change them. The response to antiresorptive therapy is generally greatest when measured with telopeptide assays, intermediate with total DPD assay, and lowest with free DPD assay.

Clinical Significance of Telopeptides and Crosslinks

Increased concentrations of urinary telopeptides and DPD have been reported in patients with (1) osteoporosis, (2) Paget disease of bone, (3) primary and secondary hyperparathyroidism, (4) hyperthyroidism, and (5) other diseases with increased bone resorption or osteolysis. Treatment of postmenopausal women or osteoporotic individuals with bisphosphonates or other antiresorptive drugs decreases bone resorption markers. Alternatively, teriparatide treatment induces minor changes in the serum concentration of telopeptides or tartrate-resistant acid phosphatase (see Figure 39-8).

Measurement of Telopeptides and Pyridinium Crosslinks

Several methods are commercially available. The most commonly used are (1) serum and urine assays for NTx and CTx, (2) serum assay for ICTP, and a (3) urine assay for DPD.

N-Telopeptide Assay. NTx in urine is measured with a commercially-available ELISA that measures both pyridolines and pyrroles but not uncross-linked precursors. A serum NTx method is also available, but mostly for technical reasons, this assay has not become as widely used as the assay for NTx in urine.

C-Telopeptide CTx Assay. The urinary CTx immunoassay is based on a synthetic peptide of the $\alpha_1(I)$ chain of type I collagen, which includes the cross-linking site. This method recognizes mainly the β-isomer of aspartic acid induced in the sequence. Serum CTx is measured using two monoclonal antibodies. With two $\alpha_1(I)$ chain telopeptides in each collagen molecule, the use of two antibodies directed against the β-isomer ensures that only the β-forms are measured.

C-Telopeptide ICTP Assay. The carboxy-terminal telopeptide of type I collagen (ICTP) assay detects collagen degradation fragments in serum. The epitope measured is vulnerable to digestion by cathepsin K. However, the method is suitable for detecting the osteolytic processes taking place in multiple myeloma or metastatic bone disease, as well as the erosion process in rheumatoid arthritis.

Deoxypyridinoline and Pyridinoline Crosslinks. **Deoxypyridinoline (DPD)** and **Pyridinoline (PYD)** have been measured by HPLC or by immunoassay using automated analyzers or manual ELISA. HPLC methods measure total DPD and total PYD, whereas the immunoassays for DPD or DPD/PYD measure primarily free forms. In urine, approximately 40% of PYD and DPD are free, and 60% is protein bound.

Specimen Requirements

Serum is collected after overnight fasting. Tests using timed or random urine have been used for PYD and telopeptide measurements. Although early studies used 24-hour urine samples, timed or early-morning voided urine samples have also been used. A second morning void, collected by 1000, is most commonly recommended. For treatment monitoring, the specimens should be collected at the same time as the baseline specimen. Peak urinary excretion of PYDs occurs at about 0500 to 0800, reflecting the nocturnal peak in bone turnover. Urinary PYDs reach a nadir between 1400 and 2300.

Reference Intervals

Serum NTx reference intervals are 8.7 to 19.8 nmol BCE/L for premenopausal women and 10.7 to 22.9 nmol BCE/L for men. For urinary NTx the reference intervals are 10 to 110 μmol BCE/mol creatinine and 11 to 103, respectively, for premenopausal women and for men. Serum CTx upper limit is ≤573 ng/L for premenopausal women and ≤584 ng/L for men and the mean of urinary CTx concentration are 220 mg/mol creatinine and 249 mg/mol creatinine, respectively, for premenopausal women and men. The reference interval for serum ICTP concentration is 1.5 to 5.0 μg/L for premenosausal women and men. The reference intervals for free DPD concentration in urine are 3.0 to 7.4 μmol/mol creatinine for premenosausal women and 2.3 to 5.4 μmol/mol creatinine for men. Concentrations are higher in children, especially during periods of rapid bone growth.

Tartrate-Resistant Acid Phosphatase

During bone resorption osteoclasts produce and secrete two tartrate-resistant acid phosphatases. *TRACP5b* is produced by the osteoclasts and *TRACP5a* from other cells. Only about 10% of TRACP circulates in enzymatically active form, and the remaining 90% circulates as inactive fragments. Two commercial immunoassays are available for TRACP5b that show similar specificity and clinical performance.

Clinical Significance

Osteoclasts number can be increased in bone disorders and decreased by antiresorptive treatment. Reflecting these changes, In response to alendronate, TRACP5b decreased 39% in response to treatment with alendronate, compared with decreases of 49% to 69% for urinary telopeptides (CTx and NTx) and 75% for serum CTx.

Specimen Requirements

The preferred sample for measuring TRACP5b is serum. Diurnal variation is minor. TRACP5b may be relatively unstable on storage, although it has been shown that TRACP5b can be stored for up to 8 hours at room temperature and up to 3 days at 4 °C. For long-term storage, it is essential that samples be stored at—80 °C.

Reference Interval

An immunoassay for TRACP5b has upper limits of reference intervals of 4.15 U/L for women and 4.82 U/L for men.

Metabolic Bone Diseases

Metabolic bone diseases result from a partial uncoupling or imbalance between bone resorption and formation.[2,6,7,9,12] Decreased bone mass, or **osteopenia**, is more common than abnormal increases of bone mass. The most prevalent metabolic bone diseases are (1) osteoporosis, (2) osteomalacia and rickets, and (3) **renal osteodystrophy**. In addition to these three diseases that affect the skeleton in general, two diseases characterized by localized bone involvement are (1) Paget disease of bone and (2) bone metastases.

Osteoporosis

Osteoporosis, the most prevalent metabolic bone disease in developed countries, is characterized by (1) loss of bone mass, (2) microarchitectural deterioration of bone tissue, and (3) increased risk of fracture. Women have a lifetime fracture risk three times that of men. One third of women older than 65 suffer vertebral crush fractures. Lifetime risk of hip fracture is 15%. Vertebral fractures occur earlier than hip fractures. Peak bone mass is attained by 30 years of age and decreases after 35 to 45 years of age. Bone loss is approximately 1% per year, but accelerates to about 2% per year after menopause.[2,6,7,12]

After decreased bone mass is documented by bone mass measurements, the diagnostic work-up is directed at determining the cause (Box 39-11). Most often the cause is attributed to age (senile osteoporosis), postmenopausal osteoporosis, or both, but it may be secondary to chronic diseases,

---

BOX 39-11   Causes of Osteoporosis

Failure to develop normal skeletal mass during growth and development because of poor nutrition or inadequate exercise
Endocrine deficiency or excess
   Estrogen or testosterone deficiency
   Cushing syndrome
   Hyperthyroidism
   Hyperparathyroidism
Immobilization or weightlessness
Hematological malignancies (multiple myeloma)
Inherited defects of collagen synthesis (osteogenesis imperfecta)
Systemic mastocytosis
Heparin therapy
Rheumatoid arthritis
Idiopathic juvenile osteoporosis

---

drug therapies, treatment with corticosteroids or thyroxine, or other causes.

In practice, bone markers are measured to assess bone turnover in patients with osteoporosis. The rate of bone turnover (spontaneous or modified by the therapy) is considered an important determinant of bone fragility in postmenopausal and older women. Elevated markers of bone turnover indicate increased bone turnover but are not diagnostic for osteoporosis. Because of the coupling between bone formation and resorption, markers for both bone resorption and bone formation are useful in monitoring the effects of antiresorptive therapy. Teriparatide treatment is best monitored by the measurement of PINP or OC, but resorption markers may change later during therapy (see Figure 39-8).

Of note, the International Osteoporosis Foundation (IOF/ http://www.iofbonehealth.org/accessed November 18, 2013) and International Federation of Clinical Chemistry and Laboratory Medicine (IFCC/ http://www.ifcc.org/accessed November 18, 2013) have recommended for osteoporosis studies one formation marker (serum PINP) and one resorption marker (serum CTx) to be used as reference markers.

Efforts are aimed at prevention of osteoporosis by (1) adequate nutrition, (2) calcium and vitamin D supplementation, and (3) exercise. Treatment of osteoporosis depends on the cause. In secondary osteoporosis, treatment is directed at the underlying condition. Most therapies for the treatment of postmenopausal osteoporosis are directed at decreasing osteoclastic bone resorption. Antiresorptive therapies include administration of (1) bisphosphonates (such as, alendronate and risedronate), (2) estrogen, (3) selective estrogen receptor modulators (raloxifene), and (4) calcitonin (nasal spray or injection). Treatment with teriparatide is the first approved therapy for stimulating bone formation.

Osteomalacia and Rickets

Osteomalacia and rickets are caused by a mineralization defect during bone formation, resulting in an increase in osteoid, the unmineralized organic matrix of bone. Defective mineralization produces rickets in children and osteomalacia in adults. Osteomalacia or rickets is usually due to either vitamin D deficiency or phosphate depletion.

The causes of decreased 25(OH)D and 1,25(OH)$_2$D are listed in Boxes 39-9 and 39-10, respectively. Breast-fed infants, the elderly, strict vegetarians, and individuals with darker skin pigmentation are at increased risk of vitamin D insufficiency. Clinical osteomalacia caused by vitamin D deficiency is uncommon in the United States, but the prevalence of subclinical or mild osteomalacia is unknown. Subclinical osteomalacia may coexist with osteoporosis in elderly patients with poor diets and little exposure to sunlight. Vitamin D deficiency may develop in patients with malabsorption caused by (1) postgastrectomy syndrome, (2) small bowel disease (e.g., celiac sprue), (3) hepatobiliary disease, or (4) pancreatic insufficiency.

Vitamin D resistance is rare. Vitamin D—dependent rickets type I is an inherited defect in 25(OH)D-1α-hydroxylase causing impaired formation of 1,25(OH)$_2$D. The disease is manifested in infancy and is treated with physiological doses of 1,25(OH)$_2$D. Vitamin D—dependent rickets type II is an inherited disorder characterized by very high serum concentrations of 1,25(OH)$_2$D. This syndrome is due to resistance to 1,25(OH)$_2$D, secondary to defects in the 1,25(OH)$_2$D receptor.

Osteomalacia and rickets may also occur because of phosphate depletion. The most common cause of rickets in the United States is hypophosphatemic osteomalacia (also known as *hypophosphatemic vitamin D—resistant rickets* and *vitamin D—resistant rickets*). This disorder is an X-linked dominant inherited trait characterized by renal phosphate wasting. Tubular phosphate wasting also has been known to occur sporadically in adults and as part of Fanconi syndrome. Certain rare mesenchymal tumors may also produce a phosphaturic factor (phosphatonin or fibroblast growth factor [FGF]-23), resulting in renal phosphate wasting and osteomalacia. In developing countries, dietary calcium deprivation may lead to the clinical picture of rickets, without clear vitamin D or phosphate deficiency.

Drugs have also been associated with osteomalacia. Anticonvulsants increase the hepatic catabolism of vitamin D metabolites, and produce end-organ resistance. Phosphate-binding antacids used for treatment of peptic ulcer disease cause osteomalacia by preventing the intestinal absorption of phosphate. Etidronate treatment (of, for example, Paget disease, osteoporosis, or hypercalcemia of malignancy) can cause a mineralization defect and result in osteomalacia.

Clinical manifestations of rickets include bowing of the extremities and short stature. In adults with osteomalacia, bone pain is the most common symptom, and stress fractures and frank skeletal fractures occur in some patients. X-rays show classic findings in rickets, and pseudofractures are common in adults.

In rickets and osteomalacia, the activity of ALP is typically increased because of the increased osteoblastic activity associated with producing unmineralized osteoid. Calcium concentrations may be low or within the reference interval in vitamin D deficiency. Phosphate may be within the healthy reference interval or low, but falls with the development of secondary hyperparathyroidism. Vitamin D nutrition is best assessed by the determination of serum 25(OH)D.

In renal tubular defects of phosphate transport, the serum calcium and PTH concentrations are usually within the healthy reference interval. Renal phosphate defects can be best assessed by studies of renal phosphate handling.

Nutritional rickets and osteomalacia are healed by treatment with physiological doses of vitamin D, whereas higher doses may be required in malabsorption. Adequate dietary intakes of calcium and phosphorus are critical during therapy. Renal phosphate-wasting syndromes require frequent pharmacological administration of oral phosphate.

Disorders of Bone and Mineral in Chronic Kidney Disease (Renal Osteodystrophy)

Renal osteodystrophy is a complex condition that develops in response to abnormalities of the endocrine and excretory functions of the kidneys. It includes all the disorders of bone and mineral metabolism associated with chronic renal failure.[2,8] The renal bone diseases include both high-turnover bone disease (osteitis fibrosa or secondary hyperparathyroidism) and low-turnover bone diseases (osteomalacia and adynamic bone disease).

Osteitis fibrosa (hyperparathyroid bone disease) is the most common high-turnover bone disease. This disorder is caused by the high concentrations of serum PTH in secondary hyperparathyroidism. Secondary hyperparathyroidism is a consequence of the hypocalcemia associated with hyperphosphatemia and 1,25(OH)$_2$D deficiency. Hyperphosphatemia is a result of the kidneys' inability to excrete phosphate. 1,25(OH)$_2$D deficiency results from the decreased renal synthesis of 1,25(OH)$_2$D because of decreased renal mass and suppression of 25(OH)D-1α-hydroxylase activity by high concentrations of phosphate. Deficiency of 1,25(OH)$_2$D leads to reduced intestinal absorption of calcium and reduced inhibition of PTH secretion by 1,25(OH)$_2$D. Skeletal resistance to PTH also contributes to the hypocalcemia and secondary hyperparathyroidism.

Low-turnover bone diseases include osteomalacia and adynamic (also known as *aplastic*) bone diseases. Osteomalacia and adynamic bone disease are distinguished by the extent of unmineralized bone matrix or osteoid that is increased in osteomalacia but low or unchanged in adynamic bone disease. Osteomalacia in chronic renal failure may reflect vitamin D deficiency because of the decreased renal synthesis of 1,25(OH)$_2$D. In the 1970s and 1980s, aluminum intoxication, from the therapeutic use of aluminum-containing antacids to reduce intestinal phosphate absorption, was a significant contributing factor to the development of osteomalacia and adynamic bone disease. Other causes of adynamic renal bone disease include (1) calcium supplementation, (2) excessive vitamin D administration, (3) treatment of hyperparathyroidism, (4) advanced age and osteoporosis, (5) diabetes, (6) corticosteroid therapy, and (7) immobilization. Today, oversuppression of parathyroid function (by calcium carbonate pills, vitamin D, and dialysate solutions with high calcium) is believed to be the main cause of adynamic renal bone disease.

Bone pain is the most common complaint of patients with renal osteodystrophy. Biochemical findings in chronic renal failure include hyperphosphatemia and hypocalcemia. PTH concentrations typically are increased and 1,25(OH)$_2$D decreased. Serum ALP is increased in patients with either hyperparathyroidism or osteomalacia. Management includes restriction of dietary phosphate, use of (aluminum-free) phosphate-binding agents, treatment with 1,25(OH)$_2$D or other active forms of vitamin D, dialysis, and ultimately, transplantation.

Paget Disease of Bone

Paget disease is a localized disease of bone characterized by osteoclastic bone resorption, followed by replacement of bone in a chaotic fashion. It may affect one or several bones. The disease has a restricted geographical distribution, being most common in (1) Europe, (2) North America, (3) Australia, and (4) New Zealand, where it can affect up to 4% of people of Anglo-Saxon descent over 40 years of age. The cause is unknown. A family history of Paget disease is reported by 20% to 30% of patients.

The (1) skull, (2) femur, (3) pelvis, and (4) vertebrae are affected most commonly. In the United States, the disease is most often diagnosed from radiographs or abnormal laboratory tests such as ALP that have been performed for another reason. Bone pain and increased warmth may occur in or over the affected bone. Advanced disease has been known to produce deformities, such as skull enlargement and bowing of the weight-bearing bones such as the femur and tibia. Complications of deformed bone include (1) arthritic symptoms, (2) nerve compression, and in rare cases (3) osteogenic sarcoma.

The most common finding leading to the diagnosis of Paget disease is increased serum activity of ALP (up to tenfold). Increases in markers of bone *resorption* reflect the osteoclastic nature of this disease. Bone markers may be useful in diagnosis and therapeutic monitoring. Radiological examination demonstrates characteristic findings. The bone scan is the most sensitive test for detecting small, early lesions.

Therapy is directed at decreasing osteoclastic bone resorption by administration of bisphosphonates or calcitonin. Surgery is used to treat skeletal deformities that limit mobility or compress nerves.

Involvement of Bone in Malignancies

Bone metastases are the most common skeletal complication of malignancy, occurring in up to 70% of patients with advanced breast or prostate cancer, and to a smaller extent in other carcinomas. Metastases can be (1) markedly osteolytic (as in breast cancer) or (2) predominantly osteoblastic (as in prostate cancer), but often they are (3) mixed. The lesions of multiple myeloma are purely osteolytic as the tumor cells secrete factors that suppress bone formation. Generalized osteoporosis is also a feature of the disease. Many biochemical bone markers, reflecting bone formation or bone resorption, have been investigated for use in early detection or treatment monitoring of bone metastases and myeloma.

Review Questions

1. In regard to calcium and phosphate regulation, the function of 1,25(OH)$_2$D in the small intestine is to
   a. increase bone resorption by inducing the formation of osteoclasts.
   b. stimulate calcium absorption in the duodenum and phosphate absorption in the jejunum.
   c. increase synthesis of alkaline phosphatase (ALP).
   d. inhibit the synthesis and secretion of parathyroid hormone (PTH) by the parathyroid gland.

2. The most important laboratory test for the differential diagnosis of hypercalcemia is
   a. calcium.
   b. phosphate.
   c. calcitonin.
   d. parathyroid hormone (PTH).

3. Which one of the following anticoagulants is acceptable for use when collecting a blood sample for magnesium measurement?
   a. Heparin
   b. Ethylenediaminetetraacetic acid (EDTA)
   c. Sodium citrate
   d. Oxalate

4. Increased transport of phosphate and glucose into cells that is induced by stimulation of insulin secretion will cause
   a. hyperphosphatemia.
   b. hypocalcemia.
   c. pseudohypoparathyroidism.
   d. hypophosphatemia.

5. The protein to which approximately 80% of protein-bound calcium is attached is
   a. calcitonin.
   b. albumin.
   c. immunoglobulin M (IgM).
   d. vitamin D.

6. Hypoparathyroidism is most commonly caused by
   a. chronic renal failure.
   b. decreased dietary intake.
   c. parathyroid gland destruction.
   d. bone tumors.

7. A disease of bone that is characterized by osteoclastic bone resorption followed by chaotic replacement of the bone of, for example, the femur and vertebrae, is
   a. osteomalacia.
   b. osteoporosis.
   c. rickets.
   d. Paget disease.

8. A mineralization defect during bone formation will result in an increase in osteoid. In adults, this will produce
   a. rickets.
   b. osteomalacia.
   c. Paget disease.
   d. osteoporosis.

9. Chronic liver disease will cause hypoproteinemia, particularly of albumin. How will this affect the total serum calcium concentration?
   a. Decrease
   b. Increase
   c. There will be no change.

10. In regard to biochemical markers of bone resorption, most markers reflect which one of the following?
    a. Osteoblast mineralization phase
    b. The amount of vitamin D activity
    c. Some aspect of the degradation of type I collagen
    d. Kidney ability to excrete calcium and phosphate

References

1. Bilezikian JP, Marcus R, Levine MA, eds. The parathyroids: basic and clinical concepts, 2nd edition. San Diego: Academic Press, 2001.

2. Bilezikian JP, Raisz LG, Martin TJ, eds. Principles of bone biology, 3rd edition. San Diego: Academic Press, 2008.

3. DeGroot LJ, Jamison JL, eds. Endocrinology, 5th edition. Philadelphia: WB Saunders, 2005.

4. Eastell R, Baumann M, Hoyle N, Wieczorek L, eds. Bone markers: biochemical and clinical perspectives. London: Martin Dunitz, 2001.

5. Feldman D, Pike JW, Adams JS, eds. Vitamin D, 3rd edition. San Diego: Academic Press, 2011.

6. Kleerekoper M, Siris ES, McClung, eds. The bone and mineral manual: A practical guide. 2nd edition. San Diego: Academic Press, 2005.

7. Marcus R, Feldman D, Nelson DA, Rosen CJ, eds. Osteoporosis, 3rd edition. San Diego: Academic Press, 2011.

8. Massry SG, Coburn JW, Hruska Ket al. National Kidney Foundation K/DOQI Guidelines for Bone Metabolism and Disease in Chronic Kidney Disease 2003, http://www.kidney.org/professionals/kdoqi/guidelines_bone/index.htm.

9. Melmed S, Polonsky KS, Larsen R, Kronenberg HM, eds. Williams textbook of endocrinology, 12th edition. Philadelphia: Saunders, 2008.

10. Rosen C, Compston J, Lian JB, eds. Primer on the metabolic bone diseases and disorders of mineral metabolism, 7th edition. Washington, DC: American Society for Bone and Mineral Research, 2008.

11 Risteli J, Winter WE, Kleerkoper M, Risteli, L. Bone and Mineral Metabolism, In: Burtis C, Ashwood E, Bruns D, eds. Tietz textbook of clinical chemistry and molecular diagnostics, 5th edition. St Louis: Saunders, 2012;1733–801.

12 Seibel MJ, Robins SP, Bilezikian JP, eds. Dynamics of bone and cartilage metabolism, 2nd edition. San Diego: Academic Press, 2006.

Disorders of the Pituitary*

Ishwarlal Jialal, M.D., Ph.D., William E. Winter, M.D., and Roger L. Bertholf, Ph.D.

Objectives

1. Define the following:

Adenohypophysis	Neurohypophysis
Diabetes insipidus	Pituitary adenoma
Gonadotropin	Pituitary gland
Hypophysis	Syndrome of inappropriate
Hypothalamus	antidiuretic hormone
	secretion (SIADH)

2. Describe the structure and function of the pituitary gland including lobes, vascular supply, target endocrine glands, and involvement in the regulation of the endocrine system.
3. List and describe the stimulating and inhibiting hormones synthesized and released by the hypothalamus, including the neurotransmitters involved and feedback loops regulate release.
4. For each of the following hormones, describe their site of synthesis and secretion, biochemistry, regulation, physiological actions, disorders caused by hyper- and hyposecretion (if any), and analytical methods used to assess:

Adrenocorticotropic hormone (ACTH)	Luteinizing hormone (LH)
Antidiuretic hormone (ADH, arginine vasovasopressin)	Oxytocin
Follicle-stimulating hormone (FSH)	Prolactin (PRL)
Growth hormone (GH)	Thyrotropin
Insulin-like growth factor (IGF)	

5. Discuss diabetes insipidus (DI), including causes, symptoms, comparison of these to diabetes mellitus, and the water-deprivation test.
6. State the need for the cosyntropin stimulation test and the insulin tolerance test, including hormones tested, hypothalamic-pituitary axis involved, and expected results.
7. Analyze and solve case studies related to pituitary gland disease and laboratory investigations of them.

Key Words and Definitions

Acromegaly A chronic disease of adults caused by hypersecretion of pituitary growth hormone and characterized by enlargement of many organs and parts of the skeleton and soft tissues.

Adenoma A benign epithelial tumor in which the cells form recognizable glandular structures or in which the cells are derived from glandular epithelium.

Adrenocorticotropic hormone (ACTH, corticotropin) A 39–amino acid peptide hormone secreted by the anterior pituitary gland that stimulates the adrenal cortex to secrete corticosteroids.

Antidiuretic hormone (ADH) A peptide hormone synthesized in the hypothalamus, but stored and released from the posterior pituitary lobe (also known as *arginine vasopressin* and *vasopressin*).

Arginine vasopressin (AVP) A peptide hormone also known as *antidiuretic hormone (ADH)* and *vasopressin (VP)* that is synthesized in the hypothalamus, but released from the posterior pituitary lobe.

beta-lipotropin (β-LPH) An 89–amino acid polypeptide hormone synthesized by the anterior pituitary; it exerts a mild peripheral lipolytic action and serves as a precursor of several hormones.

Corticotropin-releasing hormone (CRH) A neuropeptide released by the hypothalamus that stimulates release of ACTH (corticotropin) by the anterior pituitary gland.

Cushing disease A condition characterized by hyperadrenocorticism that is secondary to excessive anterior pituitary secretion of corticotropin by the pituitary.

Cushing syndrome A complex of symptoms caused by hyperadrenocorticism due either to a neoplasm of the adrenal cortex or adenohypophysis, or to excessive intake of glucocorticoids. When secondary to excessive pituitary secretion of corticotropin, it is known as *Cushing disease*.

*The authors gratefully acknowledge the contributions of Laurence Demers, Wayne Meikle, Nelson B. Watts, Ronald J. Whitley, and Mary Lee Vance on which portions of this chapter are based.

Key Words and Definitions—cont'd

Diabetes insipidus A form of diabetes in which the kidney tubules do not reabsorb sufficient water. Caused by either a deficiency of ADH or defective receptor action.

Follicle-stimulating hormone (FSH) A glycopeptide hormone secreted by the anterior pituitary gland; it has important effects on the ovaries and testes.

Ghrelin A peptide hormone, expressed primarily by the stomach, that stimulates the secretion of growth hormone and is considered a hunger-stimulating hormone.

Gonadotropin-releasing hormone (Gn-RH) Any hypothalamic factor that stimulates the release of both follicle-stimulating hormone and luteinizing hormone.

Growth hormone (GH) A polypeptide of 191 amino acids that is produced by the anterior pituitary and affects the metabolism of carbohydrates, lipids and proteins; it increases IGF-I.

Growth hormone–releasing hormone (GHRH) A hypothalamic hormone that regulates the release of growth hormone.

Hyperprolactinemia A condition characterized by increased levels of prolactin in the blood; in women it is associated with amenorrhea and galactorrhea, and in men it has been reported to cause hypogonadism, impotence, and in some cases gynecomastia.

Insulin-like growth factor (IGF) IGFs I and II (IGF-I and IGF-II) are polypeptides with considerable sequence similarity to insulin; IGF-I mediates some of the effects of growth hormone.

Kallmann syndrome A type of hypogonadotropic hypogonadism caused by failure of fetal gonadotropin-releasing hormone neurons to migrate to the hypothalamus.

Laron syndrome An autosomal recessive syndrome of skeletal growth retardation due to impaired inability to synthesize insulin-like growth factor I, usually because of growth hormone receptor defects. Also called *Laron dwarfism.*

Luteinizing hormone (LH) A glycoprotein gonadotropic hormone secreted by the anterior pituitary.

Oxytocin A nonapeptide hormone synthesized in the hypothalamus and stored in the posterior lobe of the pituitary.

Pituitary dwarfism Short stature caused by decreased synthesis or action of growth hormone.

Pituitary gigantism Excessive growth caused by increased synthesis of growth hormone before the epiphyses have fused.

Pituitary gland An elliptical body located at the base of the brain and attached by a stalk to the hypothalamus, from which it receives important neural and vascular outflow. It is divided into the anterior (adenohypophysis) and posterior (neurohypophysis) pituitary with each responsible for the production of its own unique hormones.

Polydipsia Chronic excessive intake of water as in diabetes mellitus or diabetes insipidus.

Polyuria The passage of a large volume of urine in a given period, which is a characteristic of diabetes mellitus and diabetes insipidus.

Prolactin (PRL) A lactogenic hormone synthesized by the anterior pituitary gland.

Prolactin-inhibiting hormone (PIH) A hormone released by the hypothalamus that inhibits secretion of prolactin by the adenohypophysis. Also known as *prolactin-inhibiting factor* and *prolactostatin.*

Pro-opiomelanocortin (POMC) The 31,000 dalton prohormone that is the precursor of corticotropin, the lipotropins, the melanocyte-stimulating hormones, and the endorphins, all of which are produced by posttranslational proteolytic cleavage of POMC in cell types that produce these hormones.

Somatostatin Any of several cyclic tetradecapeptides produced in the hypothalamus that inhibit release of several hormones of the pituitary.

Syndrome of inappropriate antidiuretic hormone (SIADH) A condition in which inappropriate antidiuretic hormone secretion produces dilutional hyponatremia, and increased extracellular fluid volume with an elevated urine osmolality.

Thyroid-stimulating hormone (TSH) A glycoprotein hormone synthesized by the anterior pituitary gland; also called *thyrotropin.*

Thyrotropin A glycoprotein hormone synthesized by the anterior pituitary gland that promotes the growth of the thyroid gland and stimulates the hormonal secretion by the gland. Also called *thyroid-stimulating* hormone.

Thyrotropin-releasing hormone (TRH) A tripeptide produced in the hypothalamus that stimulates the release of TSH from the anterior pituitary.

The **pituitary gland** (also known as the hypophysis) is located at the base of the skull (Figure 40-1)[10] in a bone cavity called the *sella turcica* (Turkish saddle). The gland is small—1 cm or less in height and width—and weighs approximately 500 mg. It is anatomically divided into the anterior (*adenohypophysis*) and the posterior (*neurohypophysis*) lobes. A third lobe (the intermediate lobe) is present in most vertebrates and in the human fetus; this lobe is rudimentary in the adult human.

Arterial blood reaches the pituitary gland via the superior hypophyseal artery. Venous blood, carrying neurosecretory hormones from the hypothalamus, reaches the pituitary through the hypothalamic hypophyseal portal system. These hypothalamic factors stimulate or inhibit the release of hormones from the adenohypophysis.

The pituitary gland regulates the endocrine system by integrating chemical signals from the brain with regulatory feedback from the concentration of hormones in the circulation to stimulate intermittent hormone release from target endocrine glands.[2,4,5,8] Historically the pituitary gland has been called the *master endocrine organ,* because it is intimately involved in the regulation of (1) growth, (2) development, (3) thyroid function, (4) adrenal function, (5) gonadal function, and (6) water and salt homeostasis.

The adenohypophysis secretes (1) **growth hormone (GH)**, (2) **prolactin (PRL)**, (3) **thyroid-stimulating hormone (TSH)**, (also known as **thyrotropin**), (4) **adrenocorticotropic hormone (ACTH)**, (5) **follicle-stimulating hormone (FSH)**, and (6) **luteinizing hormone (LH)**. TSH, LH, and FSH are glycoprotein hormones that possess a common alpha subunit and a distinct beta subunit that confers biologic specificity. ACTH, PRL, and GH are polypeptide hormones (Table 40-1).[10] The adenohypophysis also secretes **beta-lipotropin (β-LPH)** and a number of smaller peptides of undetermined significance. **Arginine vasopressin** (also known as antidiuretic hormone) and oxytocin are produced in the hypothalamus and are carried through the neurohypophyseal nerve axons to the neurohypophysis. Thus the neurohypophysis is not a discrete endocrine organ, but rather functions as a reservoir for these two hormones.

Of the six major hormones from the adenohypophysis, GH and PRL act primarily on diffuse target tissues with TSH, ACTH, and the gonadotropins (LH and FSH) acting primarily on specific target endocrine glands, specifically the (1) thyroid gland, (2) adrenal cortex, and (3) gonads, respectively (Table 40-2).[10] These peptide hormones originating from the pituitary and related hormones elaborated by the placenta during pregnancy have been classified based on their molecular structure and biochemical evolution.

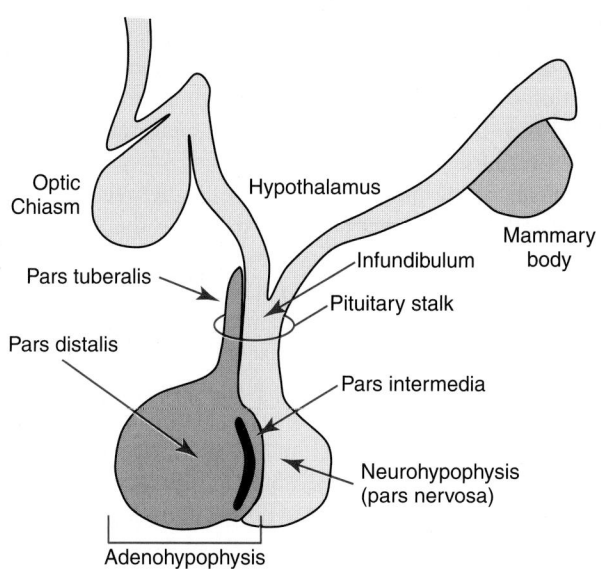

Figure 40-1 The hypophysis (pituitary gland) is composed of the adenohypophysis (the anterior lobe of the pituitary) and the neurohypophysis (the posterior lobe of the pituitary; pars nervosa). The adenohypophysis has three parts: the pars distalis, where most of the hormone-producing cells are located; the pars tuberalis, which is part of the pituitary stalk; and the pars intermedia.

TABLE 40-2	Hypothalamic Hormones and the Anterior Pituitary Hormones That They Regulate, Target Organ or Tissues Regulated by the Anterior Pituitary Hormone, and Hormonal Product of the Target Organ or Tissues

Hypothalamic Hormone(s)	Anterior Pituitary Hormone	Target Organ/Tissue	Target Hormone
CRH	ACTH	Adrenal cortex: zona fasciculata and zona reticularis	Cortisol
TRH	TSH	Thyroid follicular cell	T_4 and T_3
GHRH and Somatostatin	GH	Liver and many tissues of the body	IGF-I, IGHBP-3, and ALS
GnRH	LH, FSH	Gonad	Sex steroids and inhibins
PRIH	PRL	Breast	Not applicable

ACTH, Adrenocorticotropic hormone; *ALS,* acid-labile subunit; *CRH,* corticotropin-releasing hormone; *FSH,* follicle-stimulating hormone; *GH,* growth hormone; *GHRH,* growth hormone-releasing hormone; *GnRH,* gonadotropin-releasing hormone; *IGF-I,* insulin-like growth factor I; *IGHBP-3,* IGF binding protein-3; *LH,* luteinizing hormone; *PRIH,* prolactin release-inhibiting hormone; *PRL,* prolactin; T_3, 3, 5, 3′-triiodothyronine; T_4, thyroxine; *TRH,* thyrotropin-releasing hormone; *TSH,* thyroid-stimulating hormone.

TABLE 40-1	Hypothalamic Releasing or Inhibiting Hormones, Their Target Cells, and the Hormone That Is Regulated

Hypothalamic Hormone/Abbreviation	Amino Acids	Anterior Pituitary Target Cell	Hormone Regulated	Amino Acids	Molecular Weight
Corticotropin-releasing hormone (CRH)	41	Corticotroph	ACTH	39	4.5 kDa
Thyrotropin-releasing hormone (TRH)	3	Thyrotroph	TSH*	alpha: 92 beta: 118	28 kDa
Growth hormone-releasing hormone (GHRH)	44	Somatotroph	GH	191 176	22 kDa 20 kDa
Somatotrophin release-inhibiting hormone†	14	Somatotroph	GH	See above	see above
Gonadotropin-releasing hormone (GnRH)	10	Gonadotroph	LH* FSH*	alpha: 92 beta: 121 alpha: 92 beta: 111	32 kDa 30 kDa
Prolactin release-inhibiting hormone (PRIH)	1	Lactotroph	PRL	199	22 kDa

*All alpha glycoprotein chains are identical, including the alpha chain of human chorionic gonadotropin (hCG).
†Also known as somatostatin.
ACTH, Adrenocorticotropic hormone; *FSH,* follicle-stimulating hormone; *GH,* growth hormone; *LH,* luteinizing hormone; *PRL,* prolactin; *TSH,* thyroid-stimulating hormone.

Hypothalamic Regulation[2-5,8]

Secretion of hormones from the anterior lobe of the pituitary gland is controlled by the hypothalamus, which synthesizes small peptide hormones known as *releasing* or *inhibitory hormones* (Figure 40-2).[2,5,8-10] Several have been characterized including: (1) **corticotropin-releasing hormone (CRH)**, (2) **thyrotropin-releasing hormone (TRH)**, (3) **growth hormone–releasing hormone (GHRH)**, (4) **somatostatin**, (5) **gonadotropin-releasing hormone (GnRH)**, (also called *luteinizing hormone–releasing hormone*), and (6) **prolactin-inhibiting hormone (PIH)** that is actually the neurotransmitter dopamine. In addition, GnRH stimulates the secretion of FSH and LH. However, a separate and distinct releasing factor for FSH has not yet been established, although negative feedback control of this gonadotropin is effected by *inhibin*, a peptide of gonadal origin.

Hormones that have been used to test for pituitary hormone reserve include (1) CRH, (2) TRH, (3) GHRH, and (4) GnRH In addition, pulsatile GnRH administration is used to initiate puberty and to induce ovulation or spermatogenesis. Alternately, GnRH antagonists that inhibit the action of endogenous GnRH are used to treat patients with (1) precocious puberty, (2) endometriosis, (3) uterine fibroids, and (4) prostate carcinoma. GHRH is yet another hypothalamic peptide that is used to treat patients with GH deficiency caused by hypothalamic disease.

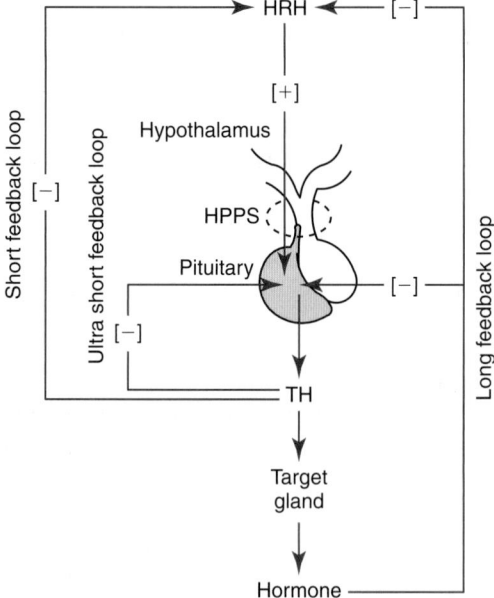

Figure 40-2 Many anterior pituitary trophic hormones (THs) (e.g., ACTH, TSH, GH, LH, and FSH) are regulated by hypothalamic releasing hormones (HRHs). Releasing hormones secreted by the hypothalamus reach the pituitary via the hypothalamic-pituitary portal system (HPPS). Long feedback loops involve negative feedback of the target cell hormone at the pituitary gland and hypothalamus. The short feedback loop involves the anterior pituitary trophic hormone feeding back at the hypothalamus, whereas the ultra-short feedback loop involves the anterior pituitary hormone feeding back at the anterior pituitary. [+], Stimulation; [–], suppression.

The neurons that elaborate hypophysiotropic hormones are themselves influenced by hypothalamic neurotransmitters, such as (1) dopamine, (2) norepinephrine, (3) serotonin, (4) acetylcholine, and (5) endorphins. These neurotransmitters also modify the secretory activity of anterior pituitary hormones. For example, (1) basal and episodic secretion, (2) diurnal rhythm, and (3) nocturnal release of pituitary hormones are all considered to be secondary to central nervous system events that are mediated through hypothalamic hormones.

In addition to higher center regulation of the hypothalamic-pituitary axis by classic neurotransmitters, chemical mediators released by inflammatory cells (cytokines) have been discovered that participate in altering the control mechanisms associated with the neuroendocrine axis. For example, modulation of the feedback loop between the hypothalamic-pituitary-adrenal axis by cytokines, such as *interleukin 1* (IL-1) and *interleukin 6* (IL-6), released as a result of infection or stress, has been shown to diminish the immune system via release of ACTH which then raises cortisol concentrations.

Control of the functional relationship between the pituitary gland and its target organs is based on the principle of feedback control. This feedback is a primarily negative one between the blood concentration of circulating hormones and the pituitary gland and hypothalamus. The effect of negative feedback is typically opposite to that of the initial stimulus. For example, an elevated concentration of cortisol (initial stimulus) reduces the synthesis and the release of CRH, resulting in decreased secretion of ACTH and, ultimately, reduced secretion of cortisol (final response). Such feedback control maintains an optimal concentration of hormone in the blood under a variety of circumstances.

Hormones of the Adenohypophysis[2-5,8]

Hormones of the adenohypophysis are listed in Table 40-2[10] and discussed below.

Growth Hormone and Insulin-Like Growth Factors

The most abundant hormone produced by the adenohypophysis is GH. **Insulin-like growth factor (IGF)** I is a polypeptide synthesized and released by the liver in response to GH. IGF-I (and IGF-II) have considerable amino acid sequence and functional similarity to insulin.

Biochemistry

GH is a single-chain polypeptide with a molecular mass of 21,500 Da that contains 191 amino acids and two intramolecular disulfide bridges. It is structurally similar to PRL and to the placental hormone chorionic somatomammotropin (hCS, placental lactogen), with which it has overlapping biological effects.

GH is synthesized by the somatotropic (acidophilic) cells of the adenohypophysis and is stored within intracellular granules. During the daytime hours, the plasma concentration of GH in healthy adults remains stable and relatively low (<2 ng/mL) with several secretory "spikes" occurring approximately

3 hours after meals and after exercise. In contrast during the evening hours, adults and children show a marked rise in GH secretory activity approximately 90 minutes after the onset of sleep; GH concentrations reach a peak value during the period of deepest sleep. This *pulsatile* pattern of GH secretion may be important to anabolic and repair processes and for proper skeletal growth.

IGFs are polypeptides with high sequence similarity to insulin. Unlike most other peptide hormones, IGFs circulate in blood complexed to specific plasma-binding proteins. Six major IGF-binding proteins have been identified in human plasma. *Insulin-like growth factor binding protein (IGFBP)-3*, a glycosylated binding protein, complexes more than 75% of the circulating IGF-I. The concentration of this binding protein is GH dependent and provides for a circulating reserve pool of IGF-I. Dissociation of the IGFs from the binding proteins occurs before passage through capillary membranes and entrance into tissue, such as cartilage.

Regulation of Release

The release of GH is thought to be controlled by hypothalamic GHRH and somatostatin. The former stimulates GH release and the latter inhibits GH release. Somatostatin is also found in the delta cells of the pancreatic islets and in many other sites in the digestive tract. It has important effects on the secretion of gastrointestinal hormones and causes inhibition of insulin and glucagon release. The hypothalamic influence on GH release appears to be primarily stimulatory through the action of GHRH. Release of these two hypothalamic factors is in turn influenced by higher centers of the brain. Thus different stimuli, such as (1) exercise, (2) physical and emotional stress, (3) hypoglycemia, (4) increased circulating amino acid concentrations (particularly arginine), and (5) hormones (such as, testosterone, estrogens, and thyroxine) evoke an increase in GH secretion. In the presence of abnormally high concentrations of glucocorticoids, GH secretion is suppressed. Other hypothalamic hormones (such as, TRH and GnRH) do not affect GH release in healthy subjects,[6] but may provoke GH release in patients with **acromegaly**.

Isolation and discovery of **ghrelin** revealed the existence of another control system for GH. Ghrelin is a small 28–amino acid peptide released from neuroendocrine cells in the gastric mucosa that binds to the GH secretagogue receptor to induce the secretion of both GHRH and GH itself. Ghrelin also induces food intake.

Physiological Actions

The overall physiological effect of GH is to promote growth in (1) soft tissue, (2) cartilage, and (3) bone. This action results from stimulation of protein synthesis that is partly induced by an increase in amino acid transport through cell membranes. The effects of GH on bone and muscle are exerted both directly and through the effects of IGF-I that is produced in the liver and other tissues under the influence of GH (e.g., bone). The increased growth of soft tissue and the skeleton is accompanied by changes in electrolyte metabolism, including a

(1) positive nitrogen and phosphorus balance, (2) rise in plasma phosphorus concentrations, and (3) fall in blood urea and amino acid concentrations. Additional responses to GH include increased intestinal absorption of calcium and decreased urinary excretion of sodium and potassium. The metabolic changes are thought to result from the increased uptake of these ions by growing tissue. GH has other effects on intermediary metabolism. For example, GH stimulates the uptake of nonesterified fatty acids by muscle and accelerates the mobilization and metabolism of fat from adipose tissue to the liver. Chronic GH excess stimulates hepatic glycogenolysis and antagonizes the effect of insulin on glucose uptake by peripheral cells leading to an increase in blood glucose concentrations. GH and insulin induce growth in a similar manner because both have protein anabolic effects and stimulate the transport of amino acids into peripheral cells. Their respective effects on glucose homeostasis, however, oppose each other. Most growth-promoting GH effects are delayed rather than immediate and are exerted primarily through IGF-I.

The most important of the IGFs is IGF-I. In addition to its growth-promoting effects on cartilage, IGF-I also shows insulin-like activity in other tissue. IGF-I increases glucose oxidation in adipose tissue and stimulates glucose and amino acid transport into diaphragmatic muscle and heart muscle. Synthesis of collagen and proteoglycans is enhanced by IGF-I, which also has positive effects on (1) calcium, (2) magnesium, and (3) potassium homeostasis.

Plasma concentrations of immunoreactive IGF-I rise during childhood and achieve adult concentrations by the time of puberty. During puberty IGF-I concentrations have been observed to be two to three times the adult concentration. Following adolescence, IGF-I concentrations show a gradual decline, reaching a steady state in the third decade of life. IGF-I concentrations are increased as expected in patients with acromegaly and are reduced in GH-deficiency states and in many other conditions including (1) growth retardation, (2) hypothyroidism, (3) chronic illness, (4) nutritional deficiency, and (5) liver disease.

Clinical Significance[2-5,8]

Clinically important states of GH excess or deficiency are relatively uncommon and often difficult to diagnose. GH concentrations vary widely under normal circumstances, so the measurement of GH under random conditions is not generally considered useful. A single GH measurement should not be used to distinguish normal fluctuations from the low or high concentrations that are seen in various disease states. GH measurements are best determined as part of dynamic testing that involves the use of pharmacological or physiological stimuli to increase or suppress GH release.

In contrast to GH, a single measurement of IGF-I is considered an accurate reflection of IGF-I production. Serum concentrations of IGF-I are influenced by nonpathological factors such as (1) age, (2) degree of sexual maturation, and (3) nutritional status. As mentioned previously, IGF-I concentrations are low in states of GH deficiency, but also in patients with acute or chronic protein or caloric deprivation as well as in hypothyroidism.

Growth Hormone Excess

Excess GH production is associated with an eosinophilic or chromophobe **adenoma** of the pituitary gland. These tumors are usually macroadenomas, that is, >10 mm in diameter. Prolonged exposure to GH excess causes an overgrowth of the skeleton and soft tissue. The acral (pertaining to or affecting a limb or other extremity) overgrowth is recognized by increasing (1) ring, (2) shoe, or (3) glove size. This occurs most commonly in adults and is known as acromegaly. When GH excess is seen before long-bone growth is complete (i.e., before epiphyseal fusion), the condition is called **pituitary gigantism**. With pituitary gigantism, in addition to the overgrowth of bone and soft tissue particularly evident in the face and extremities, there is a striking acceleration of linear growth. In severe or advanced cases of GH excess, the diagnosis is made on the basis of physical appearance alone. The physical changes are often subtle and gradual so that a high degree of clinical suspicion is needed to make an early diagnosis. The reversibility of the tissue changes depends largely on the duration of the disease. In addition to the soft-tissue changes, acromegaly may cause severe disability or death from (1) cardiac, (2) respiratory, or (3) neurological sequelae. The most important requirement for the diagnosis of acromegaly is the demonstration of inappropriate and excessive GH secretion.

GH-secreting pituitary tumors account for most of the cases of acromegaly.[3,6] Patients who have pituitary tumors that produce GH are frequently shown to release GH in response to other hypothalamic peptides (TRH and GnRH) that under normal circumstances do not elicit a release of GH. On occasion, pituitary tumors that produce excess amounts of both GH and PRL are observed in around 25% of patients with acromegaly. Few cases of acromegaly, however, are due to GHRH hypersecretion by tumors.

As many as 10% of patients with active acromegaly have random serum GH concentrations that are within the healthy reference interval. The test of choice for the diagnosis of acromegaly is a glucose tolerance test. Healthy individuals suppress their GH to very low concentrations at 60 to 120 minutes after a 75-gram oral glucose challenge. Essentially, all patients with acromegaly have an abnormal response to oral glucose. Patients with acromegaly typically show either no change in their basal concentration of GH or sometimes demonstrate a paradoxical increase in GH.

Serum IGF-I concentrations are elevated in active acromegaly. IGF-I concentrations often correlate better with the clinical severity of acromegaly than with glucose-suppressed or basal GH concentrations. In healthy nourished persons without liver or kidney disease, IGF-I concentrations reflect the integrated effect of GH at the tissue concentration and correlate with 24-hour GH concentrations. Other biochemical abnormalities in acromegaly include (1) hyperphosphatemia, (2) impaired glucose tolerance, and (3) frank diabetes.

Growth Hormone Deficiency States and Growth Retardation[2-5,8]

Children who have inadequate GH production or a GH receptor defect do not grow normally. GH deficiency may be (1) congenital or acquired, (2) idiopathic or caused by anatomical damage to the pituitary gland or hypothalamus, or (3) caused by isolated GH deficiency or associated deficiencies of other pituitary hormones. In one reversible GH deficiency state known as *psychosocial dwarfism,* environmental stress has been shown to inhibit pituitary and hypothalamic function, leading to GH suppression and growth retardation. Children with this disorder show clinical and chemical evidence of growth deficiency when first evaluated, but usually have healthy pituitary function after a few days of hospital stay. GH deficiency is not a common cause of growth retardation. About one half of the children evaluated for growth retardation have no specific organic cause. Approximately, 15% of children with growth retardation have endocrine problems, and approximately one half of these children (about 8% of all children with short stature) have GH deficiency. However, children with growth retardation or **pituitary dwarfism** with no clear explanation (including exclusion of hypothyroidism) should at least be screened for GH deficiency. With the availability of recombinant GH for therapeutic use, many children with short stature are now being selectively treated with GH to advance their growth pattern to more closely achieve their genetic potential.

GH deficiency in adults is probably the most common demonstrable abnormality in patients with large pituitary adenomas or patients who have undergone pituitary irradiation. In adults it has been known to lead to (1) premature mortality, (2) abnormal body composition, (3) impaired serum lipids, (4) decreased bone density with an increase in fracture risk, and (5) overall an impaired quality of life. Thus GH replacement therapy is an important clinical intervention in GH-deficient adults and considered the standard of care.

Resistance to GH results in growth failure despite normal or increased serum GH concentrations and decreased plasma IGF-1 concentrations as in **Laron syndrome**. Patients who have familial short stature and high serum GH concentrations represent many different defects in genetic coding for the GH receptor that result in the absence of or defective GH receptors. In affected individuals, exogenous GH fails to produce any appreciable metabolic changes or to promote growth.

In healthy individuals, the basal concentration of GH is usually low, and the half-life of circulating GH is approximately 20 minutes. Moreover, GH is secreted by the pituitary gland in short pulses or bursts. Thus assays of GH performed on a single random or fasting specimen may not distinguish patients with abnormally low concentrations from healthy subjects who have GH values at the low end of the reference interval. When evaluating GH reserve, provocative tests are frequently used to diagnose true deficiency. Although a physiological GH response to a provocative test is a strong indication for the absence of GH deficiency, no single test is considered diagnostic in this situation. For example, as many as 30% of subjects with physiological GH secretion fail to show the expected elevation in serum GH in response to a specific provocative stimulus at any given time. Consequently, to diagnose GH deficiency as a cause of growth retardation, it is necessary to demonstrate that the serum concentration of GH remains low after the use of at least two different provocative stimuli. The definition of subnormal responses, however, is arbitrarily defined and assay dependent. However, in general a GH response of 7 ng/mL or more after stimulation is considered healthy.

A number of physiological and pharmacological stimuli provoke GH release as depicted in Table 40-3.[10] In one simple screening test, the patient performs 20 minutes of vigorous exercise, and then a sample is obtained for a GH measurement. Taking advantage of the known rise in the concentration of GH that occurs with deep sleep, a sample may be obtained 60 to 90 minutes after the onset of sleep. The obvious limitation of this approach is that the patient must be in the hospital or a clinical research center for testing. Insulin-induced hypoglycemia and arginine are the standard pharmacological stimuli used to test for GH release; protocols for their use are well established and standardized (see Table 40-3).[10] Other medications used to stimulate GH release include glucagon and clonidine. GHRH administration (1.0 μg/kg) in combination with arginine has also been used to test for pituitary GH reserve directly.[5]

As expected, IGF-I concentrations are low in patients with GH deficiency and growth failure. Patients with growth failure caused by other endocrine diseases or by nonendocrine diseases often have low circulating concentrations of IGF-I; thus a low concentration of IGF-I is not specific for diagnosing a GH deficiency. The presence of a physiological concentration of IGF-I, however, does rule out severe GH deficiency.

Analytical Methodology

Immunoassays are the usual methods to measure GH and IGFs, but mass spectrometric methods have been described.[10]

Measurement of Growth Hormone

Immunoassays are used to measure GH with specific GH antibodies available commercially as part of an immunoassay kit or on automated immunoassay instruments.

With the use of highly-specific monoclonal antibodies and recombinant-derived GH, some of these assays are able to discriminate GH variants. Most immunoassays for GH use recombinant-derived GH for tracer and calibration material. The latter is usually prepared gravimetrically and verified by comparison with an international reference preparation (IRP), such as the World Health Organization's (WHO's) international standard, IRP 80/505 human growth hormone recombinant (hGHr), which has a potency of 3.3 IU/mg of hGHr, or other standard preparations, such as WHO IRP 66/217 or 88/624.

The measurement of a single basal or random concentration of GH provides little diagnostic information. Secretion of GH by the pituitary gland is both episodic and pulsatile, and transient concentrations of as much as 40 ng/mL have been observed in healthy, healthy subjects. Serum concentrations are rather low between pulses in healthy individuals, and some immunoassays may not be able to distinguish patients with abnormally low values from healthy subjects who have values that happen to fall in the low-to physiological reference interval. In some individuals, spontaneous GH secretion is best monitored by drawing specimens for GH assay every 20 to 30 minutes over a 12- to 24-hour period although cost would likely preclude such testing on a routine basis.

A number of provocative tests have been established to stimulate or suppress GH release. The insulin tolerance test, which produces a transient hypoglycemia to provoke GH release, is the most common stimulation test used to assess adequacy of GH secretion. In addition it also allows for an adequate assessment of the hypothalamic-pituitary–adrenal axis; cortisol concentrations 20 μg/dL or greater exclude any derangement of this axis. Whilst this test is considered by many as the gold standard and it allows assessment of both GH and ACTH reserve, it is important to remember that it is

TABLE 40-3	Growth Hormone Stimuli	
Growth Hormone Stimulus	**Dose**	**Growth Hormone Sampling Minutes***
Glucogen	0.03-0.1 mg/kg, IM, max 1 mg	0, 30, 60, 90, 120, 150, 180, ±240 (maximum response ≈2 to 3 hours)
L-dopa	500 mg/M² (15 mg/kg) max 500 mg (or) <15 kg: 125 mg 15-30 kg: 250 mg >30 kg: 500 mg	0, 40, 60, 90, 120
Clonidine	0.15 mg/M² <30 lbs: 0.05 mg >30 lbs: 0.1 mg (0.1 mg/tab)	0, 30, 60, 90
Arginine HCl (synthetic arginine)	0.5 g/kg, max 30 (10% solution IV over 30 min)	0, ±15, 30, 60, 90, ±120
Insulin tolerance test (ITT)	0.1 U/kg (0.05-0.15) IV push insulin	0, 10, 20, ±30, 40, 60, ±75, ±90, ±120
Arginine-insulin tolerance test (AITT)	Arginine: begin at time zero, give insulin at +60 minutes	0, 30, 60, 70, 80, 100, 120

*Experts may differ on the best interval of growth hormone (GH) measurements; ± indicates an optional time point.
IM, intramuscular; *IV,* intravenous.

contraindicated in patients with cardiovascular disease, cerebrovascular disease, and seizure disorders due to the stress of the induced hypoglycemia.

Measurement of Insulin-Like Growth Factors

IGFs and IGF-binding proteins are measured in plasma or serum by immunoassays, typically immunometric assays, with use of recombinant standards and specific monoclonal antibodies. It is important to emphasize that reference intervals vary by age and sex, and it is important to use the reference interval reported for that specific assay. At least one mass spectrometric assay is used routinely for IGF-I; the reference intervals for this assay are similar to those found by immunoassays.

Prolactin[2,4,5,8]

PRL is a hormone secreted by specialized cells within the adenohypophysis termed *lactotrophs*. PRL's primary role is to stimulate and sustain lactation in postpartum mammals. PRL has many other effects, including essential roles in the maintenance of the immune system and an important role in ovarian steroidogenesis. PRL is also known as (1) *lactogen,* (2) *lactotropin,* (3) *luteotropin,* (4) *mammotropin,* or (5) *galactopoietic, lactation, lactogenic,* or *luteotropic hormone.*

Biochemistry

PRL contains 199 amino acids and has three intramolecular disulfide bridges. It is secreted by the pituitary lactotroph cells, which are acidophilic. PRL circulates in the blood in different forms including (1) monomeric PRL, 23 kDa (referred to as *little PRL*), (2) dimeric PRL, 48 to 56 kDa (big PRL), and (3) polymeric forms of PRL >100 kDa ("big-big" PRL). The monomeric form is considered the most bioactive of the different forms found in the circulation and demonstrates the greatest response to TRH, the hypothalamic releasing hormone that stimulates the pituitary to release PRL when TRH is present in high concentrations. TRH is not typically a major regulator of PRL secretion by the pituitary. The relative number and PRL content of lactotroph cells are increased in women during pregnancy, which is also the case in fetal pituitary glands.

Secretion of PRL, as for other hormones released by the anterior lobe of the pituitary gland, falls under hypothalamic control. PRL is unique, however, among the adenohypophyseal hormones in that the primary control of its secretion is inhibitory via dopamine.

Physiological Action

PRL is the principal hormone that controls the initiation and maintenance of lactation. However, for an appropriate expression of PRL action, breast tissue requires priming by (1) estrogens, (2) progestins, (3) corticosteroids, (4) thyroid hormone, and (5) insulin. PRL also (1) induces ductal growth, 2) development of the breast lobular alveolar system, and (3) the synthesis of specific milk proteins, including casein and γ-lactalbumin. PRL has effects on the immune system and is important in the control of osmolality and various metabolic events, including (1) the metabolism of subcutaneous fat, (2) carbohydrate metabolism, (3) calcium and vitamin D metabolism, (4) fetal lung development, and (5) steroidogenesis. This last function may be related to its antigonadotropic effect.

PRL, like other pituitary hormones, binds to a specific receptor on the cell membrane of its target organs such as (1) breast, (2) adrenal, (3) ovaries, (4) testes, (5) prostate, (6) kidney, and (7) liver.

Clinical Significance[2,4,5,8]

Hyperprolactinemia is the most common hypothalamic-pituitary disorder encountered in clinical endocrinology, and prolactinomas are the most common secretory tumors of the pituitary gland. PRL concentrations also may be increased in women who have only subtle alterations of fertility, such as (1) anovulation with or without menstrual irregularity, (2) amenorrhea and galactorrhea, or (3) galactorrhea alone. PRL excess in men is frequently manifested as oligospermia or impotence, or both. In addition, men with PRL-secreting pituitary adenomas more often have macroadenomas along with visual field disturbances as a result of a larger tumor pressing on the optic chiasm. Men do not have the subtle reminder of an irregular menstrual period that frequently exposes a microadenoma in women. In both men and women, increased PRL can result in infertility. Elevated PRL concentrations are observed in as many as 30% of women with polycystic ovarian syndrome and patients with clinically silent pituitary adenomas. Other causes of PRL elevation are shown in Table 40-4[10] and should be kept in mind when evaluating patients who have an elevated concentration of PRL. There is no reliable stimulation or suppression test as with other pituitary hormones to distinguish tumor from other causes of PRL elevation.

Basal gonadotropin concentrations are low in most patients with hyperprolactinemia; most studies suggest that PRL inhibits the release of GnRH, resulting in a state of functional hypogonadotropism. Other pituitary function tests are usually normal in patients with hyperprolactinemia, except in individuals with very large macroadenomas where the tumor is pressing on normal anterior pituitary cells.

TABLE 40-4	Differential Diagnosis of Hyperprolactinemia
PRIH (dopamine) deficiency	Hypothalamic disease
	Interruption in the hypothalamic pituitary portal system
Drugs	Dopamine antagonists
	Cholinergic antagonists
	Serotonergic antagonists
Hormones	Estrogen, pregnancy
Neurogenic	Nursing (nipple stimulation)
	Chest wall disease
	Spinal cord injury
Other diseases	Hyperthyroidism (pathologically elevated TRH can release PRL)
	Chronic renal disease
	Cirrhosis

PRIH, Prolactin release-inhibiting hormone; *PRL,* prolactin; *TRH,* thyrotropin-releasing hormone.

Clinically, medications that stimulate PRL release are probably the most common cause of hyperprolactinemia. When a significant elevation of PRL is confirmed, a careful history must be recorded to rule out the possibility that medications are not the cause for the elevation in PRL.

Invariably, serial PRL concentrations higher than 200 ng/mL are sufficient evidence to support a diagnosis of a PRL-secreting adenoma especially if imaging studies demonstrate an adenoma. Rarely, "pseudoprolactinomas" do occur and are large nonsecretory tumors (such as meningiomas) that press on the pituitary stalk, disrupting the normal inhibitory flow of dopamine from the hypothalamus, resulting in modest elevations in PRL concentrations (typically between 50 and 200 µg/L). Thus imaging studies coupled with serial basal prolactin concentrations are most useful in making a diagnosis of prolactinoma. Serum prolactin concentrations can be increased also by a *macroprolactin*, which can be (1) a complex of PRL with immunoglobulins or (2) aggregates of monomeric PRL. The presence of macroprolactin explains a significant proportion of cases of increased serum PRL and should be considered when a pathological explanation for an increased serum PRL is not found.

Analytical Methodology

Human PRL is measured in serum by use of immunoassays. Two-site immunometric ("sandwich") assays that make use of two or more antibodies directed at different parts of the PRL molecule are used on automated instruments. The signal antibody is labeled with a detection molecule such as an (1) enzyme, (2) fluorophore, or (3) chemiluminescent tag. PRL calibrators have values assigned by use of reference materials with known international unit potency, such as the WHO first IRP 75/504, the second international standard (IS) 83/562, or the third IS 84/500 (http://www.nibsc.ac.uk/accessed November 20, 2013). One of the concerns with PRL immunoassays is a "hook effect" with very high prolactin concentrations that affect certain immunoassay methods, particularly one-step assays in which no washing step is included between addition of the capture and detection antibodies. When suspected, samples need to be diluted and reanalyzed.

Adrenocorticotropic Hormone and Related Peptides[2-5,8]

Adrenocorticotropic hormone (ACTH) is a peptide hormone secreted by the adenohypophysis as one of the derivatives of **pro-opiomelanocortin (POMC)**. It acts primarily on the adrenal cortex, stimulating its growth and the synthesis and secretion of corticosteroids, most importantly, cortisol. ACTH production is increased during times of stress. It is also known as *corticotropin, corticotrophin, adrenocorticotrophin,* and *adrenocorticotropin.*

Biochemistry

ACTH and related peptides originate from POMC, a large precursor molecule with a molecular weight of 31 kDa (Figure 40-3). Enzymatic cleavage of POMC to smaller peptides takes place in both the anterior and intermediate lobes of the pituitary gland. In the anterior lobe of the pituitary gland, enzymes hydrolyze POMC to β-LPH and a 22-kDa fragment known as *pro-ACTH.* This latter peptide is further processed to ACTH (a peptide consisting of 39 amino acids) and to a 16-kDa peptide, pro-γ-melanotropin (γ-MSH). In turn, β-LPH is cleaved to two smaller peptides, β-endorphin and γ-LPH. Both γ-LPH and β-endorphin are released with ACTH from the anterior lobe of the pituitary gland, but only about one third of the β-LPH is converted to β-endorphin. In contrast the intermediate lobe (when present) fully processes β-LPH to β-endorphin, cleaving pro-α-melanotropin (α-MSH) to α-melanotropin (α-MSH), and splitting ACTH to α-MSH and a corticotropin-like intermediate-lobe peptide. These smaller peptides are found in the human fetus, but only trace amounts exist in the adult human pituitary gland. The changes observed in skin pigmentation in several endocrine diseases (e.g., with adrenal insufficiency) are most likely due to the α-MSH activity of excess ACTH.

In addition to β-endorphin, β-LPH contains the amino acid sequence of another endogenous opioid, *met-enkephalin.*

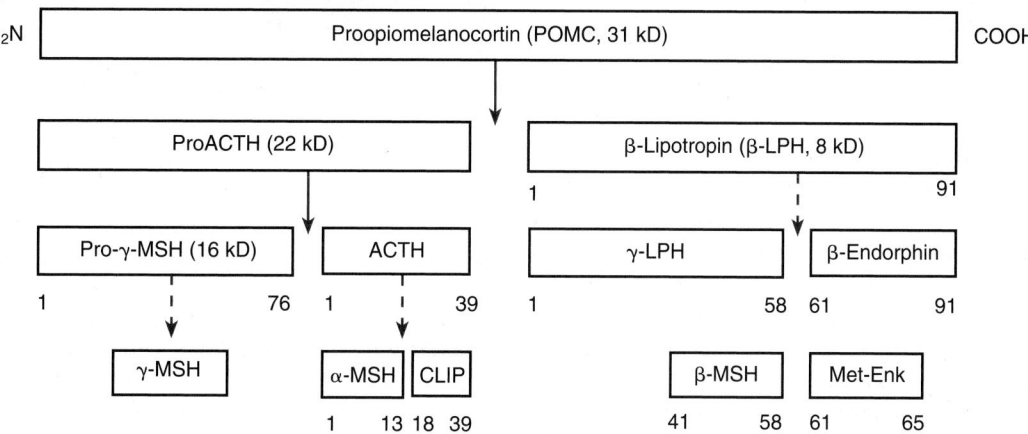

Figure 40-3 Diagrammatic representation of pro-opiomelanocortin (POMC) and its precursor relationship to adrenocorticotropic hormone (ACTH), beta-lipotropin (β-LPH), α- and β-melanotropin (MSH), and the endorphins.

However, this peptide is not the product of β-LPH breakdown, but rather arises from a precursor molecule known as *pro-enkephalin*. Pro-enkephalin is widely distributed in neurons throughout the brain and spinal cord. Some pro-enkephalin is found in the pituitary gland, but most is localized in the catecholamine-synthesizing cells of the adrenal medulla and is co-released with epinephrine and norepinephrine. A third family of endogenous opioid peptides is derived from *pro-dynorphin*, a prohormone stored primarily in the posterior lobe of the pituitary gland where it is co-released with vasopressin.

Regulation of Adrenocorticotropic Hormone Secretion

Regulation of the secretion of ACTH is described in Chapter 41.

Clinical Significance[2-5,8]

The major disorders of the pituitary gland with respect to ACTH include ACTH deficiency or secondary hypoadrenalism and excess ACTH secretion resulting in **Cushing disease** the commonest cause of **Cushing syndrome** (see Chapter 41). Briefly, for the diagnosis of Cushing syndrome/disease, useful tests include measurement of (1) the 24-hour excretion of urinary-free cortisol, (2) the dexamethasone suppression tests (both overnight with 1 mg and 48 hours with 2 mg/d), and (3) demonstration of loss of the diurnal variation with inappropriately increased cortisol concentrations in the evening as assayed by plasma or salivary cortisol. Useful tests for the diagnosis of secondary adrenal insufficiency due to CRH-ACTH deficiency include the (1) cosyntropin test, (2) overnight metyrapone test, (3) insulin tolerance tests—and, if necessary, (4) cosyntropin infusion test over several days. In the short metyrapone test a morning plasma 11-deoxycortisol >7 μg/dL excludes secondary adrenal insufficiency. Also during an insulin tolerance test if the concentration of plasma cortisol meets or exceeds a concentration of 20 μg/dL, secondary hypoadrenalism is excluded.

Gonadotropins (Follicle-Stimulating Hormone, Luteinizing Hormone)

FSH is synthesized in the adenohypophysis and (1) stimulates the growth and maturation of ovarian follicles, (2) stimulates estrogen secretion, (3) promotes the endometrial changes characteristic of the first phase (proliferative phase) of the mammalian menstrual cycle, and (4) stimulates spermatogenesis in the male. It is also called *follitropin*.

LH is also synthesized in the adenohypophysis and acts with FSH to promote ovulation and secretion of androgens and progesterone. It initiates and maintains the second (secretory) phase of the mammalian estrus and menstrual cycle. In females it is concerned with corpus luteum formation, and in males it stimulates the development and functional activity of testicular Leydig cells and testosterone production. LH is also called *interstitial cell–stimulating hormone* and *lutropin*.

Biochemistry

The glycoprotein hormones of the pituitary (LH, FSH, and TSH) and of the placenta (chorionic gonadotropin [CG]) are composed of two peptide chains (usually referred to as α- and β-subunits), each with carbohydrate substituent groups attached. The carbohydrate moiety, which accounts for 15% to 31% of the molecular weight, includes (1) fucose, (2) mannose, (3) galactose, (4) glucosamine, (5) galactosamine, and (6) sialic acid. The α-subunits of these hormones are similar to one another and are interchangeable. The β-subunits display greater differences in amino acid sequences among the various hormones that confer hormonal and immunological specificity. Isolated α-subunits are devoid of biological activity. Isolated β-subunits may have slight intrinsic biological activity, but full activity is attained when α- and β-subunits are recombined. This suggests that the presence of both subunits is important for specific receptor recognition and that the β-subunit is responsible for eliciting the specific biological response.

The gonadotropic cells of the anterior lobe of the pituitary gland secrete FSH (molecular weight 30 kDa) and LH (molecular weight 32 kDa). Because these two hormones control the functional activity of gonads, they are grouped together under the generic term *gonadotropins.*

Physiological Action

In females, FSH stimulates the growth and maturation of the ovarian follicles and, in the presence of LH, promotes secretion of estrogens by the maturing follicles. The LH surge (or "peak") in females in mid-cycle causes ovulation and release of the ovum from the ovarian follicle, which has previously ripened under the influence of FSH, and causes luteinization of the ruptured follicle to form the corpus luteum. The corpus luteum then secretes both progesterone and estradiol under the influence of pulsatile LH release. In males FSH stimulates spermatogenesis by the germ cells in the testes, and LH is responsible for the production of testosterone by the Leydig cells of the testes.

Regulation and Clinical Significance

Regulation of LH and FSH secretion and its clinical significance in reproductive endocrinology are discussed in Chapter 43. In women, a regular menstrual cycle is supportive of a normal functioning hypothalamic-pituitary-gonadal axis.

Briefly, the major clinical syndrome is deficiency of the gonadotropins LH and FSH. When there is deficiency of the gonadotropins resulting in hypogonadism, it is referred to as *hypogonadotropic hypogonadism*. These patients have low or normal concentrations of LH, FSH, and low concentrations of testosterone in males and estradiol in females. This can present as an isolated deficiency, monohypopituitarism, or part of multiple hormone deficiencies, panhypopituitarism. The best characterized isolated hormone deficiency is **Kallmann syndrome** due to a deficiency of GnRH, which is associated with impairment in smell, anosmia, or hyposmia and midline defects. In this disorder, priming with GnRH restores gonadotropin secretion and fertility. Hypogonadotropic hypogonadism can occur with (1) severe mental and physical stress, (2) anorexia nervosa, and (3) can be observed in the overtrained athlete.

Very rarely does hypogonadism result from a pituitary tumor, usually a large chromophobe adenoma.

Analytical Methodology

A number of different immunoassay methods have been developed for determining FSH and LH in blood and urine, and reliable commercial kits are widely available either for manual testing or with automated immunoassay instruments.

Currently, most immunoassays for FSH and LH show <1% cross-reactivity with TSH or human CG (hCG) or with their free α- or β-chains. For example, hCG interference in LH assays has essentially been eliminated (<0.008% cross-reactivity), and the immunometric assays found on automated instruments show precision (between-assay coefficients of variation [CVs]) of about 10% or less and limits of quantification <0.2 IU/L. The latter is especially important for use in the evaluation of prepubertal children and patients with hypothalamic disorders when LH concentrations are barely detectable.

Thyroid-Stimulating Hormone[2-5,8]

TSH is a glycoprotein hormone synthesized by the thyrotroph cells of the adenohypophysis that promotes the growth and uptake of iodine by the thyroid gland and stimulates the synthesis and secretion of thyroid hormones from the thyroid gland. It is also called *thyrotropin*. It is a peptide with a molecular weight of 26.6 kDa. A molecule of TSH consists of two noncovalently linked α- and β-subunits with the α-subunit chemically similar to the α-subunits of LH, FSH, and hCG. TSH (1) stimulates the growth and vascularity of the thyroid gland, (2) stimulates the growth of thyroid follicular cells, and (3) promotes a number of the steps involved in thyroid hormone synthesis. These include the (1) uptake of iodine, (2) organification of iodine onto tyrosine, (3) coupling of tyrosines, and (4) proteolytic release of stored thyroid hormone from thyroglobulin stores.

Regulation and Clinical Significance

The regulation of TSH secretion, its clinical significance, and methods for determining TSH are discussed in in Chapter 42. Briefly, two major clinical syndromes arise from TSH deficiency or TSH excess. TSH deficiency results in secondary hypothyroidism with low concentrations of T_4 and TSH. It needs to be emphasized that the T_4 concentrations are more reliable than TSH in the diagnosis of hypothyroidism as a result of hypothalamic-pituitary diseases, and TSH concentrations may be within the reference interval (although that is abnormal in the face of a low T_4 which should lead to TSH secretion normally and thus increased circulating TSH). A rare form of hyperthyroidism is caused by a TSH-producing tumor of the pituitary gland. Patients have clinical features of hyperthyroidism with elevated concentrations of T_4 and increased or inappropriately normal TSH concentrations.

Hormones of the Neurohypophysis[2,7-10]

The neurohypophyseal system comprises neural tissue and neurons of the supraoptic and paraventricular nuclei of the hypothalamus. These neurons are located in and travel through the median eminence and pituitary stalk with the nerve endings projecting to the posterior lobe of the pituitary gland. The cell bodies of these neurons synthesize and secrete (1) antidiuretic hormone (also known as arginine vasopressin and vasopressin) and (2) oxytocin. Both of these hormones are nonapeptides (molecular weight 1080 Da) consisting of a cyclic hexapeptide and a three–amino acid side chain. The structure of oxytocin is similar to that of **antidiuretic hormone (ADH)** but with isoleucine rather than phenylalanine at position 3 and with leucine instead of arginine at position 8.

Antidiuretic Hormone[7,9,10]

ADH is formed by neuronal cells of hypothalamic nuclei and stored in the neurohypophysis. In humans it contains arginine at position 8. (In the pig and hippopotamus, lysine is found at position 8.) ADH functions to (1) stimulate contraction of the muscles of capillaries and arterioles, raising blood pressure; (2) promote contraction of the intestinal musculature, increasing peristalsis; (3) exert contractile influence on the uterus; and (4) have a specific effect on the epithelial cells of renal collecting tubules, augmenting resorption of water independently of solutes to cause concentration of urine and dilution of blood serum. This action on the kidney is mediated by ADH binding to V2 receptors and stimulating cyclic AMP resulting in increased cell membrane expression of aquaporin-2 water channels with an increase in the reabsorption of water. ADH's rate of secretion is regulated chiefly by the osmolality of the plasma. Also a decrease in plasma volume sometimes evokes release of ADH.

Biochemistry

ADH is synthesized as part of a large precursor molecule (*preprovasopressin*) and ADH travels down axons in conjunction with a specific neurophysin-binding protein. The latter serves as a carrier protein for ADH during axonal transport and storage. Oxytocin is also synthesized as part of a preprohormone along with a separate neurophysin-binding protein. These molecular complexes are packaged into secretory granules that migrate down the nerve axons for 12 to 14 hours before reaching the posterior pituitary lobe for storage. Release of the neurohypophyseal hormones into the portal circulation occurs via calcium-dependent exocytosis on nerve cell stimulation. At the physiological pH of plasma, ADH and oxytocin circulate mainly in unbound forms.

Regulation of Secretion

Osmolality of the blood is the main regulator of ADH secretion. Osmoreceptors in the brain respond to changes in plasma osmolality. As little as a 2% increase in extracellular fluid osmolality causes shrinkage of osmoreceptor cells with stimulation of ADH release from the posterior pituitary lobe. A plasma osmolality >280 mOsm/kg is considered the osmotic threshold for ADH release.

Besides the osmoreceptor mechanism, the physiological regulation of ADH secretion also involves a pressure-volume mechanism that is distinct from the osmotic sensor. In this second process, ADH release is regulated by baroreceptors that respond to alterations in blood volume. For example, a reduction in plasma volume or arterial pressure, or both, stimulates ADH secretion. Other nonosmotic stimuli for ADH release include pain, stress, hypoglycemia, exercise, and chemical agents, such as (1) catecholamines, (2) angiotensin II, (3) opiates, (4) prostaglandins, (5) anesthetics, (6) nicotine, and (7) barbiturates. Agents such as alcohol, phenytoin, and glucocorticoids are known to inhibit ADH release, leading to a water diuresis.

The thirst center is regulated by many of the same factors that determine ADH release. This center has a higher set-point than the osmoreceptors and responds to osmolalities >290 mOsm/kg. Responses involving ADH, thirst, and the kidney are coordinated in a complex scheme to maintain plasma osmolality in healthy individuals within a narrow range (284 to 295 mOsm/kg).

Physiological Actions

The major physiological function of ADH is the control of water homeostasis, which allows the kidney to reabsorb water and concentrate urine. When released in sufficient quantity, ADH also induces a generalized vasoconstriction that leads to a rise in arterial blood pressure. ADH is believed to play an important role in the maintenance of arterial blood pressure during blood loss. Release of ADH into the pituitary portal system also augments the action of CRH in stimulating the release of ACTH from the adenohypophysis. However, ADH does not appear to affect the release of other anterior pituitary hormones.

Clinical Significance[2,7-10]

Disorders of ADH activity have been divided into hypofunction (**diabetes insipidus [DI]**) and hyperfunction (**syndrome of inappropriate antidiuretic hormone secretion [SIADH]**).

Diabetes Insipidus

Deficient production or action of ADH results in **polyuria** caused by the failure of the renal tubules to reabsorb solute-free water. Under normal circumstances, urine output is largely dependent on fluid intake. Thus an arbitrary limit for normal urine output is difficult to define. When urine output is >2.5 L/day, an investigation is usually indicated; with complete deficiency of ADH, urine output may approach 1 L/hr. If the thirst response is normal, increased ingestion of fluid (**polydipsia**) follows. If access to water is not restricted, plasma osmolality and serum electrolytes usually remain normal.

Polyuric states are divided into three main categories: (1) deficient ADH production (hypothalamic diabetes insipidus [HDI]), (2) deficient ADH action on the kidney (nephrogenic diabetes insipidus [NDI]), and (3) excessive water intake (psychogenic polydipsia). An osmotic diuresis may also produce polyuria and polydipsia. Uncontrolled diabetes mellitus with a high glucose load to the kidney is a common cause of an osmotic diuresis.

Hypothalamic Diabetes Insipidus. HDI is also called *neurogenic, central,* or *cranial diabetes insipidus*. It is caused by a failure of the pituitary gland to secrete normal amounts of ADH in response to osmoregulatory factors. The incidence of HDI is about 1 in 25,000 people. In 30% of patients, HDI occurs without apparent cause; other cases are associated with (1) tumors (pituitary area or metastatic), (2) trauma (surgery, head injury), (3) granulomatous disease (sarcoidosis, histiocytosis), (4) infections (meningitis, encephalitis), (5) vascular causes (infarction, aneurysm) and (6) inflammation (lymphocytic hypophysitis). During pregnancy, DI can result from an increase degradation of ADH by the placental cysteine aminopeptidase.

Nephrogenic Diabetes Insipidus. NDI results from the failure of the kidney to respond to typical or increased concentrations of ADH. In the majority of these patients, ADH is incapable of stimulating cyclic adenosine monophosphate (cAMP) formation. There are two major causes of congenital NDI, (1) a X-lined mutation in the v2 receptors, which accounts for 90% of cases and (2) an autosomal recessive mutation of the aquaporin-2 water channels. As an X-chromosome–linked disorder, the ADH receptor mutation form of NDI most commonly affects males. Females are more likely to have the aquaporin-2 water channel gene defect on chromosome 12, q12-13, which produces an autosomal recessive disease. Acquired forms of NDI may be caused by (1) metabolic disorders (hypokalemia, hypercalcemia, and amyloidosis), (2) drugs (lithium, demeclocycline, and barbiturates), and (3) renal diseases (polycystic disease and chronic renal failure). NDI may also be seen in the absence of these factors (idiopathic).

Psychogenic or Primary Polydipsia. A chronic, excessive intake of water suppresses ADH secretion and produces hypotonic polyuria. The polyuria and polydipsia are usually not as sustained as in HDI or NDI. Nocturnal polyuria also is less frequent. Psychogenic factors are most commonly associated with this disorder, but hypothalamic disease affecting the thirst center may be a cause. Drugs also affect the thirst center and result in primary polydipsia.

Diagnosis of Diabetes Insipidus[2,7-10]

In the classical full blown syndrome, the polyuria leads to hypertonic dehydration with hypernatremia and a serum osmolality >295 mOsm/kg. A random urine osmolality that exceeds 750 mOsm/kg excludes DI. The best provocative test to diagnose DI is the water deprivation test. This test should not be performed if (1) hypothyroidism, (2) hypoadrenalism, or (3) osmotic diuresis is present (e.g., uncontrolled diabetes mellitus). Patients are deprived of all fluids, until hourly urine osmolalities are constant and thus vary by <10%. At this point a sample is taken for plasma osmolality and ADH measurement. The test must be terminated if body weight falls by greater than 3%. Thereafter, ADH is administered (Desmopressin 2 µg subcutaneously), and serum and urine osmolality are then measured at 60 and 120 minutes post-ADH injection. In patients with psychogenic polydipsia urine osmolality after dehydration (usually >500 mOsm/kg) is greater than plasma osmolality and does not increase by greater than 10% after ADH. In partial cranial DI, urine osmolality is greater than plasma osmolality post dehydration but increases by >10% with ADH. In more severe cranial DI, urine osmolality increases by at least 50% post ADH. A plasma ADH concentration post dehydration will separate

TABLE 40-5	Causes of the Syndrome of Inappropriate Antidiuretic Hormone
CNS disease	Brain tumor
	Infection (e.g., meningitis, encephalitis, abscess)
	Prolonged seizure
	Psychiatric disease
	Stress (e.g., prolonged nausea)
Non-CNS tumor (e.g., leukemia)	
Pulmonary disease	Hypoxia (e.g., neonatal)
	Infection (e.g., pneumonia, emphysema)
Nonpulmonary infection (e.g., AIDS)	
Drugs	Drugs with CNS effects (anticonvulsants, antiparkinsonian drugs, antipsychotics, antipyretics, antidepressants)
	ACE inhibitors
	Antineoplastic drugs
	First-generation sulfonylureas

ACE, Angiotensin-converting enzyme; *AIDS,* acquired immunodeficiency syndrome; *CNS,* central nervous system.

cranial DI (concentrations low) from nephrogenic DI (concentrations high).

Syndrome of Inappropriate Antidiuretic Hormone[2,7-10]

SIADH refers to the autonomous, sustained production of ADH in the absence of known stimuli for its release. In this syndrome, plasma ADH concentrations are "inappropriately" increased relative to a low plasma osmolality and to a healthy or increased plasma volume. Causes of SIADH are shown in Table 40-5.[10] In SIADH a primary excess of ADH, coupled with unrestricted fluid intake, promotes increased reabsorption of free water by the kidney. The result is a decreased urine volume and an increased urine sodium concentration and urine osmolality. As a consequence of water retention, these patients become modestly volume expanded. The increase in intravascular volume causes hemodilution accompanied by dilutional hyponatremia and a low plasma osmolality. Volume expansion also decreases renal sodium reabsorption and thus further increases the urine sodium concentration.

The most common cause of hyponatremia in hospital patients is SIADH. However, other disorders cause dilutional hyponatremia and must be differentiated from SIADH. These conditions include (1) congestive heart failure, (2) renal insufficiency, (3) nephrotic syndrome, (4) liver cirrhosis, and (5) hypothyroidism. Hyponatremia may also occur from renal or extrarenal sodium losses (depletional hyponatremia) as a result of (1) vomiting, (2) diarrhea, (3) excessive sweating, (4) diuretic abuse, (5) salt-losing nephropathy, or (6) mineralocorticoid deficiency.

The clinical manifestations of hyponatremia are nonspecific. Weakness and apathy occur in mild cases, and central nervous system changes (lethargy, coma, and seizures) are present in more severe cases. No signs or symptoms are specific for SIADH. History, physical examination, and routine laboratory test results often suggest that hyponatremia is due to dilution or depletion.

Measurements of sodium and osmolality in blood and urine, combined with a clinical assessment of volume status, usually permit the appropriate differential diagnosis of hyponatremic conditions. The typical patient with SIADH has (1) hyponatremia, (2) hypoosmolar plasma (<280 mOsm/kg), (3) a urine osmolality >100 mOsm/kg, and (4) a urine sodium concentration that is inappropriately elevated (>40 mmol/L). Also both serum uric acid and blood urea nitrogen are decreased from free water retention. To sustain a diagnosis of SIADH, (1) hypothyroidism, (2) hypoadrenalism, (3) renal disease, and (4) diuretic use should be excluded. Patients with dilutional hyponatremia resulting from excess water intake have a hypotonic plasma, an unremarkable urine sodium concentration (<20 mmol/L), and a dilute urine. Patients with depletional hyponatremia caused by extrarenal sodium loss have (1) hypotonic plasma, (2) a low urine sodium concentration (usually <20 mmol/L), and (3) a urine osmolality that is greater than that of plasma. Patients with depletional hyponatremia caused by impaired renal conservation of sodium have similar results except that their urine sodium concentrations are elevated. Measurements of ADH in plasma are not usually needed to make a diagnosis of SIADH.

Analytical Methodology

Numerous immunoassays for measuring ADH in plasma or urine have been described.[10] With most plasma assays, a preliminary extraction procedure is required to concentrate the minute amount of hormone that is present in the specimen and remove nonspecific interfering substances. Given the rare indications for the measurement of plasma ADH, it is best to send the sample to a reference laboratory for a reliable determination.

Oxytocin[8]

Oxytocin is a nonapeptide that promotes uterine contractions and milk ejection and contributes to the second stage of labor in pregnancy.

Biochemistry

Oxytocin is synthesized in the hypothalamus as part of a preprohormone, along with a separate neurophysin-binding protein. These molecular complexes are packaged into secretory granules that migrate down the nerve axons for 12 to 14 hours before reaching the posterior pituitary lobe for storage. Release of oxytocin into the portal circulation occurs via calcium-dependent exocytosis on nerve cell stimulation. Oxytocin exists in plasma mainly in unbound forms.

Secretion

The primary stimulus for oxytocin release is suckling. Stimulation of tactile receptors located around the nipples of the breasts initiates an action potential that propagates along afferent nerve fibers through the spinal cord and midbrain to the hypothalamus. The cell bodies in the paraventricular nucleus are then stimulated, resulting in the episodic release of oxytocin. Stretch receptors in the uterus and possibly in the vaginal mucosa may also initiate action potentials in afferent nerve fibers that ultimately stimulate the release of oxytocin from the neurohypophysis. Estrogens enhance the response of oxytocin to these stimuli. The influence of other parts of the brain on the release of oxytocin has been reported. For example, emotional stress inhibits lactation.

Physiological Actions

Oxytocin is present in males and females, but its physiological effects are known only for females. Oxytocin stimulates contraction of the uterine myometrium only in the estrogen-primed uterus and activates the smooth muscles associated with milk let-down with nursing. Thus the effects of oxytocin appear limited to events of parturition and lactation. Oxytocin has been used as a therapeutic agent to induce labor, but the physiological mechanism whereby it induces uterine contractions remains obscure. There is some evidence to indicate that oxytocin stimulates prostaglandin production, which may be the vehicle through which myometrial contractility is enhanced.[10] There is evidence indicating that oxytocin may affect the central nervous system and thus modulate human behavior. Progestins are believed to counteract the actions of oxytocin. There are no major syndromes associated with oxytocin excess or deficiency in humans.

Analytical Methodology

Numerous immunoassays for measuring oxytocin in plasma or urine have been described.[10] However, their routine clinical application has been limited because of a lack of physiological relevance to human reproductive disorders.

Assessment of Anterior Pituitary Lobe Reserve

Evaluation of endocrine function is an important part of the management of patients with pituitary tumors.[1,2] Objectives of testing of pituitary function in patients with pituitary tumors are the detection of hormone deficiencies before and after treatment and recognition of hormone-producing tumors.

The assessment of anterior and posterior pituitary lobe function in patients with pituitary tumors has clinical utility for two reasons. The first is to identify clinically significant hormone deficiency states caused by the tumor itself. The second is for the re-evaluation of patients after pituitary surgery or irradiation to detect hormone deficiencies that occur as a result of invasive treatment. Testing of pituitary function is usually performed under basal conditions, but also is performed under provocative conditions to bring out subtle or mild deficiencies that are observed with disorders of the adrenal gland, thyroid, or gonads. Evaluation of pituitary reserve for PRL is usually unnecessary in adult patients because deficiency of this hormone is not believed to be clinically important.

TABLE 40-6	Summary of Pituitary Gland Assessment	
Hormone	**Deficiency**	**Excess**
GH	GH response to arginine, insulin tolerance tests, exercise, L-dopa, glucagon, GHRH IGF-I levels	IGF-I levels GH response to 75g oral glucose (glucose tolerance test)
PRL	PRL	PRL (serial measurements)
TSH	T₄, TSH	T₄, TSH, α-subunit, TSH response to TRH
Gonadotropins	Menstrual history, testosterone, estradiol, LH, FSH	LH, FSH, α-subunit
ACTH	Cortisol, cosyntropin test, metyrapone test, insulin tolerance test	Urine-free cortisol, overnight or low-dose dexamethasone suppression tests, loss of diurnal rhythm
ADH	Water deprivation test (serum and urine osmol), ADH levels at maximum dehydration	Serum and urine osmol, serum and urine Na⁺

ADH, Antidiuretic hormone; *ACTH,* adrenocorticotropic hormone; *FSH,* follicle-stimulating hormone; *GH,* growth hormone; *GHRH,* growth hormone-releasing hormone; *IGF-I,* insulin-like growth factor I; *LH,* luteinizing hormone; *PRL,* prolactin; *T₄,* thyroxine; *TRH,* thyrotropin-releasing hormone; *TSH,* thyroid-stimulating hormone.

The lowered detection limits of the newer two-site immunoassays for the measurement of pituitary hormones now make it possible to distinguish an abnormally low value from the lower end of the healthy reference interval. Although assessment of a particular aspect of pituitary function should also include clinical signs and symptoms of hormone deficiency and the measurement of hormones secreted by the pertinent endocrine gland (e.g., thyroxine, cortisol, testosterone, and estradiol), the newer, ultrasensitive assays for TSH, FSH, LH, and ACTH may allow for an accurate distinction of a true low result. Because of the importance of diagnosing and treating ACTH deficiency, invariably provocative testing is required as detailed earlier (e.g., cosyntropin, metyrapone, ITT). A summary of the assessment of pituitary function is in Table 40-6.

Hypothalamic-Pituitary-Adrenal Axis

A finding of a healthy value for a normal morning serum cortisol concentration is usually adequate evidence that the hypothalamic-pituitary-adrenal axis is intact and functioning properly. On occasion, however, the cosyntropin (a potent analogue of ACTH) stimulation test is used when the morning cortisol results are low or equivocal or when there is a strong clinical suspicion of adrenal insufficiency. This provocative test is performed by obtaining a baseline blood specimen for cortisol followed by the intravenous (IV) administration of 250 μg of cosyntropin. Specimens for cortisol are then obtained at 30 and 60 minutes after IV administration of the synthetic ACTH. A peak value for plasma cortisol of 20 μg/dL or greater is considered a healthy response to ACTH administration. Other useful tests to assess the adrenal reserve include the metyrapone test and the insulin tolerance test.

Hypothalamic-Pituitary-Thyroid Axis

When both the serum-free thyroxine concentration (FT_4) and the ultrasensitive TSH result are within their healthy reference intervals, the hypothalamic-pituitary-thyroid axis is assumed to be intact. In patients with a history of pituitary disease and secondary hypothyroidism, the serum TSH concentration is frequently within a healthy reference interval. Thus in this situation, an FT_4 concentration is the superior test to gauge normality of the hypothalamic-pituitary-thyroid axis. Lowering of the limit of quantification with third-generation TSH tests may allow for the detection of abnormalities of the hypothalamic-pituitary-thyroid axis much earlier in the disease process.

Hypothalamic-Pituitary-Gonadal Axis

History and physical examination are extremely helpful in evaluating the status of the hypothalamic-pituitary-gonadal axis; particularly in women during their reproductive years. The finding of a physiological menstrual cycle is usually indicative of an intact hypothalamic-pituitary-gonadal axis in reproductive-age women. Baseline laboratory assessment for hypothalamic-pituitary-gonadal dysregulation should include measurement of serum (1) LH, (2) FSH and (3) sex steroids (estradiol in females and testosterone in males). Provocative testing of this axis with GnRH and measurements of FSH and LH is useful in selected patients (hypogonadotropic, hypogonadism). These tests, however, are known to be unreliable in differentiating pituitary disorders from hypothalamic dysfunction; thus the physician is usually dependent on an accurate determination of LH, FSH, and sex steroids along with clinical judgment.

Review Questions

1. A function of prolactin (PRL) is to
   a. regulate respiration.
   b. stimulate uterine contraction.
   c. initiate and maintain lactation.
   d. stimulate protein synthesis.
2. A peptide hormone that modifies the body's response to stress by its action on the adrenal gland is
   a. growth hormone (GH).
   b. adrenocorticotropic hormone (ACTH).
   c. antidiuretic hormone (ADH).
   d. follicle-stimulating hormone (FSH).
3. Regulation of electrolytes and water balance is controlled in part by the renal system. Which hormone synthesized by the brain affects water balance and is regulated by the osmolality of blood?
   a. Aldosterone
   b. ACTH
   c. ADH
   d. Oxytocin

4. The anterior pituitary hormone that regulates release of thyroid hormone from the thyroid gland is
   a. TSH.
   b. ACTH.
   c. ADH.
   d. FSH.
5. An example of a hormone synthesized in the adenohypophysis would be
   a. insulin.
   b. ADH.
   c. GH.
   d. erythropoietin.
6. A second function of vasopressin (ADH) other than body water regulation is
   a. sperm growth.
   b. suppression of growth hormone (GH).
   c. inducing estrogen secretion from the ovaries.
   d. elevation of blood pressure.
7. In men, FSH functions to
   a. induce spermatogenesis.
   b. induce production of testosterone.
   c. enhance muscle mass.
   d. induce production of androstenedione.
8. If FSH and LH were decreased in a man, what is the name of the hypothalamic releasing hormone that might be involved?
   a. Thyrotropin-releasing hormone (TRH)
   b. Gonadotropin-releasing hormone (GnRH)
   c. Sheehan hormone
   d. Growth hormone-releasing hormone (GHRH)
9. Oxytocin is synthesized in the
   a. adenohypophysis.
   b. neurohypophysis.
   c. uterus.
   d. hypothalamus.
10. Regarding growth hormone (GH), hypersecretion due to a pituitary tumor would cause which one of the following disorders in an adult?
    a. Gigantism
    b. Dwarfism
    c. Acromegaly
    d. There would be no observable effect.

References

1. Ellison DH, Berl T. The syndrome of inappropriate antidiuresis. N Engl J Med 2007;356(20):2064–72.
2. Hamann K, Jialal I. Chapter 2: Laboratory investigation of disorders of the pituitary gland. In: Jialal I, Sokoll L, Winter W, eds. Handbook of diagnostic endocrinology, 2nd edition. Washington, DC: AACC Press, 2008:25–42.
3. Javorsky BR, Aron DC, Findling JW, Tyrrell JB. Chapter 4: Hypothalamus & pituitary gland. In: Gardner DG, Shoback D, eds. Basic and clinical endocrinology, 9th edition. New York, NY: McGraw-Hill Medical, 2011:65–114.
4. Melmed S, Jameson JL. Chapter 339: Disorders of the anterior pituitary and hypothalamus. In: Harrison's principles of internal medicine, 18th edition, vol. 2. DL Longo, AS Fauci, DL Kasper, SL Hauser, JL Jameson, J Loscalzo, eds. McGraw-Hill Companies Inc., 2012:2876–902.

5. Melmed S, Kleinberg DL. Chapter 8: The anterior pituitary. In: Larsen PR, Kronenberg HM, Melmed S, Polonsky KS, eds. Williams textbook of endocrinology, 10th edition. Philadelphia: WB Saunders, 2003:177–280.

6. Melmed S. Acromegaly. N Engl J Med 2006;355(24):2558–73.

7. Robertson GL. Chapter 340: Disorders of the neurohypophysis. In: Longo DL, Fauci AS, Kasper DL, et al, eds. Harrison's principles of internal medicine, 18th edition, vol 2. McGraw Hill Companies Inc., 2012;2902–11.

8. Vance ML. Hypopitutarism. N Engl J Med 1994;330(23):1651–61.

9. Verbalis JG. Disorders of body water and homeostasis. Best Pract Res Clin Endocrinol Metab 2003;17(4):471–503.

10. Winter W, Jialal I, Vance ML, Bertholf R. Chapter 53: Pituitary function and pathophysiology. In: Burtis CA, Ashwood ER, Bruns DE, eds. Tietz textbook of clinical chemistry and molecular diagnostics, 5th edition, St Louis: Elsevier, 2012;1803–45.

Disorders of the Adrenal Cortex*

Roger L. Bertholf, Ph.D., Ishwarlal Jialal, M.D., Ph.D., and William E. Winter, M.D.

Objectives

1. Define the following terms:

Androgen	Mineralocorticoid
Angiotensin	Renin
Glucocorticoid	Steroid hormone
Incidentaloma	

2. State how adrenal cortical steroid hormones are synthesized from cholesterol.
3. Describe the anatomy and physiology of the adrenal cortex.
4. For each of the following hormones, state the function, regulation (including anterior pituitary or hypothalamic hormones involved, if any), site of synthesis, circulatory transport, metabolism, and urinary metabolite:

Cortisol	Androstenedione
Aldosterone	Dehydroepiandrosterone (DHEA)

5. Describe the following dynamic test of adrenal function, including reasons for performing, protocol followed, and interpretation of results:

Adrenocorticotropic hormone (ACTH) (cosyntropin) stimulation	Metyrapone stimulation
Corticotropin-releasing hormone (CRH) stimulation	Dexamethasone suppression
Insulin-induced hypoglycemia stimulation	Mineralocorticoid stimulation/ suppression

6. Discuss the following adrenocortical disorders including hormone(s) involved, symptoms, primary/secondary/tertiary causes, and screening and suppression/stimulation tests used for assessment:

Addison disease	Cushing syndrome/Cushing disease
Conn syndrome	Congenital adrenal hyperplasia (CAH)

7. Summarize the circadian variation of cortisol and aldosterone; list the pre-analytical variables that must be considered when assessing aldosterone.
8. Diagram the renin-angiotensin-aldosterone axis.
9. List and describe the laboratory analyses used to assess adrenocortical function, including methodology, specimen type, collection, and storage requirements for the following analytes:

Cortisol (serum and urine)	Renin
Urinary free cortisol (UFC)	Angiotensin
Aldosterone	17-hydroxyprogesterone

10. Assess and solve case studies related to disorders of the adrenal cortex and their laboratory assessment.

Key Words and Definitions

Addison disease Deficiency of adrenocortical hormones secondary to disease of the adrenal glands; characterized by hypotension, and a bronzelike hyperpigmentation of the skin. Also called *primary hypoadrenalism* to distinguish from secondary hypoadrenalism (deficiency of pituitary adrenocorticotropic hormone).

Adrenal androgens A class of sex hormones that produce masculinization.

Adrenocorticotropic hormone (ACTH) A 39–amino-acid anterior pituitary hormone, that acts primarily on the adrenal cortex, stimulating its growth and the secretion of corticosteroids. Also called *corticotrophin.*

Aldosterone The major mineralocorticoid steroid hormone secreted by the adrenal cortex.

*The authors gratefully acknowledge the contribution of Ronald J. Whitley and Laurence M. Demers to the chapter in the previous edition, on which portions of this chapter are based.

Key Words and Definitions—cont'd

Androstenedione An androgenic steroid produced by the testis, adrenal cortex, and ovary.

Angiotensin II A small (eight-amino-acid) polypeptide hormone; among its functions, it stimulates release of aldosterone and other hormones, constricts blood vessels and controls arterial pressure.

Angiotensin-converting enzyme (ACE) Enzyme that catalyzes the removal of two amino acids from angiotensin I, thus converting it to the active hormone angiotensin II.

Angiotensin-converting enzyme inhibitors Pharmaceuticals that are competitive inhibitors of the angiotensin-converting enzyme. They are used in the treatment of hypertension.

Angiotensinogen A serum globulin formed by the liver that is cleaved by renin to produce angiotensin I.

Conn syndrome A condition of primary aldosteronism arising from oversecretion of aldosterone by an adrenal cortical adenoma.

Congenital adrenal hyperplasia (CAH) A group of inherited disorders in which deficiencies of enzymes that catalyze the biosynthesis of cortisol result in compensatory hypersecretion of corticotropin and subsequent adrenal hyperplasia as well as excessive androgen production.

Cortisol The major adrenal glucocorticoid synthesized in the zone fasciculata (and, to a lesser extent, the zona reticularis) of the adrenal cortex.

Cushing syndrome A condition characterized by an increased concentration of adrenal glucocorticoid hormone in the bloodstream and its effects on the body.

Dehydroepiandrosterone (DHEA) A weak androgenic steroid secreted by the adrenal cortex. It is the major androgen precursor in females.

Glucocorticoids Any of the group of C21 steroids produced by the adrenal cortex that regulate carbohydrate, fat, and protein metabolism.

Hyperaldosteronism A Condition in which the adrenal gland secretes and releases increased quantities of aldosterone.

Hypovolemia A condition characterized by an abnormal decrease in the volume of circulating blood in the body.

Multiple endocrine neoplasia A group of genetic disorders characterized by hyperplasia and hyperfunction of two or more components of the endocrine system.

Mineralocorticoids Any of the group of 21-carbon corticosteroids (principally aldosterone) that contribute to the regulation of (1) water, (2) acid-base, and (3) electrolyte balance in the body.

Renin A hydrolase enzyme that catalyzes cleavage of the leucine-leucine bond in angiotensinogen to generate angiotensin I.

Steroidogenesis The biosynthesis of steroids by the adrenal glands and gonads.

Steroidogenic acute regulatory protein (StAR) A transport protein that functions to regulate cholesterol transfer within the mitochondria.

Waterhouse-Friderichsen syndrome Adrenal gland failure caused by bleeding into the adrenal gland; it is a fulminating complication of bacterial infections, notably meningococcemia; characterized by sudden onset and short course, cyanosis with petechial hemorrhages of the skin and mucous membranes, fever, and hypotension that can lead to shock and coma.

Zona fasciculata The thick middle layer of the adrenal cortex that contains large lipid-laden cells. It is the major source of glucocorticoids and, to a lesser extent, adrenal androgens.

Zona glomerulosa The thin outer layer of the adrenal cortex. It is the source of mineralocorticoids.

Zona reticularis The inner layer of the adrenal cortex. Its cells resemble those of the zona fasciculata, except they contain less lipid. The zona reticularis is the major source of adrenal androgens and produces glucocorticoids to a lesser degree.

The adrenal gland lies at the upper pole of each human kidney (see Figure 25-1, Chapter 25, page 431). Each gland (1) is pyramidal in shape, (2) is approximately 2 to 3 cm in width, 4 to 6 cm long, 1 cm thick, and (3) weighs approximately 4 g, regardless of age, weight, or sex. Each gland consists of a yellow, outer cortex and a gray, inner medulla. Beneath the capsule of the outer cortex lies the **zona glomerulosa** that constitutes approximately 15% of the cortex (Table 41-1). The next layer is the **zona fasciculata** that composes about 75% of the cortex with large and lipid-laden cells. The innermost zone is the **zona reticularis** that contains irregular looking cells with little lipid content. The cells of the adrenal cortex synthesize steroid hormones. The cells of the adrenal medulla synthesize catecholamines, such as (1) dopamine, (2) norepinephrine, and (3) epinephrine aromatic amines, which have important consequences for blood pressure regulation. The catecholamines and their function are discussed in Chapter 26.

The human adrenal cortex secretes three major classes of *steroid* hormones that possess a wide range of physiological functions. These are the (1) **mineralocorticoids**, (2) **glucocorticoids**, and (3) **adrenal androgens**. This chapter begins with a section on general steroid biochemistry, followed by a discussion of the clinical and biological functions of the steroid hormones produced by the adrenal cortex.

General Steroid Chemistry

Steroid hormones are steroids that act as hormones. In this section, the general (1) chemical structure, (2) biochemistry, and (3) metabolism of steroids are briefly discussed.

Chemical Structure

Steroids contain a cyclopentanoperhydrophenanthrene nucleus as their basic structure (Figure 41-1). The three six-sided rings (A, B, and C) constitute the phenanthrene nucleus, to which is attached the D or cyclopentane ring. The prefix "perhydro" refers to the saturation of the compound with hydrogen atoms. This class of compounds includes such natural products as (1) sterols

TABLE 41-1	Anatomy and Products of the Adrenal Gland	
Adrenal Layer	**Major Product(s)**	**Action**
Cortex		
Zona glomerulosa	Aldosterone	Mineralocorticoid
Zona fasciculata	Cortisol	Glucocorticoid
Zona reticularis	Dehydroepiandrosterone (DHEA)	Androgens
	Androstenedione	
Medulla	Epinephrine	Catecholamine

TABLE 41-2	Trivial and Systematic Names of Some Important Steroid Hormones
Trivial Name	**Systematic Name**
Aldosterone	11β-21-Dihydroxy-3,20-dioxopregn-4-en-18-al
Androstenedione	Androst-4-ene-3,11,17-trione
Androsterone	3α-Hydroxy-5α-androstan-17-one
Cortisol	11β,17,21-Trihydroxypregn-4-ene-3,20-dione
Dehydroepiandrosterone (DHEA)	3β-Hydroxyandrost-5-en-17-one
Estradiol-17β	Estra-1,3,5(10)-triene-3,17β-diol
Estriol	Estra-1,3,5(10)-triene-3,16α,17β-triol
Estrone	3-Hydroxyestra-1,3,5(10)-trien-17-one
Etiocholanolone	3α-Hydroxy-5β-androstan-17-one
Pregnanediol	5β-Pregnane-3α,20α-diol
Progesterone	Pregn-4-ene-3,20-dione
Testosterone	17β-Hydroxy-androst-4-en-3-one
Urocortisol	3α,11β,17,21-Tetrahydroxy-(tetrahydro F) 5β-pregnan-20-one

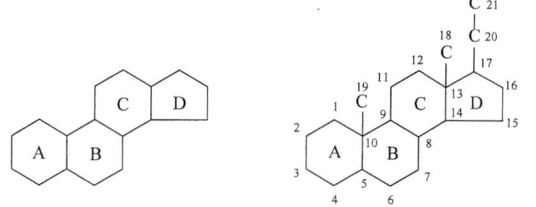

Cyclopentanoperhydrophenanthrene

Figure 41-1 Common features and numbering system of steroids.

(e.g., cholesterol), (2) bile acids (e.g., cholanic acid), (3) sex hormones (e.g., estrogens and androgens), (4) vitamin D (sterols), and (4) corticosteroids. Steroid hormones contain up to 21 carbon atoms (C21 steroids), numbered as shown in Figure 41-1.

Steroids are three-dimensional molecules. Their constituent atoms lie in different planes, which results in the creation of isomers. The direction of the (1) hydrogen atoms, (2) substituents, and (3) side chains play a much more important role in the differentiation among various steroid compound isomers than do the relative positions of the carbon atoms in the rings. Thus, the isomers resulting from fusion of two rings are identified on the basis of the spatial relationship between the hydrogen atoms or the substituents at common carbon atoms. When rings A and B are fused, two isomers are possible depending on whether the hydrogen atom at C-5 and the methyl group at C-10 are on the same or the opposite side of the plane of the rings. If the hydrogen atom points in the same direction as that of the angular methyl group at C-10, the compound is in the *cis,* or *normal,* form. However, if they are on opposite sides, the compound is in the *trans,* or *allo,* form. Depending on which side of the molecule the substituents are attached to relative to these two methyl groups, they have either an α or β orientation. For example, when the substituents are on the same side as the two methyl groups, they have a β configuration, which is indicated by a solid line (—) joining the substituents to the appropriate carbon atoms in the nucleus. Substituents on the opposite side are attached by a broken line (- -) to denote an α configuration.

Individual steroids containing the cyclopentanoperhydrophenanthrene nucleus are differentiated by the presence of double bonds between certain pairs of carbon atoms, the introduction of substituents for the hydrogen atoms, or the addition of a specific type of side chain. On the basis of such structural characteristics, the steroidal compounds are classified as derivatives of certain parent hydrocarbons such as (1) estrane for

estrogens, (2) androstane for androgens, and (3) pregnane for corticosteroids and progestins. The trivial and systematic names of several important steroid hormones are listed in Table 41-2.

Biochemistry

Human steroid hormones are synthesized primarily from cholesterol in the adrenal glands and gonads (see Chapter 23). Typically, cholesterol is acquired from the circulation in the form of low-density lipoprotein (LDL) cholesterol. The uptake of LDL takes place by way of specific cell-surface LDL receptors on the adrenal gland surface that internalize the cholesterol moiety, releasing it as substrate for **steroidogenesis.** Also, all steroidogenic cells are capable of de novo synthesis from acetyl coenzyme A. To ensure a continuous supply of free cholesterol for steroid synthesis, lipoprotein cholesterol uptake is coordinated with intracellular cholesterol synthesis and with the mobilization of intracellular cholesteryl ester pools. When the rate of cholesterol uptake exceeds the rate of steroidogenesis, intracellular cholesterol synthesis is suppressed, and cholesterol in excess of cellular needs is esterified and stored for future use.

The initial rate-limiting step in the transport of intracellular cholesterol to sites of steroidogenesis is mediated by a **steroidogenic acute regulatory protein (StAR)** that is regulated by **adrenocorticotropic hormone (ACTH)** from the pituitary gland.

The nature and quantity of steroid hormones produced by the adrenal glands and gonads are different. For example, the enzymes 11β-hydroxylase and 21-hydroxylase, present only in the adrenal glands, synthesize steroids characteristic of the adrenal glands. Similarly the ovaries and the testes contain enzymes that synthesize the male and female sex hormones (see Chapter 43). Enzymes participating in the biosynthesis of steroid hormones are broadly classified as (1) hydroxylases, (2) lyases, (3) dehydrogenases, and (4) isomerases.

Metabolism

The liver is the major site of steroid metabolism. In addition, the kidney and the gastrointestinal tract both carry out important metabolic transformation of steroids. Important biochemical steps for neutralizing the potent biological activity of hormones and facilitating their rapid elimination from the systemic circulation include (1) the introduction of an additional hydroxyl group (e.g., estradiol to estriol); (2) dehydrogenation (e.g., testosterone to **androstenedione**); (3) reduction of a double bond (e.g., **cortisol** to dihydrocortisol); and (4) conjugation of an essential hydroxyl group or groups with a chemical moiety, such as glucuronic acid (e.g., testosterone to testosterone glucuronide). The conjugation of these hormones and their metabolites with sulfuric or glucuronic acid is the most efficient single metabolic process for their excretion in the urine. Almost all steroid metabolites are excreted as water-soluble glucuronides or sulfates.

Adrenocortical Steroids

The human adrenal cortex secretes a number of steroid hormones that are involved with a wide range of metabolic processes.

Classification

Steroid hormones that are classified as adrenocortical steroids include the corticosteroids and adrenal androgens. The corticosteroids include the mineralocorticoids and glucocorticoids. These steroids are physiologically and quantitatively the most important group of adrenal steroids. The structural formulas of some of the most significant biologically active corticosteroids are shown in Figure 41-2; their trivial and systematic names are listed in Table 41-2.

Mineralocorticoids (Aldosterone)

Mineralocorticoids regulate salt homeostasis (sodium conservation and potassium loss) and extracellular fluid volume. **Aldosterone** is the most potent naturally occurring mineralocorticoid and is synthesized exclusively in the zona glomerulosa region of the adrenal cortex (Figure 41-3). This zone uniquely contains the enzyme aldosterone synthase, an obligatory enzyme in the synthetic pathway to aldosterone. It is secreted at the rate of approximately 200 μg/day.[14,15] The actions of mineralocorticoids are summarized in Table 41-3.

Mineralocorticoids bind to a cytoplasmic mineralocorticoid receptor (MR) in the (1) distal convoluted tubule (DCT) and collecting duct of the nephron, (2) colon, and (3) salivary glands to promote sodium reabsorption and potassium and hydrogen ion excretion.[20] When a mineralocorticoid binds to the MR, the complex relocates to the nucleus, where it influences cellular DNA regulating gene transcription through the transcription factor-action of the glucocorticoid-MR complex.

Other adrenocortical steroids that have mineralocorticoid properties with varying degrees of potency include (1) deoxycorticosterone (DOC), (2) 18-hydroxy-DOC, (3) corticosterone, and (4) cortisol. A large number of analogues with mineralocorticoid and glucocorticoid activity have been synthesized; some are more potent than those that occur naturally.

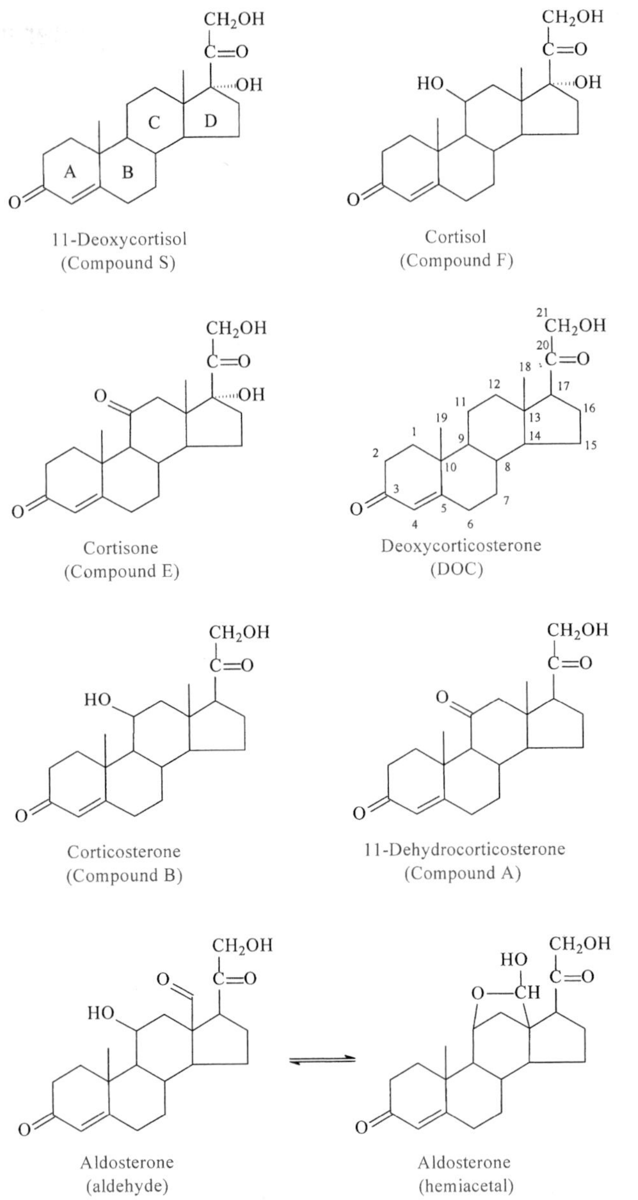

Figure 41-2 Structural formulas and trivial names of some biologically active corticosteroids. Note alphabetical ring system and the numerical system for 21 carbon atoms.

Glucocorticoids (Cortisol)

Cortisol is the major glucocorticoid synthesized from cholesterol in the zona fasciculata and reticularis of the human adrenal cortex (see Figure 41-3). It is secreted at the rate of approximately 25 mg/day. When released into the circulation, cortisol is principally bound to corticosteroid-binding globulin (CBG) and transported as such. Cortisol is metabolized and conjugated in the liver to several inactive metabolites. More than 95% of cortisol and its metabolite cortisone is conjugated to glucuronic acid and excreted into the urine as a conjugate. Less than 2% of cortisol is excreted in the urine unmetabolized as urinary free cortisol (UFC).

Glucocorticoids bind to the glucocorticoid receptor (GR) expressed in many tissues, including (1) lymphocytes, (2) hepatocytes, and (3) bone.[4] Because of the wide distribution of

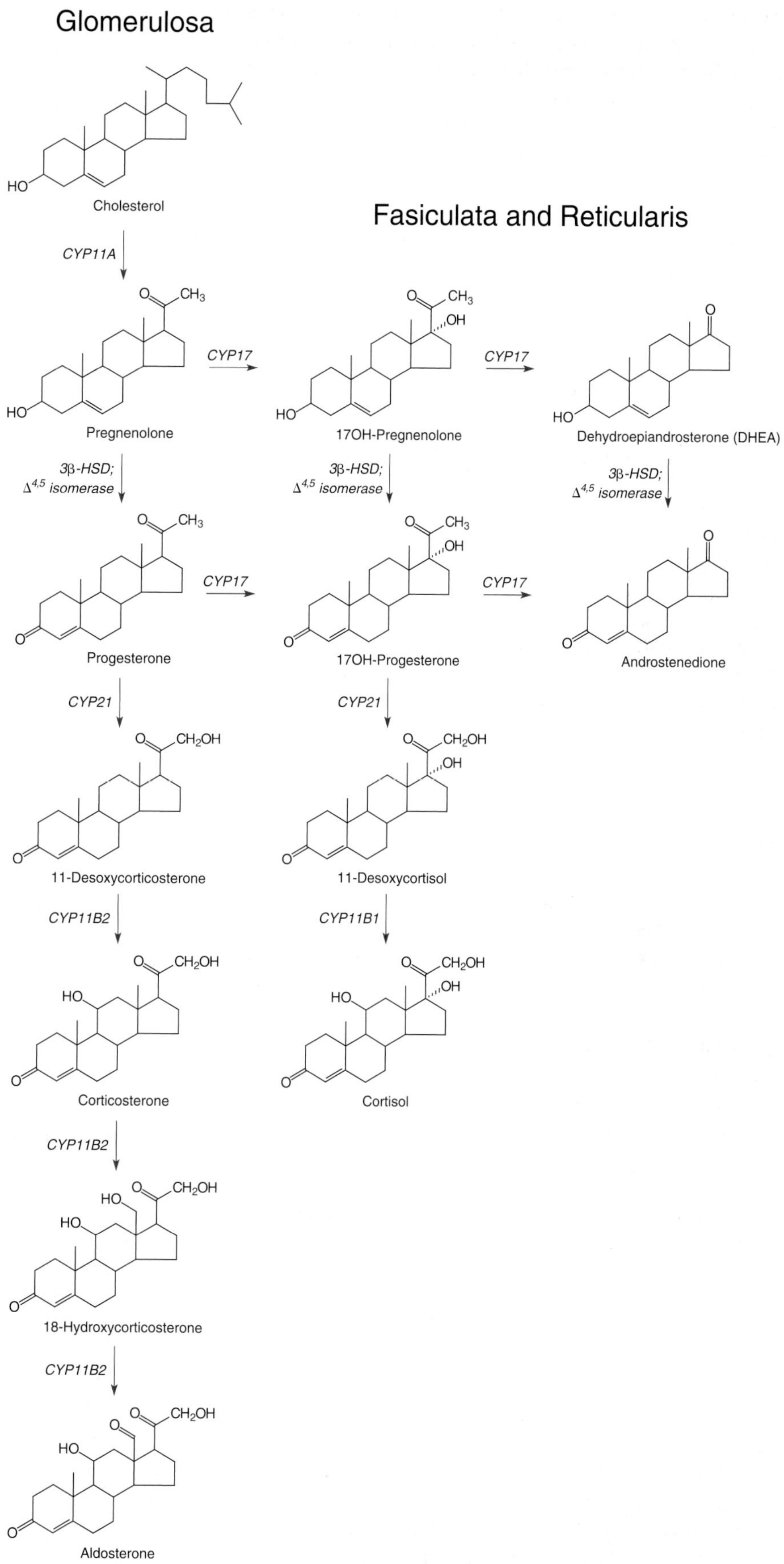

Glomerulosa

Fasiculata and Reticularis

Figure 41-3 The zona glomerulosa is the site of aldosterone synthesis. CYP11B2 is under the predominant control of angiotensin II, which controls aldosterone synthesis and secretion. In the fasciculata and reticularis layers, cortisol and the adrenal androgens dehydroepiandrosterone (DHEA) and androstenedione are produced. CYP11A, 3 beta-HSD, CYP17, CYP21, and CYP11B1 are controlled by adrenocorticotropic hormone (ACTH).

TABLE 41-3	Physiological Effects of Mineralocorticoids	
Action	Physiological Effect of Excessive Action	Physiological Effect of Deficient Action
Sodium retention*	Hypertension	Hypotension
Urinary potassium wasting	Hypokalemia	Hyperkalemia
Urinary hydrogen ion wasting	Alkalosis	Acidemia does not usually occur

*With consequent H_2O retention.

the GR, glucocorticoid effects are diverse, including changes in intermediary metabolism and immunoregulation.

Glucocorticoids have multiple effects on metabolism of glucose and carbohydrates, including (1) increased synthesis of gluconeogenic enzymes such as glucose-6-phosphatase and phosphoenol pyruvate carboxykinase that increase blood glucose, (2) increased liver glycogen content through activation of glycogen synthase, and (3) inhibition of glycogen phosphorylase, producing insulin resistance, in both muscle and adipose tissue, which further increases blood glucose concentrations.

Cortisol increases protein catabolism in multiple tissues. For example, excess cortisol produces (1) myopathy and consequent weakness, (2) thinning of the skin, (3) loss of strength in connective tissues, and (4) bone loss, which leads to fractures and compressed vertebrae.

Glucocorticoids have several effects on lipid metabolism including (1) adipose tissue redistribution centrally to the trunk, neck, and face, (2) increased adipocyte differentiation, (3) promotion of lipogenesis in these tissues, (4) increased very low-density lipoprotein (VLDL) and triglyceride concentrations, (5) decreased high-density lipoprotein (HDL) and HDL-cholesterol concentrations, and (6) increased activity of adipose tissue hormone-sensitive lipase, allowing triglyceride breakdown to free fatty acids and increased free fatty acid delivery to the liver. This provides substrate for hepatic triglyceride resynthesis and VLDL production and export. In addition, glucocorticoids increase appetite, which results in an increase in caloric intake and subsequent weight gain.

Glucocorticoids are powerful antiinflammatory hormones that suppress (1) the activity of pro-inflammatory enzymes (such as, cyclo-oxygenase 2 [COX-2]) and inducible nitric oxide synthase (iNOS), (2) various interleukins (IL-1, IL-2, and IL-6), (3) tumor necrosis factor-alpha, (4) interferon-gamma, and (5) E-selectin. (ACTH secretion is stimulated by IL-1, IL-6, and tumor necrosis factor-alpha.)

At physiological concentrations, glucocorticoids (1) help maintain vascular tone and cardiac output, (2) stabilize lysosomal membranes, and (3) suppress hypersensitivity responses by inhibiting the production of histamine by basophils and mast cells. Modest doses of glucocorticoids may improve one's mood, yet in pharmacologic concentrations, they may produce psychosis. The actions of glucocorticoids are summarized in Table 41-4.

TABLE 41-4	Major Targets of Glucocorticoid Action and Adverse Consequences of Excesses and Deficiencies	
	ADVERSE OUTCOME	
Target Tissue	Excessive Action	Deficient Action
Central Nervous System	Polyphagia	Anorexia
	Depression or psychosis	Depression
Endocrine System		
Carbohydrate metabolism	Hyperglycemia	Hypoglycemia
Glycogen synthesis, gluconeogenesis, insulin resistance	Increased	Decreased
Free fatty acids, triglycerides	Increased	NSE
Body weight	Increased	Decreased
Fat distribution	Centripital	NSE
Pituitary	Decreased TSH	NSE
Musculoskeletal and Connective Tissue		
Muscle	Atrophy (catabolism)	NSE
Skin	Thinning (catabolism)	NSE
Bone	Osteoporosis	NSE
Immune System	Immunosuppression	NSE

NSE, No specific effect.

Adrenal Androgens (Dehydroepiandrosterone and Androstenedione)

The adrenal androgens (1) **dehydroepiandrosterone (DHEA)**, (2) dehydroepiandrosterone sulfate (DHEA-S), and (3) androstenedione provide androgenic effects through their peripheral conversion to testosterone, which in turn binds to the androgen receptor (AR). Between ages 7 and 8, the urinary excretion of 17-ketosteroids (the breakdown products of adrenal androgens) increases as an early sign that puberty will begin in the coming 3 to 5 years.

In males, DHEA and androstenedione are not usually important because gonadal testosterone is a much more potent androgen. However, they are important in pubertal and adult women, because they produce axillary and pubic hair. Females with Turner syndrome (45,X, or "gonadal syndrome") illustrate the effects of adrenal androgens in women. Because of streak gonads (hypoplastic and dysfunctioning gonads mainly composed of fibrous tissue), adolescent girls with Turner syndrome do not experience ovarian gonadarchy (the period during which the ovaries begin to secrete estrogenic sex hormones), because essentially all of their ovarian follicles are atretic before birth. Estrogen deficiency during adolescence is manifested in (1) lack of breast development, (2) primary amenorrhea, and (3) failure of fat redistribution to the hips and buttocks. However, because adrenarchy (the increase in activity of the adrenal glands preceding puberty) is normal in adolescents with Turner syndrome, these girls will develop axillary and pubic hair despite their lack of estrogenization.

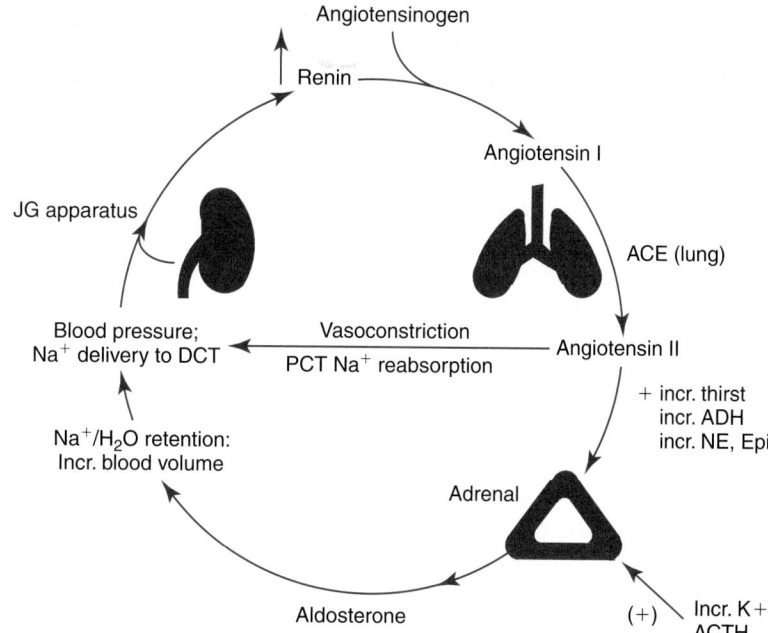

Figure 41-4 The juxtaglomerular apparatus (JGA) monitors the perfusion pressure of the glomerulus and the sodium concentration in the distal convoluted tubule (DCT). Renin is released in cases of decreased renal perfusion or decreased sodium concentration in the DCT. Renin cleaves angiotensinogen to angiotensin I. Angiotensin-converting enzyme (ACE) converts angiotensin I to angiotensin II predominantly in the lung. Angiotensin II has direct vasoconstrictive effects and stimulates sodium reabsorption by the proximal convoluted tubule (PCT); it also stimulates thirst, antidiuretic hormone (ADH) release, catecholamine release (Epi, epinephrine; NE, norepinephrine), and aldosterone synthesis and secretion. Aldosterone increases sodium reabsorption, and, as water follows salt, blood volume increases along with blood pressure. Overall these effects act to restore renal perfusion. Adrenocorticotropic hormone (ACTH) and increased potassium have minor effects in stimulating aldosterone synthesis and secretion.

Regulation of Adrenocortical Hormones

Steroid hormones are not stored in hormone-producing cells and therefore must be produced as needed. Steroids are lipophilic and therefore (1) pass through cell membranes to exit the hormone-producing cells, (2) enter the circulation to be distributed throughout the body, and (3) enter the cytoplasm of target cells where they bind to nuclear receptors. Translocation of the hormone-receptor complex to the nucleus initiates the action of the hormone. Growing evidence suggests that steroid hormones may also act independently of their effect on DNA transcription. In the case of glucocorticoids, there is evidence that the GR may be expressed on the cell surface, explaining some of the immediate effects of glucocorticoids on cellular physiology.

Aldosterone

The production and secretion of aldosterone are regulated by the renin-angiotensin system. As shown in Figure 41-4, **renin** is an enzyme that cleaves the leucine-leucine bond in **angiotensinogen** (a serum α_2-globulin secreted in the liver) to generate angiotensin I. Angiotensin I is the precursor of **angiotensin II**, a polypeptide hormone with important functions in control of arterial pressure and other physiological variables. The rate-limiting component in this system is renin release, which is regulated by the juxtaglomerular apparatus (JGA) of

the kidney (see Chapter 35). The JGA is composed of modified smooth muscle cells that synthesize and secrete renin. The JGA cells function as baroreceptors, responding to increased pressure in the arteriole leading to the glomerulus. Decreased renal perfusion pressure leads to renin release. This is the most important mechanism regulating renin concentrations in the circulation.

The macula densa consists of specialized cells that line the DCT. Compared with other tubular cells, these cells are unique in that their nuclei are near the apical (luminal) pole of the cell, whereas the Golgi apparatus is near the basolateral pole of the cell. Acting as a chemoreceptor, the macula densa monitors the sodium concentration in the DCT. If the sodium concentration declines, the macula densa signals the JGA cells, via prostacyclin, to release renin. Anatomically, the DCT passes between the afferent and efferent arterioles of the nephron, which, respectively, supply blood to, and drain blood from, the glomerular capillaries.

Decreased sodium delivery to the DCT results from hyponatremia or decreased glomerular filtration, both of which elicit renin release. Norepinephrine and dopamine stimulate renin release via sympathetic innervation of the β-adrenoreceptors located in the JCA. Thus, with upright posture and catecholamine release, renin release is enhanced. Potassium also directly stimulates renin release.

Overall, renin is physiologically released in response to (1) **hypovolemia**, (2) reduced cardiac output, (3) systemic vasodilation, (4) selectively reduced renal perfusion, (5) hyponatremia, and (6) stress (mediated by catecholamines).

Angiotensinogen is an α_2-globulin synthesized in hepatocytes. Renin cleaves angiotensinogen to form the decapeptide angiotensin I. Angiotensin I has no (1) endocrine, (2) paracrine, or (3) autocrine effects. **Angiotensin-converting enzyme** (ACE), a zinc metallopeptidase that occurs mostly in the lung, removes the two C-terminal residues from angiotensin I to generate the octapeptide angiotensin II, the most active form of the hormone. Further degradation of angiotensin II by aminopeptidase A yields the heptapeptide angiotensin III. The ratio of angiotensin II to angiotensin III is usually 4 to 1.

Angiotensin II acts to preserve circulating blood volume and maintain blood pressure through several mechanisms: (1) stimulation of aldosterone synthase (CYP11B2) to produce aldosterone; (2) direct vasoconstriction; (3) increased release of epinephrine and norepinephrine from the adrenal medulla, which will also act as vasoconstrictors; (4) stimulation of sodium reabsorption in the proximal convoluted tubule (PCT); (5) stimulation of thirst; and (6) stimulated release of antidiuretic hormone (ADH). Angiotensin III has equivalent potency in stimulating aldosterone secretion.

Cortisol

Cortisol release is controlled through a hypothalamic-pituitary-end organ negative feedback system (Figure 41-5). With this system, corticotropin-releasing hormone (CRH) secretion is stimulated by (1) stress, (2) exercise, and (3) hypoglycemia. Stress may be physiological, including (1) pain, (2) trauma, (3) surgery, and (4) hemorrhage, or psychological, due to severe anxiety and/or depression. Prolonged administration of large doses of glucocorticoids will suppress the hypothalamic-pituitary-adrenal axis, leading to adrenal atrophy. Therefore, abrupt termination of exogenous steroids may induce acute and possibly life-threatening glucocorticoid insufficiency.

CRH is secreted by cells in the paraventricular nucleus of the hypothalamus, and reaches the anterior pituitary gland through the hypothalamic pituitary portal system. Corticotrophs represent about 20% of functional anterior pituitary cells and express receptors for CRH that promote synthesis, storage, and release of adrenocorticotropin (ACTH). ACTH release from the pituitary is also stimulated by ADH, but to a lesser degree than by CRH. The pro-inflammatory cytokines (1) IL-1, (2) IL-6, and (3) tumor necrosis factor-alpha also stimulate ACTH release.

Circulating ACTH binds to receptors located on cells within the adrenal cortex, triggering activity by protein kinase A and protein kinase C, leading to (1) steroidogenesis, (2) increased size and number of adrenocortical cells, and (3) increased size and functional complexity of cellular organelles, all of which result in synthesis and release of cortisol. Cortisol feedback occurs centrally at the hypothalamus, and to a lesser degree at the anterior pituitary, to suppress

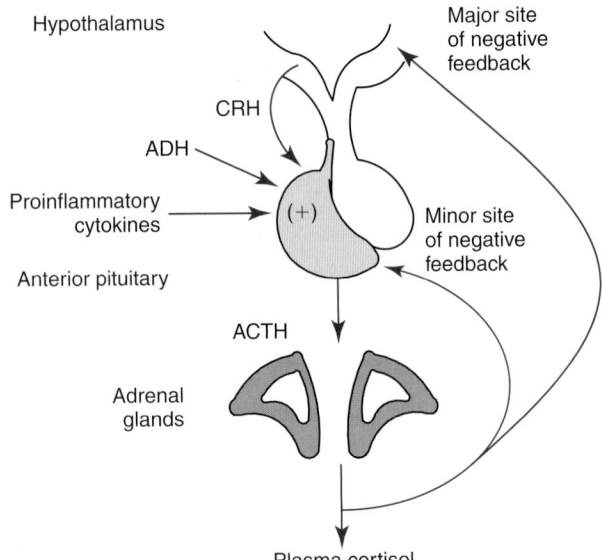

Figure 41-5 Cortisol is controlled through a traditional hypothalamic-pituitary-end organ negative feedback system. Corticotropin-releasing hormone (CRH) is released from the hypothalamus and is delivered to the anterior pituitary via the hypothalamic-pituitary portal system. CRH releases adrenocorticotropic hormone (ACTH) from anterior pituitary corticotroph cells. Increased concentrations of antidiuretic hormone (ADH) and proinflammatory cytokines (such as IL-1, IL-6, and tumor necrosis factor-alpha) can also stimulate ACTH release. ACTH stimulates the synthesis and release of cortisol from the adrenal cortex. Cortisol feeds back negatively at the pituitary, but the major site of negative feedback is the hypothalamus.

CRH and ACTH secretion, respectively. Other negative feedback loops include (1) ACTH suppression of hypothalamic CRH and (2) an ultra-short feedback loop whereby ACTH suppresses its own release.

Pulses of CRH cause the release of ACTH, which stimulates cortisol secretion. There is wide diurnal variation in the secretion of cortisol with highest concentrations in the early morning (about 2 hours before awakening) and lowest concentrations near midnight (assuming that the individual sleeps overnight).

Adrenal Androgens

The regulation of adrenal androgen synthesis and secretion is not well understood.[12] The best characterized regulator of androstenedione and DHEA secretion, however, is ACTH. A diurnal rhythm in adrenal androgen concentrations parallels cortisol variations. Nevertheless, ACTH regulation of adrenal androgens does not explain the normal prepubertal and pubertal increases in adrenal androgen synthesis that occur in both boys and girls because ACTH does not increase prior to puberty.

Circulation

Circulating adrenocortical steroid hormones are 90% to 98% bound to specific carrier proteins or albumin. Unbound steroids in the plasma are mostly conjugated to sulfate or glucuronic acid. Aldosterone is carried primarily by albumin since

(1) cortisol, (2) corticosterone, and (3) 17-hydroxyprogesterone occupy most of the binding sites on CBG. Typical concentrations of cortisol exceed those of aldosterone by many-fold, explaining why little aldosterone is carried on CBG.

Between 80% and 90% of cortisol is carried by CBG, 7% of cortisol is loosely bound to albumin, and 2% to 3% is unbound (free). When total cortisol is increased, the increased plasma free cortisol readily spills into the urine, increasing the UFC excretion. Typically, only 0.25% to 0.5% of total cortisol is excreted in the urine. Because more cortisol than aldosterone is bound to CBG (which slows clearance), the half-life of cortisol is longer (60 to 80 minutes) than the half-life of aldosterone (20 to 30 minutes). In pregnancy, CBG may increase two- to threefold in response to estrogens. Some patients with chronic active hepatitis may display increased concentrations of CBG. Conversely, CBG concentrations are decreased in (1) nephrosis (as a result of CBG loss in the urine), (2) cirrhosis (because of decreased production), (3) hyperthyroidism (due to increased metabolism), and (4) with glucocorticoid treatment (probably as a result of enhanced protein catabolism). Even with changes in total cortisol due to changes in CBG, the concentration of free cortisol remains stable if the hypothalamic-pituitary-adrenal axis is functioning normally.

DHEA and its sulfated form, DHEA-S, and estradiol are predominantly bound to albumin, whereas testosterone and dihydrotestosterone (DHT) are mostly bound to sex hormone–binding globulin (SHBG). Estrogens and thyroid hormone increase SHBG concentrations, whereas (1) insulin, (2) growth hormone, (3) glucocorticoids, (4) androgens, and (5) progestins lower SHBG concentrations. SHBG concentrations are higher in children than in adults.

Metabolism

The liver is the major site of steroid metabolism (Figure 41-6), via P450 enzymes with the kidney playing less of a metabolic role but an important excretory role. Clearance of steroid hormones involves (1) hydroxylation, (2) dehydrogenation, (3) reduction of double bonds, and (4) conjugation to sulfates or glucuronides. The reduction in steroid concentrations increases their solubility and provides functional sites (such as, hydroxyl groups) for their conjugation to sulfate or glucuronic acid; this increases their solubility in urine, promoting their excretion. Approximately 90% of conjugated steroids are excreted by the kidney.

Cortisol metabolism and clearance affect cortisol concentrations. If the clearance of cortisol is reduced, plasma cortisol concentrations increase, whereas enhanced clearance of cortisol decreases its concentrations.

Urinary Metabolites

Measurement of the urinary excretion of adrenocortical hormones may be useful in the laboratory assessment of adrenal disease. However the difficulty of accurately collecting timed urine samples remains a challenge, and serum or plasma steroid assays are often preferred. Immunoassays for the major circulating steroid hormones are widely available.

Biochemically 17-hydroxyprogesterone is reduced to pregnanetriol, which typically is measured in urine. Before the development of immunoassays for 17-hydroxyprogesterone, a 24-hour urine was collected for measurement of pregnanetriol excretion in most types of congenital adrenal hyperplasia (CAH). The urinary metabolites of 11-desoxycortisol and cortisol are classified as 17-hydroxycorticosteroids (17-OHCS). Analytically, 17-OHCS are photometrically measured by the reaction of 17,21-dihydroxy-20-oxosteroids with a phenylhydrazine-ethanol-sulfuric acid reagent, producing yellow phenylhydrazones called the *Porter-Silber chromogens*.

Collectively, the urinary metabolites are (1) 17-hydroxyprogesterone, (2) 11-desoxycortisol, and (3) cortisol are 17-ketogenic steroids (17-KGS). Ketogenic steroids have been measured using the Zimmermann reaction, in which an alkaline solution of meta-dinitrobenzene reacts with methylene groups at carbon-16 of the 17-ketosteroids.

Dynamic Tests of Adrenal Function

Several tests are used to assess adrenal function. These tests are typically designed to differentiate between primary and secondary causes of disease, or to detect abnormalities that may not be apparent in the results of static, baseline laboratory measurements. A stimulus is applied, and the release of a given hormone over a specific time frame is measured. Alternatively, suppression tests are used to determine whether physiological feedback mechanisms are intact.

Adrenocorticotropic Hormone Stimulation (Cosyntropin) Tests

ACTH stimulation tests are designed to document the functional capacity of the adrenal glands to synthesize cortisol. In the test, the adrenal glands are stimulated by cosyntropin (also called *tetracosactrin*; Synacthen and Cortrosyn are brand names), a synthetic polypeptide that is the N-terminal 24 amino acid sequence of ACTH and contains the biologically active domain of the hormone. It is a potent stimulator of cortisol secretion, and it has a very short half-life and minimal antigenicity. The test determines whether the adrenal glands are responsive to ACTH.

Corticotropin-Releasing Hormone Stimulation Test

A direct and selective test of anterior pituitary gland function is the CRH stimulation test. Injection of ovine CRH stimulates ACTH secretion in healthy subjects within 60 to 180 minutes; glucocorticoids inhibit this effect (as in cases of **Cushing syndrome** resulting from an adrenal adenoma or ectopic ACTH secretion by a tumor).

Insulin-Induced Hypoglycemia Stimulation Test

To test the integrity of the hypothalamic-pituitary-adrenal axis, indirect tests of ACTH secretion rely on the adrenal response to signals that stimulate ACTH release. In the insulin-induced hypoglycemia stimulation test, insulin is given to produce hypoglycemia which is a physiologic stimulus for release of CRH; plasma ACTH or cortisol concentrations are then measured and will be increased if the hypothalamic-pituitary-adrenal

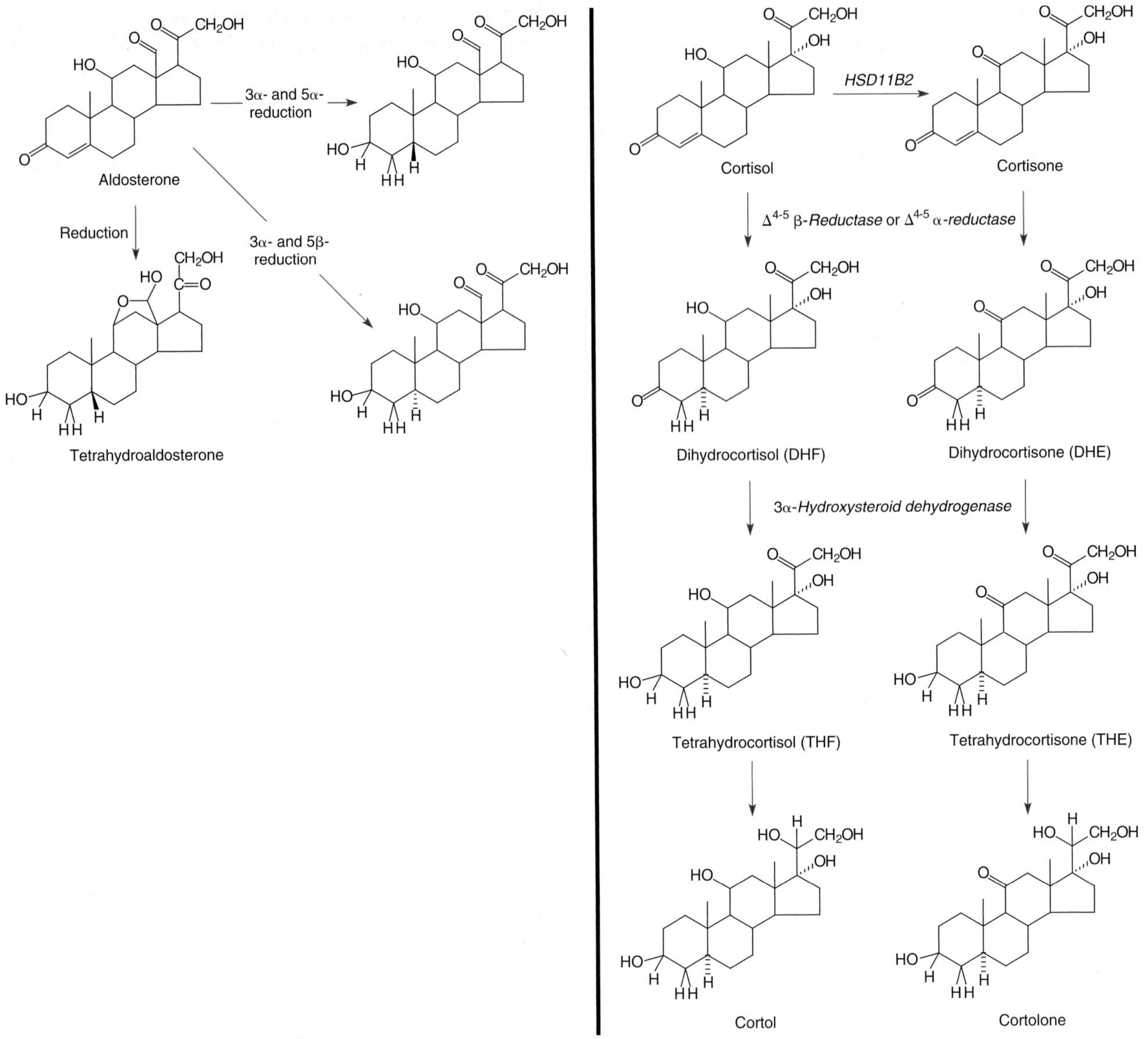

Figure 41-6 Left panel: **Aldosterone metabolism:** Aldosterone is reduced to tetrahydroaldosterone. Aldosterone is 3 alpha- and 5 alpha-reduced, or 3 alpha- and 5 beta-reduced. Right panel: **Cortisol metabolism:** Cortisone is formed from cortisol via 11-beta hydroxysteroid dehydrogenase-2 (HSD11B2). Reduction of the double bonds at carbons 4-5 via delta(4)-5 beta reductase or delta(4)-5 alpha reductase yields dihydrocortisol (DHF) and dihydrocortisone (DHE). Metabolism with reduction of the ketone groups at carbon 3 results in tetrahydrocortisol (THF) and tetrahydrocortisone (THE), which account for the major portion of cortisol clearance (≈50%). Further metabolism of THF and THE via 20-alpha hydroxysteroid dehydrogenase or 20-beta hydroxysteroid dehydrogenase produces alpha and beta cortol and cortolone (the cortoic acids), which account for ≈30% of cortisol excretion.

axis is intact. This test involves risks of hypoglycemia such as (1) obtundation/decreased mental capacity, (2) seizure, (3) coma, and (4) death; it should be performed only under carefully supervised conditions. Venous access must be maintained during the procedure to facilitate rapid administration of glucose should hypoglycemia not spontaneously resolve or a hypoglycemia-induced seizure occur requiring immediate administration of intravenous glucose.

Metyrapone Stimulation Test

A less risky indirect test of hypothalamic-pituitary-adrenal axis function involves the administration of metyrapone, an inhibitor of the 11 β-hydroxylase enzyme (CYP11B1) that converts 11-desoxycortisol to cortisol. The decrease of cortisol is expected to allow an increase in ACTH secretion. Several protocols have been designed to directly or indirectly monitor the effect of metyrapone on ACTH secretion.

Dexamethasone Suppression Test

In healthy individuals, an increase in cortisol inhibits CRH release from the hypothalamus, resulting in decreased production of ACTH and, subsequently, of cortisol. With the dexamethasone suppression test, the integrity of this feedback mechanism is assessed by administering the potent glucocorticoid dexamethasone, and measuring serum or urine cortisol concentrations to evaluate the hypothalamic response. Several dexamethasone suppression tests are available for clinical use. Dexamethasone is chosen for suppression testing, because it does not significantly cross-react in cortisol immunoassays. Patients with Cushing syndrome of any cause will fail to suppress their morning plasma cortisol concentration to less than 2 µg/dL in response to a 1-mg dose of dexamethasone administered at 22:00. This is a screening test, and confirmation of Cushing syndrome requires repeat testing or measurement of urinary cortisol on at least two separate days or some other combination of tests.

Mineralocorticoid Stimulation Tests

The renin-angiotensin-aldosterone system responds to (1) blood volume, (2) blood pressure, and (3) electrolyte balance (and imbalance). Sodium excretion and extracellular fluid volume are inversely correlated with plasma renin and aldosterone concentrations. Procedures for stimulating the renin-angiotensin system are based on volume depletion maneuvers, such as (1) sodium restriction, (2) upright posture, or (3) diuretic administration.

In the furosemide stimulation test, the diuretic furosemide (40 to 80 mg) is administered to decrease plasma volume, followed by 4 hours of upright posture. This test does not require hospitalization or special diets, although it is recommended that the patient maintain a diet with a normal salt intake. The normal response is a two- to threefold increase in plasma renin, indicating that the JGA is responding properly to decreased plasma volume.

Another simple and convenient stimulation test consists of sodium restriction and upright posture. Dietary sodium is restricted to less than 20 mmol/day for 3 to 5 days; urine is collected for creatinine and sodium measurements until equilibrium with the new diet is established. Plasma renin activity (PRA) is measured after 2 hours of standing. A normal response is a two- to threefold increase in plasma renin. In a patient with mineralocorticoid deficiency, hydration status should be assessed carefully to prevent the development of acute hypovolemia and its potential adverse consequences.

Mineralocorticoid Suppression Tests

Mineralocorticoid suppression tests use either (1) saline infusion, (2) oral salt loading, or (3) mineralocorticoid administration, each of which should suppress the secretion of aldosterone by the adrenal gland. In healthy individuals, acute expansion of plasma volume with salt increases renal perfusion, suppresses renin release, and decreases aldosterone secretion. If hypertension is present, this test can potentially raise the patient's blood pressure to undesirable levels.

Disorders of the Adrenal Cortex

Thomas Addison first reported hypofunction of the adrenal cortex in 1855.[16] Subsequently, many diseases associated with abnormal adrenal function have been discovered and studied.

Although circulating concentrations of adrenal androgens decline with advancing age, it is unclear whether this simply reflects physiological changes associated with aging, or if it is a pathological condition that should be treated. Most experts believe the former and do not recommend adrenal androgens as "treatment" for aging. Adrenal androgen deficiency occurs as part of primary adrenal failure in aging, but it has no clear pathologic consequences.

Adrenal Insufficiency (Addison Disease)

Adrenal insufficiency causing combined mineralocorticoid and glucocorticoid deficiency is a rare disorder with a prevalence of only 4 to 11 cases per 100,000. If left untreated, adrenal insufficiency can be fatal. Cortisol deficiency is classified as primary, secondary, or tertiary.

Primary adrenal insufficiency, also known as **Addison disease**, results from progressive destruction or dysfunction of the adrenal glands by (1) an autoimmune process, (2) a systemic disorder, (3) an inborn error of metabolism (endogenous causes), or (4) by an exogenous cause, such as infection (Table 41-5). Worldwide, the most common cause of primary adrenal insufficiency is infectious diseases which include (1) tuberculosis, (2) fungal infections (histoplasmosis, cryptococcosis, North and South American blastomycosis, sporotrichosis, and coccidiomycosis), and (3) cytomegalovirus infection. Syphilis produces a syphilitic gumma (a fibrotic and granulomatous lesion) that destroys the adrenal gland. In patients with AIDS, opportunistic infections with (1) cytomegalovirus, (2) fungi, (3) mycobacteria, and other microbes have been known to damage the adrenal gland. Autoimmune adrenalitis accounts for more than 70% of cases reported in developed countries, with adrenal autoantibodies measurable in more than 75% of these cases. In adrenal insufficiency the adrenal glands are atrophic with loss of cortical cells but an intact medulla.

The most common inborn errors of steroidogenesis involve defects in the the synthesis of cortisol, with or without concurrent aldosterone deficiency. Because such disorders commonly lead to excessive adrenal androgen production, they are discussed in a later section concerning hyperfunction of the adrenal cortex. The onset of clinical manifestations is usually gradual, and the degree and severity of symptoms depend on the extent of adrenal failure. In early or mild expressions of primary adrenal insufficiency, hypofunction may not be evident unless the patient is under stress (e.g., following trauma or surgery). Complete glucocorticoid deficiency manifests in a variety of ways, including (1) fatigue, (2) weakness, (3) weight loss, (4) gastrointestinal disturbance, and (5) fasting hypoglycemia. Mineralocorticoid deficiency leads to dehydration with (1) hypotension, (2) acidosis, (3) hyponatremia, and (4) hyperkalemia. Excessive pituitary synthesis and release of ACTH, unchecked by the negative feedback system, may cause

TABLE 41-5   Causes of Primary Adrenal Insufficiency or Failure of Aldosterone Production

Endogenous Causes

Autoimmune disease	Sporadic
	Autoimmune polyglandular syndrome type 1 (Addison disease, candidiasis, hypoparathyroidism, and primary gonadal failure)
	Autoimmune polyglandular syndrome type 2 (Addison disease, primary hypothyroidism, primary hypogonadism, diabetes, and pernicious anemia)
Inborn errors	Congenital adrenal hyperplasia (CAH)
	Congenital adrenal hypoplasia (DAX-1 mutation)
	Demyelinating disorders: adrenoleukodystrophies
	Childhood X-linked recessive adrenoleukodystrophy (Brown-Schilder disease)
	Neonatal autosomal recessive adrenoleukodystrophy
	X-linked recessive adrenomyeloneuropathy (sudanophilic leukodystrophy)
	Familial (isolated) glucocorticoid deficiency (degeneration of fasciculata-reticularis layers)
	Wolman disease (lysosomal acid lipase deficiency)
	Steroidogenic factor-1 (SF-1) mutations
	Mitochondrial forms of Addison disease (Kearns-Sayre syndrome)
	Smith-Lemli-Opitz syndrome (sterol delta-7-reductase mutations)
	Adrenocorticotropic hormone (ACTH) resistance syndromes
Vascular disorders	Intra-adrenal hemorrhage (Waterhouse-Friderichsen syndrome; caused by infection [especially Neisseria meningitidis, but also Pseudomonas aeruginosa, Haemophilus influenzae, Streptococcus pyogenes, or Streptococcus pneumoniae]) or anticoagulants
Glandular infiltration	Neoplastic
	Leukemia, lymphoma, carcinoma of the lung, carcinoma of the breast
	Non-neoplastic
	Amyloid
	Hemochromatosis

Exogenous Causes

Infection	Granulomatous disease
	Tuberculosis, sarcoidosis, histoplasmosis, cryptococcosis, blastomycosis (North and South American), sporotrichosis, and coccidiomycosis
	Other infections
	Cytomegalovirus, opportunistic infections in HIV
Drugs	Blockers of steroid synthesis: mitotane, aminoglutethimide, trilostane, ketoconazole, metyrapone
	Glucocorticoid receptor blockers: Mifepristone (RU-486)

Abdominal Irradiation

Bilateral adrenalectomy	Intra-adrenal thrombosis: renal vein thrombosis in neonates, heparin-induced thrombocytopenia, antiphospholipid syndrome

Causes of Deficient Mineralocorticoid Activity

Failure of Aldosterone Production (Decreased Aldosterone)

Hyperreninemic hypoaldosteronism (synthetic deficiency)	Primary adrenal insufficiency
	Selective aldosterone deficiency
	Inborn errors (e.g., CYP11B2 mutations)
	Drug-induced aldosterone suppression
	Heparin (direct inhibition of aldosterone secretion)
	Angiotensin-converting enzyme (ACE) inhibitors
	Angiotensin receptor blockers (ARBs)
	Hypoaldosteronism in critical illness/hypotension (e.g., selective zona glomerulosa injury)[2]
Hyporeninemic hypoaldosteronism (deficient aldosterone stimulation)	Renin deficiency (e.g., diabetes, renal failure)

Deficient Aldosterone Action (Resistance to Aldosterone; Increased Aldosterone)

Pseudohypoaldosteronism, type 1	Renal
	Multiple target organ defects
	Early childhood hyperkalemia

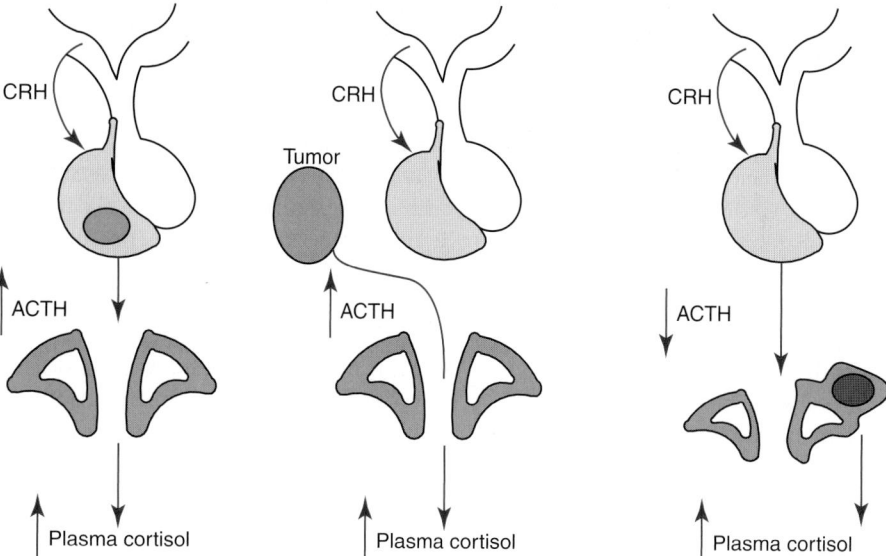

Figure 41-7 Endogenous Cushing syndrome is also classified as Cushing disease (left panel), ectopic ACTH syndrome (middle panel), or adrenal Cushing syndrome (right panel). ACTH is elevated in cases of Cushing disease and ectopic ACTH syndrome. ACTH is suppressed in cases of adrenal Cushing syndrome.

hyperpigmentation of the skin and mucous membranes due to stimulation of melanin production.

In secondary and tertiary adrenal insufficiency, inadequate cortisol production may be due to destructive processes in the hypothalamus and/or pituitary that result in a decreased ability to secrete CRH (tertiary adrenal insufficiency) or ACTH (secondary adrenal insufficiency). However, the most common cause of tertiary cortisol insufficiency is long-term administration of glucocorticoids that suppress CRH, leading to a decrease in both ACTH release and cortisol secretion due to adrenal atrophy. Clinical features of glucocorticoid deficiency in secondary and tertiary adrenal insufficiency are similar to those of primary insufficiency, except that hyperpigmentation is not present and hypotension is less severe. Mineralocorticoid deficiency, hyperkalemia, and ACTH excess are not features of secondary or tertiary adrenal insufficiency. The cosyntropin stimulation test, which tests how well the adrenal glands responde to ACTH, distinguishes primary adrenal insufficiency (impaired response to cosyntropin) from secondary or tertiary causes of adrenal insufficiency.

ACTH and cortisol concentrations often are not useful for establishing the diagnosis of secondary adrenal insufficiency. Episodic secretion and circadian variation result in ACTH and cortisol concentrations that overlap between normal subjects and individuals with secondary or tertiary adrenal insufficiency.[9] A morning cortisol is a useful screening test for adrenal insufficiency since concentrations are highest in the morning; morning cortisol in patients with adrenal insufficiency usually is below 10 μg/dL.

Although subnormal basal plasma concentrations of DHEA-S occur in (1) primary, (2) secondary, and (3) tertiary forms of adrenal insufficiency, DHEA-S measurements are of limited value in the diagnosis of adrenal insufficiency. Low concentrations of adrenal androgens are normally observed in young children (before ages 7 to 9) and in the elderly.

Measurement of adrenal autoantibodies may be useful in evaluating patients suspected of adrenal insufficiency.[3] Such autoantibodies are detected by indirect immunofluorescence (adrenal cytoplasmic autoantibodies [ACA]) or by ELISA (21-hydroxylase autoantibodies).

Hypoaldosteronism

Deficient aldosterone production also occurs in conditions other than Addison disease. For example, isolated aldosterone deficiency accompanied by normal cortisol production occurs in patients with (1) inadequate production of renin by the kidney, which leads to secondary aldosterone deficiency (hyporeninemic hypoaldosteronism); (2) inherited enzyme defects in aldosterone biosynthesis; and (3) acquired forms of primary aldosterone deficiency (post-surgical or due to heparin therapy). The resulting metabolic changes are hyperkalemia and hyponatremia. Mild or moderate volume depletion, often with postural or unprovoked hypotension, may also occur. Nevertheless, isolated aldosterone deficiency is not as common as Addison disease.

Glucocorticoid Excess (Cushing Syndrome)

Endogenous Cushing syndrome is the result of autonomous excessive production of cortisol, leading to a characteristic set of clinical features, including (1) truncal obesity, (2) moon facies, (3) a "buffalo" hump on the upper back below the neck, (4) supraclavicular fat pads, (5) purple striae, (6) myopathy, (7) hypertension, (8) hirsutism, (9) hypokalemic alkalosis, (10) carbohydrate intolerance, (11) secondary osteoporosis, (12) disturbed reproductive function, and (13) neuropsychiatric symptoms. Exogenous Cushing syndrome is caused by excessive oral or parenteral glucocorticoid therapy.

Endogenous disorders that cause hypersecretion of cortisol and Cushing syndrome (Figure 41-7) may be classified as ACTH dependent or ACTH independent. Cushing disease is the pituitary-dependent form of Cushing syndrome. In Cushing disease, hypersecretion of ACTH by an anterior pituitary tumor leads to bilateral adrenal hyperplasia and cortisol overproduction. In the ectopic ACTH syndrome, nonendocrine tumors develop the ability to secrete ACTH, resulting in (1) bilateral adrenal hyperplasia, (2) unregulated cortisol secretion, and (3) suppression of pituitary ACTH release. Rarely, does ectopic secretion of CRH occur. In ectopic ACTH syndrome, the patient's clinical presentation is usually dominated by the presence of cancer, and the patient may not display classic clinical findings of Cushing syndrome, such as centripetal obesity. Ectopic Cushing syndrome due to a bronchial carcinoid has been known to mimic classical Cushing disease and present a diagnostic dilemma requiring measurements of hormones in blood obtained from the inferior petrosal venous sinus.

Multiple endocrine neoplasia type 1 (MEN1) is part of a group of disorders that affect the endocrine system through development of neoplastic lesions in the (1) pituitary, (2) parathyroid gland, and (3) pancreas. It is an uncommon cause of Cushing syndrome. Excess cortisol production when seen in MEN1 is most commonly attributable to hypersecretion of ACTH from a pituitary microadenoma.

Cushing syndrome is an uncommon disorder, but it must be considered frequently as many of the usual signs and symptoms of this syndrome are seen commonly in patients. The initial diagnosis of Cushing syndrome, particularly in mild or early disease, rests on laboratory evidence of excessive and autonomous cortisol production. The following three screening tests are available for detecting Cushing syndrome: (1) measurement of 24-hour UFC, (2) overnight dexamethasone suppression test, and (3) midnight measurements of salivary or serum/plasma cortisol. The most reliable screening test is measurement of 24-hour urine free cortisol excretion.[7]

Congenital Adrenal Hyperplasia

CAH is the most common cause of adrenocortical insufficiency in newborns. It is discussed under adrenal hormone overproduction syndromes, because CAH commonly leads to overproduction of adrenal androgens. Thus, as noted previously, CAH presents a mixed picture of cortisol deficiency (hypofunction) and adrenal androgen overproduction (hyperfunction).

CAH results from loss-of-function mutations in specific adrenocortical enzymes that are responsible for the synthesis of cortisol. These disorders are inherited as autosomal recessive traits. Six enzymes are necessary for the conversion of cholesterol into cortisol, and deficiencies of five of these enzymes have been described. However, 95% of CAH cases are due to deficiency in CYP21, also called *21α-hydroxylase;* most of the remaining cases are due to CYP11B1 (11β-hydroxylase) deficiency. Other causes of CAH are rare. The incidence of 21α-hydroxylase CAH in Western societies varies from 1 in 5000 to 15,000 live births. Neonatal screening for 21α-hydroxylase–deficient and 11β-hydroxylase–deficient CAH in newborns by measuring 17α-hydroxyprogesterone (17-OHP) is practiced in the United States and many other countries. 17-OHP measurements are more sensitive for the detection of 21α-hydroxylase–deficient CAH than 11β-hydroxylase–deficient CAH. Because CAH produces elevations of adrenal androgens (DHEA and androstenedione) in utero, virilization of the external genitalia of the female fetus occurs, producing sexual ambiguity. Inadequate

male sexual development occurs in rare forms of CAH due to deficiencies of 3β hydroxysteroid dehydrogenase or 17-hydroxylase (CYP17).

Rarely, traumatic adrenal hemorrhage or adrenal hemorrhage from sepsis (**Waterhouse-Friderichsen syndrome**) causes adrenal failure in newborns.

Cortisol deficiency in affected individuals leads to (1) malaise, (2) failure to thrive, (3) hypoglycemia, and (4) vascular instability. In approximately one half of infants afflicted with 21α-hydroxylase–deficient CAH, insufficient aldosterone production causes (1) hyponatremia, (2) hyperkalemia, (3) acidosis, (4) dehydration, and (5) hypotension. In its most severe form, this type of "salt-losing" 21α-hydroxylase–deficient CAH patients clinically present at 10 to 14 days of age with Addisonian crisis. Untreated, mortality is very high in salt-losing 21α-hydroxylase deficiency. The non–salt-losing form of this disease is customarily referred to as *simple virilizing* 21α-hydroxylase deficient CAH.

Functioning Adrenocortical Tumors

Increased concentrations of (1) plasma DHEA-S, (2) DHEA, (3) androstenedione, and (4) testosterone are seen in patients with virilizing adrenal adenomas and Cushing syndrome. The plasma concentrations of DHEA may also be increased in women with virilizing ovarian tumors. CT scans along with MRI are useful in differentiating the sites of the tumors (e.g., ovarian versus adrenal).

Aldosterone-producing adenomas, referred to as **Conn syndrome**, are typically small microadenomas found in the zona glomerulosa that hypersecrete aldosterone, producing the syndrome characterized by low renin, hypokalemic alkalosis, and hypertension.

Adrenal carcinomas are rare, with an incidence of only 1 per million population, and occur more commonly in women than in men by a 2.5:1.0 ratio. Most adrenal carcinomas are functional, producing glucocorticoids alone or both glucocorticoids and androgens. Plasma DHEA-S, DHEA, and androstenedione concentrations are markedly increased in patients with functional adrenal carcinomas. The peripheral conversion of adrenal androgens to testosterone results in hirsutism and virilization. Concentrations of DHEA-S often exceed 10 μg/mL in patients with adrenal carcinoma and usually are diagnostic for this malignancy. Feminizing adrenocortical carcinomas are also rare. These tumors produce increased concentrations in plasma of (1) DHEA-S, (2) DHEA, (3) androstenedione, (4) estrone, and (5) estradiol, Gynecomastia and sexual dysfunction occur in males, and precocious pseudopuberty occurs in prepubertal females.

Nonfunctioning Adrenocortical Tumors

Approximately 2% of the human population has an adrenal mass; most of these tumors are nonfunctioning and benign and are called incidentalomas when found during imaging studies conducted to investigate unrelated signs and symptoms.[1] The tumors usually are found when a CT or MRI scan of the abdomen is performed that easily detects tumors 1 cm in diameter or 5 g in weight. No virilizing tumors smaller than

1 cm in diameter have been reported. Carcinomas usually weigh more than 30 g. An unexpected finding of an adrenal mass is investigated by clinical examination of the patient for signs of adrenal cortical hormone action. Laboratory evaluation includes tests for cortisol and aldosterone, plus tests to rule out tumors of the adrenal medulla.

Mineralocorticoid Excess (Hyperaldosteronism)

Primary **hyperaldosteronism**, a syndrome of adrenal hypersecretion of aldosterone by the adrenals, is an increasingly recognized, treatable cause of hypertension. In primary hyperaldosteronism, excessive aldosterone production originates within the adrenal gland. The most common causes are aldosterone producing adenoma and bilateral idiopathic hyperplasia. In secondary hyperaldosteronism, a stimulus outside the adrenal gland activates the renin-angiotensin system. The interactions of (1) renin, (2) angiotensin, and (3) aldosterone are important in the regulation of extracellular fluid volume and blood pressure, and in regulating the balance of sodium and potassium ions as well as acid-base balance.

Secondary hyperaldosteronism is suspected in patients with (1) volume depletion, (2) edema, and (3) hypokalemic alkalosis. Hypertension is present in primary hyperaldosteronism, but it is usually absent in secondary hyperaldosteronism, unless the patient has a reninoma (renin-secreting tumor) or renal artery stenosis. Measurements of renin and aldosterone concentrations are seldom needed in cases of secondary hyperaldosteronism, because precipitating circumstances that explain the patient's hypokalemia and alkalosis (e.g., secondary hyperaldosteronism is expected in congestive heart failure) are apparent. Renin and aldosterone measurements are essential, however, in the investigation of primary disturbances in the renin-angiotensin-aldosterone system and in the assessment of renal artery stenosis.

In suspected primary hyperaldosteronism a useful screening test is the plasma aldosterone concentration (PAC)/PRA ratio. If the PAC/PRA is greater than 20 to 25, the presumptive diagnosis of primary aldosteronism is established, and confirmation with dynamic tests should be sought.

Hypokalemia is the key clinical finding that primary hyperaldosteronism may be present in a patient with diastolic hypertension. To confirm the diagnosis, it is necessary to demonstrate (1) hyposecretion of renin that is not appropriately corrected during volume depletion, and (2) hypersecretion of aldosterone that fails to suppress appropriately during volume expansion. Figure 41-8 shows a suggested scheme for evaluating patients with suspected mineralocorticoid excess.

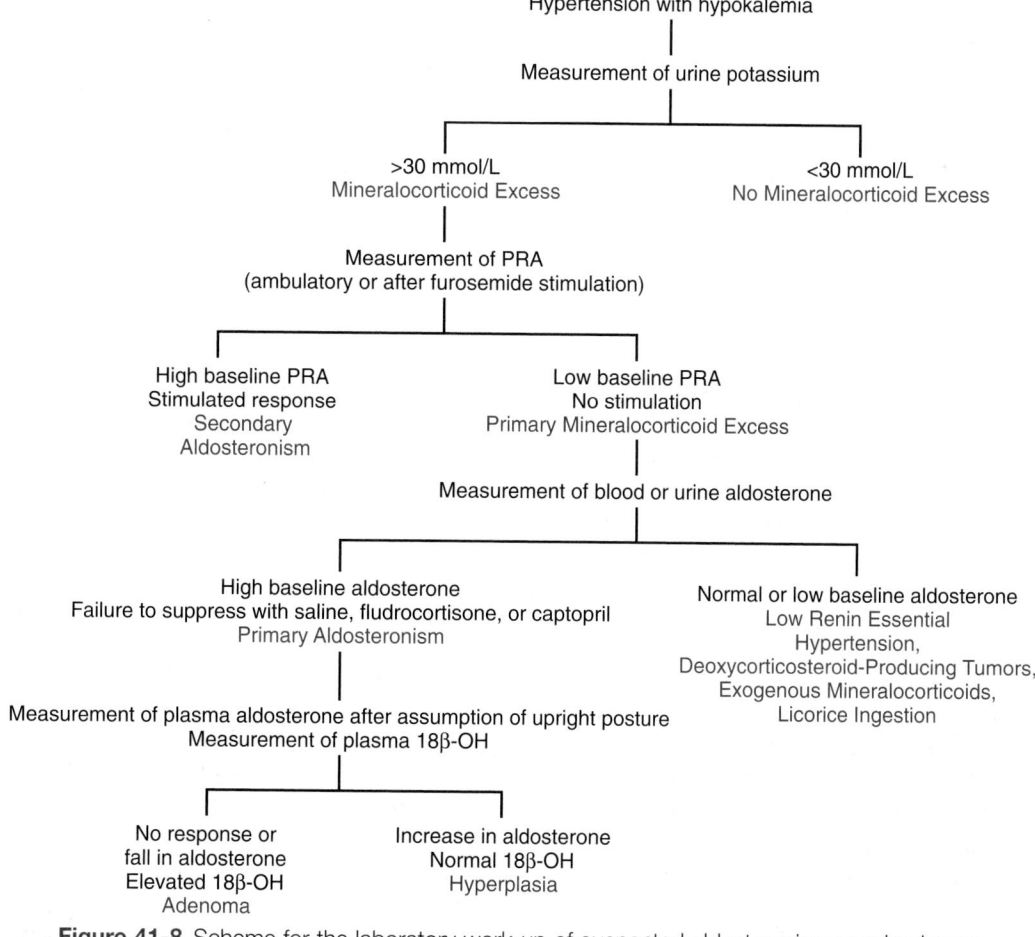

Figure 41-8 Scheme for the laboratory work-up of suspected aldosteronism causing hypertension. *18β-OH,* 18β-hydroxycorticosterone; *PRA,* plasma renin activity.

In specialized centers, measurements of aldosterone concentrations in the veins that drain the left and right adrenal glands are used before surgical treatment to determine which adrenal is responsible for the hyperaldosteronism (presumably from an adenoma), or if the secretion shows no "lateralization."

Laboratory Evaluation of Adrenocortical Function

Laboratory evaluation of adrenal cortex function centers on measurement of (1) cortisol, the primary glucocorticoid; (2) aldosterone, the primary mineralocorticoid; and (3) androgens, of which the adrenal cortex is a primary source in females and minor source in males. Chromaffin cells in the adrenal medulla are a source of catecholamines, which are discussed in Chapter 26.

Choice of Specimen

Steroid hormones are measured in (1) urine, (2) blood, (3) saliva, and (4) hair. The choice of specimen depends on the application. For clinical assessment of adrenal function, blood (plasma or serum) measurements are convenient, but conditions that cause the binding protein concentration to increase may produce clinically benign elevations in the total cortisol concentration. Urinary concentrations are helpful in determining time-integrated hormone production and provide useful estimates of free hormone concentrations in blood if an appropriately timed urine specimen collection is available. Measurement of steroid hormones in saliva has been proposed as an alternative to urinary hormone assays to estimate free hormone concentrations in blood, the principal advantage being ease of collection of saliva.[19] Hair analysis may be useful for assessing adrenal hormone production over an extended period of time, but currently hair testing is not in widespread use.

Urine

Urinary excretion of a hormone, or its metabolites, provides an approximation of the amount secreted over the time the urine is collected, typically 24 hours. Thus, urinary hormone or metabolite measurements are useful when the hormone has a very short biological half-life and/or its secretion is pulsatile or varies in predictable cycles. Timed urine collections suffer variability associated with factors, such as completeness of collection and impaired renal function.

Blood

Circulating concentrations of steroids in the blood provide the most direct measure of hormone secretion. Provocative testing (stimulation and suppression tests, discussed earlier) often require blood samples to study the rapid changes that occur in hormone concentrations. Many of the steroid hormones are released in a pulsatile or rhythmic fashion, so their concentrations in an isolated blood specimen should take into account these variables.

Mineralocorticoid and adrenal androgen secretion is circadian and episodic in nature, but the dynamic swings in concentration are not as pronounced as with cortisol. It is usually recommended, however, that blood samples for adrenal steroids be collected between 0700 and 1000 for consistency in interpreting the results, particularly when comparing to reference intervals.

Steroid hormone concentrations are nearly the same in serum and plasma. It has been suggested that steroid hormone concentrations may change in unseparated blood specimens as the result of 17β-hydroxysteroid dehydrogenase activity in red blood cells and macrophages, but stability studies of (1) estradiol, (2) cortisol, (3) testosterone, (4) progesterone, (5) 17α- hydroxyprogesterone, androstenedione, and (6) DHEA-S have failed to reveal any clinically significant changes in these hormones in whole blood specimens stored at room temperature for up to 1 week.[10]

Saliva (Oral Fluid)

Most steroids of clinical interest have been measured in saliva, and for some steroids, such as (1) cortisol, (2) estriol, and (3) progesterone, salivary concentrations appear to correlate with the free hormone concentration in plasma. For other steroids, such as (1) testosterone, (2) 17α-hydroxyprogesterone, (3) estradiol, and (4) aldosterone, the clinical usefulness of salivary measurements is yet to be established.

Measurement of steroids in saliva is attractive because specimens are simple to collect; this consideration is particularly important in pediatric patients. Several saliva collection devices using absorbent materials have been designed to collect a sufficient volume of saliva for steroid analysis. However, recovery of cortisol from these devices has been questioned. Collection of saliva specimens using cotton swabs, cotton ropes, and hydrocellulose microsponges has been reported, but cortisol measurements in saliva specimens collected with these devices are more variable than measurements in directly collected ("passive drool") saliva specimens. Salivary cortisol concentrations measured around midnight are usually <0.15 μg/dL.

Analytical Methods

Immunometric, chromatographic and combined chromatographic/mass-spectrometric methods are available for measuring steroid hormones. Methods for measuring several of these hormones are discussed below.

Measurement of Total Cortisol

Approximately 90% of circulating cortisol is bound to plasma proteins, primarily to CBG. Cortisol also binds weakly to albumin. The concentration of CBG in the plasma increases in hyperestrogenic states, including pregnancy and oral contraceptive use; therefore total cortisol in serum is increased in these conditions, although free cortisol remains within normal limits. Immunoassays for direct measurement of cortisol have mostly replaced extraction/chromatographic methods for routine cortisol determinations.

Immunoassay

Immunoassays are the most commonly used methods for measuring cortisol in serum and urine, and are widely available on various automated immunoassay platforms. Most cortisol immunoassays in routine use are heterogeneous, competitive-binding assays that require no initial extraction of steroids from the specimen. Cortisol is displaced from CBG and other endogenous binding proteins by (1) protein-binding agents, such as ANS or salicylate, (2) low pH, or (3) heat treatment. The efficiency of cortisol displacement from proteins by agents (such as, ANS) may be influenced by the concentration of binding proteins in the specimen; the amount of ANS that is adequate for plasma obtained from healthy men and nonpregnant women may be insufficient to completely displace cortisol from CBG in pregnancy when CBG concentrations are increased.

Most contemporary automated cortisol immunoassays use nonisotopic labels. Enzyme labels used in these immunoassays include (1) horseradish peroxidase, (2) alkaline phosphatase, or (3) β-galactosidase. The products generated from these assays are measured using (1) photometric, (2) fluorescent, or (3) chemiluminescent labels and detectors. Nonenzymatic approaches involve fluorescent and chemiluminescent labels, and these are the most common methods currently in use. Both heterogeneous and homogeneous designs have been developed. Most current heterogeneous immunoassays for cortisol involve chemiluminescent labels and magnetic separation. Homogeneous immunoassays for cortisol include the enzyme-multiplied immunoassay technique (EMIT) and the cloned enzyme donor immunoassay (CEDIA).

Chromatographic Methods

Chromatographic methods used to measure cortisol include (1) gas chromatography (GC), (2) thin-layer chromatography (TLC), (3) high performance liquid chromatography (HPLC), and (4) GC and HPLC coupled to mass spectrophotometric detectors (GCMS, LCMS, and LCMSMS). Methods using these latter detectors provide the most specific methods for measuring corticosteroids. Cortisol methods based on capillary electrophoresis are also available. All of these methods demonstrate high specificity for cortisol but have relatively low throughput and require sample preparation steps before analysis. For example, most HPLC methods require preanalytical extraction of cortisol with solid-phase extraction columns or liquid-liquid extraction prior to separation and detection by reversed- or normal-phase HPLC and a fluorescence or ultraviolet absorption detector. GCMS methods for cortisol typically require extraction of the hormone from plasma and conversion to the methoxime-trimethylsilyl derivative prior to analysis. Deuterated cortisol is available for use as the internal standard in MS.

Liquid chromatography/tandem mass spectrometry (LCMSMS) methods are becoming increasingly common. Liquid chromatography has the advantage of not requiring volatile derivatives, so specimen preparation is vastly simplified. LCMSMS methods have been developed that measure cortisol, corticosterone, and multiple corticosteroids.[6] LCMSMS appears poised to become the method of choice for corticosteroid measurements.

Specimen Collection and Storage

Cortisol is measured in (1) serum, (2) heparinized plasma, or (3) EDTA plasma; although some methods avoid EDTA plasma because of assay interference. In serum or plasma specimens, cortisol is stable for 7 days at room temperature or refrigerated, and it is stable for 3 months frozen at −20 °C.

Comments

Blood cortisol concentrations parallel ACTH concentrations with episodic and diurnal minima and maxima observed throughout the day. The cortisol concentration in the evening is normally less than 50% of the morning cortisol concentration. Increased cortisol is associated with (1) stress, (2) glucocorticoid therapy, (3) pregnancy, (4) depression, and (5) hypoglycemia. No significant difference in cortisol concentrations has been noted between males and females, and reference intervals for cortisol are not age dependent. The half-life of cortisol in the circulation is approximately 60 minutes, so concentrations of this hormone in blood change rapidly. In newborns, a transient increase in cortisol occurs immediately after birth, but after 12 to 48 hours, cortisol declines to concentrations below umbilical cord blood concentrations. It then increases to a stable reference interval by about 1 week of age. Renal failure does not directly affect serum cortisol, but metabolites that are not cleared in the urine have the potential to cross-react with immunoassays, causing overestimation of blood cortisol concentrations. Extraction of cortisol into an organic solvent may eliminate interference from hydrophilic metabolites. Celite chromatography has been used to "clear" the sample of possible interference before immunoassay measurements are carried out in patients with renal failure.

Measurement of Free Cortisol

Various methods have been developed to measure the free fraction of cortisol in serum, including (1) ultrafiltration, (2) equilibrium dialysis, and (3) gel filtration. These assays, however, are technically complex and expensive, and are not in general use. Algorithms have been suggested for estimating the free cortisol concentration based on CBG and albumin concentrations.[11] Measurement of urinary cortisol provides an estimate of the free hormone concentration and for many years has been considered the best screening test for Cushing related disease, although salivary (oral fluid) cortisol has been recommended as the first-line diagnostic test. Approximately 2% of total cortisol is excreted in the urine, and urinary cortisol may be used as a screening test for cortisol hypersecretion. However, β-hydroxycortisol also appears in the urine and may interfere with some immunoassays used to measure cortisol in urine.

Methods

Salivary cortisol reflects the concentration of free cortisol in blood, and measurement of cortisol in saliva (i.e., oral fluid) is a practical and convenient way to assess the free hormone concentration. Most immunoassays for total serum cortisol have been used to measure cortisol in saliva. Extraction for these assays is not required because saliva contains virtually no cortisol-binding proteins or other cortisol metabolites. The glycoproteins in saliva are precipitated by freezing and thawing followed by centrifugation, producing a clear fluid that is free of protein interference. In some protocols, 10 minutes prior to obtaining the salivary cortisol sample, the subject is required to rinse their mouths with water. Any oral bleeding can increase the salivary cortisol concentration, because blood has much higher concentrations of cortisol than saliva, reflecting the higher concentrations in blood of proteins that bind cortisol.

Immunoassays designed to measure total serum cortisol have been used to measure urinary (free) cortisol provided that cortisol metabolites and conjugates that cross-react with the anti-cortisol antibodies are first removed by liquid/liquid or solid phase extraction. Unextracted urine may be assayed for cortisol if the antibody has sufficient selectivity, although reference values may differ from those seen in methods that include an extraction step. Even with solvent extraction, most commercial assays for cortisol in urine are subject to interference and imprecision. Chromatographic procedures (such as HPLC) are more specific than immunoassays for measuring urinary cortisol; LCMSMS is the preferred method.

Specimen Collection and Storage

A 24-hour urine specimen should be collected with 10 g of boric acid to maintain the urine pH below 7.5, and the urine should be refrigerated during the collection period (for example, the sample is placed on ice in a disposable Styrofoam ice chest). After the total volume of urine is measured, a thoroughly mixed aliquot may be stored at −20 °C prior to analysis. Care should be taken to ensure an appropriately timed, complete 24-hour collection, because an incorrectly timed sample is the largest source of error with this method. Cortisol measurements on randomly collected urine specimens are not useful. One report described falsely increased urinary cortisol results attributed to interference from carbamazepine.[18] The drug interfered with the liquid chromatography method used for measuring urinary cortisol. It was also speculated that CYP3A4 induction by carbamazepine affected the results of the low-dose dexamethasone suppression test through enhanced metabolism of dexamethasone.

Cortisol is stable in saliva for 1 week at 4 °C and for 4 months when stored frozen. Freezing of specimens is recommended, because it leads to precipitation of salivary glycoproteins and produces a nonviscous liquid supernatant that makes volumetric transfer by pipette more reliable.

Measurement of Aldosterone

Measurement of aldosterone is technically challenging, because the concentration of this hormone in blood is very low, nearly one thousandth that of the cortisol concentration.

Methods

Immunoassays for measuring aldosterone in blood and urine are available. Radioimmunoassay methods for measuring aldosterone ordinarily use antibodies generated against an aldosterone-3-mono-oxime-bovine serum albumin (BSA) conjugate, an 125I-labeled ligand, and ANS at pH 3.6 to displace aldosterone from binding proteins (primarily albumin). Although RIA methods for measuring aldosterone remain relatively common, nonisotopic immunoassays are becoming increasingly available.

The cross-reactivity of anti-aldosterone antibodies with other adrenal steroids, such as desoxycortisol and corticosterone is relatively low (<0.01%). However, the concentration of potentially cross-reacting steroids sometimes is very high, requiring some purification of aldosterone before measurement. Unconjugated plasma aldosterone is extracted into an organic solvent and purified by chromatography. The addition of tritiated aldosterone as an internal standard corrects for incomplete extraction. In urine, unconjugated steroids first are extracted into an organic solvent (such as ethyl acetate or methylene chloride) after acid hydrolysis of the conjugates. The solvent is evaporated, and the dried extract is reconstituted in a buffer before analysis. Whether the specimen requires purification depends on the diagnostic kit being used and the type of patient being evaluated. For example, specificity is not a significant concern in hypertensive adults without adrenal disease, whereas greater specificity may be needed for newborns and young infants, patients with adrenal disease, and pregnant women, in whom high concentrations of potentially interfering steroids are likely.

An automated heterogeneous immunoassay for aldosterone involving a monoclonal anti-aldosterone antibody and a chemiluminescent tracer has been validated against three RIA methods.[17] This method displays minimal (<0.05) cross-reactivity with (1) corticosterone, (2) cortisol, (3) 11-desoxycorticosterone, (4) 18-hydroxycorticosterone, and (5) dexamethasone, and it has a linear range of 15 to 1200 ng/L. A time-resolved fluorescence immunoassay for measuring aldosterone in saliva is available.[15] LC/MS-MS has also been applied to aldosterone measurements; these results were in close agreement with RIA measurements. The LC/MS-MS method had a detection limit of 69 pmol/L and linearity up to 5.5 nmol/L.

Specimen Collection and Storage

If possible, the patient should be in an upright position (standing or seated) for 30 to 120 minutes before collection because reference intervals were determined with use of samples from ambulatory subjects. Plasma (heparin or EDTA) or serum is suitable for aldosterone measurement, although EDTA plasma is preferred. The aldosterone concentration in specimens stored at room temperature begins to decline after 24 hours, although little change in aldosterone was observed in unseparated blood specimens stored at 32 °C for 24 hours. The aldosterone concentration in refrigerated or frozen specimens is stable for at least 4 days. For urine assays, a 24-hour urine specimen should be collected with boric acid as a preservative.

Measurement of 17-Hydroxyprogesterone

The most common cause of CAH is a deficiency in the 21α-hydroxylase enzyme (CYP21), which converts 17-hydroxyprogesterone (17-OHP) to 11-desoxycortisol.

17-OHP may also be increased in CYP11B1-11β-hydroxylase deficiency CAH. Therefore, measurement of serum or plasma 17-OHP is used to diagnose the most common cases of CAH. In 21α-hydroxylase deficiency, 17-OHP concentrations may reach several hundred times the upper limit of the reference interval.

Methods

Radioimmunoassays for 17-OHP that use antibodies against 17-hydroxyprogesterone-3-carboxymethyloxime-BSA are available; these methods are used with (1) serum, (2) plasma, (3) saliva, and even (4) amniotic fluid. Monoclonal antibody-based methods have also been described. In addition to radioiodinated tracers, nonisotopic labels used in 17-OHP immunoassays include enzymes with (1) photometric, (2) fluorescent, or (3) chemiluminescent substrates, and fluorescence-based immunoassays using fluorescein or streptavidin-europium labels, and chemiluminescent labels. Despite the use of highly specific antisera, most immunoassays are susceptible to interference by other corticosteroids that may be present in neonatal and infant plasma specimens.

Methods for measuring 17-OHP in serum by GCMS and LCMSMS have been described. For chromatographic analysis, 17-OHP is typically extracted using a liquid-liquid (diethyl-ether/diethylacetate or methyl-tert-butyl-ether), solid-phase, or on-line extraction procedure; these methods have detection limits below 1 nmol/L. LCMSMS methods for measuring 17-OHP in dried blood spots obtained from neonates and in urine are also available.

Specimen Collection and Storage

Most reports of analytical methods for measuring 17-OHP use serum, although plasma has also been used. Specimens may be stored at 4 °C for up to 4 days or at −20 °C for up to 1 month. 17-OHP is stable in unseparated blood at room temperature for 1 week.

Screening newborns for 21α-hydroxylase deficiency has been possible since the introduction of 17-OHP immunoassays in 1977. Neonatal specimens are obtained by heel puncture and collected in capillary tubes or on filter paper. Dried blood specimens are (1) stable, (2) easily transported, and (3) are widely used to screen newborns for metabolic defects. It has been reported that the presence of EDTA in dried blood specimens may interfere with 17-OHP results measured by immunometric methods based on lanthanide fluorescence. 17-OHP may also be measured in saliva.

Measurement of 11-Desoxycortisol

Serum or plasma 11-desoxycortisol (compound S) measurements are used to detect 11β-hydroxylase (or CYP11B1 hydroxylase) deficiency or as part of the metyrapone stimulation test. Metyrapone inhibits the 11β-hydroxylase enzyme, and a 40- to 80-fold increase in plasma 11-desoxycortisol is observed after metyrapone stimulation in patients with normal pituitary-adrenal reserve. As a consequence, analytical methods for 11-desoxycortisol in the metyrapone stimulation tests do not require particularly high sensitivity.

Methods

Radioimmunoassay methods for the direct determination of plasma 11-desoxycortisol are available. Antiserum raised against 11-desoxycortisol-3-carboxymethyloxime-BSA has provided appropriate specificity with minimal cross-reactivity against other adrenal steroids. Some radioimmunoassay methods include an extraction step or column chromatography, or both. Nonisotopic methods for measuring 11-desoxycortisol in serum have been described, including (1) enzyme immunoassay, (2) fluorometric, and (3) fluorescence polarization methods. One method for measurement of 11-desoxycortisol involves the "open-sandwich enzyme immunoassay" technique, which is based on the reassociation of two cloned antibody variable regions by a bridging antigen.[13]

LCMSMS methods for measuring 11-desoxycortisol have been described, mostly as part of corticosteroid profiles. These methods typically include a liquid-liquid extraction into an organic solvent step, although solid-phase extraction has been used as well.

Specimen Collection and Storage

Most of the methods used for measuring 11-desoxycortisol have used serum, although use of plasma and urine are also used. The stability of 11-desoxycortisol in stored specimens has not been established.

Measurement of Renin Activity and Concentration

Circulating concentrations of prorenin may be as many as 100-fold greater than the concentration of renin (although a 10:1 ratio of prorenin to renin is more common); therefore even minimal cross-reactivity of prorenin with anti-renin antibodies used in direct immunoassays to measure renin is problematical.

Methods

Assays exist to measure PRA (by monitoring the production of angiotensin I) or the mass of renin by immunoassay. Each approach has advantages and disadvantages.

Renin Activity. Measuring renin activity (traditionally called *plasma renin activity*, or *PRA*) is a test of function that provides an indication of the biologically active fraction of renin in the specimen. It measures the primary function of the enzyme, which is the conversion of angiotensinogen to angiotensin I. In the test, angiotensinogen is provided by the patient's serum. Renin activity measurements, however, are difficult to standardize, and two general approaches are used to measure renin activity.

In the classic PRA method, inhibitors of angiotensinase and ACE are added to prevent the conversion of angiotensin I to angiotensin II (some methods "trap" angiotensin I with an antibody to prevent its conversion to angiotensin II), the specimen is incubated at 37 °C, and production of angiotensin I is measured. The rate of the renin-catalyzed production of angiotensin I is influenced by pH, incubation time, and, most importantly, the endogenous angiotensinogen concentration in the specimen, which is increased in (1) pregnancy, (2) glucocorticoid excess, and (3) estrogen administration. Because the angiotensinogen concentration in blood does not ordinarily exceed the Michaelis–Menten term (Km) for the renin-angiotensinogen complex, its concentration is rate limiting. Therefore, the classic PRA method produces results that vary significantly, depending on the endogenous concentration of angiotensinogen.

In practice, a typical PRA method involves the preparation of two aliquots of plasma. One of the aliquots is incubated at 37 °C for 3 hours, and the other is kept at 4 °C (renin is not active at cold temperature). Following the incubation period, angiotensin I is measured by immunoassay in both aliquots, and the difference between the two reflects the renin activity, expressed as pg of angiotensin per mL of plasma generated per unit of time. The specificity of the PRA assay can be validated using plasma from anephric patients or deangiotensinized plasma.

A second approach to measure renin activity uses exogenous angiotensinogen as substrate and thereby avoids the variability associated with endogenous angiotensinogen concentrations. (Note: This approach is sometimes called plasma renin concentration assay, which is a confusing term in that the assay still involves the measurement of activity, rather than concentration. Furthermore, the term is not consistently applied; plasma renin concentration has been used to describe immunoassays that measure the renin concentration, rather than activity.) These renin activity methods use angiotensinogen derived from plasma collected from nephrectomized sheep; it is added at a concentration that is several times the K_m for the renin-angiotensinogen complex, ensuring that the reaction rate is limited by renin activity alone. An advantage of using a consistent source of angiotensinogen is that these activity assays are calibrated against renin reference materials. An International Reference Preparation of human renin (68/356), validated by bioassay, has been available from the WHO.

Prorenin exists in two forms, depending on whether the 46 amino acid "pro" segment is in an "open" or "closed" conformation. The open conformation of prorenin has the active site of the enzyme exposed, so this form is enzymatically active. In the blood, approximately 2% of prorenin is in the open conformation, but assay conditions (such as, cooling and low pH) will sometimes cause the closed conformation of prorenin to open, which results in an overestimate of physiologic renin activity. Incubation of plasma at 22 °C for 24 hours reversibly activates (unfolds) approximately 5% of prorenin, although incubation at 37 °C promotes refolding of the "pro" segment to its closed form. In some assays, the closed prorenin is deliberately opened by acidification (pH 3.3) or incubation with trypsin, which removes the "pro" segment from prorenin altogether. These assays measure total renin and prorenin by activating all of the prorenin and follow with a standard renin activity assay.

Angiotensin I and II. All renin activity assays rely on the conversion of angiotensinogen to angiotensin I or the subsequent production from angiotensin I of angiotensin II, the active form of the angiotensin hormone. Angiotensin II has a very short half-life (1 to 2 minutes) and is difficult to measure. Monoclonal antibodies with high affinity and specificity for angiotensin II have been produced. These antibodies have been used to develop a direct immunoassay for angiotensin II; as little as 0.8 fmol of angiotensin II in 2 mL of plasma has been detected without interference from angiotensin I. When angiotensinogen and ACE are in sufficient supply, however, the concentration of the prohormone angiotensin I is a reliable proxy for the renin activity and angiotensin II concentration in blood. Most angiotensin I methods involve radioimmunoassay, but (1) enzyme immunoassays, (2) HPLC, (3) fluorescence polarization and (4) mass spectrometric methods have also been described. A 2009 report described a homogeneous immunoassay for angiotensin I that is based on luminescent oxygen channeling, a technology involving chemiluminescence stimulated by photoexcited singlet oxygen.[5]

Renin Concentration. As an alternative to the PRA assays, the concentration of renin is measured by immunoassay. (These methods are sometimes called direct renin assays or mass assays.) A variety of monoclonal immunoradiometric assays (IRMAs) for renin have been developed, some of which measure renin and prorenin in the open configuration, and others of which measure all forms of renin and prorenin. Immunochemiluminometric (ICL) methods for renin are available, and the results of these assays have been correlated with IRMA results. One such assay involves a biotinylated capture antibody (which recognizes both renin and prorenin) immobilized to streptavidin-coated magnetic particles, and an acridinium ester–labeled signal antibody that recognizes only renin.[8] The chemiluminescent assay had a limit of detection of less than 0.1 mU/L and a limit of quantification of 2.6 mU/L with a CV <20%.

Direct renin immunoassays (both IRMA and ICL) show high correlation (r = 0.98) with renin activity assays. Direct renin results are expressed in mIU/L, and PRA results are expressed in $\text{ng} \cdot \text{mL}^{-1} \cdot \text{h}^{-1}$.

Specimen Collection and Storage

EDTA plasma is typically used for PRA assays. After centrifugation, plasma should be removed and frozen at −20 °C or below, although the renin concentration is stable in unseparated blood at room temperature for up to 6 hours. Plasma for PRA can be stored frozen up to 1 month before assay, but freeze-thaw cycles should be avoided because of the possible activation of prorenin. At the time of collection, blood should not be chilled or placed on ice because irreversible cryoactivation of prorenin may occur, leading to falsely high estimates of PRA. Serum or plasma samples collected in another anticoagulant have been used as long as EDTA is added (3 mmol/L) before incubation to inhibit ACE. Cryoactivation of prorenin, however, is more likely in serum than in plasma. Hemolyzed specimens should not be used because red blood cells contain angiotensinases.

If renin deficiency is suspected, the patient should be ambulatory for 30 minutes before blood collection. A 24-hour urine specimen for sodium is often collected on the day before the renin test to verify salt intake. Specimens with high renin activity can generate considerable amounts of angiotensin I before and during storage even at −20 °C. This will not affect results, however, if angiotensin I is measured with and without incubation.

Review Questions

1. Measurement of urinary free cortisol (UFC) is typically used as a screening test for:
   a. hyperaldosteronism.
   b. cortisol hypersecretion.
   c. adrenal insufficiency.
   d. congenital adrenal hyperplasia (CAH).

2. Glucocorticoids _____ blood glucose concentrations by altering synthesis of gluconeogenic enzymes.
   a. increase
   b. decrease
   c. do not affect

3. The primary mineralocorticoid is:
   a. cortisol.
   b. dehydroepiandrosterone (DHEA).
   c. 11-deoxycortisol.
   d. aldosterone.

4. The major site of steroid hormone metabolism that involves the P450 enzyme systems is the:
   a. liver.
   b. kidney.
   c. gastrointestinal tract.
   d. adipose tissue.

5. The stimulation test that is used to assess the ability of the adrenal glands to synthesize cortisol is referred to as the:
   a. dexamethasone test.
   b. metapyrone test.
   c. cosyntropin test.
   d. salt-loading test.

6. *Primary* adrenal insufficiency is referred to as:
   a. Cushing syndrome.
   b. Addison disease.
   c. Conn syndrome.
   d. congenital adrenal hyperplasia (CAH).

7. The adrenocortical disorder that results from loss-of-function mutations in specific adrenocortical enzymes that are responsible for the synthesis of cortisol is:
   a. Cushing syndrome.
   b. Addison disease.
   c. Conn syndrome.
   d. congenital adrenal hyperplasia (CAH).

8. The anterior pituitary hormone that is responsible for increasing the size and number of adrenocortical cells and for eventual cortisol synthesis is:
   a. corticotropin.
   b. growth hormone.
   c. corticotropin-releasing hormone (CRH).
   d. aldosterone.

9. One of the main functions of the mineralocorticoids is:
   a. increasing blood glucose.
   b. increased fat breakdown.
   c. sodium retention.
   d. glycogen synthesis.

10. Which one of the following disorders is the result of autonomous excessive production of cortisol?
    a. Cushing syndrome.
    b. Addison disease.
    c. Conn syndrome.
    d. congenital adrenal hyperplasia (CAH).

References

1. Anagnostis P, Karagiannis A, Tziomalos K, Kakafika AI, Athyros VG, Mikhailidis D. Adrenal incidentaloma: a diagnostic challenge. Hormones (Athens) 2009;8:163–84.
2. Arafah BM. Hypothalamic pituitary adrenal function during critical illness: limitations of current assessment methods. J Clin Endocrinol Metab 2006;91:3725–45.
3. Betterle C, Coco G, Zanchetta R. Adrenal cortex autoantibodies in subjects with normal adrenal function. Best Pract Res Clin Endocrinol Metab 2005;19:85–99.
4. Biddie SC, Hager GL. Glucocorticoid receptor dynamics and gene regulation. Stress 2009;12:193–205.
5. Cauchon E, Liu S, Percival MD, Rowland SE, Xu D, Binkert C. Set al. Development of a homogeneous immunoassay for the detection of angiotensin I in plasma using AlphaLISA acceptor beads technology. Anal Biochem 2009;388, 134–9.
6. Cho HJ. Kim JD, Lee WY, Chung BC, Choi MH. Quantitative metabolic profiling of 21 endogenous corticosteroids in urine by liquid chromatography-triple quadrupole-mass spectrometry. Anal Chim Acta 2009;632:101–8.
7. Crapo L. Cushing's syndrome: a review of diagnostic tests. Metabolism 1979;28:955–77.
8. de Bruin RA, Bouhuizen A, Diederich S, Perschel FH, Boomsma F, Deinum J, Validation of a new automated renin assay. Clin Chem 2004;50;2111–6.
9. Deuschle M, Schweiger U, Weber B, Gotthardt U, Korner A, Schmider J, et al. Diurnal activity and pulsatility of the hypothalamus-pituitary-adrenal system in male depressed patients and healthy controls. J Clin Endocrinol Metab 1997;82:234–8.
10. Diver MJ, Hughes JG, Hutton JL, West CR, Hipkin LJ. The long-term stability in whole blood of 14 commonly-requested hormone analytes. Ann Clin Biochem 1994;31:561–5.
11. Dorin RI, Pai HK, Ho JT, Lewis JG, Torpy DJ, Urban FKIII, Qualls CR. Validation of a simple method of estimating plasma free cortisol: role of cortisol binding to albumin. Clin Biochem 2009;42:64–71.
12. Havelock JC, Auchus RJ, Rainey WE. The rise in adrenal androgen biosynthesis: adrenarche. Semin Reprod Med 2004;22:337–47.
13. Ihara M, Suzuki T, Kobayashi N, Goto J, Ueda H. Open-sandwich enzyme immunoassay for one-step noncompetitive detection of corticosteroid 11-deoxycortisol. Anal Chem 2009;81:8298–304.
14. Kai H, Kudo H, Takayama N, Yasuoka S, Kajimoto H, Imaizumi T. Large blood pressure variability and hypertensive cardiac remodeling–role of cardiac inflammation. Circ J 2009;73:2198–203.
15. Manolopoulou J, Gerum S, Mulatero P, Rossignol P, Plouin PF, Reincke M, Bidlingmaier M. Salivary aldosterone as a diagnostic aid in primary aldosteronism. Horm Metab Res 2010;42:400–5.
16. Pearce JM. Thomas Addison (1793-1860). J R Soc Med 2004;97:297–300.
17. Schirpenbach C, Seiler L, Maser-Gluth C, Beuschlein F, Reincke M, Bidlingmaier M. Automated chemiluminescence-immunoassay for aldosterone during dynamic testing: comparison to radioimmunoassays with and without extraction steps. Clin Chem 2006;52:1749–55.
18. Tiong K, Falhammar H. Carbamazepine and falsely positive screening tests for Cushing's syndrome. N Z Med J 2009;122:100–2.
19. Vining RF, McGinley RA. The measurement of hormones in saliva: possibilities and pitfalls. J Steroid Biochem 1987;27:81–94.
20. Yang J, Young MJ. The mineralocorticoid receptor and its coregulators. J Mol Endocrinol 2009;43:53–64.

Thyroid Disorders[*]

William E. Winter, M.D., Desmond Schatz, M.D., and Roger L. Bertholf, Ph.D.

Objectives

1. Define the following terms

Colloid	Iodide
Cretinism	Reverse T_3 (rT_3)
Euthyroid	Thyroglobulin (Tg)
Follicle	Thyrotoxicosis
Goiter	Thyroid storm
Hashitoxicosis	Thyrotropin-releasing
	hormone (TRH)

2. Describe the structure and function of the thyroid gland, including cell types, internal location of key hormone precursors and proteins, regulation of thyroid gland, and functions of the hormones synthesized and secreted.

3. Describe the metabolism of thyroid hormones, including synthesis, peripheral deiodination, specific effects on target tissues, and catabolism; state the full names of the thyroid hormones.

4. State the effects of increased and decreased thyroid hormones on thyroid-stimulating hormone (TSH), thyrotropin-releasing hormone (TRH), and target tissues.

5. For the following disorders, state the cause(s), symptoms, laboratory analyses, and lab results used to diagnose:

Autoimmune hypothyroidism	Primary and secondary
Graves disease	hyperthyroidism
Hashimoto thyroiditis	Primary and secondary
hCG-induced hyperthyroidism	hypothyroidism
Myxedema	Sick euthyroid syndrome
	T_3 thyrotoxicosis

6. Name and describe the thyroid autoantibodies associated with thyroid disease, including mechanism of action, specificity of autoantibody to each disease, methods of detection and interferences.

7. State the methods, specimen requirements and problems with methods used to assess total and free thyroid hormones, thyroxine-binding globulin (TBG), thyroglobulin (Tg), and TSH.

8. State the formulae for estimation of free thyroid hormone concentration; given appropriate information, calculate estimates of free hormone concentration.

9. Analyze and solve case studies related to thyroid disease and laboratory analysis of these conditions.

Key Words and Definitions

Allan-Herndon-Dudley syndrome An X-linked syndrome caused by mutations in the *SLC16A2* gene (locus: Xq13.2), which encodes a thyroid hormone transporter, and characterized by severe mental retardation, dysarthria, athetoid movements, muscle hypoplasia, and spastic paraplegia.

Apathetic hyperthyroidism A form of Graves disease that tends to affect mainly older adults who have stereotyped "senile" physical features and whose behavior is apathetic (indifferent) and inactive rather than hyperkinetic.

Autoimmune thyroid disease (AITD) Diseases in which the immune system attacks or stimulates the body's own thyroid gland.

Central hypothyroidism Refers to thyroid hormone deficiency due to a disorder of the (1) pituitary, (2) hypothalamus, or (3) hypothalamic-pituitary portal circulation.

Colloid An amorphous material found in the follicular lumen of the thyroid gland. A critical component is *thyroglobulin* (Tg).

Congenital hypothyroidism A pathological condition resulting from severe thyroid insufficiency, which may lead to cretinism or myxedema.

Cretinism An archaic term for the clinical consequences of untreated congenital hypothyroidism caused by a deficiency of thyroid hormone during prenatal development and infancy; characterized in childhood by short stature, developmental delay, dystrophy of the bones, and a low basal metabolism. Also called *congenital myxedema* which is also an archaic term.

Euthyroid Having normal thyroid function.

Euthyroid hyperthyroxinemia A condition characterized by increased concentrations of thyroxine in the blood but a normal concentration of thyroid-stimulating hormone and normal thyroid function.

[*]The authors gratefully acknowledge the contributions of Ronald J. Whitley and Laurence M. Demers to the chapter in the previous editions, on which portions of this chapter are based.

Key Words and Definitions—cont'd

Goiter An enlargement of the thyroid gland that causes a swelling in the front part of the neck.

Graves disease A disorder of the thyroid of autoimmune etiology that causes hyperthyroidism. Characterized by having at least two of the following conditions: hyperthyroidism, goiter, and exophthalmos. Also known in Europe as *Basedow disease.*

Hashimoto thyroiditis An autoimmune disorder in which the thyroid gland is attacked by a cell-mediated autoimmune process. Also known as *Hashimoto disease* and *chronic lymphocytic thyroiditis,* it is marked by (1) goiter, (2) chronic inflammation of the thyroid (*thyroiditis*), and (3) often hypothyroidism.

Hashitoxicosis Hyperthyroidism in patients with Hashimoto disease.

Hyperthyroidism A condition caused by excessive production of iodinated thyroid hormones. Symptoms and signs include increased basal metabolic rate, enlargement of the thyroid gland, rapid heart rate, high systolic blood pressure, and a number of secondary symptoms.

Hypothyroidism A condition of deficient thyroid gland activity leading to lethargy, muscle weakness, and intolerance to cold.

Myxedema A severe form of hypothyroidism in which there is accumulation of mucopolysaccharides in the skin and other tissue, leading to a thickening of facial features and a doughy induration of the skin.

Organification A process in the thyroid gland whereby iodide is oxidized and incorporated into tyrosyl residues (tyrosine) of thyroglobulin (Tg). Organification is catalyzed by the enzyme thyroperoxidase (TPO).

Pendrin A protein that is mutated in Pendred syndrome, which is an autosomal recessive disorder characterized by (1) sensorineural hearing loss, (2) goiter, and (3) a partial organification problem. Also known as the *sodium-independent chloride/iodide transporter.*

Primary hypothyroidism A condition that develops when the thyroid gland fails to produce or secrete as much thyroxine (T_4) as the body needs.

Reverse T_3 (rT_3) A biologically inert metabolite of thyroxine (T_4) with three iodine molecules attached in a configuration (L-3,3′,5′-triiodothyronine) different from that of the active thyroid hormone triiodothyronine (T_3).

Secondary hypothyroidism Hypothyroidism that arises as a consequence of inadequate secretion of thyroid stimulating hormone (TSH or *thyrotropin*) by the anterior pituitary gland.

Sick euthyroid syndrome Abnormalities of T_4, free T_4, T_3 and TSH concentrations that are seen in people with severe illness. In general, treatment with replacement thyroid hormone is not indicated.

Subclinical hyperthyroidism A biochemical condition with normal concentrations of serum thyroid hormones when the serum TSH concentration is repeatedly low in the absence of hypothalamic or pituitary disease.

T_3 Thyrotoxicosis A hyperthyroid condition in which T_3 but not T_4 is elevated.

Thyroglobulin (Tg) An iodine-containing glycoprotein of high molecular weight (663 kDa) present in the colloid of the follicles of the thyroid gland.

Thyroid follicle The secretory unit of the thyroid gland consisting of an outer layer of epithelial cells that enclose an amorphous material called colloid.

Thyroiditis A condition characterized by inflammation of the thyroid gland.

Thyroid-stimulating hormone (TSH) A polypeptide hormone synthesized by the anterior pituitary gland that promotes the growth of the thyroid gland and stimulates the synthesis and release of thyroid hormones by the thyroid gland. Also called *thyrotropin.*

Thyroid storm A life-threatening condition that develops in a minority of cases of untreated thyrotoxicosis (hyperthyroidism, or overactive thyroid).

Thyrotoxicosis A toxic condition resulting from excessive amounts of thyroid hormones in the body.

Thyrotropin-releasing hormone (TRH) A tripeptide produced in the hypothalamus that stimulates the synthesis and release of TSH from the anterior pituitary.

Thyroxine The major hormone synthesized and released by the thyroid gland that contains four iodine molecules (L-3,5,3′,5′-tetraiodothyronine).

Toxic multinodular goiter A condition in which the thyroid gland contains multiple lumps (nodules) that are overactive and that produce excess thyroid hormones. Also known as *Parry disease* and *Plummer disease.*

Transthyretin (TTR) A protein found in serum and cerebrospinal fluid that binds to and transports thyroxine (T_4). TTR complexes with retinol binding protein (RBP) to prevent its loss through the glomerulus by filtration. Was once called *prealbumin,* because it traveles faster than albumin on electrophoresis gels.

Triiodothyronine The biologically active form of thyroid hormone formed primarily outside of the thyroid gland by the peripheral deiodination of thyroxine (T_4). Has three iodine molecules attached to its molecular structure (L-3,5,3′-triiodothyronine).

The thyroid gland is a butterfly-shaped gland located in the front of the neck just above the trachea in the adult human (see Figure 25-1, Chapter 25, page 431). The fully developed thyroid gland in a human weighs approximately 15 to 20 g. However, in disease states, the gland may weigh up to several hundred grams. The thyroid is composed of two lobes with the right lobe being somewhat larger than the left lobe. The lobes are connected by the isthmus.

The **thyroid follicle** or *acinus* (Figure 42-1) is the secretory unit of the thyroid gland. Each follicle has an outer layer of epithelial cells that enclose an amorphous material called **colloid** that is s mainly composed of **thyroglobulin (Tg)**. The important reactions of thyroid hormone synthesis, such as iodination and the initial phase of hormone secretion (colloid resorption into the cells), are believed to take place at or near the surface of the epithelial cells in the colloid.

The thyroid gland also contains another type of cell known as *parafollicular* or *C cells*. These cells have been shown to produce the polypeptide hormone *calcitonin*. These cells are confined within the follicular basement lamina or exist in clusters in the interfollicular spaces.

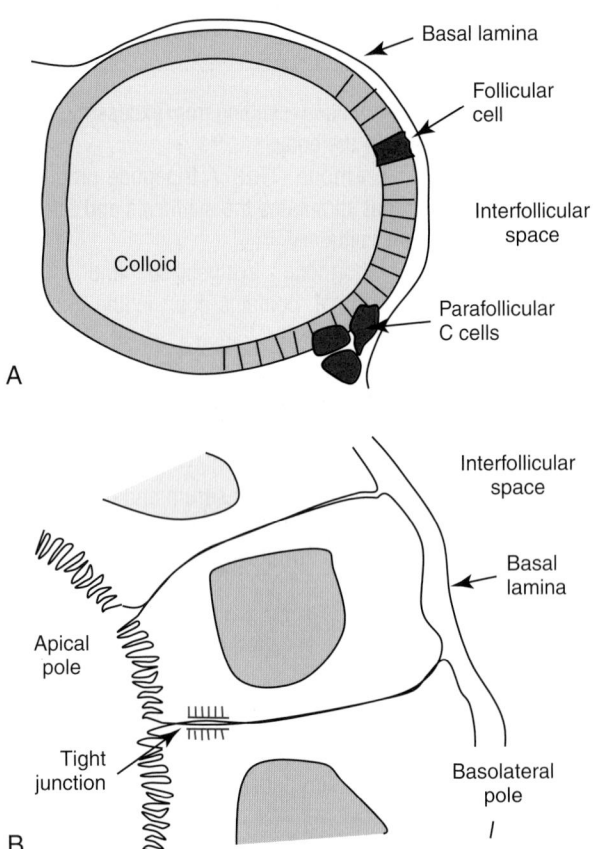

A

B

Figure 42-1 A, Basic unit of the thyroid gland. The follicle is the basic unit of the thyroid gland. It is composed of thyroid follicular cells surrounding the colloid. Outside the follicular cells is a basal lamina. Parafollicular (C cells) that secrete calcitonin can be found beneath or outside the basal lamina. *Not pictured,* between the follicles are capillaries and fibroblasts. **B** (inset image), Apical and basolateral poles of the follicular cells and tight junctions between the follicular cells.

Thyroid Hormones

The thyroid gland secretes two hormones, **thyroxine** (3,5,3′,5′-L-tetraiodothyronine) and **triiodothyronine** (3,5,3′-L-triiodothyronine), which are commonly known as T_4 and T_3, respectively (Table 42-1). In addition, the thyroid gland secretes very small amounts of biologically inactive 3,3′,5′-L-triiodothyronine (**reverse T_3 [rT_3]**) and minute quantities of monoiodotyrosine (MIT) and diiodotyrosine (DIT), which are precursors of T_3 and T_4. The structures of these compounds are shown in Figure 42-2.

Biological Function

The functions of thyroid hormones include (1) control of the basal metabolic rate and calorigenesis, (2) enhancement of mitochondrial metabolism, (3) stimulation of neural development and normal growth, (4) promotion of sexual maturation, (5) stimulation of adrenergic activity with increased heart rate

TABLE 42-1	**Nomenclature and Abbreviations for Thyroid Tests**
Hormone Concentration	
Total thyroxine	T_4
Total triiodothyronine (3,5,3′-triiodothyronine)	T_3
Free thyroxine	FT_4
Free triiodothyronine	FT_3
Thyrotropin (thyroid-stimulating hormone)	TSH
Reverse T_3 (3,3′,5′-triiodothyronine)	rT_3
Serum Binding Proteins	
Thyroxine-binding globulin	TBG
Thyroxine-binding prealbumin (transthyretin)	TBPA
Tests for Autoimmune Thyroid Disease	
Thyroglobulin autoantibodies	TgAb
Microsomal autoantibodies	TMAb
Thyroperoxidase autoantibodies	TPO Ab
TSH receptor autoantibodies	TRAb
Other Hormones and Thyroid-Related Proteins	
Thyrotropin-releasing hormone (thyrotropin)	TRH
Thyroglobulin	Tg
Calcitonin	CT

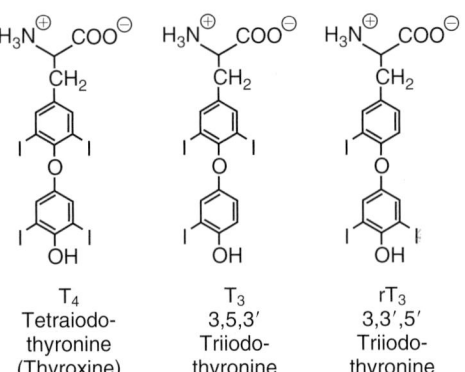

Figure 42-2 Chemical structures of thyroxine (T_4), triiodothyronine (T_3), and reverse T_3.

and myocardial contractility, (6) stimulation of protein synthesis and carbohydrate metabolism, (7) increasing the synthesis and degradation of cholesterol and triglycerides, (8) increasing the requirement for vitamins, (9) increasing the calcium and phosphorus metabolism, and (10) enhancing the sensitivity of adrenergic receptors to catecholamines. These effects are typically magnified in patients with either an overactive thyroid gland (such as in **hyperthyroidism**), or reduced in patients with reduced thyroid function (such as, **hypothyroidism**).

Biochemistry

Approximately 40% of secreted T_4 is deiodinated in peripheral tissues by enzyme deiodinases to yield T_3, and about 45% is deiodinated to yield rT_3, a biologically inactive metabolite. Therefore, with normal T_4 production of -100 nmol (approximately 80 µg) daily, approximately 40 nmol (26 µg) of T_3 and 45 nmol (29 µg) of rT_3 are produced by peripheral deiodination. From the estimated daily production rates for T_3 (30 µg) and rT_3 (30 µg) in a normal (**euthyroid**) state, at least 85% of T_3 production and essentially all of rT_3 production are accounted for by peripheral deiodination of T_4 rather than by direct secretion from the thyroid gland T_3 is at least four to five times more potent in biological systems than T_4. Because one third of all T_4 is converted to T_3 during the course of its metabolism, T_4 may be considered to be a prohormone for T_3.

The biosynthesis of thyroid hormones occurs by a process termed "**organification**" It involves the (1) trapping of circulating iodide by the thyroid gland, (2) incorporation of iodine into thyroglobulin tyrosines producing monoiodinated tyrosines and di-iodinated tyrosines, and (3) coupling of two iodinated tyrosyl residues to form the thyronines (T_4 and T_3) within the protein backbone of the thyroglobulin (Tg) protein in the follicular lumen. (Figure 42-3). Endocytosis followed by proteolytic cleavage of Tg releases the iodothyronines into the circulation.

Dietary iodine is the basic element involved in the synthesis of thyroid hormones. It is normally ingested in the form of iodide. Iodide transport to the follicles is the first and rate-limiting step in the synthetic process. The follicular cells of the thyroid concentrate iodide to some 30 to 40 times the normal plasma concentration by means of an energy-dependent pump mechanism, the sodium-iodide symporter (appoved gene name:solute carrier family 5 (sodium/iodide cotransporter), member 5; approved symbol *SLC5A5*; chromosome 19p13.11).

The synthesis of MIT and DIT (Figure 42-4), T_4 (Figure 42-5), and T_3 Figure 42-6), occurs mainly at the follicular cell–colloid interface but also within the colloid (Figure 42-3). Tg is present in highest concentrations within the colloid, where it is stored. The follicular cells engulf colloid globules by

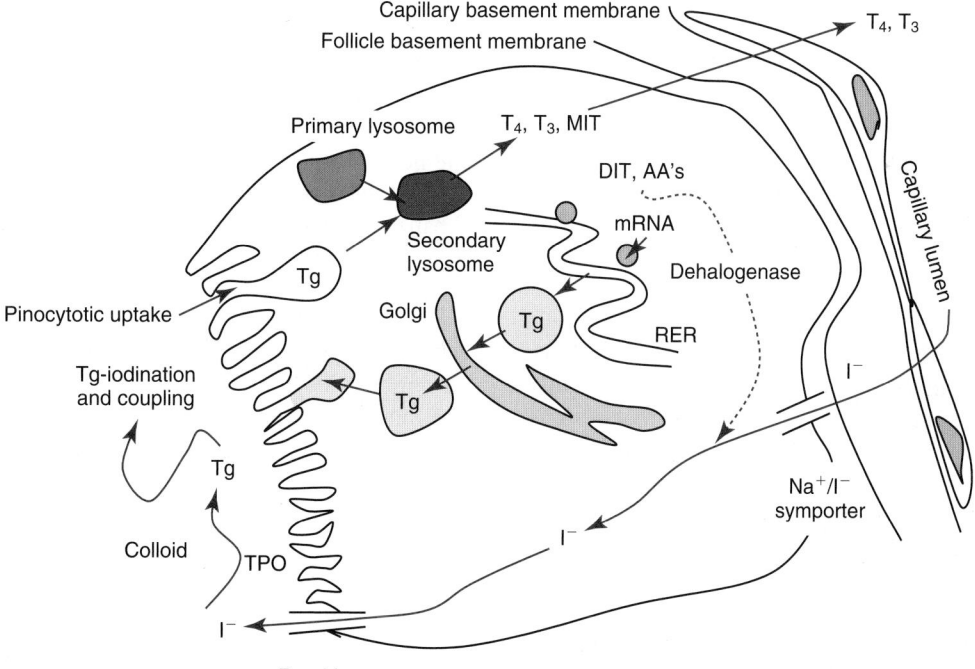

Figure 42-3 Synthesis of thyroid hormones begins with absorption of iodide by the thyroid follicular cell and the Na^+/I^- symporter (NIS). From the cytoplasm, iodide moves into the lacunae via pendrin. Within the lacunae, thyroperoxidase (TPO) and the dual oxidases [DUOX (not depicted)] convert iodide to iodine, leading to iodination of tyrosine residues on thyroglobulin (Tg). Tg is synthesized in the cell and exported to the lacunae. TPO is responsible for the coupling of monoiodotyrosine (MIT) and di-iodotyrosine (DIT) to form T_3, and di-iodotyrosine and di-iodotyrosine to form T_4. Upon uptake of iodinated Tg (containing T_4 and T_3) and fusion of this phagosome-like vesicle with a primary lysosome, Tg is degraded in a secondary lysosome, releasing T_4 and T_3 into the circulation and MIT and DIT undergo deiodination via a dehalogenase to recycle the iodine for new thyroid hormone synthesis.

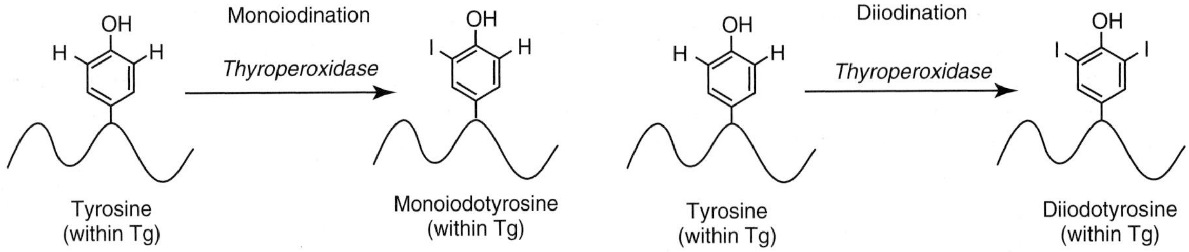

Figure 42-4 Monoiodination and di-iodination of tyrosine.

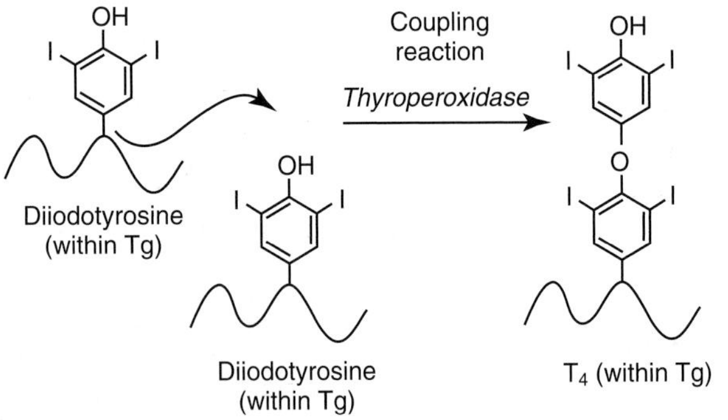

Figure 42-5 Chemical coupling of two molecules of diiodo-tyrosines (DITs) to produce a molecule of thyroxine (T_4). The reaction is catalyzed by thyroperoxidase (TPO).

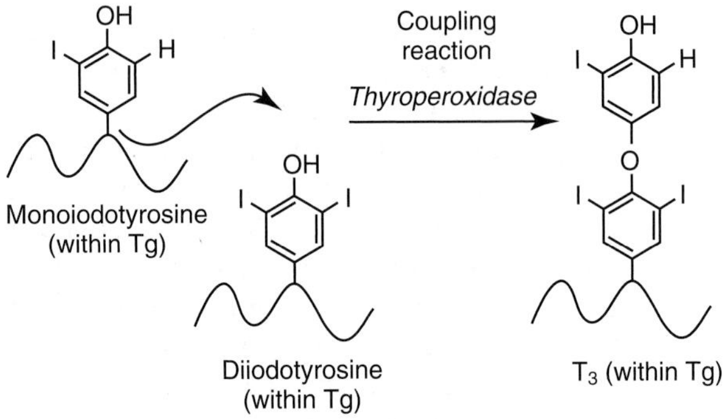

Figure 42-6 Chemical coupling of one molecule of monoiodo-tyrosine and one molecule of di-iodotyrosine to produce one molecule of T_3. The reaction is catalyzed by thyroperoxidase.

endocytosis; these globules then merge with lysosomes in the follicular cell. Lysosomal proteases break the peptide bonds between iodinated residues of Tg, and MIT, DIT, T_4, and T_3, are released into the cytoplasm of the follicular cell. T_4 and T_3 diffuse into the systemic circulation after their liberation from Tg. DIT and MIT are deiodinated by an intracellular microsomal iodotyrosine dehalogenase (approved gene name iodotyrosine deiodinase, approved symbol *IYD*; chromosome 6q25.1). The freed iodide is then reused for thyroid hormone synthesis.

Each step in the synthesis of thyroid hormones is regulated by pituitary **thyroid-stimulating hormone (TSH)**. TSH (also known as *thyrotropin*) stimulates (1) the "iodide pump," (2) Tg synthesis, and (3) colloidal uptake by follicular cells. TSH also regulates the rate of proteolysis of Tg for the liberation of T_4 and T_3. In addition, TSH induces an increase in the size and number of the thyroid follicular cells. Prolonged TSH stimulation leads to increased vascularity and eventual hypertrophic enlargement of the thyroid gland (**goiter**).

Initially, it was believed that both T_4 and T_3 entered cells by passive diffusion across the plasma membrane. However, researchers have now shown that thyroid hormones cross plasma membranes using specific transporters.[15] One important thyroid hormone transporter is monocarboxylate transporter 8 (MCT8; gene symbol *SLC16A2*; chromosome Xq13.2). MCT10 (*SLC16A10*; chromosome 6q21-q22) transports iodothyronines and aromatic amino acids across membranes, and MCT10 is likely more preferential than MCT8 in transporting T_3 over T_4 across plasma membranes. Organic anion transporting polypeptide 1C1 (OATP1C1) also has high affinity for thyroid hormone and may be an important component of the transport of T_3 and T_4.

Metabolism

Free (unbound) T_4 (FT_4) is the primary secretory product of the normal thyroid gland. T_4 undergoes peripheral deiodination of the outer ring at the 5′ position to yield T_3. This deiodination occurs in a number of tissues but primarily in the liver. rT_3, produced by removal of one iodine from the inner ring of T_4, is metabolically inactive and is an end-product of T_4 metabolism. Peripheral deiodination is a rapidly responsive mechanism of control for thyroid hormone balance. Acute or chronic stress or illness causes a shift in the direction of this deiodination, favoring formation of rT_3 rather than T_3. Various medications also shift peripheral deiodination toward the inactive product rT_3.

T_4 and T_3 in the circulation are bound reversibly and almost completely to carrier proteins. These carrier proteins are (1) thyroxine-binding globulin (TBG), (2) thyroxine-binding prealbumin (TBPA; **transthyretin [TTR]**), and (3) albumin. Collectively, these proteins bind 99.97% of T_4 and 99.7% of T_3. Thus only a very small fraction of each of these hormones is unbound and free for biological activity. Because a wide variation exists in the concentration of thyroid hormone binding proteins, even under normal circumstances, a wide variation also exists in total T_4 concentrations among individuals with normal (euthyroid) thyroid function. Total T_3 concentrations also vary with alterations in binding proteins, although usually to a lesser degree than T_4 concentrations. Circumstances in which thyroid hormone-binding protein concentrations are increased or decreased are shown in Box 42-1.

BOX 42-1   Alterations in the Concentration or Affinity of Thyroid Hormone–Binding Proteins

Increases In

A. Thyroxine-binding globulin (TBG) concentration (or affinity)
   1. Genetic (inherited) causes
   2. Nonthyroidal illness (HIV infection, infectious and chronic active hepatitis, estrogen-producing tumors, acute intermittent porphyria)
   3. Normal physiology (pregnancy, newborn)
   4. Drug use (oral contraceptives, estrogens, tamoxifen, methadone)
B. Prealbumin binding (familial euthyroid thyroxine excess)
C. Albumin binding (familial dysalbuminemic hyperthyroxinemia)
D. T_4 binding by autoantibodies (autoimmune thyroid disease, hepatocellular carcinoma)

Decreases In

A. TBG concentration
   1. Genetic (inherited) determination
   2. Nonthyroidal illness (major illness or surgical stress, chronic liver disease, protein-losing enteropathy, nephrotic syndrome)
   3. Drug use (androgens, anabolic steroids, large doses of glucocorticoids)
B. TBG-binding capacity (drugs bound to TBG, such as salicylates and phenytoin)
C. Prealbumin concentration

HIV, Human immunodeficiency virus; T_4, thyroxine; *TBG,* thyroxine-binding globulin.

Regulation and Control

Thyroid hormone synthesis and secretion are controlled by a negative feedback system (Figure 42-7) involving (1) **thyrotropin-releasing hormone (TRH)** from the hypothalamus, (2) TSH from the pituitary, and (3) thyroid hormones from the follicular cells of the thyroid glands.

Biochemistry

TRH is the modified tripeptide L-pyroglutamyl-L-histidyl-L-prolinamide secreted by the paraventricular nuclei (PVN) in the hypothalamus (Figure 42-8). Its concentrations rise in thyroid hormone deficiency with TRH declining when thyroid hormone is in excess. TRH is delivered to the anterior pituitary gland via the hypothalamic-pituitary portal system. As discussed in Chapter 40, TSH (also known as *thyrotropin*) is secreted by anterior pituitary cells known as *thyrotrophs*. In relative terms, TRH has a greater effect on TSH glycosylation than hormone release. However, glycosylation of TSH is necessary for normal TSH bioactivity. When TRH is deficient, TSH may lack potency as the result of insufficient glycosylation, yet nonglycosylated TSH may retain much of its immunoreactivity.

Chemically, TSH is a 30 kDa heterodimeric glycoprotein that shares the 14.7 kDa alpha subunit (gene location: chromosome 6q21.1-q23) with (1) luteinizing hormone (LH), (2) follicular stimulating hormone (FSH), and (3) human chorionic gonadotropin (hCG), whereas each hormone has a unique beta subunit (see Chapters 40 and 44).

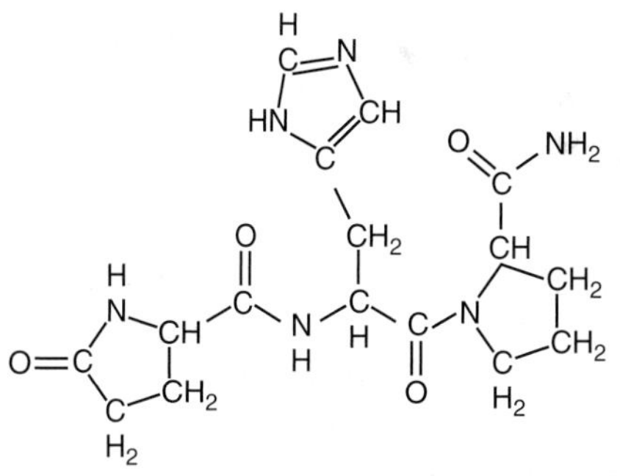

Function

The effects of TSH on the thyroid follicular cell are mediated through the TSH receptor. At physiological TSH concentrations, the second messenger system involves G_S proteins, adenylate

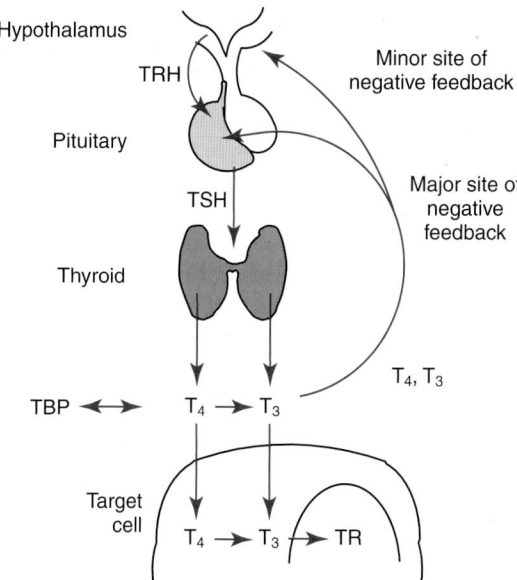

Figure 42-7 Metabolic control of thyroid hormones. Thyrotropin-releasing hormone (TRH) from the hypothalamus enters the hypothalamic-pituitary portal system to release thyroid-stimulating hormone (TSH; thyrotropin) from anterior pituitary thyrotrophs. TSH stimulates the release of thyroxine (T_4) and triiodothyronine (T_3) from the thyroid gland, although most T_3 (~80%) comes from peripheral monodeiodination of T_4 to T_3. More than 99% of T_4 and T_3 is bound to various thyroid hormone–binding proteins. T_4 and T_3 negatively feed back on the hypothalamus and, more powerfully, the pituitary. T_4 and T_3 enter into target tissues, where T_4 is converted to T_3 with T_3 binding to the thyroid hormone receptor (TR).

(pyro)Glu-His-Pro(NH$_2$)

Figure 42-8 Chemical structure of thyrotropin-releasing hormone (TRH). Note that TRH is a tripeptide (L-pyroglutamyl-L-histidyl-L-prolinamide).

cyclase and the formation of cyclic AMP. At supraphysiological concentrations (100X normal), TSH signals through the inositol-phosphate diacylglycerol cascade. The 743 amino acid glycosylated thyroid stimulating hormone receptor (TSHR/≈100 kDa) may be in either the "on" conformation, with active signaling, or the "off" conformation, where signaling does not occur. TSH binding to the TSHR places the TSHR in the "on" conformation, leading to stimulation of the thyroid gland.

Within the TSH-stimulated thyroid follicular cell, the (1) activity of the sodium-iodine symporter increases; (2) synthesis of Tg and thyroperoxidase (TPO) increases, and (3) release

TABLE 42-2   Patterns of Thyroid Dysfunction

	TSH	FT$_4$	Comments
Primary hypothyroidism	Increased	Decreased	—
Subclinical primary hypothyroidism	Increased	Normal	—
Primary hyperthyroidism	Decreased	Increased	T$_3$: increased
T$_3$ toxicosis	Decreased	Normal	T$_3$: increased
Subclinical primary hyperthyroidism	Decreased	Normal	T$_3$: normal
Thyroid hormone resistance due to defects in the thyroid hormone receptor	Normal to increased	Increased	T$_3$: increased; rT$_3$: increased
Thyroid hormone resistance due to defects in thyroid hormone metabolism of T$_4$ converted to T$_3$	Mildly increased	Increased	T$_3$: decreased; rT$_3$: increased
Thyroid hormone resistance due to defects in thyroid hormone transport into cells	Normal to increased	Normal to decreased	T$_3$: increased; rT$_3$: decreased

T$_3$, Triiodothyronine; rT$_3$, reverse T$_3$; FT$_4$, free T$_4$; T$_4$, thyroxine.

of T$_4$ and T$_3$ increases. TSH stimulation increases the size and number of thyroid follicular cells.

Thyroid Disorders

Hypothyroidism and hyperthyroidism are the two principal pathological conditions that involve the thyroid gland (Table 42-2). In addition, there are also disorders of the thyroid that are classified as nonthyroidal illnesses (NTIs).

Hypothyroidism[6]

Hypothyroidism is defined as a deficiency in thyroid hormone secretion and action. It is a common disorder that occurs in both mild and severe forms in 2% to 15% of the population. Women are afflicted more often than men, and both sexes are affected more frequently with increasing age. Clinical symptoms and physical signs of hypothyroidism are listed in Box 42-2. **Myxedema** is a severe form of hypothyroidism in which there is accumulation of mucopolysaccharides in the skin and other tissue, leading to a thickening of facial features and a doughy induration of the skin.[1] **Cretinism** is the archaic term used to describe severe hypothyroidism that develops in the newborn period. The appropriate term in this setting is "**congenital hypothyroidism.**"

Many structural or functional abnormalities of the thyroid gland lead to thyroid hormone deficiency. Diseases or treatments that directly destroy thyroid tissue or interfere with thyroid hormone biosynthesis frequently cause primary hypothyroidism. The causes of **primary hypothyroidism** are classified as endogenous or exogenous (Box 42-3).[6] Endogenous disorders are conditions that develop within the patient, such as (1) autoimmune thyroid gland dysfunction, (2) inborn errors, and (3) developmental abnormalities. Exogenous disorders are conditions that originate outside the patient, such as (1) iodine deficiency, (2) effects of excess goitrogens, (3) drug effects, and (4) postsurgical hypothyroidism or hypothyroidism following radioactive iodine treatment.

Secondary hypothyroidism occurs as a result of pituitary or hypothalamic disease and/or disorders.

BOX 42-2   Clinical Symptoms and Physical Signs of Hypothyroidism

Clinical Symptoms
Mental dullness
Somnolence
Increased sleeping
Lethargy
Easy fatigability
Hoarseness or deepening of the voice
Hair loss
Weight gain
Cold intolerance
Menstrual irregularities
Infertility
Growth failure
Delayed puberty in adolescents
Constipation
Muscle weakness or cramps
Depressed affect or frank clinical depression

Physical Signs
Bradycardia
Decreased pulse pressure
Cool and/or dry skin
Puffy eyes
Loss of the outer lateral eyebrows
Delayed relaxation phase of reflexes ("hung-up" reflexes)
Myopathy
Carotenemia
Occasional galactorrhea
Short stature in affected children
Radiologic evidence of delayed bone age in children
Congestive heart failure
Coma may rarely occur (severe hypothyroidism)

Primary Hypothyroidism

Primary hypothyroidism occurs when the production of T$_4$ and T$_3$ is impaired, either because of an extrinsic factor (e.g., iodine deficiency) or because of an intrinsic problem (e.g., **Hashimoto thyroiditis**). As a result, the positive feedback loop causes compensatory thyroid enlargement (goiter)

BOX 42-3 Causes of Primary Hypothyroidism

Endogenous Disorders

Autoimmune thyroid disease (AITD)
  Hashimoto thyroiditis
  Atrophic thyroiditis
  Late-stage Graves disease
  Postpartum thyroiditis
Inborn errors in thyroid hormone biosynthesis (dyshormonogenesis)
  Na+/Iodide pump dysfunction
  Inadequate organification/iodination—thyroperoxidase (TPO) dysfunction
  Defective thyroglobulin (Tg)
  Deiodinase deficiency
  Pendred syndrome—hypothyroidism and deafness
Developmental disorders involving the thyroid gland
  Congenital hypothyroidism: aplasia, hypoplasia
  Ectopic thyroid: lingual thyroid, thyroglossal duct cyst
Consumptive hypothyroidism (increased metabolism of T_4 and T_3 by tumors)

Exogenous Disorders

Iodine excess/deficiency
Drugs
Thionamides
Lithium
Nitroprusside
Amiodarone
Biologicals (e.g., interferon, interleukin-2)
Dietary goitrogens
Radiation-induced hypothyroidism
Surgical removal of the thyroid gland
Viral or bacterial thyroiditis

through the hypersecretion of TRH and TSH. Hashimoto **thyroiditis** is the most frequent cause of primary hypothyroidism in developed countries where iodine intake is sufficient. Worldwide, iodine deficiency is the most common cause of primary hypothyroidism. This can result from surgical removal or radioiodine ablation of the thyroid gland in the treatment of **Graves disease**. Primary hypothyroidism is frequently associated with circulating thyroid autoantibodies and may coexist with other diseases (e.g., pernicious anemia) in which autoantibodies are found. In addition, primary hypothyroidism may be one manifestation of autoimmune syndromes of polyglandular endocrine failure.[9]

Reduced concentrations and availability of T_4 and T_3 lead to hypersecretion of pituitary TSH and notable elevations in serum TSH concentrations. The elevated concentration of TSH is an important laboratory finding, particularly in the early detection of thyroid failure. In subclinical hypothyroidism,[4,9,14] thyroid hormone concentrations remain within the reference interval, but the TSH concentration is persistently elevated. The etiology of primary hypothyroidism is usually determined through (1) a detailed history, (2) a physical examination, and (3) detection of circulating thyroid autoantibodies, especially those directed againt thyroperoxidase (thyroperoxidase autoantibodies; TPOAb).

Congenital hypothyroidism is caused most commonly by the complete absence of the thyroid gland (athyreosis; thyroid gland agenesis) or partial absence (thyroid gland hypoplasia),

and, less commonly, by defects in thyroid hormone biosynthesis or, **central hypothyroidism**. Congenital hypothyroidism occurs once in every 3500 to 4000 live births, and early treatment with thyroid hormone replacement is critical if irreversible neurological damage is to be prevented.[6,10] Screening programs for congenital hypothyroidism have been developed by organizations, such as the (1) American Thyroid Association (http://www.thyroid.org, accessed December 04, 2013), (2) National Academy of Clinical Biochemistry (http://www.aacc.org, accessed December 04, 2013), and (3) Royal College of Physicians (http://www.rcplondon.ac.uk, accessed December 04, 2013). North American programs involve total T_4 screening with TSH measurement in the samples with the lowest total T_4 levels (e.g., the bottom 10% of results) whereas European screening programs measure TSH followed by T_4 measurements when TSH values exceed 20 mIU/L. Primary hypothyroidism is readily treatable by the daily administration of oral T_4. During initial treatment, serum FT_4 concentrations adjust quickly, but TSH concentrations remain high. Because the pituitary is slow to register acute changes in thyroid hormone status ("pituitary lag"), 4 to 8 weeks or more may be needed for serum TSH values to reach a new steady state after dose adjustments. Periodic monitoring of serum TSH, one to three times a year, is recommended to help maintain clinical euthyroidism and a serum TSH concentration within the reference interval. Excessive treatment with oral T_4 should be avoided to minimize the risk of accelerated bone resorption and/or atrial fibrillation.

Central Hypothyroidism

In the setting of clinical hypothyroidism with low concentrations of FT_4 and a TSH that is within or below the reference interval or only mildly elevated, central hypothyroidism is diagnosed. Central hypothyroidism is classified as secondary hypothyroidism when there is pituitary disease (with TSH deficiency) versus tertiary (with TRH defieincy) when there is disease of the hypothalamus or the hypothalamic-pituitary portal system.

Causes of central hypothyroidism include (1) a tumor, (2) hemorrhage, (3) trauma, (4) malformation, (5) postinfectious damage, and (6) postsurgical damage. Rare hereditary disorders, such as mutations in the paired-like homeodomain transcription factor-1 (previous name Pit-1; approved gene symbol *POU1F1*; chromosome 3p11) and PROphet of Pit-1 (gene name PROP paired-like homeobox 1, symbol 1PROP1; chromosome 5q35.3) transcription factors, also have been known to cause hypopituitarism and TSH deficiency. Isolated TSH deficiency is rare, and most patients with secondary hypothyroidism also have other pituitary hormone deficiencies as well (panhypopituitarism).

Other Causes of Hypothyroidism

Other causes of hypothyroidism include (1) autoimmune hypothyroidism, (2) inborn errors in thyroid hormone biosynthesis, (3) iodine deficiency or excess, (4) drug-induced,[13] (5) surgical- and radiation-induced, (6) viral or bacterial thyroiditis, (7) subclinical hypothyroidism,[4,9] and (8) the MCT8 mutation.[11]

Autoimmune Hypothyroidism

Excluding the newborn period, **autoimmune thyroid disease (AITD)** is the most common cause of thyroid disease. Hashimoto thryoiditis (chronic lymphocytic thyroiditis) leads to destruction of the thyroid follicular cells through a cell-mediated autoimmune process. Initially, the gland is usually enlarged. Over time, with destruction of the gland, it will atrophy or become firm or even fibrotic.

Inborn Errors in Thyroid Hormone Biosynthesis

Inborn errors in thyroid hormone biosynthesis (dyshormonogenesis) are rare causes of primary hypothyroidism. These defects usually present early in life and will often appear in newborns as large goiters with tracheal compression. Biochemical defects include (1) iodine transport defects from loss-of-function mutations in the sodium iodide symporter (NIS) transporter system, (2) defect in TPO function (DUOX2), and (3) defect in **pendrin** function (a protein that is mutated in Pendred syndrome), (4) Tg deficiency, and (5) iodotyrosine dehalogenase mutations (potentially causing iodine deficiency through loss of MIT, DIT, and iodine in the urine).

Iodine Deficiency or Excess

Worldwide, the most common cause of goiter is iodine deficiency producing "endemic" goiter with or without nodularity. A significant danger of iodine deficiency is maternal hypothyroidism leading to an insufficient supply of thyroid hormone to the fetus in the first half of gestation, when the fetus is entirely dependent on maternal thyroid hormone. Also maternal iodine deficiency will produce fetal iodine deficiency. Excess iodine can cause a transient state of reduced thyroid function.

Drug-Induced[13]

Various drugs effect thyroid function (Table 42-3).

Surgical and Radiation-Induced

Surgical removal of the thyroid gland will produce hypothyroidism. External irradiation of the thyroid gland (e.g., treatment of lymphoma or Hodgkin disease) or ingestion of radioactive iodine also have been known to cause hypothyroidism.

Viral or Bacterial Thyroiditis

Although rarely occurring, some (1) viral infections (such as, subacute thyroiditis or giant cell thyroiditis), or (2) bacterial infections (acute thyroiditis or abscesses)[3] of the thyroid gland will seriously damage the thyroid gland and lead to hypothyroidism.

Subclinical Hypothyroidism[4,9]

Subclinical hypothyroidism is defined by a persistent elevation in TSH (6 to 12 weeks or longer) in the setting of FT_4 concentrations that are repeatedly found within the reference interval.[9] Other conditions in which the concentration of TSH is elevated but the concentration of FT_4 is within the reference interval include (1) recent reinstitution of thyroid hormone replacement therapy, (2) poor compliance with treatment of primary hypothyroidism, (3) recovery from nonthyroidal

TABLE 42-3 Effects of Some Drugs on Tests of Thyroid Function

Cause	Drug	Effect
Inhibit TSH secretion	Dopamine	$\downarrow T_4$; $\downarrow T_3$; $\downarrow$ TSH
	L-dopa	
	Glucocorticoids	
	Somatostatin	
Inhibit thyroid hormone synthesis or release	Iodine	$\downarrow T_4$; $\downarrow T_3$; $\uparrow$ TSH
	Lithium	
Inhibit conversion of T_4 to T_3	Amiodarone	$\downarrow T_3$; $\uparrow rT_3$; $\downarrow, \rightleftharpoons, \uparrow T_4$ and FT_4; $\rightleftharpoons, \uparrow$ TSH
	Glucocorticoids	
	Propranolol	
	Propylthiouracil	
	Radiographic contrast agents	
Inhibit binding of T_4/T_3 to serum proteins	Salicylates	$\downarrow T_4$; $\downarrow T_3$; $\rightleftharpoons, \uparrow FT_4$; $\rightleftharpoons$ TSH
	Phenytoin	
	Carbamazepine	
	Furosemide	
	Nonsteroidal antiinflammatory agents	
	Heparin (in vitro effect)	
Stimulate metabolism of iodothyronines	Phenobarbital	$\downarrow T_4$; $\downarrow FT_4$; $\rightleftharpoons$ TSH
	Phenytoin	
	Carbamazepine	
	Rifampicin	
Inhibit absorption of ingested T_4	Aluminum hydroxide	$\downarrow T_4$; $\downarrow FT_4$; $\uparrow$ TSH
	Ferrous sulfate	
	Cholestyramine	
	Colestipol	
	Iron sucralfate	
	Soybean preparations	
	Kayexalate	
Increase in concentration of T_4-binding proteins	Estrogen	$\uparrow T_4$; $\uparrow T_3$; $\rightleftharpoons FT_4$; $\rightleftharpoons$ TSH
	Clofibrate	
	Opiates (heroin, methadone)	
	5-Fluorouracil	
	Perphenazine	
Decrease in concentration of T_4-binding proteins	Androgens	$\downarrow T_4$; $\downarrow T_3$; $\rightleftharpoons FT_4$; $\rightleftharpoons$ TSH
	Glucocorticoids	

$\downarrow$, Reduced serum concentration; $\uparrow$, increased serum concentration; $\rightleftharpoons$, no change. T_3, Triiodothyronine; rT_3, reverse T_3; FT_4, free T_4; T_4, thyroxine; *TSH,* thyroid-stimulating hormone.
Data from Smallridge RD. Chapter 33, Thyroid function tests. In: Becker KL, ed. Principles and practice of endocrinology and metabolism, 7th edition. Philadelphia, PA: JB Lippincott, 1995:299-306; Stockigt JR. Thyroid hormone changes in critical illness: the sick euthyroid "syndrome." Diagn Endo Metab 1997;15:39-46.

illness,[1] and (4) interfering heterophilic antibodies in immunoassays falsely raising the TSH.

Monocarboxylate Transporter 8 Mutation (Allan-Herndon-Dudley Syndrome)[11]

MCT8 is a protein is encoded by the *SLC16A2* gene.[11] MCT8 transports a variety of iodo-thyronines, including the thyroid hormones T_3 and T_4 across cell membranes. A genetic disorder of this gene causes the **Allan-Herndon-Dudley syndrome.** Symptoms of this disorder include (1) normal to slightly elevated concentrations of TSH, (2) elevated concentrations

---

BOX 42-4 Clinical Symptoms and Physical Signs of Hyperthyroidism

Clinical Symptoms
Nervousness
Erratic behavior
Emotional lability
Restlessness
Sleeplessness
Difficulty concentrating
Smooth and/or shiny hair and/or skin
Weight loss
Excessive sweating
Heat intolerance
Menstrual irregularities
Diarrhea or frequent bowel movements

Physical Signs
Tachycardia
Atrial arrhythmias
Systolic murmurs
Increased pulse pressure
Bounding pulse
Warm and/or damp skin
Softened texture of the skin
Tremor
Increased reflexes
Eyelid retraction
Other signs of ophthalmopathy in Graves disease

BOX 42-5 Causes of Hyperthyroidism

Endogenous Thyroid Disorders
Autoimmune thyroid disease (AITD)
Graves disease
Hashitoxicosis
Postpartum thyroiditis
Gain-of-function mutation in the TSH receptor
Toxic nodule
Toxic multinodular goiter
Toxic adenoma
Familial
Struma ovarii
hCG-induced hyperthyroidism
Gestational transient thyrotoxicosis
TSH receptor sensitivity to hCG
hCG-secreting tumors
Secondary hyperthyroidism (e.g., central hyperthyroidism)

Exogenous Disorders
Thyroid destruction from viral or bacterial thyroiditis
Iodine-induced hyperthyroidism
Thyroid hormone ingestion (thyrotoxicosis factitia)

---

of T_3, (3) reduced concentrations of T_4, (4) developmental delay and (5) mobility problems.

Hyperthyroidism[17]

Hyperthyroidism is defined as a hypermetabolic condition caused by excessive production of thyroid hormones. This disorder is caused by a number of conditions resulting from excess availability of thyroid hormones. Some clinicians prefer the general term **thyrotoxicosis** rather than hyperthyroidism to define the hypermetabolic state associated with increased amounts of thyroid hormone in the circulation. Clinical symptoms and physical signs of hypothyroidism are listed in Box 42-4. The causes of hyperthyroidism are listed in Box 42-5. Endogenous disorders causing hyperthyroidism include (1) intrinsic thyroid disease (primary hyperthyroidism), (2) ectopic thyroid tissue (struma ovarii), and (3) disorders of the hypothalamus or pituitary causing excess TSH secretion (central hyperthyroidism). Exogenous causes of hyperthyroidism (disease related to external factors) include (1) infectious origins (thyroid gland inflammation and destruction), (2) iodine-induced hyperthyroidism, and (3) thyroid hormone ingestion (thyrotoxicosis factitia). In North America, the most common cause of hyperthyroidism is Graves disease, an autoimmune disorder that affects 0.4% of the US population.[5]

Women are more prone to developing hyperthyroidism than men. The ratio of females to males with Graves disease is approximately 5:1. Hyperthyroidism is often easier to diagnose by clinical observation than is hypothyroidism. In some patients with hyperthyroidism, particularly individuals older than 60 years of age, the diagnosis may not be self-evident, and symptoms may be dismissed or attributed to stress or other causes.[16] This conditions is termed "**apathetic hyperthyroidism**."

The biochemical picture of primary hyperthyroidism shows increases in concentrations of T_4 and T_3 with the quantities of TSH suppressed to undetectable concentrations (or less than 0.01 mU/L). Secondary hyperthyroidism is hyperthyroidism resulting from excess TSH. Such cases include TSH-secreting pituitary adenomas and pituitary resistance to thyroid hormone with normal peripheral sensitivity.

When testing for primary hyperthyroidism, the concentration of TSH is suppressed and the serum FT_4 concentration should be determined which will typically be elevated. Finding a low TSH concentration and an elevated FT_4 concentration is usually sufficient to establish the diagnosis of hyperthyroidism in the setting of compatible symptoms. If the TSH concentration is low but the FT_4 concentration is within the reference interval, a T_3 measurement should be performed, because serum T_3 concentrations are often elevated to a greater degree than T_4 in the early phases of Graves disease and in some patients with solitary or multinodular toxic goiters (so-called T_3 **thyrotoxicosis**). A persistently suppressed concentration of serum TSH with normal concentrations of serum T_3 and FT_4 define **subclinical hyperthyroidism** (assuming conditions that suppress TSH are excluded such as the use of high dose glucocorticoids or dopamine), which is a defined biochemical entity with few or subtle clinical symptoms. Although the measurement of the free portion of T_3 (FT_3) is helpful to compensate for variations in binding proteins, measurements of total T_3 are usually sufficient because T_3 should be measured only in cases of suspected hyperthyroidism. FT_3 assays are more expensive that total T_3 measurements and total T_3 assays are more robust than FT_3 assays. A number of medications and acute and chronic illnesses do cause a transient lowering of T_3 concentrations. In patients with NTIs,[1] an early diagnosis of hyperthyroidism may not be possible until the other illness has resolved.

Occasionally, increases in serum concentrations of T_4 and T_3 will occur (1) as a result of the ingestion of large quantities of exogenous thyroid hormones, or (2) due to the release of thyroid hormones as a result of damage to the thyroid parenchyma associated with subacute thyroiditis or chronic lymphocytic thyroiditis. The increase in T_4 and T_3 concentrations may be associated with clinical findings compatible with hyperthyroidism. This diagnostic dilemma, however, is resolved by performing a radioactive iodine uptake test and finding a low radioactive iodine uptake (percent of orally administered radioactive iodine taken up by the gland at 6 or 24 hours) in cases where thyroid damage is releasing excessive thyroid hormone. When this occurs in people with pre-existing Hashimoto thyroiditis, the term "**hashitoxicosis**" can be applied. In most cases of thyroiditis with hyperthyroidism, the condition is self-limited and will resolve without residual thyroid function abnormalities. Certainly thioureas are not indicated therapeutically; beta-blockers such as propranolol can be used to diminish symptoms.

Treatments

Treatments for hyperthyroidism include (1) administration of antithyroid drugs, (2) radioiodine ablation, and (3) surgical removal of the thyroid gland. Treatment is typically designed to decrease thyroid hormone production or inhibit peripheral conversion of T_4 to T_3. At the time treatment is initiated, measurements of serum FT_4 concentrations are recommended every few weeks until symptoms abate and serum values normalize. Continuous monitoring for recurrence of hyperthyroidism is suggested two or three times a year after successful therapy. Because the pituitary gland is suppressed in hyperthyroidism, measurement of the concentration of serum TSH is not a good monitor of thyroid status in the immediate period following the start of antithyroid therapy. In fact, TSH concentrations remain suppressed for months after the patient becomes clinically euthyroid. Ablation of thyroid tissue or overtreatment with antithyroid drugs sometimes leads to clinical hypothyroidism and an increase in serum TSH. Surveillance for hypothyroidism in previously treated hyperthyroid patients must continue for the life of the patient and is best monitored with a serum TSH measurement.

Specific Causes of Hyperthyroidism

Specific causes of hyperthyroidism include (1) Graves disease,[5] (2) Hashimoto thyroiditis and postpartum thyroiditis, (3) toxic nodular or multinodular goiter, (4) gain-of-function mutations in the TSH receptor, (5) central hyperthyroidism, (6) hyperthyroidism due to human chorionic gonadotropin, (7) iodine-induced, and (8) other exogenous causes of hyperthyroidism. It should be noted that T_3 toxicosis is not a specific diagnosis. T_3 toxicosis is a descriptive term for cases where

clinical hyperthyroidism is observed in the setting of a suppressed TSH, normal FT_4 and elevated T_3. T_3 toxicosis can represent an early phase in hyperthyroidism or the case of hyperthyroidism occurring in the setting of iodine deficiency (see Table 42-2).

Thyroid storm (also known as *thyrotoxic crisis*) is an uncommon syndrome of severe and accelerating hyperthyroidism potentially manifested in (1) tachycardia, (2) restlessness, (3) high-output congestive heart failure, (4) fever greater than 41 °C (106 °F), (5) extreme irritability, (6) delirium or coma, (7) hypotension, and (8) vomiting or diarrhea. In older individuals, an unusual variant of hyperthyroidism is termed apathetic hyperthyroidism.[16] These disorders are descriptive terms and do not convey the cause of the underlying hyperthyroidism.

Likewise subclinical hyperthyroidism is not a specific etiology but the description of a clinical and biochemical variant of hyperthyroidism. A persistent depression in the concentration of TSH when FT_4 and T_3 concentrations are normal identifies subclinical hyperthyroidism. Patients with it have increased frequencies of atrial fibrillation and osteoporosis. In the absence of a clinically compatible cardiac arrhythmia or significantly reduced bone mineral density, there is little justification for the use of antithyroid drugs.

Graves Disease[5]

Graves disease is an autoimmune disease where the thyroid is overactive, producing an excessive amount of thyroid hormone. It affects approximately 0.4% of the US population and results from agonistic autoantibodies that bind to, and activate, the TSH receptor, producing hyperthyroidism. Similar to Hashimoto thyroditis, genetic susceptibility to Graves disease is polygenic. It is associated with HLA-DR3, a MHC class II cell surface receptor encoded by the human leukocyte antigen complex on chromosome 6 region 6p21.31. Other genes that influence susceptibility to AITD encode CTLA-4, PTPN22, FOXP3, CD25, CD40, thyroglobulin and the TSH receptor.

The classical clinical triad described in patients with Graves disease consists of (1) goiter and biochemical hyperthyroidism, (2) exophthalmos, and (3) nonpitting pretibial myxedema, although the latter is rarely seen.

Thyroperoxidase autoantibodies (TPOA) and Tg autoantibodies (TgA) antibodies are found in the sera of patients with both Hashimoto thyroiditis and Graves disease. However, these autoantibodies do not distinguish the two conditions. TSH receptor autoantibody (TRA) testing is available for stimulatory autoantibodies (TSIs) and receptor-binding autoantibodies (thyrotropin-binding inhibitory immunoglobulins [TBIIs]). TSI and TBII positivity is common in Graves disease and uncommon in Hashimoto thyroiditis.

Hashimoto Thyroiditis and Postpartum Thyroiditis

Hashimoto dthyroiditis (also known as *Hashimoto disease* and *chronic lymphocytic thyroiditis*) is an autoimmune disease in which the thyroid gland is attacked by a cell-mediated autoimmune processes. During the clinical course of Hashimoto thyroiditis, if a period of accelerated destruction occurs, subsequent release of thyroid hormone will produce a transient hyperthyroidism, termed *hashitoxicosis* (hyperthyroidism in patients with Hashimoto thyroiditis). Hashitoxicosis needs to be differentiated from Graves disease, because the treatments for these two conditions are different. Hashitoxicosis is self-limited, and if any treatment is required, β-blockers (such as, propranolol) are used to suppress the effects of excess catecholamines (such as, tachycardia). Patients with postpartum thyroiditis may experience a period of transient, usually self-limited, hyperthyroidism from accelerated breakdown of thyroid tissue. Alternatively postpartum thyroiditis can cause primary hypothyroidism or, sequential hyperthyroidism and then hypothyroidism or the reverse order of hypothyroidism and then hyperthyroidism. After 1 year, most women with postpartum thyroiditis enter into the euthyroid state but are at increased risk for the development of hypothyroidism later in life. Subacute (viral) or acute (bacterial) thyroiditis has also been known to produce transient hyperthyroidism.

Toxic Nodular or Multinodular Goiter
A subset of patients with nodular or multinodular goiter develop hyperthyroidism. When hyperthyroidism is caused by these lesions, the term *toxic* has been used (**toxic multinodular goiter**). In the older literature, toxic multinodular goiter is referred to as *Plummer disease.*

Gain-of-Function Mutations in the Thyroid-Stimulating Hormone Receptor
A rare familial, autosomal dominant hyperthyroidism has been known to result from gain-of-function mutations in the TSH receptor. Certain heterozygous mutations have caused infantile hyperthyroidism, whereas in infants homozygous for such mutations, potentially severe neonatal thyrotoxicosis has been observed requiring emergency thyroidectomy.

Central Hyperthyroidism
Although rare, TSH-secreting anterior pituitary adenomas have been observed. Their diagnosis is suggested by (1) clinical hyperthyroidism, (2) elevated concentrations of FT_4, (3) normal to elevated TSH concentration, and (4) evidence of a pituitary mass on a computed tomography (CT) scan or via magnetic resonance imaging (MRI).

Hyperthyroidism Due to Human Chorionic Gonadotropin
hCG–induced hyperthyroidism is observed in (1) gestational transient thyrotoxicosis, (2) TSH receptor hypersensitivity to appropriate hCG concentrations during pregnancy, and (3) hCG-secreting tumors. In gestational transient thyrotoxicosis, (1) testing for thyroid autoantibodies is negative, (2) hyperthyroidism is typically clinically mild, and (3) treatment is not usually required.[19] There is one case report of a daughter and her mother who both developed hyperthyroidism during pregnancy that were shown to express a mutant TSH receptor with increased sensitivity to normal

pregnancy-levels of hCG. Tumors that secrete hCG, such as (1) choriocarcinoma, (2) hydatidiform mole, or (3) metastatic embryonal carcinoma have been known to cause hyperthyroidism.

Iodine-Induced Hyperthyroidism
In a patient with iodine deficiency and underlying Graves disease, or nodular or multinodular goiter, iodine administration may lead to hyperthyroidism. Before iodine replenishment is provided, hyperthyroidism is likely kept in check by iodine deficiency. The phenomenon of iodine-induced hyperthyroidism is termed the *Jod-Basedow syndrome* (or phenomenon).

Other Exogenous Causes of Hyperthyroidism
Thyroid gland destruction from any cause may release excessive amounts of thyroid hormones. Intentional or unintentional ingestion of excess thyroid hormone will also produce hyperthyroidism.

When thyroid hormone is ingested or released from an inflamed or damaged thyroid gland, subsequent suppression of TSH reduces thyroidal iodine uptake, which is reflected in a reduction in the radioactive iodine uptake test. Likewise, glandular suppression or destruction lowers circulating Tg concentrations. If T_3 is ingested, hyperthyroidism may develop, producing an unusual set of biochemical abnormalities including (1) suppressed concentrations of TSH, (2) suppressed concentrations of FT_4 and total T_4, and (3) elevated total T_3 and FT_3.

Nonthyroidal Illness (Sick Euthyroid Syndrome)[8]
Many disorders are associated with variation in the concentration of thyroid hormones in the absence of definable thyroid disease (Table 42-4). For example, disorders resulting from (1) significant nutritional deprivation, (2) acute severe illness, or (3) chronic illness often result in changes in thyroid function. Collectively they are characterized as *nonthyroidal illnesses* (NTI; **sick euthyroid syndrome**).

A progressive spectrum of thyroid test result anomalies often accompany non-thyroidal illnesses in euthyroid patients. The earliest and most common changes that occur are a reduction in the serum concentrations of total and free T_3, sometimes to extremely low concentrations, and an elevation in the serum concentration of rT_3 (the "low T_3 state"). These changes have been ascribed to a block in the 5′ deiodinases that convert T_4 to T_3 in peripheral tissue. This conversion is inhibited in

TABLE 42-4	Nonthyroidal Illness[1]			
Hormone	Initial	Midcourse	Prolonged	Resolution
TSH	Normal	Normal to decreased	Decreased	Increases
T_4	Normal	Normal to decreased	Decreased	Increases
T_3	Decreased	Decreased	Decreased	Increases
	(−)	(− −)	(− − −)	
rT_3	Increased (+)	Increased (+ +)	Increased (+)	Decreases

Note: The severity of decreased T_3 is proportional to the number of (−) signs. The degree of increase in rT_3 is proportional to the number of (+) signs.
T_3, Triiodothyronine; rT_3, reverse T_3; T_4, thyroxine; *TSH*, thyroid-stimulating hormone.

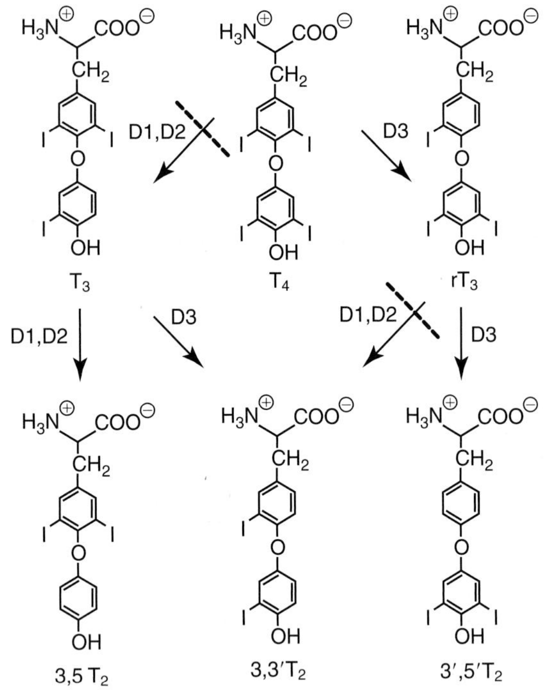

Figure 42-9 Effects of altered deiodination. In states of nonthyroidal illness (e.g., the sick euthyroid syndrome), thyroid hormone deiodination patterns are altered with reduced T_3 concentrations and elevated concentrations of rT_3.

patients with (1) acute and chronic nutritional problems, (2) poorly controlled diabetes mellitus, and (3) use of drugs such as hydrocortisone and beta blockers.

Serum TSH concentrations are usually normal in euthyroid sick patients, but may be mildly to moderately depressed with moderate to severe NTI or slightly elevated during recovery from a severe illness (Figure 42-9).[2] Causes of these transient abnormal TSH concentrations are not fully understood, but may relate to the effects of endogenous or exogenous hormones, such as glucocorticoids or dopamine, which independently suppress secretion of pituitary TSH concentrations. Other possible causes include altered nutrition or altered biological activity of immunoreactive TSH.[8] Decreased T_4 levels may result from T_4 displacement from thyroid hormone binding proteins.

As patients recover from NTIs, many of the thyroid test abnormalities revert to normal. T_4 concentrations will be corrected first followed by a rise in the concentration of T_3. Serum TSH may also transiently rebound to high concentrations for several days or weeks before returning to normal.

Thyroid Hormone Resistance

Loss-of-function mutations in the TRβ chain, or less commonly, the TRα chain, lead to two distinct and rare syndromes of thyroid hormone resistance.[2] In the autosomal dominant TRβ chain mutations, supraphysiologic concentrations of T_3 and T_4 (and FT_3 and FT_4) are required to maintain the euthyroid state. Therefore, in the absence of clinical hyperthyroidism, if the concentrations of T_4, FT_4, T_3, and FT_3 are elevated with a TSH in the upper reference

interval or mildly elevated, thyroid hormone resistance is likely. Sometimes thyroid glandular enlargement is seen. Some affected patients may even have mild clinical findings of hypothyroidism. Inappropriate treatment of thyroid hormone resistance with antithyroid drugs has been known to induce hypothyroidism.

Euthyroid Hyperthyroxinemia

Euthyroid hyperthyroxinemia exists when the total T_4 concentration is elevated, yet the patient is clinically euthyroid. Because FT_4 measurements have supplanted total T_4 measurements, this disorder is not commonly encountered in modern clinical practice.

Besides TBG elevations and the thyroid hormone resistance syndromes, euthyroid hyperthyroxinemia also result from acute illness (though the mechanism is not well understood) or autosomal dominant abnormalities in albumin (familial dysalbuminemic hyperthyroxinemia) or transthyretin (familial euthyroid thyroxine excess). In these two disorders, the concentrations of TSH, FT_4 and T_3 are within their reference intervals, whereas the concentration of total T_4 is elevated (see Table 42-4).

Analytical Methodology

In clinical practice, thyroid function tests are routinely measured to diagnose disorders of the thyroid[3,7] (see Table 42-1). For example, in combination with information obtained from a (1) a history, (2) a physical, and (3) laboratory results; patients are classified as (1) hypothyroid, (2) hyperthyroid, or (3) euthyroid (Figure 42-10).

Almost all laboratory tests for thyroid function are commercially available in either kit form or on automated immunoassay instruments. The following is a brief description of tests that are used for the evaluation of thyroid status. Package inserts that accompany commercial products also are a source of additional information. Reference intervals for the analytes discussed later are found in Table 50-1 in Chapter 50.

Measurement of Thyroid-Stimulating Hormone

Immunoassay is the method of choice for the measurement of serum TSH in the clinical laboratory. Human TSH is a 28 to 30 kDa dimeric glycoprotein consisting of a 92 amino acid alpha subunit (identical to the alpha subunit of hCG, follicle-stimulating hormone, and LH) and a 112 to 118 amino acid beta subunit. Current generation TSH assays distinguish mild to modest TSH suppression (due to, for example, overtreatment of hypothyroidism) from severely suppressed TSH levels as observed in Graves disease.

Principles of Thyroid-Stimulating Hormone Immunoassays

Essentially all current TSH methods used in clinical laboratories are two-site "sandwich" heterogeneous immunoassays involving (1) enzyme, (2) fluorometric substrate, or (3) chemiluminescent labels. These assays employ two antibodies with

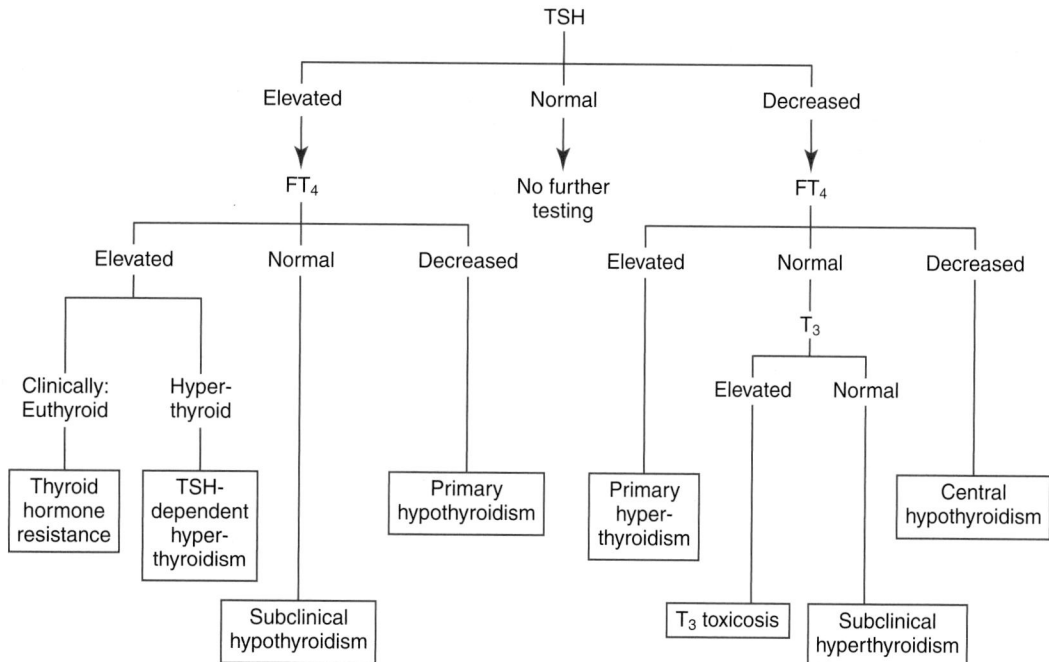

Figure 42-10 Suggested algorithm for the laboratory evaluation of thyroid function.

the capture antibody directed toward the alpha subunit and a signal antibody that recognizes an epitope on the unique beta subunit. Heterogeneous immunoassays differ in the method used to separate bound and free fractions before application of the signal antibody. In contrast to the inverse dose-response relationship in radioimmunoassay (RIA), immunometric assays generate a proportional dose-response calibration curve with higher signals corresponding to increased concentrations of analyte. Because the physiological interval of TSH concentrations is typically less than three orders of magnitude, high-dose hook effects are rarely encountered with TSH immunoassays. When compared with traditional competitive immunoassays, such as RIA, heterogeneous immunoassays for TSH offer (1) lower limits of detection, (2) rapid turnaround time, and (3) a wider linear measurement range.

Specimen Collection and Storage

Both serum and plasma are used for TSH measurements. TSH is stable for 5 days at 2 to 8 °C, and for at least 1 month when stored frozen. For newborn screening, whole blood may be collected by heel puncture 48 to 72 hours after birth.

Comments on Thyroid-Stimulating Hormone Measurements

Secretion of TSH is circadian with peak concentrations of TSH occurring between 0200 and 0400, and the lowest between 1700 and 1800. Low-amplitude oscillations occur throughout the day. TSH surges immediately after birth, reaching a peak of 25 to 160 mIU/L within 30 minutes and declining back to cord blood concentrations by postpartum day 3. TSH concentrations stabilize to near adult concentrations within the first few weeks of life. In the first trimester of pregnancy, TSH concentrations decline as hCG stimulates the maternal

thyroid gland to produce thyroid hormone, sometimes leading to a TSH concentration that is just below the lower limit of the reference interval. Reference intervals for adult TSH concentrations are the same for men and women (generally near 0.4 to 4.5 mIU/L). However, there is active discussion that the upper limit of the reference interval may be as low as 2.5 to 3.5 mIU/L if people with thyroid autoantibodies and/or abnormal thyroid ultrasound findings are excluded from the reference population.

Measurement of Total Thyroxine

T_4 is the principal hormone secreted by the thyroid, and its circulating concentration is under the control of TSH. The hormone is synthesized from tyrosine residues on Tg in the colloid of the thyroid gland. Circulating T_4 is highly (>99.9%) protein bound, and the fraction that is bound to protein is biologically inactive.

Methodology

Immunoassays and instrument-based methods are used to measure T_4 in biological fluids, predominantly serum or plasma.

Immunoassays

Many clinical laboratories measure total T_4 by using an automated competitive immunoassay. Most of these T_4 immunoassays use high-affinity polyclonal antibodies produced against an albumin-T_4 conjugate. These polyclonal antibodies are highly specific and display minimal cross-reactivity with T_3. Tg sometimes has been used as the immunogen, because it contains iodinated tyrosine residues that are the precursors of T_4 and T_3. Monoclonal antibodies against T_4 have also been developed.

Immunoassays of total T_4 measure both free and protein-bound hormone. Accurate measurement of total T_4 therefore requires dissociation of the hormone from serum proteins, such as (1) TBG, (2) albumin, and (3) transthyretin, that bind more than 99.9% of circulating T_4. Various blocking agents have been used to dissociate T_4 from TBG. The most common of these blocking agents is (1) 8-anilino-1-naphthalene-sulfonic acid (ANS), although (2) salicylate, (3) thimerosal, and (4) phenytoin have also been used for this purpose. Barbital is used to dissociate T_4 from transthyretin.

Considerable effort has been directed toward the development of immunoassays that do not require the use and measurement of radioactivity, and nonisotopic assays for T_4 are widely available for use on various automated immunoassay systems, or adaptable to automated chemistry platforms. Chemiluminescent and electrochemiluminescent assays have also been adapted for use on automated platforms.

Instrument-Based Methods

Instruments used to measure T_4 in human serum include (1) electron capture gas chromatography, (2) high-performance liquid chromatography, and (3) isotope dilution tandem mass spectrometry. The latter method has been suggested as a reference method for assay of T_4. With this technique, (1) tritium-labeled T_4 is added as an internal standard followed by (2) extraction, (3) derivatization, and (4) quantitation by combined gas chromatography–mass spectrometry.

Specimen Collection and Storage

Serum is the preferred specimen for the measurement of T_4, but plasma with ethylenediaminetetraacetic acid (EDTA) or heparin as anticoagulant has also been used. If plasma is used, repeated freeze-thaw cycles should be avoided as fibrin clots may form producing potentially spurious results due to changes in specimen viscosity. Gel barrier collection devices do not have any apparent adverse effect on T_4 methods. T_4 is a stable analyte with no appreciable change in concentration for up to 7 days at room temperature, or 30 days when frozen. Mild to moderate hemolysis and lipemia do not significantly affect most T_4 immunoassays; however, grossly hemolyzed specimens should be avoided because of dilutional effects. T_4 autoantibodies interfere with some immunoassays and may produce erroneously low or high results, depending on the method. Such interferences should be considered when there is discordance between the clinical and laboratory findings.

Heel stick capillary specimens have been used for T_4 measurement, as have dried blood specimens collected on filter paper. Dried blood specimens are stable and easily transported and are widely used in the US to screen neonates for congenital hypothyroidism. T_4 is extracted from a punched out disk of blood saturated filter paper into a buffer before assay. The filter paper should not be exposed to extreme heat or light.

Comments on Total Thyroxine Measurements

Because it reflects mostly inactive (protein-bound) hormone, the quantity of total T_4 alone provides limited clinical

information. For this reason, FT_4 measurements are preferred over total T_4 measurements for routine testing.

Cord blood T_4 concentrations are lower in preterm than in full-term neonates, and they correlate positively with birth weight in full-term infants. At birth, serum total T_4 concentrations are higher in neonates because of the maternal estrogen-induced increase in serum TBG; FT_4 concentrations are near adult concentrations. The concentration of total T_4 rises abruptly in the first few hours after birth and declines gradually until adolescence.

Measurement of Triiodothyronine

T_3 is the principal active thyroid hormone with approximately 20% of circulating T_3 secreted by the thyroid gland, and the remainder is produced by deiodination of T_4 in the peripheral tissues. Like T_4, T_3 is highly bound to protein with less than 1% of the total concentration as free active hormone. Compared with T_4, however, it is less tightly bound to serum proteins by about an order of magnitude. Consequently, the displacement of bound T_3 from proteins is essentially complete in the presence of conventional blocking agents, such as ANS. Also T_3 does not ordinarily displace T_4 from thyroid hormone–binding proteins.

Methods

Immunoassays are the techniques of choice to measure T_3 in body fluids, predominantly serum or plasma.

Radioimmunoassays

Numerous commercial RIA kits are available for measuring total T_3 concentrations in serum. Most analytical designs use a ^{125}I-T_3 tracer and incorporate antibodies bound to a solid phase, such as the wall of a cuvette or paramagnetic particles.

Nonisotopic Immunoassays

Nonisotopic immunoassays for T_3 are similar to total T_4 methods. Many of the T_3 methods have been developed for use on automated immunoassay systems, and some are compatible with chemistry platforms. Many commercial methods use enzyme labels, such as peroxidase or alkaline phosphatase, conjugated to T_3 or anti-T_3 antibodies. Enzyme activity is determined by using a variety of sensitive (1) photometric, (2) fluorescent, or (3) chemiluminescent substrates. Automated platforms that employ chemiluminescent labels are the analytical systems of choice to measure T_3. Both heterogeneous and homogeneous immunoassays for T_3 have been described.

Specimen Collection and Storage

Serum is the preferred specimen, but plasma with EDTA or heparin as anticoagulant may be used. Serum specimens should be tested within 24 hours of collection, or stored at 2 °C to 8 °C if tested beyond 24 hours. Frozen specimens are stable for at least 30 days. Turbid samples may require centrifugation before testing.

Comments on Total Triiodothyronine Measurements

Significant discrepancies have been observed when the results of different T_3 immunoassays were compared using reference sera. Interlaboratory quality assurance (proficiency testing) results also demonstrate higher analytical variance for T_3 compared with T_4 methods. Among the factors that have been suggested to account for the poorer analytical performance of T_3 immunoassays are the (1) lower concentration of T_3 in serum, (2) greater antibody cross-reactivity, (3) protein interferences, and (4) different limits of detection for T_3 methods. Total T_3 measurements are useful in the diagnosis and monitoring of hyperthyroid patients with suppressed TSH and normal FT_4 concentrations ("T_3-thyrotoxicosis"); T_3 measurements have only limited value in euthyroid and hypothyroid patients. Thyroid hormone replacement in hypothyroid patients is monitored by TSH and FT_4 measurements and is not monitored by measuring T_3.

Measurement of Reverse Triiodothyronine

Several RIA methods for measuring rT_3 have been developed and commercial assays are available. However, none of these assays have been adapted to automated platform because rT_3 measurement has limited diagnostic value. The diagnosis of NTI can usually be established without measuring rT3.

Measurement of Free Thyroid Hormones

Numerous methods have been developed for assessing the concentrations of FT_4 and FT_3 in serum. These methods include (1) direct assays that currently serve as reference methods and (2) indirect or estimate assays that are more widely available for general laboratory use.

Direct Reference Methods

Direct measurement of FT_4 (and FT_3) in serum is a technical challenge as the quantity of free hormone in normal serum is exceedingly low—typically less than 100 pmol/L (7.8 ng/dL). Reliable methods for measuring FT_4 and FT_3 in serum include those that separate free and bound hormone fractions by (1) direct equilibrium dialysis or (2) ultrafiltration. After separation, the free concentration is measured by a sensitive analytical method, such as immunoassay or mass spectrometry.

Direct Equilibrium Dialysis

In this procedure isotopically labeled T_4 or T_3 "tracer" is added to the specimen before dialysis is performed. When equilibrium is established, concentrations of the tracer on both sides of the dialysis membrane are used to calculate the ratio of bound to free hormone, so the FT_4 (or FT_3) concentration is able to be calculated based on the total T_4 or T_3 concentration. If the amount of tracer added to the specimen is small in comparison with the endogenous hormone concentration, minimal disruption of free/bound hormone is noted.

Ultrafiltration

The ultrafiltration procedure for FT_4 determination in serum is significantly less time-consuming than dialysis. In this method, the serum specimen is (1) adjusted to a pH of 7.4, (2) incubated for 20 minutes at 37 °C (to achieve equilibrium of the binding at this temperature), and then (3) applied to an ultrafiltration device for centrifugation for 30 minutes at 37 °C and 2000 × g (using a fixed-angle rotor). Subsequently the ultrafiltrate is analyzed for T_4 by immunoassay.

Comments

FT_4 assays based on ultrafiltration measure free hormone without the need for total hormone measurements. Direct equilibrium dialysis and ultrafiltration methods are unaffected by either variations in serum binding proteins or thyroid hormone autoantibodies. Mean values obtained in euthyroid healthy subjects are reported to be slightly higher when using ultrafiltration methods than when using equilibrium dialysis.

Indirect Methods for Estimating Free Thyroid Hormones

Two-step and one-step immunoassays estimate free hormone concentrations by using antibody extraction techniques. They are subdivided into *sequential two-step assays* and *simultaneous one-step ("analogue") assays*. The analogue methods are no longer used, and the sequential two-step assays are preferred. Each procedure involves the direct incubation of serum with a specific anti-T_4 or anti-T_3 antibody, during which thyroid hormones reach a new equilibrium with all of the binders present. A slight decrease in free hormone concentration occurs, but is insignificant if the antibody sequesters less than 5% of the total amount of hormone present in the specimen. Thus the amount of immunoextracted T_4 or T_3 closely approximates the undisturbed free hormone concentration that preexists in serum at equilibrium.

Comments

Estimates of FT_4 and FT_3 generally give reliable results in (1) healthy subjects, (2) hyperthyroid and hypothyroid patients, and (3) patients with only mild binding protein abnormalities. Results are comparable with those of reference methods, such as those that use direct equilibrium dialysis. In certain clinical conditions, free hormone estimate methods may give abnormal results that differ from the generally accepted reference values. These abnormalities are commonly encountered in euthyroid patients who show significant changes in T_4 or T_3 binding to serum proteins.

Measurement of Thyroxine-Binding Globulin

Modern TBG methods measure its concentration directly using a variety of immunochemical approaches. For example, one competitive, heterogeneous method measures the competition between endogenous TBG and labeled TBG for binding to an immobilized anti-TBG antibody. Another assay utilizes a solid-phase second antibody; bound conjugate that is measured by chemiluminescence after the addition of Luminol and hydrogen peroxide. A third immunoassay is based on enhanced microparticle turbidimetry, in which the presence of endogenous antigen inhibits the cross-linking of antigen-microparticle complexes by anti-TBG antibody, reducing the turbidity of the reaction mixture.

Measurement of Thyroglobulin

Both competitive and noncompetitive immunoassays have been applied to Tg measurement.[12,18] Present-day competitive immunoassays typically incubate the serum with anti-Tg antibody; this is followed by the addition of ^{125}I-labeled Tg. The Tg–anti-Tg complex is precipitated by a second antibody, separating antibody-bound from free ^{125}I-labeled Tg. Noncompetitive (sandwich) immunoassays for Tg have been developed using a variety of labels. Technical improvements in such assays have resulted in the availability of a new generation of Tg assays with enhanced lower limits of detection.[12]

A technical problem with Tg assays is interference from TGAs in the patient's blood that limits the accurate measurement of Tg. Consequently, it is standard practice to search for TGA whenever Tg is measured. When TGAs are detected, the TGA concentration may be useful as a secondary marker of the mass of thyroid tissue present in the patient. Of note is the fact that anti-Tg autoantibodies are much more common in thyroid cancer patients than in the general population.[10] For example, TGAs are reported in 15% to 35% of thyroid cancer patients. Consequently, Tg measurements should not be used as tumor markers in the clinical management of patients with demonstrated TGA.

Determination of Thyroid Autoantibodies

Increased circulating concentrations of thyroid autoantibodies are found in a variety of thyroid disorders and in other autoimmune diseases and certain malignancies. These autoantibodies are directed against several thyroid and thyroid hormone antigens, including (1) Tg (TgAb), (2) thyroid peroxidase antibody (TPOAb), (3) the TSH receptor (TRAb), (4) TSH, (5) T_4, and (6) T_3. Of these autoantibodies, measurement of TPOAb is the test most often used to evaluate thyroid autoimmune diseases.

TPOAs and Tg autoantibodies are detected by a variety of methods, including (1) indirect immunofluorescence, (2) the agar gel diffusion precipitin technique, (3) agglutination (hemagglutination or latex particle agglutination), (4) RIA, (5) complement fixation, (6) ELISA techniques, and (7) chemiluminescence-based immunometric assays.[20]

Review Questions

1. What is the most common type of laboratory assay that is widely used to assess thyroid hormone concentrations?
   a. Ultrafiltration.
   b. Immunoassay.
   c. Potentiometry.
   d. Estimation from using a formula.
2. What stimulates the uptake of iodide by the thyroid gland for thyroid hormone synthesis?
   a. Thyroid-stimulating hormone (TSH)
   b. Thyroxine (T_4)
   c. Tyrosine
   d. Thyroiditis
3. What causes primary hypothyroidism?
   a. The absence or dysfunction of the thyroid gland.
   b. Increased TSH.
   c. A pituitary disorder.
   d. A hypothalamus disorder.

4. Hyperthyroidism is also referred to as
   a. Athyreosis.
   b. Myxedema.
   c. Thyrotoxicosis.
   d. Exophthalmos.
5. What is the function of thyroid hormones?
   a. Inhibit the secretion of growth hormone.
   b. Solely regulate reproductive processes in male and females.
   c. Maintain water homeostasis.
   d. Regulate carbohydrate, lipid, and protein metabolism within cells.
6. *Secondary hypothyroidism* is indicated by which one of the following sets of lab results?
   a. Increased T_4, and decreased TSH
   b. Increased T_4, and increased TSH
   c. Decreased T_4, and increased TSH
   d. Decreased T_4, and decreased TSH
7. The thyroid gland produces all of the following hormones *except* which one of the following hormones?
   a. TSH.
   b. Calcitonin.
   c. Thyroxine (T_4).
   d. Triiodothyronine (T_3).
8. What is the amino acid precursor of T_4?
   a. Threonine.
   b. Tyrosine.
   c. Thyronine.
   d. Alanine.
9. What is the technique of choice to measure T_3 in body fluids?
   a. Nephelometry.
   b. Potentiometry.
   c. Immunoassay.
   d. Atomic absorption.
10. Which one of the following analytes is most sensitive for the early detection of primary thyroid gland failure?
    a. Thyroxine (T_4)
    b. TSH
    c. Thyroglobulin (Tg)
    d. Thyroid-binding globulin (TBO)

References

1. Adler SM, Wartofsky L. The nonthyroidal illness syndrome. Endocrinol Metab Clin North Am 2007;36:657–72.
2. Agrawal NK, Goyal R, Rastogi A, Naik D, Singh SK. Thyroid hormone resistance. Postgrad Med J 2008;84:473–7.
3. Andersen S, Bruun NH, Pedersen KM, Laurberg P. Biologic variation is important for interpretation of thyroid function tests. Thyroid 2003;13:1069–78.
4. Arrigo T, Wasniewska M, Crisafulli G, Lombardo F, Messina MF, Rulli I, et al. Subclinical hypothyroidism: the state of the art. J Endocrinol Invest 2008;31:79–84.
5. Brent GA. Clinical practice: Graves' disease. N Engl J Med 2008;358:2594–605.
6. Devdhar M, Ousman YH, Burman KD. Hypothyroidism. Endocrinol Metab Clin North Am 2007;36:595–615.
7. Dufour DR. Laboratory tests of thyroid function: uses and limitations. Endocrinol Metab Clin North Am 2007;36:579–948.

8. Farwell AP. Thyroid hormone therapy is not indicated in the majority of patients with the sick euthyroid syndrome. Endocr Pract 2008;14:1180–7.

9. Fatourechi V. Subclinical hypothyroidism: an update for primary care physicians. Mayo Clin Proc 2009;64:65–71.

10. Francis Z, Schlumberger M. Serum thyroglobulin determination in thyroid cancer patients. Best Pract Res Clin Endocrinol Metab 2008;6:1039–46.

11. Friesema EC, Ganguly S, Abdalla A, Manning Fox JE, Halestrap AP, Visser TJ. Identification of monocarboxylate transporter 8 as a specific thyroid hormone transporter". J Biol Chem 2003;278: 40128–35.

12. Giovanella L. Highly sensitive thyroglobulin measurements in differentiated thyroid carcinoma management. Clin Chem Lab Med 2008;46:1067–73.

13. Gittoes NJ, Franklyn JA. Drug-induced thyroid disorders. Drug Saf 1995;13:46–55.

14. Helfand M. Screening for subclinical thyroid dysfunction in nonpregnant adults: a summary of the evidence for the U.S. Preventive Services Task Force. Ann Intern Med 2004;140:128–41.

15. Heuer H, Visser TJ. Minireview: pathophysiological importance of thyroid hormone transporters. Endocrinology 2009;150:1078–83.

16. Mooradian AD. Asymptomatic hyperthyroidism in older adults: is it a distinct clinical and laboratory entity? Drugs Aging 2008;25:371–80.

17. Nayak B, Hodak SP. Hyperthyroidism. Endocrinol Metab Clin North Am 2007;36:617–56.

18. Pacini F, Pinchera A. Serum and tissue thyroglobulin measurement: clinical applications in thyroid disease. Biochimie 1999;81:463–7.

19. Patil-Sisodia K, Mestman JH. Graves' hyperthyroidism and pregnancy: a clinical update. Endocr Pract 2012;16:1–36.

20. Winter WE, Schatz, D, Bertholf RL. The thyroid: pathophysiology and thyroid function testing. In Burtis CA, Ashwood ER, Bruns DE, editors, Tietz textbook of clinical chemistry and molecular diagnostics. 5th edition. St Louis: Saunders, 2012:1905–44.

Reproduction-Related Disorders[*]

Mari L. DeMarco, Ph.D., and Ann M. Gronowski, Ph.D.

Objectives

1. Define the following:

   Amenorrhea

   Androgen

   Dehydroepiandrosterone sulfate (DHEAS)

   Gonadotropin-releasing hormone (GnRH)

   Gynecomastia

   Hirsutism

   Infertility

   Inhibin

   Menopause

   Polycystic ovary syndrome (PCOS)

   Precocious puberty

   Virilization

2. Describe the hypothalamic-pituitary control of the gonads.

3. For each of the hormones listed below, state and describe sites of synthesis and action on target organ, transport, physiological function, metabolism, and regulation in both males and females:

   Estrogens

   Follicle stimulating hormone

   Gonadotropin-releasing hormone (GnRH)

   Luteinizing hormone (LH)

   Progesterone

   Testosterone

4. Diagram the phases of the normal female reproductive cycle and include the specific hormones involved in each phase; describe the roles of these hormones and the control mechanisms of each phase.

5. List the hormone changes, symptoms, and causes of the following disorders:

   Amenorrhea

   Erectile dysfunction

   Hyper- and hypogonadotropic hypogonadism

   Infertility

   Kallmann syndrome

   Polycystic ovary syndrome (PCOS)

   Precocious puberty

6. Discuss the role of the clinical laboratory in the evaluation of ovulation, amenorrhea, menopause, male/female infertility, and other reproductive endocrine disorders; include specific laboratory tests used and results of these tests.

7. Assess and solve case studies related to reproductive endocrinology and disorders.

Key Words and Definitions

Androgen insensitivity syndrome (AIS) A genetic disorder in which XY male fetuses are unresponsive to androgens and are born looking externally like normal females.

Amenorrhea The absence of menstruation.

Androstenedione An androgenic steroid produced by the (1) testes, (2) adrenal cortex, and (3) ovary. It is converted metabolically to testosterone and other androgens.

Congenital adrenal hyperplasia (CAH) A genetic disorder characterized by a deficiency of any one of several enzymes needed to make cortisol from cholesterol; symptoms arise from lack of the hormones cortisol and aldosterone and altered production of sex hormones; the latter may affect sexual development before birth.

Corpus luteum A yellow glandular mass in the ovary formed by an ovarian follicle that has matured and discharged its ovum; secretes progesterone.

Corticosteroid-binding globulin An α-globulin that binds unconjugated corticosteroid and transports it in the plasma.

Dehydroepiandrosterone (DHEA) A hormone produced by the adrenal glands. After being secreted, it circulates in the bloodstream as DHEA-sulfate (DHEAS) and is converted as needed into other hormones.

Dihydrotestosterone (DHT) A powerful androgenic hormone that is formed in peripheral tissue by the action of the enzyme 5α-reductase on testosterone.

---

[*]The authors gratefully acknowledge the original contribution of R. J. Whitley, A. W. Meikle, N. B. Watts, T.S. Isbell, and E. Jungheim, on which portions of this chapter are based.

Key Words and Definitions—cont'd

Estradiol (E₂) and Estriol (E₃) Estrogenic hormones produced by the (1) ovaries, (2) corpus luteum, and during pregnancy by the (3) placenta. The adrenal glands and testes (in men) are also believed to secrete smaller quantities of estrogens.

Estrone (E₁) A natural estrogenic hormone that is a ketone found in the body chiefly as a metabolite of estradiol (E₂); it is also secreted especially by the ovaries.

Female athletic triad A group of findings commonly seen in young female athletes, consisting of (1) eating disorders, (2) amenorrhea, and (3) osteoporosis.

Follicle A pouch-like sac that is on the surface of the ovary and contains the maturing ovum (egg); also called *Graafian follicle.*

Follicle-stimulating hormone (FSH) An anterior pituitary peptide that stimulates the development of Graafian follicles in the female and spermatozoa in the male.

Gonad A gamete-producing organ (an ovary or a testis).

Gonadotropin-releasing hormone (GnRH) A peptide that is released from the brain and stimulates the pituitary gland to secrete gonadotrophic hormones that in turn act on the sex glands.

Gynecomastia Excessive development of the male mammary glands.

Hirsutism Abnormal hairiness, especially an adult male pattern of hair distribution in females.

Human chorionic gonadotropin (hCG) A hormone produced early in pregnancy by the placenta.

hCG stimulation test A test administered to assess the ability of the testes to respond to hCG and produce testosterone.

3β-Hydroxysteroid dehydrogenase deficiency An inherited disorder that affects hormone-producing glands, including the gonads (ovaries in females and testes in males) and the adrenal glands.

11β-Hydroxylase deficiency A type of congenital adrenal hyperplasia due to 11β-hydroxylase deficiency; it is one of a group of disorders (collectively called *congenital adrenal hyperplasia*) that affect the adrenal glands.

21-Hydroxylase deficiency A deficiency of this enzyme results in decreased cortisol synthesis and increased synthesis of male hormones by the adrenal; three types are described: (1) salt-wasting, (2) simple virilizing, and (3) nonclassical.

Hyperandrogenism A medical condition characterized by excessive production and/or secretion of androgens.

Hypergonadotropic hypogonadism A condition characterized by (1) defective development of ovaries or testes, (2) excess pituitary gonadotropin secretion, and (3) delayed sexual development and growth delay.

Hyperprolactinemia A condition characterized by the presence of abnormally-high levels of prolactin.

Hypertrichosis Excessive growth of hair.

Hypogonadotropic hypogonadism A condition with impaired production of the hormones (LH and FSH) that stimulate the gonads; lack of LH and FSH leads to decreased sex hormone production by the gonads and accompanying symptoms.

Infertility The inability to conceive after 1 year of unprotected intercourse.

Inhibin A peptide hormone secreted by the follicular cells of the ovary and the Sertoli cells of the testis that inhibits secretion of follicle stimulating hormone (FSH) from the anterior pituitary.

Inhibin A Ovary-produced inhibin A is an important negative feedback hormone that suppresses pituitary secretion of FSH during the late follicular and luteal phases of the menstrual cycle.

Klinefelter syndrome A condition in a male characterized by (1) two X and one Y chromosomes, (2) infertility, (3) small testicles, (4) sparse facial and body hair, and (5) enlarged breasts.

Late-onset 21-hydroxylase deficiency A condition due to 21-hydroxylase deficiency. It is a common, milder form of congenital adrenal hyperplasia (CAH) characterized by a later onset of androgen excess symptoms seen in females and precocious pseudopuberty in both sexes; also known as *non classical congenital adrenal hyperplasia.*

Leydig cell A type of cell in the testes that secretes testosterone.

LH surge A sharp increase in serum concentrations of luteinizing hormone seen near the middle of the menstrual cycle about one to two days before ovulation.

Luteinizing hormone (LH) A hormone produced by the anterior lobe of the pituitary gland that stimulates ovulation and the development of the corpus luteum in the female and the production of testosterone by the interstitial cells of the testis in the male.

Menarche The establishment or beginning of the menstrual function.

Menopause Cessation of menstruation, which usually occurs around the age of 50.

Menses The monthly flow of blood from the genital tract of women.

Müllerian duct agenesis A congenital malformation characterized by a failure of the Müllerian duct to develop, with resultant absence or malformation of the vagina and/or uterus.

Müllerian duct Either of two embryonic tubes extending along the mesonephros that become the uterine tubes, uterus, and part of the vagina in the female and that form the prostatic utricle in the male.

Oligomenorrhea Menses occurring at intervals longer than 35 days.

Ovaries The paired female reproductive organs that produce ova (eggs), estrogens and progesterone.

Placenta A fetomaternal organ that is characteristic of true mammals during pregnancy; its functions include (1) transport of nutrients to the fetus, (2) transport of waste from the fetus, and (3) exchange of gases (oxygen and carbon dioxide) between the mother and fetus.

Polycystic ovary syndrome (PCOS) A female condition that is characterized by multiple ovarian follicles and increased androgen production.

Precocious puberty Early development of secondary sex characteristics; in girls generally before age 8 and in boys before age 9.

Primary ovarian insufficiency (POI) A condition in which the ovary fails to function adequately in a woman younger than 40 years.

Progesterone The principal progestational hormone liberated by the (1) corpus luteum, (2) adrenal cortex, and (3) placenta, whose function is to prepare the uterus for the implantation and development of the fertilized oocyte.

Progestational Preceding or promoting pregnancy; the phase of the menstrual cycle after ovulation; related to the characteristic actions of progesterone.

Key Words and Definitions—cont'd

Prolactin (PRL) A pituitary hormone that stimulates and maintains the secretion of milk.

Pseudohermaphroditism The condition of having the gonads and karyotype of one sex and external genitalia that is of the other sex or is ambiguous.

Pseudoprecocious puberty Development of secondary sex characters and reproductive organs that is not associated with pubertal levels of gonadotropins and gonadotropin-releasing hormone. Also called *GnRH-independent precocious puberty.*

Pure gonadal dysgenesis An intersex disorder characterized by 46,XX chromosomes and normal external female genitalia at birth.

Sertoli cell Any of the elongated, striated cells of the seminiferous tubules of the testis, to which spermatids attach for nourishment during spermatogenesis.

Sertoli cell–only syndrome A condition characterized by congenital absence of germinal epithelium from the seminiferous tubules, which contain only Sertoli cells, resulting in sterility

due to the absence of living sperm cells in the semen. Also called *Del Castillo syndrome.*

Sex hormone–binding globulin (SHBG) A glycoprotein that binds to sex hormones, specifically androgens and estrogens.

Sperm protein SP-10 A sperm acrosomal protein, specific to the testis, that is believed to play an important role in egg-sperm binding.

Testis The male gonad, either of two oval reproductive glands located in the scrotum.

Testosterone The principal androgenic hormone, produced by the Leydig cells of the testes in response to stimulation by LH of the anterior pituitary gland.

Turner syndrome A chromosomal disorder affecting females wherein one of the two X-chromosomes is defective or completely absent.

Virilization The induction or development of male secondary sex characteristics; especially the induction of such changes in the female.

Reproductive endocrinology encompasses the hormones of the hypothalamic-pituitary-gonadal axis, as well as the adrenal glands (see Chapters 40 and 41). These hormones are crucial for reproductive function and include (1) **gonadotropin-releasing hormone (GnRH)**, (2) **luteinizing hormone (LH)**, (3) **follicle-stimulating hormone (FSH)**, and (4) a multitude of sex steroids. The sex steroids are synthesized by the (1) **ovaries**, (2) **testes**, and (3) adrenal glands and are responsible for the manifestation of primary and secondary sex characteristics.

Male Reproductive Biology

The male reproductive system consists of (1) testes, (2) a penis, and (3) related glands, such as the prostate and Cowper glands (Figure 43-1).

Biological Functions

The function of the testes is to synthesize sperm and androgens. Sertoli and Leydig cells play key roles in this process. For example, **Sertoli cells** in the seminiferous tubules of the testes have a crucial role in sperm maturation and secrete **inhibin**, a glycoprotein that inhibits the pituitary secretion of FSH.[9] Surrounding the seminiferous tubules are the interstitial **Leydig cells**, the primary site of androgen production. The principal androgen in the human male is **testosterone**, which is required for (1) sexual differentiation, (2) spermatogenesis, and (3) promotion and maintenance of sexual maturity at puberty.

Role of the Hypothalamic-Pituitary-Gonadal Axis

GnRH is a decapeptide synthesized in the hypothalamus and transported to the anterior pituitary gland, where it stimulates the release of both FSH and LH (Figure 43-1).

In adult men, (1) GnRH, (2) LH, and (3) FSH are secreted in pulsatile patterns with higher concentrations found in the

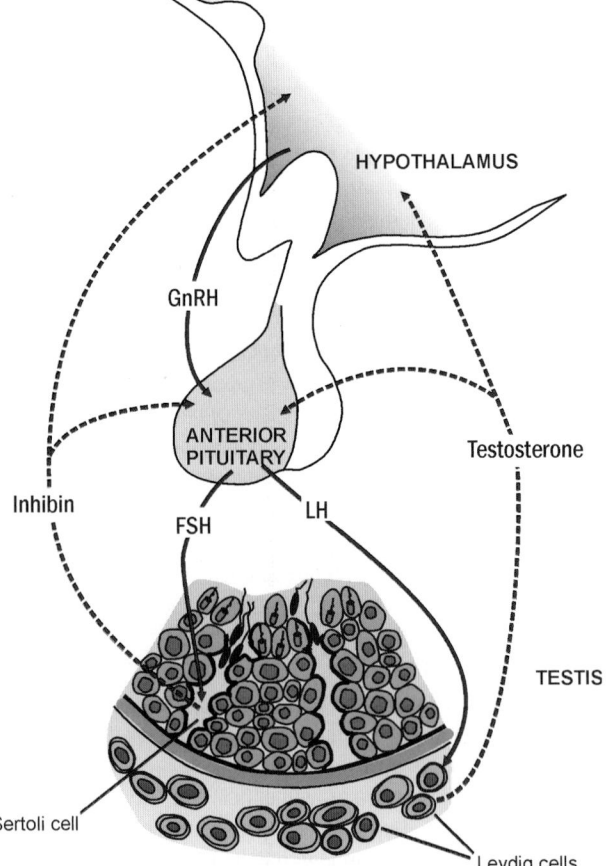

Figure 43-1 Summary of the endocrine control of the testis. *Dashed* lines indicate inhibitory effects, and *solid* lines stimulatory effects. *FSH,* Follicle-stimulating hormone; *GnRH,* gonadotropin-releasing hormone; *LH,* luteinizing hormone.

early morning hours and lower concentrations in the late evening. LH acts on Leydig cells to stimulate the conversion of cholesterol to pregnenolone. FSH acts on Sertoli cells and spermatocytes and is central to the initiation (in puberty) and maintenance (in adulthood) of spermatogenesis. Sex steroids and inhibin provide negative feedback control of LH and FSH secretion, respectively. LH secretion is inhibited by testosterone and by its metabolites, **estradiol (E_2)** and **dihydrotestosterone (DHT)**. Plasma FSH may be increased in disorders in which Sertoli cell numbers and inhibin concentrations are reduced. Likewise, a reduction in the number of Leydig cells and testosterone secretion leads to increased concentrations of LH.

Androgens

Androgens are a group of C-19 steroids (Figure 43-2) responsible for masculinization of the genital tract and development and maintenance of male secondary sex characteristics. Testosterone is the principle androgen secreted in men.

Biosynthesis of Testosterone

Testosterone is synthesized primarily by the Leydig cells of the testes (95%) and, to a lesser extent ($\approx$5%) via peripheral

Testosterone
(17β-Hydroxyandrost-4-en-3-one)

Dihydrotestosterone (DHT)
(17β-Hydroxy-5α-androstan-3-one)

Androstenediol
(3β,17β-Dihydroxyandrost-5-ene)

Androstanediol
(3α,17β-Dihydroxy-5α-androstane)

Δ4-Androstene-3,17-dione

Dehydroepiandrosterone (DHEA)

Dehydroepiandrosterone sulfate
(DHEAS)

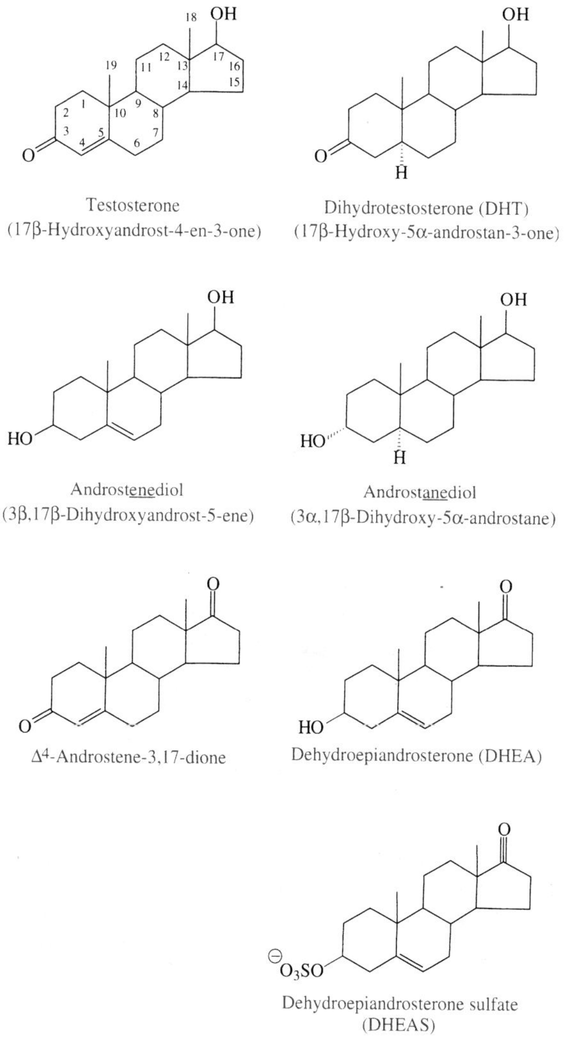

Figure 43-2 Chemical structure of androgens.

conversion from the precursors **dehydroepiandrosterone (DHEA)** and **androstenedione** (which are synthesized in the adrenal glands). Synthesis of androgens begins with formation of pregnenolone from cholesterol. Following the formation of pregnenolone, four additional enzymatic steps are required to convert cholesterol to testosterone (Figure 43-3).

Androgen Transport in Blood

Testosterone and DHT circulate in plasma freely ($\approx$2% to 3%) or bound to plasma proteins. Binding proteins include the specific **sex hormone–binding globulin (SHBG)** and nonspecific proteins, such as albumin. SHBG has low capacity for steroids but binds with very high affinity, whereas albumin has high capacity but low affinity. Testosterone and SHBG concentrations peak in the early morning (0400-0800 hours) and are at their lowest concentration in the evening (1600-2000 hours).

The biologically active fraction includes free testosterone and possibly albumin-bound testosterone. Consequently, the bioavailable testosterone (free + albumin-bound) is thought to be $\approx$35% of the total quantity.[10] Concentrations of bioavailable testosterone correlate with those of free testosterone.

Metabolism of Testosterone

Circulating testosterone serves as a precursor for the formation of two additional active metabolites. As shown in Figure 43-3, testosterone is converted to estradiol and to DHT by 5α-reductase or to estrogen by aromatase.[10]

DHT is thought to be (1) the essential androgen responsible for formation of primary sex characters in males during embryogenesis, (2) for development of most male secondary sex characters at puberty, and (3) for adult male sexual function. It is formed in androgen target tissues such as the skin and prostate, whereas aromatization occurs in many tissues, especially the liver and adipose tissue. Peripheral aromatization occurs primarily in adipose tissue (of both men and women) because of the high concentration of aromatase in this tissue. The rate of extraglandular aromatization therefore increases with body fat.

DHT is metabolized to 3α-androstanediol (see Figure 43-3) and then is conjugated to form 3α-androstanediol glucuronide. Serum concentrations of 3α-androstanediol glucuronide or 3α-androstanediol have bewen measured as markers of DHT production in peripheral tissues.

The main excretory metabolites of androstenedione, testosterone, and DHEA are shown in Figure 43-4. Except for epitestosterone, these catabolites constitute a group of steroids known as *17-ketosteroids (17-KSs);* they are excreted primarily in the urine.

Testosterone Concentrations

Fetal testes produce testosterone around the seventh week of gestation with peak serum concentrations of $\approx$250 ng/dL observed at the beginning of the second trimester and with concentrations gradually returning to baseline by birth. Shortly after birth, the concentration of testosterone begins to increase, peaking again at $\approx$250 ng/dL at 2 to 3 months of age, and then falls to baseline again by 6 to 12 months. The concentration of

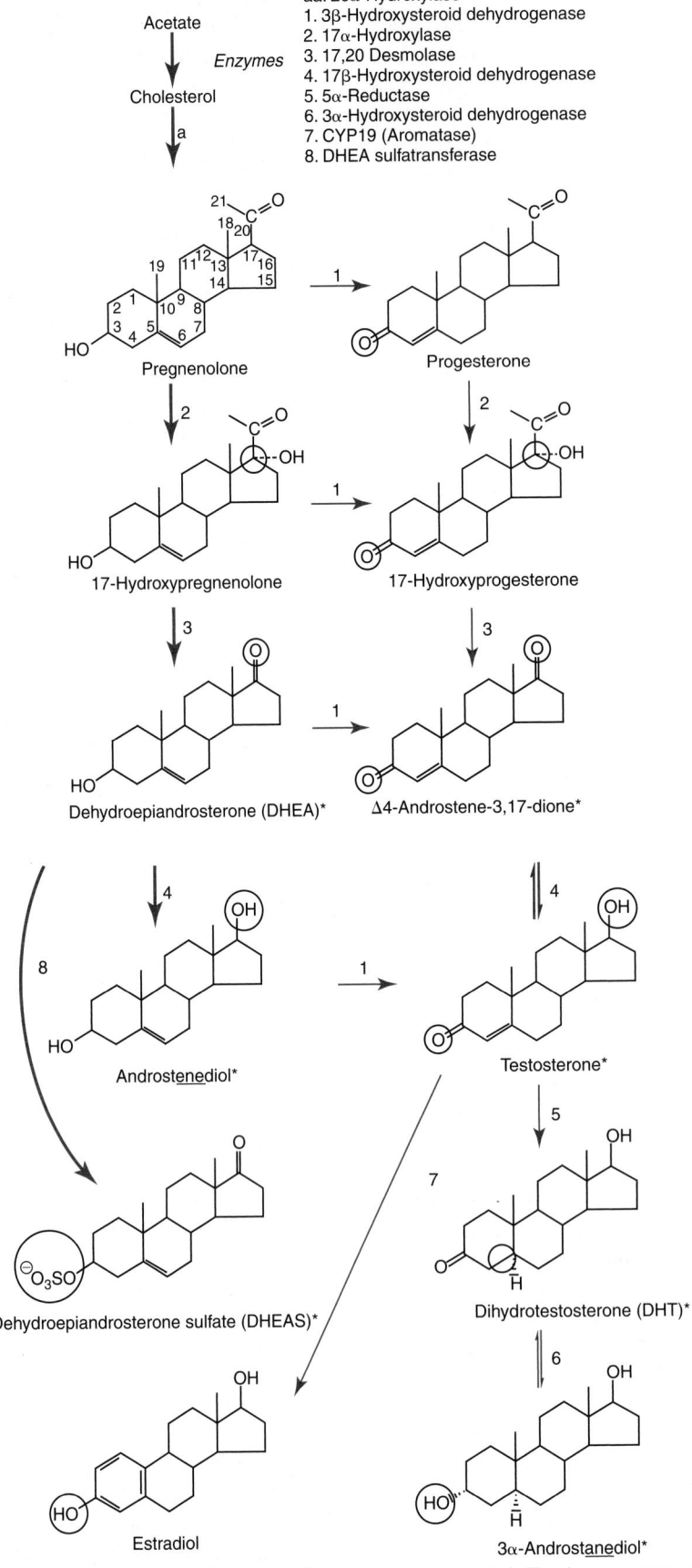

Figure 43-3 Biosynthesis of androgens (adrenal glands and testis). The *heavy arrows* indicate the preferred pathway. The *encircled areas* represents the sites of chemical change. *Denotes androgens.

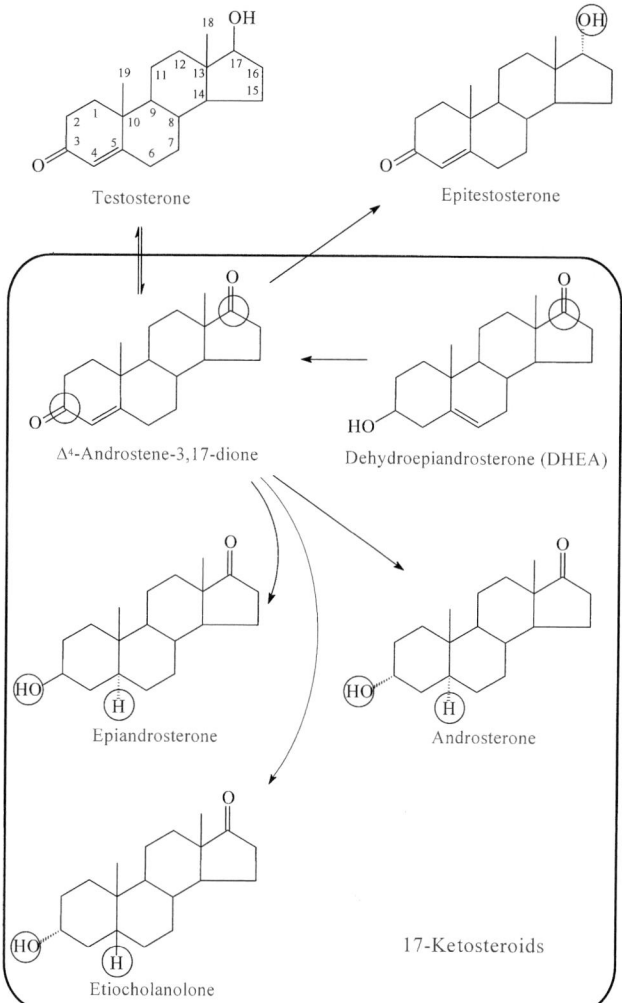

Figure 43-4 Catabolism of $C_{19}O_2$ androgens. The *circled area* represents the site of chemical change.

testosterone remains low (<50 ng/dL) until puberty, when the concentration of testosterone rises to 500 to 700 ng/dL. Testosterone remains at high concentrations through adulthood.

Men beyond the age of 30 to 40 years experience an age-dependent decrease in circulating testosterone concentration. The 1.3% decrease per year in bioavailable serum testosterone is thought to be due to (1) a decrease in Leydig cell numbers, (2) decreased GnRH pulse amplitude, and (3) increases in SHBG. These decreases in circulating concentrations of testosterone, while typical, are now viewed as therapeutic targets when associated with clinical correlates of hypogonadism. Late-onset hypogonadism (LOH), and testosterone deficiency syndrome (TDS), represent the current nomenclature for the treatable syndrome characterized by an age related decline in serum testosterone accompanied by the clinical symptoms. Clinically, patients should exhibit symptoms suggestive of testosterone deficiency, such as (1) decreased libido, (2) erectile dysfunction, (3) decreased muscle mass and strength, (4) decreased bone mineral density, and (5) changes in mood. Patients should exhibit one to three of these symptoms with a concomitant low concentration of serum testosterone to fit

various diagnostic criteria. Total serum testosterone is the most widely used biochemical parameter for assessment of hypogonadism. Measurement of free or bioavailable testosterone should be considered when total testosterone is not diagnostic despite the clinical presentation of hypogonadism. This is particularly true in the setting of obesity and advanced age, where high concentrations of SHBG may mask a true deficit in testosterone. To assess whether hypogonadism is primary or secondary, serum LH should be measured; a serum **prolactin** (PRL) measurement is indicated when serum testosterone concentrations are lower than 5.2 nmol/L (150 ng/dL), or when secondary hypogonadism is suspected.

Male Reproductive Abnormalities

A variety of abnormalities affect the male reproductive system before birth, in childhood, or in adulthood (Box 43-1). For the purposes of this chapter, they have been divided into the categories of (1) hypogonadotropic hypogonadism, (2) hypergonadotropic hypogonadism, (3) defects in androgen action, (4) erectile dysfunction, and (5) **gynecomastia.**

Hypogonadotropic Hypogonadism

Male hypogonadism is a condition caused by decreased function of the testes, which can lead to retardation of sexual development if manifested early in life. The disorder is classified as *hypogonadotropic* or *hypergonadotropic* depending on whether the pituitary gonadotropic hormones (LH and FSH) are decreased or increased.

Hypogonadotropic hypogonadism occurs when defects in the hypothalamus or pituitary prevent normal gonadal stimulation. Causative factors include (1) congenital or acquired panhypopituitarism, (2) hypothalamic syndromes, (3) GnRH deficiency, (4) **hyperprolactinemia,** (5) malnutrition or anorexia, and (6) iatrogenic causes. All of these abnormalities are associated with decreased testosterone and gonadotropin concentrations.

Kallmann syndrome, the most common form of hypogonadotropic hypogonadism, results from a deficiency of GnRH in the hypothalamus during embryonic development. It is characterized by hypogonadism and anosmia (loss of the sense of smell) in male or female patients. It is a congenital defect with several genetic causes that result in gonadotropic deficiency.

Hypergonadotropic Hypogonadism

Hypergonadotropic hypogonadism results from a primary gonadal disorder. Patients with primary testicular failure have increased concentrations of LH and FSH and decreased concentrations of testosterone. Causes for primary hypogonadism are categorized as (1) acquired causes (irradiation, castration, mumps orchitis, or cytotoxic drugs), (2) chromosome defects (such as **Klinefelter syndrome),** (3) defective androgen synthesis (20α-hydroxylase deficiency), (4) testicular agenesis, (5) seminiferous tubular disease, and (6) other miscellaneous causes. Aging is associated with gonadal failure, which leads to decreased testosterone secretion.[9]

Defects in Androgen Action

The most common and severe defect in androgen action is **androgen insensitivity syndrome (AIS),** a disorder arising from mutations in the androgen receptor (AR) gene. AIS is classified as complete (CAIS) or partial (PAIS), depending on the amount of residual receptor function. Individuals with CAIS (formerly known as *testicular feminization*) have a male karyotype (46,XY) with female external genitalia and intraabdominal testes. The circulating concentration of testosterone in these patients is greater than or equal to that of a healthy male, whereas LH concentrations are typically increased.

Males with 5α-reductase deficiency (5-ARD) have reduced efficiency of the conversion of testosterone to the more potent DHT. Because DHT leads to masculinization of external genitalia in utero, males with 5-ARD are born with ambiguous genitalia. High ratios of the circulating concentrations of testosterone to DHT are indicative of 5-ARD.

In patients with cryptorchidism or ambiguous genitalia, identification of abdominal **gonads** is essential for proper diagnosis and treatment. The presence of testicular tissue has traditionally been detected by measurement of Leydig cell testosterone production after stimulation with **human chorionic gonadotropin (hCG).** In addition, serum inhibin and plasma anti-Müllerian hormone may offer a noninvasive evaluation of seminiferous tubular integrity.

Erectile Dysfunction

Erectile dysfunction (formerly referred to as *impotence*) is the persistent inability to develop or maintain a penile erection that is sufficient for intercourse and ejaculation in 50% or more of attempts.[8] Psychogenic erectile dysfunction is the most common diagnosis. Other causes include (1) vascular disease, (2) diabetes mellitus, (3) hypertension, (4) uremia, (5) neurologic disease, (6) hypogonadism, (7) hyperthyroidism, (8) hypothyroidism, (9) neoplasms, and (10) drugs. If no obvious explanation for erectile dysfunction is found, measurement of morning serum testosterone, LH, and thyroid-stimulating hormone (TSH) concentrations has been suggested. Elevated gonadotropin concentrations indicate primary hypogonadism. Total and even free testosterone concentrations may be within reference intervals, yet still may be subnormal for a given patient if found in the presence of elevated LH or FSH.

Gynecomastia

Gynecomastia, the benign growth of glandular breast tissue in men, is a common finding among males of varied ages. Gynecomastia, which is associated with an increase in the estrogen/androgen ratio, is commonly associated with three distinct periods of life. First, transient gynecomastia is found in 60% to 90% of all newborns because of high estrogen concentrations that cross the **placenta.** The second peak occurs during puberty in 50% to 70% of healthy boys. It is usually self-limited and may be due to a (1) low serum testosterone, (2) low DHT, or (3) high estrogen/androgen ratio. The last peak is found in the adult population, most frequently among men aged 50 to 80 years. Gynecomastia may be due to (1) testicular failure, resulting in an increased estrogen/androgen ratio, or to (2) increased body fat, resulting in increased peripheral aromatization of testosterone to E_2.

Gynecomastia may also develop as the result of (1) iatrogenic causes, (2) hyperthyroidism, or (3) liver disease. In cases of striking gynecomastia in which history and physical examination point to no specific disorder, measurements of (1) hCG, (2) E2, (3) testosterone, and (4) LH concentrations are appropriate. It is important to note that prolactin plays an important role in galactorrhea (milk production), but only an indirect role in gynecomastia.

Female Reproductive Biology

The female reproductive system consists of a (1) vagina, (2) uterus, (3) fallopian tubes, and (4) ovaries. The function of the ovaries is to produce ova and secrete the sex hormones **progesterone** and estrogen.

Biological Functions

Healthy female neonates possesses approximately 400,000 primordial **follicles,** each containing an immature ovum. During

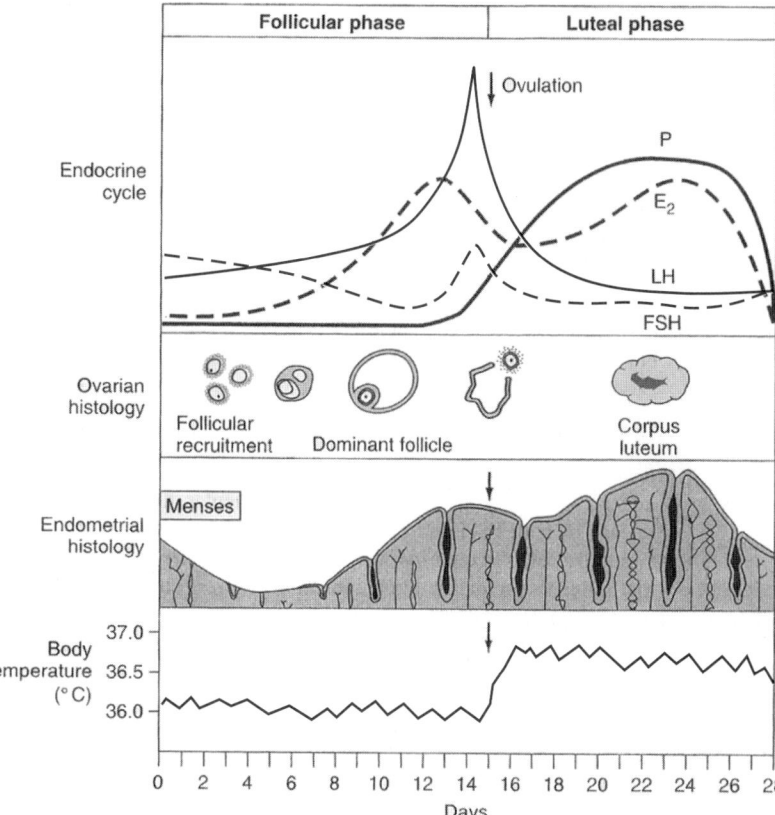

Figure 43-5 Hormonal, ovarian, endometrial, and basal body temperature changes throughout the normal menstrual cycle. *(From Carr BR, Bradshaw KD. Disorders of the ovary and female reproductive tract. In: Braunwald E, Fauci A, Kasper D, Hauser SL, Longo DL, Jameson JL eds. Harrison's principles of internal medicine, 15th edition. New York, NY: McGraw-Hill, 2001:2158; used with permission.)*

the reproductive life span of an adult woman, 300 to 400 follicles will reach maturity. A single mature follicle is produced during each normal menstrual cycle at approximately day 14 (Figure 43-5). The mature follicle undergoes ovulation by the process of rupture, thereby releasing the oocyte into the proximity of the fallopian tubes. The granulosa and theca cells of the follicle lining quickly proliferate to form the **corpus luteum** (yellow body). The luteal cells produce estrogen and progesterone. If fertilization and pregnancy occur, the corpus luteum persists and continues to produce estrogen and progesterone. If no pregnancy occurs, the corpus luteum regresses, and the next menstrual cycle begins.

During the follicular phase, the endometrial lining of the uterus increases in thickness and vascularity in response to increasing circulating concentrations of estrogen. After regression of the corpus luteum, menstruation begins, and the endometrium is shed in response to the withdrawal of progesterone.

Hypothalamic-Pituitary-Gonadal Axis

In adult women, a tightly coordinated feedback system exists between (1) hypothalamus, (2) anterior pituitary, and (3) ovaries to orchestrate menstruation. FSH serves to stimulate follicular growth, and LH stimulates ovulation and progesterone secretion from the developing corpus luteum (Figure 43-6).

Estrogens

Estrogens are responsible for the development and maintenance of female sex organs and female secondary sex

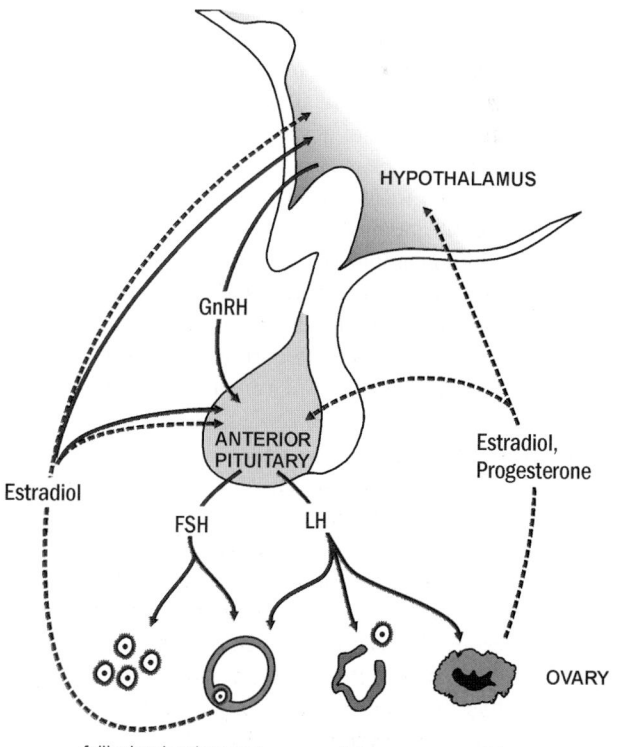

Figure 43-6 Summary of the endocrine control and changes in ovary and endometrium during the menstrual cycle. *Dashed lines* indicate inhibitory effects, and *solid lines* indicate stimulatory effects.

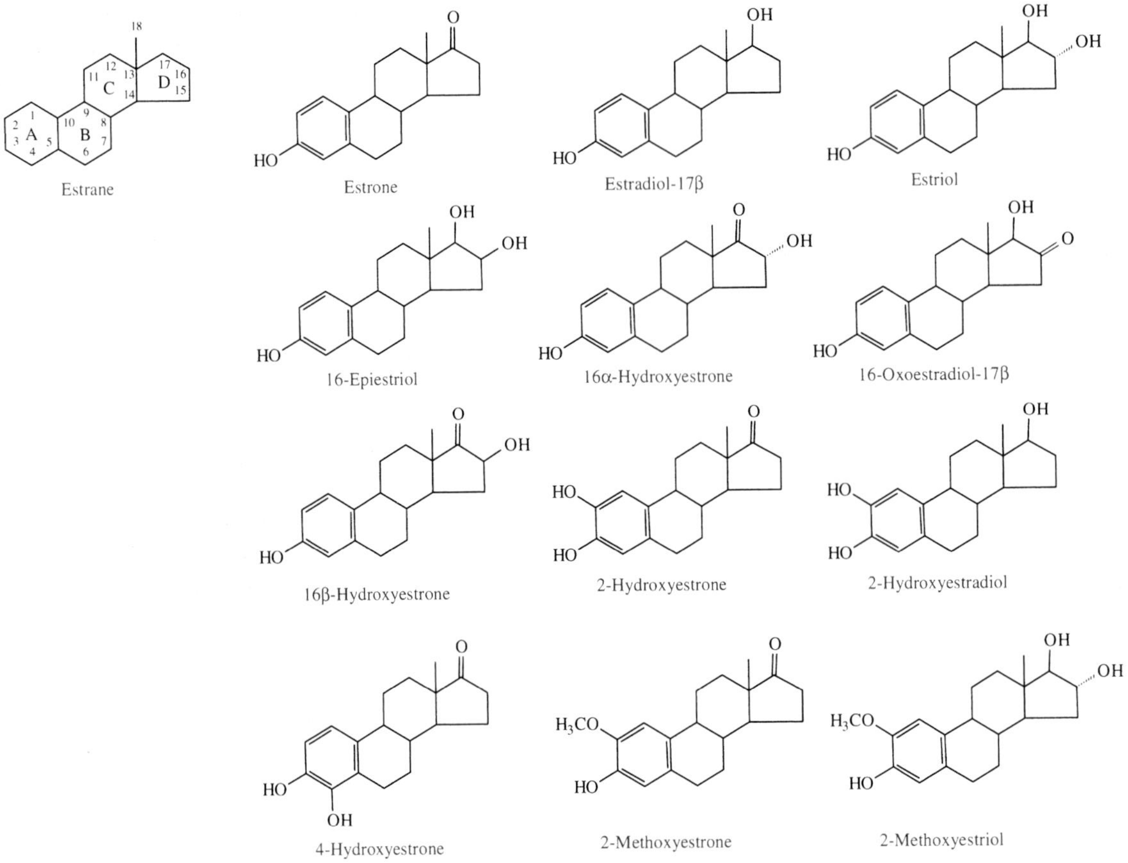

Figure 43-7 Structural formulas of important estrogens.

characteristics. In conjunction with progesterone, they participate in (1) regulation of the menstrual cycle, (2) breast and uterine growth, and (3) the maintenance of pregnancy.

Estrogens affect calcium homeostasis and have a beneficial effect on bone mass. Estrogens also increase concentrations of plasma proteins including (1) SHBG, (2) corticosteroid-binding globulin, and (3) thyroxine-binding globulin. Boys and girls have comparable concentrations of SHBG, but adult men have SHBG concentrations that are about one half those of adult women. Concentrations of plasma proteins that bind copper and iron are also elevated in response to estrogen, as are the concentrations of high-density lipoproteins.

Chemistry

The three most biologically active estrogens in order of potency are (1) **estrone** (E_1), (2) E_2, and (3) **estriol** (E_3) (Figure 43-7). Chemically, estrogens are structural derivatives of the parent hydrocarbon *estrane*. All estrogens possess a phenolic hydroxyl group at C-3, which gives the compounds acidic properties, and lack a methyl group at C-10. In addition, estrogens may possess a ketone (E_1) or hydroxyl group (E_2) at position C-17. The phenolic ring A and the hydroxyl group at C-17 are essential for biological activity.

Biosynthesis

Estrogens are secreted primarily in healthy women by the (1) ovarian follicles, (2) corpus luteum, and during pregnancy by

the (3) placenta. The adrenal glands and testes (in men) are also believed to secrete minute quantities of estrogens. The ovary synthesizes estrogens via aromatization of androgens (Figure 43-8). The healthy human ovary produces (1) estrogens, (2) progestagens, and (3) androgens. However, E_2 and progesterone are its primary secretory products. Because the ovary lacks both the 21-hydroxylase and 11β-hydroxylase enzymes, glucocorticoids and mineralocorticoids are not produced in the ovary.[3,12] More than 20 estrogens have been identified, but only 17β-estradiol and E_3 are routinely measured clinically. The most potent estrogen secreted by the ovary is 17β-estradiol. Because it is derived almost exclusively from the ovaries, its measurement is often considered sufficient for evaluation of ovarian function.

Estrogens are also produced by peripheral aromatization of androgens, primarily androstenedione. In healthy men and women, ≈1% of secreted androstenedione is converted to E_1. Although the ovaries of postmenopausal women do not secrete estrogens, these women have significant blood concentrations of E_1 originating from the peripheral conversion of adrenal androstenedione. Because a major site of this conversion is adipose tissue, E_1 is increased in obese postmenopausal women, sometimes yielding enough estrogen to produce bleeding.

Biosynthesis during Pregnancy

The biosynthesis of estrogens differs qualitatively and quantitatively in pregnant women compared with nonpregnant

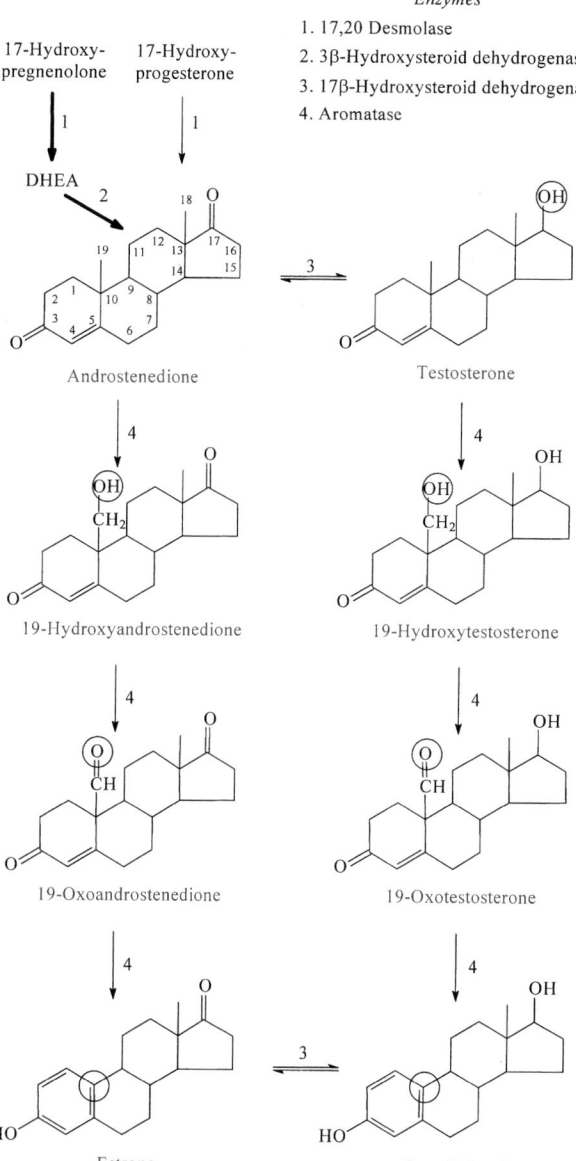

Enzymes

1. 17,20 Desmolase
2. 3β-Hydroxysteroid dehydrogenase
3. 17β-Hydroxysteroid dehydrogenase
4. Aromatase

Figure 43-8 Biosynthesis of estrogens. *Heavy arrows* indicate the Δ5-3β-hydroxy pathway. The *circled area* represents the site of chemical change. See Figure 43-4 for early synthetic steps.

ones. In pregnant women, the major source of estrogens is the placenta, whereas in nonpregnant women, the ovaries are the main site of synthesis.[3,13] In contrast to the microgram quantities secreted by nonpregnant women, the quantity of estrogens secreted during pregnancy increases to milligram amounts. The major estrogen secreted by the ovary is E_2, whereas the major product secreted by the placenta is E_3. E_3 is formed from plasma dehydroepiandrosterone sulfate (DHEAS) in the placenta. Except during pregnancy, measurements of E_3 have little clinical value because in nonpregnant women, E_3 is derived almost exclusively from E_2.

E_3 is the predominant hormone of late pregnancy. Maternal E_3 is almost entirely ($\approx$90%) derived from fetal and placental sources. It is first detected during the ninth gestational

week and gradually increases during the first and second trimesters. Plasma and salivary E_3 concentrations peak approximately 3 to 5 weeks before labor and delivery. Measurements of (1) unconjugated E_3,[8] (2) α-fetoprotein, (3) hCG, and (4) **inhibin A** are commonly used as part of the "quad" maternal screens for fetuses with Down syndrome (see Chapter 44). On average, unconjugated E_3 is 0.72 times less than normal (reference interval at 16 weeks: 0.30 to 1.50 μg/L) when fetal Down syndrome is present.

Estrogen Transport in Blood

More than 97% of circulating E_2 is bound to plasma proteins. It is bound specifically and with high affinity to SHBG, and nonspecifically to albumin. SHBG concentrations are increased by estrogens and therefore are higher in women than in men. They are also increased during (1) pregnancy, (2) oral contraceptive use, (3) hyperthyroidism, and (4) administration of certain antiepileptic drugs, such as phenytoin. SHBG concentrations may decrease in hypothyroidism, obesity, or androgen excess. Only 2% to 3% of total E_2 circulates in free form. In contrast, E_1 and estrone sulfate circulate bound almost exclusively to albumin. As with testosterone, both free and albumin-bound fractions of E_2 are thought to be biologically available, but measurement of this fraction has not been shown to be clinically important.

Metabolism

Typically, E_2 is converted to E_1 by the reversible oxidation of the C-17 β-hydroxy group. E_1 is further oxidized along two pathways leading to formation of (1) catechol estrogens, and (2) E_3 (Figure 43-9). The direction of E_1 metabolism is affected by the pathophysiologic state. For example, obesity and hypothyroidism are associated with an increase in E_3 formation, whereas low body weight and hyperthyroidism are associated with formation of catechol estrogens.[3] Although assays for catechol estrogen measurement are available, they have no known current clinical value.

Progesterone

Progesterone, similar to the estrogens, is a female sex hormone. In conjunction with estrogens, it helps to regulate the accessory organs during the menstrual cycle.[4,12] This hormone is especially important in preparing the uterus for implantation of the blastocyst and in maintaining pregnancy. In nonpregnant women, progesterone is secreted mainly by the corpus luteum. During pregnancy, the placenta becomes the major source of this hormone. Minor sources are the adrenal cortex in both sexes and the testes in men.

Chemistry

The structural formula and metabolism of progesterone (pregn-4-ene-3,20-dione), a C_{21} compound, are shown in Figure 43-10. Like corticosteroids and testosterone, progesterone contains a keto group (at C-3) and a double bond between C-4 and C-5 (Δ^4); these structural characteristics are essential for **progestational** activity.

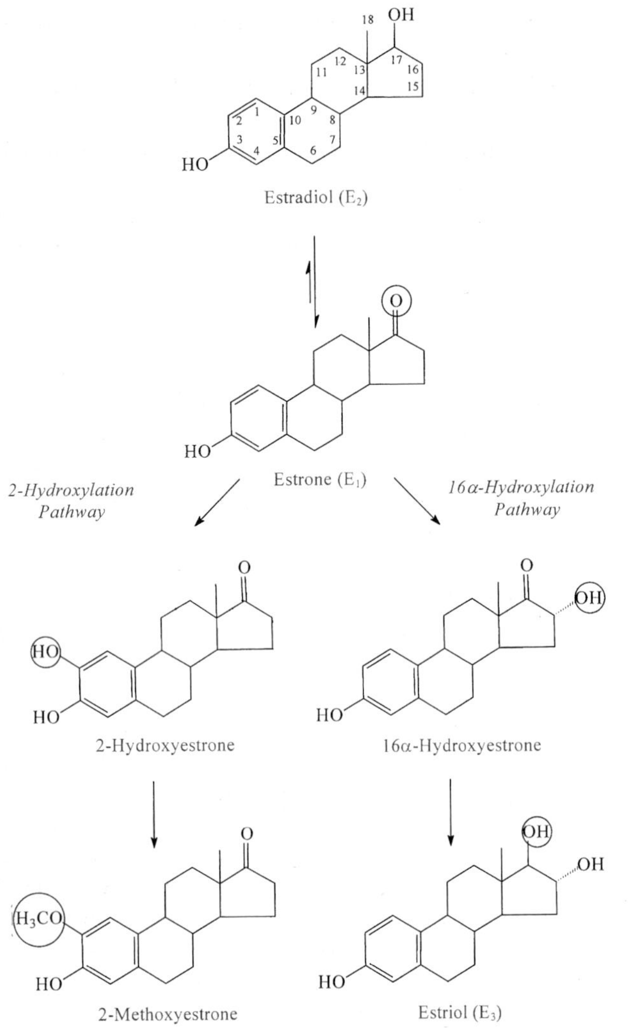

Figure 43-9 Main pathways of estradiol (E2) metabolism in humans. The *circled area* represents the site of chemical change.

Biosynthesis

Biosynthesis of progesterone in ovarian tissues follows the same path from acetate to cholesterol through pregnenolone as it does in the adrenal cortex (see Chapter 41).[3,13] Initiation and control of luteal secretion of progesterone are regulated by LH and FSH.

Transport

Progesterone does not have a specific plasma-binding protein but, similar to cortisol, is bound by corticosteroid-binding globulin. Reported concentrations for plasma free progesterone vary from 2% to 10% of total concentration, and the percentage of unbound progesterone remains constant throughout the normal menstrual cycle.

Metabolism

Reduction and conjugation are important metabolic events leading to the inactivation of progesterone (Figure 43-10). Metabolites of progesterone are classified into groups based on the degree of reduction. They include (1) pregnanediones, (2) pregnanolones, and (3) pregnanediols. Reduced metabolites

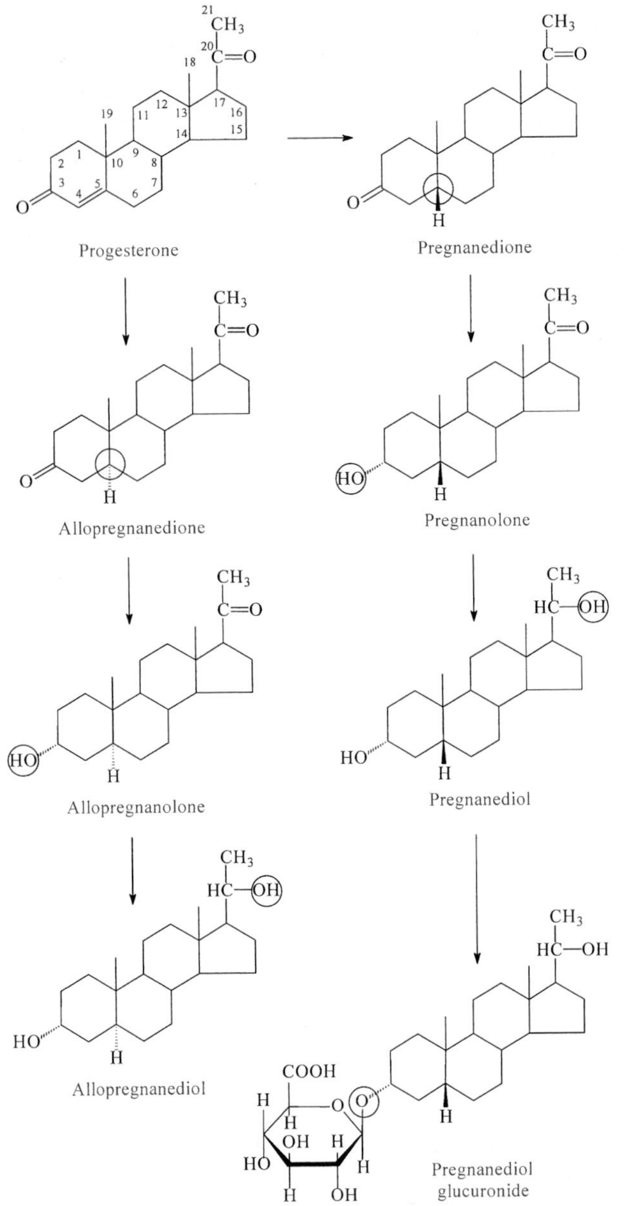

Figure 43-10 Metabolism of progesterone. The *circled area* represents the site of chemical change.

are eventually conjugated with glucuronic acid and excreted as water-soluble glucuronides.

Female Reproductive Development

Reproductive development begins with (1) anatomy during the fetal period, (2) a postnatal period of adaptation to reduced maternal sex steroids, and (3) finishes with sexual maturation during puberty.

Fetal Period

In the genotypic female, lack of testosterone and anti-Müllerian hormone result in the formation of the female reproductive tract. Gonadotropin activity in utero is suppressed because of high concentrations of circulating estrogens derived from the mother.

Postnatal Period

When the placenta separates, concentrations of fetal sex steroids drop abruptly. Serum E_2 in neonates decreases to basal concentrations within 5 to 7 days after birth and persists at this concentration until puberty. The negative feedback action of steroids is now removed, and gonadotropins are released. Postnatal peaks of LH and FSH are measurable for a few months after birth, peaking at 2 to 5 months and then dropping to basal concentrations. During childhood, circulating concentrations of sex steroids and gonadotropins are relatively low and are similar for both sexes.

Puberty

The transition from sexual immaturity appears to begin with diminished sensitivity of the pituitary gland or hypothalamus, or both, to the negative feedback effect of sex steroids. As puberty approaches, nocturnal secretion of gonadotropins occurs. Concentrations for (1) LH, (2) FSH, and (3) gonadal steroids rise gradually over several years before stabilizing at adult concentrations when full sexual maturity is reached. In girls, puberty is considered precocious if onset of pubertal development (secondary sex characteristics) occurs before the age of 8 years, and delayed if no development has occurred by the age of 13 years, or if **menarche** has not occurred by age 16.5 years. The median age of menarche in the United States is 12.43 years. Adrenarche precedes puberty by a few years. In girls, the rise in concentrations of (1) DHEA, (2) DHEAS, and (3) androstenedione begins at age 6 to 7 years. This rise in adrenal androgen concentrations lasts until late puberty. In girls, puberty is associated with elevations in estrogen secretion by the ovary in response to gonadotropin concentrations that increase in response to GnRH.

Normal Menstrual Cycle

During a normal menstrual cycle, a closely coordinated interplay of feedback effects occurs between the (1) hypothalamus, (2) the anterior lobe of the pituitary gland, and (3) the ovaries. In addition, cyclic hormone changes lead to functional and structural changes in the (1) ovaries, (2) uterus, (3) cervix, and (4) vagina.

Phases

The menstrual cycle is measured beginning on day 1 as the first day of menstrual bleeding. Each cycle consists of a (1) follicular phase followed by (2) ovulation and then a (3) luteal phase.

Follicular Phase. The follicular phase begins with the initiation of follicular growth, begins during the last few days of the previous luteal phase and terminates at ovulation. During the early part of the follicular phase, concentrations of FSH are elevated, but they decline up until ovulation (Figure 43-5).[3] LH secretion begins to increase around the middle of the follicular phase. Just before ovulation, estrogen secretion by the follicle increases dramatically; this positively stimulates the hypothalamus and triggers the **LH surge**. The LH surge is a reliable predictor of ovulation with onset of the surge for 90% of women occurring 16 to 58 hours before, and the peak

occurring 3 to 36 hours before, ovulation.[3] Ovulation occurs around day 14 of the menstrual cycle.

Ovulation. Ovulation occurs around day 14 of the menstrual cycle.

Luteal Phase. The luteal phase occurs in the last half of the cycle and is characterized by increasing production of progesterone and estrogen from the corpus luteum with consequent gradual lowering of LH and FSH concentrations. The concentration of progesterone reaches a peak at about 8 days post ovulation. If ovulation does not occur, the corpus luteum fails to form, and a cyclic rise in the concentration of progesterone is subnormal. If ovulation, fertilization and implantation occur, hCG maintains the corpus luteum and the concentration of progesterone continues to increase. In the absence of conception, the corpus luteum resolves, resulting in a decrease in estrogen and progesterone concentrations and a breakdown of the endometrium.

Role of Individual Hormones

The major hormones that influence the control and effects of the normal menstrual cycle include (1) GnRH, (2) FSH, (3) LH, (4) E_2, and (5) progesterone (Figure 43-6).

Gonadotropin-Releasing Hormone. GnRH triggers the LH surge that precedes ovulation.[3,7,13] There appear to be two separate feedback centers in the hypothalamus: (1) a tonic negative feedback center, and (2) a cyclic positive feedback center. Low concentrations of E_2, such as those that are present during the follicular phase, affect the negative feedback center, whereas high concentrations of E_2, such as those seen just before the midcycle LH peak, trigger the positive feedback center. Progesterone, in combination with estrogen, affects the negative feedback center in the luteal phase.

Follicle-Stimulating Hormone. A few days before day 1 of the cycle, FSH shows a slight but important peak (Figure 43-5). This peak in FSH initiates the growth and maturation of a cohort of ovarian follicles.[3,7,13] LH and FSH release is pulsatile throughout the cycle. As estrogen is released from the growing follicles, FSH concentrations fall again and remain low through the follicular phase. By days 5 to 7, a single follicle is selected for further growth. The effect of FSH on the maturing follicle is increased through E_2-induced changes in FSH receptors. FSH, aided by E_2, acts on the cells of the follicle to increase the responsiveness of LH receptors by the time of the midcycle surge. FSH and LH receptors respond with an increase in their number or in their affinity for corresponding gonadotropin. A rise in FSH at midcycle is triggered by progesterone. During the luteal phase, FSH is suppressed by negative feedback from E_2 until a lesser FSH peak, occurring near the end of the cycle, starts off the follicular maturation of the next cycle.

Luteinizing Hormone. LH secretion is suppressed in the follicular phase by negative feedback from E_2.[7,13] As E_2 production by the developing follicle increases, the effect of E_2 on the positive feedback center becomes important. Increasing release of GnRH from the hypothalamus and increasing the sensitivity of the anterior lobe of the pituitary gland to it lead to the midcycle surge of LH. Ovarian follicle receptors for LH, sensitized by FSH and E_2, transmit the stimulus to enhance differentiation of the theca cell and production of progesterone by the developing corpus luteum. LH production is suppressed during the luteal phase by negative feedback from progesterone combined with E_2.

Estradiol. E_2 production by the ovary decreases near the end of a cycle but begins to increase again under the influence of FSH (Figure 43-5).[3,7,13] E_2 enhances the FSH effect on a maturing follicle through changes in FSH receptors of the follicular cells, but it suppresses pituitary FSH and LH release during the follicular phase through negative feedback. Before the mid–follicular phase, estrogen concentrations are less than 50 pg/mL, but they increase rapidly as the follicle matures. E_2 production increases, reaching a midcycle peak at between 250 and 500 pg/mL. E_2 concentrations decrease abruptly after ovulation but increase again as the corpus luteum is formed, reaching concentrations of approximately 125 pg/mL during the luteal phase. Progesterone produced by the corpus luteum, combined with E_2, exerts a negative effect on the hypothalamus and anterior lobe of the pituitary gland. As a result, LH and FSH secretion is suppressed again during the luteal phase. E_2 is essential for the development of proliferative endometrium and is synergistic with progesterone for the development of changes in the endometrium that initiate shedding; the decrease in negative feedback from E_2 on the anterior lobe of the pituitary gland triggers the FSH surge that begins the development of an ovarian follicle for the next cycle.[3]

Progesterone. Progesterone is not produced in significant amounts until after the midcycle LH-surge and ovulation. LH enhances theca cell differentiation and progesterone production, which increase by a factor of 10 to 20 to a maximum about 8 days after the midcycle peak of LH. Progesterone is thought to stimulate the ovulatory peak of FSH and to promote the growth of secretory endometrium, which is necessary for implantation of the fertilized ovum.[3]

Ovulation

An intricate interplay of endocrine events contributes to follicular maturation. How an individual follicle is selected each menstrual cycle for maturation is unknown; however, the late-cycle peak in FSH concentration is likely important in this process. Once a follicle has been stimulated, E_2 production causes that specific follicle to be more receptive to effects of FSH. After ovulation, LH is suppressed by progesterone and E_2, but the effect of LH on the corpus luteum is increased.[7,13] In the event of a successful fertilization and implantation, corpus luteum function is sustained by hCG produced by trophoblastic cells of the developing embryo with high molecular homology to LH, and it is capable of binding and stimulating LH receptors. Otherwise, the declining concentration of E_2 leads to regression of the corpus luteum and to the late-cycle FSH peak that starts the process again.

Menopause

Menopause begins with the ovaries failing to produce adequate amounts of estrogen and inhibin; as a result, gonadotropin production is increased in a continued attempt to stimulate the ovary. The mean age of menopause in the United States is 51 years but varies considerably.[3,6] Ovarian failure may occur at any age, but menopause before age 40 years is considered premature.[6]

Hormonal changes begin about 5 years before the actual menopause, as the response of the ovary to gonadotropins begins to decrease and menstrual cycles become increasingly irregular. The term *perimenopausal* refers to the time interval from onset of these menstrual irregularities to menopause itself. This transition phase will last from 2 to 8 years.[6] At this time, FSH concentrations increase and E_2 concentrations decrease, whereas LH and progesterone concentrations remain unchanged, indicating that menstrual cycles are ovulatory. The decrease in estrogen concentrations gives rise to vasomotor instability and "hot flashes."

After menopause, the ovary continues to produce androgens, particularly testosterone and androstenedione, as a result of increased LH concentrations. In addition, the adrenal gland continues to secrete androgens. The resulting decrease in the estrogen/androgen ratio causes the **hirsutism** often seen in postmenopausal women.[1] Prolonged estrogen deficiency results in increased resorption and bone remodeling, leading to accelerated bone loss and osteoporosis in postmenopausal women.

It is important to note that perimenopausal and postmenopausal women secrete pituitary hCG.[5] Serum concentrations generally are low (<13 IU/L), but positive hCG results often causes confusion and delays important diagnostic tests or treatments. Pituitary versus placental hCG has been confirmed by measuring serum FSH (concentrations of FSH >45 IU/L are consistent with menopause and make pregnancy unlikely) or by 2 weeks of hormone replacement therapy (hormone replacement therapy should decrease LH, FSH, and hCG concentrations).[5]

Female Reproductive Abnormalities

A wide variety of abnormalities affect the female reproductive system and have been classified in a variety of manners. For the purposes of this chapter, they have been divided into categories of (1) **pseudohermaphroditism**, (2) precocious puberty, (3) irregular **menses**, and (4) menopause. **Infertility** from the male and female perspective is discussed in a separate section later in the chapter.

Female Pseudohermaphroditism

The female pseudohermaphrodite is an individual who is genetically female, but whose phenotypic characteristics are, to varying degrees, male. In neonates with a 46,XX karyotype and ambiguous genitalia, **congenital adrenal hyperplasia** (**CAH**) should be considered. CAH is a family of autosomal recessive disorders of adrenal steroidogenesis (see Chapter 41). Each disorder has a specific pattern of hormonal abnormalities resulting in deficiency or excess of androgens. Only deficiencies of 21-hydroxylase and 11β-hydroxylase enzymes are predominantly virilizing disorders. Deficiency of 3β-hydroxysteroid dehydrogenase is rare, but when it occurs, affected girls may exhibit **virilization**.

Diagnosis of **21-hydroxylase deficiency** is made in infants and children with excess excretion of urinary 17-KS and pregnanetriol and elevated concentrations of plasma 17-hydroxyprogesterone and androstenedione. Elevation of 17-hydroxyprogesterone concentrations in early infancy (>3000 ng/dL) confirms the diagnosis of this disorder.

An **11β-hydroxylase deficiency** is confirmed by finding (1) elevated plasma concentrations of 11–deoxycortisol and deoxycorticosterone, (2) increased concentrations of their metabolites in urine, and (3) their suppression by glucocorticoid therapy. Plasma renin activity and aldosterone concentrations are low in this deficiency.

Elevated plasma concentrations of (1) 17-hydroxypregnenolone, (2) DHEA, and (3) DHEAS are found in patients with **3β-hydroxysteroid dehydrogenase deficiency**. The ratio of 17-hydroxypregnenolone to 17-hydroxyprogesterone is strikingly elevated in these patients.

Precocious Puberty

Precocious puberty is the development of secondary sexual characteristics in girls younger than 8 years old and boys younger than 9 years old. Early puberty is manifested by the appearance of secondary sexual characteristics, such as (1) premature thelarche (premature breast development), (2) premature adrenarche (premature sexual hair development), or (3) phallic enlargement. When presented as isolated cases, these secondary sexual characteristics are not considered to be pathologic, as none progresses to full-blown puberty, nor are they associated with increased rates of bone growth and maturation. However, if a child has at least two signs of puberty and also demonstrates increased rates of bone growth and maturation, the many causes of true precocious puberty must be considered.[4]

Precocious puberty has been classified as GnRH dependent or independent. GnRH-dependent precocious puberty (also called *central precocious puberty*) is due to precocious activation of the hypothalamic-pituitary-gonadal axis. **Pseudoprecocious puberty** (also called *GnRH-independent precocious puberty*) refers to precocious sex steroid secretion that is independent of pituitary gonadotropin release. CAHs are a common cause of pseudoprecocious puberty. Other causes include tumors of the (1) adrenal gland, (2) ovaries, and (3) testes that secrete androgens or estrogens.

Diagnosis of precocious puberty is based on (1) clinical presentation, (2) a thorough pubertal history, (3) bone age determinations, and (4) laboratory tests performed to assess gonadotropin concentrations and response to exogenous GnRH. The GnRH stimulation test is the gold standard for diagnosis of GnRH-dependent precocious puberty. Pubertal responses of LH and FSH to GnRH stimulation are considered diagnostic of precocious puberty when chronological age is inappropriate for the hormone response. The GnRH stimulation test is also used to monitor the effectiveness of GnRH agonist therapy. Typically, an IV bolus of exogenous GnRH is administered followed by a single measurement (at 40 to 45 minutes) or serial measurements of LH and FSH concentrations.

Breast Cancer—Effect of Estrogens

Suspicions of estrogen-based causes in the development of human breast cancer stem from epidemiologic and experimental observations.[11] Ovarian estrogen has been assumed to be the causative factor because administration of estrogen negates the protective effects of early oophorectomy (surgical removal of an ovary or ovaries). Moreover, treatment of men with estrogen for prostatic cancer or after transsexual operations is associated with increased risk of breast cancer. Low risk for breast cancer has consistently been connected with high parity. Increased risk is associated with early menarche, late (>30 years of age) first full-term pregnancy, and late menopause. Pregnancy occurring before age 25 to 30 years has a protective effect.

Cytoplasmic estrogen receptors are important prognostic indicators that are routinely measured in samples of breast tissue after surgical removal of the tumor. Sixty percent of patients with carcinoma of the breast have tumors that are estrogen receptor positive. The greater the estrogen receptor content of the tumor, the higher is the response rate to endocrine therapy and the lower is the incidence of recurrence.

Irregular Menses

Healthy women display considerable variation in cycle length ranging from 25 to 30 days (28 days on average). **Amenorrhea,** the absence of menstrual bleeding, is traditionally categorized as (1) primary (women who have never menstruated) or (2) secondary (women in whom menstruation is present for a variable time and then ceases). Amenorrhea is a relatively common disorder with an estimated prevalence of 5%.

Primary Amenorrhea

Primary amenorrhea is defined as failure to establish spontaneous periodic menstruation by the age of 16 years regardless of whether secondary sex characteristics have developed. About 40% of phenotypic females who have primary amenorrhea (nearly always associated with absence of development of secondary sex characteristics) have **Turner syndrome** (45,X karyotype) or **pure gonadal dysgenesis** (46,XX or XY karyotype).[3] **Müllerian duct agenesis** or *dysgenesis* with absence of the vagina or uterus is the second most common manifestation, and the third most common is AIS (AR deficiency) and normal or elevated plasma testosterone concentrations if the patient is past puberty and is karyotype XY.

The differential diagnosis of primary and secondary amenorrhea is shown in Table 43-1. When puberty is delayed in a girl, plasma concentrations of serum gonadotropins are measured. Low concentrations may indicate pituitary failure, whereas concentrations elevated into the postmenopausal interval indicate definite gonadal failure. In the latter case, chromosome studies are indicated. In the former case, pituitary function testing and radiography may be helpful. Patients with short stature without Turner syndrome but with primary amenorrhea may have multiple deficiencies of pituitary hormone secretion. In these patients, a *craniopharyngioma* or *pituitary tumor* should be suspected.

The diagnosis of 17α-hydroxylase deficiency is made when the concentration of (1) serum progesterone is greater than

TABLE 43-1 Differential Diagnosis of Amenorrhea				
Causes	**FSH**	**LH**	**Estrogen (E2)**	**Uterine Bleeding After Progesterone**
Hypothalamic				
CNS—hypothalamic dysfunction				
Idiopathic	N	N	N	+
Secondary to medications	N	N	N	+
Secondary to stress	N	N	N	+
CNS—hypothalamic dysfunction or failure due to exercise	↓ or N	↓ or N	↓ or N	±
CNS—hypothalamic dysfunction or failure due to weight loss				
Simple weight loss	↓ or N	↓ or N	↓ or N	±
Anorexia nervosa	↓	↓	↓	−
CNS—hypothalamic failure				
Lesions	↓	↓	↓	−
Idiopathic	↓	↓	↓	−
CNS—hypothalamic–adreno-ovarian dysfunction (PCOS) or hyperandrogen chronic anovulation	N	↑*	N	+
Pituitary				
Destructive lesions (Sheehan syndrome)	↓	↓	↓	−
Tumor	↓	↓	↓	−
Ovarian				
Premature ovarian insufficiency	↑	↑	↓	−
Loss of ovarian function (oophorectomy, infection, cystic degeneration, chemotherapy, radiation)	↑	↑	↓	−
Uterine				
Uterine synechiae (Asherman syndrome)	N	N	N	−

CNS, Central nervous system; E$_2$, estradiol; FSH, follicle-stimulating hormone; LH, luteinizing hormone; N, value within normal reference interval; PCOS, polycystic ovary syndrome; ↓, value below reference interval; ↑, value above reference interval; ↑*, >25 mIU/mL, less than menopausal concentration; ±, positive or negative bleeding response to progesterone.
From Davajan V, Kletzky OA. Amenorrhea. In: Mishell DR, Davajan V, Lobo RA, eds. Infertility, contraception and reproductive endocrinology, 3rd edition. Boston, MA: Blackwell Scientific Publications, 1991:373.

3 ng/mL; (2) 17α-hydroxyprogesterone is less than 0.2 ng/mL; (3) aldosterone is low; and (4) 11-deoxycorticosterone is elevated. Plasma concentrations of (1) 11-deoxycortisol, (2) testosterone, (3) E$_2$, and (4) DHEAS are also low. The diagnosis is made with an adrenocorticotropic hormone (ACTH) stimulation test in which baseline concentrations of progesterone and 17α-hydroxyprogesterone are measured first, followed by administration of 0.25 mg ACTH. Diagnosis is confirmed if serum concentrations of progesterone are significantly increased and 17α-hydroxyprogesterone concentrations are unchanged at 60 minutes after ACTH administration.

Secondary Amenorrhea

Secondary amenorrhea is defined as absence of periodic menstruation for at least 6 months in women who have previously experienced menses. With few exceptions, the causes of primary and secondary amenorrhea overlap (Box 43-2). Pregnancy, the most common cause of secondary amenorrhea, must be considered first and ruled out. Elevated concentrations of prolactin—iatrogenic or induced by a prolactin-secreting tumor—can result in oligomenorrhea or amenorrhea. It is thought that hyperprolactinemia inhibits the release of LH and FSH. Both hyperthyroidism and hypothyroidism are associated with a variety of menstrual disorders because of their effects on metabolism and inter-conversion of androgens and estrogens. In practice, it is helpful to separate patients with

secondary amenorrhea into those with and without signs of hirsutism and androgen excess.

Assessment of women with secondary amenorrhea begins with a careful history that includes a complete description of menstrual patterns. In addition, the patient should be evaluated for (1) galactorrhea, (2) hot flashes, (3) abnormalities of thyroid size and function, (4) hirsutism,[1] (5) cushingoid appearance, (6) abdominal or pelvic masses, (7) pelvic or uterine trauma, (8) clitoral enlargement, (9) medications prescribed, (10) nutritional history, (11) patterns of exercise, (12) previous contraceptive use, (13) weight changes, (14) stress, (15) chronic disease, (16) visual field defects, and (17) evidence of malnutrition. Serum or urine hCG should be measured to rule out pregnancy. Because both hypothyroidism and hyperprolactinemia have been known to cause amenorrhea, they are easily excluded by measuring concentrations of serum TSH and prolactin.

A 24-hour urine cortisol or an overnight dexamethasone suppression test is performed in those patients suspected of having Cushing syndrome (see Chapter 41). A GnRH stimulation test with measurement of LH and FSH concentrations in those patients with gonadotropin deficiency assists in differentiating hypothalamic disease from pituitary disease.

Oligomenorrhea

Oligomenorrhea is infrequent menstruation that occurs fewer than nine times per year.

BOX 43-2   Causes of Amenorrhea

Primary Amenorrhea
Lower tract defects
  Vaginal aplasia
  Imperforate hymen
  Congenital vaginal atresia
Uterine disorders
  Congenital absence of the uterus
  Endometritis
  Müllerian agenesis (Mayer-Rokitansky-Kuster-Hauser syndrome)
Ovarian disorders
  XO gonadal and X dysgenesis and variants
  XX gonadal dysgenesis
  Turner syndrome
  Androgen insensitivity syndrome (AIS)
  17-Hydroxylase deficiency of the ovaries and adrenal glands
  Autoimmune oophoritis
  Resistant ovary syndrome
  Polycystic ovary syndrome (PCOS)
Adrenal disorders (congenital adrenal hyperplasia [CAH])
Thyroid disorders (hypothyroidism)
Pituitary-hypothalamic disorders
  Hypopituitarism
  Constitutional delay in the onset of menses (physiologic)
  Nutritional disorders
  Kallmann syndrome

Secondary Amenorrhea
Pregnancy/lactation
Uterine disorders
  Post-traumatic uterine synechiae (Asherman syndrome)
  Progestational agents
Ovarian disorders

Polycystic ovary syndrome (PCOS) (hypothalamic)
Ovarian tumor
Primary ovarian insufficiency (POI) (idiopathic, autoimmune, chemotherapy, radiation, injury)
  Antimetabolite therapy
Adrenal disorders
  Late-onset adrenal hyperplasia
  Cushing syndrome
  Virilizing adrenal tumors
  Adrenocorticoid insufficiency
Thyroid disorders
  Hypothyroidism
  Hyperthyroidism
Pituitary disorders
  Acquired hypopituitarism (trauma, tumor, Sheehan syndrome, lymphocytic hypophysitis)
  Physiologic or pathologic hyperprolactinemia
Hypothalamic disorders
  Tumor and infiltrative disease
  Nutritional disorders
  Hypophysitis
  Excessive exercise
  Stress
Iatrogenic
  Antipsychotics (phenothiazines, haloperidol, clozapine, pimozide)
  Antidepressants (tricyclics, monoamine oxidase inhibitors)
  Antihypertensives (calcium channel blockers, methyldopa, reserpine)
  Drugs with estrogenic activity (digitalis, flavonoids, marijuana, oral contraceptives)
  Drugs with ovarian toxicity (busulfan, chlorambucil, cisplatin, cyclophosphamide, fluorouracil)

Progesterone Challenge for Evaluating Amenorrhea

When the cause of amenorrhea is unclear after the initial assessment, relative estrogen status should be determined. Serum E_2 is measured, or a *progesterone challenge* may be performed.[3] Women with an estrogen-primed uterus have withdrawal vaginal bleeding after being administered oral progestin at concentrations of (1) 30 mg daily for 3 days, (2) 10 mg daily for 5 to 10 days, or (3) 100 to 200 mg of progesterone in oil given intramuscularly. If estrogen concentrations are adequate and the outflow tract is intact, menstrual bleeding should occur within a week of treatment. In patients with withdrawal bleeding, the plasma E_2 concentration is usually greater than 40 pg/mL. Measurement of serum E_2 is an alternative to the progesterone challenge but is not preferred because estrogen concentration fluctuates throughout the day, and withdrawal bleeding is an indication of a normal outflow tract. If bleeding fails to occur after progestin challenge, then additional laboratory tests are indicated, including measurement of LH and FSH to localize the problem to the (1) follicle, (2) pituitary, or (3) hypothalamus.

Androgen Excess

Amenorrhea due to androgen excess has been shown to be due to (1) adult-onset CAH, (2) corticotropin-dependent Cushing syndrome, or (3) **polycystic ovary syndrome (PCOS)**. Patients with androgen excess often will present with (1) acne, (2) obesity, and (3) variable degrees of excess hair on the (a) face, (b) chest, (c) abdomen, and (d) thighs. Some individuals with 21-hydroxylase deficiency do not manifest any developmental abnormalities or salt wasting, but they present with signs of androgen excess. This clinical syndrome, referred to as *nonclassic, adult-onset,* or *late-onset CAH,* may be clinically indistinguishable from PCOS.[2]

PCOS occurs in ≈4% of premenopausal women, and is clinically defined by **hyperandrogenism** with chronic anovulation in women with no other cause. This syndrome is characterized by (1) infertility, (2) hirsutism, (3) obesity, and (4) various menstrual disturbances ranging from amenorrhea to irregular vaginal bleeding (Table 43-2). Relatively low FSH and disproportionately high LH concentrations are common in PCOS. Serum androstenedione and testosterone concentrations (total and free concentrations) are elevated with mean concentrations 50% to 150% higher than normal.[3] PCOS patients have substantial estrogen production due to peripheral conversion of androgens to estrogens.

Hirsutism and Virilization[1]

Hirsutism is defined as excessive growth of terminal hair in women and children in a distribution similar to that occurring in postpubertal men. True hirsutism, which is androgen responsive, is distinguished from **hypertrichosis**, which

TABLE 43-2	Clinical Features of the Polycystic Ovary Syndrome*	
Clinical Features		**Frequency**
Hirsutism		65
Acne		26
Obesity		37
Infertility		48
Amenorrhea		35
Oligomenorrhea		42
Regular menstrual cycle		20

*Data were compiled from three studies. Two used ultrasonography as the primary method of diagnosis, one used ovarian histology. Total N=1935.
Modified from Frank S. Polycystic ovary syndrome. N Engl J Med 1995;333:1435.

BOX 43-3 Causes of Hirsutism

Ovarian
Severe insulin resistance
Hyperthecosis, hilus cell or stromal cell hyperplasia
Androgen-producing ovarian tumor
Menopause

Adrenal
Classic congenital hyperplasia
21-Hydroxylase deficiency
11-Hydroxylase deficiency
3β-Hydroxysteroid dehydrogenase deficiency
Adult or attenuated adrenal hyperplasia
Androgen-producing adrenal tumor

Familial Hirsutism

Endocrine Disorders
Polycystic ovary syndrome (PCOS)
Hyperprolactinemia
Acromegaly
Cushing syndrome

Idiopathic Hirsutism (Includes Increased Skin Sensitivity to Androgens)
Iatrogenic
Androgens
Dilantin
Diazoxide
Minoxidil
Streptomycin
Cyclosporine
Danazol
Metyrapone
Phenothiazides
Progestagens (19-nonsteroid derivatives)

---

consists of excessive growth of vellus or non–androgen-responsive hair. The causes of hirsutism are listed in Box 43-3.

Virilization is characterized by (1) clitoral hypertrophy, (2) deepening of the voice, (3) temporal hair recession, (4) baldness, (5) increased libido, (6) decreased body fat, and (7) menstrual irregularities or amenorrhea. Hirsutism is usually associated with normal or slightly elevated serum androgens, whereas virilization is associated with marked increases in ovarian or adrenal androgen production.[3]

Important screening tests used in the evaluation of women for hirsutism and virilization are the measurement of serum total or free testosterone and DHEAS.[3] Increased concentrations of DHEAS suggest an adrenal origin of androgens, whereas increased concentrations of testosterone indicate an adrenal or ovarian source. Neoplastic disease is unlikely if the (1) serum testosterone concentration is less than 2 ng/mL, (2) DHEAS concentration is less than 700 μg/dL, or (3) 17-KS concentrations are less than 30 mg/d. Regardless of the source of excess androgen production, the androstanediol glucuronide concentration is elevated in more than 90% of women with hirsutism, because it is a marker of excessive DHT production in skin.

PCOS is primarily a clinical diagnosis, and few laboratory tests are needed. Given a history of androgen excess and chronic anovulation (usually since menarche), the only condition that needs to be excluded is 21-hydroxylase–deficient nonclassic CAH; this is achieved by measuring 17-hydroxyprogesterone (early morning; follicular phase). If the result is less than 2 ng/mL, nonclassic CAH is excluded. Serum testosterone measurement is not necessary if clear hirsutism is present. Testosterone concentrations greater than 60 ng/dL are consistent with PCOS. FSH concentrations are often disproportionately normal or low. Patients with PCOS usually have E_2 concentrations greater than 40 pg/mL and therefore experience withdrawal bleeding in response to a progestin challenge.

Morning plasma 17α-hydroxyprogesterone concentrations are measured to evaluate nonclassic or **late-onset 21-hydroxylase deficiency (NCAH)**. A concentration less than 200 ng/dL (6.1 nmol/L) excludes this diagnosis, and a concentration greater than 1500 ng/dL (30 nmol/L) in nonpregnant women is confirmatory. When basal concentrations between 200 and 1500 ng/dL are found, an ACTH stimulation test should be performed. NCAH typically responds with a 17α-hydroxyprogesterone concentration greater than 1500 ng/dL, and classic CAH has a response over 2000 ng/dL. Patients with attenuated forms of CAH usually have normal concentrations of FSH and LH. About one half have elevated testosterone and androstenedione concentrations. Most of these patients also have increased concentrations of DHEAS, and more than 90% have supranormal concentrations of androstanediol glucuronide.

Other Causitive Factors
Many other factors or conditions have been observed to cause secondary amenorrhea, including disorders of the (1) ovary, (2) uterus, (4) pituitary, and (5) hypothalamus, and (6) the use of drugs.

Disorders of the ovary, such as **primary ovarian insufficiency (POI)** (formerly referred to as *premature ovarian failure [POF]*) and loss of ovarian function, have been known to cause amenorrhea. POI has been defined as failure of ovarian estrogen production that occurs in a hypergonadotropic state at any age between menarche and 40 years.[3] Autoimmune disorders have been associated with 20% to 40% of cases of POI that result in destruction of the ovary and in amenorrhea.[3] Other causes for ovarian failure include (1) oophorectomy, (2) cystic degeneration, (3) trauma, (4) infection, (5) interference with blood supply, (6) radiotherapy treatment, and (7) treatment with cytotoxic chemotherapeutic agents.

Hypothalamic dysfunction consists of those disorders that disrupt the frequency or amplitude of GnRH. Most commonly, disruption occurs in response to (1) psychological stress, (2) depression, (3) severe weight loss, (4) anorexia nervosa, or (5) strenuous exercise. A syndrome known as the **female athletic triad** has been described. This syndrome is prevalent in women who exercise vigorously, and is associated with (1) amenorrhea, (2) disordered eating, and (3) osteoporosis. Many other factors or conditions have been observed to cause secondary amenorrhea, including disorders of the (1) ovary, (2) uterus, and (3) pituitary, and the (4) use of drugs.

Infertility

Infertility is defined as the inability to conceive after 1 year of unprotected intercourse.[15] It has been estimated that 93% of healthy couples practicing unprotected intercourse should expect to conceive within 1 year, and 100% will be successful within 2 years. Primary infertility refers to couples or patients who have had no previous successful pregnancies. Secondary infertility encompasses patients who have previously conceived, but are currently unable to conceive. These types of infertility generally share common causes.

Infertility problems often arise as a result of hormonal dysfunction of the hypothalamic-pituitary-gonadal axis. Measurements of peptide and steroid hormones in the serum are therefore essential aspects of the evaluation of infertility, and are the focus of this section.

Male Infertility

A list of the most common male infertility factors is given in Box 43-4. Laboratory evaluation of male infertility should begin with evaluation of semen, which should be followed by evaluation of endocrine parameters.

Evaluation of Semen

Semen analysis measures (1) ejaculate volume, (2) pH, (3) sperm count, (4) motility, (5) forward progression, and (6) morphology.[16] Semen should be analyzed within 1 hour after collection. Although semen analysis is not a test for infertility, it is considered the most important laboratory test in the evaluation of male fertility. Reference seminal fluid values provided by the World Health Organization (WHO) guidelines have helped establish limits of adequacy.[16] If semen analysis is normal, it is unlikely that other laboratory testing will be useful. If semen analysis is abnormal, it should be repeated in ≈6 weeks. Additional investigations may include measurement of **sperm protein SP-10** via immunoassay. SP-10 is **testis**-specific, arises within the acrosomal vesicle during spermatogenesis, and is associated with the acrosomal membranes and matrix of mature sperm. A version of the test is available to check the success of vasectomy.

Evaluation of Obstruction

Obstruction of the male reproductive tract results in male infertility, and analysis of specific semen parameters has

---

BOX 43-4   Male Infertility Factors

Endocrine Disorders
Hypothalamic dysfunction (Kallmann syndrome)
Pituitary failure (tumor, radiation, surgery)
Hyperprolactinemia (drug, tumor)
Exogenous androgens
Thyroid disorders
Adrenal hyperplasia
Testicular failure

Anatomic
Congenital absence of vas deferens
Obstructed vas deferens
Congenital abnormalities of ejaculatory system
Varicocele
Retrograde ejaculation

Abnormal Spermatogenesis
Unexplained azoospermia
Chromosomal abnormalities
Mumps orchitis
Cryptorchidism
Chemical or radiation exposure

Abnormal Motility
Absent cilia (Kartagener syndrome)
Antibody formation

Psychosocial
Unexplained impotence
Decreased libido

Modified from Morell V. Basic infertility assessment. Primary Care 1997;24:195-204.

---

proved a useful adjunct to physical examination in the evaluation of male reproductive tract obstruction. Testosterone produced after administration of hCG causes the (1) seminal vesicles, (2) epididymis, and (3) prostate to increase the volume of ejaculate. An appropriate increase in serum testosterone without change in the ejaculate volume may indicate mechanical blockage.

Evaluation of Endocrine Parameters

If severe oligospermia (low sperm count) or azoospermia (no measurable sperm in semen) is found, then measurement of (1) serum testosterone, (2) LH, and (3) FSH concentrations is warranted, with or without measurement of (4) prolactin and (5) TSH concentrations. Hyperprolactinemia is a cause of secondary testicular dysfunction. If hyperprolactinemia is found, it is imperative to check for hypothyroidism, because elevated TRH concentrations result in hyperprolactinemia. Pituitary adenomas and drugs, such as (1) anxiolytics, (2) antihypertensives, (3) serotonergics, and (4) histamine H_2 receptor antagonists also increase serum prolactin. Hyperthyroidism and hypothyroidism will alter spermatogenesis. Hyperthyroidism affects both pituitary and testicular function with alterations in the secretion of releasing hormones and increased conversion of androgens to estrogens.

Patients with borderline or suppressed testosterone concentrations are evaluated with an **hCG stimulation test.** With this test, an injection of 5000 IU hCG is administered intramuscularly following collection of a basal, early morning testosterone sample. Serum testosterone is measured 72 hours later. Hypogonadal men show a depressed rise in testosterone concentration in response to this challenge. Doubling of testosterone concentration over baseline is consistent with normal Leydig cell function. Failure to increase testosterone concentrations to greater than 150 ng/dL indicates primary hypogonadism.

Hypergonadotropic Hypogonadism

Measurement of the concentration of FSH is indicated in men with sperm count lower than 5 to 10 million/mL. Elevated concentrations of FSH indicate (1) Sertoli cell dysfunction and, in azoospermic men, (2) primary germinal cell failure, (3) **Sertoli cell–only syndrome** (a condition resulting in sterility due to the absence of living sperm cells in the semen), or (4) genetic conditions, such as Klinefelter syndrome (47,XXY karyotype). Elevated FSH (>120 mIU/mL) in the setting of decreased testosterone (<200 ng/dL) and oligospermia indicate primary testicular failure.

Hypogonadotropic Hypogonadism

Decreased concentrations of testosterone (<200 ng/dL) and decreased concentrations of FSH (<10 mIU/mL) are suggestive of hypogonadotropic hypogonadism. Administering GnRH may help to distinguish between gonadal insufficiencies caused by pituitary versus hypothalamic dysfunction. One approach to this test involves the intravenous injection of 100 μg of GnRH with measurement of FSH and LH concentrations at 0, 30, 60, 120, and 180 minutes after injection. An increase in serum gonadotropins of 10 mIU/mL or more over baseline is normal. If little to no increase in gonadotropins is seen, pituitary disease is likely. Patients with hypothalamic disease demonstrate a delayed but significant increase of 7 mIU/mL or more within 180 minutes.

Female Infertility

Factors associated with common female infertility are listed in Box 43-5.

Evaluation of Female Infertility

The initial evaluation of female infertility includes a detailed history and physical examination. The physical examination should include evaluation of (1) the external genitalia and hair pattern (for signs of androgen excess including cliteromegaly, hirsutism, and virilization), (2) the pelvis (for masses, nodularity or tenderness), the (3) breasts (for signs of galactorrhea), (4) neurological findings (sense of smell and visual impairments), (5) the thyroid (for enlargement or nodules), and (6) body mass index. All abnormalities in the history and physical examination should be pursued. A thorough medical and surgical history is also necessary including an assessment of (1) the patient's gravidity and parity, (2) coital frequency, (3) duration of infertility, and (4) prior work up and treatment for infertility. Also, (1) history of sexually transmitted infections, (2) assessment of previous cervical cytologic and HPV testing and treatment, and (3) a menstrual history should be obtained. Concentrations of (1) TSH, (2) testosterone, and (3)

BOX 43-5   Female Infertility Factors

Ovarian or Hormonal Factors
Metabolic disease
  Thyroid
  Liver
  Obesity
  Androgen excess
  Polycystic ovary syndrome (PCOS)
Hypergonadotropic hypogonadism
  Menopause
  Luteal phase deficiency
  Gonadal dysgenesis
  Primary ovarian insufficiency (POI) (autoimmune, cytotoxic, chemotherapy, radiation, tumor)
  Resistant ovary syndrome
Hypogonadotropic hypogonadism
  Hyperprolactinemia (tumor, drugs)
  Hypothalamic insufficiency (Kallmann syndrome)
  Pituitary insufficiency (tumor, necrosis, thrombosis, stress, exercise, anorexia)

Tubal Factors
Occlusion or scarring
Salpingitis isthmica nodosa
Infectious salpingitis

Cervical Factors
Stenosis
Inflammation or infection
Abnormal mucous viscosity

Uterine Factors
Leiomyomata
Congenital malformation
Adhesions
Endometritis or abnormal endometrium

Psychosocial Factors
Decreased libido
Anorgasmia

Iatrogenic

Immunologic (antisperm antibodies)

Modified from Morell V. Basic infertility assessment. Primary Care 1997;24:195-204.

---

prolactin should be measured if menstrual cycles are absent or irregular or if there are signs of galactorrhoea or thyroid abnormalities. Ovulation reserve testing as discussed below should be considered in cases where diminished ovarian reserve is suspected.

Evaluation of Ovulation

Currently, laboratory tests will not confirm ovum release. However, measurement of the concentration of mid-luteal plasma progesterone does indicate that a corpus luteum was formed. Other methods such as measurement of the LH surge (to predict ovulation) and basal body temperature (to detect a rise in progesterone) have been used to assess ovulation.

Clinical Utility of Progesterone Measurements. Measurement of serum progesterone concentration is the primary assay used for the evaluation of ovulation. Beginning immediately after ovulation, serum progesterone concentrations rise and peak within 5 to 9 days during the mid-luteal phase (days 21 to 23). If ovulation does not occur, the corpus luteum fails to form, and the expected cyclic rise in progesterone concentration is subnormal. If pregnancy occurs, hCG maintains the corpus luteum, and progesterone production continues to rise. Mid-luteal progesterone concentrations greater than 3 ng/mL indicate that ovulation has taken place, although concentrations of 10 ng/mL or more are more common in conception cycles. Concentrations less than 10 ng/mL indicate the possibility of inadequate luteal phase progesterone production, or inappropriate timing of sample collection.[14]

Clinical Utility of Measurement of Basal Body Temperature. Basal body temperature charts have long been accepted as simple, cost-effective indicators of ovulation. Ovulation is associated with a rapid rise in body temperature (by 0.5 °F), which persists through the luteal phase. The rise in temperature is due to increased quantities of progesterone. However, similar to progesterone, the rise in body temperature is evident only retrospectively and therefore does not predict imminent ovulation in a way helpful for timing intercourse.

Clinical Utility of the Measurement of the Luteinizing Hormone Surge. LH appears in the urine just after the serum LH surge and 24 to 36 hours before ovulation. Measurement of LH does not confirm ovulation or provide insight into the cause of anovulation, but rather indicates when ovulation should occur and provides a guide with which to time intercourse. Home LH kits provide information as to the timing of ovulation, and may reduce stress and costs associated with infertility programs. These tests effectively predict ovulation in 70% of women.

Evaluation of Endocrine Parameters

Disorders of the (1) hypothalamus, (2) pituitary, and (3) ovary are endocrine causes of infertility in women.

Hypergonadotropic Hypogonadism

In women younger than 40 years, hypergonadotropic hypogonadism is indicated by repeatedly elevated basal FSH concentrations (>30 IU/L) or a single elevation of greater than 40 IU/L. These patients are hypoestrogenic (E_2 <20 IU/L) and do not respond to a progestin challenge because their endometrium is atrophic. Basal serum FSH has been used as an indicator of relative ovarian reserve.

Assessing Ovarian Reserve. Women in their mid to late 30s and early 40s with infertility constitute the largest portion of the total infertility population and are at increased risk for pregnancy loss. This reflects a diminished ovarian reserve as a result of follicular depletion and a decline in oocyte quality. As women age, serum FSH concentrations in the early follicular phase begin to increase.

A rise in basal FSH is an excellent indicator of ovarian aging. In general, day 3 FSH concentrations greater than 20 to 25 IU/L are considered to be elevated and associated with poor reproductive outcome. Concomitant measurement of serum E_2 concentration adds to the predictive power of an isolated FSH determination. Basal E_2 concentrations greater than 75 to 80 pg/mL are associated with poor response to ovarian stimulation and pregnancy outcome. The concentration of inhibin B has been used in conjunction with serum FSH and E_2 to assess ovarian function. Inhibin is produced by gonadal tissue and thus is thought to be a more direct marker of gonadal activity and ovarian reserve than pituitary hormones alone.

Hypogonadotropic Hypogonadism

In hypogonadotropic hypogonadism, serum E_2 concentrations are less than 40 pg/mL (110 pmol/L); therefore, there is no withdrawal bleeding with a progestin challenge. Quantities of LH (<10 IU/L) and FSH (<10 IU/L) are decreased. Hyperprolactinemia causes hypergonadotropic hypogonadic infertility. The upper limit of normal plasma prolactin in an amenorrheic, hypoestrogenic, nonpregnant woman is 400 to 500 mIU/mL (20 to 25 ng/mL). If estrogen status is normal, maximum prolactin concentrations vary from 600 to 800 mIU/mL (30 to 40 ng/mL). TSH should be measured to exclude hypothyroidism. Prolactin concentrations are elevated in patients with PCOS and those taking medications, such as (1) antidepressants, (2) cimetidine, and (3) methyldopa, and (4) in stressful conditions. Radiographic imaging of the pituitary is indicated to rule out pituitary adenoma or empty sella syndrome.

Analytical Methodology

Various methods are available for measurement of male and female reproductive and related hormones in body fluids. Reference intervals for many of these hormones are listed in Table 50-1 in Chapter 50.

Measurement of Total Testosterone in Blood

The circulating concentration of testosterone collectively includes a (1) non–protein-bound or "free" form, (2) weakly bound form, and (3) tightly bound form. The weakly bound form is associated with albumin and the tightly bound form with SHBG (also known as *testosterone/E₂-binding globulin*). The term *total testosterone* refers to a serum measurement that includes (1) free testosterone, (2) albumin-bound testosterone, and (3) SHBG-bound testosterone. Bioavailable testosterone includes circulating free testosterone and albumin-bound testosterone. Testosterone bound to SHBG is not biologically active, whereas the free form is available for target cells. Albumin-bound testosterone is also available to target tissue because testosterone dissociates from the albumin carrier and rapidly diffuses into target cells.

Methodology

Enzyme (nonisotopic) immunoassays and tandem mass spectrometry (MS/MS) are widely used techniques for measuring the concentration of circulating testosterone. Isotope-dilution gas chromatography mass spectrometry

(IDGC-MS) is the reference method for testosterone measurement,[3] and there is a candidate liquid chromatography-MS/MS method. For the measurement of testosterone in females and prepubertal subjects, mass spectrometry is the method of choice, as it is the only method that can accurately and precisely quantify testosterone concentrations below 5.2 nmol/L (150 ng/dL).[11]

. Direct (no extraction required) immunoassay methods have been reported for the determination of testosterone in serum or plasma. In such methods, testosterone must be displaced from its binding proteins (albumin and SHBG). Methods used to release it from the endogenous binding proteins include use of (1) salicylates or surfactants, (2) chemicals that alter pH, (3) techniques to change temperature, and (4) competing steroids, such as E_1 or E_2.

Fully automated immunoassays incorporating analogs labeled with enzymes, and fluorescent- or chemiluminescent-signaling molecules are commercially available for routine use. For adult male patients, these assays have demonstrated acceptable precision and recovery, and agreement with GC-MS and RIA methods. However, the use of such assays for female and prepubertal subjects is contraindicated, and a mass spectrometry method is required.[12]

Regardless of the type of immunoassay used, almost all testosterone antisera show some degree of cross-reactivity with DHT (typically 3% to 5%), but show negligible cross-reactivity with other androgens. Assays that use antisera generated against the C-19 position give maximum analytical specificity with respect to endogenous steroids. However, cross-reactions with 19-norsteroids that are used in contraceptive preparations have caused a problem. In most clinical situations, estimation of testosterone without prior separation of DHT is permitted because plasma concentrations of DHT are only 10% to 20% of those for testosterone. Moreover, testosterone and DHT are the two most important androgens in the systemic circulation. Even when a method measures the concentrations of both of them, clinically useful information about the total androgen load still is obtained. However, if specific estimation of just testosterone concentration is required, then chromatographic separation of testosterone and DHT prior to analysis is usually necessary to obtain reliable immunoassay results.

Specimen Collection and Storage

Either serum or heparinized plasma is used to measure total or free testosterone. Testosterone is subject to a diurnal variation, reaching a peak concentration between 400 and 800. Therefore morning specimens are preferred. Specimens are stable for a week (men) or 3 days (women) refrigerated and for up to 1 year at −20 °C. Medications such as (1) steroid, (2) thyroid, (3) ACTH, (4) E_2, or (5) gonadotropin drugs should not be given for 48 hours before sample collection. Most assays are standardized for serum or heparinized plasma. Other anticoagulants, such as ethylenediaminetetraacetic acid (EDTA), may give different values. In certain RIA assays, presence of EDTA can cause a 10% decrease in total testosterone concentrations.

Comments

Knowledge of the SHBG concentration in serum can be very useful for interpreting blood concentrations of testosterone. Assays for measuring SHBG include (1) binding assays, in which the quantity of a radiolabeled androgen bound to SHBG is measured; and (2) specific immunoassays for the SHBG protein.

Measurement of Free and Weakly Bound Testosterone in Blood

Several methods are available for determining the concentrations of the free or bioavailable forms of testosterone in serum or plasma. These include methods that estimate the (1) free testosterone fraction by equilibrium dialysis or ultrafiltration, (2) free hormone using a direct ("analog tracer") immunoassay, (3) combined free and weakly bound ("bioavailable") testosterone fractions by selective precipitation of the tightly bound form, (4) androgen index using indices that reflect ratios of the testosterone pools, and (5) free and weakly bound testosterone concentrations by mathematical modeling.[15] The last approach uses mass action equations to calculate free and weakly bound testosterone concentrations from the concentrations of (1) total testosterone, (2) SHBG, and (3) albumin, and from the association constants for the binding of testosterone to the two binding proteins.

Measurement of Dehydroepiandrosterone and Its Sulfate

Measurements of DHEA or its sulfated conjugate, DHEAS, in serum and plasma are important to investigations of adrenal androgen production, such as the assessment of (1) hyperplasia, (2) adrenal tumors, (3) adrenarche, (4) delayed puberty, and (5) hirsutism.[1] DHEAS in circulation originates primarily from the adrenal glands, although in men some may be derived from the testes. None is produced by the ovaries. DHEA is secreted almost entirely by the adrenal glands.

DHEA concentrations exhibit a circadian rhythm that reflects the secretion of ACTH and also varies during the menstrual cycle. DHEAS concentrations do not exhibit a circadian rhythm because of their longer circulating half-life.

Methodology

Mass spectrometry is the method of choice for measurements of DHEA and DHEAS. Other methods include (1) immunoassays, (2) double-isotope derivative methods, and (3) competitive protein-binding assays. The latter actually measures 5-androstenediol derivatives and uses SHBG as a naturally occurring binding protein. A reference method based on LC-MS/MS has been used for independent evaluation of routine methods. Immunoassays for DHEAS demonstrate significant cross-reactivity with (1) DHEA, (2) androstenedione, and (3) androsterone, yet the relative concentrations of these steroids cause a minimal effect on assay performance.

Reference intervals for serum concentrations of DHEAS and DHEA are listed in Table 50-1 in Chapter 50.

Specimen Collection and Storage

Serum or plasma (preserved with EDTA) is suitable for DHEA or DHEAS immunoassays. Medications such as (1) steroid, (2) ACTH, (3) E_2, or (4) gonadotropin drugs should not be given for 48 hours before sample collection. Early morning collection, before 1030, is preferred for DHEA. Refrigerated samples (4 °C to 8 °C) are stable for up to 14 days; those frozen at −20 °C are stable for about 1 year.

Measurement of 17-Ketosteroids in Urine

The 17-KSs are metabolites of precursors secreted by the (1) adrenal glands, (2) testes, and to some extent the (3) ovaries. In men, approximately one third of the total urinary 17-KSs represent metabolites of testosterone secreted by the testes, whereas most of the remaining two thirds are derived from the steroids produced by the adrenal glands. In women, who normally excrete smaller quantities than men, the total 17-KS concentrations are derived almost exclusively from the adrenal glands.

The bulk of the urinary 17-KSs consists of (1) androsterone, (2) epiandrosterone, (3) etiocholanolone, (4) DHEA, (5) 11-keto- and (6) 11β-hydroxyandrosterone, and (7) 11-keto- and (8) 11β-hydroxyetiocholanolone. DHEA and 11-hydroxy 17-KSs are produced only by the adrenal glands, whereas the others also arise from precursors (androstenedione and testosterone) elaborated by the **gonads**. Thus the main purpose of measuring these steroid metabolites is to assess adrenal androgen production.

Mass spectrometric methods are available for estimating the concentration of total 17-KSs in urine. Ketogenic steroids also have been measured using the Zimmermann reaction, in which an alkaline solution of meta-dinitrobenzene reacts with methylene groups at carbon-16 of the 17-ketosteroids.

Of note, various drugs interfere with the photometric 17-KS assays. Those that produce a positive interference include (1) chlorpromazine, (2) ethinamate, (3) meprobamate, (4) nalidixic acid, (5) penicillin, (6) phenaglycodol, and (7) spironolactone. Drugs that produce a negative interference include (1) chlordiazepoxide, (2) progestational agents, (3) propoxyphene, and (4) reserpine.

Measurement of Anabolic Steroids

Exogenous steroids, such as testosterone and DHT, that are used to improve athletic performance are a challenge for the laboratory to detect and quantify. The ratio of testosterone to epitestosterone has been used for detection of testosterone abuse. A ratio of testosterone to epitestosterone greater than 6:1 suggests exogenous testosterone use and further testing should be performed for confirmation. Others have suggested a ratio of testosterone to LH in the urine as an indication of testosterone doping. Mass spectrometry is commonly used for screening and confirmation.

Measurement of Estrogens in Blood

Both instrumental and immunoassay methods are used to measure estrogens in blood.

Instrumental Methods

Isotope dilution LC-MS/MS methods provide the most accurate and reliable measurement of E_2.[8] The key steps in these method are (1) solvent extraction, (2) chromatographic fractionation, (3) chemical derivatization, and (4) detection. For routine purposes, GC-MS methods have been largely replaced by immunoassays.

Immunoassay

Both indirect (extraction required) and direct (no extraction required) immunoassays are used. The most common antigen used to prepare antibodies for E_2 assays is estradiol-6-(O-carboxymethyl) oxime conjugated to bovine serum albumin. Cross-reactivity with other C_{18} steroids is usually minimal as the 3- and 17-hydroxyl groups are left free. Direct enzyme immunoassays have largely replaced RIAs for routine measurement of E_2 concentrations. Measurement of estrogen concentrations in (1) men, (2) postmenopausal women, and (3) children requires use of more sensitive RIAs. Many of the early immunoassays used organic solvents for selective extraction of E_2 from serum. This step not only removes E_2 from endogenous binding proteins but also removes other compounds that interfere with the method.

To measure E_2 directly without extraction and chromatography, the steroid must be displaced from its binding proteins. The displacing agents used in commercial methods are often not disclosed, but in some systems effective displacement is achieved by adding 8-anilino-1-naphthalene sulfonic acid (ANS) or a large excess of a competing steroid, such as DHT to the sample.

Specimen Collection and Storage

Serum or plasma (with EDTA or heparin as anticoagulant) are used in the measurement of estrogens. Samples should be centrifuged and separated within 24 hours. Samples may be stored refrigerated for 24 hours or frozen for up to 1 year. E_2 concentrations are increased in liver cirrhosis, and oral contraceptives have been found to alter concentrations. In practice, (1) steroid, (2) ACTH, (3) gonadotropin, or (4) E_2 medications should not be given within 48 hours of sample collection.

Measurement of Progesterone in Blood

Measurement of progesterone in serum or plasma is considered to be the most reliable technique to assess its rate of production.

Methodology

Double isotope derivative methods and competitive protein-binding assays have been applied to the measurement of serum progesterone. These methods require extensive purification of the steroid and are labor intensive. GC procedures using (1) flame ionization, (2) electron capture, or (3) nitrogen detection have been used to improve the accuracy of progesterone analysis. These methods also are time consuming and often require (1) solvent extraction, (2) chromatography, and (3) derivatization before the steroid is quantified. There is a candidate isotope-dilution LC-MS/MS reference method for progesterone determination.[14]

For routine measurement of progesterone, immunoassays using steroid-specific antibodies are preferred. Initial immunoassays for serum progesterone measurement used organic solvents to remove the steroid from endogenous binding proteins, such as **corticosteroid-binding globulin** (transcortin and albumin). Direct (nonextraction) measurement of progesterone in serum or plasma is considered the method of choice for routine applications. A number of different antigens have been used to prepare antisera for progesterone assays. Cross-reactivity is most prominent with 5β-pregnanediol, ranging from 6% to 11%. Both RIA and nonisotopic immunoassays are available for measuring progesterone. Enzyme immunoassays are the methods of choice for measuring progesterone.

Specimen Collection and Storage

Serum or plasma (with heparin or EDTA as anticoagulant) has been used, but should be separated within 24 hours. The patient need not be fasting, and no special handling procedures are necessary. Samples may be stored refrigerated for up to 3 days at 4 °C to 8 °C or for up to 1 year at −20 °C. Patients should not be on any (1) corticosteroid, (2) ACTH, (3) estrogen, or (4) gonadotropin medication for at least 48 hours before specimen collection.

Measurement of Luteinizing Hormone and Follicle-Stimulating Hormone

The α subunit of several pituitary hormones is homologous. These hormones include (1) LH, (2) FSH, (3) growth hormone, (4) chorionic gonadotropin, and (5) thyrotropin. Therefore, analytical methods for measuring LH and FSH must recognize the unique β subunits of these hormones.

Methodology

Two-site (double antibody) heterogeneous immunoassays are currently the methods of choice for measuring gonadotropins, and a wide variety of assays have been adapted to automated platforms. Some commercially available methods attach a capture antibody to the surface of test tubes or plastic beads, whereas others use a paramagnetic label or a microparticle to capture the antibody-antigen complexes. Numerous labels have been used for the second antibody, including (1) radioisotopes, (2) enzymes, (3) fluorophores, and (4) chemiluminescent molecules. In modern immunometric assays, (1) hCG interference has been mostly eliminated (<0.008% cross-reactivity), (2) better assay precision has been achieved (between-assay coefficient of variation [CV] <10%), and (3) detection limits have been lowered (<0.2 IU/L). A low limit of detection for LH assays is especially important in the evaluation of prepubertal children and patients with hypothalamic disorders, because LH concentrations in them are very low.

Calibration of gonadotropin assays is difficult because LH and FSH undergo post-translational modifications that produce a mixture of closely related compounds. The earliest reference material used for calibration of LH and FSH assays was the second international reference preparation (IRP) for human menopausal gonadotropins, isolated from the urine of postmenopausal women. Alterations during metabolism and excretion, however, limited the comparability of this preparation with circulating forms of the hormones, and subsequent calibrators were prepared from extracts derived from the human pituitary gland. Purified pituitary extracts, such as the first and second IRPs for FSH and LH, were available for many years but have been replaced by highly purified extracts that have minimal contamination with cross-reacting glycoproteins. Manufacturers of older immunoassays for LH and FSH used one or more pituitary-derived reference materials for their working calibrators, but recombinant gonadotropin calibrators are now available.

Biases in analytical results still exist between different immunoassay systems (most notably in LH assays), and results have been known to differ by more than 50%, even when calibrated with the same reference preparation.

Specimen Collection and Storage

Serum is the preferred specimen for gonadotropin measurements. Hemolyzed, lipemic, and/or icteric specimens should not be used. Both hormones are stable for 8 days at room temperature, and for 2 weeks at 4 °C; for longer periods, the serum specimen should be frozen at or below −20 °C. Because of (1) episodic, (2) circadian, and (3) cyclic variations in the secretion of gonadotropins, meaningful clinical evaluation of these hormones may require determinations in (1) pooled blood specimens, (2) multiple serial blood specimens, or (3) timed urine specimens. Urine specimens should not contain preservatives; storage at or below −20 °C is recommended.

Comments

Clinically, the pulsatile and episodic release of gonadotropins makes a single blood concentration of FSH or LH difficult to interpret. In adults, concentrations of gonadotropins in blood, particularly LH, may differ as much as threefold between blood specimens collected from the same individual 20 minutes apart. In addition, the lower detection limit of many FSH and LH immunoassays may be within the reference interval for these hormones in healthy adults. In prepubertal children, most blood assays are not capable of measuring normal concentrations because they are so low.

Measurement of Urinary Follicle-Stimulating Hormone and Luteinizing Hormone

To optimize detection limits for gonadotropin assays in children, urinary FSH or LH assays have been used. Some pediatric endocrinologists favor urine assays when investigating pubertal disorders of gonadotropin secretion.

Review Questions

1. In females, follicle-stimulating hormone (FSH) functions to:
   a. induce development of the ovum within the follicle.
   b. maintain bone integrity in premenopausal women.
   c. trigger release of the ovum from the follicle.
   d. induce development of the endometrium.

2. In males, luteinizing hormone (LH) functions to:
   a. induce sperm production by the Leydig cells.
   b. stimulate production of testosterone by Leydig cells.
   c. promote sperm production by the Sertoli cells.
   d. induce synthesis of testosterone by the Sertoli cells.

3. Progesterone is synthesized and secreted by the:
   a. corpus luteum.
   b. placenta.
   c. pituitary gland.
   d. Both A and B are correct.

4. Which of the following hormones is considered to be the most potent of the three biologically active estrogens?
   a. Estriol (E_3)
   b. Estradiol (E_2)
   c. Estrone (E_1)
   d. Progesterone

5. Increased production of progesterone and estrogen from the corpus luteum with gradual lowering of LH and FSH concentrations is characteristic of which phase of the reproductive cycle?
   a. Follicular
   b. Luteal
   c. Ovulatory
   d. Menopausal

6. Which ovarian disorder results in an *overall decrease* in FSH, LH, estrogen, and progesterone?
   a. Hypogonadotropic hypergonadism
   b. Hypergonadotropic hypogonadism
   c. Hypergonadotropic hypergonadism
   d. Hypogonadotropic hypogonadism

7. In a woman, failure to establish spontaneous periodic menstruation by the age of 16 regardless of whether secondary sex characteristics have developed is referred to as:
   a. primary amenorrhea.
   b. secondary amenorrhea.
   c. precocious puberty.
   d. pseudohermaphroditism.

8. In males, FSH functions to:
   a. enhance muscle mass.
   b. induce production of testosterone.
   c. stimulate spermatogenesis.
   d. induce production of androstenedione.

9. The major estrogen secreted by the ovary is ____, whereas the major product secreted by the placenta is ____.
   a. estriol; estradiol
   b. estradiol; estriol
   c. estrone; estradiol
   d. estriol; estrone

10. The most common form of hypogonadotropic hypogonadism in men results from a deficiency of GnRH in the hypothalamus during embryonic development and is referred to as:
    a. Turner syndrome.
    b. Klinefelter syndrome.
    c. Down syndrome.
    d. Kallmann syndrome.

References

1. Azziz R. The evaluation and management of hirsutism. Obstetrics & Gynecology 2003;101(5, Part 1):995–1007.
2. Azziz R, Carmina E, Dewailly D, Diamanti-Kandarakis E, Escobar-Morreale HF, Futterweit W, et al. The Androgen Excess and PCOS Society criteria for the polycystic ovary syndrome: the complete task force report. Fertility and Sterility 2009;91(2):456–88.
3. Bulun SE. Physiology and pathology of the female reproductive axis. In: Melmed S, Polonsky KS, Larsen PR, Kronenberg HM, eds. Williams textbook of endocrinology. 12th ed. Philadelphia: Saunders; 2012:581–660.
4. Carel J-C, Léger J. Precocious puberty. New England Journal of Medicine 2008;358(22):2366–77.
5. Cole LA, Sasaki Y, Muller CY. Normal production of human chorionic gonadotropin in menopause. New England Journal of Medicine 2007;356(11):1184–6.
6. Greendale GA, Lee NP, Arriola ER. The menopause. The Lancet 1999;353(9152):571–80.
7. Hall JE. Neuroendocrine control of the menstrual cycle. In: Strauss JF, Barbieri RL, eds. Yen & Jaffe's reproductive endocrinology. 6th ed. Philadelphia: Saunders; 2009:139–54.
8. Huang X, Spink DC, Schneider E, et al. Measurement of unconjugated estriol in serum by liquid chromatography—tandem mass spectrometry and assessment of the accuracy of chemilaminescent immunoassays. Clin Chem 2014;60:260–8.
9. Liu PY, Veldhuis JD. The hypothalmo-pituitary unit, testes, and male accessory organs. In: Strauss JF, Barbieri RL, eds. Yen & Jaffe's reproductive endocrinology. 6th ed. Philadelphia: Saunders; 2009:283–98.
10. Matsumoto AM, Bremner W. Testicular disorders. In: Melmed S, Polonsky KS, Larsen PR, Kronenberg HM, eds. Williams textbook of endocrinology. 12th ed. Phlladelphia: Saunders, 2012:688–777.
11. Muti P. The role of endogenous hormones in the etiology and prevention of breast cancer: the epidemiological evidence. Annals of the New York Academy of Sciences. 2004;1028(1):273–82.
12. Rosner W, Auchus RJ, Azziz R, Sluss PM, Raff H. Utility, limitations, and pitfalls in measuring testosterone: An Endocrine Society position statement. J Clin Endocrinol Metab. 2007;92(2):405–13.
13. Strauss JF, Williams CJ. The ovarian life cycle. In: Strauss JF, Barbieri RL, eds. Yen & Jaffe's reproductive endocrinology, 6th edition. Philadelphia: Saunders, 2009:155–90.
14. Tai SS, Xu B, Welch MJ, Development and evaluation of a candidate reference measurement procedure for the determination of progesterone in human serum using isotope-dilution liquid chromatography/tandem mass spectrometry. Anal Chem. 2006;78(18):6628–33.
15. Williams C, Giannopoulos T, Sherriff EA. best practice no 170. Investigation of infertility with the emphasis on laboratory testing and with reference to radiological imaging. Journal of Clinical Pathology 2003;56(4):261–7.
16. WHO. Laboratory manual for the examination and processing of human semen. 5th ed. Geneva: WHO Press; 2010.

44   Pregnancy and Prenatal Testing[*]

David G. Grenache, Ph.D., M.T. (A.S.C.P.), D.A.B.C.C., F.A.C.B.,
and Geralyn Lambert-Messerlian, Ph.D., F.A.C.B.

Objectives

1. Define the following:

Alpha fetoprotein (AFP)	Meconium
Amnion	Nuchal transparency
Amniotic fluid	Placenta
Chorion	Human placental lactogen (hPL),
Conception	or placental lactogen (PL)
Embryo	Prenatal screening
Gestation	Surfactant

2. Outline the events in the normal development of a fetus, beginning with conception and ending with birth.

3. Describe the structure and functions of the following, including hormones synthesized (if any), effect on maternal/fetal health if dysfunctional, and laboratory analyses and results used to determine health or disease:

Amnion/amniotic fluid	Corpus luteum
Blastocyst	Ovaries
Chorionic villus	Placenta

4. List the components of amniotic fluid, and state their specific functions and what laboratory analyses are used to examine amniotic fluid.

5. Describe the major biochemical changes that take place during a normal pregnancy in maternal physiological systems including renal, hemostatic, and endocrine changes.

6. State the clinical significance of the following laboratory analytes in the assessment of maternal and fetal health:

Alpha fetoprotein (AFP)	Fetal fibronectin
Human chorionic	Pregnancy-associated plasma
gonadotropin	protein A (PAPP-A)
(hCG), or chorionic	Unconjugated estriol (uE$_3$)
gonadotropin (CG)	
Inhibin A (inhA)	

7. Describe the fetal renal, gastrointestinal, hepatic, pulmonary systems, including functions, development and maturation, and how and why these systems are assessed by the laboratory.

8. For the following disorders, list the causes and symptoms, and state the laboratory analytical procedures, specimen requirements, and laboratory results used to assess and diagnose:

Anencephaly	Hemolytic disease of the
Down syndrome	newborn (HDN)
Eclampsia	Hyperemesis gravidarum
Ectopic pregnancy	Preeclampsia
HELLP syndrome	Respiratory distress syndrome
	(RDS)
	Spina bifida

9. In regard to maternal serum screening for fetal defects, describe the composition, timing during pregnancy and utility of the triple, quad, and integrated tests.

10. Analyze and solve case studies related to disorders of pregnancy and laboratory analysis of these.

Key Words and Definitions

Acute fatty liver of pregnancy A rare, life-threatening complication of pregnancy that occurs in the third trimester or the immediate period after delivery.

Alpha fetoprotein (AFP) A protein produced in the fetal liver that is measured in maternal serum for predicting risk of anencephaly, spina bifida, and Down syndrome in the fetus.

Amniotic fluid Substance derived mostly from fetal urine that protects the developing fetus.

Anencephaly A birth defect characterized by a brain, skull, and scalp that does not develop normally.

Assisted reproductive technologies (ART) Procedures involving the manipulation of eggs or sperm to establish pregnancy in the treatment of infertility.

---

*The authors gratefully acknowledge the original contributions of E.R. Ashwood and G. J. Knight on which portions of this chapter are based.

Key Words and Definitions—cont'd

Blastocyst A thin-walled hollow structure in early embryonic development that contains a cluster of cells called the *inner cell mass* from which the embryo arises.

Cholestasis of pregnancy A condition during pregnancy characterized by impaired bile flow allowing bile salts to be deposited in the skin and the placenta.

Chorionic villi One of the minute vascular projections of the fetal chorion that combines with maternal uterine tissue to form the placenta.

CLIA waived tests Tests categorized as "waived" by the FDA under the Clinical Laboratory Improvement Amendments of 1988. These tests employ methodologies that are considered to be so simple and accurate as to render the likelihood of erroneous results negligible.

Conception The union of the sperm and the ovum. Synonymous with fertilization.

Down syndrome A birth defect characterized by having three copies of chromosome 21 rather than the normal two copies. Also known as *trisomy 21.*

Eclampsia Convulsions and coma occurring in a pregnant woman or a woman who recently gave birth.

Ectopic pregnancy An embryo developing in the fallopian tube or abdomen instead of the uterus.

Embryo A developing infant that has not yet finished organ development (before 10 weeks gestation).

Endometrium The glandular mucous membrane that lines the uterus.

Expected date of confinement (EDC) The date at which an infant is expected to be born, calculated from the date of the last menstrual period (LMP). Also called *due date.*

Fetal erythroblastosis A severe hemolytic disease of a fetus or newborn infant caused by the production of maternal antibodies against the fetal red blood cells, usually involving rhesus (Rh) blood group incompatibility between the mother and fetus.

Fetal fibronectin (fFN) A protein produced during pregnancy that is thought to function as a "glue" attaching the fetal sac to the uterine lining; a test for fFN in cervicovaginal fluid is used to assess risk of preterm labor.

Fetal lung maturity (FLM) A parameter that determines the likelihood a neonate will develop respiratory distress syndrome.

Fetus A developing infant that has finished organ development (following 10 weeks gestation).

Gestation The process, state or period of carrying an embryo or fetus from conception until birth; by convention, the time is measured clinically from the first day of the last menstrual period (LMP) and reported in weeks; gestational age of the fetus is often estimated by use of ultrasound.

HELLP syndrome A life-threatening pregnancy complication usually considered to be a variant of preeclampsia and usually occurring between the 23rd and 39th weeks. The name is an acronym for the diagnostic features:

H – Hemolysis
EL – Elevated Liver enzymes
LP – Low Platelets.

Hemolytic disease of the newborn (HDN) A disease of the fetus and newborn caused by maternal antibody–mediated fetal erythrocyte destruction.

Human antimouse antibodies (HAMA) Antibodies made by humans that bind mouse proteins. Their presence in body fluids causes both positive and negative interferences in two-site mouse monoclonal antibody-based assays.

Human chorionic gonadotropin (hCG) A placental glycoprotein hormone that stimulates the ovary to produce progesterone.

Human placental lactogen (hPL) A placental hormone, similar in structure and function to growth hormone, that disappears from the blood immediately after delivery.

Hydramnios (or polyhydramnios) An abnormality of pregnancy characterized by an accumulation of excess amniotic fluid.

Hydrops fetalis A condition in which a fetus or newborn baby accumulates fluids, causing swollen arms and legs and impaired breathing.

Hyperemesis gravidarum Extreme, excessive, and persistent vomiting in early pregnancy that may lead to dehydration and malnutrition.

Insulin-like growth factors One of three protein hormones that share structural similarity to insulin.

In vitro fertilization (IVF) A procedure in which (1) eggs (ova) from a woman's ovary are removed, (2) the removed eggs are fertilized with sperm in a laboratory procedure, and (3) the fertilized egg (embryo) is returned to the woman's uterus.

Lamellar bodies Packages of phospholipids that are produced by type II alveolar cells and represent the storage form of surfactant. They are similar in size to platelets and are present in amniotic fluid.

Lamellar body count (LBC) Concentration of lamellar bodies in amniotic fluid. LBC increases as gestation advances. Most electronic cell counters will count the lamellar bodies.

Lanugo A very fine, soft, and usually unpigmented downy hair on the body of a fetus or newborn baby.

Meconium A dark green fecal material that accumulates in the fetal intestines and is discharged at or near the time of birth.

Molar pregnancy A type of pregnancy caused by abnormal proliferation of placental tissue in the uterus. Also known as a *hydatidiform mole.*

Morula A solid ball of cells resulting from division of a fertilized ovum and from which a blastula is formed.

Multiple of the median (MoM) In clinical screening, the statistic used to normalize analyte values.

Neural tube defect (NTD) A major birth defect resulting from the abnormal development of the neural tube present during embryonic life that gives rise to the central nervous system; the two most common NTDs are *spina bifida* and anencephaly.

Nuchal translucency (NT) test A measurement of the size of the translucent space behind the neck of the fetus; made using ultrasound between 10 and 14 weeks of pregnancy. NT tends to be increased in chromosome disorders, such as Turner syndrome and Down syndrome.

Key Words and Definitions—cont'd

Oligohydramnios A condition in pregnancy characterized by a deficiency of amniotic fluid.

Omphalocele A birth defect in which the infant's intestine or other abdominal organs protrude from the navel.

Ovulation The release of the ripe egg (ovum) from the ovary.

Parathyroid hormone (PTH) The hormone secreted by the parathyroid glands that controls the concentration of calcium in the blood.

Placenta A membranous vascular organ that develops in female mammals during pregnancy, lining the uterine wall and partially enveloping the fetus, to which it is attached by the umbilical cord. Following birth, the placenta is expelled.

Placental alpha microglobulin-1 (PAMG-1) A protein present in blood and the amniotic fluid and cervico-vaginal discharge of pregnant women.

Polyhydramnios (or hydramnios) The presence of excess amniotic fluid in the uterus.

Preeclampsia A disorder of widespread vascular endothelial malfunction and vasospasm that occurs after 20 weeks gestation and can present as late as 4 to 6 weeks postpartum. It is clinically defined by hypertension and proteinuria, with or without pathologic edema.

Pregnancy The period from conception to birth. It usually lasts 40 weeks, beginning from the first day of the woman's last menstrual period (LMP), and is divided into three trimesters, each lasting 3 months.

Pregnancy-associated plasma protein A (PAPP-A) A protein used in screening tests for Down syndrome.

Premature rupture of membranes (PROM) Breakage of the sac containing the developing fetus and the amniotic fluid prior to the start of labor; rupture before the 37th week of gestation is called preterm PROM (PPROM).

Preterm delivery The birth of an infant before 37 weeks gestation.

Prolactin A pituitary hormone that stimulates and maintains the secretion of milk.

Puerperium The approximate 6-week period lasting from childbirth to the return of normal uterine size.

Pulmonary surfactant A fluid secreted by the cells of the alveoli that serves to reduce the surface tension of pulmonary fluids.

Rapid plasma reagin test (RPR) test Any of a group of serologic tests for syphilis.

Respiratory distress syndrome (RDS) A disease of premature infants caused by a deficiency of lung surfactant.

Smith-Lemli-Opitz syndrome (SLOS) A congenital malformation syndrome caused by deficiency of the enzyme 7-dehydrocholesterol reductase (DHCR7), due to mutation of the DHCR7 gene on chromosome 11.

Spina bifida A congenital disorder caused by the incomplete closure of the embryonic neural tube (see *neural tube defect*); *the most common form is meningomyelocele (also called myelomeningocele).*

Triploidy A condition characterized by the individual having three times the haploid number of chromosomes in the cell nucleus.

Trisomy 18 (Edwards syndrome) A genetic disorder caused by the presence of all or part of an extra 18th chromosome (trisomy: three chromosomes).

Trophoblasts The outermost layer of cells of the blastocyst that attaches the fertilized ovum to the uterine wall and serves as a nutritive pathway for the embryo.

Umbilical cord A flexible cordlike structure containing blood vessels and attaching a human or other mammalian fetus to the placenta during gestation.

Vernix caseosa A white cheese-like protective material that covers the skin of a fetus.

Yolk sac A membranous sac attached to an embryo that provides early nourishment in the form of yolk in many animals, including humans where it functions as the circulatory system before internal circulation begins.

Zygote The fertilized ovum or diploid cell resulting from the fusion of two haploid gametes.

The clinical laboratory has an important role in managing **pregnancy**. In contrast to most clinical situations, when treating an expectant mother, a clinician must simultaneously care for both the mother and the child. This chapter reviews (1) the biology of pregnancy, (2) disorders related to pregnancy, and (3) laboratory tests used to detect, evaluate, and monitor both normal and abnormal pregnancies.

Human Pregnancy[9]

To appreciate the role of laboratory tests in pregnancy healthcare, it is necessary to understand fundamental topics, such as (1) **conception**, (2) **embryo** development, (3) fetal growth, (4) the role of the **placenta**, (5) the importance and composition of amniotic fluid, (6) maternal adaptation to pregnancy, and (7) functional maturation of the **fetus**.[9]

Conception, Embryo, and Fetus

In a normal human pregnancy, the time between **gestation** from conception to birth is approximately 40 weeks. This time period is measured from the first day of the last normal menstrual period (LMP or LNMP). The anticipated date of birth of an infant is commonly referred to as the **expected date of confinement (EDC)**. During pregnancy, a woman undergoes dramatic physiological and hormonal changes. In practice, clinicians customarily divide pregnancy into three timed intervals called *trimesters*, each of which lasts about 13 weeks. By convention, the first trimester, 0 to 13 weeks, begins on the first day of the LMP.

Ovulation occurs on approximately the 14th day of the regular menstrual cycle (see Chapter 43). If conception occurs, the ovum is fertilized, usually in the fallopian tube, and becomes a **zygote**, which is then carried down the tube into the uterus. The zygote divides, becoming a **morula**. After 50 to 60 cells are present, the morula develops into the primitive **yolk sac**. This becomes a **blastocyst,** which implants into the uterine wall about 5 days after fertilization. The cells on the exterior wall of the blastocyst, **trophoblasts,** synergistically invade the uterine **endometrium** and develop into **chorionic villi,** creating the placenta.

At this stage, the product of conception is referred to as an embryo. A cavity called the amnion forms and enlarges with the accumulation of **amniotic fluid.** Nourished by the placenta and protected by the amniotic fluid, an embryo undergoes rapid cell division, differentiation, and growth. From combinations of (1) ectoderm, (2) mesoderm, and (3) endoderm cell types, organs begin to form through a process called *organogenesis*. At 10 weeks, an embryo has developed most major structures and is now referred to as a fetus. At 13 weeks, the fetus weighs approximately 13 g and is about 8 cm long.

Rapid fetal growth occurs during the 13 to 26 weeks of the second trimester. By the end of the second trimester, the fetus weighs approximately 700 g and is 30 cm long. Many fetal organs begin to mature. The 26 to 38 weeks of the third trimester is the time interval in which fetal organs complete their prenatal maturation. During this trimester, the growth rate decelerates. At the end of the third trimester, the fetus weighs approximately 3200 g and is about 50 cm long. *Term pregnancy* is used to define the interval from 37 to 42 weeks. Normal labor, rhythmic uterine contractions, and birth occur during this period.

Placenta

The placenta and the **umbilical cord** form the primary link between fetus and mother. The placenta grows throughout pregnancy and is normally delivered through the birth canal immediately after the birth of the infant.

Function

The placenta (1) keeps the maternal and fetal circulation systems separate, (2) nourishes the fetus, (3) eliminates fetal wastes, and (4) produces hormones vital to pregnancy. It is composed of large collections of fetal vessels called *villi*, which are surrounded by intervillous spaces in which maternal blood flows. For substances to move from the maternal circulation to the fetal circulation, they must cross through the trophoblast cells and several membranes. The transfer of any substance depends largely on the (1) concentration gradient between the maternal and fetal circulatory systems, (2) presence or absence of circulating binding proteins, (3) lipid solubility of the substance, and (4) presence of facilitated transport, such as ion pumps or receptor-mediated endocytosis (Box 44-1). The placenta is an effective barrier to the movement of large proteins and hydrophobic compounds bound to plasma proteins. Maternal immunoglobulin G (IgG) crosses the placenta via receptor-mediated endocytosis. Because of its long half-life, maternally produced IgG protects a newborn for the first 6 months of life. IgG antibody assays with low limits of detection may be positive in infants up to age 18 months because of maternal antibodies.

BOX 44-1 | **Normal Placental Transport**

No Transport
Most proteins
Thyroid hormones
Maternal IgM, IgA
Maternal and fetal erythrocytes

Limited Passive Transport
Unconjugated steroids
Steroid sulfates
Free fatty acids

Passive Transport
Molecules up to a molecular weight of 5000 Da having lipid solubility
Oxygen
Carbon dioxide
Sodium and chloride
Urea
Ethanol

Active Transport across Cell Membranes
Glucose
Many amino acids
Calcium

Receptor-Mediated Endocytosis
Maternal IgG
Insulin
Low-density lipoprotein

IgA, Immunoglobulin A; IgG, immunoglobulin G; IgM, immunoglobulin M.

Placental Hormones

The placenta produces several protein and steroid hormones (Figure 44-1). The major protein hormones are **human chorionic gonadotropin (hCG)** and **human placental lactogen (hPL)**. The steroids include (1) progesterone, (2) estradiol (E_2), (3) estriol (E_3), and (4) estrone (E_1) (see Chapter 43). The placenta secretes most of its products into the maternal circulation with only small amounts reaching the fetal circulation. Generally, hormone production by the placenta increases in proportion to the increase in placental mass. Therefore concentrations of hormones derived from the placenta, such as hPL, increase in maternal peripheral blood as the placenta increases in size. An exception is hCG, which peaks at the end of the first trimester.

Human Chorionic Gonadotropin

One of the most important placental hormones is hCG. It stimulates the ovary to produce progesterone, which, in turn, prevents menstruation, thereby protecting the pregnancy. The chemistry, biochemistry, and methods for hCG are discussed later in this chapter.

Human Placental Lactogen

Human placental lactogen (hPL), also known as placental lactogen (PL), and human chorionic somatomammotropin (hCS), is a single polypeptide chain of 191 amino acids having two intra-molecular disulfide bridges and a molecular mass of 22,279 Da. The structure of PL is exceptionally homologous (96%) with growth hormone (GH) and less so with **prolactin** (67%). Placental secretion near term is 1 to 2 g/d, the largest of any known human hormone.

PL has many biological activities, including (1) lactogenic, (2) metabolic, (3) somatotropic, (4) luteotropic, (5) erythropoietic, and (6) aldosterone-stimulating effects. Although PL was used in the past to evaluate fetal health, currently no apparent clinical reason exists to measure PL.

Placental Steroids

The placenta produces a wide variety of steroid hormones, including estrogen and progesterone. These steroids are is described in Chapter 43. Maternal cholesterol is the main precursor for placental progesterone production. Biosynthesis of estrogens by the placenta differs from that of the ovaries because the placenta has no 17α-hydroxylase. Thus, each of the estrogens—estrone (E_1), estradiol (E_2), and estriol (E_3)—must be synthesized from C-19 intermediates that already have a hydroxyl group at position 17. In nonpregnant women, the ovaries secrete 100 to 600 μg/d of E_2, of which about 10% is metabolized to E_3. During late pregnancy, the placenta produces 50 to 150 mg/d of E_3 and 15 to 20 mg/d of E_2 and E_1. Secretion of estrogens and progesterone throughout pregnancy ensures (1) appropriate development of the endometrium, (2) uterine growth, (3) adequate uterine blood supply, and (4) preparation of the uterus for labor. Although measurement of E_3 in the third trimester was used in the past to assess fetal health, most obstetricians now consider this practice obsolete. E_3 measurements in the second trimester of

pregnancy are useful in predicting fetal trisomy 21 and 18 (see later discussion on prenatal screening for fetal defects).

Amniotic Fluid

Throughout intrauterine life, the fetus lives within an amniotic fluid-filled compartment that (1) provides a medium in which a fetus readily moves, (2) cushions it against possible injury, and (3) helps maintain a constant temperature. Amniotic fluid is a dynamic medium whose volume and chemical composition are controlled within relatively narrow limits.

The volume of amniotic fluid is 200 to 300 mL at 16 weeks, 400 to 1400 mL at 26 weeks, 300 to 2000 mL at 34 weeks, and 300 to 1400 mL at 40 weeks. The volume at any given moment is a function of several interrelated fluid movements, including fetal (1) swallowing of amniotic fluid, (2) urination, (3) intramembranous transport (across the amnion and into the underlying fetal vasculature), and (4) pulmonary excretion of fluid. The fetal tracheobronchial tree is filled with amniotic fluid. Although lung fluid transport contributes a small volume, fetal breathing of this fluid is the mechanism of surfactant transport from the fetal lungs into the amniotic fluid.

Pathological decreases and increases in amniotic fluid volume are encountered frequently. Intrauterine growth retardation and anomalies of the fetal urinary tract, such as bilateral renal agenesis or obstruction of the urethra, are associated with **oligohydramnios**, an abnormally low amniotic fluid volume. Increased fluid volume is known as **hydramnios** (also termed **polyhydramnios**). Conditions associated with hydramnios include (1) maternal diabetes mellitus, (2) severe **hemolytic disease of the newborn (HDN)**, (3) fetal esophageal atresia, (4) multifetal pregnancy, (5) **anencephaly**, and (6) **spina bifida**.

Early in gestation, the composition of the amniotic fluid resembles a complex dialysate of the maternal serum. As a fetus grows, the amniotic fluid changes in several ways (Table 44-1). Most notably, sodium concentration and osmolality decrease and concentrations of (1) urea, (2) creatinine, and (3) uric acid increase. The major lipids of interest are the

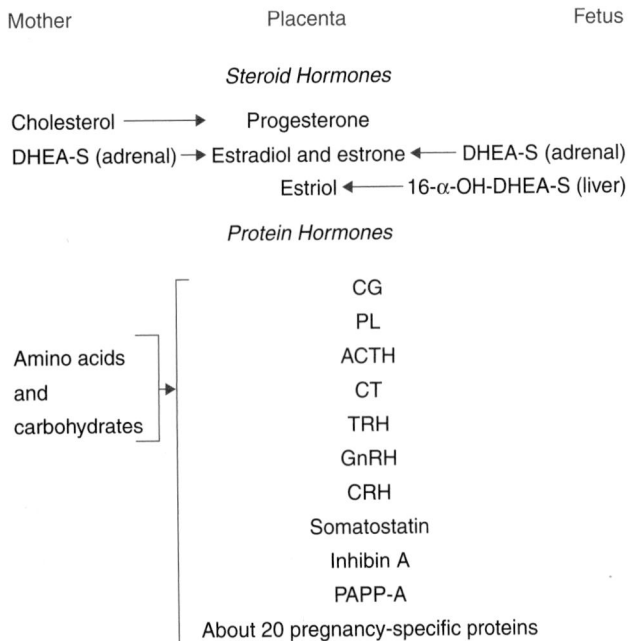

Figure 44-1 Schematic representation of steroid and protein hormone production by the placenta. *ACTH,* Adrenocorticotropic hormone; *CRH,* corticotropin-releasing hormone; *CT,* chorionic thyrotropin; *DHEA-S,* dehydroepiandrosterone sulfate; *GnRH,* gonadotropin-releasing hormone; *hCG,* human chorionic gonadotropin; *PAPP-A,* pregnancy-associated plasma protein A; *PL,* placental lactogen; *TRH,* thyrotropin-releasing hormone.

TABLE 44-1   Composition of Amniotic Fluid (Mean Values)

Component	Gestational Age (Week)		
	15	25	40
Bicarbonate, mmol/L	16	18	16
Bilirubin, mg/dL	0.13	0.14	0.04
Chloride, mmol/L	111	109	103
Creatinine, mg/dL	0.8	0.9	2.2
Glucose, mg/dL	47	39	32
Osmolality, mOsm/kg H_2O	272	272	255
Potassium, mmol/L	3.9	4.0	4.3
Sodium, mmol/L	136	138	126
Total protein, g/dL	0.5	0.8	0.3
Urea nitrogen, mg/dL	11	11	18
Uric acid, mg/dL	4.0	5.7	10.4

From Benzie RJ, Doran TA, Harkins JL, Owen VM, Porter CJ. Composition of the amniotic fluid and maternal serum in pregnancy. Am J Obstet Gynecol 1974;119:798-810.

phospholipids, whose type and concentrations reflect **fetal lung maturity (FLM)** (discussed further later). Numerous steroid and protein hormones are also present in amniotic fluid and some are useful for diagnosing congenital adrenal hyperplasia (CAH) and fetal thyroid disease.[3]

Early in pregnancy, little if any particulate matter is found in the amniotic fluid. By 16 weeks of gestation, large numbers of cells are present, having been shed from the surfaces of the (1) amnion, (2) skin, and (3) tracheobronchial tree. These cells have proved to be of great utility in antenatal diagnosis. As pregnancy continues to progress, scalp hair and **lanugo** (fine hair on the body of the fetus) are shed into the fluid and contribute to its turbidity. Production of surfactant particles in the lung, termed **lamellar bodies**, greatly increases the haziness of the fluid. At term, amniotic fluid contains gross particles of **vernix caseosa**, the oily substance composed of sebum and desquamated epithelial cells covering the fetal skin.

Normal fetuses do not defecate during pregnancy. If severely stressed, a fetus may pass stool that is called **meconium.** This heterogeneous material contains many bile pigments and therefore stains the amniotic fluid green. Meconium-stained amniotic fluid is a sign of fetal stress.

Maternal Adaptation

During pregnancy, a woman undergoes dramatic physiologic and hormonal changes. The large quantities of (1) estrogen, (2) progesterone, (3) PL, and (4) corticosteroids produced during pregnancy affect various body systems. In addition, the woman experiences an increase in resistance to angiotensin and a predominance of lipid metabolism over glucose use. As a result of such changes, many of the laboratory reference intervals for nonpregnant patients are not appropriate for pregnant patients. Mean values for selected tests during pregnancy, expressed as a percentage of control means, are presented in Table 44-2.

Hematologic Changes

Maternal blood volume increases during pregnancy by an average of 45%. Plasma volume increases more rapidly than red blood cell mass; therefore, despite augmented erythropoiesis, (1) hemoglobin concentration, (2) erythrocyte count, and (3) hematocrit all decrease during normal pregnancy. Hemoglobin concentrations at term average 12.6 g/dL, compared with 13.3 g/dL for the nonpregnant state. The leukocyte count varies considerably during pregnancy, from 4000 to 13,000/μL. During labor and **puerperium** (the interval immediately after delivery), leukocyte counts may be markedly elevated.

The concentrations of several blood coagulation factors are increased during pregnancy. For example, plasma fibrinogen increases by approximately 65%, from 275 to 450 mg/dL; this increase contributes to the increase in sedimentation rate. Other clotting factors also increase, including factors VII, VIII, IX, and X. Prothrombin and factors V and XII do not change, whereas factors XI and XIII decrease slightly. Even though the platelet count remains unchanged in most women, prothrombin and activated partial thromboplastin times decrease

| TABLE 44-2 | Mean Serum and Plasma Laboratory Values during Normal Pregnancies Expressed as a Percentage of the Nonpregnant Mean (n = 29) |

	Time of Gestation		
Analyte	12 Weeks	32 Weeks	Term
α_1-Antitrypsin	129	174	191
Activated partial thromboplastin time	95	91	93
Albumin	93	78	78
Aldosterone	—	—	1500
Alkaline phosphatase	90	203	347
Bicarbonate	85	85	81
Bilirubin, unconjugated	56	67	78
Calcium	98	94	97
Chloride	98	100	99
Cholesterol	100	144	156
Cortisol	111	301	309
Creatine kinase	87	86	135
Creatinine	71	74	81
1,25-Dihydroxyvitamin D	—	—	400
Fasting glucose	98	94	94
Fasting triglycerides	141	300	349
Ferritin	81	33	59
Fibrinogen	119	154	165
Free ionized calcium	99	101	102
Free thyroxine	98	72	74
High-density lipoprotein (HDL)-cholesterol	121	119	130
Hematocrit	94	91	97
Hemoglobin	95	90	96
Iron	112	94	94
Iron-binding capacity	95	139	144
Low-density lipoprotein (LDL)-cholesterol	80	118	146
Leukocyte count	144	167	240
Magnesium	92	87	87
Parathyroid hormone (PTH), intact	—	—	140
Phosphate	108	97	96
Platelet count	98	96	100
Potassium	95	95	100
Prolactin	—	—	800
Protein	92	83	83
Prothrombin time	99	97	97
Sodium	97	98	97
Thyroid-stimulating hormone (TSH)	111	122	139
Thyroxine (T_4)	103	107	100
Thyroxine-binding globulin (TBG)	114	155	182
Transferrin	105	160	170
Transferrin saturation	136	68	64
Triiodothyronine (T_3)	100	121	121
Urea nitrogen	77	63	77
Uric acid	68	92	120
Zinc protoporphyrin	107	109	144

Data from Lockitch G, ed. Handbook of diagnostic biochemistry and hematology in normal pregnancy. Boca Raton, FL: CRC Press, 1993.

slightly. Pregnancy increases the risk of thromboembolism to up to five times that of nonpregnant women.

Biochemical

During pregnancy, electrolytes show little change, but concentrations of serum (1) triglycerides, (2) cholesterol, (3) phospholipids, and (4) free fatty acids increase by approximately 40%. The concentration of plasma albumin is decreased to an average of 3.4 g/dL in late pregnancy and plasma globulin concentrations increase slightly. The concentrations of several of the plasma transport proteins, such as sex hormone–binding globulin (SHBG), increase markedly. Serum cholinesterase activity is reduced, whereas alkaline phosphatase activity in serum is tripled, mainly as the result of an increase in very heat-stable alkaline phosphatase of placental origin. In addition, total creatine kinase activity and the isoenzyme CKMB can increase markedly upon delivery.

Renal Function

Pregnancy increases the glomerular filtration rate (GFR) to about 170 mL/min/1.73 m^2 by 20 weeks, and therefore increases the clearance of (1) urea, (2) creatinine, and (3) uric acid. Concentrations of these three analytes are slightly decreased in serum for much of the pregnancy. As term approaches, the GFR begins to return to nonpregnant values. Urea and creatinine concentrations rise slightly during the last 4 weeks. During this time, tubular reabsorption of uric acid increases dramatically, which increases serum uric acid compared with the nonpregnant state. Increased excretion of glucose, up to 1000 mg/d, may occur owing to increased GFR, which presents more fluid to the kidney tubules and therefore lowers the renal glucose threshold. Protein loss in the urine can increase to up to 300 mg/d.

Endocrine

The action of progesterone prevents menses and thus allows pregnancy to continue. In early pregnancy, progesterone is produced by the corpus luteum of the maternal ovary in response to hCG. In later stages, the placenta directly produces enough progesterone to maintain the pregnancy.

Throughout pregnancy, the concentration of **parathyroid hormone** (PTH) is increased by approximately 40% with almost no change in the amount of free calcium, thus suggesting a new set point for the secretion of PTH. During pregnancy, calcitonin does not increase predictably, whereas 1,25-dihydroxyvitamin D is increased and promotes increased intestinal calcium absorption. These changes permit the transfer of large amounts of calcium to the developing fetus.

Elevated estrogen concentration stimulates increased hepatic production of cortisol binding globulin and the hepatic clearance of cortisol decreases. Thus, the absolute plasma concentrations of both total and free cortisol are several times higher during pregnancy. The diurnal rhythm of cortisol, higher in the morning and lower in the evening, is maintained. Plasma concentrations of aldosterone and deoxycorticosterone are increased.

Increasing estrogen concentrations throughout pregnancy increase the secretion of prolactin up to tenfold. Conversely,

high estrogen concentrations during pregnancy suppress the secretion of luteinizing hormone (LH) and follicle-stimulating hormone (FSH). Baseline concentrations of other pituitary hormones, such as thyroid-stimulating hormone (TSH), remain approximately unchanged. Although normal pregnancy is a euthyroid state, many changes occur in thyroid function.[3] For example, high concentrations of thyroxine-binding globulin (TBG) increase the concentrations of total thyroxine (T$_4$) and triiodothyronine (T$_3$), but free T$_4$ concentration decreases slightly during the second and third trimesters. Very few (0.2%) pregnant individuals develop hyperthyroidism, and hypothyroidism is also rare (~ 2%). Postpartum thyroid dysfunction is common and is frequently unrecognized. Thyroid screening in pregnancy is recommended for high-risk women but is controversial for others.[3] Thyroid hormone results should be interpreted using trimester-specific and method-specific reference intervals.

Functional Development of the Fetus

Fetal organs mature during the third trimester but not at the same rate. This section reviews the (1) lung, (2) liver, (3) kidneys, and (4) blood maturation in the fetus.

Lungs and Pulmonary Surfactant

In healthy air-breathing lungs, a substance called **pulmonary surfactant** coats the alveolar epithelium and responds to alveolar volume changes by reducing surface tension in the alveolar wall during exhalation. Surfactant is needed because surface tension is an inverse function of the radius of the airway. Thus, small alveoli have a higher collapsing force than larger alveoli. Surfactant opposes the force and keeps the small alveoli from collapsing. Specialized alveolar cells called *type II granular pneumocytes* synthesize pulmonary surfactant and package it into laminated storage granules called *lamellar bodies*. These storage granules are 1 to 5 μm in diameter and contain (1) phospholipids, (2) cholesterol, and (3) protein. Production starts as early as 20 weeks of gestation, but adequate amounts do not accumulate until about 36 weeks. Fetal breathing movements transport lamellar bodies into the amniotic fluid. The newborn lung contains 100 times more surfactant per cm^3 than the adult lung. Excessive surfactant is needed at birth as the newborn transitions from breathing amniotic fluid to breathing air. Surfactant overcomes the surface tension produced in water-filled alveoli that are admitting air for the first time.

Pulmonary surfactant is a complex mixture of lipids and proteins; less than 5% is composed of carbohydrates. Most of the lipid is phospholipid, and most of that is lecithin (phosphatidylcholine). Unlike lecithin from other tissues, pulmonary lecithin has two saturated fatty acids, usually palmitoyl groups. Other lipids present are (1) phosphatidylglycerol (PG), (2) phosphatidylinositol (PI), and (3) phosphatidylethanolamine (see Chapter 23). Sphingomyelin is present in very small amounts (2%). The protein fraction of lamellar bodies is approximately 4% and is composed of four surfactant-specific proteins: SP-A, SP-B, SP-C, and SP-D.

Liver

Hematopoiesis (formation and development of blood cells) occurs in the liver during the first two trimesters and is transferred to the fetal bone marrow during the third trimester. The liver is also responsible for (1) production of specific proteins such as albumin and clotting factors, (2) metabolism and detoxification of many compounds, and (3) secretion of substances such as bilirubin. The liver produces **alpha fetoprotein (AFP)**, which is measured as a clinically useful marker (discussed later in this chapter). Detoxification and bilirubin secretion mechanisms are immature until late in pregnancy and even in the first few months after birth. Thus premature infants often have high serum bilirubin concentrations and metabolize drugs poorly.

Kidneys

Toward the end of the first trimester, the fetal kidneys begin to produce urine, which is the main component of amniotic fluid. However, early nephrons cannot produce concentrated urine, and pH regulation is also limited. Complete maturation occurs after birth. Although kidneys are not required for fetal survival, amniotic fluid is required. Without fluid to breathe, the fetal lungs fail to develp properly. Thus newborns without kidneys die of pulmonary failure.

Fetal Blood Development

Fetal blood is produced (1) first by the embryonic yolk sac, (2) then by the liver, and (3) finally by the fetal bone marrow. The yolk sac produces three embryonic hemoglobins: Portland, Gower-1, and Gower-2. These normal embryonic hemoglobins are of little importance in clinical chemistry, because they are present in fetal blood only in the first trimester.

With the switch of erythropoiesis to the fetal liver and spleen, fetal hemoglobin (Hb F) production begins. Hb F consists of two α- and two γ-chains ($\alpha_2\gamma_2$). Small amounts of adult hemoglobin, Hb A ($\alpha_2\beta_2$), are also produced, but Hb F predominates during the remainder of fetal life. As the fetal bone marrow begins red cell production, Hb A production increases. At birth, fetal blood contains 75% Hb F and 25% Hb A. Hb F production rapidly diminishes during the first year of postnatal life. In normal adults, less than 1% of hemoglobin is Hb F. Hb F has a higher affinity for oxygen than does Hb A. Thus, in the placenta, oxygen (1) is released from the maternal Hb A, (2) diffuses into the chorionic villi, and (3) binds to the fetal Hb F. In addition, 2,3-diphosphoglycerate (2,3-DPG) does not bind Hb F and therefore cannot decrease its affinity for oxygen as occurs with Hb A.

Maternal and Fetal Health Assessment

For optimum healthcare during pregnancy, a woman should consult her physician before conception. Preconception evaluation should include (1) a medical, reproductive, and family history; (2) physical examination; and (3) laboratory tests.

Laboratory Testing

The following laboratory tests frequently are recommended as part of a preconception evaluation: (1) hematocrit, (2) blood type and Rh compatibility, (3) erythrocyte antibody screen, (4) Papanicolaou smear (or human papillomavirus [HPV] test), (5) urinalysis, (6) rubella titer, (7) **rapid plasma reagin (RPR) test**, (8) gonococcal and chlamydia DNA test, (9) cystic fibrosis carrier status, (10) human immunodeficiency virus (HIV) antibody, and (11) hepatitis B surface antigen (HBsAg). Depending on demographic risks, genetic testing for disorders such as (1) Tay-Sachs disease, (2) thalassemia, and (3) sickle cell disease may be offered. A careful diet history is warranted. Folic acid supplementation should be recommended to reduce the risk of **neural tube defects**.

Many women consult a physician a few days after a missed menses if they suspect they might be pregnant. A urine hCG test result is positive (meaning that the test detects hCG above an analytical detection limit) in over half of pregnant females on the day of the expected menses, that is, at about 2 weeks after conception. Screening for fetal neural tube defects and **Down syndrome**[10] should be offered to all pregnant patients.[8] Depending on diabetes risk, glucose tolerance testing should be performed immediately or at 24 to 28 weeks (see Chapter 33). Some physicians test selected patients for preterm labor risk at 24 to 30 weeks using a test for **fetal fibronectin (fFN)** in cervicovaginal fluid. Current methods that are used for monitoring fetal well-being include (1) maternal observation and recording of fetal movements, (2) ultrasound examination, and, based on limited evidence, (3) tests that monitor the fetal heart rate during random uterine contractions or fetal movement.

Clinical Specimens

Many different samples are used in clinical laboratory analysis before and during pregnancy. These include (1) paternal saliva, serum, and blood; (2) maternal saliva, serum, blood, and urine; (3) amniotic fluid obtained by amniocentesis or from pools of fluid in the vagina after rupture of the fetal membranes; (4) chorionic villi; (5) fetal blood obtained by percutaneous umbilical blood sampling; and (6) fetal tissue obtained by biopsy.

The technique of amniocentesis is described in Chapter 6. Additional information is found in the section on tests for evaluating FLM later in this chapter. Amniotic fluid is sometimes obtained immediately after transvaginal puncture of the bulging membranes. It is possible to use this fluid for analysis if it is not grossly contaminated with blood or vaginal secretions. Clinicians consider amniocentesis for patients with spontaneously ruptured membranes.

Small samples of placental tissue (chorionic villi) also are used for analysis. They are obtained with a catheter between 9 and 12 weeks gestation. Chorionic villi specimens have been used to (1) identify the fetal chromosomes (the karyotype), (2) determine enzyme activities, or (3) detect specific gene mutations. It is possible to perform this procedure earlier in pregnancy than amniocentesis, but it has a higher rate of fetal loss.

Diagnosis and Dating of Pregnancy

The most important aspects of pregnancy management are detection of pregnancy and establishing accurate estimates of fetal age. The most useful test for detecting pregnancy is the hCG test.

Qualitative tests for hCG in blood or urine are used primarily to screen for and diagnose pregnancy. Urine hCG tests are usually sufficient to diagnose and confirm a normal pregnancy when it has progressed beyond the first week after the missed period. However, serum hCG tests may detect pregnancy earlier than urine tests, and quantitative hCG tests are able to reveal problems in early pregnancy. In the first 8 weeks of pregnancy, the hCG concentration in maternal serum rises geometrically (Figure 44-2). Detectable amounts (~5 IU/L) are present in the serum 8 to 11 days after conception, which is in the third week of pregnancy as measured from the LMP. In practice, hCG usually becomes detectable in the urine at or around the same time it appears in the serum, although the interval is highly variable. For women aged 13 to 40, serum hCG concentrations of 5 IU/L or greater are consistent with pregnancy. Concentrations in approximately half of pregnant women reach 25 IU/L on the first day of their missed period. The peak concentration occurs at about 8 to 10 weeks and is about 100,000 IU/L. Subsequently, hCG concentrations start to decline and by the end of the second trimester, a 90% reduction from peak concentration has usually occurred. The presence of twins approximately doubles hCG concentrations.

False-positive or increased serum hCG test results have been obtained from qualitative and quantitative assays when **human antimouse antibodies (HAMA)** or other interfering antibodies are present. If suspected, investigative experiments include (1) testing a urine specimen for the presence of hCG, (2) serially diluting the serum to confirm an appropriate dose response, (3) testing the serum using a different hCG method, and (4) retesting the serum after treatment with interfering antibody blocking agents.

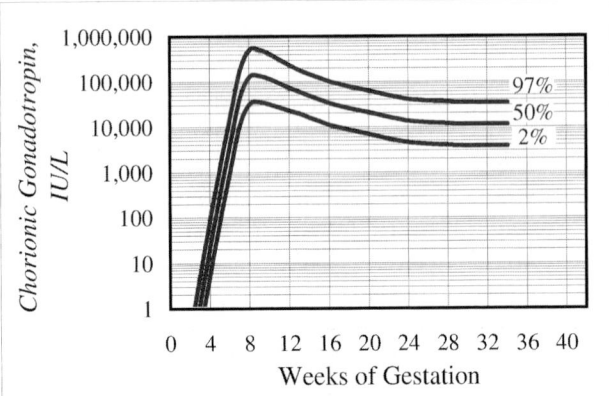

Figure 44-2 Concentration of human chorionic gonadotropin (hCG) in maternal serum as a function of gestational age. *Lines* represent the 2nd, 50th, and 97th percentiles. The maternal serum values from 14 to 25 weeks are medians calculated from 24,229 pregnancies from testing performed at ARUP Laboratories Inc. from January to October 1997. *(Redrawn from Ashwood ER. Evaluating health and maturation of the unborn: the role of the clinical laboratory. Clin Chem 1992;38:1523-1529. Permission granted from Clin Chem.)*

Complications of Pregnancy

Although most pregnancies progress without problems, complications can occur in the (1) mother, (2) placenta, or (3) fetus.

Abnormal Pregnancies

Conditions arising primarily in the mother include (1) **ectopic pregnancy**, (2) **hyperemesis gravidarum**, (3) **preeclampsia**, (4) **HELLP syndrome**, (5) liver disease, (6) Graves disease, and (7) HDN. The clinician must distinguish abnormal changes in laboratory tests from normal physiological changes induced by pregnancy (see Table 44-2).

Ectopic Pregnancy and Threatened Abortion[5]
When a fertilized egg implants in a location other than the body of the uterus, the condition is called an ectopic pregnancy. Most abnormal implantations occur in the fallopian tube; they can also occur in the abdomen, although this is rare. Tubal rupture and hemorrhage are serious and life-threatening complications of ectopic pregnancy. About 25% of individuals with an ectopic pregnancy have classic symptoms of (1) lower abdominal pain, (2) vaginal bleeding, and (3) an adnexal mass. Of all individuals with these symptoms, about 15% have an ectopic pregnancy, and a smaller percentage have incomplete or complete spontaneous abortion. A pregnant patient has about a 1 in 200 chance of dying from an ectopic pregnancy. Management of ectopic pregnancy is surgical (by laparoscopy) or medical (with intramuscular administration of methotrexate). Early detection and proper management of ectopic pregnancy are the most effective means of preventing maternal morbidity and mortality.

Preeclampsia and Eclampsia
Preeclampsia is a pregnancy condition characterized by (1) hypertension, (2) proteinuria, and often (3) edema. It occurs late in the second trimester or early in the third trimester, and affecting 5% to 10% of pregnancies. If the mother develops convulsions, the condition is called **eclampsia**. Its cause is not known but research suggests that abnormal formation of the placenta may have a role. Most maternal deaths are due to central nervous system complications, but ischemic liver damage may also occur. The only cure for preeclampsia is delivery of the placenta.

HELLP Syndrome
The HELLP syndrome (hemolysis, elevated liver enzymes, and low platelet counts in association with preeclampsia) is a life-threatening obstetric complication that occurs in 0.1% of pregnancies. Its most prominent features are thrombocytopenia and disseminated intravascular coagulation. Most cases occur between the 27th and 36th weeks of pregnancy, but the syndrome also may occur postpartum. Women typically present with (1) epigastric or right upper quadrant pain, (2) malaise, (3) nausea, (4) vomiting, (5) headache, and (6) jaundice that occurs in 5% of patients. Lactate dehydrogenase (LD) activities may be very high, and alanine aminotransferase

(ALT) and aspartate aminotransferase (AST) activities are usually 2 to 10 times their upper reference limits. Treatment is delivery. Postpartum management of the patient may require plasmapheresis or organ transplantation. Recurrence rates are 3% to 27%.

Liver Disease

Several liver disorders are unique to pregnancy. These include (1) hyperemesis gravidarum, (2) **cholestasis of pregnancy**, and (3) **acute fatty liver of pregnancy**. These disorders must be distinguished from the normal physiological changes of pregnancy (see Table 44-2). Significant changes normally seen in pregnancy include a dilutional decrease in serum albumin and elevation of alkaline phosphatase (from the placenta). Notably, (1) total bilirubin, (2) 5'-nucleotidase, (3) γ-glutamyltranspeptidase (GGT), (4) ALT, and (5) AST are unchanged in mothers with a normal pregnancy. Changes in these analytes may reflect hepatobiliary disease.

Hyperemesis Gravidarum

Hyperemesis gravidarum is characterized by nausea and vomiting and, in severe cases, dehydration and malnutrition. It typically occurs in the first trimester. When hyperemesis is severe enough to cause dehydration, abnormal liver enzyme values—usually less than four times the upper reference limit—are seen in approximately 50% of patients. Mild hyperbilirubinemia may occur. However, significant liver disease does not occur, and liver biopsy results are normal. Low birth weight babies are common, especially for women who develop malnutrition.

Cholestasis of Pregnancy

Cholestasis of pregnancy usually occurs in the third trimester and is manifested clinically by diffuse pruritus and, in 10% of patients, jaundice. Typical features of cholestasis, including pale stools and dark urine, are present and last until delivery. Women who experience cholestasis while taking oral contraceptives usually develop cholestasis of pregnancy. Serum bilirubin rarely exceeds 5 mg/dL. Alkaline phosphatase is typically two to four times the upper reference limit. Aminotransferase enzyme activities are mildly elevated. Prothrombin time may be elevated because of vitamin K malabsorption. Although many clinicians order serum bile acids in this setting, this test is rarely necessary for diagnosis. The condition itself is benign, but is associated with increased risk of premature birth and fetal death. It recurs with subsequent pregnancies.

Acute Fatty Liver of Pregnancy

Acute fatty liver of pregnancy occurs in approximately 1 in 10,000 pregnancies and is characterized by accumulation of microvesicular fat in the hepatocytes. Many cases of this maternal disorder are caused by an inherited mitochondrial fatty acid oxidation disorder in the fetus. The disease typically occurs at week 37 and is manifested clinically by rapid onset of (1) malaise, (2) nausea, (3) vomiting, and (4) abdominal pain. Mild elevations—less than six times the upper reference limits—of the aminotransferases occur, with the AST activity

typically greater than that of the ALT. Serum bilirubin is usually greater than 6 mg/dL. Life-threatening hypoglycemia may occur. Hyperuricemia, presumably from tissue destruction and renal failure, is characteristic. Liver histology shows acute fatty infiltration with little necrosis or inflammation. If untreated, fulminant hepatic failure with hepatic encephalopathy results. Treatment is immediate termination of the pregnancy, at which time rapid recovery usually occurs. Infant and maternal mortality is approximately 50% and 20%.

Non–Pregnancy-Related Liver Disease in Pregnancy

Pregnancy does not preclude the acquisition or aggravation of non–pregnancy-related liver disease. Thus, cholestasis during pregnancy may reflect the presence of (1) hepatotoxicity from drugs, (2) primary biliary cirrhosis, (3) Dubin-Johnson syndrome, or (4) cholelithiasis (see Chapter 37).

Viral hepatitis occurs with the same frequency in pregnancy as would be expected in a comparable age group. Women who acquire hepatitis B late in pregnancy or who are chronic carriers are likely to transmit the disease to their babies. This is especially so if the mother is hepatitis B e antigen (HBeAg) positive. The outcome in the infant varies from fulminant hepatitis (rare and usually in anti–HBeAg-positive mothers) to mild hepatitis to chronic hepatitis (the usual outcome in 90% of chronically infected woman). In the US, pregnant women are screened for hepatitis B with HBsAg testing. If positive, their babies are immunized with hepatitis B immune globulin and hepatitis B vaccine. Babies born to hepatitis C–positive mothers usually have the passively transmitted antibody for several months, but transmission of active hepatitis is unusual. Because there is no known treatment for the newborn, screening is not recommended for hepatitis C virus infection.

Neonatal Thyroid Function

During the first trimester of pregnancy, the fetus is dependent on the mother for its supply of thyroid hormone. Low maternal thyroid hormone concentrations (overt or subclinical hypothyroidism) have been associated with adverse outcomes, such as (1) **preterm delivery**, (2) fetal death, and (3) a reduced intelligence quotient (IQ) in children. Later in pregnancy, the fetal thyroid-pituitary axis functions independently from the mother's axis in most cases. However, if the mother has preexisting Graves disease (see Chapter 42), her autoantibodies are able to cross the placenta and stimulate the fetal thyroid gland. Thus, it is possible for the fetus to develop hyperthyroidism.

Hemolytic Disease of the Newborn

HDN is a fetal hemolytic disorder caused by maternal antibodies directed against antigen on fetal erythrocytes. Commonly used synonyms for this disorder are (1) isoimmunization disease, (2) Rh isoimmune disease, (3) Rh disease, (4) D isoimmunization, and (5) **fetal erythroblastosis**. Any of a large number of erythrocyte surface antigens, such as (1) Rh(CcDEe), (2) A, (3) B, (4) Kell, (5) Duffy, (6) Kidd, and (7) others, may be responsible for isoimmune hemolysis. In the past, disease severity was assessed by measuring the amount of bilirubin in the amniotic fluid. Presently ultrasonographic determination of middle fetal cerebral artery velocity is replacing amniotic fluid bilirubin for the assessment of fetal hemolytic anemia.

Causative Factors and Consequences

Maternal sensitization may occur in response to blood transfusion or a pregnancy in which the fetus has a blood cell antigen that the mother lacks. Antibodies against RhD are the most common cause of HDN, although antibodies against other erythrocyte antigens also cause disease. The resulting antibodies are actively transported across the placenta and into the fetus, where they cause destruction of fetal erythrocytes. The severity of the resulting hemolysis is influenced by antibody (1) specificity, (2) titer, and (3) transfer rate, as well as by the (4) functional maturity of the fetal spleen in which sensitized erythrocytes are destroyed.

With HDN, fetal erythrocytes are destroyed. The resulting anemia stimulates the fetal marrow and extramedullary erythropoiesis in the liver and spleen to replace destroyed erythrocytes. Extramedullary erythropoiesis destroys hepatocytes and leads to decreased production of serum albumin and decreased oncotic pressure in the intravascular space. When severe, these changes lead to congestive heart failure and generalized fetal edema, a condition referred to as **hydrops fetalis**, which carries a very grave prognosis. Without therapeutic intervention, intrauterine demise soon follows.

Clinical Management of Sensitized Mothers

To identify sensitized women, an alloantibody screen is performed at the first prenatal visit. If an antibody to an erythrocyte antigen is identified, the titer is determined. The *critical anti-RhD titer*, defined as the titer associated with risk for fetal hydrops, is usually 1:8 to 1:32, although studies of critical titer are quite disparate. For all sensitized women, the paternal erythrocyte phenotype is determined. If the father is RhD negative, then no follow-up studies are required. If he is D positive, then zygosity (presence of one or two copies of the gene) is determined. Although this has historically been estimated from Rh antigen phenotypes, DNA testing for RhD zygosity is more reliable. If the father is homozygous, all of his offspring are assumed to be RhD positive, negating the need for fetal RhD testing. Fetal RhD genotyping from cultured amniocytes is required if the father is heterozygous or is not available for testing. To guard against a false negative caused by a paternal RhD gene rearrangement (occurring in about 1.5% of Caucasians), the father is also genotyped. A frequent occurrence in those of African ancestry is an RhD pseudogene; the patient is RhD negative by serology, but RhD positive on genotype. If the fetus is RhD genotype positive, the mother (who is RhD negative serologically) should be tested for RhD genotype. In practice, laboratories have begun to offer fetal Rh genotyping using cell-free fetal DNA that circulates in maternal blood.

For sensitized mothers with an at-risk fetus, serial titers are performed on maternal serum every month until 24 weeks gestation, then every 2 weeks thereafter. If a critical titer anti-D is detected, ultrasound Doppler measurements are used to determine the peak velocity of blood flow in the fetal middle cerebral artery. Higher velocity is a strong indicator of fetal anemia. If Doppler velocimetry is not available, amniocentesis is performed every 10 to 14 days to assess the bilirubin concentration in amniotic fluid. The procedure to estimate the bilirubin concentration was originally called ΔOD_{450} (*change in optical density at a wavelength of 450 nm*), and that term is still encountered, but now the preferred clinical chemistry term is ΔA_{450} (*change in absorbance at a wavelength of 450 nm*). Serial testing is indicated every 10 to 14 days. Decreasing values are reassuring and indicate an unaffected or RhD-negative fetus. Values that plateau or increase suggest active hemolysis, which may require therapeutic intervention including ultrasound-guided umbilical blood sampling to determine (1) fetal blood type, (2) hemoglobin concentration, (3) presence of an antibody, (4) reticulocyte count, and (5) total bilirubin concentration. Intrauterine intravascular blood transfusion is performed if indicated. If fetal pulmonary maturation has occurred (usually 35 weeks or greater), delivery is indicated.

Trophoblastic Disease

Serum hCG determinations are very useful for monitoring patients with (1) trophoblastic disease, (2) germ cell–derived neoplasms or, rarely, (3) other hCG- producing tumors. Use of hCG in these diseases is discussed in Chapter 20.

Fetal Anomalies

Fetal anomalies that are detected by prenatal screening include (1) **neural tube defects**, (2) Down syndrome, and (3) **trisomy 18**.

Neural Tube Defects

Neural tube defects are serious abnormalities that occur early in embryonic development. By 19 days after fertilization, the area that is to form the central nervous system (brain and spinal cord) has differentiated into a plate of cells. The flat plate then rolls up, and its edges fuse into a hollow neural tube that drops into the embryo to develop just underneath what will become the skin of the back. Neural tube formation is normally complete 4 weeks after fertilization. Failure of neural tube fusion leads to permanent developmental defects of the brain, spinal cord, or both. These defects are called (1) anencephaly, (2) spina bifida (the most common defect being a meningomyelocele), and (3) encephalocele. Although many causes are known, about 90% fall into the classification of multifactorial inheritance. Folic acid deficiency is clearly associated with increased frequency of neural tube closure defects. Since 1997, grain products in the United States and Canada have been fortified with 140 µg folic acid/100 g, but the amount added is unlikely to be sufficient to reduce birth prevalence by more than about 30%. Most vitamin supplements contain 400 µg of folic acid, which is the dose recommended daily by authorities.

The birth prevalence of open neural tube defects varies with factors such as (1) geographic location (higher in the Eastern United States, lower in the West), (2) race (lower in black), (3) ethnicity (higher in Scotch-Irish), (4) family history (higher with prior births of affected individuals), and (5) maternal weight (higher in obese women). An average figure for the United States is 1 open neural tube defect per 1000 pregnancies (about 1 in 2000 for each individual defect).

Down Syndrome

Down syndrome (trisomy 21) is the most common serious disorder of the autosomal chromosomes, occurring in 1 in 700 live births. An extra copy of chromosome 21 produces a phenotype consisting of (1) moderate to severe mental retardation, (2) hypotonia (low muscle tone), (3) congenital heart defects, and (4) a flat facial profile. Most often an affected child has three copies of chromosome 21, but 5% of cases are caused by translocations (a transfer of a chromosomal segment to a new position) and 1% of cases are mosaics (the presence of two or more populations of cells with different genotypes in one individual who has developed from a single fertilized egg). A woman's risk of having a Down syndrome baby increases slowly up to age 30 and then steadily increases between ages 30 and 45 to a plateau.

Trisomy 18

Trisomy 18 (Edwards syndrome) is caused by a nondisjunction event (failure either of two homologous chromosomes to pass to separate cells during the first meiotic division or of the two chromatids of a chromosome to pass to separate cells during mitosis or during the second meiotic division) during meiosis. This results in a fetus having an extra copy of chromosome 18. Although it occurs in only 1 in 8,000 births, it is probably the most common chromosome defect at the time of conception. The dramatic change in prevalence is due to the very high fetal loss rate both before 8 weeks (>80%) and during the second and third trimesters (~70%). Approximately 25% of affected fetuses have meningomyelocele (spina bifida) or **omphalocele** (abdominal wall defect). A high cesarean section rate has been reported for undiagnosed cases. Following birth, 50% of infants die within the first 5 days and 90% die within 100 days.

Preterm Delivery

The leading cause of neonatal morbidity and mortality in the United States is preterm delivery, defined as delivery before 37 weeks gestation. Approximately 300,000 to 500,000 preterm births occur each year.[11] Rupture of the fetal membranes before the onset of uterine contractions is known as **premature rupture of membranes (PROM)**. When this occurs at less than 37 completed weeks gestation, it is referred to as preterm PROM and is responsible for nearly one third of preterm deliveries.

The cause of preterm labor is unknown, but it is likely that many factors are involved. Several mechanisms have been supported by a considerable amount of clinical and experimental evidence and include (1) pathological distention of the uterus, (2) decidual hemorrhage, (3) activation of the maternal-fetal hypothalamic-pituitary-adrenal axis, and (4) intrauterine infection or inflammation. fFN may be used for evaluating patients suspected of having preterm labor. The fFN test is described later, in the section entitled "Analytical Methodology."

Premature Rupture of Membranes

PROM is a complication in 3% of pregnancies. Risk factors for preterm PROM include (1) a history of preterm PROM, (2) genital tract infection, (3) antepartum bleeding, and (4) smoking. Most women who experience PROM will deliver their infants within 1 week. Management of preterm PROM varies according to the gestational age of the fetus and the presence or absence of maternal/fetal infection. For PROM that occurs at 34 to 36 weeks gestation, delivery of the infant has been shown to reduce maternal and fetal infection rates compared with expectant management. When it occurs at 32 to 33 weeks, FLM might assist in decision-making regarding delivery. If the fetal lungs are immature, conservative management with close fetal monitoring is necessary in conjunction with antibiotic therapy and administration of corticosteroids to accelerate lung development. Because of the high risk of severe neonatal morbidity and mortality, women with PROM at less than 32 weeks of gestation are managed conservatively in an attempt to prolong pregnancy to 32 weeks. Interventions include (1) antibiotic therapy, (2) administration of medications to suppress preterm labor (tocolytics), and (3) fetal monitoring.

Fetal Lung Maturity

Respiratory distress syndrome (RDS) is the most common critical problem encountered in clinical management of preterm newborns. The risk of RDS is inversely related to gestational age at the time of birth. Affected infants require supplemental oxygen and mechanical ventilation to remain properly oxygenated. The disorder is caused by a deficiency of *pulmonary surfactant*. In healthy lungs, surfactant coats the alveolar epithelium and responds to alveolar volume changes by reducing surface tension in the alveolar wall during expiration. When the quantity of surfactant is deficient, many of the alveoli collapse on expiration and thereby overinflate the remaining airways. The lungs become progressively noncompliant (rigid), and blood flowing through the capillary beds of collapsed alveoli fails to oxygenate. During the first few hours of life, affected infants develop (1) tachypnea with or without cyanosis, (2) nasal flaring, (3) expiratory grunting, and (4) intercostal retractions. The disease worsens during the next few days and usually is worse on the third or fourth day of life. Infants at risk for developing RDS have been treated with intratracheal administration of exogenous surfactant immediately at birth.

Prenatal Screening for Fetal Defects

Prenatal screening is the process of identifying pregnancies at sufficiently high risk of a serious birth defect, such as Down syndrome, to warrant invasive diagnostic testing.[1,12] Before 2003, most obstetricians offered amniocentesis for fetal karyotype determination to all mothers who would be 35 years of age or older at the time of birth. However, in 2002, almost 14% of pregnant women in the United States were 35 or older, and these women accounted for 51% of Down syndrome pregnancies. Therefore, if maternal age alone were used for screening, half of Down syndrome pregnancies would not be detected, and cases in younger women would not be detected at all. The risk for Down syndrome calculated using screening is more accurate than the use of maternal age alone, and it is now recommended by the American College of Obstetricians and Gynecologists (ACOG) to offer screening to women of all ages.

Terminology and Method of Risk Calculation in Prenatal Screening

Calculation of risk in prenatal screening depends on the pregnancy's prior risk and the pattern of test results.

Multiple of the Median

In clinical screening, the **multiple of the median (MoM)** is the statistic used to normalize analyte values. The initial step in calculating a MoM is to develop a set of median values for each week (or, preferably, each day) of gestation, using the laboratory's own assay values measured on the population to be screened. Individual test results are then expressed as the MoM by dividing each individual analyte value by the median at the relevant gestational age. The MoM is now universally used as a common factor for converting analyte values into an interpretative unit and serves as the starting point for calculating screening results for (1) neural tube defects, (2) Down syndrome, and (3) trisomy 18.

Calculating Individualized Patient-Specific Risks Using Multiple Biochemical Measurements

Measurements of each analyte are made on a maternal serum sample, and the results in mass units are converted to MoM for the appropriate week (or day) of gestation. This MoM value is then adjusted for other variables, such as maternal weight and race (as described later in this chapter). The individualized risk (patient-specific risk) for any given condition is determined by multiplying the *a priori* (or pre-test) risk for that condition by a likelihood ratio that is calculated using the woman's MoM values as shown in the following equation:

$$\text{Patient risk} = A \; priori \; risk \times \text{Likelihood ratio}$$

The *a priori* risk is obtained from large epidemiologic studies that ascertain the prevalence for the condition under consideration. For example, a woman's age is used to define her *a priori* risk for having a fetus with Down syndrome. The likelihood ratio is determined by calculating the ratio of the heights of the affected and unaffected overlapping population distributions for any specified MoM value. When multiple tests are used, a single likelihood ratio is calculated using the overlapping distributions for each test but with the correlation between tests taken into account. This final risk is the screening variable upon which clinical decisions are made.

Second Trimester Screening Tests

Maternal serum screening began in the 1970s with the use of second trimester serum testing for neural tube defects and progressed to include screening for Down syndrome and trisomy 18.

Neural Tube Defects

In the early 1970s, Brock and colleagues demonstrated that AFP concentrations were increased in the amniotic fluid of mothers carrying fetuses affected with an open neural tube defect. Subsequently, it was shown that AFP concentrations also were increased in the maternal serum of affected pregnancies. However, the distribution of AFP concentrations in serum in affected and unaffected pregnancies overlapped considerably indicating that maternal serum AFP would be useful only as an initial screening test to identify women at high risk for having an affected fetus. These women would then need to be referred for diagnostic procedures, such as (1) high-resolution ultrasound, (2) measurement of AFP, and (3) measurement of acetylcholinesterase in amniotic fluid to determine whether the fetus had an open neural tube defect. The use of maternal serum AFP to screen for open neural tube defects is a standard of care in the United States.

Down Syndrome

In 1984, an association between second trimester maternal serum AFP concentrations and fetal Down syndrome was reported.[4] Maternal serum AFP concentrations are about 25% lower in Down syndrome than in unaffected pregnancies. This finding resulted in the use of AFP measurements in screening programs for Down syndrome. Subsequently, (1) unconjugated estriol (uE_3), (2) hCG, and (3) inhibin A (inhA) were added to screening regiments. This resulted in the use of "quadruple test" being commonly offered and found to provide a detection rate of approximately 80% for Down syndrome.

Trisomy 18

Prenatal screening studies have found that fetal trisomy 18 has a distinctive triple marker pattern that is different from the Down syndrome pattern (Table 44-3). For example, a risk-based algorithm has demonstrated that at a second trimester risk cutoff of 1:100, 60% of trisomy 18 pregnancies could be identified with about 0.5% of women having an initial positive screen.

Other Aneuploidies

Although chromosome disorders other than trisomies 21 and 18 are not part of routine screening, the marker patterns exhibited in maternal serum for some aneuploidies are similar. For example, hydropic Turner syndrome and **triploidy** of paternal origin have serum marker patterns resembling that of a Down syndrome pregnancy and sometimes are identified as high risk using this algorithm. Similarly, Turner syndrome without hydrops and triploidy of maternal origin are sometimes identified by the trisomy 18 risk algorithm. The pattern for trisomy 13 is variable (see Table 44-3).

Newer Screening Algorithms

Following extensive use of screening tests in the second trimester, newer tests have been introduced that use maternal serum collected in the first trimester.

First Trimester Combined Test

For patients seeking early diagnosis, screening for Down syndrome in the first trimester (10 to 13 weeks gestation) is

TABLE 44-3 Conditions Associated with Various Maternal Serum Screening Result Patterns

Condition	Second Trimester				First Trimester		
	AFP	hCG	uE₃	inhA	PAPP-A	hCG	NT
Amniocentesis	Normal to high	—	—	—	—	—	—
Anencephaly	Very high	—	Very low	—	—	—	—
Congenital nephrosis, duodenal atresia, encephalocele, esophageal atresia, gastroschisis, hydrocephalus, Meckel syndrome, omphalocele, sacrococcygeal teratoma	High	—	—	—	—	—	—
Cystic hygroma	High	—	—	—	—	—	Increased
Down syndrome	Low	High	Low	High	Low	High	Increased
Fetal blood contamination	High to very high	Unchanged	Unchanged	Unchanged	—	—	—
Molar pregnancy	Very low	Very high	Very low	Normal	—	—	—
Molar pregnancy (partial)	Low to normal	Very high	Low to normal	Normal	—	—	—
Myelomeningocele (open spina bifida)	High	—	—	—	—	—	—
Normal pregnancy	Low, normal, or high	Low, normal, or high	Low, normal, or high	Low, normal, or high	—	—	—
Overestimated gestational age	Low	High	Low	Normal	—	—	—
Preeclampsia	Normal to high	High	—	—	—	—	—
Pseudocyesis (imaginary pregnancy)	Undetectable	Undetectable	Undetectable	Undetectable	—	—	—
Smith-Lemli-Opitz syndrome (SLOS)	Low	Low	Very low	—	—	—	—
Spontaneous or impending pregnancy loss	Variable	Low or high	Low	Low or high	—	—	—
Steroid sulfatase deficiency (fetal)	Unchanged	Unchanged	Very low	Unchanged	—	—	—
Triploidy (paternal)	Variable	High	Low	High	Variable	Very high	—
Triploidy (maternal)	Variable	Low	Low	Low	Variable	Very low	—
Trisomy 13	Variable	Variable	Variable	Variable	Very low	Low	High
Trisomy 18	Low	Low	Very low	Normal	Very low	Very low	High
Turner syndrome without hydrops	Low	Low	Very low	Low	Variable	Variable	High
Turner syndrome with hydrops	Low	High	Very low	High	Variable	Variable	High
Twins and other multiple gestations	High	High	High	High	High	High	—
Underestimated gestational age	High	Low	High	Normal	—	—	—

AFP, Alpha fetoprotein; *hCG*, human chorionic gonadotropin; *inhA*, inhibin A; *NT*, nuchal translucency; *PAPP-A*, pregnancy-associated plasma protein A; *uE₃*, unconjugated estriol.

available.[13] This screening involves measurement of (1) maternal serum **pregnancy-associated plasma protein-A (PAPP-A)**, (2) hCG, and (3) fetal **nuchal translucency (NT) test**, the subcutaneous space between the skin and the cervical spine.

In 2003 and 2005,[4] two independent multicenter trials demonstrated that a combination of NT and the measurements of PAPP-A and hCG (termed the *combined test*) was comparable or slightly better than the second trimester quadruple test for Down syndrome screening, detecting about 85% of cases at a 5% false-positive rate. Also, a large study with comprehensive outcome tracking suggests that the detection rate for trisomy 18 is about 80% at a 0.3% positive rate.[4]

Integrated Test
The integrated test takes advantage of first and second trimester markers and avoids most of the limitations of stand-alone first trimester screening (Figure 44-3). With this approach, measurements of NT and PAPP-A are made in the first trimester but are usually not interpreted or acted upon until testing

in the second trimester is complete. In the second trimester, a second blood sample is collected and a quadruple test performed. Results from all six tests (1) NT, (2) PAPP-A, (3) AFP, (4) uE₃, (5) hCG, and (6) inhA are then combined into a single risk estimate. This approach detects 85% of Down syndrome cases at only a 1% false-positive rate.

Follow-Up Testing for Women with Screen-Positive Results
Recommended follow-up testing depends on the types of positive results obtained.

Neural Tube Defects[14]
Women who have a positive screening test result for an open neural tube defect should be offered genetic counseling and further testing. A low-resolution ultrasound examination may verify gestational age and identify other possible reasons for the increased AFP test results such as (1) inaccurate gestational dating, (2) recent fetal demise, (3) twins. Patients who have an unexplained

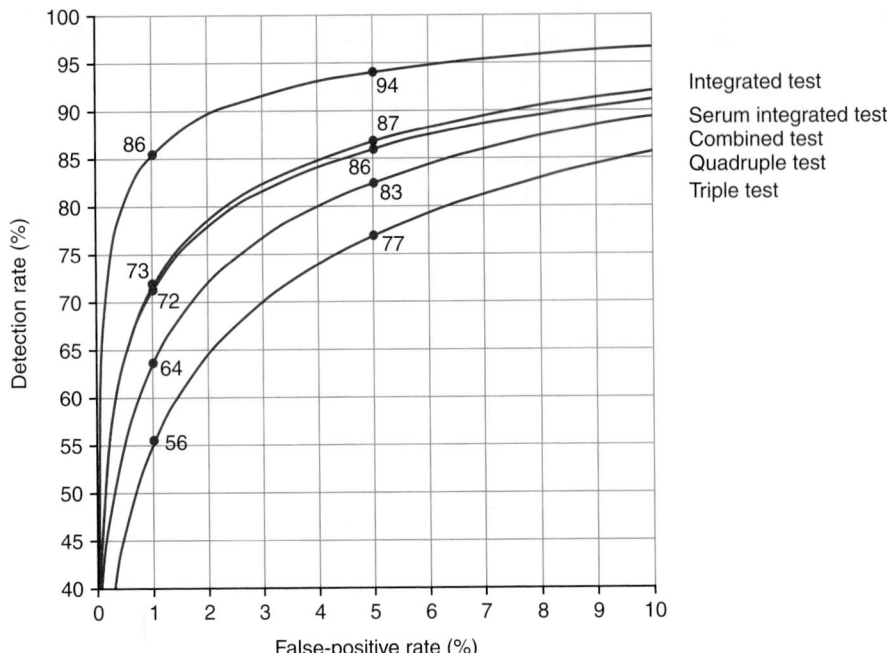

Figure 44-3 Relative performance of different prenatal screening tests.

high maternal serum AFP result are offered high-resolution ultrasound and/or amniocentesis for measurement of amniotic fluid AFP. Compared with maternal serum, the distribution of amniotic fluid AFP concentrations in pregnancies affected by open neural tube defects is far more separated from unaffected pregnancies. However, amniotic fluid AFP measurements are not by themselves diagnostic because of rare false-positive results. If the amniotic fluid is contaminated with even a small amount of fetal blood, as many as 2% to 3% of results can be falsely positive. Down syndrome. Women who have a positive screening test result for Down syndrome are usually referred for genetic counseling and further testing. A low-resolution ultrasound examination may be offered as a way to verify gestational age and to identify other possible reasons for the positive test result. One of the most common reasons for increased Down syndrome risk in the second trimester is overestimated gestational age.

Trisomy 18

In contrast to screening protocols for open neural tube defects and Down syndrome, a dating ultrasound is not recommended as the first step after a finding of increased risk of trisomy 18. The second trimester serum marker pattern (Figure 44-4) is not consistent with incorrect gestational dating, and amniocentesis should be offered. A high proportion of fetuses with trisomy 18 will have abnormal but non-diagnostic second trimester ultrasound findings (e.g., heart defects and clenched fists). Chorionic villi sampling (CVS) may be offered to patients at high risk of trisomy 18 based on first trimester screening results.

Adjustments for Factors That Influence Screening Measurements

Prenatal screening for both open neural tube defects and Down syndrome is optimized when each woman's analyte

values are compared with those of other women (the reference group). In addition to gestational age, this "similarity" extends to other factors that have been shown to affect analyte concentrations, including (1) maternal weight, (2) race, (3) insulin-dependent diabetes (IDD), (4) multiple pregnancy, and (5) use of assisted reproduction. Taking into account these factors enhances the accuracy of the interpretation.

Maternal Weight

As maternal weight increases, the average concentration of analyte values decreases, because a fixed amount of analyte is diluted in an increased maternal blood volume. Maternal weight is taken into account for all serum markers by adjusting each woman's MoM values by a factor corresponding to the expected MoM value for women with her weight. Distributions of maternal weight vary within each racial group with Asian women tending to have lower maternal weights than Caucasians and with blacks weighing more. It is optimal to apply adjustment equations for each racial group to correct marker concentrations for weight.

Maternal Race

For second trimester markers, black women have maternal serum AFP and hCG concentrations that are 10% to 15% higher than those found in Caucasian women. InhA concentrations are about 8% lower in blacks, and uE₃ concentrations are not different in these two populations.

Insulin-Dependent Diabetes

Maternal serum AFP values in women who require insulin before pregnancy have been reported to be systematically

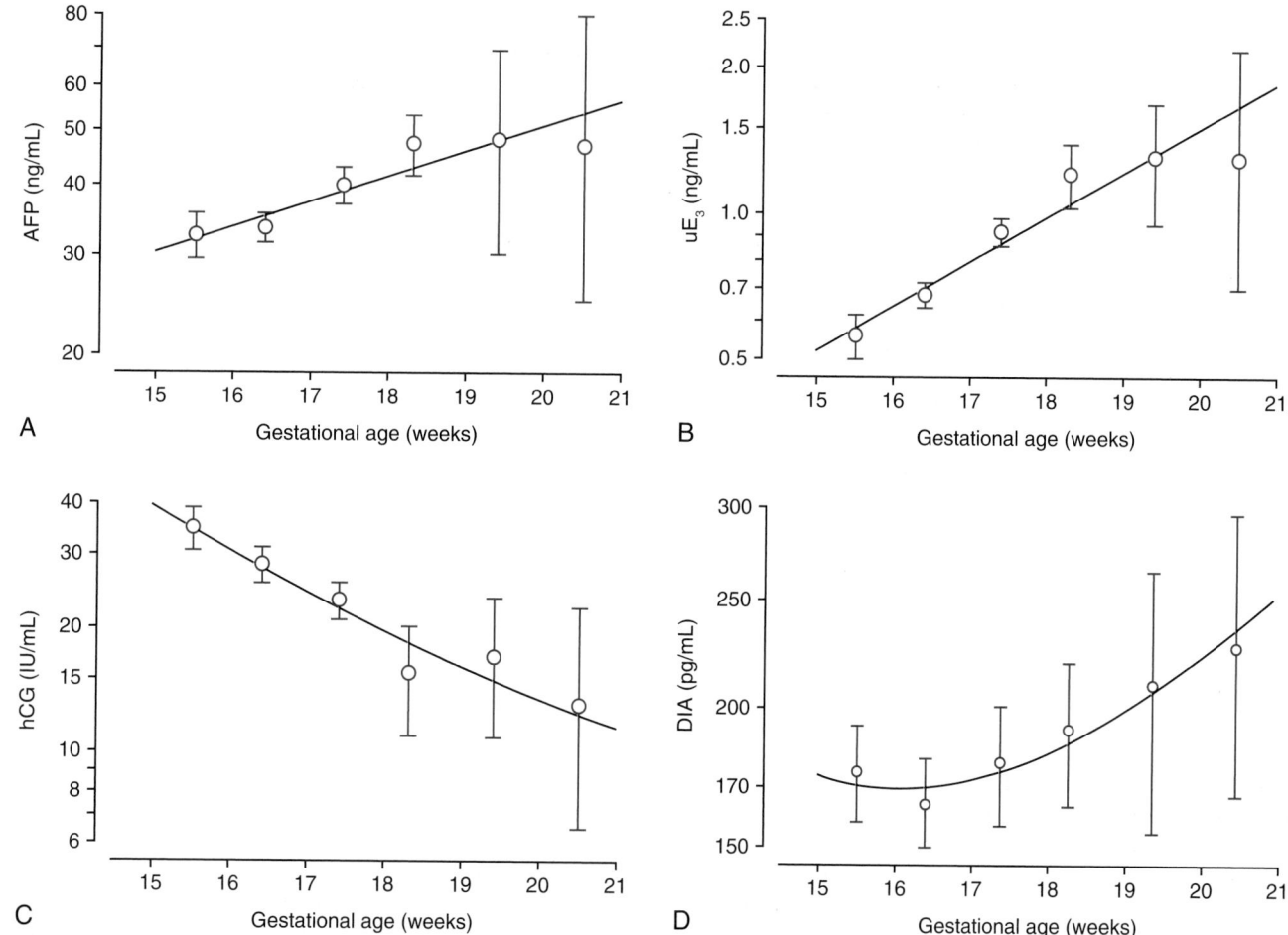

Figure 44-4 Typical median values for maternal serum alpha fetoprotein (AFP), unconjugated estriol (uE$_3$), human chorionic gonadotropin (hCG), and inhibin A (inhA) in the second trimester. The observed average gestational age is plotted on the horizontal axis, and the median of that week's marker measurements is plotted on the vertical logarithmic axis.

lower by about 20% (0.88 MoM). Women with type 2 diabetes, taking insulin or oral hypoglycemic agents, or on dietary restriction before pregnancy, also show reduced second trimester maternal serum AFP concentrations.

Twin Pregnancy

Maternal serum analyte concentrations in twin pregnancies are about twice the concentration found in singleton pregnancies. For example, the median and MoM values for the analytes measured in unaffected twin pregnancy are (1) AFP [2.0], (2) uE$_3$ [1.7], (3) hCG [1.9], (4) inhA [2.0] , and (5) PAPP-A [1.8].

Calculation of an approximate risk (sometimes called a pseudorisk) for twin pregnancy is possible. This is accomplished by dividing the MoM value for each analyte by the corresponding median found in unaffected twin pregnancies.

Pregnancies Achieved by Assisted Reproductive Technologies

As women are choosing to conceive at older ages, the use of **assisted reproductive technologies (ART)**, such as **in vitro fertilization (IVF)**, is increasing. Women who achieve pregnancy by IVF are about twice as likely to have a positive result of

second-trimester Down syndrome screening than are women who achieve pregnancy spontaneously. The increased rate is avoided with adjustment of MoM values for uE$_3$ (reduced to 0.9 MoM), hCG (increased to 1.0), and inhA (increased 1.2). These corrections restore an appropriate screen-positive rate. Pregnancies achieved by intrauterine insemination, with or without ovulation induction, show a similar trend in marker concentrations.

Analytical Methodology

In this section, methodologies for the measurement of (1) hCG, (2) AFP, (3) uE$_3$, (4) inhA, (5) PAPP-A, (6) fFN, (7) amniotic fluid bilirubin, and (8) tests for FLM are reviewed.

Human Chorionic Gonadotropin

Human chorionic gonadotropin is commonly abbreviated as hCG although it is often referred to simply as *chorionic gonadotropin (CG)*. Measurement of hCG assists in (1) diagnosing and dating pregnancy, (2) identifying ectopic pregnancies and other abnormalities, (3) managing certain neoplasms, and (4) predicting the risk of Down syndrome and trisomy 18.

Chemistry

hCG is a glycoprotein containing a protein core with branched carbohydrate sidechains that usually terminate with sialic acid. The hormone is a heterodimer composed of two nonidentical, non–covalently bound glycoprotein subunits—alpha (α) and beta (β). When the hCG dimer is dissociated, hormone activity is lost. It has a molecular weight of approximately 37,900 Da and a higher carbohydrate proportion than any other human hormone.

The hCG carbohydrate composition changes as pregnancy progresses. For example, in the first few weeks of pregnancy, more than 80% of hCG is a large molecular mass (41,000 to 42,000 Da) with additional monosaccharides in its carbohydrate chains called hyperglycosylated hCG (hCG-H). Serum concentrations of hCG-H decline rapidly after the fourth week, and the 37,900 Da molecular mass predominates for the remainder of the pregnancy. In addition to hCG and hCG-H, maternal serum includes numerous other hCG variants. To avoid confusion, the International Federation of Clinical Chemistry and Laboratory Medicine (IFCC) has recommended specific nomenclature for the identification of intact hCG and its variants. These include (1) nicked hCG (hCGn), (2) free α subunit (hCGα), (3) free β subunit (hCGβ), (4) nicked free β subunit (hCGβn), and (5) β core fragment (hCGβcf). The variant hCGn is produced from enzymatic cleavage of peptide bonds in hCGβ at position 44-45 (and, after prolonged incubation, at position 51-52) and is biologically inactive. The variant hCGβcf is the terminal degradation product of hCGβ and represents the 73 amino acid core of hCGβ. It is detected only in urine.

Biochemistry

The hCG hormone is synthesized in the syncytiotrophoblast cells of the placenta. Minute amounts may also be made by the pituitary glands of older men and women. A single gene located on chromosome 6 encodes the α subunit of all four glycoprotein hormones (TSH, LH, FSH, and hCG). Chromosome 19 contains a family of seven genes that encode the hCGβ subunit, although only three appear to be active. Separate messenger RNAs are transcribed from the respective genes, and the α and β subunits are translated from each. The subunits spontaneously combine in the rough endoplasmic reticulum and are continuously secreted into the maternal circulation.

Physiology

Physiologically, hCG stimulates the corpus luteum in the ovary to synthesize progesterone during the first weeks of pregnancy. The placenta makes inadequate amounts of progesterone during this time. No specific receptor for hCG is known; it binds to and activates the LH receptor in cells of the corpus luteum in the maternal ovary.

Methods

Measurement of hCG assists in (1) diagnosing and dating pregnancy, (2) identifying ectopic pregnancies and other abnormalities, (3) managing certain neoplasms, and (4) predicting the risk of Down syndrome and trisomy 18. Many assay techniques have been used to detect and/or measure hCG with immunoassay being the basis for the methods of choice and both qualitative and quantitative types are available.

Qualitative Methods

Numerous home (over-the-counter) kits or point-of-care (POC) devices are available for the qualitative detection of hCG in urine or serum and are widely used for the rapid identification of pregnancy. These methods for the qualitative detection of hCG in urine have been granted "**CLIA waived test**" status. These tests are designed to employ methodologies that are "so simple and accurate as to render the likelihood of erroneous results negligible." Consequently, they have found widespread applications in situations where a formally trained laboratorian is not available, such as at home and POC environments.

Regarding the latter application, POC devices are single-use methods that utilize immunochromatography for the rapid qualitative detection of hCG when its concentration exceeds a detection threshold, frequently 10 to 25 IU/L. Because qualitative hCG tests are used only for the detection of pregnancy, they are often designed to detect dimeric hCG using a combination of anti-hCGα and anti-hCGβ antibodies. However, the methods incorporated into some devices are designed to detect nondimeric hCG variants. First-morning specimens are preferred for qualitative POC urine pregnancy tests because they are the most concentrated.

Quantitative Methods

All commonly used quantitative hCG methods are immunometric assays designed to measure hCG over a wide range of concentrations. Upper limits of detection vary from 400 to 15,000 IU/L, and specimen dilution is frequently required to obtain an absolute measurement. The lowest detectable concentration of these assays varies from 1 to 2 IU/L.

Quantitative measurement of hCG is complicated by its molecular heterogeneity. Consequently, considerable variation in measured hCG concentrations is observed between the different methods due to the use of different antibody pairs in different hCG assays. For example, antibodies to hCG will recognize epitopes on the α subunit, the β subunit, or the αβ heterodimer, and consequently, analytical specificity is dependent on the specific pair of antibodies utilized. Another source of variation is the reference material used to calibrate hCG assays. Most hCG assays are calibrated against a World Health Organization (WHO) International Standard, which contains purified urinary hCG with an activity value determined by bioassay.[15] However, these materials also contain substantial amounts of hCGn and hCGβ which is problematic in that some hCG assays over- or under-recognize these variants or may not detect them at all. As a result, hCG assays currently lack harmonization and results from different hCG assays are not the same and cannot be directly compared.

CG measurements in early pregnancy generally are expressed as international units per liter (IU/L). A typical hCG concentration at 16 weeks is approximately 30,000 IU/L, and many laboratories express hCG concentrations in international units per milliliter (e.g., 30,000 IU/L is expressed as 30

IU/mL) (see Figure 44-2). A simple alternative is to use kilo-international units per liter, consistent with the international system for SI units, in which concentrations are expressed per liter.

Serum is used for quantitative hCG assays and is obtained from fasting or non-fasting women by standard phlebotomy techniques. When so collected, hCG is stable in maternal serum and can be shipped at ambient temperature and stored at 4 to 8 °C for 1 week. If testing is to be delayed beyond 1 week, serum should be stored at −20 °C.

Alpha Fetoprotein

The measurement of AFP in maternal serum and amniotic fluid is useful for detecting some serious fetal anomalies (see Table 44-3). For example, maternal serum AFP is elevated in 85% to 95% of cases of fetal open neural tube defects and is low in cases of fetal Down syndrome and trisomy 18. AFP measurement in nonpregnant patients may be used for monitoring certain cancers.

Chemistry

AFP is a glycoprotein having a molecular mass of ~70,000 Da and is synthesized from a gene on chromosome 4. The protein is composed of carbohydrate and a single polypeptide chain containing 591 amino acids. The carbohydrate composition varies depending on the organ of synthesis, the length of gestation, and the source of the specimen (fetal serum vs. amniotic fluid).

Biochemistry

AFP is produced initially by the fetal yolk sac in small quantities, and then by the fetal liver in larger quantities as the yolk sac degenerates. Trace amounts are also produced in the fetal gut and kidneys. Maximal concentration in fetal serum (~3 million µg/L) is reached at about 9 weeks gestation. The concentration then declines steadily to about 20,000 µg/L at term. The increase and decrease in concentration of AFP in the amniotic fluid roughly parallel those in the fetal serum, but the concentration is two to three orders of magnitude lower (~15,000 µg/L at 16 weeks gestation). Amniotic fluid AFP has been measured as early as 8 weeks. It rapidly decreases to its lowest point at 11 weeks, then increases to reach a second maximum at 13 weeks. The concentration then falls in a log-linear fashion until 25 weeks when the decline steepens.

In maternal serum, AFP is first detectable (~5 µg/L) at about the 10th week of gestation. The concentration increases about 15% per week to a peak of approximately 180 µg/L at 25 weeks. The concentration in maternal serum then subsequently declines slowly until term. After birth, the maternal serum AFP rapidly decreases to less than 2 µg/L. In an infant, serum AFP declines exponentially to reach adult concentrations by the 10th month of life. Factors that affect the concentration of AFP in maternal serum include (1) gestational age, (2) maternal weight, (3) the presence of insulin-dependent maternal diabetes mellitus, (4) maternal race, (5) the number of fetuses present, (6) fetal renal disorders that cause proteinuria, and (7) fetal structural anomalies.

Methods

Several commercial immunometric methods are available for the measurement of the concentration of AFP in body fluids. For example, AFP is measured in amniotic fluid using the same immunoassays as for maternal serum AFP after a suitable dilution (usually 1:50 to 1:200). Although two essentially equivalent international reference materials (WHO Reference Preparation for AFP [72-225] and British Standard [72-227]) calibrated in international units are available, most laboratories in the United States report AFP in nanograms per milliliter (micrograms per liter). The relationship between nanograms and international units usually is given as 1.21 ng = 1 IU, but conversion factors may vary by manufacturer, perhaps reflecting differences in the carbohydrate content of respective calibrators.

Serum specimens to be assayed for AFP are obtained from non-fasting women through standard phlebotomy techniques. AFP is very stable in maternal serum and can be shipped at ambient temperature and stored at 4 to 8 °C for 1 week or at −20 °C for years.

AFP in amniotic fluid is less stable than in serum, and leaving samples at room temperature for prolonged periods results in degradation of amniotic fluid AFP. As refrigeration of amniotic fluid compromises chromosome analysis, a portion of the collected fluid should be placed in the refrigerator as soon as possible after collection. Samples sent to reference laboratories should be shipped for next day delivery at ambient temperature or on ice packs if the outside temperature is high. The presence of fetal blood in amniotic fluid samples has been known to increase AFP results, and laboratories should note the presence of blood on the report. In the event of an increased amniotic fluid AFP result (usually >2.0 or 2.5 MoM), the laboratory should test for the presence of fetal blood. Laboratories that measure amniotic fluid AFP need to establish medians for each week between 13 and 25 weeks gestation.

Unconjugated Estriol

In current practice, measurement of urinary and serum estriol (E$_3$) is no longer recommended for the assessment of fetal well-being.[4] As a replacement, measurement of unconjugated estriol (uE$_3$) is now used routinely by most U.S. laboratories that provide screening for Down syndrome. This steroid, rather than total estriol (unconjugated plus conjugated estriol), is the most specific of the estrogens for identifying a fetus with Down syndrome.

Any disruption in its biosynthetic pathway will lead to very low concentrations of maternal serum uE$_3$. Conditions that cause disruption include (1) fetal anencephaly, (2) placental sulfatase deficiency, (3) fetal death, (4) chromosome abnormalities, (5) **molar pregnancy**, and (6) **Smith-Lemli-Opitz syndrome (SLOS)**. Placental sulfatase deficiency presents in the infant as X-linked ichthyosis (thick, scaly skin). It occurs in approximately 1 in every 2000 males. Because of the lack of uE$_3$, the mother often has delayed onset of labor, and the cesarean section rate is significantly higher in these mothers. SLOS is a serious, rare birth defect that is the result of an inborn error in cholesterol metabolism. Down syndrome leads to a modest decrease in uE$_3$. Molar pregnancy is an abnormal pregnancy that is caused by abnormal proliferation of placental tissue in the uterus. It is classified as a gestational trophoblastic disease that grows into a mass in the uterus that has swollen chorionic villi that resemble grapes.

Chemistry

E$_3$ is an estrogen with hydroxyl groups at positions 3, 16, and 17 (see Chapter 43). Although present in nonpregnant patients in very low concentrations, during late pregnancy this estrogen predominates. Only a minor amount (~10%) of the hormone circulates in plasma unconjugated and, because of its low solubility, this form is strongly bound to SHBG. The majority of E$_3$ exists as conjugates of glucuronate and sulfate. Conjugation occurs in the maternal liver, makes the hormone more soluble, and thus permits renal clearance.

Biochemistry

E$_3$ is produced in very large amounts during the last trimester of pregnancy. The biosynthetic pathway requires the (1) fetal adrenal gland, (2) fetal liver, and (3) placenta to be fully functioning. The fetal adrenal cortex possesses a unique zone for the production of steroids. The fetal adrenal avidly binds low-density lipoprotein to take in cholesterol, which is converted to two major steroid intermediates: pregnenolone sulfate and dehydroepiandrosterone sulfate (DHEA-S). The fetal liver, possessing 16α-hydroxylase, converts DHEA-S to 16α-hydroxy-DHEA-S, and finally, the placenta uses fetal 16α-hydroxy-DHEA-S to synthesize E$_3$. Approximately 90% of maternal serum E$_3$ is derived from this pathway. A minor amount is made using precursors from the maternal ovary. Concentrations typical for the second trimester of pregnancy are 0.70 to 2.50 µg/L, depending on the assay used.

Methods

Determination of uE$_3$ is difficult because of its low concentration. Nonisotopic, automated immunometric methods are commercially available. They are calibrated by the use of chemically pure E$_3$. E$_3$ values are reported in mass units (nanograms per milliliter or micrograms per liter) or SI units (nanomoles per liter). The equation for converting mass to SI units is:

$$1 \text{ ng/mL} \times 3.47 = 3.47 \text{ nmol/L}$$

Maternal serum specimens are obtained from fasting or non-fasting women by standard phlebotomy techniques. However, uE$_3$ is relatively unstable and the procedures for the (1) collection, (2) storage, and (3) shipment of maternal serum specimens need to be rigorously adhered to. For example, the uE$_3$ concentration increases in blood at room temperature and at 4 °C, because the conjugated forms are able to spontaneously deconjugate to form the parent hormone. Therefore collected blood should be allowed to clot, and then serum should be removed promptly. uE$_3$ is stable in serum for up to 7 days at 2 to 4 °C.

Inhibin A

In addition to the utility of inhibin A as a predictor of Down syndrome risk as discussed previously, inhibin A and B

measurements have applications in (1) ovarian cancer monitoring, (2) disorders of ovulation, and (3) early detection of viable pregnancy following IVF.

Chemistry

Inhibins are proteins consisting of dimers of dissimilar subunits (α and β) linked by disulfide bridges. The β subunit occurs in two closely related forms (β$_A$ and β$_B$), leading to two types of dimeric inhibin (inhibin A, αβ$_A$, and inhibin B, αβ$_B$). The mature form of inhibin, which has a molecular mass of approximately 32,000 Da, is produced by cleavage of larger precursor forms. Another group of related molecules, the activins, are dimers consisting of just the β subunits. InhA is the only form within the inbibin/activin family of proteins that provides sufficient discrimination to be useful in Down syndrome screening.

Biochemistry

Inhibins are members of the transforming growth factor-β (TGFβ) superfamily of proteins. They and their closely related activins are proteins that suppress or stimulate FSH secretion, respectively. In the reproductive system, inhibin and activin subunits are expressed in the (1) placenta, (2) granulosa cells of the ovary, and (3) Sertoli cells of the testis. InhA and inhibin B have distinctive serum profiles during the human menstrual cycle. InhA peaks in the luteal phase of the cycle, whereas inhibin B is maximal in serum during the mid-follicular phase with a peak at ovulation. In postmenopausal women, the concentrations of both forms of inhibin are non-detectable.

InhA is produced by the fetoplacental unit beginning in early pregnancy. InhA concentrations exhibit a complex pattern during the course of pregnancy, rising to a peak at 8 to 10 weeks gestation, declining to a minimum at 17 weeks, and then resuming to slowly increase to term. Unlike the other screening tests, average inhibin concentrations change relatively little from 15 to 20 weeks gestation. Typical values in the second trimester of pregnancy range from 50 to 400 ng/L with levels at 17 weeks gestation reaching a nadir of about175 ng/L.

Methods

Highly specific methods for measuring inhibins are available. Serum specimens to be assayed for inhibins are obtained from non-fasting women by standard phlebotomy techniques. InhA is stable in maternal serum with shipment at ambient temperature and storage at 4 to 8 °C for 1 week.

Pregnancy-Associated Plasma Protein A

Low concentrations of PAPP-A early in pregnancy have been associated with (1) Down syndrome, (2) a high rate of fetal loss, (3) poor fetal growth (intrauterine growth retardation), (4) premature delivery, (5) hypertension, and (6) preeclampsia.

Chemistry

PAPP-A is a zinc-containing metalloproteinase glycoprotein. Its gene is found on chromosome 9. It is translated into a 1,626 amino acid product, of which 1,546 amino acids compose the mature protein. Circulating PAPP-A is part of a larger molecular complex that includes two subunits of PAPP-A covalently bound to two subunits of a protein called the "pro major basic protein (pro MBP)", forming a heterotetramer. The PAPP-A complex has a molecular mass of about 500 kDa.

Biochemistry

PAPP-A t is expressed at low concentrations in many tissues, but high amounts of PAPP-A protein and mRNA are localized to placental tissues throughout gestation. PAPP-A immunoreactivity is found in syncytiotrophoblast cells.

Concentrations of maternal serum PAPP-A increase as gestation proceeds to term (Figure 44-5). These are critical to normal fetal growth because of its role as an insulin-like growth factor binding protein (IGFBP) protease. It regulates the action of **insulin-like growth factor** (II IGF-II) and predominantly cleaves IGFBP-4.

Methods

PAPP-A immunoassays are commercially available in the United States, in both manual and automated formats. However, their use is currently restricted for research use only. Serum specimens to be assayed for PAPP-A are obtained from fasting and non-fasting women by standard phlebotomy techniques. A small increase in PAPP-A concentrations has been reported for collection in plastic versus glass tubes. PAPP-A concentrations are stable in serum at 4 °C for 1 week or longer, depending on the assay used for testing.

Fetal Fibronectin

The concentration of fFN in cervical and vaginal secretions was proposed in 1991 as a test to aid in predicting preterm delivery.

Biochemistry

Fibronectin is a term for a family of ubiquitous adhesive glycoproteins that cross-link to collagen to bind cells together. These proteins are found on cell surfaces and in plasma and amniotic fluid. The fetus has a unique fibronectin that is defined by a monoclonal antibody, FDC-6. When labor begins and cellular adhesion between the placenta and the uterine wall is disrupted, the concentration of fFN in cervical and vaginal secretions increases. Mothers with more than 50 ng/mL (50 µg/L) of fFN in these secretions during the second and third trimesters have a higher risk for preterm delivery, whereas those below that cutoff are at decreased risk. A majority of patients with results greater than 50 ng/mL will, however, repair any placental disruption and successfully continue the pregnancy.

Method

In one commercial method, fFN is measured using a membrane immunoassay, which has a solid phase polyclonal goat anti-fFN antibody and an enzyme-labeled monoclonal anti-fFN. The specimen to be assayed for fFN is obtained by collecting cervical or vaginal mucus with a Dacron polyester swab. The fully saturated swab contains approximately 150 µL of fluid. The swab is placed into 750 µL of buffer. An aliquot of the diluted specimen is added to the cassette containing the antibodies and color development is measured and related to the concentration of fFN.

Placental Alpha Microglobulin-1

Placental alpha microglobulin-1 (PAMG-1) is a placental glycoprotein secreted into the amniotic fluid during pregnancy. Its concentration in amniotic fluid is 400 to 1,000 times greater than in maternal blood and up to 40,000 times greater than in cervicovaginal fluid with intact membranes. A test for PAMG-1 that exploits these large differences in concentration has been developed for clinical use as an aid for the detection of PROM.

A rapid immunochromatographic method is commercially that utilizes two monoclonal antibodies for the rapid detection of PAMG-1 in cervicovaginal fluid. The specimen is collected using a polyester swab that is placed into the vagina for 1 minute. The fluid obtained is eluted off the swab by rinsing it in a vial containing a buffer solution for 1 minute. After standing in buffer for 10 minutes, the test result is determined by visual inspection of a test and a control line on the lateral flow device. The analytical limit of detection of the test is 5 ng/mL.

This test is highly sensitive and specific for the detection of PROM. False-positive results may be caused by contamination of the specimen with large amounts of blood. False-negative results may occur if the specimen is collected 12 or more hours after a rupture that is subsequently obstructed by the fetus or is resealed.

Amniotic Fluid Bilirubin

The presence of bilirubin in amniotic fluid is an indicator of fetal erythroblastosis. As the concentration of bilirubin in amniotic fluid is generally too low (~0.01 to 0.03 mg/dL) to be measured by standard photometric techniques, a direct spectrophotometric method is used. The test is referred to as the ΔA_{450} test. In this procedure, the difference in the direct absorbance measured between 365 and 550 nm of an amniotic fluid is used to prepare a calibration curve. To interpret

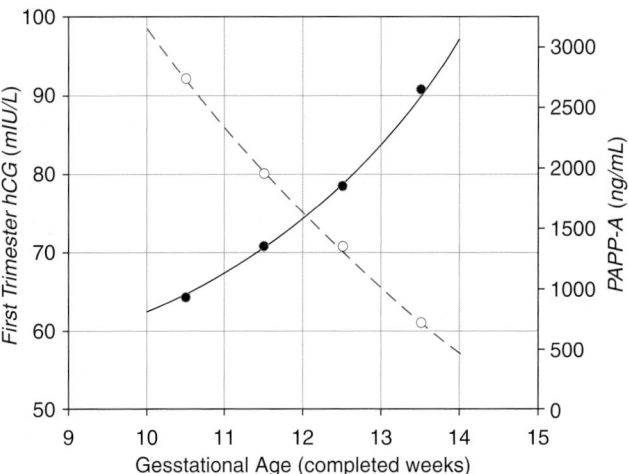

Figure 44-5 Typical median values for maternal serum pregnancy-associated plasma protein A (closed black circles) and total human chorionic gonadotropin (open red circles) in the first trimester. The observed average gestational age is plotted on the horizontal axis, and the median of that week's PAPP-A or total hCG measurements is plotted on the vertical axis.

the results obtained with this method, the gestational age of the fetus must be known as the amount of bilirubin present in amniotic fluid changes with gestational age.

Tests for Evaluating Fetal Lung Maturity[7]

Historically, FLM tests have been used to determine whether the best perinatal survival will be achieved in utero or in the nursery. Common situations in which FLM testing is requested include (1) before repeat cesarean delivery when the age of gestation is uncertain, (2) preterm labor, (3) PROM, (4) worsening maternal hypertension, (5) severe renal disease, (6) intrauterine growth retardation, or (7) fetal distress.[2]

Standards of Laboratory Practice

Several standards of laboratory practice for FLM testing have been published.[4,6] They contain recommendations regarding (1) specimen collection, (2) handling, (3) centrifugation, and (4) mixing that remain valid today. These recommendations include (1) assessment of FLM should be conducted prior to a delivery at less than 39 weeks gestation, (2) FLM tests should be selected based on sample quality, (3) hospital laboratories should offer a rapid FLM test in their laboratory or from a reference laboratory, (4) rapid FLM tests should be available daily on both a routine and emergency basis, and (5) laboratories should communicate the results of any FLM test immediately to the ordering location.

Collection and Handling of Amniotic Fluid Specimens for Fetal Lung Maturity Assessment

Amniotic fluid is obtained by transabdominal amniocentesis (see Chapter 6). In a multifetal pregnancy, there are usually separate sacs, each of which should be sampled. Vaginal pool specimens are rarely adequate for testing.

Whenever possible, the fluid should be tested immediately. If there is to be a delay of a few hours, the fluid should be refrigerated at 4 °C. The total phospholipid content of amniotic fluid does not change significantly during at least a week of storage, and lamellar bodies are stable for at least 30 days. It should be noted that a single freeze-thaw cycle decreases the **lamellar body count (LBC)**. Immediately before the fluid is tested, it should be gently inverted several times to obtain a uniform suspension.

Tests Used to Assess Fetal Lung Maturity

Tests used to assess FLM include measurement of (1) LBC, (2) PG content, and (3) Lecithin/Sphingomyelin (L/S) ratio.

Counting of Lamellar Bodies

Lamellar bodies have been counted directly using the platelet channel of whole blood cell counters. This test is termed the lamellar body count (LBC).

When counting lamellar bodies, the procedural step of centrifugation of the amniotic fluid sample is omitted. Also, mixing of the fluid is critical to obtain a homogenous suspension prior to testing. Because of different platelet identification algorithms, counts will be lower or higher on different instruments. Instruments that use similar techniques to count the

platelets (e.g., impedance) will show greater concordance than those that use different techniques.

Specimens containing mucus produce erratic results. In addition, contamination of the fluid with whole blood will decrease the LBC by presumably trapping them in a fibrin matrix. Contamination with even small amounts of meconium will produce dramatic increases in the LBC.

Clinical outcomes studies have reported that LBC has high clinical sensitivity (95% to 100%) but low clinical specificity (about 70%) for prediction of RDS.

Determination of Lecithin and Lecithin/Sphingomyelin Ratio

Chemically, lecithin is palmitate disaturated-phosphatidylcholine (DSPC). It is the major surfactant found in the lung representing 85% of total lecithins in the body.[4] Its concentration in amniotic fluid tends to rise with increasing gestational age. The concentration of lecithin in amniotic fluid is measured directly and is correlated with FLM, or its concentration is related to another lipid, sphingomyelin, and that ratio used to predict lung maturity. This L/S ratio tends to rise with increasing gestational age. This is not a uniform gradual increase; a rather sudden increase occurs at 34 to 36 weeks gestation and correlates with the development of FLM.

A conservative reference interval for lung maturity is an L/S ratio of 2.5 or greater. About 1% of babies delivered within 24 hours of obtaining an L/S ratio greater than 2.5 are expected to develop RDS. Almost half of infants with L/S ratios between 1.5 and 2.5, however, will not develop RDS.

Measurement of Phosphatidylglycerol

The detection of PG is a commonly used qualitative method used to assess FLM. Measurement of PG was classically performed in conjunction with the L/S ratio, and the combination of the two tests is known as the *lung profile*. The rapid detection of PG is typically accomplished using a commercially available immunochemical test.

The concentration of PG in amniotic fluid increases with gestational age. Most thin-layer chromatography (TLC) techniques are positive when PG exceeds about 2 μmol/L. At this cutoff, results indicating maturity are almost always correct, but results indicating immaturity are frequently incorrect.

Review Questions

1. The most severe form of hemolytic disease of the newborn (HDN) is referred to as
   a. respiratory distress syndrome (RDS).
   b. ectopic pregnancy.
   c. jaundice.
   d. erythroblastosis fetalis.
2. In a developing fetus, the major blood-forming organ until 24 weeks gestation is the
   a. bone marrow.
   b. liver.
   c. lung.
   d. kidney.

3. The trophoblast cells that surround the developing blastocyst
   a. form the amnion and amniotic fluid.
   b. synthesize glucose for the fetus.
   c. are the major blood-forming organs in early fetal life.
   d. invade the endometrium and form the placenta.

4. The composition of amniotic fluid is most typically like that of which one of the following?
   a. Extracellular fluid
   b. Intracellular fluid
   c. Cerebrospinal fluid
   d. Blood

5. Hemolytic disease of the newborn (HDN) is caused by
   a. lack of folic acid in the maternal diet.
   b. increased formation of fetal hemoglobin (Hb F).
   c. maternal antibodies against fetal erythrocytes.
   d. blockage of placental transfer of immunoglobulin A (IgA) antibodies.

6. Which one of the following fetal disorders has been demonstrated to be caused by low folic acid intake during pregnancy?
   a. Neural tube defects
   b. Trisomy 18
   c. Renal atresia
   d. Respiratory distress

7. Which of the following hormones is (are) synthesized by the placenta?
   a. Chorionic gonadotropin (CG)
   b. Estriol (E$_3$)
   c. Progesterone
   d. All of the above are synthesized by the placenta.

8. The process of identifying pregnancies at sufficiently high risk of a serious birth defect, such as Down syndrome, to warrant invasive diagnostic testing is referred to as
   a. presymptomatic testing.
   b. prenatal screening.
   c. identity testing.
   d. karyotype analysis.

9. The majority of waste produced by a fetus is in the amniotic fluid. Which one of the following structures is responsible for removal of this waste from the amniotic fluid?
   a. Fetal kidneys
   b. Fetal liver
   c. Fetal lungs
   d. Placenta

10. When a fertilized egg implants in a location other than the body of the uterus, the condition is called
    a. Down syndrome.
    b. spina bifida.
    c. ectopic pregnancy.
    d. hyperemesis gravidarum.

References

1. American College of Obstetricians and Gynecologists. ACOG Practice Bulletin No. 77: screening for fetal chromosomal abnormalities. Obstet Gynecol 2007;109:217–27.
2. American College of Obstetricians and Gynecologists. ACOG Practice Bulletin No. 97: fetal lung maturity. Obstet Gynecol 2008;112:717–26.
3. American Thyroid Association Taskforce on thyroid disease during pregnancy and postpartum. Thyroid 2011;21(10):1081–125.
4. Ashwood ER, Grenache DG, Lambert-Messerlian G. Pregnancy and its disorders. In Burtis CA, Ashwood ER, Bruns DE, eds. Tietz textbook of clinical chemistry and molecular diagnostics, 5th edition. St Louis, MO: Elsevier/Saunders, 2012:1991–2044.
5. Barnhart KT. Clinical practice. Ectopic pregnancy. New Engl J Med 2009;361:379–87.
6. CLSI. Assessment of fetal lung maturity by the lamellar body count; approved guideline. CLSI document C58-A. Wayne, PA: Clinical and Laboratory Standards Institute, 2011.
7. Grenache DG, Wilson AR, Gross GA, Gronowski AM. Clinical and laboratory trends in fetal lung maturity testing. Clin Chim Acta 2010;411;1746–9.
8. Knight GJ, Palomaki GE. Epidemiologic monitoring of prenatal screening for neural tube defects and Down syndrome. Clin Lab Med 2003;23:531–51.
9. Lockitch G, ed. Handbook of diagnostic biochemistry and hematology in normal pregnancy. Boca Raton, FL: CRC Press, 1993.
10. Malone FD, Canick JA, Ball RH, Nyberg DA, Comstock CH, Bukowski R, et al. First trimester or second trimester screening, or both, for Down's syndrome. N Engl J Med 2005;353:2001–11.
11. Muglia LJ, Katz M. The enigma of spontaneous preterm birth. N Engl J Med 2010;362:529–35.
12. Sherwin JE, Lockitch G, Rosenthal P, Ashwood ER, Geaghan S, Magee LA. Maternal-fetal risk assessment and reference values in pregnancy. National Academy of Clinical Biochemistry Laboratory Medicine practice guidelines. Washington, DC: National Academy of Clinical Biochemistry, 2006:1–75.
13. Wald NJ, Rodeck C, Hackshaw AK, Walters J, Chitty L, Mackinson AM. First and second trimester antenatal screening for Down's syndrome: the results of the Serum, Urine and Ultrasound Screening Study (SURUSS). J Med Screen 2003;10:56–104.
14. Wald NJ. Neural tube defects. In: Wald, N, Leck, I, eds. Antenatal and neonatal screening, 2nd edition. Oxford: Oxford University Press, 2000:61–80.
15. Whittington J, Fantz CR, Gronowski AM, McCudden CR, Mullins R, Sokoll L, et al. The analytical specificity of human chorionic gonadotropin assays determined using WHO International Reference Reagents. Clin Chim Acta 2010;411:81–5.

Newborn Screening and
Inborn Errors of Metabolism*

Marzia Pasquali, Ph.D., F.A.C.M.G., and Nicola Longo, M.D., Ph.D., F.A.C.M.G

Objectives

1. Define the following:

   Aminoacidopathy

   Fatty acid oxidation disorder

   Inborn error of metabolism (IEM)

   Multiplex analysis

   Newborn screening

   Organic acidemia

   Second-tier testing

   Tandem mass spectrometry (MS/MS)

   Urea cycle disorder

2. Define and describe autosomal recessive inheritance patterns including significance of this pattern in inborn errors of metabolism (IEMs), percent risk of having an affected child in each pregnancy, percent chance of having a carrier and percent chance of having an unaffected child; diagram an autosomal recessive inheritance pattern pedigree.

3. List the six components of a newborn screening program; state the criteria required of any newborn screening program.

4. Discuss the American College of Medical Genetics and Genomics (ACMG) uniform screening panel of newborn screening tests, including classifications and names of disorders.

5. State the three classes of metabolic disorders, and list an example of each class; list five disorders of amino acid metabolism, three disorders of fatty acid metabolism, and three disorders of carbohydrate metabolism.

6. For the following disorders, list causes and symptoms, treatments, available screening, and second-tier laboratory analyses and results of them:

   Alkaptonuria

   Galactosemia

   Glutaric acidemia type I

   Glycine encephalopathy

   Homocystinuria

   Maple syrup urine disease (MSUD)

   Medium-chain acyl-CoA dehydrogenase (MCAD) deficiency

   Phenylketonuria (PKU)

   Tyrosinemia

   Urea cycle disorders

7. State the principle of tandem mass spectrometry (MS/MS) and how the results of this screening analysis are interpreted with regard to inborn errors of metabolism (IEMs); state an advantage of using this type of analysis.

8. Discuss the issue of false positive results in newborn screening, including tests most commonly misinterpreted and the use and principle of second-tier tests.

9. List four types of confirmatory laboratory tests used to verify borderline newborn screening test results.

10. Analyze and solve case studies related to inborn errors of metabolism (IEMs), newborn screening, and laboratory testing related to them.

Key Words and Definitions

Alkaptonuria A genetic disorder due to deficiency of the enzyme homogentisic acid (HGA) dioxygenase.

Aminoacidopathy Any one of group of inborn errors of amino acid metabolism caused by (1) defective activity of an enzyme in the metabolic pathway of one or more amino acids or (2) a defect in a protein needed for transport of an amino acid into or out of cells; usually detected by the presence of increased concentrations of one or more amino acids in blood or urine or both.

Argininosuccinate lyase (ASL) deficiency A genetic disorder that affects the body's ability to clear the nitrogen already incorporated into the urea cycle as argininosuccinate. This disorder often presents with rapid-onset hyperammonemia in the newborn period. Also known as *argininosuccinic aciduria*.

Argininosuccinate synthetase (ASS) deficiency A genetic disorder characterized by a deficiency of argininosuccinate and an increase in the ammonia concentration in the blood. Also known as *citrullinemia type I*.

Autosomal recessive disorder A disorder characterized by the requirement that both copies of a gene are abnormal (see following definition for *autosomal recessive inheritance*).

Autosomal recessive inheritance A Mendelian inheritance pattern in which (1) nonsex chromosomes (autosomes) carry a DNA sequence (gene) for the inherited trait and (2) two copies of the DNA sequence must be present for the trait to appear in an individual; heterozygous parents have a 25% chance of having an affected offspring.

*The authors gratefully acknowledge the contributions of Dr. Barbara Sawyer to the previous edition of this chapter on which portions of this chapter are based.

Key Words and Definitions—cont'd

Citrullinemia type II An autosomal recessive disease characterized by increased concentrations of citrulline in serum and urine. Ammonia intoxication is another manifestation. This disorder is characterized by neuropsychiatric symptoms, including abnormal behaviors, loss of memory, seizures, and coma.

Dihydropteridine reductase (DHPR) An enzyme that catalyzes the reversible formation of tetrahydrobiopterin (BH_4) from dihydrobiopterine; deficiency of BH_4 results in malignant hyperphenylalaninemia.

Disorders of amino acid metabolism A group of disorders of amino acid metabolism caused by defective activity of an enzyme leading to increased amino acids in blood (and urine).

Disorders of carbohydrate metabolism A group of disorders caused by loss of an enzyme in the metabolic pathway of a carbohydrate, leading to increased concentrations of that carbohydrate in blood or its accumulation within organs and tissues.

Disorders of fatty acid oxidation A group of disorders caused by deficiency of an enzyme in the oxidation pathway of fatty acids, leading to inability to use fat as an energy source.

Dried blood spot (DBS) A form of biosampling where blood samples are blotted and dried on filter paper.

Galactosemia An inherited disease in which the transformation of galactose to glucose is blocked, allowing galactose to increase to toxic concentrations in the body.

Glucose-6-phosphate dehydrogenase (G-6-PD) deficiency An X-linked recessive hereditary disease characterized by abnormally low quantities of the enzyme G-6-PD involved in the pentose phosphate pathway, especially important in red blood cell metabolism.

Glutaric acidemia type I (GAI) An inherited disorder in which an affected individual is unable to completely metabolize (1) lysine, (2) hydroxylysine, and (3) tryptophan. Excessive quantities of glutaric acid (GA) and related compounds accumulate and damage the brain.

Glycogen storage diseases Genetic diseases, also known as *glycogenoses*, that involve the enzymes regulating glycogen accumulation and breakdown.

Guthrie test A semiquantitative microbiological assay for the determination of amino acids in blood or urine.

Homocystinuria A condition characterized by the excretion of excess homocystine in the urine; this biochemical abnormality has a variety of autosomal recessive genetic causes as well as nongenetic causes.

Hyperornithinemia-Hyperammonemia-Homocitrullinuria (HHH) syndrome An autosomal recessive syndrome characterized by increased plasma concentrations of ornithine, postprandial hyperammonemia and homocitrullinuria, and aversion to protein ingestion; the affected gene codes for the mitochondrial ornithine transporter, ornithine translocase.

Inborn error of metabolism (IEM) Inherited disorder due to deficiency of an enzyme or transporter impairing the transformation of body chemicals.

Isovaleric academia A metabolic disorder which disrupts or prevents normal metabolism of the branched-chain amino acid leucine. It is characterized by acidosis, coma, and an unpleasant body odor.

Long-chain 3-hydroxyacyl-CoA dehydrogenase (LCHAD) deficiency A metabolic disease characterized by defective fatty acid oxidation due to a defect in an enzyme in the β-oxidation pathway.

Maple syrup urine disease (MSUD) An autosomal recessive metabolic disorder affecting branched-chain amino acids (leucine, isoleucine, and valine). The urine of affected individuals smells like maple syrup.

Marfan syndrome A congenital disorder of connective tissue characterized by long limbs and casued by abnormal fibrillin metabolism; it affects various structures, notably heart valves and aorta.

Medium-chain acyl-CoA dehydrogenase (MCAD) deficiency A disorder of fatty acid oxidation that impairs the body's ability to break down medium-chain fatty acids into acetyl-CoA.

Methylmalonic acidemia An autosomal recessive metabolic disorder resulting from defects in the metabolic pathway in which methylmalonyl-coenzyme A (CoA) is converted into succinyl-CoA by the enzyme methylmalonyl-CoA mutase.

Microcephaly A condition characterized by an abnormally small head circumference; associated with a small brain (microencephaly).

Multiplex analysis Simultaneous assessment of multiple analytes in a single sample.

Nonketotic hyperglycinemia (NKHG) A usually fatal autosomal-recessive aminoacidopathy with accumulation of glycine in body fluids, particularly the blood, urine, and cerebrospinal fluid.

Ochronosis A condition characterized by an accumulation of dark pigment in cartilage and other connective tissue that indicates alkaptonuria or phenol poisoning.

Organic acidemia A disorder of intermediary metabolism in which lack of an enzyme leads to buildup of an organic acid (from deamination of the amino acid) as opposed to the buildup of the parent amino acid.

Ornithine translocase deficiency Ornithine translocase transports ornithine into the liver where it enters the urea cycle. When ornithine translocase is deficient, the concentration of ornithine and ammonia increases in the blood.

Phenylketonuria (PKU) A disorder characterized by the accumulation of phenylalanine in blood that results from the absence of phenylalanine hydroxylase activity leading to production of phenylketones that are excreted in urine.

Propionic acidemia An organic acid disorder due to deficiency of an enzyme involved in amino acid and fatty acid catabolism. It is characterized by excess of propionic acid in the blood and urine,

Tandem mass spectrometry (MS/MS) A spectrometric method of analysis where two mass spectrometers are connected in series. It involves separation and identification of substances and chemicals based on their mass to charge (m/z) ratio.

Tyrosinemia A genetic disorder involving the metabolism of the tyrosine. Affected individuals have high concentrations of tyrosine in blood (hypertyrosinemia) and urine (tyrosinuria).

Urea cycle disorder Any disorder in which the body is unable to excrete waste nitrogen–ammonia, resulting in mental and behavioral dysfunction, coma, and death.

Inborn errors of metabolism (IEM) are genetically determined biochemical disorders affecting an individual's ability to convert nutrients or to use them for energy production. They are caused by the impaired function of (1) enzymes, (2) transporters, or (3) cofactors and result in accumulation of abnormal metabolites (substrates) proximal to the metabolic block or by lack of necessary products (path A to D, Figure 45-1). Abnormal by-products can also be generated when alternative pathways are used to dispose of the excess metabolites (path A to F, Figure 45-1).

Typically, IEMs present in the newborn period or in infancy. Some diseases, however, such as fatty acid oxidation defects or milder variants of classic metabolic disorders, may not be detected until adulthood. Despite the long asymptomatic period, their consequences are still devastating and may result in death. Therefore, it is critical to identify and treat these diseases before irreversible damage occurs. The frequency of individual diseases is rare, varying from 1:10,000 to 1:200,000 or even rarer. Their cumulative frequency, however, is substantial and approaches a frequency of 1:2,000.

Inheritance Pattern of Metabolic Disorders

Metabolic disorders are caused by mutations in genes that code for specific enzymes or transporters involved in metabolic pathways. The majority of metabolic disorders have **autosomal recessive inheritance,** in which affected individuals have a mutation in both alleles encoding for a specific enzyme or transporter (Figure 45-2). Because the mutation is in a gene on a nonsex chromosome (autosome), girls are affected as often as boys. In most cases, the parents of children with one of these metabolic conditions are carriers of the condition, that is, they carry one normal allele and one mutant allele, and they do not show clinical signs of the condition. In each singleton pregnancy when both parents are carriers, there is (1) a 25% chance that the child is affected, (2) a 50% chance that the child is a carrier like the parents, and (3) a 25% chance that the child has two normal alleles (Figure 45-2).

Clinical Presentation of Metabolic Disorders

The medical consequences of IEMs vary from failure to thrive to acute illness leading in some cases to (1) brain damage, (2) coma, and (3) death. In many cases the acute presentation is preceded by a symptom-free period that is variable in length depending on the specific disease. In most cases, there is a treatment available for these disorders consisting of special diets (formulas) that do not contain the specific nutrients that the patients are unable to metabolize. The treatment is effective if begun early before symptoms occur, but damage that has already occurred is usually irreversible. Thus, the ideal time for identifying patients with metabolic disorders is at birth or earlier.

Biochemical Diagnosis

The biochemical diagnosis of IEMs and treatment monitoring involve analysis of (1) metabolites, (2) enzymatic activity, and/or (3) DNA sequence. Because of technological advances (such as, the introduction of **tandem mass spectrometry (MS/MS)**, allowing the simultaneous detection of multiple analytes), many IEMs are now included in newborn screening programs.

Newborn Screening

Newborn screening is a public health activity aimed at early identification of conditions for which timely intervention is expected to result in elimination or reduction of (1) morbidity, (2) mortality, and (3) disabilities.

Background

Newborn screening was originally instituted in the 1960s as a result of the pioneering efforts of Robert Guthrie and his colleagues, who developed a screening assay (known as the **Guthrie test**) for measuring the phenylalanine content of a **dried blood spot (DBS)** on filter paper collected from the blood of newborn babies.[5,6]

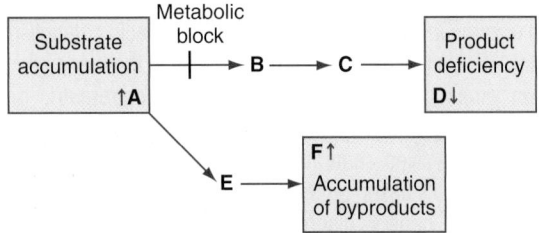

Figure 45-1 Schematic of metabolic pathway. The substrate *A* is converted by a series of reactions into product *D.* If one of the enzymes *(arrows)* is defective (metabolic block), the substrate of the reaction will accumulate (*A* in this case) and can enter alternative pathways of metabolism, leading to the formation of byproducts (*E* and *F* in this case). At the same time, the concentration of the product of the reaction *(D)* will decrease.

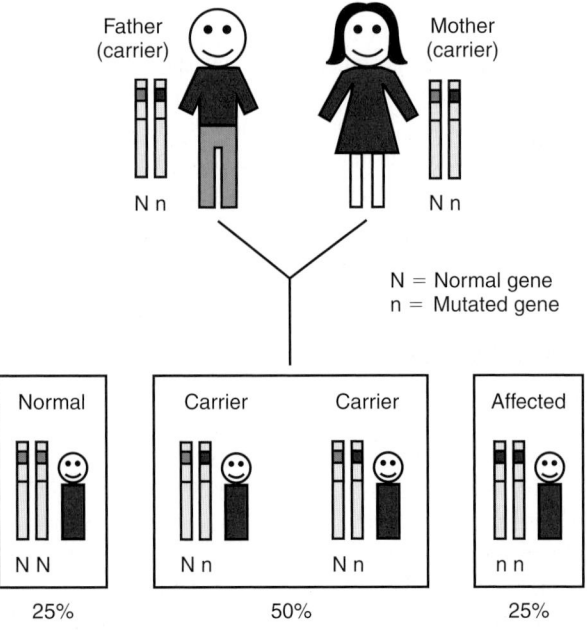

Figure 45-2 Autosomal recessive inheritance pattern.

Criteria of Newborn Screening Programs

Newborn screening tests must fit specific criteria that evaluate the (1) characteristics of the disease, (2) test used to screen for it, and (3) newborn screening program. The disease to be screened must (1) be serious, (2) be fairly common, (3) have a natural history that is understood, and (4) have helpful treatment or genetic counselling (in the case of genetic disease) available. In addition, the screening test must be (1) acceptable to the public, (2) reliable, (3) valid, and (4) affordable. The newborn screening program requires the availability of expedient diagnosis and treatment of the disease and effective communication of results. Newborn screening programs must be effectual public health approaches to the diagnosis of treatable disorders early in life. Because newborn screening is a program, its efficacy depends on the integration and collaboration among its different components, involving (1) organizations of public health, (2) screening and diagnostic laboratories, (3) physicians, and (4) families of affected children.

Steps to be Followed in a Newborn Screening Program

The different steps that need to be coordinated and tracked in a newborn screening program are:

1. Screening (sample collection and delivery, laboratory testing)
2. Follow-up (complete demographic information, satisfactory specimens, abnormal screening results)
3. Diagnosis (confirmatory tests, clinical consultation)
4. Clinical management (medical home, specialist physician, genetic counselor, dietitian)
5. Education (healthcare professionals, parents)
6. Quality assurance: analytical (proficiency testing, quality controls, standards), efficiency of follow-up system, efficacy of treatment, long-term outcome

Each of these components should have specifically-written protocols that deal directly with the performance of the tasks involved. To assist laboratories in writing such protocols and procedures, the Clinical and Laboratory Standards Institute has published guidelines for newborn Screening, including guidelines on (1) blood collection on filter paper (LA 4-A5/new code NBS01-A6), (2) laboratory testing by tandem mass spectrometry (NBS04-A), (3) follow-up activities (I/LA27-A/new code NBS02-A6), and (4) document preparation (QMS02-A6). These documents describe the basic principles, scope, and range of activities within a newborn screening program and how to prepare the prerequisite documents. They are available at http://www.clsi.org/; (accessed December 31. 2013).

Second-Tier Testing

One of the major pitfalls in newborn screening is the number of false-positive results associated with certain screening tests. To reduce the number of infants requiring additional confirmatory testing, second-tier tests have been developed. These second-tier tests involve further analysis of the same blood spot that produced an abnormal result targeting different, more specific analytes and, often, using a methodology different from the one used in the primary screening test. They include (1) DNA analysis for cystic fibrosis[10] (see Chapter 24),

(2) MS/MS steroid profiling for congenital adrenal hyperplasia[11] (see Chapter 41), and (3) other biochemical tests, such as thyroid stimulating hormone for congenital hypothyroidism[8] (see Chapter 42). Second-tier testing has become a crucial component of newborn screening programs to increase the sensitivity and the specificity of the screening test.

Although metabolic disorders identified by MS/MS represent the largest group of diseases identifiable by newborn screening, more traditional screening methods can identify other IEMs and endocrine and hematologic disorders such as, (1) **galactosemia**, (2) biotinidase deficiency, (3) cystic fibrosis, (4) congenital hypothyroidism, (5) congenital adrenal hyperplasia, (6) hemoglobinopathies, and (7) severe combined immunodeficiency. Such tests include (1) enzyme assays, (2) immunoassays, (3) electrophoresis, and (4) DNA tests. Advances in therapeutic interventions for IEMs are continuously expanding the role of newborn screening. Of note, newborn screening does not identify all metabolic disorders, and some patients are missed. Therefore a symptomatic patient, at any age, should be investigated despite normal newborn screening results.

Inborn Errors of Metabolism

In this section, disorders of metabolism of (1) amino acids, (2) fats, and (3) carbohydrates are discussed in general, with selected individual disorders of each class reviewed in more detail as examples. An online database containing a catalog of human genetic disorders is found at www.ncbi.nlm.nih.gov/omim/ (accessed December 31, 2013. This database is entitled "Online Mendelian Inheritance in Man" (OMIM) and is a comprehensive and authoritative compendium of human genes and genetic phenotypes. In this database, individual disorders are assigned a specific OMIM number.

Disorders of Amino Acid Metabolism

Disorders of amino acid metabolism collectively affect approximately 1 in 8000 newborns. Almost all are transmitted as autosomal recessive traits and result from a lack of a specific enzyme in the metabolic pathway of an amino acid. This leads either to the accumulation of (1) the parent amino acid, (2) its by-products or (3) the catabolic products (organic acids), depending on the location of the enzyme block. Disorders of amino acid metabolism are divided into two groups: (1) **aminoacidopathies**, in which the parent amino acid accumulates in excess in blood and spills over into urine; and (2) **organic acidemias**, in which products in the catabolic pathway of certain amino acids accumulate.

An example of an aminoacidopathy is **phenylketonuria (PKU)**, a disorder of phenylalanine metabolism caused in the majority of cases by deficiency of phenylalanine hydroxylase, the enzyme responsible for the conversion of phenylalanine to tyrosine. Other examples include (1) **maple syrup urine disease (MSUD)**, (2) **homocystinuria**, and (3) **tyrosinemia**.

Glutaric acidemia type I is an example of an organic acidemia that is a disorder of lysine and tryptophan metabolism. Others include (1) **isovaleric acidemia**, (2) **methylmalonic acidemia**, and (3) **propionic acidemia** (Table 45-1).

TABLE 45-1 Uniform Screening Panel recommended for every Newborn Screening Program by the American College of Medical Genetics and Genomics: Core Conditions*

ACMG Code	Core Condition	Metabolic Disorder			Endocrine Disorder	Hemoglobin Disorder	Other Disorder
		Organic Acid Condition	Fatty Acid Oxidation Disorders	Amino Acid Disorders			
PROP	Propionic acidemia	X					
MUT	Methylmalonic acidemia (methylmalonyl-CoA mutase)	X					
Cbl A,B	Methylmalonic acidemia (cobalamin disorders)	X					
IVA	Isovaleric acidemia	X					
3-MCC	3-Methylcrotonyl-CoA carboxylase deficiency	X					
HMG	3-Hydroxy-3-methyglutaric aciduria	X					
MCD	Holocarboxylase synthase deficiency	X					
βKT	β-Ketothiolase deficiency	X					
GAI	Glutaric acidemia type I	X					
CUD	Carnitine uptake defect (carnitine transport defect)		X				
MCAD	Medium-chain acyl-CoA dehydrogenase deficiency		X				
VLCAD	Very long-chain acyl-CoA dehydrogenase deficiency		X				
LCHAD	Long-chain 3-hydroxyacyl-CoA dehydrogenase deficiency		X				
TFP	Trifunctional protein deficiency		X				
ASA	Argininosuccinic aciduria			X			
CIT	Citrullinemia type I			X			
MSUD	Maple syrup urine disease			X			
HCY	Homocystinuria			X			
PKU	Phenylketonuria			X			
TYR-I	Tyrosinemia type I			X			
CH	Congenital hypothyroidism				X		
CAH	Congenital adrenal hyperplasia				X		
Hb SS	S,S disease (Sickle cell anemia)					X	
Hb S/βTh	S, βeta-thalassemia					X	
Hb S/C	S,C disease					X	
BIOT	Biotinidase deficiency						X
CCHD	Critical congenital heart disease						X
CF	Cystic fibrosis						X
GALT	Galactosemia						X
HEAR	Hearing loss						X
SCID	Severe combined immunodeficiencies						X

*The nomenclature for conditions is based on data from reference 12.[12]
ACMG, American College of Medical Genetics and Genomics.
Modified from American College of Medical Genetics and Genomics. Newborn screening: towards a uniform screening panel and system. Genetic Med 2006;8(5) Suppl:S12-S252.

The clinical manifestations of the organic acidemias vary from no observable clinical consequences to neonatal mortality. Conditions, such as (1) developmental retardation, (2) seizures, (3) alterations in sensorium, or (4) behavioral disturbances, occur in more than half the disorders. Metabolic ketoacidosis, often accompanied by hyperammonemia, is a frequent finding in organic acidemias. The compound(s) accumulated depend on the (1) site of the enzymatic block, (2) reversibility of the reactions proximal to the lesion, and (3) availability of alternative pathways of metabolic "runoff."

Phenylketonuria

PKU (OMIM #261600) is a disorder of phenylalanine metabolism that results from the absence of phenylalanine hydroxylase activity leading to the accumulation of phenylalanine and production of phenylketones that are excreted in urine.

Phenylalanine is an essential amino acid, constituting 4% to 6% of all dietary protein. Phenylalanine that is not used in protein synthesis is converted to tyrosine by the enzyme phenylalanine hydroxylase and further degraded via a ketogenic pathway (Figure 45-3). The frequency of hyperphenylalaninemia/PKU is 1:10,000 to 1:20,000 live births. The majority (98%) of cases of PKU are caused by mutations in the phenylalanine hydroxylase gene with the remaining 2% being caused by defects in biosynthesis or recycling of tetrahydrobiopterin (BH_4), the cofactor for phenylalanine hydroxylase.

Primary or secondary (due to a deficiency of the cofactor) impairment of phenylalanine hydroxylase causes (1) increased phenylalanine, (2) increased phenylketones, (3) increased phenylamines, and (4) a deficiency of tyrosine (Figure 45-3). The greatly increased concentration of phenylalanine impairs brain development and function, affecting other organs minimally. Patients with classic PKU are clinically asymptomatic at birth with developmental delays and neurological manifestations typically becoming evident at several months of life when brain damage has already occurred. Untreated PKU patients develop (1) **microcephaly**, (2) eczematous skin rash, (3) "mousy" odor (due to accumulation of phenylacetate), and (4) severe mental retardation. The treatment of PKU includes a diet (1) low in protein and phenylalanine and (2) supplemented with tyrosine, minerals, vitamins, and other nutrients to sustain normal growth. Treatment should be continued for life.

Newborn screening leads to early detection and therapy of patients with PKU with prevention of mental retardation. Ideally, treatment should start before 2 weeks of age. Pregnant women with PKU should adhere to a strictly controlled diet that is low in phenylalanine and proteins, because phenylalanine is teratogenic and results in an increased risk of spontaneous abortions or of having a child with (1) growth retardation, (2) microcephaly, (3) significant developmental delays, and (4) birth defects.

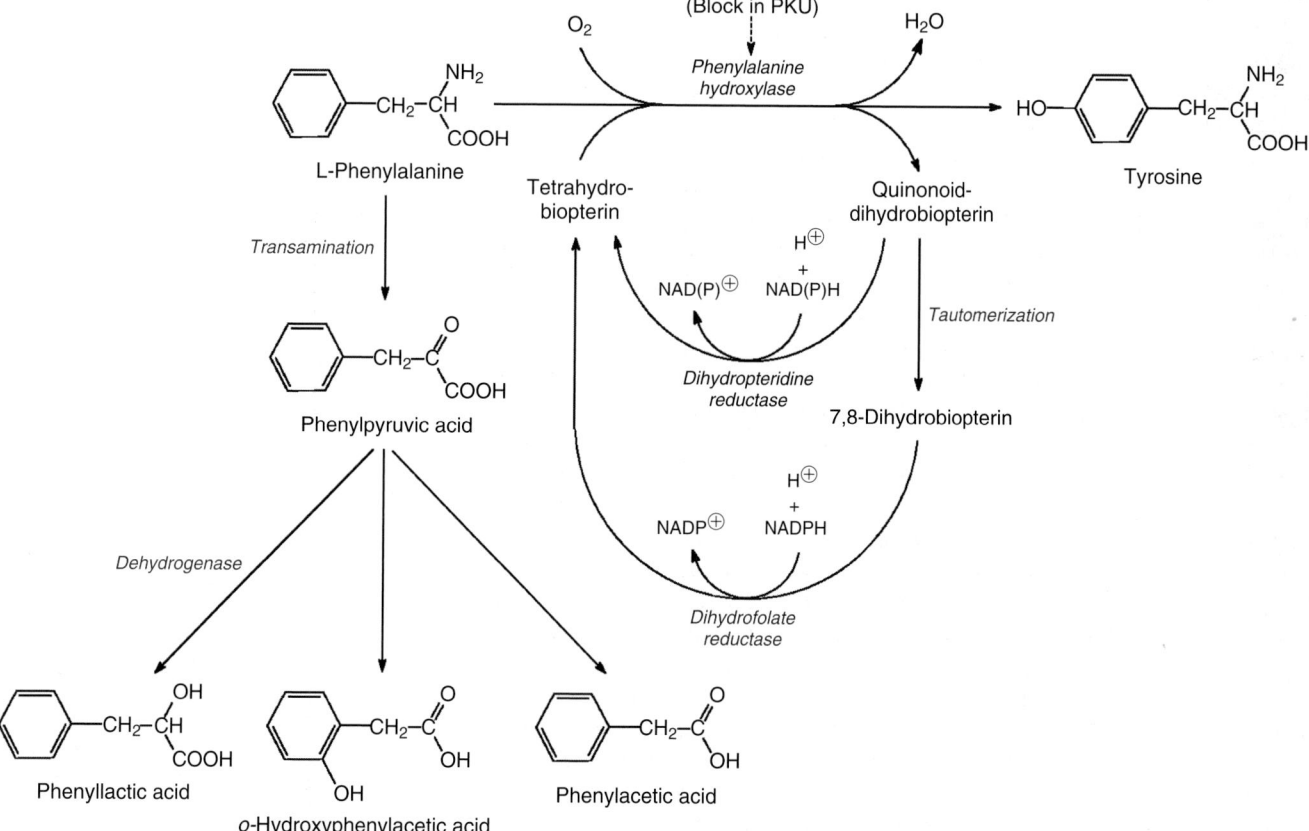

Figure 45-3 Metabolism of phenylalanine and tyrosine.

The diagnosis of PKU is confirmed biochemically by demonstration of increased plasma phenylalanine and an increased phenylalanine:tyrosine ratio. Urine specimens from affected individuals contain increased concentrations of phenylketones (hence the name *phenylketonuria*). Enzymatic confirmation of phenylalanine hydroxylase deficiency is not usually performed (the enzyme is expressed only in the liver), but mutational analysis of the gene is increasingly used because there is a correlation between severity of the mutation and phenylalanine tolerance. All children with hyperphenylalaninemia should be screened for defects in BH_4 synthesis or recycling. This is performed by measuring the urinary pterin profile and by measuring the enzyme activity of **dihydropteridine reductase (DHPR)** in blood spotted on filter paper. Deficiency of BH_4 affects the synthesis of several neurotransmitters, including dopamine and serotonin, because it is a cofactor of (1) phenylalanine hydroxylase, (2) tyrosine hydroxylase, (3) tryptophan hydroxylase, and (4) nitric oxide synthase. Patients with a defect in BH_4 synthesis or recycling have neurological symptoms and developmental regression in the first few months of life, despite adequate control of phenylalanine intake and plasma concentrations. They can develop seizures and have a characteristic hypotonia of the trunk with hypertonia of the extremities. These patients require therapy with BH_4 and appropriate neurotransmitters. They may or may not require a low phenylalanine diet once BH_4 therapy is initiated.

Tyrosinemia

Tyrosinemia is a genetic disorder characterized by increased blood concentrations of tyrosine. There are three types of tyrosinemia (I-III); each is caused by the deficiency of a different enzyme (Figure 45-4). Tyrosinemia type I (TYR-I) is the most severe form and is caused by a deficiency of fumarylacetoacetate hydrolase. Tyrosinemia type II is caused by a deficiency of tyrosine aminotransferase, and tyrosinemia type III is caused by a deficiency of 4-hydroxyphenylpyruvate dioxygenase.

The incidence of TYR-I is approximately 1 in 100,000 with a clustering of cases in the Lac-St. Jean region of Quebec (Canada). Patients with TYR-I present, usually before 6 months of age, with severe liver involvement, or with (1) chronic failure to thrive, (2) mild hepatocellular dysfunction, (3) renal involvement, and (4) rickets due to renal Fanconi syndrome. They have extreme irritability caused by peripheral neuropathy mimicking acute intermittent porphyria. Untreated patients develop liver cirrhosis and are at very high risk for liver cancer.

Patients with TYR-I have increased concentrations of tyrosine in the plasma, but this increase usually is not as marked as in patients with other forms of tyrosinemia. Increased tyrosine can also be seen in (1) tyrosinemia types II and III, (2) transient tyrosinemia of the newborn, (3) prematurity, (4) liver disease from any cause, (5) mitochondrial DNA depletion syndrome, and (6) diets very rich in proteins. The biochemical diagnosis of TYR-I is based on the detection in urine organic-acid testing of succinylacetone, derived from fumarylacetoacetic acid, the intermediate immediately upstream of the enzyme defect. TYR-1 is identified by newborn screening only when succinylacetone is used as the primary marker, because tyrosine usually is not elevated in the newborn period in these patients. Therapy consists of (1) low dietary tyrosine, (2) low dietary phenylalanine, and (3) drug therapy with 2-(2-nitro-4-trifluoro-methylbenzoyl)-1,3-cyclohexanedione (NTBC), an inhibitor of 4- hydroxyphenylpyruvate dioxygenase (see Figure 45-4). NTBC prevents the synthesis of succinylacetone, which disappears almost immediately from urine organic-acid testing after initiation of treatment. The adequacy of the diet is monitored by measuring the plasma amino acids and urine organic acids which will show disappearance of succinylacetone. Measurement of alpha fetoprotein is also used to monitor these patients, because liver cancer is a complication of this condition. Liver transplantation is indicated in patients who progress to liver failure and in those acquiring liver cancer.

Alkaptonuria

Alkaptonuria is caused by deficiency of the enzyme homogentisic acid (HGA) dioxygenase (see Figure 45-4). Deficiency of this enzyme leads to (1) the presence of HGA and its oxide (called *alkapton*) in the urine, (2) bluish-black pigmentation in connective tissue (**ochronosis**), (3) arthritis, and (4) urine that turns dark with standing or alkalinization. The accumulation of HGA in tissues causes cartilage damage in their joints, specifically in the spine, leading to low back pain at a young age. The pigment can also accumulate in cardiac valves causing their failure.

Treatments that reduce the complications of alkaptonuria are not available. However, treatment with NTBC prevents formation of homogentisic acid and is being explored as a potential therapy.

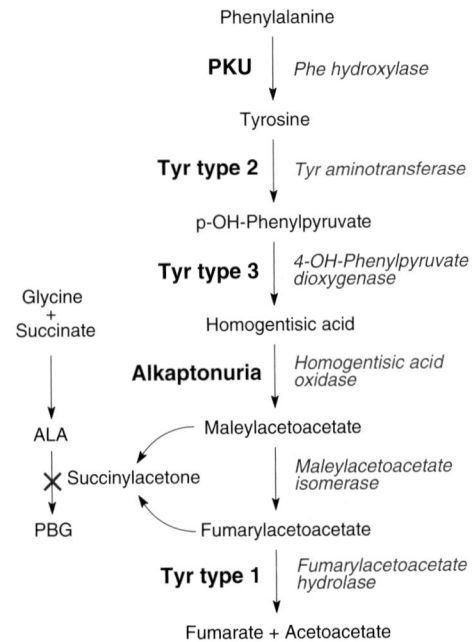

Figure 45-4 Disorders of inborn errors of metabolism (IEMs) resulting from deficiency of key enzymes required in the metabolic catabolism of phenylalanine. Specific disorders are shown in *bold letters*.

Homocystinuria

Homocystinuria is characterized by increased concentrations of the sulfur-containing amino acid, homocysteine, in blood and urine (Figure 45-5). It is caused by at least seven genetically different disorders. The most common disorder is classic homocystinuria that is caused by reduced activity of cystathionine β-synthase. The worldwide incidence is approximately 1:300,000 live births with a very high incidence in the country of Qatar (1:1800). Clinical manifestations are nonspecific at first and may include failure to thrive and developmental delay. Patients usually develop lens dislocation (often requiring surgery) and a body habitus like that seen in **Marfan syndrome**. (Homocysteine interferes with disulfide formation in fibrillin, the protein defective in Marfan syndrome). Patients whose blood homocysteine concentration continues to increase are at risk of blood clots, which are a life-threatening complication of the condition.

The biochemical diagnosis of homocystinuria is obtained by plasma amino acid analysis showing increased plasma concentrations of methionine (especially in children) and the presence of the disulfide homocystine. Classic homocystinuria is detected in newborn screening by increased concentrations of methionine in whole blood spots. Therapy for classic homocystinuria requires (1) high doses of pyridoxine (the cofactor of cystathionine β-synthase), (2) a special diet low in methionine, and (3) administration of betaine that donates a methyl group to homocysteine to generate methionine.

Maple Syrup Urine Disease

Maple syrup urine disease (MSUD) is an **autosomal recessive disorder** with an incidence of approximately 1:250,000 live births. It is caused by a deficiency of the branched-chain alpha-keto acid dehydrogenase complex (BCKDC), leading to a buildup of the branched-chain amino acids leucine, isoleucine, and valine and their toxic ketoacids in the blood and urine (Figure 45-6). The disease is named for the presence of sweet-smelling urine with an odor similar to that of maple syrup. Several forms of this disease may occur, depending on the gene affected and the severity of the mutations. The enzyme complex consists of four subunits designated $E_1\alpha$, $E_1\beta$,

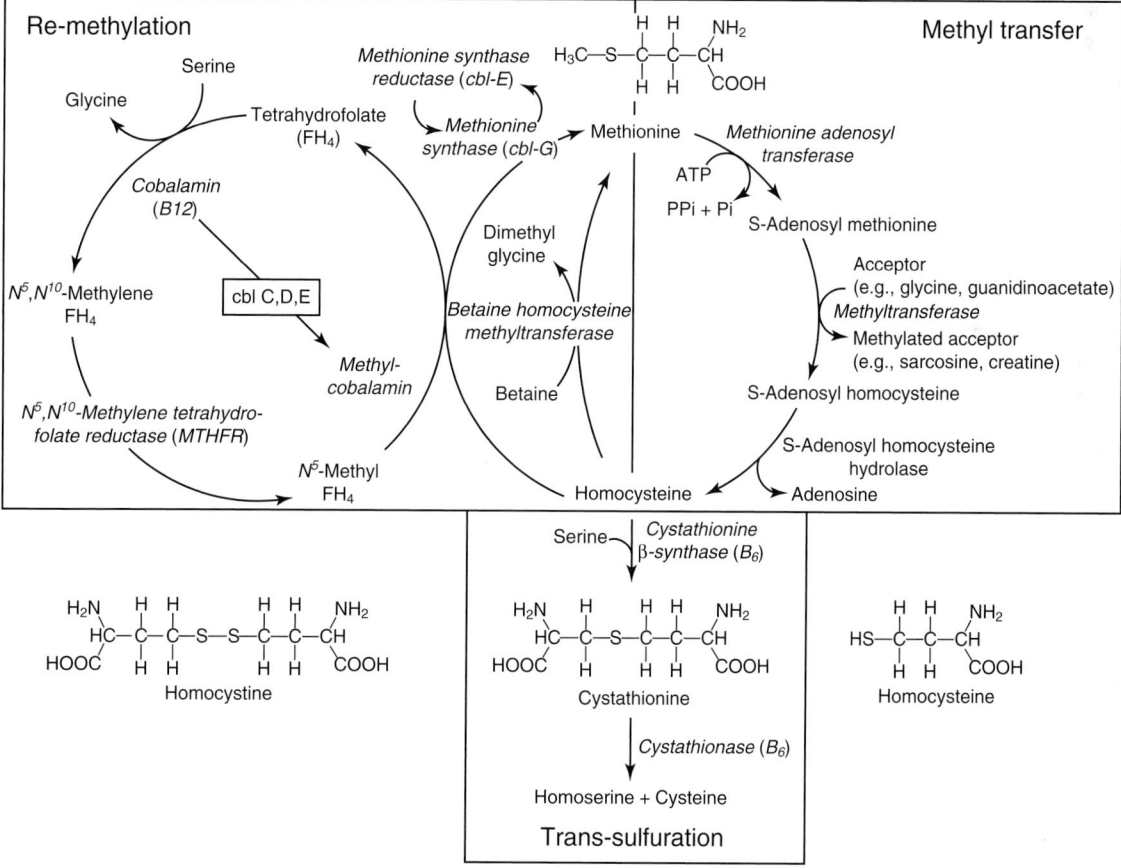

Figure 45-5 Sulfur amino acid metabolism. Methionine transfers a methyl group during its conversion to homocysteine. Defects in methyl transfer or in the subsequent metabolism of homocysteine by the pyridoxal phosphate (vitamin B_6)–dependent cystathionine β-synthase increase plasma methionine concentrations. Homocysteine is transformed into methionine via remethylation. This reaction is catalyzed by methionine synthase and requires methylcobalamin and folic acid. Deficiencies in these enzymes or lack of cofactors is associated with decreased or normal methionine concentrations. In an alternative pathway, homocysteine is remethylated by betaine:homocysteine methyl transferase. The chemical structures of homocystine and homocysteine are also shown.

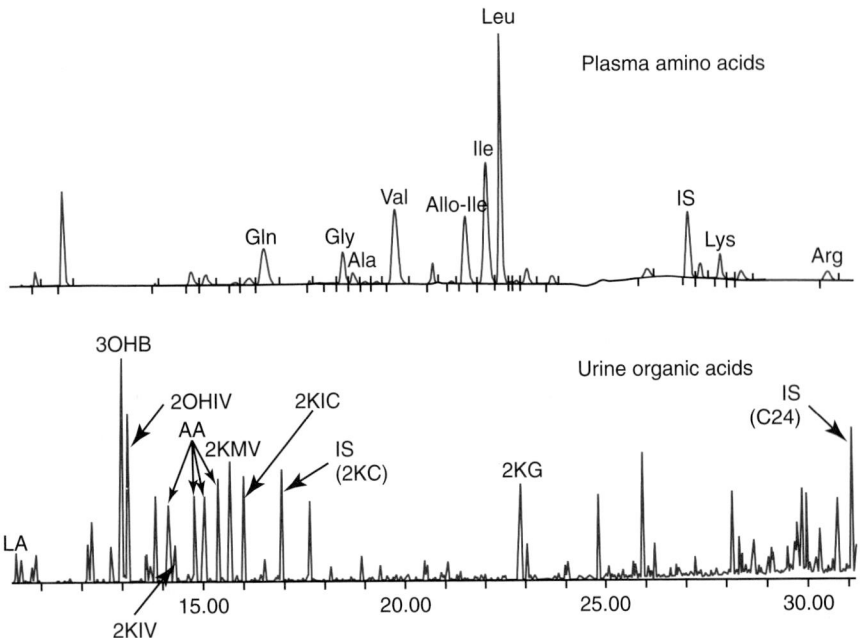

Figure 45-6 Profiles of plasma amino acids and urine organic acids in maple syrup urine disease (MSUD) as measured by ion-exchange chromatography and gas chromatography mass spectrometry (GCMS) respectively. *Top,* All three branched-chain amino acids (leucine, valine, and isoleucine) are increased in MSUD. Alloisoleucine (an amino acid not normally present) is also seen in this condition. *Bottom,* Urine organic acids show the presence of the characteristic metabolites 2-OH-isovaleric acid (2OHIV), 2-ketoisovaleric acid (2KIV), 2-ketomethylvaleric acid (2KMV), and 2-ketoisocaproic (2KIC). Lactic acid (LA) and ketones (3-OH-butyric acid [3OHB] and acetoacetate [AA]) are also increased in the catabolic state. 2-ketocaproic acid (2KC) and tetracosane (C24) are used as internal standards.

E_2, and E_3. MSUD results from mutations in any of the genes that code for the enzyme subunits.

Individuals with classic MSUD present with poor feeding and vomiting during the first week of life followed by lethargy and coma within a few days. This usually follows a normal birth and an uneventful first few days of life. Routine laboratory work is mostly unremarkable except for the presence of ketones in urine. Diagnosis is established by measuring plasma amino acids and finding increased branched chain amino acids and the presence of alloisoleucine, which is characteristic of this disease.

Cornerstones of treatment include diets that have a restricted content of branched-chain amino acids and include supplementation with (1) high-dose thiamine and, in many patients, low doses of (2) valine and (3) isoleucine.

Urea Cycle Disorders

A **urea cycle disorder**, or urea cycle defect, is caused by a deficiency of one of the enzymes or a transporter in the urea cycle, which is responsible for removing ammonia from the blood stream. The urea cycle involves a series of biochemical steps in which nitrogen derived from protein metabolism is removed from the blood and converted to urea, which is then excreted in urine. In urea cycle disorders, the nitrogen accumulates in the form of ammonia, a toxic substance, and is not removed from the body.

Urea cycle disorders can result in (1) mental and behavioral dysfunction, (2) coma, and (3) death. The urea cycle disposes of the nitrogen groups of amino acids before their carbon skeleton is metabolized to gluconeogenic (most amino acids) or ketogenic precursors (leucine and lysine), or both (isoleucine, phenylalanine, tyrosine, and tryptophan). This cycle requires the combined action of different enzymes and mitochondrial transporters (Figure 45-7). Deficiency of any of these enzymes

or transporters impairs the function of the urea cycle, causing hyperammonemia.

Newborn screening can identify **argininosuccinate synthetase deficiency** (ASS deficiency **or citrullinemia type I**), **citrullinemia type II** (mitochondrial aspartate transporter/citrin deficiency), **argininosuccinate lyase (ASL) deficiency,** and arginase deficiency. Increased ornithine and homocitrulline, theoretically, are the markers for the syndrome of **hyperammonemia-hyperornithinemia-homocitrullinuria syndrome (HHH) syndrome** (also known as **ornithine translocase deficiency**). Patients with urea cycle defects may have symptoms at any age. In the neonatal period, there is usually a brief interval between birth and clinical manifestations with the most severe cases having symptoms before the results of newborn screening are available. Hyperammonemia and the accumulation of glutamine in the brain lead to (1) poor feeding, (2) vomiting, (3) lethargy, or (4) irritability progressing to coma and death.

Diagnosis is accomplished by measuring plasma amino acids and identifying the compound present in excess. Patients are treated by a diet low in proteins and administration of nitrogen scavengers, such as sodium benzoate and phenylacetate, which bind and remove glycine and glutamine, respectively.

Glycine Encephalopathy (Nonketotic Hyperglycinemia)

Glycine encephalopathy, or **nonketotic hyperglycinemia (NKHG)**, is a severe condition caused, in most cases, by a defect in the P, T, and H proteins of the glycine cleavage system. Patients with the classic form of the disease have symptoms within the first days of life with (1) lethargy, (2) poor suckling, (3) severe hypotonia, (4) hiccups, (5) seizures, and (6) apnea. Most of these patients die in the first few months of life or survive with profound developmental delays. Atypical

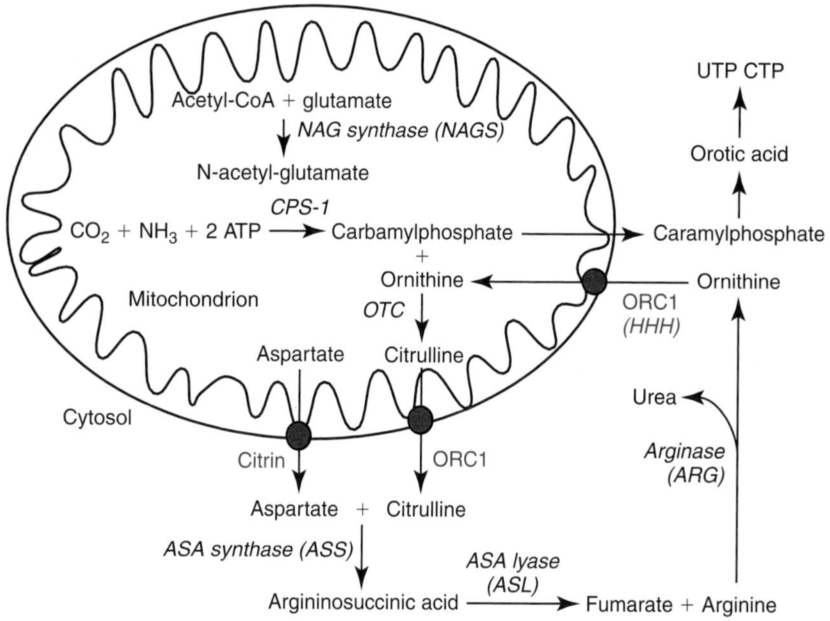

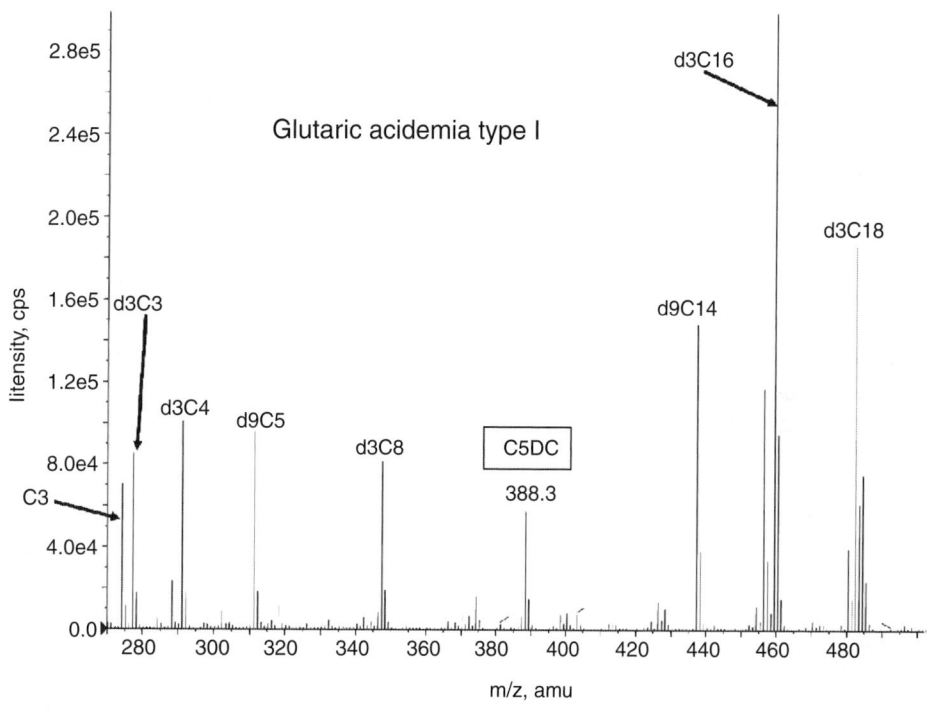

Figure 45-7 The urea cycle. In this cycle, urea is formed starting from ammonia (NH_3). It requires several enzymes and mitochondrial transporters, any of which can be defective and may impair the function of the urea cycle. *ASL,* Argininosuccinate lyase; *ASS,* argininosuccinate synthase; *ARG,* arginase; *citrin,* aspartate/glutamate exchanger; *CP,* carbamylphosphate; *CPS-1,* carbamyl phosphate synthase 1; *CTP,* cytidine triphosphate; *NAGS,* N-acetylglutamate synthase; *ORC1,* ornithine/citrulline mitochondrial transporter; *OTC,* ornithine transcarbamylase; *UTP,* uridine triphosphate.

Figure 45-8 Acylcarnitine profile (by tandem mass spectrometry [MS/MS]) in glutaric acidemia type I (GAI). Glutaryl (C5-DC)-carnitine is the diagnostic metabolite in GAI. Internal standards (deuterated) are indicated by the number of deuterium atoms (d) and the length of the carbon chain (C) attached to carnitine.

variants of NKHG have been diagnosed in patients with rather disparate manifestations who have in common, in most cases, seizures and delays of different degrees of severity.

Glutaric Acidemia Type I

Glutaric acidemia type I (GAI) (OMIM #231670) is an autosomal recessive disorder of the metabolism of (1) lysine, (2) hydroxylysine, and (3) tryptophan; it is caused by deficiency of glutaryl-CoA dehydrogenase. In this condition, glutaric acid (GA) and 3-hydroxyglutaric acid (3-OH-GA), formed in the catabolic pathway of the earlier amino acids, accumulate especially in urine. Affected patients have brain atrophy and macrocephaly (head circumference often increases

dramatically following birth), and they can develop acute dystonia secondary to degeneration of the corpus striatum (a component of the motor system in the brain). In most cases this is triggered by an infection, with fever, between 6 and 18 months of age.[6]

GAI is identified by an increased concentration of glutarylcarnitine (C5DC) on newborn screening (Figure 45-8). The diagnosis is biochemically confirmed by urine organic acid analysis that indicates the presence of excess 3-OH-GA, and the urine acylcarnitine profile shows glutarylcarnitine as the major peak. Therapy consists of (1) carnitine supplementation to remove GA, (2) a diet restricted in amino acids capable of producing GA, and (3) prompt administration of

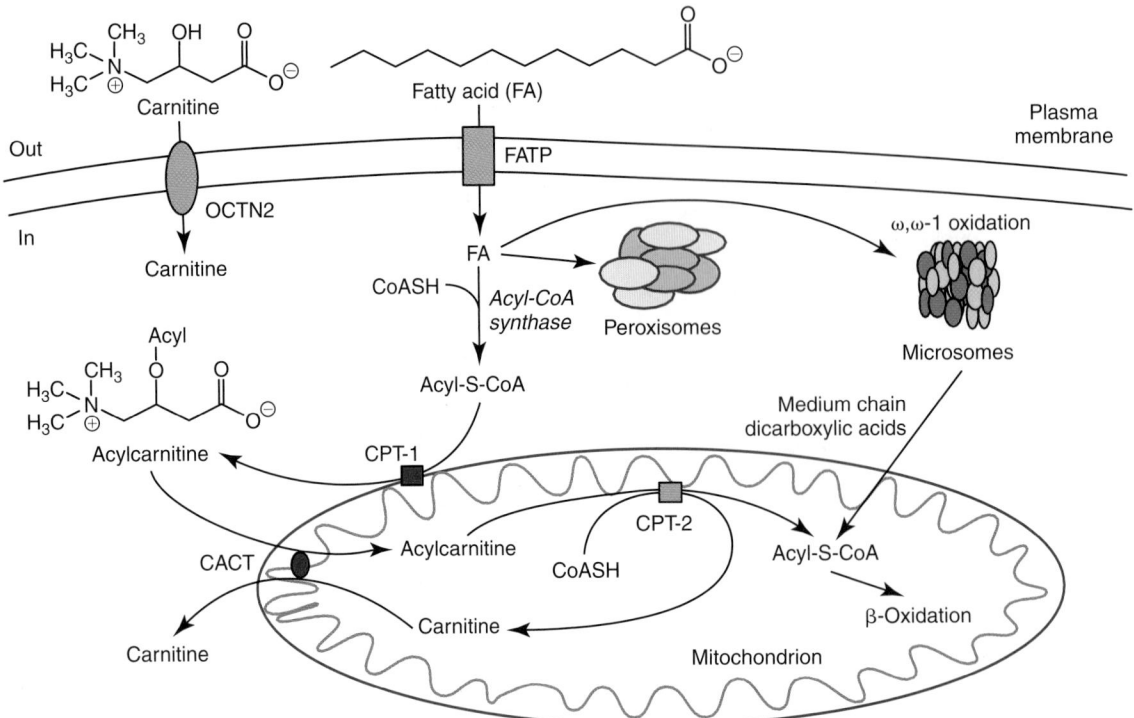

Figure 45-9 The carnitine cycle in fatty acid oxidation. The carnitine cycle is responsible for delivering long-chain fatty acid to the mitochondrial matrix for subsequent beta oxidation. *CACT,* Carnitine acyl carnitine translocase; *CPT-1,* carnitine palmitoyl transferase 1; *CPT-2,* carnitine palmitoyl transferase 2; *FA,* fatty acid; *FATP,* fatty acid transporter protein. *(Modified from Longo N, Amat di San Filippo C, Pasquali M. Disorders of carnitine transport and the carnitine cycle. Am J Med Genet C Semin Med Genet 2006;142:77-85.)*

intravenous calories in the child who is unable to eat for any reason such as (1) infections, (2) fever, and (3) gastroenteritis. Early diagnosis and therapy reduce the risk of acute dystonia in patients with GAI.[13]

Treatment of Organic Acidemias and Aminoacidopathies

As with the treatment regimens for acidemias, therapy for organic acid disorders consists of (1) special diets restricting the compounds (usually amino acids) that result in the formation of the abnormal organic acid or the accumulation of high concentrations of amino acids, (2) supplementation with vitamins specific for each disorder, (3) carnitine supplements, and (4) sometimes avoidance of fasting. For some of these conditions, aggressive therapy of illnesses with intravenous fluids containing glucose is essential to avoid catabolism that aggravates clinical symptoms.

Disorders of Fatty Acid Oxidation

Fatty acids are metabolized within mitochondria to produce energy. Carnitine and the carnitine cycle are required to transfer long-chain fatty acids into mitochondria for subsequent beta-oxidation (Figure 45-9).[7] There, long-chain fatty acids are progressively shortened of two carbon units at each cycle to generate acetyl CoA, which is used by the Krebs cycle to produce energy (Figure 45-10). **Disorders of fatty acid oxidation,** such as **medium-chain acyl-CoA**

dehydrogenase (MCAD) deficiency, occur when an enzyme is missing in the metabolic pathway and fatty acids fail to undergo oxidation to supply energy. These disorders are usually silent and become evident only when the body needs energy from fat during times of (1) fasting, (2) infections, or (3) fever. In this case, apparently healthy children with these disorders (1) become acutely sick, (2) lose consciousness, (3) become comatose, and (4) may die. When symptomatic, patients with fatty acid oxidation disorders develop hypoglycemia and might show increased serum transaminases indicating liver damage. Some fatty acid oxidation disorders (such as **long-chain 3-hydroxyacyl-CoA dehydrogenase [LCHAD] deficiency**) also (1) affect skeletal muscle, (2) affect cardiac muscle, and (3) affect the mother during pregnancy. Other disorders include carnitine transporter defect and very long-chain acyl-CoA dehydrogenase deficiency (see Table 45-1).

Medium-Chain Acyl-CoA Dehydrogenase Deficiency

MCAD (OMIM #201450) deficiency is the most common disorder of fatty acid oxidation with a frequency of 1:6000 to 1:10,000 births among Caucasians.[9] The symptoms of the disease are (1) asymptomatic, (2) hypoglycemia, (3) lethargy, (4) coma, and (5) sudden death, which is usually triggered by prolonged fasting, acute illness, or both. The majority of patients have symptoms in the first year of life, but clinical symptoms can occur at any time during life, and often the

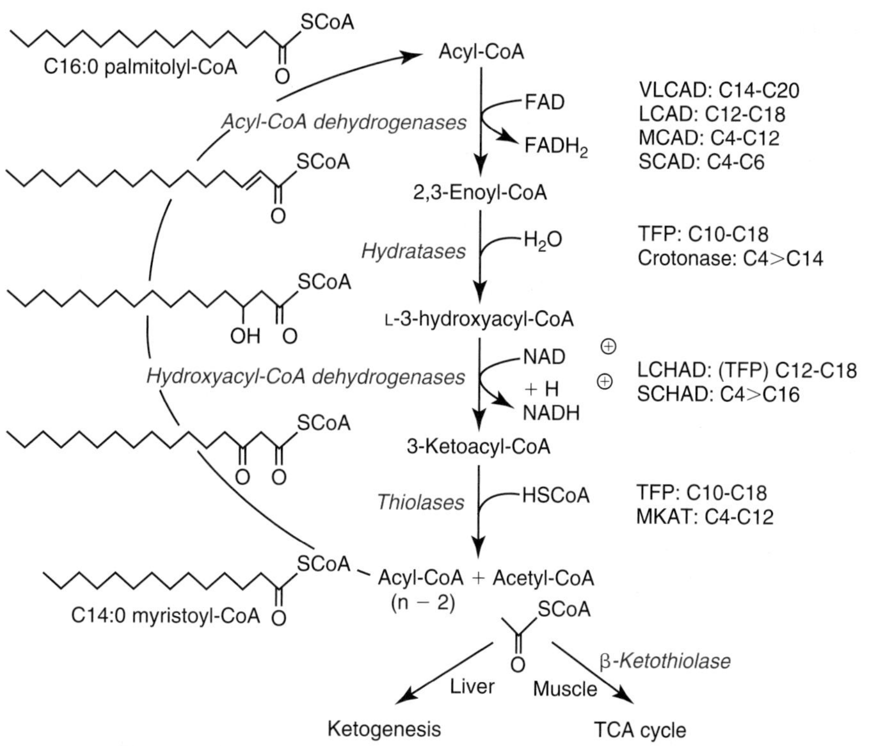

Figure 45-10 Beta oxidation of fatty acids. In the mitochondrial matrix, long-chain fatty acids undergo a series of steps to progressively shorten the fatty acids of two carbon units (acetyl-CoA) through a series of enzymatic reactions. Dehydrogenases that are specific for fatty acids with different carbon chain lengths (*LCAD,* long-chain acyl-CoA dehydrogenase; *MCAD,* medium-chain acyl-CoA dehydrogenase; *SCAD,* short-chain acyl-CoA dehydrogenase; *VLCAD,* very long-chain acyl-CoA dehydrogenase) introduce a double bond between C2 and C3. A trifunctional protein (TFP) adds water and cleaves two carbon atoms from the long-chain fatty acid. This is done through sequential action of a hydratase (enoyl-CoA hydratase), a L-3-hydroxyacyl-CoA dehydrogenase (*LCHAD,* long-chain 3-hydroxyacyl-CoA dehydrogenase), and a thiolase (acyl-CoA acetyltransferase). The two carbon units generated can be completely oxidized in the muscle to CO2 or can generate ketone bodies in the liver that may be exported to other organs to provide energy.

first episode is fatal. The treatment consists of (1) avoidance of fasting, (2) consumption of low-fat foods, (3) carnitine supplementation, and (4) institution of an emergency plan in case of illness or other metabolic stress. Early diagnosis through newborn screening and early initiation of treatment leads to a favourable prognosis.[14] Patients with MCAD deficiency are identified by MS/MS newborn screening because of the characteristic acylcarnitine profile with increased concentrations of (1) C6- (hexanoyl), (2) C8- (octanoyl), and (3) C10:1- (decenoyl) carnitine and increased C8/C2 and C8/C10 ratios.

The diagnosis of MCAD is confirmed biochemically by urine organic acid and acylglycine analysis showing (1) excess hexanoylglycine, (2) plasma acylcarnitine profile (confirming increased C6-, C8-, and C10:1 carnitine), and by (3) DNA analysis.[9] Two common mutations have been identified in the *ACADM* gene of patients with MCAD deficiency. The most common mutation is a single-nucleotide A-to-G change in exon 11 (c.985A>G) that results in a lysine-for-glutamate amino acid change in the protein (p.K304E). This mutation is prevalent in symptomatic patients (80% of symptomatic patients are homozygous for this mutation, 98% carry at least one copy) A second mutation, which changes a tyrosine to a histidine (p.Y42H), has been found in asymptomatic newborns identified through MS/MS newborn screening.

Treatment of Fatty Acid Oxidation Disorders

Treatment of fatty acid oxidation disorders consists of (1) avoidance of fasting, (2) adherence to a low-fat diet, and (3) carnitine supplementation. For some disorders of fatty acid oxidation, a diet is indicated that is supplemented with medium chain triglycerides (oil) that enter mitochondria independently from carnitine and bypass the metabolic block. In addition, conditions that increase catabolism such as (1) fever, (2) vomiting, and (3) infections need to be aggressively treated with antibiotics (if necessary) and antipyretics and with intravenous glucose.

Disorders of Carbohydrate Metabolism

Enzyme deficiency in the metabolic pathways for carbohydrates results in accumulation of sugars within organs or tissues impairing their function, inability to obtain energy from them, or toxicity from the excess of monosaccharides or their derivatives (phosphorylated sugars). **Disorders of carbohydrate metabolism** include the (1) **glycogen storage diseases**, (2) **glucose-6-phosphate dehydrogenase (G-6-PD) deficiency**, and (3) classic galactosemia.

Glycogen storage disorders affect primarily the liver or the skeletal muscle. The accumulation of glycogen impairs organ function and, if the liver is affected, prevents release of glucose with resulting hypoglycemia. They are usually treated with avoidance of fasting and a special diet devoid of simple sugars and supplements with uncooked cornstarch. Glucose-6-phosphate dehydrogenase deficiency affects red blood cells, causing them to break down (hemolysis). It can cause mild to severe jaundice in newborns and in some cases hemolytic anemia. Symptoms can be triggered by (1) infections, (2) certain drugs (some antibiotics and medications used to treat malaria), or (3) exposure to fava beans (a reaction called favism). The gene for this condition is on the X chromosomes and the condition affects mostly males. Avoidance of stressors can mitigate or avoid symptoms.

Classic galactosemia results from absence of galactose-1-phosphate uridyl transferase.[4] Galactose is derived from the disaccharide lactose found in milk. In galactosemia, galactose is phosphorylated to galactose-1-phosphate, but it is not further metabolized. Increased concentrations of galactose-1-phosphate in cells are toxic. Infants have (1) failure to thrive, (2) jaundice, (3) liver failure, and (4) predisposition to sometimes life-threatening infections with *E. coli* and other Gram-negative bacteria. The treatment of galactosemia involves removal of lactose (contained in human or animal-derived milk, but not in soy milk) and avoidance of all foods containing galactose. In galactosemia, intervention early in life provides the best prognosis although some long-lasting effects may continue to be observed, particularly in girls who for unknown reasons develop ovarian failure. Learning disorders are occasionally observed in treated individuals as well.

Diagnostic Tests for Inherited Disorders of Metabolism

A newborn screening result highly suggestive of a metabolic disorder typically leads to an immediate evaluation using confirmatory tests and a referral of the newborn to a metabolic center.

Types of Confirmatory Tests

In asymptomatic patients, the confirmation of diagnosis relies on specific tests, such as (1) ion-exchange chromatography, (2) liquid chromatography-tandem mass spectrometry (LC-MS/MS) for amino acids analysis, (3) gas chromatography-mass spectrometry (GC-MS) for organic acids analysis, and (4) MS/MS with or without liquid chromatographic separation for acylcarnitines and acylglycines analyses. The combination of these tests is the key in the confirmation of abnormal newborn screening results, especially for those with borderline values.

DNA testing and enzyme assays are available for further confirmation of most of these conditions.

These techniques are described in Chapters 12, 13, and 18. Tandem mass spectrometry (MSMS) is a technique of choice in newborn screening programs.

Tandem Mass Spectrometry

The introduction of tandem mass spectrometry (MSMS) as a routine laboratory technique has dramatically increased the number of disorders amenable to newborn screening since multiple metabolites are detected simultaneously in the same blood spot (**multiplex analysis**). This, allows the identification of several disorders at once, whereas traditional screening techniques were based on one test for one disorder.[2]

Application

In 2005, the American College of Medical Genetics and Genomics (ACMG) released a report, commissioned by the Maternal and Child Health Bureau (MCHB) of the Health Resources and Services Administration (HRSA) with recommendations for a uniform panel for newborn screening (www.acmg.net/; accessed December 17, 2013)[1] This panel is periodically updated by the Secretary's Advisory Committee on Heritable Disorders in Newborns and Children (www.hrsa.gov/; accessed December 17, 2013). Current recommendations for the uniform screening panel of core conditions include at least (1) five fatty acid oxidation disorders, (2) nine organic acidemias, (3) six aminoacidopathies, (4) two endocrinopathies, (5) three hemoglobinopathies/thalassemias, and (6) six other disorders (see Table 45-1) two of which (hearing loss and critical congenital heart disease) are tested directly in the birth facility. In addition, many secondary conditions have been identified using MS/MS and are routinely reported by most newborn screening programs (Table 45-2).

Methodological Details

MS/MS measures the ratio of the mass (m) of a chemical to its charge z (see Chapter 13 for details of technique). For newborn screening, a tandem mass spectrometer is configured to measure only acylcarnitines and amino acids using the information about their mass and fragmentation pattern. Labelled internal standards are added to the extraction mixtures to quantify the different species.

Interpretation

With MS/MS screening, several analytes are detected at the same time and the interpretation of the results is based heavily on pattern recognition, whereas the measurement of the concentration of the different metabolites supports the interpretation.[3] The ability to detect multiple metabolites by MS/MS allows the use of ratios of metabolites to define whether an increased value is due to a metabolic derangement or to the clinical and nutritional status of the newborn.

Assessment of congenital disorders at the appropriate time after birth is crucial. For example, although amino acid concentrations do not change significantly with newborn

TABLE 45-2 Uniform Screening Panel: Secondary Conditions as Recommended by the Discretionary Advisory Committee on Heritable Disorders in Newborns and Children*

| ACMG* Code | Secondary Condition | Metabolic Disorder | | | | |
		Organic Acid Condition	Fatty Acid Oxidation Disorders	Amino Acid Disorders	Hemoglobin Disorder	Other Disorder
Cbl C,D	Methylmalonic acidemia with homocystinuria	X				
MAL	Malonic acidemia	X				
IBG	Isobutyrylglycinuria	X				
2MBG	2-Methylbutyrylglycinuria	X				
3MGA	3-Methylglutaconic aciduria	X				
2M3HBA	2-Methyl-3-hydroxybutyric aciduria	X				
SCAD	Short-chain acyl-CoA dehydrogenase deficiency		X			
M/SCHAD	Medium/short-chain L-3-hydroxyacl-CoA dehydrogenase deficiency		X			
GA2	Glutaric acidemia type II		X			
MCAT	Medium-chain ketoacyl-CoA thiolase deficiency		X			
DE RED	2,4 Dienoyl-CoA reductase deficiency		X			
CPT IA	Carnitine palmitoyltransferase type I deficiency		X			
CPT II	Carnitine palmitoyltransferase type II deficiency		X			
CACT	Carnitine acylcarnitine translocase deficiency		X			
ARG	Argininemia			X		
CIT II	Citrullinemia type II			X		
MET	Hypermethioninemia			X		
H-PHE	Benign hyperphenylalaninemia			X		
BIOPT (BS)	Biopterin defect in cofactor biosynthesis			X		
BIOPT (REG)	Biopterin defect in cofactor regeneration			X		
TYR-II	Tyrosinemia type II			X		
TYR-III	Tyrosinemia type III			X		
Var Hb	Various other hemoglobinopathies				X	
GALE	Galactoepimerase deficiency					X
GALK	Galactokinase deficiency					X
	T-cell related lymphocyte deficiencies					X

*Note: These disorders are detected in the differential diagnosis of core disorders listed in Table 45-1. The nomenclature for conditions is based on data from reference 12.[12]
ACMG, American College of Medical Genetics and Genomics.
Adopted from American College of Medical Genetics and Genomics. newborn screening: towards a uniform screening panel and system. Genetic Med 2006;8(5) Suppl:S12-S252.

age, acylcarnitine concentrations vary significantly. For most acylcarnitines, the concentrations are highest in the first week of life and decrease rapidly afterwards. In some states, a second screening test is mandated at 1 to 4 weeks of age. Age-appropriate cutoff values for all screening tests should be used for the interpretation of newborn screening results.

Review Questions

1. An inherited disorder that affects the conversion of nutrients into energy is referred to as a(n)
   a. aminoacidopathy.
   b. autosomal recessive disorder.
   c. inborn error of metabolism (IEM).
   d. hemolytic disease of a newborn.
2. Tandem mass spectrometry (MS/MS) involves

   a. an ultraviolet laser to ionize small amounts of matrix and analyte that are directed into the mass analyzer.
   b. screening a large number of infants for disorders of amino acid metabolism using different growth antagonists.
   c. an ion trap designed to trap ions in three dimensions instead of two dimensions.
   d. assessment of the mass-to-charge ratio of a chemical.
3. An inborn disorder of metabolism that is triggered by prolonged fasting and/or acute illness and that is confirmed by abnormal acylcarnitine concentrations is
   a. galactosemia.
   b. medium-chain acyl-CoA dehydrogenase (MCAD) deficiency.
   c. phenylketonuria (PKU).
   d. glutaric acidemia type I (GAI).

4. Deficiency of an enzyme that results in excess of monosaccharides in the blood of a newborn leads to a specific disorder of metabolism. An example of this type of disorder would be
   a. galactosemia.
   b. medium-chain acyl-CoA dehydrogenase (MCAD) deficiency.
   c. phenylketonuria (PKU).
   d. glutaric acidemia type I (GAI).

5. The disorder that is identified by increased serum glutarylcarnitine and urine glutaric acid (GA) on newborn screening is characterized by dysfunctional metabolism of
   a. hydroxylysine and phenylalanine.
   b. tyrosine and tryptophan.
   c. tryptophan, hydroxylysine, and lysine.
   d. cystine and hydroxylysine.

6. In a disorder that has an autosomal recessive inheritance pattern, what is the risk of two carrier parents having an affected child with that disorder?
   a. 0%
   b. 25%
   c. 50%
   d. 100%

7. In relation to newborn screening for inborn errors of metabolism (IEMs), second-tier testing is done to
   a. assess the parents of the newborn for possible carrier status.
   b. assess the siblings of the newborn for similar symptoms or disorders.
   c. determine the number of false negatives that might have occurred with initial screening.
   d. further assess a positive screening test result by targeting more specific analytes.

8. The disorder of amino acid metabolism in which the parent amino acid accumulates in blood and spills over into urine is classified as
   a. an organic acidemia.
   b. an aminoacidopathy.
   c. a carbohydrate disorder.
   d. a disorder of fatty acid oxidation.

9. The simultaneous analysis of multiple analytes using a single sample, such as a blood spot from a newborn, is referred to as
   a. multiplex analysis.
   b. newborn screening.
   c. tandem mass spectrometry (MS/MS).
   d. multiple of means.

10. The enzyme that is absent in the aminoacidopathy phenylketonuria (PKU) is
    a. phenylalanine decarboxylase.
    b. ornithine translocase.
    c. phenylalanine hydroxylase.
    d. succinyl-coenzyme A (CoA) mutase.

References

1. American College of Medical Genetics. Newborn screening: toward a uniform screening panel and system. Genet Med 2006;8 Suppl 1:1S–252S.
2. Chace DH. Mass spectrometry in newborn and metabolic screening: historical perspective and future directions. J Mass Spectrom 2009;44:163–70.
3. Chace DH, Kalas TA, Naylor EW. Use of tandem mass spectrometry for multianalyte screening of dried blood specimens from newborns. Clin Chem 2003;49:1797–817.
4. Elsas LJ. Galactosemia. In: Pagon RA, Adam MP, Bird TD, et al, eds. GeneReviews™ [Internet]. Seattle (WA): University of Washington, Seattle; 1993-2013. 2000 Feb 04 [updated 2010 Oct 26].
5. Guthrie R, Susi A. A simple phenylalanine method for detecting phenylketonuria in large populations of newborn infants. Pediatrics 1963;32:338–43.
6. Hedlund GL, Longo N, Pasquali M. Glutaric acidemia type 1. Am J Med Genet C Semin Med Genet 2006;142C(2):86–94.
7. Longo N, Amat di San Filippo C, Pasquali M. Disorders of carnitine transport and the carnitine cycle. Am J Med Genet C Semin Med Genet 2006;142C:77–85.
8. Maniatis AK, Taylor L, Letson GW, et al. Congenital hypothyroidism and the second newborn metabolic screening in Colorado, USA. J Pediatr Endocrinol Metab 2006;19:31–8.
9. Matern D, Rinaldo P. Medium-chain acyl-coenzyme a dehydrogenase deficiency. In: Pagon RA, Adam MP, Bird TD, et al, eds. GeneReviews™ [Internet]. Seattle (WA): University of Washington, Seattle; 1993-2013. 2000 Feb 04 [updated 2010 Oct 26].
10. Rock MJ, Hoffman G, Laessig RH, et al. Newborn screening for cystic fibrosis in Wisconsin: nine-year experience with routine trypsinogen/DNA testing. J Pediatr 2005;147:S73–7.
11. Schwarz E, Liu A, Randall H, et al. Use of steroid profiling by UPLC-MS/MS as a second tier test in newborn screening for congenital adrenal hyperplasia: the Utah experience. Pediatr 2009;Res 66:230–35.
12. Sweetman L, Millington DS, Therrell BL, et al. Naming and counting disorders (conditions) included in newborn screening panels. Pediatr 2006;117:S308–14.
13. Viau K, Ernst SL, Vanzo RJ, et al. Glutaric acidemia type 1: outcomes before and after expanded newborn screening. Mol Genet Metab 2012;106:430–38.
14. Wilcken B. Fatty acid oxidation disorders: outcome and long-term prognosis. J Inherit Metab Dis 2010;33:501–6.

Pharmacogenetics

Gwendolyn A. McMillin, Ph.D., D.A.B.C.C. (C.C., T.C.)

Objectives

1. Define the following:

   Adverse drug reaction (ADR)   Pharmacogenetics
   Cytochrome P450 (CYP)   Pharmacokinetics
   Haplotype   Phase I/II enzyme
   Metabolizer   Prodrug
   Pharmacodynamics   Single-nucleotide
                                    polymorphism

2. List and describe three characteristics of a drug-gene pair that contribute to successful clinical implementation of a pharmacogenetic test.

3. Compare genotyping and phenotyping in regard to pharmacogenetic testing, including how each is determined, limitations in testing, and the continued need for therapeutic drug monitoring.

4. List the general actions that Phase I and Phase II enzymes have on substrates.

5. For each of the following enzymes, state whether it is a Phase I or Phase II enzyme, list the specific substrates of each enzyme, and state whether the substrate is a prodrug and the action of the enzyme on that substrate:

   Cytochrome P450 2C19   N-acetyltransferase 2
     (CYP2C19)   (NAT2)
   Cytochrome P450 2C9   Thiopurine
     (CYP2C9)   S-methyltransferase
   Cytochrome P450 2D6   (TPMT)
     (CYP2D6)   UDP-Glucuronosyltransferase
   Dihydropyrimidine   1A1 (UGT1A1)
     dehydrogenase (DPD)   Vitamin K epoxide reductase
   N-acetyltransferase 1   (VKOR)
     (NAT1)

6. For the *HLA-B* gene and the *HLA-B*5701* allele, describe the relationship of allelic variants with drug hypersensitivity, including associated phenotypes and laboratory analysis.

7. Analyze and resolve case studies related to pharmacogenetic testing in the laboratory.

Key Words and Definitions

Acute lymphoblastic leukemia (ALL) An acute, rapidly progressing form of leukemia that is characterized by the presence in the blood and bone marrow of large numbers of unusually immature white blood cells destined to become lymphocytes.

Adverse drug reaction (ADR) Any undesirable side effect or toxic reaction that is caused by the administration of a drug.

Allele One of the alternative versions of a gene at a given location (locus) along a chromosome. An individual inherits two alleles for each gene, one from each parent. If the two alleles are the same, the individual is homozygous for that gene. If the alleles are different, the individual is heterozygous. The term now also refers to variation among non-coding DNA sequences in addition to genes.

Cytochrome P450 (CYP) A large family of metabolic enzymes that catalyze the oxidations of organic substrates. They are important in metabolism of drugs, steroid hormones, fatty acids, and other substances.

Drug metabolism The process by which drugs are chemically modified in the body.

Gene duplication A process by which a chromosome or a portion of DNA is duplicated, resulting in an additional copy of a gene. Also referred to as *chromosomal duplication* or *gene amplification*.

Genotype The genetic makeup of an individual or a group of individuals. An individual's genotype codes for that individual's phenotype. The genotype for a specific gene requires knowledge of both *alleles* of the gene.

Genotyping Laboratory testing designed to detect specific genetic variants that are used to identify and classify variant alleles. The alleles are reported together as a genotype that may or may not be predictive of a phenotype.

Gilbert syndrome A common hereditary cause of increased bilirubin; found in up to 5% to 10% of the population.

Haplotype A combination of alleles (for different genes) that are located closely together on the same chromosome and that tend to be inherited together.

Key Words and Definitions—cont'd

International normalized ratio (INR) A method of reporting prothrombin time results for patients receiving oral anticoagulant therapy

Irinotecan A DNA topoisomerase inhibitor used as an antineoplastic drug in the treatment of colorectal carcinoma.

Metabolizer classification A classification of four drug-metabolism phenotypes as they relate to an individual's metabolic efficiency for processing a specific therapeutic drug. The four types are (1) poor metabolizers (PMs), (2) ultra-rapid metabolizers (UMs), (3) extensive metabolizesr (EMs), and (4) intermediate metabolizers (IMs).

N-acetyltransferase (NAT) A family of metabolic enzymes that acetylate drugs.

National Institutes of Health (NIH) Pharmacogenomics Research Network (PGRN) A network of scientists focused on understanding how a person's genes affect his or her response to medicines.

Pharmaceutical drug Any chemical substance intended for use in the (1) medical diagnosis, (2) cure, (3) treatment, or (4) prevention of disease. Also referred to as a *medicine* or *medication.*

Pharmacodynamics A process that defines how a drug acts on its target and its mechanisms of action.

Pharmacogenetics Study of the variations in single genes or small groups of related genes that affect the response to a drug, including its metabolism.

Pharmacogenomics The study of how combinations of variations in several genes, potentially extended to the complete genome, influence the pharmacology of a drug(s).

Pharmacogenomics Knowledge Base (PharmGKB) An integrated resource about how variation in human genetics leads to variation in response to drugs; database of information about genes (pharmacogenes) involved in modulating the response to drugs.

Pharmacokinetics A process describing how a drug is (1) absorbed, (2) distributed, (3) metabolized, and (4) eliminated.

Phenocopying The alteration of a phenotype through a non-genetic, environmental mechanism.

Phenotype The observable physical or biochemical characteristics of an individual, as determined by their genetic makeup and environmental influences.

Phenotyping Laboratory testing designed to measure or predict the reaction or response of an individual to a stimulus (such as, a specific drug). A drug-related phenotype is based upon an individual's genes, but it is also influenced by non-genetic factors, such as concomitant medications, liver function, and renal function.

Prodrug A drug that is administered in an inactive or poorly-active form and is converted to an active drug by metabolism.

Pseudogene A defective segment of DNA that resembles a gene but cannot be transcribed.

Severe cutaneous adverse reaction syndromes (SCARS) A group of serious skin conditions that are characterized by blisters and epidermal detachment.

Single-nucleotide polymorphism (SNP) (Pronounced "snips.") A DNA sequence variation that occurs at appreciable frequency in the population.

Star (*)-allele nomenclature A nomenclature developed to standardize genetic polymorphism annotation for the cytochrome P450 genes.

Stevens-Johnson syndrome (SJS) A serious allergic reaction with a characteristic rash involving the skin and mucous membranes. The hypersensitive (allergic) reaction may be initiated by drugs, infectious agents, or other stimuli.

Thiopurine S-methyltransferase (TPMT) A metabolic enzyme that methylates and thereby inactivates certain antimetabolites, such as 6-mercaptopurine (6-MP) (cancer therapeutic).

Toxic epidermal necrolysis (TEN) A rare condition that causes large portions of the epidermis (the skin's outermost layer) to detach from the layers of skin below.

Uridine 5′-diphosphate (UDP)-glucuronosyltransferase (UGT) A family of metabolic enzymes that conjugate compounds with glucuronide molecules.

Pharmacogenetics is a term originating from merging the expressions *pharmacology* (the study of drugs) and *genetics* (the study of inherited traits). *Pharmacogenetic testing* is a term describing a process that predicts or explains how an individual (based on their **genotype**) will respond to (1) **pharmaceutical drugs,** (2) medicines, and (3) other pharmacologically or toxicologically active compounds. Related work associating drug handling and response with the entire genome is known as **pharmacogenomics,** although some use that term and pharmacogenetics interchangeably.

Genotype and phenotype are terms of particular relevance to the understanding of the discipline of pharmacogenomics. Biologically, the genotype of an individual is the inherited set of instructions one carries within his or her genetic code. This code is expressed through one's **phenotype** (the composite of one's observable characteristics or traits). Relating these definitions to the practice of administering pharmaceutical drugs,

pharmacogenomics is based on the premise that one's genotype carries the code for how one metabolizes and utilizes a particular drug or group of drugs, and subsequently one's phenotype is a reflection of how this genetic code is executed. Therefore, if basic studies have provided the necessary genotypic and phenotypic data for a particular drug's metabolism and utilization, then pharmacogenetic testing of an individual will provide the information that then would be used to predict their phenotype and ultimately guide drug and dose selection for that individual.[10] For example, predicted phenotype information would be medically useful for (1) selecting or avoiding a specific drug(s), (2) selecting the optimal dose, (3) selecting the optimal dosing interval for a given patient, (4) avoiding and minimizing the incidence of **adverse drug reactions (ADR),** and (5) avoiding and minimizing drug hypersensitivity.

Approximately 10% of all drug labels now include references to pharmacogenetic findings, and several pharmacogenetic tests are available clinically that are designed to identify patients that may be genetically predisposed to ADRs or therapeutic failure.[3] However, incorporation of pharmacogenetics into routine prescribing decisions for most drugs requires further development and validation of specific dosing guidelines and algorithms.

This chapter presents a general introduction to pharmacogenomics and human pharmacogenetic testing and several polymorphic genes and specific applications to drug selection/avoidance decisions are discussed.

Defining Pharmacogenetic Targets

Response to drugs, whether desirable (therapeutic) or undesirable (toxic), depends on many variables, such as (1) drug formulation, (2) route of administration, (3) clinical status, (4) age, (5) sex, (6) co-medications, and (7) genetics. However, most drugs are historically dosed according to population-derived recommendations. Dosing is typically optimized through trial and error, based on how a patient handles and responds to a drug. Minimizing this process of trial and error is one of several tactics proposed to reduce the incidence of ADRs and improve rates of response.[10] Specifically, pharmacogenetic testing is used to understand and predict some aspects of **pharmacokinetics** and **pharmacodynamics**. These processes are described briefly in the next two paragraphs; see Chapter 30 of this textbook for further discussion and detail.

Pharmacokinetics describes how the body acts on a drug, including (1) absorption, (2) distribution, (3) metabolism, and (4) elimination. Pharmacokinetic targets may therefore represent genes that code for (1) transport proteins, (2) metabolic enzymes, and (3) drug-binding proteins. Pharmacokinetics is often evaluated by measuring drugs and their metabolites in biological fluids that are collected at specific times relative to the time of drug administration. From these results, time-versus-concentration curves are generated, and parameters (such as, clearance) are calculated. Metabolic ratios (such as, metabolite concentration divided by parent drug concentration) are also used to evaluate variation in pharmacokinetics.

Pharmacodynamics describes how a drug elicits responses and whether the response is desirable or undesirable. Pharmacodynamic targets may represent genes that code for (1) enzymes, (2) receptors, (3) ion channels, and (4) other signaling proteins. Response to a drug may or may not show a relationship to drug dose or to the concentration of drug in blood. Pharmacodynamics are measured for some drugs with biomarkers or clinical measurements.

The first recognized pharmacogenetic targets described variation in **drug metabolism** (pharmacokinetics). The early focus on drug metabolism reflects the fact that measurements of drug and drug metabolite concentrations in biological fluids define a phenotype, and that biological fluids (usually blood or urine) are reasonably accessible for testing. Several metabolic phenotypes were (1) characterized, (2) found to cluster within families, and (3) later explained by specific gene variants.

Metabolic phenotypes reflect either poor or rapid drug metabolism. Metabolism of a drug either inactivates or activates

the drug. Each metabolite exhibits unique pharmacokinetic and pharmacodynamic phenotypes as well and may undergo subsequent metabolic reactions. As such, there may be several important metabolites to consider for a single drug; each metabolite may be more or less active than the parent drug, and it may be eliminated more rapidly or more slowly than the parent drug.

Currently, most drug-gene associations are not sufficiently studied to be used routinely for directing clinical therapy. And, it is (1) not practical, (2) medically indicated, nor (3) cost-effective to provide pharmacogenetic profiles for every protein known to be associated with every drug. Based on successful applications to date, pharmacogenetic targets are most likely to be successful clinically when they:

1. Define a major pathway for metabolism of, or response to, a specific drug, thereby providing clear guidance for drug selection or avoidance.
2. Are associated with a clinically significant and actionable effect on the relationship between dose and plasma drug concentration or a measurable biomarker.
3. Predict dosing for a drug that is known to be clinically challenging, such as due to (1) a narrow therapeutic index, (2) limited temporal opportunity to exert efficacy, or (3) a requirement for a long period of taking the drug to determine if the drug is effective in that patient.

The utility of pharmacogenetic testing may be compromised when (1) alternative drugs are not available, (2) incorporation of pharmacogenetic testing does not clearly improve patient care, (3) less sophisticated or less expensive tools or tests are sufficient for making prescribing decisions, or (4) accommodations to specific dose or dosing strategies are not available. Some specific gene-drug relationships for which the drug labeling includes pharmacogenetic information are shown in Table 46-1. Although these gene-drug examples apply to specific areas of medicine, other areas of medicine are likely to benefit from pharmacogenetic testing as well.

Approaches to Pharmacogenetic Testing

In practice, pharmacogenetic testing is a tool that a clinician uses to predict that a patient is likely to (1) fail therapy, (2) suffer an ADR, or (3) exhibit altered pharmacokinetics. This knowledge then assists the clinician in (1) selection/avoidance of a drug, (2) establishing a drug dosage, and (3) establishing a dosing frequency with intent to improve success of therapy.

Pharmacogenetic testing may be accomplished through phenotype or genotype testing. Table 46-2 compares characteristics of the phenotype and the genotype. **Phenotyping** can be done before or after administration of a drug. Phenotyping before administration of a drug can be accomplished by various techniques, such as measurement of metabolic ratios in blood or urine after administration of a probe drug, or use of functional tests that reflect key enzymes or proteins involved in drug metabolism or response. Such testing is not common today. Post-therapeutic phenotyping, however, particularly therapeutic drug monitoring, is used to personalize

TABLE 46-1   Examples of Germline Pharmacogenetic Relationships in Medicine Today

Drug	Relevant Area of Medicine	Approximate Rate of ADRs or Resistance	Gene or Allele	Other Drugs with Pharmacogenetic Relationship
6-Mercaptopurine	Oncology	Up to 10% ADRs	TPMT	Azathioprine, 6-thioguanine
Irinotecan	Oncology	Up to 40% ADRs	UGT1A1	Topotecan, nilotinib, protease inhibitors
5-Fluorouracil	Oncology	20% ADRs	DYPD	Capecitabine
Tamoxifen	Oncology	30% resistant	CYP2D6	Risperidone, fluoxetine, codeine, atomoxetine, amiodarone, doxorubicin
Nortriptyline	Psychiatry	Up to 10% ADRs		
Abacavir	Infectious disease	Up to 10% ADRs	HLA-B*5701	
Warfarin	Cardiology	Up to 40% ADRs	CYP2C9, VKORC1	
Clopidogrel	Cardiology	30% resistant	CYP2C19	Voriconazole, omeprazole, diazepam, antidepressants

ADRs, Adverse drug reactions.

TABLE 46-2   Comparing Phenotype and Genotype Testing Strategies

	Phenotype	Genotype
Represents	"State" represents current response; may not represent inheritance	"Trait" represents inheritance; may not be consistent with the phenotype
Sensitive to gene expression	Yes	No
Sensitive to protein function	Yes	No
Requires collection of multiple specimens	Commonly	No
Requires administration of a probe drug	Possibly	No
Other limitations	• Timing of specimen collection may be critical • May not be appropriate for patients who recently received a blood transfusion • May be influenced by co-medications (drug-drug interactions)	• May not detect all clinically relevant genes and/or alleles • Genotype-phenotype relationship (interpretation) may not be known

drug therapy and should help to adjust for pharmacogenetic or other sources of variation in drug handling and/or drug response.

The value of **genotyping** depends on a strong genotype-phenotype correlation. In the simplest scenario, a genotype result accounts for 100% of the anticipated phenotype. Unfortunately, completely definitive genotype-phenotype relationships (100% certainty) are rare—a fact that creates controversy surrounding the value of a single-gene association. Limitations in testing and the possibility of false-negative results due to the targeted nature of most pharmacogenetic testing may also reduce the clinical utility of genotyping, as will inter-individual variation in gene expression, and non-genetic factors, such as drug-drug or drug-food interactions. As such, genetic testing may guide initial drug and dose selection, but post-therapeutic monitoring that evaluates the patient "state" may be required to verify or further optimize dose of that drug. Indeed, neither phenotyping nor genotyping is intended to replace the need for clinical assessments of drug response.

Clinical Applications of Pharmacogenetic Testing

Pharmacogenetic testing is clinically useful only when information is sufficient to clearly guide drug and/or dose selection.

While many examples of this type of information are found in the peer-reviewed literature, most of the available data came from retrospective studies. The **Pharmacogenomics Knowledge Base (PharmGKB)**[4] is a publicly available Internet research tool developed by Stanford University with funding from the **National Institutes of Health (NIH)** and is part of the **NIH Pharmacogenomics Research Network (PGRN)**, a nationwide collaborative research consortium (http://www.nigms.nih.gov/;accessed December 18, 2013). Its aim is to aid researchers in understanding how genetic variation among individuals contributes to differences in reactions to drugs. This regularly updated database is an excellent source of genetic and clinical information derived from research studies at various medical centers worldwide.[8] Organized registries for clinical studies (such as, http://clinicaltrials.gov; accessed December 18, 2013) are also good resources. It is anticipated that drugs previously removed from development because of ADRs will be reconsidered if genetic tests identify individuals at high risk for ADRs, who could avoid use of that drug. Thus, companion diagnostics and pharmacogenetic-based dosing guidelines are likely to be introduced. Indeed, the US Food and Drug Administration (FDA) has published a draft guidance for companion diagnostics, and several such products are currently cleared and referenced on their website (http://www.fda.gov/;accessed December 18, 2013).

Some of the most successful pharmacogenetics tests in existence today support diverse medical disciplines, including (1) oncology, (2) psychiatry and neurology, (3) cardiology, and (4) infectious disease. Each of these clinical disciplines utilizes medications that exhibit substantial inter-individual variability in response and toxicity profiles. Although pharmacogenetic test results do not guarantee selection of the best drug at the best dose for an individual patient, testing does provide information that is used to guide pharmacotherapy decision-making and help identify whether individual patients are suitable or unsuitable candidates for a particular drug. Pharmacogenetic testing may also help identify patients that may require additional monitoring, relative to generalized population-based recommendations. A number of common drugs and genes that serve as examples of successful pharmacogenetic applications are listed in Table 46-1. These specific genes and how they predict or explain variation in pharmacokinetics and/or pharmacodynamics of certain drugs are discussed later in the next paragraphs.

Drug Metabolism and Pharmacogenomics

Metabolism of drugs is often described in terms of phase I and phase II reactions. Most phase I reactions are oxidative and are mediated by **cytochrome P450 enzymes (CYPs)**. They are the major enzymes involved in drug metabolism and bioactivation, accounting for about 75% of the total number of different metabolic reactions. Phase II reactions typically involve enzymes that conjugate drug analytes with (1) acetyl, (2) glucuronosyl, (3) amino acyl, or (4) sulfate groups. Despite the name, phase II reactions may occur before or after phase I reactions, or independently.

Phase I Cytochrome P450 Enzymes

CYPs are heme-containing enzymes that are synthesized from a superfamily of CYP genes, classified into families, and further classified into subfamilies, based on amino acid homology.* They were originally termed *P450 cytochromes* with the "450" referring to the 450-nanometer absorption maximum of a carbon monoxide binding pigment found in the microsomes of liver.

The major CYPs involved in drug metabolism are (1) cytochrome P450 1A2 (CYP1A2), (2) cytochrome P450 2B6 (CYP2B6), (3) cytochrome P450 2C9 (CYP2C9), (4) cytochrome P450 2C19 (CYP2C19), (5) cytochrome P450 2D6 (CYP2D6), (6) cytochrome P450 2E1 (CYP2E1), and the (7) cytochrome P450 3A family, particularly CYP3A4 and CYP3A5.[17] CYP2D6, CYP2C9, and CYP2C19, are discussed in more detail later. Genetic variants of the CYPs are associated with changes in enzyme (1) activity, (2) stability, and (3) substrate affinity that leads to clinically significant phenotypes. In addition to genetic variability, many CYP isoenzymes are susceptible to dramatic differences in expression (more than 1000-fold), based on (1) age, (2) clinical status, and (3) food/drug interactions.

The relationship of CYPs as drug (1) substrates, (2) inhibitors, and (3) inducers is described in the package labeling for individual drugs and summarized in many books, websites, and other resources. Only selected drug examples, which have thoroughly-described pharmacogenetic targets, will be discussed here, but all the CYP families exhibit genetic variation that could influence optimal prescribing practices for drugs that are substrates for them.

Alleles for all CYP genes are described according to an international consensus classification termed the **Star (∗)-allele nomenclature**.[6,15] For example, the "star 1" allele is the normal allele and codes for a protein predicted to function with full enzymatic activity and to be expressed in typical quantities. Often ∗1 describes a situation where no variant alleles are detected. Therefore, the true accuracy of a ∗1 allele designation is dependent on whether the assay used to make that call is comprehensive. All alleles are described with a star followed by a number, and possibly a letter to describe an allele subtype. Subtypes have not been shown to influence the clinical phenotype, thus far, but could be important for future **haplotype** assignment or to support research studies. Numerical assignments of other alleles (after ∗1) are based largely on chronology of identification, wherein alleles identified earliest in time have the lowest numbers.

Common alleles for *CYP2D6, CYP2C9,* and *CYP2C19* are shown in Table 46-3. A **single-nucleotide polymorphism (SNP/**pronounced "snip") that is frequently used to detect each allele is bolded, but in many cases detection of other SNPs is required to accurately classify an allele. The effects of the genetic variation are shown, where known, both in vitro and in vivo. A model for assignment of estimated phenotype predictions from genotype is illustrated for CYP2D6 in Figure 46-1, which in principle, applies to other CYPs as well. As shown in the figure and discussed in more detail later, the genotype predicts phenotype based on the presumed composite of the alleles detected, and it must be considered relative to other factors that could influence the phenotype.

Cytochrome P450 2D6

CYP2D6, originally named *debrisoquine hydroxylase,* is known to metabolize more than 100 drugs and environmental toxins.[14] It frequently is implicated in ADRs and has been the subject of many US FDA-issued public health advisories. Metabolic phenotypes of CYP2D6 are best described as a continuum that varies from no activity to very high activity. For ease of characterization, CYP2D6 activity is classified according to the **metabolizer classification**. This scheme contains four phenotypes: (1) *ultra-rapid metabolizers (UMs),* (2) *extensive (normal) metabolizers (EMs),* (3) *intermediate metabolizers (IMs),* and (4) *poor metabolizers (PMs).* Translation of a phenotype to a clinical application is somewhat difficult because the actual phenotype is dependent not only on the genetic makeup of CYP2D6, but also on (1) expression of CYP2D6, (2) whether drug-drug interactions affect the phenotype, and (3) whether CYP2D6 activates or inactivates the drug of interest. CYP2D6 is inhibited by several compounds, some of which are also substrates. For example, when a CYP2D6

---

*By convention, names of genes are italicized. For example, *CYP2E1* is the gene that encodes the cytochrome CYP2E1.

TABLE 46-3 Common CYP2D6, CYP2C9, and CYP2C19 Alleles*

Allele	Nucleotide Changes (cDNA)	Effect	Enzyme Activity In Vivo	In Vitro
CYP2D6*1A	None		Normal	Normal
CYP2D6* xN	Based on alleles duplicated	N active genes	Increased for functional alleles	
CYP2D6*2A	**−1584C→G**; −1235A→G; −740C→T; −678G→A; CYP2D7 conversion in intron 1; 1661G→C; 2850C→T; 4180G→C	R296C; S486T	Normal	Normal
CYP2D6*3A	2549delA	Frame shift	None	None
CYP2D6*4A	**100C→T**; 974C→A; 984A→G; 997C→G; 1661G→C; **1846G→A**; 4180G→C	P34S; L91M; H94R; splicing defect; S486T	None	None
CYP2D6*5	Gene deletion		None	
CYP2D6*10A	**100C→T**; 1661G→C; 4180G→C	P34S; S486T	Decreased	Decreased
CYP2D6*17	**1023C→T**; 1661G→C; 2850C→>T; 4180G→C	T1071; R296C; S486T	Decreased	Decreased
CYP2D6*41	−1584C −1235A→G; −740C→T; −678G→A; CYP2D7 conversion in intron 1; 1661G→C; 2850C→T **2988G→A**; 4180G→C	R296C; splicing defect; S486T	Decreased	Decreased
CYP2C9*1A	None		Normal	Normal
CYP2C9*2	**430C→T**	R144C		Decreased
CYP2C9*3	1075A→C	I359L	Decreased	Decreased
CYP2C19*1A	None		Normal	Normal
CYP2C19*2A	99C→T; **681G→A**; 990C→T; 991A→G	Splicing defect; I331V	None	
CYP2C19*3A	**636G→A**; 991A→G; 1251A→C	W212X; I331V	None	
CYP2C19*17	−806C>T (promoter, not c.DNA); 99C→T; 991A→G	Expression	Increased	Increased

*Commonly used analytical target for genotyping is bolded.
Modified from the Human Cytochrome P450 (CYP) Allele Nomenclature Committee. Available at: http://www.CYPalleles.ki.se/; accessed on February 6, 2014. Reproduced with permission of Sarah C. Sim, Webmaster.
No information regarding enzyme activity is listed in the above table when none was present at this reference.

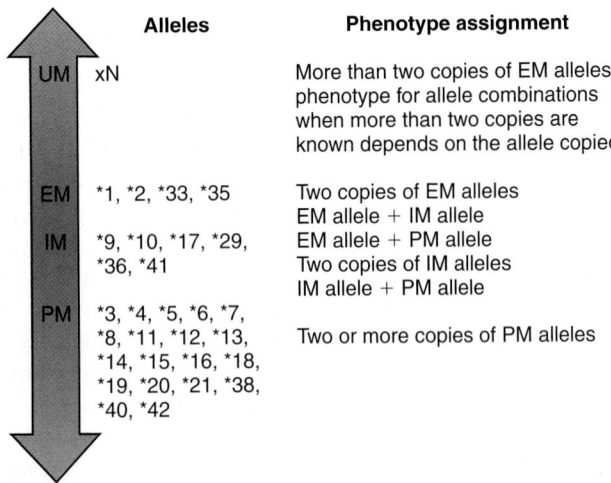

Alleles	Phenotype assignment
UM xN	More than two copies of EM alleles phenotype for allele combinations when more than two copies are known depends on the allele copied
EM *1, *2, *33, *35	Two copies of EM alleles EM allele + IM allele
IM *9, *10, *17, *29, *36, *41	EM allele + PM allele Two copies of IM alleles IM allele + PM allele
PM *3, *4, *5, *6, *7, *8, *11, *12, *13, *14, *15, *16, *18, *19, *20, *21, *38, *40, *42	Two or more copies of PM alleles

Figure 46-1 CYP2D6 phenotype is estimated based on the combination of alleles detected. Shown here is a continuum of metabolic phenotypes: poor metabolizer (PM), extensive metabolizer (EM, normal), intermediate metabolizer (IM), and ultra-rapid metabolizer (UM). The alleles that correspond to enzyme activity are also listed, adjacent to the formulas for establishing a clinical phenotype, based on the combination of two or more alleles.

inhibitor is administered along with a CYP2D6 substrate, the phenotype for the patient may appear impaired. This process, known as **phenocopying**, is defined as the alteration of a phenotype through a non-genetic, environmental, mechanism. It is of clinical relevance for CYP2D6.

The relationship between function of the CYP2D6 enzyme (phenotype) and the CYP2D6 genotype has been extensively characterized, but it is still not well defined for all genotypes, particularly genotypes that predict the impact of IM phenotype. More than 100 allelic variants have been described in the CYP2D6 gene, including complete gene deletions and duplications. Examples of the most common CYP2D6 alleles, listed with associated nucleotide changes and known effects on enzyme activity of CYP2D6, are shown in Table 46-3. Effects on enzyme activity are used to group the alleles according to the predicted phenotype, assuming that two alleles were inherited. However, the actual phenotype reflects a sum of the alleles and non-genetic factors. Among Caucasians, approximately 2% are genetically UM, and 10% are PM. Only 1% to 3% of Blacks and Asians are PMs, but many are IMs.

The CYP2D6 phenotype that is most simple to characterize is the PM phenotype, for which essentially zero CYP2D6 activity is anticipated. The PM phenotype is expected when two or more copies of PM alleles are inherited (see Figure 46-1). Other phenotype assignments are based on the highest functioning phenotype prediction. For example, at least one functional EM allele is thought to generate a phenotype that falls within the limits of normal. The UM phenotype is assigned when more than two copies of functional EM alleles are identified (xN); this is often referred to as a **gene duplication**. Duplication of PM alleles has no effect on the phenotype, and duplication of IM alleles may or may not affect the phenotype.

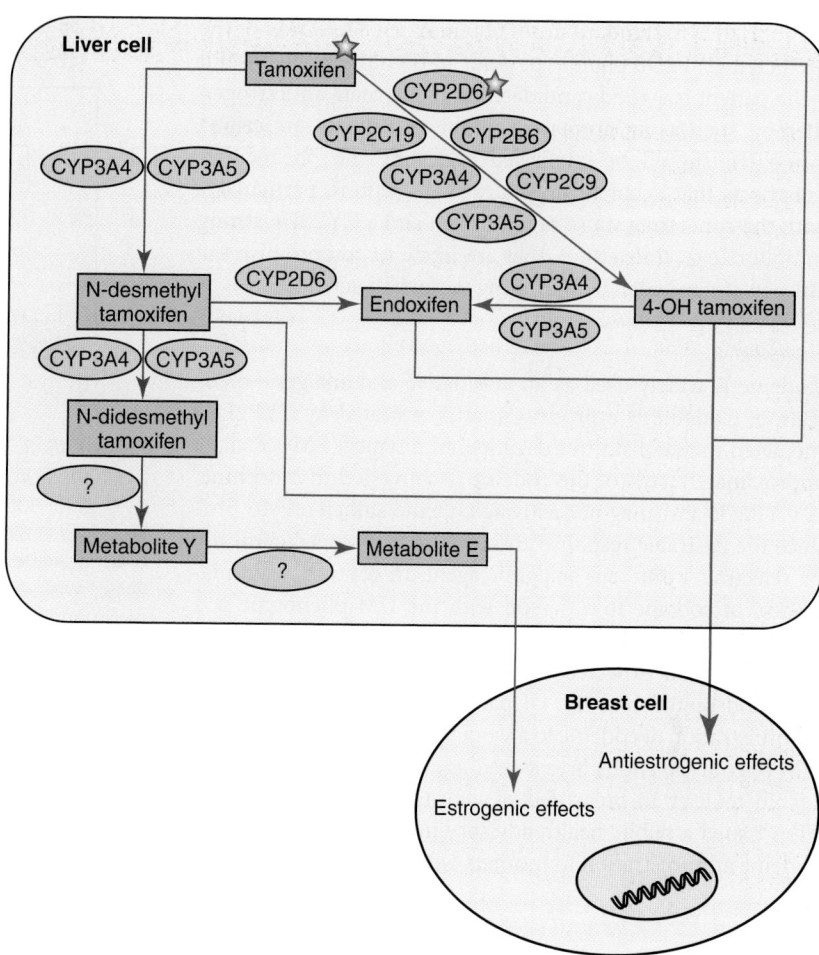

Figure 46-2 Illustrated pharmacokinetic and pharmacodynamic pathways for tamoxifen. Cytochrome P450 (CYP) isozymes are involved in the activation and inactivation of tamoxifen, and cytochrome P450 2D6 (CYP2D6) is key to production of the active metabolite, endoxifen. Most of the antiestrogenic effects of tamoxifen are attributed to endoxifen. Many additional factors in the pharmacokinetics and pharmacodynamics of tamoxifen are not known. *(Reproduced by permission from PharmGKB and Stanford University.)*

The *CYP2D6* gene, like many other CYP genes, is challenging to genotype because of (1) the presence of the **pseudogenes**, (2) the sheer number of genetic variants, (3) the complexity of the genetic variants, and (4) the need for identification of gene dose, specifically, duplications and deletions of the gene. *CYP2D6* pharmacogenetic screening protocols vary tremendously in ability to accurately detect gene dose and to detect many versus only a few of the most common variants. It is important that an assay identify a sufficient number of variants to accurately classify an allele. For example, both the *CYP2D6*10* and *CYP2D6*4* alleles contain the 100C →T variant.* Because the phenotype predictions differ for the two alleles, it is clinically relevant to determine which allele is present. The pattern of additional SNPs unique to each allele helps distinguish the two and suggests the likelihood that both alleles could be present. Examples of how pharmacogenomic testing of *CYP2D6* would have clinical utility in guiding the administration of (1) tamoxifen, (2) codeine, and (3) antidepressants are presented later.

Examples of the pharmacogenomics application of CPY2D6 are in the administration of tamoxifen, codeine and nortriptyline.

*A form of nomenclature that indicates a replacement of a cytosine molecule for a thymidine molecule at position 100 in a gene.

Tamoxifen

Tamoxifen is widely used to treat and prevent breast cancer. Tamoxifen mediates its therapeutic effects through modulation of estrogen receptors, leading to suppression of estrogen-mediated cell proliferation. Therefore, hormone-sensitive breast tumors (estrogen receptor–positive) are most likely to respond to tamoxifen. A meta-analysis of the Early Breast Cancer Trialist Collaborative Group showed that 5 years of tamoxifen reduced the recurrence rate by 50% and the mortality rate by a third.[13] However, the success of tamoxifen therapy is variable, and 30% to 45% of patients on tamoxifen relapse or die from recurrent cancer.

Tamoxifen is a **prodrug** and must be metabolized to the active principles to elicit the desired therapeutic effect (Figure 46-2). The lack of efficacy with tamoxifen is explained, in part, by inter-individual differences in the metabolic activation of tamoxifen. The metabolite of tamoxifen with the greatest therapeutic effect is endoxifen, which is formed largely by a reaction mediated by CYP2D6. Patients with impaired CYP2D6 produce less endoxifen than patients with a CYP2D6 EM phenotype.

An individual's CYP2D6 phenotype could be used clinically to qualify patients as good candidates for tamoxifen therapy.[11] For example, patients with a PM genotype are not expected to convert tamoxifen to endoxifen, and they may not respond appropriately to standard doses of tamoxifen. Detection of the predicted CYP2D6 phenotype prior to therapy may be useful if the patient is a good candidate for an alternate antiestrogen therapy, such as an aromatase inhibitor. Patients prescribed tamoxifen should be counseled regarding the phenocopying effects that occur through drug interactions, particularly with the concomitant use of tamoxifen and a CYP2D6 strong inhibitor (e.g., fluoxetine), that are likely to compromise the efficacy of tamoxifen by inhibiting tamoxifen activation.

Codeine

Codeine is widely used as an antitussive and analgesic medication. Codeine is a prodrug that is activated by CYP2D6-mediated metabolism to morphine. In a typical EM scenario, approximately 10% of the codeine is converted to morphine. A CYP2D6 PM may not activate codeine sufficiently to produce the desirable response and may be best served clinically by selecting a different analgesic agent. In contrast, administration of codeine to a person with the UM phenotype is a significant safety concern, because higher concentrations of morphine than expected lead to risk of unintentional overdose and opioid toxicity. Of particular concern clinically is administration of codeine to a woman who exhibits a CYP2D6 UM phenotype and is breast-feeding. After clinical reports of opioid toxicity in breast-fed newborns of UM mothers, the FDA issued a public health advisory in 2007 warning against codeine administration to mothers with a CYP2D6 UM.[2]

Antidepressant Therapy— Nortriptyline

Antidepressant therapy is challenging because it may require several weeks of drug administration to assess efficacy, and optimizing dose may require many months of trial and error. Most of the antidepressants available today are substrates of CYP2D6, and many are also inhibitors; many case reports of CYP2D6-related toxicity and death have been published. A well-characterized example relates to the tricyclic antidepressants, such as nortriptyline. Nortriptyline is an active drug (and an active drug metabolite of amitriptyline) that is inactivated by CYP2D6-mediated metabolism. When CYP2D6 is impaired, nortriptyline accumulates. High concentrations of nortriptyline are associated with an anticholinergic toxidrome and life-threatening ADRs. Clearance of amitriptyline, nortriptyline, and other tricyclic antidepressants is reduced by at least 50% in PMs of CYP2D6. As shown in Figure 46-3, an individual with a CYP2D6 PM phenotype requires lower doses of nortriptyline than a patient with an EM phenotype to produce similar serum concentrations of active drug.[17]

Cytochrome P450 2C9

CYP2C9 is a member of the CYP2C family, which includes (1) CYP2C8, (2) CYP2C9, (3) CYP2C18, and (4) CYP2C19. Examples of drugs metabolized by CYP2C9 include (1) warfarin, (2) anticonvulsants, (3) nonsteroidal antiinflammatory drugs (NSAIDs), (4) antidiabetic agents, (5) cholesterol-lowering drugs, and (6) drugs used to treat infection. Like other CYPs, CYP2C9 is subject to inhibition through drug-drug interactions, which affects the phenotype (phenocopying).[14,17]

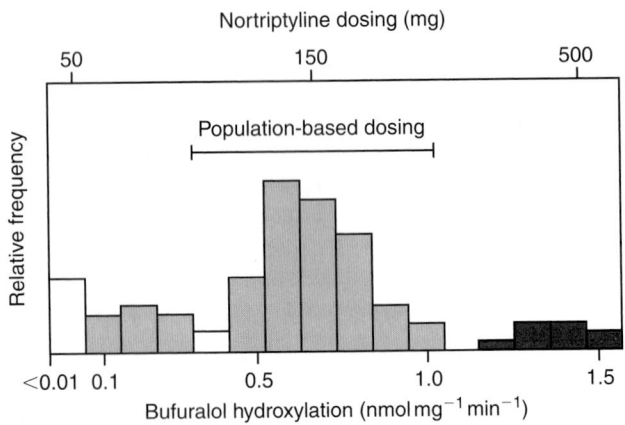

Figure 46-3 Variation in drug metabolism and nortriptyline dosing in the European population, based on cytochrome P450 2D6 (CYP2D6) activity (hydroxylation of bufuralol). Within the population, four phenotypes are identified: (1) poor metabolizers (PMs), who lack the functional enzyme; (2) intermediary metabolizers (IMs), who are heterozygous for one functional allele or have two partially defective alleles encoding the enzyme; (3) extensive metabolizers (EMs), who have two normal alleles; and (4) ultra-rapid metabolizers (UMs), who carry duplicated or multi-duplicated functional CYP2D6 genes. The relative frequency of these phenotypes refers to the European population as a whole. The doses of nortriptyline that are required to achieve therapeutic concentrations in all phenotypes are given. Despite this variation in metabolizing capability, population-based dosing is used today and is based on the average plasma concentrations obtained in a given population for a given dose. *(From Ingelman-Sundberg M. Pharmacogenetics of cytochrome P450 and its applications in drug therapy: the past, present and future. Trends Pharmacol Sci 2004;25:193-200. Reproduced with permission from Elsevier.)*

The *CYP2C9* gene is highly polymorphic, and more than 50 allelic variants have been described.[4] However, two variant alleles, *CYP2C9*2* and *CYP2C9*3*, account for most impaired CYP2C9 PM phenotypes. The *2 allele is identified by R144C (430C→T), and the *3 allele is identified by I359L (1075A→C). The allelic frequency of *CYP2C9*2* is approximately 15% in Caucasians, and less than 5% in other populations. This allele has not been detected in Asians. The allelic frequency of *CYP2C9*3* has been reported as approximately 10% in Caucasians, up to 5% in Asians, and less than 2% in black people. The clinical impact of a *CYP2C9*3* variant is more significant than that of a *CYP2C9*2* variant due to the greater loss of enzymatic activity associated with the *CYP2C9*3* variant. No UM genotype or phenotype has been described for CYP2C9.

Several protocols have been published or are available commercially for detecting variants in this gene. Most focus on detection of only the *2 and *3 alleles, as well as the common promoter variant of another gene, *VKORC1*, due to the complimentary utility in identification of patients at risk for warfarin sensitivity. The warfarin application of *CYP2C9* genotyping is described in more detail later, with *VKORC1*, a gene associated with pharmacodynamics of warfarin response. Other clinical applications of *CYP2C9* and *VKORC1* genotyping are not routine.

Cytochrome P450 2C19

CYP2C19 is involved in the metabolism of a number of therapeutic drugs, including (1) clopidogrel, (2) citalopram, (3) diazepam, (4) omeprazole, (5) propranolol, and (6) proguanil. Known metabolizer phenotypes are (1) PM, (2) IM, (3) EM, and (4) UM.[3,5,14,17] With CYP2C9, there are two common alleles, CYP2C19*2 and CYP2C19*3, that account for nearly all PMs. The PM phenotype occurs in 2% to 5% of Caucasian and Black populations, and 10% to 23% of Asian populations. The CYP2C19*2 arises from a 681G→A mutation, which results in a splicing defect and essentially no enzyme activity. The second most common CYP2C19 allele (CYP2C19*3) associated with the PM phenotype results from a single nucleotide substitution, 636G→A, which produces a premature stop codon and no active enzyme product, but allele frequencies are less than 1% in most populations. The CYP2C19*17 arises from a promoter variant in the gene (-806C→T); it is present in nearly 40% of Caucasians, Blacks, and Asians; and is associated with a UM phenotype. Several protocols have been published for detecting variants in CYP2C19, most of which focus on detection of the *2, *3, and *17 alleles.

Examples of the pharmacogenomic application of CYP2C19 are in the administration of clopidogrel and antidepressants.

Clopidogrel

Clopidogrel is a common drug prescribed to inhibit platelet aggregation, often in combination with aspirin. Approximately one third of patients do not respond to clopidogrel. One explanation for drug resistance is that clopidogrel is a prodrug that requires metabolism to the active metabolite, prasugrel. Carriers of the CYP2C19*2 and *3 alleles have reduced formation of the active metabolite, and they have a higher incidence of major thrombotic events. It is recommended that patients who carry one or more copies of the CYP2C19*2 allele consider an alternative therapy, such as prasugrel itself.[16]

Antidepressant

Genotyping of CYP2C19 may be complimentary to genotyping of CYP2D6 for explaining inappropriate responses to antidepressant medications. For example, CYP2C19 is the primary enzyme responsible for converting amitriptyline to its active metabolite nortriptyline. Monitoring serum or plasma concentrations of both amitriptyline and nortriptyline is also used to guide amitriptyline therapy. Although CYP2D6 is thought to be more relevant clinically than CYP2C19 for most antidepressants, CYP2C19 becomes very important for a drug that is a substrate of both CYP2D6 and CYP2C19 when CYP2D6 is impaired or deficient, particularly if the CYP2C19*17 is present.

Phase II Enzymes

Phase II reactions typically involve enzymes that conjugate drug analytes with (1) acetyl, (2) glucuronyl, (3) amino acyl, or (4) sulfate groups. In general, these enzymes are not typically induced or inhibited to the same degree as CYPs. However, exhausting the substrates or cofactors that are transferred prevents the corresponding transferase reactions from occurring.

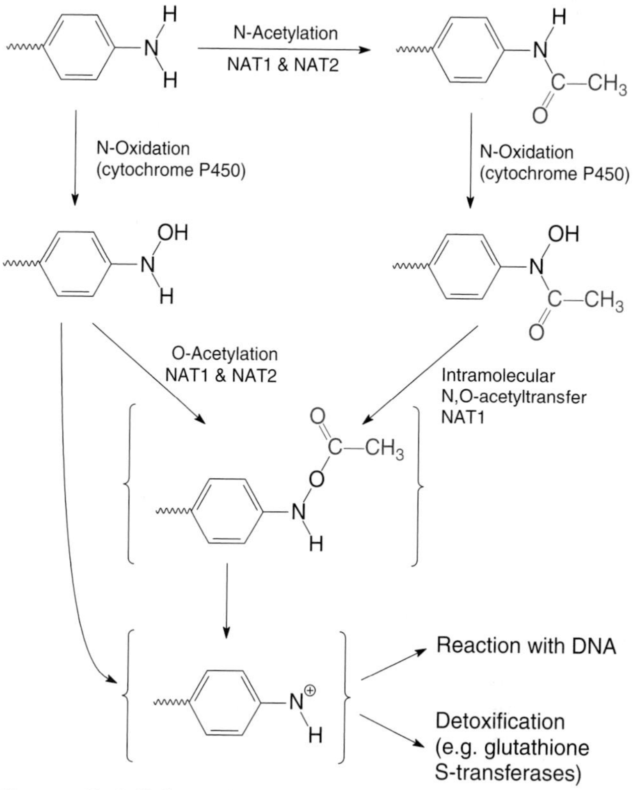

Figure 46-4 Schematic view of the role of N-acetyltransferase (NAT) enzymes in the metabolism of aromatic amines. N-acetylation might be a detoxification reaction in a number of cases; however, after N-hydroxylation of aromatic amines (e.g., by cytochrome P450 [CYP] enzymes), NAT enzymes are able to bioactivate these intermediates by O-acetylation or by intramolecular N,O-acetyltransfer, leading to the formation of nitrenium ions, which might react with DNA or alternatively be detoxified by, for example, glutathione s-transferase enzymes. It is shown that a number of other biotransformation enzymes are involved in the metabolism of aromatic amines as well. (Redrawn from Wormhoudt LW, Commandeur JNM, Vermeulen NPE. Genetic polymorphisms of human N-acetyltransferase, cytochrome P450, glutathione-S-transferase, and epoxide hydrolase enzymes: relevance to xenobiotic metabolism and toxicity. Crit Rev Toxicol 1999;29:59-124. Reproduced by permission from Taylor and Francis, Inc.)

Like phase I enzymes, phase II enzymes are synthesized from genes that are classified into families and further into subfamilies based on homology. These include (1) **N-acetyltransferases (NATs)**, (2) **thiopurine S-methyltransferases (TPMTs)**, (3) **uridine 5'-diphosphate (UDP) glucuronosyltransferases (UGTs)**, and (4) dihydropyrimidine dehydrogenases (DPDs).

N-acetyltransferase

The N-acetyltransferases (NAT) slow acetylator is one of the earliest-described pharmacogenetic phenotypes. NAT1 and NAT2 are two thoroughly-characterized isoforms that catalyze the transfer of an acetyl moiety from acetyl-coenzyme A (CoA) to homocyclic and heterocyclic arylamines and hydrazines (Figure 46-4). Substrates of these phase II reactions include (1) drugs, (2) carcinogens, (3) toxicants, and (4) possibly endogenous compounds. NAT status has been implicated in predisposing to ADRs, and it has also been associated with risk of diseases, including immunologic disorders and several cancers. NAT substrates also have been related to (1) cigarette smoking, (2) some medications, and (3) occupational exposures.

The *NAT1* and *NAT2* genes share 87% nucleotide sequence identity and 81% amino acid sequence identity. Many variant alleles have been described, and a consensus nomenclature has been published.[18] *NAT1*3* and *NAT2*4* are considered the wild-type alleles. The *NAT1*10* is the most common variant *NAT1* allele in many human populations, but the phenotype-genotype relationship is not well defined. For *NAT2*, the (1) *5, (2) *6, (3) *7, (4) *13, and (5) *14 alleles are thought to account for more than 99% of slow acetylator phenotypes.

NAT2 slow acetylators are common in many populations, including approximately 80% of Egyptians; 50% of Caucasians, Europeans, and Blacks; 20% of Asians; and 5% of Canadian Inuits.[17] Genotyping and phenotyping methods predict NAT phenotype; neither genotyping nor phenotyping methods are widely available to support routine clinical testing today.

Thiopurine S-Methyltransferase

Thiopurine S-methyltransferase (TPMT) is a phase II metabolic enzyme that catalyzes the inactivation of 6-mercaptopurine (6-MP) by S-methylation, thus preventing it from forming the thioguanine nucleotides (TGNs) that are responsible for the activity of 6-MP. It also affects azathioprine (AZA) metabolism, because AZA is another prodrug that is metabolized to 6-MP (Figure 46-5). Endogenous substrates for TPMT are currently unknown. AZA and 6-MP are used in the therapeutic management of leukemia, particularly **acute lymphoblastic leukemia (ALL)** in children, but they are also used to treat a diverse range of conditions, including treatment of autoimmunce conditions (such as rheumatoid arthritis and inflammatory bowel disease) and prevention and treatment of rejection of transplanted solid organs. These agents are cytotoxic, acting via incorporation of TGN into DNA. Outside the bone marrow, these agents are oxidatively inactivated by xanthine oxidase or methylated by TPMT. In hematopoietic tissue, however, the effect of xanthine oxidase is negligible, leaving TPMT as the only significant inactivation pathway. Hematopoietic tissues are therefore susceptible to damage in cases in which TPMT activity is very low. TPMT activity is highly variable in all large populations studied to date; approximately 90% of individuals have high activity, 10% have immediate activity, and 0.3% have low or undetectable enzyme activity. Numerous studies have shown that TPMT-deficient patients are at high risk for severe, and sometimes fatal, toxicity.[17]

The (1) *2, (2) *3A, (3) *3B, and (4) *3C alleles of TPMT, account for 80% to 95% of intermediate or low enzyme activity cases in most ethnic groups (see Figure 46-5). The *3A allele is most common in Caucasians, and *3C is most common in Blacks and in Asian populations. The *TPMT*2* and *3B* alleles are rare in comparison with *TPMT*3A* or *3C*. The relationship between phenotype and genotype is very good for most patients, as illustrated in Figure 46-6.

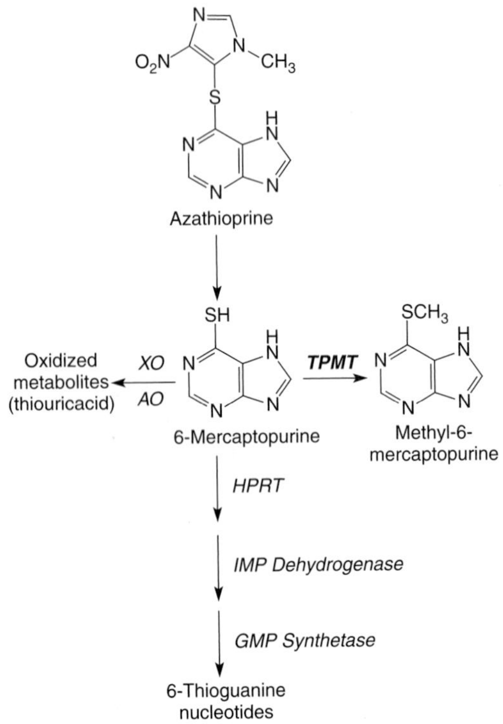

Figure 46-5 Simplified metabolic pathway for prodrug thiopurines, azathioprine (AZA) and 6-mercaptopurine (6-MP). *AO,* Aldehyde oxidase; *GMP,* guanine monophosphate; *HPRT,* hypoxanthine phosphoribosyltransferase; *IMP,* inositol monophosphate; *TPMT,* thiopurine S-methyltransferase; *XO,* xanthine oxidase.

There are at least three approaches to TPMT testing: (1) biochemical phenotyping by determination of TPMT activity within erythrocytes from the patient before administration of drug, (2) metabolic phenotyping by measurement of the concentrations of 6-MP and metabolites in the blood after drug administration, or (3) genotyping. Biochemical phenotyping is limited to patients who have not received a blood transfusion over the weeks previous to TPMT testing and who have healthy red blood cells at the time of testing (often not the case at the time ALL is diagnosed). Metabolic phenotyping requires that AZA or 6-MP be administered before testing. This approach is therefore most useful for optimizing dose once steady-state concentrations have been achieved, or for troubleshooting for patients who have experienced toxicity or an ADR. Genotyping is valid anytime, as long as the patient genotype is detected by the analytical technique employed.

The influence of *TPMT* genotype on hematopoietic toxicity is most dramatic for homozygous variant patients, but it is also of clinical relevance for heterozygous individuals. The labeling for 6-MP was revised in 2004 to include TPMT testing options. It is advised that patients who are TPMT PMs either seek alternative therapies, or receive only 5% to 10% of the conventional dose with careful monitoring. For patients who are predicted to be TPMT IMs, a dose reduction of 30% to 70% has been recommended, depending on the specific clinical scenario.

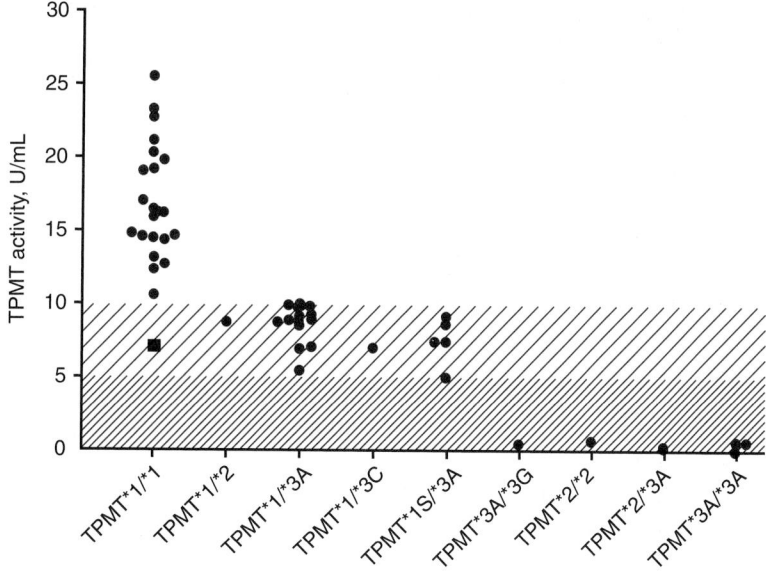

Figure 46-6 Thiopurine S-methyltransferase (TPMT) activity as related to genotypes determined by mutation-specific polymerase chain reaction methods. The *heavily shaded area* depicts the range of TPMT activity in erythrocytes that defines TPMT deficiency (5 U/mL of packed red blood cells); the *lightly shaded area* depicts intermediate activity that defines TPMT heterozygous phenotypes (5 to 10 U/mL of packed red blood cells); and the *nonshaded area* depicts the range of TPMT activity in patients who have homozygous wild-type phenotypes. *Red circles* indicate patients with concordant genotype and phenotype; the black square indicates one patient with discordant genotype and phenotype (TPMT*1/*1). *(From Yates CR, Krynetski EY, Loennechen T, Fessing MY, Tai HL, Pui CH, et al. Molecular diagnosis of thiopurine S-methyltransferase deficiency: genetic basis for azathioprine and mercaptopurine intolerance. Ann Intern Med 1997;126:608-14. Reproduced with permission from the American College of Physicians.)*

UDP-Glucuronosyltransferase 1A1

The mammalian uridine 5′-diphosphate (**UDP**)-**glucuronosyl transferase** (**UGT**) is a superfamily comprised of more than 100 members. The UGT1 and UGT2 families are most efficient at glucuronidation of drugs and toxicants in humans. The UDP-glucuronosyltransferase 1A1 (UGT1A1) isoform has been of greatest interest clinically. The primary goal of glucuronidation is to increase the water solubility of a compound, which typically inactivates that compound and promotes its elimination. An important endogenous substrate for UGT1A1 is bilirubin. Impairment of UGT1A1 leads to accumulation of bilirubin. UGT1A1 is also involved in the glucuronidation of drugs. Impairment of UGT1A1-mediated glucuronidation of drugs was first recognized in patients with **Gilbert syndrome** who were administered **irinotecan**. An inverse relationship between expression of UGT1A1 and bilirubin concentration was recognized in patients with Gilbert syndrome and ultimately led to recognition of variation in the promoter region of the gene.[17]

UGT1A1 is the most 3′ of the UGT1A isoform genes. More than thirty SNPs that lead to nonfunctional UGT1A1 have been identified, but the number of TA repeats found in the TATA sequence of the *UGT1A1* promoter region dramatically affects expression of the gene. The number of TA repeats in unaffected Caucasians is 6, which is described as (TA)6 or *UGT1A1*1*. The most common variant of this sequence is the presence of seven repeats, known as (TA)7 or *UGT1A1*28*, and this leads to a 30% reduction in promoter activity of the UGT1A1 and a subsequent reduction in transcription.[9] Tests for detection of *UGT1A1*28* are commercially available. Both (TA)5 and (TA)8 variants of this sequence, although relatively rare, are recognized to exist and correlate with higher and lower expression, respectively, than the (TA)6. Genotypes are typically referred to as 6/6 for no variants, or 7/7 for homozygosity of *UGT1A1*28*. The *UGT1A1*28* allele is observed in approximately 40% of Caucasians and blacks.

A thoroughly-studied example of a pharmacogenetic application for *UGT1A1*28* genotyping is seen with irinotecan. Irinotecan is widely used in metastatic colorectal cancer and in other tumors, such as lung and liver. It is a prodrug and is converted to its active, cytotoxic metabolite SN-38. Approximately 20% to 35% of patients accumulate SN-38 and experience dose-limiting and potentially life-threatening (grade 3 or 4) diarrhea and/or neutropenia when treated with irinotecan. A major route for inactivation of SN-38 is formation of the glucuronide conjugate by UGT1A1. Individuals possessing variant TA repeats in *UGT1A1* are susceptible to toxicity with irinotecan. It is generally recommended that patients with the TA7/7 genotype receive a reduced dose of irinotecan, although specific dosing guidelines are lacking, and the effect is probably most relevant only in "high dose" irinotecan regimens.

Dihydropyrimidine Dehydrogenase

DPD, coded from *DPYD,* is the initial and rate-limiting enzyme in the three-step pathway of uracil and thymidine catabolism and in the pathway leading to formation of β-alanine. It is also responsible for degrading fluoropyrimidines, such as the commonly-used cancer chemotherapeutic drugs, fluorouracil and capecitabine. Under typical metabolic conditions, approximately 80% of 5-fluorouracil is inactivated by DPD. Patients who are homozygote for deleterious *DPYD* variants should seek alternative treatment, or reduce the dose of 5-flurouracil significantly, to minimize the incidence of severe and sometimes life-threatening toxicity.[17]

Genes Associated with Pharmacodynamics

Vitamin K Epoxide Reductase Complex 1

Vitamin K epoxide reductase (VKOR), a key enzyme in the vitamin K cycle, is encoded by the gene named VKOR complex, subunit 1 *(VKORC1).* VKOR converts vitamin K epoxide to vitamin K and is the primary site of action for the commonly-used oral anticoagulant warfarin. VKOR thus is a component of warfarin pharmacodynamics, rather than of warfarin metabolism. Impairment of VKOR therefore limits activation of the vitamin K–dependent coagulation factors and explains the anticoagulation effect of warfarin. The amount of VKOR expressed, which may be genetically controlled, dictates a person's sensitivity to warfarin.

More than thirty *VKORC1* variants have been described, but most clinical testing detects only the promoter variant of *VKORC1* (−1639G→A). The variant is strongly linked (through linkage disequilibrium; see Chapter 47) with known warfarin-sensitive genotypes and haplotypes.

Warfarin is an anticoagulant drug given to control the formation of blood clots. Individual response to warfarin is highly variable, and the drug is implicated in life-threatening adverse events. Administration of excess warfarin leads to bleeding, and too little warfarin fails to prevent blood clots. In routine clinical practice, the dose for individual patients is adjusted to achieve a target therapeutic **International Normalized Ratio (INR)**, usually between 2 and 3. INR is calculated from the prothrombin (clotting) time (PT) of blood samples. Factors known to affect warfarin dose requirements include (1) clinical factors, (2) dietary factors, (3) concomitant medications, and (4) genetics. These sources of variability are discussed in detail in the 2008 practice guidelines published by the American College of Chest Physicians, as well as in the product labeling for the popular formulation of warfarin sold as Coumadin.[1]

Genetic variants of *VKORC1,* representing sensitivity in response to warfarin, and of *CYP2C9,* representing pharmacokinetics of warfarin inactivation, are thought to account for approximately one third of the variability among patients. When the genetic variants are combined with common clinical factors and early INR data, up to 70% of the variability seen among patients is thought to be explained. Among the many mathematical algorithms published for predicting warfarin dose, consistently included predictors (covariates) include age, gender, an index of body size, the three common genetic variants: *CYP2C9*2, CYP2C9*3,* and the promoter variant of *VKORC1* (−1639G→A). Some algorithms account for factors such as (1) smoking status, (2) common interfering co-medications (e.g., amiodarone), (3) liver disease, and (4) existing INR data. Comparisons of several published algorithms demonstrate good agreement in predicting maintenance dose requirements, and the International Warfarin Pharmacogenetics Consortium indicates that pharmacogenetics-guided management offers improved outcomes over fixed dose or clinical monitoring alone, particularly for people who require low doses.[7] Clinical consensus has not been achieved, however, for application of pharmacogenetic data and related dosing algorithms in routine warfarin initiation and management.

Human Leukocyte Antigen Complex, Class I, B

The HLA complex is a cornerstone for the immune system because of its involvement in identification of foreign proteins. HLA is the human version of the major histocompatibility complex (MHC), a gene family common to many species. The HLA proteins produced from these genes are expressed on the surface of nearly all cells, where they bind to peptides that are exported from the cell. These peptides are thereby captured and displayed to the circulating cells of the immune system. If the immune system recognizes the peptides as foreign (e.g., viral or bacterial peptides), it responds by triggering the infected cell to self-destruct. This process contributes to the toxicity of drugs such as abacavir.

The MHC in humans consists of more than 200 genes that are categorized into three groups: class I, class II, and class III. Humans have three major class I genes, known as *HLA-A, HLA-B,* and *HLA-C.* It is the *HLA-B* gene, and in particular, the *HLA-B*5701* allele, that has been best characterized from the perspective of pharmacogenetics, based on association of variants with drug hypersensitivity phenotypes. *HLA-B* gene variants are also associated with risk of disease, particularly immune-mediated inflammatory disease.

Severe cutaneous adverse reaction syndromes (SCARS), such as **Stevens-Johnson syndrome (SJS)** and **toxic epidermal necrolysis (TEN)**, lead to extremely painful rashes that sometimes are life-threatening. Drug-induced hypersensitivity reactions like SCARS are associated with several drugs. A thoroughly-characterized HLA-drug association is the one between *HLA-B*5701* and abacavir. Abacavir is a reverse transcriptase inhibitor used to treat HIV infection. Approximately 10% of Indian, 5% to 8% of Caucasians, and 2% to 3% of black people treated with abacavir develop a SCARS-like reaction during the first 6 weeks of therapy. Abacavir binds to the peptide binding groove of HLA-B*5701, and the binding changes the self-peptides that are presented to the immune system. The change leads to immune-mediated destruction of the cells. The reaction to abacavir is not dose-dependent and requires permanent discontinuation of the drug. Future exposure to abacavir, in a sensitive individual that was previously exposed, may precipitate a life-threatening reaction due to sensitization.

Genetic testing to detect the *HLA-B*5701* allele varies among laboratories, ranging from complete gene sequencing to identification of single SNPs in related genes (genes in linkage disequilibrium with *HLA-B*5701*, such as *HCP5*). Phenotyping for abacavir is also available, such as through flow cytometric analysis. Due to the high positive predictive value of *HLA-B*5701* identification, pre-therapeutic testing to detect patients at risk for abacavir hypersensitivity was incorporated into the 2008 guidelines for the use of antiretroviral agents in HIV-1 infected adults and adolescents, published by the Office of AIDS Research Advisory Council, and it has been shown to be medically useful and cost-effective.[5,12]

Review Questions

1. The acronym "SNP" stands for
   a. single-nucleotide polymorphism.
   b. single native protein.
   c. singlet nuclear proteomic.
   d. single-gene normal phenotype.

2. Pharmacogenetics is defined as
   a. entry level human genetics for pharmacists.
   b. the study of genetic polymorphisms as revealed by drug responses.
   c. the study of the genetics of human drug metabolism.
   d. the study of human disease susceptibility genes.

3. The response to which one of the following drugs is affected by the cytochrome P450 2D6 (CYP2D6) polymorphism?
   a. Warfarin
   b. Omeprazole
   c. Codeine
   d. Nicotine

4. A phase II enzyme acts on a substrate to
   a. conjugate it with an acetyl or sulfate group.
   b. oxidize it.
   c. stabilize it so that metabolism will not occur.
   d. modulate its binding to a receptor.

5. A drug that is administered in an inactive form that must be metabolized before it has an effective action is referred to as a(n)
   a. cytochrome P450 (CYP) enzyme.
   b. poor metabolizer (PM).
   c. antidrug.
   d. prodrug.

6. The acronym "ADR" stands for
   a. ability to drive reaction.
   b. allelic diversity response.
   c. adverse drug reaction.
   d. allele-driven result.

7. An example of a phase I enzyme is
   a. thiopurine S-methyltransferase (TPMT).
   b. cytochrome P450 2C9 (CYP2C9).
   c. *N*-acetyltransferase 1 (NAT1)
   d. human leukocyte antigen complex, class I, B (HLA-B)

8. How a drug elicits responses and whether the response is desirable or undesirable is described by which one of the following?
   a. Pharmacodynamics
   b. Pharmacokinetics
   c. Phenocopying
   d. Pharmacogenetics

9. The inherited instructions an individual carries within their genetic code is referred to as their
   a. phenotype.
   b. phenocopy.
   c. genotype.
   d. metabolizer status.

10. Nonsteroidal antiinflammatory drugs (NSAIDs), such as ibuprofen or aspirin, are metabolized by which one of the following enzymes?
    a. *N*-acetyltransferase 2 (NAT2)
    b. UDP-glucuronosyltransferase 1A1 (UGT1A1)
    c. cytochrome P450 2C19 (CYP2C19)
    d. cytochrome P450 2C9 (CYP2C9)

References

1. Ansell J, Hirsh J, Hylek E, Jacobson A, Crowther M, Palareti G. Pharmacology and management of the vitamin K antagonists: American College of Chest Physicians evidence-based clinical practice guidelines, 8th edition. Chest 2008;133:160S–198S.

2. Crews KR, Gaedigk A, Dunnenberger HM, Klein TE, Shen DD, Callaghan JT, et al. Clinical pharmacogenetics implementation consortium (CPIC) guidelines for codeine therapy in the context of cytochrome P450 2D6 (*CYP2D6*) genotype. Clinical Pharmacol Therap 2012;91(2):321–6.

3. Frueh FW, Amur S, Mummaneni P, Epstein RS, Aubert RE, DeLuca TM, et al. Pharmacogenomic biomarker information in drug labels approved by the United States Food and Drug Administration: prevalence of related drug use. Pharmacotherapy 2008;28:992–8.

4. Hernandez-Boussard T, Whirl-Carrillo M, Hebert J M, Gong L, Owen R, Gong M, et al. The pharmacogenetics and pharmacogenomics knowledge base: Accentuating the knowledge. Nucleic Acids Res 2008; 36: D913–D918.

5. Hughes DA, Vilar FJ, Ward CC, Alfirevic A, Park BK, Pirmohamed M. Cost-effectiveness analysis of *HLA B*5701* genotyping in preventing abacavir hypersensitivity. Pharmacogenetics 2004;14: 335–42.

6. Ingelman-Sundberg M, Oscarson M, Daly AK, Garte S, Nebert DW. Human cytochrome *P-450 (CYP)* genes: a web page for the nomenclature of alleles. Cancer Epidemiol Biomarkers Prev 2001;10:1307–8.

7. Klein TE, Altman RB, Eriksson N, Gage BF, Kimmel SE, Lee MT, et al. Estimation of the warfarin dose with clinical and pharmacogenetic data. N Engl J Med 2009;360:753–64.

8. Klein TE, Chang JT, Cho MK, Easton KL, Fergerson R, Hewett M, et al. Integrating genotype and phenotype information: an overview of the PharmGKB project. Pharmacogenetics Research acetyltransferases. Pharmacogenetics 1995;5:1–17.

9. Lankisch TO, Moebius U, Wehmeier M, Behrens G, Manns MP, Schmidt RE, et al. Gilbert's disease and atazanavir: from phenotype to UDP-glucuronosyltransferase haplotype. Hepatology 2006;44: 1324–32.

10. Lesko LJ and Schmidt S. Individualization of drug therapy: history, present state, and opportunities for the future. Clinical Pharmacol Therap 2012;92(4):458–66

11. Lyon E, Foster JG, Palomaki GE, Pratt VM, Reynolds K, Sabato MF, et al. Laboratory testing of *CYP2D6* alleles in relation to tamoxifen therapy. Genetics Med, online publication 6 September, 2012.

12. Mallal S, Phillips E, Carosi G, Molina JM, Workman C, Tomazic J, et al. HLA-B*5701 screening for hypersensitivity to abacavir. N Engl J Med 2008;358:568–79.

13. Osborne CK. Tamoxifen in the treatment of breast cancer. N Engl J Med 1998;339:1609–18.

14. Rendic S, Di Carlo FJ. Human cytochrome P450 enzymes: a status report summarizing their reactions, substrates, inducers, and inhibitors. Drug Metab Rev 1997;29:413–580.

15. Robarge JD, Li L, Desta Z, Nguyen A, Flockhart DA. The star-allele nomenclature: retooling for translational genomics. Clin Pharmacol Ther. 2007 Sep;82(3):244–8.

16. Scott SA, Sangkuhl K, Gardner EE, Stein CM, Hulot J-S, Johnson JA, et al. Clinical pharmacogenetics implementation consortium guidelines for cytochrome P450-2C19 (*CYP2C19*) genotype and clopidogrel therapy. Clinical Pharmacol Therap 2011;90(2):328–32.

17. Tomalik-Scharte D, Lazar A, Fuhr U, Kirchheiner J. The clinical role of genetic polymorphisms in drug-metabolizing enzymes. Pharmacogenomics J 2008;8:4–15.

18. Vatsis KP, Weber WW, Bell DA, Dupret JM, Evans DAP, Grant DM, et al. Nomenclature for *N*-acetyltransferases. Pharmacogenetics 1995;5:1–17.

Principles of Molecular Biology

Y. M. Dennis Lo, M.A., D.M., D. Phil., F.R.C.P., F.R.C. Path., F.R.S., and Rossa W. K. Chiu, M.B.B.S., Ph.D., F.R.C.P.A., FHKAM (Pathology)

Objectives

1. Define the following:

Allele	Genetic code
Chromatin	Genome
Chromosome	Genotype
Circulating nucleic acids	Intron
Codon	Nucleic acid
Epigenetics	Nucleotide
Exon	Phenotype
Gene	Semiconservative

2. Describe the essential aspects of molecular biology, including functions of DNA and RNA, transfer of genetic information from parent to daughter cell, content of the human genome, and uses of genotyping and phenotyping.

3. Discuss the similarities and differences between DNA and RNA, including physical and chemical structure, physiologic function, and uses in clinical diagnostic testing; compare the structure and functions of messenger RNA (mRNA), transfer RNA (tRNA), and ribosomal RNA (rRNA).

4. State the structure, chemical composition, and chemical bonds (if any) of purines and pyrimidines, bases and base-pairs, nucleotides and DNA strands; calculate the percentage of nucleotides present in a genome given appropriate information.

5. Draw a nuclear chromosome, including position of telomeres and centromeres; compare telomeres and centromeres, including function and location on a chromosome.

6. Describe the physical structure and chemical composition of chromatin during its dynamic changes during the cell cycle and including histone interaction with DNA; state the importance of chromatin in packing of DNA into chromosomes; compare euchromatin and heterochromatin, including structure, function, and specific location in a chromosome.

7. For each of the following processes, list the steps of the process, where they occur within a eukaryotic cell, the proteins involved, and events occurring in each step:
   DNA replication
   RNA transcription and processing
   mRNA translation

8. State the specific physiologic functions of DNA polymerase and RNA polymerase II.

9. For each of the following epigenetic phenomena, state the function, biochemical interactions, and significance in gene expression:
   DNA methylation
   Histone modification
   Nucleosome positioning and remodeling

10. Describe non-coding RNAs, including biogenic pathway (if known), structure, and known or purported function.

11. Compare the mitochondrial genome to nuclear DNA, including structure, cellular location, inheritance, and packaging.

12. For the following projects, list the general aims and current state of completion or outcome:

1000 Genomes Project	Human Genome Project
ENCODE	International HapMap
Human Epigenome Project	Project

Key Words and Definitions

Allele One of the alternative versions of a gene at a given location (locus) along a chromosome. An individual inherits two alleles for each gene, one from each parent. Alleles may demonstrate sequence variations that determine variations in the functional characteristics of a gene product (e.g., translated protein).

Argonaute proteins Proteins of the RNA-induced silencing complex (RISC), the complex responsible for the gene silencing process known as RNA interference (RNAi).

Autosome A nonsex chromosome; there are 22 pairs of autosomes in the human genome.

Key Words and Definitions—cont'd

Base pair A purine and a pyrimidine nucleotide bound by hydrogen bonds; in DNA base pairing, adenine binds to thymine and guanine pairs with cytosine; in RNA, uracil replaces thymidine for base pairing.

CentiMorgan (cM) A unit of measure that refers to the distance between two gene loci determined by the frequency with which recombination occurs between them. Two loci are said to be one cM apart if recombination is observed between them in 1% of cell division cycles.

Centromere A primary constriction in a chromosome; centromeres play an important role in directing the movement of chromosomes between daughter cells during cell division.

Chromatin Nuclear DNA and its associated structural proteins; chromatin is arranged and organized in a hierarchical fashion in which the degree of its condensation increases with higher levels of structural organization.

Chromosome A highly-ordered structure of a single double-stranded DNA (dsDNA) molecule, compacted many times with the aid of structural DNA-binding proteins.

Codon A three-nucleotide sequence that "codes" for an amino acid during translation; there are 64 possible codons in nuclear DNA.

Deoxyribonucleic acid (DNA) A molecule that carries genetic information and is a double-stranded polymer of nucleotides.

DNA-binding proteins Proteins that recognize and bind to specific DNA sequences. Some DNA-binding proteins are involved in the regulation of DNA transcription.

DNA methylation The addition of a methyl group typically to the fifth carbon position of cytosine residues in CpG dinucleotides; this epigenetic process is implicated in growth and development of organisms.

DNA methyltransferase (DNMT) Any of a group of enzymes that catalyze the transfer of a methyl group from S-adenosylmethionine to a specific nucleotide in a DNA molecule, with different enzymes acting on specific nucleotides and positions of methylation.

Drosha A Class 2 RNase III enzyme responsible for processing of microRNA (miRNA).

Epigenetics Processes that alter gene function or its interpretation by mechanisms other than those that rely on changes in DNA sequences; these processes include DNA methylation, genomic imprinting, histone modification, and chromatin remodeling.

Euchromatin Genomic regions that are rich in genes and are, in general, less compactly organized during interphase.

Eukaryote Organisms such as higher plants and animals, fungi, protozoa, and most algae; they have a true nucleus bounded by a nuclear membrane within which lie the chromosomes.

Exon The coding region of a gene that will be expressed as protein following translation.

Exonuclease A nuclease that releases one nucleotide at a time (serially) beginning at one end of a nucleic acid; exonuclease activity excises incorrectly paired nucleotides during replication.

Gene A unit of DNA that specifies production of proteins and RNA molecules required for cellular function.

Genetic code The complete list of nucleotide codons and the amino acids or actions they "code" for.

Gene expression The process responsible for the flow of genetic information from gene to protein.

Genome The complete set of chromosomes; the total complement of hereditary information; the human genome contains two copies, termed *alleles,* of each autosomal gene. One half of the genome is inherited from each parent and is termed the *haploid genome.* The complete genome inherited from both parents is termed the *diploid genome.*

Genotype The primary nucleotide sequences of the two gene alleles.

Heterochromatin Genomic regions that are gene poor or span transcriptionally silent genes and are more densely packed during interphase.

Heteroplasmy The presence of more than one population of mitochondrial DNA sequences in a cell consequent to the accumulation of sequence variations.

Histones A class of structural proteins involved in the three-dimensional organization of nuclear DNA.

Homoplasmy The presence of a homogeneous population of mitochondrial genomes in a cell.

Human Genome Project A project undertaken by the International Human Genome Sequencing Consortium to decipher the three billion base pairs in the human genome; the project was completed in 2003.

Interphase The period between cell divisions.

Intron A noncoding region of a gene, locked between exons, that will not be translated into protein.

Leber's hereditary optic neuropathy (LHON) A neuropathy transmitted from mother to children that is characterized by a degeneration of retinal ganglion cells (RGCs) and their axons that leads to a loss of central vision.

Linkage disequilibrium Nonrandom association of alleles at different loci; the rate reflects rates of recombination and is used as a measure of distance between the loci. See **centiMorgan**.

MicroRNA (miRNA) Short noncoding RNA (ncRNA) molecules around 22 nucleotides in length that play a role in regulation of gene expression by interfering with effective translation of mRNA to proteins.

Mitochondrial DNA The circular DNA within a mitochondrial organelle that codes for polypeptides involved in the oxidative phosphorylation pathway; this DNA is typically transmitted across generations by maternal inheritance.

Nucleases Enzymes that catalyze the hydrolysis of nucleic acid by cleaving chains of nucleotides into smaller units.

Nucleic acid A polymer made of nucleotide monomers (a sugar moiety, a phosphoric acid, and purine or pyrimidine bases); examples are deoxyribonucleic acid (DNA) and ribonucleic acid (RNA).

Nucleosome A unit of chromatin consisting of nucleosome core particles (146 base pairs of double-stranded DNA [ds-DNA]) wound around a core of eight histone proteins; technically, a nucleosome also includes a linker DNA between nucleosomes, but the word often is used to mean the core particle.

Nucleotide A unit of DNA or RNA, consisting of one chemical base (purine or pyrimidine) plus a sugar molecule (deoxyribose or ribose) and at least one phosphate group.

Key Words and Definitions—cont'd

Okazaki fragment A relatively short fragment of DNA (with no RNA primer at the 5′ terminus) created on the lagging strand of DNA during DNA synthesis.

Phenotype The observable characteristics of an organism, including visible features (eye color, height) and chemical and behavioral characteristics; reflects interaction of genes and environment.

Polymerase Enzymes involved in DNA replication and transcription; DNA polymerase epsilon reads a parent DNA template and attaches nucleotides to a growing daughter strand according to the base-pairing rules of double-stranded DNA (ds-DNA); RNA polymerase II binds to a promoter region of a DNA strand to initiate transcription.

Polymerase chain reaction (PCR) An in vitro method for exponentially amplifying DNA.

Prokaryote Oganisms (such as bacteria) that are characterized by the absence of a distinct, membrane-bound nucleus or membrane-bound organelles and by DNA that is not organized into chromosomes.

Promoter A regulatory region of DNA that serves to bind RNA polymerase II that in turn binds other substances that will lead to initiation of transcription; promoters and the substances that bind to them control the rate and timing of tRNA synthesis and thus of synthesis of the coded protein.

Purine A base containing two carbon-nitrogen rings; adenine and guanine are purines.

Pyrimidine A base containing one carbon-nitrogen ring; cytosine, thymine, and uracil are pyrimidines.

Recombination The process of exchange of genes or segments of DNA between chromosomes; recombination produces gametes with chromosomes that are different from the parent's. Reombination of DNA segments is also done in the laboratory as a step in prodcing *recombinant* proteins (see centiMorgan).

Replication The faithful reproduction of the DNA content from parent to daughter cells during cell division.

Ribonucleic acid (RNA) A biological substance similar to DNA with the exceptions of being single stranded, containing ribose as the sugar moiety, having an extra hydroxyl group, and containing uracil instead of thymine; there are different functional types of RNA, including messenger (coding) RNA (mRNA), ribosomal RNA (rRNA), transfer RNA (tRNA), and other small noncoding RNAs (ncRNAs), such as microRNA (miRNA).

Ribosome A large molecular structure comprised of ribosomal RNA and protein that is found in the cytoplasm of cells that serves as the site of protein synthesis.

Spliceosome A large ribonucleoprotein complex, composed of various small nuclear ribonucleoproteins (snRNP) as well as other protein factors; it attaches to specific sites on pre-mRNA and catalyzes splicing out of their introns in the formation of mature mRNA.

Telomere The DNA sequences at the end of a chromosome; telomeres contain repetitive nucleotide sequences that protect the ends of chromosomes from recombination with other chromosomes.

Tiling arrays A subtype of microarray that functions by hybridizing labeled DNA or RNA target molecules to probes fixed onto a solid surface.

Transcription The process of transferring sequence information from the gene regions of DNA to a messenger RNA molecule.

Translation The process whereby an mRNA sequence forms an amino acid sequence with the help of tRNA and eventual enzymatic peptide bond formation between amino acids to synthesize polypeptides; translation occurs on cytoplasmic ribosomes.

Molecular diagnostics represents one of the most rapidly developing areas within many diagnostic disciplines, including (1) clinical chemistry, (2) clinical hematology, (3) clinical immunology, (4) clinical microbiology, and (5) tissue pathology. Advances in the field have been made possible by improved understanding of molecular biology and genetics and of their relationships with human diseases and the development of powerful technologies for the analysis of **nucleic acids**. The fundamental concepts in molecular biology are reviewed in this chapter.

Landmark Developments in Genetics and Molecular Diagnostics

Significant events that occurred in the late 20th century include (1) decoding of the human **genome**, (2) cloning of organisms, and (3) progress in stem cell research and **gene** therapy. Many of these advances would not have been possible without the

many earlier landmark discoveries that unveiled the mysteries of genetics and paved the way for modern molecular diagnostics.[5] Genetics began modestly when Mendel experimented with garden peas. His findings, published in 1866 and suggesting the concepts of **alleles** and genes as discrete units of heredity, essentially captured the most fundamental concepts in inheritance. In 1910 Morgan revealed that the units of heredity are contained within **chromosomes**, but it was Avery in 1944 who confirmed through studies on bacteria that it was **deoxyribonucleic acid (DNA)** that carried the genetic information. Franklin and Wilkins studied DNA by x-ray crystallography, which subsequently led to unraveling of the double-helical structure of DNA by Watson and Crick in 1953. In the 1960s Smith demonstrated that DNA can be cleaved by restriction enzymes, which Arber had discovered earlier. This facilitated the subsequent development of recombinant DNA technologies. Nathans furthered the work on restriction enzymes and was the first to construct a genetic map. In 1975 the Southern blot was invented, which allowed the detection of specific DNA sequences. Soon after, in 1977, DNA-sequencing methods were developed, and the first complete DNA sequence of an organism, a bacteriophage, was published. Prenatal genetic diagnosis of sickle cell disease was first shown to be feasible by Kan and Chang in 1978. In 1985 Mullis and co-workers developed the **polymerase chain reaction (PCR)**, which provided a rapid way to make many copies of a DNA molecule. The existence of functional small *noncoding RNAs* (ncRNAs) in organisms was first realized in 1993. DNA microarrays, which allow the simultaneous interrogation of many DNA/cDNA loci by nucleic acid hybridization, became a reality in 1996. Remarkably the draft human genome sequence was released in 2001 and completed in 2003. Massively parallel sequencing became an accessible laboratory tool from 2005, and genomic scale analysis has become possible in diagnostic laboratories.

In brief, the explosive accumulation of genetic knowledge has translated into escalating clinical demands for molecular diagnostics in clinical laboratories. Consequently, An understanding of the fundamental aspects of molecular biology, as outlined in this chapter, is required for the effective implementation and interpretation of molecular diagnostics. In addition, the readers should note that discussions in this chapter refer primarily to **eukaryotes** (such as humans whose cells have a true nucleus bounded by a nuclear membrane) and not to **prokaryotes** (such as bacteria whose cells do not).

The Essentials

On the simplest level, genes are defined as segments of DNA that encode for proteins or **ribonucleic acid (RNA)** products with biological functions. DNA is a biological substance that carries genetic information and is a polymer of **nucleotides** or bases. Genetic information is reproduced from parent to daughter cells during cell division through the process of DNA **replication**. When genes are expressed ("switched on"), the DNA sequence is transcribed into RNA. RNA molecules are polymers of ribonucleotides that exist in a number of functional forms. RNA molecules that act as intermediates for protein production are termed *messenger RNA (mRNA)*. RNA molecules that serve a direct biological function without coding for a protein are collectively termed *ncRNAs*.[13] mRNA is the product of a transcribed nucleotide sequence and is in turn translated into a protein, which is a polymer of amino acids. Each amino acid is encoded by a triplet nucleotide code, termed a **codon**. The human **genetic code** comprises 64 codons encoding for 21 amino acids and 3 stop codons. mRNA codons are read by the anticodon regions of transfer RNA (tRNA) molecules, which are small RNAs that bring the corresponding amino acid to the growing polypeptide chain. The polypeptide chain is synthesized by **ribosomes**, which are macromolecular complexes containing ribosomal RNA (rRNA) and a protein component with catalytic function.

Most human cells contain two full copies/versions of the haploid human genome, which is organized and packaged into 23 pairs of chromosomes (diploid genome). A chromosome is a highly ordered structure of a single DNA molecule with specialized structural features, namely, one **centromere** and two **telomeres**. Every individual inherits one copy/version of the human genome from his or her father and another from the mother. Thus, the human genome contains two copies, termed *alleles*, of each autosomal gene. Although a gene sequence may encode for a specific protein or RNA with defined functions, alleles of genes may demonstrate sequence variations that in turn contribute to variations in the functional characteristics of the gene product between individuals. The primary nucleotide sequences of the two gene alleles form the **genotype**, whereas the expressed function or biological effect of the gene product is termed the **phenotype**. Thus one could study a human disease or trait at the genetic level through determination of the allelic sequence of a gene by genotyping or at the functional level by phenotyping. Examples of phenotyping include the investigation of (1) enzyme concentrations or activities, (2) ABO blood groups, (3) electrophoretic mobility of hemoglobin variants, (4) RNA expression levels, and (5) others. The choice of genotyping or phenotyping for making a diagnosis depends on the specific diagnostic application and the strength of the association between a genotype and its consequential phenotype.

Nucleic Acid Structure and Organization

An intimate relationship has been observed between nucleic acid structure and function. The physiological function of nucleic acid is facilitated by its structure. Although an alteration in the structure of nucleic acids would lead to an altered function, an altered function, on the other hand, may be seen as an altered structure. Thus, a discussion of nucleic acid structure is pertinent to further discussion on nucleic acid function.

Molecular Compositions and Structures of DNA and RNA

DNA

The physicochemical properties and functions of nucleic acids are largely governed by the compositions and structures of DNA and RNA. A single molecule of DNA is a polymer consisting of a backbone of invariant composition and side groups arranged in a variable sequence (Figures 47-1 and 47-2). The polymer is synthesized from monomers (nucleotides) composed of the sugar deoxyribose, a phosphate residue, and a **purine** or **pyrimidine** base. The purines are adenine (A) and guanine (G), and the pyrimidines are cytosine (C) and thymine (T) (see Figure 47-1). The four nucleotide building blocks of DNA are (1) deoxyadenosine triphosphate (dATP), (2) deoxyguanosine triphosphate (dGTP), (3) deoxycytidine triphosphate (dCTP), and (4) deoxythymidine triphosphate (dTTP). Nucleotides are joined by phosphodiester bonds that link the 5′-phosphate group of one to the 3′-hydroxyl group of the next (see Figure 47-2). No 3′-3′ or 5′-5′ linkages are present; thus the sugar and phosphate moieties compose the non-specific portions of the molecule. The sequence of the bases

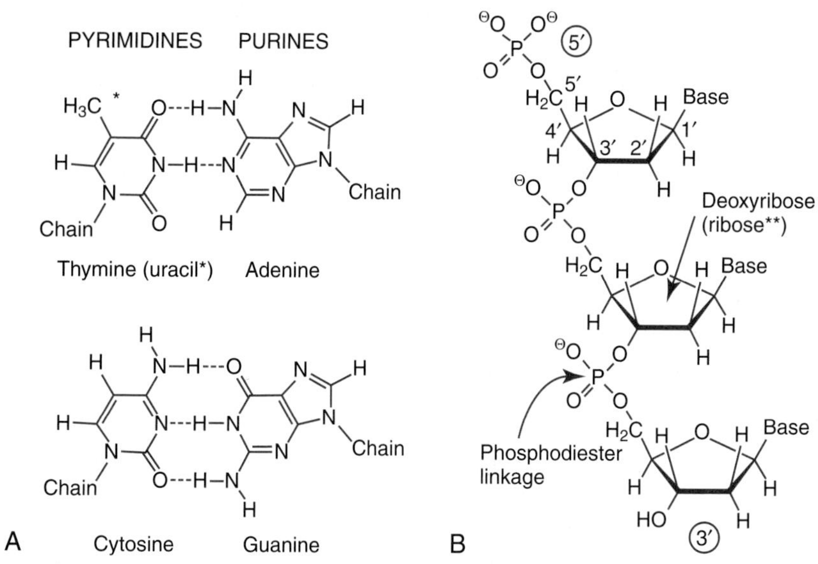

Figure 47-1 A, Purine and pyrimidine bases and the formation of complementary base pairs. *Dashed lines* indicate hydrogen bonds. (In RNA, thymine is replaced by uracil, which differs from thymine only in its lack of the methyl group.) **B,** A single-stranded DNA chain. Repeating nucleotide units are linked by phosphodiester bonds that join the 5′ carbon of one sugar to the 3′ carbon of the next. Each nucleotide monomer consists of a sugar moiety, a phosphate residue, and a base. (In RNA, the sugar is ribose, which adds a 2′-hydroxyl to deoxyribose.) *(Modified from Piper MA, Unger ER. Nucleic acid probes: a primer for pathologists. Chicago, IL: ASCP Press, 1989.)*

varies from molecule to molecule and uniquely identifies each DNA polymer, which, as discussed later, determines the identity and function of the protein or RNA products that the DNA encodes.

Although the purines and pyrimidines are of different compositions and sizes, when in the proper orientation, adenine forms two hydrogen bonds with thymine, and guanine forms three hydrogen bonds with cytosine, to form planar structures of similar dimensions (see Figure 47-1). This combined with the fact that the base portion of each nucleotide is hydrophobic contributes to the energetically favorable secondary structure of DNA as it is found in its native form a right-handed, double-stranded helix. The planar base pairs stack in the inside of the helix, ten bases per turn, whereas the hydrophilic sugar-phosphate backbone forms noncovalent bonds with surrounding water molecules. For the two DNA polymers to form the proper hydrogen bonds between the bases, two requirements must be fulfilled: the polymers must run in opposite directions (antiparallel) as defined by the free hydroxyl groups at each end (3′-5′ vs. 5′-3′), and the sequences of each molecule must be such that A:T and G:C hydrogen bonds are always formed (base pairing). Two DNA strands that meet this requirement are called *complementary.*

Owing to base pairing and the double-helical conformation, double-stranded DNA (ds-DNA) is an exceptionally stable molecule. Retention of **base pairs** in the inner portion of the helix prevents disruption by water molecules. The helical conformation places each monomer in an identical orientation within the molecule and forms the same secondary bonds as every other monomer. This secondary bonding contributes to the overall stability. Because the base pairs are of similar size, the helix retains a constant angle of rotation and avoids distortion. All of these features dictate that all ds-DNA molecules, regardless of base sequence, retain the same shape and size within a pH range of approximately 4 to 9. Outside these limits, the base pair bonds are disrupted and the helix unwinds.

RNA

RNA is chemically very similar to DNA but differs in important ways. For example, the sugar unit is ribose with an added hydroxyl group at the 2′ position, and the methylated pyrimidine uracil (U) replaces thymine. RNA exists in various functional forms but mostly as a single-stranded polymer that is much shorter than DNA and that has an irregular three-dimensional structure. Despite their irregular shape, RNA conformations are not random structures, and the folding mechanism of RNA molecules is complex. The secondary structure adopted by an RNA molecule is to a large extent related to its nucleotide sequence. RNA molecules fold sequentially from 5′ to 3′ to form stable submotifs dictated by their primary sequence. One such example is the hairpin loop structure of precursor **microRNAs (miRNAs)** (see later section on ncRNAs). RNA molecules may adopt further tertiary folding. An RNA molecule has the potential to be folded into a number of different conformations, but usually only one conformation is functional. The folding process is influenced by (1) ions, (2) cofactors, and (3) proteins. Once an RNA molecule adopts a conformation most favored by its immediate cellular environment, it rarely switches to another conformation. RNA molecules also will further interact with other RNA or protein molecules to form complex quaternary structures, such as ribonucleoproteins, that are essential to certain cellular processes.

Chromosome Structure

DNA molecules are extremely long and in the eukaryotic cell are maintained in orderly and compact three-dimensional structures. Each diploid human cell contains two full sets of the human genome with each copy consisting of approximately 3.2 billion nucleotides. This vast amount of genetic material is organized into 23 homologous chromosome pairs with each pair contributed by a homolog of maternal origin and one of paternal origin. The two chromosomes of each pair are similar (homologous) and, except for the sex chromosomes (X and Y),

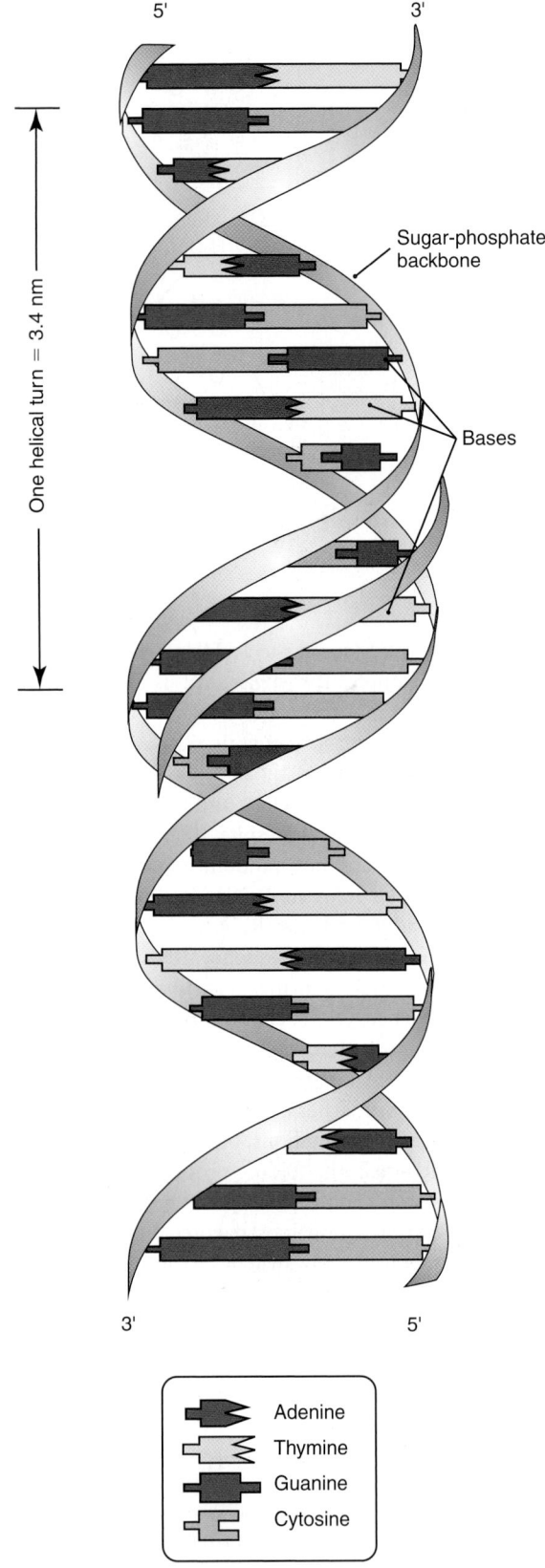

5'　3'

One helical turn = 3.4 nm

Sugar-phosphate backbone

Bases

3'　5'

	Adenine
	Thymine
	Guanine
	Cytosine

Figure 47-2 The DNA double helix with sugar-phosphate backbone and pairing of the bases in the core-forming planar structures.

contain the same genes arranged in the same sequence. Each chromosome is a highly ordered structure of a single ds-DNA molecule, compacted many times with the aid of structural **DNA-binding proteins** such as **histones** (Figure 47-3). The chromosomes are in their most compact state and appear as finger-like structures during metaphase of the cell cycle. A primary constriction, the centromere, is also notable on each chromosome. The ends of the chromosomes are termed the telomeres (see Figure 47-3). Both centromeres and telomeres have specialized functions, which are discussed later. The non-sex chromosomes, the **autosomes**, in the human genome are numbered in order of decreasing size (except chromosomes 21 and 22). Chromosome 1 contains 250 million base-pairs (megabase pairs or Mbp), and chromosome 21 is 48 Mbp long. The chromosomal arrangement of human DNA not only allows packaging of the vast human genome into the limited physical dimensions of the cell nucleus, but also governs one of the Mendelian laws of inheritance on independent assortment whereby genes located on different chromosomes recombine at random from one generation to the next.

Chromatin Packing

Nuclear DNA in conjunction with its associated structural proteins, including histone and nonhistone proteins, is known as **chromatin**. Chromatin is arranged and organized in a hierarchical fashion whereby the degree of packing or condensation increases with higher levels of structural organization. The **nucleosome** represents the most basic level of chromatin organization and is present as repeated units along the full length of each chromosome. Each nucleosome unit consists of a nucleosome core particle and 20 to 80 base pairs of linker DNA, which spans between adjacent nucleosomes, resembling what has been referred as "beads on a string" (Figure 47-4). A nucleosome core particle involves 146 base pairs of ds-DNA tightly wound 1.65 times around an octamer of histone proteins, two each of four histone proteins, namely, H2A, H2B, H3, and H4. Amino termini or "tails" of these histone molecules protrude from the nucleosomal core. The histone tails are subjected to covalent modifications, including (1) acetylation, (2) methylation, (3) phosphorylation, and (4) ubiquitination (a process that features the attachment of ubiquitin a small regulatory protein).[7] The linker DNA segments are associated with the linker histone H1. Nucleosomes are further packed in successive levels of complexity by up to a factor of 10,000[3]; in the most compact stage, chromatin appears as discrete mitotic chromosomes seen in the metaphase of a cell cycle, as described earlier. The orderly process of chromatin condensation involves **DNA methylation**, histone modifications, ncRNAs, and sequence-specific **DNA-binding proteins**.

Chromatin packing serves the function of containing the genome within the nucleus, but this could potentially render the genetic code inaccessible to various cellular machineries.[3] However, this does not occur because chromatin condensation is not a static process but a dynamic one that changes in a coordinated fashion during the cell cycle. In general, chromatin is much less condensed during **interphase**, at which time DNA is replicated. The extent of chromatin condensation during

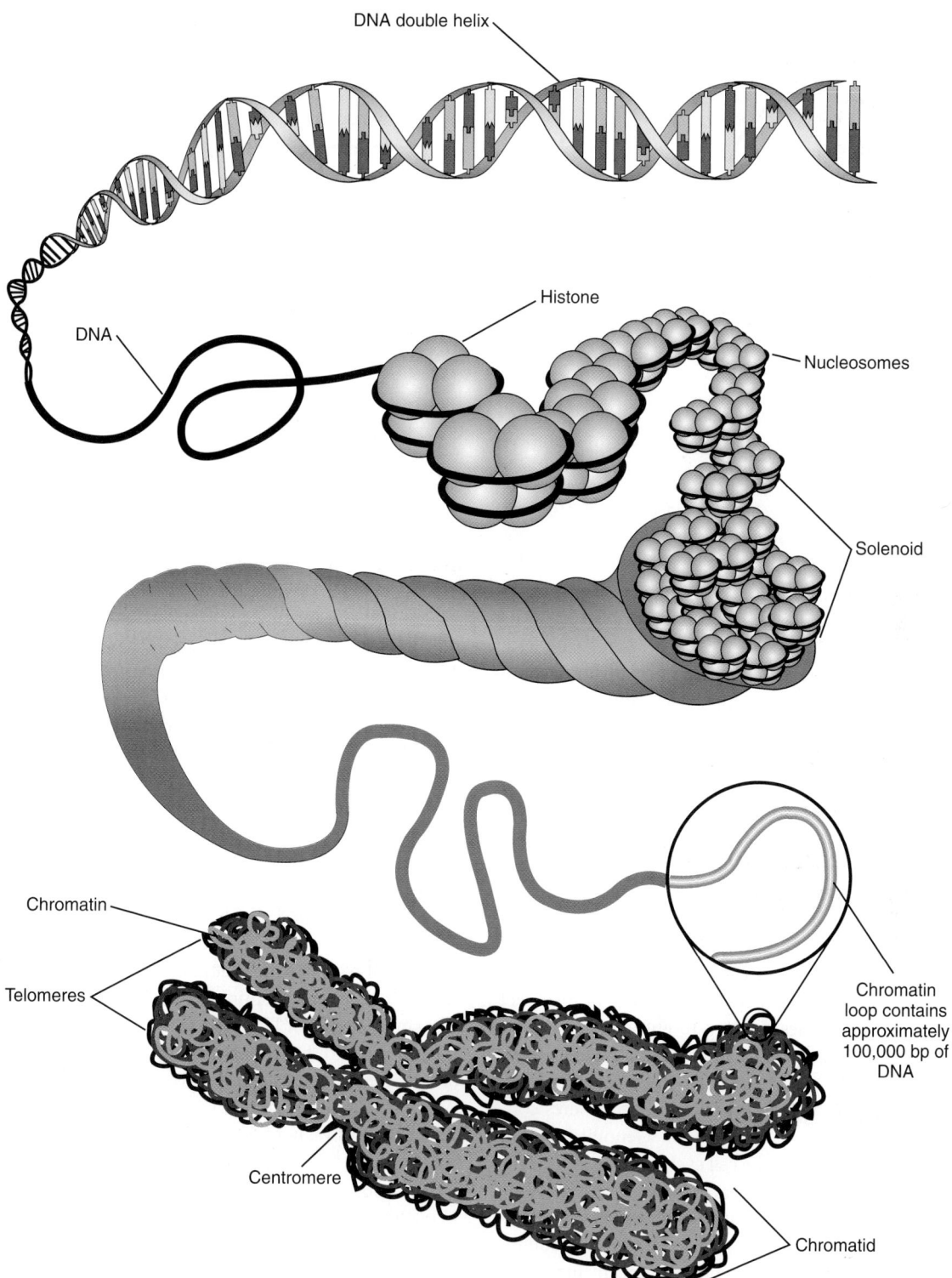

Figure 47-3 Structural organization of human chromosomal DNA. Double-stranded DNA (dsDNA) is wound around histones to form nucleosomes. Nuclear DNA in conjunction with its associated structural proteins is known as *chromatin*. Chromatin in its most compact state forms chromosomes. The primary constriction of a chromosome is the centromere, and the chromosome's ends are the telomeres.

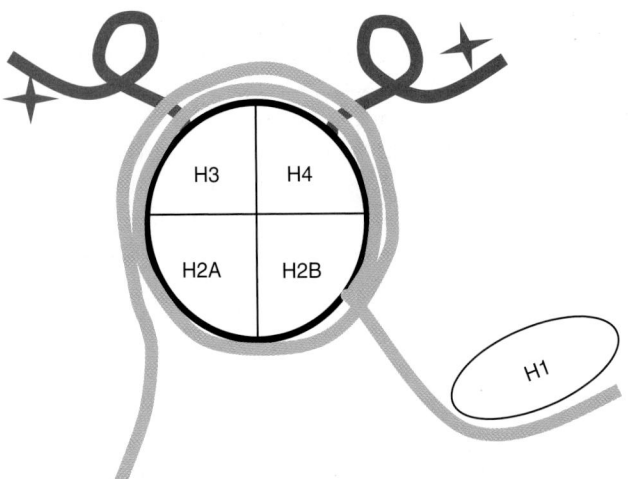

Figure 47-4 Schematic illustration of a nucleosome unit. A segment of DNA is wound around a nucleosome core particle consisting of an octamer with two of each of the histone proteins H2A, H2B, H3, and H4. Tails with modifications (*indicated by a red star*) are shown to protrude from H3 and H4. Adjacent nucleosomes are separated by a segment of linker DNA and the linker histone, H1.

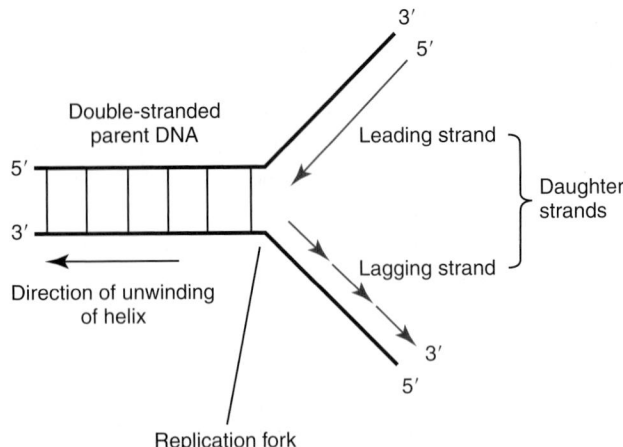

Figure 47-5 DNA replication. Double-stranded DNA is separated at the replication fork. The leading strand is synthesized continuously, while the lagging strand is synthesized discontinuously but is joined later by DNA ligase.

interphase varies among regions of the genome. Genomic regions that are rich in genes generally open up to become less compactly organized during interphase and are termed **euchromatin.** Regions that are gene-poor or that span transcriptionally silent genes remain mostly densely packed and are called **heterochromatin.** This material is important for (1) maintenance of specialized chromatin structures, (2) inactivation of the X chromosome in females, and (3) maintenance of genome stability by stabilizing repetitive DNA sequences.[2] Eukaryote chromosomes contain two specialized regions of heterochromatin, namely, centromeres and telomeres. Centromeres play an important role in directing the movement of chromosomes between daughter cells during cell division. Poor execution of this process could result in incorrect segregation of chromosomes, leading to chromosomal gains or losses in the daughter cells. Telomeres contain repetitive nucleotide sequences that are located on and protect the ends of chromosomes. Alterations in the lengths of telomeres contribute to aging and cancer development. Genomic regions that remain condensed during the cell cycle such as (1) centromeres, (2) telomeres, and (3) the inactivated X chromosome in female cells are termed *constitutive heterochromatin.* Also, some other heterochromatin domains are scattered throughout the genome and are able to respond dynamically in various cellular states. Those regions are termed *facultative heterochromatin* and are associated with regulation of gene expression.[2] Functional implications of the structural organization of chromatin will be discussed further in the following sections.

Nucleic Acid Physiology and Functional Regulation

Nucleic acids form the repository for hereditary information and provide the means of translating that information into the cellular machinery of life. **Gene expression** refers to the process of transforming the genetic blueprint into functional products that participate in various biological processes of a cell. Faithful reproduction of the DNA content from parent to daughter cells during cell division is termed replication. A gene is expressed through **transcription** of its DNA sequence into RNA. mRNAs encode for proteins, and a polypeptide is synthesized through **translation** of the mRNA base sequence into the corresponding amino acid sequence.

Replication

Each time a cell divides, the entire DNA content of that cell must be faithfully duplicated so that the total complement of hereditary information (the human genome) is retained in each daughter cell. This process is called *replication.* Owing to the laws of base pairing that mandates that adenine pairs only with thymine, and guanine only with cytosine, the sequence of a single strand of DNA dictates the sequence of its complementary strand. In replication, each of the two parent strands of a ds-DNA molecule serves as the template for the synthesis of a daughter strand (Figure 47-5). The process is called *semiconservative,* because each of the duplicated dsDNA molecules produced in this manner is composed of one parent (conserved) strand and one daughter strand. For replication to occur, the original double-stranded helix must be separated. This is an energetically unfavorable event that is accomplished with a combination of DNA-specific proteins and enzymes, and synthesis of both daughter strands proceeds as the parent strands separate. Replication is initiated at multiple sites (origins of replication) during this process, but each origin of replication is used only once during a single cell cycle.

Daughter strands are synthesized by DNA polymerase III, an enzyme that reads the parent template and attaches nucleotides to the growing daughter strand according to the base pairing rules of ds-DNA. DNA **polymerase** III begins synthesis at the replication fork (see Figure 47-5), the point of strand separation, with a short RNA primer that base pairs to the parent template. Later, this primer is excised and replaced with DNA by the DNA repair enzyme, DNA polymerase I. Because DNA polymerase epsilon synthesizes DNA only in the 5′-3′ direction, one daughter strand, the leading strand, is synthesized continuously, whereas the other, the lagging strand known as an **Okazaki fragment**, must be synthesized discontinuously in short segments (see Figure 47-5). Fragments on the discontinuous strand are then joined by the DNA ligase enzyme. Many other proteins are involved (1) in unwinding and stabilizing the parent strands for synthesis, (2) in protecting single-stranded regions, (3) in recognizing initiation sites, and (4) in synthesizing the RNA primer. In addition to synthetic capabilities, the DNA polymerases possess an **exonuclease** or "proofreading" function: when an incorrect nucleotide is added to the growing polymer, a conformational change brings the chain in contact with the exonuclease portion of the enzyme, which cuts out ("excises") the incorrect nucleotide. This helps maintain the integrity of the original DNA sequence, and it has been estimated that one nucleotide error could occur for every 10^5 nucleotides incorporated into the growing strand. However, the proofreading function of DNA polymerase works in concert with a set of DNA repair mechanisms that detect and correct DNA replication errors in such a way that the resultant error rate of DNA replication is reduced to one error per 10^9 to 10^{10} nucleotides replicated. Given that 3 billion base pairs are present in the human genome, about 0.3 to 3 errors occur per cell division.

Transcription

DNA carries information that specifies the production of RNA molecules and proteins that can execute biological functions. The segment of the genome that specifies the production of a functional product, such as a protein or ncRNA, is termed a *gene*. In short, a gene is a functional unit of the genome. On the most basic level, the span of a gene encompasses the nucleotide sequence that specifies its ncRNA product or the amino acid sequence of its protein product. However, a series of processes determines the timing and rate of expression of each gene. Those processes that control gene expression act via regulatory regions of the genome. Thus, it is customary to define a gene to be inclusive of such associated regulatory elements. An important regulatory region is the **promoter** of a gene, which, as will be discussed later, is the genomic region where regulatory factors act in concert to activate expression of that gene. Previously, it was generally thought that the promoter region was located immediately 5′ to the start of the protein-coding portion of a gene. Yet, recent evidence demonstrates that regions showing properties of a promoter could be found within the protein-coding portion of genes, toward the 3′ end, or lying at a substantial distance between coding sequences. In addition, the same promoter region could trigger the expression of different DNA segments both 5′ or 3′ to it. Hence, it has become increasingly difficult to precisely define the physical boundaries of individual genes.

When a gene is expressed, the DNA sequence is first transcribed into RNA. The process of transferring the sequence information from DNA to RNA is called transcription.

Regulation of transcription is the primary mechanism that cells use to control gene expression. Similar to replication, transcription requires separation of duplex DNA strands and uses a polymerase to copy the template DNA strand. For transcription, the polymerase is RNA polymerase II, which first binds to specific sequences in the promoter, called the *core promoter*, upon initiation of gene expression. Core promoters that have been identified to date generally occur within a hundred bases around the initiation site of transcription, known as the *transcription start site*, where the first ribonucleotide unit is paired with the template DNA (uracil pairs with adenine). Several nucleotide sequence motifs or patterns have now been recognized among core promoters. For example, one of the best studied core promoter motifs, the TATA box, refers to a short stretch of nucleotides rich in thymine and adenine in repeating patterns. It is typically located about 25 nucleotides "upstream" at the 5′ end of the transcription start site. Some other core promoter elements are located just downstream to the transcription start site. Research has suggested that the various core promoter elements may have different strength and efficiency in activating gene expression.

To initiate transcription, a series of protein cofactors, known as *general transcription factors*, is required to bind to RNA polymerase II to form an assembly known as the *preinitiation complex*, which, in turn, acts on the gene by interacting with the core promoter. Other regions of DNA known as *activators* or *co-activators* may interact with the preinitiation complex to stimulate or repress transcription.

Once transcription is activated, RNA polymerase II moves along and unwinds the DNA double helix. The growing RNA transcript pairs with one of the DNA strands, called the *template*, where RNA polymerase II adds complementary ribonucleotide triphosphates in a 5′ to 3′ direction. It is now known that both DNA strands of the double helix can act as a template for RNA transcription. For example, when the growing RNA transcript pairs with the antisense (−) DNA strand, the resultant RNA molecule is a copy of the sense (+) strand of DNA, and vice versa. Natural antisense transcripts such as RNA transcripts that are copies of the antisense DNA strand have been better known only in recent years. Both protein-coding and non–protein-coding RNAs have been reported to be natural antisense RNAs.

RNA elongation continues until chain termination occurs. The precise signaling mechanism for chain termination still is not well understood. The RNA transcript quickly detaches from the template DNA because restoration of the DNA-DNA duplex is energetically more favorable than is retention of the DNA-RNA hybrid or a segment of single-stranded DNA. The newly synthesized RNA molecule then undergoes further modification depending on its functional class. We shall discuss the fate of the ncRNAs in a later section of this chapter. Here we focus on describing subsequent processing of the protein-coding RNAs, which are referred to as mRNA. First, the 5′ end of the RNA molecule is modified by the addition of 7-methylguanosine residues to form a structure called a *cap* (Figure 47-6). The 3′ end is modified by the addition of multiple adenine bases, called the *poly(A) tail* (see Figure 47-6). Both the

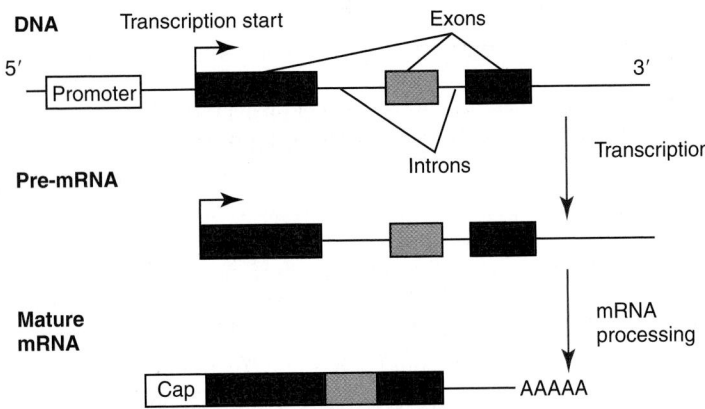

Figure 47-6 DNA transcription and mRNA processing. A gene that encodes for a protein contains a promoter region with variable numbers of introns and exons. Transcription commences at the transcription start site. Pre-mRNA is processed by capping, polyadenylation, and intron splicing and becomes a mature messenger RNA (mRNA).

TABLE 47-1   The Genetic Code (Translation of Messenger RNA to Amino Acids during Protein Synthesis)

		Nucleotide Position in the Codon			
		Third			
First	Second	U	C	A	G
U	U	Phenylalanine	Phenylalanine	Leucine	Leucine
	C	Serine	Serine	Serine	Serine
	A	Tyrosine	Tyrosine	Stop	Pyrrolysine*
	G	Cysteine	Cysteine	Selenocysteine*	Tryptophan
C	U	Leucine	Leucine	Leucine	Leucine
	C	Proline	Proline	Proline	Proline
	A	Histidine	Histidine	Glutamine	Glutamine
	G	Arginine	Arginine	Arginine	Arginine
A	U	Isoleucine	Isoleucine	Isoleucine	Methionine
	C	Threonine	Threonine	Threonine	Threonine
	A	Asparagine	Asparagine	Lysine	Lysine
	G	Serine	Serine	Arginine	Arginine
G	U	Valine	Valine	Valine	Valine
	C	Alanine	Alanine	Alanine	Alanine
	A	Aspartic acid	Aspartic acid	Glutamic acid	Glutamic acid
	G	Glycine	Glycine	Glycine	Glycine

*The codon UGA can code for selenocysteine or stop, and the codon UAG can code for pyrrolysine or stop.

cap and the tail are necessary for translation of mRNA into protein, and they protect the mRNA molecule from degradation by exonucleases. The coding region of a gene that contributes to the amino acid sequence of the protein is termed an **exon**. Interspersed between exons are noncoding regions termed **introns** (see Figure 47-6). The number and size of introns and exons differ among genes. Excision or splicing of the noncoding introns is carried out by a molecular complex termed a **spliceosome**. These complexes are composed of multiple small nuclear ribonucleoprotein particles. Spliceosomes mediate the cleavage and ligation of RNA at specific recognition sequences, termed *splicing donor* and *acceptor sequences*. After the introns have been removed, the exons are juxtaposed to each other, forming a mature mRNA molecule (see Figure 47-6) that is transported into the cytoplasm, where protein translation takes place.

Translation

Translation is the process whereby the mRNA sequence directs the amino acid sequence during protein synthesis. To date,

22 amino acids have been reported in nature. Each amino acid is specified by a three-nucleotide sequence known as a *codon*. Because 64 possible codons are known, most amino acids are specified by more than one codon. One codon, UAA, does not code for amino acids but always signals termination of protein synthesis (a stop codon). UGA codes for a stop or for selenocysteine, and UAG codes for a stop or for pyrrolysine, depending on adjacent sequences or RNA-binding proteins. With the exception of pyrrolysine, which is the most recently identified amino acid and so far has been found in proteins of bacteria and archaea only, all other amino acids are involved in human protein synthesis. The full menu of codon sequences forms the genetic code, which is shown in Table 47-1.

Translation takes place on ribosomes, which are ribonucleoprotein complexes that function as protein synthesis factories. A ribosome binds to the initiation site on mRNA to form an initiation complex. Protein synthesis begins at the translation initiation codon, AUG, which codes for the amino acid, methionine. The region of the mRNA molecule preceding the

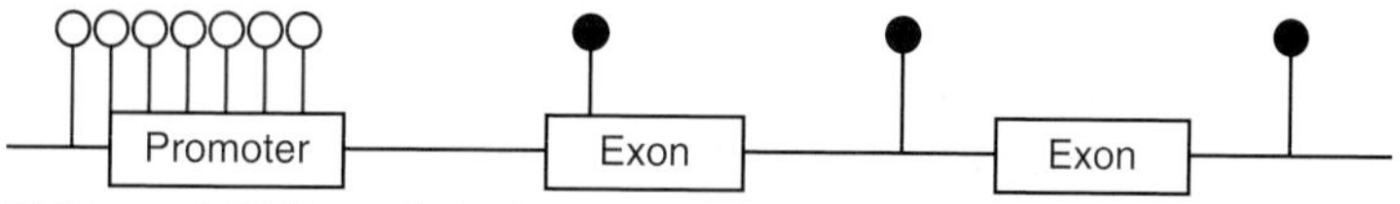

Figure 47-7 Normal DNA methylation pattern in the human genome. Sites of CpG dinucleotides are indicated by *circles*. CpG islands in association with gene promoters are generally unmethylated, but isolated CpG dinucleotides are methylated. *Filled circles,* methylated; *open circles,* unmethylated.

initiation codon is termed the *5′ untranslated region (5′UTR).* The initiation codon and each subsequent codon are "read" by tRNA, short RNA molecules that have a sequence complementary to an amino acid codon (anticodon) and are bound to the amino acid molecule specified by the codon. As synthesis proceeds, the appropriate tRNA anticodon forms base pairs with the next mRNA codon and thus brings this amino acid bound to it into close proximity of the growing peptide chain. An enzyme on the ribosome then catalyzes the formation of a peptide bond between the amino acid and the growing peptide chain. The previous tRNA is released and the appropriate tRNA (with its amino acid) is attached to the next codon. The ribosome moves along the mRNA until a stop codon is reached and synthesis is complete. The ribosome and the protein product are then dissociated from the mRNA. More than one ribosome can move along an mRNA molecule at a time, forming a polyribosome. The rest of the mRNA molecule downstream to the stop codon is termed the *3′ untranslated region (3′UTR).*

Genetics and Epigenetics

Genetic and **epigenetic** phenomena are intimately related and work in concert to bring about the normal development and functioning of each cell and the whole organism. In general, genetic events are related to the sequence information of DNA, and include the consequences of transmission of a particular DNA sequence (e.g., inheritance of DNA mutations or polymorphisms) or of acquisition of DNA sequence variations (e.g., accumulation of somatic mutations in aging or cancer development). These pathologies are discussed in Chapter 49. On the other hand, a broad definition of epigenetics encompasses processes that alter gene function or its interpretation by mechanisms other than those that rely on DNA sequence change. Practically, epigenetics has evolved to include the study of (1) DNA methylation, (2) genomic imprinting, (3) histone modifications, (4) chromatin remodeling, (5) ncRNA regulation, and (6) other processes. Most of these processes add another dimension to gene expression control and thus play a role in all fundamental cellular events, including (1) cell differentiation, (2) cell growth, (3) cell death, and (4) DNA repair.

DNA Methylation

DNA methylation is possibly the most widely studied epigenetic phenomenon. It refers to the addition of a methyl group to the fifth carbon position of cytosine residues in CpG dinucleotides. CpG dinucleotides are present throughout the genome and may exist singly as an isolated CpG site or in clusters,

termed *CpG islands* (Figure 47-7). Most CpG dinucleotides in the human genome are methylated; these include CpG sites that are (1) within genes, (2) within intergenic regions, and (3) in DNA repeat elements (see Figure 47-7).[12] Unmethylated regions of the human genome are mostly found at CpG islands located (1) at the 5′ ends, (2) in promoters or first exons of genes, and occasionally (3) in some intergenic (a stretch of DNA sequences located between genes) CpG islands.[12] However, it is noteworthy that not all gene promoters are associated with CpG islands, and not all promoter-associated CpG islands are unmethylated. About 56% of human genes have promoters with CpG islands.[12] Some 10% of promoter CpG islands are methylated.

It has been well accepted that DNA methylation mediates the silencing of gene transcription. The methylation of gene promoters hinders the association of methylation-sensitive transcription factors, thus preventing gene activation. Consequently, the promoters of actively transcribed genes are generally unmethylated, while silenced genes are associated with methylated promoters. Because gene expression varies between cell types, the profile of DNA methylation differs between cell and tissue types. Furthermore, a CpG island may be composed of varying numbers of methylated and unmethylated CpG sites. Hence, a genomic region can be further described in relative degree of methylation using the term *hypomethylated* or *hypermethylated.* It has been suggested that stably silenced genes tend to be associated with densely methylated promoters, and hypomethylated gene promoters can potentially be activated.[12] Methylation of the nonpromoter regions of genes, however, is thought to suppress inadvertent transcription.[12] Furthermore, methylation of repeat elements in the genome helps to maintain chromosome stability by preventing translocations and insertions of transposons, which are repeat sequences that could randomly insert into the genome, causing gene disruptions.

Because DNA methylation has implications for gene expression, aberrant changes in DNA methylation profiles may cause pathologies. For example, aberrant hypermethylation of gene promoters, particularly those of tumor suppressor genes, contributes to cancer development. Hence, it is important that the DNA methylation pattern of a cell should be faithfully propagated to its daughter cells upon cell division. This process is executed by maintenance **DNA methyltransferases (DNMT).** DNMT1 is said to perform a "maintenance" role because the DNA methylation patterns inherited by somatic cells were originally laid down by other de novo DNA methyltransferases (DNMT3a and DNMT3b) in the early embryo.

After embryo fertilization, the genome becomes demethylated (except imprinted loci; see discussion later in this chapter) to pave the way for the establishment of developmentally related patterns of DNA methylation by de novo DNMTs. Genomic imprinting and gene dosage compensation of X-linked genes in females, termed *X-inactivation* or *lyonization,* are also mediated by DNA methylation.

X chromosome inactivation is an epigenetic phenomenon that occurs in female cells. Each female cell has two X chromosomes, and each male cell has only one X chromosome. The function of one of the X chromosomes in female cells is epigenetically silenced, so the dosage of X chromosome genes in female and male cells is the same. Gene silencing on the inactive X chromosome is maintained by dense methylation of CpG island promoters. Within each female cell, either of the X chromosomes could be chosen for inactivation.

Genomic imprinting refers to the phenomenon whereby the function of each of the two alleles of a gene is determined by its parental origin. Differential methylation of the imprinted locus from the time of germ cell development allows recognition of the parental origin of imprinted alleles by cellular processes. The human insulin-like growth factor-2 H19 (IGF2-H19) locus on chromosome 15 is an example of an imprinted locus in which a maternal allele is unmethylated and a paternal allele is methylated. Inheritance of two copies of the paternal or maternal allele (rather than one allele from each parent) is called *disomy* and results in significantly different clinical outcomes, namely, Prader-Willi and Angelman syndromes, respectively.

Histone Modifications

Hypermethylated CpG dinucleotides are also known to attract the binding of methyl-CpG binding proteins, such as methyl-CpG binding protein 2 (MECP2) and methyl-CpG binding domain proteins (MBD1 and MBD2), which further block the association of a number of transcription factors and thus block transcription.[7] It is now appreciated that these methyl-CpG binding proteins have the ability to recruit histone deacetylases, a phenomenon that leads to deacetylation of histones and ultimately represses transcription.

As discussed, histones are an integral part of nucleosomes, the basic repeating structural unit of chromatin. The amino termini of histone proteins can be modified post-translationally by processes that include (1) acetylation, (2) methylation, (3) phosphorylation, and (4) ubiquitination (see sites of modifications in Figure 47-4).[7] Acetylation of the lysines on amino termini of histones H3 and H4 by histone acetyltransferases decreases histone-DNA interaction and improves accessibility of DNA to transcriptional activation. On the contrary, histone deacetylation by histone deacetylases promotes the formation of compact nucleosomes, leading to repression of transcription. Histone deacetylation is in fact a key component of the assembly of heterochromatin, the transcriptionally inactive chromatin.[2] Methylation of the ninth amino acid residue, lysine, on histone H3 generates a binding site for heterochromatin protein (HP1) and thus is another key event in heterochromatin formation. Phosphorylation of the tenth amino acid, serine, on histone H3 is important for chromosome condensation and mitosis.

Nucleosome Positioning and Remodeling

Besides histone modifications, the position of nucleosomes is known to affect the transcriptional activity of the corresponding region of DNA. It is now known that the positioning of histones is not an entirely random process. It has been demonstrated that nucleosome-free regions are present at the 5′ and 3′ ends of genes. The 5′ nucleosome-free region is thought to be the assembly point of the preinitiation complex for transcription, and the 3′ one is the location of transcription termination.[3] A nucleosome unit is located just upstream to the 5′ nucleosome-free region, and another nucleosome is located just downstream to it, close to the transcription start site. The location of the nucleosome nearest to the transcription start site is predictable and consistent.[3] Positioning of the nucleosomes farther downstream through the gene, however, is more random. In summary, it seems that mechanisms control the positioning of nucleosomes so that their presence will not be inhibitory to the initiation of transcription.

During transcription, the nucleosomes along a gene undergo a series of changes successively. First, histones H2A and H3 are replaced by the histone variants, H2A.Z and H3.3. The histone tails are acetylated and methylated. The nucleosome would then be repositioned laterally and ultimately evicted to clear the DNA for access by the transcription machinery.[3] The nucleosome may then return to the DNA after RNA polymerase II has passed through. Consequently, nucleosomes are dynamic structures that can be remodeled according to the transcriptional demands of the cell.

Noncoding RNAs

It was once thought that much of the transcriptional activity of the human genome was directed toward the production of proteins, but exons of protein-coding genes occupy only 1% to 2% of base pairs in the human genome. Thus, the rest of the genome was previously thought to be "junk" DNA, serving no function, and was merely a fossil of our evolutionary past. The availability of innovative technologies in recent years has enabled researchers to study transcriptional activity or RNA expression on a genome-wide scale.[4] These studies revealed that almost the entire genome is transcribed. Transcription takes place in both sense and antisense directions. The same genomic region could serve as the template for many non-overlapping or overlapping transcription units. Most transcription units do not result in the production of a protein product. Researchers became aware that some of the transcribed RNA molecules serve a direct biological function. An increasing number of classes of such functional RNA molecules have been described; they are collectively termed *ncRNAs.*[13] In retrospect, rRNA and tRNA are the earliest classes of ncRNAs described. Most recently, a class of short ncRNAs, miRNAs, has become the focus of much research interest.

MicroRNA

Mature, functional miRNAs are 21 to 24 nucleotides long. The first step in the miRNA biogenesis pathway involves the initial transcription of an RNA molecule in the nucleus by RNA polymerase II. The first transcript, termed the *primary miRNA,* may be derived from short introns or a longer primary transcript that subsequently gives rise to multiple mature miRNAs. Regions of the primary miRNA that ultimately contribute to sequences of the mature miRNA are typified by their adoption of a stem-loop, also known as *hairpin configuration,* with imperfect base pairing between sequences on both sides of the stem. The primary miRNA is cleaved by **Drosha**, a Class 2 RNase III enzyme. The resultant RNA molecule, which is approximately 70 nucleotides long, is termed the *precursor miRNA.* The precursor miRNA is exported to the cytoplasm of the cell, where another RNase III–like enzyme, *Dicer,* cleaves at the loop end of the molecule, thus generating a double-stranded RNA product. The double-stranded product of Dicer is 21 to 24 nucleotides long, consisting of a mature miRNA paired with its imperfect complementary strand, termed *miRNA*.* Some evidence suggests that miRNA* may serve some biological function, and the conclusion awaits further investigation.

The mature miRNA detaches from its partner and is incorporated into the RNA-silencing complex (RISC), which includes one or more **Argonaute proteins** that are responsible for the gene silencing process known as RNA interference (RNAi). The biological function of miRNA is effected through RISC. The miRNA pairs with the 3′ untranslated region of mRNAs, leading to (1) repression of protein translation or (2) mRNA degradation. The actual biological consequence is determined by the degree of complementarity base pairing between the miRNA and the target mRNA. mRNAs that can be influenced by a particular miRNA are referred to as the target mRNAs of the corresponding miRNA. More than 850 human mature miRNAs have now been discovered. Because miRNAs can function via imperfect base pairing to mRNA, each miRNA can have an effect on multiple target mRNAs.

miRNAs modulate gene expression at the post-transcriptional level. Therefore, they are involved in many biological processes, including development and cell differentiation. They regulate (1) cell proliferation, (2) apoptosis, and (3) maturation. Because of their important regulatory role, aberrant expression of miRNAs has been reported for a myriad of diseases involving, for example, the (1) cardiovascular, (2) neurologic, (3) musculoskeletal, (4) endocrinologic, and (5) immunologic systems. Moreover, aberrant miRNA expression has been implicated in carcinogenesis. The association of miRNAs with pathologies, coupled with recognition of the presence of miRNAs in plasma and serum, makes them attractive candidate biomarkers for disease diagnosis and monitoring.

Other Noncoding RNAs

Besides miRNA, several other novel classes of ncRNAs have been discovered. In general, the ncRNA classes are subdivided into short and long ncRNAs based on their nucleotide lengths, using an arbitrary cutoff of 200 bases.[13] The group of short ncRNAs includes the miRNAs described earlier and several other species. Small interfering RNAs (siRNAs) are 21 to 22 nucleotides long and are produced by Dicer cleavage (an endoribonuclease in the RNase III family) of perfectly complementary double-stranded RNA molecules. siRNAs form

complexes with certain Argonaute proteins and are involved in (1) gene regulation, (2) transposon control, and (3) viral defense.[13] Piwi-interacting RNAs (piRNAs) are 26 to 30 nucleotides long and function in the germline to regulate transposon activity and the chromatin state.[13] piRNAs are derived not from Dicer cleavage but from successive Argonaute cleavage of long ncRNAs. Promoter-associated RNAs (PASRs) and transcription initiation RNAs (tiRNAs) are 20 to 200 nucleotides and 18 nucleotides long, respectively.[13] They are transcribed from promoters and transcription start sites and may be involved in regulating gene expression.

Long ncRNAs include a broad range of transcripts longer than 200 nucleotides and may be as long as 100 kb.[13] Some of these long ncRNAs could be (1) 5′ capped, (2) 3′ polyadenylated, and (3) spliced like mRNAs. Because this is a heterogeneous group of transcripts, their reported functions are varied and include (1) modulation of chromatin architecture, (2) regulation of gene expression, and (3) others.[13] Long ncRNAs have been shown to regulate expression of protein-coding genes by modulating histone methylation and chromatin accessibility.[13] Long ncRNAs may exert biological effects directly or as an intermediary by acting as the precursor of multiple small ncRNAs. For example, the long ncRNA *Xist* is a transcript that is expressed exclusively from the inactive X chromosome with a key role in initiating the process of X chromosome inactivation. *Xist* literally coats the X chromosome that is destined to be inactivated and suppresses transcriptional activity. However, besides acting directly, the corresponding transcript in mice, *Xist,* has been shown to anneal with its antisense partner, *Tsix,* another long ncRNA. The *Xist-Tsix* duplex is further cleaved by Dicer to produce siRNAs, which, in turn, are involved in epigenetic modifications that maintain gene silencing on the inactive X chromosome.

Beyond the Nuclear Genome

The Mitochondrial Genome

Up to this point, this chapter has focused attention on the nuclear genome, but the mitochondrial genome is also an important genetic component of eukaryotic cells. The human mitochondrial genome is a circular piece of DNA 16.5 kb in length. **Mitochondrial DNA** is transmitted between generations by maternal inheritance with the mitochondria coming from the oocytes and typically not from sperm. Multiple copies of mitochondrial DNA are present within each mitochondrion, and each cell contains a variable number of mitochondria, depending on the energy requirements of the particular cell type. Thus, certain cell types may contain up to several thousand copies of mitochondrial DNA. This greater abundance, compared with that of nuclear DNA, makes mitochondrial DNA attractive for tests for which sample DNA is limited (e.g., crime scenes, pathogen detection, and paleontology). Mitochondrial DNA is double-stranded for most of its length, except at the replication and transcription control region (the D-loop). Unlike the nuclear genome, the mitochondrial genome is not packaged into nucleosomal units. Instead, it has a unique structural organization. It codes for (1) 13 polypeptides, all involved in the oxidative phosphorylation pathway; (2) two rRNAs; and (3) all of the 22 tRNAs required for mitochondrial protein synthesis. Several other proteins are also required for normal mitochondrial function and are encoded by nuclear genes.

The mutation rate of mitochondrial DNA is ten to twenty times higher than that of nuclear DNA. This high rate has been viewed as resulting from the poor fidelity of mitochondrial DNA polymerase. Germline mutations in the mitochondrial genome generally lead to neurodegenerative and/or myopathic disease, such as MELAS (myopathy, encephalopathy, lactic acidosis, and strokelike episodes) and **Leber's hereditary optic neuropathy**. Somatic mutations, on the other hand, are associated with aging and cancer development. Consequent to the accumulation of sequence variations, more than one population of mitochondrial DNA sequences may be present in a cell. This state is termed **heteroplasmy** as opposed to **homoplasmy**, in which the cell contains a homogeneous population of mitochondrial genomes. When genetic analysis is performed for mitochondrial DNA, a note of caution is warranted on potential problems related to the presence of nuclear pseudogenes, which are DNA segments in the nuclear genome with significant homology to the mitochondrial genome. The close resemblance of the nuclear and mitochondrial DNA segments may result in false-positive detection of mitochondrial DNA sequences; thus the specificity of PCR systems for mitochondrial DNA detection needs to be carefully evaluated.

Circulating Nucleic Acids

Besides being confined within cellular boundaries, nucleic acid molecules are present in the blood circulation. Cell-free DNA and RNA molecules exist in plasma of healthy humans. DNA, RNA, miRNA, and methylated DNA sequences derived from (1) tumors, (2) the unborn fetus, (3) transplant donors, and (4) traumatized tissues have been found in the plasma of 1) cancer patients, 2) pregnant women, 3) transplant recipients, and (4) patients suffering acute pathologies, respectively. Because cell-free nucleic acid molecules could be sampled simply through collection of a peripheral blood sample, the potential for developing molecular diagnostic applications based on their detection is vast. A number of reviews have been published on this topic.[1, 9, 10]

Understanding Our Genome

Evident from the previous discussions, understanding of the structure and function of the human genome has vastly expanded over the past decade. This is a consequence of the availability of high-throughput technologies that allow scientists to study almost every aspect of the human genome on a genome-wide scale. For example, both sequencing and hybridization techniques that allow the interrogation of nucleic acid pools from the entire genome have been extensively employed in research. In terms of sequencing, the so-called next-generation sequencers decode millions to billions of nucleotide fragments in a massively parallel fashion and

are capable of producing giga (10^9) bases of sequence output in a matter of days. Regarding hybridization techniques, high-density microarrays with probes carpeting the entire genome, referred to as **tiling arrays**, are readily available. Both sequencing and hybridization techniques can be coupled with various sample preparation protocols for analysis of pools of DNA, RNA, or complementary DNA (DNA generated by reverse-transcribing RNA) from the entire genome or subsets enriched with (1) exon sequences, (2) transcription factor–binding sites, (3) methylated CpG sites, (4) short RNAs, (5) polyadenylated RNAs, and (6) others. Each of these experiments generates vast quantities of data. Basic management and analysis and further interpretation of such large data sets require the use of high-throughput computing. Hence, the field of bioinformatics has flourished and become an essential and fundamental component of life science research.

The first of the whole-genome-scale projects addressed by humankind was the **Human Genome Project**. It is the biggest biological project completed to date. Apart from its ambitious goal of deciphering the 3 billion base pairs that make up the human genetic code, it also represents a model for the (1) planning, (2) organization, and (3) execution of large-scale biological projects. The first serious discussion of the feasibility of such a project can be traced back to the mid-1980s. It was visionary of early proponents to conceive of the project before the advent of high-throughput sequencing technologies. In fact, the proposal was suggested just years after the invention of DNA sequencing in 1977. Based on technology available at the time, sequencing of the human genome would be a mammoth task, requiring a multinational effort. In 1988, a special committee of the US National Research Council of the US National Academy of Sciences formulated a 15-year human genome project, costing some $200 million a year. A genetic map with one **centiMorgan** (cM) resolution was accomplished in September 1994. A physical map involving 52,000 sequence-tagged sites (STSs) was completed in October 1998. The final journey to completion of this project was marked by a highly publicized race between a publicly funded group of investigators and a private effort. The public effort, undertaken by the International Human Genome Sequencing Consortium, consisted of investigators from twenty centers located in six countries: the (1) United States, (2) United Kingdom, (3) Japan, (4) China, (5) France, and (6) Germany. Completion of a draft sequence was announced on June 26, 2000, and it was published in two landmark papers, one from the public team and one from the private team, in February 2001.[6, 14] The final sequence was accomplished in April 2003 with 99.99% sequencing accuracy.

The Human Genome Project has far reaching implications. Technologically, it accelerated the pace of development of (1) sequencing technologies, (2) computational tools for alignment of stretches of DNA reads, and (3) organization of the data. Biologically, the human race has produced a copy of its genetic code. However, many more questions stem from having the reference human genome sequence. For example, how different is the genome between individuals? With the reduction in the cost of genome sequencing and a reduction in its technical complexity, sequencing of the genomes of a handful of individuals, including that performed by Watson[15] and Venter,[8] the pioneers of the Human Genome Project, has been completed. Cross-comparisons have been made between the sequences of these genomes.

To enhance understanding of human genomic diversity on a broader scale, two large-scale projects were launched. The first one, the International HapMap Project (http://www.hapmap. ncbi.nlm.nih.gov/; accessed December 26, 2013), was launched to study heritable variations such as (1) polymorphisms, (2) patterns of **linkage disequilibrium**, and (3) haplotypes across the human genome. The HapMap Project primarily focuses on one class of genome variations, namely, single-nucleotide polymorphisms (SNPs). Cataloguing genetic variations between different ethnic populations is useful for understanding the ancestral relationships between those populations. Once identified, a catalog of SNPs is also useful in providing landmarks of genomic locations for identification of disease-causing genes. If a SNP allele is found to be associated with a particular disease, the SNP allele serves as a marker for assessment of an individual's susceptibility (statistical probability) of developing said disease.

The second project, the 1000 Genomes Project (http://www .1000genomes.org/; accessed December 26, 2013), also aims to study genomic diversity and disease-causing genes in humans. The approach is based on whole genome sequencing of 1000 individuals, and the analysis is not limited to SNPs. Most recently, researchers have embarked on another approach to identify disease-causing genes through whole genome sequencing of families. This approach entails the comparison of genomic sequences between affected and unaffected relatives within families known to propagate a hereditary disease under investigation.

After the alphabets of the human genome have been spelled out, another obvious follow-up would be to decode the meaning of the 3 billion nucleotides that are the functional aspects of the human genome). This led to the launch of the Encyclopedia of DNA Elements (ENCODE) Project (http://www.genome.gov/ENCODE/; accessed December 26, 2013), which aims to identify all functional elements within the human genome. A feasibility study targeting 1% of the human genome has been done. Data from just this 1% of the genome have already led to many surprises that overturned many of our earlier simplistic views of the genome. Just to name a few of these surprises, as discussed earlier, other than the 1% to 2% of the genome that was previously annotated as protein-coding and much of the entire genome is transcribed. Promoters that activate transcription are not limited to the 5′ ends of genes but instead are distributed at various locations of the transcription unit. Transcription takes place on both sense and antisense strands with highly overlapping units. Such new information redefines many previously established concepts including very fundamental ones, for example, what is a gene? Our renewed understanding has brought about our appreciation of the highly sophisticated and complex nature of the workings of the human genome.

All this new information is facilitated by the advent of high-throughput technologies, as discussed earlier. Our macroscopic view of some functional aspects of the human genome is now improving. However, a long journey lies ahead before we attain a full understanding of each of the specific cellular and molecular mechanisms. Although our current understanding of the wonders of the genome is very limited, it is hoped that ultimately, humankind will have a better grasp of the causative mechanisms of pathologies to facilitate our efforts in (1) predicting, (2) diagnosing, (3) monitoring, and (4) treating disease.

Other large-scale projects that researchers are currently tackling include the Human Epigenome Project (http:// http:// www.epigenome.org/; accessed December 26, 2013), which aims to identify, catalog, and interpret genome-wide DNA methylation patterns of all human genes in all major tissues. This would represent yet another major challenge because only one reference human genome is known and many methylomes are present, given the different DNA methylation profiles between cells. Besides genetic polymorphisms such as SNPs, it is now known that structural variations between individuals are characterized by comparatively large regions of gains and losses in DNA and are known as *copy number variations*. Hence, a copy number variation project aims to catalog and interpret the functional implications of copy number variations.[11]

In conclusion, it is expected that our understanding of the human genome will continue to expand at an unimaginable rate. This will continue to drive changes in the way medicine and diagnostics is practiced. An emerging theme shows that each individual is a unique being, and much heterogeneity is seen even within the same disease entity. Thus, it is possible that *personalized medicine* with *individualized therapies* will be the standard of the future.

Review Questions

1. What are the four bases found in RNA?
   a. Adenine, cytosine, guanine, thymine
   b. Asparagine, cysteine, glycine, threonine
   c. Adenine, cytosine, guanine, uracil
   d. Adenylate, cytosol, guanidil, uracil
2. DNA polymerase is necessary for
   a. adding new nucleotides to a growing DNA strand.
   b. forming an messenger RNA (mRNA) strand from a DNA strand.
   c. releasing the tension in the double helix as replication progresses.
   d. synthesizing protein from messenger RNA (mRNA).
3. Which is true about RNA splicing?
   a. The RNA is spliced to the growing polypeptide chain.
   b. The exons are snipped out and discarded while the introns are spliced together.
   c. The introns are excised while the exons are spliced together.
   d. The promoter sequence is snipped out and the introns and exons are spliced together.

4. How many *total* chromosomes are found in a normal human somatic cell?
   a. 22
   b. 23
   c. 44
   d. 46
5. What type of bond connects complementary bases between DNA strands?
   a. Hydrogen
   b. Covalent
   c. Phosphodiester
   d. Van der Waals
6. Euchromatin
   a. maintains specialized chromatin structures.
   b. becomes less compactly organized during interphase of the cell cycle.
   c. contains transcriptionally silent genes and is densely packed.
   d. directs movement of chromosomes between daughter cells.
7. Following the attachment of a number of factors to a strand of DNA, the enzyme required for the actual process of *transcription* to occur is
   a. RNase.
   b. DNA polymerase
   c. RNA polymerase
   d. transcriptase.
8. A nucleic acid is
   a. a nucleotide.
   b. DNA or RNA.
   c. a base pair.
   d. a trinucleotide sequence.
9. The conversion of messenger RNA (mRNA) nucleotide sequences and their attached amino acids into a peptide is referred to as
   a. replication.
   b. transcription.
   c. conversion.
   d. translation.

10. The "Genetic Code" refers to
    a. the relationship between a trinucleotide sequence of RNA and the corresponding amino acid.
    b. the statement that genes are perpetuated as nucleic acid but function in the form of protein.
    c. the relationship between a nucleotide sequence of DNA and the corresponding sequence of RNA.
    d. the complementary pairing of bases along a double strand of DNA.

References

1. Chiu RWK, Lo YMD. Clinical applications of maternal plasma fetal DNA analysis: translating the fruits of 15 years of research. Clin Chem Lab Med 2013;61:197–204.
2. Grewal SI, Jia S. Heterochromatin revisited. Nat Rev Genet 2007;8:35–46.
3. Jiang C, Pugh BF. Nucleosome positioning and gene regulation: advances through genomics. Nat Rev Genet 2009;10:161–72.
4. Kapranov P, Cheng J, Dike S, Nix DA, Duttagupta R, Willingham AT, et al. RNA maps reveal new RNA classes and a possible function for pervasive transcription. Science 2007;316:1484–8.
5. Kumar D. Genomic medicine: a new frontier of medicine in the twenty first century. Genomic Med 2007;1:3–7.
6. Lander ES, Linton LM, Birren B, Nusbaum C, Zody MC, Baldwin J, et al. Initial sequencing and analysis of the human genome. Nature 2001;409:860–921.
7. Latham JA, Dent SY. Cross-regulation of histone modifications. Nat Struct Mol Biol 2007;14:1017–24.
8. Levy S, Sutton G, Ng PC, Feuk L, Halpern AL, Walenz BP, et al. The diploid genome sequence of an individual human. PLoS Biol 2007;5:e254.
9. Lo YMD. Transplantation monitoring by plasma DNA sequencing. Clin Chem 2011;57:941–2.
10. Pathak AK, Bhutani M, Kumar S, Mohan A, Guleria R. Circulating cell-free DNA in plasma/serum of lung cancer patients as a potential screening and prognostic tool. Clin Chem 2006;52:1833–42.
11. Redon R, Ishikawa S, Fitch KR, Feuk L, Perry GH, Andrews TD, et al. Global variation in copy number in the human genome. Nature 2006;444:444–54.
12. Suzuki MM, Bird A. DNA methylation landscapes: provocative insights from epigenomics. Nat Rev Genet 2008;9:465–76.
13. Taft RJ, Pang KC, Mercer TR, Dinger M, Mattick JS. Non-coding RNAs: regulators of disease. J Pathol 2010;220:126–39.
14. Venter JC, Adams MD, Myers EW, Li PW, Mural RJ, Sutton GG, et al. The sequence of the human genome. Science 2001;291:1304–51.
15. Wheeler DA, Srinivasan M, Egholm M, Shen Y, Chen L, McGuire A, et al. The complete genome of an individual by massively parallel DNA sequencing. Nature 2008;452:872–6.

Nucleic Acid Techniques
and Applications

CHAPTER

48

Carl T. Wittwer, M.D., Ph.D., and Noriko Kusukawa, Ph.D.

Objectives

1. Define the following:

Amplicon	Melting analysis
Amplification	Primer
Blot	Probe
Hybridization	Single-nucleotide variant (SNV)
Label	

2. For each of the following nucleic acid enzymes, state the enzyme's action, its physiologic function and biological source, and its use in laboratory applications (if any):

Ligase	Reverse transcriptase
Nuclease	Polymerase
Restriction endonuclease	

3. Compare target amplification, signal amplification, and probe amplification techniques, including what is amplified in each and how each is used in a clinical laboratory.

4. List and describe the steps involved in a polymerase chain reaction (PCR) including enzymes and other components required, what occurs in each step, issues with and controls for contamination and/or inhibition.

5. For each of the following target amplification techniques, state the principle of the amplification, components required, differences from conventional PCR, equilibrium quantification methods, and uses of each technique in a molecular diagnostics laboratory:

Allele-specific PCR	Ligase chain reaction (LCR)
Asymmetric PCR	Transcription mediated
Digital PCR	amplification (TMA)
	Whole genome/transcriptome amplification

6. For each of the following nucleic acid detection methods, state the principle of the method and what is measured by the method:

   Fluorometry
   UV spectrophotometry

7. Describe basic nucleic acid electrophoresis, including separation principles, types and uses of gels, and uses of electrophoresis in the molecular diagnostics laboratory.

8. State the principles of the following techniques and their use in a molecular diagnostics laboratory:

Branched-chain signal amplification	Pyrosequencing
Conformation-sensitive scanning	Restriction fragment length polymorphism (RFLP)
Dideoxy-termination sequencing for DNA	Rolling circle amplification (RCA)
High-throughput sequencing	Single nucleotide extension (SNE)
Mass spectrometry	Southern blotting
Oligo ligation	

9. Discuss the uses of hybridization techniques in the molecular diagnostics laboratory, including the principle of basic hybridization, probes and controls used, microarrays, and quantification methods; state the difference between solid-phase hybridization and solution-phase hybridization assays, and give one example of each.

10. For real-time PCR, state the reason it is considered a hybridization assay; list the components used in a real-time assay, including fluorescent dyes, primers and probes available, detection methods, and quantification of product.

11. Describe high resolution melting curve analysis for genotyping and scanning, including principle of melting, uses in single-nucleotide variant (SNV) genotyping, and for heterozygote variant scanning.

12. Analyze and solve case studies related to nucleic acid techniques used in a molecular diagnostics laboratory.

Key Words and Definitions

Allele-specific PCR A version of polymerase chain reaction (PCR) in which specific alleles or DNA sequence variants are amplified at the same locus.

Amplicon The product of an amplification reaction.

Amplification methods Techniques to amplify the amount of target, signal, or probe so that specific sequences are readily observed.

Antisense RNA (asRNA) A single-stranded RNA that is complementary to a messenger RNA (mRNA) strand transcribed within a cell.

Key Words and Definitions—cont'd

Array An ordered linear, two-dimensional, or three-dimensional arrangement of a multiplicity of discrete objects, such as individual deposits (spots or lines) of DNA or reaction chambers.

Asymmetric PCR A version of PCR that preferentially amplifies one strand of the target DNA.

Base pair A purine/pyrimidine pair linked by hydrogen bonds that connects the complementary strands of DNA or of hybrid molecules joining DNA and RNA. The base pairs are adenine-thymine and guanine-cytosine in DNA, and adenine-uracil and guanine-cytosine in RNA.

Branched-chain signal amplification A molecular probe technique that utilizes branched DNA (bDNA) as a means to amplify the hybridization signal.

Calibration An analytical process to determine the functional relationship between measured values and analytical quantities.

Cloning In biology, cloning is the process of producing similar populations of genetically identical individuals. In molecular diagnostics, cloning is the process used to create copies of DNA fragments (molecular cloning), cells (cell cloning), or organisms.

Comparative genomic hybridization (CGH) A cytogenetic technique in which reference and test DNA are respectively labeled with green- and red-fluorescing fluorochromes. Genetic abnormalities are detected by changes in the green-to-red ratio.

Conformation-sensitive gel electrophoresis (CSGE) A type of electrophoretic mutation scanning in which a segment of DNA is screened for mismatch pairing between normal and mutated base pairs.

Copy number variant (CNV) A segment of DNA in which copy-number differences have been found by comparison of two or more genomes.

Denaturing gradient gel electrophoresis (DGGE) An electrophoretic method for separating DNA fragments according to their mobilities under increasing denaturing conditions (usually increasing formamide or urea concentrations).

Deoxyribonucleic acid (DNA) A nucleic acid that carries the genetic information in the cell. It consists of two long chains of nucleotides twisted into a double helix and joined by hydrogen bonds between the complementary bases adenine and thymine or cytosine and guanine. The sequence of nucleotides determines individual hereditary characteristics.

Deoxyribonucleotide triphosphates (dNDT) The building blocks of DNA (typically dATP, dCTP, dGTP, and dTTP).

Detection methods In molecular diagnostics, these are the techniques used to detect nucleic acid sequences, usually after purification and amplification.

Dideoxy-termination sequencing A method of DNA sequencing based on the selective incorporation of chain-terminating dideoxynucleotides by DNA polymerase during in vitro DNA replication. Also known as *Sanger sequencing*.

Digital polymerase chain reaction A modification of conventional PCR where the sample is separated into a large number of partitions and the amplification is carried out in each partition individually. Also known as dPCR.

DNA microarray An array of microscopic spots of different DNA molecules attached to a solid surface Also known as *DNA chip* or *biochip*.

Electrophoresis Movement caused by an electrical field, often through a gel matrix. Polyacrylamide and agarose are common matrices used to separate DNA and RNA under an electric field.

Endonuclease An enzyme that hydrolyzes an internal phosphodiester bond, splitting a nucleic acid into two or more parts.

Exome The part of the genome that codes for exons, the sequences that remain in the mature RNA after transcription and removal of introns by RNA splicing. It differs from a transcriptome in that it consists of only DNA that is transcribed into mature RNA, excluding transfer RNA, ribosomal RNA, and other non-coding RNA.

Exonuclease An enzyme that removes terminal nucleotides from a polynucleotide.

Flow cytometry A technique for counting cells suspended in fluid as they flow one at a time past a focus of exciting light.

Fluorescence A physical property of some molecules to emit light at a longer wavelength when excited at a shorter wavelength.

Fluorescence in situ hybridization (FISH) A genetic mapping technique using fluorescent tags for analysis of chromosomal aberrations and genetic abnormalities. *Chromosome painting* is a form of FISH

Heteroduplex A DNA duplex with internal mismatches or loops.

Hetero-duplex analysis (HDA) A type of mutation scanning in which a segment of DNA is screened by gel or capillary electrophoresis for mismatch pairing between normal and mutated base pairs.

High-resolution melting analysis An indirect method of observing DNA dissociation by using dyes that fluoresce in the presence of double-stranded DNA but not single-stranded DNA.

Homoduplex A perfectly matched DNA duplex.

Hybridization The annealing or pairing of two DNA strands.

Insertion An extra DNA sequence that is present in one sample compared with a reference sequence.

Intron DNA sequence within a gene that is spliced out during messenger RNA (mRNA) processing.

Label A modification that renders a molecule observable.

Ligases Enzyme that covalently joins two DNA strands.

Ligase chain reaction (LCR) A DNA amplification technique that uses four primers instead of two and uses the ligase to ligate or join two segments of DNA.

Loop-mediated amplification (LAMP) A single tube technique for the amplification of DNA that uses a single-temperature incubation.

Melting curve analysis A direct measurement of double-stranded DNA (dsDNA) dissociation during heating. As the temperature is raised, the double strand dissociates resulting in an increase in the absorbance of the solution containing the DNA.

Melting temperature (T_m) The temperature at which 50% of the DNA strands are in the random coil or single-stranded (ssDNA) state. It depends on the length of the DNA molecule and its specific nucleotide sequence.

Key Words and Definitions—cont'd

Microtiter plate A flat plate containing a two-dimensional array of multiple "wells" used as small reaction chambers. Such plates typically have 6, 24, 96, 384, or even 1536 sample wells arranged in a rectangular array.

Multiplex ligation-dependent probe amplification (MLPA) A variation of PCR that permits multiple targets to be amplified with only a single primer pair.

Northern blot A technique for identifying specific sequences of RNA in which RNA molecules are sequentially (1) separated by electrophoresis, (2) transferred to nitrocellulose, and (3) identified with a suitable probe.

Nuclease An enzyme that degrades nucleic acid.

Nucleic acid A complex compound found in all living cells and viruses, composed of (1) purines, (2) pyrimidines, (3) carbohydrates, and (4) phosphoric acid.

Nucleic acid analogs Compounds that are analogous (structurally similar) to naturally occurring RNA and DNA. They are used in medicine and in molecular biology research.

Oligonucleotide A short single-stranded polymer of nucleic acid.

Oligonucleotide ligation assay (OLA) A technique for determining the presence or absence of a specific nucleotide pair within a target gene, often indicating whether the gene is wild type (normal) or mutant (defective).

Peptide nucleic acid (PNA) An artificially synthesized polymer similar to DNA or RNA. The term is somewhat of a misnomer, because PNA is not an acid.

Plasmid An extrachromosomal self-replicating structure found in bacterial cells that carries genes for a variety of functions not essential for cell growth. Plasmids consist of cyclic double-stranded DNA molecules, replicating independently of the chromosomes and transmitting through successive cell divisions.

Polymerases Enzymes that sequentially adds nucleotides onto a growing polynucleotide, usually requiring a primer and a template.

Polymerase chain reaction (PCR) An in vitro method for exponentially amplifying DNA.

Primer An oligonucleotide that serves to initiate polymerase-catalyzed addition of nucleotides by annealing to a template strand.

Probe A nucleic acid used to identify a target by hybridization.

Pseudogene A genetic element that does not result in a functional gene product, usually because of accumulated mutations.

Pyrosequencing A method of DNA sequencing based on the "sequencing by synthesis" principle that relies on the detection of pyrophosphate (PPi) release on nucleotide incorporation.

Real-time PCR Observation of PCR during amplification at least once each cycle.

Restriction endonuclease An endonuclease, usually from bacteria, that cuts nucleic acid in a sequence-specific manner.

Restriction fragment length polymorphism (RFLP) A genetic polymorphism revealed by changes in the sizes of DNA fragments after restriction enzyme digestion and electrophoresis.

Retrovirus A family of RNA viruses containing a reverse transcriptase enzyme that allows the viruses' genetic information to become part of the genetic information of the host cell upon replication.

Reverse transcriptase A polymerase that catalyzes synthesis of DNA from an RNA template.

Ribonucleic acid (RNA) A polymeric biochemical consisting of a long, usually single-stranded chain of alternating phosphate and ribose units with one of four bases bonded to the ribose; the bases are (1) adenine, (2) guanine, (3) cytosine, and (4) uracil.

Rolling circle amplification (RCA) A probe amplification method where, in the presence of template, a linear probe is ligated to form a circle that is replicated continuously by a polymerase and one or more primers.

Sanger sequencing A method of DNA sequencing based on the selective incorporation of chain-terminating dideoxynucleotides by DNA polymerase during in vitro DNA replication. Also known as dideoxy-termination sequencing.

Sequencing Any method that determines the exact order of bases in a DNA fragment.

Serial invasive signal amplification A signal enhancing technique that combines two invasive signal amplification reactions in series in a single-tube format. The cleaved 5′ arm from the target-specific primary reaction is used to drive a secondary invasive reaction.

Single-base primer extension (SBE) assay An assay performed by annealing a primer to ssDNA immediately adjacent to the single base variant.

Signal amplification Any method that increases the signal resulting from a molecular interaction that does not involve target amplification or probe amplification.

Single-nucleotide variant (SNV) Any change in a nucleic acid that involves only a single nucleotide, including base changes, and single base deletions/ insertions. Now favored over the related term "single nucleotide polymorphism" (SNP) and not limited to variants present at a frequency of >1% as is SNP.

Single-stranded conformational polymorphism (SSCP) A gel electrophoresis technique where single-stranded DNA (ssDNA) segments are identified by their abnormal migration patterns.

Southern blot A method for detecting DNA sequence variants after restriction enzyme digestion and size separation by electrophoresis.

Strand displacement amplification (SDA) An amplification technique that uses two types of primers and DNA polymerase and restriction endonuclease to exponentially produce single-stranded amplicons asynchronously.

Target amplification Any method for increasing the amount of target nucleic acid.

Temperature-gradient gel electrophoresis (TGGE) A form of electrophoresis that uses temperature to denature the sample as it moves across an acrylamide gel.

Template A nucleic acid molecule the sequence of which serves as a pattern to be copied by a polymerase to produce a DNA or RNA with a complementary sequence.

Thermocycler A laboratory apparatus used in the amplification of segments of DNA via the PCR. Often, the device has a thermal block with holes where tubes holding the reaction mixtures are inserted. The cycler then raises and lowers the temperature of the block in discrete, pre-programmed steps.

Thermus aquaticus (Taq) DNA polymerase A thermostable DNA polymerase named after the thermophilic bacterium *Thermus aquaticus*. It is often abbreviated to "Taq Pol" or "Taq" and is frequently used in PCR.

Key Words and Definitions—cont'd

Transcription mediated amplification (TMA) An amplification method that uses RNA polymerase and reverse transcriptase to produce an RNA amplicon from a target nucleic acid. TMA can use either RNA or single-stranded DNA as a template.

Transcriptome The set of all RNA molecules, including (1) messenger RNA (mRNA), (2) ribosomal RNA (rRNA), (3) transfer RNA (tRNA), and (4) other non-coding RNAs produced in one or a population of cells.

Virtual karyotyping A technique used to analyze a short sequence of DNA from specific loci all over a genome to obtain information that reflects a karyotype.

Whole genome amplification (WGA) A non-specific amplification technique that produces an amplified product that represents the initial starting material (whole genome).

Molecular diagnostics requires techniques to detect sequence variations that are minute changes in complex genomes.[3,12] A multitude of molecular tools have been developed that make such analysis easier. In general, molecular diagnostics typically requires: (1) selection and amplification of the **nucleic acid** of interest, (2) visualization of the amplified nucleic acids, and (3) specific identification and often quantification of individual nucleic acid species. Original research references for many of the techniques described here are available elsewhere.[14]

Nucleic Acid Enzymes

Nucleic acid enzymes are critical tools in molecular diagnostics. Common enzymes that act on nucleic acids include those that synthesize longer polymers and those that degrade nucleic acid into shorter fragments. These enzymes are critical for **deoxyribonucleic acid (DNA)** replication and for transcription and must be present in all cells that replicate. In addition to general-function enzymes, a variety of unique enzymes, found in bacteria and viruses, act on specific nucleic acid sequences. Many of these enzymes have been purified and synthesized in vitro. Some have been "engineered" with alterations that improve their performance or stability. The ability to manipulate nucleic acids in vitro with these enzymes has made modern molecular biology possible. Enzymes are also used extensively in nucleic acid diagnostics, including (1) sample preparation, (2) **probe** labeling, (3) signal generation, and (4) amplification.

Nucleases

Nucleases are enzymes that hydrolyze one or more phosphodiester bonds in nucleic acid polymers. They may cleave nucleotides one at a time from the ends (**exonucleases**), or may act only on internal bonds (**endonucleases**). For example, some probe methods are based on 5'-exonuclease activity that cleaves nucleic acids between two fluorescent **labels**. Nucleases are either DNA or **ribonucleic acid (RNA)** specific and may act on only double- or single-stranded polymers. For example, DNAse I digests double-stranded DNA (dsDNA), and S1 nuclease acts only on single-stranded DNA (ssDNA). DNAse I has been used to specifically degrade DNA in nucleic acid mixtures when only RNA is of interest. RNAses are very stable enzymes that are difficult to remove. As common laboratory contaminants, they make RNA analysis difficult.

Restriction Endonucleases

Restriction endonucleases are found in bacteria; these enzymes degrade foreign DNA. Their action is sequence specific, requiring recognition sequences of usually 4 to 10 nucleotides on a dsDNA molecule. At each location where this sequence is found, the enzyme cuts both strands in a reproducible manner, resulting in either staggered or blunt-end cuts. For example, EcoRI is a restriction enzyme from *E. coli* that recognizes the six-base sequence GAATTC and cuts between the G and the A on both strands, producing a staggered cut:

$$5' \cdots G/AATTC \cdots 3'$$

$$3' \cdots CTTAA/G \cdots 5'$$

Note that "blunt-end" cuts would be produced if the enzyme hydrolyzed the bond between A and T.

Restriction enzymes are used for digesting large fragments of DNA into smaller pieces and for preparing DNA from different sources to be joined together in **cloning** procedures. Nicking enzymes are restriction enzymes that cut only one strand of double-stranded nucleic acid. Methylation-sensitive enzymes are restriction enzymes that distinguish between cytosine and 5-methylcytosine. In humans, methylation of cytosine is a common epigenetic modification of DNA and is important because it affects gene expression (see Chapter 47).

Ligases

Ligases catalyze the formation of phosphodiester linkages between two nucleic acid chains. DNA ligases are not sequence specific and require the presence of a complementary **template**. In contrast, RNA ligases used in messenger RNA (mRNA) processing do not require a template but are sensitive to sequence.

Polymerases

Polymerases catalyze the synthesis of complementary nucleic acid polymers using a parent strand as a template. In vitro, these enzymes extend an **oligonucleotide primer** that is annealed to a template strand. Extension requires that the 3'OH of the extending end is free and that nucleotide triphosphates (NTPs) are present. Extension ends if you run out of template or NTPs or if no 3'OH groups are available at the extending end. Thermostable polymerases, such as **Thermus aquaticus (Taq) DNA polymerase**, are essential reagents for the automation of many nucleic acid amplification procedures because of their stability at high temperatures. Some DNA polymerases also have 3′ to 5′, exonuclease activity, 5′ to 3′ activity, or both. A polymerase with 3′ to 5′ exonuclease activity is able to correct mismatched **base pairs** at the 3′-end of the extending chain. Such proofreading activity increases polymerase *fidelity* by decreasing the number of errors or misincorporated bases. A polymerase with 5′ to 3′ exonuclease activity is able to increase the process ability of a polymerase by cleaving any blocking probes or secondary structures, thereby increasing the number of bases incorporated during each extension.

Reverse Transcriptase

Reverse transcriptase is found in **retroviruses** and catalyzes the synthesis of DNA from either an RNA or a DNA template. Retroviruses have RNA genomes, and reverse transcriptase activity is required as part of their replication. In vitro, reverse transcriptase is used to make complementary DNA (cDNA) copies of RNA and may be used for (1) cloning, (2) probe preparation, and (3) nucleic acid assays.

Amplification Techniques

Techniques that increase (1) the amount of the nucleic acid target, (2) the detection signal, or (3) the probe are referred to as **amplification methods**. Examples of amplification methods are listed in Table 48-1. In **target amplification**, the sequence of interest is copied many times by in vitro methods. Areas outside the target are not amplified. In **signal amplification**, the amount of target stays the same, but the signal is increased. Finally, in probe amplification, the probe is amplified only in the presence of the target. In practice, amplification techniques may achieve more than a million-fold amplification in less than an hour.

Polymerase Chain Reaction

When the amount of target nucleic acid is increased by synthetic in vitro methods, target amplification occurs. The **polymerase chain reaction (PCR)**[8] is the most widely known and applied target amplification method.

Methodological Details

PCR requires (1) a thermostable DNA polymerase, (2) deoxynucleotides of each base (collectively referred to as **dNTPs**), (3) the target sequence, and (4) a pair of oligonucleotides (referred to as primers) complementary to opposite strands flanking the sequence to be amplified. In the first step, target duplexes are denatured into single strands by heat (Figure 48-1). When the mixture is cooled, primers provided in great excess (usually more than a million times the concentration of the initial target) specifically anneal to complementary sequences on the target. Once the primers are annealed, the action of the polymerase synthesizes two additional DNA strands containing the primers as the 5′ ends. The primers are placed close enough together so that the polymerase extends each strand far enough to include the priming site of the other primer. Usually the optimum temperature for polymerization is at an intermediate temperature between the denaturation and annealing temperatures. The second cycle also begins with denaturation, but now there are twice as many strands (the original genomic DNA and the extension products from the first cycle) available for primer annealing and subsequent extension. The temperature cycling is typically continued among three temperatures: (1) a high temperature sufficient to denature the target sequence, (2) a low temperature that allows annealing of the primers to the target, and (3) a third temperature that is optimum for polymerase extension. The instrument that takes samples through the multiple steps of changing temperature is known as a **thermocycler**.

Repetitive thermocycling results in the exponential accumulation of the short product (consisting of primers and all intervening sequences). If the efficiency of each cycle is optimal, the number of target sequences doubles each cycle (efficiency expressed as 1.0 or 100%). PCR efficiency depends on (1) the concentrations of the primers and polymerase, (2) the temperature-cycling protocol, and (3) any polymerase inhibitors. Amplified products accumulate exponentially in the beginning cycles of PCR. At some point, however, the efficiency of amplification falls, and eventually the amount of product plateaus (Figure 48-2) either from (1) exhaustion

TABLE 48-1 Common Amplification Techniques

Method	Abbreviation	Type	Enzymes Required
Polymerase chain reaction	PCR	Target	DNA polymerase
Reverse transcriptase PCR	RT-PCR	Target	Reverse transcriptase, DNA polymerase
Transcription mediated amplification	TMA	Target	Reverse transcriptase, RNAse H, RNA polymerase
Ligase chain reaction	LCR	Target	DNA ligase
Strand displacement amplification	SDA	Target	DNA polymerase, restriction enzyme
Loop-mediated amplification	LAMP	Target	DNA polymerase
Whole genome amplification	WGA	Target	Processive DNA polymerase
Antisense RNA amplification	asRNA	Target	Reverse transcriptase, RNAse H DNA polymerase, RNA polymerase
Branched DNA	bDNA	Signal	Alkaline phosphatase
Serial invasive signal amplification	SISAR	Signal	Structure-specific 5′-nuclease
Rolling circle amplification	RCA	Probe	DNA ligase processive DNA polymerase

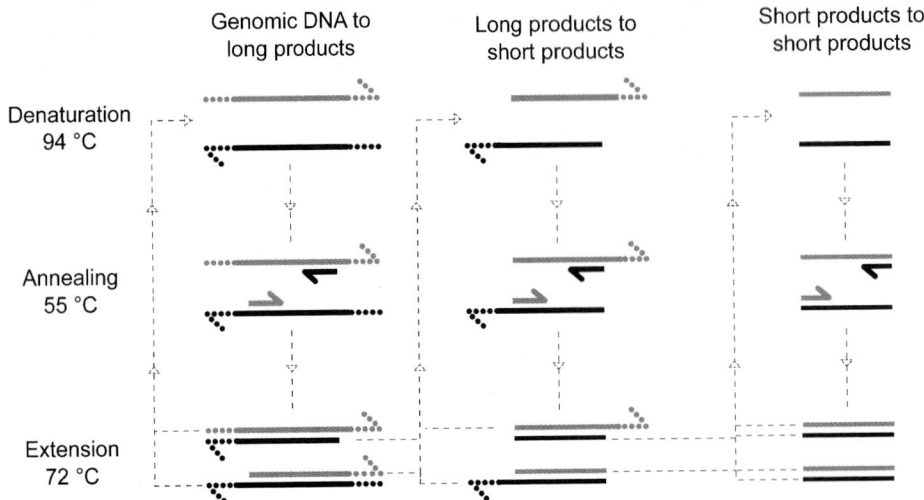

Genomic DNA to long products   Long products to short products   Short products to short products

Denaturation 94 °C

Annealing 55 °C

Extension 72 °C

Figure 48-1 Schematic diagram of the polymerase chain reaction (PCR). Repetitive cycles of denaturation, annealing, and extension are paced by temperature cycling of the reaction. Two primers (indicated as *short segments with half arrowheads*) anneal to opposite template strands *(long heavy lines)* to define the region to be amplified. Extension occurs from the 3′ ends (indicated with *half arrowheads*). In each cycle, genomic DNA is denatured and annealed to primers that extend in opposite directions across the same region, producing long products of undefined length. Long products generated by extension of one of the primers anneal to the other primer during the next cycle, producing short products of defined length. Any short products present also produce more short products. After n cycles, 2^n new copies of the amplified region (n long products + $[2^n - n]$ short products) are generated from each original genomic copy. A similar approach is used to amplify RNA targets by initial reverse transcription of the RNA template to produce the DNA template.

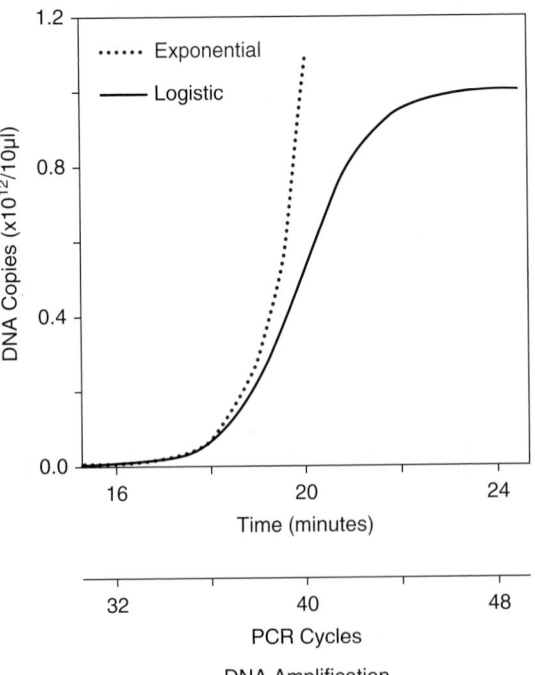

DNA Amplification

Figure 48-2 Exponential and logistic curves for DNA amplification by polymerase chain reaction (PCR). A doubling time of 30 seconds is assumed for PCR. That is, given the equation $N_t = N_0 e^{rt}$, in which N_t is the amount of DNA at time t and N_0 is the initial amount of the DNA, r is 1.386 min^{-1} for PCR. A carrying capacity of 10^{11} copies of PCR product per microliter was used, assuming that the reaction is primer limited at one third the primer concentration (initially at 0.5 8 mol/L, or 10^{11} primer molecule pairs per microliter). Starting with one target copy, it takes 23 minutes (46 cycles) to amplify the target to saturation. *(Modified with permission of the publisher from Wittwer CT, Kusukawa N. Real-time PCR and melting analysis. In Persing DH, Tenover FC, Tang YW, Versalovic J, Nolte FS, Hayden RT, Belkum AV [eds.], Molecular microbiology: diagnostic principles and practice, 2nd edition, Washington, DC: ASM Press, 2011:63-82. © 2011 ASM Press.)*

of components or (2) from competition between primer and product annealing as the single strands of product are at such high concentrations that they anneal to each other rather than to the primers. The S-curve shape is similar to the logistic model for population growth. In a typical PCR reaction using 0.5 μmol/L of each primer, the maximum DNA concentration achievable is about 10^{11} copies/μL.

After amplification, the products are detected by various methods. Simple gel **electrophoresis** with ethidium bromide staining provides an approximate size of the PCR product. When greater accuracy is required, one of the primers is fluorescently labeled so that after PCR the fragments are able to be sized on a DNA **sequencing** device. Alternatively, some form of **hybridization** assay is used to verify or analyze the amplified product. Automated methods are available, and closed-tube methods are particularly advantageous in the clinical laboratory. Adding a fluorescent dye or probe before amplification allows thermocyclers equipped with optical detection to analyze the reaction as it progresses (**real-time PCR**) or after the reaction is complete (end point or equilibrium measurement) without need to process the sample for a separate analysis step.

Kinetics and Rapid Cycling

A typical cycle of PCR requires (1) denaturation of double-stranded target, (2) annealing of primers to their targets, and (3) extension of the DNA strand from the primer. In practice, each of these steps occur at a selected temperature, for example, (1) denaturation at 94 °C, (2) annealing at 55 °C, and (3) extension at 72 °C, and for a chosen duration. Standard thermocycling instruments focus on accurate temperature control at equilibrium, not on the dynamic control of the sample temperature during transitions. As a result, long cycle times have become standard to ensure that the sample reaches target temperatures and PCR may require hours to complete typical 30-cycle amplifications.

However, the kinetics of PCR suggest that controlled transitions between temperatures with minimal or no pauses (temperature plateaus) are optimum for PCR amplification (Figure 48-3). Thus, denaturation, annealing, and extension are very rapid reactions. The use of temperature "spikes" at denaturation and annealing, instead of extended temperature plateaus, allows for *rapid cycling*. The actual time required for PCR depends on the size of the product, but when it is less than 500 base pairs (bp), a 30-cycle amplification is easily completed in 15 to 30 minutes. Furthermore, rapid amplification improves specificity. Figure 48-4 shows PCR amplification of a 536-bp fragment of β-globin amplified at different cycling speeds. With conventional slow cycling, many nonspecific products are generated (cycling profile A). These products disappear as the cycling time is decreased (profiles B, C, and D). In fact, amplification yield and product specificity are optimal when denaturation and annealing times are minimal. Most PCR is slow because of instrument limitations. In contrast, the biochemical components of PCR are rapid, and extremely fast PCR is now feasible (<1 min).[14]

Detection Limits

When PCR is performed under optimal conditions, it is possible to detect a single copy of the target. In practice, however, the chance of getting one or more copies from a dilute template solution into individual reactions must be considered. The Poisson distribution (a discrete probability distribution) indicates that if, on average, one target copy will be present per

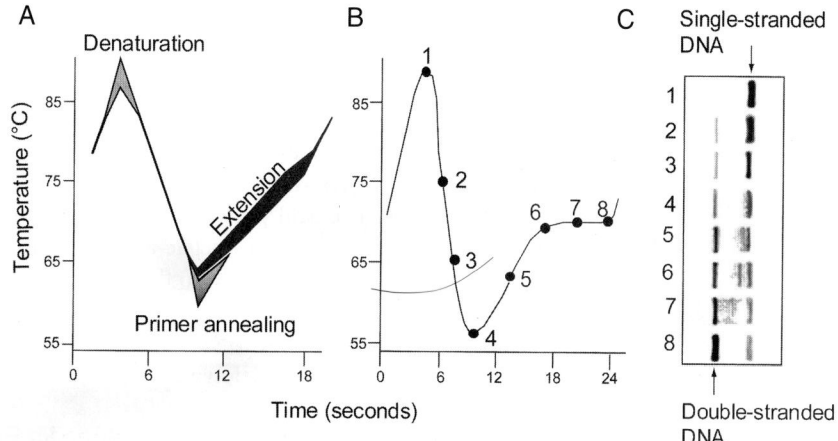

Figure 48-3 A visual demonstration of polymerase chain reaction (PCR) kinetics. The three phases of PCR (denaturation, annealing, and extension) occur as the temperature is continuously changing (*panel A*). Toward the end of PCR temperature cycling, the reaction contains single- and double-stranded PCR products. When different points of the cycle are sampled (by snap cooling the mixture in ice water, *panel B*) and analyzed, the transition from denatured single-stranded DNA (ssDNA) to double-stranded DNA (dsDNA) is revealed as a continuum (*panel C*). Progression of the extension reaction can be followed by additional bands appearing between the ssDNA and dsDNA (time points 5 to 7). (*Modified with permission from Wittwer CT, Herrmann MG: Rapid thermal cycling and PCR kinetics. In Innis M, Gelfand D, Sninsky J, eds. PCR applications, San Diego: Academic Press, 1999:211-229. © 1999 Academic Press.*)

tube, 37% of the tubes will have no target, 37% will have one target, and the remainder will have more than one. If there is an average of two copies per tube, approximately 14% of the tubes will have no template and will provide a false-negative result. About five copies on average are necessary for 99% of the tubes to include at least one copy. In practice, single-molecule PCR has been used to overcome these sensitivity limits.

Single-molecule PCR/Digital Polymerase Chain Reaction[5]

Single-molecule PCR (also known as **digital polymerase chain reaction** (digital PCR)) is a technique that limits the amount of template that is distributed across many reaction compartments so that some compartments have no template. Digital PCR depends on an on-off signal resulting from either the presence or absence of template in each of many reactions. Instead of conventional tubes, these compartments may be (1) very small droplets in a water-in-oil emulsion (emulsion PCR),

(2) PCR colonies (polonies) within a gel, (3) on the surface of a flowcell, or (4) on microbeads. When thousands of reactions are analyzed, it is possible to obtain very exact quantification. For example, copy number changes and rare mutations in a population of tumor cells are easily quantified.[14] The clonal nature of digital PCR allows one to assess whether multiple variants are on the same or different chromosomes. Single-molecule PCR is also used as the first step for many of the high-throughput sequencing methods reviewed later in this chapter.

Contamination Control (False-Positive)

Because PCR is able to detect a single molecule of target sequence, a small amount of contamination in a sample easily produces a false-positive result. The greatest potential for contamination comes from the product of the amplification reaction, referred to as the **amplicon** (used interchangeably with *PCR product*). After amplification, each reaction mixture may contain as many as 10^{12} copies of the amplicon. Thus minute aerosol droplets contain more than enough target for robust amplification. Amplicons contaminate (1) reagents, (2) pipettes, and (3) glassware. Simple laboratory precautions that have been utilized to minimize contamination by amplicons include the use of (1) physically separated areas for preamplification and postamplification steps, (2) positive-displacement pipettes to minimize aerosol contamination, and (3) prealiquoted reagents. The most effective way of all is to contain the product in a closed tube and not let any escape. Even with these precautions, a negative control or blank (all reactants minus target DNA) is an important feature of a quality control program for monitoring PCR.

Inhibition Control (False-Negative Results)

An advantage of PCR is that it does not require highly purified nucleic acid to achieve a successful amplification. In practice, however, clinical samples may contain unpredictable amounts of impurities that could inhibit polymerase activity. Consequently to ensure reliable amplification in clinical analyses, some form of nucleic acid purification is often used. The diverse nature of PCR inhibitors within clinical specimens requires demonstration that the sample (or preparation of nucleic acid purified from it) will allow amplification. Typically, a control nucleic acid sequence, usually different from the target, is added to the sample (or to nucleic acid extracted from the sample). Failure to amplify this control indicates that further purification of the sample is required to remove inhibitors of the reaction.

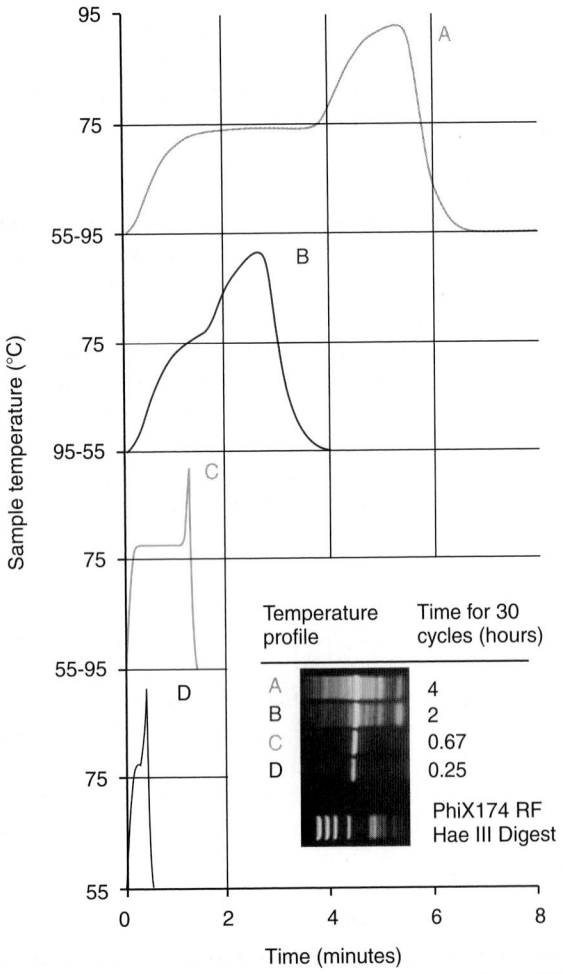

Figure 48-4 Rapid polymerase chain reaction (PCR) improves product specificity. Samples were cycled 30 times through profiles *A, B, C,* and *D*. Increased specificity of amplification of a 534 bp β-globin fragment is seen with faster cycles (*C* and *D*). *(Reprinted by permission of the publisher from Wittwer CT, Garling DJ: Rapid cycle DNA amplification: time and temperature optimization. BioTechniques 1991, 10:76-83. © 1991 Eaton Publishing.)*

Asymmetric and Allele-Specific Polymerase Chain Reaction

Conventional PCR uses primers that are present in equal amounts, thereby ensuring that the majority of the products are double-stranded amplicons. **Asymmetric PCR** uses different concentrations of the two primers to generate more of one strand than of the other so that the single stranded product is able to be directly hybridized to probes without denaturation.

Another variant method called **allele-specific PCR** enables preferential amplification of one genetic allele over another. The 3′ end of one primer is placed at the polymorphic site and is extended readily only if it is completely complementary to the target. This strategy is useful for distinguishing a gene from its **pseudogenes** and for genotyping of SNVs.

Additional Amplification Methods

In addition to PCR, many other methods for amplification have been developed, and some are briefly described below. Citations to the original literature are available elsewhere.[14]

Transcription Mediated Amplification

Transcription mediated amplification (TMA) is modeled after the replication of retroviruses. The target is isothermally amplified without temperature cycling and a reverse transcriptase, RNAse H, and RNA polymerase are required. As illustrated in Figure 48-5, the method may be applied to single-stranded RNA or dsDNA targets. As in PCR, all reagents are included and amplification is exponential with completion

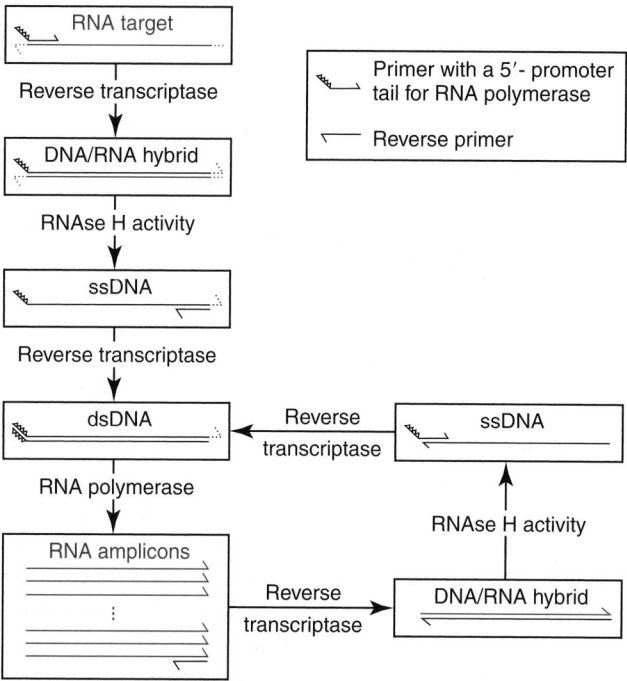

Figure 48-5 Schematic diagram of transcription mediated amplification (TMA). Starting with a single-stranded RNA target, a primer with an RNA polymerase promoter on its 5′-end is extended by reverse transcriptase to form a DNA/RNA hybrid. The reverse transcriptase also has RNAse H activity that subsequently degrades the RNA strand to leave single-stranded DNA (ssDNA). A second primer then binds to the ssDNA, and extension forms double-stranded DNA (dsDNA) with the attached RNA polymerase promoter. RNA polymerase then makes 100 to 1000 copies of RNA, some of which are again primed by the second primer. Repeated cycles of reverse transcription, DNA/RNA hybrid degradation by RNAse H activity, ds-DNA formation by reverse transcriptase, and further transcription by RNA polymerase exponentially produce ssRNA amplicons. Single-stranded targets are amplified isothermally, while double-stranded targets are first denatured to single strands.

in less than an hour. Unlike PCR, temperature cycling is not required, although an initial heat denaturation is needed if a dsDNA template is used. The method is particularly advantageous when the target is a viral RNA from patients carrying the human immunodeficiency virus [HIV] or hepatitis C virus [HCV] in blood bank nucleic acid testing.

Additional Target Amplification Techniques

Additional target amplification techniques include (1) the **ligase chain reaction (LCR)**, (2) **strand displacement amplification (SDA)**, and (3) **loop-mediated amplification (LAMP)**. In the LCR, a ligase replaces the polymerase of PCR, resulting in exponential ligation during temperature cycling. In SDA, strand displacement is used instead of thermal denaturation, allowing isothermal amplification. LAMP also uses strand displacement and is isothermal, producing a myriad of looped structures of different sizes. All target amplification methods increase the concentration of target sequences so that they are easier to detect.

Whole Genome, Transcriptome, or Exome Amplification

Instead of specific amplification of one target to improve sensitivity, methods that amplify all nucleic acids of a specific class are useful when the target is in short supply. For example, **whole genome amplification (WGA)** uses random hexamers and a highly processive polymerase to amplify DNA nonspecifically. Similarly, it is possible to generically select, amplify and sequence an **exome** or **transcriptome** by first isolating the respective RNAs. For example, it is possible to reverse transcribe mRNA by use of a poly(T) primer modified with an RNA polymerase promoter. After reverse transcription, second-strand DNA synthesis, and transcription, **antisense RNA (asRNA)** is produced that is then used in expression studies. Whole genome, transcriptome and exome amplification are useful to enrich and amplify before detection or sequencing

Branched-Chain Signal Amplification

The **branched-chain signal amplification technique** creates branched DNA (bDNA) by hybridizing the target nucleic acid to multiple capture probes affixed to a microtiter well. This is followed by hybridization to a series of (1) "extender," (2) "preamplifier," and (3) amplifier probes. The final, highly-branched amplifier probe includes multiple copies of signal-generating enzymes that act on a chemiluminescent substrate to produce light.

Signal and Probe Amplification Methods

Signal and probe amplification methods are also used in molecular diagnostics. For example, **serial invasive signal amplification** is a target-dependent signal amplification method used for SNV genotyping that generates **fluorescence** by recycling the cleavage of primary and secondary probes. **Rolling circle amplification (RCA)** is a probe amplification method. In the presence of template, a linear probe is ligated to form a circle that is replicated continuously by a polymerase and one or more primers. The amplified probe is then detected and indicates the presence of the target.

Quantification after Amplification

Quantitative analysis at the end of amplification usually requires **calibration** with known amounts of target or a target mimic. Quantification is accomplished by comparison to an internal standard that is added at the time of sample processing to control for losses during nucleic acid purification. Examples of internal standards are (1) DNA fragments, (2) plasmids, and (3) RNA packaged into synthetic phage or virus particles to mimic the assay of real viruses ("armored" RNA). If the competitor template is amplified by the target primers but generates an amplicon with a sequence or size different from the target amplicon, any variation in reaction activity affects both products identically. Thus, both are amplified. Real-time PCR, however, is a simpler and more powerful approach to quantification than end-point assays. The reaction is monitored each cycle, and the profiles of the curves are used to calculate initial target concentrations. Details of **real-time PCR** are described later in this chapter.

Detection Techniques

Molecular diagnostics relies on both generic and specific **detection methods** for nucleic acids. Generic techniques measure the total amount of nucleic acid, whereas specific techniques measure a particular sequence often by the use of nucleic acid probes.

Generic Measurement and Visualization

To generically measure or visualize nucleic acids, ultraviolet (UV) spectrophotometry and fluorometry combined with fluorescent staining dyes are commonly used.

Ultraviolet Spectrophotometry

Nucleic acid molecules absorb UV light maximally at 260 nm, a property that is often used to measure the nucleic acid content of a solution. If a dsDNA preparation is pure, a 50 mg/L solution has an absorbance of 1.0 at 260 nm. Also, the purity of a nucleic acid preparation can be assessed by its absorbance ratio at 260 nm and 280 nm (260:280 ratio). In contrast to nucleic acids, proteins absorb maximally at 280 nm. A pure DNA sample should have a 260:280 ratio of 1.7-2.0. Lower values suggest significant protein contamination.

Fluorometry and Fluorescent Staining

Although absorbance measurements are simple and precise, they often are not sensitive enough for generic measurement and visualization applications. Consequently, fluorometric and fluorescent staining techniques are often used to measure nucleic acids as they are 1000 to 10,000 times more sensitive than absorbance measurements. A widely used fluorescent nucleic acid dye is ethidium bromide, a positively charged, intercalating dye for dsDNA and to a lesser extent, ssDNA and RNA. Cyanine dyes, such as SYBR Green I, are also popular stains for nucleic acids because they do not fluoresce unless they are bound to nucleic acids, thus providing very low background. With the

appropriate optics, it is possible to visualize single molecules of DNA with cyanine-based nucleic acid stains.[6]

Sequence Specific Labels

Sequence-specific labels are used to discriminate between different nucleic acid sequences, and many types of labels have been covalently attached or incorporated into nucleic acid to form probes. The first probes used in nucleic acid detection were radioactively labeled. Radioactive labels are still favored in some research settings because of the sensitivity obtained with probes of high specific activity. However, radioactive probes are limited by isotopic decay and radiolysis of the nucleic acid. This inherent instability, along with concerns of radioisotope safety and disposal, restricts the use of radioactive probes in the clinical laboratory.

Biotin or digoxigenin are commonly used nonradioactive probes that are usually labeled at the 3′ or 5′ end of the molecule to minimize interference with hybridization. Such affinity labels do not generate signals on their own, but require high-affinity binding partners like antibodies or streptavidin. These high affinity binding molecules are often linked to enzymes with substrates that produce (1) chemiluminescent, (2) spectrophotometric, or (3) fluorescent signals.

In practice, affinity labels have been used to capture and localize targets to a solid support. For example, biotinylated probes may be affixed to a streptavidin-coated surface. After incubation with the target nucleic acid, a second probe is added, which is either directly labeled with a fluorescence chemical or conjugated through an affinity label to an enzyme. Any background or nonspecific localization of reagents results in amplification of an undesired signal along with the desired signal, and these methods usually require multiple separation and washing steps to decrease the background.

Advances in oligonucleotide synthesis and fluorescence detection have made fluorescene-labeled probes the preferred reporter for nucleic acid analysis. Many fluorescent labels are now available, allowing color multiplexing for applications, such as (1) DNA sequencing, (2) fragment length analysis, (3) DNA **arrays**, and (4) real-time PCR (all reviewed later in this chapter). Techniques such as (1) fluorescence polarization, (2) fluorescence resonance energy transfer (FRET), and (3) fluorescence quenching provide additional detection specificity.

Discrimination Techniques

Widely-used general categories of nucleic acid discrimination are:

- Electrophoretic separation: Provides physical separation of individual nucleic acid species based on molecular weight and shape.
- Discrimination by size or sequence without use of electrophoresis. Examples are (1) high-performance liquid chromatography (HPLC), (2) mass spectrometry, and (3) high throughput sequencing.
- Hybridization assays: Provides visualization of specific nucleic acids out of a background, usually with probes. Some techniques use both electrophoresis and hybridization.

Electrophoresis

Electrophoresis (see Chapter 11) is the most commonly used method for separating molecules of DNA and RNA. Both DNA and RNA are negatively charged and will migrate toward the positively charged electrode when an electrical field is present within an appropriately buffered solution. Separation of different nucleic acids occurs when mixtures are allowed to travel through a neutral sieving polymer under the electrical field. Separation is primarily based on molecular weight with smaller molecules traveling faster through the polymer than larger ones (Figure 48-6). When very large molecules (≥50 kb) have to be separated, pulsed electrical fields are employed to help move these molecules through the polymer matrix. Separation also occurs based on the physical conformation, or shape, of the molecule. For instance, single-stranded molecules may fold into secondary structures, and double-stranded molecules may form (1) **heteroduplexes**, (2) nicked strands, or (3) superhelical circular structures. Separation based on shape provides useful information, but sometimes confuses size-based analysis. For instance, because RNA generally has a high degree of secondary structure, electrophoresis of RNA is usually performed under denaturing conditions to abolish these secondary structures. Electrophoresis of DNA is performed under native or denaturing conditions depending on the application.

RNA electrophoresis is commonly performed as a quality control check before transcript quantification or microarray expression analysis. As RNA is degraded easily by tissue or environmental RNAses, it is important to assess the quality of the RNA used in these methods. Because RNA often has

secondary structure, electrophoresis is usually performed under denaturing conditions to eliminate them. Microfluidic chips with integrated microelectrophoresis are commercially available to rapidly assess RNA integrity by inspection of ribosomal RNA peaks (Figure 48-7). In practice, only small amounts of starting RNA are needed by this method. However, it does not detect specific transcripts.

Agarose gels and polyacrylamide are the two types of polymeric support medias commonly used in electrophoresis. Agarose gels are able to separate nucleic acid fragments as small as 20 bp to more than 10 Mb (10,000 kb), including chromosomes of (1) yeast, (2) fungi, and (3) parasites. However, the resolution of separations in agarose is limited, usually to a size difference of 2% to 5%. Polyacrylamide polymers are suited for high-resolution separation (down to about a 0.1% size differences) of short molecules (up to about 2 kb) and are the primary polymer for single-stranded nucleic acid separation, such as DNA sequencing. Table 48-2 lists common electrophoresis-based techniques described further in this section.

Polymerase Chain Reaction Product Length

The analysis of PCR product by electrophoresis is frequently used to assess the quality and specificity of PCR amplification. PCR products are visualized by staining the gel with a fluorescent DNA-binding dye, such as ethidium bromide. In some situations, the presence of an amplification product is directly diagnostic, such as the detection of sequences found only in a (1) bacterium, (2) virus, or (3) fungus in a human sample. The specificity of the amplification reaction is verified by the known size of the fragment. Internal negative and positive controls are used to control for potential contamination and to establish detection sensitivity.

Monitoring of the PCR product length on gels allows detection of (1) small **insertions**, (2) deletions, (3) rearrangements,

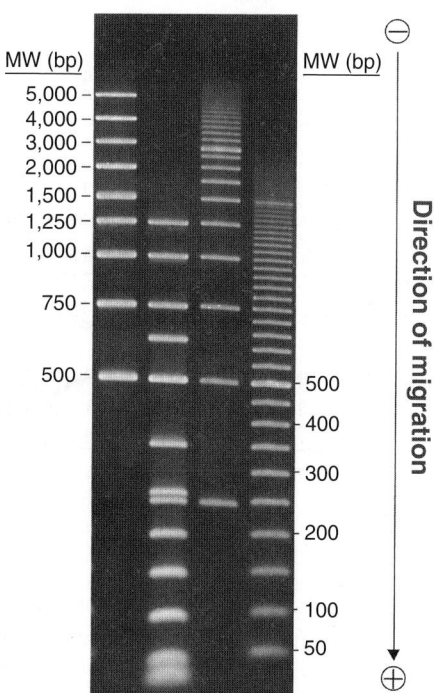

Figure 48-6 A photograph of multiple DNA fragments after agarose gel electrophoresis (1% w/v, SeaKem LE agarose gel) showing the separation of dsDNA molecules by size. *(Photograph courtesy of Lonza Bioscience, Rockland, ME.)*

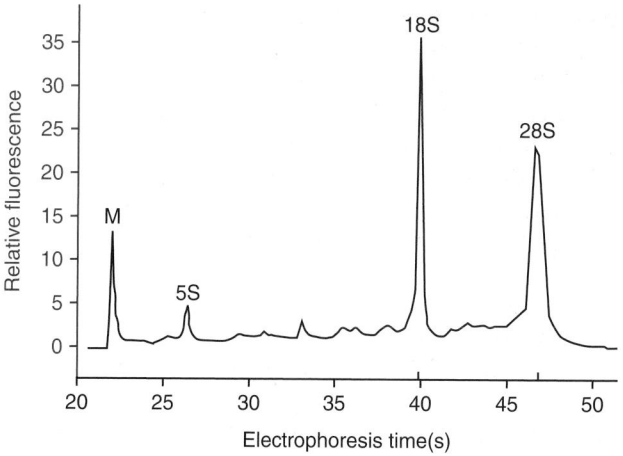

Figure 48-7 Microelectrophoresis of human white blood cell RNA. After isolation of white blood cells and extraction of total RNA, samples were denatured, stained with a fluorescent dye, and applied to a commercial microelectrophoresis platform for assessment of RNA quality. Prominent 18S and 28S bands of ribosomal RNA suggest the RNA is largely intact. Also indicated are a reference marker (M) and the 5S ribosomal band. Note that electrophoresis was performed in less than 1 minute.

and (4) changes in the number of repeated sequences. Length differences may be large and easily detected with agarose gel electrophoresis, or they may be small enough to require a denaturing polyacrylamide support matrix. Fluorescent primers may be incorporated into the product during PCR to simplify detection of fragment lengths. These techniques are commonly used in the diagnosis of inherited diseases and in identity assessment.

Restriction Fragment Length Polymorphism

DNA extracted from a cell is extremely long and is usually cut into shorter fragments before electrophoresis to aid the analysis. For example, restriction endonucleases cut dsDNA into fragments of reproducible size and the same enzyme produces the same fragments in different specimens if the specimens contain the same DNA sequence. If an alteration in the DNA abolishes or creates a cleavage site recognized by the enzyme (or changes the spacing between two cleavage sites), then the digested fragments will have different lengths: hence, the name **restriction fragment length polymorphism (RFLP)**. However, restriction digestion produces thousands of fragments. To be useful, specific fragments need to be visualized.

The **Southern blot** technique separates restriction fragments by agarose gel electrophoresis and transfers by blotting them to a membrane for selective visualization by labeled probes. The hybridized probes then are visualized by autoradiography or chemiluminescence. Southern blotting detects RFLPs, including large structural alterations, such as (1) deletions, (2) duplications, (3) insertions, and (4) rearrangements. The procedure was named after its inventor, E. M. Southern, and it was the first discrimination method with adequate sensitivity and specificity for DNA analysis of single-copy genes in complex genomes. However, it requires large amounts of DNA (10-50 μg/lane)

and is labor intensive and time consuming. Today, it has largely been replaced by PCR-based assays.

Polymerase chain reaction/Restriction Fragment Length Polymorphism

PCR can be used to amplify regions of DNA that contain known sequence alterations that alter restriction-enzyme cleavage sites. After PCR, the products are digested with one or more restriction enzymes and analyzed by electrophoresis. For example, if a sample has a variant (such as a mutation) that disrupts a restriction-enzyme recognition site, this is distinguished from a sample that does not have the variant. Such an assay will produce one uncut PCR fragment when the mutation is present and two shorter fragments when the mutation is absent (Figure 48-8). If the variant is present as a heterozygote (e.g., one normal and one mutant copy of DNA), then one long and two shorter fragments will be observed. Typically the assay is designed such that the fragments are easily resolved by agarose electrophoresis and visualized by staining the gel with a fluorescent DNA-binding dye, such as ethidium bromide. One variant of this technique uses reverse-transcribed mRNA, which lacks the **introns** that would be present in the DNA. It is possible to analyze multiple exons in one PCR.

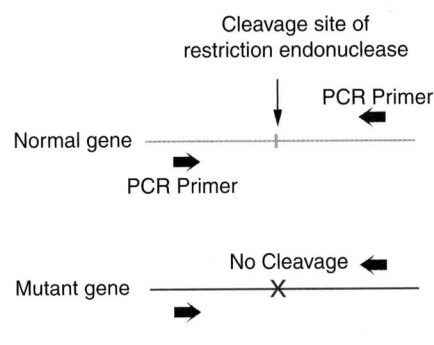

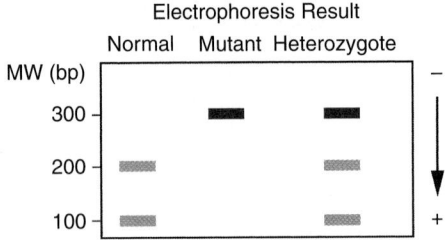

Figure 48-8 An example of polymerase chain reaction–restriction fragment length polymorphism (PCR–RFLP). A DNA fragment amplified by PCR carries a site (a unique sequence of generally four or more bases) that is recognized and cleaved by a specific restriction endonuclease. If a mutation is present, this site is altered and is no longer recognized by the enzyme. Electrophoresis reveals that the fragment from a normal specimen was indeed cut by the enzyme, generating two fragments shorter than the original length, whereas the fragment from a homozygous mutant was not cut, and the original length of the amplicon was preserved. In a heterozygous mutant, both the original fragment and the shorter fragments are visible.

TABLE 48-2   Commonly Used Electrophoresis-Based Techniques

Technique	Abbreviation	Use
PCR product length		Detection
Southern blotting		Detection, Quantification
PCR/Restriction fragment length polymorphism	PCR/RFLP	Genotyping
Conformation-sensitive gel electrophoresis	CSGE	Scanning
Denaturing gradient gel electrophoresis	DGGE	Scanning
Temperature gradient gel electrophoresis	TGGE	Scanning
Single-stranded conformational polymorphism	SSCP	Scanning
DNA sequencing (dideoxy termination/Sanger sequencing)		Sequencing
Single-nucleotide extension assay	SNE	Genotyping
Oligo ligation assay	OLA	Genotyping
Multiplex ligation-dependent probe amplification	MLPA	Quantification

Conformation-Sensitive Scanning Techniques

Several electrophoretic methods detect sequence variants within PCR products. For example, **hetero-duplex analysis (HDA)** that is also called **conformation-sensitive gel electrophoresis (CSGE)**, reveals the presence of mutations by the altered mobility of a dsDNA fragment that contains one or more mismatched bases (a heteroduplex) versus one that is perfectly matched (a **homoduplex**). Heteroduplexes usually migrate more slowly than homoduplexes during electrophoresis (Figure 48-9). **Denaturing gradient gel electrophoresis (DGGE)** and **temperature-gradient gel electrophoresis (TGGE)** detect heteroduplexes by their lower stability. As the temperature or denaturing gradients are increased, heteroduplexes melt at lower temperatures, and eventually the strands separate, altering the gel migration. CSGE, DGGE, and TGGE depend on altered **heteroduplex** migration. Homozygous variants are not detected unless mixed with a homozygous normal to form heteroduplexes.

Single-stranded conformational polymorphism (SSCP) analysis is another electrophoresis technique used to scan for unknown variants in nucleic acids. After PCR and denaturation, the single DNA strands fold into three-dimensional structures depending on their sequence. Electrophoretic mobility is a function of size and shape of the folded single-stranded molecules. If the sequence of a reference sample differs from that of the fragment being tested, the molecules adopt different conformations and exhibit unique banding patterns. Unlike the heteroduplex methods, homozygous changes are also detected with SSCP.

Scanning methods are useful when a wide variety of sequence alterations might be present. Particularly when most of the samples tested are wild type ("normal"), an initial scan for the presence of mutations before targeted genotyping or sequencing is more efficient.

Dideoxy-Termination Sequencing

Dideoxy-termination sequencing is a method of DNA sequencing based on the selective incorporation of chain-terminating dideoxynucleotides by DNA polymerase during in vitro DNA replication. It is also known as **Sanger sequencing** and is now routinely performed in the clinical laboratory. In addition, it is possible to sequence RNA after conversion to DNA with reverse transcriptase. Using Sanger sequencing, base changes resulting in (1) different amino acid codons, (2) stop codons, (3) deletions, or (4) insertions are identified. The most common sequencing strategy uses PCR in the first step to amplify the region of interest, followed by a variation of the chain-termination reaction developed by F. Sanger in the late 1970s.[9] This reaction generates fragments that are terminated at various lengths by the incorporation of one of the four dideoxynucleotide base analogs (Figure 48-10) during extension from the sequencing primer (Figure 48-11). Dideoxynucleotides lack the 3′ hydroxyl group (OH) and the 2′ OH on the pentose ring. Because DNA chain growth requires the addition of deoxynucleotides to the 3′ OH, incorporation of a dideoxynucleotide terminates chain growth. The most common method for generating these terminated fragments is cycle sequencing by repeating the temperature-controlled steps of (1) annealing, (2) chain extension with termination, and (3) denaturation, similar to PCR. The fragments generated are (1) labeled with fluorescent dyes on the terminating dideoxynucleotides, (2) separated by capillary electrophoresis, and (3) detected by fluorescence as the fragments travel past a detector (Figure 48-12). Dideoxy-termination DNA sequencing in the clinical laboratory is commonly used in infectious disease testing, such as genotyping of HIV to detect mutation

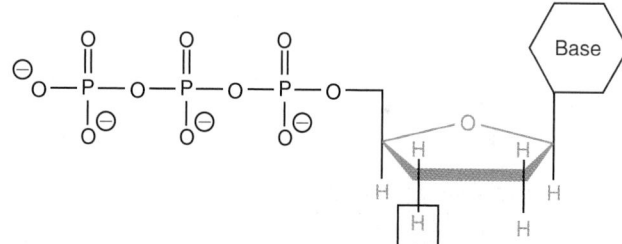

Figure 48-10 A dideoxynucleotide. Notice the absence of the 3′-OH that is usually present in standard deoxynucleotides. Without a 3′-OH, polymerase extension cannot occur.

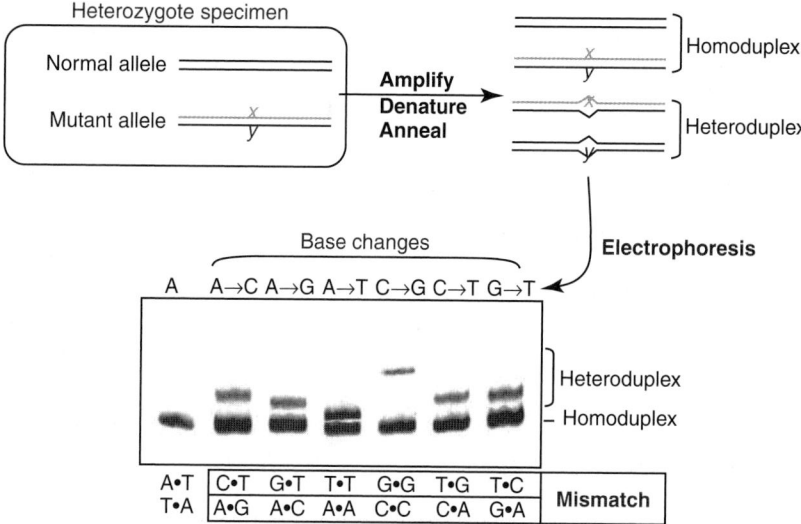

Figure 48-9 A schematic of heteroduplex migration analysis. When amplified DNA from a heterozygous specimen is denatured and cooled, the fragments anneal in four combinations. Electrophoresis on a polyacrylamide gel reveals the presence of heteroduplexes as extra band(s) appearing above the homoduplex band.

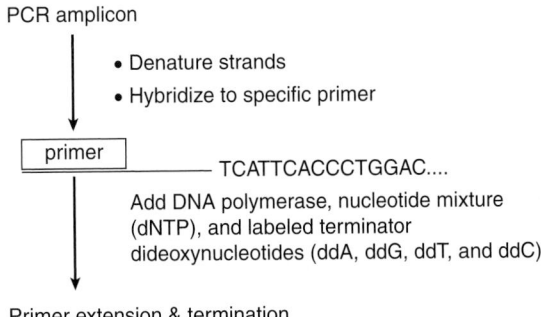

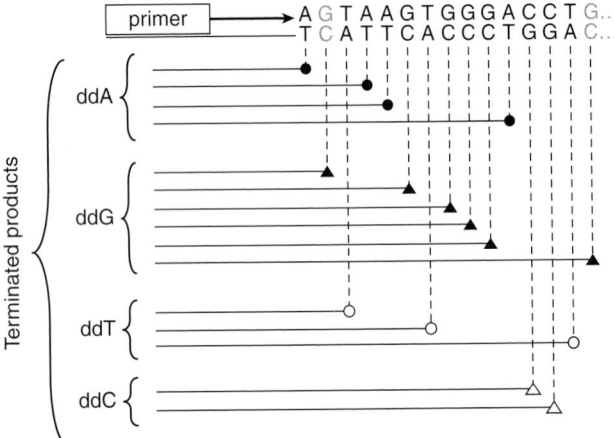

Figure 48-11 The dideoxy-termination reaction for sequencing. A polymerase chain reaction (PCR) amplicon is denatured and then hybridized to a specific oligonucleotide primer. As the DNA polymerase extends the primer by incorporating bases (dNTPs) complementary to the template, it occasionally incorporates a terminator base analog (ddA, ddG, ddT, or ddC) that stops further extension. The result is a mixture of extended products with varying lengths. Each terminator base may be labeled with one of four different fluorescent tags (shown as *symbols with different shapes [circles, triangles] and colors in the diagram*). The original procedure incorporated a radioactive dNTP during extension, allowing monochromatic detection of the truncated fragments that were electrophoresed in four separate lanes, one lane for each of the terminator bases.

in HIV RNA that convey drug resistance and of HCV to identify mutations that affect prognosis and influence the choice of therapy.

Single Nucleotide Extension

Single nucleotide extension (SNE) assays (also known as **single-base primer extension (SBE)** or *minisequencing assays)* are performed by annealing a primer to ssDNA immediately adjacent to the single base variant. The primer is then extended by the polymerase with dideoxynucleotide terminators in the absence of dNTPs. Each of the four terminators is labeled with a unique label so that it is possible to identify the incorporated base. SNE assays have been multiplexed on automated DNA sequencing instruments by varying the lengths of the primers so that each SNV is resolved by size in one electrophoresis run. There are also many SNE detection methods other

than electrophoresis, including (1) photometric detection on microtiter plates, (2) product-capture detection systems on **DNA microarrays**, (3) bead hybridization assays detected by **flow cytometry**, (4) solution-based fluorescence polarization detection systems, and (5) mass spectrometry. SNE assays are useful when a moderate number of disease-causing SNVs need to be genotyped. They do not work well if there are polymorphisms in the primer-binding site. Also, they are not designed to detect variants at positions other than immediately adjacent to the primer.

Oligo Ligation

Another assay format for SNV detection is the **oligonucleotide ligation assay (OLA)**. With this assay, two oligonucleotide probes are hybridized to adjacent sequences of amplified target DNA with the known SNV site positioned at the end of one probe (Figure 48-13). DNA ligase covalently joins the two probes only if both are perfectly hybridized to the target. A probe matching the normal base and another probe matching the mutant base are usually prepared with different length tails that modify their electrophoretic mobility. The probe hybridizing to both alleles is fluorescently labeled. Multiplexing of SNV genotyping is achieved by attaching different fluorescent labels to the common probes and also varying the tail lengths on the allele-specific probes. Following ligation, probes for multiple SNV sites are separated on a sequencing gel.

Multiplex Ligation-Dependent Probe Amplification

Muliplex ligation-dependent probe amplification (MLPA)[11] is a convenient method for relative quantification of 10 to 50 targets. The method is particularly useful to screen for deletions or duplications of multiple exons within a gene. For each target, two probes are designed that hybridize adjacent to each other so that they are in position to be ligated. The two probes have unique sequence tails that do not hybridize to the target and that are the same between targets. After hybridization and ligation, the probes are amplified by PCR with a common primer pair (complementary to the tails). One of the primers is fluorescently labeled at its 5′ end. Because probes of different lengths are used, multiple PCR products of different sizes are produced and separated on a sequencing gel. The relative peak heights or areas of each target are compared for relative quantification.

Discrimination by Mass or Sequence without Electrophoresis

Newer technologies that replace assays traditionally performed by electrophoresis are emerging. Some of these are attractive alternatives for the clinical laboratory because they are amenable to automation. These approaches include (1) mass spectrometry, (2) pyrosequencing, and (3) high-throughput sequencing.

Mass Spectrometry

Matrix-assisted laser-desorption ionization time-of-flight (MALDI-TOF) mass spectrometry (see Chapter 13) is used to genotype sequence variants. With mass spectrometry, no

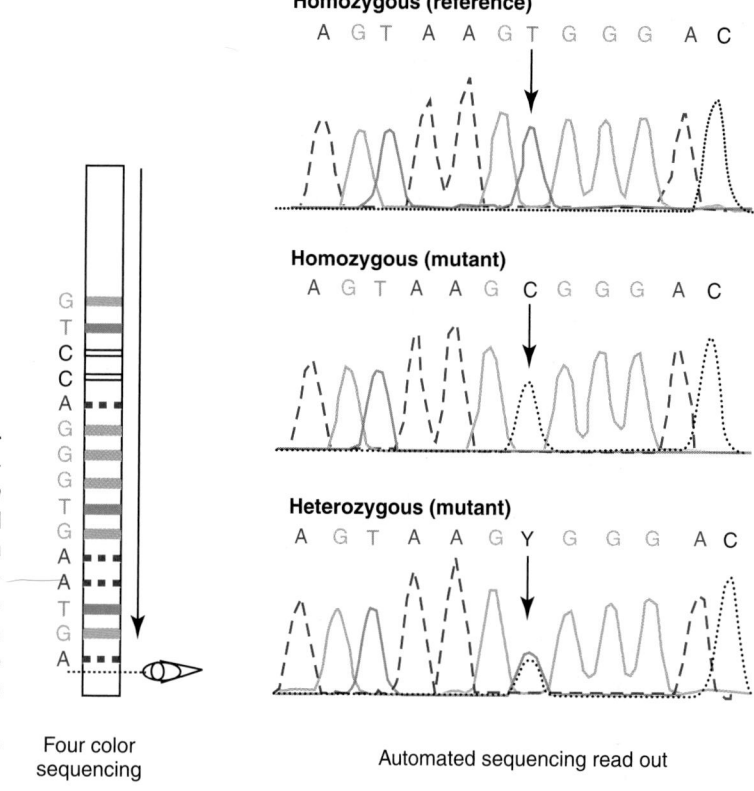

Figure 48-12 Schematic of targeted DNA sequencing. Extension products generated by the chain-termination reaction with *different colors for each terminating base* are separated by polyacrylamide gel electrophoresis. Automated fluorescence detection (shown by *the eye icon*) identifies each base during capillary electrophoresis. The direction of fragment migration is from top to bottom. The sequence is read from bottom to top in the gels and from left to right for the automated sequence. Examples of a reference sample (homozygous *T* at the polymorphic site), a mutant sample (homozygous *C*), and a heterozygous mutant sample (*T* and *C*) are shown. *Y* indicates a pyrimidine (*T* or *C*).

Four color sequencing

Automated sequencing read out

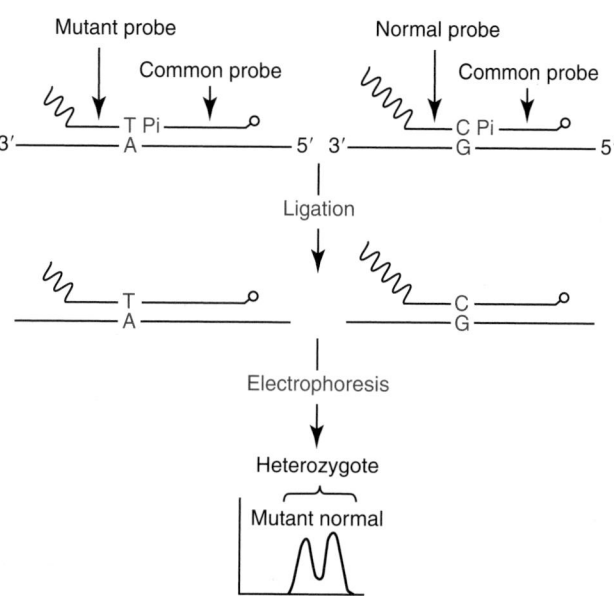

Figure 48-13 Oligo ligation assay (OLA). A probe specific to the normal allele *(C)* is shown hybridized onto a normal DNA sample *(G)*. This probe also is attached to a mobility modifying tail. Hybridized next to the normal-allele probe is the common probe that is labeled with a fluorescent tag. In the presence of ligase, the two probes are covalently joined to generate a longer probe. The mutant-allele-specific probe *(T)* with a shorter tail also hybridizes to the normal DNA sample, but it is not ligated to the common probe because of the mismatched base at its 3′ end. Electrophoresis and end-point, laser-induced detection reveals the ligated normal-allele probe, which is differentiated from the significantly shorter common probe alone (not shown on the graph) or from a ligated mutant-allele probe because of the different lengths of their tails. Multiple single-nucleotide variant (SNV) sites can be analyzed in one electrophoresis assay by varying the tail lengths (e.g., SNV site 2 in the graph) or by use of multicolor fluorescence tags.

label is necessary, because the alleles differ in mass. A DNA fragment including the variant site is amplified by PCR. After removal of the primers and dNTPs, an extension primer is hybridized directly or closely adjacent to the polymorphic site. Appropriate unlabeled deoxynucleotides and/or dideoxy-nucleotides are incorporated to generate allele-specific diagnostic products of different masses. Salt is removed from the sample, and approximately 10 nL of it is spotted onto an array and the mass of the extension products used to determine the genotype (Figure 48-14). Despite its complexity, automated systems are available that are capable of processing 384 to 1536 samples in a batch.

Pyrosequencing

Pyrosequencing determines the nucleic acid sequence of short segments without electrophoresis. With this technique, a sequencing primer is first hybridized to a single-stranded template previously generated by PCR. Four enzymes and two substrates are included in the reaction mixture (Figure 48-15). Next, one of the four dNTPs is added. If the base is complementary to the template strand, DNA polymerase catalyzes its incorporation and releases pyrophosphate (PPi). PPi release generates visible light through linked enzyme reactions. The process is repeated by adding one dNTP at a time to determine the nucleotide sequence. Because the technique has been automated, it is useful when the sequences of a large number of short segments need to be determined.

High Throughput Sequencing with Amplification

The need to understand genome-wide human variation has led to the development of new high-throughput sequencing techniques.[13] Most of these techniques typically are initiated by randomly fragmenting DNA into small pieces, usually less than 1 kb, and many between 100 and 500 bases. Short adapter sequences are ligated to each fragment to provide priming sites that initiate massively parallel sequencing reactions. Adapters also facilitate initial capture of DNA fragments onto solid surfaces to spatially restrict clonal amplification onto beads or spots on an array surface. Clonal amplification is performed by one of several methods, including the following:

- Emulsion PCR, in which one strand of the template fragment is captured on one bead and clonally amplified inside a water-in-oil droplet, generating a bead tethered by single-stranded amplicons (Figure 48-16). The beads are then deposited onto a glass surface or into discrete wells on a fiberoptic slide.
- Bridge amplification, which generates clusters of single-stranded amplicons tethered to the surface of a planar flow-cell (Figure 48-17).[4]
- RCA, which generates *concatemers* (intermediate structures formed during the replication of some DNA molecules) of templates that self-assemble into DNA balls in solution and are deposited onto ordered spots on a silicon array.

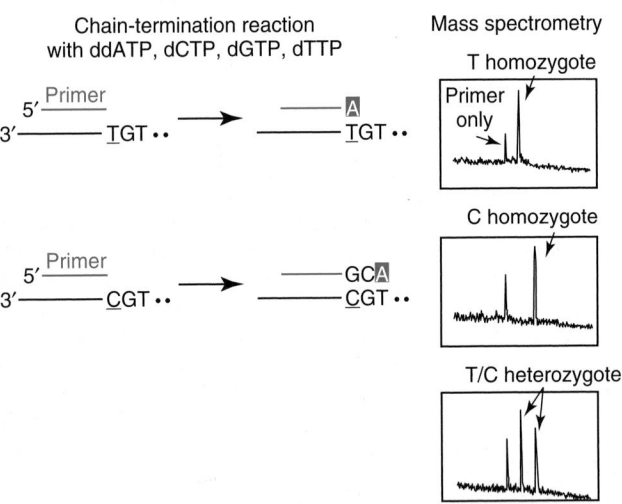

Figure 48-14 Sequence polymorphism analysis by mass spectrometry. The underlined base is the polymorphic site in the template (*T* or *C*). The single-stranded template is primed and extended in the presence of three dNTPs and one ddNTP, producing fragments of different mass depending on the sequence. The boxed *"A"* in this example indicates the incorporated terminator adenine base. The mass of terminated products is precisely measured by matrix-assisted laser-desorption ionization time-of-flight (MALDI-TOF) mass spectrometric data (relative intensity versus m/z).

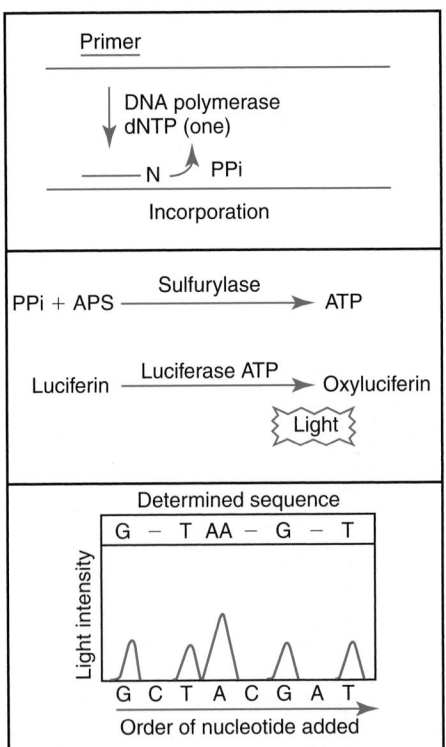

Figure 48-15 Schematic of pyrosequencing. Individual dNTPs are added one by one to the single-stranded template, a primer, and a polymerase. Pyrophosphate (PPi) is generated if the dNTP is complementary to the next base on the template (*top*). Any PPi produced reacts with adenosine-5′-phosphosulfate (APS) to produce ATP, which in turn generates light in the presence of luciferase (*middle*). The sequence can be determined from the order of dNTP addition and the intensity of light produced.

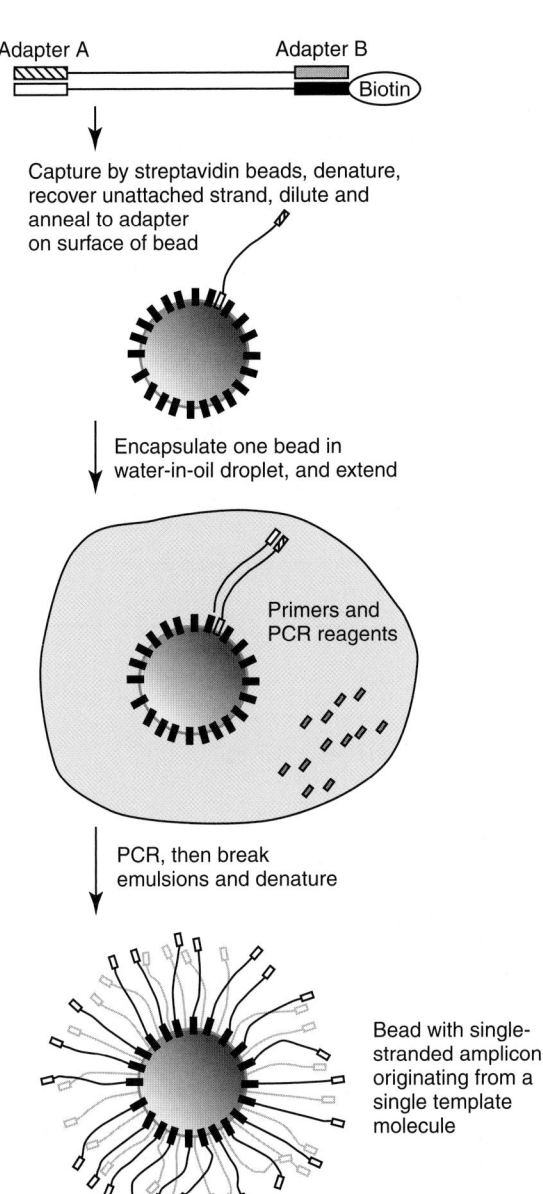

Figure 48-16 Emulsion polymerase chain reaction (PCR). Two adapters (adapters A and B) are randomly ligated to DNA fragments. Adapter B has a biotin on its 5′ end. Fragments with adapter B on one or both ends are captured by streptavidin beads, while fragments with only adapter A are washed away (not shown). Then fragments are denatured, and the free strand with adapter A and adapter B at each end is collected (fragments with adapter B on both ends will not be released from the streptavidin bead). One molecule of the single-stranded template is then captured on a bead coated with adapter and is encapsulated inside a water-in-oil droplet that contains PCR reagents and primers. After PCR, the emulsion is broken and the DNA is denatured. This generates a bead with a large number of clonal single strands tethered to it. The bead is then deposited into one of many wells on a fiberoptic slide, or onto a glass slide for sequence analysis (not shown).

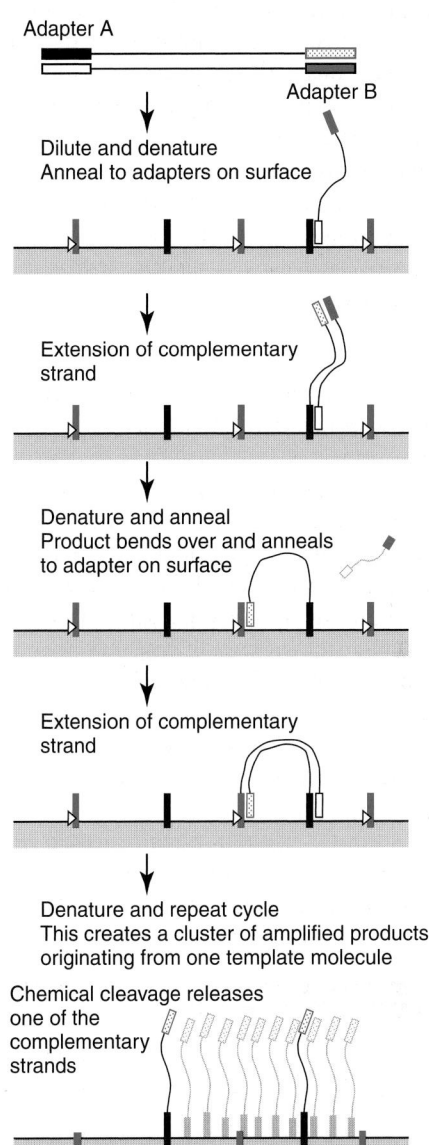

Figure 48-17 Bridge amplification. Two adapters (A and B) are ligated to a DNA template. Once diluted and denatured into single strands, the template is captured onto a flow cell surface by annealing to one of the two surface-bound primers that share sequences with adapter A or B. The polymerase reagent introduced into the flow cell extends the primer and generates the complementary strand of the template. The denaturant (usually sodium hydroxide) is introduced to the flow cell to release the original template strand. The free end of the newly synthesized strand anneals to a nearby primer by bending over, and a second round of reagent addition catalyzes the synthesis of another complementary strand. By repeating many of these cycles, a clonal cluster that consists of about 1000 copies of single-stranded template tethered to the surface is generated. This cluster is still a mixture of both complementary strands. One of the strands is selectively eliminated by treatment with periodic acid that cleaves the diol linkage present in one of the surface-bound primers (open triangle on red primer). The cluster now contains only one of the template strands and is ready for sequence analysis.

Sequence determination of nucleic acids is performed on these clonally amplified templates in a massively parallel fashion using sequencing by synthesis. In the presence of polymerase and a primer, one dNTP is added at a time and incorporation detected by pyrosequencing, fluorescence, or pH changes (semiconductor sequencing).

High-Throughput Sequencing without Amplification

Some high-throughput sequencing methods do not require amplification. With these techniques, sensitive optical techniques are used to observe incorporation of fluorescent nucleotides during strand synthesis on single template molecules. One such method observes real-time DNA synthesis by a single polymerase molecule immobilized inside a nanostructure array. The method uses four-color dNTPs whose label cleaves off as nucleotides are incorporated into the newly synthesized DNA strand. Each addition of a base is observed as a short pulse of one of the colors representing one of four bases. Long contiguous reads are possible. When high accuracy is achieved, single molecule methods have advantages of (1) efficient sequence assembly, (2) analyses of repetitive sequences, and (3) de novo sequencing. In contrast, many of the other high-throughput sequencing methods generate short sequence reads (30 to 70 bases long) that have to be aligned and analyzed to derive a consensus, then stitched together and compared with reference genome sequences. Accurate assembly of sequence data relies on sufficient coverage or redundancy across the sequenced region and informatics tools for this process are rapidly evolving.

Hybridization Assays

Principles

Hybridization assays are based on the ability of single-stranded nucleic acids to form specific double-stranded hybrids. The process requires that (1) probe and target nucleic acids are mixed under conditions that allow for complementary base pairing and (2) there is a method to detect any resulting double-stranded nucleic acids. A "probe" is a nucleic acid whose identity and sequence is known and is used to hybridize to a complementary *target* nucleic acid whose identity or abundance is revealed by the hybridization. In some of the methods discussed below, hybridization occurs between a target in solution and a probe that is attached ("tethered") to a solid surface. In homogeneous or real-time techniques, both the probes and the targets are in solution, and hybridization and detection occur without washing steps. Some of the homogeneous methods also monitor the dissociation of hybridized duplexes under controlled heating, revealing the identities of the hybridized duplexes by melting curve signatures.

As with any assay, both positive and negative controls are necessary for validation of the analytical phase of hybridization assays. Positive controls contain sequences complementary to the probe that are used to assess assay sensitivity, and they ensure that conditions are right for the probe to hybridize to the target under the assay conditions. Negative controls without target sequence assess assay specificity and will detect positive contamination if present.

Hybridization Thermodynamics

The favored structure of DNA under physiological conditions is an ordered double-stranded helix held together by noncovalent interactions (see Chapter 47). The duplex structure is most stable when all opposing bases are complementary, allowing for maximal hydrogen bonding and base stacking. The noncovalent binding between two DNA strands is (1) specific, (2) sequence dependent, and (3) reversible. Denaturing conditions, such as

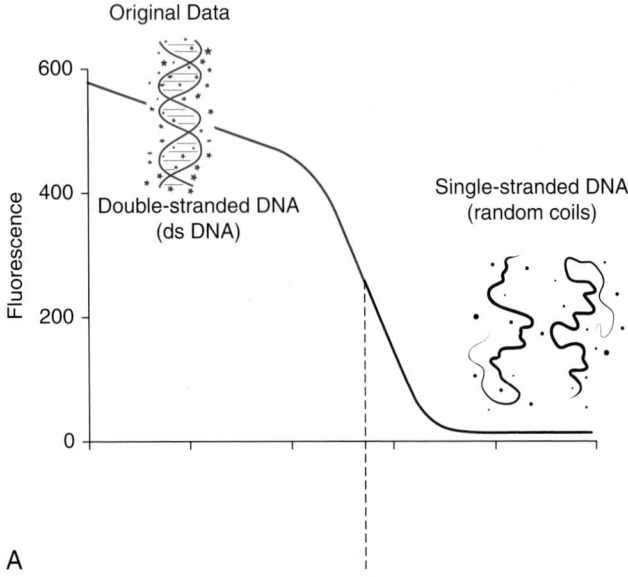

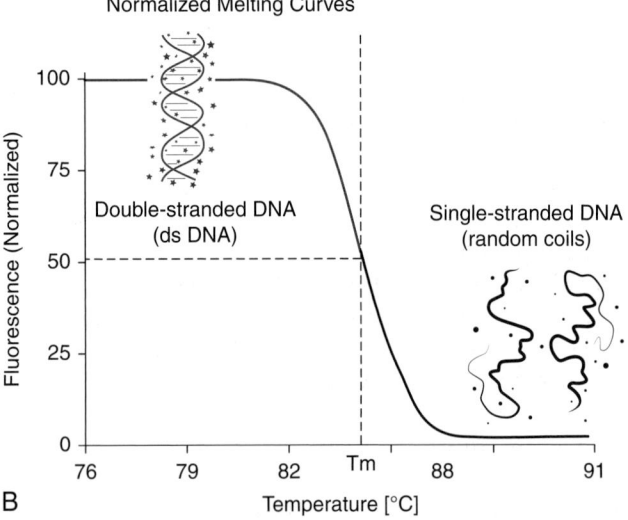

Figure 48-18 Fluorescence melting curve of a polymerase chain reaction (PCR) product. PCR-amplified DNA was melted in the presence of the cyanine dye, LCGreen Plus. In *panel A,* fluorescence gradually decreases as the temperature is increased until a more rapid decrease occurs centered at the DNA melting temperature (Tm) of the PCR product. In *panel B,* the data are normalized between 0% and 100% after removal of background fluorescence to obtain constant fluorescence outside of the transition. *(Modified with permission of the publisher from Wittwer CT, Kusukawa N. Real-time PCR and melting analysis. In Persing DH, Tenover FC, Tang YW, et al, eds. Molecular microbiology: diagnostic principles and practice, 2nd edition, Washington, DC: ASM Press, 2011:63-82. © 2011 ASM Press.)*

(1) high temperature (>90 °C), (2) presence of formamide, or (3) extremes of pH, favor dissociation of the double-stranded molecule into two separate random coils (Figure 48-18). On removal of the denaturant, single strands attempt to rejoin to form duplexes; rejoining strongly favors interactions that maximize complementary base pairing. Because temperature is the denaturant most easily manipulated, the **melting temperature** (T_m) of a DNA molecule is defined as the temperature at which 50% of the DNA molecules dissociate or "melt" from a double strand configuration to a single-strand configuration. Molecules with mismatched base pairs are less stable than those with a perfect sequence match and thus melt at a lower temperature. The reverse process, in which two complementary strands recombine to form a stable duplex molecule, is referred to as *annealing* or *hybridization*. Hybridization occurs between (1) DNA strands, (2) RNA strands, and (3) strands of **nucleic acid analogs** (such as **peptide nucleic acids [PNAs]**), in all combinations.

Hybridization Kinetics

The rate kinetics of solution-phase hybridizations is second order, being proportional to the concentrations of both hybridizing strands. The rate-limiting step is nucleation, where a small number of base pairs are formed in the correct orientation, followed by a rapid "zippering" of complementary sequences. In the case of a probe present in great excess to the target, hybridization proceeds as a pseudo–first order reaction, depending only on the concentration of the target. However, the time required to hybridize the probe to a given fraction of the target is proportional to the probe concentration. For example, during a PCR the concentration of primers is much greater than that of the target, and the reaction rate during each annealing step depends on the concentration of available single-stranded product, but the time required to anneal primers to a certain fraction of the target is proportional to the primer concentration.

The availability of nucleic acids for hybridization also is an issue. As the temperature cools during thermocycling, PCR primer annealing competes with the formation of double-stranded product. As the concentration of product increases during a PCR, some double-stranded product is formed before primer annealing occurs (see Figure 48-3). Similarly, when double-stranded probes are used at high concentrations, probe self-annealing interferes with probe-target hybridization. Available hybridization sites also are limited by intramolecular secondary structure of the probe or target, such as seen in SSCP.

Hybridization rates are influenced by many factors in the reaction environment, most notably temperature and ionic strength. Above the Tm, no stable hybrids are present, although transient complexes may form. As the temperature is lowered below the Tm, hybridization rates increase until a broad maximum occurs about 20 °C to 25 °C below the Tm. Hybridization rates also increase with an increase with the ionic strength of a solution. Divalent cations, such as Mg^{+2}, have a much stronger effect than monovalent cations, such as Na^+ or K^+.

Probes

In a hybridization assay, the probe is analogous in its role and importance to the antibody in an immunoassay. As discussed earlier, a probe is the nucleic acid whose identity is known and is used to reveal the identity or abundance of a target. Like antibodies in immunoassays, probes are either unlabeled or labeled with one of a variety of reporter molecules. Probes may be (1) cloned (recombinant), (2) generated by PCR, or (3) synthesized (oligonucleotides). They may be (1) DNA, (2) RNA, or (3) PNA, and single stranded or double stranded. Selection, purification, and labeling of probes are crucial to success of hybridization assays.

Cloned Probes

Cloned probes consist of a known segment of DNA inserted into a **plasmid** vector that is propagated by growth in a bacterium. Many different plasmid vectors are now available; pBR322 was one of the first in common use. The entire plasmid DNA (insert plus vector sequences) may be used as a probe, or the insert may be purified first from the vector sequences. The latter method is obviously more cumbersome, but may result in reduced background. The resulting probe is a dsDNA probe, and it must be denatured before use.

Some vectors contain RNA promoter regions adjacent to the inserted DNA sequence. These regions permit generation of RNA transcripts from the DNA insert. Because only one strand is copied during the RNA synthesis, single-stranded RNA probes are generated. Controlling the orientation of the insert in relation to the promoter region allows the production of transcripts in the "sense" direction (same as mRNA) or "antisense" direction (complementary to mRNA).

Polymerase Chain Reaction-Generated Probes

PCR-generated probes are simple to prepare. During amplification, the PCR product typically is labeled with nucleotides that are (1) radioactive, (2) fluorescent, or (3) have attached affinity labels. If desired, single-stranded probes are obtained by using a biotin-labeled primer, followed by solid-phase separation with streptavidin.

Oligonucleotide Probes

Oligonucleotide probes are even easier to synthesize or acquire than PCR-generated probes. These probes are usually 15 to 45 bases of single-stranded nucleic acid that are chemically synthesized as a specific base sequence. Most commonly, they are DNA, but RNA and PNA oligonucleotides also are used. Methods of synthesis that are (1) automated, (2) efficient, and (3) accurate continue to lower the cost of producing probes. Sequence information is now routinely available in public databases, such as the National Institutes of Health (NIH) genetic sequence database GenBank[1], and a similarity check for probe sequence is performed using public algorithms, such as the Basic Local Alignment Search Tool (BLAST; http://blast.ncbi.nlm.nih.gov/;accessed December 30, 2013). In practice, probe sequences must be carefully chosen to minimize cross-hybridization with pseudogenes (eukaryotes) or related species (bacteria and viruses). The Tm of the probe should allow both favorable hybrid stability and discrimination between related sequences. Oligonucleotide probes are often prepared with covalent attachment of a reporter molecule (such as fluorescent dyes) or affinity labels that allow them to be attached to solid supports. Probes used in real-time PCR are usually oligonucleotides with a fluorescent label.

Estimating Melting Temperature of Oligonucleotide Probes

Nearest-neighbor stability calculations allow probe Tm estimation to within 2 °C. A unified thermodynamic database has been compiled, and new parameters for all possible single mismatches and dangling ends have been estimated. Many software programs and websites are available to estimate Tm by computer simulation.[14]

Purity of Labeled Oligonucleotide Probes

The purity of labeled oligonucleotide probes is important for hybridization assays and critical in real-time PCR. Commercial oligonucleotides with a fluorescent label are of variable quality, and their concentration and purity should be assessed before use. Mass spectrometry and/or co-elution of absorbance at 260 nm (A_{260}) and fluorescence peaks on reversed-phase HPLC also are indicative of probe purity.

Quantitative estimates of probe purity are also obtained by simple absorbance measurements of fluorophore and the oligonucleotide and use of their molar absorptivities. The ratio of the concentrations of fluorophore and oligonucleotide should be nearly 1.0. Acceptable ratios are between 0.8 and 1.2. Ratios less than 0.8 suggest incomplete labeling or destruction of the attached dye. Ratios greater than 1.2 suggest the presence of free dye. Note, however, that a ratio near 1 is a necessary but not a sufficient criterion of a pure probe.

Hybridization Assays: Examples

Hybridization reactions are divided into two broad categories: (1) solid-phase, in which either probe or target is tethered to a solid support while the other is in solution, and (2) solution-phase, in which both are in solution (Table 48-3).

Solid-Phase Hybridization Assays

Solid-phase assays are of particular utility as multiple samples are processed together, which facilitates (1) control, (2) washing, and (3) separation procedures. Hybridization on a solid support is, however, less efficient than solution-hybridization, and the kinetics are slower and more difficult to predict. Both solid-phase and liquid-phase assays are used routinely in the clinical laboratory. Solid-phase assays include (1) dot blot assays, (2) line probe assays, (3) assays using arrays, (4) in situ hybridization assays, (5) **Southern blot** assays and (6) **Northern blot** assays.

Dot-Blot and Line-Probe Assays

Conventional hybridization assays on membranes are known as *dot blots* or *line probes,* depending on the geometry of the individual spots. The nucleic acids are applied with suction, forming a shape that is either round (dot) or elongated (line or slot). After immobilization the membrane is incubated with complementary nucleic acid at a constant temperature, followed by one or more washes to discriminate matched from mismatched nucleic acid. The method allows multiple simultaneous hybridizations under identical conditions.

Two general formats are used for these assays. In one, multiple samples are affixed to the solid support and interrogated by a small number of probes ("sample-down"). In the other, multiple probes are attached to the support and a small number of samples are added ("probe-down"). Results of dot-blot and line-probe assays are usually qualitative: if hybridization has occurred, a signal is generated at the specified spot and a simple yes or no interpretation is given.

Medium-Density Arrays

Dot-blot and line-probe assays have largely been replaced by medium-density arrays that typically analyze 20 to 500 spots. Medium-density arrays are useful for testing multiple mutations in specimens for (1) genetic disease, (2) oncology, and (3) pharmacogenetics. These arrays do not need to be attached to a two-dimensional surface as long as their location or "address" is able to be decoded. For example, microspheres can be used with flow cytometers, with the microspheres analogous to the spots on a two-dimensional surface. The microspheres can be coded by fluorescence intensity of dyes within them (which are detected by "channels" in the flow cytometer) while fluorescence in another channel monitors hybridization. All channels are then read simultaneously using a flow cytometer.

Microarrays

Increasing further the density of hybridization assays, microarrays (also called *DNA arrays, DNA chips,* or *biochips*) were introduced in the mid-1990s.[10] Compared with medium density arrays, spot sizes in microarrays are decreased (typically to less than 200 microns in diameter) such that one array contains thousands to millions of spots. This dimensional change requires specialized (1) detection equipment, (2) software, and (3) informatics to analyze the data. Because of their high density, microarrays have attracted intense interest among researchers who wish to monitor the whole genome for (1) **single-nucleotide variants (SNVs)** (2) gene expression, and (3) **copy number variants (CNVs).**

Because SNVs represent the most common genetic difference between individuals, much effort has focused on correlating SNV genotypes to phenotype and disease association. Microarrays that analyze human SNVs (SNV chips) provide the technology to genotype most known human SNVs in one experiment. Nearby SNV alleles tend to cluster together as haplotypes, so disease association by haplotype simplifies the analysis.

TABLE 48-3 Hybridization Assays	
Solid-Phase Hybridization	• Dot-blot and line-probe assays • Arrays (microarrays and medium-density arrays) • In situ hybridization • Southern and Northern blotting
Solution-Phase Hybridization	• Real-time PCR • PCR melting analysis • Single molecule visualization • Other classical techniques

Gene expression microarrays quantify the relative amounts of different mRNAs in test and reference samples. An example of a two-color microarray for gene expression is shown in Figure 48-19. Because the human genome is completely sequenced, mRNA probes are usually directly synthesized on microarrays. Modern gene expression arrays have been used to measure the mRNA transcribed from all human genes in one experiment.[15] They have been applied to almost every conceivable human condition, including (1) neoplastic, (2) inflammatory, and (3) psychiatric conditions. In oncology, gene expression microarrays have led to new diagnostic and prognostic markers in (1) breast cancer, (2) bladder cancer, (3) leukemia, and (4) sarcoma, among others.[14] Currently in the clinical laboratory, expression arrays are used directly in only a limited number of diagnostic or prognostic tests. Most

arrays are used in marker discovery projects and for selection of a smaller panel of expression targets that are then analyzed by other quantitative methods (such as real-time PCR) that provides greater precision and dynamic range.

Another important clinical application of microarrays is the genome-wide analysis of deletions and duplications, referred to as copy number variants. CNV analysis using microarrays is replacing much of the traditional cytogenetic chromosome analysis (karyotyping) and **fluorescence in situ hybridization (FISH)** analysis. Similar to gene expression arrays, many of the CNV arrays use two-color comparative hybridization to determine the gene dosage in a specimen compared with a normal reference genome by the technique of **comparative genomic hybridization (CGH)**. Arrays for CGH use oligonucleotide probes for very high resolution and data density. An example

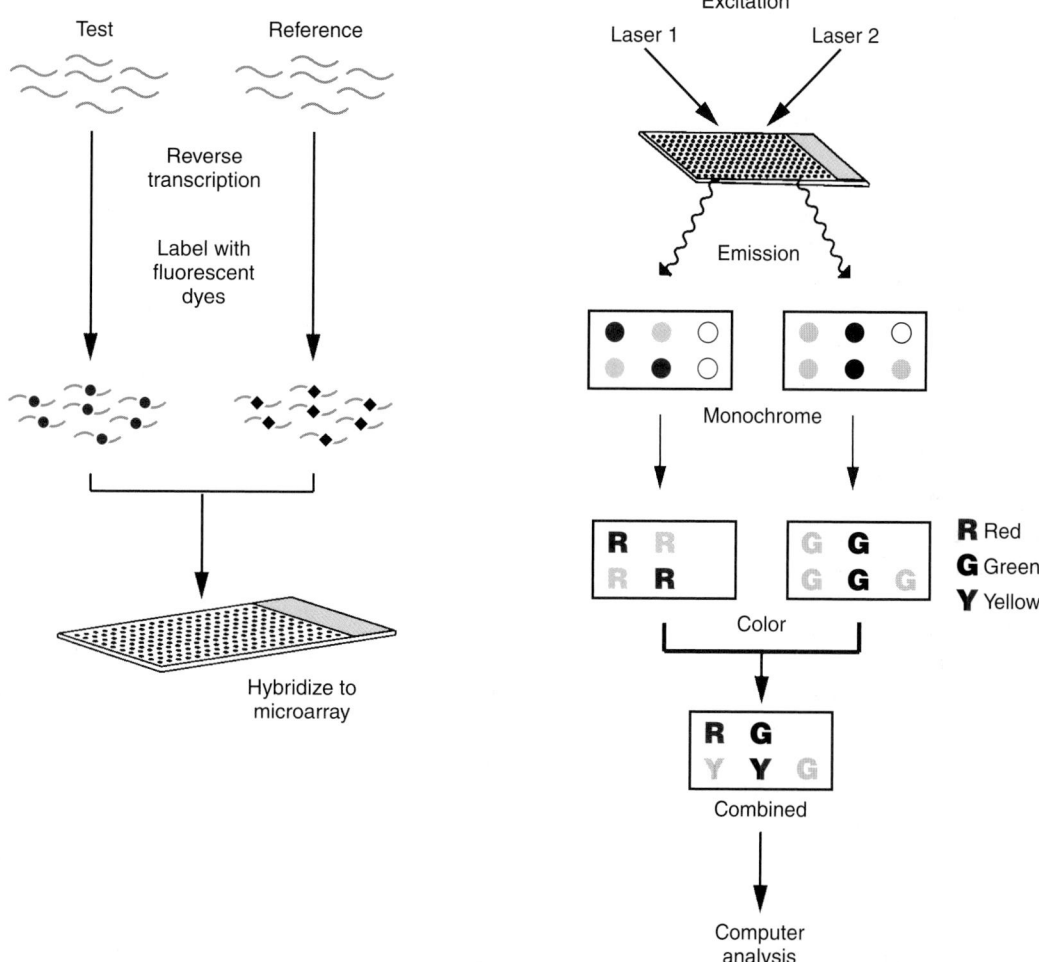

Figure 48-19 A two-color microarray experiment. An array of DNA oligonucleotides complementary to messenger RNA (mRNA) sequences is affixed to a glass slide. The mRNAs in the test and reference specimen are converted into differentially labeled cDNA by reverse transcription and incorporation of two different fluorescent dyes. The two samples are hybridized together onto the array. The array is washed, and the image is captured twice, each time with a laser of a wavelength that excites one of the dyes but not the other. The monochromatic images are then converted to two colors (green for the test sample [G], and red for the reference [R]), and the images are combined. If the abundance of cDNA is the same in each of the two samples, then the composite spot will be shown as yellow (Y). If one is in greater abundance, then that color will be preserved. Up-regulation and down-regulation of gene expression are then analyzed by software.

of CNV analysis using a CGH array is shown in Figure 48-20. SNV arrays also are used to detect copy number changes by loss of heterozygosity (this method is sometimes referred to as **virtual karyotyping**). Unlike CGH, SNV arrays have the advantage of analyzing the specimen without the need to mix in a reference genome. SNV arrays also are able to detect copy number neutral changes caused by inversions or uniparental disomy (a chromosome abnormality in which both chromosomes in a pair are inherited from the same parent) that are not detected by CGH methods.

Solution-Phase Hybridization Assays

Several classical hybridization methods use probe-target hybridization in solution. For example, hybrid capture

employs an antibody that is specific for RNA-DNA hybrid molecules that are formed during solution-phase hybridization of a DNA sample and an unlabeled RNA probe. The assay also has been adapted to a **microtiter plate** format for automation of washing and detection. In addition, solution hybridization has been combined with (1) amplification, (2) detection, and (3) quantification steps all in the same tube. Such closed-tube, real-time assays do not require any additions, washing, or separation steps.

Single-Copy Visualization

If a nucleic acid probe is labeled with many fluorescent molecules, it is possible to optically visualize a single copy of a nucleic acid target by fluorescent microscopy. One technique

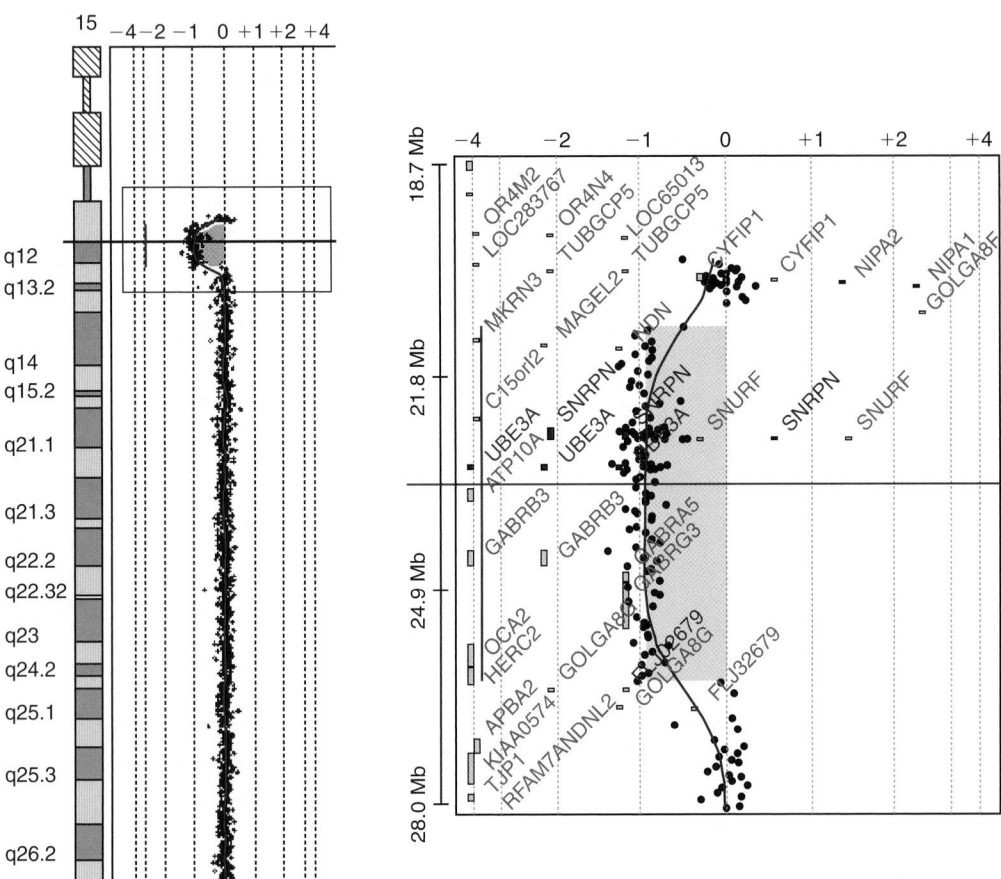

Figure 48-20 Copy number variation identified with a comparative genomic hybridization (CGH) array made from oligonucleotides. DNA from a subject is fragmented, labeled with Cy5, and hybridized onto a microarray, together with Cy3-labeled reference DNA. On the array are nearly 44,000 oligonucleotide probes, each about 60 bases long and tiled across the whole genome at an average spacing of 75 kb. The left panel shows results of probes on chromosome 15 (all other chromosomes are analyzed in this assay but are not shown). Each dot represents a specific probe to which the subject's DNA hybridizes. Their positions (0, −1, +1, etc.) reflect the dosage of the subject's DNA relative to the reference DNA. A majority of the probes line up on "0," indicating no quantitative difference compared with the reference DNA. Probes in the 15q11 to 15q13 region, however, are on the "−1" line, indicating that the subject has a deletion of that region in one of the chromosomes. A closer view of that region (right panel) shows that among the deleted genes are *UBE3A*, which causes Angelman syndrome, and *SNRPN*, which causes Prader-Willi syndrome. Because the method does not distinguish the methylation status of the deleted alleles, this result alone cannot determine which of the two disorders the subject has. *(Courtesy Sarah South, Ph.D., ARUP Laboratories.)*

uses reporter probes that are labeled with a long string of multicolored fluorescent labels. Several tandem color segments have been placed on the reporter probe with each segment consisting of about a hundred fluorophores. The sequence of different color segments uniquely identifies the target. The target nucleic acid is hybridized in solution with the reporter probe together with a capture probe and is (1) washed, (2) immobilized, (3) stretched, and (4) oriented on the surface of an optical slide. Each captured target is then identified by the color code of the reporter and is counted (Figure 48-21). Although the sensitivity of this technique is not as high as that of real-time PCR (see next section), up to 150 reporter probes have been multiplexed in one reaction. One application of this technique is direct measurement of mRNA expression in tissue specimens prepared from formalin-fixed paraffin blocks without the need for cDNA preparation or PCR.

Real-Time Polymerase Chain Reaction

Real-time PCR and melting analysis are considered "dynamic" hybridization assays in which the formation or dissociation of the probe-target duplex (or product duplex) is monitored in real time. With this technique, data elements are collected during the nucleic acid amplification step rather than at the end of it. The technique uses fluorescent dyes or probes and instrumentation that records fluorescence during thermal cycling. The data obtained provide information on the identity and quantity of the nucleic acid sample. During the entire process, the same reaction tube is used for amplification and fluorescence monitoring, and there are no (1) sample transfers, (2) reagent additions, or (3) gel separation steps required. This eliminates the risk of product contamination in subsequent reactions. Because the process is simple and fast, real-time PCR is replacing many older molecular techniques in the clinical laboratory.

Real-time PCR was first described using ethidium bromide to monitor the accumulation of a double-stranded PCR product.[2] If target DNA is present, the fluorescence signal increases. How early during PCR one begins to see a signal depends on the initial amount of target DNA, and this provides a systematic method of quantification. Further, when fluorescence is continuously monitored as the temperature is increased, a melting curve is generated. Often the first derivative of this melting curve is plotted to visually aid the analyst in determining the position of the Tm. Melting analysis is used to verify the identity of the amplified product and to detect sequence variants down to a single base (Figure 48-22).

Dyes and Probes for Real-Time Polymerase Chain Reaction

Many different fluorescent reporters are used in real-time PCR, and some of the more common ones are shown in Figure 48-23. Fluorescent probes have sequences complementary to the target, whereas dsDNA dyes and fluorescently-labeled primers rely on the specificity of the PCR primers. Some

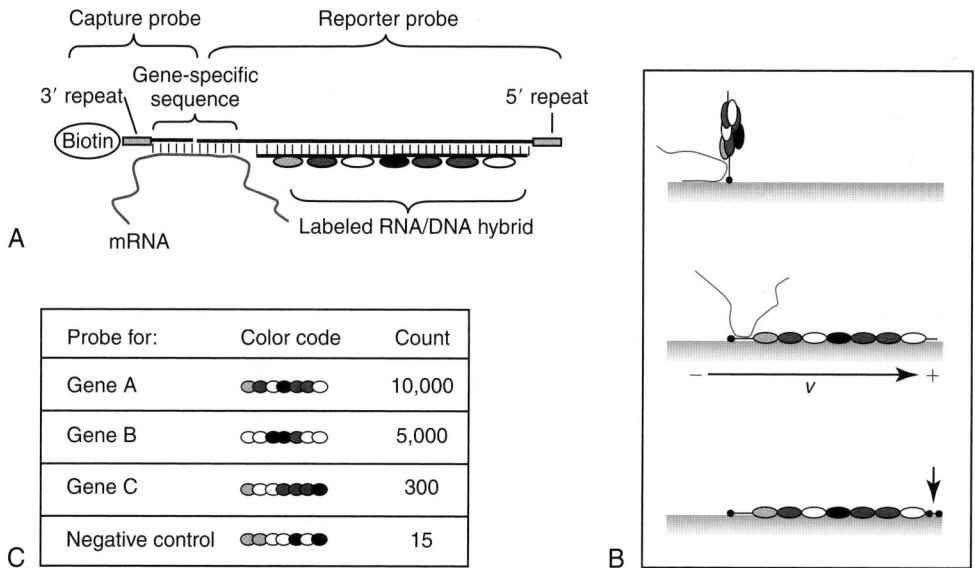

Figure 48-21 Single-copy visualization. A pair of probes (capture probe and reporter probe) hybridize to the messenger RNA (mRNA) target in solution through gene-specific probe sequences *(A)*. The reporter probe has seven color segments, each segment made of ≈900 RNA bases that are labeled with about a hundred fluorophores of one color. The labeled portion of the probe is a DNA/RNA hybrid that can be observed as a ≈3 nm fluorescent spot. Excess probes and unbound DNA are removed and the target complex is immobilized on a streptavidin-coated slide through the biotin on the capture probe *(B, top)*. An electrical current is applied, and the complex is stretched *(B, middle)*. The reporter probe is immobilized in extended form by biotin-labeled oligonucleotides complementary to its 5′ repeat sequence *(B, bottom)*. The color code of the probe is read by an epi-fluorescent microscope (a microscope where excitation of the fluorophore and detection of fluorescence are accomplished through the same light path), and each unique probe is counted *(C)*. Normally, a number of negative control probes are present in the hybridization solution to establish nonspecific background counts.

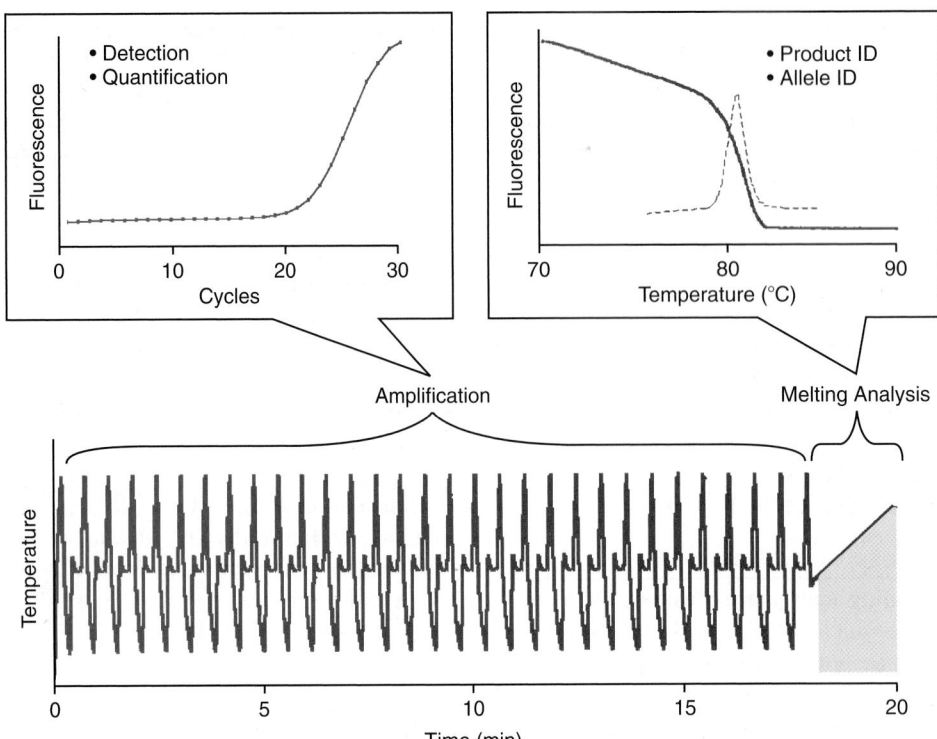

Figure 48-22 Real-time monitoring during amplification and melting analysis. The *bottom panel* shows a typical rapid-cycle temperature profile that is followed by a temperature ramp for melting analysis. When fluorescence is monitored during amplification once each cycle *(dotted lines)*, information is provided on the presence or absence of specific target sequences and allows quantification of the target. When fluorescence is monitored continuously through the melting phase *(shaded area)*, information can be provided that verifies target identification or establishes genotype. *(Modifed with permission of the publisher from Wittwer CT, Kusukawa N. Real-time PCR. In: Persing DH, Tenover FC, Versalovic J, et al, eds. Molecular microbiology: diagnostic principles and practice. Washington, DC: ASM Press, 2004:71-84.)*

methods include the option of melting analysis to verify the Tm of the probe or product.

Double-Stranded DNA Binding Dyes

Certain dyes increase their fluorescence in the presence of double-stranded DNA (ds-DNA) (see Figure 48-23, row one). Currently, SYBR Green I is the most common dye used in real-time PCR. It is popular in the research setting when the specificity of a probe is not needed, and the lower cost is attractive. The dsDNA dyes also allow melting analysis at the end of PCR for product identification and some dyes even allow SNV genotyping by **high-resolution melting analysis (HRMA)** of PCR products.

Fluorescently Labeled Primers

Labeled primers also are used to monitor PCR. In one system, a primer with a 5′ hairpin is labeled with a fluorophore and a quencher so that fluorescence is quenched in the hairpin conformation. When the primer straightens out during the PCR process, fluorescence increases (see Figure 48-23, row six). One advantage of fluorescently labeled primers over dsDNA dyes is that multiplexing by color is possible. However, with both dsDNA dyes and labeled primers, reaction specificity

depends completely on the primers. Any double-stranded product that is formed will be detected. Therefore, methods that increase specificity, such as **melting curve analysis**, are helpful to confirm the presence of the desired product.

Probe-Specific Detection

The use of fluorescent probes in PCR provides an additional level of specificity. Fluorescent probes that hybridize to PCR products during amplification change fluorescence by two possible mechanisms: (1) a covalent bond between two dyes is broken by hydrolysis, or (2) the fluorescence change follows reversible hybridization of the probe to the target. Following this distinction, when covalent bonds are broken, the probes are called *hydrolysis probes*. When probes reversibly change fluorescence on duplex formation, they are called *hybridization probes*. One major difference between the two probe types is that melting analysis is possible with hybridization probes, but not with hydrolysis probes.

Hybridization Probes. These probes change fluorescence upon hybridization, usually by FRET. Two interacting fluorophores may be placed on adjacent probes (see Figure 48-23, row two), or one may be placed on a primer and the other on a probe (see Figure 48-23, row three). Only one probe with one

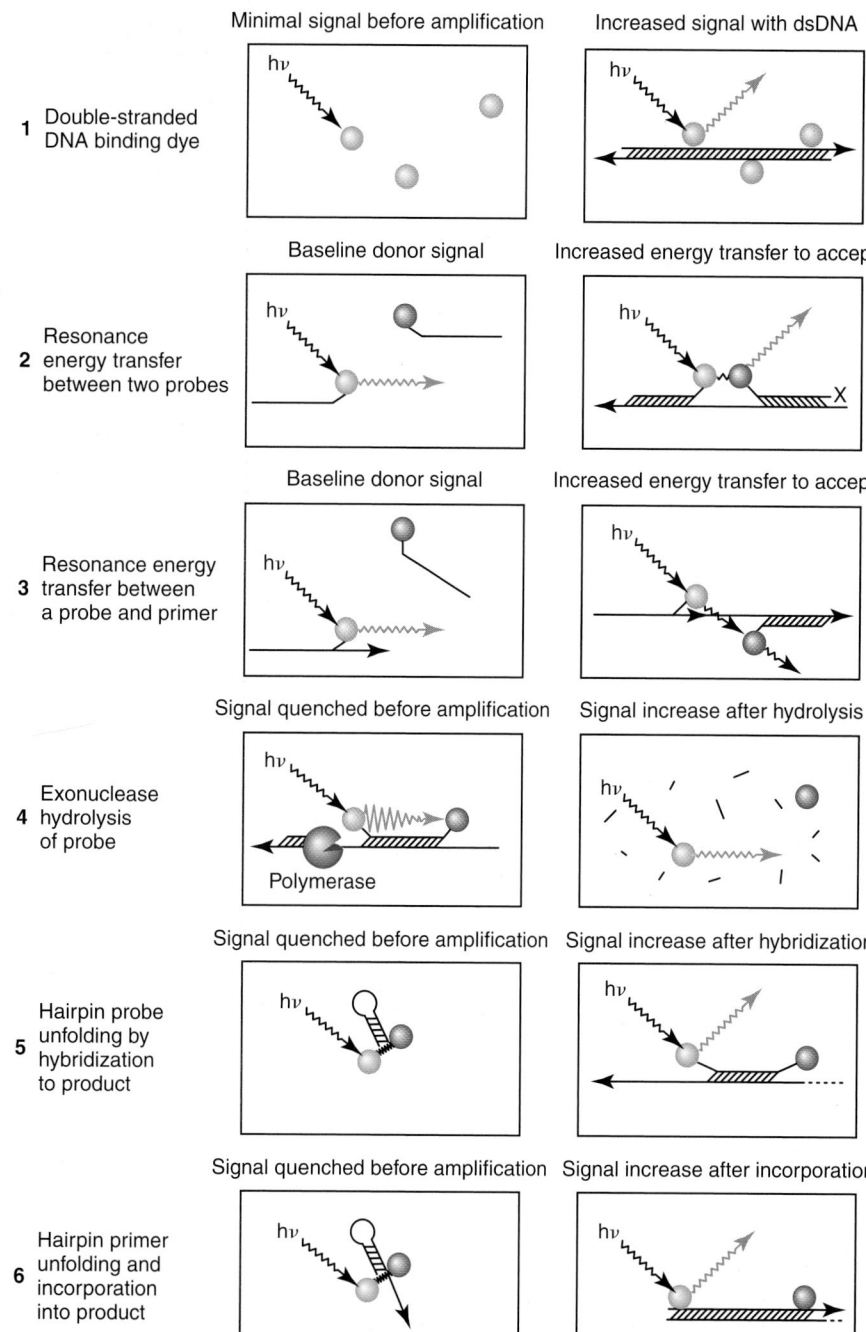

Figure 48-23 Common probes and dyes for real-time polymerase chain reaction (PCR). *(1)* Double-stranded DNA (dsDNA) dyes show a significant increase in fluorescence when bound to DNA (*hv* = excitation light). *(2)* Adjacent hybridization probes. Fluorescence resonance energy transfer (FRET) is illustrated between a donor and acceptor fluorophore. The *"x"* indicates termination of the 3′-end of the probe to prevent polymerase extension. *(3)* FRET between a labeled primer and a single hybridization probe. *(4)* Hydrolysis probes are cleaved between a fluorescent reporter and a quencher, resulting in increased fluorescence. *(5)* Hairpin probes are quenched in the native conformation, but increase in fluorescence when hybridized. *(6)* Hairpin primers retain their native, quenched conformation until they are incorporated into a double-stranded product. *(Modified with permission of the publisher from Pritham GH, Wittwer CT. Continuous fluorescent monitoring of PCR. J Clin Lig Assay 1998;21:404-12. © 1998 Clinical Ligand Assay Society Inc.)*

fluorophore may be necessary if the fluorescence is quenched by deoxyguanosine residues. Another single-labeled probe design uses thiazole orange attached to a PNA. In each of these designs, the fluorescence change with hybridization is reversible with melting.

Hydrolysis Probes. Fluorescent probes have been synthesized with a quencher molecule positioned to quench the fluorescence of another label. If the probe is hydrolyzed between the fluorophore and the quenching molecule during the PCR, fluorescence will increase. The most common implementation uses the 5′-exonuclease activity of the DNA polymerase to hydrolyze the probe and dissociate the labels (see Figure 48-23, row four). This method has been simplified by putting the

labels on opposite ends of the probe. Hybrid-stabilizing agents, such as a minor-groove (a shallow "furrow" in the molecular structure of a DNA double helix) binder, have been added to the probe to make the system more robust. Dual-labeled probes also have been cleaved using a DNAzyme (a DNA molecule that acts as a catalyst) generated during PCR. Hydrolysis probes generate fluorescence by breaking covalent bonds. The change in fluorescence is irreversible, and melting analysis of the hydrolyzed probe is not possible.

Mixed Mechanism Probes. Several probe systems appear to function by both hydrolysis and hybridization mechanisms. These include (1) hairpin probes, (2) self-probing amplicon primers, and (3) displacement probes. A hairpin probe functions similarly to a hairpin primer in that it is designed to increase the fluorescence signal when the distance between the quencher and the reporter increases upon target hybridization (see Figure 48-23, row five). Similarly, primers that result in self-probing amplicons have a hairpin that separates quencher from reporter when hybridized. Competitive displacement probes separate quencher and reporter by competitive hybridization. However, in all three cases, polymerases with exonuclease activity are usually used, and the labeled probes are potential substrates for exonuclease cleavage. Indeed, the fluorescence versus cycle number plots often resemble irreversible hydrolysis rather than reversible hybridization (Figure 48-24). Conversely, many hydrolysis probes, especially probes labeled on each end, show significant hybridization signals.

Detection and Quantification in Real-Time Polymerase Chain Reaction

When fluorescence is monitored once each cycle in the presence of SYBR Green I, the data closely follow the expected S-shaped logistic curve (see Figures 48-2 and 48-24, *top left*). However, with hydrolysis probes, fluorescence is cumulative and continues to increase even after the amount of product reaches a plateau (see Figure 48-24, *top middle*). In contrast, reactions monitored with hybridization probes may show a decrease in fluorescence at high cycle number (see Figure 48-24, *top right*). Despite differences in curve shape, all real-time systems follow the amount of product being produced during PCR, and this information is used for detection and quantification.

Detection

A fluorescent signal that increases during PCR and follows one of the expected curve shapes suggests that the specific target is present and was amplified. In contrast, if the background signal remains constant even after 40 to 50 PCR cycles suggests that the target is absent and that no amplification has occurred. Algorithms that analyze the entire curve are more robust than simple threshold methods. Positive controls (to rule out inhibitory factors) and negative controls (to rule out product contamination and nonspecific signal generation) are necessary. If the fluorescent signal is reversible with hybridization, melting analysis is useful to verify the expected Tm of the probe or product.

A note of caution: When specificity of the assay depends only on the primers ("primer-specific detection," as is the case when DNA dyes or labeled primers are used), the possibility of unexpectedly amplifying other targets or primer-dimers is a concern. One technique to eliminate or decrease the detection of unexpected targets is to acquire fluorescence during each cycle at a temperature just below the melting transition of the expected target. To illustrate the concept, Figure 48-25 shows a first-derivative melting curve of products at the end of a PCR that generated unexpected products along with the desired product. The signal was generated with SYBR Green I, a dye that detects all dsDNA. The plot reveals both lower Tm species that are unexpected products and a single Gaussian-shaped peak that is centered on the target's predicted Tm. If fluorescence is acquired during each cycle at (in this case) 85 °C, the unexpected products will be denatured and will not contribute to the signal.

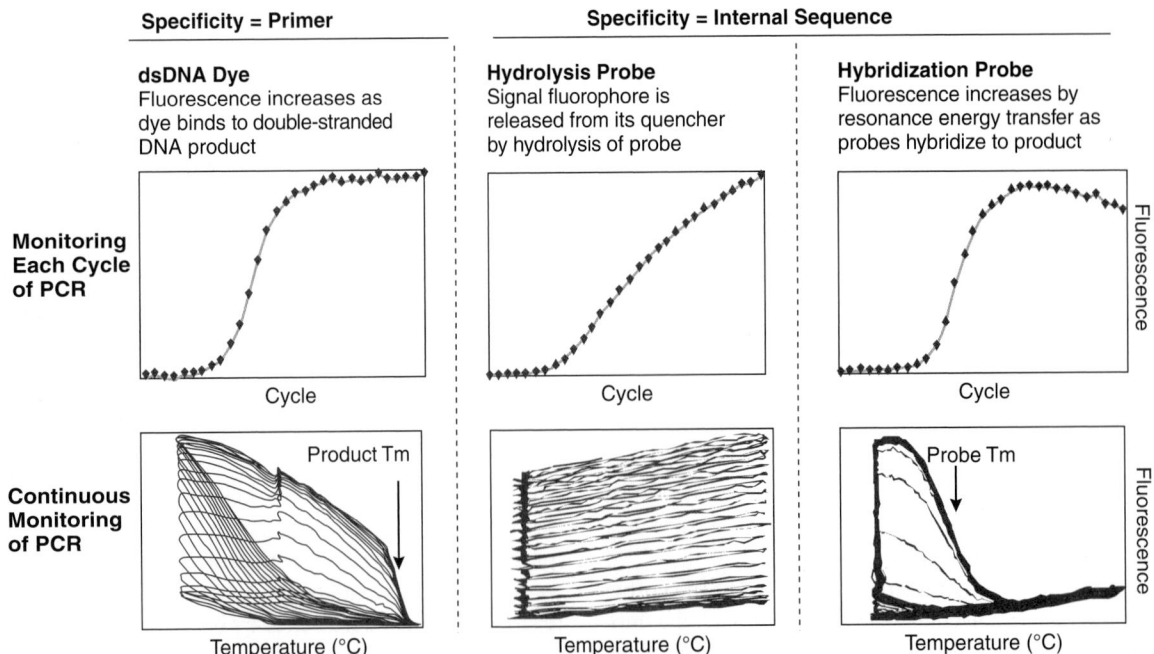

Figure 48-24 Monitoring in real time. The *top row* shows data collected once each polymerase chain reaction (PCR) cycle, and the *bottom row* shows data collected continuously (five times per second) during all PCR cycles. Three different reporter systems are shown. *(Modified with permission of the publisher from Wittwer CT, Kusukawa N. Real-time PCR. In: Persing DH, Tenover FC, Versalovic J, et al, eds. Molecular microbiology: diagnostic principles and practice. Washington, DC: ASM Press, 2004:71-84.)*

Multiplexing of detection is possible with probes that are labeled with different-color dyes or with probes that have different Tm's. Examples in the clinical laboratory include probe multiplexing to detect the presence of more than one infectious organism or to discriminate an internal control template from the target.

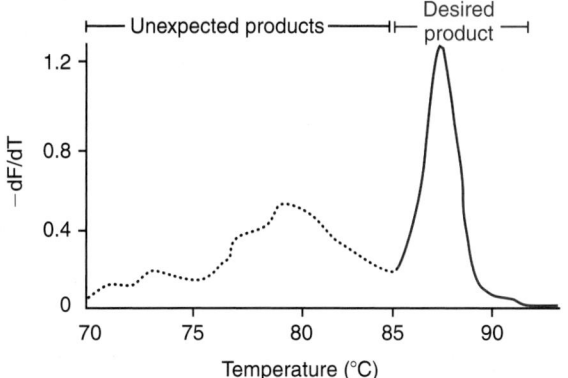

Figure 48-25 First-derivative melting curve showing the target (at high Tm, *solid line*) and nonspecific polymerase chain reaction (PCR) products (at lower Tm's, *dotted line*). *(Modified by permission of the publisher from Morrison TB, Weiss JJ, Wittwer CT. Quantification of low-copy transcripts by continuous SYBR Green I monitoring during amplification. Biotechniques 1998;24:954-63. © 1998 Eaton Publishing.)*

Quantification

Real-time PCR offers a convenient and systematic approach to quantify by monitoring the amount of product produced each cycle. For example, real-time PCR is widely used for the assessment of viral load, particularly for HIV, and other amplification systems, particularly transcription-based and bDNA methods, are also used. Additional quantitative applications of real-time PCR include quantification of mRNAs (after reverse transcription) in gene-expression studies and assessment of gene dosage in genetics and oncology.

One of the advantages of real-time PCR is its large dynamic range. Figure 48-26, *Panel A,* shows an extended range of external calibrators in a typical real-time PCR. As the initial template concentration increases, the curves shift to earlier cycles. The extent of the shift depends on the PCR efficiency (Table 48-4). The cycle at which fluorescence rises above background correlates inversely with the log of the initial template concentration (Figure 48-26, *Panel B*). This "cycle" is actually a *virtual* cycle that includes a fractional component determined by interpolation, which is calculated by several methods. One method uses the maximum second derivative of the curve to determine the cycle number (Figure 48-27). The second derivative is derived from the shape of the curves, and adjustment of baselines and normalization of fluorescence values are not required. Alternatively, in threshold analysis, a fluorescence level is selected that intersects with the amplification curves, and the fractional cycle numbers are found by interpolation.

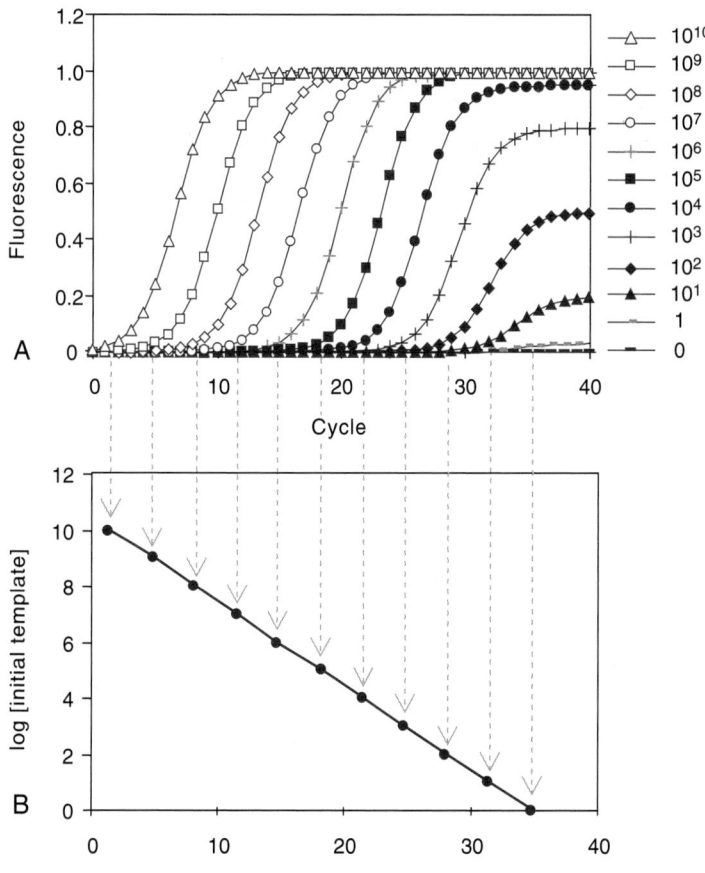

Figure 48-26 Quantification by real-time polymerase chain reaction (PCR). Shown are typical real-time curves for amplification reactions of varying initial target concentrations *(A),* and the log of the initial concentration plotted against the quantification cycle *(B)* as calculated by the second derivative maximum. *(Modified with permission of the publisher from Wittwer CT, Kusukawa N. Real-time PCR. In: Persing DH, Tenover FC, Versalovic J, et al, eds. Molecular microbiology: diagnostic principles and practice. Washington, DC: ASM Press, 2004:71-84.)*

TABLE 48-4	Correlation between Polymerase Chain Reaction Efficiency and Amplification Curve Spacing
PCR Efficiency	**Cycles/Log [DNA]***
2.0	3.32
1.9	3.59
1.8	3.92
1.7	4.34
1.6	4.90
1.5	5.68

From Wittwer CT, Kusukawa N. Real-time PCR and melting analysis. In Persing DH, Tenover FC, Tang YW, et al, eds., Molecular microbiology: diagnostic principles and practice, 2nd edition, Washington, DC: ASM Press, 2011:63-82. © 2011 ASM Press.

*The number of cycles that separates each decade difference in initial template concentration (Cycles/log [DNA]) is 1/log (E+1), where E is the PCR efficiency.

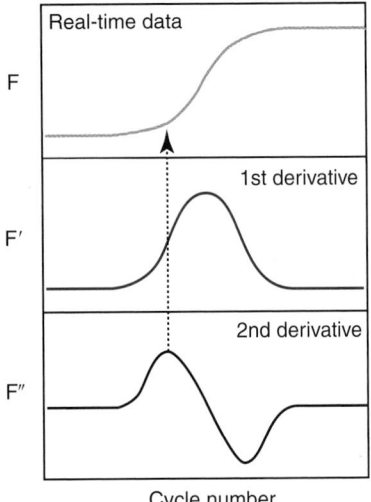

Figure 48-27 Finding the fractional cycle number for quantification. Real-time fluorescence data *(F)* from the amplification reaction are shown with the first *(F′)* and second *(F″)* derivatives. The maximum of the second derivative provides one way to determine the quantification cycle, Cq. *(Modified with permission of the publisher from Wittwer CT, Kusukawa N. Real-time PCR. In: Persing DH, Tenover FC, Versalovic J, et al, eds. Molecular microbiology: diagnostic principles and practice. Washington, DC: ASM Press, 2004:71-84.)*

Accuracy and Precision

The accuracy of real-time PCR quantification depends not only on the method chosen to analyze the curves but also on the quality of calibrators used. Purified PCR products quantified by spectrophotometry are available and easily obtained. When serially diluted, such products are used as calibrators. Alternatively, purified plasmids or genomic DNA have been used as calibrators. The precision of quantitative real-time PCR depends on the copy number. When the initial target concentration is low, imprecision is high. At least part of the variance comes from stochastic limitations as defined by the Poisson distribution as described earlier.

Melting Curve Analysis

Homogeneous hybridization has been used for (1) amplification, (2) detection, (3) quantification, and (4) obtaining detailed genotyping information. In practice, genotyping is preferably performed in the same tube by monitoring the melting of hybridized duplexes during controlled heating, producing a *melting curve signature* for the duplex. Such a signature monitors duplex binding over a range of temperatures in contrast to the single-temperature analysis of conventional hybridization techniques, such as dot blots or microarrays. The advantages of complete melting curves also apply when considering only homogeneous techniques. For example, methods that rely on hydrolysis for signal generation and/or those that acquire data only at one temperature generally result in more genotyping errors. Real-time amplification and melting analysis constitute a powerful combination of techniques that only requires temperature control and sampling of fluorescence. Many other genotyping techniques require complex separation and/or detection equipment after PCR. Real-time PCR with melting curve analysis allows (1) amplification, (2) detection, (3) quantification, and (4) genotyping (see Figure 48-22) without ancillary processing or additional equipment. The entire process can be completed in <30 minutes depending on the instrumentation used.

When fluorescence is monitored continuously within each cycle of PCR, the hybridization characteristics of PCR products and probes can be observed (see Figure 48-24, bottom panels). Using SYBR Green I dye, the melting characteristics of the amplified DNA is used to identify the product. No hybridization information is revealed with hydrolysis probes, whereas the melting of hybridization probes is readily apparent. Probe melting occurs at a characteristic temperature that is exploited to confirm target identity and to analyze sequence alterations under the probe. For routine testing in the clinical laboratory, a single melting curve is usually performed at the end of PCR instead of monitoring hybridization throughout the entire PCR process (see Figure 48-22). Immediately after the last PCR cycle, samples are momentarily denatured (94 °C), cooled to about 10 °C below the lowest temperature of interest, and heated at a rate of 0.1 to 0.3 °C/s, while fluorescence is continuously monitored. When hybridization probes are used, rapid cooling maximizes formation of probe-target duplexes while minimizing formation of the duplex PCR product. Primer asymmetry and use of 5′-exonuclease–deficient polymerases may augment the probe signal.

Genotyping of Single-Nucleotide Variants by Melting Curve Analysis

A hybridization probe-pair placed over a heterozygous polymorphism is shown in Figure 48-28. The reporter probe is complementary to the normal allele. As the temperature is increased, the mismatched mutant hybrid dissociates first, giving the first transition, followed by the matched normal hybrid. The Tm's of both hybrids are easily seen in derivative plots. A well-optimized probe design will provide a Tm difference of 4 °C to 10 °C for a single base mismatch under the probe.

SNV genotyping by melting curve analysis has been achieved with a variety of probe and dye methods.[14] Figure 48-29, *A*, shows the design of traditional hybridization probe pairs and the results

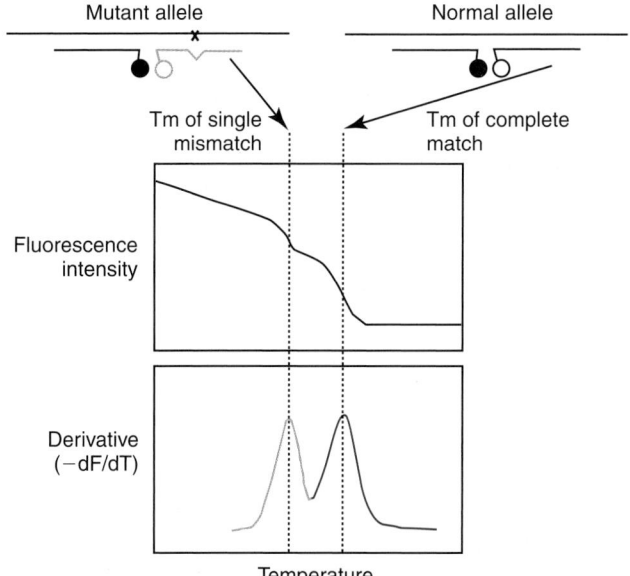

Figure 48-28 Melting curve single-nucleotide variant (SNV) genotyping. A heterozygous specimen with an SNV under the probe is amplified and melted. Two temperature transitions are visible: one from the mutant allele that is mismatched with the probe and melts at a lower temperature, and one from the normal allele that is completely matched with the probe and melts at a higher temperature. The derivative plot shows the melting temperatures of both the mutant-probe and the normal-probe duplexes as peaks. *(Modified with permission of the publisher from Bernard PS, Pritham GH, Wittwer CT. Color multiplexing hybridization probes using the apolipoprotein E locus as a model system for genotyping. Anal Biochem 1999;273:221-228. © 1999 Academic Press.)*

of (1) homozygous wild-type, (2) mutant, and (3) heterozygous samples that are well discriminated from each other. Virtually the same result is achieved with a single hybridization probe in which the fluorescent signal is quenched on the free probe but increased when it forms a hybrid with the target (Figure 48-29, B). Figure 48-29, C, illustrates genotyping with an unlabeled probe and a saturating DNA binding dye. Both probe and amplicon melting transitions are present. Figure 48-29, D, shows similar results using a snapback primer, an unlabeled probe attached as a 5′-tail to one of the primers. The advantage of these last two methods is that they do not require fluorescently labeled probes. Finally, SNV genotyping is possible by amplicon melting alone if a saturating DNA binding dye is used (Figure 48-29, E). However, the temperature difference between genotypes may be small, and high-resolution melting may be required for accurate genotyping.

High Resolution Melting Curve Analysis

Melting curve analysis with saturating dyes detects single base changes with high sensitivity and does not require processing or separation. Although conventional fluorescent melting analysis can distinguish PCR products with Tm's that differ by 1 °C to 2 °C, high-resolution melting instruments now provide a precision and resolution improvement of at least ten-fold and require only a few minutes. Typically, melting data are normalized between 0% and 100% fluorescence with the background

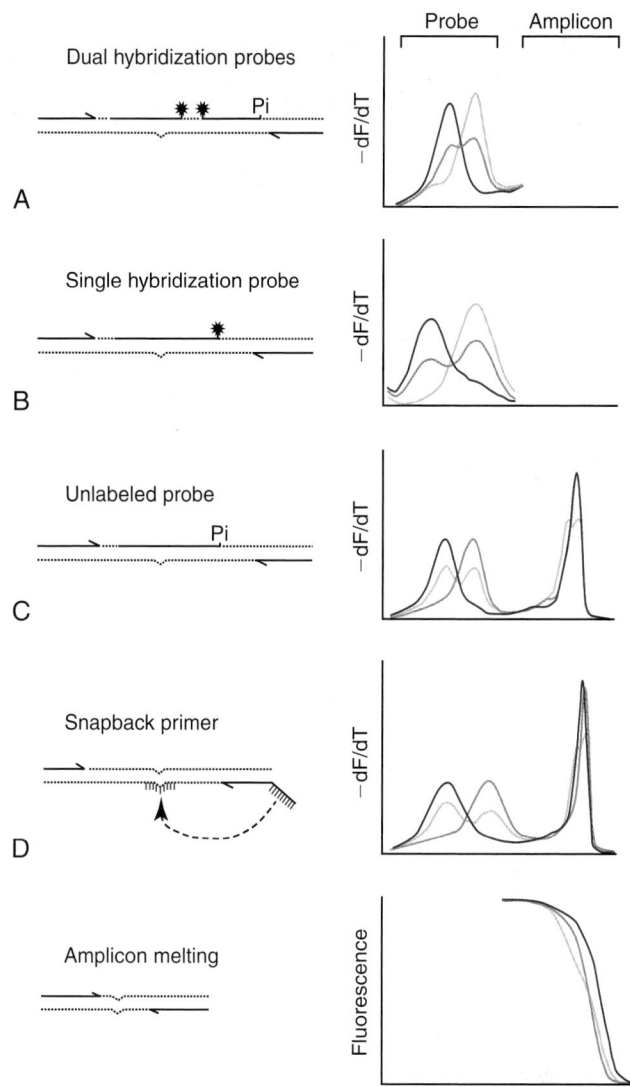

Figure 48-29 Five designs for single-nucleotide variant (SNV) genotyping and corresponding melting curve results. The traditional dual hybridization probe design *(A)* uses a pair of probes: one labeled with an acceptor fluorophore and the other with a donor fluorophore. The single hybridization probe design *(B)* lacks the second probe. The unlabeled probe design *(C)* does not require a covalently attached fluorescent label, using instead a saturating DNA binding dye in solution. Snapback primers *(D)* are similar to unlabeled probes with the probe attached to one primer as a 5′-tail. Finally, amplicon melting *(E)* uses only two regular polymerase chain reaction (PCR) primers, relying on high-resolution melting analysis to distinguish the small differences between genotypes. The two homozygotes are differentiated by melting temperature (Tm), and the heterozygote differs in shape from the contribution of heteroduplexes. Pi indicates a 3′-phosphate or other blocker that prevents polymerase extension.

removed to better match predicted helicity. Different homozygotes are distinguished by Tm and heterozygotes are identified by a change in shape. For example, SNV genotyping within a two-domain melting curve is shown in Figure 48-30. Major applications of high-resolution melting include (1) genotyping, (2) mutation scanning, and (3) sequence matching.

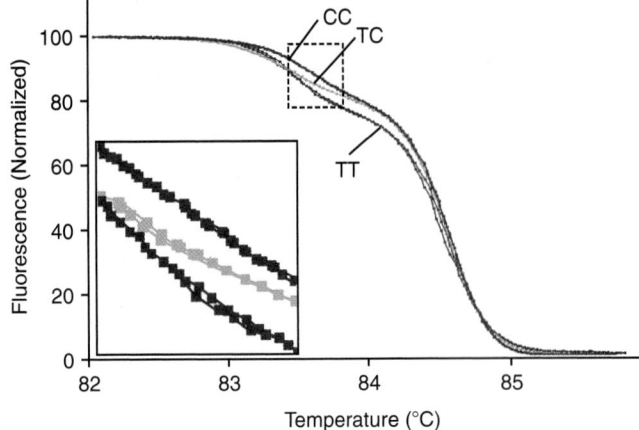

Figure 48-30 A single base change in a 544 bp fragment detected by melting analysis. Shown are high-resolution melting curves of polymerase chain reaction (PCR) amplicons from the gene *HTR2A* carrying a single-nucleotide variant (SNV). Results are shown for six individuals, two different individuals for each of the three genotypes: wild-type homozygote (TT), mutant homozygote (CC), and heterozygote (TC). Two melting domains are present because of differing GC content. The SNV was present in the lower melting domain. The *inset* magnifies a portion of the data, showing that all three genotypes can be discriminated. *(Modified by permission of the publisher from Wittwer CT, Reed GH, Gundry CN, et al. High-resolution genotyping by amplicon melting analysis using LC Green. Clin Chem 2003;49:853-60. © AACC.)*

TABLE 48-5	Comparison of Homogeneous Single-Nucleotide Variant Genotyping Methods (In Order of Increasing Complexity)		
Method	**Oligonucleotides**	**Modifications**	**Comments**
Amplicon melting	2	0	Simplest and least expensive
Snapback primers	2	1	Self-complementary 5′ tail
Allele-specific PCR (real time)	3	0	One well for each allele
Unlabeled probes	3	1	3′-block on probe
Allele-specific PCR (melting)	3	1-2	GC clamps as 5′ tails
Single hybridization probe	3	1-2	3′ block if the fluorescent label is 5′
Dual hybridization probes	4	3	Two fluorescent labels and one 3′ block
Hydrolysis probes	4	4	Two fluorescent labels and two quenchers
Hairpin probes	4	4	Two fluorescent labels and two quenchers
Self-probing amplicon	3-4	6	
Minor groove binder hydrolysis	4	6	
Serial invasive signal amplification	5	4	

Comparison of Homogeneous Single-Nucleotide Variant Genotyping Methods

Methods for closed-tube homogeneous SNV genotyping differ greatly in their level of complexity (Table 48-5). For example, the five simplest methods do not use fluorescently labeled probes. Amplicon melting requires only two primers and a heteroduplex-detecting DNA dye (see Figure 48-29, *E*). The snapback primer system also requires only two primers—one with a self-probing 5′-tail (see Figure 48-29, *D*). Unlabeled probe genotyping requires two primers and one 3′-blocked probe (see Figure 48-29, *C*). Allele-specific PCR requires three primers and is based on a preference by the polymerase to extend only a perfectly matched primer. In practice, genotyping is either performed in two wells by monitoring fluorescence at each cycle or in one well by incorporating GC-clamp(s) so that alleles will be differentiated at the end of PCR by their melting temperatures.

Intermediate in complexity are hybridization probe melting assays. Designs with single or dual hybridization probes are shown in Figure 48-29, *A* and *B*.

The more complex closed-tube methods for SNV genotyping are equilibrium type assays. Allele-specific hydrolysis and hairpin probes are commonly used. Self-probing amplicons and minor groove binder hydrolysis probes both require three modifications on two probes for SNV typing. Finally, serial invasive signal amplification is a method of homogeneous genotyping that does not require PCR.

Review Questions

1. The correct sequence of events during thermal cycling in a polymerase chain reaction (PCR) is
   a. anneal, extend, denature.
   b. denature, anneal, extend.

c. extend, anneal, denature.

d. extend, denature, anneal.

2. Regarding DNA electrophoresis, the type of gel that is used to separate nucleic acid fragments with low resolution between 20 bp up to 10,000 kilobases in length is
   a. agarose gel.
   b. polyacrylamide gel.
   c. polyimide gel.
   d. sucrose gradient gel.

3. In the determination of nucleic acid purity following isolation, the most acceptable A260/280 ratio for DNA is:
   a. 1.2
   b. 1.4
   c. 1.8
   d. 2.1

4. Which component is *not* part of PCR amplification?
   a. Taq polyermase
   b. Magnesium
   c. dNTPs
   d. Restriction enzyme

5. Another name for a restriction enzyme is
   a. an exonuclease.
   b. an endonuclease.
   c. a polymerase.
   d. a telomerase.

6. An amplification control in an infectious disease molecular assay
   a. is used to quantify unknowns.
   b. can signal a false negative result.
   c. indicates whether there is contamination.
   d. serves as a molecular weight standard.

7. The process of transferring the electrophoresed DNA out of a gel and onto a nylon paper is referred to as
   a. Southern blotting.
   b. Northern blotting.
   c. Western blotting.
   d. hybridization.

8. One of the major advantages of real-time polymerase chain reaction (PCR) compared to conventional PCR is that
   a. there is no need for specialized instruments.
   b. primers are not required.
   c. it can be used to quantify nucleic acid.
   d. it does not require the use of fluorescent compounds.

9. In the polymerase chain reaction (PCR), which one of the following components initiates extension of the sequence of interest by allowing polymerase to "see" single strands of DNA and begin adding nucleotides?
   a. Probe
   b. Ligase
   c. Promoter
   d. Primer

10. Differences observed in the sizes and number of fragments generated by restriction enzyme digestion of DNA is called
    a. restriction fragment length polymorphism (RFLP).
    b. variable number of tandem repeats.
    c. hybridization.
    d. strand displacement.

References

1. Benson DA, Cavanaugh M, Clark K, Karsch-Mizrachi I, Lipman DJ, Ostell J, et al. GenBank. Nucleic Acids Res 2013;41:D36–42.
2. Higuchi R, Fockler C, Dollinger G, Watson R. Kinetic PCR analysis: real-time monitoring of DNA amplification reactions. Biotechnology (N Y) 1993;11:1026–30.
3. Lander ES, Linton LM, Birren B, Nusbaum C, Zody MC, Baldwin J, et al. Initial sequencing and analysis of the human genome. Nature 2001;409:860–921.
4. Margulies M, Egholm M, Altman WE, Attiya S, Bader JS, Bemben LA, et al. Genome sequencing in microfabricated high-density picolitre reactors. Nature 2005;437:376–80.
5. Mitra RD, Butty VL, Shendure J, Williams BR, Housman DE, Church GM. Digital genotyping and haplotyping with polymerase colonies. Proc Natl Acad Sci U S A 2003;100:5926–31.
6. Perkins TT, Quake SR, Smith DE, Chu S. Relaxation of a single DNA molecule observed by optical microscopy. Science 1994;264:822–6.
7. Reed GH, Wittwer CT. Sensitivity and specificity of single-nucleotide polymorphism scanning by high-resolution melting analysis. Clin Chem 2004;50:1748–54.
8. Saiki RK, Gelfand DH, Stoffel S, Scharf SJ, Higuchi R, Horn GT, et al. Primer-directed enzymatic amplification of DNA with a thermostable DNA polymerase. Science 1988;239:487–91.
9. Sanger F, Nicklen S, Coulson AR. DNA sequencing with chain-terminating inhibitors. Proc Natl Acad Sci U S A 1977;74:5463–7.
10. Schena M, Shalon D, Davis RW, Brown PO. Quantitative monitoring of gene expression patterns with a complementary DNA microarray. Science 1995;270:467–70.
11. Schouten JP, McElgunn CJ, Waaijer R, Zwijnenburg D, Diepvens F, Pals G. Relative quantification of 40 nucleic acid sequences by multiplex ligation-dependent probe amplification. Nucleic Acids Res 2002;30:e57.
12. Stenson PD, Ball EV, Howells K, Phillips AD, Thomas NS, et al. Human Gene Mutation Database: 2008 update. Genome Med 2009;1:13.
13. Voelkerding KV, Dames SA, Durtschi JD. Next-generation sequencing: from basic research to diagnostics. Clin Chem 2009;55:641–58.
14. Wittwer CT, Kusukawa N. Nucleic acid techniques. In Burtis CA, Ashwood ER, Bruns DE, eds. Tietz textbook of clinical chemistry and molecular diagnostics, 5th ed. St Louis: Elsevier Saunders, 2012:401–42.
15. Witwer KW. Data submission and quality in microarray-based micro-RNA profiling. Clin Chem 2013 Feb;59(2):392–400.

Genomes and Nucleic Acid Variations

Carl T. Wittwer, M.D., Ph.D., and Noriko Kusukawa, Ph.D.

Objectives

1. Describe the human genome including size and composition; state the size contribution and function (if known) of each of the following genomic elements:

Genes	Segmental duplications
Intergenic DNA	Structural DNA
Mitochondrial DNA	Transposons

2. Compare microsatellite sequences (short tandem repeats [STRs]) to minisatellite sequences (variable-number tandem repeats [VNTRs]), including size, genomic location, role in human disease, and use in nucleic acid testing.

3. Compare single-nucleotide variants (SNVs) to copy number variants (CNVs), including composition, genomic frequency, and role in human disease.

4. For the following, state the specific DNA alteration and how it relates to human disease or gene expression:

Copy number variants (CNVs)	Insertion
Deletion	Missense
Epigenetic alterations	Nonsense
Indel	

5. Compare the human genome to bacterial, viral, and fungal genomes, including size, complexity, and percent of expressed genes.

Key Words and Definitions

Copy number variant (CNV) A structural variant of a large region of the genome that has been deleted or duplicated.

Deletion A DNA sequence that is missing in one sample compared with another. Deletions may be as small as one nucleotide or as large as an entire chromosome.

Heteroplasmy A condition in which a continuously variable proportion of DNA alleles is possible in a cell; for example, within a single cell, there is a mixture of mitochondria, some containing mutant mitochondrial DNA and some containing normal mitochondrial DNA.

Indel A sequence variant arising from both an insertion and a deletion.

Insertion An extra DNA sequence that is present in one sample compared with a reference sequence.

Intergenic DNA sequence between genes.

Microsatellites Short segments of DNA (1 to 13 bases long) that are repeated end to end. Also known as *short tandem repeats (STRs).*

Minisatellites Repeated segments of DNA that are 14 to 500 bases long. Also known as *sequences with a variable number of tandem repeats (VNTRs).*

Missense A nucleotide substitution that changes a codon to the code for a different amino acid. Although these sequence changes are commonly referred to as missense "mutations," this is strictly a misnomer, because they may be benign and cause no disease.

Mutation A disease-causing sequence variation.

Nonsense A nucleotide substitution that results in a stop codon, prematurely terminating the protein.

Oligonucleotide A short single-stranded polymer of nucleic acid.

Plasmid An extrachromosomal ring of double-stranded, closed DNA found in bacteria.

Pseudogene A genetic element that does not code for a functional gene product, usually because of accumulated sequence variations.

Short tandem repeats (STRs) Short segments of DNA (1 to 13 bases long) that are repeated end to end. Also known as *microsatellites.*

Simple sequence repeats (SSRs) Any sequence repeated over and over again in tandem, such as microsatellites and minisatellites.

Single-nucleotide polymorphism (SNP) A benign single-nucleotide variant (SNV) (substitution, deletion, or insertion) that occurs in the population at a frequency of at least 1%.

Single-nucleotide variant (SNV) Genetic variation of a single nucleotide (substitution, deletion, or insertion). SNVs may be benign or may cause disease.

Transposon A mobile genetic element that can delete and insert itself variably into the genome.

Variable-number tandem repeats (VNTRs) Repeated segments of DNA that are 14 to 500 bases long. Also known as *minisatellites.*

Variation A change in DNA sequence. It may be benign or may cause disease.

Molecular diagnostics focuses on medically important sequence **variations** within a background of complex genomic structure. This chapter reviews the organization of human, bacterial, viral, and fungal genomes and the spectrum of variations in nucleic acids that are of medical concern.

Genomes and Nucleic Acid Variations

In what follows, the structures of human, bacterial, viral, and fungal genomes are reviewed. Nucleic acid alterations of medical interest are introduced, emphasizing concepts relevant to molecular diagnostics.

Human Genome

Each human cell contains two copies of a 3.08-billion sequence code of nucleic acid bases spread across 46 chromosomes. Box 49-1 lists statistics for the human genome and the types of variations that are important in clinical diagnostics.

Three quarters of human DNA is **intergenic** or between genes. More than 60% of this intergenic sequence consists of "parasitic" DNA regions of transposable elements 100 to 11,000 bases in length. Between 2 million and 3 million of these **transposons** are present in each copy of the genome. They contribute to genetic recombination and chromosome structure and provide an evolutionary record of sequence variation and selection.

Segmental duplications constitute 5.3% of the human genome. They are over 1 kilobase (a thousand bases, or kb) in length and have a sequence identity of at least 90%; they are not transposable. Segmental duplications are common in the human genome and are prone to **deletion** and/or rearrangement, often with medical consequences.

Intergenic DNA also carries most of the **simple sequence repeats (SSRs)** present in the genome. These repeats are known as **microsatellites** or **short tandem repeats (STRs)** when the repeat unit is 1 to 13 bases and **minisatellites** or **variable-number tandem repeats (VNTRs)** when the repeat unit is 14 to 500 bases. SSRs are critical markers in genetic linkage studies and in forensic or medical identity testing. They are formed by slippage during replication and are highly polymorphic between individuals. The most common SSRs are dinucleotide repeats, such as ACACAC and ATAT. On average approximately one SSR has been found every 2000 bases.

Approximately 2% of DNA is required to maintain the structure of chromosomes and is located at chromosome centers (centromeres) and ends (telomeres). Centromeric DNA consists of many tandem copies of nearly identical 171 base pair (bp) repeats encompassing 0.24 to 5.0 Mb per chromosome. Each chromosome end is capped with several kb of the telomeric 6 base repeat TTAGGG.

Although intergenic DNA does not code for protein and was originally considered "junk," much of this DNA is transcribed to RNA, producing a complex "transcriptome" network of RNA control elements whose function and mechanics are active areas of investigation.[1]

One quarter of the human genome consists of genes. There are about 20,000 to 25,000 genes in the human genome. The

---

BOX 49-1	The Human Genome and Its Sequence Variation[4,5,11,12]

The Human Genome

3.08 billion base pairs in 23 chromosomes (46-244 million base pairs per chromosome)

Genes (25%)	Intergenic Sequences (75%)
23% Intron sequence	45% Parasitic (transposon-derived repeats)
1.9% Exon sequence	5% Segmental duplications
1.2% Coding	3% Simple sequence repeats
0.7% Untranslated	2% Structural (centromers, telomers)
	20% Other

Number of genes: 20,000 to 25,000
Average gene: 27,000 base pairs
    10.4 exons
    9.1 transcribed exons
    1340 bases of coding sequence
    446 amino acids
Sequence variation: 99.9% identity (1 difference every 1250 bases between randomly selected haploid genomes)
Single-nucleotide variants (SNVs): identified every 100 to 300 bases
    97% Noncoding (average of 126 within each gene)
    3% Within exons (average of 5 within the coding regions of each gene)
    Copy number variants (CNVs) constitute 5% to 12% of the genome

Disease-Causing Variants
68% SNVs
    45% Missense (amino acid substitution)
    11% Nonsense (termination)
    10% Splicing
    1%-2% Regulatory
    24% Small insertions and/or deletions
    8% Structural (large insertions/deletions, rearrangements, copy number)

Epigenetic Alterations
    Variable initiation
    Alternative splicing
    Cytosine methylation (regulation)
    Histone phosphorylation, methylation, acetylation

---

average gene covers 27,000 bases, but only about 1300 of these bases code for amino acid sequences. The primary RNA transcript is processed by splicing to retain exons that are interspersed throughout the gene and have higher proportions of guanine and cytosine than noncoding regions have. On average, 95% of a gene is excised as introns, retaining a mean of 10.4 exons, of which 9.1 are translated into proteins. Exons make up only 1.9% of the total genome with 1.1% of the genome coding for proteins. Some important genes are present in many copies, so overall protein expression is not affected if a chance variation occurs in one copy. If extra copies of genes lose their function, they are known as **pseudogenes**. At least as many pseudogenes as functional genes are present in the human genome. It is important to distinguish pseudogenes from functional genes because sequence variations in pseudogenes are seldom of clinical importance.

Even though 99% of the genome does not code for protein, most of it is transcribed into noncoding RNA. At least 93% of the genome is transcribed,[1] producing more than ten times the amount of RNA that is produced from the coding segments of genes.[2] Both strands of DNA may be transcribed, and long noncoding transcripts may overlap coding regions, producing a complex transcriptome of functional RNA molecules that may variably regulate (1) transcription of coding regions, (2) RNA processing, (3) messenger RNA (mRNA) stability, (4) translation, (5) protein stability, and (6) secretion. In addition to long noncoding RNA, ribosomal RNA, and transfer RNA, specific classes of noncoding RNAs include (1) small nuclear RNAs critical for splicing, (2) small nucleolar RNAs that modify rRNA, (3) telomerase RNAs for maintenance of telomeres, (4) small interfering RNAs, and (5) microRNAs (miRNAs) that regulate gene expression.[8,9] The miRNAs[3] are discussed in more detail in Chapter 47.

Sequence Variation within the Human Genome

Consider the genome as a book. Nucleotides (bases) are the individual letters, and three-base words code for each amino acid. The words are organized into sentences or exons that are separated by periods or introns. Each sentence is further organized into paragraphs or genes. Many paragraphs constitute a chapter or chromosome, and several chapters make up a book or genome. If the DNA of any two individuals is compared, on average one spelling difference is noted every 1250 bases (i.e., approximately 99.9% of the sequence is identical between randomly chosen copies of the genome). However, different individuals (copies of the same book) vary in a subtler way. Some of the pages are copied more than once and may be scattered throughout the book. Such **copy number variants (CNVs)** involve a greater amount of text than the spelling differences with 0.5% of the genome differing on average between two individuals when 50 kb pages are considered,[7] (that is, between individuals, at least five times as many bases are affected by copy number changes as by small sequence differences).

Any sequence change (compared to a reference sequence) is called a *sequence variant* or variation. Many variations do not affect human health and are benign or silent. For example, most (1) copy-number variations, (2) **single-nucleotide variants (SNVs)**, and (3) SSRs found between genes are seldom associated with disease. Similarly, most of the SNVs within introns, except for splicing and regulatory variants, are not known to affect gene function. In addition, some of the SNVs within exons are silent alterations that do not code for a change in amino acid sequence because of the redundancy in the genetic code. Still other SNVs in exons code for amino acid changes that do not affect protein function. Even such silent SNVs nonetheless may be of interest as genetic markers.

The most common sequence variations are single base changes, also known as SNVs. Millions of SNVs have been described, and many new SNVs continue to be reported. Some SNVs are common in the population, with allele frequencies of 0.1 to 0.5 (i.e., present in 10 to 50 of every 100 copies studied), though other single base changes are very rare. Although an SNV has been identified every 100 to 300 bases, many of these are not found frequently in the population. The vast majority of SNVs (97%) occur in noncoding regions; only 3% of SNVs are associated with exons.

Although SNVs are the most common sequence variant, copy number variants (CNVs) cover more of the genome than SNVs. These CNVs occur in stretches of DNA that may range from 100 bases up to several Mb (megabases, or million bases) in size. CNVs may be duplicated in tandem or may involve complex gains or losses of homologous sequences at multiple sites in the genome. CNV regions exist in every chromosome and involve 5% to 12% of the human genome.[7,10] Most CNVs are inherited and biallelic, similar to **single-nucleotide polymorphism (SNPs)**. More than 6000 CNV loci have been reported, and many of them overlap with genes. Individuals differ on average at more than 200 CNV loci, and these overlap the transcribed regions of more than 100 genes.

Variations That Cause Human Disease

Sequence alterations that are known to cause disease are often called **mutations** or, "disease-causing variants." About 68% of known disease-causing variants involve only a single base. Most of the remaining disease-causing variants (24%) are small insertions or deletions. The remainder (8%) are more complex structural variations.

Single-Nucleotide Variants

Most SNVs that cause disease are **missense** and result in an amino acid substitution, whereas significantly fewer are **nonsense** variants that result in a termination codon and premature polypeptide chain termination. Approximately 10% of disease-causing variants are SNVs that affect splicing sites and result in altered concatenation of coding sequences. Finally, less than 2% of known disease-causing variants are SNVs that affect the regulatory efficiency of transcription by altering promoter and/or enhancer regions in introns or the stability of the RNA transcript.

Small Insertions and Deletions

Small insertion and/or deletion variants account for 24% of variants that cause disease. An **insertion** refers to the presence of extra bases, whereas deletion implies the absence of certain bases in comparison with a reference sequence. Insertions and deletions often cause a shift of the codon reading frame, resulting in altered amino acid sequence downstream of the variation—commonly followed by chain termination from a nonsense codon. An **indel** implies both an insertion and a deletion at the same locus (e.g., replacement of TG with AGGTC).

Structural Variants

The remaining 8% of variants that relate to health and disease are mostly structural variants, including (1) duplications or deletions of entire exons or genes, (2) chromosomal translocations, (3) inversions, (4) SSR expansions (e.g., an increased number of trinucleotide repeats), (5) gene rearrangements (e.g., rearrangements of immunoglobulin genes in B cells that are required for production of antibodies), (6) complex polymorphic loci related to health and disease (e.g., human leukocyte antigen [HLA]), and (7) CNVs.

Interest in CNVs in relation to disease has increased recently as the extent of variation has become clear.[13] CNVs can involve genes or contiguous sets of genes. When the normal dosage of the gene is two, but more than two functional copies of a gene are present, then the gene is "amplified." If a dosage-sensitive gene, such as HER-2-neu (*ERBB2*), is amplified, this usually leads to overexpression of messenger RNA and protein, resulting in cellular abnormalities and possible progression to diseases such as cancer. When the normal gene dosage is two, and loss of one of the functional copies of the gene occurs, disorders such as mental retardation and developmental delay may result. Structural variants can be determined by cytogenetic techniques, including (1) karyotyping, (2) fluorescent in situ hybridization, (3) comparative genomic hybridization, and (4) virtual karyotyping by SNV microarrays.

Alterations in Mitochondrial DNA and Hemizygous Genes

Most human genetic material is present in two copies with the exception of the unpaired sex chromosome in males and mitochondrial DNA. The presence of only a single copy of genes on the X and Y chromosome in males leads to well-known sex-linked disorders. In contrast, the 16,500-bp mitochondrial genome is present in more than 1000 copies per cell, constituting about 0.3% of human DNA. Allele fractions may vary over a wide range when all mitochondria in a cell are considered. That is, mitochondrial DNA demonstrates **heteroplasmy** meaning that the ratio of the wild-type allele to a variant allele within a cell can vary almost continuously, sometimes resulting in a wide range of symptoms even when only one sequence variant is involved.

Human Epigenetic Alterations[6]

In addition to the sequence variants considered earlier, epigenetic alterations, including alternative splicing and methylation, affect gene expression. Even though the number of genes may be limited to less than 25,000, variable transcription initiation and exon splicing produce about 90,000 messenger RNA transcripts and protein products.

Methylation of cytosine to 5-methylcytosine occurs frequently; about 70% of cytosine-guanine dinucleotides (CpG) in the human genome are methylated. Although not inherited, interest in this "5th base" has increased as correlations with cancer have been reported. CpG islands are about 1000 bases in length and are often found near the 5′ end of genes. These regions consist of clusters of CpG dinucleotides that are usually not methylated in normal cells. However, CpG methylation correlates with condensed chromatin structure and promoter inactivation; an important example occurs in tumor-suppressor genes.

Since DNA is associated with proteins in nucleosomes, gene expression can be altered by histone phosphorylation, acetylation, and methylation. See Chapter 47 for further discussion of nucleosomes, histone modifications, and other epigenetic alterations and their relation to disease.

Bacterial Genomes

Bacterial genomes are considerably less complex than human or other eukaryotic genomes. Common bacteria have only one chromosome, usually a circular DNA double helix of 4 million to 5 million base pairs, about 1000 times less than the amount of DNA in a human cell. About 90% of the DNA in bacteria codes for protein. There are no introns, but there are multiple small intergenic regions of repetitive sequences that are dispersed throughout the genome. The common bacterium, *Escherichia coli,* includes about 4300 genes.

In addition to the large circular chromosome that carries essential genes, bacteria also carry accessory genes in smaller circles of double-stranded DNA (ds-DNA) known as **plasmids**. Plasmids range in size from 1000 to more than 1 million base pairs. Plasmids are important in molecular diagnosis of bacterial infections, because they often encode pathogenic factors and antibiotic resistance.

The bacterial repertoire of DNA can be altered by: (1) gain or loss of plasmids; (2) single-base changes, small insertions and deletions as in eukaryotic genomes; and (3) larger segmental rearrangements, including inversions, deletions, and duplications. Some genes, such as those for ribosomal RNA, are present in many copies and have been used to identify species of bacteria. In addition, the intergenic repetitive sequences serve as multiple targets for **oligonucleotide** probes, enabling the generation of unique DNA profiles or fingerprints for individual bacterial strains.

Viral Genomes

Viral genomes are considerably less complex than bacterial genomes. Common viruses that infect humans vary in size from about 5000 to 250,000 bases, or 20 to 1000 times less than the amount of nucleic acid in *E. coli*. Because viruses use the host's cellular machinery, they do not need as many genes as bacteria do. Small viruses may encode only several genes, but the larger viruses can encode hundreds. The viral genome consists of either DNA or RNA, and the nucleic acid may be single stranded or double stranded, linear, or circular with one or multiple fragments and/or copies per viral particle. As in bacteria, there are no introns. In fact, in some viruses the exons overlap with different reading frames coding different products from the same nucleic acid sequence. Noncoding regions are usually present at the terminal ends of linear genomes. Repeat segments are often found as terminal or internal repeats and may be inverted.

Sequence alterations in viruses are common. Areas of high sequence variation may be interspersed between conserved domains. Higher frequencies of variation have been correlated with lower polymerase fidelity and may allow escape from antibody recognition and from antiviral drugs. Common sequence variants in viruses include single base changes, insertions, and deletions. Sequence diversity within a viral species may be so great that consensus sequences for molecular typing are difficult to find.

Fungal Genomes

Fungi are eukaryotes, and their genomes are more complex than the genomes of bacteria or viruses. Common fungi that cause human disease have genome sizes of 7.5 to 30 million bases and 8 to 14 chromosomes, as well as mitochondrial genomes. Some fungi have diploid genomes, and others have haploid genomes. Many of their genes have introns. For instance, *Aspergillus fumigatus* (a fungus that causes allergic reactions and systemic disease with a high mortality rate) has a haploid genome of about 30 million bases with more than 9900 predicted genes on eight chromosomes. Its genes are smaller than human genes, with an average length of 1400 bp and 2.8 exons per gene.

Review Questions

1. A mutation is defined as
   a. the location of a particular sequence on a chromosome.
   b. a proofreading error that occurs during translation.
   c. a disease-causing variant.
   d. a repeated sequence found in an intron within a segment of genomic DNA.

2. If the nucleotide "A" were inserted into the following mRNA strand at the point where the asterisk (*) is, how would sequence change?

   mRNA strand: AAC CGA CUC *UCC AGG UAA GAG

   a. There would be no change in the sequence.
   b. AAC CGA CUC AUC CAG GUA AGA…
   c. ACC CGA CUCA UCC AGG UAA GAG
   d. ACC CGA CUC AUC AGG UAA GAG

3. True or false: 99% of the human genome codes for protein.
   a. True
   b. False

4. The absence of certain bases in a DNA sequence in comparison with a reference sequence is referred to as a(n)
   a. aneuploidy.
   b. deletion.
   c. translocation.
   d. isochrome formation.

5. True or false: Bacterial genomes are more complex than human genomes because of the presence of more genes.
   a. True
   b. False

6. An example of an epigenetic alteration that would affect gene expression is
   a. methylation of cystosine in a cytosine-guanine dinucleotide.
   b. an insertion of an extra base in a gene.
   c. a chromosomal translocation
   d. heteroplasmy.

7. Simple sequence repeats, such as short tandem repeats (STRs) or variable number of tandem repeats (VNTRs), that are highly polymorphic between individuals are formed by
   a. transcription errors.
   b. frameshift mutations.
   c. capping by a six base repeat.
   d. slippage during replication.

8. Regions of the human genome that provide an evolutionary record of sequence variation and selection are referred to as
   a. genes.
   b. chromosomes.
   c. transposons.
   d. transcriptomes.

9. Sequence variations between wild-type alleles and variant alleles in mitochondrial DNA within a cell can vary continuously. This is
   a. heteroplasmy.
   b. translocation.
   c. insertion.
   d. methylation.

10. The explanation as to why not all single-nucleotide variants (SNVs) affect human health and are benign is that
    a. SNVs are unrelated to gene expression.
    b. they involve complex losses of homologous sequences that are unimportant in disease.
    c. they are deleted during replication.
    d. the vast majority of SNVs occur in noncoding regions of the genome.

References

1. Amaral PP, Dinger ME, Mercer TR, et al. The eukaryotic genome as an RNA machine. Science 2008;319:1787–9.
2. Carninci P, Kasukawa T, Katayama S, et al. The transcriptional landscape of the mammalian genome. Science 2005;309:1559–63.
3. Griffiths-Jones S, Saini HK, van Dongen S, et al. miRBase: tools for microRNA genomics. Nucleic Acids Res 2008;36:D154–8.
4. International Human Genome Consortium. Finishing the euchromatic sequence of the human genome. Nature 2004;431:931–45.
5. Lander ES, Linton LM, Birren B, et al. Initial sequencing and analysis of the human genome. Nature 2001;409:860–921.
6. Lopez J, Percharde M, Coley HM, et al. The context and potential of epigenetics in oncology. Br J Cancer 2009;100:571–7.
7. McCarroll SA, Kuruvilla FG, Korn JM, et al. Integrated detection and population-genetic analysis of SNPs and copy number variation. Nat Genet 2008;40:1166–74.
8. Mendes Soares LM, Valcarcel J. The expanding transcriptome: the genome as the "Book of Sand." EMBO J 2006;25:923–31.
9. Mercer TR, Dinger ME, Mattick JS. Long non-coding RNAs: insights into functions. Nat Rev Genet 2009;10:155–9.
10. Redon R, Ishikawa S, Fitch KR, et al. Global variation in copy number in the human genome. Nature 2006;444:444–54.
11. Stenson PD, Mort M, Ball EV, et al. The human gene mutation database: 2008 update. Genome Med 2009;1:13.
12. Venter JC, Adams MD, Myers EW, et al. The sequence of the human genome. Science 2001;291:1304–51.
13. Wain LV, Armour JA, Tobin MD. Genomic copy number variation, human health, and disease. Lancet 2009;15:15.

Reference Information for the Clinical Laboratory*

Gwendolyn A. McMillin, Ph.D., D.A.B.C.C. (C.C., T.C.), Carl A. Burtis, Ph.D., and David E. Bruns, M.D.

Contents

*The authors gratefully acknowledge the contributions of William L. Roberts, Edward R. Ashwood, Pennell C. Painter, June Y. Cope, and Jane L. Smith, upon which portions of this chapter are based.

TABLE 50-1   Reference Intervals and Values

Results of laboratory tests have little practical utility until clinical studies have ascribed various states of health and disease to intervals of values. Reference intervals are useful because they attempt to describe the typical results found in a defined population of apparently healthy people. Different methods may yield different values, depending on calibration and other technical considerations. Hence, different reference intervals and results may be obtained in different laboratories. Variability among methods is particularly characteristic of methods that use antibodies to detect the material of interest, and when results are reported as relative units of activity. Values from apparently "healthy" and diseased people may overlap significantly. Therefore reference intervals, although useful as a guide for clinicians, should not be used as absolute indicators of health and disease (see Chapter 5). The reference intervals presented in this chapter are for *general informational purposes only.* Guidelines for defining and determining reference intervals have been discussed in Chapter 5 and published in the 2010 CLSI C28-A3 guideline ("How to Define and Determine Reference Intervals in the Clinical Laboratory; Approved Guideline—Third Edition"). As stated in several chapters in this textbook, *each individual laboratory should generate its own set of reference intervals.*

Where both exist, reference intervals are listed in both conventional and international units and are for use in adults in the fasting state unless otherwise stated. Values for other age groups, when included, are clearly identified. Most of the values listed were obtained from chapters in this book. Some were extracted, however, from *Tietz clinical guide to laboratory tests,* 4th edition, by Alan H. B. Wu (Philadelphia, WB Saunders/Elsevier, 2006), and *Tietz textbook of clinical chemistry and molecular diagnostics,* 5th edition, by Burtis CA, Ashwood ER, and Bruns DE (St Louis, Saunders/Elsevier, 2012). For several of the specific proteins, reference intervals—obtained after calibration of the analytical system with the international protein reference RPPHS/CRM-470—are listed in Chapter 18.

A valuable source for reference intervals for older methods is http://cclnprod.cc.nih.gov/dlm/testguide.nsf/ (accessed June 17, 2013).

For convenience and to preserve space, we have used the standard abbreviations listed below:

Abbreviation	Term
Amf	Amniotic fluid
CSF	Cerebrospinal fluid
EDTA	Ethylenediaminetetraacetic acid
F⁻	Fluoride ion
F⁻/Ox	Fluoride ion and oxalate
Hep	Heparin
Occup. exp.	Occupational exposure
Ox	Oxalate
P	Plasma
Plt	Platelets
RBC	Red blood cells
S	Serum
Sal	Saliva
U	Urine
WB	Whole blood

Analyte	Specimen	Condition	REFERENCE INTERVALS Conventional Units	REFERENCE INTERVALS Conversion Factor	REFERENCE INTERVALS SI Units
α₁-Acid glycoprotein			mg/dL		g/L
	S	Adult (20-60 y)	50-120	0.01	0.5-1.2
Adipoylcarnitine					mmol/mol creatinine
	U	0-7 d			0.04-0.40
		8 d-7 y			0.01-0.81
		>7 y			0.00-0.13
Adrenocorticotropic hormone			pg/mL		pmol/L
	P, EDTA	Cord	50-570	0.22	11-125
		Newborn	10-185		2.2-41
		Adult (0800-0900)	<120		<26
		Adult (24 h, supine)	<85		<19
β-Alanine			mg/dL		μmol/L
	P		<0.44	112.2	<49
			<0.26		<29
			mg/d		μmol/d
	U, 24 h	3-16 y	<3.8	11.2	<42
		Adult	<8.3		<93
			mg/g creatinine		mmol/mol creatinine
			11	1.27	14

TABLE 50-1 Reference Intervals and Values—cont'd

Analyte	Specimen	Condition	REFERENCE INTERVALS Conventional Units	Conversion Factor	SI Units
Alanine aminotransferase (ALT, SGPT) IFCC, 37 °C	S	Adult male	U/L <45	0.017	µkat/L <0.77
		Adult female	<34		<0.58
Albumin	S	0-4 d	g/dL 2.8-4.4	10	g/L 28-44
		4 d-14 y	3.8-5.4		38-54
		14-18 y	3.2-4.5		32-45
		Adult (20-60 y)	3.5-5.2		35-52
		60-90 y	3.2-4.6		32-46
		>90 y	2.9-4.5		29-45
	U, 24 h		mg/d 3.9-24.4	1	mg/d 3.9-24.4
	CSF, lumbar		mg/dL 17.7-25.1	10	mg/L 177-251
Aldolase	S	Child	U/L		µkat/L
		10-24 mo	10-40	0.017	0.17-0.68
		25 mo to16 y	5-20		0.09-0.34
		Adult	2.5-10.0		0.04-0.13
Aldosterone	S	Cord blood	ng/dL 40-200	0.0277	nmol/L 1.11-5.54
		Premature infants	19-141		0.53-3.91
		Full-term infants and children			
		3 d	7-184		0.19-5.10
		1 wk	5-175		0.03-4.85
		1-12 mo	5-90		0.14-2.49
		1-2 y	7-54		0.19-1.50
		2-10 y (supine)	3-35		0.08-0.97
		2-10 y (upright)	5-80		0.14-2.22
		10-15 y (supine)	2-22		0.06-0.61
		10-15 y (upright)	4-48		0.11-1.33
		Adults			
		supine	3-16		0.08-0.44
		upright	7-30		0.19-0.83
	U, 24 h		µg/d	nmol/d	µg/g creatinine
		Newborns (1-3 d)	0.5-5	2.771-14	20-140
		Prepubertal children 4-10 y	1-8	3-22	4-22
		Adults	3-19	8-51	1.5-20
Aluminum	S, P		µg/L <5.51	0.0371	µmol/L <0.2
		Patients on hemodialysis	20-550		0.74-20.4
		Al medication	<30		<1.11
	U		5-30		0.19-1.11
Ammonia nitrogen	P (Hep)		µg N/dL		µmol N/L
		Newborn	90-150	0.714	64-107
		0-2 wk	79-129		56-92
		>1 mo	29-70		21-50
		Adult	15-45		11-32
	U, 24 h		mg N/d		mmol N/d
		Infant	560-2900	0.0714	40-207
		Adult	140-1500		10-107
Amylase IFCC, 37 °C	S	Adult	U/L 28-100	0.017	µkat/L 0.48-1.70

Continued

TABLE 50-1   Reference Intervals and Values—cont'd

Analyte	Specimen	Condition		Conventional Units (REFERENCE INTERVALS)	Conversion Factor	SI Units
3α-Androstanediol glucuronide				ng/dL		nmol/L
		Child, prepubertal		10-60	0.0213	0.2-1.3
	S	Adult, M		260-1500		5.5-32
		Adult, F		60-300		1.3-6.4
Androstenedione				ng/dL		nmol/L
	S	Child, prepubertal		<5	0.0349	<0.2
		Adults		75-205		2.6-7.2
		Adult, F postmenopausal		82-275		3.0-9.6
Antidiuretic hormone (ADH)		mOsm/kg		ng/L		pmol/L
	P, EDTA	270-280		<1.5	0.926	<1.4
		280-285		<2.5		<2.3
		285-290		1-5		0.9-4.6
		290-294		2-7		1.9-6.5
		295-300		4-12		3.7-11.1
Antimony				μg/dL		nmol/L
	P (Hep)			0.014-0.090	82.1	1.15-7.39
				μg/L		nmol/L
	U			<10	8.21	<82.1
				mg/L		μmol/L
		Toxic		>1		>8.21
α₁-Antitrypsin	S			mg/dL		g/L
		Adult (20-60 y)		90-200	0.01	0.9-2.0
Apolipoprotein A-1				mg/dL		g/L
	S	4-5 y	M	109-172	0.01	1.09-1.72
			F	104-163		1.04-1.63
		6-11 y	M	111-177		1.11-1.77
			F	110-166		1.10-1.66
		12-19 y	M	99-165		0.99-1.65
			F	105-180		1.05-1.80
		20-29 y	M	105-173		1.05-1.73
			F	111-209		1.11-2.09
		30-39 y	M	105-173		1.05-1.73
			F	110-189		1.10-1.89
		40-49 y	M	103-178		1.03-1.78
			F	115-195		1.15-1.95
		50-59 y	M	107-173		1.07-1.73
			F	117-211		1.17-2.11
		60-69 y	M	111-184		1.11-1.84
			F	120-205		1.20-2.05
		>69 y	M	109-180		1.09-1.80
			F	118-199		1.18-1.99
Apolipoprotein B				mg/dL		g/L
	S	4-5 y	M	58-103	0.01	0.58-1.03
			F	58-104		0.58-1.04
		6-11 y	M	56-105		0.56-1.05
			F	57-113		0.57-1.13
		12-19 y	M	55-110		0.55-1.10
			F	53-119		0.53-1.19
		20-29 y	M	59-130		0.59-1.30
			F	59-132		0.59-1.32
		30-39 y	M	63-143		0.63-1.43
			F	70-132		0.70-1.32
		40-49 y	M	71-152		0.71-1.52
			F	75-136		0.75-1.36
		50-59 y	M	75-160		0.75-1.60
			F	75-168		0.75-1.68

TABLE 50-1   Reference Intervals and Values—cont'd

Analyte	Specimen	Condition		REFERENCE INTERVALS		
				Conventional Units	Conversion Factor	SI Units
Apolipoprotein B, cont'd		60-69 y	M	81-156		0.81-1.56
			F	75-173		0.75-1.73
		>69 y	M	73-152		0.73-1.52
			F	79-168		0.79-1.68
Arsenic				µg/L		µmol/L
	WB (Hep)			2-23	0.0133	0.03-0.31
		Chronic poisoning		100-500		1.33-6.65
		Acute poisoning		600-9300		7.98-124
				µg/d		µmol/d
	U, 24 h			5-50		0.07-0.67
Ascorbic acid (*see* Vitamin C)						
Aspartate aminotransferase	S			U/L		µkat/L
(AST, SGOT)		Adult male		<35		<0.60
IFCC, 37 °C		Adult female		<31	0.017	<0.53
Beryllium	U, 24 h			µg/L		µmol/L
		Negative		None detected	0.111	None detected
		Toxic		>20		>2.22
Bilirubin				mg/dL		µmol/L
Total	S	Cord (premature)		<2.0	17.1	<34.2
		Cord (full term)		<2.0		<34.2
		0-1 d (premature)		1.0-8.0		17-187
		0-1 d (full term)		2.0-6.0		34-103
		1-2 d (premature)		6.0-12.0		103-205
		1-2 d (full term)		6.0-10.0		103-171
		3-5 d (premature)		10.0-14.0		171-240
		3-5 d (full term)		4.0-8.0		68-137
		Adult		0-2.0		0-34
	U			Negative		Negative
	Amf	28 wk		<0.075		<1.28
				$\Delta A_{450} < 0.048$		
		40 wk		<0.025		<0.43
				$\Delta A_{450} < 0.02$		
Conjugated	S			0.0-0.2		0.0-3.4
Biotin	WB	Healthy				0.5-2.20 nmol/L
		Deficiency				<0.5 nmol/L
BNP (see Chapter 34)						
	U					0.1-2.0
Cadmium	WB (Hep)			µg/L		nmol/L
		Nonsmokers		0.3-1.2	8.897	2.7-10.7
		Smokers		0.6-3.9		5.3-34.7
				µg/L		µmol/L
	U, 24 h	Toxic range		100-3000		0.9-26.7
Calcitonin	S, P			pg/mL		ng/L
		Men		<8.8	1.0	<8.8
		Women		<5.8		<5.8
		Athyroidal		<0.5		<0.5
Calcium, ionized (free)	S, P (Hep)			mg/dL		mmol/L
		Adults		4.6-5.3	0.25	1.15-1.33
Calcium, total	S, P (Hep)			mg/dL		mmol/L
		Adults		8.6-10.3	0.25	2.15-2.57
β-Carotene	S			µg/dL		µmol/L
HPLC				10-85	0.0186	0.19-1.58
Cancer antigen 15-3				U/mL		kU/L
	S			<30	1.0	<30

Continued

TABLE 50-1   Reference Intervals and Values—cont'd

Analyte	Specimen	Condition	Conventional Units	Conversion Factor	SI Units
Cancer antigen 19-9			U/mL		kU/L
	S		<37	1.0	<37
Cancer antigen 27.29			U/mL		kU/L
	S		<37.7	1.0	<37.7
Cancer antigen 125			U/mL		kU/L
	S		<35	1.0	<35
Carbon dioxide, partial pressure			mm Hg		kPa
PCO_2	WB, arterial (Hep)	Newborn	27-40	0.133	3.59-5.32
		Infant	27-41		3.59-5.45
		Adult, M	35-48		4.66-6.38
		Adult, F	32-45		4.26-5.99
Carbon dioxide, total (tCO_2)			mEq/L		mmol/L
		Cord blood	14-22	1.0	14-22
	P, S	Adult	23-30		23-30
		>60 y	23-31		23-31
		>90 y	20-29		20-29
	P, Capillary	Premature, 1 wk	14-27		14-27
		Newborn	13-22		13-22
		Infant	20-28		20-28
		Child	20-28		20-28
		Adult	22-28		22-28
	Whole blood				
	Arterial		19-24		19-24
	Venous		22-26		22-26
Carbon monoxide	WB (EDTA)		% HbCO		HbCO fraction
		Nonsmokers	0.5-1.5	0.01	0.005-0.015
		Smokers			
		1-2 packs/d	4-5		0.04-0.05
		>2 packs/d	8-9		0.08-0.09
		Toxic	>20		>0.20
		Lethal	>50		>0.5
Carcinoembryonic antigen (CEA)			ng/mL		µg/L
	S	Nonsmokers	<3	1.0	<3
		Smokers	<5		<5
Catecholamines					
Epinephrine	P	Adults	pg/mL		pmol/L
		Supine (30 min)	<50	5.46	<273
		Sitting (15 min)	<60		<328
		Standing (30 min)	<90		<491
Norepinephrine	P	Adults	pg/mL		pmol/L
		Supine (30 min)	110-410	5.91	650-2423
		Sitting (15 min)	120-680		709-4019
		Standing (30 min)	125-700		739-4137
Dopamine	P	Adults	pg/mL		pmol/L
		Supine (30 min)	<87	6.53	<475
		Sitting (15 min)	<87		<475
		Standing (30 min)	<87		<475
Epinephrine	U, 24 h		µg/d		nmol/d
		0-1 y	0-2.5	5.46	0-14
		1-2 y	0-3.5		0-19
		2-4 y	0-6.0		0-33
		4-7 y	0.2-10		1-55
		7-10 y	0.2-10		1-55
		10-15 y	0.5-20		3-109
		>15 y	0.5-20		3-109

TABLE 50-1   Reference Intervals and Values—cont'd

Analyte	Specimen	Condition	REFERENCE INTERVALS Conventional Units	Conversion Factor	SI Units
Norepinephrine	U, 24 h		µg/d		nmol/d
		0-1 y	0-10	5.91	0-59
		1-2 y	1-17		6-100
		2-4 y	4-29		24-171
		4-7 y	8-45		47-266
		7-10 y	13-65		77-384
		10-15 y	15-80		89-473
		>15 y	15-80		89-473
Dopamine	U, 24 h		µg/d		nmol/d
		0-1 y	0-85	6.53	0-555
		1-2 y	10-140		65-914
		2-4 y	40-260		261-1697
		4-7 y	65-400		424-2612
		7-10 y	65-400		424-2612
		10-15 y	65-400		424-2612
		>15 y	65-400		424-2612
Ceruloplasmin			mg/L		g/L
	P	Cord (term)	50-330	0.001	0.050-0.33
		Birth-4 mo	150-560		0.15-0.56
		Adult (male)	220-400		0.22-0.40
		Adult (female), no contraceptive	250-600		0.25-0.60
		Adult (female), contraceptives (estrogen)	270-660		0.27-0.66
		Adult, pregnant female	300-1200		0.30-1.20
			mg/dL		g/L
	S	Adult (20-60 y)	20-60	0.01	0.2-0.6
Chloride (Cl)	S, P		mEq/L		mmol/L
		Cord	96-104	1.0	96-104
		Premature	95-110		95-110
		0-30 d	98-113		98-113
		Adult	98-107		98-107
		>90 y	98-111		98-111
			mEq/d		mmol/d
	U, 24 h	Infant	2-10		2-10
		Child <6 y	15-40		15-40
		6-10 y			
		M	36-110		36-110
		F	18-74		18-74
		10-14 y			
		M	64-176		64-176
		F	36-173		36-173
		Adult	110-250		110-250
		>60 y	95-195		95-195
	Sweat (iontophoresis)		mEq/L		mmol/L
		Infancy			
		≤6 months age			
		Cystic fibrosis unlikely	≤29	1.0	≤29
		Intermediate	30 to 59		30 to 59
		Indicative of cystic fibrosis	≥60 mmol/L		≥60 mmol/L
		Beyond infancy			
		≥6 months age			
		Cystic fibrosis unlikely	≤39		≤39
		Intermediate	40 to 59		40 to 59
		Indicative of cystic fibrosis	≥60		≥60

Continued

TABLE 50-1   Reference Intervals and Values—cont'd

Analyte	Specimen	Condition		Conventional Units	Conversion Factor	SI Units
						REFERENCE INTERVALS
Cholesterol				mg/dL 5th-95th percentile		mmol/L 5th-95th percentile
	S	0-4 y	M	114-203	0.0259	2.96-5.26
			F	112-200		2.90-5.18
		5-9 y	M	125-189		3.23-4.89
			F	131-197		3.39-5.10
		10-14 y	M	124-204		3.21-5.29
			F	125-205		3.24-5.31
		15-19 y	M	118-191		3.06-4.95
			F	119-208		3.08-5.39
		20-24 y	M	118-212		3.06-5.49
			F	121-237		3.14-6.14
		25-29 y	M	130-234		3.37-6.06
			F	130-231		3.37-5.99
		30-34 y	M	142-258		3.68-6.68
			F	133-227		3.45-5.87
		35-39 y	M	147-267		3.81-6.92
			F	139-249		3.60-6.45
		40-44 y	M	150-260		3.89-6.74
			F	146-259		3.78-6.71
		45-49 y	M	163-275		4.22-7.12
			F	148-268		3.83-6.94
		50-54 y	M	156-274		4.04-7.10
			F	163-281		4.22-7.28
		55-59 y	M	161-280		4.17-7.25
			F	167-294		4.33-7.61
		60-64 y	M	163-287		4.22-7.43
			F	172-300		4.46-7.77
		65-69 y	M	166-288		4.30-7.46
			F	167-291		4.33-7.54
		>69 y	M	144-265		3.73-6.87
			F	173-280		4.48-7.25
	Coronary heart disease risk					
	Child	Desirable		<170	0.0259	<4.4
		Borderline high		170-199		4.40-5.15
		High		>199		>5.15
	Adult	Desirable		<200		<5.18
		Borderline high		200-239		5.18-6.19
		High		>239		>6.19
Cholinesterase (37 °C)				U/L		μkat/L
	S	Male		40-78	0.017	0.68-1.33
		Female		33-76		0.56-1.29
Chorionic gonadotropin intact molecule				mIU/mL		IU/L
	S	Male and nonpregnant female		<5.0	1.0	<5.0
		Female				
		Pregnancy (weeks of gestation)				
		4 wk		5-100		5-100
		5 wk		200-3000		200-3000
		6 wk		10,000-80,000		10,000-80,000
		7-14 wk		90,000-500,000		90,000-500,000
		15-26 wk		5000-80,000		5000-80,000
		27-40 wk		3000-15,000		3000-15,000
				Values based on the Second International Standard for CG		
		Trophoblastic disease		>100,000		>100,000

TABLE 50-1   Reference Intervals and Values—cont'd

Analyte	Specimen	Condition	REFERENCE INTERVALS Conventional Units	Conversion Factor	SI Units
Chorionic gonadotropin intact molecule, cont'd	U		Negative		Negative
			One half of pregnancies are detected on the first day of the missed menstrual period		One half of pregnancies are detected on the first day of the missed menstrual period
Chromium			µg/L		nmol/L
	WB (Hep)		0.7-28.0	19.23	14-538
	S		0.1-0.2		2-3
			µg/d		nmol/d
	U, 24 h		0.1-2.0		1.9-38.4
			µg/L		nmol/L
	RBC		20-36		384-692
Chymotrypsin (37 °C)	F		12 U/g stool	1	12 U/g stool
Citric acid					mmol/mol creatinine
	U	0-1 mo			<1046
		1-6 mo			104-268
		6 mo-5 y			0-656
		>5 y			87-639
Cobalt			µg/L		nmol/L
	S		0.11-0.45	16.97	1.9-7.6
	U		1-2		17.0-34.0
			µg/kg		nmol/kg
	RBC		16-46		272-781
Complement C3	S		mg/dL		g/L
		Adult (20-60 y)	90-180	0.01	0.9-1.8
Complement C4	S		mg/dL		g/L
		Adult (20-60 y)	10-40		0.1-0.4
Copper	S		µg/dL		µmol/L
		Birth-6 mo	20-70	0.157	3.14-10.99
		Deficiency	<30		<5
		6 y	90-190		14.13-29.83
		12 y	80-160		12.56-25.12
		Adult			
		Male	70-140		10.99-21.98
		Female	80-155		12.56-24.34
		Deficiency	50		8
		Pregnancy, at term	118-302		18.53-47.41
		Blacks	Blacks 8%-12% higher		Blacks 8%-12% higher
	U, 24 h	Adults	<60 µg/24 h	0.0157	1.0 µmol/24 h
		Wilson disease	>200 µg/24 h		>3 µmol/24 h
Cortisol, free			µg/dL		nmol/L
	S	0800 h	0.6-1.6	27.6	17-44
		1600 h	0.2-0.9		6-25
			ng/mL		nmol/L
	Sal	0700 h	1.4-10.1	2.76	4-30
		2200 h	0.7-2.2		2-6
			µg/d		nmol/d
	U, 24 h	Child			
		1-10 y	2-27		6-74
		2-11 y	1-21		3-58

Continued

TABLE 50-1   Reference Intervals and Values—cont'd

Analyte	Specimen	Condition	REFERENCE INTERVALS Conventional Units	Conversion Factor	SI Units
Cortisol, free, cont'd		11-20 y	5-55		14-152
		12-16 y	2-38	2.76	6-105
		Adult			
		Extracted	20-90		55-248
		Unextracted	75-270		207-745
Cortisol, total			µg/dL		nmol/L
	S	Cord blood	5-17	27.6	138-469
		Infant (1-7 d)	2-11		55-304
		Child (1-16 y)			
		0800 h	3-21		83-580
		Adult			
		0800 h	5-23		138-635
		1600 h	3-16		83-441
		2000 h	<50% of 0800 values		<50% of 0800 values
C-Reactive Protein (CRP)	S		mg/dL		mg/L
		Adult (20-60 y)	<0.5	10	<5
CRP (high-sensitivity)	S		mg/L		mg/L
		American males	0.3-8.6	1.0	0.3-8.6
		White American males	0.2-12.3		0.2-12.3
		African American males	0.1-8.2		0.1-8.2
		Mexican American males	0.2-6.3		0.2-6.3
		European males	0.3-8.6		0.3-8.6
		Japanese males	<7.8		<7.8
		American females	0.2-9.1		0.2-9.1
		European females	0.3-8.8		0.3-8.8
Creatine kinase (CK)	S		U/L		µkat/L
IFCC, 37 °C		Male	46-171	0.017	0.78-2.90
		Female	34-145		0.58-2.47
Creatine kinase isoenzymes	S	Fraction 2 (MB)	<5.0 µg/L	1.0	<5.0 µg/L
		Relative index	<3.9%	0.01	<0.039
Creatinine enzymatic					
	S		mg/dL		µmol/L
		0-1 y	0.04-0.33	88.4	4-29
		2-5 y	0.04-0.45		4-40
		6-9 y	0.20-0.52		18-46
		10 y	0.22-0.59		19-52
		Adult male	0.62-1.10		55-96
		Adult female	0.45-0.75		40-66
Jaffe	S		mg/dL		µmol/L
		Cord	0.6-1.2	88.4	53-106
		Newborn (1-4 d)	0.3-1.0		27-88
		Infant	0.2-0.4		18-35
		Child	0.3-0.7		27-62
		Adolescent	0.5-1.0		44-88
		18-60 y			
		Male	0.9-1.3		80-115
		Female	0.6-1.1		53-97
		60-90 y			
		Male	0.8-1.3		71-115
		Female	0.6-1.2		53-106
		>90 y			
		Male	1.0-1.7		88-150
		Female	0.6-1.3		53-115

TABLE 50-1	Reference Intervals and Values—cont'd				

			REFERENCE INTERVALS		
Analyte	**Specimen**	**Condition**	**Conventional Units**	**Conversion Factor**	**SI Units**
IDMS traceable	S		mg/dL	88.4	μmol/L
		Male	0.72-1.18		64 to 104
		Female	0.55-1.02		49-90
Jaffe, manual	U, 24 h		mg/kg/d		μmol/kg/d
		Infant	8-20	8.84	71-177
		Child	8-22		71-194
		Adolescent	8-30		71-265
		Adult			
		Male	14-26		124-230
		Female	11-20		97-177
	U, excretion		mg/kg/day		μmol/kg/day
		Male	14 to 26		124 to 230
		Female	11 to 20		97 to 177
Creatinine clearance (*see* Glomerular filtration rate)					
C-Telopeptide	S		ng/L		ng/L
		Men	<1009	1.0	<1009
		Premenopausal women	<574		<574
			mg/mol creatinine		mg/mol creatinine
	U	Men	0-505		0-505
		Premenopausal women	0-476		0-476
Cyanide	WB (Ox)		mg/L		μmol/L
		Nonsmokers	<0.2	38.5	<7.7
		Smokers	<0.4		<15.4
		Nitroprusside therapy	Up to 100 without toxicity		Up to 3850
		Toxic	>1		>38.5
Dehydroepiandrosterone, unconjugated			ng/dL		nmol/L
	S	Children			
		6-9 y, M	13-187	0.0347	0.45-6.49
		6-9 y, F	18-189		0.62-6.55
		10-11 y, M	31-205		1.07-7.11
		10-11 y, F	112-224		3.88-7.77
		12-14 y, M	83-258		2.88-8.95
		12-14 y, F	98-360		3.40-12.5
		Adult			
		Male	180-1250		6.25-43.4
		Female	130-980		4.51-34.0
Dehydroepiandrosterone sulfate			μg/dL		μmol/L
	S	Children			
		1-5 d, M	12-254	0.027	0.3-6.9
		1-5 d, F	10-248		0.3-6.7
		1 mo-5 y, M	1-41		0.03-1.1
		1 mo-5 y, F	5-55		0.1-1.5
		6-9 y, M	2.5-145		0.07-3.9
		6-9 y, F	2.5-140		0.07-3.8
		10-11 y, M	15-115		0.4-3.1
		10-11 y, F	15-260		0.4-7.0
		12-17 y, M	20-555		0.5-15.0
		12-17 y, F	20-535		0.5-14.4
		Pubertal levels, Tanner stage			
		1 M	5-265		0.1-7.2
		1 F	5-125		0.1-3.4
		2 M	15-380		0.4-10.3

Continued

TABLE 50-1 Reference Intervals and Values—cont'd

			REFERENCE INTERVALS		
Analyte	**Specimen**	**Condition**	**Conventional Units**	**Conversion Factor**	**SI Units**
Dehydroepiandrosterone, cont'd		2 F	15-150	0.027	0.4-4.0
		3 M	60-505		1.6-13.6
		3 F	20-535		0.5-14.4
		4 M	65-560		1.8-15.1
		4 F	35-485		0.9-13.1
		5 M	165-500		4.4-13.5
		5 F	75-530		2.0-14.3
		Adults			
		18-30 y, M	125-619		3.4-16.7
		18-30 y, F	45-380		1.2-10.3
		31-50 y, M	5-532		1.6-12.2
		31-50 y, F	12-379		0.8-10.2
		51-60 y, M	20-413		0.5-11.1
		61-83 y, M	10-285		0.3-7.7
		Postmenopausal, F	30-260		0.8-7.0
11-Deoxycortisol			ng/dL		nmol/L
	S	Cord blood	295-554	0.0289	9-16
		Children and adults	20-158		0.6-4.6
Deoxypyridinoline			µmol/mol creatinine		µmol/mol creatinine
	U	Men	2.3-5.4	1.0	2.3-5.4
		Premenopausal women	3.0-7.4		3.0-7.4
Dihydrotestosterone			ng/dL		nmol/L
	S	Child, prepubertal	<3	0.0344	<0.10
		Adult, M	30-85		1.03-2.92
		Adult, F	4-22		0.14-0.76
Dopamines	P, S	Normotensive adults	pg/mL		nmol/L
L-Dopa			1042-2366	0.0051	5.3-12.0
DHPG (3, 4-dihydroxyphenylglycol)			797-1208	0.0059	4.7-7.1
Estradiol (E$_2$)			pg/mL		pmol/L
	S	Children			
		1-5 y, M	3-10	3.69	11-37
		1-5 y, F	5-10		18-37
		6-9 y, M	3-10		11-37
		6-9 y, F	5-60		18-220
		10-11 y, M	5-10		18-37
		10-11 y, F	5-300		18-1100
		12-14 y, M	5-30		18-110
		12-14 y, F	24-410		92-1505
		15-17 y, M	5-45		18-165
		12-17 y, F	40-410		147-1505
		Adults			
		Male	10-50		37-184
		Female			
		Early follicular phase	20-150		73-550
		Late follicular phase	40-350		147-1285
		Midcycle	150-750		550-2753
		Luteal phase	30-450		110-1652
		Postmenopausal	<21		<74
		Pubertal levels, Tanner stage			
		1, M	3-15		11-35
		1, F	5-10		18-37
		2, M	3-10		11-37
		2, F	5-115		18-422
		3, M	5-15		18-55

TABLE 50-1 | Reference Intervals and Values—cont'd

Analyte	Specimen	Condition	REFERENCE INTERVALS Conventional Units	Conversion Factor	SI Units
Estradiol (E$_2$), cont'd		3, F	5-180	3.69	18-660
		4, M	3-40		11-147
		4, F	25-345		92-1267
		5, M	15-45		55-165
		5, F	25-410		92-1505
Estriol, free (unconjugated, uE$_3$)			ng/mL		nmol/L
	S	Males and nonpregnant females	<2.0	3.47	<6.9
		Pregnancy (weeks of gestation)			
		16	0.30-1.05		1.04-3.64
		18	0.63-2.30		2.19-7.98
		34	5.3-18.3		18.4-63.5
		35	5.2-26.4		18.0-91.6
		36	8.2-28.1		28.4-97.5
		37	8.0-30.1		27.8-104.0
		38	8.6-38.0		29.8-131.9
		39	7.2-34.3		25.0-119.0
		40	9.6-28.9		33.3-100.3
	Amf	Pregnancy (weeks of gestation)			
		16-20	1.0-3.2		3.5-11
		20-24	2.1-7.8		7.3-27
		24-28	2.1-7.8		7.3-27
		28-32	4.0-13.6		14-47
		32-36	3.6-15.5		12-54
		36-38	4.6-18.0		16-62
		38-40	5.4-19.8		19-69
Estriol, total (E$_3$)			ng/mL		nmol/L
	S	Pregnancy (weeks of gestation)			
		34	38-140	3.47	132-486
		35	31-140		108-486
		36	35-330		121-1145
		37	45-260		156-902
		38	48-350		167-1215
		39	59-570		205-1978
		40	95-460		330-1596
			µg/d		nmol/d
	U, 24 h	Male	1.0-11.0	3.47	3.5-38.2
		Female			
		Follicular phase	0-15.0		0-52.0
		Ovulatory phase	13.0-54.0		45.1-187.4
		Luteal phase	8.0-60.0		27.8-208.2
		Postmenopausal	0-11.0		0-38.2
		Pregnancy			
		1st trimester	0-800		0-2776
		2nd trimester	800-12,000		2776-41,640
		3rd trimester	5000-50,000		17,350-173,500
			ng/mL		nmol/L
	Amf	Weeks of gestation			
		21-32	5-50		17-174
		33-35	90-240		312-833
		36-41	150-213		521-739

Continued

TABLE 50-1 Reference Intervals and Values—cont'd

Analyte	Specimen	Condition	REFERENCE INTERVALS Conventional Units	Conversion Factor	SI Units
Estrone (E$_1$)			pg/mL		pmol/L
	S	Male	15-65	3.69	55-240
		Female			
		Early follicular phase	15-150		55-555
		Late follicular phase	100-250		370-925
		Luteal phase	15-200		55-740
		Postmenopausal	15-55		55-204
Ethanol	WB (Ox)		mg/dL		mmol/L
		Impairment	50-100	0.217	11-22
		Depression of CNS	>100		>21.7
		Fatalities reported	>400		>86.8
	U				0.4-17
Ferritin	S		ng/mL		µg/L
		Newborn	25-200	1.0	25-200
		1 mo	200-600		200-600
		2-5 mo	50-200		50-200
		6 mo-15 y	7-140		7-140
		Adult			
		Male	20-250		20-250
		Female	10-120		10-120
α-Fetoprotein (AFP)	S		mg/L		g/L
		Fetal, 1st trimester	200-400	0.01	2.0-4.0
		Cord blood	<5		<0.05
			ng/mL		µg/L
		Child, 1 y	<30	1.0	<30
		Adult (85% of population)	<8.5		<8.5
		Adult (100% of population)	<15		<15
			ng/mL		µg/L
	Maternal serum	Weeks of gestation	(median)		(median)
		14	25.6		25.6
		15	29.9		29.9
		16	34.8		34.8
		17	40.6		40.6
		18	47.3		47.3
		19	55.1		55.1
		20	64.3		64.3
		21	74.9		74.9
	S	Tumor marker	ng/mL		µg/L
		Early marker	10-20		10-20
		Cancer	>1000		>1000
			µg/mL		mg/L
	Amf	Weeks of gestation	(median)		(median)
		15	16.3		16.3
		16	14.5		14.5
		17	13.4		13.4
		18	12.0		12.0
		19	10.7		10.7
		20	8.1		8.1
Fluoride	S		mg/L		µmol/L
			0.2-3.2	52.6	10.5-168
Folate			µg/L		nmol/L
	S		2.6-12.2	2.265	6.0-28.0
	Erythrocyte		103-411		237-948
	S Deficiency		<1.4		<3.2
	Erythrocyte deficiency		<110		<252

TABLE 50-1 Reference Intervals and Values—cont'd

Analyte	Specimen	Condition	Conventional Units	Conversion Factor	SI Units
Follicle-stimulating hormone (FSH)			mIU/mL		IU/L
	S	Males (23-70 y)	1.4-15.4	1.0	1.4-15.4
		Female			
		Follicular phase	1.4-9.9		1.4-9.9
		Midcycle peak	0.2-17.2		0.2-17.2
		Luteal phase	1.1-9.2		1.1-9.2
		Postmenopausal	19.3-100.6		19.3-100.6
Fructosamine	S	Child	5% below adult levels		
		Adult	205-285 μmol/L	1.0	205-285 μmol/L
Glomerular filtration rate (endogenous)			mL/min/1.73 m²		mL/s/m²
	S or P and U	Males			
		17-24 y	93-131	0.00963	0.90-1.26
		25-34 y	78-146		0.75-1.41
		35-44 y	74-138		0.71-1.33
		45-54 y	74-129		0.72-1.24
		55-64 y	69-122		0.67-1.18
		65-74 y	61-114		0.59-1.10
		75-84 y	52-102		0.50-0.98
		Females			
		40-49 y	65-123		0.63-1.19
		50-59 y	58-110		0.56-1.06
		60-69 y	50-111		0.48-1.07
		70-79 y	46-105		0.44-1.01
		80+ y	48-85		0.46-0.82
Glucagon			ng/L		ng/L
	P (Hep or EDTA)	Adult	70-180	1.0	70-180
	Amf	Midgestation	23-63		23-63
		Term	41-193		41-193
Glucose	S, fasting		mg/dL		mmol/L
		Cord	45-96	0.0555	2.5-5.3
		Premature	20-60		1.1-3.3
		Neonate	30-60		1.7-3.3
		Newborn			
		1 d	40-60		2.2-3.3
		>1 d	50-80		2.8-4.5
		Child	60-100		3.3-5.6
		Adult	74-100		4.1-5.6
		>60 y	82-115		4.6-6.4
		>90 y	75-121		4.2-6.7
	WB (Hep)	Adult	65-95		3.5-5.3
	CSF	Infant, child	60-80		3.3-4.5
		Adult	40-70		2.2-3.9
	U		1-15		0.1-0.8
	U, 24 h		<0.5 g/d	5.55	<2.8 mmol/d
Glucose-6-phosphate dehydrogenase (G-6-PD) in erythrocytes, WHO, and ICSH	WB (ACD, EDTA, or Hep)		7.9-16.3 U/g Hb	64.5	510-1050 U/ mmol Hb
			230-470 U/10¹² RBC	10⁻³	0.23-0.47 nU/RBC
			2.69-5.53 U/mL RBC	1.0	2.69-5.53 kU/L RBC
γ-Glutamyltransferase IFCC, 37 °C	S		U/L		μkat/L
		Male	<55	0.017	<0.94
		Female	<38		<0.65

Continued

TABLE 50-1   Reference Intervals and Values—cont'd

Analyte	Specimen	Condition		Conventional Units	Conversion Factor	SI Units
Glutaric acid						mmol/mol creatinine
	U					0.5-13
Glycated hemoglobin (HbA$_{1c}$)				% Total Hb		mmol/mol
	WB (EDTA, Hep, or Ox)	Cut off for diagnosis.		<6.5		20 to 38
		Reference Interval (NGSP)		4-5.6		
Growth hormone	S			ng/mL		µg/L
		Basal		2-5	1.0	2-5
		Insulin tolerance test		>10		>10
		Arginine		>7.5		>7.5
		L-Dopa		>7.5		>7.5
Haptoglobin	S			mg/dL		g/L
		Children		20-160	0.01	0.2-1.6
		Adult (20-60 y)		30-200		0.3-2.0
High-density lipoprotein cholesterol (HDL-C)				mg/dL		mmol/L
				5th-95th percentile		5th-95th percentile
	S	5-9 y	M	38-75	0.0259	0.99-1.94
			F	36-73		0.93-1.89
		10-14 y	M	37-74		0.96-1.92
			F	37-70		0.96-1.82
		15-19 y	M	30-63		0.78-1.63
			F	35-74		0.91-1.92
		20-24 y	M	30-63		0.78-1.63
			F	33-79		0.86-2.05
		25-29 y	M	31-63		0.81-1.63
			F	37-83		0.96-2.15
		30-34 y	M	28-63		0.73-1.63
			F	36-77		0.94-2.00
		35-39 y	M	29-62		0.75-1.61
			F	34-82		0.88-2.13
		40-44 y	M	27-67		0.70-1.74
			F	34-88		0.88-2.28
		45-49 y	M	30-64		0.78-1.66
			F	34-87		0.88-2.26
		50-54 y	M	28-63		0.73-1.63
			F	37-92		0.96-2.39
		55-59 y	M	28-71		0.73-1.84
			F	37-91		0.96-2.36
		60-64 y	M	30-74		0.78-1.92
			F	38-92		0.99-2.39
		65-69 y	M	30-75		0.78-1.95
			F	35-96		0.91-2.49
		>69 y	M	31-75		0.80-1.95
			F	33-92		0.86-2.39
	ATP III classification			mg/dL		g/L
	S	Low		<40	0.01	<0.40
		High		>59		>0.59
Homocysteine, total				µmol/L		µmol/L
	S, P	Folate supplemented diet				
		<15 y		<8	1.0	<8
		15-65 y		<12		<12
		>65 y		<16		<16
		No folate supplementation				
		<15 y		<10		<10
		15-65 y		<15		<15
		>65 y		<20		<20

TABLE 50-1 Reference Intervals and Values—cont'd

Analyte	Specimen	Condition	REFERENCE INTERVALS Conventional Units	Conversion Factor	SI Units
Homogentisic acid					mmol/mol creatinine
	U				<11
Homovanillic acid (HVA)	U, 24 h		mg/d		µmol/d
		3-6 y	1.4-4.3	5.49	8-24
		6-10 y	2.1-4.7		12-26
		10-16 y	2.4-8.7		13-48
		16-83 y	1.4-8.8		8-48
	U		mg/g creatinine		mmol/mol creatinine
		0-6 mo	<40	0.571	<23
		6 mo-5 y	<10		<6
		3-6 y	5.4-15.5		3.4-9.6
		6-10 y	4.4-11.5		2.7-7.1
		10-16 y	3.3-10.3		2.0-6.4
3-Hydroxybutyric acid					mmol/mol creatinine
	U	0-5 y			<6
		>5 y			<11
5-Hydroxyindoleacetic acid			ng/L		nmol/L
	P		5.2-13.4	5.23	27-70
			mg/g creatinine		mmol/mol creatinine
	U	0-5 y	<21	0.592	<13
		>5 y	<16		<10
17-Hydroxyprogesterone			ng/dL		nmol/L
		Cord blood	900-5000	0.03	27.3-151.5
		Premature	26-568		0.8-17.0
		Newborn, 3 d	7-77		0.2-2.7
		Prepubertal child	3-90		0.1-2.7
		Puberty			
		Tanner stage			
		1. Male	3-90		0.1-2.7
		Female	3-82		0.1-2.5
		2. Male	5-115		0.2-3.5
		Female	11-98		0.3-3.0
		3. Male	10-139		0.3-4.2
		Female	11-155		0.3-4.7
		4. Male	29-180		0.9-5.4
		Female	18-230		0.5-7.0
		5. Male	24-175		0.7-5.3
		Female	20-267		0.6-8.0
		Adults			
		Male	27-199		0.8-6.0
		Female			
		Follicular phase	15-70		0.4-2.1
		Luteal phase	35-290		1.0-8.7
		Pregnancy	200-1200		6.0-36.0
		Post ACTH	<320		<9.6
		Postmenopausal	<70		<2.1
Immunoglobulin A			mg/dL		g/L
	S	Neonate (4 d)	0-2.2	0.01	0.0-0.02
		Adult (20-60 y)	70-400		0.7-4.0
		Adult (>60 y)	90-410		0.9-4.1
	CSF		0.0-0.6		0.0-0.006
	Saliva		<11		<0.11
Immunoglobulin D			IU/mL		kIU/L
	S	Adult (20-60 y)	0-160	1.0	0-160
			ng/mL		µg/L
			0-384	1.0	0-384

Continued

TABLE 50-1 Reference Intervals and Values—cont'd

Analyte	Specimen	Condition	Conventional Units	Conversion Factor	SI Units
Immunoglobulin E			kIU/L		µg/L
	S	Adult (20-60 y)	0-160	2.4	0-380
Immunoglobulin G			mg/dL		g/L
	S	Newborn (4 d)	700-1480	0.01	7.0-14.8
		Adult (20-60 y)	700-1600		7.0-16.0
		Adult (>60 y)	600-1560		6.0-15.6
	CSF		0-5.5		0-0.055
Immunoglobulin M			mg/dL		g/L
	S	Newborn (4 d)	5-30	0.01	0.05-0.30
		Adult (20-60 y)	40-230		0.4-2.3
		Adult (>60 y)	30-360		0.3-3.6
	CSF		0.0-1.3		0.0-0.013
Inhibin A			pg/mL		ng/L
	S	Males	1.0-3.6	1.0	1.0-3.6
		Females (Cycling; days of cycle)			
		Early follicular phase (−14 to −10 d)	5.5-28.2		5.5-28.2
		Midfollicular phase (−9 to −4 d)	7.9-34.5		7.9-34.5
		Late follicular phase (−3 to −1 d)	19.5-102.3		19.5-102.3
		Midcycle (day 0)	49.9-155.5		49.9-155.5
		Early luteal (1 to 3 d)	35.9-132.7		35.9-132.7
		Midluteal (4 to 11 d)	13.2-159.6		13.2-159.6
		Late luteal (12 to 14 d)	7.3-89.9		7.3-89.9
		IVF, peak levels	354-1690		354-1690
		PCOS, ovulatory	5.7-16.0		5.7-16.0
		Postmenopausal	1.0-3.9		1.0-3.9
	S, maternal	Pregnancy, wk	pg/mL (median)		ng/L (median)
		15	174		174
		16	170		170
		17	173		173
		18	182		182
		19	198		198
		20	222		222
Insulin	S		µIU/mL		pmol/L
		Adult	2-25	6.00	12-150
Insulin-like growth factor-I (IGF-1)	S		ng/mL		µg/L
		1-2 y			
		Male	31-160	1.0	31-160
		Female	11-206		11-206
		3-6 y			
		Male	16-288		16-288
		Female	70-316		70-316
		7-10 y			
		Male	136-385		136-385
		Female	123-396		123-396
		11-12 y			
		Male	136-440		136-440
		Female	191-462		191-462
		13-14 y			
		Male	165-616		165-616
		Female	286-660		286-660

TABLE 50-1   Reference Intervals and Values—cont'd

Analyte	Specimen	Condition		Conventional Units	Conversion Factor	SI Units
				REFERENCE INTERVALS		
Insulin-like growth factor-I (IGF-1), cont'd		15-18 y				
		Male		134-836		134-836
		Female		152-660		152-660
		19-25 y				
		Male		202-433		202-433
		Female		231-550		231-550
		Adult (25-85 y)				
		Male		135-449		135-449
		Female		135-449		135-449
Insulin-like growth factor-II (IGF-2)	S			ng/mL		μg/L
		Child				
		Prepubertal		334-642	1.0	334-642
		Pubertal		245-737		245-737
		Adult		288-736		288-736
		GH deficiency		51-299		51-299
Iron (see Chapter 28)						
l-Lactate				mg/dL		mmol/L
	WB (Hep)	At bed rest				
		Venous		5-12	0.111	0.56-1.39
		Arterial		3-7		0.36-0.75
	CSF	Child		16-17		1.78-1.88
	U, 24 h	Adult		496-1982 mg/d	0.0111	5.5-22 mmol/d
						mmol/mol creatinine
		0-1 mo				46-348
		1-6 mo				57-346
		6 mo-5 y				21-38
		>5 y				20-101
	Gastric fluid			Negative		Negative
Lactate dehydrogenase (LD)				U/L		μkat/L
Total L → P	S	24 mo-12 y		180-360	0.017	3.1-6.1
IFCC, 37 °C		12-60 y		125-220		2.1-3.7
Lead				μg/dL		μmol/L
	WB (Hep)	Child		<25	0.0483	<1.21
		Adult		<25		<1.21
		Toxic		>99		>4.78
				μg/L		μmol/L
	U, 24 h			<80		<0.39
Lipase, 37 °C				U/L		μkat/L
	S	Adult		<38	0.017	<0.65
Low-density lipoprotein cholesterol (LDL-C)				mg/dL		mmol/L
				5th-95th percentile		5th-95th percentile
	S	5-9 y	M	63-129	0.0259	1.63-3.34
			F	68-140		1.76-3.63
		10-14 y	M	64-133		1.66-3.44
			F	68-136		1.76-3.52
		15-19 y	M	62-130		1.61-3.37
			F	59-137		1.53-3.55
		20-24 y	M	66-147		1.53-3.81
			F	57-159		1.48-4.12
		25-29 y	M	70-165		1.81-4.27
			F	71-164		1.84-4.25
		30-34 y	M	78-185		2.02-4.79
			F	70-156		1.81-4.04

Continued

TABLE 50-1 | Reference Intervals and Values—cont'd

| | | | | REFERENCE INTERVALS | | |
| | | | | Conventional Units | Conversion Factor | SI Units |
Analyte	Specimen	Condition				
Low-density lipoprotein cholesterol (LDL-C), cont'd		35-39 y	M	81-189		2.10-4.90
			F	75-172		1.94-4.45
		40-44 y	M	87-186		2.25-4.82
			F	74-174		1.92-4.51
		45-49 y	M	97-202		2.51-5.23
			F	79-186		2.05-4.82
		50-54 y	M	89-197		2.31-5.10
			F	88-201		2.28-5.21
		55-59 y	M	88-203		2.28-5.26
			F	89-210		2.31-5.44
		60-64 y	M	83-210		2.15-5.44
			F	100-224		2.59-5.81
		65-69 y	M	98-210		2.54-5.44
			F	92-221		2.39-5.73
		>69 y	M	88-186		2.28-4.82
			F	96-206		2.49-5.34
	Risk coronary heart disease			mg/dL		mmol/L
		Optimal		<100	0.0259	<2.59
		Near/above optimal		100-129		2.59-3.34
		Borderline high		130-159		3.37-4.12
		High		160-189		4.15-4.90
		Very high		>189		>4.90
L/S ratio	Amf			Ratio		Ratio
		State of fetal maturity				
		Immature		<1.5	1.0	<1.5
		Transitional		1.6-2.4		1.6-2.4
		Mature		>2.5		>2.5
		Diabetic		>2.5		>2.5
Luteinizing hormone (LH)				mIU/mL		IU/L
		Males (23-70 y)		1.2-7.8	1.0	1.2-7.8
		Female				
		Follicular phase		1.7-15.0		1.7-15.0
		Midcycle peak		21.9-56.6		21.9-56.6
		Luteal phase		0.6-16.3		0.6-16.3
		Postmenopausal		14.2-52.3		14.2-52.3
α_2-Macroglobulin	S			mg/dL		g/L
		Adult (20-60 y)		130-300	0.01	1.3-3.0
Magnesium AAS				mg/dL		mmol/L
	S	Newborn, 2-4 d		1.5-2.2	0.4114	0.62-0.91
		5 mo-6 y		1.7-2.3		0.70-0.95
		6-12 y		1.7-2.1		0.70-0.86
		Adults		1.7 to 2.4		0.66 to 1.07
				mg/24h		mEq/24h
	U, 24 h			12-291	0.083	1.0-24.0
Magnesium, free	S			mmol/L		mmol/L
				0.45-0.60	1.0	0.45-0.60
Manganese				µg/L		nmol/L
	WB (Hep)			5-15	18.0	90-270
	S			0.5-1.3		9-24
	U, collect in metal free container			0.5-9.8		9.1-178
		Toxic conc.		>19		>342
Mercury				µg/L		nmol/L
	WB (EDTA)			0.6-59	4.99	3.0-294.4
	U, 24 h			<20		<99.8

TABLE 50-1 | Reference Intervals and Values—cont'd

Analyte	Specimen	Condition	REFERENCE INTERVALS Conventional Units	Conversion Factor	SI Units
Mercury, cont'd		Toxic conc.	>150		>748.5
		Lethal conc.	>800		>3992
Metanephrines					
Free normetanephrine	S, P		pg/mL		nmol/L
		Hypertensive adults	24-145	0.0054	0.13-0.79
		Normotensive adults	18-101		0.10-0.55
		Normotensive children	22-83		0.12-0.45
Metanephrine	S, P		pg/mL		nmol/L
		Hypertensive adults	12-72	0.0050	0.06-0.37
		Normotensive adults	12-67		0.06-0.34
		Normotensive children	10-95		0.05-0.48
Total normetanephrine	S, P		pg/mL		nmol/L
		Hypertensive adults	755-5623	0.0054	4.1-30.7
		Normotensive adults	624-3041		3.4-16.6
		Normotensive children	851-2398		4.7-13.1
Metanephrine	S, P		pg/mL		nmol/L
		Hypertensive adults	327-2042	0.0050	1.7-10.4
		Normotensive adults	328-1837		1.7-9.3
		Normotensive children	380-1995		1.9-10.1
Metanephrines (total)					
Metanephrine	U, 24 h		µg/d		nmol/d
		0-3 mo	5.9-37	5.07	30-188
		4-6 mo	6.1-42		31-213
		7-9 mo	12-41		61-210
		10-12 mo	8.5-101		43-510
		1-2 y	6.7-52		34-264
		2-6 y	11-99		56-501
		6-10 y	54-138		275-701
		10-16 y	39-242		200-1231
		Adult	74-297		375-1506
Metanephrine	U		µg/g creatinine		mmol/mol creatinine
		0-3 mo	202-708	0.574	116-407
		4-6 mo	156-572		89-328
		7-9 mo	150-526		86-302
		10-12 mo	148-651		85-374
		1-2 y	40-526		23-302
		2-6 y	74-504		42-289
		6-10 y	121-319		69-183
		10-16 y	46-307		26-176
Normetanephrine	U, 24 h		µg/d		nmol/d
		0-3 mo	47-156	5.46	257-852
		4-6 mo	31-111		171-607
		7-9 mo	42-109		230-595
		10-12 mo	23-103		127-562
		1-2 y	32-118		175-647
		2-6 y	50-111		274-604
		6-10 y	47-176		255-964
		10-16 y	53-290		289-1586
		Adult	105-354		573-1933
Normetanephrine	U		µg/g creatinine		mmol/mol creatinine
		0-3 mo	1535-3355	0.617	947-2070
		4-6 mo	737-2194		454-1354
		7-9 mo	592-1046		365-645
		10-12 mo	271-1117		167-689
		1-2 y	350-1275		216-787

Continued

TABLE 50-1 Reference Intervals and Values—cont'd

Analyte	Specimen	Condition	Conventional Units	Conversion Factor	SI Units
		2-6 y	104-609		64-376
		6-10 y	103-452		63-279
		10-16 y	96-411		59-254
Methanol			mg/L		mmol/L
	WB (F⁻/Ox)		<1.5	0.0312	<0.05
		Toxic	>200		>6.24
	U	Occup. exp.	<50		<1.56
			ppm		mmol/L
	Breath		0.8		0.03
		Occup. exp.	2.5		0.08
Methemoglobin (MetHb)			g/dL		µmol/L
	WB (EDTA, Hep, or ACD)		0.06-0.24	155	9.3-37.2
			% of total Hb		Mass fraction of total Hb
			0.04-1.52	0.01	0.0004-0.0152
β₂-Microglobulin			mg/dL (mean)		mg/L (mean)
	S	Neonates	0.30	10	3.0
		0-59 y	0.19		1.9
		60-69 y	0.21		2.1
		>70 y	0.24		2.4
Molybdenum			µg/L		nmol/L
	S		0.1-3.0	10.42	1.0-31.3
	U, 24 h		40-60 µg/d		416-625 nmol/d
Mucin-like carcinoma-associated antigen (MCA)			U/mL		kU/L
	S		<14	1.0	<14
Niacin			mg/d		µmol/d
	U, 24 h		2.4-6.4	7.30	17.5-46.7
Nickel			µg/L		nmol/L
	S or P (Hep)		0.14-1.0	17	2.4-17.0
	WB		1.0-28.0		17-476
			µg/d		nmol/d
	U, 24 h		0.1-10		2-170
N-telopeptide			nmol BCE/L		nmol BCE/L
	S	Men	5.4-24.2	1.0	5.4-24.2
		Premenopausal women	6.2-19.0		6.2-19.0
			nmol BCE/mmol creatinine		nmol BCE/mmol creatinine
	U	Men	3-63		3-63
		Premenopausal women	5-65		5-65
Nuclear matrix protein 22 (NMP-22)			U/mL		kU/L
	S		<10	1.0	<10
Orotic acid					mmol/mol creatinine
	U	0-1 mo			1.4-5.3
		1-6 mo			1.0-3.2
		6 mo-5 y			0.5-3.3
		>5 y			0.4-1.2
Osteocalcin			ng/mL		µg/L
	S	Adult male	3.0-13.0	1.0	3.0-13.0
		Adult female			
		Premenopausal	0.4-8.2		0.4-8.2
		Postmenopausal	1.5-11.0		1.5-11.0
Oxalic acid					mmol/mol creatinine
	U	0-1 mo			51-931
		1-6 mo			7-567

TABLE 50-1   Reference Intervals and Values—cont'd

Analyte	Specimen	Condition	REFERENCE INTERVALS Conventional Units	Conversion Factor	SI Units
Oxalic acid, cont'd		6 mo-5 y			7-352
		>5 y			<188
2-Oxoglutaric acid					mmol/mol creatinine
	S	0-1 mo			22-567
		1-6 mo			63-552
		6 mo-5 y			36-103
		>5 y			41-82
Oxygen, partial pressure (PO_2)			mm Hg		kPa
	Cord blood				
	Arterial		5.7-30.5	0.133	0.8-4.0
	Venous		17.4-41.0		2.3-5.5
	WB, arterial				
		Birth	8-24		1.06-3.19
		5-10 min	33-75		4.39-9.96
		30 min	31-85		4.12-11.31
		1 h	55-80		7.32-10.64
		1 d	54-95		7.18-12.64
		2 d-60 y	83-108		11.04-14.36
		>60 y	>80		>10.64
		>70 y	>70		>9.31
		>80 y	>60		>7.98
		>90 y	>50		>6.65
Oxygen, saturation (sO_2)	WB, arterial		Percent saturation		Fraction saturation
		Newborn	40-90	0.01	0.40-0.90
		Thereafter	94-98		0.94-0.98
Oxytocin	P, EDTA		µU/mL		mU/L
		Males	1.1-1.9	1.0	1.0-1.9
		Females			
		Nonpregnant	1.0-1.8		1.0-1.8
		Second stage of labor	3.2-5.3		3.2-5.3
Pantothenic acid	WB		344-583 µg/L	0.0046	1.57-2.66 µmol/L
	U, 24 h		1-15 mg/d	4.53	5-68 µmol/d
Parathyroid hormone, intact	S		pg/mL		ng/L
			10-65	1.0	10-65
		1-84 fragment	6-40	1.0	6-40
Parathyroid hormone-related peptide (PTHrP)	S		pmol/L <1.4		pmol/L <1.4
pH (37 °C)	WB, arterial		pH		pH
		Cord blood			
		Arterial	7.18-7.38	1.0	7.18-7.38
		Venous	7.25-7.45		7.25-7.45
		Newborn			
		Premature, 48 h	7.35-7.50		7.35-7.50
		Full term			
		Birth	7.11-7.36		7.11-7.36
		5-10 min	7.09-7.30		7.09-7.30
		30 min	7.21-7.38		7.21-7.38
		1 h	7.26-7.49		7.26-7.49
		1 d	7.29-7.45		7.29-7.45
		Children, adults			
		Arterial	7.35-7.45		7.35-7.45
		Venous	7.32-7.43		7.32-7.43
		Adults			
		60-90 y	7.31-7.42		7.31-7.42
		>90 y	7.26-7.43		7.26-7.43

Continued

TABLE 50-1   Reference Intervals and Values—cont'd

Analyte	Specimen	Condition	REFERENCE INTERVALS Conventional Units	Conversion Factor	SI Units
Phosphate	S, P (Hep)		mg/dL		mmol/L
		Children	4.0-7.0	0.323	1.29-2.26
		Adults	2.5-4.5		0.81-1.45
	U, 24 h		g/d		mmol/d
		Adults	0.4-1.3	32.3	12.9-42.0
Phosphatase, acid tartrate resistant 37 °C	S		U/L		μkat/L
		Children	3.4-9.0	0.017	0.05-0.15
		Adult	1.5-4.5		0.03-0.08
Phosphatase, alkaline IFCC, 37 °C	S		U/L		μkat/L
		4-15 y (male)	54-369	0.017	0.91-6.23
		4-15 y (female)	54-369		0.91-6.23
		20-50 y (male)	53-128		0.90-2.18
		20-50 y (female)	42-98		0.71-1.67
		>60 y (male)	56-119		0.95-2.02
		>60 y (female)	53-141		0.90-2.40
Phosphatase, alkaline (bone specific, by immunoabsorption)			U/L		U/L
	S	Men	15.0-41.3	1.0	15.0-41.3
		Premenopausal women	11.6-29.6		11.6-29.6

Phosphatase, alkaline isoenzymes

Percentage of total activity	<1 y	1-15 y	Adult	Pregnant women	Postmenopausal women
Biliary	3-6	2-5	1-3	1-3	0-12
Liver	20-34	22-34	17-35	5-17	17-48
Bone	20-30	21-30	13-19	8-14	8-21
Placental	8-19	5-17	13-21	53-69	7-15
Renal	1-3	0-1	0-2	3-6	0-2
Intestinal	0-2	0-1	0-1	0-1	0-1
Fraction activity	<1 y	1-15 y	Adult	Pregnant women	Postmenopausal women
Biliary	0.03-0.06	0.02-0.05	0.01-0.03	0.01-0.03	0.0-0.12
Liver	0.20-0.34	0.22-0.34	0.17-0.35	0.05-0.17	0.17-0.48
Bone	0.20-0.30	0.21-0.30	0.13-0.19	0.08-0.14	0.08-0.21
Placental	0.08-0.19	0.05-0.17	0.13-0.21	0.53-0.69	0.07-0.15
Renal	0.01-0.03	0.0-0.01	0.0-0.02	0.03-0.06	0.0-0.02
Intestinal	0.0-0.02	0.0-0.01	0.0-0.01	0.0-0.01	0.0-0.01

Analyte	Specimen	Condition	Conventional Units	Conversion Factor	SI Units
Porphobilinogen			mg/L		μmol/L
	U, 24 h		<2.26	4.42	<10
Porphyrins, total					nmol/L
	U, 24 h				20-320
					nmol/L g dry weight
	Feces				10-200
					μmol/L erythrocytes
	Erythrocytes				0.4-1.7
Potassium (K)			mEq/L		mmol/L
	S	Premature cord	5.0-10.2	1.0	5.0-10.2
		Premature, 48 h	3.0-6.0		3.0-6.0
		Newborn cord	5.6-12.0		5.6-12.0
		Newborn	3.7-5.9		3.7-5.9
		Infant	4.1-5.3		4.1-5.3
		Child	3.4-4.7		3.4-4.7
		Adults	3.5-5.1		3.5-5.1
	P (Hep)	Male	3.5-4.5		3.5-4.5
		Female	3.4-4.4		3.4-4.4

TABLE 50-1   Reference Intervals and Values—cont'd

Analyte	Specimen	Condition	Conventional Units	Conversion Factor	SI Units
Potassium (K), cont'd			mEq/d		mmol/d
	U, 24 h	6-10 y			
		Male	17-54		17-54
		Female	8-37		8-37
		10-14 y			
		Male	22-57		22-57
		Female	18-58		18-58
		Adult	25-125		25-125
Proinsulin	S		pmol/L		pmol/L
			1.1-6.9	1.0	1.1-6.9
Prolactin			ng/mL		μg/L
	S	Cord blood	45-539	1.0	45-539
		Children, Tanner stage 1			
		Male	<10		<10
		Female	3.6-12		3.6-12
		Children, Tanner stage 2-3			
		Male	<6.1		<6.1
		Female	2.6-18		2.6-18
		Children, Tanner stage 4-5			
		Male	2.8-11		2.8-11
		Female	3.2-20		3.2-20
		Adult			
		Male	3.0-14.7		3.0-14.7
		Female	3.8-23.0		3.8-23.0
		Pregnancy, third trimester	95-473		95-473
Propionylcarnitine					μmol/L
	P	0-7 d			0.07-1.85
		8 d-7 y			0.17-1.27
		>7 y			0.17-1.49
	WB spots				0.55-8.01
	Bile spots				0.36-8.10
					mmol/mol creatinine
	U	0-7 d			0.01-0.20
		8 d-7 y			0.01-1.20
		>7 y			0.00-0.06
Prostate-specific antigen (PSA)			ng/mL		μg/L
	S	Males			
		40-49 y	0-2.5	1.0	0-2.5
		50-59 y	0-3.5		0-3.5
		60-69 y	0-4.5		0-4.5
		70-79 y	0-6.5		0-6.5
Protein, total			g/dL		g/L
	S	Cord	4.8-8.0	10	48-80
		Premature	3.6-6.0		36-60
		Newborn	4.6-7.0		46-70
		1 wk	4.4-7.6		44-76
		7 mo-1 y	5.1-7.3		51-73
		1-2 y	5.6-7.5		56-75
		>2 y	6.0-8.0		60-80
		Adult, ambulatory	6.4-8.3		64-83
		Adult, recumbent	6.0-7.8		60-78
		>60 y	Lower by <0.2		Lower by <2.0
			mg/dL		mg/L
	U, 24 h	Adult	1-14		10-140

Continued

TABLE 50-1   Reference Intervals and Values—cont'd

Analyte	Specimen	Condition	REFERENCE INTERVALS Conventional Units	Conversion Factor	SI Units
Protein, total, cont'd		Excretion	mg/d		g/d
		Adult	<100	0.001	<0.1
		Pregnancy	<150		<0.15
			mg/dL		g/L
	CSF	Premature	15-130	10	150-1300
		Full-term newborn	40-120		400-1200
		<1 mo	20-80		200-800
		>1 mo	15-40		150-400
		Ventricular fluid	5-15		50-150
		Cisternal fluid	15-25		150-250
			g/dL		g/L
	Amf	Early pregnancy	0.2-1.7		2.0-17.0
		Late pregnancy	0.175-0.705		1.8-7.1
Retinol-binding protein (RBP)			mg/dL		g/L
	S	Birth	1.1-3.4	0.01	0.011-0.034
		6 mo	1.8-5.0		0.018-0.05
		Adult	3.0-6.0		0.03-0.06
Reverse triiodothyronine (rT$_3$)			ng/dL		nmol/L
	S	Cord (>37 wk)	130-300	0.0154	2.00-4.62
		Children			
		1 d	83-194		1.28-2.99
		2 d	107-209		1.65-3.22
		3 d	102-166		1.57-2.56
		1 mo-20 y	10-35		0.15-0.54
		Adult	10-28		0.15-0.43
		Maternal serum			0.17-0.51
		(15-40 wk)	11-33		
		Amniotic serum			
		(17-22 wk)	163-599		2.51-9.22
Riboflavin (vitamin B$_2$)			µg/dL		nmol/L
	S		4-24	26.6	106-638
	Erythrocytes		10-50		266-1330
	U		>80 µg/g creatinine	0.3	>24 µmol/mol creatinine
	U, 24 h		>100 µg/d	2.66	>266 nmol/L
Selenium			µg/L		µmol/L
	S	Neonates	<8.0 (deficiency)	0.0127	<0.10 (deficiency)
		<2 y	16-71		0.2-0.9
		2-4 y	40-103		0.5-1.3
		4-16 y	55-134		0.7-1.7
		Adults	63-160		0.8-2.0
	WB (Hep)		58-234		0.74-2.97
	U, 24 h		7-160		0.09-2.03
		Toxic conc.	>400		>5.08
Serotonin			ng/mL		nmol/L
	WB		50-200	5.68	280-1140
			ng/10^9 platelets		nmol/10^9 platelets
	WB		88-1230	0.00568	0.5-7.0
			ng/mL		nmol/L
	S		30-200	5.68	170-1140
			µg/d		nmol/d
	U, 24 h		60-167		340-950
			µg/g creatinine		µmol/mol creatinine
	U		38-101	0.653	25-66
			ng/mL		nmol/L
	CSF		1.0-2.1	5.68	5.7-12.0

TABLE 50-1   Reference Intervals and Values—cont'd

Analyte	Specimen	Condition	Conventional Units	Conversion Factor	SI Units
Serotonin, cont'd			ng/10⁹ platelets		nmol/10⁹ platelets
	Platelet-rich serum		370-970	0.00568	2.07-5.55
	Isolated platelets		ng/10⁹ platelets		nmol/10⁹ platelets
			154-1086		0.88-6.16
	Platelet-poor plasma		ng/mL		nmol/L
			0-3.60	5.68	0-22.5
Sodium (Na)	S		mEq/L		mmol/L
		Premature cord	116-140	1.0	116-140
		Premature, 48 h	128-148		128-148
		Newborn cord	126-166		126-166
		Newborn	133-146		133-146
		Infant	139-146		139-146
		Child	138-145		138-145
		Adult	136-145		136-145
		>90 y	132-146		132-146
	U, 24 h		mEq/d		mmol/L
		6-10 y			
		Male	41-115		41-115
		Female	20-69		20-69
		10-14 y			
		Male	63-177		63-177
		Female	48-168		48-168
		Adult			
		Male	40-220		40-220
		Female	27-287		27-287
Testosterone, bioavailable	S		ng/dL		nmol/L
		Adult, M	66-417	0.0347	2.29-14.5
		Adult, F	0.6-5.0		0.02-0.17
Testosterone, free	S		pg/mL		pmol/L
		Cord, M	5-22	3.47	17.4-76.3
		Cord, F	4-19		13.9-55.5
		Newborn, 1-15 d, M	1.5-31.0		5.2-107.5
		Newborn, 1-15 d, F	0.5-2.5		1.7-8.7
		1-3 mo, M	3.3-8.0		11.5-62.5
		1-3 mo, F	0.1-1.3		0.3-4.5
		3-5 mo, M	0.7-14.0		2.4-48.6
		3-5 mo, F	0.3-1.1		1.0-3.8
		5-7 mo, M	0.4-4.8		1.4-16.6
		5-7 mo, F	0.2-0.6		0.7-2.1
		6-9 y, M	0.1-3.2		0.3-11.1
		6-9 y, F	0.1-0.9		0.3-3.1
		10-11 y, M	0.6-5.7		2.1-19.8
		10-11 y, F	1.0-5.2		3.5-18.0
		12-14 y, M	1.4-156		4.9-541
		12-14 y, F	1.0-5.2		3.5-18.0
		15-17 y, M	80-159		278-552
		15-17 y, F	1.0-5.2		3.5-18.0
		Adult, M	50-210		174-729
		Adult, F	1.0-8.5		3.5-29.5
Testosterone, total			ng/dL		nmol/L
	S	Cord, M	13-55	0.0347	0.45-1.91
		Cord, F	5-45		0.17-1.56
		Premature, M	37-198		1.28-6.87
		Premature, F	5-22		0.17-0.76
		Newborn, M	75-400		2.6-13.9
		Newborn, F	20-64		0.69-2.22

Continued

TABLE 50-1 | Reference Intervals and Values—cont'd

Analyte	Specimen	Condition	REFERENCE INTERVALS Conventional Units	Conversion Factor	SI Units
Testosterone, total, cont'd		Prepubertal child			
		1-5 mo, M	1-177		0.03-6.14
		1-5 mo, F	1-5		0.03-0.17
		6-11 mo, M	2-7		0.07-0.24
		6-11 mo, F	2-5		0.07-0.17
		1-5 y, M	2-25		0.07-0.87
		1-5 y, F	2-10		0.07-0.35
		6-9 y, M	3-30		0.10-1.04
		6-9 y, F	2-20		0.07-0.69
		Puberty, Tanner stage			
		1, M	2-23		0.07-0.80
		1, F	2-10		0.07-0.35
		2, M	5-70		0.17-2.43
		2, F	5-30		0.17-1.04
		3, M	15-280		0.52-9.72
		3, F	10-30		0.35-1.04
		4, M	105-545		3.64-18.91
		4, F	15-40		0.52-1.39
		5, M	65-800		9.19-27.76
		5, F	10-40		0.35-1.39
		Adult, M	260-1000		9-34.72
		Adult, F	15-70		0.52-2.43
Thallium			µg/L		nmol/L
	WB (Hep)		<5	4.89	<24.5
			mg/L		µmol/L
		Toxic	0.1-8.0		0.5-390
			µg/L		nmol/L
	U, 24 h		<2.0		<9.8
			mg/L		µmol/L
		Toxic	1.0-20.0		4.9-97.8
Thiocyanate			mg/dL		µmol/L
	S	Nonsmokers	<0.4	172.4	<69
		Smokers	<1.2		<207
		Nitroprusside therapy	0.6-2.9		103-500
		Toxic	>5		>862
Thyroglobulin (Tg)			ng/mL		µg/L
	S	Adult euthyroid	3-42	1.0	3-42
		Athyroidic patient	<5		<5
Thyrotropin (thyroid-stimulating hormone) (TSH)			µIU/mL		mIU/L
	S	Premature, 28-36 wk	0.7-27.0	1.0	0.7-27.0
		Cord blood (>37 wk)	2.3-13.2		2.3-13.2
		Children			
		Birth-4 d	1.0-39.0		1.0-39.0
		2-20 wk	1.7-9.1		1.7-9.1
		21 wk-20 y	0.7-6.4		0.7-6.4
		Adults			
		21-54 y	0.4-4.5		0.4-4.5
		55-87 y	0.4-4.5		0.4-4.5
		Pregnancy			
		First trimester	0.3-4.5		0.3-4.5
		Second trimester	0.5-4.6		0.5-4.6
		Third trimester	0.8-5.2		0.8-5.2
	Whole blood (heel puncture)	Newborn screen	<20		<20

TABLE 50-1   Reference Intervals and Values—cont'd

Analyte	Specimen	Condition	REFERENCE INTERVALS Conventional Units	Conversion Factor	SI Units
Thyroxine-binding globulin (TBG)			mg/dL		mg/L
	S	Cord	3.6-9.6	10	36-96
		Children			
		4-12 mo	3.1-5.6		31-56
		1-5 y	2.9-5.4		29-54
		5-10 y	2.5-5.0		25-50
		10-15 y	2.1-4.6		21-46
		Adult			
		Male	1.2-2.5		12-25
		Female	1.4-3.0		14-30
		Female (oral contraceptive)	1.5-5.5		15-55
Thyroxine (T$_4$)			µg/dL		nmol/L
	S	Cord	7.4-13.1	12.9	95-168
		Children			
		1-3 d	11.8-22.6		152-292
		1-2 wk	9.9-16.6		126-214
		1-4 mo	7.2-14.4		93-186
		4-12 mo	7.8-16.5		101-213
		1-5 y	7.3-15.0		94-194
		5-10 y	6.4-13.3		83-172
		1-15 y	5.6-11.7		72-151
		Adults (15-60 y)			
		Males	4.6-10.5		59-135
		Females	5.5-11.0		65-138
		>60 y	5.0-10.7		65-138
		Newborn screen			
		1-5 d	>7.5		>97
		6 d	>6.5		>84
Thyroxine, free (FT$_4$)			ng/dL		pmol/L
	S	Newborns (1-4 d)	2.2-5.3	12.9	28.4-68.4
		Children (2 wk-20 y)	0.8-2.0		10.3-25.8
		Adults (21-87 y)	0.8-2.7		10.3-34.7
		Pregnancy			
		First trimester	0.7-2.0		9.0-25.7
		Second and third trimesters	0.5-1.6		6.4-20.6
Thyroxine, free index (FT$_4$)			µg/dL		nmol/L
	S	Cord	6.0-13.2	12.9	77-170
		Infants			
		1-3 d	9.9-17.5		128-226
		1 wk	7.5-15.1		97-195
		1-12 mo	5.0-13.0		65-168
		Children			
		1-10 y	5.4-12.8		70-165
		Pubertal child and adult	4.2-13.0		54-168
Transferrin			mg/dL		g/L
	S	Newborn	117-250	0.01	1.17-2.5
		20-60 y	200-360		2.0-3.6
		>60 y	160-340		1.6-3.4
Transketolase, erythrocyte	Erythrocytes		0.75-1.30 U/g Hb	64.53	48.4-83.9 kU/mol Hb
Transthyretin (prealbumin)	S		mg/dL		g/L
		Adult (20-60 y)	20-40	0.01	0.2-0.4
Triglycerides			mg/dL 5th-95th percentile		mmol/L 5th-95th percentile

Continued

| TABLE 50-1 | Reference Intervals and Values—cont'd | | | | | |

Analyte	Specimen	Condition	REFERENCE INTERVALS		
			Conventional Units	Conversion Factor	SI Units
Triglycerides, cont'd	S	0-4 y, M	29-99	0.0113	0.33-1.12
		0-4 y, F	34-112		0.39-1.27
		5-9 y, M	28-85		0.32-0.96
		5-9 y, F	32-126		0.36-1.43
		10-14 y, M	33-111		0.38-1.26
		10-14 y, F	39-120		0.44-1.36
		15-19 y, M	38-143		0.43-1.62
		15-19 y, F	36-126		0.41-1.43
		20-24 y, M	44-165		0.50-1.87
		20-24 y, F	37-168		0.42-1.90
		25-29 y, M	45-204		0.57-2.31
		25-29 y, F	42-159		0.48-1.80
		30-34 y, M	46-253		0.52-2.86
		30-34 y, F	40-163		0.45-1.84
		35-39 y, M	52-316		0.59-3.57
		35-39 y, F	40-205		0.45-2.32
		40-44 y, M	56-318		0.63-3.60
		40-44 y, F	45-191		0.51-2.16
		45-49 y, M	56-279		0.64-3.16
		45-49 y, F	44-223		0.50-2.52
		50-54 y, M	63-313		0.71-3.54
		50-54 y, F	53-223		0.60-2.52
		55-59 y, M	60-261		0.68-2.95
		55-59 y, F	59-279		0.67-3.16
		60-64 y, M	56-240		0.64-2.71
		60-64 y, F	57-256		0.65-2.90
		65-69 y, M	54-256		0.61-2.90
		65-69 y, F	56-260		0.64-2.94
		>69 y, M	63-239		0.71-2.70
		>69 y, F	60-289		0.68-3.27
	Recommended cutoff points		mg/dL		mmol/L
		Normal	<150	0.0113	<1.70
		High	150-199		1.70-2.25
		Hypertriglyceridemic	200-499		2.26-5.64
		Very high	>499		>5.64
Triiodothyronine (T_3), free			pg/dL		pmol/L
	S	Cord	15-391	0.0154	0.2-6.0
		Child and adult	210-440		3.2-6.8
		Pregnancy	200-380		3.1-5.9
Triiodothyronine (T_3), total			ng/dL		nmol/L
	S	Cord (>37 wk)	5-141	0.0154	0.08-2.17
		Children			
		1-3 d	100-740		1.54-11.40
		1-11 mo	105-245		1.62-3.77
		1-5 y	105-269		1.62-4.14
		6-10 y	94-241		1.44-3.28
		11-15 y	82-213		1.26-3.28
		Adolescents			
		16-20 y	80-210		1.23-3.23
		Adults			
		20-50 y	70-204		1.08-3.14
		50-90 y	40-181		0.62-2.79
		Pregnancy			
		First trimester	81-190		1.25-2.93
		Second and third trimesters	100-260		1.54-4.00

TABLE 50-1   Reference Intervals and Values—cont'd

Analyte	Specimen	Condition	Conventional Units	Conversion Factor	SI Units
Troponins (see Chapter 34)					
Urea nitrogen	S		mg/dL		mmol/L
		Cord	21-40	0.357	7.5-14.3
		Premature (1 wk)	3-25		1.1-8.9
		Newborn	4-12		1.4-4.3
		Infant/child	5-18	0.357	1.8-6.4
		Adult	6-20		2.1-7.1
		Adult >60 y	8-23		2.9-8.2
			g/d		mol/d
	U, 24 h		10-20	0.0357	0.43-0.71
Uric acid					
Phosphotungstate	S		mg/dL		mmol/L
		Adult			
		Male	4.4-7.6	0.059	0.26-0.45
		Female	2.3-6.6		0.13-0.39
		>60 y			
		Male	4.2-8.0		0.25-0.47
		Female	3.5-7.3		0.20-0.43
Uricase		Child	2.0-5.0	0.060	0.12-0.32
		Adult			
		Male	3.5-7.2		0.21-0.42
		Female	2.6-6.0		0.15-0.35
	U, 24 h		mg/d		mmol/L
		Purine-free diet			
		Male	<420	0.0059	<2.48
		Female	Slightly lower		Slightly lower
		Low-purine diet			
		Male	<480		<2.83
		Female	<400		<2.36
		High-purine diet	<1000		<5.90
		Average diet	250-750		1.48-4.43
	U				mmol/mol creatinine
		0-1 mo			359-2644
		1-6 mo			359-2644
		6 mo-5 y			185-1134
		>5 y			199-1034
Vanillylmandelic acid (VMA)	U, 24 h		mg/d		μmol/d
		3-6 y	1-2.6	5.05	5-13
		6-10 y	2.0-3.2		10-16
		10-16 y	2.3-5.2		12-26
		16-83 y	1.4-6.5		7-33
	U		mg/g creatinine		mmol/mol creatinine
		0-1 mo	<27	0.571	<16
		1-6 mo	<19		<11
		6 mo-5 y	<13		<8
		3-6 y	4.0-10.8		2.3-6.2
		6-10 y	4.0-7.5		2.3-4.3
		10-16 y	3.0-8.8		1.7-5.0
Vitamin A	S		μg/dL		μmol/L
		1-6 y	20-40	0.0349	0.70-1.40
		7-12 y	26-49		0.91-1.71
		13-19 y	26-72		0.91-2.51
		Adult	30-80		1.05-2.8
Vitamin B$_1$ (thiamine diphosphate)	WB		90-140 nmol/L	1.0	90-140 nmol/L
	Erythrocytes		280-590 ng/g Hb	0.146	40.3-85.0 μmol/mol Hb

Continued

TABLE 50-1	Reference Intervals and Values—cont'd

Analyte	Specimen	Condition	REFERENCE INTERVALS		
			Conventional Units	Conversion Factor	SI Units
Vitamin B$_2$ (*see* Riboflavin)					
Vitamin B$_6$	P (EDTA)		ng/mL		nmol/L
			5-30	4.046	20-121
		Deficiency	<5		<20.2
Vitamin B$_{12}$			ng/L		pmol/L
	S		206-678	0.733	151-497
		Acceptable (WHO)	>201		>147
		Deficiency (WHO)	<150		<110
Vitamin C (ascorbic acid)			mg/dL		µmol/L
	S		0.4-1.5	56.78	23-85
		Deficiency	<0.2		<11
	Leukocyte		20-53 µg/10^8 leukocytes	0.057	1.14-3.01 fmol/10^8 leukocytes
		Deficiency	<10 µg/10^8 leukocytes		<0.57 fmol/10^8 leukocytes
Vitamin D	S		ng/mL		nmol/L
25(OH)D			10-65	2.50	25-162
			pg/mL		pmol/L
1,25(OH)$_2$D			15-60	2.4	36-144
Vitamin E	S		mg/dL		µmol/L
		Premature neonates	0.1-0.5	23.2	2.3-11.6
		Children	0.3-0.9		7-21
		Teenagers	0.6-1.0		14-23
		Adults	0.5-1.8		12-42
Vitamin K	S		ng/mL		nmol/L
			0.13-1.19	2.22	0.29-2.64
Zinc			µg/dL		µmol/L
	S		80-120	0.153	12-18
		Deficiency	<30		<5
	U, 24 h		0.2-1.3 mg/24 h	15.3	3-21 µmol/24 h

AAS, Atomic absorption spectroscopy *ACD,* Acid Citrate Dextrose anticoagulant; *ACTH,* adrenocorticotropic hormone; *ALT,* alanine aminotransferase; *AST,* aspartate aminotransferase; *ATP,* adenosine triphosphate; *BCE,* bone collagen equivalents; *BNP,* B-type natriuretic peptide; *CK,* creatine kinase; Creatine phosphokinase MB isoenzyme; *GH,* growth hormone; *Hb,* Hemoglobin; *HbCO,* carbon monoxide hemoglobin; *HPLC,* high-performance liquid chromatography; *ICSH,* International Council for Standardization in Hematology; *IDMS,* Isotope Dilution Mass Spectrometry; *IFCC,* International Federation of Clinical Chemistry and Laboratory Medicine; *IVF,* in vitro fertilization; *PCOS,* polycystic ovary syndrome; *SGOT,* Serum glutamic oxaloacetic transaminase; *SGPT,* Serum glutamic pyruvic transaminase; *WHO,* World Health Organization.

TABLE 50-2	Therapeutic and Toxic Levels of Drugs

Therapeutic drug monitoring and detection of drug overdose have become increasingly important aspects of the role of the laboratory in patient care. The information given for drugs in this table has been gathered from published sources. These examples are intended to complement Chapter 30 of this book and do not represent all drugs for which drug testing may be useful. In addition, knowledge and drug measurement methodologies are continuously improving; therefore it may be necessary to supplement the information given here with information obtained from other sources as it becomes available for these and other drugs. Reliable drug analysis information depends on a well-coordinated sample collection, assay methodology characteristics, and patient-associated considerations, such as age, disease state, concomitant drug administration, and clinical procedures that the patient may have undergone. In practice, each organization *should have its own set of therapeutic and toxic levels for the drugs it measures.*

Many tests for therapeutic drugs require careful timing between administration and sample collection if the measured concentration of the measured drug is to be of optimal use clinically. Drugs are listed by their chemical or generic name, followed by an example of a commercial brand name for the drug (where appropriate). Unless otherwise indicated, target concentrations reflect steady-state, predose (trough) sampling. These targets, as well as toxic thresholds provided, are intended to serve as guidelines and should not be used to optimize drug dosing independently of clinical factors. See Chapter 30 for detailed information about therapeutic drug monitoring regarding these and additional drugs.

TABLE 50-2   Therapeutic and Toxic Levels of Drugs—cont'd

Conversion factors provided represent the free-base form of the parent drug only—not metabolites, unless otherwise indicated. Active metabolites are indicated for many drugs as "+," but therapeutic or toxic concentrations are not routinely provided. Note that calculated conversions to SI units are rounded, unless the value is less than 1.0. For convenience and to preserve space, standard abbreviations commonly used in laboratory medicine are used. Less common abbreviations and some nonstandard abbreviations are given in the following paragraph. Whenever plasma or whole blood is indicated, the recommended preservative is presumed to be ethylenediaminetetraacetic acid (EDTA), although heparin may be acceptable. Separator gel blood collection tubes for serum or plasma are not recommended for drug testing because of possible adsorption of drugs and/or drug metabolites to the gel itself, contributing to the risk of falsely low drug concentrations. Some drugs (e.g., busulfan, olanzapine) are labile and require special handling. Consult laboratory validation data and current literature sources for specific handling recommendations and anticipated stability guidelines.

Abbreviation	Term
AUC	Area under the plasma drug concentration versus time curve
EDTA	Ethylenediaminetetraacetic acid
MIC	Minimum inhibitory concentration
P	Plasma
S	Serum
Therap	Therapeutic
U	Urine
WB	Whole blood

Drug	Specimen	Status	REFERENCE VALUES		
			Conventional Units	Conversion Factor	SI Units
Acetaminophen (Tylenol)	S or P		μg/mL		μmol/L
		Therap	10-30	6.62	66-199
		Toxic			
		4 h after dose	>200		>1324
		12 h after dose	>50		>331
Amikacin (Amikin)	S or P		μg/mL		μmol/L
		Therap			
		Peak	25-35	1.71	43-60
		Trough			
		Less severe infection	1-4		2-7
		Severe infection	4-8		7-14
		Toxic			
		Peak	>40		>68
		Trough	>10		>17
		Peak/MIC	>10		>17
Aminocaproic acid (Amicar)	S or P		μg/mL		μmol/L
		Therap			
		Trough	100-400	7.62	762-3048
Amiodarone (Cordarone)	S or P		μg/mL		μmol/L
		Therap	0.5-2.0	1.47	1-3
		Toxic	>2.5		>4
Amitriptyline (Elavil) + nortriptyline	S or P		ng/mL		nmol/L
		Therap	80-200	3.61	289-722
		Toxic	>300 (sum)		>1083
Amobarbital (Amytal) sodium	S or P		μg/mL		μmol/L
		Therap	1-5	4.03	4-20
		Toxic	>10		>40
Amoxapine (Asendin) +8-hydroxy amoxapine	S or P		ng/mL		nmol/L
		Therap	200-600	3.19	638-1914
		Toxic	>600		>1914
Amphetamine (Adderall)	S or P		ng/mL		nmol/L
		Therap	20-30	7.40	148-222
		Toxic	>200		>1480

Continued

TABLE 50-2   Therapeutic and Toxic Levels of Drugs—cont'd

Drug	Specimen	Status	REFERENCE VALUES Conventional Units	Conversion Factor	SI Units
Bromide as bromine	S or P		µg/mL		mmol/L
		Therap	750-1500	0.0125	9-19
		Toxic	>1250		>16
Bupropion (Wellbutrin, Zyban)	S or P		ng/mL		nmol/L
		Therap	25-100	3.62	91-362
		Toxic	>100		>362
Caffeine	S or P		µg/mL		µmol/L
		Therap	8-20	5.15	41-103
		Toxic	>20		>103
Carbamazepine (Tegretol)	S or P		µg/mL		µmol/L
		Therap	4-12	4.23	17-51
		Toxic	>15		>63
Carbamazepine-10,11-epoxide (carbamazepine metabolite)	S or P		µg/mL	3.97	µmol/L
		Therap	0.4-4		2-16
		Toxic	>8		>32
Carbenicillin (Geocillin)	S or P		µg/mL		µmol/L
		Therap	Dependent on MIC of specific organism	2.64	
		Toxic	>250 (neurotoxicity)		>660
Chloral hydrate (Noctec) as trichloroethanol	S or P		µg/mL		µmol/L
		Therap	2-12	6.69	13-80
		Toxic	>20		>134
Chloramphenicol sodium succinate (Chloromycetin)	S or P		µg/mL		µmol/L
		Therap	10-25	2.25	22-56
		Toxic	>25		>56
		Gray baby syndrome	>40		>124
Chlordiazepoxide (Librium) + nordiazepine	S or P		ng/mL		µmol/L
		Therap	700-1000	0.003	2-3
		Toxic	>5000		>17
Chlorpromazine (Thorazine)	S or P		ng/mL		nmol/L
		Therap			
		Adult	30-300	3.14	94-942
		Child	40-80		126-251
		Toxic	>750		>2355
Cimetidine (Tagamet)	S or P		µg/mL		µmol/L
		Therap			
		Trough	0.5-1.2	3.96	2-5
		Toxic	>1.3		>5
Ciprofloxacin (Cipro)	S or P		µg/mL		µmol/L
		Therap			
		Peak (oral dose)	0.5-1.5	3.02	2-5
		Peak (IV dose)	<5.0		<15
		Toxic	>5.0		>15
		Gram-positive AUC/MIC	>30		
		Gram-negative AUC/MIC	>125		

TABLE 50-2   Therapeutic and Toxic Levels of Drugs—cont'd

Drug	Specimen	Status	REFERENCE VALUES Conventional Units	Conversion Factor	SI Units
Clomipramine (Anafranil) + norclomipramine	S or P		ng/mL		nmol/L
		Therap	230-430	3.18	731-1431
		Toxic	>450 (sum)		>1431
Clonazepam (Klonopin)	S or P		ng/mL		nmol/L
		Therap	20-70	3.17	63-222
		Toxic	>80		>254
Clonidine (Catapres)	S or P		ng/mL		nmol/L
		Therap	1.0-2.0	4.35	4-9
Clorazepate (Tranxene) (*see* Nordiazepam)					
Clozapine (Clozaril)	S or P		ng/mL	3.06	nmol/L
		Therap	350-600		1071-1836
		Toxic	>1000		>3000
Codeine	S or P		ng/mL		nmol/L
		Therap	10-100	3.34	33-334
		Toxic	>1100		>3340
Cyclosporin A (Sandimmune)	WB		ng/mL		nmol/L
		Therap 12 h after dose	50-350	0.83	42-291
		Toxic	>350		>291
Delavirdine (Rescriptor)			µg/mL		µmol/L
	S or P	Therap			
		Trough	3-8	1.80	5-14
		Peak	14-16		25-29
		Toxic	>16		>29
Desipramine (Norpramin)	S or P		ng/mL		nmol/L
		Therap	100-300	3.75	375-1126
		Toxic	>300		>1125
Diazepam (Valium) + nordiazepine	S or P		ng/mL		nmol/L
		Therap	100-1000	3.51	351-3512
		Toxic	>5000		>17,559
Digitoxin	S or P		ng/mL		nmol/L
		Therap ≥8 h after dose	10-30	1.31	13-39
		Toxic	>45		>59
Digoxin (Lanoxin)	S or P		ng/mL		nmol/L
		Therap ≥12 h after dose	0.5-2.0	1.28	0.6-3
		In heart failure	0.5-0.8		0.6-1
		Toxic	>3.0		>3.8
Disopyramide (Norpace)	S or P		µg/mL		µmol/L
		Therap	2-5	2.95	6-15
		Toxic	>7		>21
Doxepin (Sinequan, Adapin) + nordoxepin	S or P		ng/mL		nmol/L
		Therap	50-150	3.58	179-537
		Toxic	>500		>1790
Efavirenz (Sustiva)	S or P		µg/mL		µmol/L
		Therap	1-4	3.16	3-13
		Toxic	>4		>13
Ephedrine (Ectasule)	S or P		µg/mL		µmol/L
		Therap	0.05-0.10	6.05	0.3-0.6
		Toxic	>2		>12
Ethchlorvynol (Placidyl)	S or P		µg/mL		µmol/L
		Therap	2-8	6.92	14-55
		Toxic	>20		>138

Continued

TABLE 50-2 Therapeutic and Toxic Levels of Drugs—cont'd

Drug	Specimen	Status	REFERENCE VALUES Conventional Units	Conversion Factor	SI Units
Ethosuximide (Zarontin)	S or P		µg/mL		µmol/L
		Therap	40-100	7.08	283-708
		Toxic	>150		>1062
Everolimus (Zortress)	WB		ng/mL		nmol/L
		Therap	3-15	1.04	3-16
		Toxic	>15		>16
Felbamate (Felbatol)	S or P		µg/mL		µmol/L
		Therap	30-60	4.20	126-252
		Toxic	>120		>504
Fenoprofen (Nalfon)	S or P		µg/mL		µmol/L
		Therap	20-65	4.12	82-268
Flecainide (Tambocor)	S or P		µg/mL		µmol/L
		Therap	0.2-1.0	2.41	0.5-2
		Toxic	>1.0		>2
5-Flucytosine (Ancobon)	S or P		µg/mL		µmol/L
		Peak	>25	7.75	>194
		Toxic	>100		>775
Fluoxetine (Prozac) + norfluoxetine	S or P		ng/mL		nmol/L
		Therap	120-500	3.23	388-1615
		Toxic	>1000		>3230
Fluphenazine (Modecate)	S or P		ng/mL		nmol/L
		Therap	1-10	2.29	3-30
		Toxic	>15		>35
Flurazepam (Dalmane)	S or P		µg/mL		µmol/L
		Toxic	>0.2	2.58	>0.5
Gabapentin (cNeurontin)	S or P		µg/mL		µmol/L
		Therap	2-20	5.84	12-117
		Toxic	>12		>70
Gentamicin (Garamycin)	S or P		µg/mL		µmol/L
		Therap			
		Peak	5-12	2.09	11-25
		Less severe infection	5-8		11-17
		Severe infection	8-10		17-21
		Trough			
		Less severe infection	<1		<2
		Moderate infection	<2		<4
		Severe infection	<4		<8
		Toxic			
		Peak	>10		>21
		Trough	>2		>4
		Peak/MIC	>10		>21
Glutethimide (Doriden)	S or P		µg/mL		µmol/L
		Therap	2-6	4.60	9-28
		Toxic	>5		>23
Haloperidol (Haldol)	S or P		ng/mL		nmol/L
		Therap	1-10	2.66	3-30
		Toxic	>15		>40
Hydromorphone (Dilaudid)	S or P		ng/mL		nmol/L
		Therap	1-3	3.50	4-11
		Toxic	>100		>350
Ibuprofen (Motrin)	S or P		µg/mL		µmol/L
		Therap	10-50	4.85	49-243
		Toxic	>200		>970

TABLE 50-2 Therapeutic and Toxic Levels of Drugs—cont'd

Drug	Specimen	Status	REFERENCE VALUES		
			Conventional Units	Conversion Factor	SI Units
Imipramine (Tofranil) + desipramine	S or P		ng/mL		nmol/L
		Therap	175-300	3.57	624-1071
		Toxic	>300 (sum)		>1071
Indinavir (Crixivan)	S or P		µg/mL		µmol/L
		Therap			
		Trough	>0.1	1.41	>0.14
		Peak	8-10		11-14
		Toxic	>10		>14
Isoniazid (Hyzyd, Nydrazid)	S or P		µg/mL		µmol/L
		Therap	1-7	7.29	7-51
		Toxic	>20		>146
Itraconazole (Sporanox) + hydroxyitraconazole	S or P		µg/mL		µmol/L
		Therap	>1.5	1.42	>2
Kanamycin (Kantrex)	S or P		µg/mL		µmol/L
		Therap			
		Peak	25-35	2.06	52-72
		Trough			
		Less severe infection	1-4		2-8
		Severe infection	4-8		8-17
		Toxic			
		Peak	>35		>72
		Trough	>10		>21
		Peak/MIC	>10		>21
Lamivudine (Epivir, 3TC)	S or P		µg/mL		µmol/L
		Therap	>0.4	4.36	>2
Lamotrigine (Lamictal)	S or P		µg/mL		µmol/L
		Therap	2.5-15	3.91	10-59
Levetiracetam (Keppra)	S or P		µg/mL		µmol/L
		Therap	12-46	5.88	71-270
Lidocaine (Xylocaine)	S or P		µg/mL		µmol/L
		Therap ≥45 min following bolus dose	1.5-5	4.27	6-21
		Toxic	>6		>26
Lithium (Eskalith)	S or P		mEq/L		mmol/L
		Therap	0.5-1.2	1.0	0.5-1
		Toxic	>1.2		>1
Lorazepam (Ativan)	S or P		ng/mL		nmol/L
		Therap dose	50-240	3.11	156-746
Maprotiline (Ludiomil)	S or P		ng/mL		nmol/L
		Therap	125-200	3.60	450-720
		Toxic	>300		>1080
Meperidine (Demerol)	S or P		ng/mL		nmol/L
		Therap	70-500	4.04	283-2020
		Toxic	>1000		>4004
Mephobarbital (Mebaral)	S or P		µg/mL		µmol/L
		Therap	1-7	4.06	4-28
		Toxic	>15		>61
Meprobamate (Equanil)	S or P		µg/mL		µmol/L
		Therap	6-12	4.58	28-55
		Toxic	>60		>275
Methadone (Dolophine)	S or P		ng/mL		nmol/L
		Therap	100-400	3.23	320-1280
		Toxic	>2000		>6460

Continued

TABLE 50-2   Therapeutic and Toxic Levels of Drugs—cont'd

Drug	Specimen	Status	REFERENCE VALUES Conventional Units	Conversion Factor	SI Units
Methamphetamine (Desoxyn)	S or P		µg/mL		µmol/L
		Therap	0.01-0.05	6.70	0.07-0.34
		Toxic	>0.5		>3
Methaqualone (Quaalude)	S or P		µg/mL		µmol/L
		Therap	2-3	4.00	8-12
		Toxic	>10		>40
Methotrexate (Trexall, Rheumatrex)	S or P		µmol/L		µmol/L
		Toxic			
		24 h after high-dose therapy	≥10	2.20	≥22
		48 h after high-dose therapy	≥1		≥2
		72 h after high-dose therapy	≥0.1		≥0.2
Methsuximide (Celontin) as normethsuximide	S or P		µg/mL		µmol/L
		Therap	10-40	5.29	53-212
		Toxic	>40		>212
Methyldopa (Aldomet)	S or P		µg/mL		µmol/L
		Therap	1-5	4.73	5-24
		Toxic	>7		>33
Methyprylon (Noludar)	S or P		µg/mL		µmol/L
		Therap	8-10	5.46	43-55
		Toxic	>50		273
Mexiletine (Mexitil)	S or P		µg/mL		µmol/L
		Therap	0.5-2	5.58	3-11
		Toxic	>2.0		>11
Morphine	S or P		ng/mL		nmol/L
		Therap	10-80	3.50	35-280
		Toxic	>200		>700
Mycophenolate mofetil (CellCept) as mycophenolic acid	S or P		µg/mL		µmol/L
		Therap	1.3-3.5	3.12	4-11
		Toxic	>12		>38
Nefazodone (Serzone)	S or P		ng/mL		nmol/L
		Therap	25-2500	2.13	53-5325
		Toxic	>2500		>5325
Nelfinavir (Viracept)	S or P		µg/mL		µmol/L
		Therap	>1	1.76	>2
		Toxic	>6		>11
Netilmicin (Netromycin)	S or P		µg/mL		µmol/L
		Therap			
		Peak			
		Less severe infection	5-8	2.10	10-17
		Severe infection	8-10		17-21
		Trough			
		Less severe infection	<1		<2
		Moderate infection	<2		<4
		Severe infection	<4		<8
		Toxic			
		Peak	>10		>21
		Trough	>2		>4

TABLE 50-2   Therapeutic and Toxic Levels of Drugs—cont'd

Drug	Specimen	Status	REFERENCE VALUES Conventional Units	Conversion Factor	SI Units
Nevirapine (Viramune)	S or P		µg/mL		µmol/L
		Therap	>3.5	3.76	<13.2
		Toxic	>12		>45.1
Nordiazepine, active metabolite of several benzodiazepines	S or P		ng/mL		nmol/L
	S or P	Therap	100-500	3.76	376-1880
		Toxic	>500		>1880
Nortriptyline (Aventyl)	S or P		ng/mL		nmol/L
		Therap	70-170	3.80	266-646
		Toxic	>300		>1140
Olanzapine (Zyprexa)	S or P		ng/mL		nmol/L
		Therap	20-80	3.20	64-256
		Toxic	>150		>480
Oxazepam (Serax)	S or P		µg/mL		µmol/L
		Therap	0.2-1.4	3.49	0.7-5
Oxcarbazepine (Trileptal) as monohy-droxyoxcarbazepine (MHD)	S or P		µg/mL		µmol/L
	S or P	Therap	3-35	3.97	12-139
		Toxic	>40		>159
Oxycodone (Percodan)	S or P		ng/mL		nmol/L
		Therap	10-100	3.17	32-317
		Toxic	>200		>634
Paraldehyde (Paral)	S or P		µg/mL		µmol/L
		Therap			
		Sedation	10-100	7.57	76-757
		Anesthesia	>200		>1514
		Toxic	>200		>1514
		Lethal	>500		>3785
Paroxetine (Paxil)	S or P		ng/mL		nmol/L
		Therap	30-120	3.04	91-365
Pentazocine (Talwin)	S or P		µg/mL		µmol/L
		Therap	0.05-0.2	3.5	0.2-0.7
		Toxic	>1.0		>4
Pentobarbital (Nembutal)	S or P		µg/mL		µmol/L
		Therap			
		Hypnotic	1-5	4.42	4-22
		Therap coma	20-50		88-221
		Toxic	>10		>44
Perphenazine (Apo-Perphenazine)	S or P		µg/mL		µmol/L
		Therap	0.6-2.4	2.48	2-6
		Toxic	>5		>12.4
Phenacetin	S or P		µg/mL		µmol/L
		Therap	1-30	5.58	6-167
		Toxic	50-250		279-1395
Phenobarbital (Luminal)	S or P		µg/mL		µmol/L
		Therap	10-40	4.31	43-173
		Toxic			
		Slowness, ataxia, nystagmus	35-80		151-345
		Coma, with reflexes	65-117		280-504
		Coma, without reflexes	>100		>431
Phensuximide (Milontin) + norphensuximide	S or P		µg/mL		µmol/L
		Therap	40-60	5.29	212-317

Continued

TABLE 50-2	Therapeutic and Toxic Levels of Drugs—cont'd

Drug	Specimen	Status	Conventional Units	Conversion Factor	SI Units
				REFERENCE VALUES	
Phenylbutazone (Butazolidin)	S or P		µg/mL		µmol/L
		Therap	50-100	3.24	162-324
		Toxic	>100		>324
Phenytoin (Dilantin)	S or P		µg/mL		µmol/L
		Therap	10-20	3.96	40-79
		Free	1.0-2.0		4-8
		Toxic	>20		>79
Posaconazole (Noxafil)	S or P		µg/mL		µmol/L
		Therap	>1.25	1.43	>2
Primidone (Mysoline) + phenobarbital	S or P		µg/mL		µmol/L
		Therap	5-10	4.58	23-46
		Toxic	>15		>69
Procainamide (Pronestyl) + N-acetylprocainamide (NAPA)	S or P		µg/mL		µmol/L
		Therap	4-8	4.25	17-34
			10-20 (NAPA)	3.61	36-72
		Toxic	>10		>43
			>40 (NAPA)		>144
Propafenone (Rythmol)	S or P		µg/mL		µmol/L
		Therap	0.5-2.0	2.93	1.5-6
		Toxic	>2		>6
Propoxyphene (Darvon)	S or P		µg/mL		µmol/L
		Therap	0.1-0.4	2.95	0.3-1
		Toxic	>0.5		>2
Propranolol (Inderal)	S or P		ng/mL		nmol/L
		Therap	20-100	3.86	77-386
Protriptyline (Vivactil)	S or P		ng/mL		nmol/L
		Therap	70-260	3.80	266-988
		Toxic	>500		>1900
Quetiapine (Seroquel)	S or P		mg/L		µmol/L
		Therap	0.7-1.7	2.58	2-4
		Toxic	>200		>516
Quinidine (BioQuin)	S or P		µg/mL		µmol/L
		Therap	2-5	3.08	6-15
		Toxic	>6		>19
Risperidone (Risperdal) + 9-hydroxyrisperidone	S or P		ng/mL		nmol/L
		Therap	20-60	2.44	49-146
Ritonavir (Norvir)	S or P		µg/mL		µmol/L
		Therap	>2	1.39	>3
		Toxic	>22		>31
Salicylates as salicylic acid	S or P		µg/mL		mmol/L
		Therap		0.00727	
		Analgesia, antipyresis	<100		<0.7
		Anti-inflammatory	150-300		1-2
		Toxic	>100		>0.7
		Lethal, 24+ h after a dose or with chronic ingestion	>500		>4
Saquinavir (Fortovase, Invirase)	S or P		µg/mL		µmol/L
		Therap	>0.25	1.49	>0.4
		Toxic	>6.0		>9
Secobarbital (Seconal)	S or P		µg/mL		µmol/L
		Therap	1-2	4.20	4.2-8.4
		Toxic	>5		>21.0

TABLE 50-2 Therapeutic and Toxic Levels of Drugs—cont'd

Drug	Specimen	Status	REFERENCE VALUES Conventional Units	Conversion Factor	SI Units
Sertraline (Zoloft)	S or P		ng/mL		nmol/L
		Therap	10-50	3.27	33-164
		Toxic	>300		>981
Sirolimus (Rapamune, Rapamycin)	WB		ng/mL		nmol/L
		Therap	4-20	1.10	4-22
		Toxic	>20		>22
Sotalol (Betapace, Sorine)	S or P		μg/mL		μmol/L
		Therap	1-3	3.67	4-11
Streptomycin	S or P		μg/mL		μmol/L
		Therap			
		Trough	<5	1.72	<9
		Peak	20-30		34-52
		Peak/MIC	>10		>17.2
		Toxic	>50		>86
Sulfonamides as sulfanilamide	S or P		mg/mL		mmol/L
		Therap	5-15	5.81	29-87
		Toxic	>20		>116
Tacrolimus (FK 506, Prograf)	WB		ng/mL		nmol/L
		Therap	3-20	1.24	4-25
		Toxic	>20		>25
Teicoplanin (Targocid)	S or P		μg/mL		μmol/L
		Peak	>10	0.53	>5
Theophylline (Uniphyl)	S or P		μg/mL		μmol/L
		Therap			
		Bronchodilator	8-20	5.55	44-111
		Prem apnea	6-13		33-72
		Toxic	>20		>111
Thiopental (Pentothal)	S or P		μg/mL		μmol/L
		Hypnotic	1-5	4.13	4-21
		Coma	30-100		124-413
		Anesthesia	7-130		29-536
		Toxic	>10		>41
Thioridazine (Mellaril)	S or P		μg/mL		μmol/L
		Therap	0.1-2.0	2.70	0.3-5
		Toxic	>10		>27
Tiagabine (Gabitril)	S or P		ng/mL		nmol/L
		Therap	20-200	2.66	53-532
		Toxic	>520		>1383
Tobramycin (Nebcin)	S or P		μg/mL		μmol/L
		Therap			
		Peak			
		Less severe infection	5-8	2.14	11-17
		Severe infection	8-10		17-21
		Trough			
		Less severe infection	<1		<2
		Moderate infection	<2		<4
		Severe infection	<4		<9
		Toxic			
		Peak	>10		>21
		Trough	>2		>4
		Peak/MIC	>10		>21
Tocainide (Tonocard)	S or P		μg/mL		μmol/L
		Therap	6-15	5.20	31-78
		Toxic	>15		>78

Continued

TABLE 50-2 Therapeutic and Toxic Levels of Drugs—cont'd

Drug	Specimen	Status	REFERENCE VALUES Conventional Units	Conversion Factor	SI Units
Tolbutamide (Orinase)	S or P		μg/mL		μmol/L
		Therap	90-240	3.70	333-888
		Toxic	>640		>2368
Topiramate (Topamax)	S or P		μg/mL		μmol/L
		Therap	5-20	2.95	15-59
		Toxic	>12		>36
Trazodone (Desyrel)	S or P		ng/mL		nmol/L
		Therap	700-1000	2.68	1876-2680
		Toxic	>1200		>3216
Trimipramine (Surmontil)	S or P		ng/mL		nmol/L
		Therap	150-350	3.40	510-1190
		Toxic	>500		>1700
Valproic acid (Depakene)	S or P		μg/mL		μmol/L
		Therap	50-100	6.93	346-693
		Toxic	>100		>693
Vancomycin (Vancocin)	S or P		μg/mL		μmol/L
		Therap			
		Peak	20-40	0.69	14-28
		Trough	>10		>7
		Toxic	>80		>55
Venlafaxine (Effexor) + desmethylvenlafaxine	S or P		ng/mL		nmol/L
		Therap	100-400	3.61	361-1444
		Toxic	>800 (sum)		>2888
Vigabatrin (Sabril)	S or P		μg/mL		μmol/L
		Therap	0.8-36	7.74	6-279
Voriconazole (Vfend)	S or P		μg/mL		μmol/L
		Therap	1-6	2.86	3-17
		Toxic	>6		>17
Warfarin (Coumadin)	S or P		μg/mL		μmol/L
		Therap	1-10	3.24	3-32
		Toxic	>10		>32
Zidovudine (AZT, Retrovir)	S or P		μg/mL		μmol/L
		Therap	>0.2	3.74	>0.8
Zonisamide (Zonegran)	S or P		μg/mL		μmol/L
		Therap	10-40	4.71	47-188

References

1. DrugBank: open drug & drug target database. http://www.drugbank.ca (accessed February 16, 2014).
2. Drug information handbook, 19th edition. Hudson, OH: Lexi-Comp, 2010.
3. O'Neil MJ, ed. The Merck index online (accessed February 16, 2014).
4. Physicians' desk reference online (accessed February 16, 2014).
5. Porter RS, ed. The Merck manual of diagnosis and therapy, Whitehouse Station: NJ; Merck & Co, 2011.
6. Schulz M, Schmoldt A. Therapeutic and toxic blood concentrations of more than 800 drugs and other xenobiotics. Pharmazie 2003;58:447-74.
7. Snozek CLH, McMillin GA, Moyer TP. Chapter 34. Therapeutic drugs and their management. In: Burtis CA, Ashwood ER, Bruns DE, eds. Tietz textbook of clinical chemistry and molecular diagnostics, 5th edition, St Louis: MO, 2012:1057-108.

TABLE 50-3 Critical Values

Critical values, also known as *panic* or *alert values,* are laboratory results that indicate a life-threatening situation for the patient. Because of their critical nature, urgent notification of a critical value to the appropriate healthcare professional is necessary. Table 50-3 has been adapted from extensive national surveys. The median or average critical limit determined by these surveys is shown. In practice, each organization should have *its own set* of critical limits and physician notification policy.

Test	Units	Lower Limit	Upper Limit	Comments
Blood Gases				
pH		7.2	7.6	Arterial, capillary
PCO_2	mm Hg	20	70	Arterial, capillary
PO_2	mm Hg	40	—	Arterial
PO_2 (children)	mm Hg	45	125	Arterial
PO_2 (newborn)	mm Hg	35	90	Arterial
Chemistry				
Albumin (children)	g/dL	1.7	6.8	Serum or plasma
Ammonia (children)	μmol/L	—	109	Plasma
Bilirubin (newborn)	mg/dL	—	15	Serum or plasma
Calcium	mg/dL	6.0	13	Serum or plasma
Calcium (children)	mg/dL	6.5	12.7	Serum or plasma
Calcium, ionized	mmol/L	0.75	1.6	Plasma
Carbon dioxide, total	mmol/L	10	40	Serum or plasma
Chloride	mmol/L	80	120	Serum or plasma
Creatinine	mg/dL	—	5.0	Serum or plasma
Creatinine (children)	mg/dL	—	3.8	Serum or plasma
Glucose	mg/dL	40	450	Serum or plasma
Glucose (children)	mg/dL	46	445	Serum or plasma
Glucose (newborn)	mg/dL	30	325	Serum or plasma
Glucose, CSF	mg/dL	40	200	CSF
Glucose, CSF (children)	mg/dL	31	—	CSF
Lactate	mmol/L	—	3.4	Plasma
Lactate (children)	mmol/L	—	4.1	Plasma
Magnesium	mg/dL	1.0	4.7	Serum or plasma
Osmolality	mOsm/kg	250	325	Serum or plasma
Phosphorus	mg/dL	1.0	8.9	Serum or plasma
Potassium	mmol/L	2.8	6.2	Serum or plasma
Potassium (newborn)	mmol/L	2.8	7.8	Serum or plasma
Protein (children)	g/dL	3.4	9.5	Serum or plasma
Protein, CSF (children)	mg/dL	—	188	CSF
Sodium	mmol/L	120	160	Serum or plasma
Urea nitrogen	mg/dL	—	80	Serum or plasma
Urea nitrogen (children)	mg/dL	—	55	Serum or plasma
Uric acid	mg/dL	—	13	Serum or plasma
Uric acid (children)	mg/dL	—	12	Serum or plasma
Hematology				
Hematocrit				
Adult	%	20	60	First report only
Newborn	%	33	71	
Hemoglobin				
Adult	g/dL	7	20	First report only
Newborn	g/dL	10	22	
WBC				
Adult	$\times10^3/\mu L$	2.0	30	First report only
Children	$\times10^3/\mu L$	2.0	43	
Platelets	$\times10^3/\mu L$	40	1000	
Blasts	Any seen (first report only)			
Drepanocytes	Presence of sickle cells or aplastic crisis			
Coagulation				
Fibrinogen	mg/dL	100	800	
Prothrombin time	s	—	30	
Partial thromboplastin time	s	—	78	

Continued

TABLE 50-3   Critical Values—cont'd

Test	Units	Lower Limit	Upper Limit	Comments
Urinalysis	Presence of pathological crystals (urate, cysteine, leucine, or tyrosine)			
Microscopic	Strongly positive glucose and ketones			
Chemical				
Cerebrospinal Fluid				
WBC (0-1 y)	Cells per μL	—	>30	
WBC (1-4 y)	Cells per μL	—	>20	
WBC (5-17 y)	Cells per μL	—	>10	
WBC (>17 y)	Cells per μL	—	>5	
Malignant cells, blasts, or microorganisms		Any	Applies to other sterile body fluids	

References

1. Dighe AS, Rao A, Coakley AB, et al. Analysis of laboratory critical value reporting at a large academic medical center. Am J Clin Pathol 2006;12:758–64.
2. Don-Wauchope AC, Wang L, Grey V. Pediatric critical values: laboratory-pediatrician discourse. Clin Biochem. 2009 Nov;42(16-17):1658–61.
3. Emancipator K. Critical values: ASCP practice parameter. Am J Clin Path 1997;108:247–53.
4. Genzen JR, Tormey CA. Pathology consultation on reporting of critical values. Am J Clin Pathol 2011;135:505–13.
5. Hortin GL, Csako G. Critical values, panic values, or alert values? Am J Clin Pathol 1998;109:496–8.
6. Howanitz PJ, Steindel SJ, Heard NV. Laboratory critical values policies and procedures: a College of American Pathologists Q-probes study in 623 institutions. Arch Pathol Lab Med 2002;126:663–9.
7. Kost GJ. Table of critical limits. MLO Med Lab Obs. 2004 Aug;36(13 Suppl):6–7.
8. Kost GJ. The significance of ionized calcium in cardiac and critical care: availability and critical limits at U.S. medical centers and children's hospitals. Arch Pathol Lab Med 1993;117:890–6.
9. Kost GJ. Using critical limits to improve patient outcome. Med Lab Observ 1993;23:22–7.
10. Kost GJ, Hale KN. Global trends in critical values practices and their harmonization. Clin Chem Lab Med. 2011 Feb;49(2):167–76.
11. Liebow EB, Derzon JH, Fontanesi J, et al. Effectiveness of automated notification and customer service call centers for timely and accurate reporting of critical values: a laboratory medicine best practices systematic review and meta-analysis. Clin Biochem. 2012 Sep;45(13-14):979–87.
12. Parl FF, O'Leary MF, Kaiser AB, et al. Implementation of a closed-loop reporting system for critical values and clinical communication in compliance with goals of The Joint Commission. Clin Chem 2010;56:417–23.
13. Piva E, Sciacovelli L, Zaninotto M, Laposata, M, Plebani, M. Evaluation of effectiveness of a computerized notification system for reporting critical values. Am J Clin Pathol 2011;131:432–41.
14. Tillman J, Barth JH, ACB National Audit Group. A survey of laboratory "critical (alert) limits" in the UK. Ann Clin Biochem 2003;40:181–4.

Glossary

Absorbance (A) The amount of light absorbed as incident light passes through a sample, which is equivalent to log (1/T) or −log (T), where T is transmittance.

Absorptivity (a) A proportionality constant for a compound that is the measure of the absorption of radiant energy at a given wavelength as it passes through a solution of that compound at a concentration of 1 g/L; expressed mathematically as absorbance divided by the product of the concentration of a substance in g/L and the sample path length in centimeters (a = A/bc).

Acid phosphatase All phosphatases with optimal activity below pH 7.0 that catalyze the cleavage of orthophosphate from orthophosphoric monoesters; most of the activity in serum is of a tartrate-resistant type.

Acid-base balance The homeostatic maintenance of acids and bases within the body to achieve a physiological pH (approximately 7.40).

Acidemia An arterial blood pH <7.35.

Acidosis Accumulation of acid and hydrogen ions or depletion of the alkaline reserve (bicarbonate content) in the blood and body tissues.

Acrodermatitis enteropathica A hereditary disorder due to defective zinc uptake.

Acromegaly A chronic disease of adults caused by hypersecretion of pituitary growth hormone and characterized by enlargement of many organs and parts of the skeleton and soft tissues.

Activator Small molecule or ion that increases the rate of an enzyme-catalyzed reaction by promoting formation of the most active state of the enzyme or of other reactants such as the substrate.

Active center/Active site That part of an enzyme formed by the tertiary structure at which the noncovalent binding of substrate occurs to form the intermediate enzyme/substrate complex.

Activity (Ion) The concentration of free, unbound ions in solution.

Acute coronary syndrome (ACS) A sudden cardiac disorder that varies from angina (chest pain on exertion with reversible tissue injury), to unstable angina (with minor myocardial injury), and to myocardial infarction (with extensive tissue necrosis, which is irreversible).

Acute fatty liver of pregnancy A rare, life-threatening complication of pregnancy that occurs in the third trimester or the immediate period after delivery.

Acute kidney injury (AKI) A rapid decline in kidney function that occurs over hours and days.

Acute lymphoblastic leukemia (ALL) An acute, rapidly progressing form of leukemia that is characterized by the presence in the blood and bone marrow of large numbers of unusually immature white blood cells destined to become lymphocytes.

Acute myocardial infarction (AMI) An acute infarction (obstruction of circulation) of the heart muscle occurring during the period when circulation to a region of the heart is obstructed and necrosis is occurring.

Acute nephritic syndrome The sudden onset of hematuria, proteinuria, diminished urine production, azotemia, hypertension, and edema.

Acute pancreatitis A sudden inflammation of the pancreas that is usually accompanied with severe upper abdominal pain.

Acute phase reaction (APR) A response of the body to inflammation that results in an increase or decrease in the plasma concentrations of a class of proteins known as acute phase reactants.

Acute porphyrias Inherited disorders of heme biosynthesis, characterized by acute attacks of neurovisceral symptoms; potentially life threatening; diagnosed by elevated urine PBG.

Acute intermittent porphyria (AIP) An autosomal dominant hepatic porphyria caused by mutation in the *HMBS* gene (locus: 11q23.3), which encodes hydroxymethylbilane synthase.

Acute poststreptococcal glomerulonephritis (APSGN) Inflammation of the kidney glomeruli, following a streptococcal infection; also called postinfectious glomerulonephritis.

Acute tubular necrosis Acute renal failure with mild to severe damage or necrosis of tubule cells.

Acute-phase response Body's response to injury or inflammation.

Acylglycerol (glycerol ester) A three-carbon alcohol that contains a hydroxyl group on each of its carbons and is classified by the number of fatty acyl groups present; triglycerides are the predominant form of glycerol ester in plasma.

Addison disease Deficiency of adrenocortical hormones secondary to disease of the adrenal glands; characterized by hypotension, and a bronzelike hyperpigmentation of the skin. Also called primary hypoadrenalism to distinguish from secondary hypoadrenalism (deficiency of pituitary adrenocorticotropic hormone).

Additives Compounds added to biological specimens to prevent them from clotting or to preserve the constituents of a specimen.

Adenocarcinoma A carcinoma derived from glandular tissue.

Adenohypophysis The anterior glandular lobe of the pituitary gland.

Adenoma A benign epithelial tumor in which the cells form recognizable glandular structures or in which the cells are derived from glandular epithelium.

Adenylate cyclase An enzyme of the lyase class that catalyzes the formation of 3′,5′-cyclic adenosine monophosphate (cAMP) from ATP.

Adrenal androgens A class of sex hormones that produce masculinization.

Adrenocorticotropic hormone (ACTH, corticotropin) A 39-amino-acid peptide hormone secreted by the anterior pituitary gland that stimulates the adrenal cortex to secrete corticosteroids.

Adsorption chromatography A separation mechanism based on the differential adsorption of analytes on the surface of a stationary phase and using hydrogen bonding and hydrophobic interactions as the forces behind the separation.

Advanced glycation end products (AGE) Proteins that have been irreversibly modified by nonenzymatic attachment of glucose; may contribute to the chronic complications of diabetes.

Adverse drug reaction (ADR) Any undesirable side effect or toxic reaction that is caused by the administration of a drug.

Adverse Reaction to Metal Debris (ARMD) A condition characterized by severe hip pain that results from metal released when the ball and joint of the prosthesis used in a hip replacement are both metal.

Adynamic bone disease (ABD) A type of renal osteodystrophy characterized by reduced osteoblasts and osteoclasts, and low turnover of bone.

Affinity Energy of interaction of a single antibody-combining site and its corresponding epitope on the antigen.

Affinity chromatography A separation mechanism in which one component of a specifically matched pair (such as antigen/antibody or hormone/receptor) is immobilized in a stationary phase and is used to capture the other component of the pair that is in the mobile phase.

Alcoholic hepatitis An acute or chronic degenerative and inflammatory lesion of the liver in the alcoholic that is potentially progressive though sometimes reversible.

Alcoholic liver disease Liver injury caused by excessive ethanol (alcohol) ingestion.

Aldehyde An organic compound with a carbonyl group (a carbon atom double-bonded to an oxygen) at the end of the carbon chain bonded to hydrogen and an R group (usually an alkyl group).

Aldolase An enzyme that catalyzes cleavage of fructose-1,6-disphosphate into dihydroxyacetone-phosphate and glyceraldehyde 3-phosphate in the glycolytic breakdown of glucose to lactate.

Aldosterone The major mineralocorticoid steroid hormone secreted by the adrenal cortex.

Alkalemia An arterial blood pH >7.45.

Alkaline phosphatase A hydrolase that catalyzes the alkaline hydrolysis of a large variety of naturally occurring and synthetic substrates.

Alkaptonuria A genetic disorder of phenylalanine and tyrosine metabolism that is caused by a deficiency of the enzyme homogentisic acid (HGA) dioxygenase.

Allan-Herndon-Dudley syndrome An X-linked syndrome caused by mutations in the *SLC16A2* gene (locus: Xq13.2), which encodes a thyroid hormone transporter, and characterized by severe mental retardation, dysarthria, athetoid movements, muscle hypoplasia, and spastic paraplegia.

Allele One of the alternative versions of a gene at a given location (locus) along a chromosome. An individual inherits two alleles for each gene, one from each parent. If the two alleles are the same, the individual is homozygous for that gene. If the alleles are different, the individual is heterozygous. The term now also refers to variation among noncoding DNA sequences in addition to genes.

Allele-specific PCR A version of polymerase chain reaction (PCR) in which specific alleles or DNA sequence variants are amplified at the same locus.

Alpha fetoprotein (AFP) A protein produced in the fetal liver that is measured in maternal serum for predicting risk of anencephaly, spina bifida, and Down syndrome in the fetus.

5-Aminolevulinic acid (ALA) Immediate precursor of porphobilinogen; two molecules of ALA combine to form one molecule of porphobilinogen.

Amenorrhea The absence of menstruation.

Amino acid An organic compound containing both amino (−NH2) and carboxyl (−COOH) functional groups.

Aminoacidopathy Any one of a group of inborn errors of amino acid metabolism caused by (1) defective activity of an enzyme in the metabolic pathway of one or more amino acids or (2) a defect in a protein needed for transport of an amino acid into or out of cells. They are usually detected by the presence of increased concentrations of one or more amino acids in blood or urine or both.

Aminoaciduria An excess of amino acids in the urine.

Aminotransferases A subclass of enzymes of the transferase class that catalyze the transfer of an amino group from a donor (generally an amino acid) to an acceptor (generally a 2-oxo acid). Most of these enzymes are pyridoxyl phosphate proteins. Alanine and aspartate aminotransferase are examples that are of significant clinical utility.

Amniotic fluid Substance derived mostly from fetal urine that protects the developing fetus.

Amperometry An electrolytic electrochemical process in which current is monitored at a fixed (controlled) voltage between working and reference electrodes in an electrochemical cell.

Amphetamine A sympathomimetic amine that has a stimulating effect on the central and peripheral nervous systems.

Ampholyte A molecule that is positively or negatively charged on the basis of the pH of the solution in which it resides;

proteins, because they contain many ionizable amino and carboxyl groups, behave as ampholytes in solution and are considered amphoteric.

Amplicon The product of an amplification reaction.

Amplification methods Techniques to amplify the amount of target, signal, or probe so that specific sequences are readily observed.

α-Amylase An enzyme that catalyzes the hydrolysis of 1,4-alpha-glycosidic linkages in starch, glycogen, and related polysaccharides and oligosaccharides.

Amyloidosis A metabolic disease characterized by abnormal deposits of amyloid in the body.

Analgesics Agents that relieve pain without causing loss of consciousness.

Analyte The substance being analyzed in an analytical procedure.

Analytical sensitivity The ability of an analytical method to assess small variations in the concentration of analyte.

Analytical specificity The ability of an assay procedure to determine specifically the concentration of the target analyte in the presence of potentially interfering substances or factors in the sample matrix.

Androgen insensitivity syndrome (AIS) A genetic disorder in which XY male fetuses are unresponsive to androgens and are born looking externally like normal females.

Androstenedione An androgenic steroid produced by the testis, adrenal cortex, and ovary.

Anemic hypoxia Hypoxia (a reduced supply of oxygen to the tissues) resulting from a decrease in amount of hemoglobin or number of erythrocytes in the blood.

Anencephaly A birth defect characterized by a brain, skull, and scalp that does not develop normally.

Angina A condition marked by severe pain in the chest, often also spreading to the shoulders, arms, and neck, caused by an inadequate blood supply to the heart.

Angiotensin II A small (eight-amino-acid) polypeptide hormone; it stimulates release of aldosterone and other hormones, constricts blood vessels, and controls arterial pressure.

Angiotensin-converting enzyme (ACE) Enzyme that catalyzes the removal of two amino acids from angiotensin I, thus converting it to the active hormone angiotensin II.

Angiotensin-converting enzyme inhibitors Pharmaceuticals that are competitive inhibitors of the angiotensin-converting enzyme. They are used in the treatment of hypertension.

Angiotensinogen A serum globulin formed by the liver that is cleaved by renin to produce angiotensin I.

Anion gap (AG) The difference between the serum sodium concentration and the sum of the serum chloride and bicarbonate concentrations; the anion gap is high in some forms of metabolic acidosis.

Antibody Immunoglobulin (Ig) class of molecule (e.g., IgA, IgG, IgM) that binds specifically to an antigen or hapten.

Anticholinergic agent An agent that opposes the effects of impulses conveyed by adrenergic postganglionic fibers.

Anticoagulant Any substance that prevents blood from clotting.

Antidiuretic hormone (ADH; vasopressin) An octapeptide hormone formed by the neuronal cells of the hypothalamic nuclei and stored in the posterior lobe of the pituitary gland (neurohypophysis). It has both antidiuretic and vasopressor actions.

Antigen Any material capable of reacting with an antibody without necessarily being capable of inducing antibody formation.

Antihistamines Antagonists of the H1 or H2 histamine receptors that are used to treat allergic reactions or gastric hyperacidity.

Antiporter A membrane transport protein that mediates the cotransport of substances in opposite directions.

Antisense RNA (asRNA) A single-stranded RNA that is complementary to a messenger RNA (mRNA) strand transcribed within a cell.

Apathetic hyperthyroidism A form of Graves disease that tends to affect mainly older adults who have stereotyped "senile" physical features and whose behavior is apathetic (indifferent) and inactive rather than hyperkinetic.

Apoenzyme The protein component of an enzyme.

Apolipoproteins The major protein components of lipoproteins.

Apoptosis Programmed cell death as signaled by the nuclei in normally functioning human and animal cells when age or state of cell health and condition dictates.

Arginine vasopressin (AVP) A peptide hormone also known as antidiuretic hormone (ADH) and vasopressin (VP) that is synthesized in the hypothalamus, but released from the posterior pituitary lobe.

Argininosuccinate lyase (AL) deficiency A genetic disorder that affects the body's ability to clear the nitrogen already incorporated into the urea cycle as argininosuccinate. This disorder often presents with rapid-onset hyperammonemia in the newborn period. Also known as argininosuccinic aciduria.

Argininosuccinate synthetase (ASS) deficiency A genetic disorder characterized by a deficiency of argininosuccinate and an increase in the ammonia concentration in the blood. Also known as citrullinemia type I.

Argonaute proteins Proteins of the RNA-induced silencing complex (RISC), the complex responsible for the gene silencing process known as RNA interference (RNAi).

Argyria A permanent ash gray discoloration of the skin, conjunctiva, and internal organs that results from long-continued use of silver salts.

Array An ordered linear, two-dimensional, or three-dimensional arrangement of a multiplicity of discrete objects, such as individual deposits (spots or lines) of DNA or reaction chambers.

Arrhythmia Any variation from the normal rhythm of the heartbeat; alternative (and broader) term: dysrhythmia, especially to indicate an abnormally slow or fast heartbeat which may have rhythmic beating.

Ascites Fluid accumulation in the abdominal cavity.

Assisted reproductive technologies (ART) Procedures involving the manipulation of eggs or sperm to establish pregnancy in the treatment of infertility.

Asymmetric PCR A version of PCR that preferentially amplifies one strand of the target DNA.

Atherosclerosis A pathogenic process that is the underlying cause of the common cardiovascular disorders of (1) myocardial infarction, (2) cerebrovascular disease, and (3) peripheral vascular disease.

Atherosclerotic plaque A pearly white area within the wall of an artery that causes the intimal (interior) surface to bulge into the lumen; composed of lipid, cell debris, smooth muscle cells, collagen, and sometimes calcium; also known as an atheroma; vulnerable to rupture that causes the formation of a platelet- and fibrin-rich thrombus leading to myocardial infarction and ischemic stroke.

Atomic absorption (AA) spectrophotometry An emission technique in which an element in a sample is dissociated from its chemical bonds (atomized) and placed in an unexcited or ground state (neutral atom); the atom at low energy is able to absorb radiation and the radiant energy given off as the element returns to its ground state is measured.

ATSDR Agency for Toxic Substances and Disease Registry.

Autocrine A mode of hormone action in which a cell secretes a hormone that binds to autocrine receptors on that same cell, leading to changes in the cell.

Autoimmune hepatitis (AIH) A form of hepatitis, usually with hypergammaglobulinemia and serum autoantibodies.

Autoimmune thyroid disease (AITD) Diseases in which the immune system attacks or stimulates the body's own thyroid gland.

Automation The process whereby an analytical instrument performs many tests with only minimal involvement of an analyst; also defined as the controlled operation of an apparatus, process, or system by mechanical or electronic devices without human intervention.

Autosomal recessive disorder A disorder characterized by the requirement that both copies of a gene are abnormal (see following definition for autosomal recessive inheritance).

Autosomal recessive inheritance A Mendelian inheritance pattern in which (1) nonsex chromosomes (autosomes) carry a DNA sequence (gene) for the inherited trait and (2) two copies of the DNA sequence must be present for the trait to appear in an individual; heterozygous parents have a 25% chance of having an affected offspring.

Autosome A nonsex chromosome; there are 22 pairs of autosomes in the human genome.

Avidity Overall strength of binding of antibody and antigen; includes the sum of the binding affinities of all individual combining sites on the antibody.

Avitaminosis A disease condition, described as a deficiency syndrome, that results from lack of a vitamin.

Azotemia An excess of urea or other nitrogenous compounds in the blood.

Bandpass The range of wavelengths passed by a filter or a monochromator at one-half the peak transmittance of that filter.

Barbiturate Any of a class of sedative-hypnotic agents derived from barbituric acid or thiobarbituric acid and classified into long-, intermediate-, short-, and ultrashort-acting classes.

Bartter syndrome Hypertrophy and hyperplasia of the juxtaglomerular cells, producing hypokalemic alkalosis and hyperaldosteronism.

Base pair A purine/pyrimidine pair linked by hydrogen bonds that connects the complementary strands of DNA or of hybrid molecules joining DNA and RNA. The base pairs are adenine-thymine and guanine-cytosine in DNA, and adenine-uracil and guanine-cytosine in RNA.

Base peak The ion with the highest abundance in the mass spectrum; it is assigned a relative abundance of 100%.

Batch analysis Type of analysis in which many specimens are grouped in the same analytical session.

Beer's law A mathematical equation that states that the con of a substance is directly proportional to the amount of light absorbed or is inversely proportional to the logarithm of the transmitted light; mathematically expressed as A = abc.

Bence-Jones proteins Small light chains of immunoglobulin found in the urine.

Benign prostatic hyperplasia (BPH) A noncancerous enlargement of the prostate gland.

Benzodiazepines Any of a group of minor tranquilizers that have a common molecular structure and similar pharmacological activity, including antianxiety, sedative, hypnotic, amnestic, anticonvulsant, and muscle-relaxing effects.

Beriberi A disease caused by a deficiency of thiamine (vitamin B1) and characterized by polyneuritis, cardiac pathology, and edema.

Berylliosis A hypersensitivity response to beryllium, usually involving the lungs and less often the skin, subcutaneous tissues, lymph nodes, liver, or other structures. Two varieties are distinguished: acute b. and chronic b. Called also beryllium poisoning.

beta-Lipotropin (β-LPH) An 89-amino-acid polypeptide hormone synthesized by the anterior pituitary; it exerts a mild peripheral lipolytic action and serves as a precursor of several hormones.

Bezoar A concretion of foreign material found in the gastrointestinal tract or urinary tract.

Bias In an analytical method, the difference between the average value and the true value that is expressed numerically and is inversely related to the trueness.

Bile A greenish-yellow fluid secreted by the liver and stored in the gallbladder.

Biliary atresia A condition characterized by failure of a fetus to develop an adequate pathway for bile to drain from the liver to the intestine.

Biliprotein The conjugated bilirubin-protein complex (also known as delta-bilirubin).

Bilirubin A yellow bile pigment that is a breakdown product of heme mainly formed from the degradation of erythrocyte hemoglobin in reticuloendothelial cells.

Bioavailability The degree to which a drug or other substance becomes available to the target tissue after administration.

Bioluminescence The emission of light when an electron returns from an excited or higher energy level to a lower energy level in which the excitation event is caused by a biochemical reaction and not by photo illumination; a special form of chemiluminescence in which an enzyme or a photoprotein increases the efficiency of the light emission.

Biomarker In medicine, a biomarker is a biological compound that is used as an indicator of a particular disease state or some other physiological state of an organism.

Biosensor A type of chemical sensor consisting of a biological recognition element and a physicochemical transducer, often an electrochemical or an optical device.

Biotransformation The series of chemical alterations of a compound (for example, a drug) that occurs within the body, as by enzymatic activity.

Blank A solution used in photometry/spectrophotometry that is identical to calibrating or unknown solutions except for the substance to be measured.

Blastocyst A thin-walled hollow structure in early embryonic development that contains a cluster of cells called the inner cell mass from which the embryo arises.

Blood gases The partial pressures of carbon dioxide (PCO_2) and oxygen (PO_2) measured in whole blood.

Blood group antigen Antigen containing a major carbohydrate component usually found on the surface of cells or secreted by cells.

Bone alkaline phosphatase (BALP) An isoenzyme of alkaline phosphatase found in bone and a biochemical marker of bone formation.

Bowman capsule The double-walled globular kidney structure that forms the beginning of a renal tubule and surrounds the glomerulus.

Branched-chain signal amplification A molecular probe technique that utilizes branched DNA (bDNA) as a means to amplify the hybridization signal.

Breath tests Tests that detect products of bacterial metabolism in the gut or products of human metabolism by measuring, most commonly, CO_2 and H_2 in the breath.

Buffer solution A solution containing either a weak acid and its salt or a weak base and its salt, which is resistant to changes in pH.

BUN (blood urea nitrogen) Obsolete term used to report results of a urea assay, particularly in the United States.

Calcitonin A 32-amino-acid polypeptide hormone elaborated by the parafollicular cells of the thyroid gland in response to hypercalcemia.

Calibration In relation to analytical methods, a function that describes the relationship between instrument signal and concentration of analyte.

Cancer A relative autonomous growth of tissue.

Cancer staging The process by which cancer is divided into groups of early and late disease; useful for prognosis and for guiding therapy.

Capillary electrophoresis A method in which the classic techniques of electrophoresis are carried out in a small-bore, fused silica capillary tube coated with a polymeric covering.

Carbohydrate Aldehyde or ketone derivatives of polyhydroxy alcohols composed of carbon, hydrogen, and oxygen in a ratio of 1:2:1.

Carbohydrate markers Carbohydrate-related tumor markers may be (1) antigens on the tumor cell surface or (2) secreted by the tumor cells.

Carboxyhemoglobin A form of hemoglobin in which the sites usually bound to oxygen are bound to carbon monoxide.

Carcinoembryonic antigen (CEA) A glycoprotein secreted into the glycocalyx coating the luminal surface of gastrointestinal epithelia.

Carcinogen Any cancer-producing substance.

Carcinoid syndrome A syndrome due to carcinoid tumors and characterized by attacks of severe cyanotic flushing of the skin—lasting from minutes to days—and by diarrheal watery stools, bronchoconstrictive attacks, sudden drops in blood pressure, edema, and ascites. Symptoms are caused by secretion from the tumor of serotonin, prostaglandins, and other biologically active substances.

Carcinoid tumor A yellow circumscribed tumor arising from enterochromaffin cells, usually in the small intestine, appendix, stomach, or colon, and less commonly in the bronchus; sometimes used alone to refer to the gastrointestinal tumor (called also argentaffinoma).

Carcinoma A malignant new growth made up of epithelial cells tending to infiltrate the surrounding tissues and give rise to metastases.

Cardiac biomarker A biological compound whose measurement is useful in the diagnosis of cardiac disease; used to (1) detect cardiac disorders, (2) detect risk of developing cardiac disorders, (3) monitor the disorder, or (4) predict the response of a disorder to a treatment.

Cardiomyopathy A general diagnostic term designating primary noninflammatory disease of the heart muscle.

Carry-over The transport of a quantity of analyte or reagent from one specimen reaction into and contaminating a subsequent one.

Catalyst A substance that modifies and increases the rate of a chemical reaction without being permanently changed or consumed; an enzyme is a protein catalyst of biological origin.

Catecholamine One of a group of biogenic amines having a sympathomimetic action, the aromatic portion of whose molecule is catechol, and the aliphatic portion an amine; examples include dopamine, norepinephrine, and epinephrine.

Catecholamine metabolites Products of catecholamine metabolism, such as dihydroxyphenylacetic acid, methoxytyramine, homovanillic acid, dihydroxyphenylglycol, methoxyhydroxyphenylglycol, normetanephrine, metanephrine, and vanillylmandelic acid.

Catechol-O-methyltransferase (COMT) An enzyme that degrades catecholamines.

Celiac disease A disease caused by the destructive interaction of gluten with the intestinal mucosa causing malabsorption. In most cases, the mucosal damage is reversed by withdrawing all gluten-containing foods from the diet. Also called gluten-sensitive enteropathy.

CentiMorgan (cM) A unit of measure that refers to the distance between two gene loci determined by the frequency with which recombination occurs between them. Two loci are said to be one cM apart if recombination is observed between them in 1% of cell division cycles.

Central hypothyroidism Refers to thyroid hormone deficiency due to a disorder of the (1) pituitary, (2) hypothalamus, or (3) hypothalamic-pituitary portal circulation.

Centrifugation The process of using centrifugal force to separate the lighter portions of a solution from the heavier portions; a centrifuge is a device by which centrifugation is effected.

Centromere A primary constriction in a chromosome; centromeres play an important role in directing the movement of chromosomes between daughter cells during cell division.

CERCLA Comprehensive Environmental Response, Compensation, and Liability Act.

Chelation therapy Administration of chelating agents to remove metals from the body.

Chemical hygiene plan (CHP) An Occupational Safety and Health Administration (OSHA)-required listing of responsibilities for laboratory employers, employees, and a chemical hygiene officer, and including a complete chemical inventory that is updated annually, along with a copy of the Material Safety Data Sheet (MSDS) that defines each chemical as toxic, carcinogenic, or dangerous, and that must be on file and available to all employees 24 hours a day, 7 days a week.

Chemical speciation Refers to the molecular form of atoms of an element or a cluster of atoms of different elements in a given matrix.

Chemiluminescence The emission of light when an electron returns from an excited or higher energy level to a lower energy level, in which the excitation event is caused by a chemical reaction and not by photo illumination; the excitation event is caused by the oxidation of an organic compound.

Chemosensor A sensor design in a point-of-care testing device that detects intrinsic properties of an analyte or that is combined with a transducing element to detect signals produced by the analyte binding to some indicator.

Cholecystitis A painful inflammation of the gallbladder.

Cholecystokinin (CCK) A 33-amino-acid peptide secreted by the upper intestinal mucosa and also found in the central nervous system. It causes gallbladder contraction and release of pancreatic exocrine (or digestive) enzymes, and affects other gastrointestinal (GI) functions.

Cholestasis of pregnancy A condition during pregnancy characterized by impaired bile flow allowing bile salts to be deposited in the skin and the placenta.

Cholestasis Suppression of the normal flow of bile.

Cholesterol A steroid alcohol with 27 carbon atoms that are arranged in a tetracyclical sterane ring system, with a C-H side chain and a polar hydroxyl group on its A-ring, making it an amphipathic molecule.

Cholinergic toxidrome A toxidrome that represents the acute phase of cholinesterase inhibitor poisoning.

Cholinesterase An enzyme of the hydrolase class that catalyzes the cleavage of the acyl group from various esters of choline, including acetylcholine, and some related compounds.

Chorionic villi One of the minute vascular projections of the fetal chorion that combines with maternal uterine tissue to form the placenta.

Chorionic villus sampling A prenatal test to detect birth defects that is performed at an early stage of pregnancy and involves retrieval and examination of tissue from the chorionic villi. Also called chorionic villus biopsy.

Chromaffin cell Neuroendocrine cell derived from embryonic neural crest found in the medulla of the adrenal gland and in other ganglia of the sympathetic nervous system; so-named because of the presence of cytoplasmic granules that give a brownish reaction with chromium salts.

Chromatin Nuclear DNA and its associated structural proteins; chromatin is arranged and organized in a hierarchical fashion in which the degree of its condensation increases with higher levels of structural organization.

Chromatogram A plot of detector response as a function of time or mobile phase volume.

Chromatography A group of separation techniques that separate analytes by differential distribution between a stationary phase and a mobile phase.

Chromosome A highly ordered structure of a single double-stranded DNA (dsDNA) molecule, compacted many times with the aid of structural DNA-binding proteins.

Chronic hepatitis A collective term for a clinical and pathological syndrome that has several causes and is characterized by varying degrees of hepatocellular necrosis and inflammation for at least 6 months.

Chronic kidney disease (CKD) Abnormalities of kidney structure or function, present for greater than 3 months, with implications for health.

Chronic myelocytic leukemia (CML) Chronic leukemia characterized by granular leukocytes.

Chronic obstructive pulmonary disease (COPD) Any disorder characterized by persistent or recurring obstruction of bronchial air flow, such as chronic bronchitis, asthma, or pulmonary emphysema.

Chronic pancreatitis An inflammatory disease characterized by persistent and progressive destruction of the pancreas.

Chyme Food that has been acted upon by the churning action of the stomach and by stomach juices and expelled by the stomach into the duodenum.

Circadian rhythms Rhythmic repetition of certain phenomena in living organisms at about the same time each day.

Cirrhosis Liver disease characterized pathologically by loss of the normal microscopic lobular architecture with fibrosis and nodular regeneration.

Citrullinemia type II An autosomal recessive disease characterized by increased concentrations of citrulline in serum and urine. Ammonia intoxication is another manifestation. This disorder is characterized by neuropsychiatric symptoms, including abnormal behaviors, loss of memory, seizures, and coma.

CLIA waived tests Tests categorized as "waived" by the FDA under the Clinical Laboratory Improvement Amendments of 1988. These tests employ methodologies that are considered to be so simple and accurate as to render the likelihood of erroneous results negligible.

Clinical audit A review of case histories of patients against the benchmark of current best practice; used as a tool to improve clinical practice.

Clinical enzymology The branch of medical science that deals with the biochemical nature and activity of enzymes of clinical relevance.

Clinical Laboratory Improvement Amendments of 1988 (CLIA-88) United States federal regulatory standards that apply to all clinical laboratory testing performed on humans in the United States, except clinical trials and basic research.

Clinical practice guidelines Systematically developed statements to assist practitioner and patient decisions about appropriate healthcare for specific clinical circumstances; in the laboratory, goals for accuracy, precision, and turnaround times of tests are included.

Clinical reference standard The best available method for establishing the presence or absence of the target condition; also, the suspected condition or disease for which the target is to be applied.

Clinical sensitivity The proportion of subjects with disease who have positive test results.

Clinical specificity The proportion of subjects without disease who have negative test results.

Clinical toxicology A subdivision of toxicology that involves the analysis of drugs, heavy metals, and other chemical agents in body fluids and tissues for the purpose of patient care.

Cloning In biology, cloning is the process of producing similar populations of genetically identical individuals. In molecular diagnostics, cloning is the process used to create copies of DNA fragments (molecular cloning), cells (cell cloning), or organisms.

CLSI The Clinical and Laboratory Standards Institute (formerly the National Committee for Clinical Laboratory Standards, or NCCLS) that guides the development and implementation of standards and guidelines that help all laboratories fulfill their goals.

Coagulation (clotting) The sequential process by which the multiple coagulation factors of blood interact in the coagulation cascade, resulting in formation of an insoluble fibrin clot.

Cocaine A crystalline alkaloid, obtained from leaves of Erythroxylon coca (coca leaves) and other Erythroxylon species, or by synthesis from ecgonine or its derivatives.

Codon A three-nucleotide sequence that "codes" for an amino acid during translation; there are 64 possible codons in nuclear DNA.

Coenzyme An organic nonprotein molecule that binds with the protein molecule (apoenzyme) to form the active enzyme (holoenzyme).

Cofactor A natural reactant, usually a metal ion or a coenzyme, that is required in an enzyme-catalyzed reaction.

Colligative properties Properties of solutions that depend on the number of particles in the solution; examples include (1) osmotic pressure, (2) boiling point elevation, (3) freezing point depression, and (4) vapor pressure lowering.

Colloid An amorphous material found in the follicular lumen of the thyroid gland. A critical component is thyroglobulin (Tg).

Column chromatography A separation method in which the stationary phase is packed into a tube or is coated onto the inner surface of the tube.

Column packing Particulate matter packed into a column used for chromatographic techniques.

Commutability The equivalence of the mathematical relationships between the results of different measurement procedures for a reference material and for representative samples from healthy and diseased individuals.

Comparative genomic hybridization A cytogenetic technique in which reference and test DNA are respectively labeled with green- and red-fluorescing fluorochromes. Genetic abnormalities are detected by changes in the green-to-red ratio.

Compensated metabolic acidosis A state of acidosis in which the pH of the blood has been returned toward normal by respiratory compensation.

Competitive immunoassay An immunoassay in which all reactants are simultaneously or sequentially mixed together and unlabeled antigen competes with labeled antigen for binding sites on the antibody; no separation step is included in this assay.

Complement system Complex system of proteins found in blood that combines with antibodies to destroy pathogenic bacteria and other foreign cells.

Complete blood count (CBC) The determination of the quantity of each type of blood cell in a mL of blood, often including the amount of hemoglobin, the hematocrit, and the proportions of various white cells.

Conception The union of the sperm and the ovum. Synonymous with fertilization.

Conductometry An electrochemical technique used to determine the quantity of an analyte present in a mixture by measuring its effect on the electrical conductivity of the mixture.

Confirmatory testing As used in programs that test for drugs of abuse, confirmatory tests are used to confirm a positive or sometimes negative result that had been presumptively classified as positive for a specific drug.

Conformation-sensitive gel electrophoresis (CSGE) A type of electrophoretic mutation scanning in which a segment of DNA is screened for mismatch pairing between normal and mutated base pairs.

Congenital adrenal hyperplasia (CAH) A group of inherited disorders in which deficiencies of enzymes that catalyze the biosynthesis of cortisol result in compensatory hypersecretion of corticotropin and subsequent adrenal hyperplasia as well as excessive androgen production.

Congenital erythropoietic porphyria (CEP) An autosomal recessive porphyria due to mutation in the *UROS* gene (locus: 10q25.2-q26.3), which encodes uroporphyrinogen-III synthase.

Congenital hypothyroidism A pathological condition resulting from severe thyroid insufficiency, which may lead to cretinism or myxedema.

Congestive heart failure (CHF) or heart failure A clinical syndrome due to heart disease, characterized by breathlessness and abnormal sodium and water retention, often resulting in edema.

Conjugated bilirubin Bilirubin that has been taken up by the liver cells and conjugated to form the water-soluble bilirubin diglucuronide.

Conn syndrome A condition of primary aldosteronism arising from oversecretion of aldosterone by an adrenal cortical adenoma.

Connectivity In a clinical laboratory, the linking of an analytical device via an electronic interface to a laboratory information system computer.

Continuous ambulatory peritoneal dialysis (CAPD) A common method of peritoneal dialysis, involving the continuous presence of dialysis solution in the peritoneal cavity.

Continuous-flow analysis Type of analysis in which each specimen in a batch passes through the same continuous stream at the same rate and is subjected to the same analytical reactions.

Control procedure Statistical and/or nonstatistical check protocols implemented in a clinical laboratory to assess the performance of an analytical method.

Control rules Decision criteria that define when an analytical run is judged acceptable ("in control") or unacceptable ("out of control").

Coproporphyrin A porphyrin with four methyl and four propionic acid sidechains attached to the tetrapyrrole backbone.

Copy number variant (CNV) A structural variant of a large region of the genome that has been deleted or duplicated.

Core laboratory A laboratory that provides all of the high-volume and emergency testing in many hospitals.

Cori cycle The mechanism by which lactate produced by muscles is carried to the liver, converted back to glucose via gluconeogenesis, and returned to the muscles.

Coronary arteries The two main arteries that provide blood to the heart, surrounding the heart like a crown, coming out of the aorta, arching down over the top of the heart, and dividing into two branches.

Coronary heart disease A narrowing of the small blood vessels that supply blood and oxygen to the heart.

Corpus luteum A yellow glandular mass in the ovary formed by an ovarian follicle that has matured and discharged its ovum; secretes progesterone.

Corticosteroid-binding globulin (transcortin) An α-globulin that binds unconjugated corticosteroid and transports it in the plasma.

Corticotropin-releasing hormone (CRH) A neuropeptide released by the hypothalamus that stimulates release of ACTH (corticotropin) by the anterior pituitary gland.

Cortisol The major adrenal glucocorticoid synthesized in the zona fasciculata (and, to a lesser extent, the zona reticularis) of the adrenal cortex.

Coulometry An electrochemical technique that measures the electrical charge passing between two electrodes in an electrochemical cell, with the amount of charge passing between the electrodes being directly proportional to oxidation or reduction of an electroactive substance at one of the electrodes.

C-Peptide A 31-amino-acid protein that connects insulin's A-chain to its B-chain in the proinsulin molecule.

Crack cocaine The freebase form of cocaine that can be smoked.

Creatine kinase A dimeric transferase enzyme that catalyzes the reversible phosphorylation of creatine by ATP. CK has four forms: CK-MM, CK-MB, CK-BB, and mitochondrial CK.

Creatinine A nonprotein nitrogen compound derived from the spontaneous hydrolysis of creatine or the cyclization of phosphocreatine; creatinine production is relatively constant, is related to muscle mass, and is often used as a marker of the glomerular filtration rate of the kidneys.

Cretinism An archaic term for the clinical consequences of untreated congenital hypothyroidism caused by a deficiency of thyroid hormone during prenatal development and infancy; characterized in childhood by short stature, developmental delay, dystrophy of the bones, and a low basal metabolism. Also called congenital myxedema, which is also an archaic term.

Crigler-Najjar syndrome An autosomal recessive form of nonhemolytic jaundice due to the absence of the hepatic enzyme glucuronosyltransferase.

Crohn disease A chronic inflammatory disease that may affect any part of the intestine from the mouth to the anus.

CTx An antigen produced when type I collagen is digested by the proteinase cathepsin K yielding cross-linked carboxy-terminal telopeptide of type I collagen; a serum marker for bone resorption and action of cathepsin K.

Cushing disease A condition characterized by hyperadrenocorticism that is secondary to excessive anterior pituitary secretion of corticotropin by the pituitary.

Cushing syndrome A condition characterized by an increased concentration of adrenal glucocorticoid hormone in the bloodstream and its effects on the body.

Cutaneous porphyrias Disorders of heme biosynthesis in which accumulations of porphyrins in the skin cause skin damage on exposure to sunlight.

Cyclic adenosine monophosphate (cAMP) A cyclic nucleotide that serves as an intracellular and, in some cases, extracellular "second messenger" mediating the action of many peptide or amine hormones.

Cystic fibrosis (CF) An inherited disease caused by genetic alteration of a cystic fibrosis transmembrane conductance regulator (CFTR) protein that leads to chronic pancreatic and obstructive pulmonary disease.

Cystic fibrosis transmembrane conductance regulator (CFTR) A transmembrane protein produced by the *CFTR* gene.

Cytochrome P$_{450}$ (CYP) A large family of metabolic enzymes that catalyze the oxidations of organic substrates. They are important in metabolism of drugs, steroid hormones, fatty acids, and other substances. Note: Often abbreviated as CYP usually followed by an arabic numeral, a letter, and another arabic numeral (e.g., CYP 2D6).

Cytokeratin One of the two types of keratin normally found in human tissue, constituting a group of proteins; these are normally found in keratin filaments.

Dehydroepiandrosterone (DHEA) A hormone produced by the adrenal glands. After being secreted, it circulates in the bloodstream as DHEA-sulfate (DHEAS) and is converted as needed into other hormones. It is the major androgen precursor in females.

Deletion A DNA sequence that is missing in one sample compared with another. Deletions may be as small as one nucleotide or as large as an entire chromosome.

Denaturing gradient gel electrophoresis (DGGE) An electrophoretic method for separating DNA fragments according to their mobilities under increasing denaturing conditions (usually increasing formamide or urea concentrations).

Densitometry A measuring technique that uses an optical system to scan and quantify electrophoretic fractions separated on a gel or other medium.

Dent disease Tubulopathy of the proximal renal tubules with low molecular weight proteinuria, hypercalciuria, hypokalemia, nephrocalcinosis, rickets, and progressive renal failure.

Deoxypyridinoline (DPD) A deoxypyridinoline crosslink of type I collagen present in bone that is excreted, free or protein-bound, in urine and serves as a marker of bone resorption.

Deoxyribonucleic acid (DNA) A nucleic acid that carries the genetic information in the cell. It consists of two long chains of nucleotides twisted into a double helix and joined by hydrogen bonds between the complementary bases adenine and thymine or cytosine and guanine. The sequence of nucleotides determines individual hereditary characteristics.

Deoxyribonucleotide triphosphates (dNDT) The building blocks of DNA (typically dATP, dCTP, dGTP, and dTTP).

Depletional hyponatremia A condition characterized by low plasma concentration of sodium associated with low total body sodium and normal blood volume; called also euvolemic hyponatremia.

Derivatization Labeling of or chemical addition to an analyte performed to increase the column retention or detectability of that analyte.

Detection methods In molecular diagnostics, these are the techniques used to detect nucleic acid sequences, usually after purification and amplification.

Detector A device that responds to the presence of analyte in the mobile phase, the magnitude of which is used to identify and quantify analytes; universal units detect most analytes and selective devices detect only analytes with specific properties.

Diabetes Control and Complications Trial (DCCT) A medical study of diabetic patients conducted in the United

States and Canada in 1983-1993 by the National Institute of Diabetes and Digestive and Kidney Diseases (NIDDK).

Diabetes insipidus Any of several types of polyuria in which the volume of urine exceeds 3 liters per day, causing dehydration and great thirst, as well as sometimes emaciation and great hunger. Caused by either a deficiency of ADH or defective receptor action.

Diabetes mellitus A group of metabolic disorders of carbohydrate metabolism in which glucose is underutilized, producing hyperglycemia.

Diabetic nephropathy The nephropathy that commonly accompanies later stages of diabetes mellitus. It begins with hyperfiltration, renal hypertrophy, albuminuria, and hypertension.

Diabetic retinopathy The retinal changes associated with diabetes mellitus.

Diabetogenes Genes that contribute to the development of diabetes; a genetic basis is identified in less than 5% of individuals with type 2 diabetes.

Diagnostic accuracy The closeness of agreement between values obtained from a diagnostic test (index test) and those of reference standard (gold standard) for a specific disease or condition; these results are expressed in a number of ways, including sensitivity and specificity, predictive values, likelihood ratios, diagnostic odds ratios, and areas under receiver operating characteristic (ROC) curves.

Dialysis The removal of certain elements from the blood by virtue of the difference in the rates of their diffusion through a semipermeable membrane, for example, by means of a hemodialysis (HD) machine or filter.

Diarrhea The passage of loose or liquid stools more than three times daily and/or a stool weight greater than 200 g/day.

Dideoxy-termination sequencing A method of DNA sequencing based on the selective incorporation of chain-terminating dideoxynucleotides by DNA polymerase during in vitro DNA replication. Also known as Sanger sequencing.

Difference plot A bias plot that shows the dispersion of observed differences between the measurements of two methods as a function of the average concentration of the measurements; also referred to as a "Bland-Altman plot."

Digestion The conversion of food, in the stomach and intestines, into soluble and diffusible products, capable of being absorbed.

Digestive process A three-phase process—neurogenic, gastric, and intestinal. The neurogenic (vagal) phase is initiated by the sight, smell, and taste of food. The gastric phase is initiated by the distention of the stomach by the entry of food. The intestinal phase begins when the partly digested food enters the duodenum from the stomach.

Digital Polymerase Chain Reaction A modification of conventional PCR where the sample is separated into a large number of partitions and the amplification is carried out in each partition individually. Also known as dPCR.

Digital rectal examination (DRE) A technique used for the early detection of prostate cancer. It is performed by inserting a gloved, lubricated finger into the rectum and feeling for abnormalities.

Dihydropteridine reductase (DHPR) An enzyme that catalyzes the reversible formation of tetrahydrobiopterin (BH_4) from dihydrobiopterine; deficiency of BH_4 results in malignant hyperphenylalaninemia.

Dihydrotestosterone (DHT) A powerful androgenic hormone that is formed in peripheral tissue by the action of the enzyme 5α-reductase on testosterone.

3,4-Dihydroxyphenylglycol (DHPG) The metabolite produced within the peripheral sympathetic or central nervous system noradrenergic nerves by deamination of norepinephrine (can also be formed from epinephrine); O-methylated to methoxyhydroxyphenylglycol in extraneuronal tissues.

Dilutional hyponatremia A condition characterized by low plasma concentration of sodium resulting from loss of sodium from the body with nonosmotic retention of water.

Dipsticks Single- or multi-pad measurement devices that quantify from one to several analytes.

Direct bilirubin The fraction of bilirubin that reacts with the diazo reagent in the absence of alcohol.

Discrete analysis Type of analysis in which the sample is aspirated into the sample probe and then is delivered, often with reagent, through the same orifice into a reaction cup or another container.

Disorders of amino acid metabolism A group of disorders of amino acid metabolism caused by defective activity of an enzyme leading to increased amino acids in blood (and urine).

Disorders of carbohydrate metabolism A group of disorders caused by loss of an enzyme in the metabolic pathway of a carbohydrate, leading to increased concentrations of that carbohydrate in blood or its accumulation within organs and tissues.

Disorders of fatty acid oxidation A group of disorders caused by deficiency of an enzyme in the oxidation pathway of fatty acids, leading to inability to use fat as an energy source.

Diuresis Increased excretion of urine.

Diurnal variation Variation that occurs in the amount of a substance during a 24-hour period.

DNA methylation The addition of a methyl group typically to the fifth carbon position of cytosine residues in CpG dinucleotides; this epigenetic process is implicated in growth and development of organisms.

DNA methyltransferase (DNMT) Any of a group of enzymes that catalyze the transfer of a methyl group from S-adenosylmethionine to a specific nucleotide in a DNA molecule, with different enzymes acting on specific nucleotides and positions of methylation.

DNA microarray An array of microscopic spots of different DNA molecules attached to a solid surface. Also known as DNA chip or *biochip*.

DNA-binding proteins Proteins that recognize and bind to specific DNA sequences. Some DNA-binding proteins are involved in the regulation of DNA transcription.

Dopamine A catecholamine formed in the body by the decarboxylation of L-dopa; an intermediate product in the synthesis of norepinephrine; acts as a neurotransmitter in the central nervous system, produced peripherally and acts on peripheral receptors.

Dot blotting A blotting technique in which the biomolecules to be detected are applied directly on a membrane as dots.

Down syndrome A birth defect characterized by having three copies of chromosome 21 rather than the normal two copies. Also known as trisomy 21.

Dried blood spot (DBS) A form of biosampling where blood samples are blotted and dried on filter paper.

Drosha A Class 2 RNase III enzyme responsible for processing of microRNA (miRNA).

Drug facilitated sexual assault (DFSA) The use of (1) alcohol, (2) drugs, and/or (3) chemical agents to incapacitate an individual and facilitate sexual assault.

Drug half-life Time required for one-half of an administered drug to be lost through metabolism and elimination.

Drug interactions The effects of a drug on absorption, metabolism, or action of another drug.

Drug metabolism The process by which drugs are chemically modified in the body.

Drug monitoring The process of studying the effects of a chemical substance administered to an individual.

Drug-induced liver injury (DILI) Damage to the liver that is caused by prescribed medications, over-the-counter medications, vitamins, hormones, herbs, illicit ("recreational") drugs, and environmental toxins.

Drugs of abuse Drugs that are repeatedly and deliberately used in a way other than prescribed or socially sanctioned (i.e., a drug that is taken for nonmedicinal reasons).

Dubin–Johnson syndrome An autosomal recessive disorder that causes an increase of conjugated bilirubin in the serum.

Dumping syndrome Following gastric surgery, hyperosmolar chyme is "dumped" into the small intestine causing rapid hypovolemia and hemoconcentration.

Eclampsia Convulsions and coma occurring in a pregnant woman or a woman who recently gave birth.

Ectopic pregnancy An embryo developing in the fallopian tube or abdomen instead of the uterus.

Ectopic syndrome Production of a hormone by nonendocrine cancerous tissue that normally does not produce the hormone (e.g., ACTH production by small-cell lung carcinoma).

Electrocardiogram (ECG) A graphic recording of the electrical activity produced by the heart.

Electrochemical cell An electrochemical device that consists of two electrodes (electron or metallic conductors) that are connected by an electrolyte solution that conducts ions (galvanic cell), or an electrochemical device in which an external voltage is applied to a polarizable working electrode with the resulting cathodic or anodic current of the cell being monitored (electrolytic cell).

Electrochemiluminescence The emission of light when an electron returns from an excited or higher energy level to a lower energy level, in which the excitation event is a reaction generated electrochemically on the surface of an electrode.

Electrode A half-cell that consists of a single metallic conductor in contact with an electrolyte solution; the indicator (measuring) electrode is one half-cell and the reference electrode is the second half-cell.

Electrode potential The reduction potential for a redox couple that is measured with respect to a standard hydrogen electrode set at zero; the electromotive force of an electrochemical cell.

Electrolyte exclusion effect Electrolytes are excluded from the fraction of total plasma volume that is occupied by solids, which leads to underestimation of electrolyte concentration by some methods.

Electrolytes Charged low-molecular-mass molecules present in plasma and cytosol, usually ions of (1) sodium, (2) potassium, (3) calcium, (4) magnesium, (5) chloride, (6) bicarbonate, (7) phosphate, (8) sulfate, and (9) lactate.

Electropherogram A densitometric display of protein zones on a support material after separation and staining.

Electrophoresis The migration of charged solutes or particles within a liquid medium under the influence of an electrical field.

Electrophoretic mobility (μ) The rate of migration (cm/s) of a charged solute in an electrical field, expressed per unit field strength (volts/cm).

Electrospray ionization A commonly used technique in which a sample is ionized at atmospheric pressure before introduction into the mass analyzer.

Embryo A developing infant that has not yet finished organ development (before 10 weeks gestation).

Enantiomer A molecule that exhibits stereoisomerism through the presence of one or more chiral centers (i.e., stereoisomers that are nonsuperimposable mirror images).

Endocrine system The system of glands that release their secretions (hormones) directly into the circulatory system. In addition to the endocrine glands, included are the chromaffin and the neurosecretory systems.

Endocrinology The scientific study of the function and pathology of the endocrine glands.

Endometrium The glandular mucous membrane that lines the uterus.

Endonuclease An enzyme that hydrolyzes an internal phosphodiester bond, splitting a nucleic acid into two or more parts.

Endosmosis (electroendosmotic flow) Preferential movement of water in one direction through an electrophoresis medium due to selective binding of one type of charge on the surface of the medium.

End-stage renal disease (ESRD) A condition where renal function is inadequate to support life.

Enteric nervous system (ENS) An independent and integrated system of neurons and supporting cells.

Enzyme A protein with catalytic properties.

Enzyme induction Increased synthesis of an enzyme in response to an inducer or other stimulus.

Enzyme inhibition Decreased enzymatic activity due to substrate competition or the presence of a compound that reduces enzyme function.

Epigenetics Processes that alter gene function or its interpretation by mechanisms other than those that rely on changes in DNA sequences; these processes include DNA methylation, genomic imprinting, histone modification, and chromatin remodeling.

Epinephrine (adrenaline) A catecholamine hormone secreted by the adrenal medulla.

Ergonomics The study of capabilities in relationship to work demands completed by defining postures that minimize unnecessary static work and reduce the forces working on the body.

Erythropoietic protoporphyria (EPP) An autosomal dominant disorder due to mutation in the *FECH* gene (locus: 18q21.3), which encodes ferrochelatase, causing a partial deficiency of the enzyme.

Erythropoietin A glycoprotein hormone secreted chiefly by the kidney in the adult; it increases the production of red blood cells.

Essential amino acids Amino acids that are not synthesized by humans and therefore are essential dietary constituents for maintaining health or growth.

Essential nutrients Nutrients (proteins, minerals, carbohydrates, lipids, vitamins) necessary for growth, normal functioning, and maintenance of life; they must be supplied by food because they cannot be synthesized by the body.

Estimated average requirement (EAR) The daily intake of a specific nutrient estimated to meet the requirement in 50% of healthy people in an age- and gender-specific group. The EAR is used to calculate the recommended dietary allowance.

Estradiol (E_2) and Estriol (E_3) Estrogenic hormones produced by the (1) ovaries, (2) corpus luteum, and during pregnancy by the (3) placenta. The adrenal glands and testes (in men) are also believed to secrete smaller quantities of estrogens.

Estrone (E_1) A natural estrogenic hormone that is a ketone found in the body chiefly as a metabolite of estradiol (E_2); it is also secreted especially by the ovaries.

Ethics Rules or standards governing the conduct of an individual or the members of a profession.

Ethylene glycol An ethylene compound with two hydroxy groups located on adjacent carbons. It is a common ingredient in antifreeze and is highly toxic if ingested.

Euchromatin Genomic regions that are rich in genes and are, in general, less compactly organized during interphase.

Eukaryote Organisms such as higher plants and animals, fungi, protozoa, and most algae; they have a true nucleus bounded by a nuclear membrane within which lie the chromosomes.

Euthyroid Having normal thyroid function.

Euthyroid hyperthyroxinemia A condition characterized by increased concentrations of thyroxine in the blood but a normal concentration of thyroid-stimulating hormone and normal thyroid function.

Evidence-based laboratory medicine The application of principles and techniques of evidence-based medicine to laboratory medicine; the conscientious, judicious, and explicit use of best evidence in laboratory medicine investigations to assist decision making about the care of individual patients.

Evidence-based medicine The conscientious, judicious, and explicit use of best evidence in making decisions about the care of individual patients.

Exome The part of the genome that codes for exons, the sequences that remain in the mature RNA after transcription and removal of introns by RNA splicing. It differs from a transcriptome in that it consists of only DNA that is transcribed into mature RNA, excluding transfer RNA, ribosomal RNA, and other non-coding RNA.

Exon The coding region of a gene that will be expressed as protein following translation.

Exonuclease A nuclease that releases one nucleotide at a time (serially) beginning at one end of a nucleic acid; exonuclease activity excises incorrectly paired nucleotides during replication.

Expected date of confinement (EDC) The date at which an infant is expected to be born, calculated from the date of the last menstrual period (LMP). Also called due date.

Exposure control plan An Occupational Safety and Health Administration (OSHA)-required plan that ensures the protection of laboratory workers against potential exposure to bloodborne pathogens, while ensuring that medical wastes produced by the clinical laboratory are managed and handled in a safe and effective manner.

External quality assessment Procedures and programs that provide information about systematic errors and maintenance of long-term accuracy of analytical methods.

Extracellular fluid (ECF) A general term for all the body fluids outside the cells, including the interstitial fluid, plasma, lymph, and cerebrospinal fluid (CSF); this fluid provides a constant external environment for the cells.

Extracted ion profile The sum of ions over a limited m/z ranged displayed as a function of time.

Facilitative glucose transporters A group of membrane proteins that facilitate the transport of glucose over a plasma membrane.

Familial hypophosphatemic rickets Any of several inherited disorders of proximal renal tubular function causing phosphate loss, hypophosphatemia, and skeletal deformities, including rickets and osteomalacia.

Fanconi syndrome A rare recessive disorder with a poor prognosis, characterized by pancytopenia, bone marrow hypoplasia, and patchy brown skin and multiple congenital anomalies of the musculoskeletal and genitourinary systems.

Fasting Abstinence from all food and drink except water for a prescribed period.

Fatty acid Any straight-chain monocarboxylic acid with an alkyl chain generally classed as saturated fatty acids with no double bonds; monounsaturated fatty acids with one double bond; and polyunsaturated fatty acids—those with multiple double bonds.

Female athletic triad A group of findings commonly seen in young female athletes, consisting of (1) eating disorders, (2) amenorrhea, and (3) osteoporosis.

Ferritin The iron/apoferritin complex, which is one of the chief forms in which iron is stored in the body; it occurs in the (1) gastrointestinal mucosa, (2) liver, (3) spleen, (4) bone marrow, and (5) reticuloendothelial cells.

Ferrochelatase A mitochondrial enzyme of the lyase class that catalyzes the insertion of ferrous iron into protoporphyrin IX to form protoheme IX, the heme of hemoglobin.

Fetal erythroblastosis A severe hemolytic disease of a fetus or newborn infant caused by the production of maternal antibodies against the fetal red blood cells, usually involving rhesus (Rh) blood group incompatibility between the mother and fetus.

Fetal fibronectin (fFN) A protein produced during pregnancy that is thought to function as a "glue" attaching the fetal sac to the uterine lining; a test for fFN in cervicovaginal fluid is used to assess risk of preterm labor.

Fetal lung maturity (FLM) A test that estimates the likelihood a neonate will develop respiratory distress syndrome.

Fetus A developing infant that has finished organ development (following 10 weeks gestation).

First messenger A factor or hormone that binds to a receptor on the external surface of a cell and sets off a series of reactions that eventually convert a precursor into a second messenger.

First-order kinetics In an enzymatic reaction, a phase of first-order dependence on substrate concentration when the rate of the reaction is proportional to the concentration of substrate or when the enzyme concentration is fixed and the substrate concentration is varied.

First-pass metabolism Extensive hepatic metabolism of a drug before it reaches the systemic circulation.

Flow cytometry The measurement of a physical or chemical characteristic of cells or particles made while the cells or particles pass singly through a measuring apparatus in a flowing fluid stream.

Fluorescence A physical property of some molecules to emit light at a longer wavelength when excited at a shorter wavelength.

Fluorescence in situ hybridization (FISH) An in situ hybridization technique in which DNA probes are labeled with fluorescent tags and hybridized to DNA to identify and localize specific sequences. Chromosome painting is a form of FISH.

Fluorescence The emission of electromagnetic radiation that occurs when a molecule absorbs light at one wavelength and reemits light at a longer wavelength, when it returns to ground state with the excitation event being caused by photo illumination.

Fluorometry The measurement of emitted fluorescence light that occurs when a molecule absorbs light at one wavelength and reemits light at a longer wavelength.

Follicle A pouch-like sac that is on the surface of the ovary and contains the maturing ovum (egg); also called Graafian follicle.

Follicle-stimulating hormone (FSH) An anterior pituitary peptide that stimulates the development of Graafian follicles in the female and spermatozoa in the male.

Fragment ion An ion formed by dissociation of a molecular ion, by convention often limited to fragmentation prior to mass analysis.

Fulminant hepatic failure A condition characterized by the development of severe liver injury with impaired synthetic capacity and encephalopathy in patients with previous normal liver or at least well-compensated liver disease.

Fulminant hepatitis A rare and frequently fatal form of acute hepatitis B in which the patient's condition rapidly deteriorates with hepatic encephalopathy, necrosis of the hepatic parenchyma, coagulopathy, renal failure, and coma.

Galactosemia An inherited disease in which the transformation of galactose to glucose is blocked, allowing galactose to increase to toxic concentrations in the body.

Gallstone A solid formation in the gallbladder, most commonly composed of cholesterol and bile salts.

Gamma-hydroxybutyrate (GHB) A potent sedative, hypnotic, euphorigenic agent that is illicitly ingested for its pleasurable effects.

Gas chromatography (GC) Column chromatography in which the mobile phase is a gas.

Gas chromatography-mass spectrometry (GC-MS) A combined technique in which a mixture of analytes is separated into individual components by gas chromatography, followed by the ionization of the separated compounds in the ion source of a mass spectrometer.

Gastrin A group of peptide hormones secreted by gastrointestinal (GI) mucosa cells in response to mechanical stress or high pH, both of which are produced by the presence of food in the stomach. Gastrin stimulates the stomach parietal cells to produce hydrochloric acid (HCl).

Gastrinoma A tumor of the pancreatic islet cells that results in an overproduction of gastric acid, leading to fulminant ulceration of the esophagus, stomach, duodenum, and jejunum. Gastrinoma may also occur in the stomach, duodenum, spleen, and regional lymph nodes.

Gastritis Mucosal inflammation of the stomach.

Gastroenteropancreatic neuroendocrine tumor (GEP-NET) Encompasses neuroendocrine tumors of the digestive system and pancreas but also covers neuroendocrine pulmonary tumors and includes carcinoid tumorss.

Gene A unit of DNA that specifies production of proteins and RNA molecules required for cellular function.

Gene duplication A process by which a chromosome or a portion of DNA is duplicated, resulting in an additional copy of a gene. Also referred to as chromosomal duplication or gene amplification.

Gene expression The process responsible for the flow of genetic information from gene to protein.

Generic form A drug not protected by a trademark. Also, the scientific name as opposed to the proprietary, brand name.

Genetic code The complete list of nucleotide codons and the amino acids or actions for which they "code."

Genetic Information Nondiscrimination Act of 2008 (GINA) Legislation enacted by the Congress of the United States that prohibits the use of genetic information in health insurance and employment.

Genome The complete set of chromosomes; the total complement of hereditary information; the human genome contains two copies, termed alleles, of each autosomal gene. One half of the genome is inherited from each parent and is termed the haploid genome. The complete genome inherited from both parents is termed the diploid genome.

Genotype The genetic makeup of an individual or a group of individuals. An individual's genotype codes for that individual's phenotype. The genotype for a specific gene requires knowledge of both alleles of the gene.

Genotyping Laboratory testing designed to detect specific genetic variants that are used to identify and classify variant alleles. The alleles are reported together as a genotype that may or may not be predictive of a phenotype.

Gestation The process, state or period of carrying an embryo or fetus from conception until birth; by convention, the time is measured clinically from the first day of the last menstrual period (LMP) and reported in weeks; gestational age of the fetus is often estimated by use of ultrasound.

Gestational diabetes mellitus (GDM) A condition of diabetes mellitus that sometimes occurs during pregnancy.

Ghrelin A peptide hormone, expressed primarily by the stomach, that stimulates the secretion of growth hormone and is considered a hunger-stimulating hormone.

Gilbert syndrome An inborn error of bilirubin metabolism.

Gitelman syndrome A syndrome of hypertrophy of juxtaglomerular cells similar to Bartter syndrome but with hypocalciuria and hypomagnesemia.

Gleason Score A grading system used to help evaluate the prognosis of men with prostate cancer.

Glioma A malignant tumor of the glial tissue of the nervous system.

Globulin Proteins that precipitate in water and redissolve when the salt concentration is raised.

Glomerular filtration rate (GFR) The rate in milliliters per minute at which small molecules are filtered through the kidney's glomeruli. It is a measure of the number of functioning nephrons.

Glomerulonephritis Nephritis accompanied by inflammation of the capillary loops of the glomeruli of the kidney. It occurs in acute, subacute, and chronic forms.

Glomerulus A tuft of blood vessels found in each nephron of the kidney that are involved in the filtration of the blood.

Glucagon A polypeptide hormone secreted by the alpha cells of the islets of Langerhans in response to hypoglycemia or the presence of acetylcholine, certain amino acids, or growth hormone. It helps to maintain blood glucose concentration by increasing blood glucose through glycogenolysis.

Glucocorticoids Any of the group of C21 steroids produced by the adrenal cortex that regulate carbohydrate, fat, and protein metabolism.

Glucose A six-carbon monosaccharide derived from the breakdown of carbohydrates in the diet or in body stores; also can be endogenously synthesized from protein or the glycerol moiety of triglyceride.

Glucose-dependent insulinotropic peptide (GIP, gastric inhibitory polypeptide) A peptide hormone (42 amino acids) that stimulates insulin release and at supraphysiological concentrations inhibits the release of gastric acid and pepsin.

Glucose-6-phosphate dehydrogenase (G-6-PD) deficiency An X-linked recessive hereditary disease characterized by abnormally low quantities of the enzyme G-6-PD involved in the pentose phosphate pathway, especially important in red blood cell metabolism.

Glucose tolerance test, oral (OGTT) A test whereby glucose is ingested into a fasting stomach and measurements of plasma glucose are taken over time; if glucose levels do not fall below specified cutpoints within 2 to 2.5 hours the patient may have impaired glucose tolerance or diabetes mellitus.

γ-Glutamyltransferase A transferase enzyme that reversibly catalyzes the transfer of a glutamyl group from a glutamyl-peptide and an amino acid to a peptide and a glutamyl-amino acid.

Glutaric acidemia type I (GAI) An inherited disorder in which an affected individual is unable to completely metabolize (1) lysine, (2) hydroxylysine, and (3) tryptophan. Excessive quantities of glutaric acid (GA) and related compounds accumulate and damage the brain.

Glycated hemoglobin Hemoglobin that has a sugar residue attached; HbA1c is the major fraction of glycated hemoglobin; also known as glycohemoglobin.

Glycogen An extensively branched polysaccharide containing many glucose residues and found particularly in muscle and liver cells for glucose storage.

Glycogen storage disease A group of rare inborn errors of metabolism caused by defects in specific enzymes or transporters involved in the metabolism of glycogen (also known as Von Gierke disease).

Goiter An enlargement of the thyroid gland that causes a swelling in the front part of the neck.

Gonad A gamete-producing organ (an ovary or a testis).

Gonadotropin Any hormone that stimulates the gonads.

Gonadotropin-releasing hormone (GnRH) A peptide hormone that is released from the hypothalmus where it stimulates the pituitary gland to secrete follicle-stimulating hormone and luteinizing hormone.

Gout A group of disorders of purine metabolism due to primary (inherited) or secondary causes such as chronic kidney disease.

G-protein–coupled receptors (GPCR) A large superfamily of membrane receptors whose intracellular effects are mediated by G proteins.

G-proteins Guanine nucleotide-binding proteins (G-proteins) are a family of proteins involved in transmitting chemical signals outside the cell, and causing changes inside the cell. They communicate signals from many hormones, neurotransmitters, and other signaling factors.

Graves disease A disorder of the thyroid of autoimmune etiology that causes hyperthyroidism. Characterized by having at least two of the following conditions: hyperthyroidism, goiter, and exophthalmos. Also known in Europe as Basedow disease.

Growth hormone (GH) A polypeptide of 191 amino acids that is produced by the anterior pituitary and affects the metabolism of carbohydrates, lipids, and proteins; it increases IGF-I.

Growth hormone–releasing hormone (GHRH) A hypothalamic hormone that regulates the release of growth hormone.

Gucagonoma A type of islet cell tumor of the alpha cells of the pancreas that secretes glucagon; some are malignant.

Gucose tolerance factor A biologically active complex of chromium and nicotinic acid that facilitates the reaction of insulin with receptor sites on tissues.

Guthrie test A semiquantitative microbiological assay for the determination of amino acids in blood or urine.

Gynecomastia Excessive development of the male mammary glands.

Half-life In endocrinology, the time required for a hormone to fall to half its original concentration in the specified fluid or blood.

Haplotype A combination of alleles (for different genes) that are located closely together on the same chromosome and that tend to be inherited together.

Hapten A chemically defined determinant that, when conjugated to an immunogenic carrier, stimulates the synthesis of antibody specific for the hapten.

Hartnup disease An inborn error of metabolism characterized by a massive aminoaciduria involving a group of neutral monoaminomonocarboxylic amino acids sharing a common renal reabsorption mechanism.

Hashimoto thyroiditis An autoimmune disorder in which the thyroid gland is attacked by a cell-mediated autoimmune process. Also known as Hashimoto disease and chronic lymphocytic thyroiditis, it is marked by (1) goiter, (2) chronic inflammation of the thyroid (thyroiditis), and (3) often hypothyroidism.

Hashitoxicosis Hyperthyroidism in patients with Hashimoto disease.

hCG stimulation test A test administered to assess the ability of the testes to respond to hCG and produce testosterone.

Helicobacter pylori A bacterium found in the mucous layer of the stomach. All strains secrete (1) proteins that cause inflammation of the mucosa and (2) the enzyme urease that produces ammonia from urea; some strains produce toxins that injure the gastric cells.

HELLP syndrome A life-threatening pregnancy complication usually considered to be a variant of preeclampsia and usually occurring between the 23rd and 39th weeks. The name is an acronym for the diagnostic features: H – Hemolysis; EL – Elevated Liver enzymes; LP – Low Platelets.

Hematuria Blood in the urine.

Heme Any quadridentate chelate of iron with the four pyrrole groups of a porphyrin, further distinguished as ferroheme or ferriheme, referring to the chelates of Fe(II) and Fe(III), respectively.

Hemin A porphyrin chelate of Fe3+ derived from red blood cells.

Hemochromatosis A rare genetic disorder caused by deposition of hemosiderin in the parenchymal cells, resulting in tissue damage and dysfunction of the liver, pancreas, heart, and pituitary. Also called iron overload disease.

Hemodiafiltration A type of hemofiltration with a dialytic component added. With it, blood flow is accelerated to twice that of conventional dialysis.

Hemoglobin The oxygen-carrying pigment of the erythrocytes, formed by the developing erythrocyte in bone marrow. It is a conjugated protein containing four heme groups and globin, with the property of reversible oxygenation.

Hemoglobinopathy Any inherited disorder caused by abnormalities of hemoglobin, resulting in conditions such as sickle cell anemia, hemolytic anemia, or thalassemia.

Hemolysis Disruption of the red cell membrane causing release of hemoglobin and other components of red blood cells.

Hemolytic disease of the newborn (HDN) A disease of the fetus and newborn caused by maternal antibody-mediated fetal erythrocyte destruction.

Hemosiderin An intracellular storage form of iron; the granules consist of an ill-defined complex of ferric hydroxides, polysaccharides, and proteins having an iron content of about 33% by weight.

Hemosiderosis A focal or general increase in tissue iron stores without associated tissue damage. Hepatic and pulmonary forms of hemosiderosis are characterized by abnormal quantities of hemosiderin in the liver and lungs, respectively.

Henderson-Hasselbalch equation An equation that defines the relationship among pH, bicarbonate, and the partial pressure of dissolved carbon dioxide gas.

Hepatic encephalopathy A condition caused by the deleterious effects of liver failure on the central nervous system. Features include confusion ranging to unresponsiveness (coma).

Hepatic failure A condition of severe liver dysfunction that is accompanied by a loss of normal liver functions.

Hepatitis Inflammation of the liver. Typically divided into acute (duration of weeks to months) and chronic (lasting for more than 6 months).

Hepatocellular carcinoma (HCC) A cancer arising from hepatocytes.

Hepatocyte An epithelial liver cell that performs most of the synthetic and metabolic functions of the liver.

Hepcidin A hormone produced by liver cells, in response to signals from a complex pathway, that decreases iron mobilization across intestinal and macrophage membranes, preventing excess iron in the blood.

Hereditary angioedema (HAE) Genetic disorder characterized by recurrent episodes of severe swelling.

Hereditary coproporphyria (HCP) An autosomal dominant hepatic porphyria caused by mutations of the *CPOX* gene (locus: 3q12) that result in partial deficiency of coproporphyrinogen oxidase activity.

Hereditary hemochromatosis A genetically heterogeneous group of inherited disorders of iron metabolism characterized by failure to prevent excessive amounts of iron from entering the circulatory pool and accumulating in the tissues.

Hereditary persistence of fetal hemoglobin A condition characterized by continued production of fetal hemoglobin beyond the point when it is normally replaced by hemoglobin A.

Heterochromatin Genomic regions that are gene poor or span transcriptionally silent genes and are more densely packed during interphase.

Heteroduplex A DNA duplex with internal mismatches or loops.

Hetero-duplex analysis (HDA) A type of mutation scanning in which a segment of DNA is screened by gel or capillary electrophoresis for mismatch pairing between normal and mutated base pairs.

Heterogeneous immunoassay An immunochemical reaction in which it is assumed that the formation of the antigen/antibody complex occurs more quickly than the breakdown of the complex into antigen and antibody; in this assay, the antigen is labeled and separation of the free from the bound labeled antigen is required.

Heteroplasmy The presence of more than one population of mitochondrial DNA sequences in a cell consequent to the accumulation of sequence variations.

High-performance liquid chromatography (HPLC) Liquid chromatography that uses columns containing small particles of stationary phase and requiring high pressure to push the mobile phase past the stationary phase.

High-resolution melting analysis (HRMA) An indirect method of observing DNA dissociation by using dyes that fluoresce in the presence of double-stranded DNA but not single-stranded DNA.

Hirsutism Abnormal hairiness, especially an adult male pattern of hair distribution in females.

Histones A class of structural proteins involved in the three-dimensional organization of nuclear DNA.

Holoenzyme Active enzyme formed by combination of a coenzyme and an apoenzyme.

Homeostasis The maintenance of equilibrium of internal body functions in response to external changes.

Homocystinuria A condition characterized by the excretion of excess homocystine in the urine; this biochemical abnormality has a variety of autosomal recessive genetic causes as well as nongenetic causes.

Homoduplex A perfectly matched DNA duplex.

Homogeneous immunoassay An immunochemical reaction in which the activity of the label attached to the antigen is modulated directly by antibody binding; this assay does not require a separation.

Homoplasmy The presence of a homogeneous population of mitochondrial genomes in a cell.

Homovanillic acid (HVA) A product of dopamine metabolism; elevated urinary concentrations are used to diagnose neuroblastoma.

Hook effect A phenomenon occurring with certain immunoassays due to very high concentrations of a particular analyte; it results in a false negative result. The hook effect mostly affects one-step immunometric assays.

Hormone A chemical substance that has a specific regulatory effect on the activity of a certain organ or organs on cell types.

Human antimouse antibodies (HAMA) Antibodies made by humans that bind mouse proteins. Their presence in body fluids causes both positive and negative interferences in two-site mouse monoclonal antibody-based assays.

Human chorionic gonadotropin (hCG) A placental glycoprotein hormone that stimulates the ovary to produce progesterone.

Human Genome Project A project undertaken by the International Human Genome Sequencing Consortium to decipher the three billion base pairs in the human genome; the project was completed in 2003.

Human placental lactogen (hPL) A placental hormone, similar in structure and function to growth hormone, that disappears from the blood immediately after delivery.

Humoral hypercalcemia of malignancy (HHM) A malignancy caused by bone resorption mediated by circulating factors released from distant tumor cells.

Hybridization The annealing or pairing of two DNA strands.

Hydramnios (or polyhydramnios) An abnormality of pregnancy characterized by an accumulation of excess amniotic fluid.

Hydrops fetalis A condition in which a fetus or newborn baby accumulates fluids, causing swollen arms and legs and impaired breathing.

5-Hydroxyindoleacetic acid (5-HIAA) A metabolite of serotonin (5-hydroxytryptamine) that is excreted in large amounts by patients with carcinoid tumors.

11β-Hydroxylase deficiency A type of congenital adrenal hyperplasia due to 11β-hydroxylase deficiency; it is one of a group of disorders (collectively called congenital adrenal hyperplasia) that affect the adrenal glands.

21-Hydroxylase deficiency A deficiency of this enzyme results in decreased cortisol synthesis and increased synthesis of male hormones by the adrenal; three types are described: (1) salt-wasting, (2) simple virilizing, and (3) nonclassical.

3β-Hydroxysteroid dehydrogenase deficiency An inherited disorder that affects hormone-producing glands, including the gonads (ovaries in females and testes in males) and the adrenal glands.

Hyperaldosteronism A condition in which the adrenal gland secretes and releases increased quantities of aldosterone.

Hyperandrogenism A condition characterized by excessive production and/or secretion of androgens.

Hyperbilirubinemia Excessive concentrations of bilirubin in the blood, which may lead to jaundice; the hyperbilirubinemias are classified as conjugated or unconjugated, according to the present form of bilirubin in the blood.

Hypercalcemia Increased concentration of calcium in plasma; manifestations include fatigability, muscle weakness, depression, anorexia, nausea, and constipation; most commonly caused by primary hyperparathyroidism or malignancy.

Hypercalcemia-associated malignancy (HAM) A malignancy characterized by hypercalcemia.

Hyperemesis gravidarum Extreme, excessive, and persistent vomiting in early pregnancy that may lead to dehydration and malnutrition.

Hyperglycemia Increased glucose concentrations in the blood.

Hypergonadotropic hypogonadism A condition characterized by (1) defective development of ovaries or testes, (2) excess pituitary gonadotropin secretion, and (3) delayed sexual development and growth delay.

Hyperkalemia A concentration of serum potassium above the reference interval limit of 5.0 mmol/L.

Hypermagnesemia A condition characterized by abnormally high concentrations of magnesium in blood plasma.

Hypernatremia A concentration of serum sodium above the reference interval limit of 150 mmol/L.

Hyperornithinemia-Hyperammonemia-Homocitrullinuria (HHH) syndrome An autosomal recessive syndrome characterized by increased plasma concentrations of ornithine, postprandial hyperammonemia and homocitrullinuria, and aversion to protein ingestion; the affected gene codes for the mitochondrial ornithine transporter, ornithine translocase.

Hyperphosphatemia A condition characterized by abnormally high concentrations of phosphates in blood plasma.

Hyperprolactinemia A condition characterized by increased levels of prolactin in the blood; in women it is associated with amenorrhea and galactorrhea, and in men it has been reported to cause hypogonadism, impotence, and in some cases gynecomastia.

Hypertension A medical condition characterized by high arterial blood pressure.

Hyperthyroidism A condition caused by excessive production of iodinated thyroid hormones. Symptoms and signs include increased basal metabolic rate, enlargement of the thyroid gland, rapid heart rate, high systolic blood pressure, and a number of secondary symptoms.

Hypertrichosis Excessive growth of hair.

Hyperuricemia An excess of uric acid or urates in the blood with many causes; it is a prerequisite for the development of gout and may lead to renal disease.

Hypervitaminosis An unhealthy condition resulting from excessive amounts of a vitamin.

Hypervolemia Abnormal increase in the volume of circulating fluid (plasma) in the body.

Hypocalcemia A condition characterized by a low concentration of calcium in plasma.

Hypoglycemia Decreased glucose concentrations in the blood.

Hypogonadotropic hypogonadism A condition with impaired production of the hormones (LH and FSH) that stimulate the gonads; lack of LH and FSH leads to decreased sex hormone production by the gonads and accompanying symptoms.

Hypokalemia A concentration of serum potassium below the reference interval limit of 3.5 mmol/L.

Hypomagnesemia A condition characterized by a low concentration of magnesium in blood.

Hyponatremia A concentration of serum sodium below the reference interval limit of 136 mmol/L.

Hypoparathyroidism The condition produced by greatly reduced function of the parathyroid glands.

Hypophosphatemia A condition characterized by a low concentration of phosphate in blood.

Hypothyroidism A condition of deficient thyroid gland activity leading to lethargy, muscle weakness, and intolerance to cold.

Hypouricemia Decreased uric acid concentration in the blood, secondary to a number of underlying conditions such as severe hepatocellular disease and defective renal tubular reabsorption.

Hypovitaminosis An unhealthy condition resulting from too little of a vitamin; interchangeable with avitaminosis.

Hypovolemia A condition characterized by an abnormal decrease in the volume of circulating blood in the body.

Icterus A condition characterized by hyperbilirubinemia and deposition of bile pigments in the skin, mucous membranes, and sclera, with resulting yellow appearance of the patient; called also jaundice.

ICTP An antigen produced when type I collagen is digested by matrix metalloproteinases, yielding cross-linked carboxy-terminal telopeptide of type I collagen; a serum marker for bone resorption.

Idiopathic postprandial syndrome Repeated occurrence of the clinical manifestations of hypoglycemia after meals.

IgA nephropathy A common, chronic form of glomerulonephritis marked by hematuria and proteinuria and by deposits of immunoglobulin A in the mesangial areas of the renal glomeruli.

Immunoassay An assay based on the reaction of an antigen with an antibody specific for the antigen.

Immunogen A substance capable of inducing an immune response.

Immunoglobulin superfamily (IgSF) A large group of cell surface and soluble proteins that are involved in the recognition, binding, or adhesion processes of cells.

Immunoglobulins A family of proteins also known as antibodies that contain highly specific antigen-binding sites consisting of two identical heavy (H) chains encoded on chromosome 14 and two identical light (L) chains encoded on chromosome 2.

Immunostrip (immunosensor) A point-of-care device in which the recognition element is an antibody that binds to the analyte; the binding event is typically detected by an optical mechanism.

Immunosuppression The prevention or diminution of the immune response by irradiation or by administration of antimetabolites, antilymphocyte serum, or specific antibody.

Impaired glucose tolerance (IGT) A term denoting values of fasting plasma glucose or results of an oral glucose tolerance test that are abnormal but not high enough to be diagnostic of diabetes mellitus.

In vitro fertilization (IVF) A procedure in which (1) eggs (ova) from a woman's ovary are removed, (2) the removed eggs are fertilized with sperm in a laboratory procedure, and (3) the fertilized egg (embryo) is returned to the woman's uterus.

Inborn error of metabolism (IEM) Inherited disorder in which a specific enzyme defect causes a metabolic block in the individual at birth or in later life.

Incretin Any of various gastrointestinal hormones and factors that act as potent stimulators of insulin secretion, such as gastric inhibitory polypeptide.

Indel A sequence variant arising from both an insertion and a deletion.

Index test In diagnostic accuracy studies, the "new" test or the test of interest.

Indirect bilirubin Free bilirubin that has not been conjugated with glucuronic acid.

Infertility The inability to conceive after one year of unprotected intercourse.

Informatics In a clinical sense, the design, management, and study of systems that store and communicate medical information; in the clinical laboratory, this refers to the communication and management of information related to laboratory testing and test interpretation.

Inhibin A peptide hormone secreted by the follicular cells of the ovary and the Sertoli cells of the testis that inhibits secretion of follicle stimulating hormone (FSH) from the anterior pituitary.

Inhibin A Ovary-produced inhibin A is an important negative feedback hormone that suppresses pituitary secretion of FSH during the late follicular and luteal phases of the menstrual cycle.

Inhibitor A substance that reduces the rate of an enzymatic reaction and is classified as reversible or irreversible.

Insertion An extra DNA sequence that is present in one sample compared with a reference sequence.

Insulin A protein hormone produced by β-cells of the pancreas that decreases blood glucose concentrations.

Insulin resistance Impairment of normal biologic responses to insulin.

Insulinlike growth factors (IGF) Serum peptides with insulin-like actions, formerly called somatomedins.

Intergenic DNA sequence between genes.

International normalized ratio (INR) A method of reporting prothrombin time results for patients receiving oral anticoagulant therapy

International System of Units (SI) A system of units for analytical results that is based on the cubic meter as the reference volume and is an internationally (except in the United States) adopted system of measurement. The units of the system are called SI units.

International unit The quantity of enzyme that catalyzes one micromole of substrate per minute.

Interphase The period between cell divisions.

Interstitial nephritis Primary or secondary disease of the renal interstitial tissue.

Intoxication A state of impaired mental or physical functioning resulting from ingestion of alcohol or drug.

Intracellular fluid (ICF) The portion of the total body water (TBW) with its dissolved solutes that is within the cell membranes.

Intron A noncoding region of a gene, located between exons, that will not be translated into protein. It is spliced out during messenger RNA (mRNA) processing.

Ion An atom that has acquired an electrical charge by losing or gaining one or more electrons.

Ion trap A component of a trapping-type mass spectrometer where ions are held in a spatially confined region of space using, for example, a magnetic or electrostatic field; manipulation of the traps allows m/z measurements to be performed.

Ion-exchange chromatography A separation mechanism that is based on the exchange of ions between a charged stationary phase and oppositely charged ions in the mobile phase.

Ionization The production of an ion from a neutral atom or molecule using various techniques including but not limited to chemical ionization or electrospray ionization; ionization is required for all mass spectrometry techniques.

Ion-selective electrode An electrode that selectively interacts with a single ionic species; the potential produced at the membrane/sample solution interface is proportional to the logarithm of the ionic activity or the concentration of the ion in question.

Irinotecan A DNA topoisomerase inhibitor used as an antineoplastic drug in the treatment of colorectal carcinoma.

ISO 9000 A set of four standards used to ensure quality management and quality assessment developed by the International Organization for Standardization.

Isoelectric focusing An electrophoretic technique that separates amphoteric compounds within a medium that possesses a stable pH gradient.

Isoelectric point (pI) The pH at which a molecule has no net charge and will not migrate during electrophoresis.

Isoenzyme A molecular form of an enzyme that originates at the level of the genes that encode the structures of the enzyme proteins in question.

Isoform A form of an enzyme that is modified by post-translational processing.

Isotope A variant of a chemical element; each variant differs in the number of neutrons in the nucleus and therefore in atomic weight from other isotopes of the same element.

Isotope dilution mass spectrometry (IDMS) An analytical technique used to quantify a compound relative to an isotopic species of known or fixed concentration using isotopically labeled internal standards.

Isovaleric acidemia A metabolic disorder which disrupts or prevents normal metabolism of the branched-chain amino acid leucine. It is characterized by acidosis, coma, and an unpleasant body odor.

Jaffe reaction The reaction of creatinine with alkaline picrate to form a colored compound.

Jaundice A clinical finding characterized by hyperbilirubinemia and deposition of pigment in the skin, mucous membranes, and sclera with resulting yellow appearance; also called icterus.

Juxtaglomerular apparatus (JGA) A complex in the kidney whose function is the autoregulation of the glomerular filtration rate.

Kallmann syndrome A type of hypogonadotropic hypogonadism caused by failure of fetal gonadotropin-releasing hormone neurons to migrate to the hypothalamus.

Kashin–Bek disease (KBD) A chronic, endemic osteochondropathy (disease of the bone).

Katal The quantity of an enzyme that catalyzes a reaction rate of one mole of substrate per second.

Kernicterus A clinical syndrome of the neonate resulting from high concentrations of unconjugated bilirubin that passes the immature blood-brain barrier of the newborn and causes degeneration of cells of the basal ganglia and hippocampus.

Keshan disease A fatal, congestive cardiomyopathy caused by deficiency of essential trace elements in the diet.

Ketoacidosis A condition characterized as acidosis accompanied by the accumulation of ketone bodies (ketosis) in the body tissues and fluids.

Ketone An organic compound that has a carbonyl group (carbon atom double-bonded to an oxygen atom) at any position other than at the end of the carbon chain.

Klinefelter syndrome A condition in a male characterized by (1) two X and one Y chromosomes, (2) infertility, (3) small testicles, (4) sparse facial and body hair, and (5) enlarged breasts.

Kwashiorkor A form of protein-energy malnutrition produced by severe protein deficiency.

Label Any substance with a measurable property attached to an antigen, antibody, or binding substance.

Laboratory medicine A component of laboratory science that is involved in the selection, provision, and interpretation of diagnostic testing of individual specimens.

Laboratory testing A process conducted in a clinical laboratory to rule in or rule out a diagnosis, to select and monitor disease treatment, to provide a prognosis, to screen for a disease, or to determine the severity of and monitor a physiological disturbance.

Lactate An intermediary product in glucose metabolism that accumulates in the blood predominantly when tissue oxygenation is decreased, as during strenuous exercise; an increased blood lactate concentration is called lactic acidosis.

Lactate dehydrogenase An oxidoreductase enzyme that reversibly catalyzes the reduction of pyruvate to L-lactate, using NADH (reduced form of nicotinamide adenine dinucleotide) as an electron donor.

Lactose intolerance A condition due to lactase deficiency leading to malabsorption of lactose and causing symptoms of flatulence, abdominal discomfort, bloating, or diarrhea after ingesting milk or foods containing lactose.

Lamellar bodies Packages of phospholipids that are produced by type II alveolar cells and represent the storage form of surfactant. They are similar in size to platelets and are present in amniotic fluid.

Lamellar body count (LBC) Number of lamellar bodies in amniotic fluid. LBC increases as gestation advances. Most electronic cell counters will count the lamellar bodies.

Lanugo A very fine, soft, and usually unpigmented downy hair on the body of a fetus or newborn baby.

Laron syndrome An autosomal recessive syndrome of skeletal growth retardation due to impaired ability to synthesize insulin-like growth factor I, usually because of growth hormone receptor defects. Also called Laron dwarfism.

Late-onset 21-hydroxylase deficiency (NCAH) A condition due to 21-hydroxylase deficiency. It is a common, milder form of congenital adrenal hyperplasia (CAH) characterized by a later onset of androgen excess symptoms seen in females and precocious pseudopuberty in both sexes. Also known as nonclassical congenital adrenal hypoplasia.

L-Dopa An amino acid—3,4-dihydroxyphenylalanine—produced by oxidation of tyrosine by tyrosine hydroxylase; the precursor of dopamine and an intermediate product in the biosynthesis of norepinephrine, epinephrine. Can also be formed in melanocytes by the actions of tyrosinase as part of the production of melanin.

Lean production A quality process that is focused on creating greater value by eliminating activities that are considered waste.

Leber's hereditary optic neuropathy (LHON) A neuropathy transmitted from mother to children that is characterized by a degeneration of retinal ganglion cells (RGCs) and their axons that leads to a loss of central vision.

Levey-Jennings control chart A graphical display with observed control values plotted against an acceptable range of values, indicated on the chart by lines for upper and lower control limits, commonly indicated as the mean control value plus or minus three standard deviations.

Leydig cell A type of cell in the testes that secretes testosterone.

LH surge A sharp increase in serum concentrations of luteinizing hormone seen near the middle of the menstrual cycle about one to two days before ovulation.

Liddle syndrome A rare autosomal dominant syndrome resulting from epithelial sodium channel mutations that lead to abnormally increased channel function.

Ligandin An hepatic transport protein; measurement of it in serum and urine may be a means of estimating the severity of hepatocellular necrosis.

Ligase An enzyme that covalently joins two DNA strands.

Ligase chain reaction (LCR) A DNA amplification technique that uses four primers instead of two and uses the ligase to ligate or join two segments of DNA.

Light Energy transmitted via electromagnetic waves that are characterized by frequency and wavelength; light is composed of photons whose energy is inversely proportional to the wavelength.

Light scattering A physical phenomenon that results from the interaction of light with particles in solution.

Likelihood ratio The probability of occurrence of a specific test value given that the disease is present divided by the probability of the same test value if the disease was absent.

Limit of detection An assay characteristic defined as the lowest value that significantly exceeds the measurements of a blank sample.

Lineweaver-Burk plot A plot of the reciprocal of the velocity of an enzyme catalyzed reaction (ordinate; y-axis) against the reciprocal of the substrate concentration (abscissa; x-axis).

Linkage disequilibrium Nonrandom association of alleles at different loci; the rate reflects rates of recombination and is used as a measure of distance between the loci. See also centiMorgan.

Lipase A hydrolase that hydrolyzes glycerol esters of long-chain fatty acid.

Lipids A class of compounds that are soluble in organic solvents but are nearly insoluble in water and that contain nonpolar carbon-hydrogen bonds.

Lipoprotein(a) A lipoprotein structurally similar to low-density lipoprotein but containing a carbohydrate-rich protein and that carries only a relatively small fraction of total cholesterol; it is considered particularly pro-atherogenic.

Lipoprotein-associated phospholipase A2 An enzyme member of the phospholipase A2 superfamily that cleaves oxidized phosphatidylcholine components of lipoprotein particles.

Lipoproteins Spherical particles involved in the transport of lipids with nonpolar neutral lipids (triglycerides and cholesterol esters) in their core and more polar amphipathic lipids (phospholipids and free cholesterol) at their surface.

Liquid chromatography (LC) Column chromatography using a liquid mobile phase.

Liquid chromatography–mass spectrometry (LC-MS) An analytical process that uses a liquid chromatograph coupled to a mass spectrometer.

Lithotripsy The crushing of a calculus within the urinary system or gallbladder, followed at once by the washing out of the fragments; it is done either surgically or by several different noninvasive methods.

Long-chain 3-hydroxyacyl-CoA dehydrogenase (LCHAD) deficiency A metabolic disease characterized by defective fatty acid oxidation due to a defect in an enzyme in the β-oxidation pathway.

Loop of Henle The U-shaped part of the renal tubule, extending through the medulla from the end of the proximal convoluted tubule to the beginning of the distal convoluted tubule.

Loop-mediated amplification (LAMP) A single tube technique for the amplification of DNA that uses a single-temperature incubation.

Lucey-Driscoll syndrome A potentially fatal disorder characterized by severe hyperbilirubinemia present at birth, which accumulates in the brain.

Luteinizing hormone (LH) A hormone produced by the anterior lobe of the pituitary gland that stimulates ovulation and the development of the corpus luteum in the female and the production of testosterone by the interstitial cells of the testis in the male.

Lymphoma Any neoplastic disorder of the lymphoid tissue.

Lysergic acid diethylamide (LSD) A derivative of an alkaloid found in certain fungi that has hallucinogenic properties.

Malabsorption An abnormality in the absorption of nutrients.

MALDI Acronym for matrix-assisted laser desorption/ionization. It is a soft ionization technique that allows the analysis of biomolecules and large organic molecules which tend to be fragile and fragment when ionized by more conventional ionization methods.

Maldigestion An abnormality of the digestive process due to dysfunction of the pancreas or small intestine.

Maple syrup urine disease (MSUD) An autosomal recessive metabolic disorder affecting branched-chain amino acids (leucine, isoleucine, and valine). The urine of affected individuals smells like maple syrup.

Marasmus A form of protein-energy malnutrition predominantly due to prolonged severe caloric deficit.

Marfan syndrome A congenital disorder of connective tissue characterized by long limbs and caused by abnormal fibrillin metabolism; it affects various structures, notably heart valves and aorta.

Marijuana A crude preparation of the leaves and flowering tops of *Cannabis sativa* plants, usually used in cigarettes and inhaled as smoke for its euphoric properties.

Mass analysis The process by which a mixture of ionic species is identified according to the mass-to-charge (m/z) ratios (ions).

Mass spectrometer An analytical instrument that first ionizes a target molecule and then separates and measures the mass-to-charge (m/z) ratio of these molecules or their fragments; this instrument interfaces with other instruments including but not limited to a second mass spectrometer or a gas chromatograph.

Mass spectrometry Study of matter through the formation of gas-phase ions that are characterized by their mass, charge, structure, and/or physico-chemical properties.

Mass spectrum A plot of the relative abundance of each ion plotted as a function of its mass-to-charge (m/z) ratio.

Mass-to-charge ratio (m/z>) The quantity formed by dividing the mass of an ion by its charge.

Material Safety Data Sheet (MSDS) A technical bulletin that contains information about a hazardous chemical, such as chemical composition, chemical and physical hazard, and precautions for safe handling and use.

Matrix In relation to analytical methods, human serum that contains analytes.

MDA (3,4-methylenedioxyamphetamine) A psychedelic drug of the phenethylamine and amphetamine classes of drugs.

MDMA (3,4-methylenedioxy-N-methylamphetamine) A drug of the phenethylamine and amphetamine classes of drugs. Known as "ecstasy."

Measurand See Analyte.

Measuring interval The analyte concentration range over which measurements are within the declared tolerances for imprecision and bias; also referred to as "reportable range."

Mechanism of action The mechanism by which a pharmacologically active substance produces an effect on a living organism or in a biochemical system.

Meconium A dark green fecal material that accumulates in the fetal intestines and is discharged at or near the time of birth.

Medium-chain acyl-CoA dehydrogenase (MCAD) deficiency A disorder of fatty acid oxidation that impairs the body's ability to break down medium-chain fatty acids into acetyl-CoA.

Medullary thyroid cancer (MTC) A slow-growing tumor associated with multiple endocrine neoplasia (MEN) syndromes.

Mees' lines Lines of discoloration across the nails of the fingers and toes.

Megaloblastic anemia Any anemia characterized by megaloblasts in the bone marrow, such as pernicious anemia.

Melatonin A hormone synthesized by the pineal gland in many species of animals; its secretion increases during exposure to light.

Melting curve analysis A direct measurement of double-stranded DNA (dsDNA) dissociation during heating. As the temperature is raised, the double strand dissociates resulting in an increase in the absorbance of the solution containing the DNA.

Melting temperature (Tm) The temperature at which 50% of the DNA strands are in the random coil or single-stranded (ssDNA) state. It depends on the length of the DNA molecule and its specific nucleotide sequence.

Menarche The establishment or beginning of the menstrual function.

Menkes disease An X-linked recessive disorder of copper metabolism caused by mutations in the *ATP7A* gene (locus: Xq12- q13), which encodes a copper transporter.

Menopause Cessation of menstruation, which usually occurs around the age of 50.

Menses The monthly flow of blood from the genital tract of women.

Mesothelioma A tumor derived from mesothelial tissue (peritoneum, pleura, pericardium); both benign and malignant varieties exist. Malignant varieties are often the result of excessive exposure to asbestos.

Metabolic acidosis Any of the various kinds of acidosis in which the acid-base status of the body shifts toward the acid side because of loss of base or retention of acids other than carbonic acid.

Metabolic alkalosis A pathological process that leads to the accumulation of base that raises the bicarbonate concentration and increases the pH; also known as primary bicarbonate excess.

Metabolizer classification A classification of four drug-metabolism phenotypes as they relate to an individual's metabolic efficiency for processing a specific therapeutic drug. The four types are (1) poor metabolizers (PMs), (2) ultra-rapid metabolizers (UMs), (3) extensive metabolizers (EMs), and (4) intermediate metabolizers (IMs).

Metanephrine A catecholamine metabolite resulting from O-methylation of epinephrine; formed mainly within adrenal chromaffin cells; excreted mainly in the urine as a sulfate-conjugated metabolite; measurements of the free and conjugated metabolites provide useful tests for diagnosis of pheochromocytoma.

Metastasis The spread of cancer from one part of the body to another.

Methadone A synthetic opioid analgesic, possessing pharmacologic actions similar to those of morphine and heroin and similar potential for addiction; used as an analgesic and as a narcotic abstinence syndrome suppressant in the treatment of heroin addiction.

Methamphetamine (Ritalin) A sympathomimetic amine closely related chemically to both amphetamine and ephedrine, having actions similar to those of amphetamine.

Methemoglobin A form of hemoglobin where its iron atom is changed from the ferrous to the ferric state.

Method comparison Comparison of measurements by two methods that is carried out objectively using statistical procedures and graphics displays.

Methoxyhydroxyphenylglycol (MHPG) A metabolite of epinephrine and norepinephrine formed primarily from O-methylation of dihydroxyphenylglycol and in smaller amounts from deamination of normetanephrine and metanephrine; found in brain, blood, CSF, and urine, where its concentration is used to measure catecholamine turnover.

Methylmalonic acidemia An autosomal recessive metabolic disorder resulting from defects in the metabolic pathway in which methylmalonyl-coenzyme A (CoA) is converted into succinyl-CoA by the enzyme methylmalonyl-CoA mutase.

Methylphenidate A central stimulant used in the treatment of attention-deficit/hyperactivity disorder, narcolepsy, and certain forms of depression

Metric system A system of weights and measures based on the meter as a standard unit of length, the liter as a standard unit of volume, and the gram as a standard unit of mass.

Michaelis-Menten constant (Km) A constant for a given enzyme acting under given conditions; the experimentally determined substrate concentration at which the enzymatic reaction velocity equals ½ of the maximum velocity of the enzymatic reaction.

Microarray-based genotyping A molecular technique used to simultaneously screen hundreds to thousands of genetic markers per individual.

Microcephaly A condition characterized by an abnormally small head circumference; associated with a small brain (microencephaly).

Microchip electrophoresis An electrophoretic technique whereby separation is conducted in fluidic channels on a microchip and detection occurs through laser-induced fluorescence.

MicroRNA (miRNA) Short noncoding RNA (ncRNA) molecules around 22 nucleotides in length that play a role in regulation of gene expression by interfering with effective translation of mRNA to proteins.

Microsatellites Short segments of DNA (1 to 13 bases long) that are repeated end to end. Also known as short tandem repeats (STRs).

Microtiter plate A flat plate containing a two-dimensional array of multiple "wells" used as small reaction chambers.

Such plates typically have 6, 24, 96, 384, or even 1536 sample wells arranged in a rectangular array.

Minamata disease A condition characterized by symptoms of alkyl mercury poisoning that were seen between 1953 and 1958 among individuals who ate seafood from a bay in Japan that was polluted with alkyl mercury compound.

Mineralization The process by which the body uses minerals to build bone structure.

Mineralocorticoids Any of the group of 21-carbon corticosteroids (principally aldosterone) that contribute to the regulation of (1) water, (2) acid-base, and (3) electrolyte balance in the body.

Minisatellites Repeated segments of DNA that are 14 to 500 bases long. Also known as sequences with a variable number of tandem repeats (VNTRs).

Miosis Constriction of the pupil of the eye, resulting from a normal response to an increase in light or caused by certain drugs or pathological conditions.

Missense A nucleotide substitution that changes a codon to the code for a different amino acid. Although these sequence changes are commonly referred to as missense "mutations," this is strictly a misnomer, because they may be benign and cause no disease.

Mitochondrial DNA The circular DNA within a mitochondrial organelle that codes for polypeptides involved in the oxidative phosphorylation pathway; this DNA is typically transmitted across generations by maternal inheritance.

Mixed acid-base disturbance The occurrence of more than one acid-base disorder simultaneously; the blood pH may be low, high, or within the reference interval.

Mnemonics A mnemonic or mnemonic device is any learning technique that aids information retention.

Mobile phase A gas or a liquid that flows in a chromatographic system and carries the sample past the stationary phase.

Model for End-Stage Liver Disease (MELD) Score A scoring system for assessing the severity of chronic liver disease.

Molar absorptivity (ε) A proportionality constant for a compound that is the measure of the absorption of radiant energy at a given wavelength as it passes through a solution of that compound at a concentration of 1 mol/L; expressed mathematically as absorbance divided by the product of the concentration of a substance in mol/L and the sample path length in centimeters ($\varepsilon = A/bc$).

Molar pregnancy A type of pregnancy caused by abnormal proliferation of placental tissue in the uterus. Also known as a hydatidiform mole.

Molecular diagnostics Use of molecular biology techniques for the purposes of prevention, diagnosis, and follow-up or prognosis of disease; and selection, optimization, and monitoring of therapies.

Monoclonal gammopathy of undetermined significance (MGUS) A condition in which a paraprotein is found in an individual's blood.

Morula A solid ball of cells resulting from division of a fertilized ovum and from which a blastula is formed.

Mucin A high-molecular-weight glycoprotein complex.

Müllerian duct Either of two embryonic tubes extending along the mesonephros that become the uterine tubes, uterus, and part of the vagina in the female and that form the prostatic utricle in the male.

Müllerian duct agenesis A congenital malformation characterized by a failure of the Müllerian duct to develop, with resultant absence or malformation of the vagina and/or uterus.

Multiple endocrine neoplasia (MEN) A group of genetic disorders characterized by hyperplasia and hyperfunction of two or more components of the endocrine system such as the parathyroid and other hormonal glands.

Multiple myeloma A cancer in which antibody-producing plasma cells grow in an uncontrolled and malignant manner.

Multiple of the median (MoM) In clinical screening, the statistic used to normalize analyte values.

Multiple-channel analysis Type of analysis in which each specimen is subjected to multiple analytical processes so that a set of test results is obtained on a single specimen; similar to random-access analysis.

Multiplex analysis Simultaneous assessment of multiple analytes in a single sample.

Multiplex ligation-dependent probe amplification (MLPA) A variation of PCR that permits multiple targets to be amplified with only a single primer pair.

Mutation A disease-causing sequence variation.

Myeloperoxidase An enzyme that catalyzes the conversion of chloride anion and hydrogen peroxide to hypochlorite, a metal chlorinating oxidant with a potent microbicidal activity.

Myocardial ischemia Deficiency of blood supply to the heart muscle due to obstruction or constriction of the coronary arteries.

Myocardium The middle and thickest layer of the heart wall, composed of cardiac muscle.

Myoglobin A heme-containing protein found in red skeletal muscle.

Myxedema A severe form of hypothyroidism in which there is accumulation of mucopolysaccharides in the skin and other tissue, leading to a thickening of facial features and a doughy induration of the skin.

N-acetyltransferase (NAT) A family of metabolic enzymes that acetylate drugs.

National Institutes of Health (NIH) Pharmacogenomics Research Network (PGRN) A network of scientists focused on understanding how a person's genes affect his or her response to medicines.

Necrosis The sum of the morphological changes indicative of cell death and caused by the progressive degradative action of enzymes; it may affect groups of cells or part of a structure or an organ.

Nephelometry The detection and measurement of light energy scattered or reflected toward a detector that is not in the direct path of the transmitted light.

Nephritis Inflammation of the kidney with focal or diffuse proliferation or destructive processes that may involve the glomerulus, tubule, or interstitial renal tissue.

Nephrolithiasis A condition marked by the presence of renal calculi (stones).

Nephron The anatomical and functional unit of the kidney, consisting of the (1) renal corpuscle, (2) proximal convoluted tubule, (3) descending and ascending limbs of loop of Henle, (4) distal convoluted tubule, and (5) collecting tubule.

Nephrotic syndrome General name for a group of diseases involving defective kidney glomeruli, characterized by massive proteinuria and lipiduria with varying degrees of edema, hypoalbuminemia, and hyperlipidemia.

Nernst equation The equation used to determine the reduction potential for a given redox couple and used to correlate chemical energy with the electrical potential of an electrochemical cell.

Neural tube defect (NTD) A major birth defect resulting from the abnormal development of the neural tube present during embryonic life that gives rise to the central nervous system; the two most common NTDs are spina bifida and anencephaly.

Neuroblastoma A sarcoma consisting of malignant neuroblasts, usually arising in the autonomic nervous system (sympathicoblastoma) or in the adrenal medulla; considered a type of neuroepithelial tumor that affects mostly infants and children up to 10 years of age.

Neuroendocrine tumors (NET) Neoplasms that arise from cells of the endocrine and peripheral nervous systems, most commonly in the digestive tract, but also found in the lung, pancreas, pituitary, thyroid, and other tissues.

Neurofibromatosis 1 (NF1) An autosomal dominant disorder due to mutation in the *NF1* gene.

Neurohypophysis The posterior lobe of the pituitary gland, making up the neural portion that secretes various hormones.

NIOSH U.S. National Institute for Occupational Safety and Health.

Non-alcoholic fatty liver disease (NAFLD) A condition characterized by the buildup of extra fat in liver cells that is not caused by alcohol.

Non-alcoholic steatohepatitis (NASH) An inflammatory disease of the liver of uncertain pathogenesis.

Noncompetitive immunoassay An immunoassay in which a capture antibody is bound to a surface with subsequent antigen binding followed by the addition of a second labeled antibody that reacts with the initial antigen/antibody complex.

Nonketotic hyperglycinemia (NKHG) A usually fatal autosomal-recessive aminoacidopathy with accumulation of glycine in body fluids, particularly the blood, urine, and cerebrospinal fluid.

Nonparametric analysis A statistical approach to reference value analysis that requires no assumptions about the nature of the distribution; thus, it can be applied to distributions that are Gaussian or non-Gaussian.

Nonsense A nucleotide substitution that results in a stop codon, prematurely terminating the protein.

Non-ST segment elevation myocardial infarction (NSTE-MI) A myocardial infarction in which the ST segment is not elevated in one lead or several leads of the EKG.

Norepinephrine (noradrenaline) A major neurotransmitter produced by some brain neurons and peripheral sympathetic nerves that acts on α- and β_1-adrenergic receptors; produced in the adrenal chromaffin cells as a precursor for epinephrine.

Normetanephrine An O-methylated metabolite of norepinephrine produced in extraneuronal cells and the adrenal medulla.

Northern blot A technique for identifying specific sequences of RNA in which RNA molecules are sequentially (1) separated by electrophoresis, (2) transferred to nitrocellulose, and (3) identified with a suitable probe.

N-telopeptide (NTx) A biochemical marker of bone resorption.

Nuchal translucency (NT) test A measurement of the size of the translucent space behind the neck of the fetus; made using ultrasound between 10 and 14 weeks of pregnancy. NT tends to be increased in chromosome disorders, such as Turner syndrome and Down syndrome.

Nuclease An enzyme that degrades nucleic acid.

Nucleic acid A polymer made of nucleotide monomers (a sugar moiety, a phosphoric acid, and purine or pyrimidine bases); examples are deoxyribonucleic acid (DNA) and ribonucleic acid (RNA).

Nucleic acid analogs Compounds that are analogous (structurally similar) to naturally occurring RNA and DNA. They are used in medicine and in molecular biology research.

Nucleosome A unit of chromatin consisting of nucleosome core particles (146 base pairs of double-stranded DNA [ds-DNA]) wound around a core of eight histone proteins; technically, a nucleosome also includes a linker DNA between nucleosomes, but the word often is used to mean the core particle.

5′-Nucleotidase A phosphatase that acts only on nucleoside-5′-phosphates, such as adenosine-5′-phosphate (AMP), releasing inorganic phosphate.

Nucleotide A unit of DNA or RNA, consisting of one chemical base (purine or pyrimidine) plus a sugar molecule (deoxyribose or ribose) and at least one phosphate group.

Nutriture The status of the body in relation to nutrition, generally or with regard to a specific nutrient such as a trace element.

Obstructive uropathy Uropathy resulting from an obstruction in the tract.

Ochronosis A condition characterized by an accumulation of dark pigment in cartilage and other connective tissue that indicates alkaptonuria or phenol poisoning.

Odds ratio The probability of the presence of a specific disease divided by the probability of its absence.

Okazaki fragment A relatively short fragment of DNA (with no RNA primer at the 5′ terminus) created on the lagging strand of DNA during DNA synthesis.

Oligohydramnios A condition in pregnancy characterized by a deficiency of amniotic fluid.

Oligomenorrhea Menses occurring at intervals longer than 35 days.

Oligonucleotide A short single-stranded polymer of nucleic acid.

Oligonucleotide ligation assay (OLA) A technique for determining the presence or absence of a specific nucleotide pair within a target gene, often indicating whether the gene is wild type (normal) or mutant (defective).

Oliguria Diminished urine production and excretion.

Omphalocele A birth defect in which the infant's intestine or other abdominal organs protrude from the navel.

Oncofetal antigen Protein produced during fetal life that decreases to low or undetectable levels after birth; reappears in some forms of cancer as the result of reactivation of genes in transformed malignant cells.

Oncogene A mutated normal cellular gene (proto-oncogene) that causes the malignant transformation of normal cells when activated.

Operator interface The part of a device that the operator is required to use for the device to work (e.g., switch on a reader, entry of a patient or sample identification, calibration of the device).

Opiate/Opioid Opiate refers to any of a group of naturally occurring (poppy plant) or semi-synthetic narcotic alkaloids with pharmacological actions and chemical structure similar to morphine. Opioid is a general term that is applied to all substances with morphine-like properties, regardless of origin or chemical structure.

Optode An optical sensor that measures specific substances such as pH, blood gases, and electrolytes using dye immobilization, fluorescence quenching, or phosphorescence.

Oral glucose tolerance test (OGTT) The most common kind of glucose tolerance test in which glucose is ingested by a fasting patient and their concentration of plasma glucose measured over time.

Ordinary least-squares regression (OLR) analysis A method used to estimate the unknown parameters in a linear regression assessment performed to minimize the sum of squared vertical distances between observed responses and responses predicted by linear approximation.

Organic acidemia A disorder of intermediary metabolism in which lack of an enzyme leads to buildup of an organic acid (from deamination of the amino acid) as opposed to the buildup of the parent amino acid.

Organification A process in the thyroid gland whereby iodide is oxidized and incorporated into tyrosyl residues (tyrosine) of thyroglobulin (Tg). Organification is catalyzed by the enzyme thyroperoxidase (TPO).

Ornithine translocase deficiency Ornithine translocase transports ornithine into the liver where it enters the urea cycle. When ornithine translocase is deficient, the concentrations of ornithine and ammonia increase in the blood.

OSHA Occupational Safety and Health Administration, formed by the federal government of the United States to formally regulate the oversight of employee safety.

Osmolal gap A difference between the observed and calculated osmolalities in serum analysis. The calculated osmolar values include sodium concentration multiplied by 1.86, plus glucose and blood urea nitrogen, plus 9.

Osmometry Technique for measuring the concentration of dissolved solute particles in a solution.

Osmotic pressure The pressure required to stop osmosis through a semipermeable membrane between a solution and pure solvent.

Osteitis fibrosa A complication of hyperparathyroidism in which the bones are soft and often deformed; also called osteitis fibrosa cystica

Osteoblasts Cells responsible for formation of bone, including synthesis of type I collagen and noncollagenous proteins and mineralization of osteoid.

Osteocalcin (OC) A protein found in the extracellular matrix of bone and dentin and involved in regulating mineralization in the bones and teeth.

Osteoclasts Large, multinuclear cells responsible for resorption of bone.

Osteomalacia Inadequate or delayed mineralization of osteoid; the adult equivalent of rickets (interruption in the development and mineralization of the growth plate in children).

Osteopenia A condition characterized by decreased bone density occurs that is often predecessor to osteoporosis. It is diagnosed with a bone density test.

Osteoporosis A condition characterized by reduction in bone mass, leading to fractures with minimal trauma; postmenopausal osteoporosis occurs in women after menopause; senile osteoporosis occurs in both men and women later in life.

Ouchterlony technique A technique in which both antigen and antibody are allowed to diffuse to each other in a gel in a precipitation reaction.

Outcomes Results related to the quality or quantity of life of patients; examples include mortality, functional status, quality of life, and well-being.

Outcomes studies Studies performed to determine whether a medical intervention (such as a specific laboratory test) will improve patient outcomes.

Ovaries The paired female reproductive organs that produce ova (eggs), estrogens, and progesterone.

Ovulation The release of the ripe egg (ovum) from the ovary.

Oximetry A technique used to determine the oxygen saturation of arterial blood.

Oxygen dissociation curve The sigmoidal curve obtained when SO_2 of blood is plotted against PO_2.

Oxygen saturation The fraction (percentage) of functional hemoglobin that is saturated with oxygen.

Oxyhemoglobin An hemoglobin that contains bound O_2.

Oxytocin A nonapeptide hormone synthesized in the hypothalamus and stored in the posterior lobe of the pituitary.

P50 PO_2 for a given blood sample at which the hemoglobin of the blood is half saturated with O_2; P50 reflects the affinity of hemoglobin for O_2.

Paget disease A localized, not metabolic bone disease characterized by osteoclastic bone resorption followed by replacement of bone in a chaotic fashion.

Paracrine A type of hormone function in which hormone synthesized in and released from endocrine cells binds to its receptor in nearby cells of a different type and affects their function.

Paraganglioma A tumor of the tissue composing the paraganglia.

Parallel analysis Type of analysis in which all specimens are subjected to a series of analytical processes at the same time and in a parallel fashion.

Parametric analysis A statistical approach to reference value analysis that requires specific distributional assumptions. For example, it usually requires that the distribution of values be Gaussian (or that the values be mathematically manipulated so that they become Gaussian).

Paraprotein A monoclonal immunoglobulin produced in excessive amounts in disorders such as multiple myeloma.

Parathyroid hormone (PTH) The hormone secreted by the parathyroid glands that controls the concentration of calcium in the blood.

Parathyroid hormone–related protein (PTHrP) A protein that mimics many actions of PTH, but is a product of a different gene that is expressed in many normal tissues and overexpressed by tumors in most cases of humoral hypercalcemia of malignancy (HHM).

Parkinson disease A slowly progressive disorder affecting the basal ganglia, usually occurring in late life, with an average age of onset of 60 years.

Paroxysmal nocturnal hemoglobinuria (PNH) Disease of the blood characterized by complement-induced intravascular hemolytic anemia, red colored urine, and thrombosis.

Partial pressure The substance (mole) fraction of gas times the total pressure; i.e., the partial pressure of oxygen, PO_2, is the fraction of oxygen gas times the barometric pressure.

Partin tables A statistical model developed by Alan W. Partin, M.D., Ph.D. at the Johns Hopkins University School of Medicine that shows the probability that the cancer is confined to the prostate and likely to be cured with surgery.

Partition chromatography A separation mechanism that is based on the differential distribution of solutes between two immiscible liquids.

Partitioning The use of specific criteria in the subclassification of reference groups to reduce the biological variation in each group; the most commonly used criteria are age and sex.

Peak concentration The highest concentration achieved within the dosing cycle.

Pellagra A clinical deficiency syndrome due to deficiency of niacin (or failure to convert tryptophan to niacin) and characterized by dermatitis, inflammation of mucous membranes, diarrhea, and psychic disturbances.

Pendrin A protein that is mutated in Pendred syndrome, which is an autosomal recessive disorder characterized by (1) sensorineural hearing loss, (2) goiter, and (3) a partial organification problem. Also known as the sodium-independent chloride/iodide transporter.

Peptic ulcer disease The collective name given to duodenal and gastric ulceration.

Peptide A compound consisting of two or more amino acids linked in a chain via peptide bonds.

Peptide bond The amide bond formed between the carboxyl group of one amino acid and the amino group of another.

Peptide nucleic acid (PNA) An artificially synthesized polymer similar to DNA or RNA. The term is somewhat of a misnomer, because PNA is not an acid.

Percutaneous coronary intervention (PCI) The management of coronary artery occlusion by any of various catheter-based techniques.

Peritoneal dialysis (PD) Diffusion of solutes and convection of fluid through the peritoneal membrane. The dialyzing solution is introduced into and removed from the peritoneal cavity as either a continuous or an intermittent procedure.

Pernicious anemia A deficiency in the production of red blood cells through a lack of vitamin B12.

pH A measure of acidity and alkalinity of a solution. (The negative logarithm of hydrogen ion activity.)

Pharmaceutical drug Any chemical substance intended for use in the (1) medical diagnosis, (2) cure, (3) treatment, or (4) prevention of disease. Also referred to as a *medicine* or *medication.*

Pharmacodynamics A process that defines how a drug acts on its target and its mechanisms of action.

Pharmacogenetics (PD) Study of the variations in single genes or small groups of related genes that affect the response to a drug, including its metabolism.

Pharmacogenomics The study of the inherited variations in genes that dictate drug response and the way these can be used to predict individual responses to a drug, using a genome-wide approach.

Pharmacogenomics Knowledge Base (PharmGKB) An integrated resource about how variation in human genetics leads to variation in response to drugs; database of information about genes (pharmacogenes) involved in modulating the response to drugs.

Pharmacokinetics (PK) A process describing how a drug is (1) absorbed, (2) distributed, (3) metabolized, and (4) eliminated.

Phencyclidine A potent veterinary analgesic and anesthetic, sometimes used as a drug of abuse by humans but capable of causing serious psychological disturbances.

Phenocopying The alteration of a phenotype through a non-genetic, environmental mechanism.

Phenotype The observable physical or biochemical characteristics of an individual, as determined by their genetic makeup and environmental influences.

Phenotyping Laboratory testing designed to measure or predict the reaction or response of an individual to a stimulus (such as, a specific drug). A drug-related phenotype is based upon an individual's genes, but it is also influenced by non-genetic factors, such as concomitant medications, liver function, and renal function.

Phenylketonuria (PKU) A disorder characterized by the accumulation of phenylalanine in blood that results from the absence of phenylalanine hydroxylase activity leading to production of phenylketones that are excreted in urine.

Pheochromocytoma A usually benign, well-encapsulated, lobular, vascular tumor of chromaffin tissue of the adrenal medulla or sympathetic paraganglia.

Philadelphia chromosome An abnormality of chromosome 22 present in marrow cells of most patients with chronic granulocytic leukemia. It is generally a reciprocal translocation between chromosomes 9 and 22 that results in expression of a fusion gene (called *BCR-ABL*) that acts as an oncogene.

Phlebotomist One who practices phlebotomy; the individual drawing a specimen of blood.

Phlebotomy The puncture of a blood vessel to collect blood; literally, "the letting of blood in the treatment of disease."

Phospholipase C Any esterase that catalyzes the hydrolysis of the phosphoric ester bond of a membrane phospholipid, generating a phosphorylated alcohol and diacylglycerol.

Phospholipid A polar amphipathic lipid located on the surface of a lipoprotein; phospholipids are also found at the aqueous interface of biological membranes.

Photometry/Spectrophotometry The measurement of the luminous intensity of light or the amount of luminous light falling on a surface from such a source; spectrophotometry is the measurement of the intensity of light at selected wavelengths.

Pilocarpine iontophoresis Noninvasive method that uses electricity to force the drug pilocarpine into the skin for the purpose of inducing sweating at the site.

Pipette Device used for the transfer of a volume of liquid from one container to another.

Pituitary dwarfism Short stature caused by decreased synthesis or action of growth hormone.

Pituitary gigantism Excessive growth caused by increased synthesis of growth hormone before the epiphyses have fused.

Pituitary gland An elliptical body located at the base of the brain and attached by a stalk to the hypothalamus, from which it receives important neural and vascular outflow. It is divided into the anterior (adenohypophysis) and posterior (neurohypophysis) pituitary with each responsible for the production of its own unique hormones.

Placenta A membranous vascular organ that develops in female mammals during pregnancy, lining the uterine wall and partially enveloping the fetus, to which it is attached by the umbilical cord. Following birth, the placenta is expelled. Its functions include (1) transport of nutrients to the fetus, (2) transport of waste from the fetus, and (3) exchange of gases (oxygen and carbon dioxide) between the mother and fetus.

Placental alpha microglobulin-1 (PAMG-1) A protein present in blood and the amniotic fluid and cervico-vaginal discharge of pregnant women.

Planar chromatography A separation technique in which the stationary phase is on a thin support such as paper or a glass plate.

Plasma The noncellular component of anticoagulated whole blood; plasma contains clotting factors.

Plasma proteins Proteins present in blood, including carrier proteins, fibrinogen and other coagulation factors, complement components, immunoglobulins, enzyme inhibitors, and many others; most are found in other body fluids but in lower concentrations.

Plasmid An extrachromosomal ring of double-stranded, closed DNA found in bacteria.

Pneumoconiosis Deposition of large amounts of dust or other particulate matter in the lungs.

Point-of-care testing (POCT) Clinical testing that occurs next to the patient, usually with a handheld device and an unprocessed specimen collected immediately before testing.

Poison Any substance that, when relatively small amounts are ingested, inhaled, or absorbed, or when it is applied to, injected into, or developed within the body, has chemical action that may cause damage to structure or disturbance of function, producing symptoms, illness, or death.

Polycystic kidney disease The most common renal cystic condition, with deterioration of renal function.

Polycystic ovary syndrome (PCOS) A female condition that is characterized by multiple ovarian follicles and increased androgen production.

Polydipsia Chronic excessive intake of water as in diabetes mellitus or diabetes insipidus.

Polyhydramnios (or hydramnios) The presence of excess amniotic fluid.

Polymerase chain reaction (PCR) An in vitro method for exponentially amplifying DNA.

Polymerases Enzymes that sequentially add nucleotides onto a growing polynucleotide, usually requiring a primer and a template.

Polyuria The passage of a large volume of urine in a given period.

Population In relation to analytical methods, the complete set of all observations that might occur as the result of performing a particular procedure according to specified conditions.

Porphobilinogen (PBG) Immediate precursor of the porphyrins; a pyrrole ring with acetyl, propionyl, and aminomethyl sidechains; four molecules of PBG condense to form one molecule of 1-hydroxymethylbilane, which is then converted successively to uroporphyrinogen-III, coproporphyrinogen-III, protoporphyrinogen-IX, protoporphyrin-IX, and heme.

Porphyria cutanea tarda (PCT) The most common form of porphyria, characterized by cutaneous photosensitivity. Porphyrin precursors ALA and PBG, the biosynthetic intermediates, are metabolized to porphyrinogens and porphyrins.

Porphyrias A group of mainly inherited metabolic disorders that result from partial deficiencies of the enzymes of heme biosynthesis, which cause increased formation and excretion of porphyrins, their precursors, or both.

Porphyrins Any of a group of compounds containing the porphyrin structure; four pyrrole rings connected by methylene bridges in a cyclical configuration, to which a variety of sidechains are attached.

Portal hypertension Any increase in the pressure in the portal vein (which carries venous blood from the intestines and spleen to the liver) due to anatomical or functional obstruction (for example, cirrhosis) to blood flow in the portal venous system.

Postgastrectomy syndrome A syndrome following surgery for peptic ulcer disease that includes the dumping syndrome, diarrhea, maldigestion, weight loss, anemia, bone disease, and gastric cancer.

Potential difference The work required to move an electrical charge and measured in volts.

Potentiometry An electrochemical technique that measures an electrical potential difference between two electrodes (half-cells) in an electrochemical cell.

Preanalytical errors Factors that affect specimens before tests are performed and that can lead to error if not controlled; they are classified as controllable or uncontrollable.

Precocious puberty Early development of secondary sex characteristics; in girls generally before age 8 and in boys before age 9.

Predictive value The predictive value of a positive laboratory test is the number of true positive results divided by the total number of positive results (true positives plus false positives); the negative predictive value is the number of true negative results divided by the total number of negative results (true negatives plus false negatives).

Predictive value of a negative test The proportion of subjects with a negative test who do not have the disease.

Predictive value of a positive test The proportion of subjects with a positive test who have the disease.

Preeclampsia A disorder of widespread vascular endothelial malfunction and vasospasm that occurs after 20 weeks gestation and can present as late as 4 to 6 weeks postpartum. It is clinically defined by hypertension and proteinuria, with or without pathologic edema.

Pregnancy The period from conception to birth. It usually lasts 40 weeks, beginning from the first day of the woman's last menstrual period (LMP), and is divided into three trimesters, each lasting 3 months.

Pregnancy-associated plasma protein A (PAPP-A) A protein used in screening tests for Down syndrome.

Premature rupture of membranes (PROM) Breakage of the sac containing the developing fetus and the amniotic fluid prior to the start of labor; rupture before the 37th week of gestation is called preterm PROM (PPROM).

Preservative A substance or preparation added to a specimen to prevent changes in the constituents of a specimen.

Preterm delivery The birth of an infant before 37 weeks gestation.

Prevalence The frequency of disease in the population examined.

Primary biliary cirrhosis (PBC) A rare form of liver disease that results in the irreversible destruction of the small bile ducts within the liver.

Primary hypothyroidism A condition that develops when the thyroid gland fails to produce or secrete as much thyroxine (T_4) as the body needs.

Primary ovarian insufficiency (POI) A condition in which the ovary fails to function adequately in a woman younger than 40 years.

Primary sclerosing cholangitis (PSC) A chronic, nonbacterial inflammatory narrowing of the bile ducts (usually the larger ducts outside of the liver).

Primer An oligonucleotide that serves to initiate polymer**ase**-catalyzed addition of nucleotides by annealing to a template strand.

Probe A nucleic acid used to identify a target by hybridization.

Procollagen type I carboxy-terminal propeptide (PICP) A biochemical marker of bone formation.

Procollagen type I N-terminal propeptide (PINP) A biochemical marker of bone formation.

Prodrug A drug that is administered in an inactive or poorly-active form and is converted to an active drug by metabolism.

Product The substance produced by the enzyme catalyzed conversion of a substrate.

Product ion A fragment ion formed when a molecular ion breaks into smaller pieces; in a tandem mass spectrometer, the fragmentation process takes place after ions have been separated by the *m/z* value in a first stage of mass spectrometry.

Proficiency testing (PT) A process in which simulated patient specimens made from a common pool are analyzed by laboratories to determine the "quality" of laboratories' performance; considered to be part of external quality assessment.

Progestational Preceding or promoting pregnancy; the phase of the menstrual cycle after ovulation; related to the characteristic actions of progesterone.

Progesterone The principal progestational hormone liberated by the (1) corpus luteum, (2) adrenal cortex, and (3) placenta, whose function is to prepare the uterus for the implantation and development of the fertilized oocyte.

Prognosis A prediction of the future course and outcome of a patient's disease based on currently known indicators (e.g., age, sex, tumor stage, tumor marker level).

Proinsulin A precursor of insulin, with a molecular weight of 8,000 to 10,000; it has minimal hormonal activity and is converted to insulin by removal of the connecting C peptide, leaving the two (A and B)-chain, active insulin molecule.

Prokaryote Organisms (such as bacteria) that are characterized by the absence of a distinct, membrane-bound nucleus or membrane-bound organelles and by DNA that is not organized into chromosomes.

Prolactin A pituitary hormone that stimulates and maintains the secretion of milk.

Prolactin-inhibiting hormone A hormone released by the hypothalamus that inhibits secretion of prolactin by the adenohypophysis. Also known as prolactin-inhibiting factor and prolactostatin.

Promoter A regulatory region of DNA that serves to bind RNA polymerase II that in turn binds other substances that will lead to initiation of transcription; promoters and the substances that bind to them control the rate and timing of tRNA synthesis and thus of synthesis of the coded protein.

Pro-opiomelanocortin (POMC) The 31,000 dalton prohormone that is the precursor of corticotropin, the lipotropins, the melanocyte-stimulating hormones, and the endorphins, all of which are produced by posttranslational proteolytic cleavage of POMC in cell types that produce these hormones.

Propionic acidemia An organic acid disorder due to deficiency of an enzyme involved in amino acid and fatty acid catabolism. It is characterized by excess of propionic acid in the blood and urine.

Prostaglandin Any of a group of compounds derived from unsaturated 20-carbon fatty acids (primarily arachidonic acid) via the cyclo-oxygenase pathway; these compounds are involved in a number of physiological processes.

Prosthetic group A tightly-bound, non-peptide structure required for the activity of an enzyme.

Protein A polymer of amino acids linked by peptide bonds with a specific sequence that folds into a defined structure; any of a group of complex organic compounds that contain carbon, hydrogen, oxygen, nitrogen, and usually sulfur (the characteristic element being nitrogen).

Proteinuria Excessive serum proteins in the urine, such as in renal disease, after strenuous exercise, and with dehydration.

Proteome The total complement of proteins expressed by the genetic material of an organism under a given set of environmental conditions.

Proteomics The identification and quantification of proteins and their posttranslational modifications in a given system or systems.

Protoporphyrin A porphyrin with four methyl, two vinyl, and two propionic acid sidechains attached to the tetrapyrrole backbone.

Pseudogene A genetic element that does not code for a functional gene product, usually because of accumulated sequence variations.

Pseudohermaphroditism The condition of having the gonads and karyotype of one sex and external genitalia that is of the other sex or is ambiguous.

Pseudohypoaldosteronism type 1 (PHA1) A hereditary disorder of infancy characterized by severe salt wasting, failure to thrive, and other signs of aldosterone deficiency.

Pseudoprecocious puberty Development of secondary sex characters and reproductive organs that is not associated with pubertal levels of gonadotropins and gonadotropin-releasing hormone. Also called GnRH-independent precocious puberty.

Puerperium The approximate 6-week period lasting from childbirth to the return of normal uterine size.

Pulmonary surfactant A fluid secreted by the cells of the alveoli that serves to reduce the surface tension of pulmonary fluids.

Pure gonadal dysgenesis An intersex disorder characterized by 46 XX chromosomes and normal external female genitalia at birth.

Purine A base containing two carbon-nitrogen rings; adenine and guanine are purines.

Pyelonephritis An inflammation of the kidney and its pelvis as a result of infection.

Pyridium crosslinks A family of molecules that links collagen molecules to each other; the breakdown products are excreted in the urine with attached crosslinks including-pyridinoline (PYD) and deoxypyridinoline (DPD).

Pyrimidine A base containing one carbon-nitrogen ring; cytosine, thymine, and uracil are pyrimidines.

Pyrosequencing A method of DNA sequencing based on the "sequencing by synthesis" principle that relies on the detection of pyrophosphate (PPi) release on nucleotide incorporation.

Pyruvate An organic acid formed from glucose through glycolysis.

Quality assessment A quality laboratory process that is concerned primarily with broader measures and monitors of laboratory performance such as turnaround times and test utility.

Quality Conformance to the requirements of users or customers and the satisfaction of their needs and expectations.

Quality control A quality laboratory process that involves statistical analysis of internal control procedures through use of control materials for method performance assessment and nonstatistical check procedures such as linearity studies and reagent checks.

Radial immunodiffusion An immunodiffusion technique used to determine the quantity of an antigen by measuring the diameters of circles of precipitin complexes surrounding samples of the antigen.

Random error Error that arises from imprecision of measurement of the type that is described by a Gaussian distribution (e.g., caused by pipetting variability, signal variability).

Random-access analysis The most common configuration of an automated analyser, in which analyses are performed on a collection of specimens sequentially and each specimen is analyzed for a different selection of tests.

Randomized controlled trial An experimental study in which study participants are randomly allocated to an intervention (treatment) group or an alternative treatment (control) group.

Rapid plasma reagin test (RPR test) Any of a group of serologic tests for syphilis.

Rapidly progressive glomerulonephritis Acute glomerulonephritis marked by a rapid progression to end-stage renal disease.

Reaction cell The location in a point-of-care testing device where the analytical reaction takes place.

Reagent Chemical used in many high-purity applications.

Real-time PCR Observation of PCR during amplification at least once each cycle.

Receiver operating characteristic plot A graph of sensitivity versus 1 minus specificity for all possible cutoff values of a diagnostic test; used to display sensitivity and specificity for various decision cutoffs.

Receptor A molecular structure within a cell or on the surface characterized by (1) selective binding of a specific substance and (2) a specific physiological effect that accompanies the binding; examples include cell surface receptors for peptide hormones, neurotransmitters, antigens, complement fragments and immunoglobulins, and cytoplasmic receptors for steroid hormones.

Recognition element A chemosensor with a transducing element that recognizes the analyte to be measured and produces a signal.

Recombination The process of exchange of genes or segments of DNA between chromosomes; recombination produces gametes with chromosomes that are different from the parent's. Recombination of DNA segments is also done in the laboratory as a step in producing recombinant proteins. (see CentiMorgan.)

Recommended dietary allowance (RDA) The amount of nutrient and calorie intake per day considered necessary for maintenance of good health, calculated for males and females of various ages and recommended by the Food and Nutrition Board of the U.S. National Research Council. Popularly called recommended daily allowance.

Redox couple A conjugate pair of substances that consists of any substance that accepts electrons (the oxidant) and any substance that donates electrons (the reductant); redox processes take place only between two redox couples, with electrons transferred from a reductant to an oxidant.

Reference individual An individual selected as the basis for comparison with individuals under clinical investigation through the use of defined criteria.

Reference interval (population-based) A set of values usually defined by an upper reference limit and a lower reference limit, representing a specified proportion of the reference population; this is frequently the central 95% of values from the reference population.

Reference interval (subject-based) A set of values usually defined by an upper reference limit and a lower reference limit, representing a specified proportion of the values from a reference individual; this is frequently the central 95% of values from the reference individual.

Reference material A material or substance, one or more physical or chemical properties of which are sufficiently well established to be used for the calibration of an apparatus, the verification of a measurement method, or the assigning of values to materials. Certified, primary, and secondary are types of reference materials.

Reference measurement procedure A procedure of highest analytical quality that has been shown to yield values having an uncertainty of measurement commensurate with its intended use, especially in assessing the trueness of other measurement procedures for the same quantity and in characterizing reference materials.

Reference population An undefined number of individuals that represent the demographic for which the reference intervals will be used. Reference individuals are chosen, preferably at random, from this larger population to provide reference samples for the establishment of a reference interval.

Reference value A value obtained by observation or measurement of a particular type of quantity on a reference individual; results of a certain type of quantity obtained from a single individual or group of individuals corresponding to a stated description.

Reflectance photometry A spectrophotometric technique in which diffused light illuminates a reaction mixture in a carrier containing a substance of interest, and the intensity of the reflected light is measured.

Regan isoenzyme Isoenzyme of alkaline phosphatase that has been observed in the plasma of patients with malignant tumors.

Regression analysis A statistical analysis that compares measurement relations between two analytical methods.

Relative centrifugal force or field (RCF) Force required to separate two phases (liquid and solid) in a centrifuge.

Renal clearance The volume of plasma from which a given substance is completely cleared by the kidneys per unit of time.

Renal osteodystrophy Bone diseases associated with chronic renal failure, including high turnover (osteitis fibrosa or secondary hyperparathyroidism) and low turnover (osteomalacia and adynamic bone) diseases.

Renal replacement therapy (RRT) Any treatment that replaces kidney function, including dialysis and transplantation.

Renal tubular acidosis (RTA) A variety of metabolic acidosis resulting from impairment of renal function.

Renin An enzyme of the hydrolase class that catalyzes cleavage of the leucine-leucine bond in angiotensinogen to generate angiotensin I.

Replication The faithful reproduction of the DNA content from parent to daughter cells during cell division.

Resolution A measure of the separation of two adjacent chromatographic peaks; resolution equals the difference in retention time for two components divided by the average of their peak widths.

Respiratory acidosis A pathological process that leads to the accumulation of carbon dioxide that raises the $P\,CO_2$ and decreases the pH; usually caused by emphysema or hypoventilation.

Respiratory alkalosis A pathological process that leads to the excessive elimination of carbon dioxide which lowers the $P\,CO_2$ and increases the pH; caused by hyperventilation.

Respiratory distress syndrome (RDS) A disease of premature infants caused by a deficiency of lung surfactant.

Restriction endonuclease An endonuclease that cuts nucleic acid in a sequence-specific manner.

Restriction fragment length polymorphism (RFLP) A genetic polymorphism revealed by changes in the sizes of DNA fragments after restriction enzyme digestion and electrophoresis.

Retention time The time interval between specimen injection and solute reaching the detector; retention time helps identify and quantify analyte.

Retrovirus A family of RNA viruses containing a reverse transcriptase enzyme that allows the viruses' genetic information to become part of the genetic information of the host cell upon replication.

Reverse T_3 (rT_3) A biologically inert metabolite of thyroxine (T_4) with three iodine molecules attached in a configuration (L-3,3′,5′-triiodothyronine) different from that of the active thyroid hormone triiodothyronine (T_3).

Reverse transcriptase A polymerase that catalyzes synthesis of DNA from an RNA template.

Reversed-phase chromatography A partitioning type of chromatography in which the mobile phase is polar relative to the nonpolar stationary phase.

Reye syndrome A sudden, sometimes fatal, disease of the brain (encephalopathy) caused by specific forms of acute injury to the liver.

Ribonucleic acid (RNA) A biological substance similar to DNA with the exceptions of being single stranded, containing ribose as the sugar moiety, having an extra hydroxyl group, and containing uracil instead of thymine; there are different functional types of RNA, including messenger (coding) RNA (mRNA), ribosomal RNA (rRNA), transfer RNA (tRNA), and other small noncoding RNAs (ncRNAs), such as microRNA (miRNA).

Ribosome A large molecular structure comprised of ribosomal RNA and protein that is found in the cytoplasm of cells that serves as the site of protein synthesis.

Rickets A disorder in children caused by a lack of vitamin D, calcium, or phosphate that leads to softening and weakening of the bones. In adults it is known as osteomalacia.

Risk stratification A statistical process used to determine detectable characteristics associated with an increased chance of experiencing unwanted outcomes.

Rolling circle amplification (RCA) A probe amplification method where, in the presence of template, a linear probe is ligated to form a circle that is replicated continuously by a polymerase and one or more primers.

Rotor syndrome A type of chronic familial nonhemolytic jaundice that differs from Dubin-Johnson syndrome in the lack of liver pigmentation.

Sanger sequencing A method of DNA sequencing based on the selective incorporation of chain-terminating dideoxynucleotides by DNA polymerase during in vitro DNA replication. Also known as dideoxy-termination sequencing.

SARA Superfund Amendments and Reauthorization Act. The Superfund Amendments and Reauthorization Act (SARA) amended the Comprehensive Environmental Response, Compensation, and Liability Act (CERCLA) on October 17, 1986.

Screening test An initial test that is used to "screen" specimens to eliminate "negative" ones from further consideration and to identify presumptively positive specimens that then require confirmatory testing.

Scurvy A condition due to deficiency of ascorbic acid (vitamin C) in the diet.

Second messenger Any of several classes of intracellular signals that translate electrical or chemical messages from the environment (first messengers) into cellular responses.

Secondary hyperparathyroidism Excessive secretion of parathyroid hormone (PTH) in response to low plasma calcium that, in turn, is caused by another condition; seen in patients with chronic renal failure and in people with inadequate vitamin D.

Secondary hypothyroidism Hypothyroidism that arises as a consequence of inadequate secretion of thyroid stimulating hormone (TSH or thyrotropin) by the anterior pituitary gland.

Secretin A peptide hormone of the gastrointestinal (GI) tract (27 amino acids) found in the mucosal cells of the duodenum. Among its multiple functions, secretin increases water and bicarbonate secretion to buffer the incoming protons of the acidic chyme. It has considerable homology with GIP, vasoactive intestinal polypeptide (VIP), and glucagon.

Sedative A drug that depresses activity of the central nervous system and reduces anxiety and induces sleep.

Selected ion monitoring (SIM) A MS technique where only specified ions of interest are monitored.

Selection criteria A set of criteria that define the desired characteristics of a reference individual. The specific criteria chosen will depend of the purpose of the reference interval and the specific population the RI is intended to represent.

Self-monitoring of blood glucose (SMBG) A procedure whereby diabetic patients collect their own blood specimens, which are then analyzed for their glucose content.

Sensitivity The proportion of subjects with disease who have a positive laboratory test result.

Sensor A component of a point-of-care testing device that identifies a signal produced by the presence of an analyte.

Sequencing Any method that determines the exact order of bases in a DNA fragment.

Sequential analysis Type of analysis in which each specimen in a batch enters the analytical process one after another, and each result or set of results emerges in the same order as the specimens are entered.

Serial invasive signal amplification A signal enhancing technique that combines two invasive signal amplification reactions in series in a single-tube format.

Seroconversion Development of antibodies in blood serum as a result of infection or immunization.

Serotonin (5-hydroxytryptamine) A monoamine vasoconstrictor synthesized in the intestinal enterochromaffin cells or in central or peripheral neurons; found in high concentrations in many body tissues, including intestinal mucosa, pineal body, and central nervous system.

Sertoli cell Any of the elongated, striated cells of the seminiferous tubules of the testis, to which spermatids attach for nourishment during spermatogenesis.

Sertoli cell–only syndrome A condition characterized by congenital absence of germinal epithelium from the seminiferous tubules, which contain only Sertoli cells, resulting in sterility due to the absence of living sperm cells in the semen. Also called Del Castillo syndrome.

Serum The watery portion of blood that remains after coagulation has occurred; it is obtained after centrifugation.

Severe cutaneous adverse reaction syndromes (SCARS) A group of serious skin conditions that are characterized by blisters and epidermal detachment.

Sex hormone binding globulin (SHBG) A glycoprotein that binds to sex hormones, specifically androgens and estrogens.

Sharps Any object which could readily puncture or cut the skin of an individual when encountered.

Sharps container A container designed for the disposal of sharps; required and regulated by the Occupational Safety and Health Administration (OSHA).

Short tandem repeats (STRs) Short segments of DNA (1 to 13 bases long) that are repeated end to end. Also known as microsatellites.

Sick euthyroid syndrome Abnormalities of T_4, free T_4, T_3, and TSH concentrations that are seen in people with severe illness. In general, treatment with replacement thyroid hormone is not indicated.

Sickle cell anemia An autosomal dominant type of hemolytic anemia that is caused by the presence of hemoglobin S with abnormal sickle-shaped erythrocytes (sickle cells).

Side chain A chemical group that is attached to a core part of the molecule.

Signal amplification Any method that increases the signal resulting from a molecular interaction that does not involve target amplification or probe amplification.

Simple sequence repeats (SSRs) Any sequence repeated over and over again in tandem, such as microsatellites and minisatellites.

Single-base primer extension (SBE) assay An assay performed by annealing a primer to ssDNA immediately adjacent to the single base variant.

Single-channel analysis Type of analysis in which each specimen is subjected to a single process so that only results for a single analyte are produced; similar to batch analysis.

Single-nucleotide polymorphism (SNP) A benign single-nucleotide variant (SNV) (substitution, deletion, or insertion) that occurs in the population at a frequency of at least 1%.

Single-nucleotide variant (SNV) Any change in a nucleic acid that involves only a single nucleotide, including base changes, and single base deletions/ insertions. Now favored over the related term "single nucleotide polymorphism" (SNP) and not limited to variants present at a frequency of >1% as is SNP. SNVs may be benign or may cause disease.

Single-stranded conformational polymorphism (SSCP) A gel electrophoresis technique where single-stranded DNA (ssDNA) segments are identified by their abnormal migration patterns.

Six Sigma process control A quantitative framework for evaluating process performance and providing more objective evidence for process improvement, with a goal of having Six Sigmas or six standard deviations of process variation fitting within the tolerance limits of the process.

Size-exclusion chromatography A separation mechanism that separates solutes on the basis of the molecular size of the solutes in a solution.

Sjögren syndrome A systemic autoimmune disease in which immune cells attack and destroy the glands that produce tears and saliva.

Skimmer A cone with a central orifice that is designed to intercept the center of a spray or jet expansion so as to sample the central portion of the expansion.

Skin puncture Collection of capillary blood usually from a pediatric patient by making a thin cut in the skin, usually at the heel of the foot.

Smith-Lemli-Opitz syndrome (SLOS) A congenital malformation syndrome caused by deficiency of the enzyme 7-dehydrocholesterol reductase (DHCR7), due to mutation of the *DHCR7* gene on chromosome 11.

Sodium–hydrogen exchanger (NHE) A membrane protein that is primarily responsible for maintaining the balance of sodium; also called the sodium–hydrogen antiporter.

Somatostatin Any of several cyclic tetradecapeptides produced in the hypothalamus that inhibit release of several hormones of the pituitary.

Southern blot A method for detecting DNA sequence variants after restriction enzyme digestion and size separation by electrophoresis.

Speciation methods Techniques used to separate the chemical complexes of individual elements present in any particular medium.

Specificity The proportion of subjects without disease who have a negative laboratory test result.

Specimen A sample or portion of body fluid or tissue collected for examination, study, or analysis.

Spectral bandwith The width in nanometers of the spectral transmittance curve at a point equal to one-half of the peak transmittance; used to describe the spectral purity of a filter or other monochromator.

Sperm protein SP-10 A sperm acrosomal protein, specific to the testis, that is believed to play an important role in egg-sperm binding.

Spina bifida A congenital disorder caused by the incomplete closure of the embryonic neural tube (see neural tube defect); the most common form is meningomyelocele (also called myelomeningocele).

Spliceosome A large ribonucleoprotein complex, composed of various small nuclear ribonucleoproteins (snRNP) as well as other protein factors; it attaches to specific sites on pre-mRNA and catalyzes splicing out of their introns in the formation of mature mRNA.

Sprue A chronic form of malabsorption syndrome occurring in tropical and nontropical forms.

ST segment elevation myocardial infarction (STEMI) Any type of myocardial infarction in which the ST segment is elevated in one lead or several leads of the EKG.

Star (*)-allele nomenclature A nomenclature developed to standardize genetic polymorphism annotation for the cytochrome P_{450} genes.

STARD Standards for Reporting of Diagnostic Accuracy; a project designed to improve the quality of reporting of the results of diagnostic accuracy studies.

Stationary phase A solid or a liquid phase that interacts with components of the mobile phase.

Steatorrhea A condition of excessive fat in feces (more than 5 g/day).

Stereoisomer One of a group of compounds differing only in the spatial arrangement of their atoms.

Steroidogenesis The biosynthesis of steroids by the adrenal glands and gonads.

Steroidogenic acute regulatory protein (StAR) A transport protein that functions to regulate cholesterol transfer within the mitochondria.

Stevens-Johnson syndrome (SJS) A serious allergic reaction with a characteristic rash involving the skin and mucous membranes. The hypersensitive (allergic) reaction may be initiated by drugs, infectious agents, or other stimuli.

Strand displacement amplification (SDA) An amplification technique that uses two types of primers and DNA polymerase and restriction endonuclease to exponentially produce single-stranded amplicons asynchronously.

Subclinical hyperthyroidism A biochemical condition with normal concentrations of serum thyroid hormones when the serum TSH concentration is repeatedly low in the absence of hypothalamic or pituitary disease.

Substrate A reactant in an enzyme-catalyzed reaction that binds to the active center of an enzyme.

Superfund A program of the U.S. Government to clean up the nation's uncontrolled hazardous waste sites. Under the Superfund program, abandoned, accidentally spilled, or illegally dumped hazardous waste that poses a current or future threat to human health or the environment is cleaned up.

Superoxide dismutase An enzyme of the oxidoreductase class that catalyzes the reduction of superoxide anions to hydrogen peroxide, protecting cells against dangerous levels of superoxide (oxygen).

Survivin A protein that neutralizes caspase activity and thus inhibits apoptosis, expressed during the G2/M phase of the cell cycle in many tumors but not in most normal differentiated adult tissues.

Sweat chloride The concentration of chloride in sweat; increased sweat chloride is characteristic of cystic fibrosis.

Syndrome of inappropriate antidiuretic hormone (SIADH) A condition in which inappropriate antidiuretic hormone secretion produces dilutional hyponatremia, and increased extracellular fluid volume with an elevated urine osmolality.

Systematic error Error in measurement that arises from calibration bias or nonspecificity of an assay and, in the course of a number of analyses of the same analyte, remains constant (y-intercept deviation from zero) or varies in a proportional way (slope deviation from unity) based on the analyte concentration.

Systematic review A methodical and comprehensive review of all published and unpublished information about a specific topic to answer a precisely defined clinical question.

Systemic inflammatory response syndrome (SIRS) The systemic inflammatory response to a wide variety of severe clinical insults.

Systemic lupus erythematosus (SLE or lupus) A condition that can affect any part of the body.

T_3 Thyrotoxicosis A hyperthyroid condition in which T_3 but not T_4 is elevated.

Tandem mass spectrometer A mass spectrometer capable of successive separation of ions in an ion beam according to m/z value (tandem in space) or separation of a set of trapped ions in an ion trap according to m/z value (tandem in time).

Tandem mass spectrometry (MS/MS) A spectrometric method of analysis where two mass spectrometers are connected in series. It involves separation and identification of substances and chemicals based on their mass to charge (m/z) ratio.

Target amplification Any method for increasing the amount of target nucleic acid. A target-specific primary reaction is used to drive a secondary invasive reaction.

Tartrate-resistant acid phosphatase 5b (TRACP5b) An enzyme derived from osteoclasts; it is a marker of bone resorption.

Telomere The DNA sequences at the end of a chromosome; telomeres contain repetitive nucleotide sequences that protect the ends of chromosomes from recombination with other chromosomes.

Temperature-gradient gel electrophoresis (TGGE) A form of electrophoresis that uses temperature to denature the sample as it moves across an acrylamide gel.

Template A nucleic acid molecule the sequence of which serves as a pattern to be copied by a polymerase to produce a DNA or RNA with a complementary sequence.

Testis The male gonad, either of two oval reproductive glands located in the scrotum.

Testosterone The principal androgenic hormone, produced by the Leydig cells of the testes in response to stimulation by LH from the anterior pituitary gland.

Thalassemia A heterogeneous group of hereditary hemolytic anemias having a decreased rate of synthesis of one or more hemoglobin polypeptide chains and classified according to the chain involved (α, β, δ); the two major categories are α- and β-thalassemia.

Thalassemia major The homozygous form of β-thalassemia, a severe condition evident from the neonatal period with complete absence of hemoglobin A.

Thalassemia minor The heterozygous form of β-thalassemia; it is usually asymptomatic, although hemoglobin A synthesis may be retarded and there is sometimes moderate anemia and splenomegaly.

Therapeutic drug monitoring/management (TDM) A process used to measure blood drug levels so that the most effective dosage is maintained and toxicity prevented.

Therapeutic range The interval between the minimum and maximum doses of a drug.

Thermocycler A laboratory apparatus used in the amplification of segments of DNA via the PCR. Often, the device has a thermal block with holes where tubes holding the reaction mixtures are inserted. The cycler then raises and lowers the temperature of the block in discrete, preprogrammed steps.

Thermus aquaticus (Taq) A thermostable DNA polymerase named after the thermophilic bacterium Thermus aquaticus. It is often abbreviated to "Taq Pol" or "Taq" and is frequently used in PCR.

Thiopurine S-methyltransferase (TPMT) A metabolic enzyme that methylates and thereby inactivates certain antimetabolites, such as 6-mercaptopurine (6-MP) (cancer therapeutic).

Threshold limit value (TLV) The maximum concentration of a chemical allowable for repeated exposure without producing adverse health effects.

Thrombolysis Lysis of a thrombus or thrombi.

Throughput The number of specimens processed by an analyzer during a given period of time, or the rate at which an analytical system processes specimens.

Thyroglobulin (Tg) An iodine-containing glycoprotein of high molecular weight (663 kDa) present in the colloid of the follicles of the thyroid gland.

Thyroid follicle The secretory unit of the thyroid gland consisting of an outer layer of epithelial cells that enclose an amorphous material called colloid.

Thyroid storm A life-threatening condition that develops in a minority of cases of untreated thyrotoxicosis (hyperthyroidism, or overactive thyroid).

Thyroiditis A condition characterized by inflammation of the thyroid gland.

Thyroid-stimulating hormone (TSH) A polypeptide hormone synthesized by the anterior pituitary gland that promotes the growth of the thyroid gland and stimulates the synthesis and release of thyroid hormones by the thyroid gland. Also called thyrotropin.

Thyrotoxicosis A toxic condition resulting from excessive amounts of thyroid hormones in the body.

Thyrotropin A glycoprotein hormone synthesized by the anterior pituitary gland that promotes the growth of the thyroid gland and stimulates the hormonal secretion by the gland. Also called thyroid-stimulating hormone.

Thyrotropin-releasing hormone (TRH) A tripeptide produced in the hypothalamus that stimulates the release of TSH from the anterior pituitary.

Thyroxine (T_4) The major hormone synthesized and released by the thyroid gland that contains four iodine molecules (L-3,5,3′,5′-tetraiodothyronine).

Tiling arrays A subtype of microarray that functions by hybridizing labeled DNA or RNA target molecules to probes fixed onto a solid surface.

Torr A non-SI unit of pressure with the ratio of 760 to 1 standard atmosphere, chosen to be roughly equal to the fluid pressure exerted by a millimeter of mercury. For example, a pressure of 1 torr is approximately equal to 1 mm of mercury.

Total body water (TBW) Any of various estimates of the water content of the human body, taking into consideration the person's height, weight, and age.

Total ion chromatogram (TIC) The sum of all ions produced displayed as a function of time.

Total parenteral nutrition (TPN) The practice of feeding a person intravenously, circumventing the gut.

Total quality management (TQM) A management philosophy and approach that focuses on processes and their improvement as the means to satisfy customer needs and requirements; a quality system that is implemented to ensure quality.

Total testing process A broad definition of the laboratory testing and reporting process that includes preanalytical, analytical, and postanalytical phases.

Toxic epidermal necrolysis (TEN) A rare condition that causes large portions of the epidermis (the skin's outermost layer) to detach from the layers of skin below.

Toxic metals Metals that are elements with high molecular weight and generally toxic in low concentrations to plant and animal life. Note: The International Union of Pure and Applied Chemistry (IUPAC) considers the term "heavy metal" to be both meaningless and misleading and recommends that it no longer be used.

Toxic multinodular goiter A condition in which the thyroid gland contains multiple lumps (nodules) that are overactive and that produce excess thyroid hormones. Also known as Parry disease and Plummer disease.

Toxic nephropathy Kidney damage caused by the effects of a nephrotoxin.

Toxidrome A syndrome caused by a dangerous concentration of toxins in the body.

Toxins Poisonous substances that are produced by living cells or organisms and are capable of causing disease when introduced into the body tissues and are often capable of inducing neutralizing antibodies or antitoxins.

Trace elements Inorganic molecules found in human and animal tissues in milligram per kilogram amounts or less.

Traceability In relation to analytical methods, a concept based on a chain of comparisons of measurements that lead to a known reference value done to ensure reasonable agreement between measurements of routine methods.

Transcription The process of transferring sequence information from the gene regions of DNA to a messenger RNA molecule.

Transcription mediated amplification (TMA) An amplification method that uses RNA polymerase and reverse transcriptase to produce an RNA amplicon from a target nucleic acid. TMA can use either RNA or single-stranded DNA as a template.

Transcriptome The set of all RNA molecules, including (1) messenger RNA (mRNA), (2) ribosomal RNA (rRNA), (3) transfer RNA (tRNA), and (4) other non-coding RNAs produced in one or a population of cells.

Transducing element A component of a point-of-care testing device such as a chemical indicator or a binding molecule that recognizes the analyte of interest and produces an electrical or optical signal.

Transferability or Transference The adoption by a laboratory of previously established reference intervals established elsewhere. Procedures for validation of reference intervals must be completed by the adopting laboratory prior to the use of the transferred RI to ensure that they are appropriate to the laboratory's patient population and laboratory methods.

Transferrin A beta globulin that carries iron in the blood.

Translation The process whereby an mRNA sequence forms an amino acid sequence with the help of tRNA and eventual enzymatic peptide bond formation between amino acids to synthesize polypeptides; translation occurs on cytoplasmic ribosomes.

Transmittance The intensity of a transmitted light beam divided by the intensity of an incident (incoming) light beam passed through a square cell containing a solution of a compound that absorbs light at a specific wavelength stated as $T = I/I_0$; when compared with a reference cell, the transmitted light is divided by the incident light ($T = I/I_R$). A reference cell is used to set an arbitrary value of 100 which corresponds to 100% transmittance.

Transposon A mobile genetic element that can delete and insert itself variably into the genome.

Transthyretin (TTR) A protein found in serum and cerebrospinal fluid that binds to and transports thyroxine (T4). TTR complexes with retinol binding protein (RBP) to prevent its loss through the glomerulus by filtration. Was once called prealbumin, because it travels faster than albumin on electrophoresis gels.

Triglyceride A glycerol ester consisting of three molecules of fatty acid esterified to glycerol and constituting 95% of tissue storage fat.

Triiodothyronine (T_3) The biologically active form of thyroid hormone formed primarily outside of the thyroid gland by the peripheral deiodination of thyroxine (T_4). Has three iodine molecules attached to its molecular structure (L-3,5,3′-triiodothyronine).

Triploidy A condition characterized by the individual having three times the haploid number of chromosomes in the cell nucleus.

Trisomy 18 (Edwards syndrome) A genetic disorder caused by the presence of all or part of an extra 18th chromosome (trisomy: three chromosomes).

Trophoblasts The outermost layer of cells of the blastocyst that attaches the fertilized ovum to the uterine wall and serves as a nutritive pathway for the embryo.

Trough concentration The lowest concentration achieved just before the next dose.

Trueness A qualitative term that describes the closeness of agreement between the average value obtained from a large series of results of measurements and a true value.

Tumor marker A substance produced by a tumor found in blood, body fluids, or tissue that may be used to predict the presence and size of the tumor and monitor its response to therapy.

Tumor-suppressor gene A gene involved in the regulation of cellular growth; loss of a tumor-suppressor gene has the potential to allow autonomous growth.

Turbidimetry The detection and measurement of a decrease in intensity of an incident beam of light as it passes through a solution of particles.

Turnaround time (TAT) The time between when a test is ordered or a specimen is submitted for analysis and when the test results are reported.

Turner syndrome A chromosomal disorder affecting females wherein one of the two X-chromosomes is defective or completely absent.

Type 1 diabetes mellitus (T1DM) One of the two major types of diabetes mellitus. It is an autoimmune disease that results in the destruction of beta cells of the pancreas, leading to loss of the ability to secrete insulin. Also called insulin-dependent diabetes, type 1A diabetes.

Type 2 diabetes mellitus (T2DM) One of the two major types of diabetes mellitus, characterized by peak age of onset between 50 and 60 years.

Tyrosinemia A genetic disorder involving the metabolism of the tyrosine. Affected individuals have high concentrations of tyrosine in blood (hypertyrosinemia) and urine (tyrosinuria).

Ulcerative colitis Recurrent inflammatory disease of the large bowel that involves the rectum and spreads to involve a variable amount of colon. Ulcerative colitis, like Crohn disease, is a form of inflammatory bowel disease (IBD).

Ultratrace elements Inorganic molecules found in human and animal tissues in microgram per kilogram amounts or less.

Umbilical cord A flexible cordlike structure containing blood vessels and attaching a human or other mammalian fetus to the placenta during gestation.

Uncertainty A parameter characterizing the range of values within which the value of the quantity being measured is expected to lie.

Unconjugated bilirubin Free bilirubin that has not been conjugated with glucuronic acid.

Universal Precautions Approach to infection control that treats all human blood and certain human body fluids as if they were known to be infectious for bloodborne pathogens.

Unstable angina An angina that occurs unpredictably or suddenly increases in severity or frequency.

Upregulation A process that results in an increase in the number of receptors on the surface of target cells, making the cells more sensitive to a hormone or another agent. *Downregulation* is an decrease in the number of receptors on the surface of target cells.

Urea The major nitrogen-containing metabolic product of protein catabolism in humans.

Urea cycle disorder Any disorder in which the body is unable to excrete waste nitrogen–ammonia, resulting in mental and behavioral dysfunction, coma, and death.

Urease methods Enzymatic assays that initially involve the hydrolysis of urea by urease to generate ammonia, which is quantified by a variety of methods.

Uremia An excess in the blood of urea, creatinine, and other nitrogenous end products of protein and amino acid metabolism; also referred to as azotemia.

Uremic syndrome The spectrum of symptoms accompanying uremia.

Uric acid A nitrogenous compound derived from the catabolism of purine nucleosides.

Uricase methods A group of enzymatic assays that initially involve oxidation of uric acid by uricase to eventually produce a chromogen that is spectrophotometrically measured to determine uric acid concentration.

Uridine 5′-diphosphate (UDP)-glucuronosyltransferase (UGT) A family of metabolic enzymes that conjugate compounds with glucuronide molecules.

Urobilinogen A colorless compound formed in the intestines by the reduction of bilirubin.

Uroporphyrin A porphyrin with four acetic acid and four propionic acid sidechains attached to the tetrapyrrole backbone.

Vanillylmandelic acid (VMA) The main end-product of norepinephrine and epinephrine metabolism excreted in the urine; formed primarily in the liver from oxidation of methoxyhydroxyphenylglycol.

Variable-number tandem repeats (VNTRs) Repeated segments of DNA that are 14 to 500 bases long. Also known as minisatellites.

Variation A change in DNA sequence. It may be benign or may cause disease.

Varices Enlarged and tortuous veins, most commonly found in the esophagus (termed esophageal varices).

Variegate porphyria (VP) An autosomal dominant hepatic porphyria due to mutation in the *PPOX* gene (locus: 1q22), which encodes protoporphyrinogen oxidase.

Vasoactive intestinal polypeptide (VIP) A peptide of 28 amino acids found in the central and peripheral nervous systems where it acts as a neurotransmitter. It is located in the enteric nerves in the gut. It relaxes smooth muscle in the gut and increases water and electrolyte secretion from the gut.

Venipuncture All of the steps involved in obtaining an appropriate and identified blood specimen from an individual's vein.

Venous occlusion Obstruction of the return of venous blood to the heart and distention of the veins; in phlebotomy, this is a temporary blockage caused by application of pressure, usually from a tourniquet.

Ventricles (right and left) The two lower chambers of the heart, responsible, respectively, for pumping blood into the lungs via the pulmonary artery and into the systemic circulation via the aorta.

Vernix caseosa A white cheese-like protective material that covers the skin of a fetus.

Viral hepatitis Liver inflammation caused by viruses. Specific hepatitis viruses have been labeled A, B, C, D, and E.

Viral load The measurement of the amount of virus in the blood. It is expressed as the copies of virus per milliliter of body fluid and used to guide treatment decisions and monitor response to treatment.

Virilization The induction or development of male secondary sex characteristics; especially the induction of such changes in the female.

Virtual karyotyping A technique used to analyze a short sequence of DNA from specific loci all over a genome to obtain information that reflects a karyotype.

Vitamer Term used to describe any of a number of compounds that possess a given vitamin activity.

Vitamin An essential organic micronutrient that must be supplied exogenously and in many cases is the precursor to a metabolically derived coenzyme.

Vitamin D Fat-soluble vitamin produced by skin upon exposure to sunlight (vitamin D3, also called cholecalciferol) or adsorbed from foods that contain it (vitamin D2 or ergocalcaliferol); deficiency causes rickets in children and osteomalacia in adults.

Voltammetry An electrolytic electrochemical process in which a specific oxidation or reduction reaction occurs at the surface of the working electrode; it is the charge transfer at this interface (current flow) that provides analytical information.

Waived test A test that (1) employs methodologies that are so simple and accurate as to render the likelihood of erroneous results negligible; (2) poses no reasonable risk of harm to the patient if the test is performed incorrectly; and (3) has been cleared by the Food and Drug Administration for home use.

Waldenström's macroglobulinemia A chronic cancer of the immune system characterized by hyperviscosity, or thickening, of the blood.

Water homeostasis The body process that maintains a balance of water intake and output.

Waterhouse-Friderichsen syndrome Adrenal gland failure caused by bleeding into the adrenal gland; it is a fulminating complication of bacterial infections, notably meningococcemia; characterized by sudden onset and short course, cyanosis with petechial hemorrhages of the skin and mucous membranes, fever, and hypotension that can lead to shock and coma.

Wavelength A characteristic of electromagnetic radiation; the distance between two wave crests that is measured in nanometers.

Western blotting Membrane-based assay in which proteins are separated by electrophoresis, which is followed by transfer to a membrane and probing with a labeled antibody.

Westgard multirules A series of control rules used to interpret quality control data.

Whipple's triad A collection of three criteria suggesting a patient's symptoms result from hypoglycemia.

WHO World Health Organization.

Whole genome amplification (WGA) A non-specific amplification technique that produces an amplified product that represents the initial starting material (whole genome).

Wick flow Movement of water from the buffer reservoirs toward the center of an electrophoresis gel or strip to replace water lost by evaporation.

Wilson disease An autosomal recessive disorder associated with excessive quantities of copper in the tissue, particularly the liver and central nervous system.

Workstation A clinical laboratory workstation dedicated to a defined task and containing appropriate laboratory instrumentation to carry out that task.

Xenobiotics Chemical substances foreign to the biological system. They include naturally occurring compounds, drugs, environmental agents, carcinogens, insecticides, etc.

X-linked hypophosphatemia A form of familial hypophosphatemic rickets, with X-linked dominant inheritance.

X-linked protoporphyria A rare genetic disorder characterized by an abnormal sensitivity to the sun (photosensitivity).

Yolk sac A membranous sac attached to an embryo that provides early nourishment in the form of yolk in many animals, including humans where it functions as the circulatory system before internal circulation begins.

Zero-order kinetics In an enzymatic reaction, when the reaction rate is constant at maximum value, the reaction rate depends only on enzyme concentration and is independent of substrate concentration; the rate of reaction is proportional to the zero power of the substrate concentration.

Zinc finger A finger-shaped fold in a protein that is created by the binding of specific amino acids in the protein to a zinc atom. Zinc-finger proteins regulate the expression of genes as well as nucleic acid recognition, reverse transcription, and virus assembly.

Zinc protoporphyrin (ZPP) A normal but minor by-product of heme biosynthesis found in the red blood cell; when insufficient Fe^{2+} is available for heme biosynthesis, increased ZPP is formed.

Zollinger-Ellison (Z-E) syndrome A condition resulting from a gastrin-producing tumor (gastrinoma) that results in an overproduction of gastric acid, leading to ulceration of the esophagus, stomach, duodenum, and jejunum, and causing hypergastrinemia, diarrhea, and steatorrhea.

Zona fasciculata The thick middle layer of the adrenal cortex that contains large lipid-laden cells. It is the major source of glucocorticoids and, to a lesser extent, adrenal androgens.

Zona glomerulosa The thin outer layer of the adrenal cortex. It is the source of mineralocorticoids.

Zona reticularis The inner layer of the adrenal cortex. Its cells resemble those of the zona fasciculata, except they contain less lipid. The zona reticularis is the major source of adrenal androgens and produces glucocorticoids to a lesser degree.

Zygote The fertilized ovum or diploid cell resulting from the fusion of two haploid gametes.

Index

Page numbers followed by f indicate figures; t, tables; b, boxes